RADIOLOGY OF CONGENITAL HEART DISEASE

Radiology of Congenital Heart Disease

KURT AMPLATZ, M.D.
Professor of Radiology
Division of Cardiovascular and Interventional Radiology
University of Minnesota
Minneapolis, Minnesota

JAMES H. MOLLER, M.D.
Professor of Pediatrics and Paul F. Dwan
Professor of Education in Pediatric Cardiology
University of Minnesota
Minneapolis, Minnesota

Illustrated by:
Martin A. Finch, M.A.
Photography by:
Michael W. Carlin

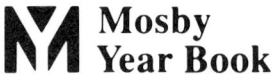

St. Louis Baltimore Boston Chicago London Philadelphia Sydney Toronto

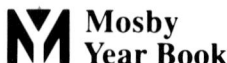
Mosby
Year Book
Dedicated to Publishing Excellence

Sponsoring Editor: Anne S. Patterson
Assistant Editor: Dana Battaglia/Maura K. Leib
Assistant Director, Manuscript Services: Frances M. Perveiler
Production Manager: Nancy C. Baker
Proofroom Manager: Barbara M. Kelly

Copyright © 1993 by Mosby–Year Book, Inc.
A C.V. Mosby imprint of Mosby–Year Book, Inc.

Mosby–Year Book, Inc.
11830 Westline Industrial Drive
St. Louis, MO 63416

All rights reserved. No part of this publication may be reproduced, stored in a retrieval system, or transmitted, in any form or by any means, electronic, mechanical, photocopying, recording, or otherwise, without prior written permission from the publisher. Printed in the United States of America.

Permission to photocopy or reproduce solely for internal or personal use is permitted for libraries or other users registered with the Copyright Clearance Center, provided that the base fee of $4.00 per chapter plus $.10 per page is paid directly to the Copyright Clearance Center, 21 Congress Street, Salem, MA 01970. This consent does not extend to other kinds of copying, such as copying for general distribution, for advertising or promotional purposes, for creating new collected works, or for resale.

1 2 3 4 5 6 7 8 9 0 CL/SE/MV 97 96 95 94 93

Library of Congress Cataloging-in-Publication Data
Amplatz, Kurt, 1924-
    Radiology of congenital heart disease / Kurt Amplatz, James H. Moller.
      p.   cm.
    Includes bibliographical references and index.
    ISBN 0-8016-7433-6
    1. Congenital heart disease in children—Imaging. I. Moller, James H., 1933- . III Title.
    [DNLM: 1. Heart Defects, Congenital—radiography. WG 220 A526ra]
    RJ426.C64A57   1992
    616.1′2043—dc20   92-49972
    DNLM/DLC   CIP
    for Library of Congress

*To the Variety Club of the Northwest (Tent 12)
and Our Teachers*

CONTRIBUTORS

HUGH D. ALLEN, M.D.
Professor and Vice Chairman of Pediatrics
Ohio State University College of Medicine
Director and Chief
Division/Section of Cardiology
OSU/Children's Hospital
Columbus, Ohio

KURT AMPLATZ, M.D.
Professor of Radiology
Division of Cardiovascular and Interventional Radiology
University of Minnesota
Minneapolis, Minnesota

ROBERT J. BOUDREAU, PH.D., M.D.
Associate Professor and Director of Nuclear Medicine
Department of Radiology
Univesity of Minnesota
Minneapolis, Minnesota

MICHAEL W. CARLIN
Westwood, New Jersey

STEVEN C. CASSIDY, M.D.
Assistant Professor of Pediatrics
Ohio State University College of Medicine
Member, Division/Section of Cardiology
OSU/Children's Hospital
Columbus, Ohio

WILFRIDO R. CASTAÑEDA-ZÚÑIGA, M.D.
Professor of Radiology
Director of Cardiovascular and Interventional Radiology
University of Minnesota
Minneapolis, Minnesota

CLAUDIA M. ENGELER, M.D.
Medical Fellow Specialist
Department of Radiology
University of Minnesota
Minneapolis, Minnesota

MARTIN E. FINCH, M.A.
Director, Biomedical Graphics Communications Department
Associate Professor
Division of Surgical Sciences
Department of Surgery
University of Minnesota
Minneapolis, Minnesota

AUGUSTIN G. FORMANEK, M.D.
Professor Emeritus
Department of Radiology
Wake Forest University
Bowman Gray School of Medicine
Winston-Salem, North Carolina

WAYNE H. FRANKLIN, M.D.
Assistant Professor of Clinical Pediatrics and Internal Medicine
Ohio State University College of Medicine
Member, Division/Section of Cardiology
OSU/Children's Hospital
Columbus, Ohio

ANTOINETTE S. GOMES, M.D.
Associate Professor of Radiology and Medicine
Department of Radiology
UCLA Medical Center
Los Angeles, California

JAMES H. MOLLER, M.D.
Professor of Pediatrics and Paul F. Dwan
Professor of Education in Pediatric Cardiology
University of Minnesota
Minneapolis, Minnesota

G. WAYNE MOORE, B.SC.
Eaglewood, Colorado

FOREWORD

The time was April 5, 1951, and the place was the University of Minnesota Hospitals. The stage was set for what promised to be a dramatic milestone in the evolution of thoracic surgery; namely, the application, for the first time, of a pump oxygenator with total cardiopulmonary bypass to correct an intracardiac (atrial secundum) defect under direct vision. Despite two preoperative heart catheterizations, and a thoracotomy with finger exploration through the left atrium 4 months earlier, the surgeons unexpectedly and unfortunately were confronted with an atrioventricularis communis malformation in its complete form. Unfamiliarity with this complex anatomy resulted in a failed repair and death of the patient.

Not long thereafter, Dr. John Gibbon of Philadelphia, after 15 years of intensive research on cardiopulmonary bypass, operated on his first patient who was in severe cardiac distress due to a presumed atrial secundum septal defect. After Dr. Gibbon instituted cardiopulmonary bypass and opened the heart, the patient exsanguinated from uncontrollable hemorrhage from an undiagnosed and widely patent ductus arteriosus. At autopsy, there were no intracardiac lesions.

As these two historical vignettes so vividly portray, a correct and precise preoperative diagnosis has always played an all important role in the success (or failure) of open heart surgery.

Today, open heart surgery is performed so effortlessly and with such a low risk at all ages—from neonates to octogenarians—that it may not be evident to the present generation of cardiologists and cardiac surgeons that the painful vignettes cited herein were not isolated events, but were repeated worldwide many times over in the decades of the 1950s and 1960s in the many centers then venturing into this new therapeutic field of open heart surgery.

Thus, with the advent of open intracardiac procedures, for the first time in cardiological history, precise anatomic diagnoses became absolutely crucial to the success of the treatment. Heretofore, exact anatomic (and physiologic) diagnoses had been largely the province of the handful of pathologists knowledgeable about the heart and the myriads of congenital malformations possible.

The authors of this comprehensive and all inclusive work, *Radiology of Congenital Heart Disease,* are uniquely qualified by their extensive experience drawn from the large number of patients with congenital heart disease attracted to the University of Minnesota Hospitals and Variety Heart Hospital in Minneapolis where a number of the early successes in the field of open heart surgery were recorded.[1-3]

This writer has personally worked with the authors for many years beginning in the 1950s when we shared the burden, with many poignant memories, of unraveling preoperatively the multiplicity of morphologic abnormalities possible in the many patients with congenitally deformed hearts needing correction at that time. In the years that have followed, the combined efforts in many parts of the world by cardiologists, radiologists, surgeons, physiologists, and pathologists have made it possible for the operating surgeon to have an accurate anatomic blueprint preoperatively. This accomplishment has contributed importantly to the spectacular progress over the past 40 years that has made virtually every type or combination or types of congenital heart malformations correctable at minimal risks.

Now that this period of explosive growth in new

knowledge and new techniques has begun to level off, it is particularly appropriate and timely for the publication of this text concentrating upon diagnosis and typing together in a single source the complete knowledge and expertise of the authors.

In this work they have expertly combined not only all aspects of radiology, but also the physical findings, electrocardiography and echocardiography for each of the lesions. In addition, the findings and role of invasive studies such as cardiac catheterizations are described and evaluated. The multidisciplinary experience and superb qualifications of the three authors give these volumes a uniform high quality often lacking in multiple authored texts. The excellence of the harmonizing artwork by Martin Finch adds significantly to the clarity and teaching value of this work.

To the authors, I heartily extend my gratitude for their skilled and untiring assistance to me and my surgical colleagues both in preoperative and postoperative evaluations of the many hundreds of patients that we've collaborated upon. And for me, it has been a special privilege to have this opportunity to review and to be able to highly recommend this superlative work.

C. Walton Lillehei, Ph.D., M.D.
Former Professor of Surgery
University of Minnesota Medical Center and Variety Club Heart Hospital
Minneapolis, Minnesota
Formerly Surgeon-in-Chief
Cornell Medical Center
New York, New York
Past President, American College of Cardiology

REFERENCES

1. Goor DA, Lillehei CW: *Congenital malformations of the heart: embryology, anatomy and operative considerations,* New York, 1975, Grune and Stratton.
2. Lillehei CW: A personalized history of extracorporeal circulation, *Am Soc Artif Intern Organs* 28:4–17, 1982.
3. Lillehei CW, Varco RL, Cohen M, et al: The first open-heart corrections of ventricular septal defect, atrioventricular communis, and tetralogy of Fallot utilizing extracorporeal circulation by cross-circulation: a 30-year follow-up, *Ann Thorac Surg* 41:4–21, 1986.

FOREWORD

"A teacher affects eternity." The ideal student-teacher relationship is of a special nature; not only does the student learn from the teacher, but he or she is given the means by which to go forward, even beyond the position of the teacher.

This book, strong on facts and precise in words, offers readers of all levels an encyclopedic array of important facts on the subject of congenital heart disease. While the primary emphasis of this work is in the field of radiology, the authors have broadly covered the study of congenital heart disease, including morphology and all other clinical parameters. This approach amply supports the concept that no branch of medicine can adequately operate alone in a vacuum.

Thus the authors have skillfully provided a stimulus to students based on the logical integration of clinical and radiologic modalities—and even more importantly provided a basis for exciting the imagination. It is through stimulating the mind that new investigation is conceived and supported.

The major accomplishments of the authors should project this work into the future as a well-recognized vehicle achieving the ideal teacher-student relationship—encouraging continued advances and meeting of challenges in this field of study.

Jesse E. Edwards, M.D.
Clinical Professor of Pathology Emeritus
University of Minnesota
Minneapolis, Minnesota

FOREWORD

It has been my sustained good fortune to have benefited in many academic, professional and personal ways from a career during the years that spawned a rapid generation of knowledge in several medical sciences responsible for creating accurate diagnostic and sound therapeutic procedures. During this time, steps were developed that became essential to the safe management of various types of congenital heart disease.

From the very beginning of the modern therapeutic era there had arisen the critical need for roentgen techniques which would reveal, unequivocally, those precise aspects of each lesion under diagnostic scrutiny. This glaringly evident challenge, therefore, loomed as a dominant incentive for those capable of achieving, and motivated to make, future advances in diagnostic radiology. In turn, and with even better methodology consistently revealing even the most complex cardiac lesions, those who were responsible for directing correctional or curative therapy were thereby challenged to utilize that newly derived knowledge in the fashion wisest for each particular patient.

So teams of human biologists have continued with their mental leap frogging from improved technology to innovative therapies. Each new step, after due trial and error, eventually taught students of this field a bit more about how best—in that particular time frame—to cope with a wide variety of congenital cardiovascular problems. Thus, both excitement and frustration have led them seductively from the early (and easiest) solutions to the more difficult and on to the present complex efforts which now deal with those complicated configurations currently managed in highly specialized centers. Today, a few remaining anomalies have yet to yield to some therapeutic intervention. These achievements overall have resulted from the combined and sustained efforts of many disciplines but particularly from those of cardiology, radiology, surgery and pathology. *Radiology of Congenital Heart Disease* demonstrates a major serious effort by dedicated teachers striving to help others move ahead with greater confidence in their field of common interest.

We are all therefore in their debt, as are future workers, for the broad understanding as revealed by the cumulative efforts of collaborative contributors Kurt Amplatz and James Moller. Thereby, they too become worthy members of that illustrious lineage that assists each generation as it moves from where it is toward where it wishes to be.

Richard L. Varco, M.D.
Professor of Surgery Emeritus
University of Minnesota
Minneapolis, Minnesota

FOREWORD

A roentgenologist and a pediatric cardiologist have collaborated and they brought to the task an extensive clinical experience and a record of innovative approaches for the accurate diagnosis of congenital malformations of the heart. The profession is well served to have the advances over the recent decades documented, and to have the accumulated radiological changes characterizing the varied morphological abnormalities recorded.

In the first half of this century, roentgenology contributed sparsely to the diagnosis of specific cardiac malformations, although the method rendered it possible to speak authoritatively for the first time of the size of the heart and of its different chambers. This is not meant to belittle the significant advances which were made during that time, such as careful measurements of the heart silhouette in different projections. Homage is due to many cardiologists worldwide who developed outstanding skills in the fluoroscopy of the heart.

The first textbook pertaining to cardiac roentgenology recommended to me was written by Hugo Roesler, a Viennese emigre, published in 1937. The chapter on congenital cardiovascular malformations consisted of only 20 pages. It begins with the discouraging affirmation: "The diagnostic aid derived from roentgenological study is comparatively slight in infants." Actually, this was the same year that the term "angiocardiography" was coined by Castellanos and co-workers, and Robb and Steinberg were independently exploring selective opacification techniques.

The fact that the heart could be safely "catheterized," demonstrated by Forsmann in 1929, was knowledge which lay dormant for about a decade. In the 1940s, rapid development and widespread implementation of the cardiac catheterization technique occurred in subjects with congenital heart disease. To the physiologist and the clinician, the measurements of pressures and of blood flows unveiled the basic hemodynamic faults; to the morphologist and surgeon, the selective injection of radiopaque material revealed the living structural abnormality. These two approaches complemented one another, resulting in an exploding revolutionary period wherein monumental developments in the understanding and management of congenital heart disease occurred. The senior authors of this volume were in the vanguard of those developing the new knowledge, and have here recorded their collated experiences in what will be a useful and authoritative text, relating the clinical, physiological and radiological aspects of congenital heart malformations. The organization is attractive and the illustrations clear and relevant. The explanatory sketches have a Vesalian quality and function as diagrams to aid in the interpretation of roentgenograms and angiocardiograms.

Howard B. Burchell, M.D., Ph.D.
Emeritus Professor of Medicine
University of Minnesota School of Medicine
Cardiovascular Section
Minneapolis, Minnesota

PREFACE

We have had the opportunity to work closely and collaboratively through the years in solving clinical problems presented by infants and children with congenital heart disease. Whether viewing chest films, working in the cardiac catheterization laboratory, or studying angiograms, we have combined the training of cardiovascular radiologists, the experience of pediatric cardiologists, and a common knowledge of hemodynamics to understand congenital cardiac malformations of individual patients.

Our collaboration occurred in the favorable environment which has existed at the University of Minnesota, an environment which lacks strong departmental lines that can tend to separate people, an environment of openness and a climate of questioning and thereby learning, a setting in which individuals can grow intellectually and professionally. Since the pioneering efforts of Dr. C. Walton Lillehei, and Dr. Richard Varco first in closed and then open-heart surgery, there has been excitement and a stimulus to learn about congenital heart disease. And we learned from each other. Dr. Ray C. Anderson and Dr. Paul Adams shared this interest in learning, and taught from their extensive experience with patients. Dr. Jesse Edwards for the last 40 years has provided a source of strength and wisdom and has often been a final arbiter in discussion regarding diagnosis.

We feel fortunate to have learned and worked in this creative environment and hope that it will continue in our institution. Through the years, many residents, fellows, and staff have been associated with us in the Variety Club Heart Hospital. Fortunately they have asked challenging questions which have forced us to think, consider, and perhaps change our thoughts or biases. They have brought forth new ideas and knowledge.

From this collaboration and from our teachers, colleagues, and students we have learned much and have attempted to organize and express this knowledge in this work, which is based on a vast clinical, radiographic, and surgical experience. We hope that our effort reflects favorably on all who have contributed to our understanding and knowledge.

Finally, we hope that in our environment at the University of Minnesota there is the germ of an idea, or the development of a new collaborative effort which will result. Then our work as teachers will be complete.

Kurt Amplatz, M.D.
James H. Moller, M.D.

ACKNOWLEDGMENTS

Our work is supported by the William Cook Foundation, The 3M Research Foundation, and the Paul F. Dwan Family Fund.

The authors express their appreciation to Mary Jo Antinozzi, Linda Boche, Debra Doi, Carla Nelson, and Joan Watkins for their assistance in the prepartion of the manuscript.

Kurt Amplatz, M.D.
James H. Moller, M.D.

CONTENTS

Forewords   ix

Preface   xvii

Color Plates   follows page 212

PART ONE: GENERAL INTRODUCTION   1

1 / Development of the Heart   3

2 / Cardiac Anatomy   13

3 / Radiation Safety   49

4 / Classification and Hemodynamics of Congenital Heart Disease   55

5 / Plain-Film Diagnosis of Congenital Cardiac Disease   61

6 / Cardiac Catheterization   115

7 / Angiographic Equipment   131

8 / Angiography   157

9 / Cardiac Ultrasound   195
   by G. Wayne Moore, Steven C. Cassidy, Wayne H. Franklin, and Hugh D. Allen

10 / Isotope Scanning   215
   by Robert J. Boudreau and Claudia M. Engeler

11 / Magnetic Resonance Imaging   229
   by Antoinette S. Gomes and Gustav Formanek

PART TWO: CARDIAC CONDITIONS ASSOCIATED WITH A LEFT-TO-RIGHT SHUNT   241

12 / Ventricular Septal Defect   243

13 / Ventricular Septal Defect With Aortic Insufficiency or Aortic Stenosis   273

14 / Aneurysm of the Membranous Ventricular Septum   279

15 / Left Ventricular—Right Atrial Communication   285

16 / Patent Ductus Arteriosus   291

17 / Aorticopulmonary Septal Defect (Window)   309

18 / Origin of Pulmonary Artery From Ascending Aorta (Hemitruncus)   315

19 / Atrial Septal Defect   321

20 / Raghib Syndrome and Other Coronary Sinus Anomalies Allowing Intracardiac Shunts   339

21 / Partial Anomalous Pulmonary Venous Connection   345

22 / Scimitar Syndrome   357

23 / Endocardial Cushion Defect   365

24 / Sinus of Valsalva Aneurysm   395

25 / Coronary Artery Fistula   407

PART THREE: INTRODUCTION TO OUTFLOW OBSTRUCTIVE LESIONS   415

26 / Aortic Stenosis   417

27 / Aortico—Left Ventricular Tunnel   461

28 / Coarctation of the Aorta   469

29 / Pulmonary Stenosis   499

PART FOUR: CYANOSIS AND DECREASED PULMONARY ARTERIAL VASCULATURE   537

30 / Tetralogy of Fallot   541

31 / Tetralogy of Fallot With Pulmonary Atresia   583

32 / Tetralogy of Fallot With Absent Pulmonary Valve *599*

33 / Tricuspid Atresia With Normally Related Great Vessels *607*

34 / Pulmonary Atresia With Intact Ventricular Septum *625*

35 / Isolated Hypoplasia of Right Ventricle *647*

36 / Ebstein's Malformation *653*

37 / Primary Tricuspid Insufficiency *665*

PART FIVE: CYANOSIS AND INCREASED PULMONARY ARTERIAL VASCULATURE *671*

38 / Complete Transposition of the Great Vessels *675*

39 / Congenital Corrected Transposition of Great Vessels: L-Transposition of Great Vessels *709*

40 / Clinical Transposition: Ventricular Inversion With Nontransposition or Isolated Ventricular Inversion *727*

41 / Double-Outlet Ventricle *731*

42 / Single Ventricle *753*

43 / Tricuspid Atresia With Transposition of Great Vessels *767*

44 / Double-Inlet Ventricle *777*

45 / Truncus Arteriosus *787*

46 / Total Anomalous Pulmonary Venous Connection *805*

47 / Single Atrium (Common Atrium) *827*

48 / Pulmonary Arteriovenous Fistula *833*

PART SEVEN: CYANOSIS AND INCREASED PULMONARY VENOUS VASCULATURE *845*

49 / Atresia of the Common Pulmonary Vein *847*

50 / Hypoplastic Left Ventricle Syndrome *853*

51 / Mitral Atresia *867*

PART EIGHT: CARDIAC CONDITIONS ASSOCIATED WITH INCREASED PULMONARY VENOUS VASCULATURE WITHOUT CYANOSIS *873*

52 / Mitral Stenosis *875*

53 / Supravalvar Stenosing Ring of Left Atrium *889*

54 / Cor Triatriatum *891*

55 / Stenosis of the Individual Pulmonary Veins *905*

56 / Cardiomyopathy *911*

57 / Anomalous Origin of Coronary Arteries From the Pulmonary Trunk *929*

58 / Malposition of the Heart *945*

59 / Criss-Cross Heart *977*

60 / Ectopia Cordis *987*

61 / Toracopagus (Conjoined Twins, Siamese Twins) *991*

PART TEN: ANOMALIES OF MAJOR BLOOD VESSELS *993*

62 / Anomalies of the Aortic Arch System *995*

63 / Abnormalities of the Venae Cavae *1051*

64 / Coronary Artery Anomalies *1061*

65 / Kawasaki Disease *1087*

66 / Systemic Arteriovenous Fistulas *1093*

PART ELEVEN: OTHER CONDITIONS *1099*

67 / Marfan Syndrome (Cystic Medial Necrosis) *1101*

68 / Mitral Valve Prolapse *1119*

69 / Abnormalities of the Mitral Valve *1127*

70 / Congenital Diverticulum of the Ventricles *1131*

71 / Aneurysm of Atrial Appendage *1141*

72 / Pericardial Defect *1145*

73 / Cardiac Tumors *1153*

74 / Complete Heart Block *1165*

75 / Pulmonary Hypertension *1171*

76 / Fetal Circulatory Problems *1179*

Index *1181*

PART ONE

General Introduction

The first eight chapters provide general information about congenital heart disease and its radiographic investigation. The first chapter reviews the normal embryologic development of the heart, as background for subsequent chapters about individual cardiac anomalies, in which abnormal development results in the cardiac malformations.

The second chapter describes details of cardiac anatomy pertinent to the cardiologist and radiologist. In this chapter, the radiologic implications of cardiac anatomy are described, and correlations with thoracic roentgenograms and angiocardiograms made.

A chapter on radiation safety is included. Although this information should be familiar to radiologists, it is included to enhance the knowledge of cardiologists. Not only is the patient but also technicians and physicians are exposed to radiation during diagnostic procedures in catheterization laboratories. The risks of radiation and methods to safeguard against those risks are described.

Thoracic roentgenograms provide valuable clues in the diagnosis and management of patients with congenital heart disease. Correct diagnosis from roentgenograms requires obtaining proper films free of confusing artifacts. It is necessary to recognize when a film has been improperly obtained and how these factors affect the interpretation of the film. Data about pulmonary vasculature, cardiac chamber and great vessel size, and cardiac contour can be gathered, which, when combined with pertinent clinical data, can lead usually to a correct diagnosis of the underlying condition.

Understanding the basic hemodynamics of various forms of congenital heart disease helps the radiologist and cardiologists in many ways. Classifications of congenital heart disease, including the one around which this work is organized, are based on hemodynamics. The clinical features, age of presentation, and laboratory features can easily be understood by knowledge of hemodynamics. Through cardiac catheterization, the hemodynamics of various anomalies are determined. Finally, knowledge of patterns of blood flow and intracardiac pressures helps the radiologists and cardiologists in many decisions about the delivery of contrast medium for angiography and in interpretation of angiographic films.

Cardiac catheterization, in addition to providing a route for angiography, yields important information about cardiac anatomy and physiology. Radiologists need an appreciation of the type of data that the cardiologist is seeking and how these data are used to derive cardiac output, shunt size, vascular resistance, and stenotic valve areas.

A variety of equipment is used during cardiac catheterization, such as cardiac catheters, contrast material, image intensifiers, and cine angiographic equipment. When properly maintained and used, they can provide high-quality films with maximal information for diagnosis. Improperly maintained and misused, such equipment may needlessly prolong studies and provide substandard films that may make diagnosis difficult, doubtful, or incorrect.

CHAPTER 1

Development of the Heart

This chapter discusses the development of the heart and fetal circulation and the hemodynamic changes that occur in the neonate. We hope this information will be helpful in understanding the embryogenesis of various congenital cardiac malformations and the disturbances of the transitional circulation.

EMBRYOLOGY OF THE HEART

At 18 days of gestation, paired cardiac cords form in the thoracic region of the embryo, which later canalize to become the paired (right and left) cardiac tubes. These endothelial-lined tubes begin to fuse cranially, with fusion progressing caudally to form a single cardiac tube by 21 days of gestation (Fig 1–1). Two processes then take place:

1. The tube develops constrictions that demarcate several cardiac segments. From caudad to craniad these are the sinus venosus, which receives the umbilical, vitelline, and common cardinal veins; the atrium; the ventricularis; the bulbus cordis; the truncus arteriosus; the aortic sac; and the aortic arches.
2. The cardiac tube elongates. Because the tube is fixed at both the sinus venosus and the arterial end, it bends on itself as it elongates, forming an S. The bulbus cordis and the ventricularis are displaced anteriorly and to the right, whereas the atrium and sinus venosus are displaced posteriorly to lie behind the ventricles.

Subsequently, the ventricularis migrates to the left, and the bulk of the cardiac mass then lies in the left hemithorax.

The discussion of the subsequent development of each portion of the heart starts with the systemic venous system.

Systemic Venous System

Early in embryonic development, there are three systems of paired veins: the cardinal, the umbilical, and the vitelline (Fig 1–2). The cardinal system drains the body of the embryo, the umbilical veins drain the developing placenta, and the vitelline veins drain the yolk sac. Because most anomalies form within the cardinal system, this system is discussed in detail, whereas the umbilical and vitelline system are not discussed further.

The cardinal venous system consists of two sets of paired veins: the precardinal veins, which drain the cephalic portion of the embryo, and the posterocardinals, which drain the caudal portion of the body. These cardinal veins join to form the common cardinal veins, which enter the sinus venosus part of the heart (see Fig 1–2).

The precardinal veins (also called the anterior cardinal veins) receive blood from the head and neck and pass caudally to the common cardinal vein. During the seventh week of development, an anastomotic channel develops between the two venous systems (see Fig 1–2,B). As this channel enlarges, the left precardinal vein loses its communication with the left common cardinal vein and involutes. The only normal remnant of this system is a cardiac vein that flows into the coronary sinus. The right anterior cardinal vessel becomes the superior vena cava, and the anastomotic channel becomes the left brachiocephalic vein (see Fig 1–2,C).

The posterior cardinal system also undergoes a series of changes. Below the diaphragm, there is a succession of two additional paired veins, the subcardinals and supracardinals, which, together with the posterior cardinal vein, are responsible for the venous drainage from the viscera, abdominal wall, and legs. These three venous systems develop anastomoses and undergo changes, during which the left-sided cardinal veins largely involute. The principal

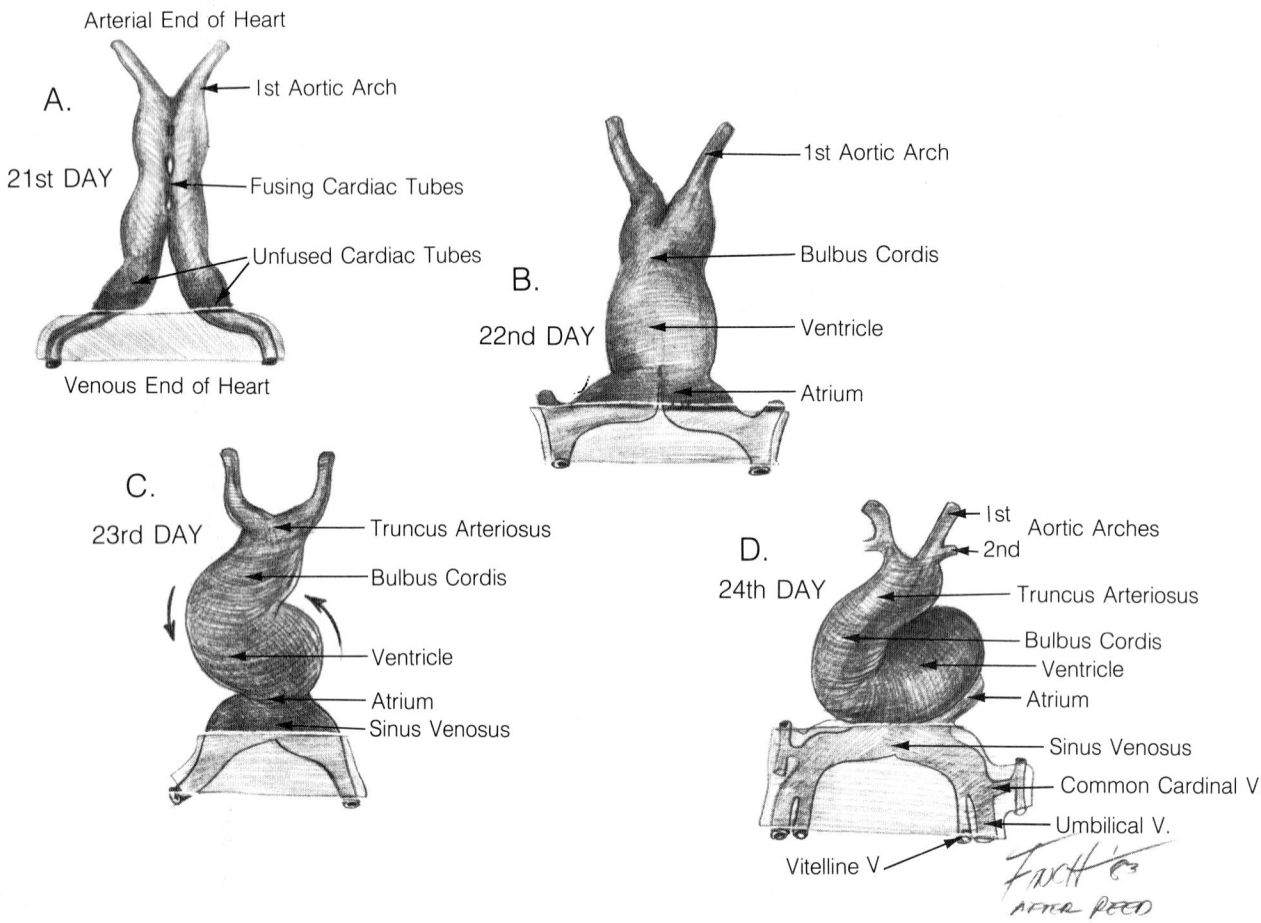

FIG 1–1.
Development of cardiac tube. **A,** day 21 of development; paired cardiac tubes fusing in cranial-to-caudal direction. **B,** day 22; cardiac tubes fused, with beginning of differentiation of portions of tube. **C,** day 23; elongation and twisting of cardiac tube. **D,** day 24; S-shaped cardiac tube, with external differentiation of portions of tube and formation of second aortic arch.

venous structure in the abdomen, the inferior vena cava, is formed from four venous structures; the hepatic segment is derived from the hepatic sinusoids; the prerenal segment, which is located between the hepatic segment and the kidneys, is derived from the subcardinal venous system; the renal segment, which includes the renal veins, represents an anastomosis between the subcardinal and supracardinal venous systems; and, finally, the segment below the renal veins is derived from the supracardinal system and joins with the iliac veins, which are derivatives of the posterior cardinal system.

Sinus Venosus

The sinus venosus is a primitive portion of the vascular system that receives the common cardinal vein through two structures, the left and right horns of the sinus venosus (Fig 1–3,A). The sinus venosus opens dorsally into the right side of the atrium. During early fetal life, the size of the left horn decreases as the venous blood in the precardinal systems is progressively diverted into the right precardinal system. Between the sixth and eighth weeks, the atria enlarge, and the right horn of the sinus venosus is incorporated into the posterior wall of the right atrium. Consequently, the orifices of the superior and inferior vena cava connect separately with the atrium (Fig 1–3,C). The area between the original right atrium and the sinus venosus is marked externally by the terminal sulcus. The opening of the primitive sinus venosus is guarded by the right and the left valves of the sinus venosus. Ultimately the left valve fuses with the septum secundum, and the right valve in the superior portion of the right atrium forms the crista terminalis and caudally forms the valves of the inferior vena cava and the coronary sinus (Fig 1–3,B).

Atrium

The primitive atrium communicates with the primitive ventricle through the atrioventricular canal, which lies predominately between the future left atrium and left ventri-

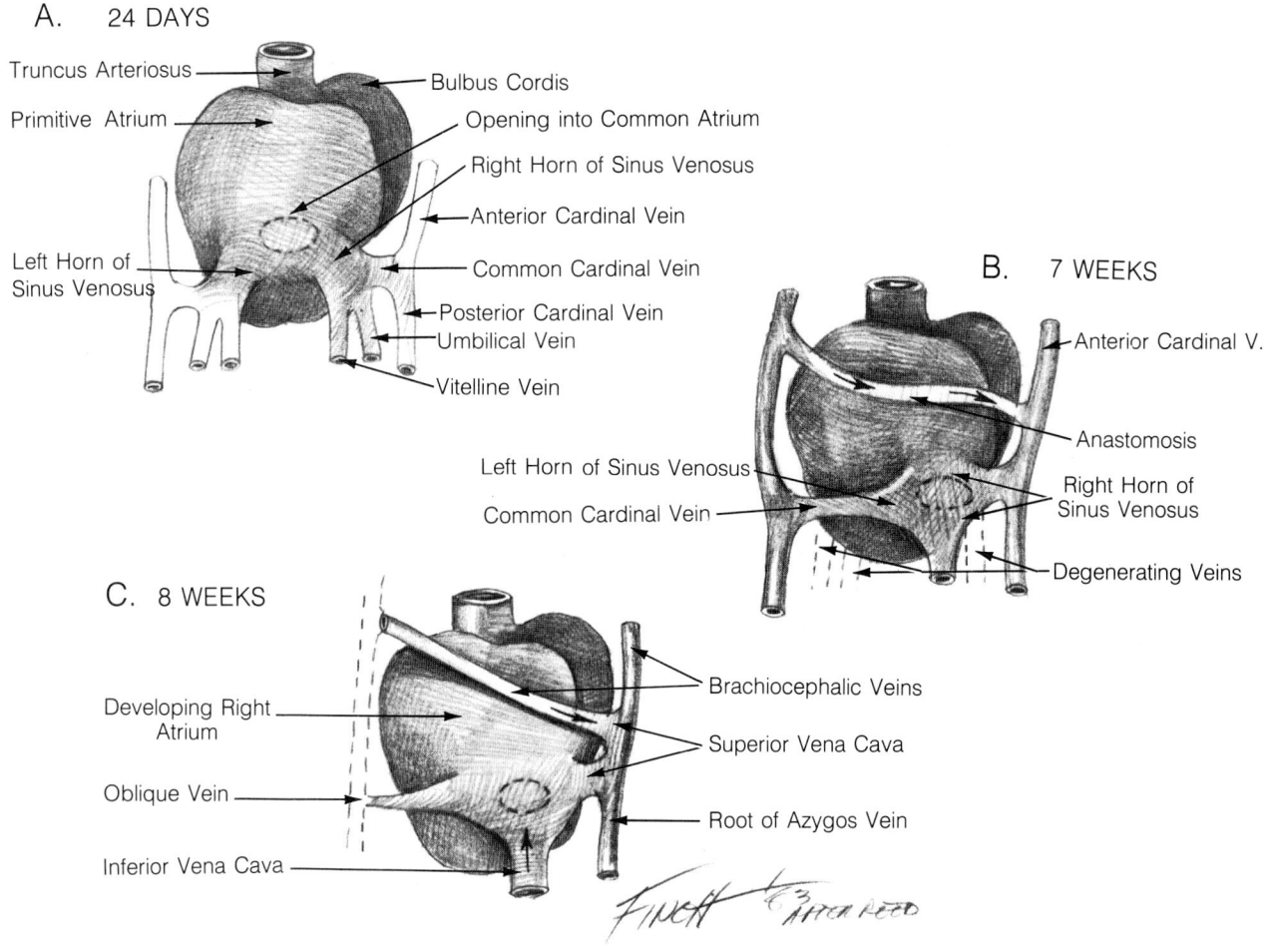

FIG 1–2.
Development of major venous systems and sinus venosus (primitive atrium viewed from behind.) **A,** day 24; paired vitelline, umbilical, posterior cardinal, and anterior cardinal veins join paired common cardinal veins and enter horns of sinus venosus. **B,** 7 weeks; anastomosis between anterior cardinal veins. **C,** 8 weeks; involution of left anterior cardinal vein and formation of inferior vena cava; sinus venosus being incorporated into right atrium.

cle. Gradually the atrioventricular canal migrates toward the right, so that it lies beneath both atria and above both ventricles. As this migration occurs, the bulbus cordis is expanding to develop into the right ventricle, and the ventricularis differentiates into the left ventricle (Fig 1–4).

The primitive atrioventricular canal is then divided into two channels, one connecting the right atrium to the right ventricle and the other the left atrium to the left ventricle. This division occurs by means of the formation of a ventral and a dorsal endocardial cushion. These tissue masses grow toward each other through the center of the atrioventricular canal, eventually meeting and fusing and thus dividing the canal. The septal surfaces of the endocardial cushion tissue differentiate further to form the septal leaflets of the mitral and the tricuspid valves, At this time, the other leaflets of the atrioventricular valves differentiate from tissue surrounding the atrioventricular annuli.

The primitive atrium is divided in a series of steps involving the formation of two septa and two foramina (Fig 1–5). A thin crescent-shaped septum forms from the cranial aspect of the primitive atrium (see Fig 1–5,A). This structure, the septum primum, generally grows toward the fused endocardial cushions, until eventually it fuses with them (see Fig 1–5,B–D). The opening between the crescent-shaped leading edge of this septum and the fused endocardial cushions is called the ostium primum and is gradually obliterated. Before the septum primum fuses with the endocardial cushion, several perforations develop in its midportion that enlarge and coalesce to form a single large opening, the ostium secundum. Thus, both ostia are in the septum primum.

Another septum, the septum secundum, then develops along the cranial and posterior wall of the right atrium (see Fig 1–5,D and E). This septum, which also has a cres-

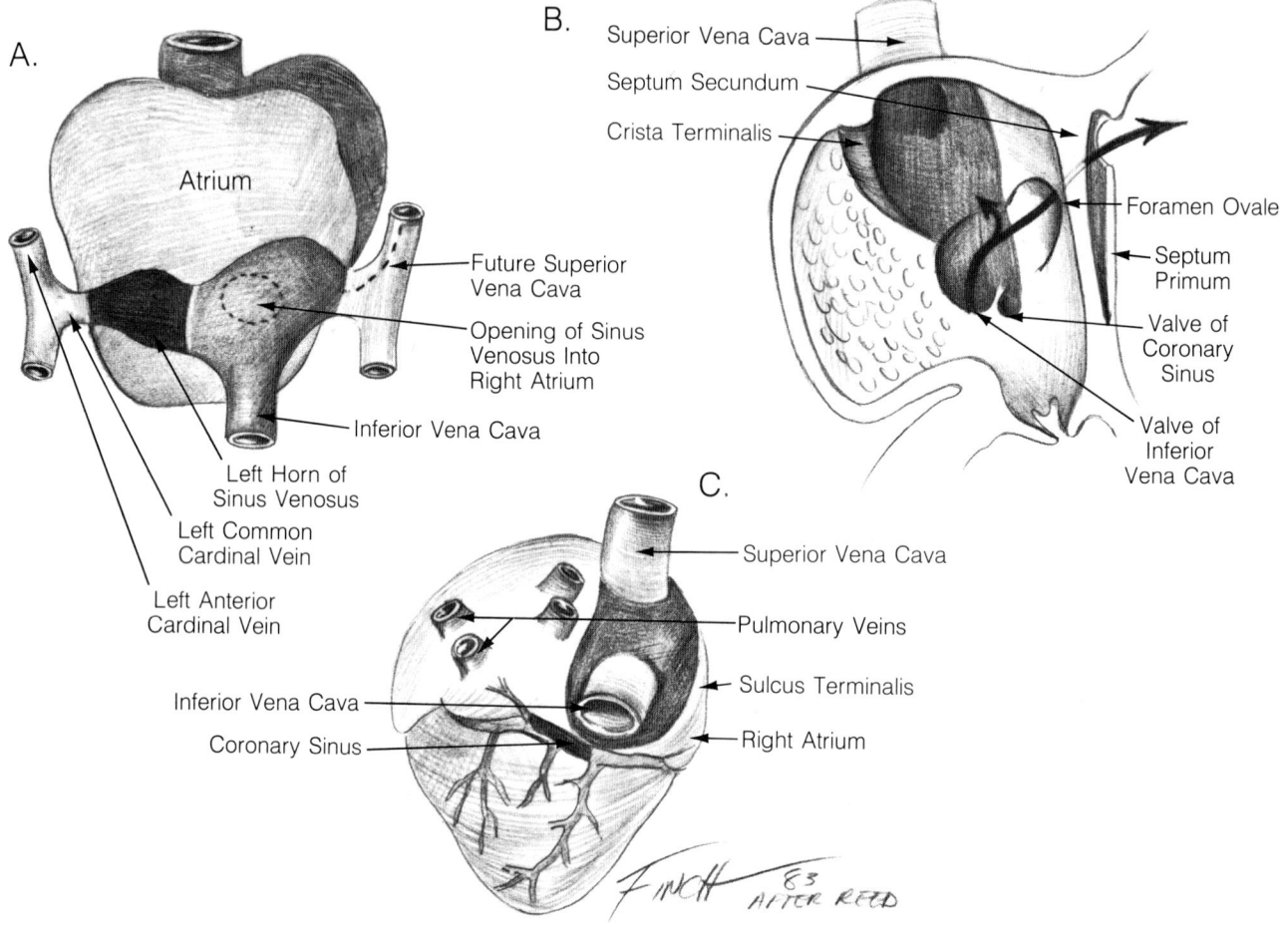

FIG 1–3.
Incorporation of sinus venosus into right atrium. **A,** major veins join sinus venosus, which opens into right atrium. **B,** internal view looking toward posterior wall of right atrium, with sinus venosus becoming incorporated into its posterior wall and right valve of sinus venosus forming valves of coronary sinus and inferior vena cava. Crista terminalis marks junction of sinus venosus and primitive atrium. **C,** external view; separate superior vena cava and inferior vena cava enter portions of posterior right atrial wall formed from sinus venosus *(shaded area).*

cent-shaped leading edge, grows downward toward the endocardial cushions but never fuses with them (see Fig 1–5,F and G). It extends midway along the septum primum, and its crescent-shaped lower margin forms the foramen ovale. Usually the septum secundum covers the ostium secundum (see Fig 1–5,H).

Ventricles

Simultaneously the primitive ventricle is being divided while the bulbus cordis expands on one side into the right ventricle and the ventricularis expands on the other side into the left ventricle. There is a space, the interventricular foramen, between the developing ventricular septum and the fusing endocardial cushions. This foramen is closed partly by endocardial cushion tissue and partly by the bulboventricular ridges, which are also responsible for dividing the primitive truncus arteriosus.

Great Arteries

The truncus arteriosus and bulbus cordis are divided by a pair of ridges of tissue resembling endocardial cushions, the bulbar ridges, which grow toward the center of the truncus arteriosus and fuse in the midline, thus dividing the truncus into an equal-sized aorta and pulmonary artery. The septum is thought to develop in a spiral, thus creating the normally entwined relation between the great vessels. The bulbar ridges develop across the junction between the truncus and ventricular mass; and as they do, they divide the truncal valve into separate aortic and pulmonary orifices, each guarded by three semilunar cusps. The bulbar ridges extend further and aid in closing the interventricular foramen, as indicated earlier.

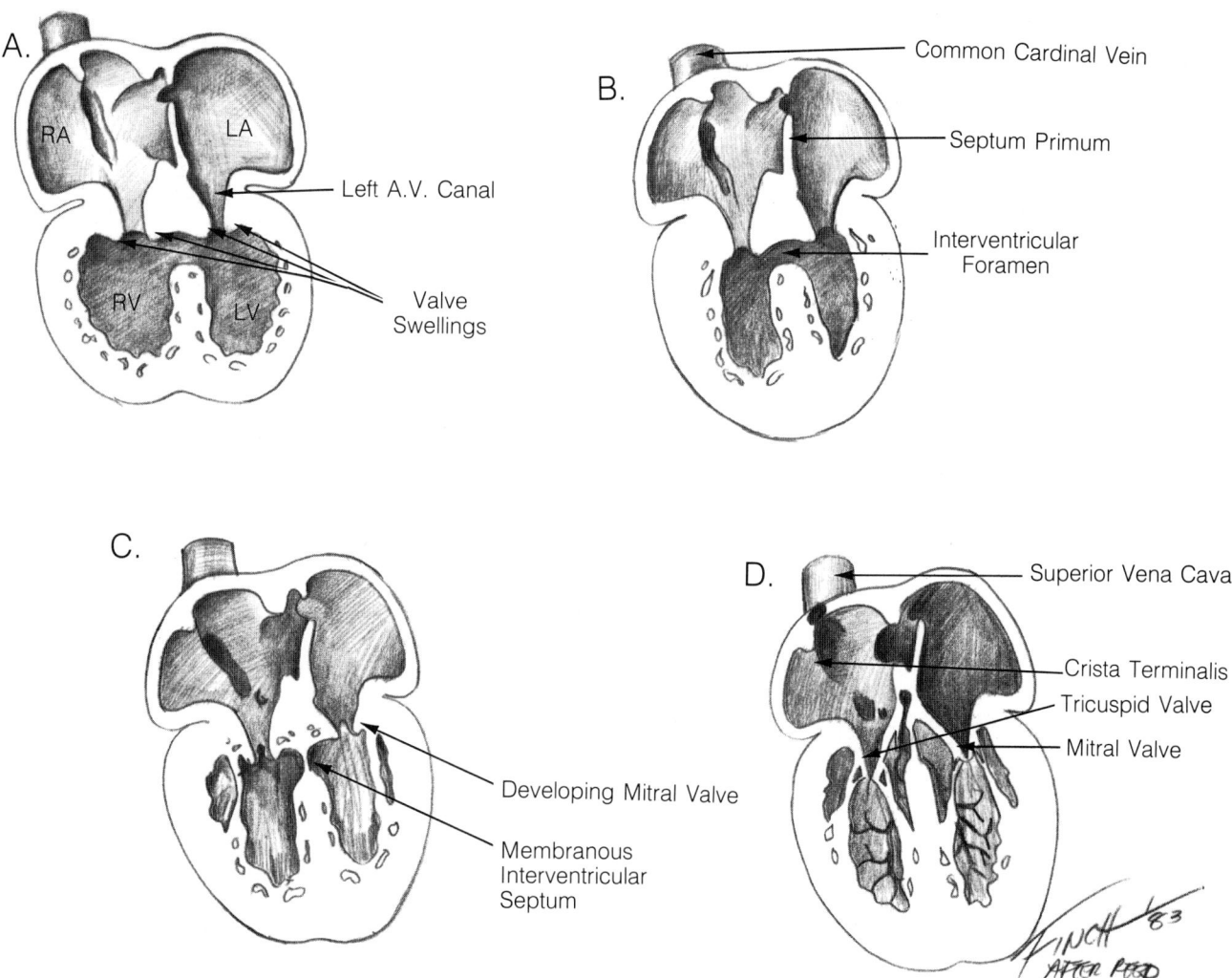

FIG 1–4.
Development of cardiac septa. **A,** endocardial cushion tissue has separated primitive atrioventricular canal into separate right and left atrioventricular *(AV)* canals; tissue beginning to differentiate into atrioventricular valvular tissue. **B,** communication below endocardial cushions between ventricles through interventricular foramen. **C,** ventricular septum sealed; valvular tissue continues to differentiate. **D,** distinct mitral and tricuspid valve leaflets.

Pulmonary Veins

The incorporation of the pulmonary veins into the left atrium is a complex process. The lungs form as outpouchings of the foregut, so their early venous return is to the cardinal and splanchnic systems. As the lungs differentiate, so do the venous channels within their mass leading to formation of individual pulmonary veins. These veins unite into a confluence immediately behind the left atrium, and venous channels pass from the confluence to the cardinal and umbilical venous systems.

The left atrium initiates the process by which it incorporates the pulmonary venous system. A projection, the common pulmonary vein, forms and expands until it makes contact with the venous confluence (Fig 1–6). An opening develops between the common pulmonary vein and the confluence and widens until the individual pulmonary veins join the left atrium. The pulmonary venous confluence thus forms the posterior wall of the left atrium.

Aortic Arches

The truncus arteriosus connects with the aortic sac, which, in turn, connects with paired aortic arches, which pass, one on the right side of the trachea and esophagus and the other on the left side of these two structures, to connect with the right and left dorsal aortae, which lie along the posterior aspect of the embryo.

A series of six paired arches form in succession, developing and involuting in a cranial to caudal direction. At any one time, perhaps only two pairs exist (Fig 1–7). During this time, the paired dorsal aortae begin to fuse into a single dorsal aorta in the abdomen. This process progresses toward the thorax, leading eventually to a left-sided descending aorta. Portions of these aortic arches may persist, the derivatives in the postnatal circulation being:

Aortic Arch	Derivative
I	Part of maxillary arteries
II	Part of stapedial arteries
III	Common carotid arteries
IV	Left aortic arch and part of right subclavian artery
V	None
VI	Left: Proximal part forms proximal portion of left pulmonary artery; distal part forms ductus arteriosus.
	Right: Proximal part forms proximal portion of right pulmonary artery; distal part, if it persists, forms rightsided ductus arteriosus.

FETAL CIRCULATION

During fetal life, the circulation differs from that of an infant or adult in both circulatory pattern and anatomy.

In the normal infant, circulation is serial, that is, dur-

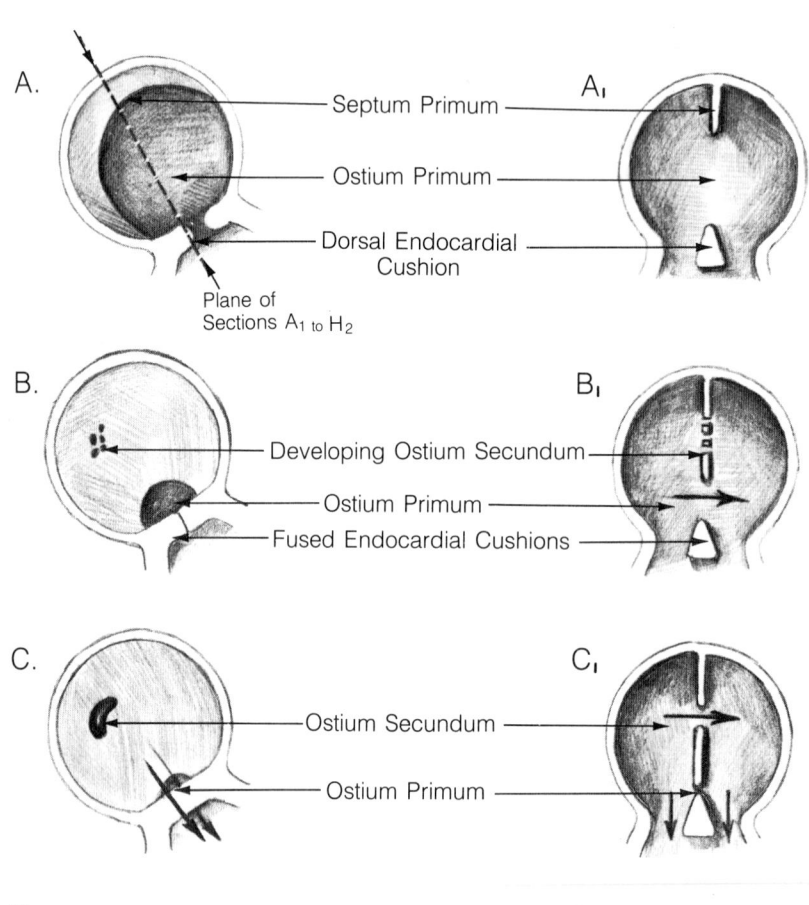

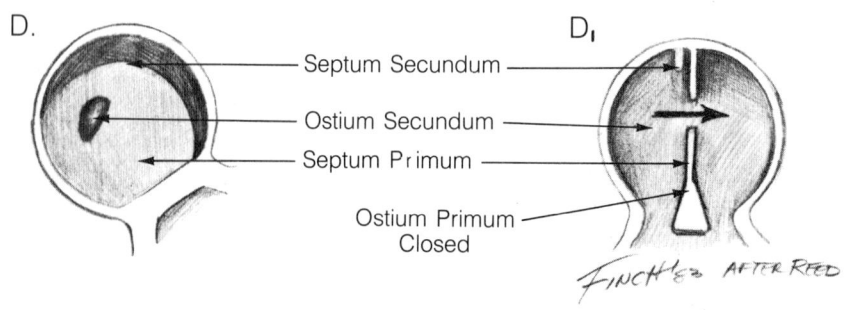

FIG 1–5.
Differentiation of atrial septum viewed from right side (lateral) and anteroposterior direction *(subscript letter)*: **A** and **A₁**, beginning of septum primum. **B** and **B₁**, growth of septum primum toward fused endocardial cushions; perforations developing as early ostium secundum. **C** and **C₁**, septum primum nearly fused to endocardial cushions. Coalesced perforations form ostium secundum. **D** and **D₁**, ostium primum closed; beginning of septum secundum. *(Continued.)*

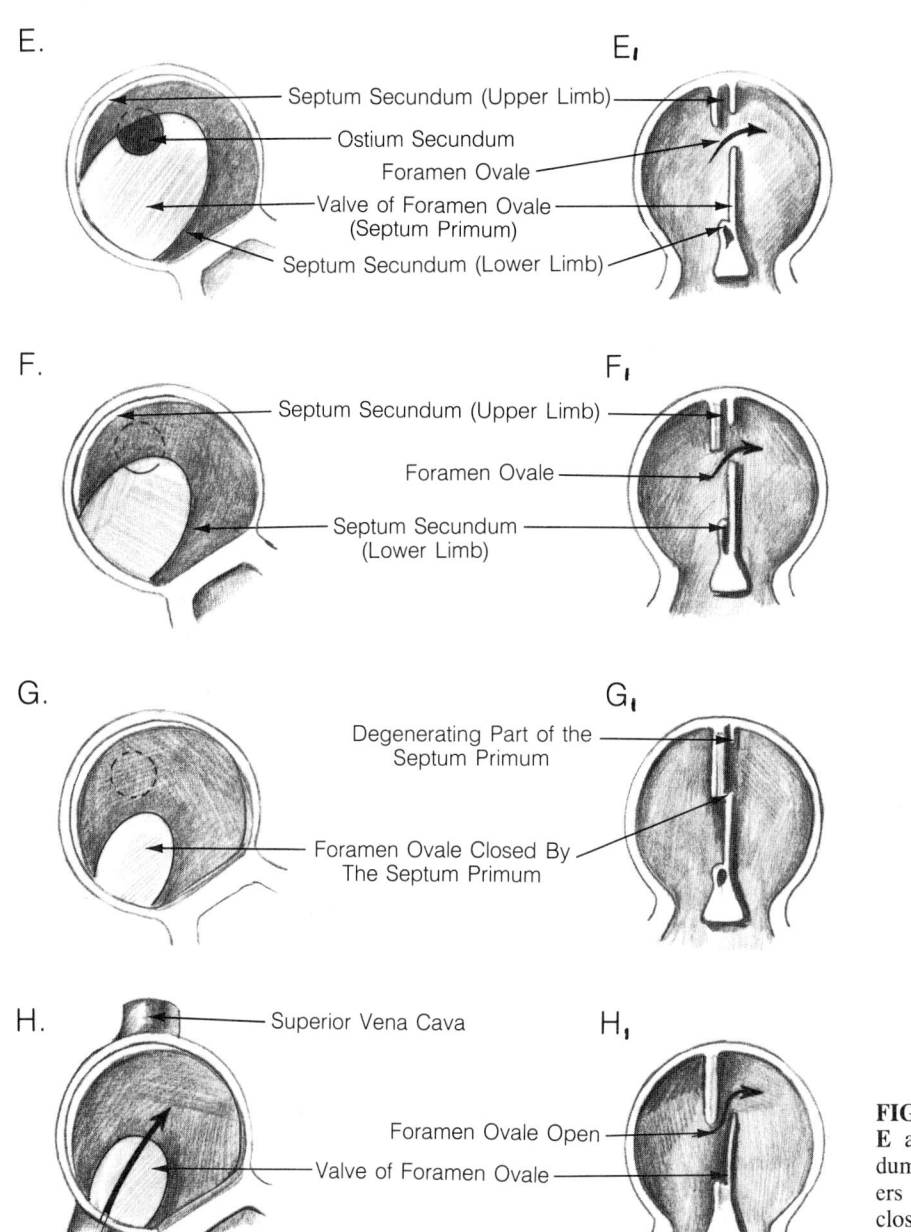

FIG 1–5 (cont.).
E and **E₁**, growth of septum secundum. **F** and **F₁**, septum secundum covers ostium secundum; foramen ovale closed. **G** and **G₁**, continued growth of septum secundum; closure of foramen ovale. **H** and **H₁**, relation between inferior vena cava and valve of foramen ovale.

ing one circuit, the blood passes through both ventricles. This indicates that systemic venous blood returns only to the right atrium, and only the left ventricle ejects blood into the aorta.

In contrast, the fetus has a parallel circulatory pattern; blood does not necessarily pass through both ventricles and the lungs before ejection into the body. The systemic venous return enters both ventricles, both of which eject blood into the aorta. In the first 24 hours of life, major changes occur that convert this parallel pattern to a serial one.

In the fetus, four unique anatomic structures maintain the fetal circulation (Fig 1–8). Normally, these disappear or are excluded within minutes or days of birth.

Placenta

The placenta is the principal site of oxygenation in the fetus and receives 20% of the combined ventricular output through paired umbilical arteries, which arise from the iliac arteries and pass in the anterior abdominal wall into the umbilical cord. Placental blood returns through a single

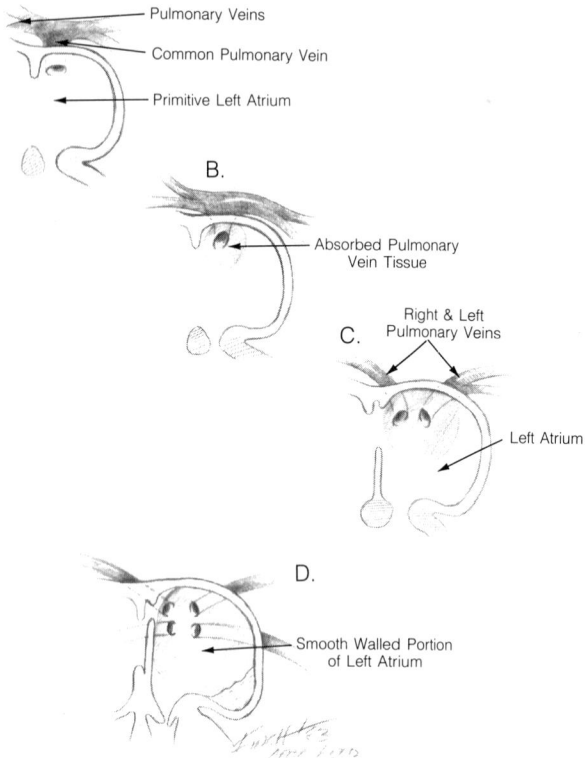

FIG 1–6.
Incorporation of pulmonary veins into left atrium. **A,** common pulmonary vein has made contact with confluence of pulmonary veins. **B** and **C,** progressive absorption of common pulmonary vein and pulmonary venous confluence into posterior left atrial wall. **D,** individual pulmonary veins join left atrium; absorbed pulmonary venous tissue forms part of left atrial wall *(shaded area)*.

umbilical vein, which passes cranially in the anterior abdominal wall. This blood has the highest oxygen content in the fetal circulation.

Ductus Venosus

Most of the umbilical blood bypasses the liver through the ductus venosus, a venous channel that lies on the visceral surface of the liver and joins the left hepatic vein at the junction with the inferior vena cava. The ductus venosus communicates with the portal vein, and a small portion of placental blood flow is diverted to the right hepatic lobe.

Foramen Ovale

The blood returning to the heart through the inferior vena cava is diverted primarily into the left atrium through an opening in the atrial septum termed the foramen ovale. The inferior margin of the septum secundum, the crista dividens, virtually straddles the orifice of the inferior vena cava, helping to divert the blood. In the left atrium, the blood mixes with a small volume of unoxygenated blood returning from the lungs. This mixture passes through the left ventricle into the ascending aorta, flowing predominately to the head and arms. Thus, the brain is perfused with well-oxygenated blood. Only a small portion of left ventricular output traverses the aortic arch to enter the descending aorta. The blood returning through the superior vena cava to the right atrium passes principally into the right ventricle and then to the pulmonary artery.

Patent Ductus Arteriosus

The right ventricular output passes predominately through the ductus arteriosus into the descending aorta; only a small portion passes through the lungs. Most of the blood flowing into the descending aorta passes to either the placenta or the kidneys.

Relative vascular resistances play a significant role in the distribution of fetal blood flow and particularly that through the ductus arteriosus. In the fetus, systemic vascular resistance is low because of the placenta, which is, in effect, a large arteriovenous fistula. In contrast, pulmonary vascular resistance is elevated to approximately twice the systemic vascular resistance. The pulmonary arterioles have a thick-walled media and a narrow lumen, because the relative fetal hypoxia is a vasoconstrictive stimulus to the pulmonary arterioles. Because the pulmonary vascular resistance exceeds the systemic vascular resistance, approximately 90% of the blood in the pulmonary trunk passes right to left through the ductus and only 10% through the lungs, even though the aortic and pulmonary arterial pressures are the same.

THE TRANSITIONAL CIRCULATION

Immediately after birth, profound hemodynamic changes occur in the circulation; and these are followed by structural changes initiated in the immediate postnatal period, although they may not be complete for days or even months (Fig 1–9).

At birth, two significant changes take place. First, the placenta is eliminated from the circulation, and this doubles the systemic vascular resistance. Second, at the same time, the neonate initiates respiration, the lungs expand, and the degree of systemic oxygenation improves dramatically. These two changes are associated with a sharp fall in pulmonary vascular resistance, and because of this fall, the volume of pulmonary blood flow increases. Therefore, the volume of blood returning from the pulmonary veins to the left atrium is increased, displacing the septum primum against the septum secundum and functionally closing the foramen ovale.

FETAL DEVELOPMENT OF THE ARTERIAL TRUNK AND BRACHIOCEPHALIC ARTERIES

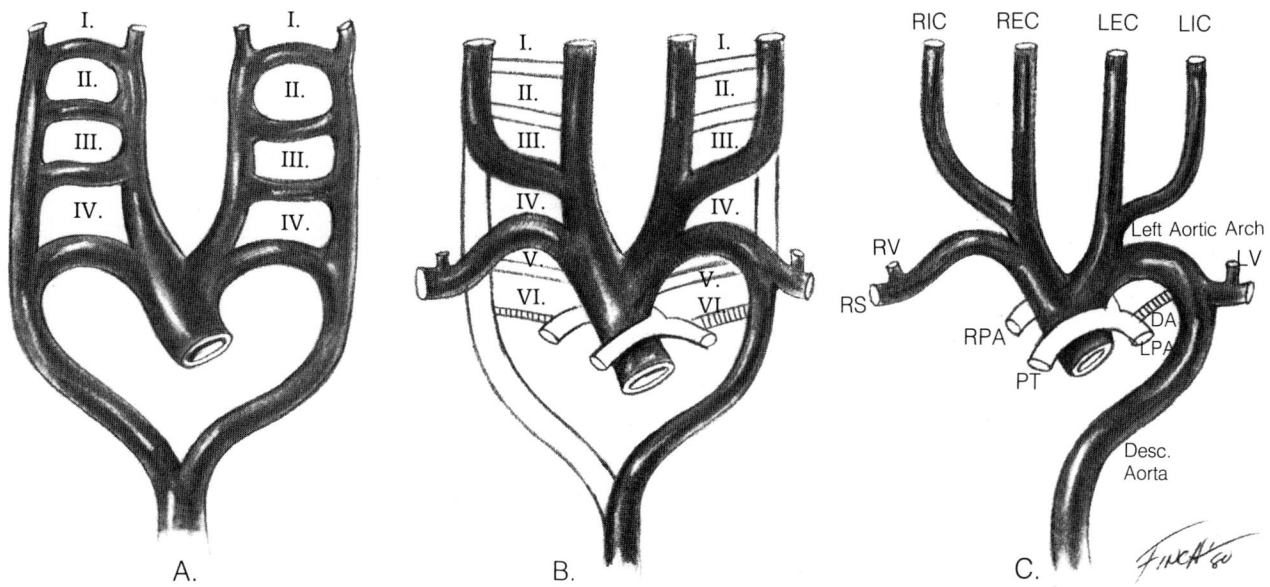

FIG 1–7.
Development of aortic arch system. **A,** early embryonic stage; four paired arches *(I, II, III,* and *IV)* join to form descending aorta. **B,** later stage; paired first *(I)* and second *(II)* arches have involuted, whereas paired third *(III)* arches persist as common carotid arteries. Right fourth *(IV)* arch has contributed to formation of right subclavian artery; left fourth arch has formed aortic arch. Connection of right arch system to descending aorta has disappeared, and primitive truncus arteriosus has been divided into separate ascending aorta and pulmonary trunk. Left sixth *(VI)* aortic arch present. **C,** at birth; *DA* = ductus arteriosus; *LEC* = left external carotid artery; *LIC* = left internal carotid artery; *LS* = left subclavian artery; *LV* = left vertebral artery; *PT* = pulmonary trunk; *REC* = right external carotid artery; *RIC* = right internal carotid artery; *RS* = right subclavian artery; *RV* = right vertebral artery.

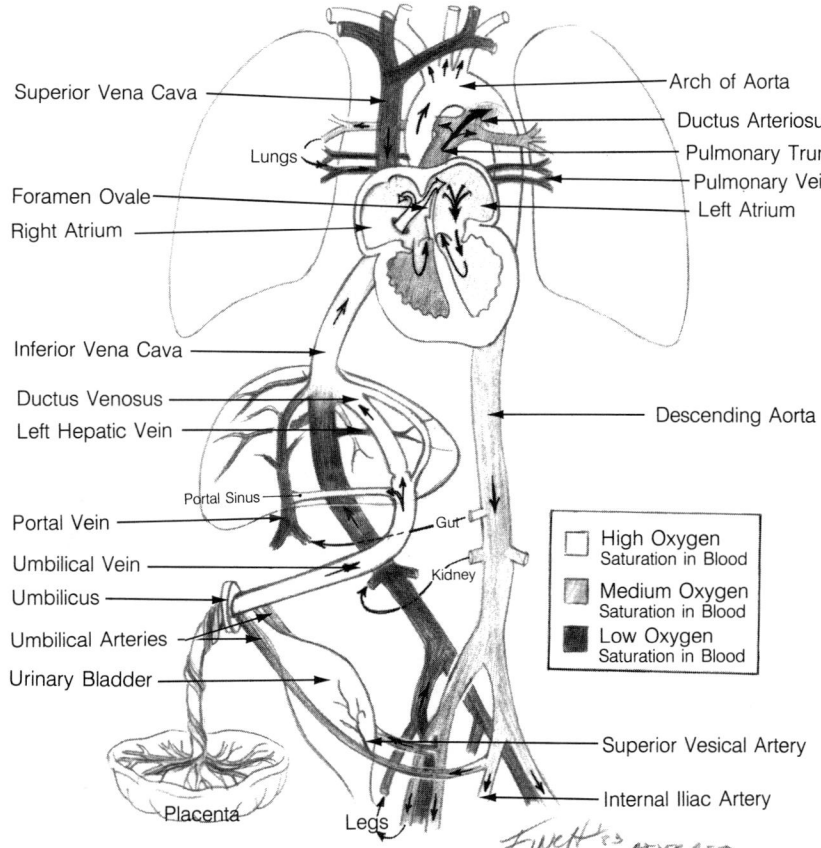

FIG 1–8.
Fetal circulation: oxygen-rich blood from placenta bypasses liver through ductus venosus to enter inferior vena cava; this stream flows preferentially through foramen ovale into left side of heart, predominately to head and arms. Blood from head and arms returns to right atrium, joining a portion of inferior vena caval blood to flow into right ventricle. From pulmonary trunk, most blood flows through patent ductus arteriosus into descending aorta, mostly to placentas. Small volume of blood in pulmonary artery flows through unexpanded lungs and returns to left atrium.

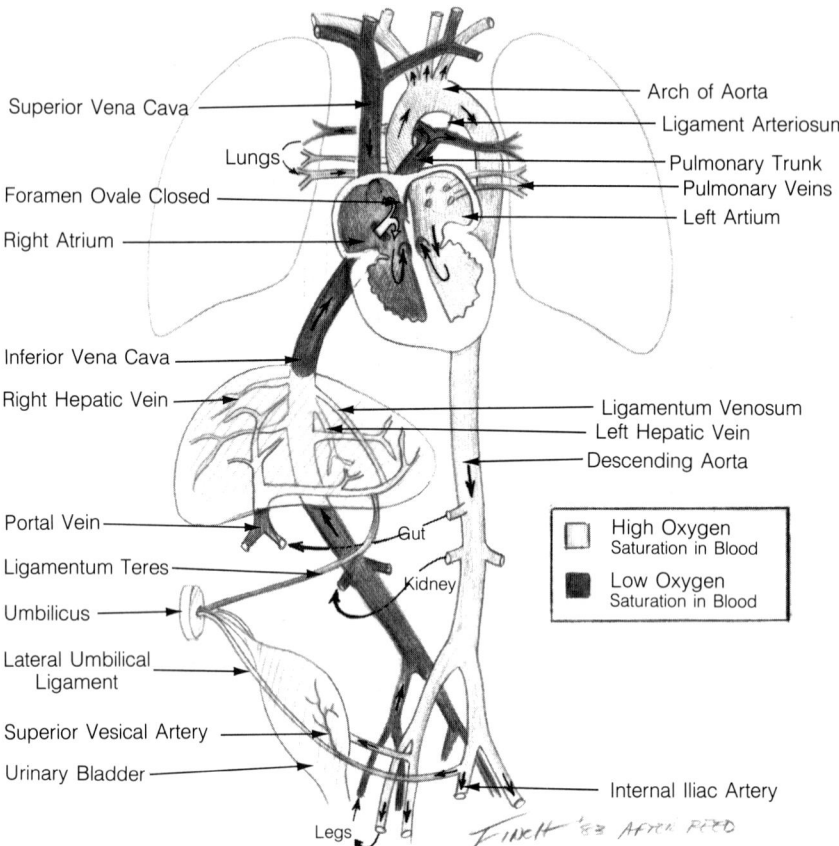

FIG 1-9.
Postnatal circulation: placenta eliminated from circulation, lungs expanded, ductus venosus and ductus arteriosus closed, and patent foramen ovale functionally closed. Course of blood flow as in adult: systemic venous blood returns to right side of heart and is delivered to lungs while oxygen-rich blood from lungs returns to left side of heart and is delivered through systemic circulation.

The fall in pulmonary vascular resistance and the rise in systemic vascular resistance also affect blood flow through the ductus arteriosus. In the first 6 hours of life, until ductal closure occurs, blood flow is bidirectional and left to right.

ANATOMIC CLOSURE

The ductus arteriosus is functionally closed by 18 to 24 hours after birth but is not anatomically closed until about 1 month of age. The improved fetal oxygenation is a major factor tending to constrict the ductus arterious. Thus, in the presence of hypoxemia or other abnormal states, the ductus may reopen for the first week or so of postnatal life.

The foramen ovale, although closed functionally soon after birth, closes anatomically at a slower rate than does the ductus arteriosus; by 1 year of age, only 75% are anatomically sealed. In patients with an unsealed foramen ovale, blood flow may occur in either direction when the pressure in one atrium greatly exceeds that in the other.

After separation from the placenta, the umbilical arteries and veins involute. The ductus venosus is closed by 3 days of age in one half of neonates and by 1 week in the remainder.

CHAPTER 2

Cardiac Anatomy

Cardiac anatomy is discussed only insofar as it is important for the understanding of angiocardiography and cardiac catheterization.

POSITION OF THE HEART IN THE THORAX

The heart is surrounded by the lungs and has an oblique position in the thoracic cavity, with the cardiac apex in the left hemithorax. The long axis of the heart and the inclination of the atrial and posterior ventricular septa lie at approximately 45 degrees to both the sagittal and the coronal planes (Fig 2–1). Deviation from this position significantly influences the radiographic appearance. Rotation of the heart about its long axis may be either clockwise or counterclockwise as the heart is viewed from below.

The orientation of the heart in relation to the horizontal plane varies considerably and is largely dependent on the position of the diaphragm. In younger or slender individuals, the heart tends to be more vertical (Fig 2–2), whereas it tends to be more horizontal in an obese patient. Usually, the inclination to the horizontal plane is approximately 45 degrees. Also, when the heart is viewed from the lateral aspect of the thorax (Fig 2–3), the inclination of its long axis is dependent largely on the position of the diaphragm, but this also is approximately 45 degrees. Thus, the heart typically is inclined 45 degrees to each major body plane.

The heart has three major surfaces. In situ the anterior surface faces ventrally and corresponds principally to the anterior wall of the right ventricle. The posterior wall consists primarily of the left atrium. The inferior, or diaphragmatic, surface is made up mainly of left ventricular wall.

That is, because the cardiac septa lie in an axis of about 45 degrees to the frontal plane, the right atrium and ventricle lie anteriorly and to the right of the posteriorly located left atrium and left ventricle.

These are the features of the heart in situ; once the organ has been removed from the thorax, as for pathologic examination, the pathologist rotates the heart in a left anterior position, which establishes a right to left orientation rather than the more anterior to posterior relation seen in situ (Fig 2–4). This orientation of the isolated heart has had a confusing effect on the nomenclature of the leaflets of the pulmonary and aortic valves. Thus, two nomenclatures have been derived:

	Heart in Situ	*Isolated Heart*
Aortic valve cusps:	Right	Posterior or non-coronary
	Anterior	Right (anterior)
	Left posterior	Left (anterior)
Pulmonary valve cusps:	Left anterior	Anterior
	Right anterior	Right (posterior)
	Posterior	Left (posterior)

Although the nomenclature of the heart in situ is more useful for the angiographer, the nomenclature of the isolated heart, as defined by the pathologist, is most widely accepted.

Within the thorax, the heart lies within the pericardial sac, a serofibrous membrane that forms a cavity enclosing the heart. The sac consists of two layers, an outer fibrous layer and a smooth, serous lining. The outer layer blends into the adventitia of the roots of the great vessels (superior vena cava, aorta, and pulmonary trunk) superiorly and fuses with the central tendon of the diaphragm. It also ex-

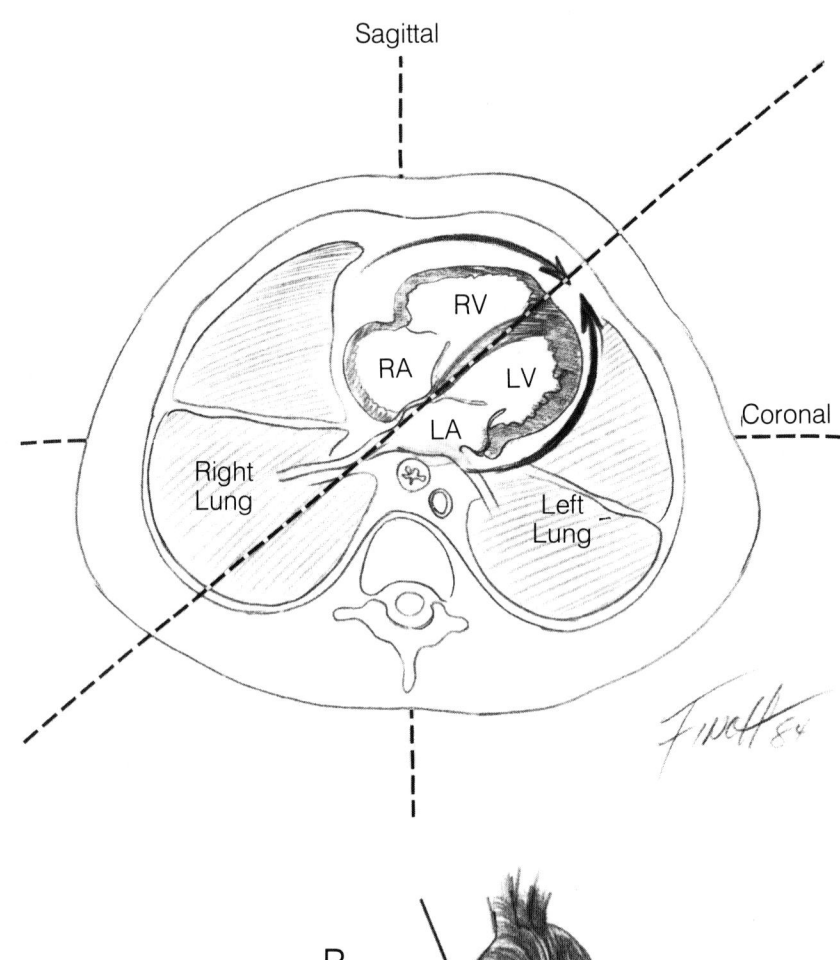

FIG 2-1.
Cross-section through thorax viewed from below; CT images are also viewed from below. Average inclination of the cardiac septa is 45 degrees; deviation from this angle is indicated as clockwise and counterclockwise rotation *(curved arrows)*. *LA* = left atrium; *LV* = left ventricle; *RA* = right atrium; *RV* = right ventricle.

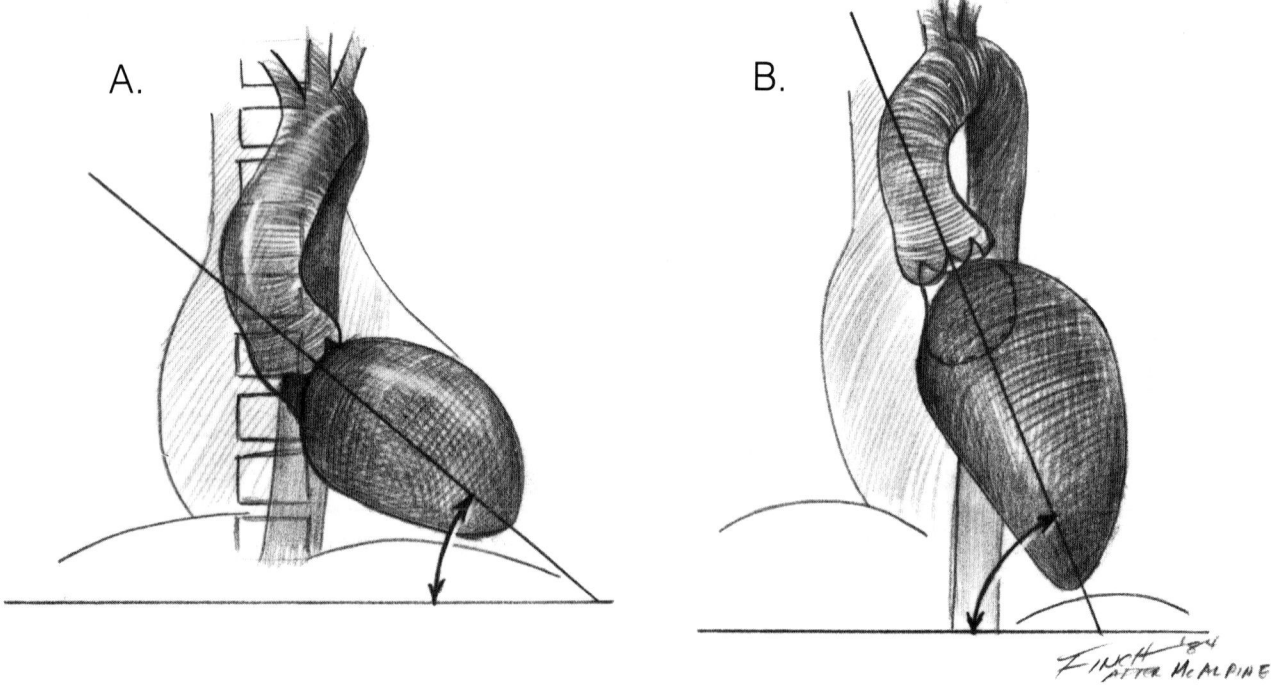

FIG 2-2.
A, position of heart with elevated diaphragm during expiration. **B,** position of heart with depressed diaphragm during deep inspiration. Angle of long axis of left ventricle and diaphragm shown.

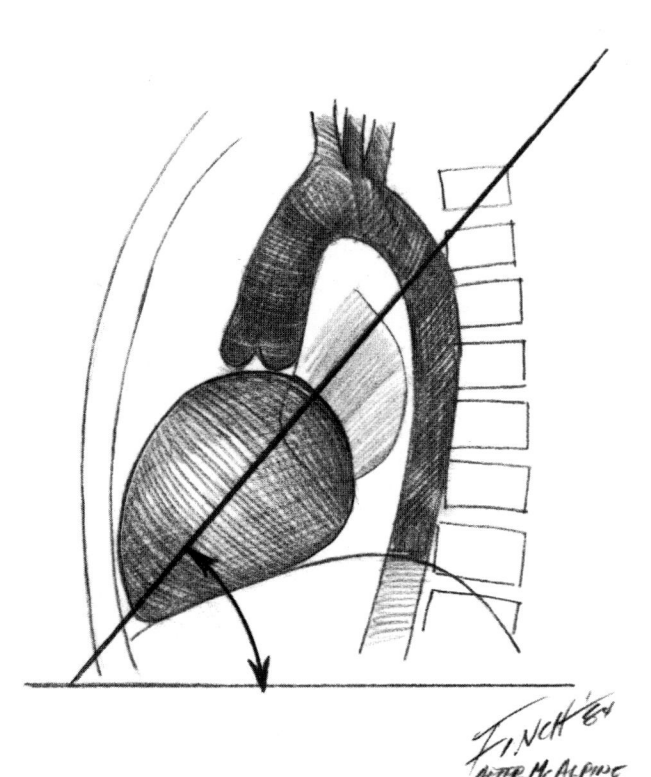

FIG 2-3.
Position of heart viewed from lateral aspect; inclination of long axis (usually 45 degrees) is largely dependent on position of diaphragm.

PATHOLOGIST'S VIEW OF HEART

FIG 2-4.
View of isolated heart as examined by a pathologist; long axis is perpendicular to coronal plane, and cardiac structures are in right-left relation. Two nomenclatures for semilunar valve cusps. **A,** heart removed from thorax, and, **B,** heart in situ.

(Continued.)

TWO COMMON SYSTEMS OF NAMING THE SEMILUNAR VALVES

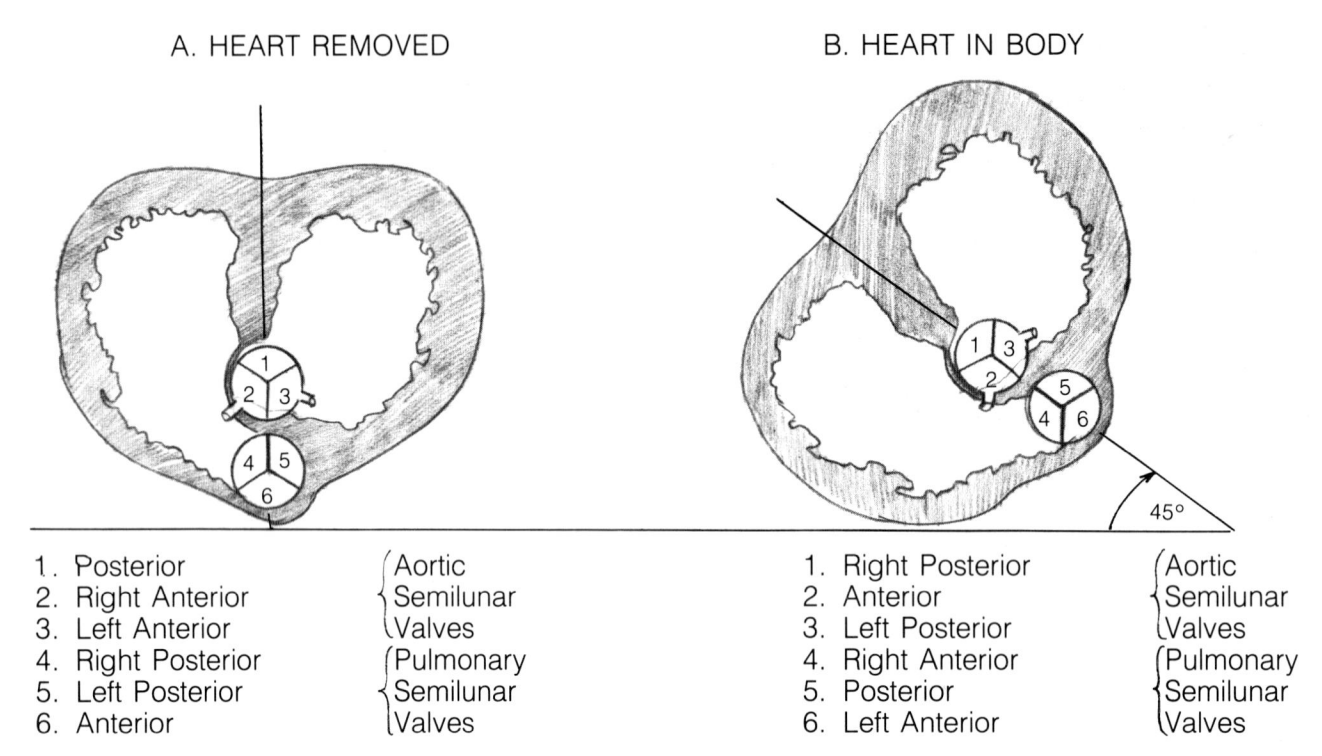

A. HEART REMOVED

1. Posterior
2. Right Anterior
3. Left Anterior
} Aortic Semilunar Valves

4. Right Posterior
5. Left Posterior
6. Anterior
} Pulmonary Semilunar Valves

B. HEART IN BODY

1. Right Posterior
2. Anterior
3. Left Posterior
} Aortic Semilunar Valves

4. Right Anterior
5. Posterior
6. Left Anterior
} Pulmonary Semilunar Valves

FIG 2–4 (cont.).
Orientation of heart in chest, demonstrating 45-degree orientation to coronal plane; atrial and ventricular septa and cardiac valves are now in right anterior and left posterior relation. Although less useful for angiographer and surgeon, the terminology for cardiac structures, particularly the semilunar valves, as described by the pathologist is the more widely accepted.

tends over the roots of the great vessels as a tubular investment (Fig 2–5). The lateral surfaces of the pericardium adhere to the parietal pleura, forming the pleuropericardial membrane, which forms the lateral borders of the anterior mediastinum. The pericardium also extends across the midline behind the sternum.

The superior vena cava has a distinct intrapericardial segment, whereas the inferior vena cava lies almost entirely extrapericardially except for the portions above the diaphragm. If the hepatic veins join the inferior vena cava above the diaphragm, the proximal portions of the hepatic veins lie within the pericardial sac. In the upper pericardial sac, there are the aortic recess and the pulmonary recess, which contain the proximal portions of the aorta and pulmonary trunk, respectively (see Fig 2–5).

The serous layer of the pericardium is reflected over the left pulmonary veins on the left side of the pericardial sac and on the right, over the right pulmonary veins, where the reflection blends with the venae cavae. The reflection from the right to the left pulmonary veins arches superiorly along the posterior atrial wall. Thus, it forms a cul-de-sac, the oblique pericardial sinus.

In an adult, the pericardial sac contains about 25 mL of fluid, which is an ultrafiltrate of serum. The blood supply to the pericardium is derived largely from the pericardiophrenic artery (a branch of the internal mammary artery) and from small pericardial branches from the thoracic aorta. The pericardium may be partially or completely absent (see Chapter 72).

VENAE CAVAE AND RIGHT ATRIUM

Anatomic Features

Systemic venous return flows to the heart through the superior and inferior venae cavae, which lie on the right side of the spine. The superior vena cava is formed by the confluence of the right and left innominate veins, which lie in front of the brachiocephalic arteries (Fig 2–6).

The superior and inferior venae cavae enter the posterior aspect of the right atrium through separate, largely unguarded orifices. Consequently, during right atriography, there is some reflux of contrast medium into the inferior vena cava and hepatic veins during systole. However, the inferior vena cava may have a medially located, crescent-shaped valve, the eustachian valve (Fig 2–7), named after

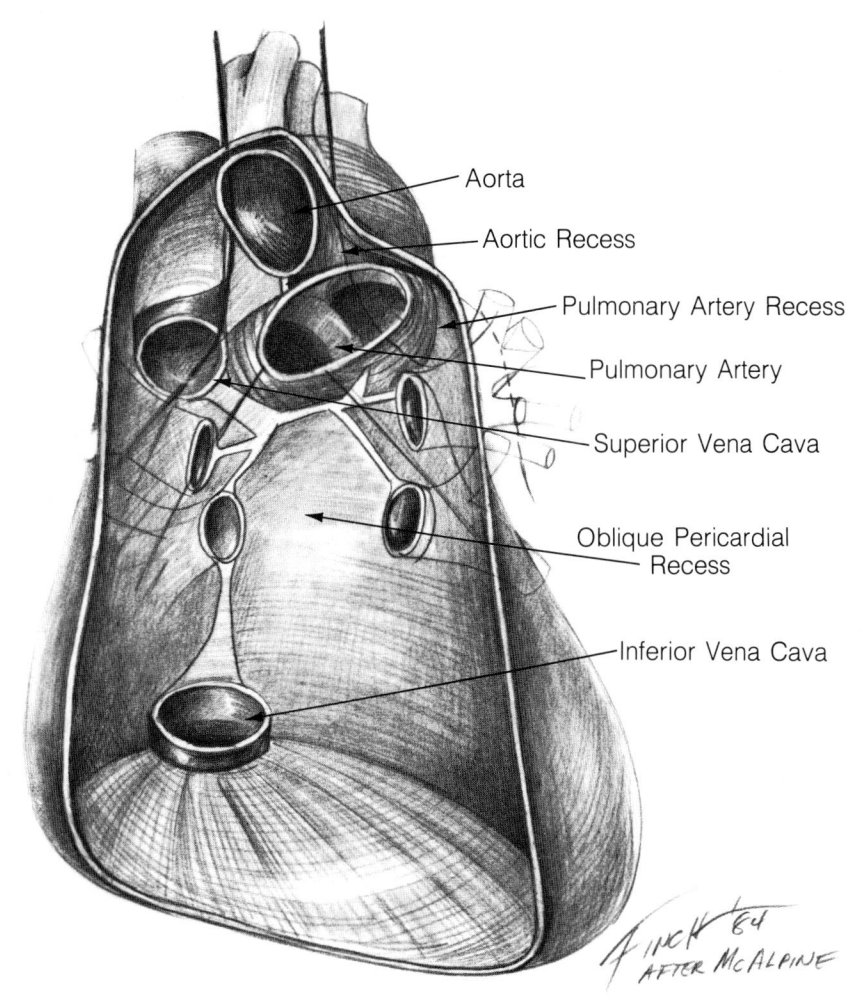

FIG 2-5.
Anatomy of pericardium after removal of heart showing pericardial attachments to cardiovascular structures and the pericardial recessed.

Bartolommeo Eustachius, a 16th century Italian anatomist. A prominent eustachian valve may cause difficulty in passage of a catheter or vena caval umbrella. The venae cavae enter the portion of the right atrium that is smooth walled and derived from the embryonic sinus venous. This portion is separated by a muscular ridge, the crista terminalis, from the thin-walled, trabeculated portion that is derived from the embryonic right atrium. The crista terminalis, which occurs in an anatomic right atrium, is most prominent superiorly, where it lies adjacent to the superior vena cava. It gradually fades toward the right of the inferior vena caval orifice (see Fig 2-7).

A number of parallel pectinate muscles pass anteriorly and laterally from the crista terminalis. Between these muscles, the atrial wall is thin and translucent. The muscles extend into the right atrial appendage, which is triangular and lies superiorly and anteriorly adjacent to the aorta. The coronary sinus enters the smooth portion of the right atrium posteriorly and medially near the tricuspid valve orifice.

In the right atrium, there are two venous valves: the eustachian valve guards the inferior vena caval orifice, and the thebesian valve guards the coronary sinus (Fig 2-8). These valves are derived from the right valve of the sinus venosus. Their size varies, and they may be absent or perforated. Rarely (2% of autopsies), remnants of either valve form strands, called a Chiari (named after Hans Chiari, a 19th century German pathologist) network (see Fig 2-7), that attach to either the atrial wall or atrial septum. Functionally, a Chiari network probably has no significance, although pulmonary embolism has been attributed to formation of thrombi on the network. It is more likely, however, that thrombi from the legs are caught in the network. The network may be seen by cardiac ultrasound

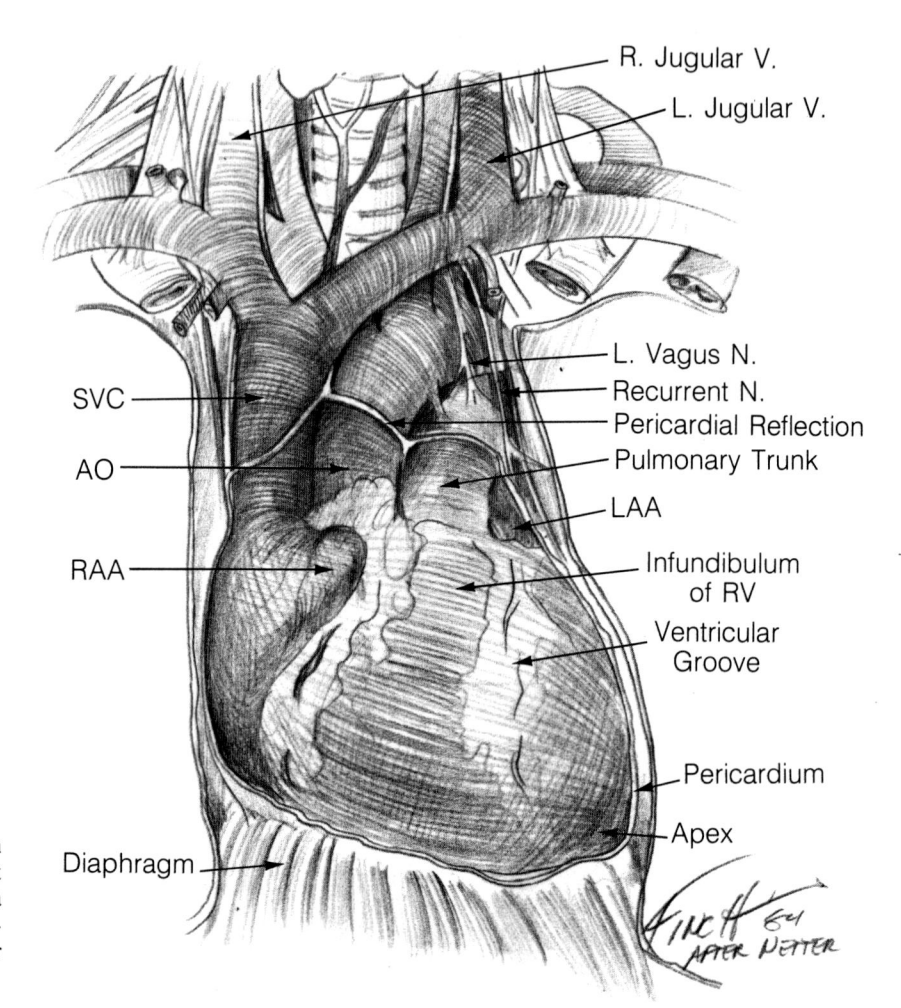

FIG 2–6.
Cardiovascular structures in thorax with pericardium opened and attachment to great vessels demonstrated. Right superior vena cava is formed by confluence of the two innominate veins, which lie anterior to major arteries.

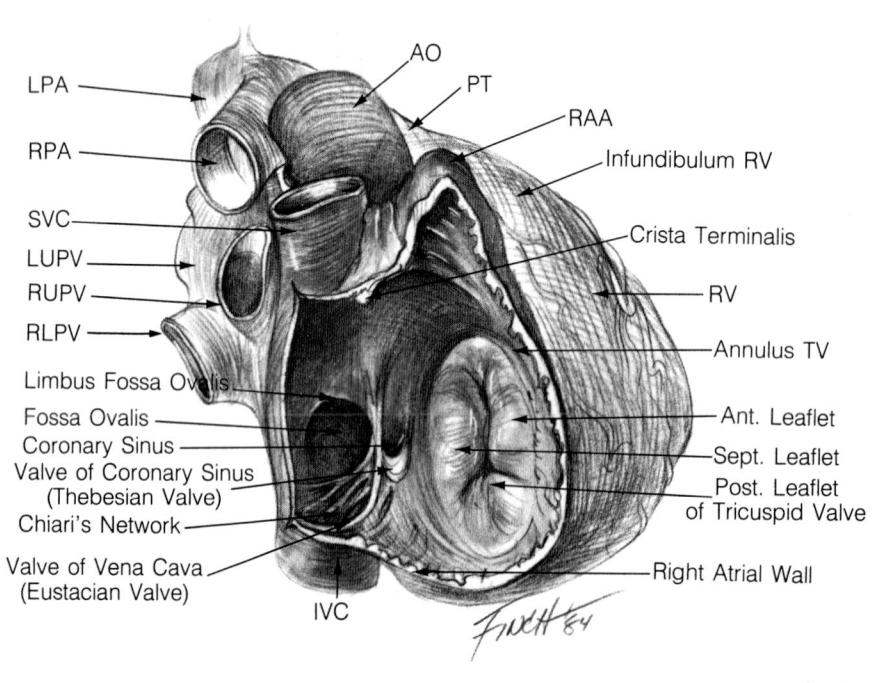

FIG 2–7.
Anatomy of right atrium with anterior wall removed. *Ao* = aorta; *IVC* = inferior vena cava; *LPA* = left pulmonary artery; *LPV* = left pulmonary vein; *PT* = pulmonary trunk; *RAA* = right atrial appendage; *RPA* = right pulmonary artery; *RPV* = right pulmonary vein; *SVC* = superior vena cava.

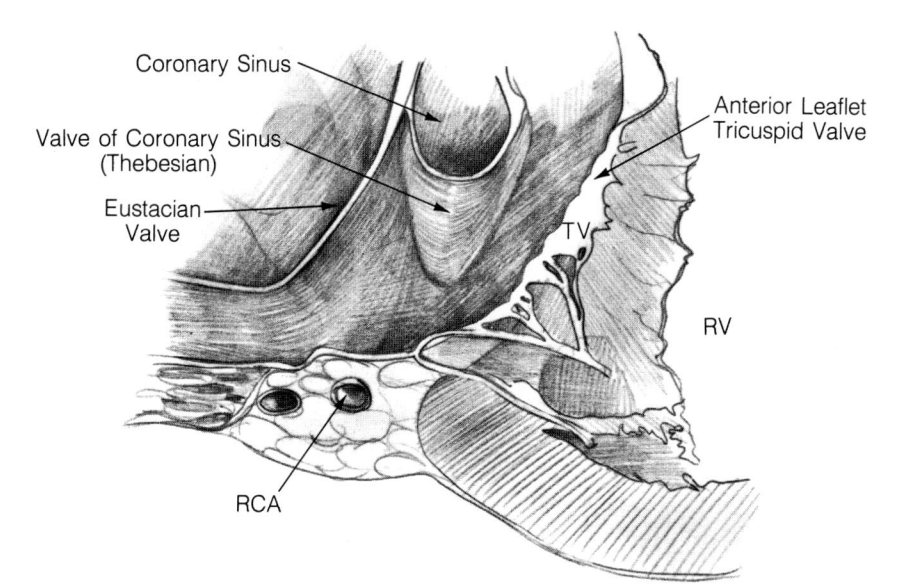

FIG 2–8.
Close-up view of valves of inferior vena cava (eustachian) and coronary sinus (thebesian); both may make passage of catheter into the inferior vena cava and coronary sinus difficult or impossible. CS = coronary sinus; RA = right atrium; RCA = right coronary artery; RV = right ventricle; TV = tricuspid valve.

and may interfere with the catheter insertion of an inferior vena caval filter, because it may prevent passage of the capsule from the right atrium into the inferior vena cava. A prominent network may cover the ostium of the coronary sinus, making catheterization of the coronary sinus impossible.

The medial wall of the right atrium is formed by the atrial septum, which is smooth and has a central, circular depression, the fossa ovalis. The margin of the septum surrounding the fossa is thickened and elevated and is called the "limbus of the fossa ovalis" (see Fig 2–7).

As left atrial pressure increases after birth, the foramen ovale seals (Fig 2–9,A), but a potential for patency between the right and left atria may persist as a probe-patent foramen ovale. Thus, at autopsy, a blunt probe can be passed underneath the superior limbus of the foramen ovale into the left atrium in 25% of hearts. Probe patency of the foramen is an important source of paradoxical emboli (Fig 2–9,C). Whenever the right atrial pressure increases, as during the Valsalva maneuver or coughing or in the presence of many right-sided obstructive cardiac lesions, a right-to-left shunt can occur through a probe-patent foramen ovale.

The limbus of the fossa ovalis (see Fig 2–9,A) facilitates the passage of a curved catheter from the right atrium into the left atrium. If the catheter is passed from below, its tip catches on the limbus, and even slight pressure may force the flap open (see Fig 2–9,B). If buckling of the catheter is prevented by the insertion of a transeptal needle, the catheter invariably passes from right to left below the limbus. Because it lies in the center of the atrial septum, the limbus facilitates radiographic localization of se-

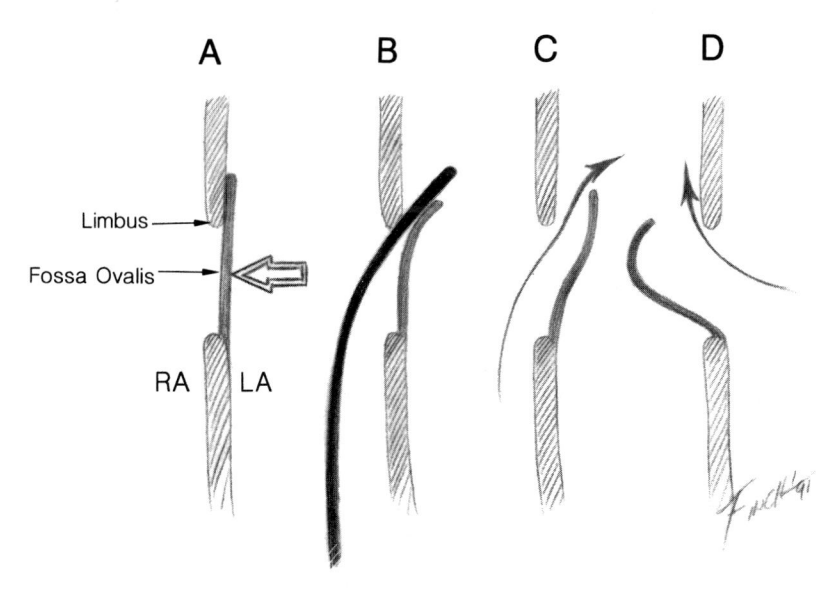

FIG 2–9.
Diagram of fossa ovalis. **A,** sealed foramen ovale; left atrial (LA) pressure is normally higher than right atrial (RA), pressure sealing even a probe-patent foramen. One-way check-valve mechanism indicated by arrow. **B,** probe-patent foramen ovale; mechanism of catheter passage from right to left atrium. **C,** right-to-left shunt through probe-patent foramen ovale when right atrial pressure exceeds left atrial pressure. **D,** with marked elevation of left atrial pressure, check-valve mechanism fails and the flap herniates, allowing a left-to-right shunt. This herniation results in a septal aneurysm (see Chapter 50).

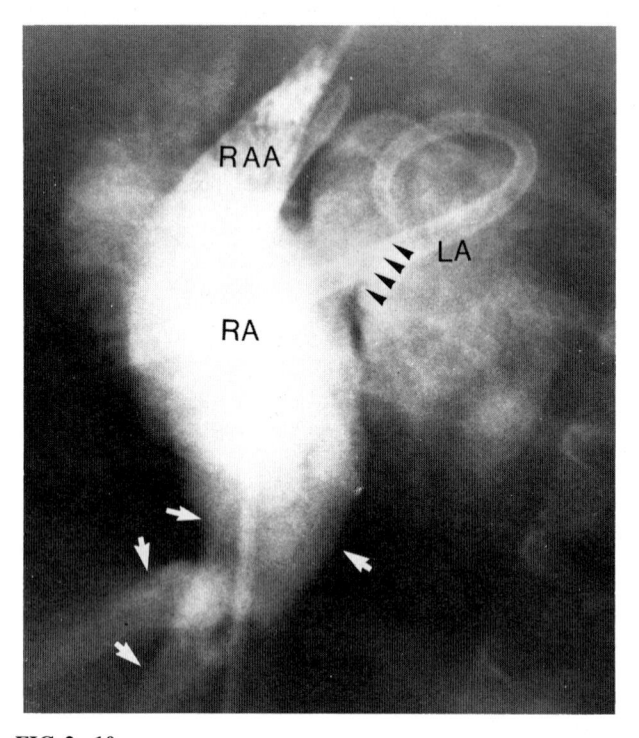

20 General Introduction

FIG 2–10.
Right atriogram in shallow left anterior oblique position with cranial beam angulation shows tricuspid atresia, resulting in shunt from right atrium *(RA)* to left atrium *(LA)*. Flap of fossa ovalis *(small black arrows)* is open toward left atrium. Reflux *(white arrows)* into hepatic veins and inferior vena cava is normal, because venae cavae possess no valves. Typical triangular right atrial appendage *(RAA)*.

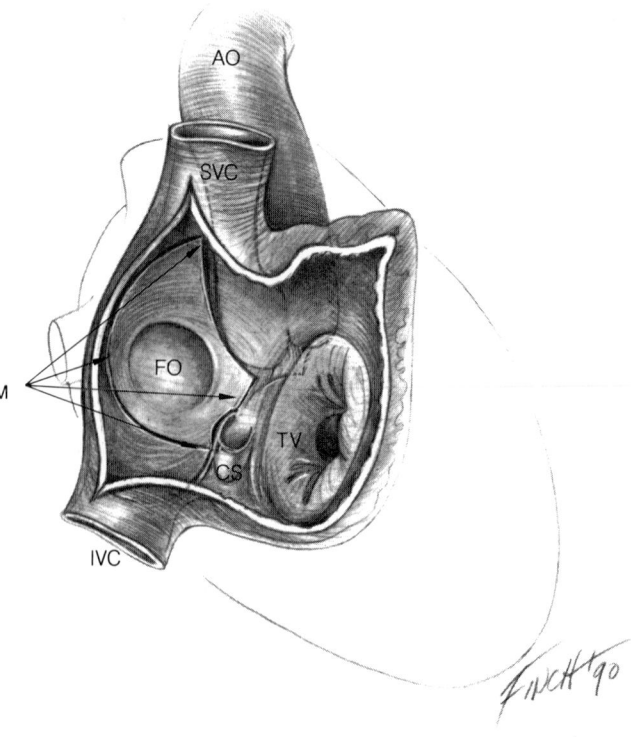

FIG 2–11.
Atrial septum as viewed through the opened right atrium. It has a blade shape and does not extend all the way to the tricuspid annulus and inferior vena cava orifice. The fossa ovalis lies in the center of the atrial septum, facilitating safe needle puncture and transseptal catheterization.

cundum-type atrial defects by characteristic catheter passage (see Chapter 19).

With the normally small pressure difference between the left and right atria, the valve remains competent, and a left-to-right shunt does not occur. If left atrial pressure increases markedly, as in left atrioventricular valve atresia, the foramen may be forced open, and the check-valve mechanism fails. This failure is associated with marked ballooning (herniation) of the fossa ovalis into the right atrium (Fig 2–9,D).

The flap-valve mechanism of the fossa ovalis can be demonstrated angiographically by injecting the right atrium and filming with the patient in a shallow left anterior oblique position and with cranial angulation (Fig 2–10).

A clear concept of the location of the atrial septum is important in cardiac catheterization. The fossa ovalis lies in the center of the atrial septum, which is blade shaped, extending from the aorta toward the inferior vena cava (Fig 2–11). The septum is separated from the inferior vena cava orifice by a small section of free wall of the right atrium. At the level of the limbus, the valve of the foramen ovale is only loosely attached to the muscular atrial septum, which allows passage of a stiff catheter even through a non–probe patent foramen. Because of the 45-degree inclination of the atrial septum, it is foreshortened in the anteroposterior projection that is most commonly used during catheterization (see Fig 2–11). The fossa ovalis lies more or less in the center of the septum. At the

ANATOMY OF THE ATRIAL SEPTUM

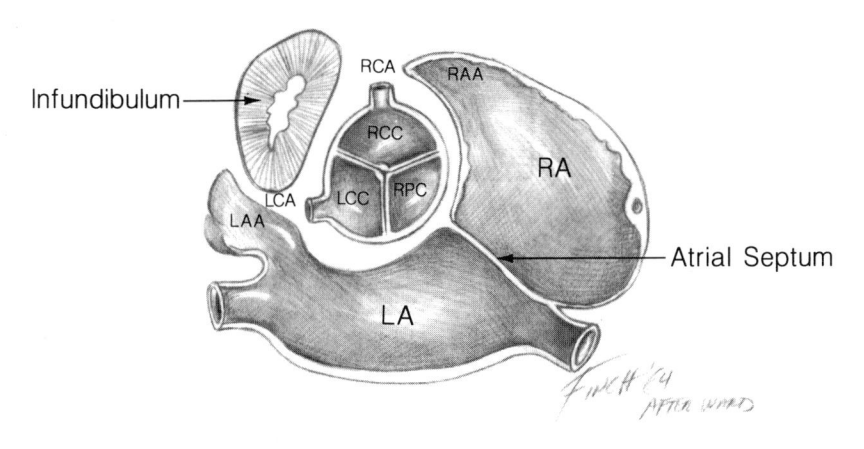

FIG 2-12.
Cross-section through heart at level of aortic valve; atrial septum is inclined (45 degrees) and straight. Anatomic relations of aorta, right atrium, left atrium, and infundibulum demonstrated.

level of the aortic valve, the septum is straight and forms about a 45-degree angle with the sagittal plane (Fig 2–12). Above the fossa ovalis, the septum has a distinct bulge, the torus aorticus, which is formed by the aortic sinuses of Valsalva (Fig 2–13). The inclination of the atrial septum varies, depending on the extent of clockwise or counterclockwise rotation of the heart. Consequently, the degree of leftward angulation of the catheter has to be varied.

During transseptal catheterization, the curved catheter with a stiffening cannula is withdrawn slowly from the superior vena cava along the atrial septum. Because of the inclination of the septum, the catheter tip must be pointed posteriorly and leftward. The tip passes first over the torus aorticus, where the transmitted aortic pulsations can be felt with the catheter. Puncture of the torus with the transseptal needle is one of the complications of this technique. As soon as the catheter passes over the limbus of the fossa ovalis, a small "jump" can be observed. The catheter can then be advanced safely through the flap of the fossa ovalis into the left atrium.

The right side of the atrial septum is demonstrated angiographically using a shallow left anterior oblique projection and a cranial beam angulation. The angle of the septum to the sagittal and coronal planes is approximately 45

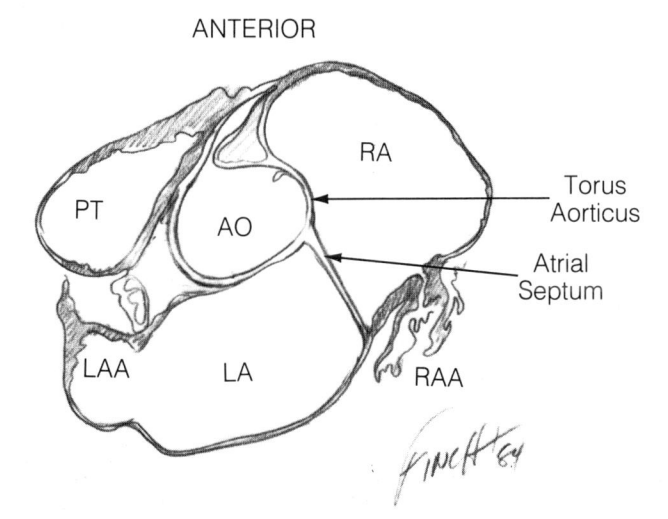

FIG 2-13.
Cross-section through heart above level of foramen ovale. Bulge in atrial septum formed by ascending aorta; this torus aorticus is an important landmark in transseptal catheterization, because aorta may be punctured accidentally at this site.

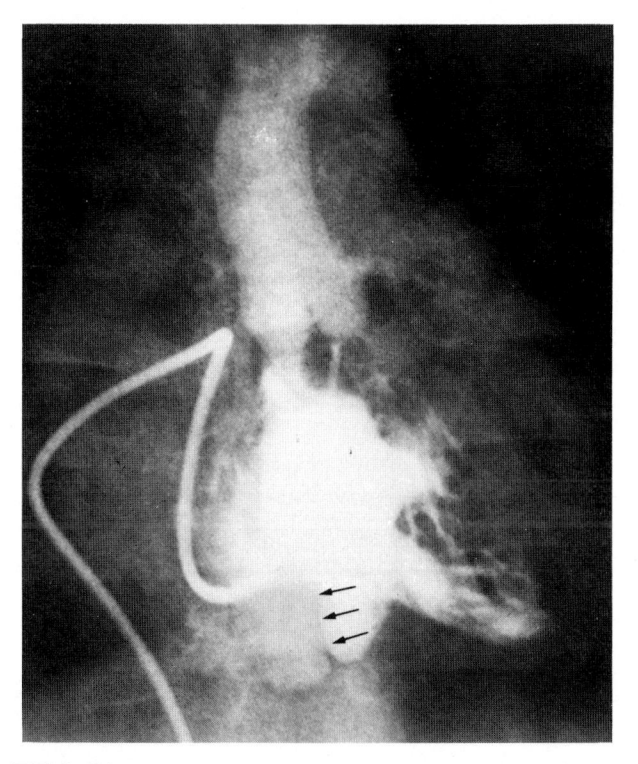

FIG 2-14.
Right ventriculogram in transposition of great vessels; tricuspid reflux partially outlining right atrium and thebesian valve *(arrows)*. (Named after Adam Thebesius, 18th century German physician).

degrees, similar to that of the posterior portion of the ventricular septum (see Fig 2–1).

Angiographic Identification of the Right Atrium

In patients with cardiac malposition and complex congenital heart disease, it is crucial to identify the anatomic right atrium. Although this chamber contains characteristic anatomic features, such as the crista terminalis, the fossa ovalis, and the coronary sinus, these structures usually are not seen by angiography. Rarely, the thebesian valve can be recognized (Fig 2–14). The anatomic right atrium can be identified angiographically in two ways:

1. By opacifying the inferior vena cava, which almost invariably connects with the right atrium (venoatrial concordance). This can be accomplished by direct injection of contrast medium, but this usually is unnecessary, because there is reflux into the inferior vena cava after injection into the right atrium. Rarely the inferior vena cava drains into the left atrium.

2. By identifying the right atrial appendage, which differs anatomically from the left atrial appendage. The former has a broad base and a triangular contour and resembles the ear of a dog (Fig 2–15,A). On an anteroposterior angiogram, it lies medially and in front of the right superior vena cava and aorta (see Figs 2–6 and 2–7), whereas on a lateral view, it projects anteriorly and overlies the right ventricular outflow tract (Fig 2–16).

However, either atrial appendage may be in an abnormal position, as in juxtaposition of atrial appendages (see Chapter 33).

Another reliable way to identify the right and left atria is based on determination of the bronchial situs, because almost invariably, bronchial situs corresponds to atrial situs. The right and left mainstem bronchi can be identified on thoracic roentgenograms or by laminography. The left mainstem bronchus is almost twice as long as the right (Fig 2–17) and lies below the left pulmonary artery (hyparterial bronchus). The right mainstem bronchus is much shorter and lies behind and above the pulmonary artery (eparterial bronchus).

RIGHT VENTRICLE

Anatomic Features

Blood leaves the right atrium through the tricuspid valve, which is located anteriorly and medially at the atrioventricular junction (Fig 2–18). Cuspis (Latin) indicates point, so the tricuspid valve has three points, or leaflets. However, the anatomy of this valve is variable, and the size and degree of differentiation of the three leaflets vary. The three leaflets are the anterior, septal (medial), and posterior; the spatially correct terms for the latter two are the anterosuperior (septal) and the inferior, respectively. There are three papillary muscles: The first is the papillary muscle of the conus (the muscle of Lancisi, named after Giovanni Lancisi, a 17th century Italian physician), which receives chordae tendineae from the anterior and septal leaflets; this muscle may be absent in tetralogy of Fallot (see Chapter 30). The second is the anterior papillary muscle, which is larger and originates from the moderator band and receives chordae tendineae from the anterior and posterior leaflets. The third is the posterior papillary muscle (see Fig 2–18). In addition, there are numerous direct chordal attachments to the septum with or without small papillary muscles. From the posterior leaflet, which blends with the septal leaflet, numerous short chordae tendineae

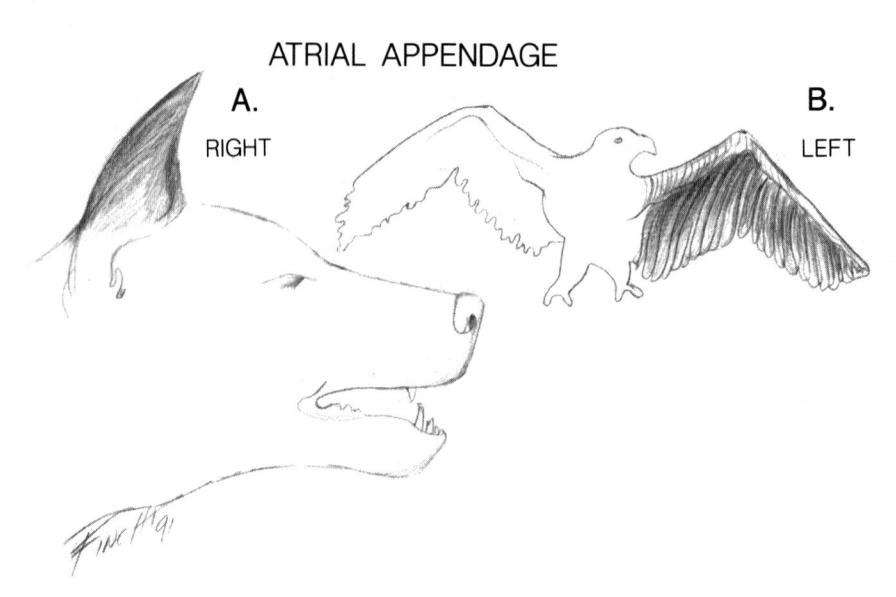

FIG 2–15.
A, drawing of dog ear resembles angiographic appearance of right atrial appendage. **B,** drawing of bird wing resembles left atrial appendage.

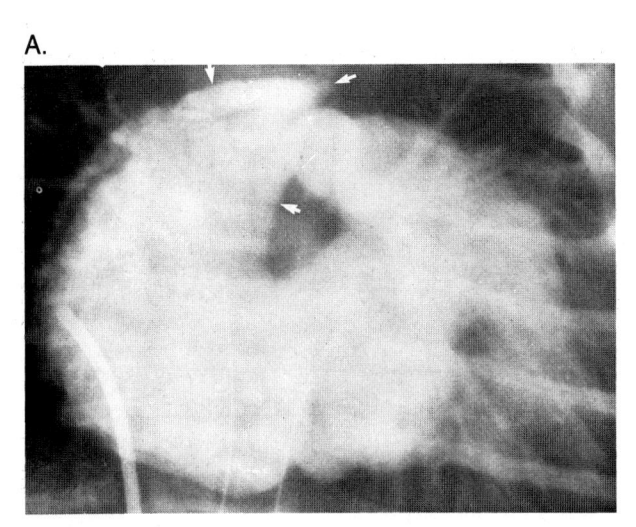

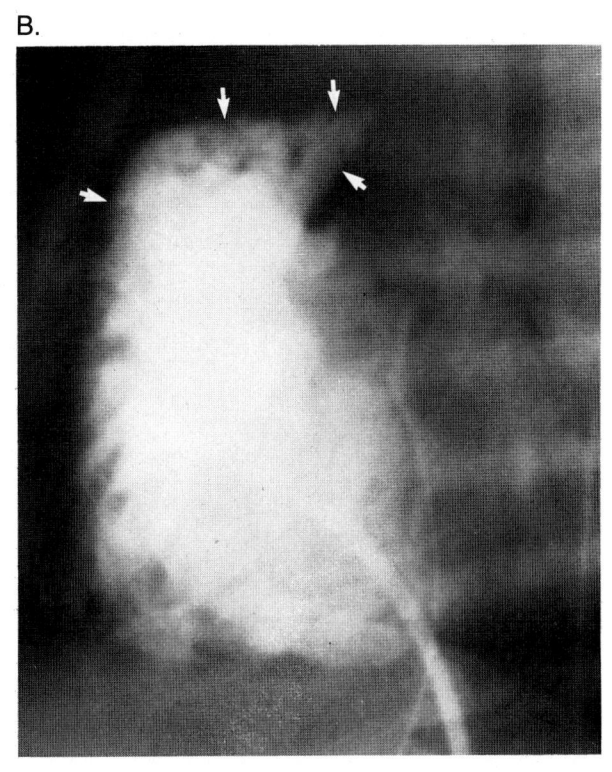

FIG 2–16.
Right atrial angiogram in tricuspid insufficiency. **A,** anteroposterior projection; characteristic broad-based right atrial appendage *(arrows),* with smooth internal architecture. **B,** lateral projection; right atrial appendage overlies right infundibulum. Triangular shape is apparent.

pass to small papillary muscles along the diaphragmatic portion of the right ventricle.

The right ventricle has two portions:

1. The inferior portion, also called the sinus, or inflow, portion, is heavily trabeculated, particularly in its apical region. The heavy trabeculations of the apex (apical recess) are of practical importance during angiography and cardiac catheterization, because cardiac catheters may become trapped in them. Perforations of the right ventricle during angiography or by pacing catheters usually occur in this region. The muscular fascicles forming the trabeculations are called trabeculae carneae (Latin: trabecula beam, carnis flesh).

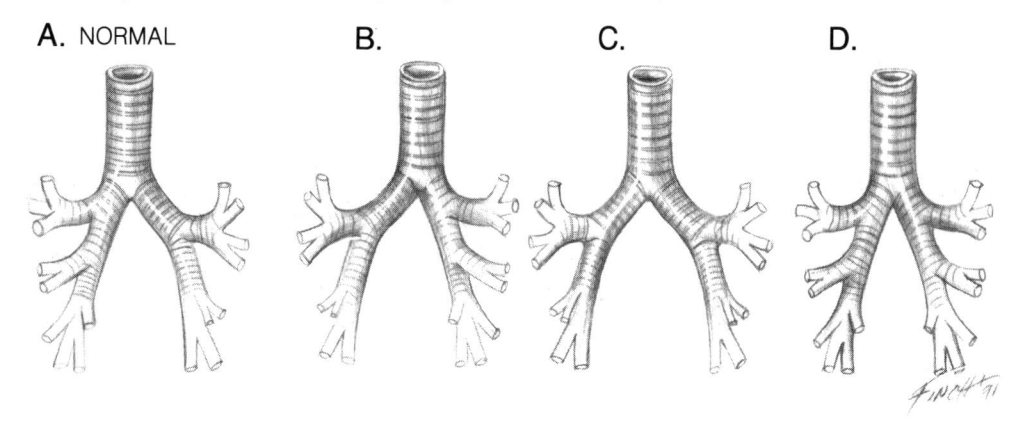

FIG 2–17.
Bronchial situs, which reflects atrial situs. **A,** situs solitus. Short right eparterial bronchus, long left hyparterial bronchus. **B,** situs inversus, mirror image of situs solitus. **C,** left atrial isomerism. Bilateral long hyparterial bronchi. Bilateral left sidedness (see Chapter 58). Two left atrial. **D,** right atrial isomerism. Bilateral short eparterial bronchi, two right atria (bilateral right sidedness; see Chapter 58).

ANATOMY OF RIGHT VENTRICLE

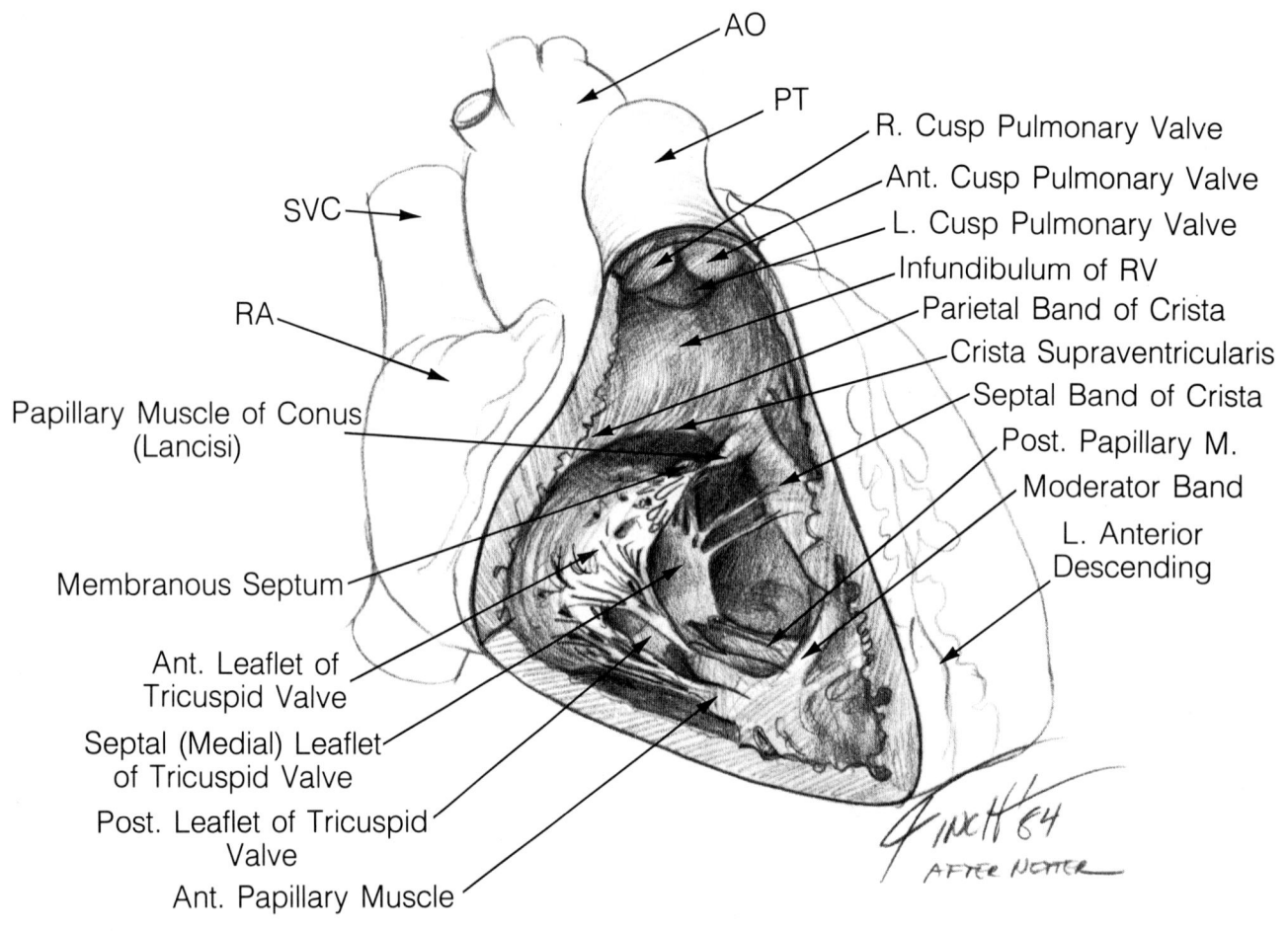

FIG 2–18.
Drawing of the right ventricle with anterior wall removed. *A* = anterior; *AO* = aorta; *IVC* = inferior vena cava; *L* = left; *LA* = left atrium; *LV* = left ventricle; *PT* = pulmonary trunk; *R* = right; *RA* = right atrium; *RV* = right ventricle; *SVC* = superior vena cava; *TV* = tricuspid valve.

2. The anterosuperior portion is also called the outflow, conus, or infundibular portion. It is less heavily trabeculated, and in the area below the pulmonary valve, it is smooth (Fig 2–19,A).

The two portions of the right ventricle lie at right angles to one another and are separated by the crista supraventricularis. This well-developed muscular ridge lies on the septal wall of the right ventricle and has two muscular extensions: the parietal band, which extends onto the free wall of the right ventricle; and the septal band, which extends inferiorly onto the ventricular septum (see Fig 2–18). The septal band, containing the right bundle of His, is continuous with the moderator band and extends into the anterior papillary muscle. In a lateral view, the inflow and outflow portions of the ventricle can be seen to form a gentle curve (Fig 2–19,B).

A more practical division of the right ventricle is into three rather than two components: an inlet zone, a heavily trabeculated apical zone, and an infundibular (outlet) zone (Fig 2–20). The trabeculated apical portion of the right ventricle is an important angiographic and anatomic landmark that allows differentiation from the anatomic left ventricle, which shows fine trabeculation in its apical region. The tripartite division of the right ventricle is particularly well demonstrated in pulmonary atresia with intact septum (see Chapter 34). With malformed right ventricles, the trabeculated apical portion remains preserved even when the inflow or outflow portions are absent. This division of the right ventricle into three components is of practical importance because muscular ventricular septal defects in the apical zone require a left ventriculotomy for surgical repair.

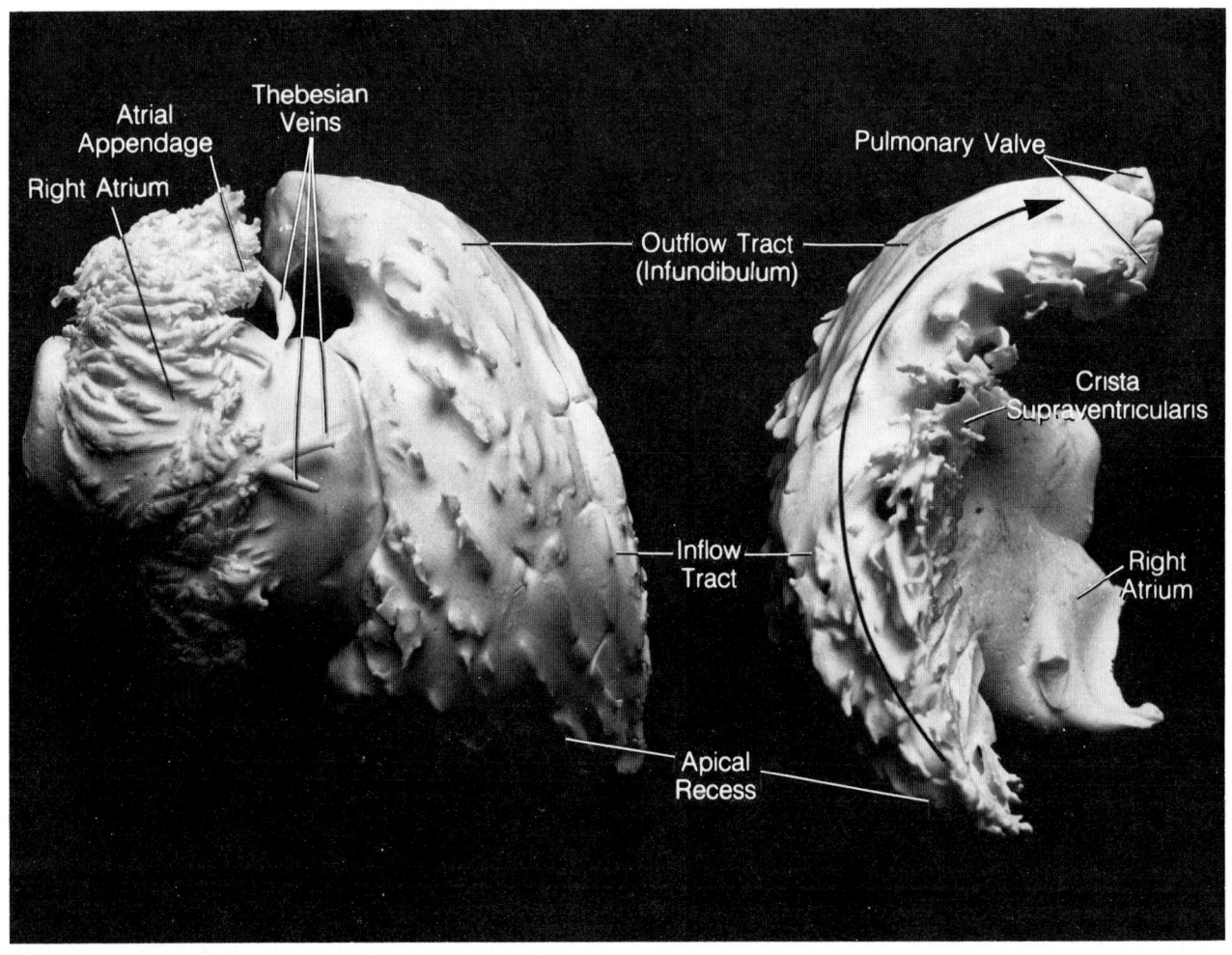

FIG 2–19.
Cast of right atrium and ventricle. **A,** right anterior oblique projection; sinus portion and conus (infundibulum) are at right angles. Apical portion has prominent trabeculations. In apical recess, catheters may become entrapped, and ventricular perforations may occur. Transventricular migration of pacing catheters also may occur at apical recess. **B,** lateral projection shows gentle curvature between inflow portion and infundibulum.

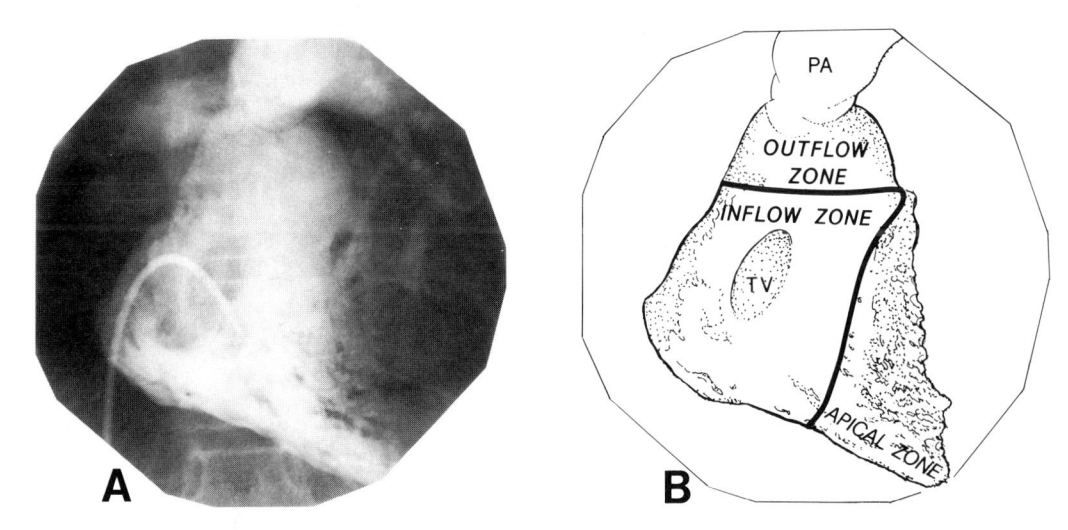

FIG 2-20.
A, a selective right ventriculogram. Diastole. Tricuspid annulus outlined by incoming unopacified blood *(arrow)*. Tripartite division of right ventricle well demonstrated **B,** explanatory diagram. The inflow (Sinus) portion of the right ventricle is relatively smooth. The apical portion is heavily trabeculated. Outflow zone (infundibulum) is smooth, separated from the inflow portion by the crista supraventricularis.

Angiographic Features

The right ventricle is usually examined in the anteroposterior, right anterior oblique, and lateral projections. In the anteroposterior plane, the ventricle is foreshortened because of the oblique position of the heart within the thorax. In this projection, the right ventricle has a triangular shape and is trabeculated (see Fig 2–20).

During diastole, when the tricuspid valve opens, incoming blood causes a radiolucency that outlines the tricuspid anulus, because contrast medium is trapped behind the valve leaflets (Fig 2–21,A). This diastolic view of the tricuspid valve is useful in understanding complex congenital heart disease, because it helps the observer determine the position of the tricuspid valve in relation to the ventricular septum and the semilunar valves. The papillary muscles and individual leaflets of the valve cannot be identified except in ventricular septal defect, when the septal (medial) leaflet is usually well seen. A perimembranous ventricular septal defect (see Chapter 12) lies close to or behind the septal leaflet of the tricuspid valve. In ventricular septal defect, contrast medium is trapped between the septum and the septal leaflet of the valve during diastole. This can be seen clearly on cine angiography (Fig

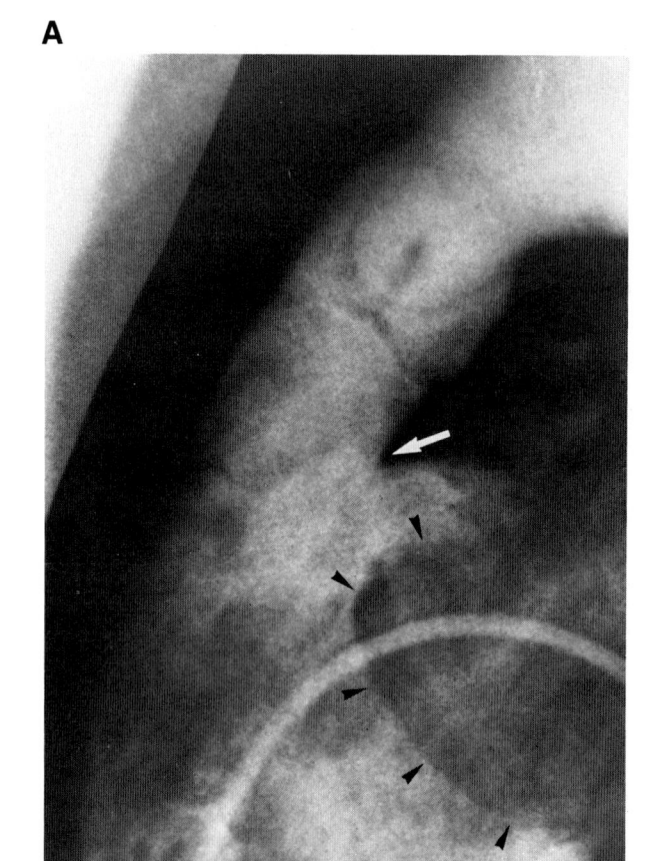

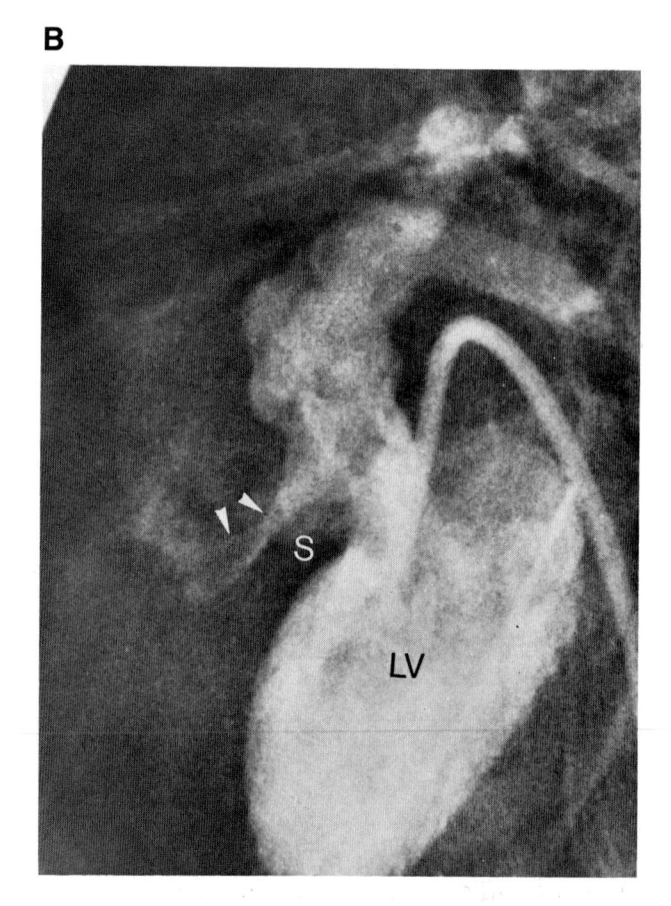

FIG 2–21.
Right ventriculogram in lateral projection during diastole; tricuspid valve is open. Nonopacified blood enters from right atrium and outlines tricuspid anulus *(black arrows)*. Individual valve leaflets, chordae tendineae, and papillary muscles cannot be seen. Crista supraventricularis demonstrated *(white arrow)*. **B,** left ventriculogram *(LV)* in steep left anterior oblique projection shows ventricular septal defect. Contrast medium trapped beneath tricuspid valve *(white arrows)* and ventricular septum *(S)* during diastole. Septal leaflet of tricuspid valve clearly seen *(arrows)*.

2–21,B). If the septal leaflet of the tricuspid valve is partially adherent to the ventricular septal defect, it will balloon during systole, forming a so-called aneurysm of the membranous septum (see Chapter 14).

Unless cranial tube angulation is used, the infundibulum is foreshortened in both the anteroposterior and right anterior oblique projections, because it forms a shallow angle with the coronal plane.

The infundibulum, crista supraventricularis, and pulmonary valve are best seen on a lateral projection (Fig 2–22). The crista forms a posterior ridge that becomes more prominent during systole. The crista is particularly prominent in patients with right ventricular outflow obstruction, because this causes generalized right ventricular hypertrophy and forceful contraction of the infundibulum. During systole, the sinus portion of the right ventricle contracts slightly sooner than the infundibulum. During diastole, the crista supraventricularis disappears or becomes less obvious angiographically, because the infundibulum has relaxed.

Angiographic Identification

Angiographic identification of the anatomy of a right ventricle is vital in the analysis of complex congenital heart disease. If the morphology of the right ventricle cannot be determined with certainty, it is preferable to speak of the ventricle that receives the systemic venous return as the "systemic venous ventricle," regardless of its morphology. In most cases, the morphologic right and left ventricles can be identified angiographically with a high degree of certainty, particularly if each ventricle is injected with contrast medium.

The characteristic angiographic features of an anatomic right ventricle are as follows:

1. The right atrioventricular valve is tricuspid, whereas the left is bicuspid. Unfortunately, angiographic differentiation between the two valves is generally impossible.

2. The papillary muscles in the right ventricle usually are not seen angiographically, because they are small and hidden by the trabeculations. If two papillary muscles are clearly demonstrated, the ventricle is probably a morphologic left ventricle.

3. The normal right ventricle has a coarse trabecular pattern in contrast to the left ventricle, which has a fine trabecular pattern and looks relatively smooth angiographically. However, this finding is not absolutely reliable and is most useful if the appearance of the ventricles can be compared.

4. The inflow and outflow portions of the right ventricle are clearly separated by a prominent muscular ridge, the crista supraventricularis.

5. The infundibulum of the right ventricle separates the pulmonary from the tricuspid valve. However, it is not always present. The crista supraventricularis represents developmentally conal tissue and may be hypoplastic or absent even in a right ventricle. Furthermore, each ventricle may have tissue separating the semilunar and atrioventricular valves; the latter condition is called double coni, most commonly seen in transposition of the great vessels (see Chapter 38).

PULMONARY VALVE AND ARTERIES

The right ventricle ends at the pulmonary valve. This semilunar valve has three cusps, usually called the anterior, right, and left, although in situ the position of the cusps corresponds to posterior, right anterior, and left anterior (see Fig 2–18). The pulmonary valve lies in a more

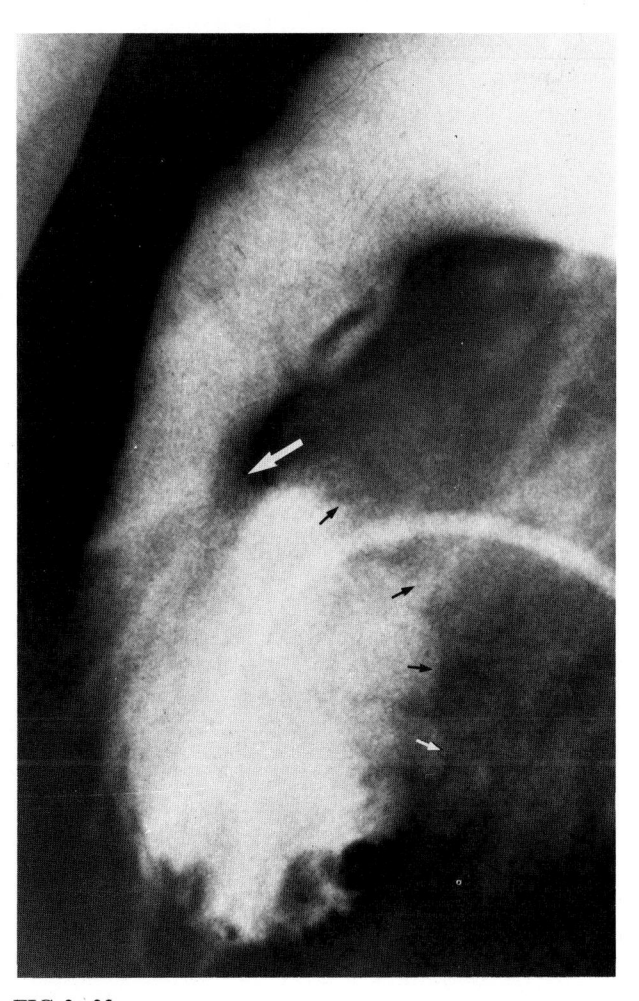

FIG 2–22.
Right ventriculogram in lateral projection during systole; tricuspid valve closed *(black arrows),* forming posterior border of opacified right ventricle. Crista supraventricularis clearly seen *(white arrow)* and is much more prominent than during diastole.

cephalad plane than the aortic valve, the right ventricle having an infundibulum that separates the right atrioventricular valve from the semilunar valve.

In a lateral view, there is a sharp angulation between the axis of the right ventricular outflow tract and the pulmonary trunk (Fig 2–23). The pulmonary trunk forms a 25- to 30-degree angle with the horizontal plane. The pulmonary valve anulus is tilted slightly in relation to the long axis of the pulmonary trunk (see Fig 2–23), and because of this angulation, on an anteroposterior angiogram of the heart, the pulmonary trunk is markedly foreshortened and the pulmonary valve is seen en face (Fig 2–24). The foreshortening of the pulmonary trunk can be minimized by cranial angulation of the x-ray beam (Fig 2–25).

During systole, all three leaflets are open completely (Fig 2–26). However, in a condition associated with decreased right ventricular stroke volume, such as cardiac myopathies or ventricular extrasystoles, the semilunar valves may not open completely, and furthermore, the pulmonary valve may open only partially because of a jet of blood through the subvalvar obstruction (see Chapter 26.)

Although the semilunar valves usually have three leaflets, the number varies; there may be a single leaflet (unicuspid valve) or two leaflets (bicuspid valve). These two types of semilunar valves are hemodynamically abnormal, creating turbulent blood flow and causing pressure gradients (see Chapters 26 and 29). A semilunar valve with four leaflets is called quadricuspid and is considered a normal variant, because it does not cause hemodynamic changes. Quadricuspid pulmonary valves are found incidentally in 0.02% of postmortem examinations. The fourth cusp tends to be rudimentary, and we have not identified a quadricuspid pulmonary valve angiographically, although we have identified a quadricuspid aortic valve, which is even less common. In patients with truncus arteriosus, the semilunar valve may have more than three leaflets.

The marked foreshortening of the pulmonary trunk in the anteroposterior view has important implications for cardiac catheterization. For example, the position of the catheter tip within the pulmonary artery cannot be determined by its height, because the artery has an almost horizontal course, particularly when the patient is supine or has a high position of the diaphragm. Thus, precise location of the catheter tip in the pulmonary trunk requires lateral fluoroscopy.

The pulmonary trunk divides into the right and left pulmonary arteries. The right artery arises at almost a right angle and passes transversely behind the ascending aorta and in front of the right mainstem bronchus. The left pulmonary artery is an extension of the pulmonary trunk and passes posteriorly over the left mainstem bronchus (see Figs 2–23 and 2–24). Therefore, on a lateral projection, the right pulmonary artery is seen as a round density in front of the bronchus, whereas the left pulmonary artery is seen in profile, passing over the left bronchus.

The proximity of the right pulmonary artery to the ascending aorta is used by surgeons to create a communication (Waterston shunt) between the two vessels for palliation of tetralogy of Fallot. The right atrium lies in front of the right pulmonary artery, so a surgical communication can be made between the right atrium and the right pulmonary artery. Known as a Fontan operation, it is used for tricuspid atresia and other cyanotic conditions.

The fact that the left pulmonary artery arises higher than the right facilitates its identification on a lateral projection (see Fig 2–23). Because it passes over the left mainstem bronchus, enlargement of the left pulmonary artery may compress the bronchus from above while the left

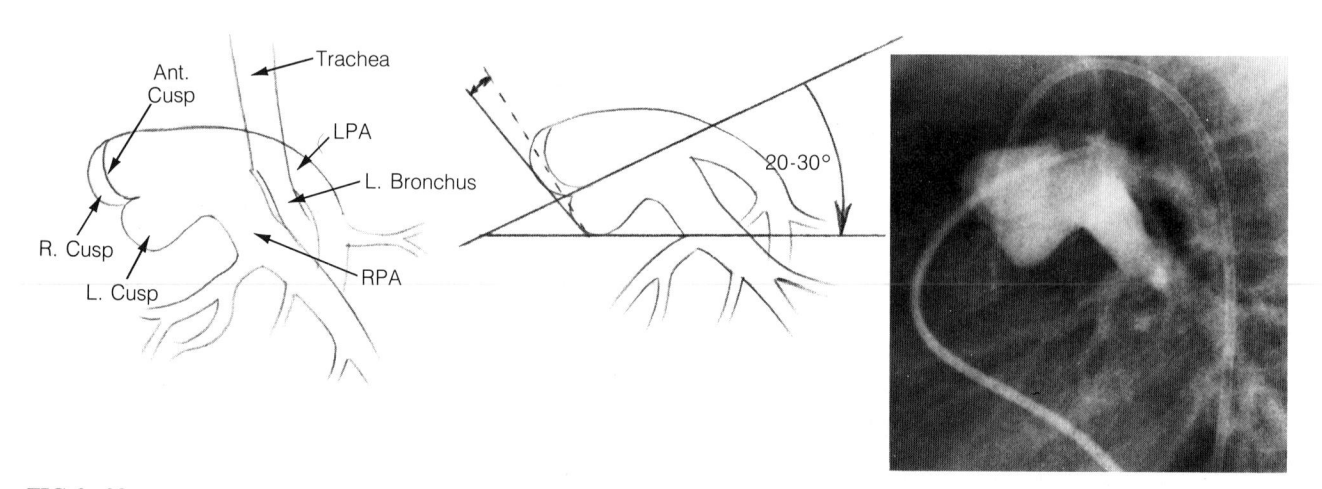

FIG 2–23.
Pulmonary arteriogram in lateral projection during diastole; right cusp and anterior cusps are superimposed. Long axis of pulmonary artery only a 20- to 30-degree angulation with horizontal plane; pulmonary valve plane slightly tilted and not at right angle with long axis of pulmonary artery. *L* = left; *LPA* = left pulmnary artery; *R* = right; *RPA* = right pulmonary artery.

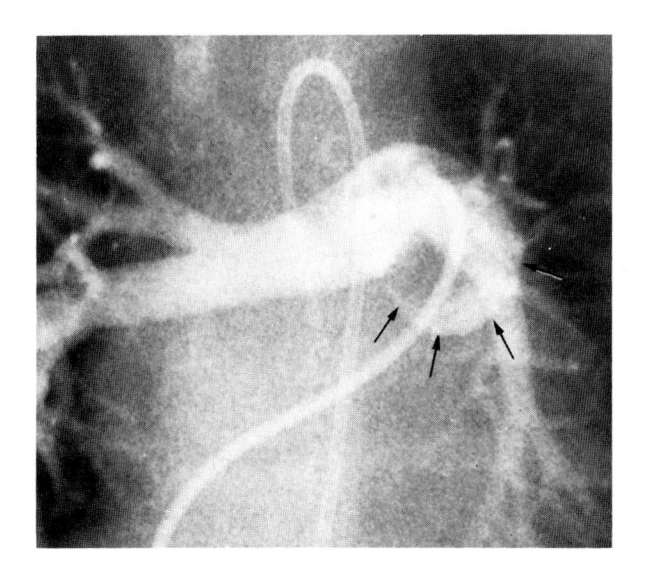

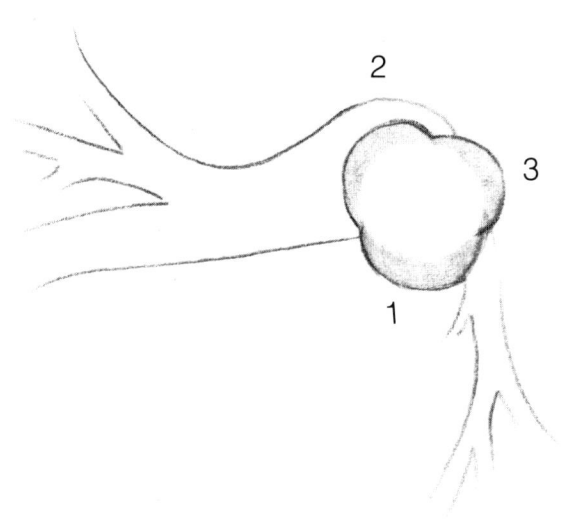

FIG 2–24.
Pulmonary arteriogram in anteroposterior projection during systole shows pulmonary valve, with leaflets seen en face *(left)*. Contrast medium is trapped behind open valve leaflet *(small black arrows)*. Other two leaflets are not seen, because they are superimposed on foreshortened main pulmonary artery. *1*, left cusp; *2*, right cusp; *3*, anterior cusp.

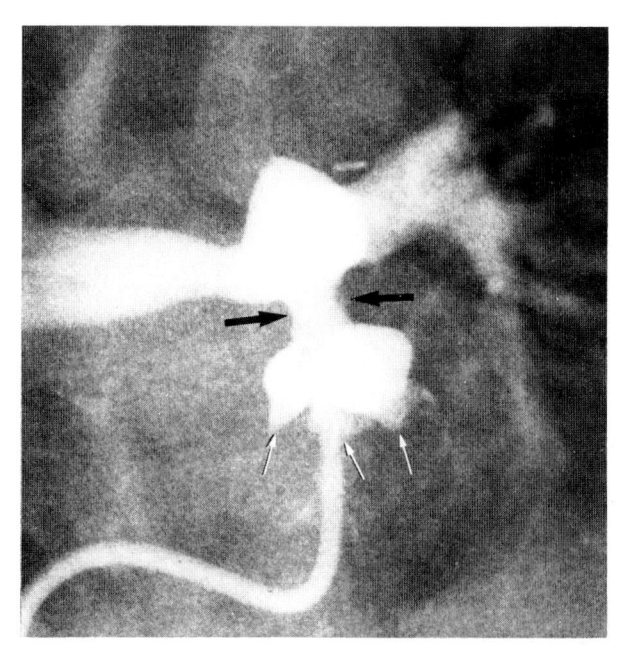

FIG 2–25.
Pulmonary arteriogram in anteroposterior projection with cranial tube angulation; main pulmonary artery and a surgically placed band *(black arrows)* well seen. Three cusps of pulmonary valve distinctly identifiable *(white arrows)*.

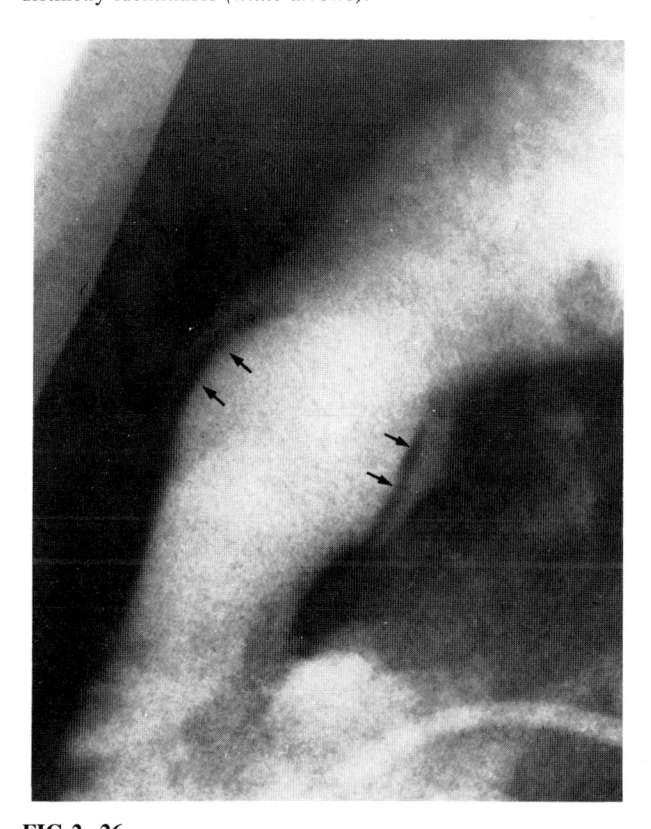

FIG 2–26.
Right ventriculogram in lateral projection during systole shows slightly thickened pulmonary valve that is completely open. Left (posterior) and right cusp seen in profile *(arrows)*.

atrium may narrow it from below (hemodynamic vise) (Figs 2–27 and 2–33). Because the left pulmonary artery is a direct extension of the pulmonary trunk, cardiac catheters tend to enter the left artery in preference to the right one, which arises at an acute angle. The ligamentum arteriosum extends from the superior aspect of the proximal portion of the left pulmonary artery to the distal aortic arch.

Angiographic demonstration of the bifurcation of the pulmonary trunk is particularly important in tetralogy of Fallot because of the common occurrence of stenosis of the proximal left and right pulmonary arteries.

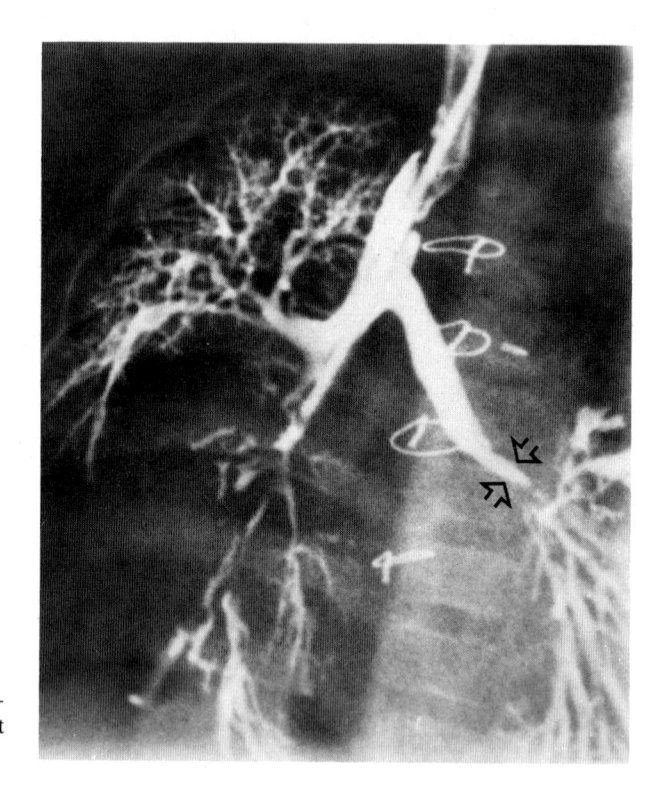

FIG 2–27.
Bronchogram in left anterior oblique projection; in patient with pulmonary hypertension. Large left pulmonary artery compresses left stem bronchus from above against left atrium below *(arrows)*.

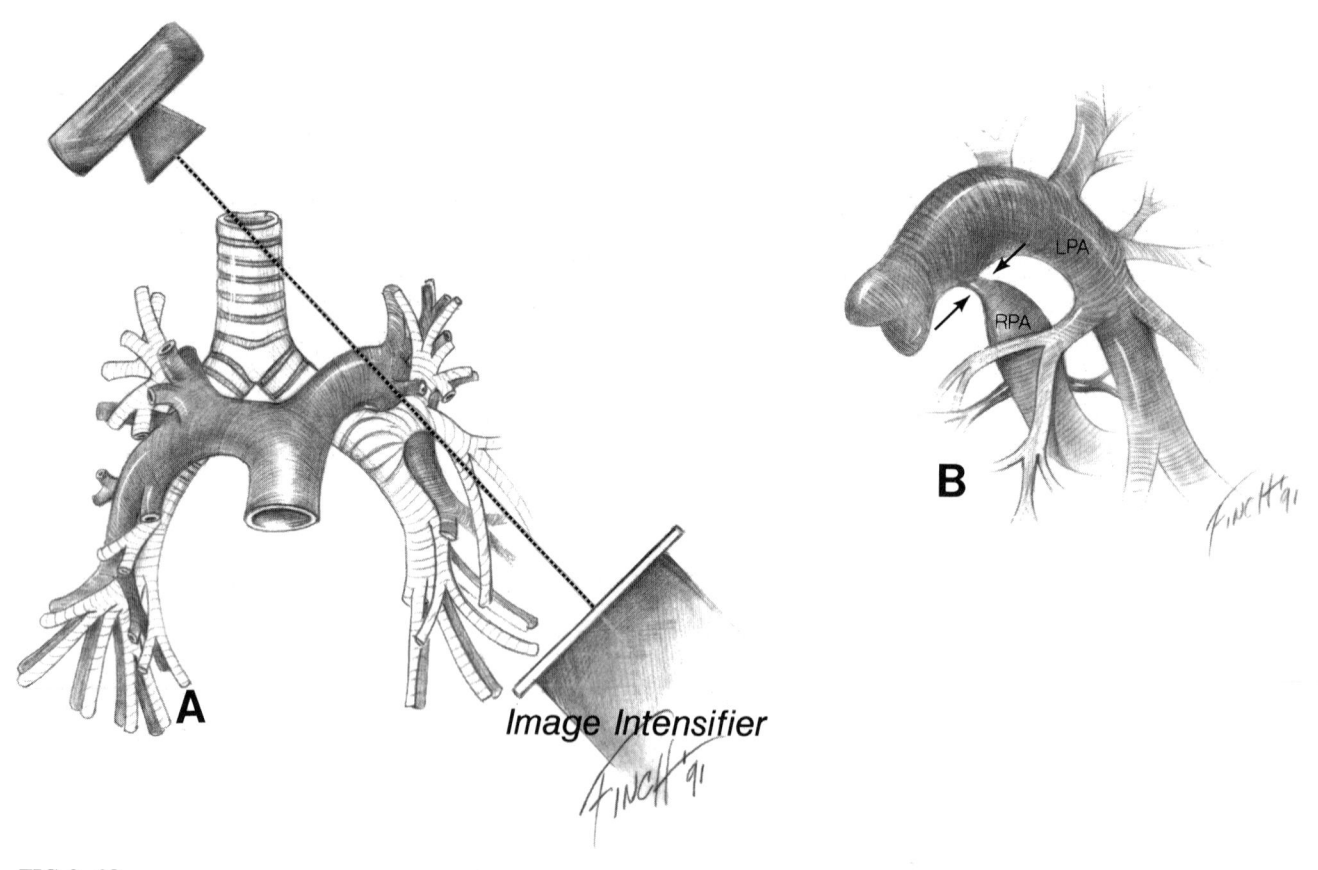

FIG 2–28.
A, diagram demonstrating caudal beam angulation (looking up) through a steep left anterior oblique view. The left pulmonary artery is projected above the right pulmonary artery as seen in **B. B,** steep left anterior oblique view of pulmonary artery with caudal beam angulation. The stenosis of the right pulmonary artery is no longer superimposed on the main pulmonary artery.

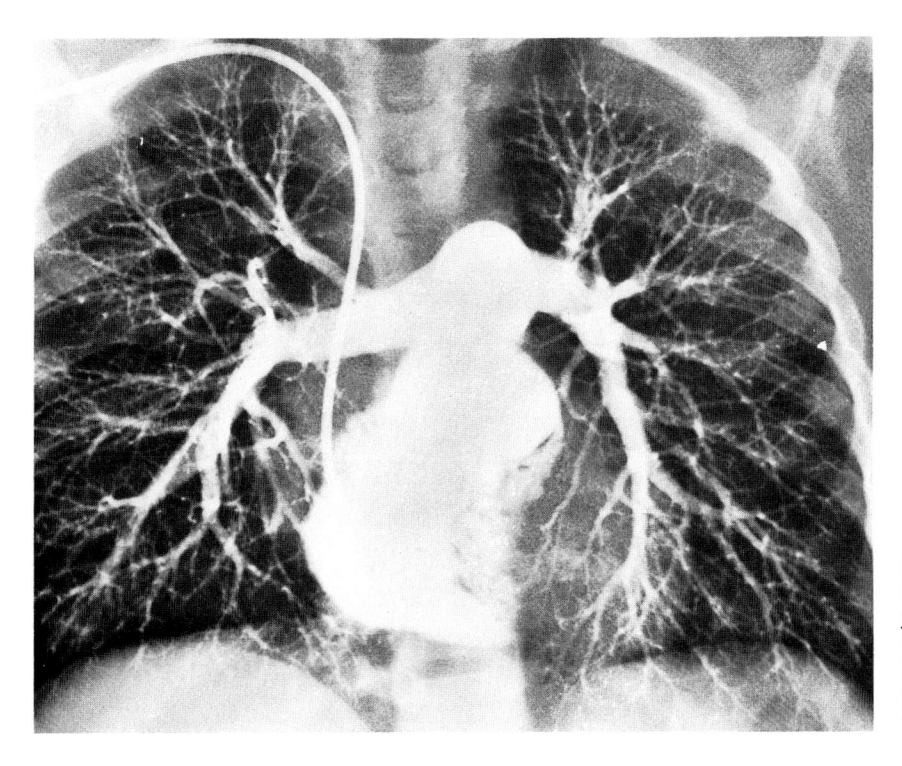

FIG 2-29.
Right ventriculogram in anteroposterior projection shows normal pulmonary arterial tree. Arteries radiate in orderly fashion from both hila and parallel the bronchial tree. Left pulmonary artery projects higher than right.

Projections

A slight right anterior oblique view with maximal cranial beam angulation demonstrates the main and the origin of the right pulmonary artery (see Fig 2–25). Sometimes also the left pulmonary artery is demonstrated (see Fig 2–25). A steep left anterior oblique or lateral projection using maximal caudal angulation demonstrates the origins of both pulmonary arteries (Fig 2–28,A). A stenosis of the right pulmonary artery can be clearly demonstrated by this projection (Fig 2–28,B; see also Chapter 30). In situs inversus, cranial beam angulation has to be used.

In the right and left hila, the pulmonary arteries divide in an orderly radial fashion into branches that closely parallel the bronchi (Fig 2–29). This arrangement of the pulmonary arterial branches allows their angiographic differentiation from the bronchial arteries, which follow a much more irregular course. The lower-lobe branches of the pulmonary arteries are the largest and form characteristic comma-shaped densities on thoracic roentgenograms.

PULMONARY VEINS AND LEFT ATRIUM

In contrast to the systemic veins, the pulmonary veins are unpaired and do not parallel the course of arteries (venae comitantes). Because they are separated from the arteries by pulmonary tissue, they can be seen as distinct vessels on a thoracic roentgenogram (Fig 2–30).

The pulmonary veins lie in front of and laterally to the pulmonary arteries (Fig 2–31). In about 50% of cases, the

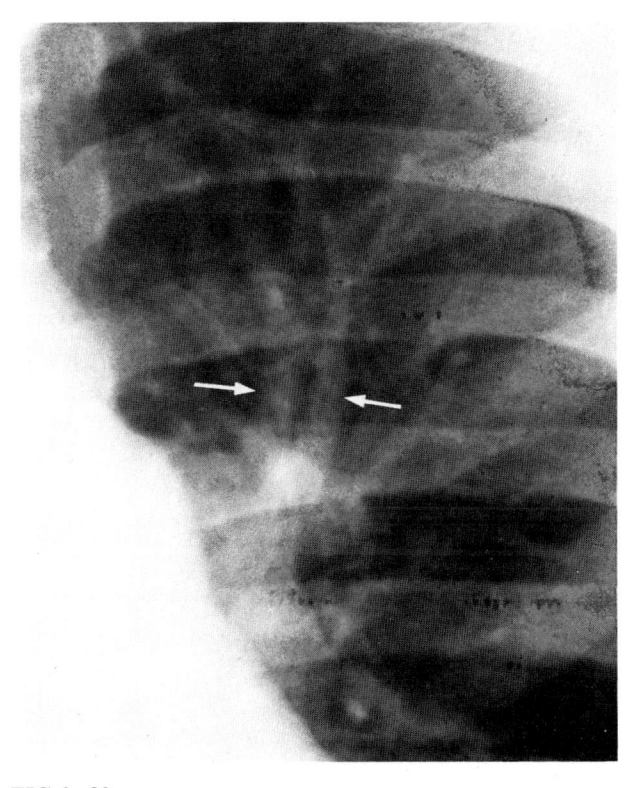

FIG 2-30.
Close-up view of left upper lobe; both pulmonary artery and pulmonary vein *(arrows)* are seen distinctly, because they are separated by pulmonary parenchyma. Pulmonary artery lies medially to pulmonary vein.

ANATOMY OF PULMONARY ARTERY AND VEINS

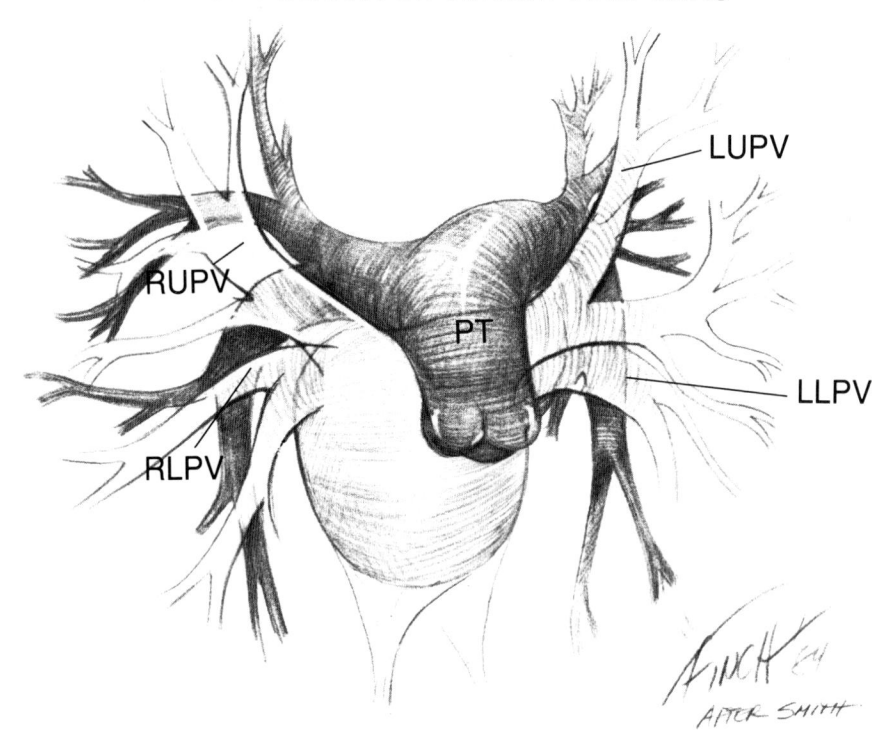

FIG 2–31.
Pulmonary arterial and venous trees. Pulmonary veins course in front of pulmonary arteries and join left atrium *(LA)* as four major trunks: *RUPV* = right upper pulmonary vein; *RLPV* = right lower pulmonary vein; *LUPV* = left upper pulmonary vein; and *LLPV* = left lower pulmonary vein; *PT* = pulmonary trunk.

upper pulmonary veins are difficult to see on thoracic roentgenograms because they are superimposed on the arteries. However, the lower-lobe veins can almost always be identified by their characteristic almost horizontal course toward the heart. The pulmonary veins have no valves.

There are two right and two left pulmonary veins, joining the posterior aspect of the left atrium. The right pulmonary veins enter close to the atrial septum, an arrangement that is of hemodynamic importance. In patients with an atrial septal defect, pulmonary venous blood from the right lung drains preferentially into the right atrium (see Chapter 19). The two left pulmonary veins frequently join the left atrium as a single trunk.

Selective injection of the pulmonary veins provides the best angiographic demonstration, although in most cases, the opacification of the pulmonary veins that follows injection of contrast medium into the pulmonary artery is adequate (Fig 2–32). Failure to enter a pulmonary vein during cardiac catheterization does not necessarily indicate an abnormality.

The atrium that receives the pulmonary veins has been termed the left atrium, although this chamber is located posteriorly in the body. It can be approached surgically through either a right or left thoracotomy and lies below the carina and in front of the esophagus (Fig 2–33). The transverse diameter of the left atrium is greater than either its anteroposterior or vertical diameter, and the wall is

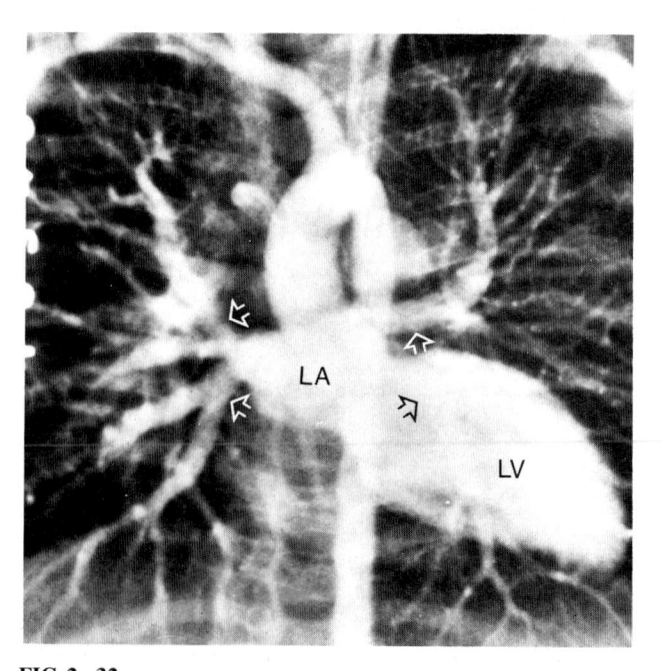

FIG 2–32.
Intravenous angiocardiogram in late phase shows anatomy of pulmonary veins. Four major veins *(open arrows)* join normal-sized left atrium *(LA)*. *LV* = left ventricle.

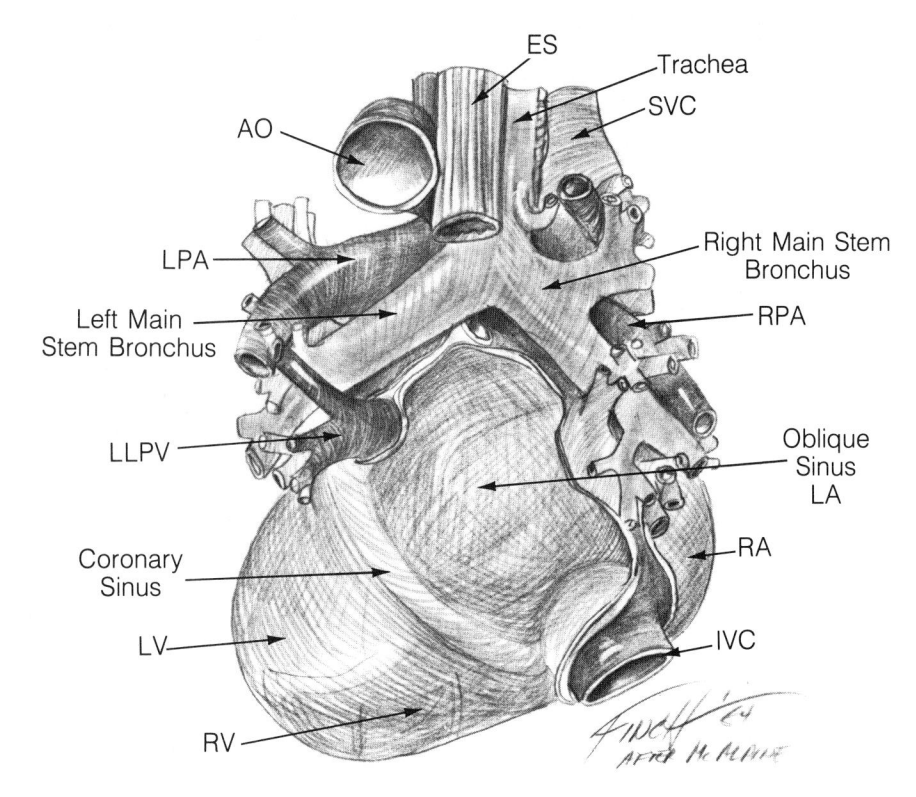

FIG 2–33.
Posterior aspect of heart showing anatomic relations of left atrium to carina and esophagus, which has been partly removed. Enlargement of left atrium splays carina and displaced esophagus. Note anatomic relationship of left mainstream bronchus to left atrium and left pulmonary artery. Enlargement of either structure may pinch left bronchus (hemodynamic vise).

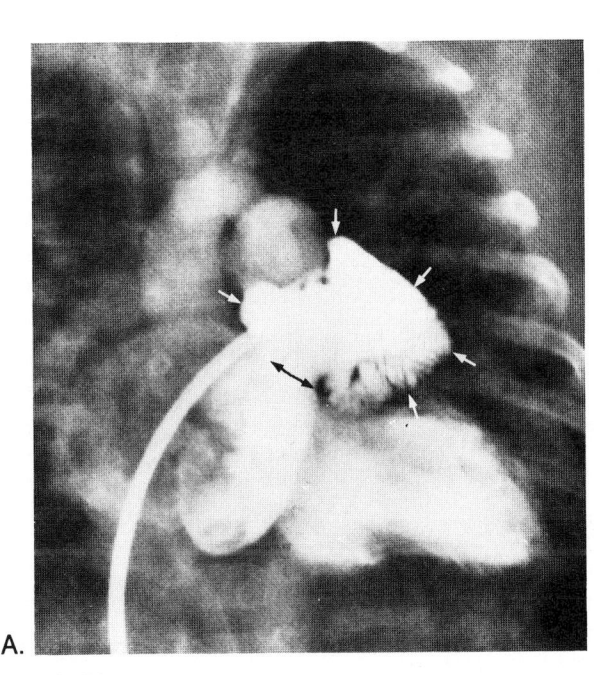

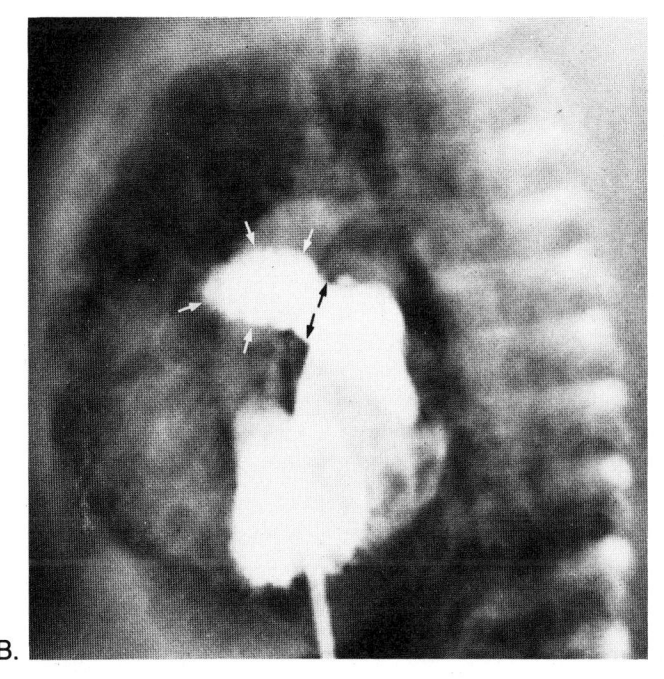

FIG 2–34.
Selective injection of left atrial appendage. **A,** anteroposterior projection; wing-shaped appendage, immediately beneath pulmonary artery, is more trabeculated than right appendage. There is a neck *(black arrows)* at junction with left atrium itself. **B,** lateral projection; neck of narrowed appendage *(black arrows)* seen. Appendage projects over ascending aorta in center of heart and is wing shaped.

thicker and smoother than that of the right atrium. The left atrial appendage is long and wing shaped (see Fig 2–15) and contains few pectinate muscles. The atrial appendage passes anteriorly around the left cardiac border below the level of the pulmonary trunk (Fig 2–34). The left surface of the atrial septum is smooth. The valve of the foramen ovale overlies the area of the fossa ovalis. The inferior border, which represents a remnant of the septum primum, may be scalloped.

The anatomic left atrium can be identified in two ways:

1. By observation of the pulmonary veins, which connect with the left atrium except in anomalous pulmonary venous connection. This exception makes the pulmonary veins a less reliable indicator of the anatomic left atrium than the inferior vena cava is for the right atrium.

2. By identifying the left atrial appendage, which is much longer than its counterpart on the right and has a much narrower connection with the atrium (see Fig 2–34,A). The shape of the left atrial appendage resembles a finger or the wing of a bird (see Fig 2–15,B). On a lateral projection, the left atrial appendage projects over the aorta and projects within the center of the cardiac contour (see Fig 2–34,B).

MITRAL VALVE

Anatomic Features

Blood flows anteriorly and laterally from the left atrium to the left ventricle through the mitral valve. The anterior location of this valve is of practical importance during cardiac catheterization; after the catheter tip has traversed the oblique atrial septum, it points always posteriorly and tends to enter a pulmonary vein or the left atrial appendage. To pass through the mitral valve, the tip must be turned sharply anteriorly, a technically difficult maneuver.

The mitral valve, like the tricuspid valve, is attached to a common fibrous annulus (Fig 2–35). The term mitral is derived from miter, a tall double-pointed headdress worn by bishops. The mitral valve has two leaflets: the anterior (septal) leaflet, which lies anteriorly and parallels the ventricular septum, and the posterior leaflet, which lies along the posterior wall of the left ventricle. The anterior leaflet is in fibrous continuity (aortic-mitral fibrosa, see Fig 2–37) with the aortic valve, because the left ventricle normally does not have an infundibulum (Fig 2–36,A). The continuity between the two valves is important in identifying the anatomic left ventricle. This fibrous continuity lies beneath the entire left coronary cusp and about one half of the noncoronary cusp (Figs 2–36,B and 2–43).

The anterior leaflet is wider than the more variably sized posterior leaflet. It attaches to the aortic-mitral intervalvar fibrosa (fibrous continuity) (see Fig 2–37), which is the immobile portion of the mitral valve. The posterior leaflet attaches to a tiny fibrous structure that lies at the junction of the left atrium and left ventricle, the so-called mitral annulus. The circumference of the posterior leaflet is larger and is partially wrapped around the anterior leaflet. The attachment of the posterior leaflet of the mitral valve may be visible on plain radiographs, because the mitral annulus may calcify, particularly in older

HEART IN SYSTOLE (ATRIA REMOVED)

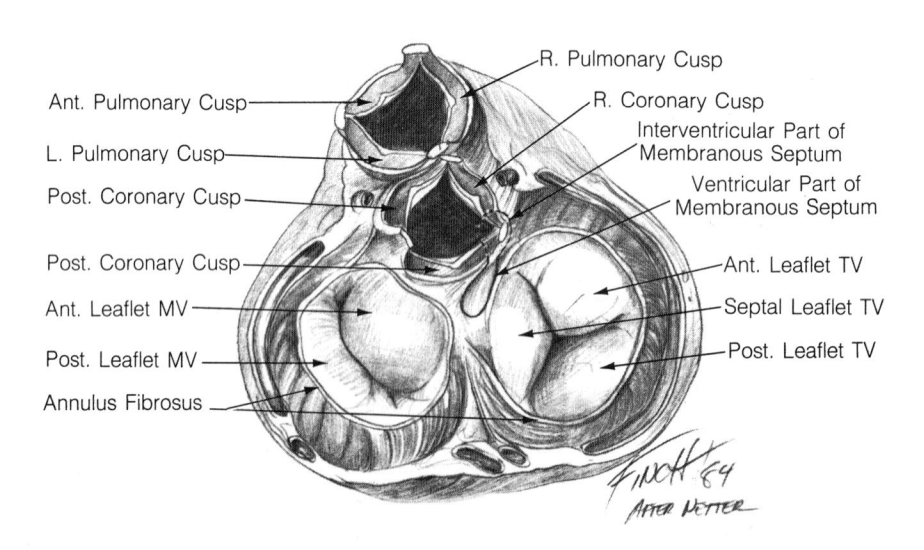

FIG 2–35.
Anatomic relations of four cardiac valves during systole. Tricuspid *(TV)* and mitral *(MV)* valve attach to common anulus fibrosus and are closed; pulmonary and aortic valves are open. The membranous ventricular septum and its atrial component are shown. *ANT* = anterior; *L* = left; *R* = right; *POST* = posterior.

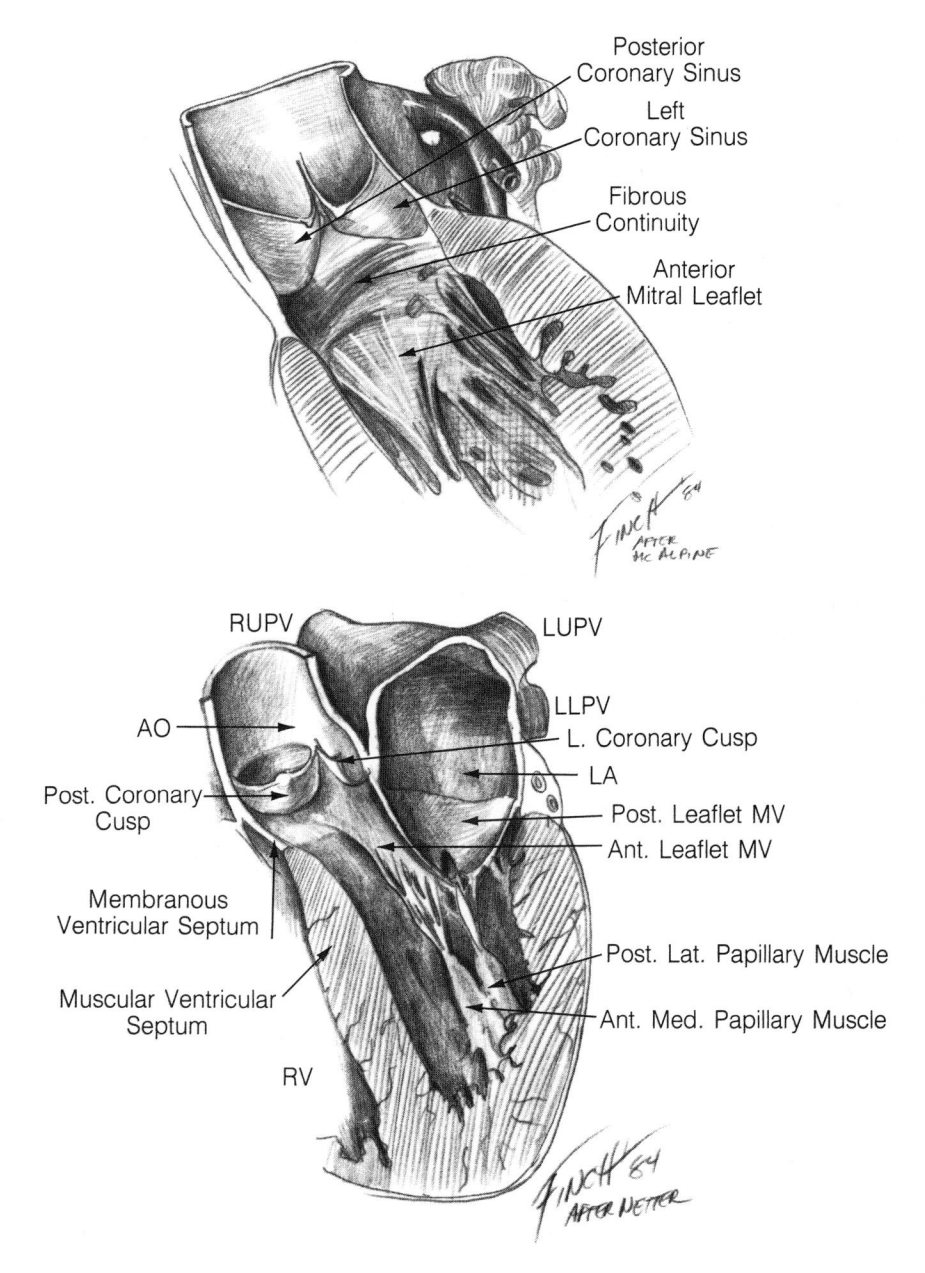

FIG 2–36.
Left ventricle. **A,** fibrous continuity of anterior leaflet of mitral valve with left coronary cusp. **B,** part of noncoronary cusp; this fibrous continuity is important in identifying anatomic left ventricle.

women. Characteristically, this calcified mitral annulus forms a C- or horseshoe-shaped density. About 60% of the mitral orifice is formed by the mitral annulus and about 40% by the intervalvar fibrosa. There are two papillary muscles, the anterolateral and the posteromedial, which receive chordae tendineae from each of the leaflets (Fig 2–37).

A rare anomaly is duplication of the mitral valve, and duplication of the tricuspid valve is even rarer. Only 14 cases of duplication of these atrioventricular valves have been described.

Angiographic Features

The mitral valve is best seen on a 70- to 80-degree left anterior oblique projection with cranial beam angulation. The leaflets are best seen if a left atriogram is performed, because contrast medium will be present on both sides of the leaflets. The anterior leaflet is usually well seen in profile, but the posterior leaflet is difficult to identify. The leaflets can also be seen after left ventriculography, when they are outlined by contrast medium on their ventricular aspect (Fig 2–38,A). In this projection, the anterior leaflet

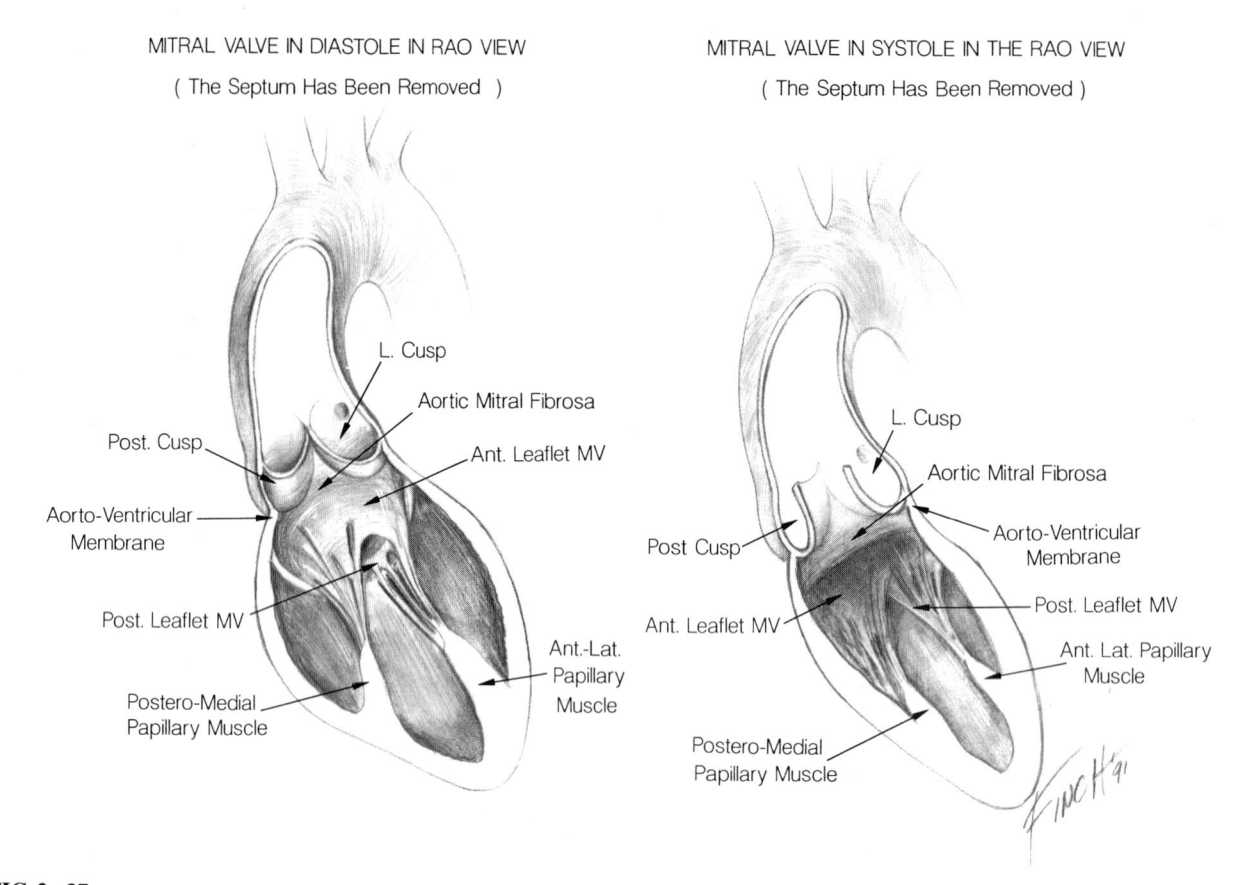

FIG 2–37.
Mitral valve *(MV)* in right anterior oblique projection during diastole **(A)** and systole **(B)**. Each leaflet attaches by chordae tendineae to each papillary muscle. Relation to aortic cusps seen. *Ant.lat.* = anterolateral; *Ant.* = anterior; *L* = left; *Post.* = posterior.

of the open mitral valve can be seen in profile during diastole as it moves toward the ventricular septum. The leaflet does not touch the septum. This normal diastolic anterior motion of the valve narrows the left ventricular outflow tract (see Fig 2–38,A).

During systole, the mitral valve leaflets close and move posteriorly. This normal systolic posterior motion of the valve widens the left ventricular outflow tract to approximately the diameter of the aorta (Fig 2–38,B).

An en face view of the mitral valve is obtained on a 30- to 40-degree right anterior oblique projection, which is at right angles to the left anterior oblique projection (Figs 2–37 and 2–39). The two leaflets are superimposed and cannot be individually identified, an important angiographic characteristic of the normal mitral valve. When there is a cleft in the anterior leaflet, the split anterior leaflet can be seen in profile on the right anterior oblique projection during diastole (see Chapter 23).

During diastole, unopacified blood enters the left ventricle, causing an ill-defined radiolucency (see Fig 2–39,A) caused by mixing of contrast medium with the incoming blood. Contrast medium trapped beneath the leaflets of the mitral valve then outlines the annulus (see Fig 2–39,A). When the commissures of the mitral valve are fused (mitral stenosis), the ballooning valve produces a more prominent filling defect in the left ventricular outflow tract because it displaces more contrast medium than does the normal mitral valve (see Fig 2–39,B).

The mitral annulus can be identified radiographically in two ways:

1. It has usually a slightly scalloped configuration, whereas the aortic mitral fibrosa is smooth and not visible.
2. It is always close to the circumflex branch of the left coronary artery and coronary sinus, regardless of obliquity.

During systole, when the mitral valve closes, its angiographic image disappears (see Fig 2–39,C). During this phase of the cardiac cycle, two distinct filling defects (the papillary muscles) appear in the left ventricular cavity (see Fig 2–39,C). These muscles are best observed in patients with a small end-systolic volume of the left ventricle, as occurs in left ventricular hypertrophy. With ventricular dilation, the papillary muscles may not be visible. Identification of the papillary muscles allows angiographic identification of the anatomic left ventricle. On a left ante-

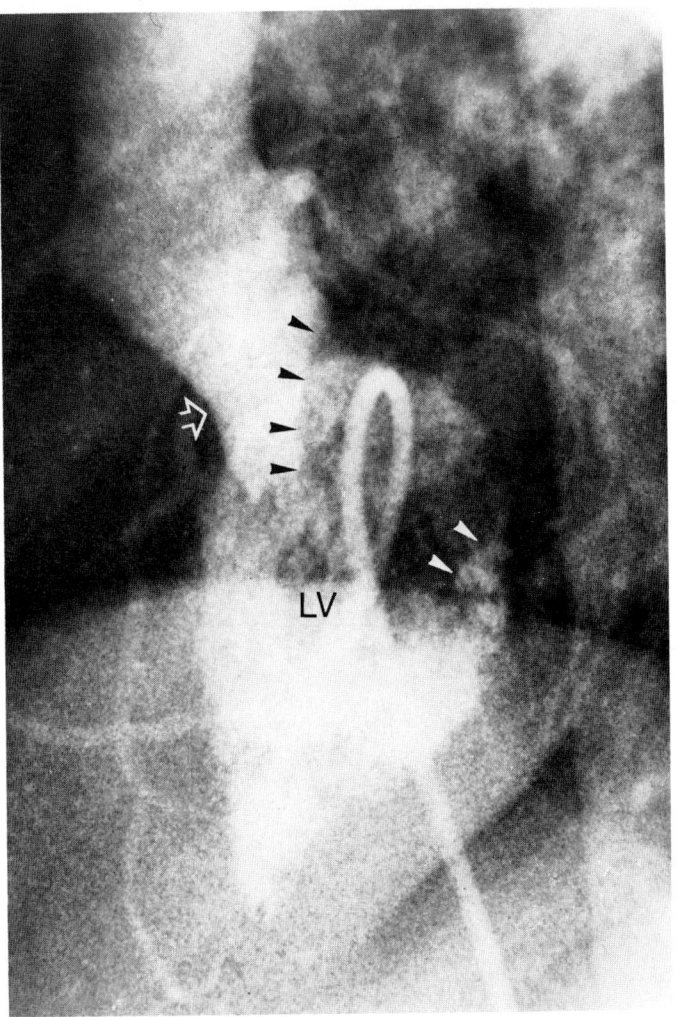

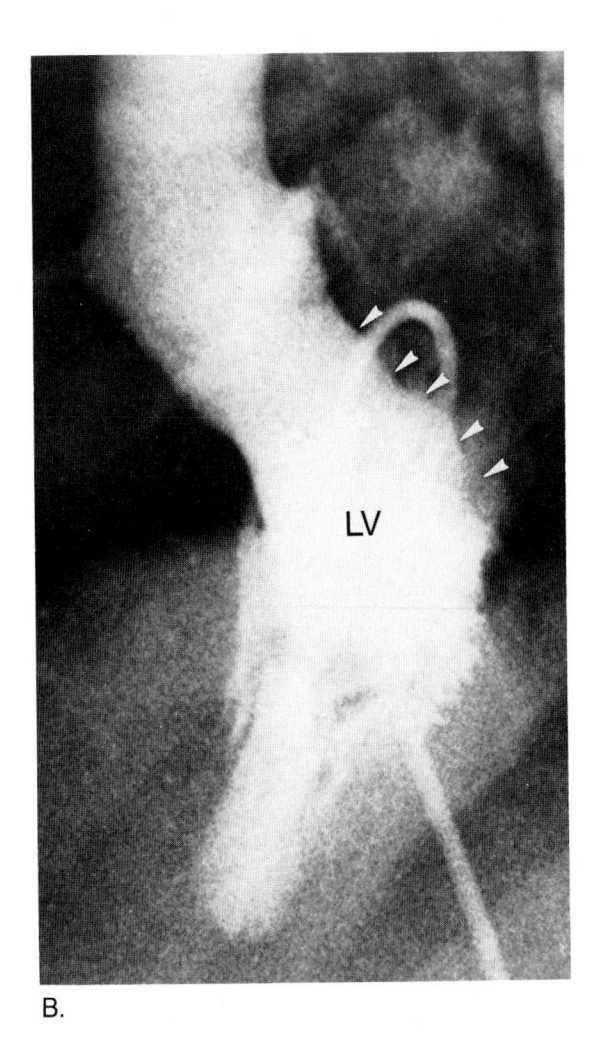

FIG 2–38.
Left ventricle in left anterior oblique and angled projection. **A,** diastole; open mitral valve. Anterior leaflet visible *(black arrows);* posterior leaflet not well demonstrated *(white arrows).* Anterior leaflet does not touch ventricular septum. Ventricular septum (anteriorly) and anterior mitral leaflet (posteriorly) slightly narrow the outflow tract *(open arrow).* Nonopacified blood entering left ventricle creates radiolucency. **B,** systole; two leaflets of mitral valve coapted, forming slightly scalloped posterior border of left ventricle. Valve does not extend beyond mitral anulus; left ventricular outflow tract is approximately as wide as the aorta.

rior oblique projection with caudal beam angulation, the papillary muscles form two distinct round filling defects (Fig 2–40).

LEFT VENTRICLE

The anterior leaflet of the mitral valve separates the left ventricle into two portions: the inflow portion, lying posteriorly to the leaflet; and the outflow portion, lying anteriorly to the leaflet. The left ventricle is conical, thick, and relatively smooth walled. Fine trabeculations may be present, but the septum is nearly smooth.

The left ventricular outflow tract is formed by the anterior leaflet of the mitral valve on one side and the ventricular septum on the other three sides. The subaortic area lies behind the outflow area of the right ventricle, because these two outflow tracts cross at nearly right angles (Fig 2–41). The right ventricular outflow area is partly wrapped around the subaortic area (Fig 2–42).

The curved ventricular septum separates the left from the right ventricle (see Fig 2–42). The septum has a muscular and a membranous portion. The membranous ventricular septum is a small diamond-shaped area located in the angle between the posterior and right aortic cusps (Fig 2–43). It is thin and translucent. Despite its small size (approximately 1–2 cm^2), it is important, because many ventricular septal defects involve a portion of the membra-

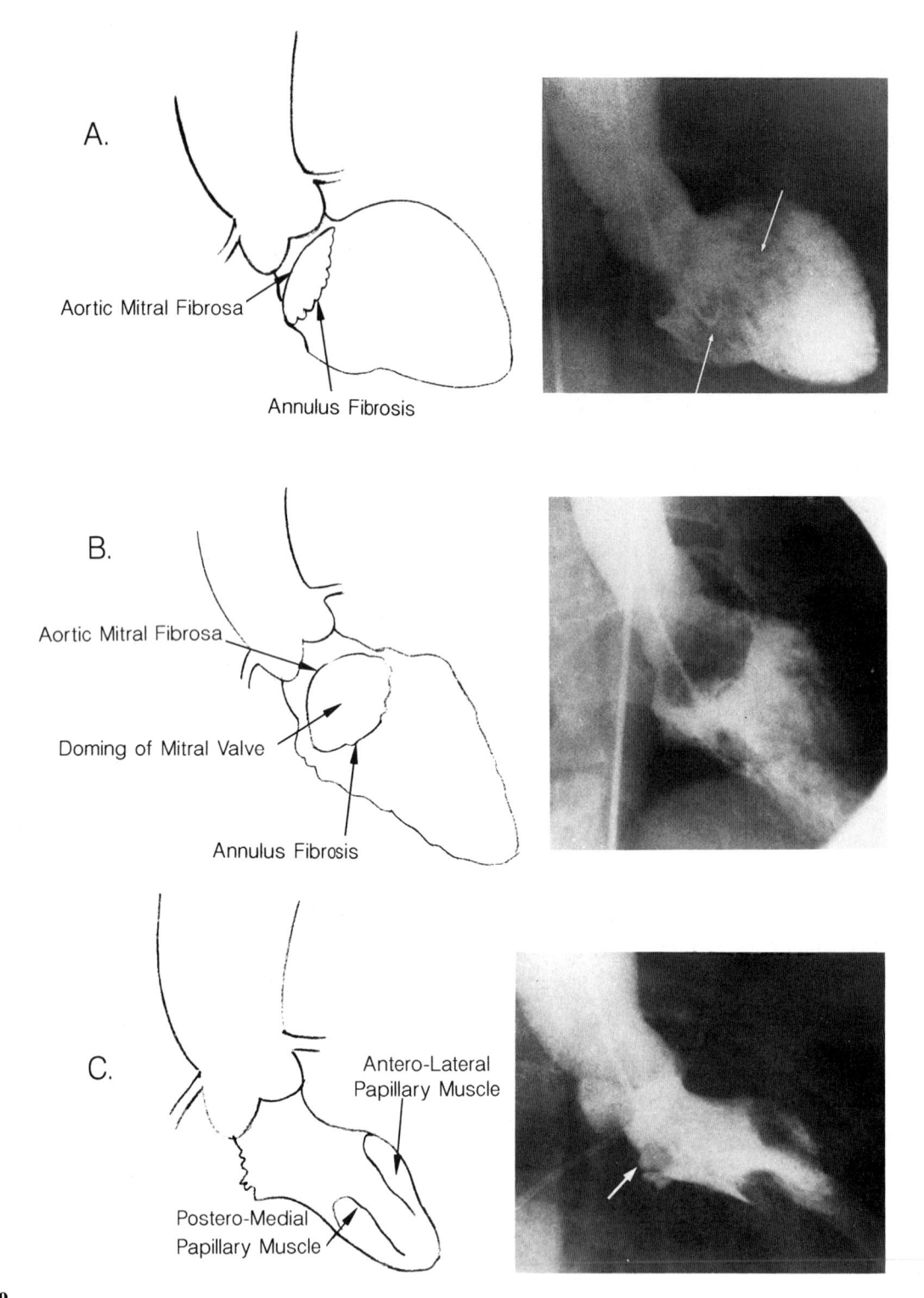

FIG 2-39.
A, left ventriculogram in right anterior oblique projection during diastole. Individual leaflets of mitral valve are seen en face and cannot be distinguished. Ill-defined radiolucency *(arrows)* is produced by incoming blood from left atrium *(arrows)*. Papillary muscles not seen. Mitral valve is open; contrast medium trapped behind posterior leaflet outlines posterior anulus, which is slightly scalloped. (See drawing of the mitral valve in diastole, Fig 2–37,**A**). **B,** left ventriculogram in right anterior oblique projection showing mitral stenosis. Doming of fused valvular leaflets causes well-defined, prominent filling defect in outflow tract; mitral anulus is sharply outlined. **C,** left ventriculogram during systole; closed mitral valve forms posterior aspect of opacified left ventricle (see Fig 2–37,**B**). Image of mitral anulus has disappeared. Valves project slightly beyond muscular ventricular wall *(arrow),* because valve anulus does not attach directly to muscle of left ventricle but to aortoventricular membrane. This normal angiographic appearance should not be confused with prolapse of posterior leaflet.

Cardiac Anatomy 39

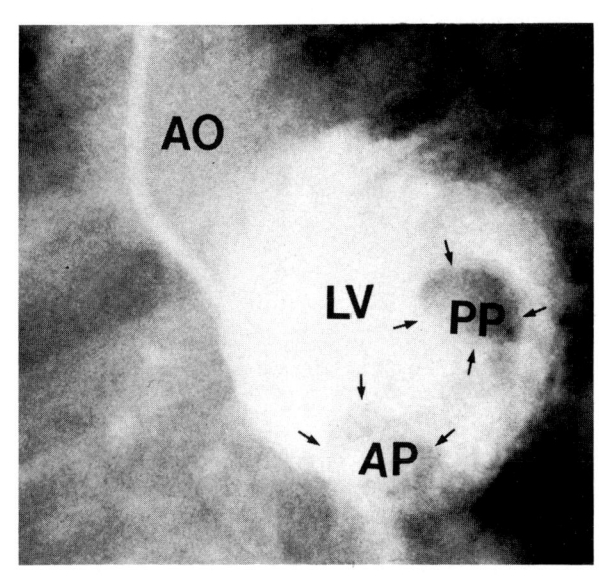

FIG 2-40.
Left ventriculogram caudal beam angulation with the lateral image tube (looking up). The anterolateral papillary muscle *(AP)* and the posteromedial papillary muscle *(PP)* form two distinct filling defects *(arrows)*.

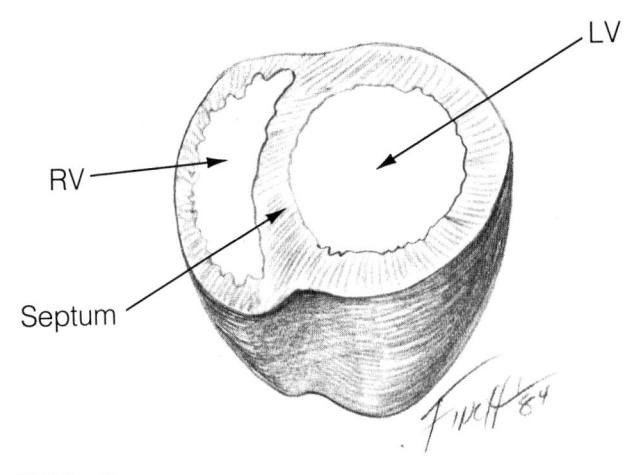

FIG 2-42.
Cross-section through ventricles showing curved ventricular septum. Left ventricle *(LV)* is round; right ventricle *(RV)* is flat and wrapped around *LV*.

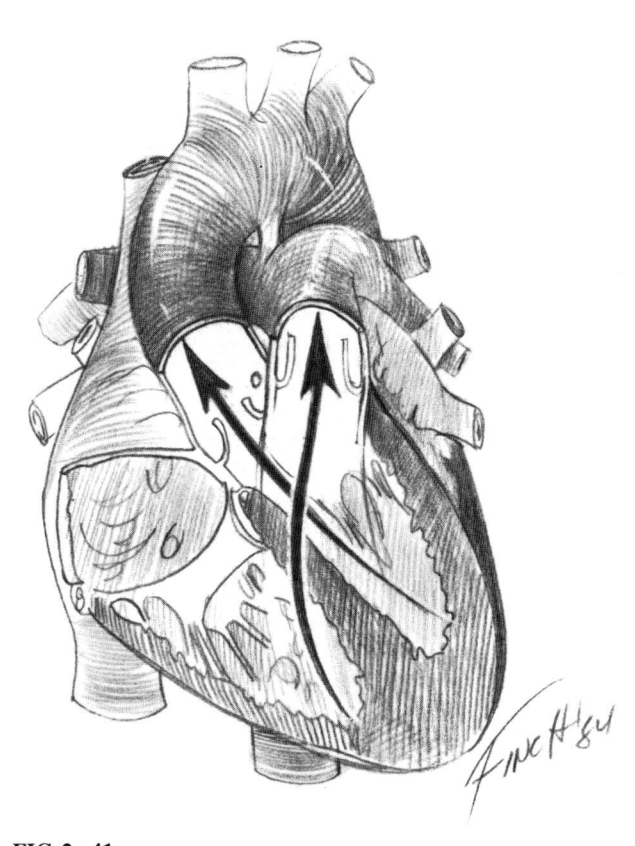

FIG 2-41.
Diagram showing crossing of right and left ventricular outflow tracts.

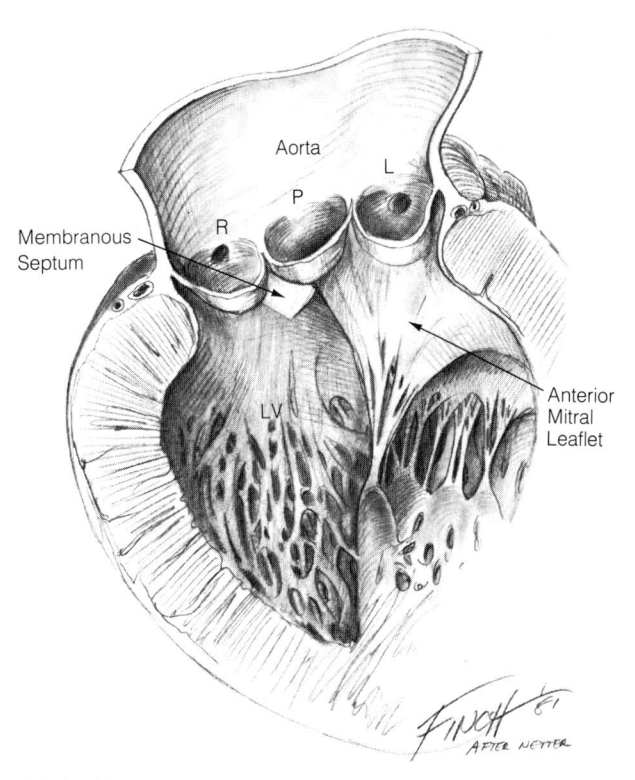

FIG 2-43.
Ventricular septum viewed from left *(LV)* side; small diamond-shaped membranous septum lies at junction of right *(R)* and posterior aortic cusps. Part of posterior cusp *(P)* and the left cusp *(L)* are in continuity with mitral valve.

40 *General Introduction*

nous septum and are consequently classified as membranous or, more correctly, perimembranous (see Chapter 12). The membranous ventricular septum also involves a small portion of the atrial septum. On the right side of the heart, most of the membranous septum lies in the atrial septum immediately above the tricuspid annulus, and a small portion lies beneath the tricuspid valve in the ventricular septum (Fig 2–44). Thus, the tricuspid annulus is slightly lower than the mitral annulus. (For detailed anatomy of the membranous septum, see Chapter 12.)

Angiographic Identification of the Anatomic Left Ventricle

Certain angiographic features permit the identification of an anatomic left ventricle, regardless of whether it receives systemic or pulmonary venous blood.

1. The left ventricle has a conical shape and is relatively smooth with fine trabeculations.
2. The left ventricle has two papillary muscles, which can be demonstrated angiographically (see Figs 2–39,C and Fig 2–40).
3. There is fibrous continuity between the atrioventricular and semilunar valves, indicating that there is no infundibulum (see Fig 2–36). This angiographic sign is not invariable, however, because in some cases of congenital heart disease, the anatomic left ventricle also may have myocardial tissue separating the mitral and semilunar valves (double coni), most commonly seen in various transpositions.

AORTIC VALVE

The normal aortic valve usually has three leaflets, although rarely a quadricuspid aortic valve is seen (Fig 2–45). This normal variant has no hemodynamic consequences. The three cusps are called the posterior (noncoronary), the right, and the left, although in situ, the right coronary cusp is a true anterior cusp, whereas the left cusp is a left posterior cusp (Figs 2–46 and 2–47) and the noncoronary is a right cusp.

The aortic root has three bulbous swellings, the sinuses of Valsalva (Fig 2–48) (Antonio Valsalva was a 17th century Italian anatomist). The upper limit of the sinus is a plane drawn through the free margin of the closed aortic valve cusps (see Fig 2–48). The transition between the bulbous and tubular portion of the aorta is called the sinotubular ridge and lies above the sinuses of Valsalva. The coronary arteries rarely arise from the sinuses; usually they arise from the aorta, above the sinuses and immediately below the sinotubular ridge. During diastole, the aortic leaflets approximate, preventing reflux of blood into the

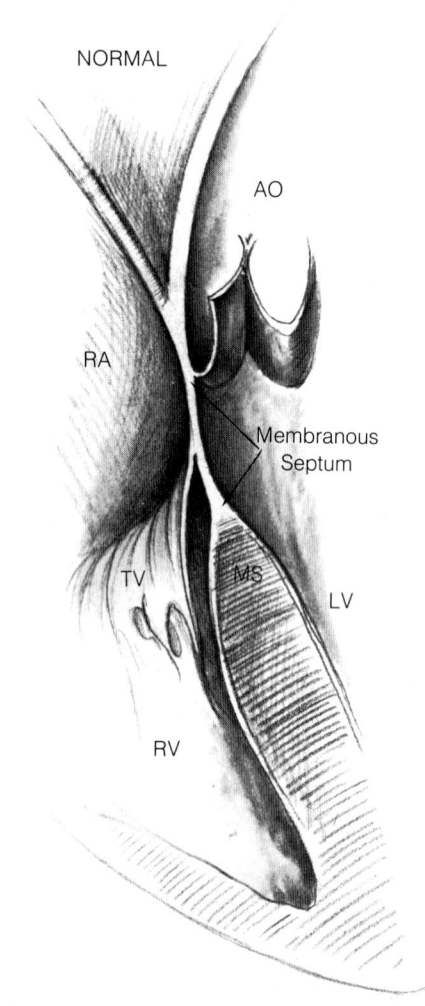

FIG 2–44.
Anatomy of membranous septum in relation to tricuspid valve *(TV)*; most of membranous septum is above tricuspid anulus in atrial septum. Defect in membranous septum can result in communication between left ventricle *(LV)* and right atrium *(RA)*. Mitral anulus is slightly higher than tricuspid anulus. *AO* = aorta; *MS* = muscular septum; *TV* = tricuspid valve.

left ventricle (Fig 2–49,C). The free margin of each leaflet is slightly thickened. Apposition is reinforced by fibrous nodules, described by Arantius (Julius Arantius, Italian anatomist) in the sixteenth century, which are located in the midportion of the free margins (see Fig 2–48). During systole, the leaflets open completely, provided the left ventricle develops a full stroke volume (Fig 2–49,A). With decreased stroke volume, as in ventricular extrasystoles and markedly dilated aortas, opening of the valve may be incomplete (Fig 2–49,B); and in subaortic obstruction, which produces a subvalvar jet, the valve opens asymmetrically and flutters (see Chapter 26).

The right ventricular outflow tract wraps around the root of the aorta (see Fig 2–46). The entire right cusp and

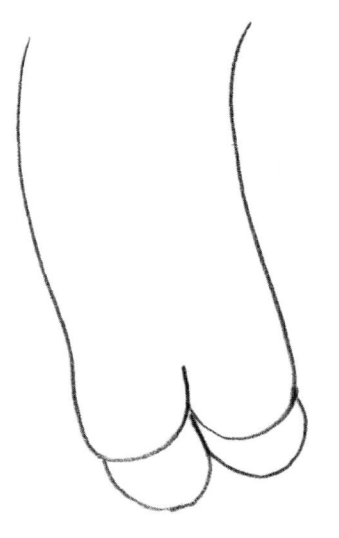

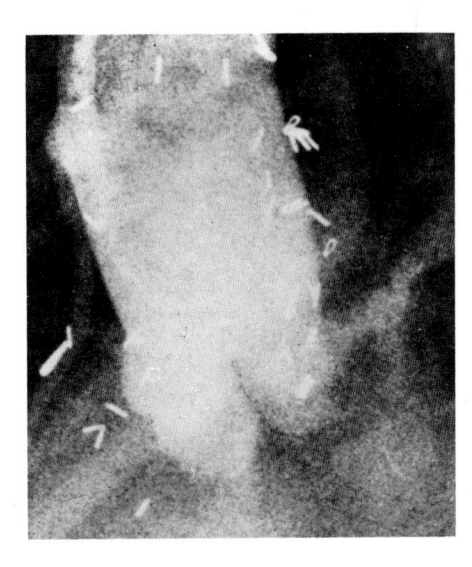

FIG 2–45.
Angiogram shows quadricuspid aortic valve, a hemodynamically insignificant variation. One leaflet is usually hypoplastic.

the left anterior half of the noncoronary (posterior) cusp are adjacent to the right ventricle. The left sinus and the posterior half of the noncoronary sinus are adjacent to the anterior leaflet of the mitral valve (see Fig 2–43).

Angiographic Features

In an anteroposterior projection, the aortic valve plane is tilted approximately 30 degrees to the horizontal plane (see Fig 2–47). The tilt varies, and it increases with age because of uncoiling of the aorta. In the anteroposterior projection, the three leaflets may be at the same level (see Fig 2–47,A), or there may be an anterior tilt (see Fig 2–47,B) that projects the right cusp lower. This is the most common, particularly in the aged. A posterior tilt of the valve plane, which projects the right coronary cusp slightly higher than the other two (see Fig 2–47,C), is common in a double-outlet right ventricle or transposition of the great vessels, as well as in normal children.

A clear understanding of the tilt of the aortic valve is important for the angiographic demonstration of subvalvar membranes, which usually lie parallel to the aortic valve plane (see Chapter 26). On an aortogram in the anteroposterior projection, the posterior and left cusps lie along the lateral borders of the aorta, whereas the right cusp, being perpendicular to the x-ray beam, may be superimposed on the aorta, depending on the tilt of the valve plane (Fig 2–50). Therefore, during systole, the posterior and left leaflets are seen in profile whereas the right leaflet is seen en face (see Fig 2–50,C). Because of the tilt of the valve in relation to the horizontal plane, in a lateral view the posterior cusp is projected considerably lower (Fig 2–51,A). During diastole, each of the three aortic sinuses is well seen. During systole, the right valve leaflet is seen in profile, and the left and posterior valve leaflets are seen end on (Fig 2–51,B). In the adult, particularly the aged, the aortic valve plane is tilted anteriorly. A slight posterior tilt (corresponding to anteroposterior projection in Fig

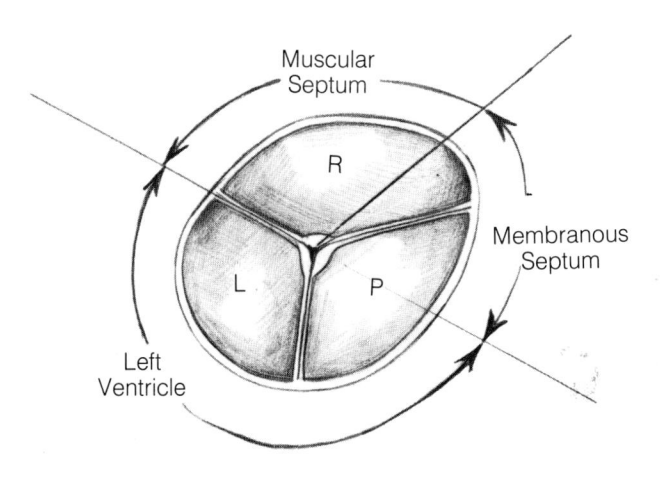

FIG 2–46.
Spatial relation of aortic cusps to surrounding cardiac structure; right *(R)* and left *(L)* cusps are related to respective ventricles, whereas posterior *(P)* cusp is related to both ventricles.

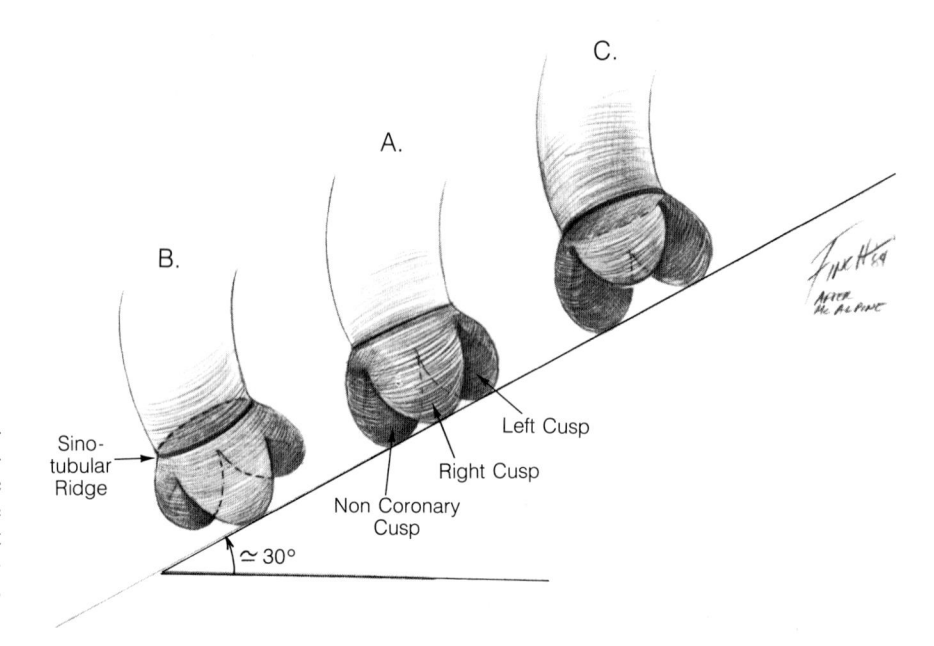

FIG 2–47.
Aortic valve in anteroposterior projection; average tilt of aortic valve, 30 degrees, increases with age. Valve plane tilted to horizontal plane. **A,** valve plane parallel to x-ray beam. **B,** anterior tilt common in older individuals. **C,** Posterior tilt occurs in younger individuals and in transposition of great vessels.

2–47,C) may be seen in children (see Fig 2–51). A significant anterior tilt of the valve plane on a lateral projection is highly suspicious for double-outlet right ventricle.

CORONARY ARTERIES

The coronary arteries arise from the aorta immediately below the sinotubular ridge and above the sinuses of Valsalva. Occasionally they also arise from the sinuses or from the tubular portion of the ascending aorta. The left coronary artery usually originates above the left aortic cusp and the right coronary artery above the right aortic cusp, although variations exist.

The left coronary artery passes behind the pulmonary artery and divides into two major branches: the anterior descending branch and the circumflex branch (Fig 2–52). The circumflex branch crosses posteriorly beneath the left atrial appendage in the left atrioventricular groove and parallels the coronary sinus in each projection. This branch gives off muscular branches, called obtuse marginal branches, and also gives rise to left atrial branches (see Fig 2–52,B), which are particularly prominent in patients with mitral stenosis. If the left coronary artery is dominant (as it

FIG 2–48.
Aortic cusp demonstrating nodules of Arantius. Space below free margin of cusps is sinus of Valsalva; junction between bulbous portion of aortic root and tubular ascending aorta is sinotubular ridge. Coronary arteries usually arise above sinus of Valsalva and Below sinotubular ridge. However, exceptions exist. (Julius Caesar Arantius, 16th century Italian anatomist.)

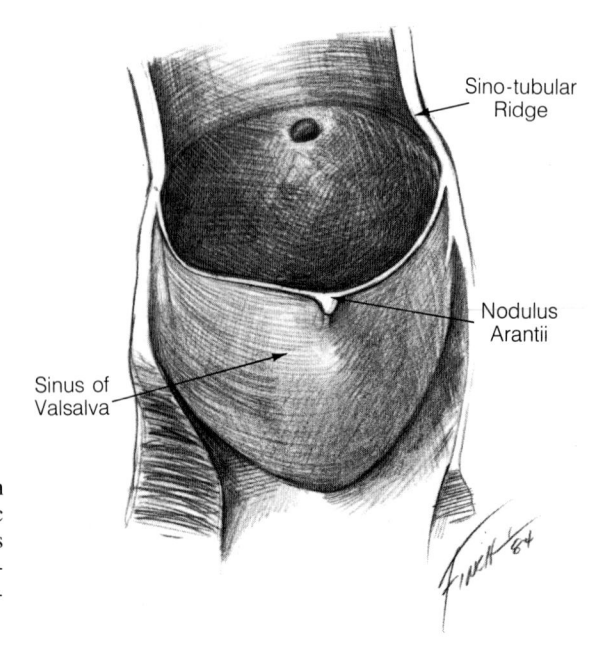

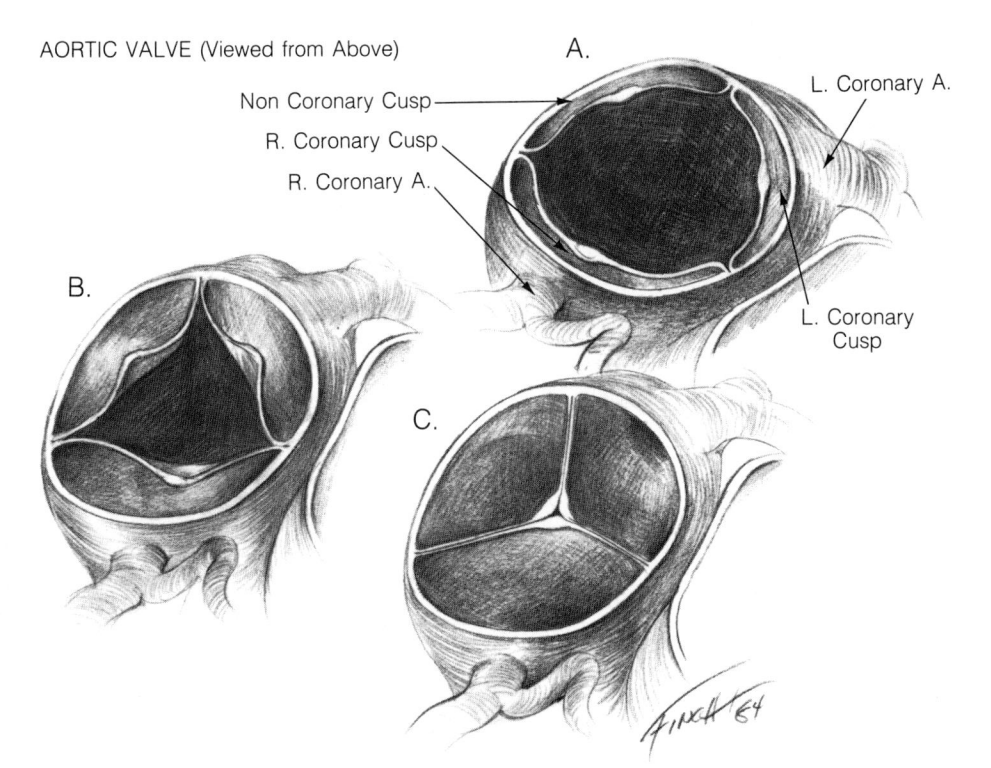

AORTIC VALVE (Viewed from Above)

FIG 2-49.
Normal aortic valve viewed from above showing three cusps. **A,** during systole, valve is completely open. **B,** valve partially open because of diminished stroke volume of left ventricle. **C,** during diastole, valve leaflets closed. A = artery; L = left; R = right.

is in 20% of persons), the circumflex artery gives rise to a posterior descending branch. The left anterior descending branches pass downward in the anterior interventricular groove and give off muscular diagonal branches. The first branch of the left anterior descending artery serves the right ventricle and is called the left conal branch (see Fig 2–52). Although small, it is important, because it may become a significant collateral pathway to the larger right conal branch, which arises from the right coronary artery. The left anterior descending branch also supplies a significant portion of the ventricular septum and gives rise to anterior septal branches, the longest being about 8 cm long and communicate with the shorter (2 cm) posterior septal branches, which arise from the posterior descending branch (see Fig 2–52).

The right coronary artery originates above the right

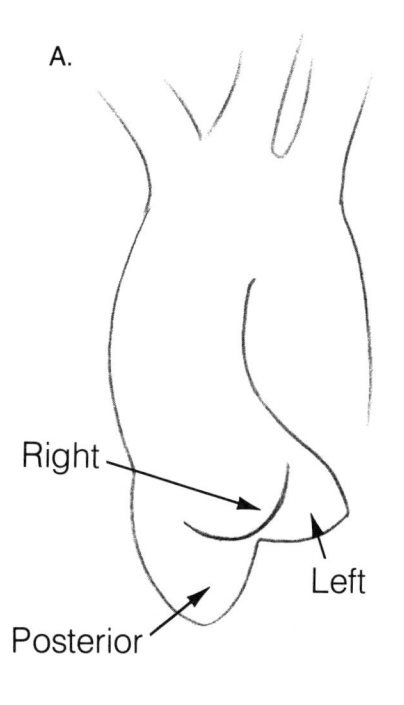

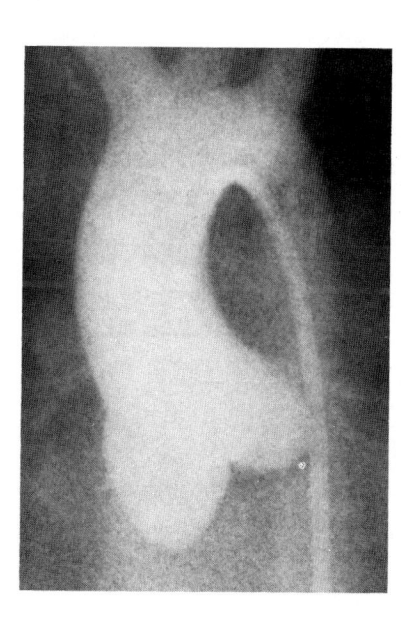

FIG 2-50.
Aortogram. **A,** anteroposterior projection during diastole; posterior cusp on right, and left cusp on left, of aortic root. Right cusp superimposed on aortic root because of minimal posterior tilt of valve plane.
(Continued.)

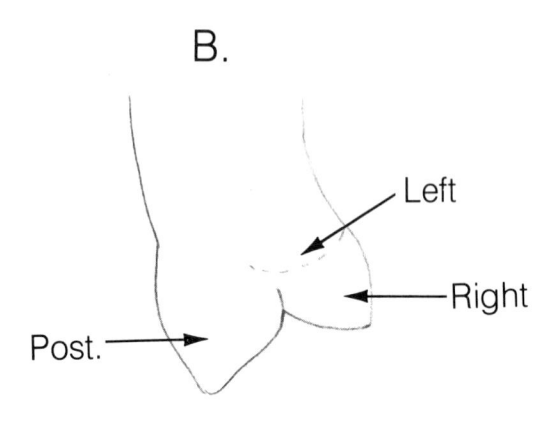

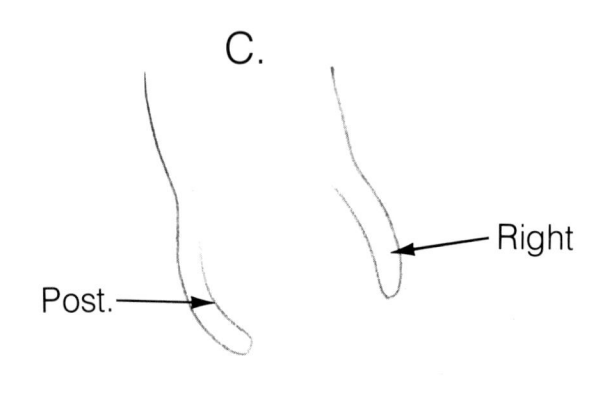

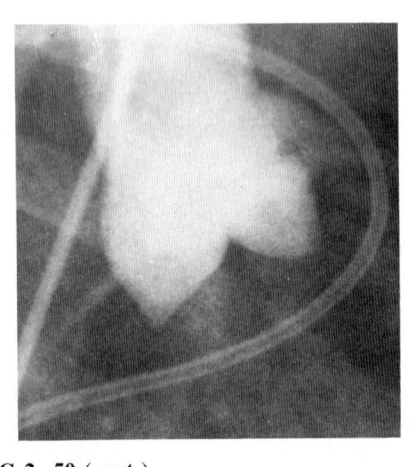

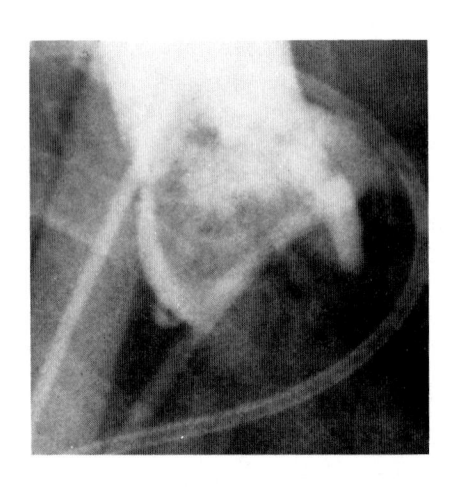

FIG 2-50 (cont.).
B, right anterior oblique projection; right aortic cusp on left, since it is related to right ventricular outflow tract. Posterior cusp forms right border of aortic root. Left cusp higher superimposed on aortic root. **C,** systole; Right anterior oblique projection; posterior and right cusps seen in profile with valve completely open.

aortic sinus and passes in the right atrioventricular groove, giving off muscular branches to the right ventricle. The first muscular branch of the right coronary artery is the right conal branch, which supplies the right ventricular outflow tract. The right conal branch anastomoses with the left conal branch, which arises from the left anterior descending branch (Figs 2-52 and 2-53). In cases of coronary artery occlusion, this communication may become an important collateral pathway, the arc of Vieussen (named for a 17th century French anatomist). Commonly, the right conal artery originates as a separate branch directly from the aorta and immediately above the orifice of the right coronary artery. Most individuals, therefore, have three, not two, individual coronary arteries. The right coronary artery also gives off small branches to the sinoatrial node and the right atrium (see Fig 2-53), although its major branches are to the right ventricle.

A fairly consistent branch of the right coronary artery lies at the acute margin of the right ventricle and is termed, appropriately, the acute marginal branch (see Fig 2-53). At the level of the posterior ventricular groove, the right coronary artery dips deep into the epicardial fat and forms a loop, or U turn (see Fig 2-53,B), from which arises a short, small, straight artery that supplies the atrioventricular node. The atrioventricular node artery anastomoses with the Kugel artery.

The right coronary artery terminates as the posterior descending artery, which supplies the posterior portion of the ventricular septum through short straight septal branches. If the right coronary artery is dominant (as it is in 80% of persons), it continues beyond the crux (Latin: crux:cross) and gives rise to muscular branches that supply the posterior aspect of the left ventricle through posterolateral branches. The most important branches of the posterior descending artery are the posterior septal branches, which communicate with the much longer anterior septal branches (see Fig 2-53). The atrioventricular node artery also communicates with a small branch that usually originates from either the right or the left circumflex coronary artery and passes along the atrial and ventricular septum.

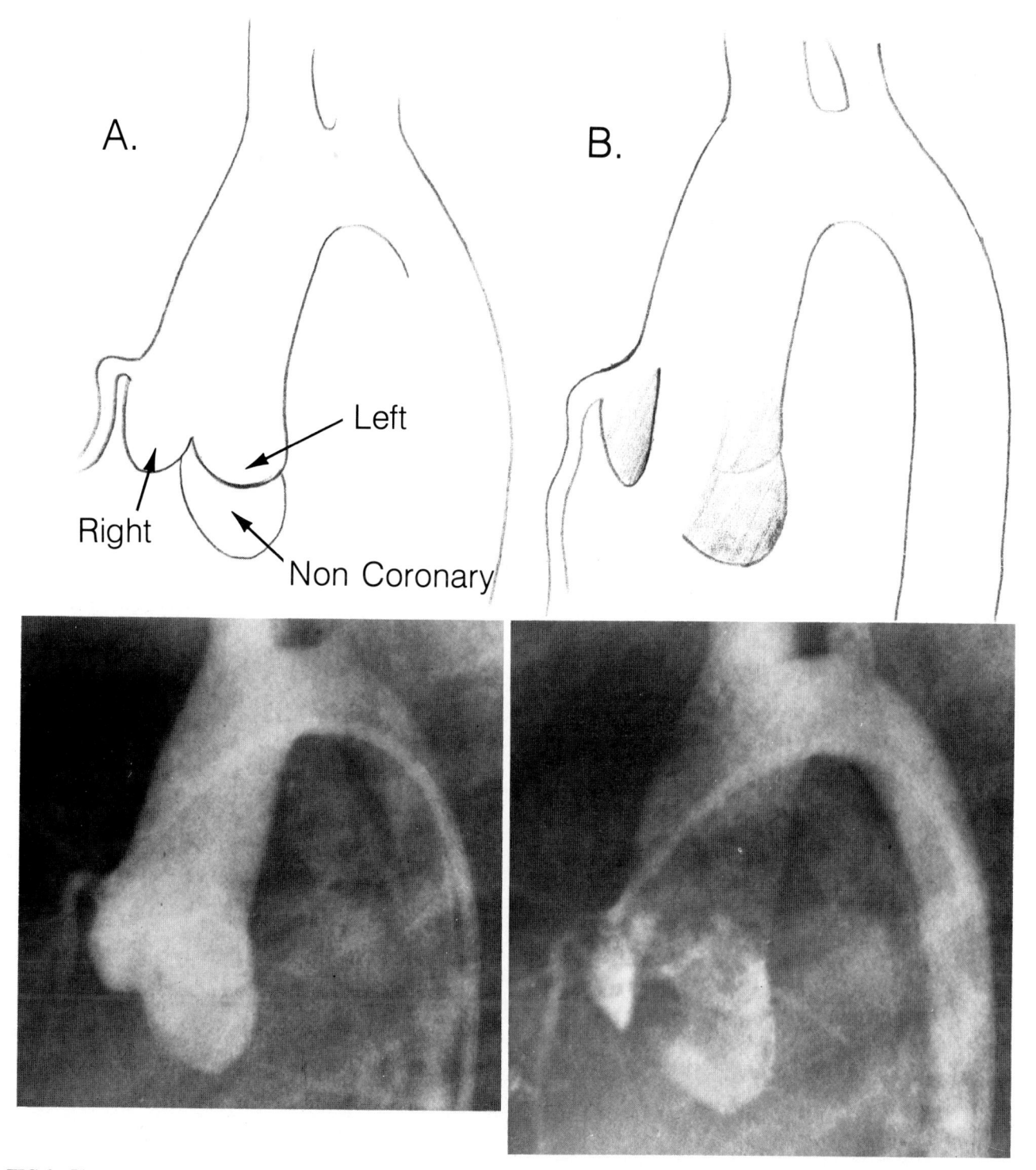

FIG 2–51.
Aortogram in lateral projection. **A,** three cusps of aorta; because of 30° tilt of valve in anteroposterior plane, noncoronary cusp is projected much lower than the other two. **B,** Aortic valve in systole. Right cusp in profile; left and posterior cusps en face.

46 *General Introduction*

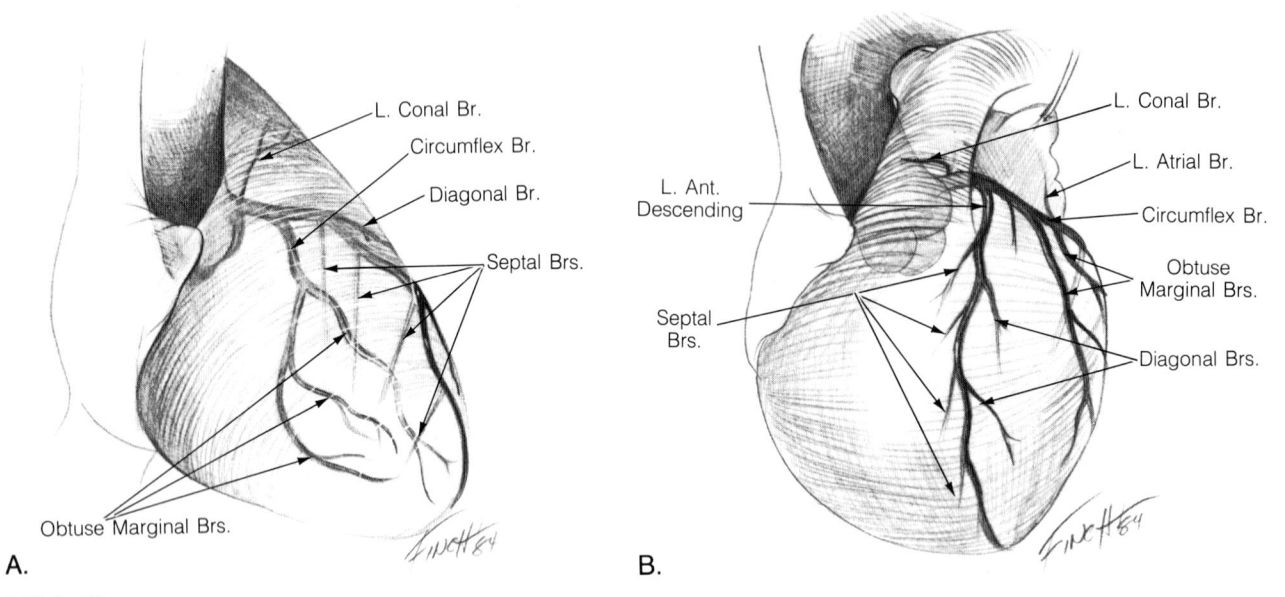

FIG 2-52.
Left coronary arterial system. **A,** right anterior oblique projection. **B,** left anterior oblique projection. *Ant.* = anterior; *Br.* = branch; *Brs.* = branches; *L* = left.

This is Kugel's artery. Although minute, it can be seen in cases of coronary obstruction. It is never an important collateral pathway.

For angiographic orientation, it is important to realize that there are two circumflex arteries, the left and the right (or right coronary artery), which together encircle the atrioventricular groove. These arteries meet near the crux, in other words, at the junction of the atrioventricular and posterior ventricular grooves. In addition, two arteries, the anterior descending and the posterior descending branches, encircle the ventricular grooves and meet at the cardiac apex. The fact that both arteries meet at the apex is impor-

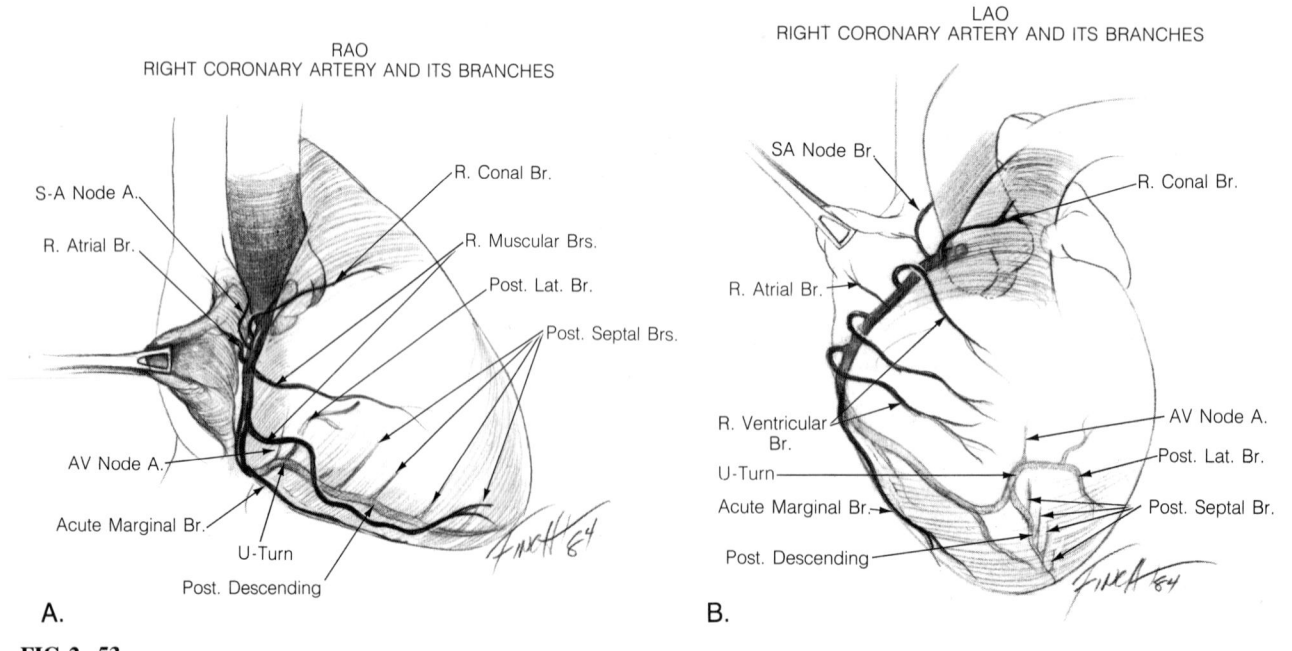

FIG 2-53.
Right coronary arterial system. **A,** right anterior oblique *(RAO)* projection. **B,** left anterior oblique *(LAO)* projection. *A* = artery; *AV* = atrioventricular; *Br.* = branch; *Brs.* = branches; *Lat.* = lateral; *Post.* = posterior; *R* = right; *S-A* = sinoatrial.

tant for the proper identification of the posterior descending branch. Muscular coronary arterial branches located on the surface of the heart can be identified because of their undulating course. They are embedded in epicardial fat and so change their contour during ventricular contraction. On the other hand, the septal branches retain their straight course between systole and diastole and tend to run parallel.

Venous drainage of the left coronary tree, including the posterior descending, is into the coronary sinus. The right coronary arterial tree drains directly into the right atrium via thebesian veins (Adam Thebesius, 17th century German physician).

AORTA

The ascending aorta passes superiorly and slightly to the right, adjacent to the superior vena cava, and forms a gentle arch. From the aortic arch, the brachiocephalic vessels, innominate artery, left carotid, and left subclavian artery arise (see Fig 2–6). The aortic arch lies to the left of the trachea, which is thereby indented and slightly displaced. Beyond the arch, the descending aorta passes beside the spine in the left hemithorax.

Prominence of the ascending aorta as seen on plain chest radiographs is an important diagnostic finding. This prominence may be caused by:

1. Enlargement of the ascending aorta as a result of dilatation, as in aortic stenosis, and cystic medial necrosis.
2. Increased flow, as from a large patent ductus.
3. Counterclockwise rotation of the heart, as from left ventricular enlargement.
4. Left anterior oblique rotation of the chest.

The aorta tends to be *inconspicuous* because of:

1. Rotation of the chest.
2. Small size, as in critical aortic stenosis, and large intracardiac shunts.
3. Clockwise rotation of the heart, as from right-sided enlargement such as atrial septal defects and Ebstein's malformation.

With increasing age the aorta becomes more prominent because of increasing left ventricular predominance and aortic elongation by atherosclerosis.

CARDIAC LYMPHATICS

Little is known about the lymphatics of the heart. The study of this system is limited by the techniques of investigation. The small size of these vessels and the histologic similarity to capillaries have made it difficult to identify these vessels microscopically. The presence of valves has made it difficult to identify cardiac lymphatics by direct injection. Studies of cardiac lymphatics has depended on injection of vital dyes cleared by lymphatics and on the topical application of hydrogen peroxide. The oxygen thereby released distends the lymphatics, allowing the identification.

Lymphatics are thin walled, transparent, and superficial. Their contour is irregular because of the presence of bulbous swellings related to the valves. Lymphatic networks have been found in the subepicardial and subendocardial regions and within the myocardium. The subepicardial network is composed of vessels 15 to 20 μm in diameter. These networks are loosely arranged and interlacing. In the subendocardial area, lymphatics are present over the ventricular surfaces, including the septum and papillary muscles. These are located in the subendocardial region and course parallel to the myocardial fibers. The drainage of the subendocardial network is toward the atrioventricular sulcus. Below the aortic and tricuspid valves, the diameter of the lymphatic channels reaches 250 μm in diameter. The presence of lymphatics in normal cardiac valves is disputed, but certainly they have been demonstrated in certain conditions such as rheumatic carditis and endocardial fibroelastosis.

From these networks, larger channels pass to the major drainage channels of the heart. The largest of these is the anterior lymph channel, which courses with the anterior coronary artery. This channel receives channels from the left anterior ventricular and right anterior ventricular lymphatic channels. Another large lymph channel parallels the posterior descending coronary artery and runs in the atrioventricular sulcus, where it receives lymphatics from the atria. Each of these major lymph channels unites into a common channel that crosses the left main coronary artery and under the arch of the main and left pulmonary arteries to leave the pericardial sac and join the left mediastinal plexus of lymph vessels. The lymph flow from the heart is through mediastinal lymph nodes into the thoracic duct to the left subclavian vein.

The pericardial lymphatic plexus is located predominately in the parietal pericardium but also in the pericardial reflections of the major blood vessels lying within the pericardial sac. The flow from pericardial lymphatics is into the anterior mediastinum along the internal mammary arteries. The connection is through clavicular nodes to both the thoracic duct and the right lymphatic trunk.

CHAPTER 3

Radiation Safety

Users of radiographic equipment, particularly cardiologists, may not be familiar with the physical principles and hazards of ionizing radiation. Nonetheless, it is important that they be familiar with the hazards and principles of radiation protection. Cardiac catheterization, particularly with cine radiography, involves the highest dose used in diagnostic radiology (Table 3–1); and for the catheterization laboratory staff, exposure extends over many years. The following basic remarks should help acquaint the inexperienced operator with radiation safety.

Radiographic equipment must comply with national standards and is tested by officers of the department of environmental health. Also, before use, new radiographic units, including those in the catheterization laboratory, must pass extensive evaluation by a radiation safety officer. The tests include measurements of half-value layers (HVLs; also called half-value thicknesses), radiation outputs, interlocks, collimation, linearity, reproducibility of exposures, automatic exposure terminations, radiographic timer, and tube leakage. Only if the results comply with the safety standards of the regulatory agencies is the equipment approved for clinical use. Thereafter, it is operated only by trained x-ray technologists supervised by a radiologist.

The safe permissible dose of radiation for persons operating radiographic equipment is unknown, but some guidelines have been developed by state radiation protection programs that are similar to the federal guidelines. Thus, the operator must remember that these exposure levels are arbitrary; exposure should always be minimized. Exposure exceeding the guidelines poses significant risk to the operator.

BASIC PRINCIPLES OF RADIATION PROTECTION

Nature of Ionizing Radiation

The diagnostic usefulness of x-rays rests on their ability to pass through matter; the attenuation of the x-ray beam by body components produces the radiographic image. This stoppage (absorption) of x-rays has a potential for harm, however. Basically, this complex process involves the formation of charged atoms (ions) within cells, which can cause biologic harm. (Of course, x-rays are only one of the relevant forms of ionizing radiation; others are γ-rays, β-rays, and neutrons.) The amount of x-ray radiation is measured by the capacity to produce ions. The internationally accepted unit of quantity of x-ray radiation is the roentgen (R), which is defined as the amount of ion production in 1 cm^3 of atmospheric air at 0°C and 760 mm Hg. Other units of radiation measurement are the rad and the rem, which, in the range of radiation used for diagnostic x-rays, are interchangeable with the roentgen.* Radiation exposure of the personnel is monitored in one of these units, usually milliroentgens (mR):

$$mR = \frac{R}{1,000}$$

There are no guidelines for radiation exposure to patients, since they are exposed only occasionally. There are guidelines for radiation exposure for radiologic personnel, who are exposed to radiation repeatedly over many years.

During their passage through the body, x-rays produce not only ions but also new x-rays with longer wavelengths. These secondary (or scattered) x-rays emanate from the radiation field in all directions and are the primary factor in the exposure of the staff in the catheterization laboratory (Fig 3–1). Because the cells of various tissues have different sensitivities to ionizing radiation, different amounts are required to damage various organs. Furthermore, a single

---

*The introduction of the Système International d'Unités (SI) has changed these units of measurement; e.g., the ion dose (R) is now expressed as coulomb/kilogram and the energy and equivalent dose (rad and rem) are expressed in joule/kilogram, or gray units (Gy). Because of the unfamiliarity of these units, we have retained the older ones in our discussion.

TABLE 3–1.
Typical Radiation Doses for Diagnostic Procedures (Skin Entrance Exposure of an Average Adult)

Chest (anteroposterior and lateral)	30 mR
Lumbar spine, lateral	1 R
Digital fluoroscopy (15 sec)	3–7 R
Fluoroscopy (5 min)	5–10 R
Abdominal computed tomography scan	3–5 R
Cine angiography (per minute)	20–40 R

exposure to radiation usually has only an acute and temporary effect, because the damaged cells are repaired or regenerated (tissue recovery).

Effects of Repeated Exposure to Ionizing Radiation

The effects of repeated exposure to ionizing radiation are of concern to the staff of cardiac catheterization laboratories. These radiation hazards are dose dependent, but the dose-effect relations are difficult to assess.

Genetic Effects

Ionizing radiation can produce chromosomal aberrations and mutations in both somatic and germ cells. The result can be obvious immediately, for example, in the death of somatic cells, or it may be long delayed, as in the case of mutations in the germ cells, which appear only in the descendants of the exposed individual. Little is known about the relation of the dose of ionizing radiation to genetic effects in humans, especially the effects on progeny.

Carcinogenic Effects

A significant risk of long-term exposure to ionizing radiation is an increased incidence of cancer, especially of leukemia or lymphoma, which is not evident until many years after the exposure. The information available about this effect is derived primarily from patients treated with x-rays for benign diseases, such as ankylosing spondylitis, hyperthyroidism, thymic enlargement, and from survivors of the Hiroshima or Nagasaki atomic bomb explosions. Significant amounts of data are now beginning to appear from large numbers of patients irradiated for the treatment of malignancies, particularly the lymphomas and testicular germ-cell tumors. As yet, available data reveal no clear dose-response curve but do suggest that any dose of radiation, no matter how small, carries some risk.

Effect on Prenatal Development

Before implantation, an irradiated embryo may die. The fetus is particularly sensitive to the effects of ionizing radiation, which may cause malformations. Furthermore, the incidence of malignant disease, particularly of leukemia and tumors of the central nervous system, is higher during the first years of life in children exposed to ionizing radiation in utero. Again, the dose-response relation in humans is unknown. Consequently, pregnant women should not be exposed to x-rays, particularly during the first trimester.

Monitoring Requirements

Persons regularly exposed to ionizing radiation, such as the staff of a cardiac catheterization laboratory, must be monitored continuously and their radiation exposure kept on record indefinitely. Persons receiving 25% of the dose standards are required by law to wear monitoring equipment.

The most widely used and convenient monitoring

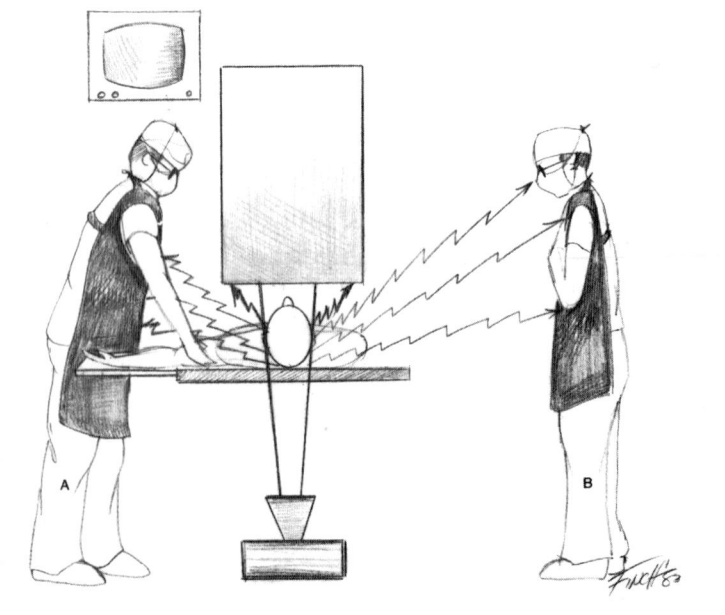

FIG 3–1.
Emission of secondary radiation during cine fluorography. Cardiologist A cannot see the radiation field and therefore his eyes and thyroid gland are completely protected by the image intensifier. Observer B receives less radiation to the body, but he can see the radiation field; therefore, secondary radiation strikes his eyes and thyroid gland. The principle is to stand either very close to or as far as possible from the radiation field. In-between positions result in high radiation doses to thyroid gland and eyes.

equipment are film badges, which are worn beneath the lead apron to monitor the exposure of blood-forming organs and gonads and on the collar or the surgical cap to monitor exposure to the eyes and thyroid gland. To monitor exposure of the operator's hands, a ring badge can be worn (Fig 3–2), and this device is recommended for persons in cardiac catheterization laboratories, particularly those involved with catheterization of infants, when the operator's hands are close to the primary x-ray beam. Periodically, the film in the badges is developed. From them, the radiation dose can be determined with an accuracy of ±10%. The radiation dosage of each staff member is recorded by the institution's department of environmental health, which makes a report to the supervising radiation physicists, who are required to notify individuals with exposure exceeding the recommended standards. These maximum permissible radiation levels are given by the Occupational Safety and Health Administration (OSHA) and the Bureau of Radiological Health (BRH) and are designed to minimize the deleterious biologic effects of ionizing radiation. As indicated earlier, these recommendations are only guidelines, because the safe level for radiation (if any) is not known. Consequently, it is wise to minimize exposure, in part by taking all protective measures described as follows.

The OSHA regulations state that the radiation exposure to operating personnel in a 3-month period should not exceed 1.25 rem to the whole body (head and trunk, active blood-forming organs, lens of eyes, and gonads), 18.75 rem to the hands and forearms and feet and ankles, and 7.5 rem to the skin of the entire body. In contrast, the National Committee on Radiation Protection recommends that a radiation worker's exposure should be limited to not more than 3 rem in any 13 consecutive weeks. The cumulative lifetime exposure should not exceed the dose given by the formula $5(N - 18)$ rems, where N is the patient's age in years. Clearly, recommendations vary even at a national level, as well as from state to state.

RADIATION PROTECTION IN CATHETERIZATION LABORATORIES

Protective Barriers

Heavy metals, particularly lead, are effective, inexpensive protective barriers because of their high absorption of ionizing radiation. Personnel in the catheterization laboratory are required to wear protective aprons, which should have a lead equivalency of at least 0.25 mm, preferably 0.5 mm. These aprons are made of lead-impregnated rubber covered by a fabric. The aprons crack as the rubber ages; consequently, they should be inspected fluoroscopically once each year. Pinhole defects are of no consequence, but large cracks significantly decrease the protective value of the apron.

Lead aprons are protective only in the direction of the x-ray beam. Thus, radiologists and cardiologists facing the radiation field wear their aprons in the front, whereas technicians recording the data commonly turn their backs to the radiation field and so should either wear lead aprons on their backs or use a wraparound apron, which provides protection in all directions (Figs 3–2 and 3–3). Protective aprons of leaded rubber also may be attached to the image intensifier, although in cardiac catheterization laboratories, this is seldom done because it interferes with sterility of the catheterization site.

The x-ray exposure of personnel is caused primarily by secondary (scattered) radiation from the fluoroscopic field, although rarely are the operator's hands placed in the direct beam. The irradiated area of the patient is another source of scattered radiation, which is emitted in all directions. However, because x-rays travel only in a straight line, radiation cannot reach the observer's eyes unless he or she can see the fluoroscopic field. Consequently, the

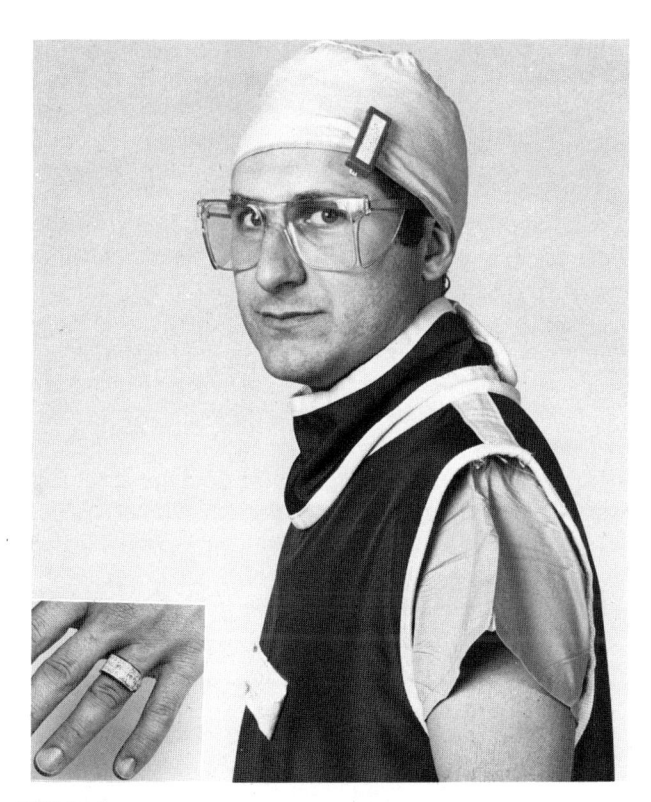

FIG 3–2.
Photograph of physician wearing lead wraparound apron of 0.5-mm lead equivalent, thyroid shield, and lead glasses with side flaps. Exposure to head and neck is monitored by film badge and exposure of hand by a ring dosimeter. Wraparound aprons are important for persons not facing the radiation field, whereas cardiologists performing catheterizations are protected adequately by regular aprons.

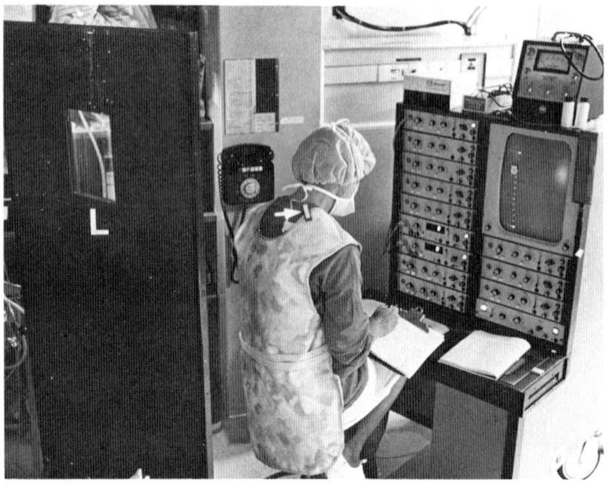

FIG 3–3.
Medical technologist recording data in a catheterization laboratory. Lead shield *(L)* provides radiation protection. In addition, a lead wraparound apron is worn over the back, and radiation is monitored by a collar badge *(arrow)*.

operator performing the cardiac catheterization should stand as close as possible to the image intensifier, which provides virtually 100% protection for the eyes and thyroid gland. If the image intensifier is tilted as with oblique projections, this protection is lost. However, more distant observers who can see the irradiated area of the patient will receive secondary radiation to their eyes and thyroid gland (see Fig 3–1), so they should stand back as far as possible to take advantage of the protection afforded by distance according to the inverse-square law. During cine recording, all uninvolved persons should step behind a radiation shield or leave the room. If manual injections are used, as in coronary angiography, the operator can step behind a lead shield. Also, lead-impregnated eyeglasses or radiation helmets may be worn, which absorb 90% of the secondary radiation. However, such glasses are protective only if the observer is looking at the radiation field. Far more often, he or she is observing the TV monitor, in which case scattered radiation will strike the eyes unless the glasses have side flaps. The thyroid gland can be protected by a thyroid shield (see Fig 3–2).

Normally, cardiologists performing catheterization procedures are close enough to the patient that secondary radiation does not strike the head and neck. A tall operator is less likely to receive secondary radiation to the face than is a short observer.

Protection by Distance

Ionizing radiation decreases by the square root of the distance from the radiation site. This inverse-square law indicates then, that if the distance is doubled, the radiation exposure decreases by a factor of four. Application of the inverse-square law is a simple and effective means of radiation protection, particularly for operating personnel, and should be remembered when cardiac catheterization laboratories are designed. Technicians recording data should be as distant from the radiation field as possible.

Shielding Against Secondary Radiation

Stationary radiation shields can be used in addition to lead aprons. Shields made of heavy lead with lead-glass inserts provide virtually 100% protection against secondary radiation and can be used by radiologists and cardiologists making manual angiographic injections, as well as to protect persons recording data.

Protection by Proper Coning

The amount of secondary radiation is directly proportional to the size of the field of radiation. Also, with increasing field size and the resulting increase in secondary radiation, the diagnostic quality of a fluoroscopic image deteriorates. Therefore, a small field obtained by proper coning improves image quality while protecting the staff. For example, increasing a fluoroscopic field from 3 by 3 in. to 4 by 4 in. causes a 90% increase in secondary radiation! In addition, proper coning significantly decreases the radiation exposure of the patient.

EXPOSURE OF WOMEN OF REPRODUCTIVE POTENTIAL

During pregnancy, exposure to ionizing radiation should be minimized, and x-ray examinations should be carried out only when there is an unquestionable need. Pregnant women should not perform cardiac catheterizations, and any pregnant women in the laboratory should be placed as far from the catheterization table as possible and should wear a wraparound apron or, preferably, two lead aprons, each of 0.5-mm lead equivalency.

SUMMARY

1. Fluoroscopy and cine fluorography result in the highest radiation doses of any diagnostic procedure both to patient and operating personnel.
2. The harmful biologic effects of ionizing radiation are well known, although the dose-response relation of repeated exposures is not clear.
3. Radiation exposure of the cardiac catheterization staff should be kept to a minimum.
4. Laboratory staff are required to wear protective aprons and radiation monitoring equipment.

5. Fluoroscopy should be as brief as possible, with optimal coning.
6. Fluoroscopy should be performed intermittently and only when the operator is observing the screen.
7. Fluoroscopy should not be routinely carried out in the magnification mode, because this requires much more radiation.
8. The cardiologist performing the procedure should stand close to the image intensifier.
9. A frame rate of 60/sec should be used only if important additional information is obtained.
10. If the image intensifier is tilted away from the operator, as with certain oblique views, protection can be provided by distance or a lead shield.
11. Observers and personnel recording data should be as far from the radiation field as feasible.
12. Staff members who do not face the radiation field should wear wraparound aprons.
13. A lead radiation shield should be used during cine recording.
14. Cine recording should be made in the biplane mode only if important information is expected from the second plane.
15. Optional protective barriers such as thyroid shields and glasses increase safety; glasses should have side flaps.
16. The safe operation of the x-ray equipment is the responsibility of a radiation physicist, the radiologist, and the x-ray technologist.

BIBLIOGRAPHY

Buschong SC: *The development of radiation protection in diagnostic radiology,* Boca Raton, Fla, 1973, CRC Press.

Dalrymple GV, Gaulden ME, Kollmorgen GM, et al: *Medical radiation biology,* Philadelphia, 1973, Saunders.

Hall EJ: *Radiobiology for the radiologist,* Philadelphia, 1973, Harper & Row.

National Council on Radiation Protection and Measurements: *Basic radiation protection criteria,* Washington, DC, 1971, NCRP Report no 39.

Pizzarello DJ, Witcofski RL: *Basic radiation biology,* ed 2, Philadelphia, 1975, Lea & Febiger.

Schultz RJ: *Primer of radiation protection,* ed 2, New York, 1969, GAF Corporation X-Ray Products.

CHAPTER 4

Classification and Hemodynamics of Congenital Heart Disease

METHODS OF CLASSIFICATION

Congenital heart disease can be classified in various ways, such as on the basis of anatomic features, age at presentation, hemodynamic pattern, and frequency of occurrence, but these classifications are not necessarily helpful clinically. We propose to classify congenital cardiac malformations on the basis of two easily obtained pieces of clinical information: the presence or absence of cyanosis and the pattern of the pulmonary vasculature as observed on a thoracic roentgenogram.

Cyanosis

Cyanosis is the bluish color imparted to the skin (particularly nonpigmented skin) when more than 5 g/dL of reduced hemoglobin is present in capillary blood. In patients with a congenital cardiac anomaly, this degree of desaturation of capillary blood can have several mechanisms. Cyanosis can be broadly divided into two categories: peripheral and central.

Peripheral cyanosis, also called acrocyanosis, is the more common of the two. In this form, the blood leaving the heart is fully saturated, but flow through capillaries is sluggish, so that extraction of oxygen is prolonged, thus lowering the oxygen saturation of the capillary blood and causing acrocyanosis (Greek acro, meaning summit). The term peripheral or acrocyanosis reflects the fact that this type generally involves the extremities and spares the trunk. It commonly occurs in the hands and feet of normal newborns or infants when they are exposed to cold, or in school-aged children, who often exhibit circumoral cyanosis when exposed to cold. It may be observed in a single extremity, often after a venous cutdown has been made. In patients with cardiogenic shock or other generalized circulatory problems that are associated with markedly reduced cardiac output and inadequate peripheral perfusion, cyanosis of the peripheral type may develop.

The second type of cyanosis is called central and is associated with a lower than normal oxygen saturation as measured in aortic blood. The blood reaching the aorta may be desaturated in pulmonary parenchymal diseases that interfere with oxygenation of blood passing through the lungs; commonly, these are conditions that cause localized perfusion-ventilation abnormalities or diffuse disorders of the alveoli, such as pulmonary edema. Thus, pulmonary parenchymal disease or pulmonary edema complicating any form of congenital cardiac disease may cause cyanosis, which disappears after treatment of the pulmonary disorder.

Central cyanosis also occurs in some types of congenital heart disease. Persistence of cyanosis in a patient with a congenital cardiac anomaly but without pulmonary disease indicates a right-to-left shunt, meaning that a portion of the systemic venous return reaches the aorta without passing through the lungs. The cardiac conditions leading to a right-to-left shunt can be subdivided into two categories: those in which there is a common cardiac chamber in which mixing of the systemic and pulmonary venous returns occurs, and those in which there is obstructed pulmonary blood flow in addition to a cardiac defect through which blood is shunted away from the lungs into the body.

Patterns of Pulmonary Vasculature

The radiographic appearance of the pulmonary vasculature can also give diagnostic information about the cardiac malformation, particularly when the presence or absence of cyanosis is also considered. There are seven patterns of pulmonary vascularity (see also Chapter 5):

1. Normal arterial and venous vascularity: The proximal right and left pulmonary arteries are observed in their respective hila on the posteroanterior and lateral projections. The vessels taper gradually through the middle third of the lung fields.

2. Increased arterial vascularity: The right and left main pulmonary arteries are enlarged, and vessels are seen in the outer third of the lung fields.

3. Decreased arterial vasculature: The right and left main pulmonary arteries are small, the peripheral pulmonary arteries are stringy, and the lung fields may appear hyperlucent.

4. Increased venous vascularity: The pulmonary veins in the upper lobes are enlarged (cephalization), and there may be a pattern of pulmonary edema, a granular pattern, or Kerley-B lines. The venous pulmonary vasculature is more hazy than the more distinct arterial vasculature.

5. Bronchial arterial vascularity: In certain patients with atresia of the pulmonary valve, the chief source of pulmonary blood may be the aorta, through vessels called bronchial collateral arteries that join the pulmonary arterial system at various locations within the lungs. On the radiograph, no discrete main right or left pulmonary arteries are observed, or the hila may be tiny. An unusual vascular pattern may be evident at other sites in the lung, lacking the normal orientation of the pulmonary arterial tree.

6. Discrepancy in vascularity between the two lung fields or within the same lung: Examples involving an entire lung occur in conditions such as atresia of the origin of a pulmonary artery or proximal interruption of a sixth aortic arch, also called absent pulmonary artery. A relative decrease in vascularity of the left upper lobe is found in tetralogy of Fallot and in patent ductus arteriosus. Other regional differences in pulmonary vascularity are discussed in the chapters on the specific cardiac anomalies in which they are seen.

7. Abnormal vascular structures in the lung: Rarely, a thoracic radiograph shows a vascular structure that follows an abnormal course within a lung field. Usually, these structures are venous. Examples are found in anomalous pulmonary venous connection, either partial or total, in scimitar syndrome, pulmonary arteriovenous fistulas and pulmonary varix.

Subclassification of Congenital Heart Disease

On the basis of observations of skin color and pulmonary vascularity, several subcategories of congenital cardiac disease can be developed into which the various anomalies can be classified:

I. Normal pulmonary vascularity—no cyanosis
   A. Outflow tract obstruction
      1. Aortic stenosis
      2. Pulmonary stenosis
      3. Coarctation of aorta
   B. Cardiomyopathy without congestive cardiac failure

II. Normal pulmonary vascularity—cyanosis (rare)
   A. Small diffuse pulmonary arteriovenous fistulas
   B. Left superior vena cava connecting with left atrium
   C. Inferior vena cava connecting with left atrium
   D. Right superior vena cava connecting with left atrium

III. Increased pulmonary arterial vascularity—no cyanosis
   A. Left-to-right shunts
      1. Shunt at ventricular level
         a. Ventricular septal defect
         b. Ventricular septal defect and aortic insufficiency
         c. Left ventricular-right atrial shunt
      2. Shunt at great-vessel level
         a. Patent ductus arteriosus
         b. Aorticopulmonary septal defect
         c. Aortic origin of a pulmonary artery
      3. Shunt at atrial level
         a. Atrial septal defect
         b. Shunts involving abnormalities of the coronary sinus
         c. Partial anomalous pulmonary venous connection, including scimitar syndrome
      4. Shunts at more than one level: endocardial cushion defect
      5. Obligatory shunt
         a. Ruptured aneurysm of sinus of Valsalva
         b. Coronary arteriovenous fistula

IV. Increased pulmonary arterial vascularity—cyanosis (admixture lesions)
   A. Truncus arteriosus
   B. Single ventricle
   C. Single atrium
   D. Total anomalous pulmonary venous connection
   E. Tricuspid atresia without pulmonary stenosis
   F. Complete transposition of great vessels

V. Decreased pulmonary vascularity—no cyanosis; there are no conditions in this category, although for many technical reasons, the pulmonary vasculature may appear reduced radiographically

VI. Decreased pulmonary vascularity—cyanosis; intracardiac defect and obstruction to pulmonary blood flow

A. With pulmonary vascular disease (Eisenmenger's syndrome)
   1. Ventricular septal defect and right-to-left shunt
   2. Atrial septal defect and right-to-left shunt
   3. Patent ductus arteriosus and right-to-left shunt
   4. Endocardial cushion defect and right-to-left shunt
B. With anatomic obstruction
   1. Right-to-left shunt at ventricular level
      a. Tetralogy of Fallot
      b. "Tetrad variants"
   2. Right-to-left shunt at atrial level
      a. Pulmonary atresia
      b. Severe pulmonary stenosis
      c. Tricuspid atresia
      d. Ebstein's malformation
      e. Tricuspid insufficiency in neonates
VII. Increased pulmonary venous vascularity—no cyanosis
   A. With cardiomegaly
      1. Cardiomyopathy with congestive cardiac failure
      2. Left ventricular failure from congenital heart disease
   B. Without cardiomegaly
      1. Mitral stenosis
      2. Supravalvular stenosing mitral ring
      3. Cor triatriatum
      4. Stenosis of individual pulmonary veins
VIII. Increased pulmonary venous vascularity—cyanosis
   A. Normally connecting pulmonary veins
      1. Aortic atresia
      2. Mitral atresia
   B. Abnormally connecting pulmonary veins
      1. Total anomalous pulmonary venous connection with obstruction
      2. Atresia of common pulmonary vein

Incidence of Congenital Heart Disease

When this classification of congenital cardiac anomalies is applied, it is also helpful for the radiologist to know the relative frequencies of these anomalies, the incidence of which is almost 1% in newborn infants. The various types account for the following percentages overall:

Isolated ventricular septal defect	25
Ventricular septal defect; associated patent ductus arteriosus or coarctation of aorta	5
Tetralogy of Fallot	10
Atrial septal defect, secundum type	10
Patent ductus arteriosus	10
Coarctation of the aorta	6
Complete transposition of the great vessels	6
Pulmonary stenosis	5
Aortic stenosis	5
Endocardial cushion defect	4
Mitral or aortic atresia	2
Anomalous pulmonary venous connection, total or partial	2
Tricuspid atresia	1
Pulmonary atresia	1
Rare or complex malformations	8

However, the relative distribution of malformations depends on the age of the patient. Because about one third of infants with congenital heart disease die within the first year of life, and because this high early mortality is caused predominately by only a few lesions, the prevalence of lesions changes with age. For example, in the first month of life, five malformations cause serious clinical problems and produce the highest death rate: aortic atresia (hypoplastic left-heart syndrome), transposition of the great vessels, coarctation of the aorta, pulmonary atresia or severe stenosis, and severe tetralogy of Fallot.

In neonates (i.e., younger than 28 days), the lesions most commonly causing severe symptoms or death, with their percentages, are:

Hypoplastic left ventricle	37
Transposition of the great vessels	25
Multiple serious defects	18
Coarctation and ventricular septal defect	16
Tetralogy of Fallot	12
Pulmonary stenosis or atresia	11

Ventricular septal defect, patent ductus arteriosus, and atrial septal defect are more common overall than these data show, but often they are not revealed until later in infancy. In school-aged children and adults, the percentages are:

Atrial septal defect	17
Ventricular septal defect	17
Patent ductus arteriosus	15
Tetralogy of Fallot	15
Pulmonary stenosis	13
Coarctation	7
Aortic stenosis	5
Other	10

The radiologist also may derive diagnostic clues from the presenting symptoms and the sex of the patient.

For example, the two most significant presenting clinical features of congenital heart disease are cyanosis and congestive cardiac failure. Cyanosis in the neonatal period is usually related to transposition of the great vessels, whereas in older children, tetralogy of Fallot or a variant thereof is the most common cause. Indeed, after the age 2 years, tetralogy of Fallot accounts for three fourths of the cases of cyanosis. Of children presenting with congestive cardiac failure, 80% are in the first year of life; and most of these have a congenital cardiac malformation. Of the 20% who present after 1 year of age, one half have congenital cardiac malformations and the other half acquired cardiac conditions such as occur in myocarditis, acute rheumatic fever, and glomerulonephritis. Further, within the first week of life, conditions such as aortic stenosis and complete transposition of the great vessels are the most common cause of congestive cardiac failure. Between 1 week and 1 month of age, coarctation of the aorta is the most common cause, and it frequently coexists with other lesions such as ventricular septal defect. After 2 months of age, the most common causes of cardiac failure are conditions associated with shunts at either the ventricular or the great-vessel level, such as ventricular septal defect or patent ductus arteriosus.

The overall incidence of congenital heart disease is slightly greater in males than in females. Aortic stenosis, coarctation of the aorta, and complete transposition of the great vessels occur twice as commonly in males as in females, whereas patent ductus arteriosus and atrial septal defect occur about twice as often in females as in males.

HEMODYNAMICS OF CONGENITAL HEART DISEASE

Although there are many types of cardiac malformations, there are only a few ways in which they affect the heart and only a few hemodynamic principles are involved. Earlier in the chapter, we classified congenital heart disease on the basis of the pattern of pulmonary vascularity and the presence or absence of cyanosis; we now consider a hemodynamic classification.

Classification by Hemodynamics

1. Shunts at the ventricular or great-vessel level. The hemodynamic principle governing a shunt through a communication at the ventricular or at the great-vessel level is the same regardless of anatomic form. Thus, the factors governing a shunt in such a diverse group of conditions as ventricular septal defect, patent ductus arteriosus, tetralogy of Fallot, truncus arteriosus, and single ventricle is the same.

In a large communication (i.e., one ≥75% of the size of the aortic anulus), the direction and magnitude of shunt depends on the relative impedance to the outflow into the pulmonary and systemic circulations. In a large communication, the systolic pressures in the right and left ventricles are equal. The impedence to outflow depends on the sites of obstruction, such as pulmonary or aortic stenosis or coarctation of the aorta, and the resistances of the pulmonary and systemic vascular beds. Vascular resistance is determined principally by the caliber and number of arterioles comprising these two vascular beds. (A more detailed discussion is presented later.) In contrast, if the communication is small (i.e., <75% of the diameter of the aortic anulus), the left ventricular systolic pressure exceeds the right ventricular systolic pressure, and this difference is the driving force through the defect.

2. Shunts at the atrial level. Regardless of the anatomic form, the magnitude and direction of blood flow through an atrial communication depends largely on the relative impedance to ventricular filling. Most atrial septal communications are large and allow free communication, so the atrial pressures are equal. If the atrioventricular valves are normal, both atria are in free communication with both ventricles. Therefore, the amount of blood flowing into each of the ventricles depends on their relative compliances. Ventricular compliance is determined principally by the thickness of the wall (degree of hypertrophy) and the stiffness of the wall, which, in turn, is affected by myocardial alterations, such as fibrosis or storage disease. Because the right ventricular systolic pressure is less than the left ventricular systolic pressure, the right ventricle is thinner than the left. Therefore, in most atrial communications, the compliance of the right ventricle is greater, and the shunt occurs from left to right. If, however, the right ventricle is severely hypertrophied, as it may be in a patient with pulmonary stenosis and atrial septal defect, the shunt occurs from right to left.

If one of the atrioventricular valves is stenotic or atretic, this alters ventricular filling and influences the shunt. Thus, in patients with tricuspid atresia, the shunt occurs from right to left through the defect, whereas in mitral atresia the opposite is true. Mitral stenosis and tricuspid stenosis would increase and decrease the left-to-right shunt, respectively.

3. Obstruction to blood flow. Regardless of the type or site of an obstructive lesion, the effects on the heart are similar. The pressure in the chamber proximal to the obstruction increases when the valve is open, the extent of the increase depending on the size of the stenotic orifice and the volume of blood passing through the valve. Thus, in aortic and pulmonary stenosis, the pressure is increased in the respective ventricles during systole, and in mitral and tricuspid stenosis, a gradient develops across the valve during diastole. Furthermore, in physiologic states, such as exercise, which increases flow across a valve, the pressure proximal to the valve increases.

The primary anatomic change in response to the elevated pressure generally is hypertrophy of the chamber wall, not dilatation. Dilatation of the chamber proximal to an obstruction most often occurs with either severe obstruction or chronic high pressure.

4. Insufficient cardiac valve. In such a case, the chambers on either side of the valve dilate. Also, the ventricular wall may become slightly thickened, because it develops higher tension.

Physical Principles

The ability of the two ventricles to react to workloads depends in part on their shape. The normal left ventricle is conical, whereas the normal right ventricle has a crescentic cross-section. As a result, the left ventricle is well equipped to handle pressure but not volume loads, whereas the reverse is true of the right ventricle. This can be explained by reference to LaPlace's and Starling's laws. LaPlace's law states that in a closed cylinder, the wall tension (T) is equal to the product of the radius (r) and the internal pressure (P): $T = rP$. Starling's law states that the force of cardiac contraction, and thus cardiac output, is directly proportional to the end-diastolic length of the cardiac fibers and hence to the end-diastolic ventricular volume.

The normal left ventricle develops a high systolic pressure and has a relatively small radius; thus, in accordance with LaPlace's law, sudden increases in the systolic pressure are well tolerated, because the proportional change in pressure is relatively small. In contrast, an increase in left ventricular volume causes a large change in the normally small radius and thus a large change in the tension. As a result, conditions such as aortic stenosis generally are well tolerated, whereas lesions such as aortic insufficiency or ventricular septal defect that increase left ventricular volume (and hence the radius) are poorly tolerated. In this case, the left ventricle cannot develop sufficient tension to maintain adequate pressure-volume relations, and congestive heart failure develops. Additional understanding can be obtained by considering the ventricular response to workloads. If Starling's law is applied to the left ventricle as a whole, as the myocardial fibers are stretched, ventricular function increases until it reaches a maximum, where upon it decreases as the fibers are stretched beyond that point. Thus, with left ventricular volume load and dilatation, myocardial fibers may become overstretched, leading to cardiac failure.

The right ventricle reacts in the opposite way to pressure and volume loads; it tolerates volume loads well but pressure loads poorly. As indicated, the right ventricle is essentially a crescent-shaped appendage to the left ventricle, giving it a large internal surface relative to its volume (a large radius) and a low systolic pressure. Applying LaPlace's law to the right ventricle shows that when this chamber is subjected to a volume load, as by an atrial level shunt, the increase in its already large radius creates only a small proportional change. Therefore, only slight changes in wall tension are required to maintain the pressure-volume relations. Thus, conditions that place a volume overload on the right ventricle, such as atrial septal defect or pulmonary insufficiency, are well tolerated. In contrast, when there is an acute increase in right ventricular systolic pressure, as from a pulmonary embolus, right ventricular failure occurs. In this situation, the relatively low resting pressure increases by a large amount proportionally, and because the radius of the right ventricle is large, a large change in wall tension will be required to maintain the pressure-volume relations.

Clinical Implications

The right ventricle of a neonate differs from that of an adult. During fetal life, the pressure in this chamber is the same as that in the systemic circulation, because it pumps blood from the pulmonary artery through the ductus arteriosus into the descending aorta. Thus, at birth the right ventricle is a thick-walled cone, similar to the left ventricle, and, in fact, it weighs more than the left ventricle. Normally, as the pulmonary arterial systolic pressure declines after birth, the right ventricle thins, and by 1 month of age the ventricular weights are equal. Later, the left ventricular weight exceeds the right ventricular weight and the right ventricle assumes its normal crescent shape. If, after birth, right ventricular systolic pressure stays elevated, as it is in patients with tetralogy of Fallot, the morphologic features of the heart at term are maintained; that is, the right ventricle remains a thick-walled cone. This permits it to tolerate the elevated systolic pressure, so congestive cardiac failure does not ensue from this specific cause.

Pulmonary Hemodynamic Considerations

The natural history, complications, and management of many forms of congenital cardiac anomalies are related to changes in the pulmonary vasculature. At birth, the pulmonary vascular resistance is high and the pulmonary arterioles have a thick medial coat and a narrow lumen, the narrowing resulting in part from pulmonary arteriolar vasoconstriction secondary to the normal fetal hypoxemia. With the onset of breathing after birth, hypoxemia improves and pulmonary vasoconstriction is released, so pulmonary arteriolar resistance falls quite dramatically in the first few days of life (although not to what will later be considered normal). Thereafter, at least two additional changes produce a more gradual decline in pulmonary arteriolar resistance. One change is a thinning of the medial musculature, with consequent widening of the arteriolar lumen. The other change is an increase in the total cross-sectional area of the pulmonary arteriolar bed as the lungs develop. Usually, by 3 months of age, pulmonary arteriolar resistance is at the normal level, although a slight decline may continue until 4 years of age.

This decline in pulmonary vascular resistance has an effect in cardiac malformations with a communication at the ventricular or great-vessel level. In these anomalies, the relative pulmonary and systemic vascular resistances influence the magnitude and direction of blood flow. For example, in patients with a large ventricular septal defect, there is little shunting through the defect in the neonatal period because of the elevated pulmonary arteriolar resistance. However, as this resistance declines, there is a progressively larger left-to-right shunt, such that the volume of pulmonary blood flow increases over 2 to 3 months. This explains why most patients with conditions such as ventricular septal defect, in which cardiac failure results from large volumes of pulmonary blood flow, typically do not have signs and symptoms until they are a few months old.

In patients with large volumes of pulmonary blood flow because of a high-pressure shunt (e.g., those with a large ventricular septal defect), pulmonary arteriolar resistance does not fall along the normal curve but generally falls along a parallel but slightly higher curve. The reasons for this are unknown, but elevated left atrial pressure, mild hypoxemia, and, perhaps, the perfusion pressure itself are believed to be factors.

Patients with large volumes of pulmonary blood flow may develop pulmonary vascular disease, a process that may begin as early as 6 months of age or may be delayed for decades. The genesis of the vascular disease is unknown. Progressive medial hypertrophy and intimal proliferation occur, which narrow the lumen of the arterioles and may eventually obliterate them. As a result, pulmonary arteriolar resistance rises, and this limits the left-to-right shunt. Eventually, pulmonary arteriolar resistance may exceed the systemic arteriolar resistance, so the shunt becomes right to left. This has been called Eisenmenger's syndrome and is irreversible.

CHAPTER 5

Plain-Film Diagnosis of Congenital Cardiac Disease

The radiologic examination of the heart without contrast medium is a simple noninvasive method to assist in diagnosis. The radiographic diagnosis of congenital heart disease is based on evaluation of the pulmonary vasculature, cardiac size, and cardiac configuration.

TECHNICAL AND PHYSIOLOGIC CONSIDERATIONS

On a thoracic roentgenogram, the appearance of the pulmonary vasculature and the cardiac size and contour can be distorted by various technical factors. A basic understanding of radiographic technique thus is essential.

Pulmonary Vasculature

The radiographic appearance of the pulmonary vasculature depends on many technical factors including kilovoltage, film characteristics, exposure time, and the degree of lung inflation. Even an experienced radiologist has great difficulty interpreting a technically inadequate radiograph.

The best results are obtained by using a latitude film such as the Trimax GT or Kodak OC, which record a long scale of grays. These latitude films, especially those developed for chest radiography, are less sensitive to overexposure than are high-contrast films, and overexposure is the most common cause of underestimation of the pulmonary vasculature. Underexposure of a thoracic radiograph, on the other hand, accentuates the pulmonary vascular markings. Thus, the pulmonary vasculature of the same patient may be read one day as increased and the following day as decreased solely because of technical variations (Fig 5–1). A high-kilovoltage technique can further increase the latitude of a radiographic system and also is useful for demonstrating the trachea, which helps in locating the aortic arch. On the other hand, high kilovoltage (i.e., > 100 kV[p]) decreases overall contrast. The degree of inspiration affects the appearance of pulmonary vessels; a film obtained on expiration accentuates the vasculature, particularly at the lung bases.

The exposure time of a chest radiograph also affects the appearance of pulmonary vasculature. The exposure time should be $1/120$ of a second (8 msec), particularly in infants because of their rapid cardiac and respiratory rates. With longer exposure, arterial pulsations and diaphragmatic motion blur the pulmonary vasculature. Portable radiographic equipment has much longer exposure times than do the stationary and larger x-ray machines in a radiology department, so the pulmonary vasculature may appear decreased on a chest film made with portable equipment and normal by standard radiograph technique.

A final consideration is that premature infants have sparse (decreased) vasculature. There are two reasons, the first of which is technical: the size of the pulmonary arteries approaches the resolving power of the radiographic system. The second reason is that premature infants have fewer peripheral pulmonary arteries per gram of lung tissue than does a full-term neonate (Fig 5–2). To establish a radiographic diagnosis, one must rate the pulmonary vasculature as "normal," "increased," or "decreased." Differentiation between arterial and venous vasculature is difficult but very important.

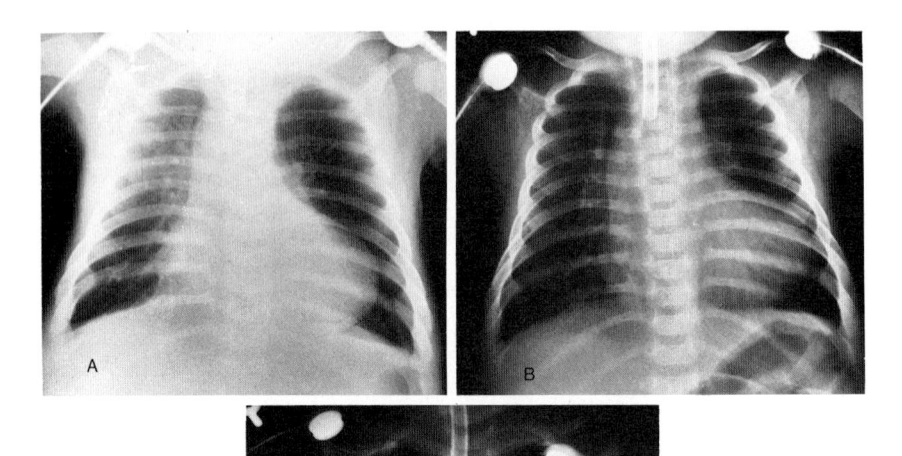

FIG 5–1.
Thoracic roentegenograms, posteroanterior projection, show change in appearance of pulmonary vasculature in the same patient because of variations in film exposure. **A,** slightly underexposed; the pulmonary vasculature appears increased. **B,** slightly overpenetrated; normal appearance of the pulmonary vasculature. **C,** considerable overpenetration; pulmonary vasculature appears decreased.

Increased Pulmonary Venous Vasculature

Three physiologic facts can be applied to understanding the effects of elevated pulmonary venous pressure on the lungs:

1. In a normal person in an upright position, relatively little blood flows through the upper lobes, largely because of gravity. Alveolar air pressure thus tends to collapse the upper lobe veins, whereas the lower lobe veins are distended by the higher venous pressure.

2. Transcapillary fluid exchange helps keep the lung free of edema. Normally the pulmonary capillary pressure is 7 to 12 mm Hg, whereas the plasma colloidal osmotic pressure is 25 to 30 mm Hg. This difference tends to force fluid into the capillary. The pulmonary capillary pressure may rise by 15 to 20 mm Hg before this force is attenuated so that pulmonary edema occurs.

3. The interstitial compartment of the lung lies between the pulmonary capillary and the alveoli, and, together with the lymphatics, it helps trap and remove fluid from the alveoli. The amount of interstitial fluid can increase sixfold before it is visible radiographically.

The first change within the lung in response to increased pulmonary venous pressure is redistribution of blood flow away from the bases and toward the apices (Fig 5–3, B and C). The reason is unknown, although it may be caused by increased resistance to flow through the lower lobes as a result of interstitial edema, by alveolar hypoxia, or by vasoconstriction of the arterioles by reflexes originating from the left atrium or pulmonary vein.

The next change secondary to increased pulmonary venous pressure is progressive accumulation of interstitial edema in the interlobular septa and subpleural spaces and around bronchi. With elevation of the pulmonary capillary pressure to 30 mm Hg, edema fluid forms within the alve-

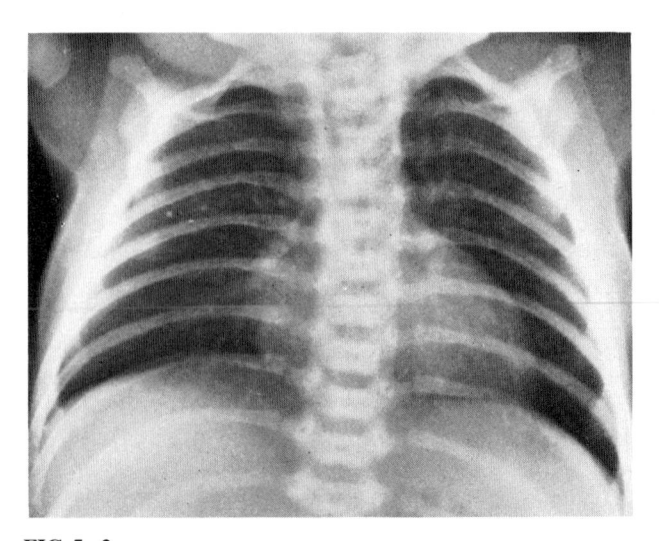

FIG 5–2.
Thoracic roentgenogram of premature infant; sparse pulmonary vasculature is normal for these infants, probably in large part because of small size of vessels.

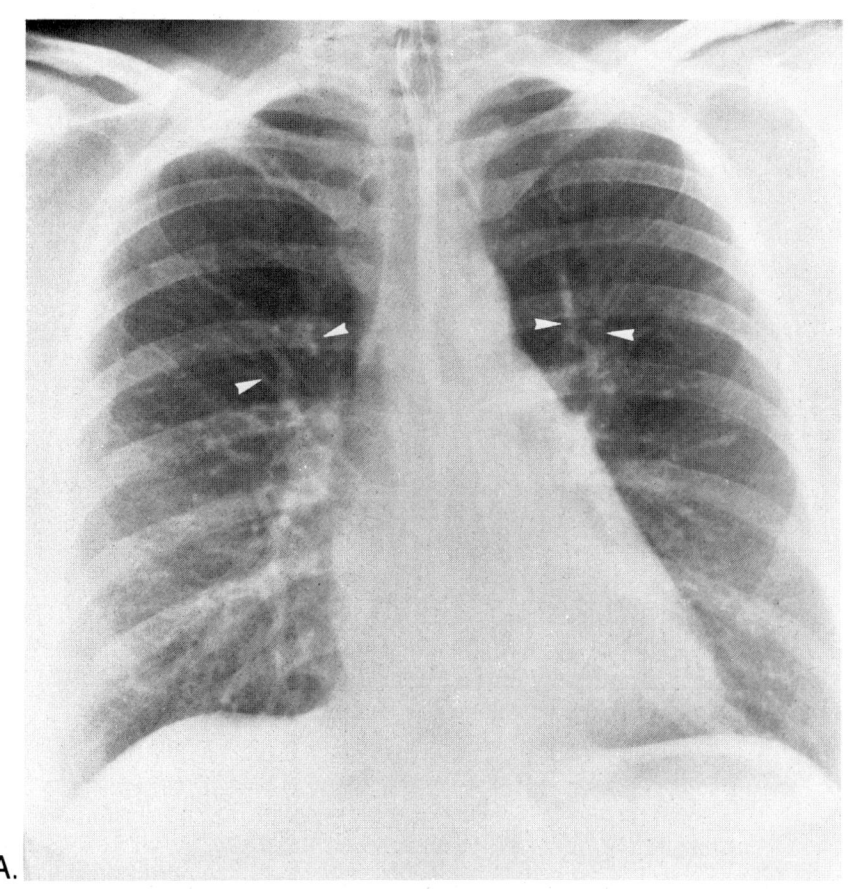

FIG 5–3.
Thoracic roentgenograms. **A,** posteroanterior projection in patients with long-standing pulmonary venous hypertension; redistribution of blood flow through upper lobe arteries and veins *(arrows)* and constriction of the lower lobe vasculature. REASON: Additional hydrostatic pressure in upright position and, probably, a reflex attenuation of lower lobe vessels. **B,** and **C,** anteroposterior and lateral left pulmonary arteriogram in patient with long-standing venous pulmonary hypertension; small contracted lower lobe arteries are still densely filled when there is filling of a large upper lobe pulmonary vein *(arrows)*. Angiogram confirms redistribution of blood flow to the upper lobe pulmonary circulation, and delay of circulation through the lower lobe vessels.

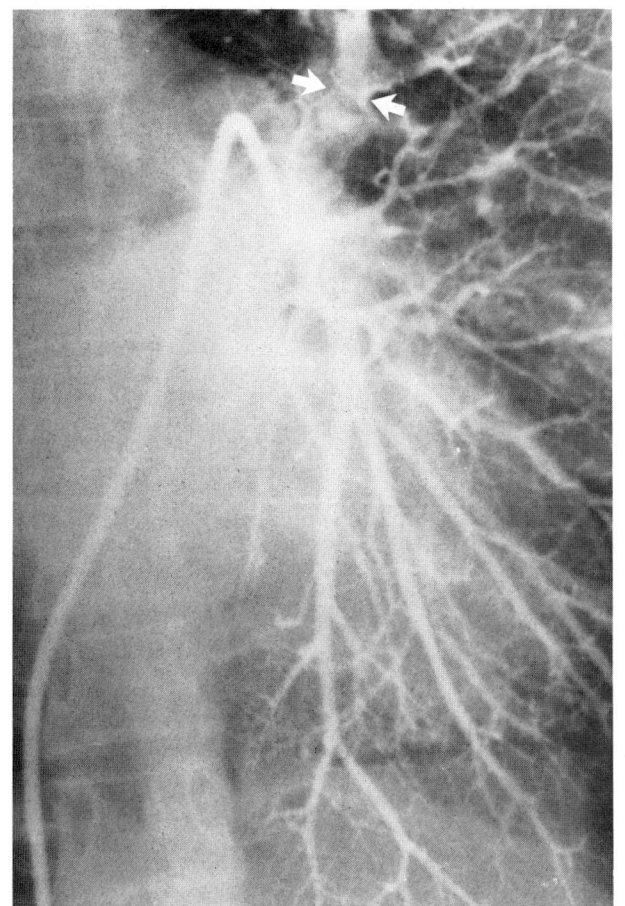

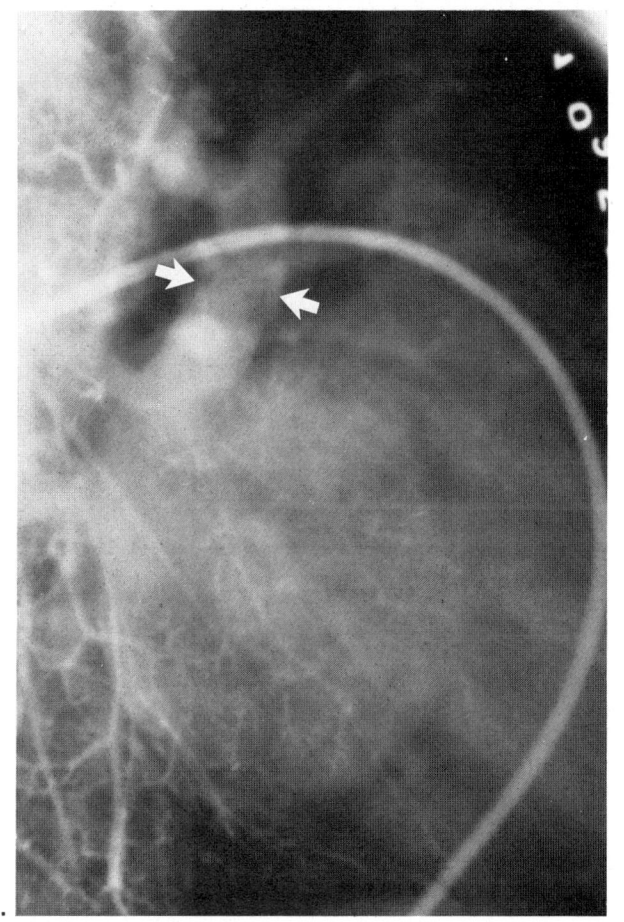

oli faster than it can be removed by the interstitial compartment and lymphatics.

An increase of the pressure in the pulmonary venous circulation (i.e., pulmonary venous obstruction) thus eventually causes fairly characteristic radiographic findings that usually permit accurate diagnosis. Sometimes, distinguishing between increased pulmonary arterial and venous vasculature is difficult, but this distinction must be made; and the radiologist should not speak loosely of "increased markings" except perhaps in the newborn and infant, in whom radiographic differentiation may not be possible.

The following clues are helpful in differential diagnosis:

1. If the pulmonary vessels are clearly seen and have well-defined margins, the vascular pattern probably is arterial.

2. If the increased vasculature is hazy and indistinct, the pattern is probably venous. This pattern results from transudation of fluid into the interstitial perivascular spaces. Transudation and edema of the central pulmonary septa may cause radiating linear densities, Kerley A lines (Fig 5-4).

3. If the pulmonary vasculature and cardiac size are both significantly increased in an infant or child, the pulmonary vasculature is much more likely to be arterial than venous. REASON: Most conditions that cause pulmonary venous obstruction are located proximal to the mitral valve and cause right ventricular hypertrophy but little cardiomegaly.

4. If the left atrium is enlarged out of proportion to the increase in the pulmonary vasculature, the vasculature is much more likely to represent pulmonary venous obstruction than increased pulmonary blood flow associated with left atrial enlargement. REASON: In conditions with increased pulmonary blood flow, the enlargement of the left atrium is proportional to the volume of flow. If the atrium is enlarged because of a shunt, pulmonary flow tends to be enormous.

5. Increased pulmonary vasculature with prominence of the main pulmonary artery strongly suggests that the increase is arterial. REASON: When a condition enlarges the peripheral pulmonary arterial vessels, the main pulmonary artery is dilated as well, whereas in pulmonary venous obstruction, dilation of the pulmonary artery is secondary and delayed. In children, no gross enlargement of the main pulmonary artery is seen.

6. If the heart is markedly enlarged and the pulmonary vasculature is slightly accentuated, the problem is most likely left ventricular failure with some congestion, so the accentuation represents increased pulmonary venous rather than arterial vasculature.

7. Kerley B lines or pleural transudation are a good sign that the increased vasculature is venous.

The radiographic picture of pulmonary venous hypertension varies with the severity of venous obstruction. With a slight elevation of the venous pressure, blood flow is redistributed, resulting in prominence of the upper lobe vessels. At the same time, the lower lobe arteries and veins are constricted. Redistribution of pulmonary blood flow is a subtle and commonly overread radiographic finding. It usually is not seen in infants and young children. Once the patient assumes an upright position, redistribu-

FIG 5-4.
Thoracic roentgenogram, posteroanterior projection, in patients with pulmonary venous obstruction. Pulmonary vasculature hazy and indistinct. Fine concentric linear densities radiating from hila are due to edema of the central pulmonary septa, deep within lungs. These densities, referred to as Kerley A lines, are seen whenever the pulmonary septa are thickened from causes such as edema secondary to venous pulmonary hypertension or lymphatic spread of tumor.

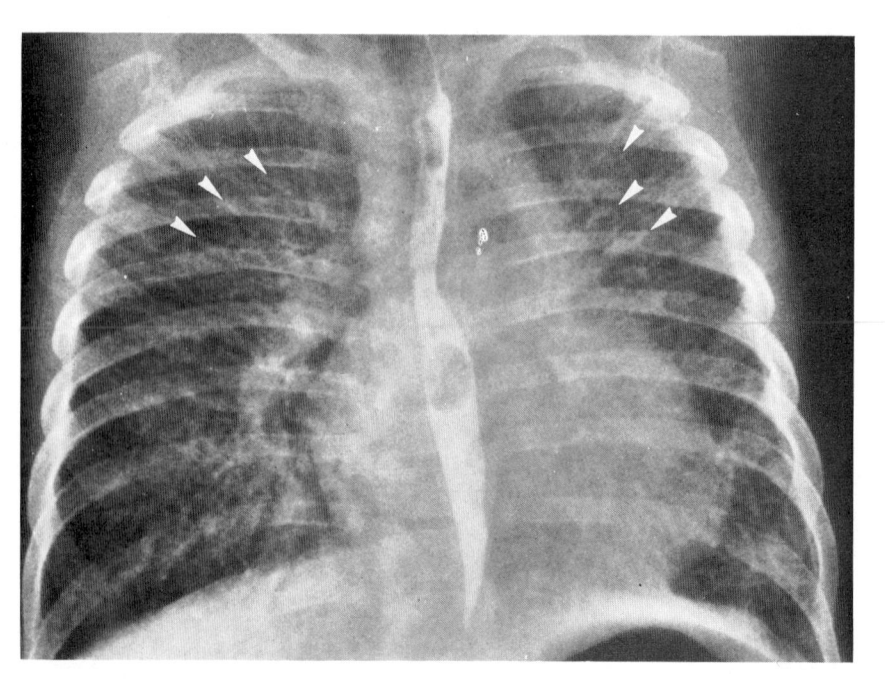

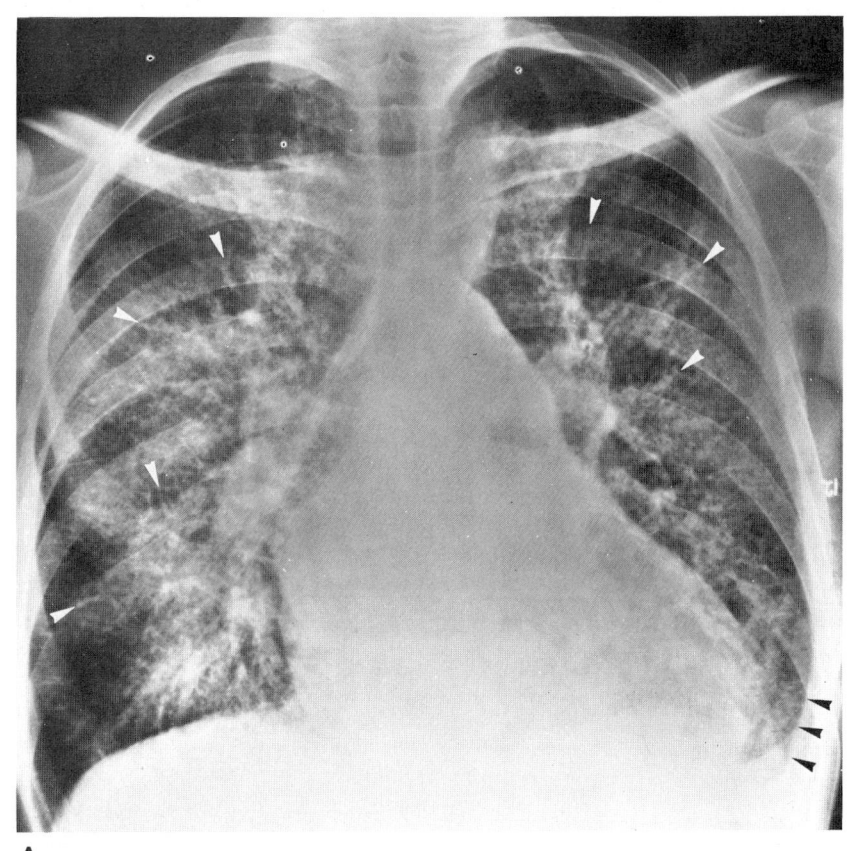

FIG 5–5.
Thoracic roentgenograms in patient with pulmonary venous hypertension. **A,** posteroanterior projection; pulmonary vasculature indistinct because of transudation of fluid into perivascular spaces. Radiating pattern from hila is due to Kerley A lines *(white arrows).* Vasculature in upper lobes more prominent than in lower lobes. Transudation of fluid into left pleural space *(black arrows);* fluid layer is tangential to x-ray beam, and fluid gravitates to lung bases when patient is upright.

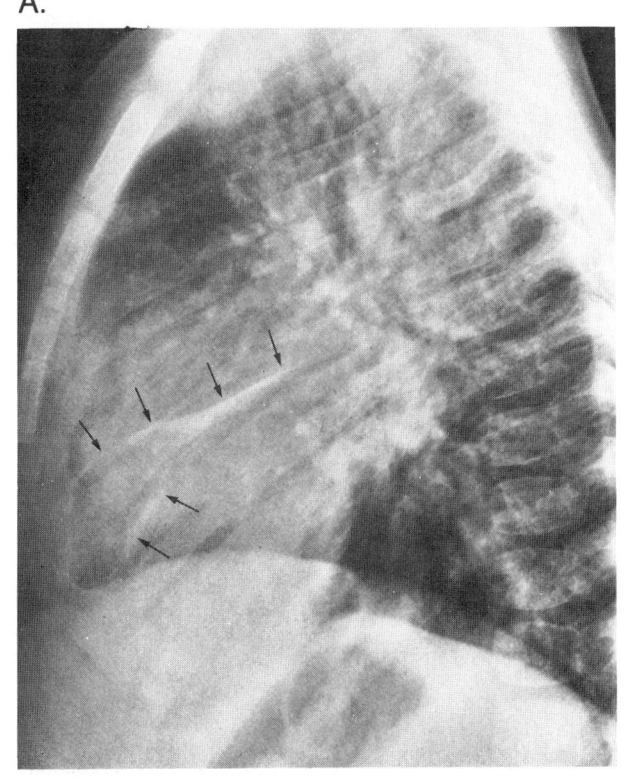

B, lateral projection; small amount of fluid in horizontal fissure *(arrows)* or, more likely, subpleural edema. The fluid is well seen, because it lies in the direction of the x-ray beam.

tion of the pulmonary blood flow can be seen on a chest film (see Fig 5–3,A). The delay of blood flow and constriction of the lower lobe pulmonary arteries can also be demonstrated angiographically. The upper lobe pulmonary arteries are dilated, and the large upper lobe veins fill early (see Fig 5–3,B and C).

With a further increase in pulmonary venous pressure, fluid transudates into interstitial spaces, making the pulmonary vessels appear less distinct. Pleural fluid may accumulate. This appearance is common in adults with left ventricular failure. However, a large pleural effusion secondary to left ventricular failure is rare in infants and young children, for unknown reasons. A small amount of transudate can best be seen at the base of the lungs or in the pulmonary fissures. The latter are seen best on the lateral view, because the fluid layer is then viewed tangentially. In many cases, the densities along the fissures are actually areas of subpleural edema (Fig 5–5).

With further increase in pulmonary venous pressure, the interlobular and subpleural septa become so edematous that they may be visible on a chest film (Fig 5–6). These septal, or Kerley B, lines cause characteristic horizontal densities that are most visible at the lung bases because of hydrostatic pressure. Kerley B lines are a reliable radiographic sign of marked pulmonary venous hypertension and suggest that the pressure exceeds 20 mm Hg. Edema in the interlobular septal may be transient, and consequently Kerley B lines may disappear when pulmonary venous pressure falls. Although Kerley B lines may occur in left ventricular failure, they are much more common in mitral obstructive disease because of the much higher pulmonary venous pressure. If severe pulmonary venous hypertension persists for a long time, fibrosis and hemosiderin deposits develop in the interlobular septa, making the Kerley B lines more prominent and permanent (Fig 5–7). The hemosiderin nodules create a granular appearance in the lung fields. Rarely, these nodules ossify and simulate healed granulomatous disease (Fig 5–8). The mechanism is not understood, because osteocytes normally are not present in the lungs, but the reaction is true ossification, with histologic proof of bone formation. In comparison with calcified granulomata, ossified hemosiderin nodules are more numerous, and they tend to be larger at the lung bases because of the increased hydrostatic pressure. Still, radiographic differentiation of these nodules from calcified granulomata may be difficult.

In contrast to Kerley B lines, Kerley A lines are not important as a predictor of cardiac disease. They are caused by edema of the deep interlobular septa and therefore radiate from the hila (see Fig 5–4).

For unknown reasons, Kerley B lines are uncommon in infancy and early childhood. When they are present, they always indicate marked pulmonary venous hyperten-

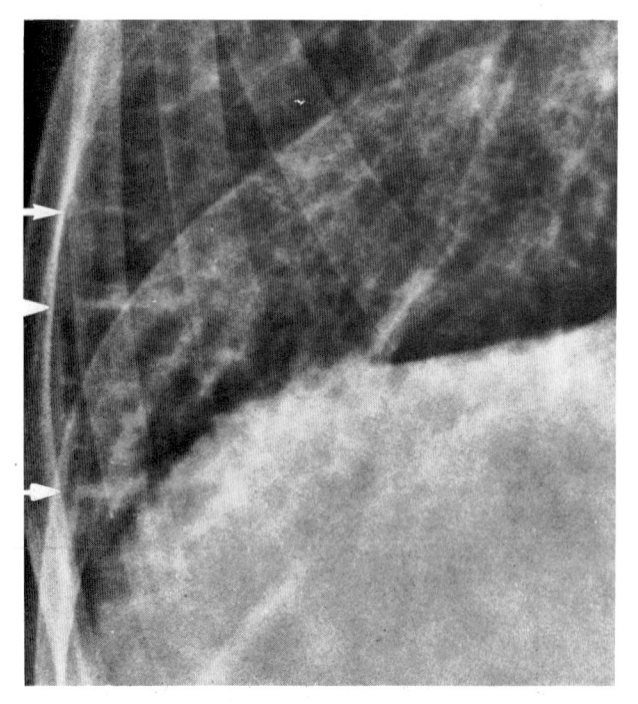

FIG 5–6.
Thoracic roentgenogram; magnified right base in patients with increased pulmonary venous pressure. Characteristic fine subpleural linear densities *(arrows)* are Kerley B lines, which suggest that the pulmonary venous pressure is above 20 mm Hg. Definite radiographic finding of pulmonary venous hypertension.

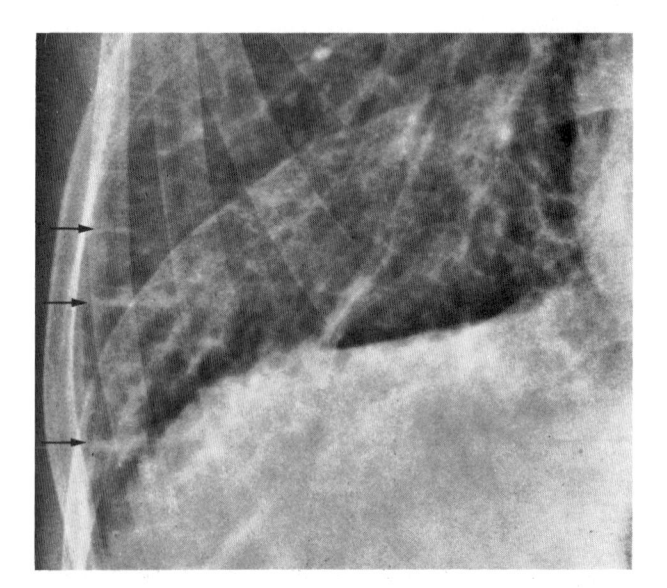

FIG 5–7.
Thoracic roentgenogram; magnified right base, in patient with long-standing severe pulmonary venous hypertension. Kerley B lines are obvious *(arrows)*, probably because of fibrosis and hemosiderin deposits in interlobular septa, which will cause these lines to persist after correction of pulmonary venous hypertension.

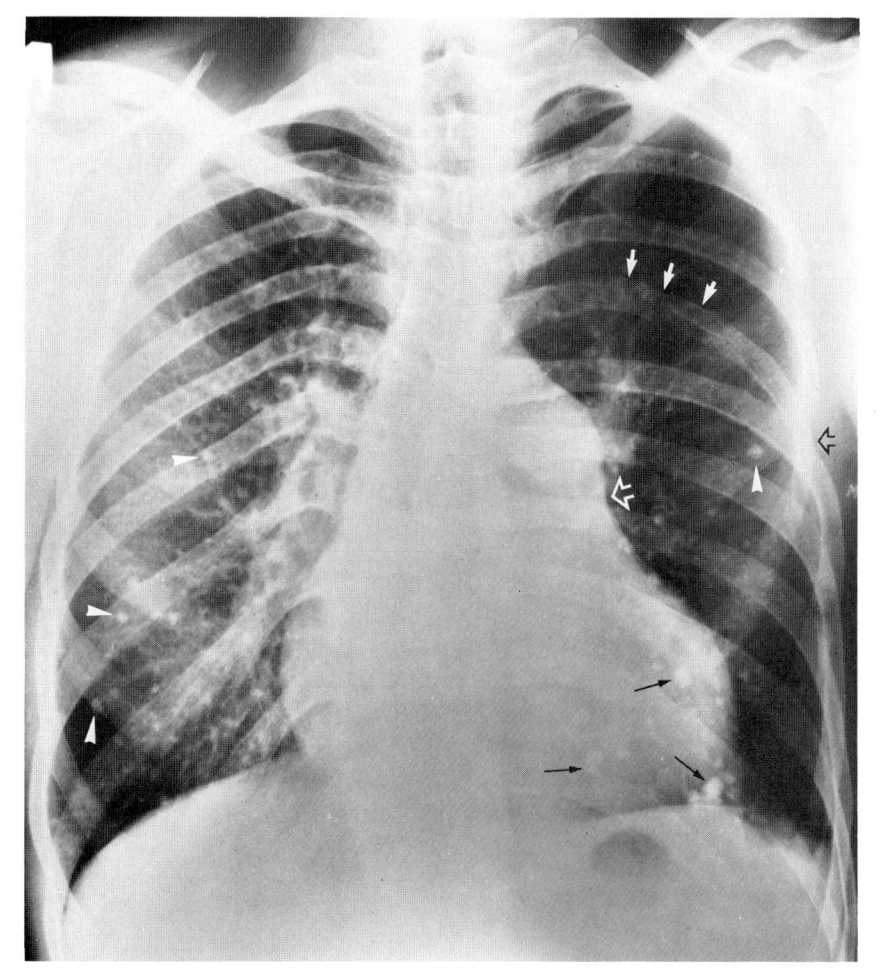

FIG 5–8.
Thoracic roentgenogram, posteroanterior projection, in patient with long-standing mitral stenosis. Previous rib resection *(white arrows)* indicates old mitral commissurotomy. Prominent main pulmonary artery segment because left atrial appendage has been resected *(open arrow)*. Consequently, "mitral" configuration of heart is lost. Calcific densities scattered throughout both lungs *(small arrows)*, more numerous at bases. Nodules that are larger at the bases suggest ossified hemosiderin rather than healed granulomatous disease.

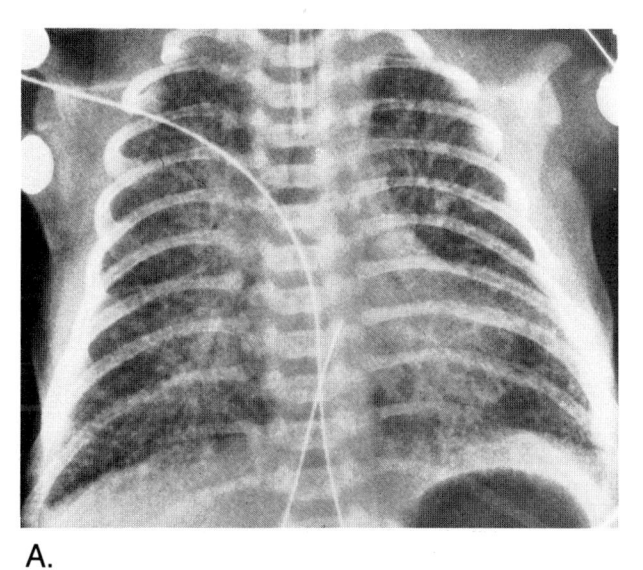

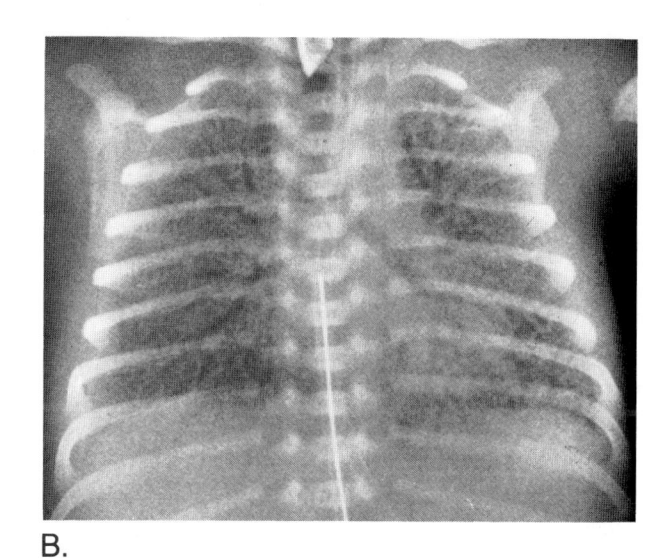

A.

B.

FIG 5–9.
Thoracic roentgenograms; posteroanterior projection. **A,** infant; severe pulmonary venous hypertension as a result of total anomalous venous return below diaphragm. Conditions with pulmonary venous obstruction usually cause only right ventricular hypertrophy. Therefore, cardiac size is normal. Fine granular pattern throughout lung fields is indistinguishable from appearance of hyaline membrane disease. No air bronchogram is present. **B,** infant with hyaline membrane disease; diffuse granular pattern throughout both lung fields, indistinguishable from radiographic appearance in Figure 5–8. However, air bronchogram strongly suggests pulmonary rather than cardiac disease.

sion. They do not occur in patients with increased blood flow, who often have a slight elevation of the left atrial pressure (relative mitral stenosis).

In infancy, for unknown reasons, severe pulmonary venous obstruction results in an unusual, but fairly characteristic, granular pattern throughout both lung fields, a radiographic picture that is virtually indistinguishable from that of hyaline membrane disease (Fig 5–9,A). Although the conditions may be identical radiographically, the presence of an air bronchogram strongly suggests pulmonary rather than cardiac disease (Fig 5–9,B). Plain-film differential diagnosis of these conditions is important, because angiography may be dangerous in neonates with hyaline membrane disease. The presence of a small pleural effusion also favors venous pulmonary hypertension.

With the sudden onset of severe pulmonary venous hypertension, the alveoli of the lungs fill with fluid (pulmonary edema). The transition from severe pulmonary venous congestion to early pulmonary edema is not sharply defined. Edema may be evidenced radiographically by an ill-defined haziness throughout both lung fields. Because the anteroposterior diameter of the chest is greatest in the region of the hilar areas, the greatest radiographic densities are produced centrally, resulting in the "butterfly" pattern often characteristic of pulmonary edema. The transudation of fluid into the alveoli is determined by the venous pulmonary pressure and the hydrostatic pressure, which, in turn, depends on gravity and consequently varies with position. Therefore, atypical patterns of pulmonary edema, such as patchy, unilateral, lobar, or basilar, may

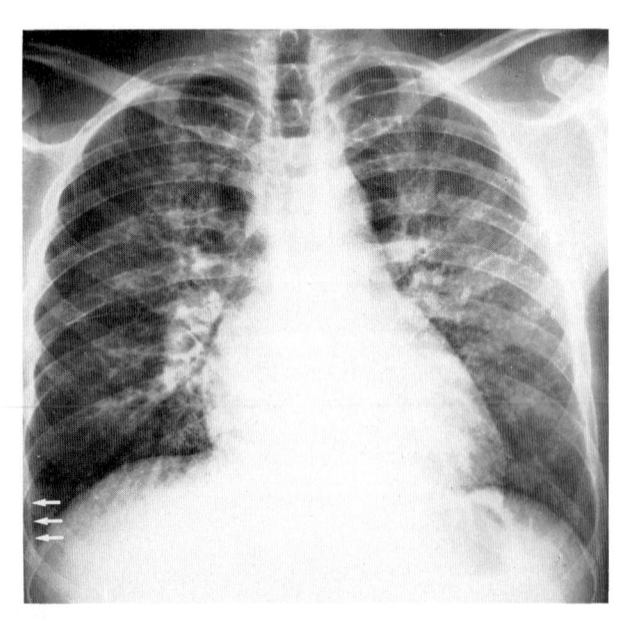

FIG 5–10.
Posteroanterior roentgenogram in pulmonary edema; both central lung fields are hazy because of accumulation of edema fluid in the alveoli. There is small pleural effusion at the right base *(arrows)*.

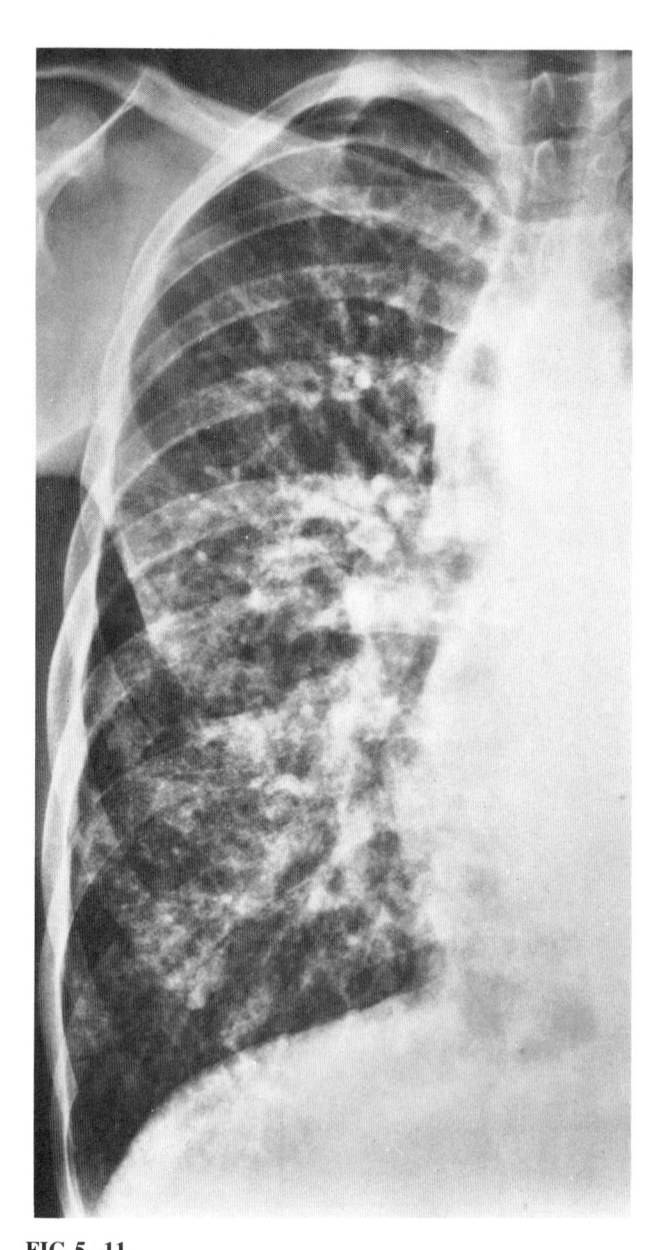

FIG 5–11.
Thoracic roentgenogram (magnified view), of right lung shows admixture-type pulmonary vasculature. Increased vasculature has unusual indistinct, fluffy appearance suggesting admixture lesion rather than left-to-right shunt.

be seen. Frank pulmonary edema is more common in adults than in children (reason unknown) (Fig 5–10).

Occasionally, differentiation of pulmonary edema from pneumonia may be difficult. A helpful finding is the much more rapid clearing of edema than of inflammatory lung disease.

The Admixture Pulmonary Vasculature

Admixture lesions are classified as cyanotic congenital heart disease with increased pulmonary blood flow. In most cases, the radiographic pattern of increased pulmonary flow is indistinguishable from that occurring in acyanotic conditions with a left-to-right shunt. However, in some cases the pattern of pulmonary vasculature is sufficiently characteristic to suggest the presence of cyanotic heart disease caused by an admixture lesion.

The admixture pulmonary vasculature appears less well defined, "fuzzier," compared with the well-delineated pulmonary arteries in patients with a left-to-right shunt (Fig 5–11). The reason for this bizarre fluffy appearance probably is the concomitant increase in the bronchial circulation. Hypoxemia is a strong stimulus for bronchial capillary growth, so in cyanotic forms of congenital heart disease, the bronchial circulation is well developed. Consequently, the admixture-type vasculature is most easily identified in older patients with a well-developed bronchial circulation. The hypothesis that the radiographic appearance of the admixture-type pulmonary vasculature is the result of enlarged pulmonary arteries plus numerous bronchial arteries is supported by the similar radiographic picture present in pulmonary atresia (tetralogy of Fallot) with huge bronchial arteries (Fig 5–12).

Decreased Pulmonary Vasculature

In congenital heart disease, the pulmonary vasculature may be frankly decreased, although this can be diagnosed radiographically only in patients with markedly decreased pulmonary flow. However, even in most patients with diminished pulmonary blood flow, the radiographic appearance of the pulmonary vasculature is still in the range of normal, although it may be classified as "decreased" to arrive at a radiographic diagnosis. Decreased pulmonary vasculature is caused by congenital lesions with a septal defect and pulmonary outflow obstruction, resulting in decreased pulmonary perfusion. In most cases, the radiographic diagnosis of decreased pulmonary vasculature is made on the basis of the clinical finding of cyanosis. Radiographically, decreased pulmonary vasculature is most impressive if there is a discrepancy between an enlarged heart and the appearance of the vasculature (Fig 5–13).

Bronchial Vasculature

Whereas the pulmonary arteries radiate from the hila, bronchial arteries have an irregular and unpredictable course. Consequently, the radiographic appearance of increased bronchial circulation is bizarre. The commalike densities of the right and left pulmonary arteries in the hila are absent, and numerous vessels are seen on-end because of the irregular course of bronchial arteries (see Fig 5–12).

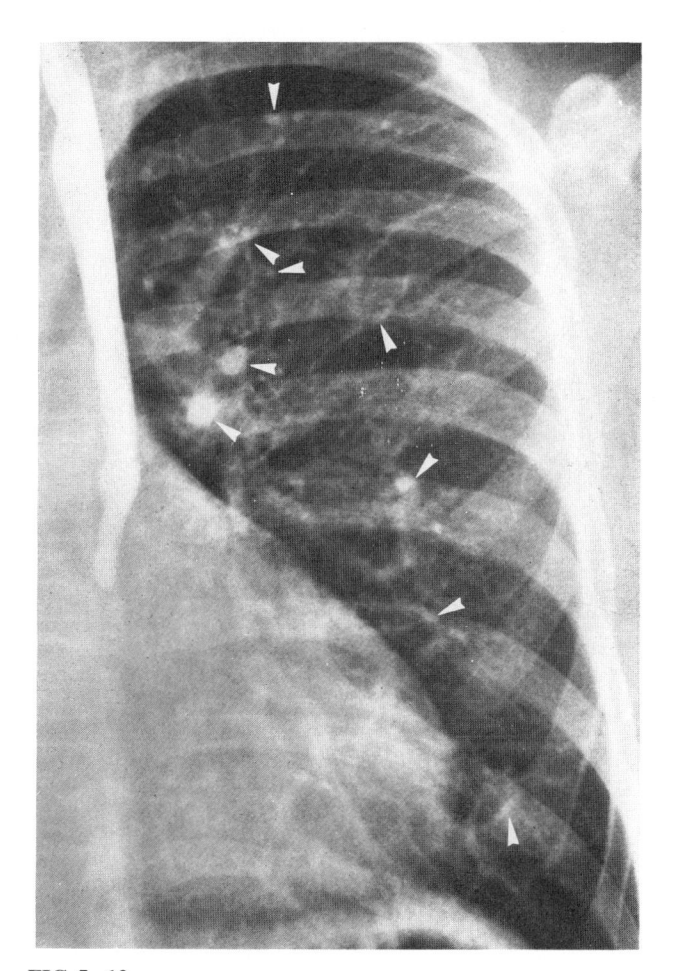

FIG 5–12.
Thoracic roentgenogram (magnified view) of left lung in patient with pulmonary atresia and markedly enlarged bronchial arteries. Because of the tortuous course of the bronchial arteries, more vessels than normally are seen on-end *(arrows)*. The "comma" density of a normal left lower lobe pulmonary artery is absent.

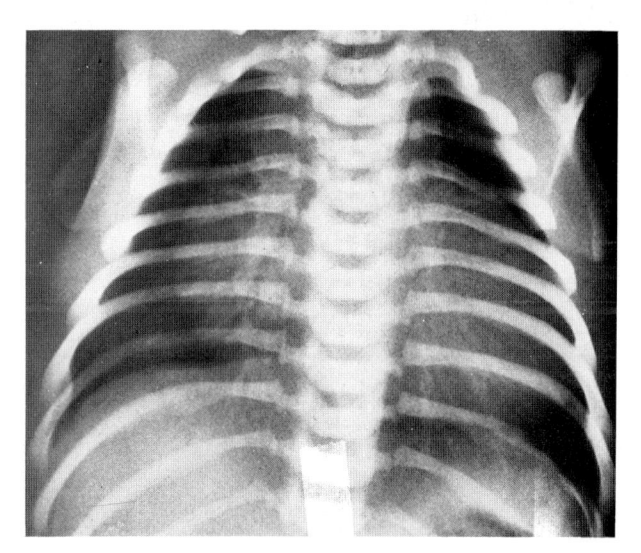

FIG 5–13.
Thoracic roentgenogram, posteroanterior projection in cyanotic patient; marked cardiomegaly and frankly decreased pulmonary vasculature. Right and left pulmonary arteries obscured by enlarged heart; peripheral pulmonary arteries sparse.

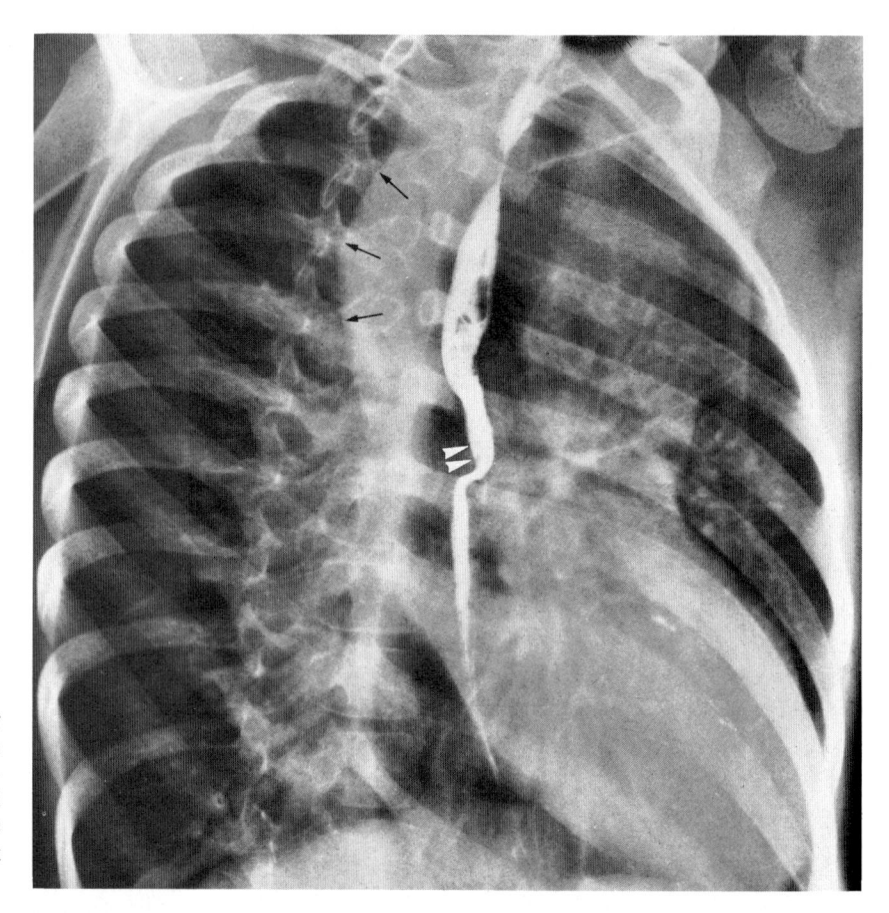

FIG 5–14.
Thoracic roentgenogram, right anterior oblique projection in cyanotic patient with large bronchial arteries. Posterior indentations *(white arrows)* of barium-filled esophagus; note density to the right of the esophagus *(black arrows)*, which is a right aortic arch.

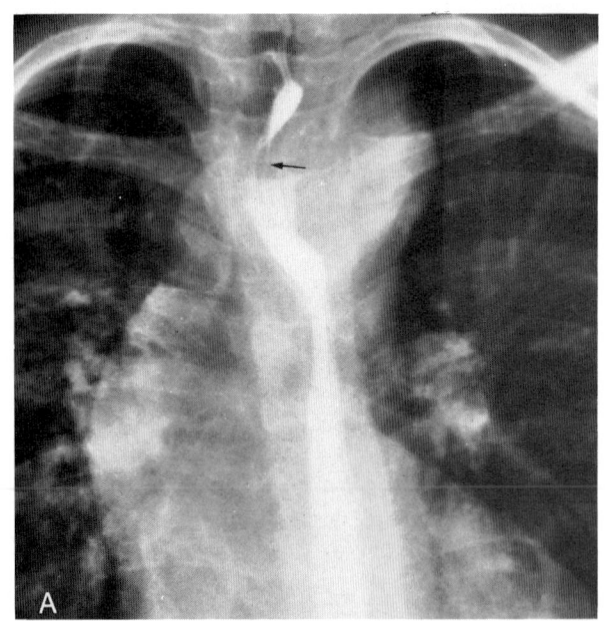

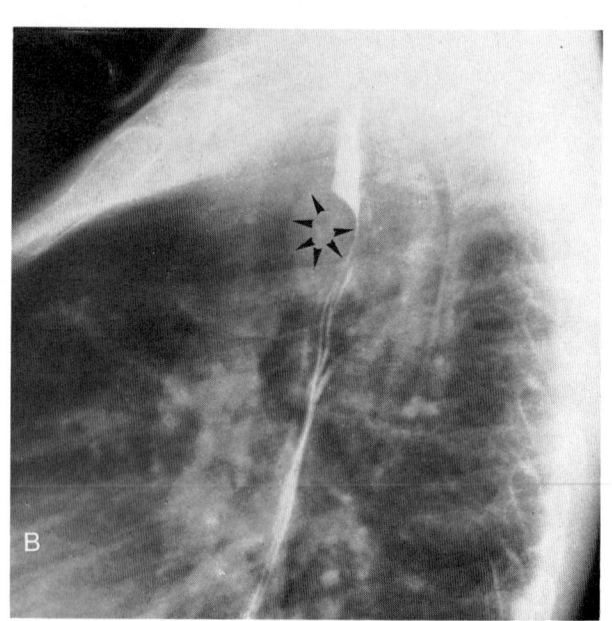

FIG 5–15.
Thoracic roentgenogram in patient with pulmonary atresia and large bronchial arteries. **A,** posteroanterior projection; barium-filled esophagus indented by bronchial artery *(arrow)*. **B,** lateral projection; indentation of barium-filled esophagus by bronchial artery *(arrow)*, which crosses between esophagus and trachea. This is extremely rare; almost invariably, bronchial arteries pass behind esophagus. The only vascular structure passing between esophagus and trachea is a vascular sling (origin of left pulmonary artery from right pulmonary artery; see Chapter 62).

Large bronchial arteries may cross behind the esophagus, causing characteristic indentations of the barium-filled passage (Fig 5–14). In rare cases, a bronchial artery passes between the esophagus and the trachea (Fig 5–15). Clinically bronchial arteries are best heard over the patient's back.

Cardiac Size

In the evaluation of patients with congenital heart disease, one of the main reasons for obtaining a chest radiograph is to estimate cardiac size. Chest radiography is also the most convenient method for detecting any *change* in cardiac size.

Effects of Technical Factors

Many factors influence the apparent cardiac size on a thoracic radiograph. For example, the cardiac silhouette appears larger on an anteroposterior projection than on a posteroanterior projection because of the divergence of the x-ray beam and the greater distance of the heart from the film in the anteroposterior projection (Fig 5–16). Cardiac size is also influenced by focus-film distance: the shorter the distance, the greater the magnification. Ideally the x-ray tube should be moved to infinity, thus resulting in a parallel beam, but because this is not possible, an upright posteroanterior view of the thorax obtained at a 2-m (6-ft) focal-film distance has become accepted international standard for evaluation of cardiac size. However, even this distance results in about a 15% enlargement of the cardiac silhouette. Radiographs obtained with portable equipment also cause apparent enlargement, because patients are usually supine and radiographs are made at a short focus-film distance (Fig 5–17).

Orthodiagraphy (orthodiascopy) is a radiographic technique that eliminates the magnification. A small bundle of a virtually parallel x-ray beam is moved along the cardiac contour, and the image is traced on the fluoroscopic screen. Although this technique measures heart size more accurately, it has been abandoned because a 15% enlargement of the cardiac silhouette is of no practical importance.

Change in Cardiac Size With Breathing

Because the heart is attached by the pericardial sac to the diaphragm, the heart moves with diaphragmatic motion. During exhalation or with the patient supine, the higher diaphragmatic position gives the heart a more transverse orientation and makes it appear larger. During deep inhalation or with the patient upright, the diaphragm is lower, so the heart assumes a more vertical position and has a smaller radiographic silhouette (Fig 5–18). Therefore, in patients with an elevated diaphragm, the radiographs show a larger cardiac silhouette than in those with a depressed diaphragm, such as patients with emphysema. A change in position of the diaphragm causes a shift of the

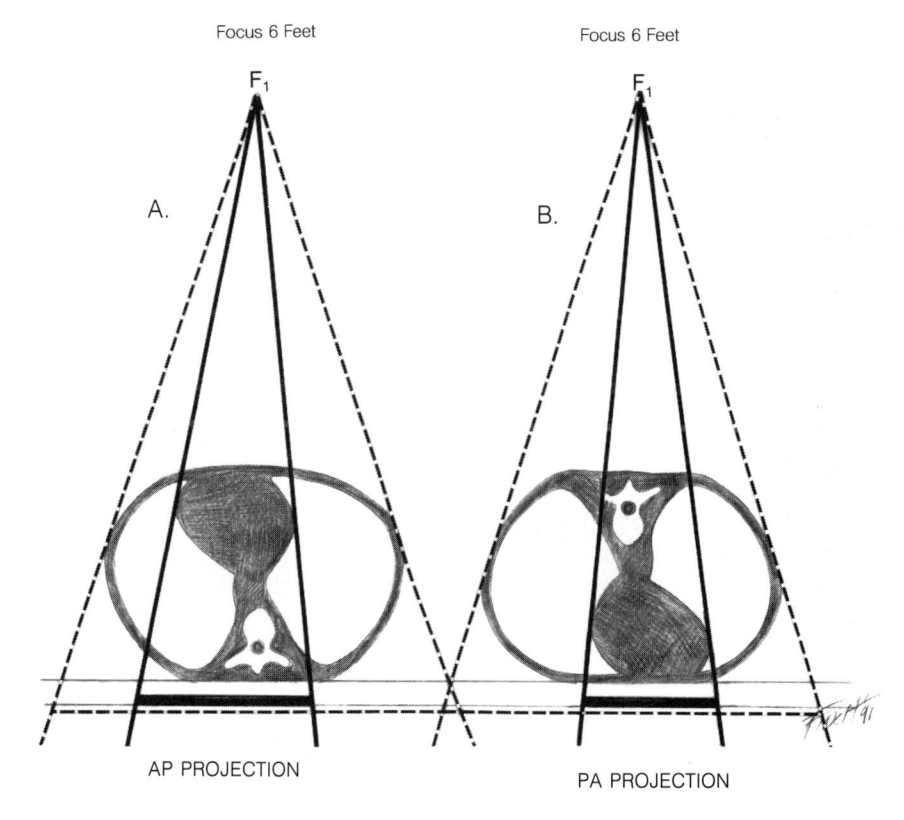

FIG 5–16.
Diagram demonstrating the difference between the anteroposterior (**A**) and posterior projection (**B**). Because of the divergence of the x-ray beam, the thoracic cage and heart are magnified. Magnification of the thorax is similar in **A** and **B,** but marked enlargement of the heart is seen in the anteroposterior projection because the heart is further away from the radiographic cassette.

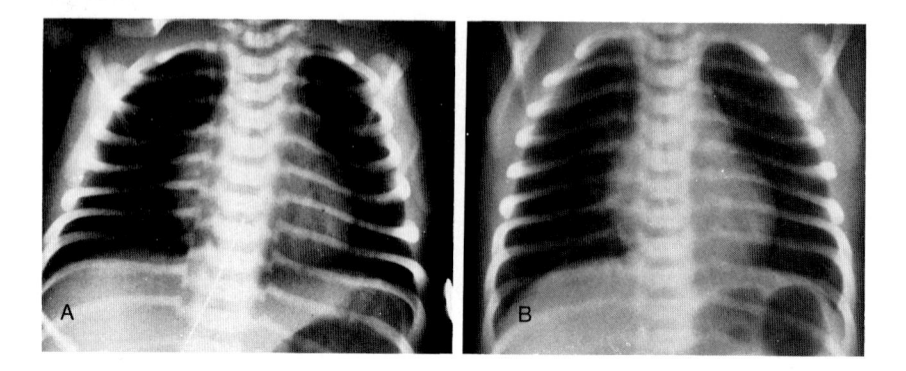

FIG 5-17.
Thoracic roentgenograms. Anteroposterior projections, in neonate made with portable apparatus (**A**) and standard equipment (**B**). Cardiac silhouette is much larger in **A** because of the shorter tube-film distance and the supine position of the patient which tends to elevate the diaphragm. Pulmonary vasculature appears decreased because of comparatively long exposure time and slight overpenetration. **B,** heart and lungs appear normal because of the 6-ft target-film distance and the upright posteroanterior projection.

long axis of the heart and results in either a "horizontal" or a "vertical" heart (Fig 5–19).

Before evaluating cardiac size on a thoracic roentgenogram, the radiologist should determine the degree of inspiration, which is best done by comparing the level of the diaphragm in relation to the posterior ribs (see Fig 5–18). The degree of inhalation is considered satisfactory for interpretation of the films when the diaphragm is at the level of the ninth or tenth rib.

Cardiac Contours

On an anteroposterior chest roentgenogram, the cardiac contour varies considerably with the angulation of the

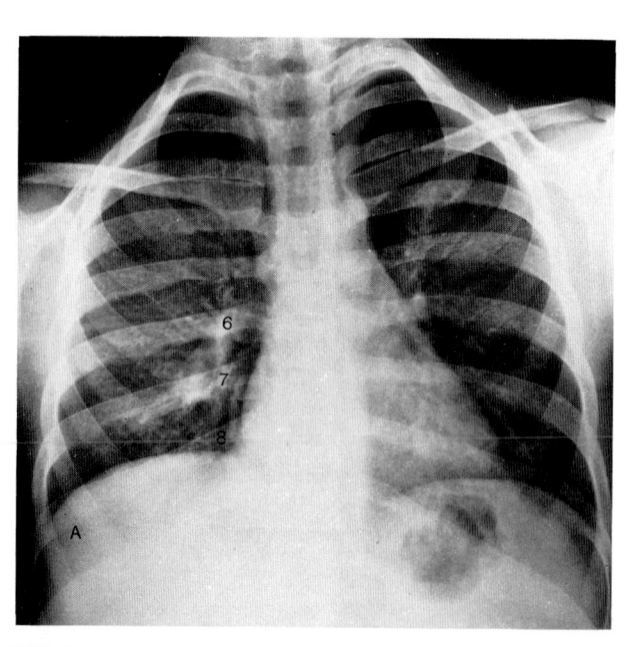

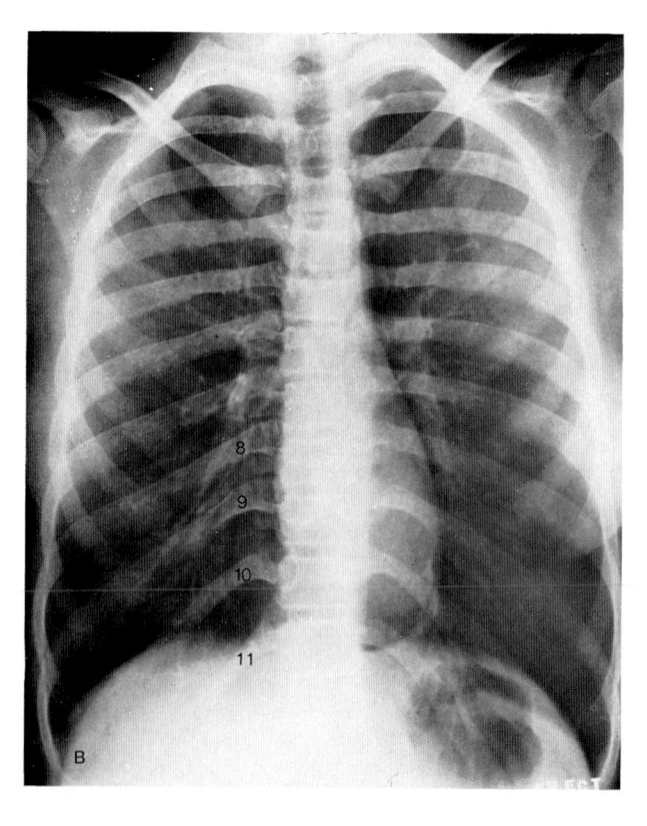

FIG 5-18.
Thoracic roentgenogram, posteroanterior projection; effect of breathing in same patient. **A,** exhalation; increased density of lung fields and transverse position of the heart. **B,** deep inhalation; vertical position of heart, which appears much smaller in relation to the thoracic cage. Degree of inhalation is indicated by counting the posterior ribs.

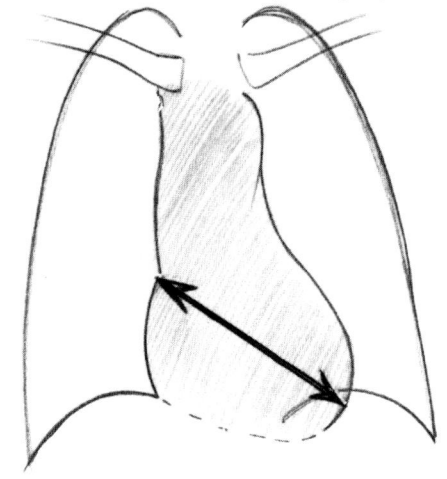

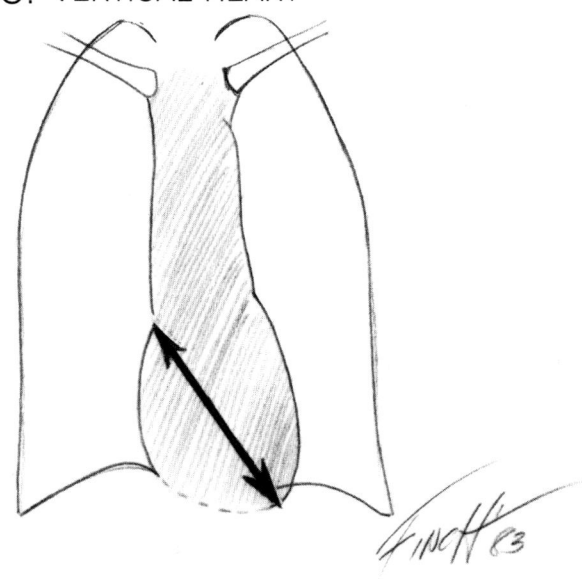

FIG 5–19.
Diagram of influence on cardiac size of the position of the diaphragm. **A,** long axis of normal oblique heart forms an approximately 45-degree angle with the horizontal and sagittal planes. **B,** the transverse heart, seen primarily in patients with elevated diaphragm, particularly obese patients; the long axis has more than a 45-degree inclination. **C,** a vertical heart, in which the angle of the long axis with the sagittal plane is less than 45 degrees, apppears small; this is seen primarily in asthenic individuals or patients with emphysema. It has also been referred to as "drop heart," but it is of anatomically normal size.

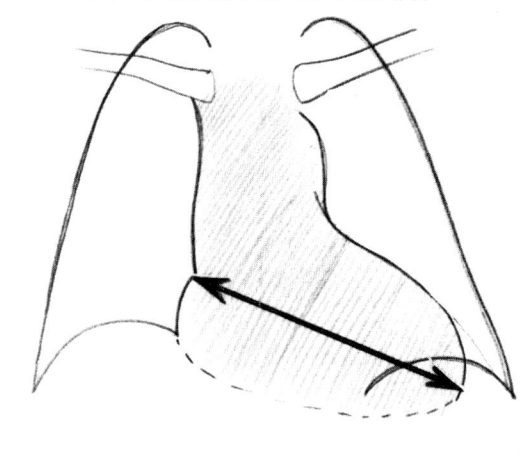

x-ray beam in a cranial-caudad direction. For example, a change in the angulation of the beam can transform a left ventricular configuration into a boot-shaped heart.

Thus, in evaluating cardiac size and configuration, the radiologist must determine the cranial-caudad inclination of the beam, which is best accomplished by observing the level of the clavicle in relation to the posterior ribs and the inclination of the anterior ribs (Fig 5–20). Caudal angulation results in a more lordotic view of the thorax, projecting the clavicle above the apex of the lung (see Fig 5–20,B). This view was used advantageously for many years in the radiographic examination of apical pulmonary disease, particularly tuberculosis. Most thoracic roentgenograms of neonates or infants are lordotic, sometimes to an extreme degree in which the anterior ribs project above the posterior ribs. This lordotic view is the principal rea-

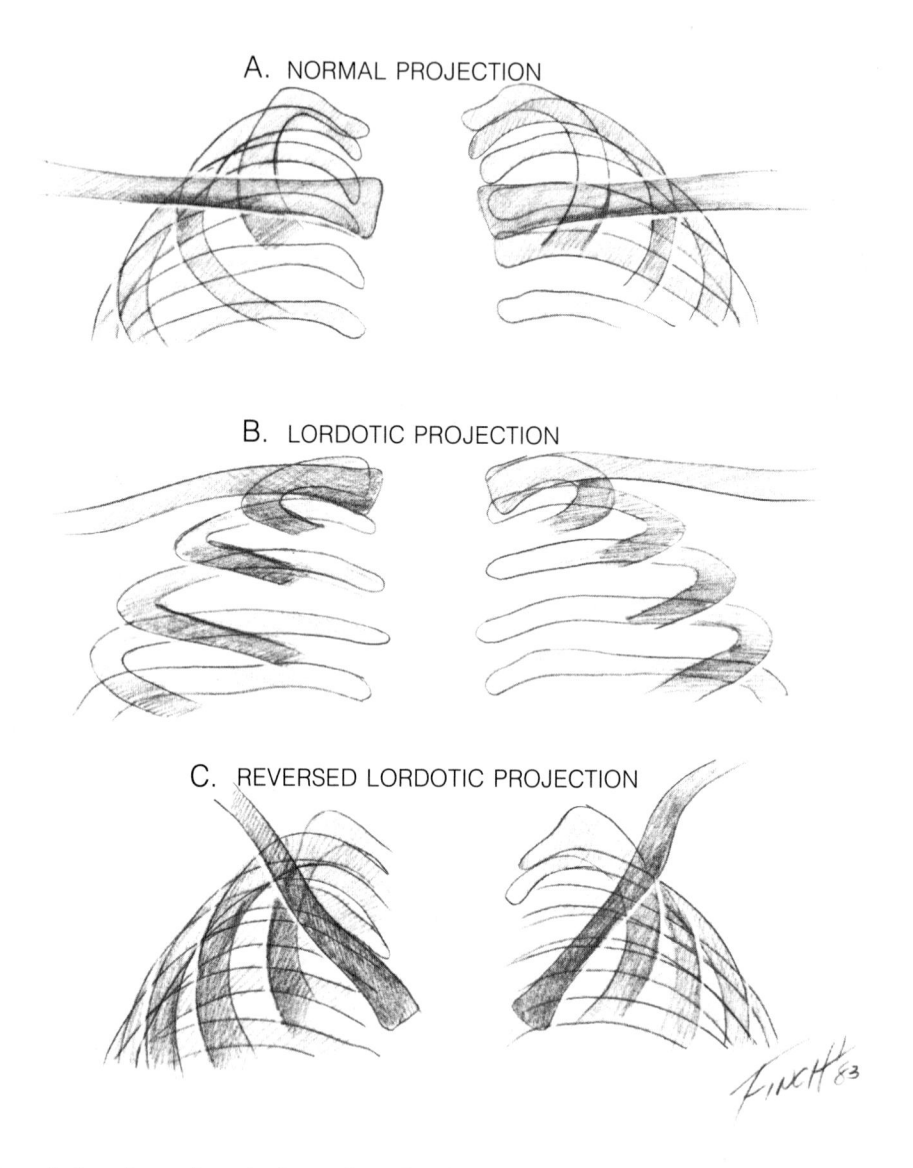

A. NORMAL PROJECTION

B. LORDOTIC PROJECTION

C. REVERSED LORDOTIC PROJECTION

FIG 5–20.
Diagram of effect of angulation of x-ray beam in the craniocaudad direction on the relations of the clavicle to the posterior ribs and the inclination of the clavicle. **A,** normal inclination, with clavicles at level of the fourth posterior rib. **B,** lordotic projection with caudad tube angulation; clavicles projected over the first rib. This is the normal projection in infants. **C,** reversed lordotic view; cranial angulation clavicles at the level of the sixth posterior rib.

son why the cardiac contour of neonates appears "globular" compared with that of older children or adults. The presence of the thymus also contributes to a different radiographic appearance of the heart of a neonate.

On a lordotic projection, all cardiac structures located anteriorly are projected up in relation to the posterior cardiac structures (Fig 5–21). The clavicles and anterior ribs shift to the greatest degree. Because the cardiac apex lies anteriorly to the dome of the diaphragm, the apex is projected upward in relation to the diaphragm, giving an appearance of an elevated apex. Because the pulmonary artery lies more anteriorly than the aortic arch, the pulmonary arterial segment is more prominent and the aortic knob less conspicuous than normal. The appearance of the pulmonary vasculature also changes, because more vessels lie in the direction of the x-ray beam and are therefore seen on-end (Fig 5–22). Consequently, there is a tendency to overread the pulmonary vasculature on lordotic views. In addition, the contour of the cardiac silhouette, particularly the right atrial and ventricular configuration, changes. The posterior aspect of the right atrium forms a small arc between the superior and inferior vena cavae (Fig 5–23), whereas on a normal radiographic projection, this portion of the right atrium forms the inconspicuous right cardiac

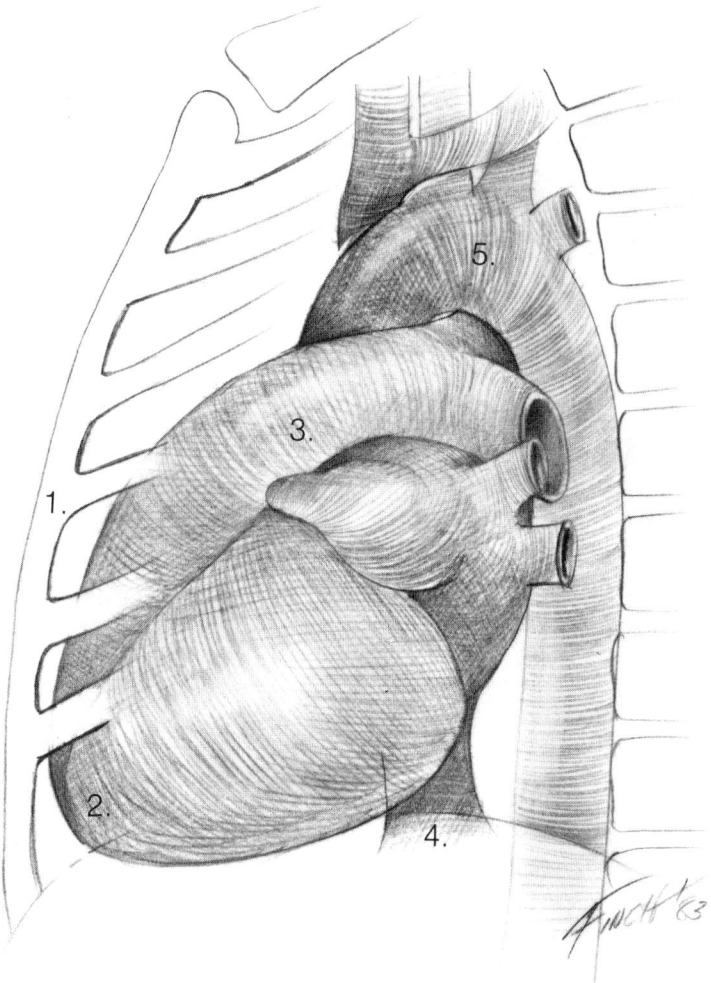

FIG 5–21.
Diagram of lateral side of chest demonstrating the spatial relation of various cardiac structures. On a lordotic posteroanterior view, the anterior structures will be elevated in relation to the posterior structures. The anterior ribs *(1)* are more anterior than the apex *(2)*, the pulmonary artery *(3)*, the dome of the diaphragm *(4)*, and the aortic arch *(5)*.

(atrial) border. On a lordotic projection, the right cardiac border and entire cardiac shadow (see Figs 5–22,B and 5–23) are enlarged because the anterior portion of the right atrium forms a large arc.

In the opposite projection, the reversed lordotic view, the posterior cardiac structures are more prominent. The aortic knob is more prominent, the pulmonary artery segment less conspicuous, and the left ventricle projects below the dome of the diaphragm. This apparent elongation of the left ventricle may erroneously be interpreted as left ventricular enlargement (Fig 5–24). The radiographic projection is therefore very important in the assessment of cardiac size and contour.

Change of Cardiac Size and Contour With Rotation

Because the long axis of the heart passes obliquely to the sagittal plane of the thorax, it is not seen in its greatest dimension on a posteroanterior chest roentgenogram (Fig 5–25,A). The degree of foreshortening of the heart depends on the angle of the cardiac axis to the sagittal plane, which varies but is usually about 45 degrees. Clockwise rotation of the heart increases the apparent cardiac size, whereas counterclockwise rotation foreshortens the long axis and decreases the apparent cardiac size (Fig 5–25 B and C). Rotation is defined by looking at the heart from below.

On the lateral view of the chest, the heart is also foreshortened. Clockwise rotation (Fig 5–26,A) produces a small cardiac dimension on the lateral view (Fig 5–26, B), whereas counterclockwise rotation (Fig 5–26,C), which produces a small cardiac dimension on the posteroanterior projection, causes a larger dimension on a lateral view. Rotation of the heart about its axis, therefore, has opposite effects on the radiographic appearances of cardiac size on

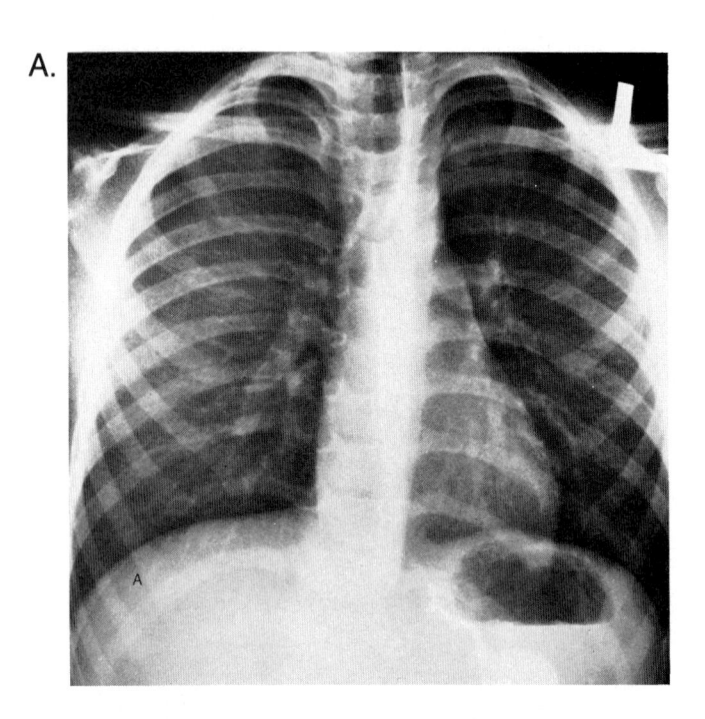

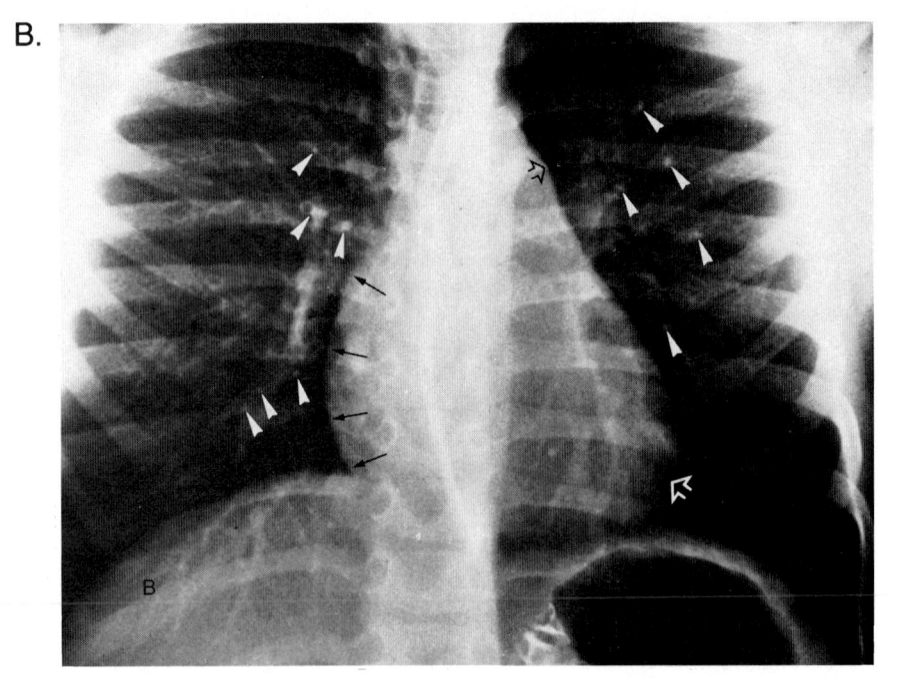

FIG 5-22.
Thoracic roentgenogram, posteroanterior projection; normal projection (**A**) and lordotic view (**B**). **A,** contour of the heart and pulmonary vasculature are normal. **B,** the heart appears large primarily because of the visibility of the more anterior portion of right atrium where it forms a larger arch *(small black arrows)*. Pulmonary artery segment is more prominent *(open black arrow)*. Cardiac apex *(open white arrows)* elevated, simulating boot-shaped heart. More pulmonary arteries *(small white arrows)* seen on-end than in **A**. The cardiac contour has assumed a globular configuration normally seen in babies because of the lordotic projection.

Plain-Film Diagnosis of Congenital Cardiac Disease 77

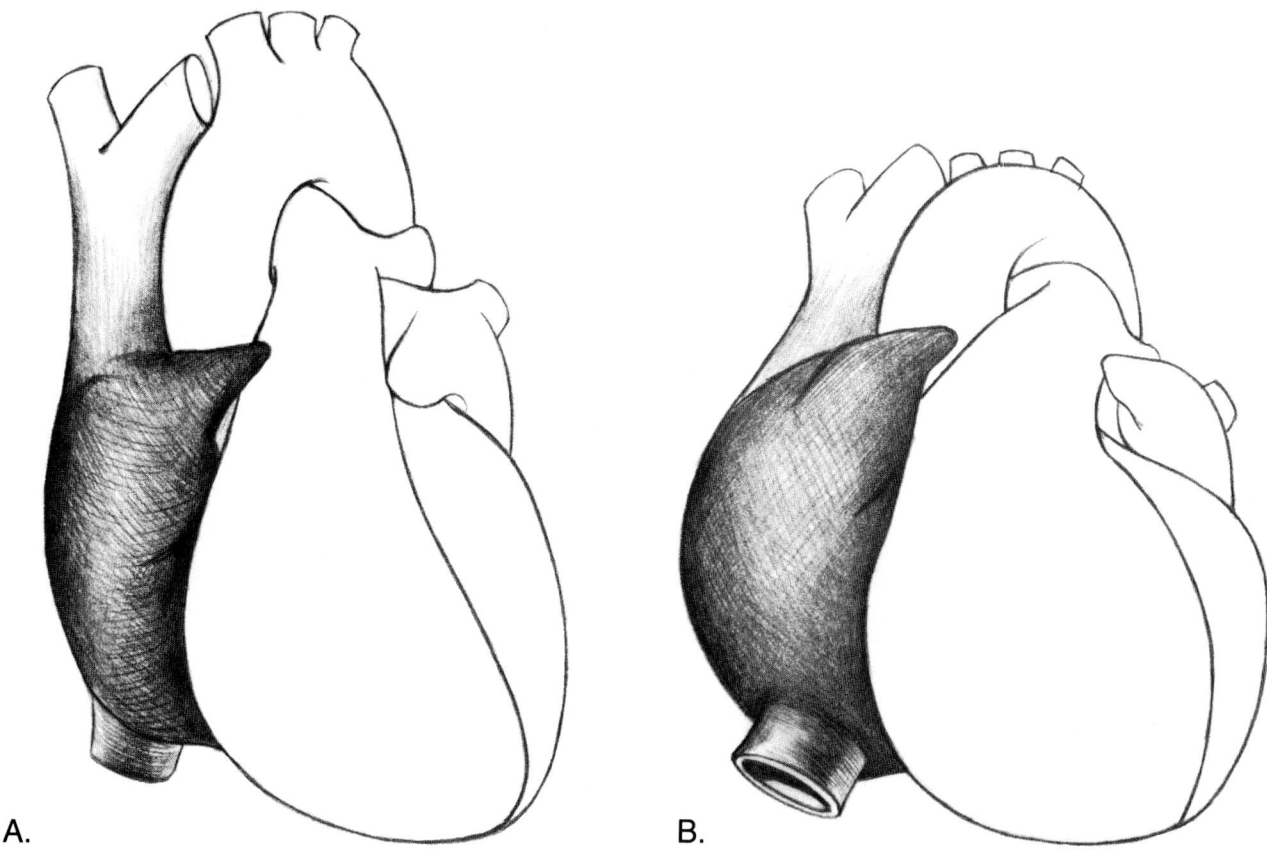

A.   **B.**

FIG 5–23.
Diagram of right atrium in posteroanterior projection. **A,** normal projection; posterior area of right atrium near the junction of the superior and inferior venae cavae is seen in profile. This portion of right atrium has a small diameter. **B,** lordotic projection; more anterior portion of the right atrium is seen. It has a larger diameter, and this alters the contour, enlarges the cardiac silhouette, and creates globular shape.

the posteroanterior and the lateral projections, so cardiac size can be estimated only if at least two views at right angles are available. A truly enlarged heart is large in both of these projections, whereas a heart that appears enlarged because of rotation about its long axis is smaller on one of the right-angle views.

Rotation about the cardiac axis also alters cardiac configuration. Clockwise rotation increases the prominence of the pulmonary arterial segment (Fig 5–26), whereas counterclockwise rotation causes prominence of the ascending aorta. Rotation may occur as a primary anomaly as a consequence of altered hemodynamics from congenital or acquired cardiac disease or as a consequence of external factors such as pneumonectomy, pneumonthorax, chest deformities with a narrow anteroposterior diameter or pectus excavatum deformity. Pectus excavatum also causes displacement of the heart into the left hemithorax (Fig 5–27).

These changes in cardiac size and configuration secondary to cardiac rotation can also be caused by slight rotation of the patient while the posteroanterior thoracic roentgenogram is being obtained. Improper positioning of the patient is common and can be recognized by observing the relations between the anterior ribs or the anterior ends of the clavicle and the thoracic spine (Fig 5–28). The changes observed in cardiac size and shape are identical to those of cardiac rotation. In the patient with scoliosis, the relations between the clavicles and the spine are affected, thus making it impossible to determine rotation and cardiac size.

Summary

Before evaluating cardiac films, the observer thus must consider many technical factors that could alter the appearance of the chest film:

1. Was the radiograph made with the patient in the upright or the supine position?
2. Was the radiograph made with a portable apparatus?

FIG 5–24.
Thoracic roengenogram, posteroanterior projection; reversed lordotic view. Projection of the cardiac apex *(white arrows)* well below the level of the diaphragm, simulating left ventricular enlargement.

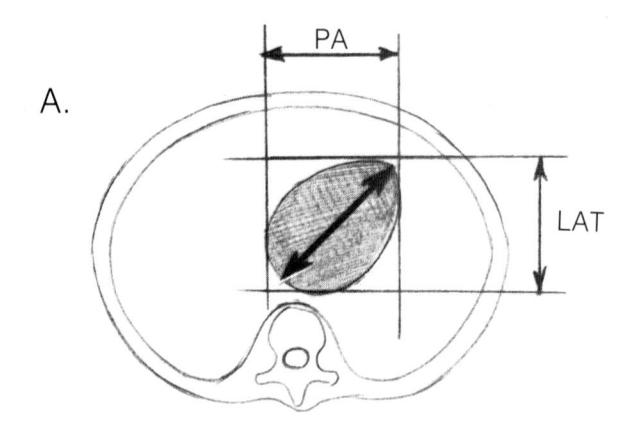

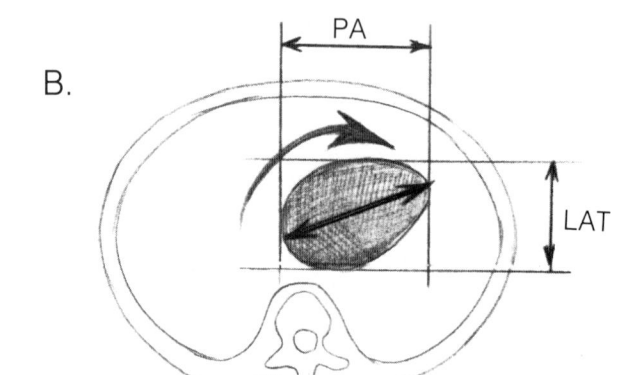

FIG 5–25.
Diagram of influence of cardiac rotation on apparent cardiac size; the longest axis of the heart and its projection are demonstrated in the posteroanterior *(PA)* and lateral *(LAT)* projections. The minor divergence of the x-ray beam has been ignored. **A,** average inclination of the long axis with the sagittal plane (about 45 degrees) produces posteroanterior and lateral dimensions of equal size. **B,** clockwise rotation of heart *(curved arrow)* produces an enlargement on the posteroanterior projection but a foreshortening on the lateral film. **C,** counterclockwise rotation *(curved arrow)* minimizes heart size in the posteroanterior projection but results in a large cardiac silhouette on the lateral projection. Estimates of cardiac size must consider both views. To measure the cardiothoracic ratio is therefore meaningless.

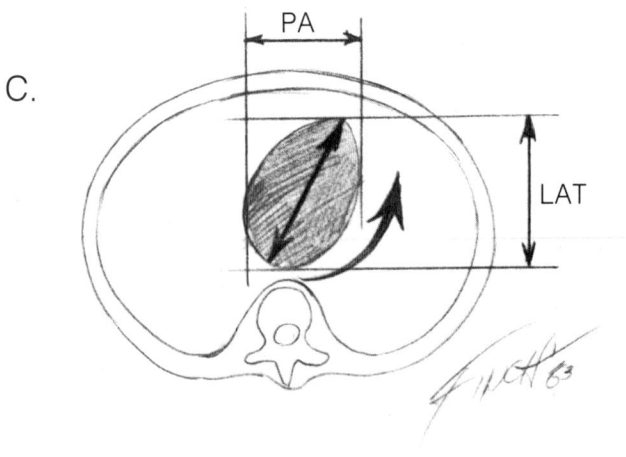

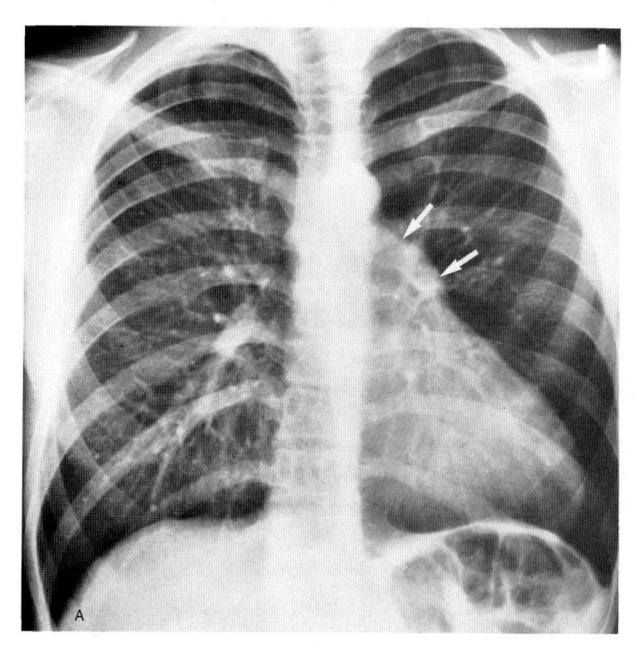

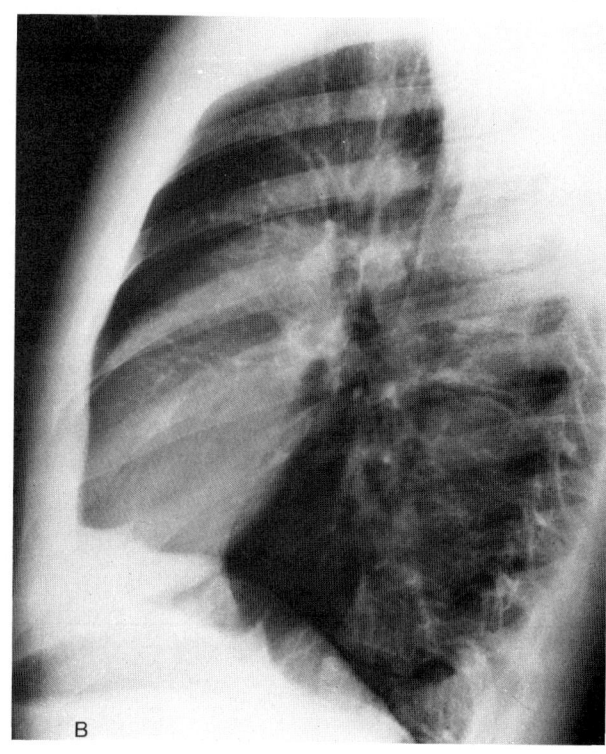

FIG 5–26.
Thoracic roentgenograms in posteroanterior (**A**) and lateral (**B**) projections of patient with clockwise rotation of the heart. **A**, cardiac silhouette appears fairly large. Distinct prominence of the main pulmonary artery segment *(arrows)*. The ascending aorta and right superior vena cava are inconspicuous. **B**, cardiac silhouette appears small on the lateral view because of clockwise rotation of the heart.

3. What was the exposure time?
4. What was the target-film distance?
5. Is the projection posteroanterior or anteroposterior?
6. Is the radiograph properly exposed (i.e., overpenetrated or underpenetrated)?
7. Was the radiograph made during deep inspiration or expiration, and what is the position of the diaphragm in relation to the posterior ribs?
8. Is the film straight, or is there rotation?
9. Was there tube angulation, resulting in a lordotic or reverse lordotic projection?

After all of these questions have been answered, one can attempt to evaluate cardiac films intelligently and estimate heart size by examining posteroanterior and lateral projections.

THE PULMONARY VASCULATURE

Analysis of the pulmonary vasculature is a key step in the radiographic evaluation of a patient with congenital heart disease. When the findings are combined with information about cardiac size and configuration and data about the presence or absence of cyanosis, a specific diagnosis can usually be made. Correct interpretation of pulmonary vasculature requires considerable experience and cannot simply be learned from a book. However, knowledge of the physiology of various cardiac lesions and their effect on the pulmonary vasculature will assist in the radiographic interpretation.

Important hemodynamic conclusions can be drawn from careful study of the pulmonary arteries and veins visible on a thoracic roentgenogram. As with the systemic vascular bed, the size of pulmonary arteries varies with the volume of blood flow and the intravascular pressure. If, for instance, the blood flow through an artery is increased by the creation of an arteriovenous fistula, the artery supplying the fistula increases dramatically in size and carries an increased volume. Conversely, with obliteration of the arteriovenous malformation, the artery decreases to normal size. The physiologic mechanism for this adaptive phenomenon is unknown; perhaps the involved artery senses the altered speed of blood flow.

A process similar to an arteriovenous fistula occurs when a left-to-right shunt is created experimentally or develops suddenly by a rupture of the ventricular septum secondary to myocardial infarction. The volume and speed of pulmonary blood flow increase suddenly. In several weeks, the pulmonary arterial tree has responded to this

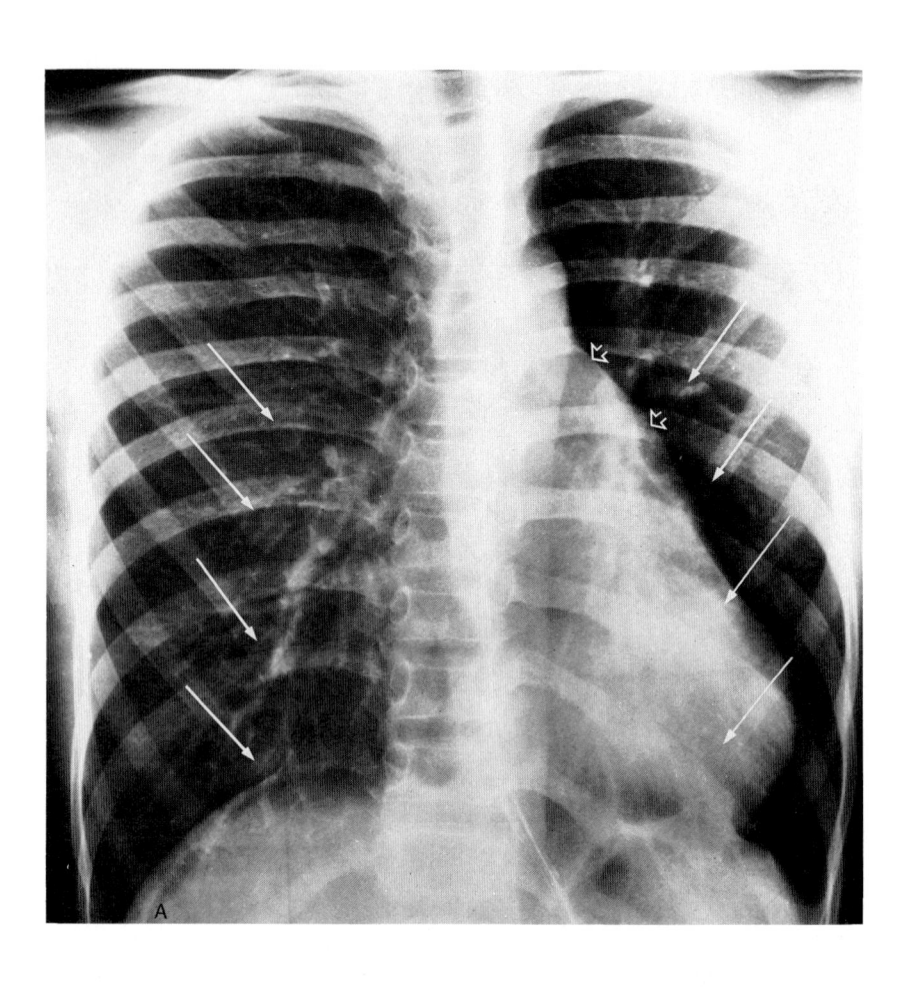

FIG 5–27.
Thoracic roentgenograms in posteroanterior (**A**) and lateral (**B**) projections in severe pectus excavatum. **A,** steep course of the anterior lower ribs *(long arrows)* is characteristic of this thoracic deformation (note fairly lordotic film obtained). Heart rotated clockwise, causing marked prominence of main pulmonary arterial segment *(open arrows)*. Displacement of heart into left side of thoracic cavity superimposes right superior portion of mediastinum on spine. **B,** severe deformity of sternum *(white arrows)* resulting in posterior displacement of heart.

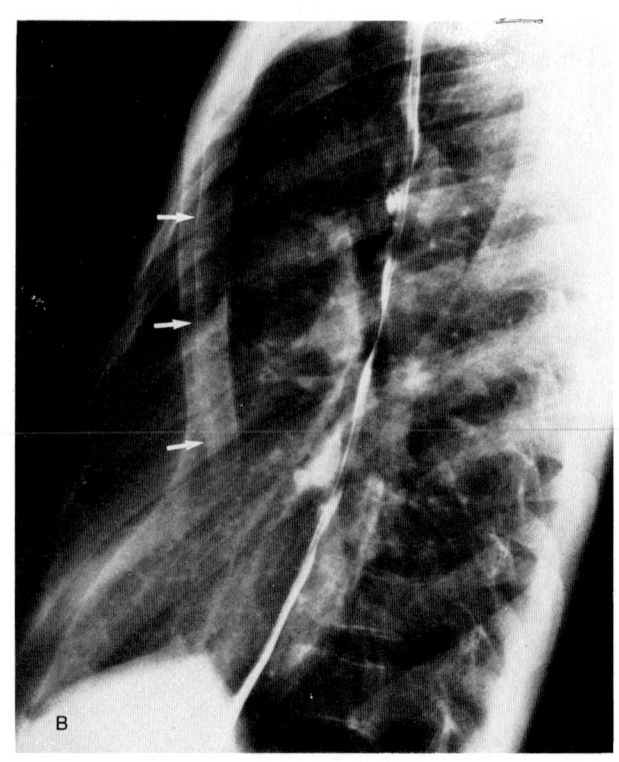

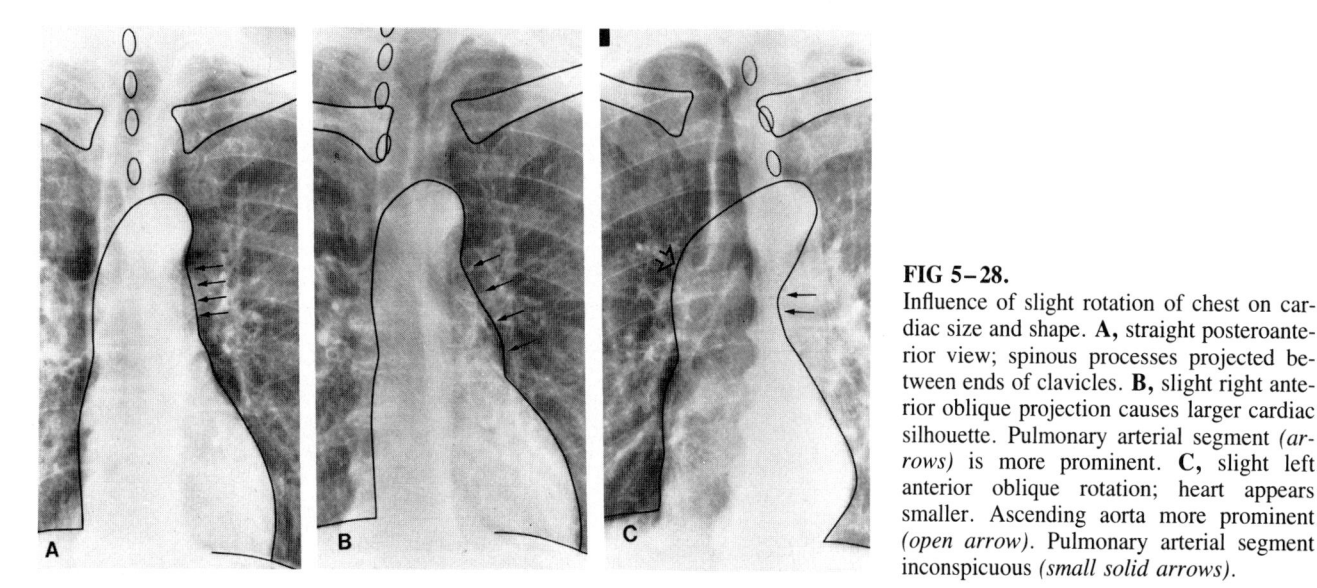

FIG 5-28.
Influence of slight rotation of chest on cardiac size and shape. **A,** straight posteroanterior view; spinous processes projected between ends of clavicles. **B,** slight right anterior oblique projection causes larger cardiac silhouette. Pulmonary arterial segment *(arrows)* is more prominent. **C,** slight left anterior oblique rotation; heart appears smaller. Ascending aorta more prominent *(open arrow)*. Pulmonary arterial segment inconspicuous *(small solid arrows)*.

stimulus, and dilatation of pulmonary arteries appears, manifested radiographically as "increased pulmonary vascularity." If the shunt is closed surgically, the size of the pulmonary arteries regresses to normal or almost normal.

Any condition, such as anemia, pregnancy, thyrotoxicosis, or systemic arteriovenous fistulas, that increases pulmonary blood flow can cause an increased pulmonary vasculature on a thoracic roentgenogram. The increased pulmonary blood volume is ejected by the ventricles; consequently, cardiac size also increases. Therefore, a relation exists between the degree of increase in pulmonary vasculature and cardiac size. If the heart is markedly enlarged and the pulmonary vasculature is only slightly increased, the cardiac enlargement is probably not caused by increased pulmonary blood flow but perhaps by myopathy; in such a case, the increased vasculature probably is venous.

The increased blood flow enlarges not only the pulmonary arteries but also the pulmonary veins. The extent of enlargement of the veins is less marked, however, because there are four veins and only two arteries. Pulmonary venous enlargement from increased blood flow is usually less obvious radiographically, but the increased pulmonary blood flow through the left atrium causes distention and enlargement of this chamber, which is readily detectable radiographically.

An increase in the pulmonary vasculature is only an accentuation of the normal radiographic appearance. Thus, because considerable variations of pulmonary vasculature exist normally, radiographic detection of increased pulmonary flow is relatively insensitive: The normal flow must be doubled before it is detectable on a thoracic roentgenogram. Therefore, a small left-to-right shunt ($\leq 50\%$), and sometimes even a moderate-sized shunt, cannot be diagnosed radiographically. Rarely, as in patients with atrial septal defect, a huge left-to-right shunt may exist with radiographically normal pulmonary vascularity (see Chapter 19). In such patients, for some unknown reason, the increased velocity of blood flow does not stimulate enlargement of the pulmonary arteries. Therefore, normal pulmonary vascularity on a thoracic roentgenogram does not definitely exclude a large left-to-right shunt, particularly among patients with an atrial septal defect who have normal pulmonary artery pressures.

In addition to increased volume and speed of blood flow, the pulmonary arteries may also enlarge because of increased pressure (pulmonary hypertension). Pressure dilatation involves primarily the larger pulmonary arteries. For some unknown reason, dilatation sometimes does not occur in spite of severe pulmonary hypertension. In our experience, this is found in patients who have had high pulmonary resistance since birth (see Chapter 75).

After the technical factors that may alter the radiographic appearance of the pulmonary vasculature are considered, the central and the peripheral vasculature must be analyzed. Because most of the left pulmonary artery is obscured by the cardiac silhouette, more information is derived by studying the arteries in the right lung. The appearance of the pulmonary vessels in the left lung, however, must also be observed through the cardiac shadow, because a discrepancy may exist between the right and the left pulmonary blood flow. In young patients with a large thymus, the radiographic evaluation of the pulmonary vasculature is particularly difficult, because both hila may be obscured, and only a small peripheral portion of the lung may be visible.

The pulmonary arteries radiate in an orderly fashion from the right hilum and the right lower lobe pulmonary artery forms a characteristic comma-shaped density that is easily seen. It has been measured to diagnose the presence of a left-to-right shunt, but such measurements are not better than the intuitive judgment of an experienced observer. The characteristic orderly fan-shaped emanation of pulmonary arteries from the right hilum allows radiographic differentiation of pulmonary from the bronchial arteries, which have a random distribution (see Fig 5–12).

On a satisfactory thoracic roentgenogram, both the artery and vein of the right lower lobe are clearly seen (Fig 5–29). The right upper lobe pulmonary vein lies laterally to the upper lobe artery, but usually it cannot be seen distinctly, although it is commonly pointed out and retouched in textbooks. In at least 50% of the cases, the right upper lobe pulmonary artery and vein are superimposed.

On a posteroanterior projection, the confluence of the right lower lobe pulmonary vein may be enlarged and simulate a mass lesion (Fig 5–30). Also, in a left anterior oblique projection, the right lower lobe pulmonary vein may be observed end-on and simulate a nodule (Fig 5–31). In contrast to a true mass, the density caused by a pulmonary

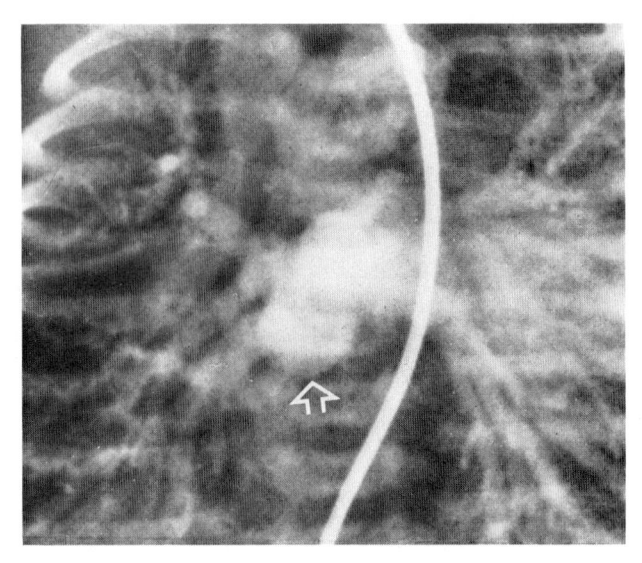

FIG 5–30.
Levophase of a pulmonary arteriogram; normal prominence of confluence of pulmonary veins simulates mass *(open arrow)*. This "structure" may also be seen in adults on a plain roentgenogram and should not be confused with a true mass.

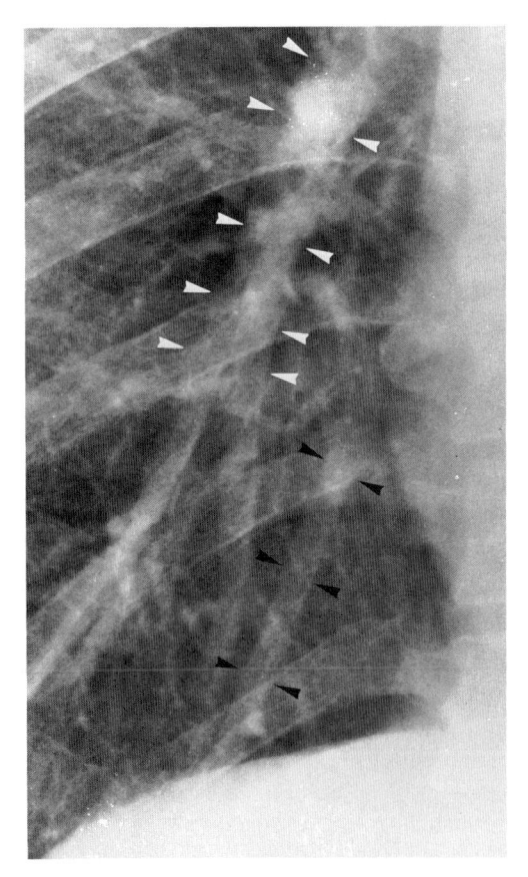

FIG 5–29.
Thoracic roentgenogram, posteroanterior projection, of right lower lung field (magnified view). "Comma" shadow of right lower pulmonary artery *(white arrows)*. Right lower lobe pulmonary vein *(black arrows)* has a lower and more medial course.

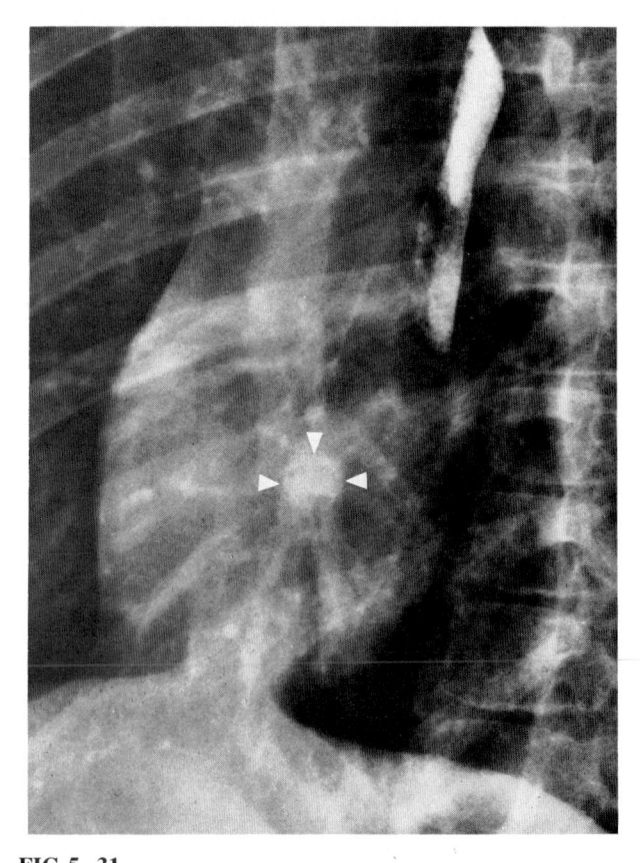

FIG 5–31.
Thoracic roentgenogram, left anterior oblique projection; right lower lobe pulmonary vein *(white arrows)* on-end view of right lower lobe pulmonary vein simulates pulmonary nodule. However, this nodular density disappears with different obliquities; a true mass density does not.

vein disappears in different oblique views, whereas the density of a mass lesion remains.

Normally the pulmonary arteries are not tortuous, so few vessels are seen end-on. The end-on view of the artery and bronchus to the anterior segment of the upper lobes can be used advantageously to judge the size of the pulmonary arteries. The diameter of the normal pulmonary artery is similar to that of the adjacent bronchus (Fig 5–32), whereas in a left-to-right shunt, the pulmonary artery is larger than the bronchus. In venous pulmonary hypertension the arterial diameter is also larger than the bronchus due to redistribution of blood flow. If interstitial pulmonary edema is present due to increased pulmonary venous pressure, the external diameters of both bronchi and arteries will change due to peribronchial "cuffing."

In addition to the analysis of the pulmonary vascularity in the right lung on a posteroanterior projection, observation of the right pulmonary artery on a lateral projection is valuable. On such a projection, the right pulmonary artery lies in the same direction as the x-ray beam, and consequently the artery is seen on-end. Without opacification, only the portion of the vessel that is surrounded by lung can be observed. In the right hilum, the artery forms a sharply defined round density in front of the bronchial bifurcation. Enlargement of the right pulmonary artery may be an important clue in the diagnosis of a left-to-right shunt, particularly if the condition of the pulmonary vascularity is unclear or if the right pulmonary artery is partially obscured by the heart on the posteroanterior projection (Fig 5–33).

The plain-film density of the right hilum is also important in the interpretation of hilar mass lesions, which create abnormal added densities on oblique and lateral projections.

Any large communication between the systemic and the pulmonary circulations, except for shunts at the atrial level, also causes increased pulmonary arterial pressure. This condition, pulmonary hypertension, cannot be diagnosed with certainty radiographically. However, it does induce increased tortuosity of the pulmonary arteries and increases the number of pulmonary blood vessels seen end-on. In many cases, however, pulmonary artery pressure cannot be predicted from the radiograph.

As pulmonary vascular disease and thus pulmonary arterial resistance increase, as in Eisenmenger's complex, the radiographic findings become more definite, and a discrepancy appears between the size of the central and peripheral pulmonary arteries (Fig 5–34). "Pruning" of the peripheral pulmonary arterial vasculature is a fairly consistent radiographic sign of hypertension secondary to increased vascular resistance. Unfortunately for the radiologist, some adults with atrial septal defect and normal pulmonary artery pressure also reveal pruning of the peripheral pulmonary vasculature.

Increased pulmonary arterial pressure may by itself enlarge the central pulmonary arteries. The radiographic findings of a left-to-right shunt with severe pulmonary hypertension (Eisenmenger's physiology) and primary pulmonary hypertension (no previous left-to-right shunt) may be identical.

In the occasional patient with a ventricular septal defect who never develops a significant left-to-right shunt because of persistence of the elevated fetal pulmonary vascular resistance, as well as in some patients with primary pulmonary hypertension, the pulmonary arteries may not enlarge at all (see Chapter 75). Consequently, a normal radiographic appearance of the pulmonary arterial tree does not exclude severe pulmonary hypertension or a large left-to-right shunt.

The most reliable and definitive radiographic sign of long-standing pulmonary hypertension is pulmonary ath-

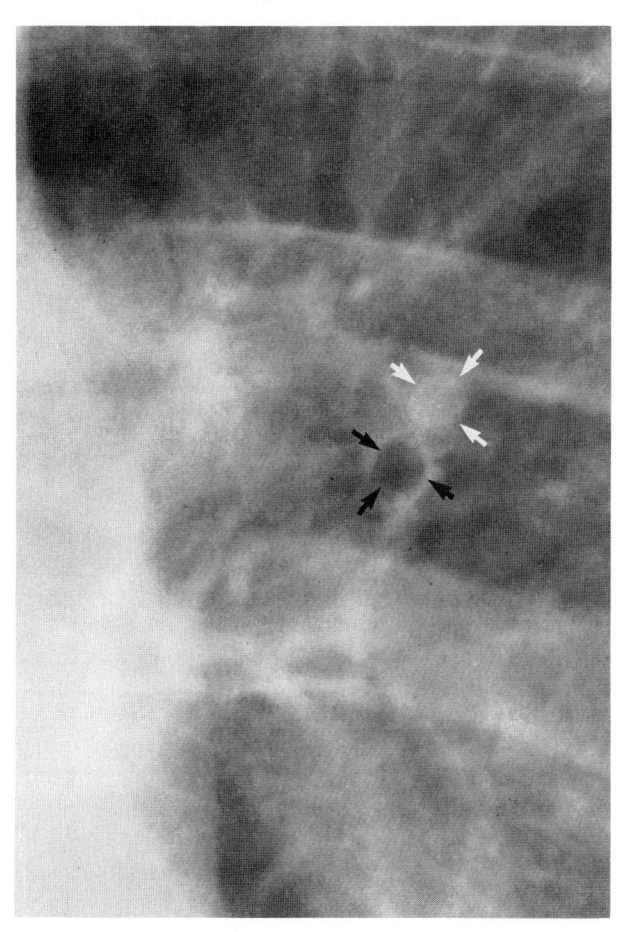

FIG 5–32.
Thoracic roentgenogram, posteroanterior projection in patient with normal pulmonary flow. End-on view of the pulmonary arterial branch and bronchus to anterior segment of left upper lobe; artery *(white arrows)* and bronchus *(black arrows)* are of almost equal size.

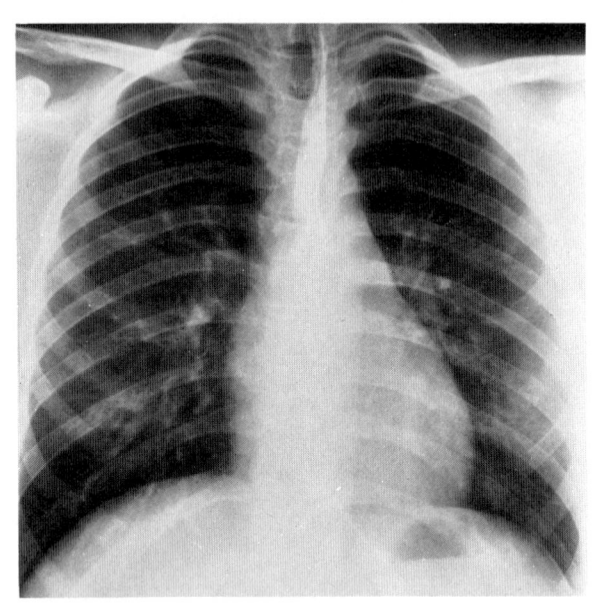

FIG 5-33.
Thoracic roentgenogram in patients with moderate left-to-right shunt **A,** posteroanterior projection; radiographic findings are at upper limits of normal. **B,** lateral projection; characteristic density of right pulmonary artery *(arrows)* in front of trachea is enlarged, suggesting a left-to-right shunt. This is a helpful but not pathognomonic finding, because other vessels in the hilum may enlarge the right pulmonary artery density on a lateral view.

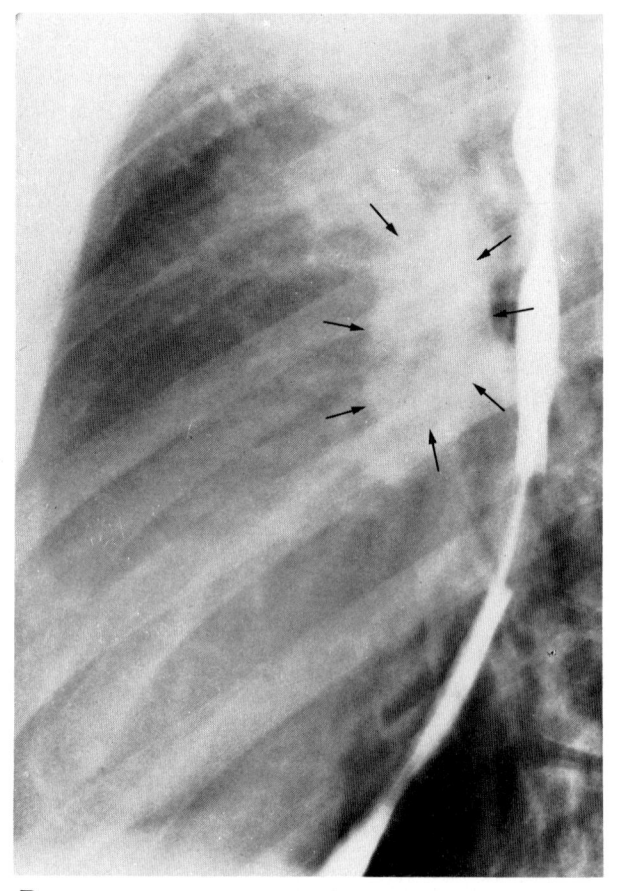

erosclerosis. Normally atherosclerosis is confined to the systemic circulation, the pulmonary arterial bed being spared because of the normally low pressure. However, with long-standing severe pulmonary hypertension, atherosclerotic plaques develop in the pulmonary arteries. When they calcify, the plaque can be seen radiographically, and this is a reliable sign of long-standing pulmonary hypertension (Fig 5-35). Although rarely a jet lesion in valvular pulmonary stenosis may calcify, these plaques are located on the anterior wall of the main pulmonary artery rather than in the right or left pulmonary arteries.

THE THORAX IN CONGENITAL HEART DISEASE

Cardiac films must be interpreted systematically. In patients with cardiac disease, the heart should not be analyzed initially just because it lies in the center of the film, because experience has shown that once the interest of the observer is focused on a central structure such as the heart or mediastinum, information on the periphery of the radiograph is missed. A logical and practical approach to chest interpretation is to sweep the periphery of the film first in either a clockwise or counterclockwise direction (Fig 5-36). The following important observations should be made during this initial step:

1. Are the L or R markers, indicating left or right, in the proper locations? If not, has the technician made a mistake, or does the patient have an abnormal body situs, which is commonly associated with congenital heart disease?
2. Is the liver in the normal position? A liver located in the right upper quadrant confirms a normal situs, whereas a midline position is virtually diagnostic for abdominal heterotaxia (see Chapter 58).
3. Is the gastric air bubble in the normal position in the left upper quadrant? If not, this strongly suggests abdominal heterotaxia.

After these observations have been made, the bony thorax should be examined by looking at each of the ribs in a systematic way. Study of the bony cage may be helpful in three ways:

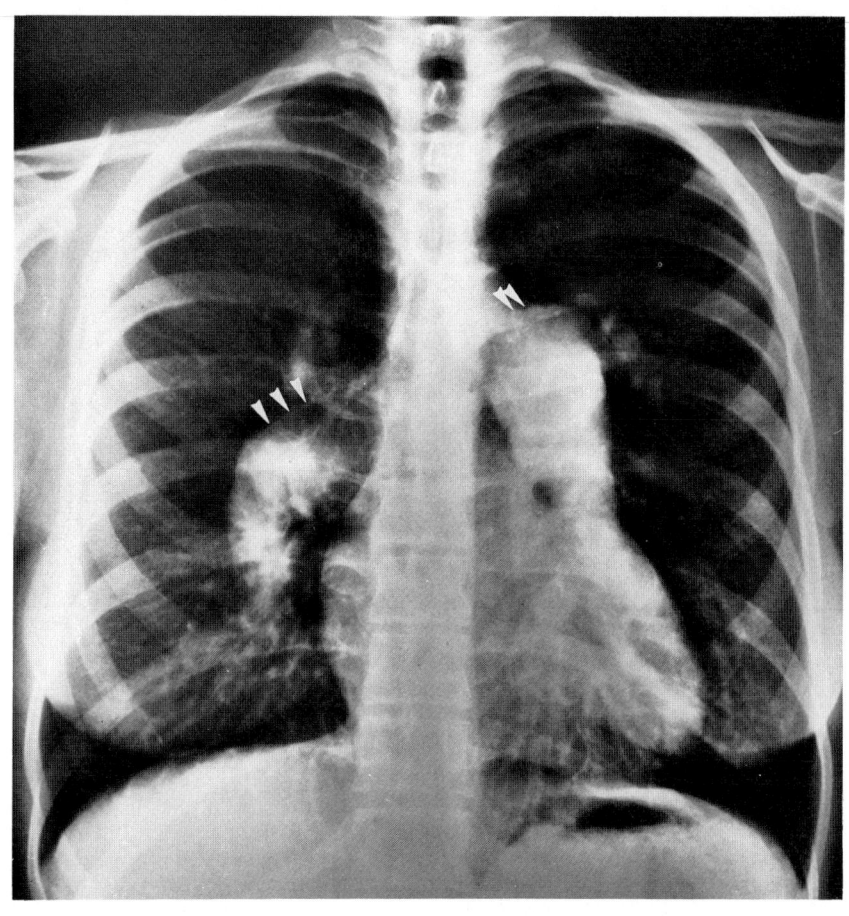

FIG 5-34.
Thoracic roentgenogram, posteroanterior projection, in patient with severe long-standing pulmonary hypertension shows enlarged central pulmonary arteries and normal or decreased size of peripheral arteries ("pruning"). Calcifications in the pulmonary arteries are visible faintly *(arrows)*.

1. The incidence of rib anomalies is higher in patients with congenital heart disease.

2. Notching of the lower rib margins indicates enlargement and collateral blood flow through the intercostal arteries (or rarely, caused by enlarged veins or nerves), which occurs in coarctation of the aorta, after cardiac operations in which the subclavian artery is divided and in certain other cardiac anomalies with the pulmonary circulation derived from collateral arteries.

3. Observation of the rib cage permits identification of previous cardiac operations. The site of operation suggests the type; thus, the cardiac condition can be predicted with a high degree of accuracy from the roentgenogram alone, thereby stunning the referring physician.

Bony Abnormalities in Congenital Heart Disease

Bony changes are common in patients with congenital heart disease and may suggest the type of cardiac abnormality. For example, whereas clubbing of the fingers is common in cyanotic heart disease, pulmonary osteoarthropathy is exceedingly rare (1 in 850 patients). Also, a higher incidence of gout has been reported, particularly in patients with cyanotic heart disease and an elevated hemoglobin level. These patients also have elevated serum uric acid concentrations that roughly correlate with the hemoglobin level.

A significantly higher incidence of congenital vertebral anomalies, such as faulty segmentation and hemivertebra formation, occurs in patients with congenital heart disease (Fig 5-37), and these anomalies contribute to the higher incidence of scoliosis. Although hemivertebrae may be associated with scoliosis in infancy and childhood, during adolescence idiopathic scoliosis may be present in 66% of cyanotic patients. In acyanotic patients, the incidence is much lower (about 20%).[1]

In patients with a congenital cardiac malformation, skeletal maturation is delayed or, rarely, accelerated. One of the more characteristic deformities is premature fusion of the sternal ossification centers, which occurs in about

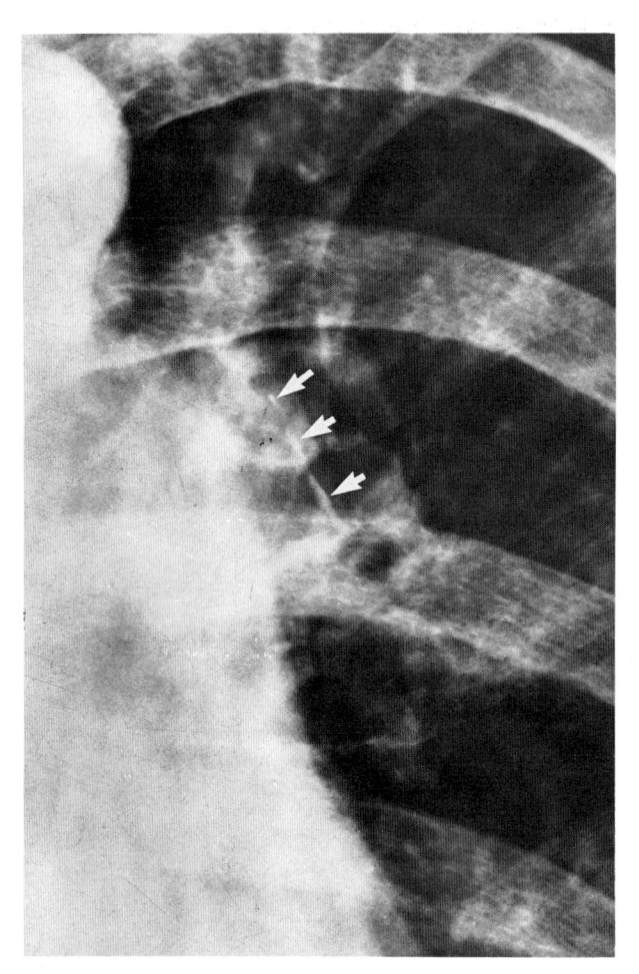

FIG 5-35.
Thoracic roentgenogram, magnified view in patient with longstanding pulmonary hypertension. Calcified atherosclerotic plaques *(arrows)* are visible in the left pulmonary artery.

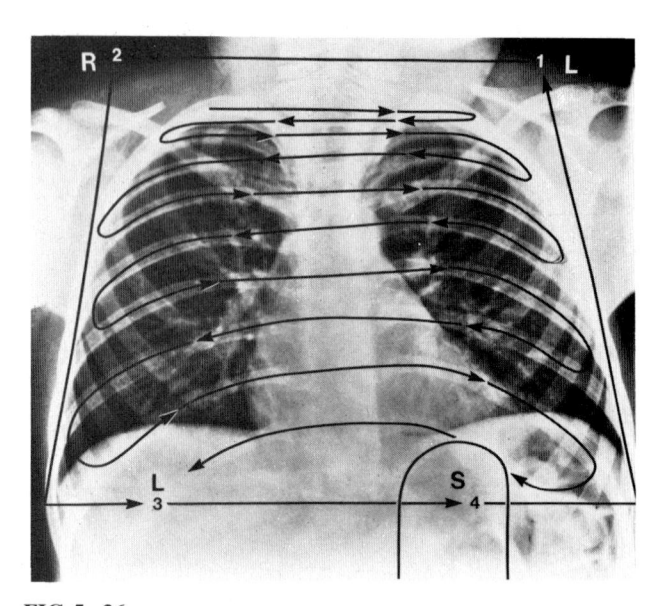

FIG 5-36.
A useful pattern for systematic evaluation of a chest roentgenogram. The observer starts in the right upper corner and moves to the left upper corner, observing the *R* and *L* markers (*1* and *2*, respectively). The lateral ribs along right chest wall and liver *(L)* are observed *(3)*. Scan continues toward the stomach *(S) (4)*. Searching sweep completed along left lateral rib cage, returning to left upper corner. Next, each posterior rib is scanned. Finally, the pulmonary vasculature and cardiac silhouette are analyzed.

50% of cyanotic patients, particularly in those with tetralogy of Fallot, compared with 2% in the normal population. The resulting pectus carinatum deformity ranges from mild to severe (Fig 5-38). Anterior bowing of the sternum also occurs with right atrial and ventricular enlargement as in atrial septal defect (see Chapter 19).

In 75% of patients with Down syndrome, the number of ossification centers in the sternum is increased (hypersegmentation of the sternum) (Fig 5-39). In the normal population, this occurs in 17%.

Rarely, a specific diagnosis of the cardiac disease can be made just on the basis of bone involvement, except for mucopolysaccharidoses (Fig 5-40).

The Postoperative Thorax in Congenital Heart Disease

The surgeon gains access to the heart either through the sternum (sternotomy) or through the right or left side

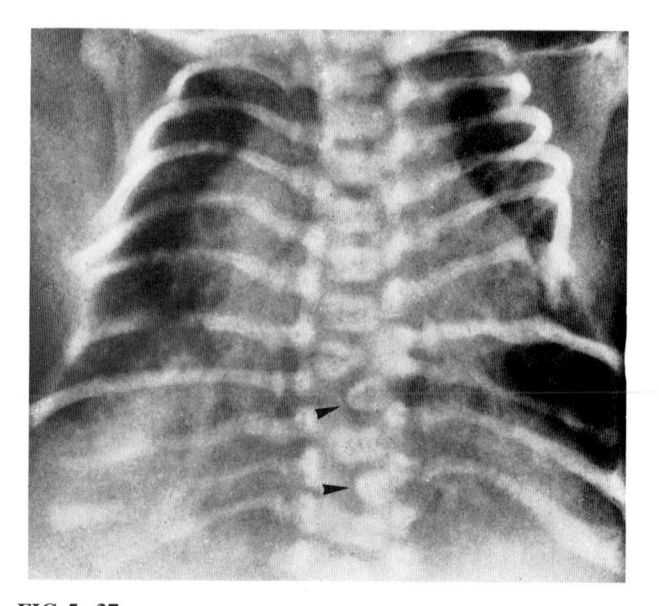

FIG 5-37.
Thoracic roentgenograph, posteroanterior projection, showing enlarged heart. Numerous hemivertebrae and rib deformities are visible. Early scoliosis.

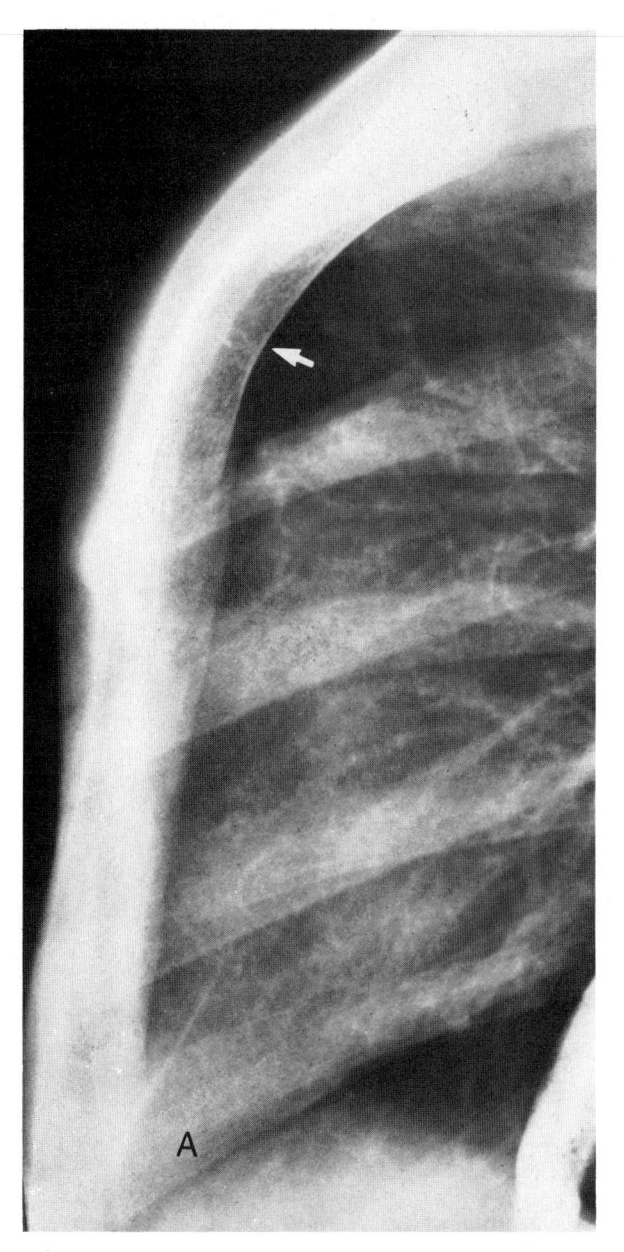

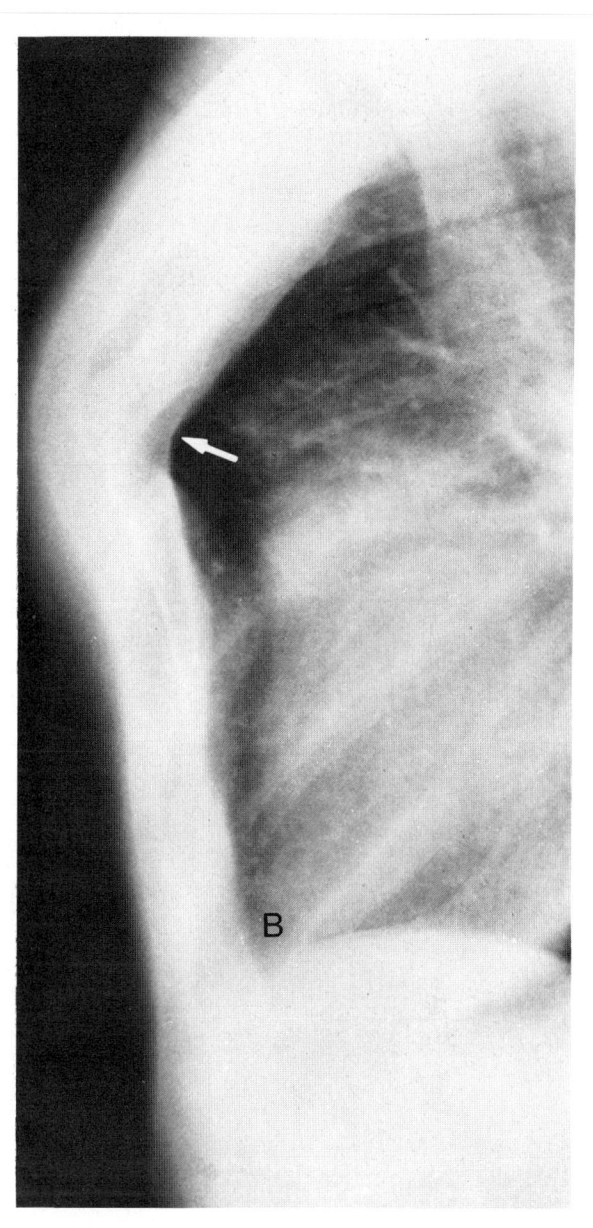

FIG 5–38.
Thoracic roentgenogram, lateral view, showing sternum in patient with tetralogy of Fallot. **A,** premature fusion of manubrial-sternal junction *(arrow);* ossification centers of body of sternum are fused. **B,** premature fusion of the manubrial-sternal junction *(arrow),* causing severe pectus carinatum deformity.

of the rib cage (thoracotomy). The sternum can be split transversely or longitudinally. Formerly, transverse sternotomies were widely used, but this caused considerable thoracic deformities. Currently, the preferred technique is a longitudinal sternotomy. At the completion of the operation, the sternum is closed by either wires or metal bands, which are readily visible on a radiograph, particularly on the lateral view (Fig 5–41).

There are two types of thoracotomy. In one, adjacent ribs are forcefully spread and the thoracic cavity entered between them. At the end of the operation, the surgeon ties the two ribs together with either suture material (nonopaque) or metal bands (radiopaque). In either case, the distance between the separated ribs is usually decreased, and this narrowed interspace can be observed on the roentgenogram (Fig 5–42). With the other technique, a rib is resected, totally in which case the permanent absence is noted radiographically, or the rib is resected subperi-

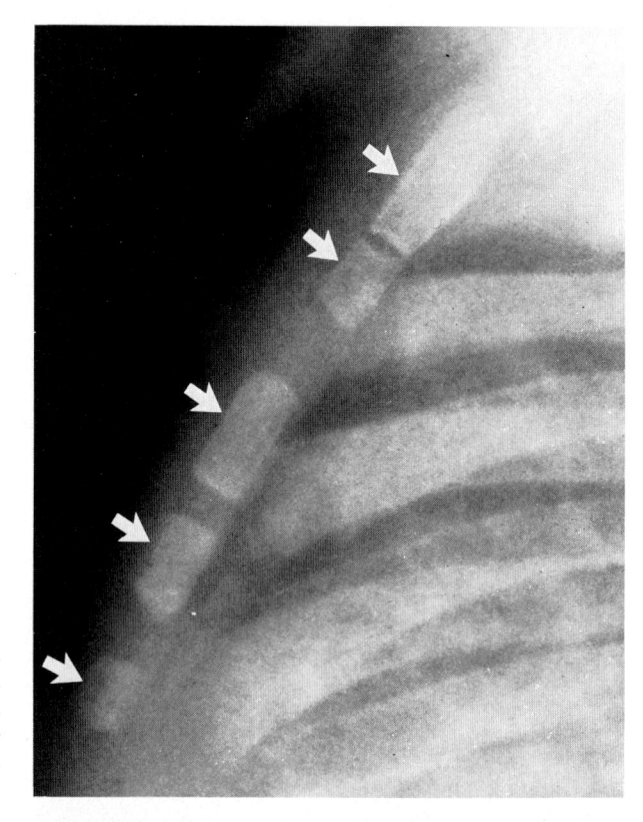

FIG 5–39.
Thoracic roentgenogram, lateral projection, shows sternum in patient with trisomy 21 (Down syndrome) and atrioventricular canal. Increased number of ossification centers *(arrows);* this finding is present in 75% of patients with Down syndrome. Normally there are only four ossification centers. (Courtesy of Hugh Williams.)

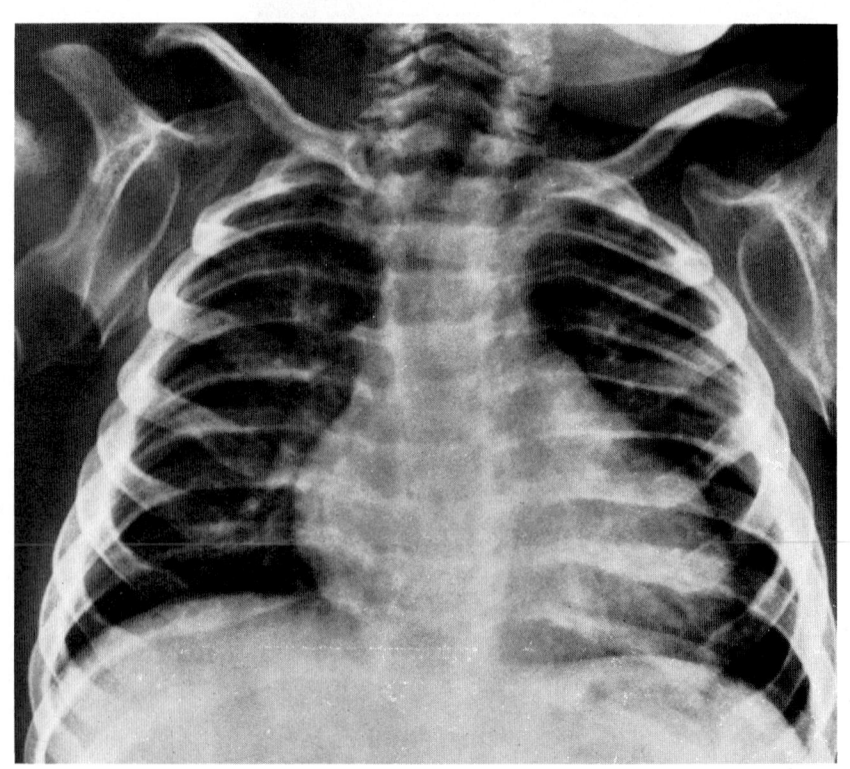

FIG 5–40.
Patient with cardiomegaly and normal pulmonary vasculature. Because of the characteristic bony changes involving the ribs, clavicles, and scapulae, a diagnosis of cardiac involvement by mucopolysaccharoidosis can be ventured.

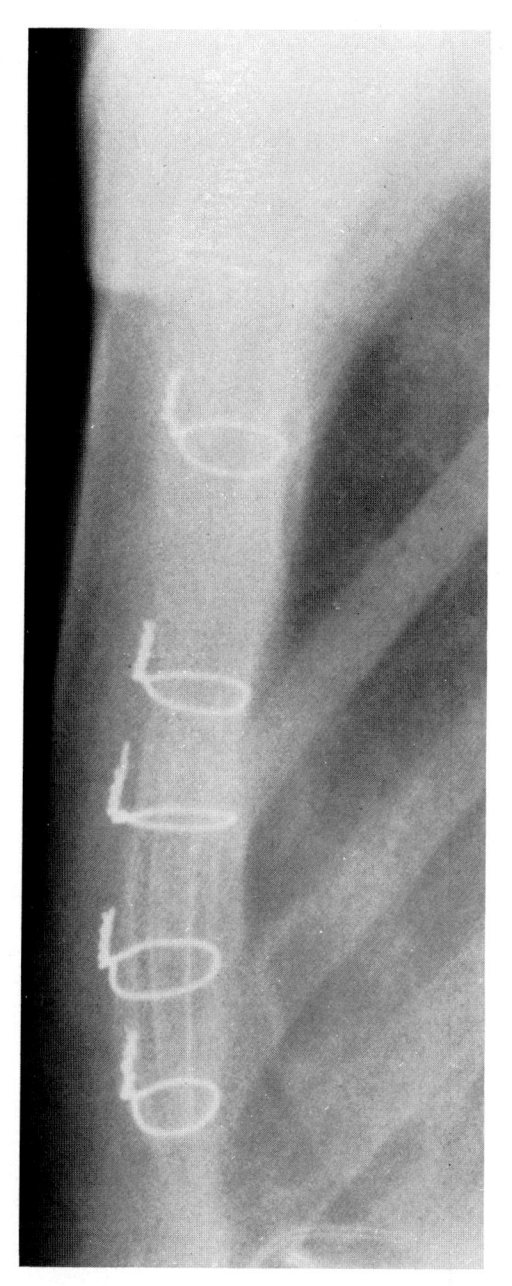

FIG 5–41.
Thoracic roentgenogram showing sternum in patient who has undergone a corrective cardiac operation through a longitudinal sternotomy. Sternum is closed by wire sutures.

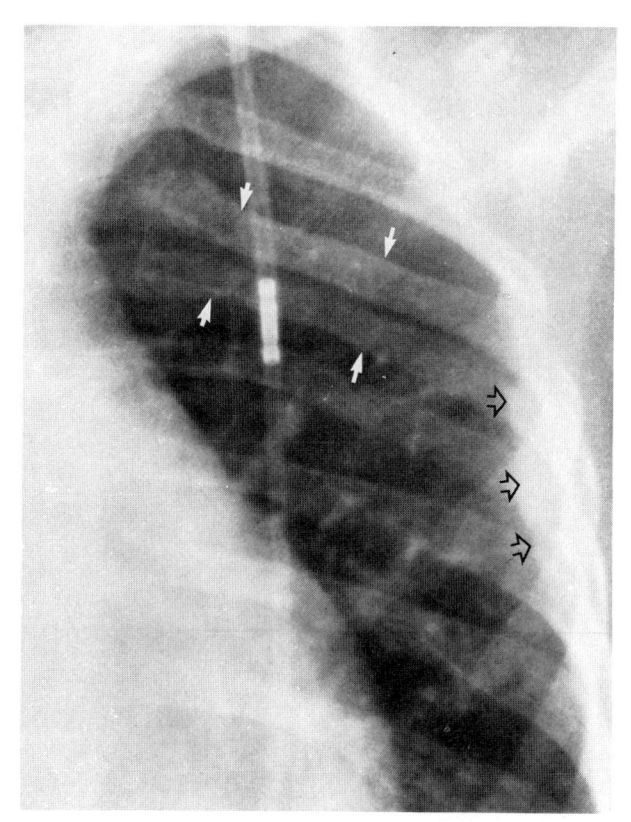

FIG 5–42.
Left thoracic cage after correction of coarctation of aorta during which left fourth and fifth ribs were tied together. Distance between the two ribs *(white arrows)* is decreased. Residual pleural changes along left lateral chest wall *(black arrows)* indicate that operation was recent.

osteally, in which case the rib regenerates. Radiographically, the latter is evident as an irregular rib contour (Fig 5–43); but after many years, these irregularities disappear, so the previous rib resection may not be evident radiographically. A recent thoracotomy also can be diagnosed radiographically by observing the residual pleural fluid and soft tissue swelling at the site of incision (see Fig 5–42).

Except for corrective surgery for coarctation of the aorta, patent ductus arteriosus, and anomalous origin of coronary arteries from pulmonary trunk, a thoracotomy is usually performed for a palliative procedure, whereas a sternotomy is used for corrective surgery. One exception to the latter rule is the insertion of a central shunt in a cyanotic infant.

The operative approach to various cardiac procedures is well established. Therefore, a basic knowledge of cardiac surgery is valuable in radiographic interpretation and diagnosis.

Left-Sided Thoracotomy

1. Patent ductus arteriosus is usually ligated and divided through a left thoracotomy because it is located in the midthorax. It can also be ligated through a sternotomy, although this is more difficult and so is used only if a midline sternotomy is required to repair another cardiac condition simultaneously.

2. Repair of coarctation of the aorta. The thoracic aorta lies posteriorly and can be easily exposed through this approach.

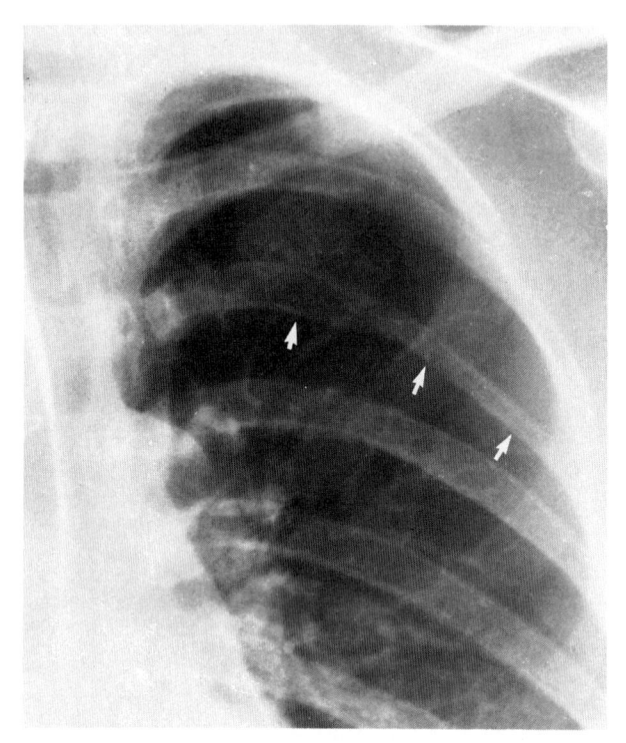

FIG 5-43.
Thoracic roentgenogram after repair of coarctation of aorta. Left fourth rib was resected subperiosteally and has regenerated in irregular fashion *(arrows)*. A previous left thoracotomy is obvious. Patent ductus arteriosus or coarctation is the most likely diagnosis.

3. Pulmonary artery banding procedures can be performed by either a left thoracotomy or a midline sternotomy.

4. Surgery for aberrant coronary artery.

5. Blalock-Taussig shunts usually in patients with right aortic arch (see Chapter 30).

5. Systemic-to-pulmonary arterial shunts such as left-sided Blalock-Taussig shunts, Potts anastomoses, or shunts with synthetic grafts. Blalock-Taussig shunts are usually performed on the side opposite the aortic arch, so the subclavian artery originating from the innominate artery does not tend to kink as it is brought down to the pulmonary artery. However, this rule is not absolute, because a shunt is sometimes performed on the same side as the aorta, and in some cases bilateral shunts may be necessary.

6. Closed mitral commissurotomy. Patients with mitral stenosis are usually adult and female. Radiographically there are clues to the presence of a mitral commissurotomy; the pulmonary artery segment is prominent because the surgeon resects the left atrial appendage. Therefore, the cardiac silhouette no longer has the typical "mitral" configuration.

Right-Sided Thoracotomy

1. Systemic-to-pulmonary artery shunts in cyanotic heart disease, usually in patients with a left-sided aortic arch and shunts using synthetic grafts.

2. Waterston shunts. In this procedure, a communication is created between the right pulmonary artery and the ascending aorta.

3. Glenn procedure. In this procedure, the superior vena cava is anastomosed to the pulmonary artery.

4. Closed atrial septostomy using the Blalock-Hanlon technique.

5. Mitral valve procedures, such as valve replacement or open commissurotomy. Because the left atrium is posteriorly located, it can also be approached from the right thorax. Usually, however, mitral valves are replaced through a midline sternotomy.

Radiographic evidence of both a thoracotomy and a sternotomy strongly suggests a previous palliative procedure, followed by a corrective operation. Therefore, not only can the underlying cardiac condition be diagnosed, but the operative history of the patient can be predicted. For example, a left-sided thoracotomy and a midline sternotomy in a patient with a right aortic arch are virtually diagnostic of a previous systemic-pulmonary shunt, followed by corrective surgery for tetralogy of Fallot (Fig 5-44). A left-sided thoracotomy and sternotomy suggest

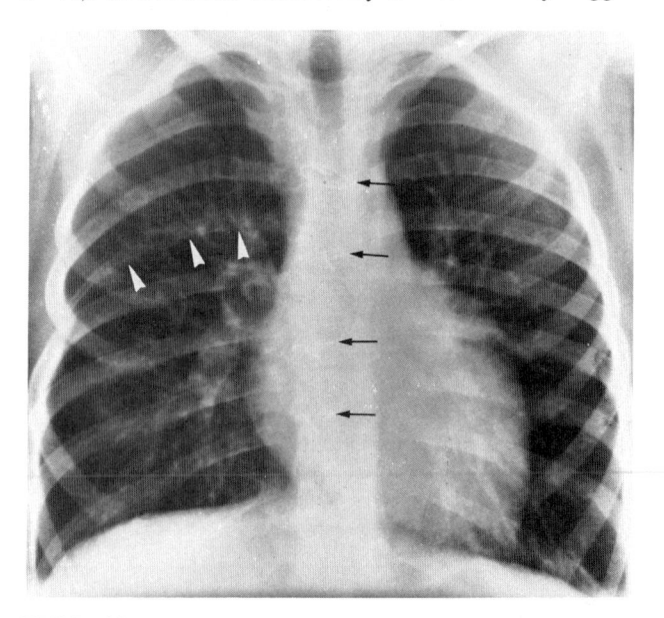

FIG 5-44.
Previous right thoracotomy *(white arrows)* and corrective surgery *(black arrows)* with left aortic arch. Likely histories: right Blalock-Taussig shunt opposite the arch and correction of the tetralogy or previous Blalock-Hanlon operation and correction for transposition. Cardiac contour supports the latter diagnosis.

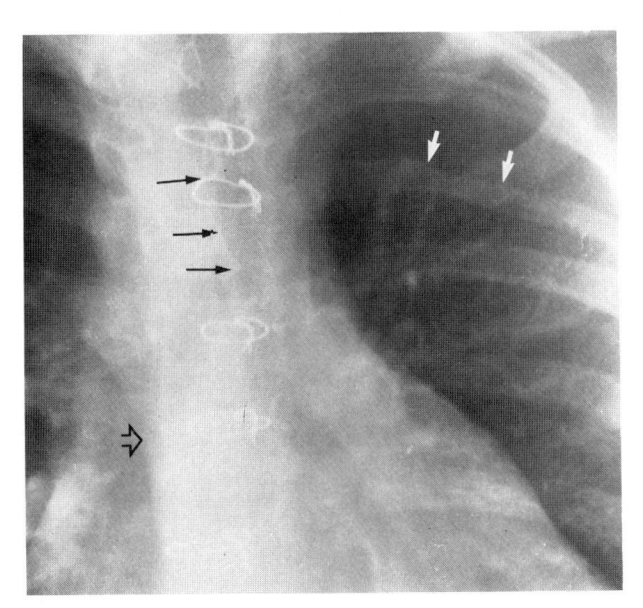

FIG 5–45.
Thoracic roentgenogram, posteroanterior projection; surgical history determined by roentgenogram. Patient has right aortic arch, tracheal deviation to the left *(black arrows)*, descending aorta on the right *(open arrow)*, regenerated left fourth rib, and sternal sutures. Diagnosis: tetralogy of Fallot, previous left Blalock-Taussig shunt, and subsequent corrective surgery.

previous repair of either a coarctation or a patent ductus arteriosus, followed by corrective surgery of an intracardiac condition, probably congenital aortic stenosis or ventricular septal defect. A right-sided thoracotomy, midline sternotomy, and left aortic arch suggest either a previous Blalock-Hanlon operation and a corrective operation for transposition of the great vessels (Fig 5–45) or a systemic pulmonary shunt and corrective surgery for tetralogy of Fallot.

ESTIMATION OF HEART SIZE

Once all the technical factors that alter apparent cardiac size and configuration have been studied, one may proceed with an estimate of cardiac size. Because of the oblique position of the heart within the thorax, its long axis is foreshortened on both the posteroanterior and lateral views. Cardiac length, therefore, depends largely on the position of the heart in the thorax and the degree of inspiration. Consequently, the radiologic estimate of cardiac size is just that: an estimate.

A large amount of literature has accumulated about cardiac measurements and volume determinations. Nonetheless, experience has shown that such measurements are impractical in everyday radiography and that the experienced radiologist may be as accurate in his or her esti-

mates as are complex calculations. Still, the inexperienced physician prefers measurements with a ruler over judgment, and the simplest and most popular measurement is the cardiothoracic ratio: The transverse diameter of the cardiac silhouette is measured at the level of the diaphragm on a posteroanterior projection and related to the transverse diameter of the chest. However, this ratio is dependent largely on the position of the heart in the chest and on the position of the diaphragm. Furthermore, it ignores information from the lateral view. Therefore, it gives inaccurate information in patients with a rotated heart or with a large thoracic cavity. Rotation of the heart may result in an "enlarged" cardiac silhouette in one view but a normal or small silhouette on the right-angle view (see Fig 5–26). The correlation between thoracic size and cardiac size is poor, although the cardiothoracic ratio compensates somewhat for patient's size, because a larger patient tends to have a larger thorax and heart.

For an accurate estimate of cardiac size, two views obtained at right angles, preferably the posteroanterior and lateral projection, must be available, because if the heart is enlarged in one projection because of axis rotation, it will appear normal or small on the right-angle projection (see Fig 5–26). Thus, if both views are considered, the cardiac volume can be estimated. Because cardiac size is an estimate, it should not be expressed numerically. It is adequate to describe the heart size as "normal," "borderline" or "questionably enlarged," "slightly enlarged," "moderately enlarged," and "severely enlarged." Semiquantitative grading on a 1 to 4+ scale is also acceptable and indeed is valuable clinically. It correlates well with cardiac measurements derived from echocardiography or postmortem examination.

In summary, whereas the cardiothoracic ratio gives only a single linear measurement of the cardiac silhouette, right-angle views permit estimates of cardiac volume and are therefore much more meaningful.

FOUR VIEWS OF THE HEART

The views of the heart are made with the image receptor (radiographic film, imaging intensifier, fluoroscopic screen) either in front or in back of the patient. In chest radiography, the radiographic film is in front of the patient to minimize enlargement of the cardiac silhouette (see Fig 5–16). This projection is posteroanterior, meaning that the anterior side of the chest is close to the radiographic film. Posteroanterior and anteroposterior projections are identical, but the heart will appear larger on the anteroposterior view. By placing the patient obliquely with the right side close to the image receptor, one may obtain a right anterior oblique view that is identical to a left posterior oblique projection.

Similarly, the lateral view of the chest can be made with the image receptor on the left or on the right side. Most commonly, the left side of the patient will be placed against the radiographic film to minimize magnification, because the heart is located primarily in the left thoracic cavity. This projection is a left lateral view, meaning that the left side of the patient is close to the radiographic film. If the right side of the patient is placed against the image receptor, an identical right lateral view will be obtained.

There are two true views of the heart: (1) the en face view, which requires about 45 degrees of chest rotation (right anterior oblique or left posterior oblique) and the heart is portrayed in its longest dimension; and (2) the end-on view, which requires approximately a 60-degree chest rotation (left anterior oblique and right posterior oblique) and results in the greatest foreshortening of the long axis of the heart. All other projections, including the posteroanterior and lateral, are oblique views of the heart.

A "complete cardiac series" consists of four projections, each of which is valuable. However, because of cost and amount of radiation exposure of a complete series, commonly only the posteroanterior and lateral views are obtained. The concern about radiation exposure is unjustified, because the dose of a single posteroanterior chest x-ray in an average adult is only about 20 mR. In contrast, the dose from biplane cineradiography is about 40,000 mR/min, or 2,000 times more. The posteroanterior view is the most informative, but it should be supplemented at least by a left lateral projection. Both views should be obtained during a barium swallow, because this permits a more accurate evaluation of left atrial size and demonstrates important features such as coarctation of the aorta, vascular sling, bronchial collaterals, and the location of the aortic arch. Barium in the esophagus does not interfere with the interpretation of cardiac films.

On conventional x-ray films, the cardiac silhouette is formed by the interface between the heart and the air in the lungs, so only the cardiac structures bordering the lungs are demonstrated. Intracardiac structures are not seen unless they are calcified, although rarely some faintly radiolucent epicardial fat is seen. Epicardial fat can sometimes be seen on fluoroscopy or, better, on cine fluorography. If visible, it can be used to diagnose pericardial effusion, because the fat will be separated from the pericardium by fluid. Cardiac fat may accumulate near the apex or in the right or left cardiophrenic angle, forming a "fat pad" that should not be confused with cardiomegaly. Fat pads are less common in children (Fig 5–46).

Major vascular structures and cardiac chambers form characteristic bulges because they are outlined by air in the

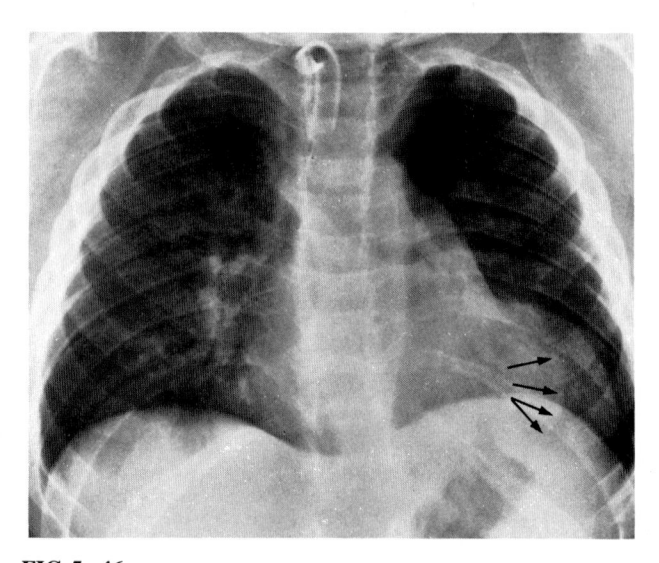

FIG 5–46.
Thoracic roentgenogram, posteroanterior projection, shows large left pericardial fat pad. Interface *(arrows)* between the ventricle and the more radiolucent fat is well seen *(arrows)*. A fat pad should not be confused with true cardiomegaly. If there is doubt, a more definitive diagnosis can be made by laminography, computed tomography, or nuclear magnetic resonance.

lungs. These bulges are best referred to as "segments." It is therefore more correct to speak, for example, of a "prominent pulmonary artery segment" than of an "enlarged pulmonary artery," because the bulge where the pulmonary artery is normally located may not be caused by the pulmonary artery at all.

Because only those portions of the vascular structures bordering the lungs are visible, no conclusions can be drawn about their size. The aortic segment (aortic knob) or pulmonary segment can be prominent radiographically but yet of normal size anatomically, because prominence depends not only on the size of the vessel but also on its position in relation to the lung. Similarly, the aorta or pulmonary artery may be greatly enlarged but not prominent on a thoracic roentgenogram.

It must also be remembered that prominence does not necessarily indicate pathology, because the normal heart may have prominent segments whenever a vascular structure protrudes further into a lung field so that more of it is outlined by air. However, in contrast to the reading of thoracic roentgenograms of patients without cardiac conditions, the films of patients with congenital heart disease are deliberately overread to make a diagnosis. In many cases the findings are still within the range of normal. Thus, a "prominent pulmonary artery segment" is suggestive of valvar pulmonary stenosis but is still within the range of normal, because normal persons may have a prominent pulmonary artery, particularly if they are adolescents or have clockwise cardiac rotation (see Fig 5–28).

The Posteroanterior View (Figs 5–47 and 5–48)

The heart rests on the anterior portion of the diaphragm. Consequently, the undersurface of the heart is not outlined by air and is invisible unless there is a large amount of gas in the gastric fundus. The highest portion of the dome of the diaphragm usually lies posterior to the heart (see Fig 5–49). Therefore, through the cardiac shadow, the diaphragm can be seen, sharply outlined by the lung (see Fig 5–48). With marked cardiomegaly, the heart may extend so far posteriorly that the dome of the diaphragm and therefore the diaphragmatic silhouette disappear. In a patient with an unusually shaped diaphragm, as well as on a lordotic projection, the left hemidiaphragm may be invisible. Thus, because cardiac films of infants are generally in a lordotic projection, the dome of the left hemidiaphragm may be invisible even with a normal-sized heart. Pulmonary consolidation or pleural fluid are the most common causes of nonappearance of the dome of the diaphragm through the heart in the adult.

The right upper cardiac border is formed by the right innominate vein and the superior vena cava. With enlargement and elongation of the aorta, as in patients with aortic stenosis, the elderly, and persons with rotation of the heart, the right cardiac border may be formed by the ascending aorta (see Figs 5–47 and 5–48). The lower right cardiac border is formed by the right atrial segment. Only a small posterior portion of the right atrium is visible, outlined by air. With deep inspiration, the supradiaphragmatic portion of the inferior vena cava may be seen (see Fig 5–48).

The left upper border of the cardiac silhouette is formed by the aortic knob, which anatomically is the posterior portion of the aortic arch. In older patients, the entire descending thoracic aorta is usually seen through the mediastinum as a straight double density extending to the

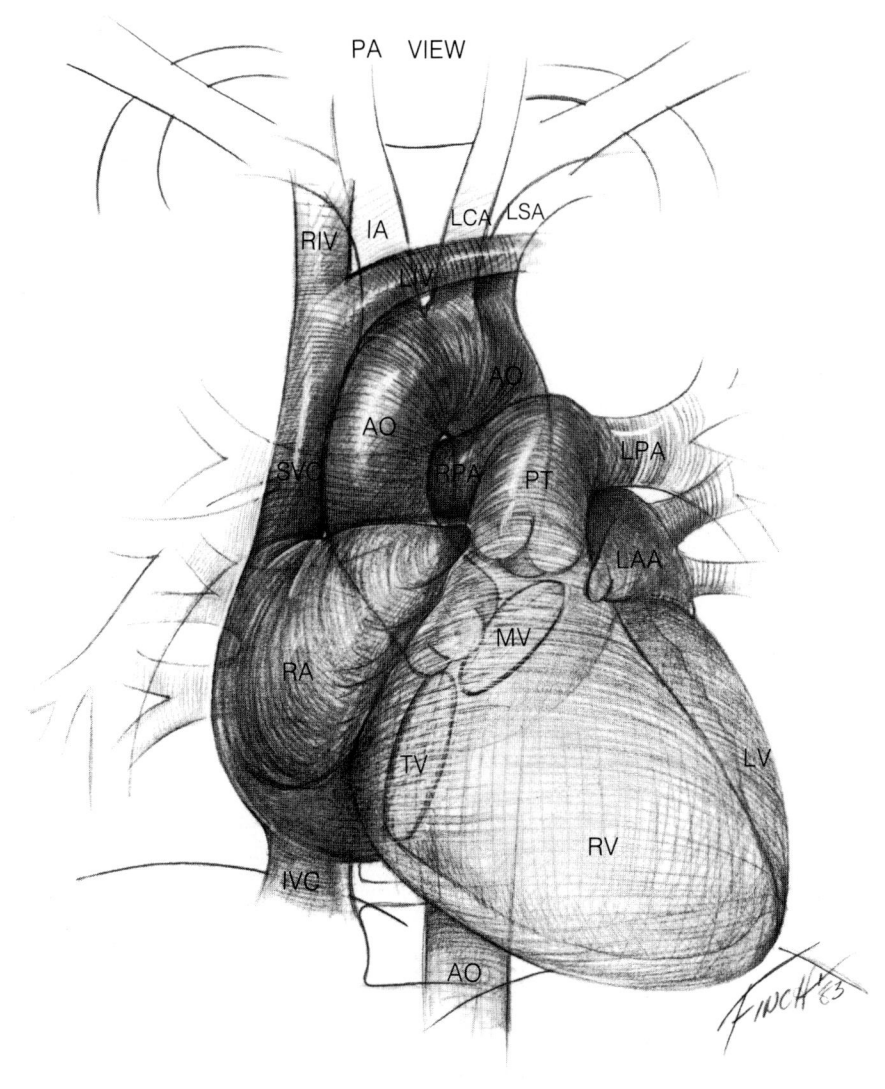

FIG 5–47.
Posteroanterior projection of the heart. *RIV* = right innominate vein; *LIV* = left innominate vein; *SVC* = superior vena cava; *RA* = right atrium; *IVC* = inferior vena cava; *AO* = aorta; *TV* = tricuspid valve; *MV* = mitral valve; *PT* = pulmonary trunk; *LAA* = left atrial appendage; *RV* = right ventricle; *LV* = left ventricle.

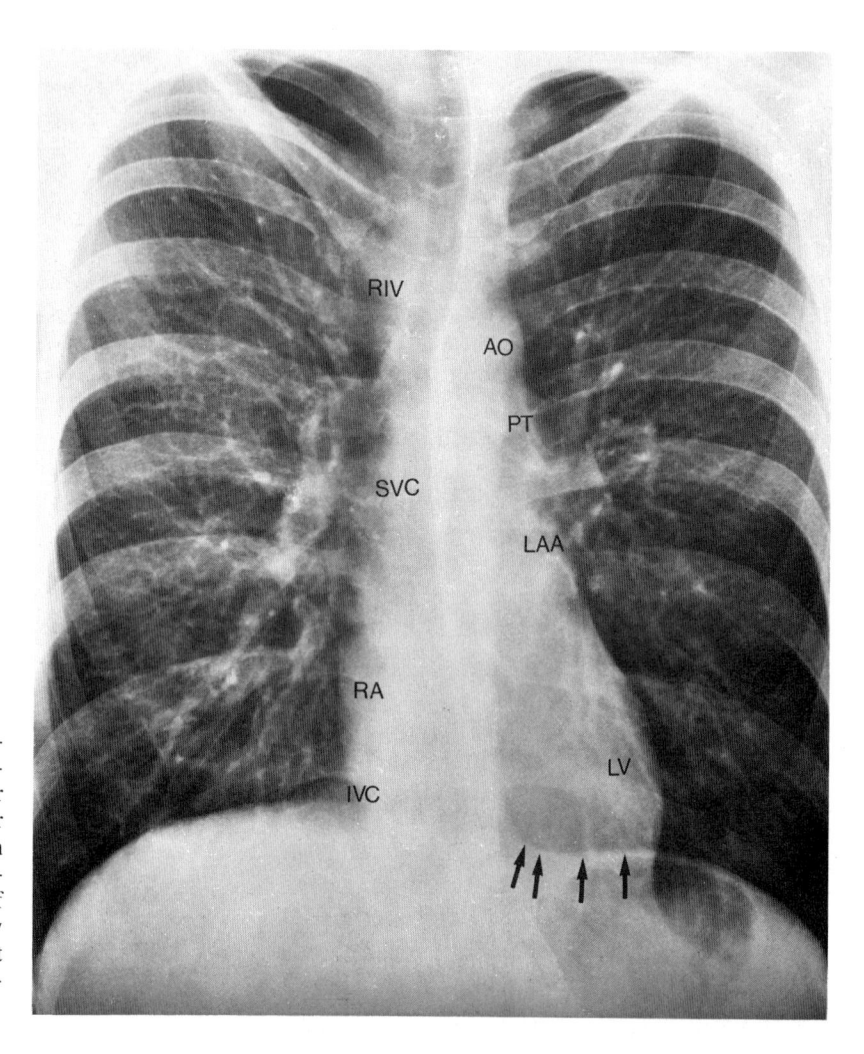

FIG 5–48.
Thoracic roentgenogram, posteroanterior projection, of normal heart. Left hemidiaphragm *(arrows)* seen through heart. Right cardiac border (interface between air and the lung and vascular structures) formed by right innominate vein *(RIV)*, superior vena cava *(SVC)*, or, in older patients, ascending aorta. Contour of left side of heart formed by aortic arch *(AO)*, pulmonary trunk *(PT)*, left atrial appendage *(LAA)*, and left ventricle *(LV)*. *(RA* = right atrium; *IVC* = inferior vena cava.

level of the diaphragm. At that point, it is no longer outlined by air and so disappears. In infants and children, the descending aorta may lie in front of the spine and may not be seen. In the older adult, the descending aorta usually is tortuous and dense because of atherosclerosis. The aortic arch indents the trachea and displaces it slightly toward the side opposite the arch. Seen best on high-kV(p) films, tracheal deviation is more pronounced on expiration films, particularly in infancy, because the trachea buckles away from the arch. This displacement of the trachea is used to locate the aortic arch.

Occasionally an additional faint straight mediastinal shadow may be seen above the aortic knob. It represents a persistent left superior vena cava.

The pulmonary segment, formed by the main pulmonary artery (pulmonary trunk), lies below the aortic segment along the left cardiac border. Only the portion of the main pulmonary artery bordering the lung is seen. The size of the pulmonary artery segment varies considerably with cardiac and thoracic rotation and with radiographic projection. In infancy, the main pulmonary artery segment is obscured by thymic tissue.

Below the pulmonary segment lies the left atrial appendage, which is usually not seen as a separate bulge. With left atrial enlargement, particularly from mitral disease, a distinct left atrial segment is formed. For unknown reasons, it almost never occurs in left-to-right shunts associated with left atrial enlargement. The left atrial appendage may be enlarged without left atrial enlargement, a condition termed idiopathic dilatation or aneurysm of the left atrial appendix (see Chapter 71).

The lower-most segment of the anterior cardiac border is formed by the ventricles, usually the left ventricle. However, in patients with clockwise rotation of the heart caused by right ventricular enlargement, the ventricular segment may be formed partly or completely by the right ventricle.

The air-containing trachea is readily seen. The right and left mainstem bronchi form the carina. The angle of the tracheal bifurcation varies somewhat, but it is usually about 60 degrees. Observation of the carina (Latin for the keel of a ship) is important in the diagnosis of left atrial enlargement because it lies immediately beneath the tracheal bifurcation. The right cardiac contour is formed by the superior vena cava and right atrium. In older patients with aortic enlargement, the ascending aorta becomes border forming. The right superior mediastinum becomes inconspicuous or invisible with clockwise rotation of the heart as in atrial septal defect (see Chapter 19).

It is important to realize the oblique position of the heart in the chest. A posteroanterior view of the chest therefore is a foreshortened oblique view of the heart.

The Right Anterior Oblique View (Figs 5–49 and 5–50)

The right anterior oblique view is the only projection that does not foreshorten the long axis of the heart. A 35- to 45-degree right anterior oblique projection of the thorax places the long axis of the ventricles more or less parallel to the radiographic film. Because this view is the best for detecting left atrial enlargement, it should always be obtained with barium in the esophagus.

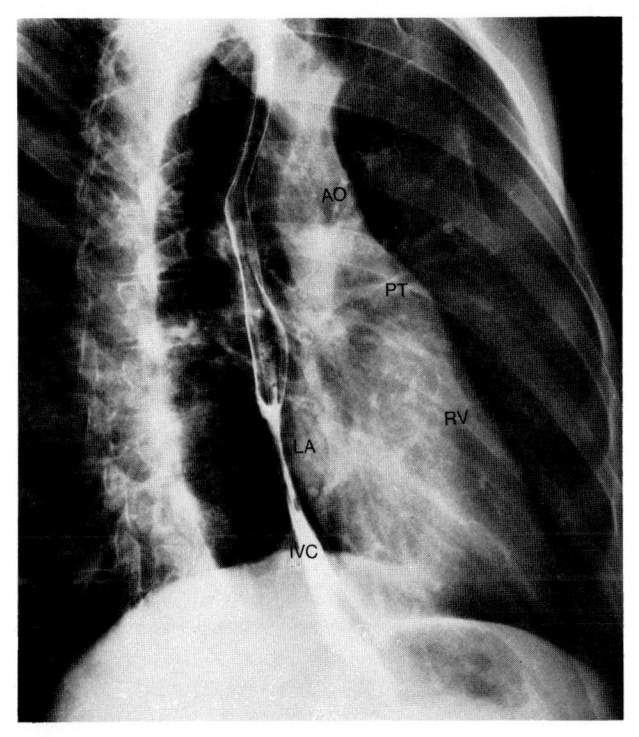

FIG 5–49.
Thoracic roentgenogram, right anterior oblique projection. Anterior cardiac border formed by aortic arch *(AO)*, pulmonary trunk *(PT)*, and right ventricle *(RV)*. Posterior border formed by barium-filled esophagus in contact with aortic arch and left atrium *(LA)*. Near diaphragm, supradiaphragmatic portion of inferior vena cava *(IVC)* is visible.

The anterior cardiac border is formed (from above downward) by the aortic arch, the pulmonary artery segment, and the ventricular segment (see Figs 5–49 and 5–50). Usually the right ventricle forms this border, but with marked left ventricular enlargement and the resultant counterclockwise rotation of the heart, part of this border may be attributable to the left ventricle. The posterior cardiac border usually is formed by the left atrium, which is in contact with the barium-filled esophagus, although, depending on the degree of rotation, the right atrium may form this border. At the base of the heart, the supradiaphragmatic portion of the inferior vena cava is seen. Because the ventricles are not foreshortened, the heart is well penetrated by the x-ray beam. Consequently, the right anterior oblique projection is the most sensitive for fluoroscopic observation of cardiac calcifications.

The Left Anterior Oblique View (Figs 5–51 and 5–52)

Rotation of the chest to approximately a 45- to 50-degree left anterior oblique view projects the heart on-end. Most commonly, the left anterior oblique view is obtained with a 60-degree rotation of the thorax, thereby eliminating the overlap of the left ventricle and the spine. Whether barium should be given for this view is debatable. However, because the barium-filled esophagus does not interfere with the interpretation and is very useful in the demonstration of important anomalies, such as coarctation or bronchial collaterals, barium should be administered. In this projection, the ventricles are maximally foreshortened, and the ventricular septum lies more or less perpendicular to the plane of the film. Thus, the cardiac silhouette is divided by the ventricular septum into an anterior portion of the "right heart" and a posterior half of the "left heart." This view is very informative for chamber analysis. It is also the best view for identifying aortic and mitral valvar calcifications.

The vascular structures forming the borders are inconstant, varying with both cardiac rotation and the degree of the left anterior oblique projection (see Fig 5–52). Anteriorly, the upper cardiac border is formed by the superior vena cava. In a steeper projection and with enlargement of the ascending aorta, as in poststenotic dilatation, the ascending aorta forms this border. Near the diaphragm, the supradiaphragmatic portion of the inferior vena cava can be seen as a linear density through the cardiac shadow. The lower segment is formed by the right atrium. With a steeper (60-degree) left anterior oblique projection, the right ventricle forms the border. Because it is impossible to determine whether the right atrium or the right ventricle forms this segment of the cardiac silhouette, it is

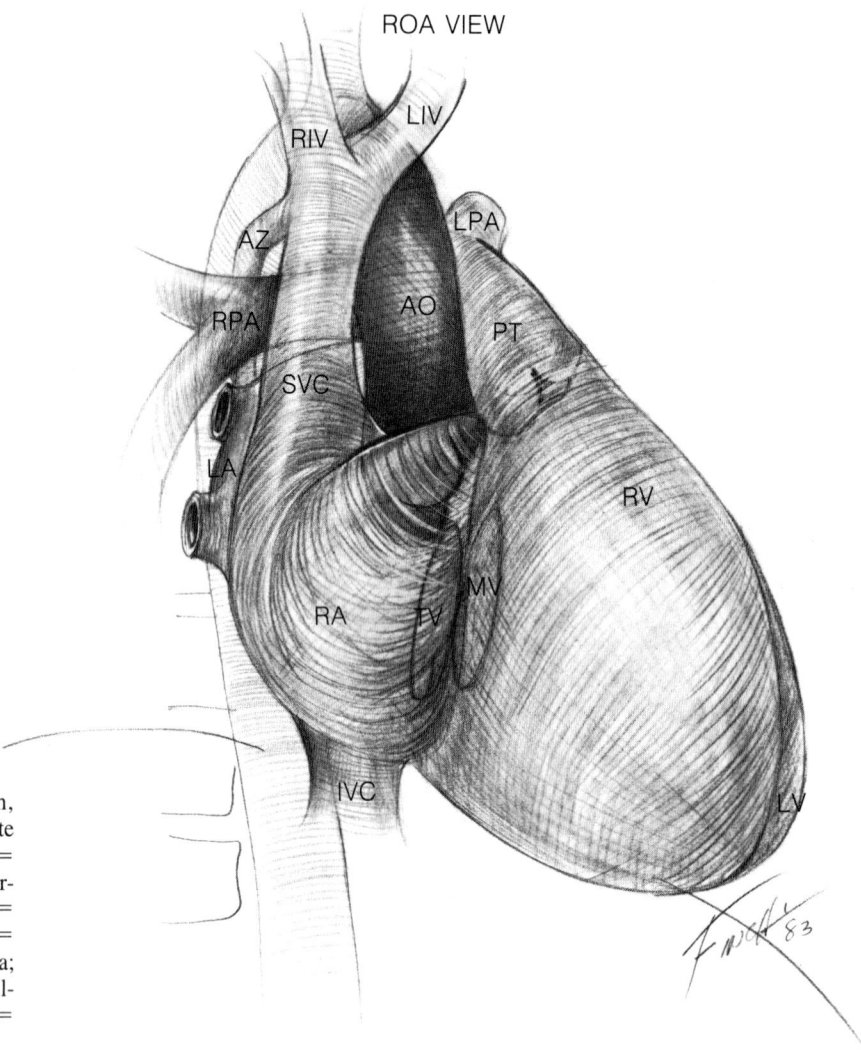

FIG 5–50.
Diagram, right anterior oblique projection, of normal heart. *RIV* = right innominate vein; *LIV* = left innominate vein; *AZ* = azygous vein; *RPA* = right pulmonary artery; *LPA* = left pulmonary artery; *SVC* = superior vena cava; *LA* = left atrium; *RA* = right atrium; *IVC* = inferior vena cava; *RAA* = right atrial appendage; *PT* = pulmonary trunk; *RV* = right ventricle; *TV* = tricuspid valve; *MV* = mitral valve.

common to speak only of the "right heart" in this projection.

Posteriorly, the aortic arch and descending aorta are seen, particularly in the elderly, because of the increased radiographic density and tortuosity of the aorta. The right and left mainstem bronchi are well demonstrated, and the left pulmonary artery crosses above the left mainstem bronchus. The right artery can be seen through the cardiac shadow as a round increased density (see insert, Fig 5–51). The left atrium is located below the left mainstem bronchus. Normally, a clear space is present between the left atrium and left mainstem bronchus. An enlarged left atrium encroaches on this space, so the left anterior oblique view is excellent for detecting left atrial enlargement. With significant left atrial enlargement, the left mainstem bronchus is elevated and displaced posteriorly.

The lower posterior segment is formed by the left ventricle. Depending on left ventricular size and the degree of cardiac and thoracic rotation, the left ventricular shadow may overlap the spine. Left ventricular enlargement is best seen in this projection, which also gives valuable information of chamber size. This view therefore has been termed the strategic view of the heart.

The Lateral Projection (Figs 5–53 and 5–54)

There are two main views of the heart: the right anterior and left anterior oblique projections. The right anterior oblique view is an en face projection of the heart, whereas the left anterior oblique view is on-end. The lateral and posteroanterior views are intermediate projections, namely 45 degrees more rotation than the right anterior oblique or left anterior oblique projections, respectively. The posteroanterior view resembles the left anterior oblique view, and the lateral view resembles the right anterior oblique view. The lateral view of the chest is part of the cardiac evaluation, because it can be obtained conveniently (see Fig 5–53).

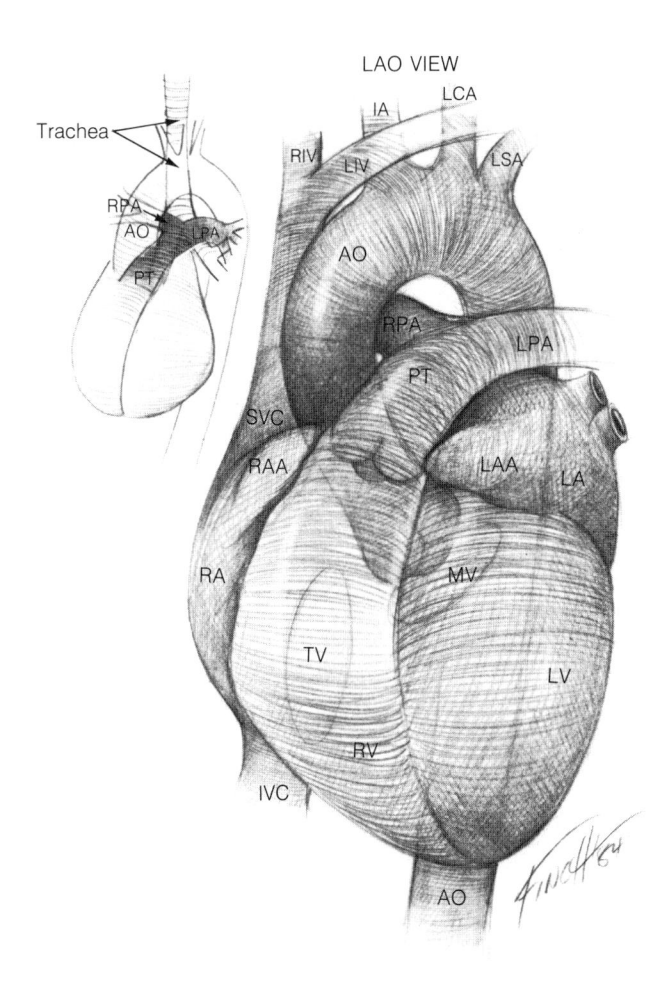

Plain-Film Diagnosis of Congenital Cardiac Disease 97

Although the heart is in contact with the sternum, the retrosternal space normally is not encroached upon unless there is right ventricular or right atrial enlargement. The anterior surface of the heart is formed by the right ventricle and right atrium. Because it is impossible to distinguish these two superimposed chambers, the use of the term "right heart" is preferable. The lower portion of the anterior cardiac contour is formed by the body of the right ventricle and the upper portion by the right ventricular outflow tract. The right atrial appendage is usually superimposed on the outflow tract. In elderly individuals with a dense aorta, the entire aortic arch may be well seen, but in younger patients, it is difficult to identify. The left and right mainstem bronchi are evident. The left mainstem bronchus normally projects slightly behind the right bronchus. With significant left atrial enlargement, the left bronchus may be displaced posteriorly, elevated, or even narrowed. The major portion of the posterior surface of the heart is formed by the left atrium, which is in direct contact with the esophagus. Normally the left atrium indents

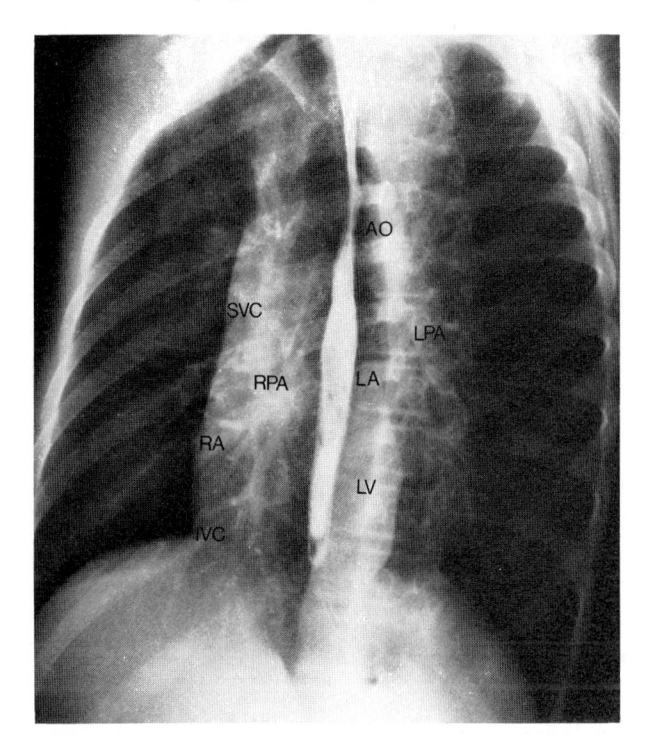

FIG 5–51.
Left anterior oblique projection. *RIV* = right innominate vein; *LIV* = left innominate vein; *SVC* = superior vena cava; *RAA* = right atrial appendage; *RA* = right atrium; *IVC* = inferior vena cava; *RV* = right ventricle; *TV* = tricuspid valve; *AO* = aorta; *IA* = innominate artery; *LC* = left carotid; *LSA* = left subclavian artery; *PT* = pulmonary trunk; *RPA* = right pulmonary artery; *LPA* = left pulmonary artery; *LAA* = left atrial appendage; *LA* = left atrium; *MV* = mitral valve; *LV* = left ventricle. Insert shows the anatomic relations of the right and left pulmonary arteries to the carina.

When combined with the posteroanterior view, the lateral projection provides useful information for evaluation of cardiac size; because it is the right-angle projection of a posteroanterior view, it allows estimation of cardiac volume. Because the cardiac apex of the heart is located closer to the left lateral chest wall, a left lateral projection is preferred (i.e., the left side of the patient is placed against the radiographic cassette), thereby minimizing magnification of the heart. The right lateral projection represents a mirror image of the left lateral view.

Because the heart rests on the anterior half of the diaphragm, it blends with the anterior left diaphragm, whereas the right side of the diaphragm is sharply outlined by the air in the lung (see Fig 5–54).

FIG 5–52.
Thoracic roentgenogram, left anterior oblique view, of normal heart in approximately 50-degree rotation. The anterior contour is formed by the superior vena cava *(SVC)*, right atrium *(RA)*, and short segment of the supradiaphragmatic portion of the inferior vena cava *(IVC)*. The posterior contour is formed by the distal aortic arch *(AO)*, left atrium *(LA)* beneath the left mainstem bronchus, and left ventricle *(LV)*. The left pulmonary artery *(LPA)* is seen as it crosses over the left mainstem bronchus. In the 60% left anterior oblique projection, the left ventricle is no longer superimposed on the spine, and the anterior upper contour is formed by the ascending aorta.

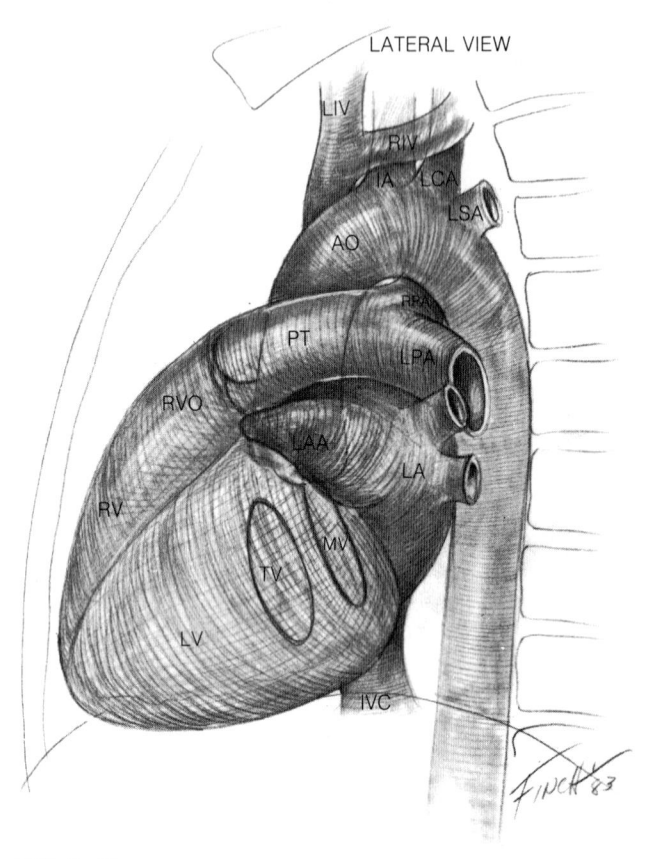

FIG 5-53.
Lateral projection of normal heart. *RV* = right ventricle; *RVO* = right ventricular outflow; *PT* = pulmonary trunk; *RP* = right pulmonary artery; *LP* = left pulmonary artery; *RIV* = right innominate vein; *LIV* = left innominate vein; *SVC* = superior vena cava; *RIA* = right innominate artery; *LCA* = left carotid artery; *LSC* = left subclavian artery; *LAA* = left atrial appendage; *LA* = left atrium; *MV* = mitral valve; *TV* = tricuspid valve; *LV* = left ventricle; *IVC* = inferior vena cava.

the anterior wall of the esophagus, particularly when the esophagus is fully distended by air or barium. This indentation therefore does not indicate true left atrial enlargement. Displacement of *both* walls of the esophagus posteriorly indicates left atrial enlargement, provided the radiograph is taken during deep inspiration.

A small segment near the diaphragm is formed by the posterior wall of the left ventricle. With significant left ventricular enlargement, this contribution becomes more obvious (see Fig 5-54).

The main right pulmonary artery in the hilum (surrounded by lung) is seen on-end as a round density located anteriorly to the trachea. The left pulmonary artery forms a characteristic commalike density above the left mainstem bronchus. Near the diaphragm, the supradiaphragmatic portion of the inferior vena cava forms a characteristic curvilinear density, which normally lies at about the same level as the left ventricle.

Summary

The four views of the heart are obtained by rotating the thorax in 45-degree increments. The right anterior oblique view is an en face view of the heart, demonstrating its long axis without foreshortening. The left anterior oblique view is an end-on view and has maximal foreshortening. The posteroanterior and lateral views are intermediate projections.

THE THYMUS

The thymus can cause difficult diagnostic problems, because it may simulate cardiac enlargement or mimic congenital heart disease or mediastinal tumors. Despite the difficulties, a firm radiographic diagnosis of persistent thymic tissue must be established.

The thymus is large at birth and decreases gradually during early childhood, so that by the age of 5 years, the amount of residual thymic tissue is small. The size and location of thymic tissue varies greatly. Thymic size decreases rapidly during stress, such as febrile episodes or starvation. Many forms of congenital heart disease, particularly with severe cyanosis, are stressful, and consequently these infants have little or no thymus. It is the absence of the thymus shadow in patients with admixture lesions that is largely responsible for the narrow mediastinum. Often, after correction of a cardiac malformation, the thymus regrows in a few weeks.

The thymus, a very soft organ, lies in the anterior mediastinum and blends with the cardiac silhouette. The size of the thymus varies markedly with breathing. During inspiration the thymus collapses (Fig 5-55,A), whereas during exhalation, the thymus enlarges markedly (Fig 5-55,B). It is this change that can be used advantageously for diagnostic purposes. In doubtful cases, a fluoroscope can be used and the infant stimulated to cry, which induces prolonged expiration during which the thymus may overshadow both lungs. During the deep inhalation that follows, the thymus collapses, and the lung fields become visible again. It is this characteristic marked variability of thymic size that is the most reliable diagnostic radiographic sign.

Usually the thymus develops symmetrically, and it can extend into both lung fields and simulate an anterior mediastinal mass. Because of the softness of thymic tissue, the anterior ribs indent the thymus, giving it a wavy contour, an appearance not seen in mediastinal tumors, which are usually harder (Fig 5-56). Sometimes, however, thymic tissue grows asymmetrically, being more obvious along one of the cardiac borders (Fig 5-57). Along the left border, the tissue may obscure the pulmonary artery segment, thus yielding a cardiac contour closely mim-

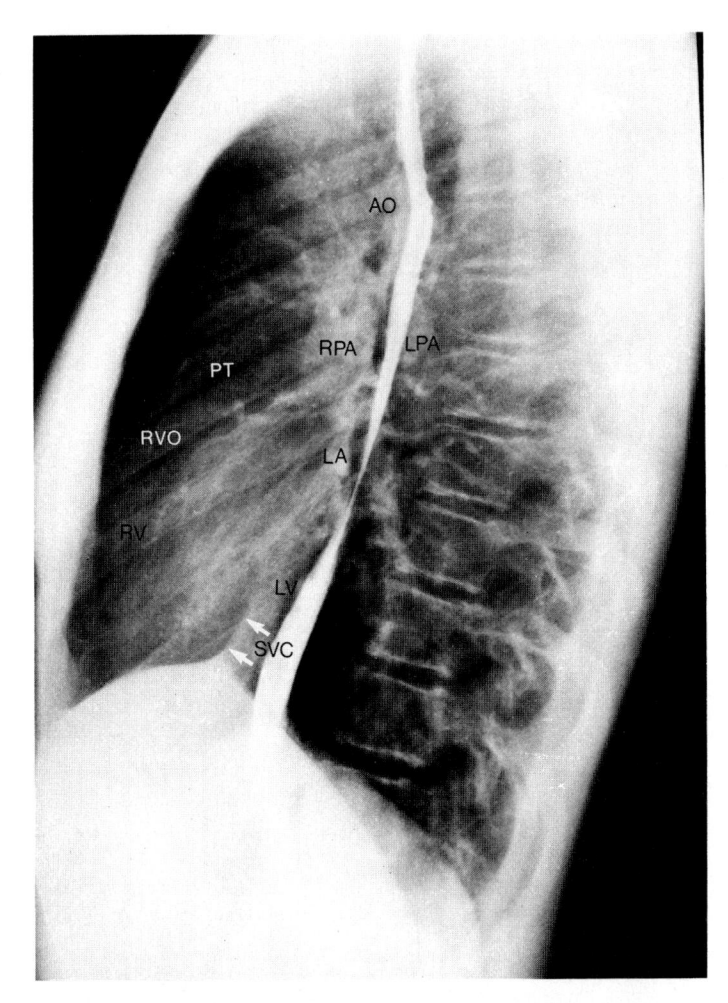

FIG 5–54.
Thoracic roentgenogram, lateral view of normal heart. Right hemidiaphragm *(open arrows)* sharply outlined by air, whereas density of left hemidiaphragm *(black arrow)* disappears because heart rests on anterior left hemidiaphragm. Lower portion of the right ventricle *(RV)* is close to sternum but retrosternal space not encroached on. Upper cardiac contour is formed by right ventricular outflow tract *(RVO)* and pulmonary trunk *(PT)*. AO = distal aortic arch. Right pulmonary artery *(RPA)* forms characteristic round density in front of trachea. Left pulmonary artery *(LPA)* seen as a commalike density above and behind left mainstem bronchus. Left atrium *(LA)* contacts barium-filled esophagus. Below left atrium, part of the left ventricle *(LV)* is visible. Supradiaphragmatic portion of inferior vena cava *(IVC) (white arrows)* forms characteristic curvilinear density.

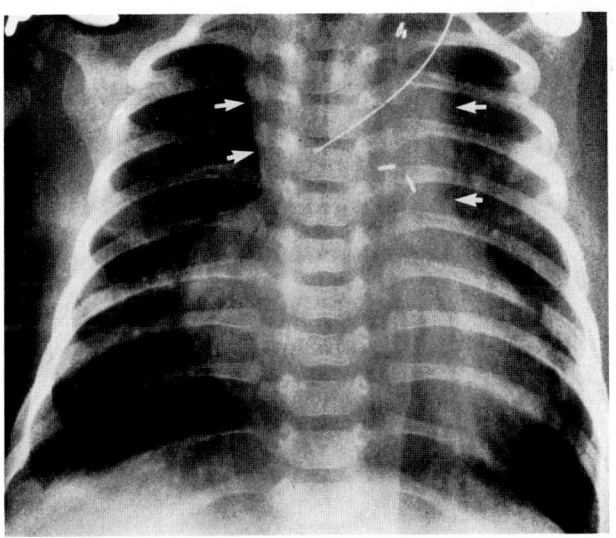

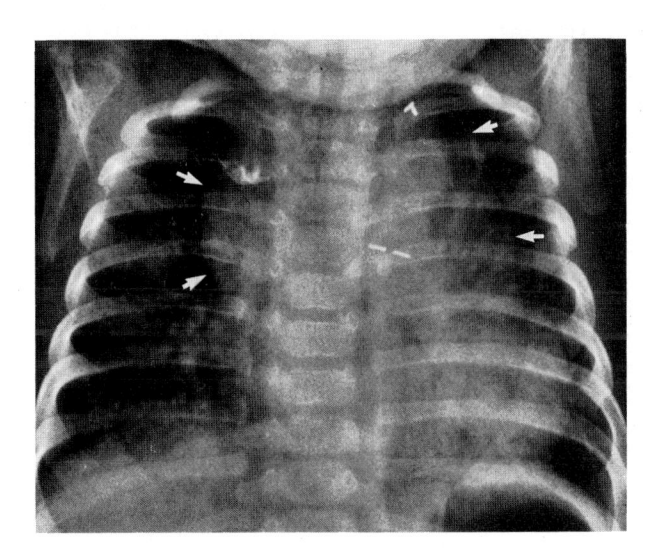

A.

B.

FIG 5–55.
Thoracic roentgenograms, posteroanterior projections, in patient with cardiomegaly. Superior mediastinal mass *(arrows)*. **A,** deep inhalation. **B,** exhalation marked increase in size of mediastinal mass *(arrows)*, indicating normal thymic tissue. Change in size, particularly during crying, establishes the diagnosis of enlarged thymus.

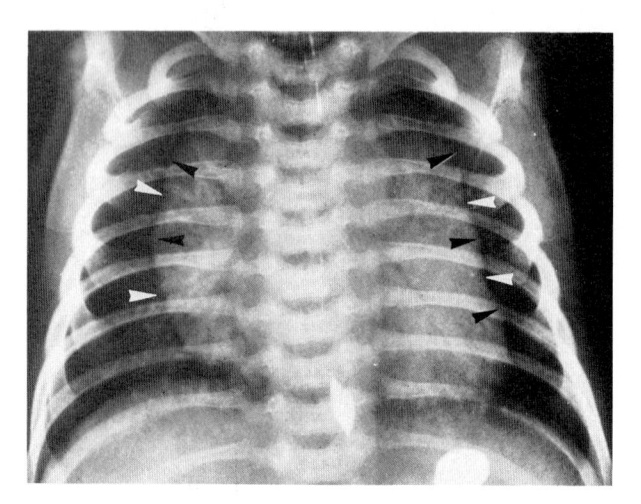

FIG 5-56.
Thoracic roentgenogram, posteroanterior projection showing typical symmetric enlarged thymus. Anterior ribs form characteristic indentations *(white arrows)*. Slight bulges *(black arrows)* between indentations correspond to intercostal spaces. This waviness is diagnostic of thymic tissue.

icking the configuration of corrected transposition (see Fig 5-57,B). Thymic tissue usually blends with the heart, but sometimes a characteristic notch is present between heart and thymus ("sail" sign). This is seen better on either a left anterior oblique (Fig 5-58,A) or posteroanterior view (Fig 5-58,B) or, rarely, on a lateral projection (Fig 5-58,C). The entire retrosternal space is generally filled in by thymus on a lateral projection, and thymic tissue cannot be differentiated from the heart (Fig 5-59).

Thymic tissue may closely mimic cardiac silhouettes of congenital heart disease (see Fig 5-57) and cause radiographic misdiagnoses. If the thymus is located primarily in the upper mediastinum and is symmetric, it closely mimics total anomalous venous return to a persistent left superior vena cava (Fig 5-60). Under those circumstances, however, the pulmonary blood flow is not increased unless there is marked venous obstruction and the characteristic locations of the caval densities are not observed on a lateral view (see Fig 5-59) (see Chapter 46).

CHAMBER ENLARGEMENT

Cardiac films are a simple and convenient means to study the size of the chambers and were particularly important before the development of echocardiography. However, although it is possible to estimate cardiac chamber size with considerable accuracy in older patients, the method is difficult and unreliable in infants because of the overlying thymic tissue.

Three noninvasive techniques are available to estimate

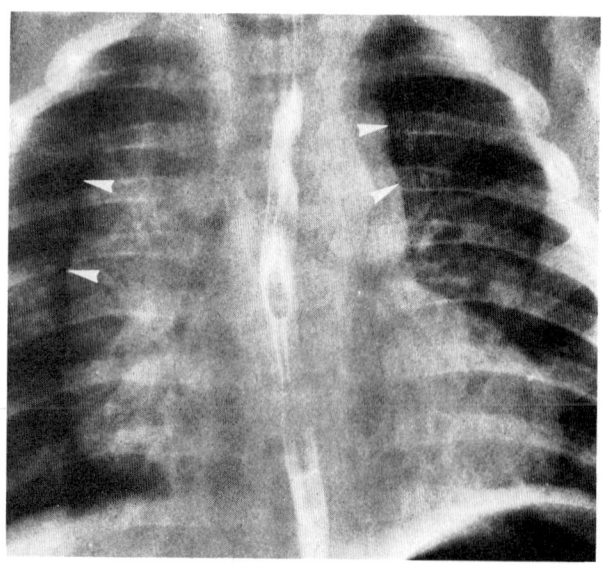

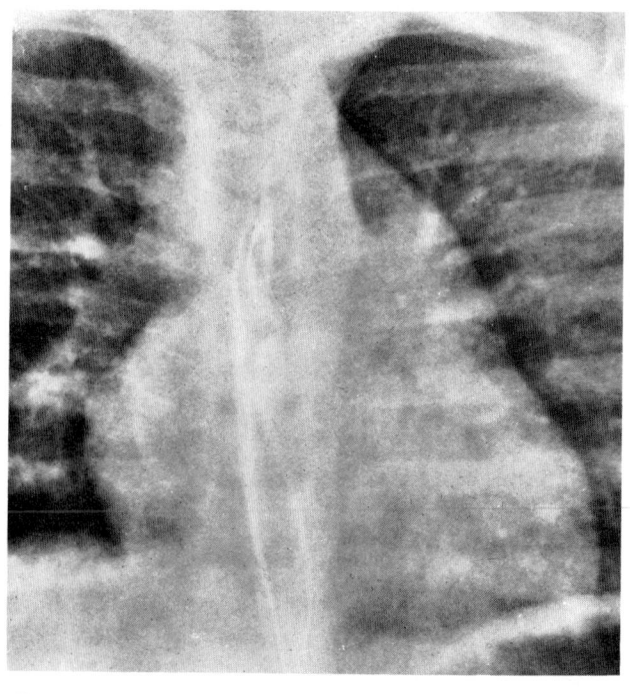

FIG 5-57.
Thoracic roentgenograms, posteroanterior projection, of asymmetric thymus. **A,** thymic prominence primarily along right cardiac border. Wavy border *(arrows)* typical of thymic tissue. **B,** thymic enlargement along left cardiac border, altering cardiac shape. Slightly wavy contour suggests thymus. Cardiac conformation mimics that of corrected transposition.

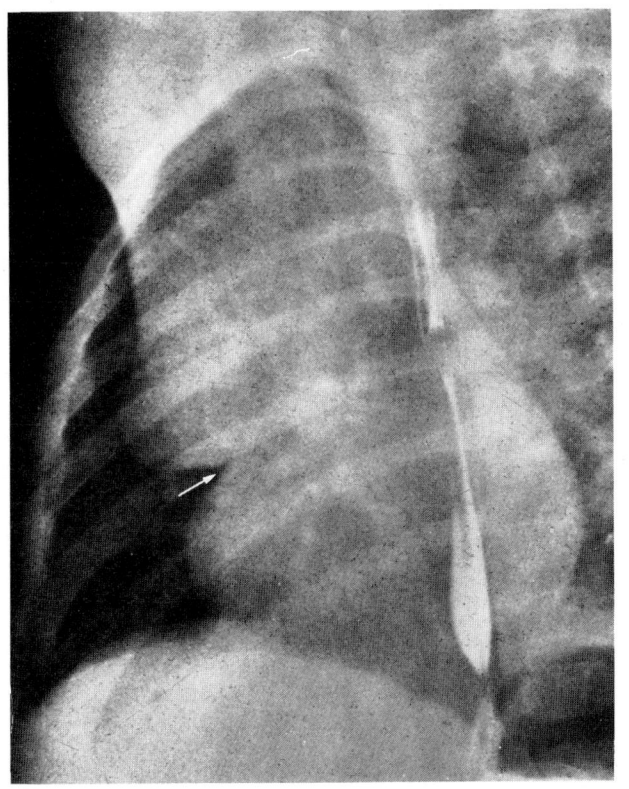

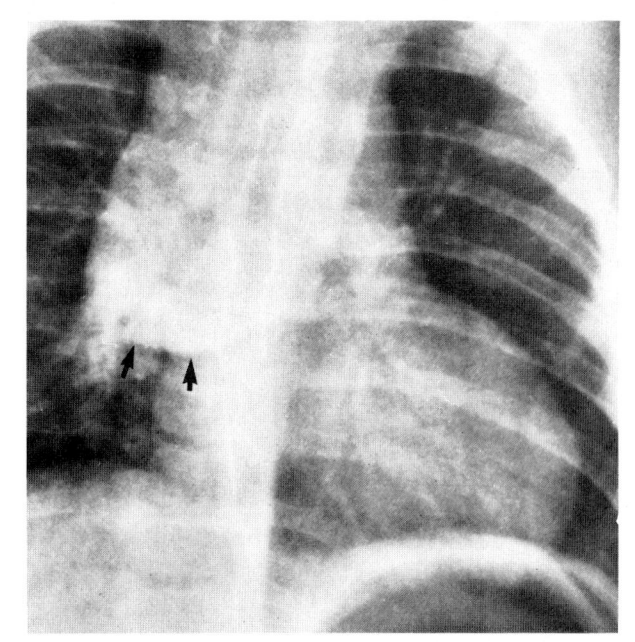

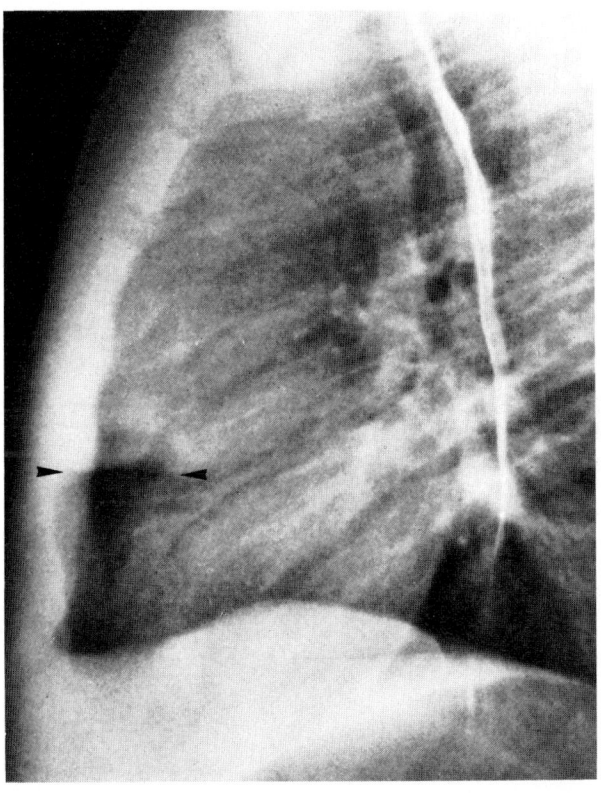

FIG 5–58.
Thoracic roentgenograms in enlarged thymus. **A,** left anterior oblique projection; sharp demarcation *(arrow)* between thymus and cardiac contour, yielding "sail" sign. **B,** posteroanterior projection, atypical thymus; pronounced sail sign *(arrows)*. **C,** lateral projection; characteristic sail sign *(arrows)*. In most cases, entire retrosternal space is filled with thymus. Sharp demarcation between thymus and heart typically is absent on lateral projection.

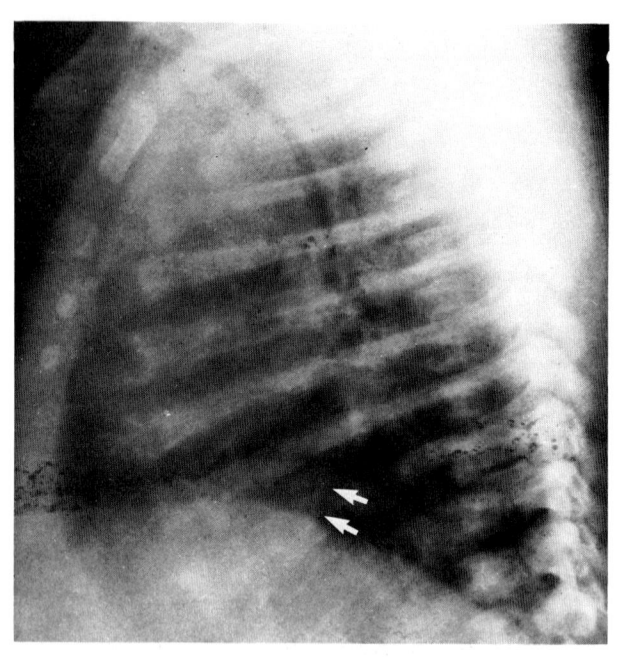

FIG 5–59.
Typical appearance of thymus on the lateral view. The thymus fills in the anterior mediastinum and blends with the heart. Only posteriorly can the heart contour be seen *(arrows)*. It is not displaced, indicating a normal heart size.

cardiac chamber size: echocardiography, electrocardiography, and roentgenography. The methods are complementary, but echocardiography has taken the lead in recent years. Thus, roentgenography is comparatively inaccurate in assessing ventricular hypertrophy (pressure overload) but more diagnostic in ventricular dilatation (volume overload).

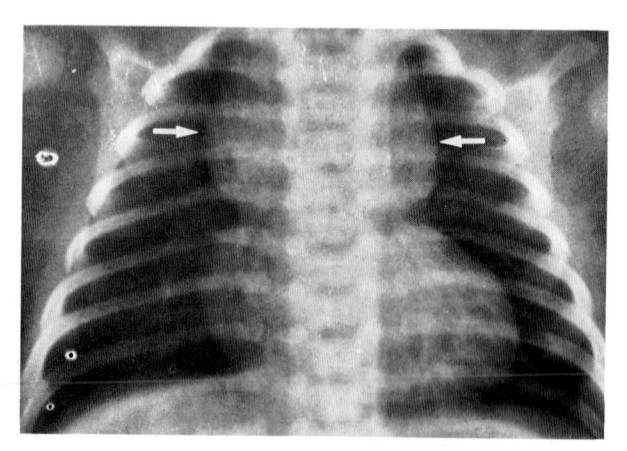

FIG 5–60.
Thoracic roentgenograms showing symmetric enlargement of superior mediastinum by thymus. Posteroanterior projection; appearance identical to that of total anomalous pulmonary venous connection to left superior vena cava ("snowman's heart"). However, normal cardiac size and pulmonary vascularity make this diagnosis unlikely. Densities of superior venae cavae not seen on lateral projection (see Chapter 46).

On the other hand, electrocardiography is more reliable in the diagnosis of ventricular hypertrophy, and echocardiography allows measurement of ventricular hypertrophy and dilatation. Consequently, the radiologic technique has lost some of its importance in evaluating cardiac size, and cardiac fluoroscopy is no longer performed, although previously it played an important role in the cardiac evaluation.

Radiographic evaluation of cardiac chamber size is more reliable in patients with acquired cardiac disease in which all chambers are normally developed and are then altered by the condition. Assessment of individual chamber enlargement is more difficult in congenital heart disease, but some of the same radiographic rules still apply. Concentric hypertrophy without ventricular enlargement (pressure overload) may cause only a subtle increased roundness of the ventricular contour. The radiographic findings are much more obvious with ventricular dilatation (volume overload).

Right Atrial Enlargement

Isolated right atrial enlargement occurs only in tricuspid stenosis, a rare condition. In all other instances, there is concomitant right ventricular enlargement, and this causes displacement of the heart, as discussed in the next section.

The right atrium casts a round density on a posteroanterior or shallow left anterior oblique projection. The right atrium enlarges concentrically, and one would assume that the right atrial segment should always be increased on a posteroanterior projection. Unfortunately, this often is not observed because the entire heart may be rotated and displaced toward the left because of the associated right ventricular enlargement. Therefore, right atrial enlargement is difficult to assess radiographically, and it is preferable to describe this appearance as right-sided enlargement. Furthermore, right-sided enlargement does not mean the heart extends more into the right hemithorax on a posteroanterior roentgenogram, because the heart rotates toward the left from ventricular enlargement. This clockwise rotation makes the right superior vena cava inconspicuous and causes the right ventricle, rather than the left ventricle, to form the left cardiac border. The resulting cardiac contour can easily be mistaken for left ventricular enlargement (Fig 5–61).

Radiographic signs of right atrial enlargement are as follows:

1. The right atrial segment tends to be more prominent and extends more into the right lung field. (Unfortunately, this is not invariably true.)
2. The superior vena cava and ascending aorta are inconspicuous or invisible on the posteroanterior film (Figs

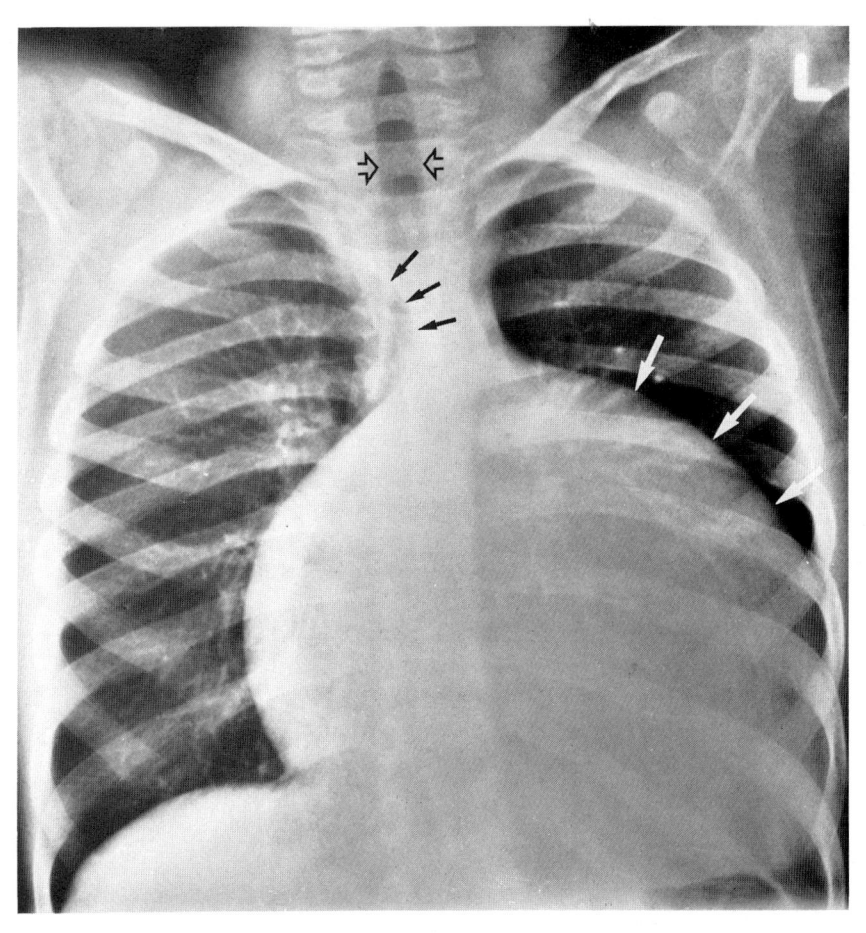

FIG 5–61.
Posteroanterior roentgenogram of patient with enormous right atrial enlargement caused by Ebstein's malformation. The roentgenogram is perfectly straight (*open arrows* outline trachea). The right atrial segment is increased but not as much as expected because of the marked clockwise rotation of the heart. The right superior vena cava density has disappeared *(small black arrows)*. The right ventricle *(white arrows)* forms the left cardiac border, simulating left ventricular enlargement.

5–61 and 5–62 [arrow]). This is caused by a shift of the heart toward the left and clockwise rotation from the right ventricular enlargement or enlargement of the right atrium against the sternum.

3. The diameter of the right atrial segment may be increased on the posteroanterior and left anterior oblique views (Fig 5–62).

4. On the lateral view, the retrosternal space is filled in by the right atrium and its enlarged appendage. The normal-sized left ventricle may be displaced posteriorly. This appearance is indistinguishable from that of right ventricular enlargement.

5. In the right anterior oblique projection, the retrosternal space tends to be obliterated (see Fig 5–62).

Not all of these signs are present in an individual patient. The most reliable view for right-sided enlargement is the left anterior oblique projection (Fig 5–63).

Right Ventricular Enlargement

Radiographic signs of right ventricular enlargement are more reliable than those of right atrial enlargement. In isolated right ventricular hypertrophy, the cardiac films may be normal. As the right ventricle enlarges, it expands anteriorly toward the sternum, and in young patients, it can cause sternal bowing. The right ventricular impulse may be felt and seen clinically as "precordial heave" (see Chapter 19). Once the retrosternal space is filled in, the heart rotates clockwise and is displaced posteriorly and toward the left (Fig 5–64).

Radiographic signs of right ventricular enlargement are as follows:

1. With slight enlargement, the posteroanterior projection is normal.
2. With severe enlargement, the cardiac silhouette is

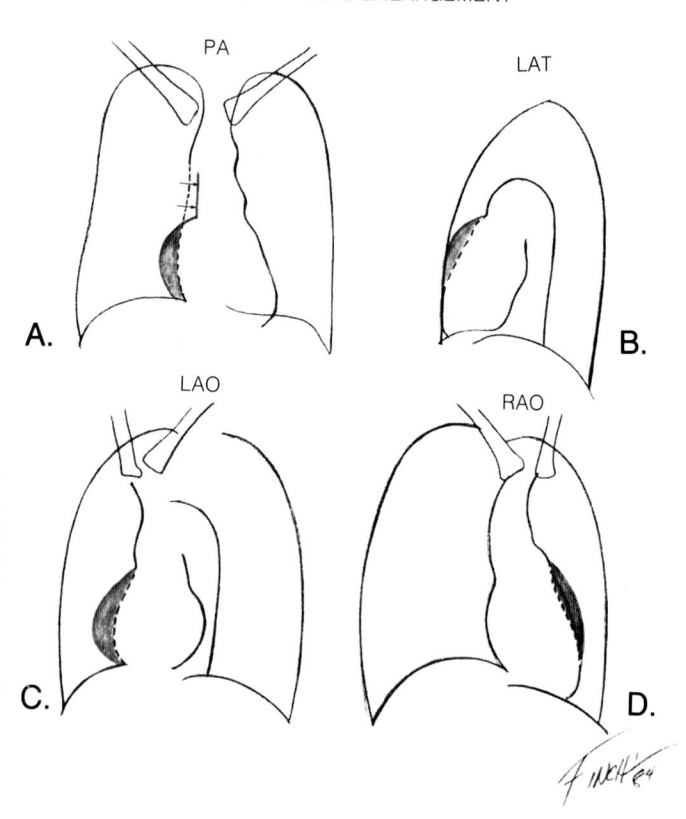

RIGHT ATRIAL ENLARGEMENT

FIG 5–62.
Diagrams of right atrial enlargement. **A,** posteroanterior projection; right atrial density protrudes more into right lung field, and its diameter is increased. Superior vena cava and ascending aorta inconspicuous because of clockwise cardiac rotation and displacement of heart toward left. **B,** lateral projection; retrosternal space obliterated by right atrial or right ventricular enlargement, which usually coexist. **C,** left anterior oblique projection; diameter and prominence of anterior cardiac contour increased. **D,** right anterior oblique projection; enlarged right atrium impinges on retrosternal space. Identical radiographic findings occur with right ventricular enlargement. Right atrial and right ventricular enlargement usually coexist ("right-sided heart enlargement").

enlarged, and the contour resembles that of left ventricular enlargement, although the apex does not extend significantly below the diaphragm because the right ventricle rests anteriorly on the diaphragm (Fig 5–65).

3. The displacement of the heart toward the left makes the density of the superior vena cava inconspicuous or invisible and projects it over the spine.

4. Because enlargement of the right ventricle is arrested not only by the sternum anteriorly but also by the diaphragm inferiorly, elongation of the right ventricle

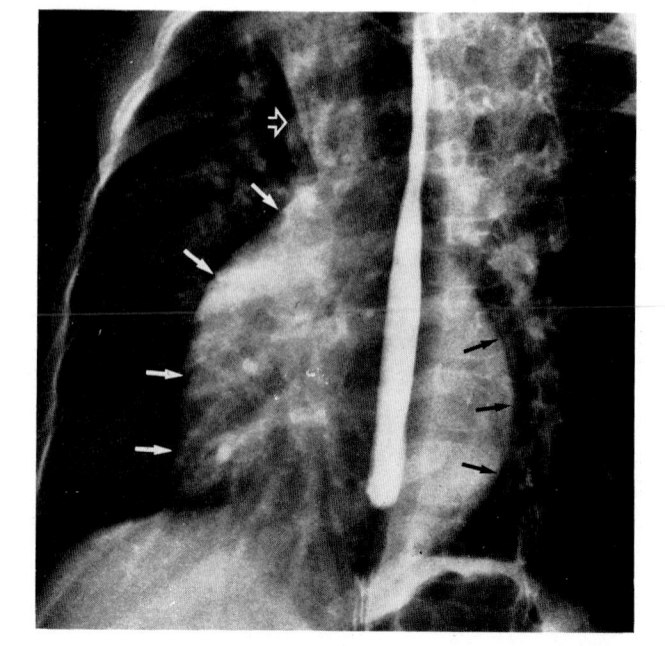

FIG 5–63.
"Right-sided heart enlargement"; left anterior oblique projection. Anterior border *(white arrows)* formed by right side of heart shows increased diameter and prominence. Superior vena cava *(open arrow)* is inconspicuous. Ascending aorta, normally visible in this projection, is not seen because of clockwise cardiac rotation. Left ventricle is elevated and displaced posteriorly and overlies spine *(black arrow)* ("pseudo left ventricular enlargement").

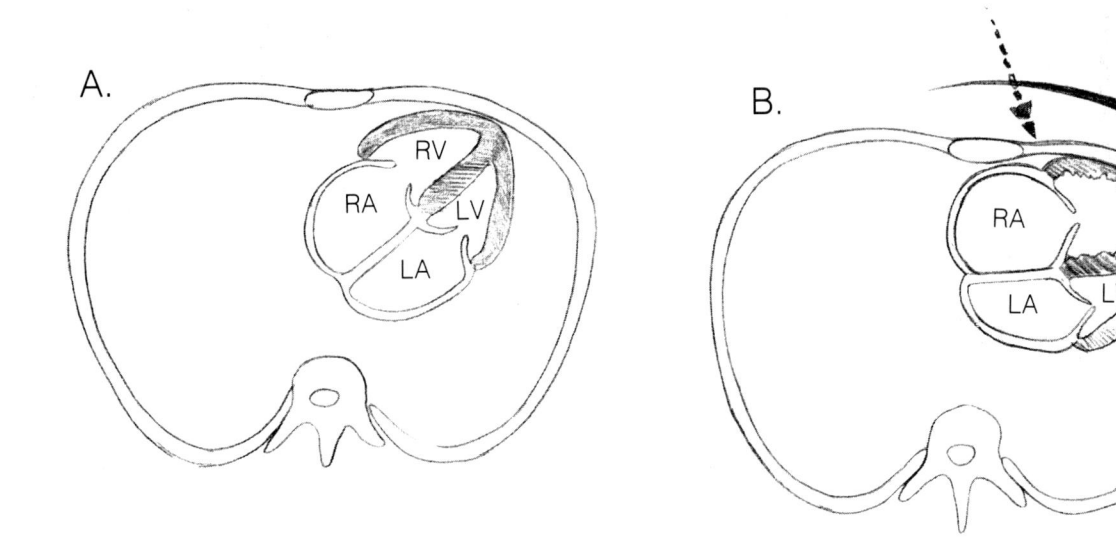

FIG 5–64.
Diagram of CT scan of heart as viewed from below. **A,** normal heart is inclined 45 degrees with sagittal plane. **B,** right-sided enlargement against the thoracic cage and sternum results in clockwise rotation *(curved arrow)* and displacement of heart into left hemithorax *(broken arrow).* This displacement minimizes the prominence of the right atrial segment on posteroanterior projection and results in an inconspicuous superior vena cava and ascending aorta. In spite of concomitant right atrial enlargement, the right atrium may appear radiographically normal or even small on the posteroanterior film.

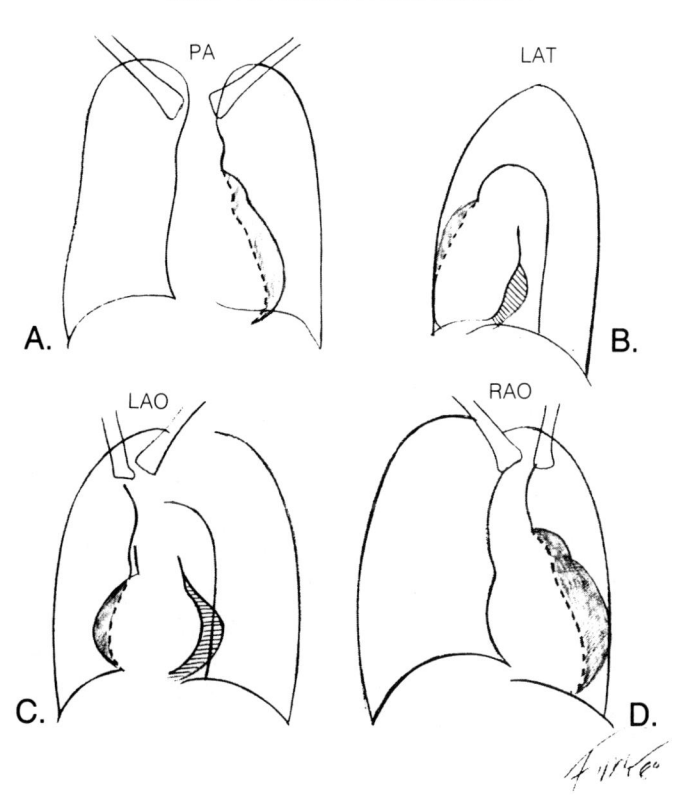

RIGHT VENTRICULAR ENLARGEMENT

FIG 5–65.
Diagrams of right ventricular enlargement. **A,** posteroanterior projection; left cardiac border is round, resembling that seen in left ventricular enlargement, but cardiac apex does not extend below dome of diaphragm. Pulmonary trunk is prominent and elevated. **B,** lateral projection, retrosternal space obliterated. Left ventricle displaced posteriorly and elevated. **C,** left anterior oblique projection; anterior cardiac border of increased prominence. Ascending aorta and superior vena cava are inconspicuous because of clockwise rotation. Left ventricle is elevated and displaced posteriorly; it may overlap spine. **D,** right anterior oblique projection; retrosternal space obliterated. Prominent and elevated pulmonary trunk caused by clockwise rotation and elongation of enlarged right ventricle.

causes elevation and prominence of the pulmonary trunk.

5. The left ventricle is elevated and displaced posteriorly so that on a 60-degree left anterior oblique projection, it may overlap the spine (pseudo left ventricular enlargement).

6. The left atrium is displaced posteriorly, indenting the barium-filled esophagus (pseudo left atrial enlargement). With severe right ventricular enlargement, even the carina may be splayed (Fig 5–66).

7. A steep left anterior oblique view is the most sensitive projection and shows an increased diameter of the right cardiac border (see Fig 5–65,C).

8. In the right anterior oblique view, the ventricular arc is increased.

9. On the lateral projection, the extent of contact between the heart and the sternum is increased, as occurs with right atrial enlargement. This sign can be appreciated only in patients without thymic tissue. The left ventricle is displaced posteriorly and upward and may not clear the spine (pseudo left ventricular enlargement).

Concentric right ventricular hypertrophy commonly causes counterclockwise rotation (see Chapter 29), whereas ventricular dilatation causes clockwise rotation (see Chapter 19). The concept of rotation of the heart is important, because it changes the appearance of the entire cardiac contour. The axis about which the heart rotates is located in the vicinity of the junction of the left atrium and left ventricle. Structures such as the pulmonary artery and aortic arch, which are most distant from this axis, show the most distortion (Fig 5–67).

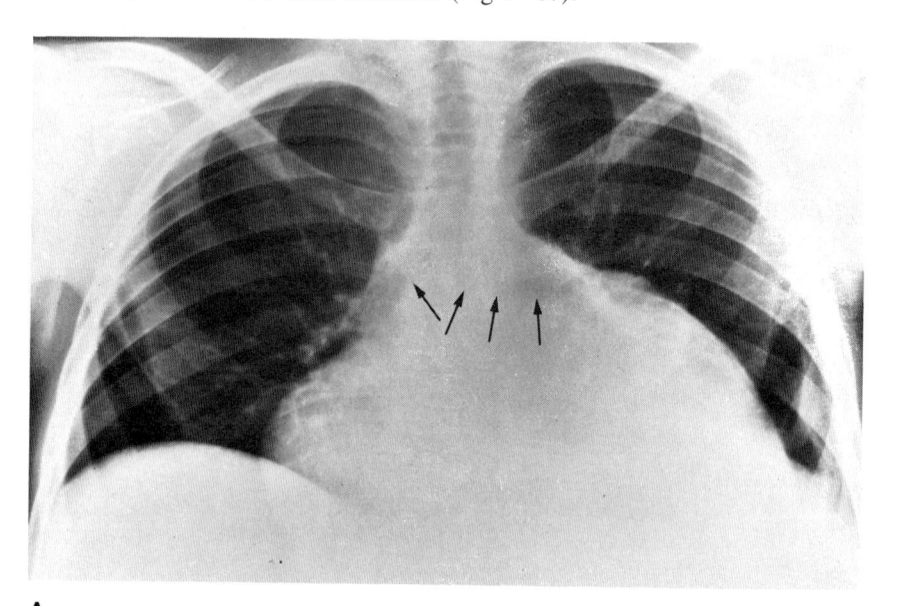

FIG 5–66.
Thoracic roentgenogram of patient with severe right atrial and right ventricular enlargement and normal-sized left chambers proved by echocardiography and postmortem examination. **A,** posteroanterior projection; right atrial segment only slightly prominent, although right atrium was found to be huge. Cardiac enlargement toward left, simulating left ventricular enlargement (shift and clockwise rotation of the heart). Superior displacement of normal-sized left atrium, splaying the carina ("pseudo enlargement of left atrium"). **B,** lateral projection; posterior displacement of left mainstem bronchus by the normal-sized left atrium (pseudo enlargement). Retrocardiac space obliterated by enormous right chambers.

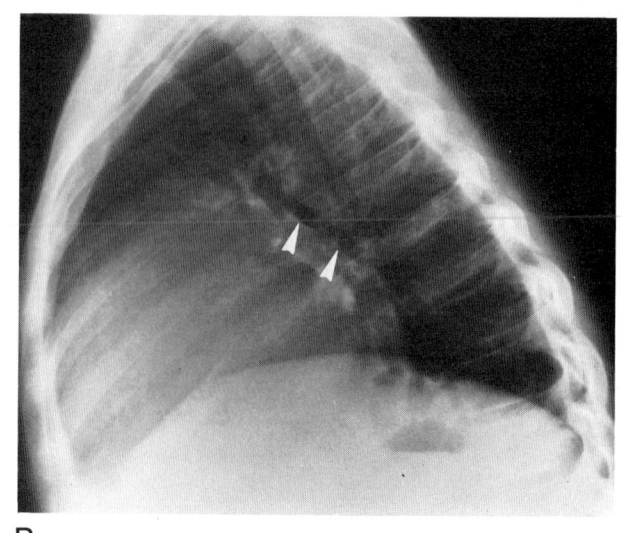

NORMAL CLOCKWISE ROTATION COUNTERCLOCKWISE ROTATION

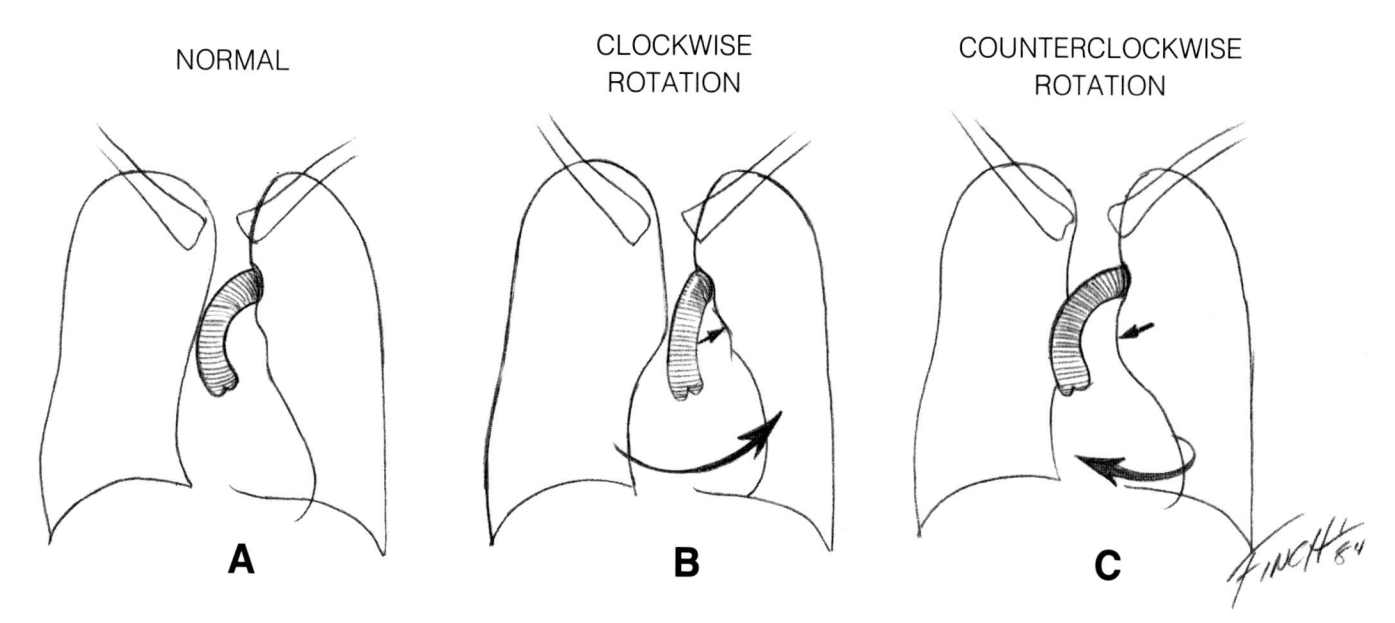

A   B   C

FIG 5–67.
Effect of cardiac rotation on radiographic cardiac contour; posteroanterior projection. **A,** normal position of heart. **B,** clockwise rotation; prominent pulmonary artery and inconspicuous ascending aorta. **C,** counterclockwise rotation; concave pulmonary arterial segment and prominent ascending aorta. This appearance is normal for older patient and is usually referred to as a "aortic" or "left ventricular" configuration.

Left Ventricular Enlargement

The heart changes its configuration during life. In children and adolescents, the pulmonary artery segment is normally prominent (Fig 5–68), whereas later the left ventricle becomes more prominent and the heart assumes a more horizontal position because of elongation (uncoiling) of the aorta. This change induces a counterclockwise rotation and results in a more medial position of the pulmonary artery, causing a more concave pulmonary artery segment (Fig 5–69). This cardiac configuration is normal in the aged and is best termed left ventricular configuration. The counterclockwise rotation of the heart that occurs with left ventricular hypertrophy results in the same cardiac configuration. Therefore, when the left ventricle is evaluated, the patient's age must be considered.

Enlargement of the right ventricle is affected by its contact with the diaphragm and sternum; the left ventricle, because it lies posteriorly, can elongate without impediment below the diaphragm. It is this downward extension of the left ventricle that is the most diagnostic sign of enlargement. However, identification of downward extension is very dependent on a proper radiographic projection; for instance, a reversed lordotic view projects even the normal left ventricle below the level of the diaphragm.

Radiographic signs of left ventricle hypertrophy or dilatation are as follows:

1. Isolated left ventricular hypertrophy causes only a rounder contour of the left ventricular border on the posteroanterior and left anterior oblique projections.

2. With left ventricular dilatation, the cardiac contour extends below the dome of the diaphragm in each projec-

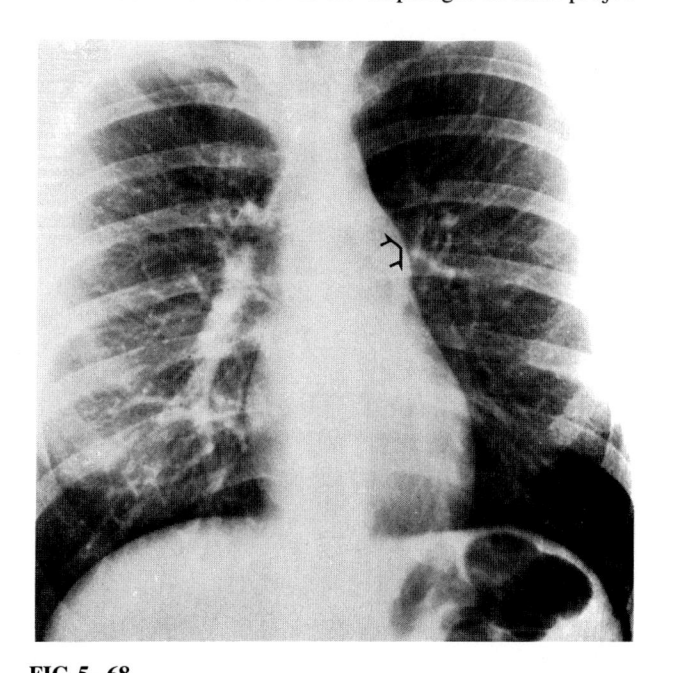

FIG 5–68.
Thoracic roentgenogram, posteroanterior projection, in normal child. Pulmonary artery *(arrow)* is prominent. Slight prominence of pulmonary vasculature is also normal.

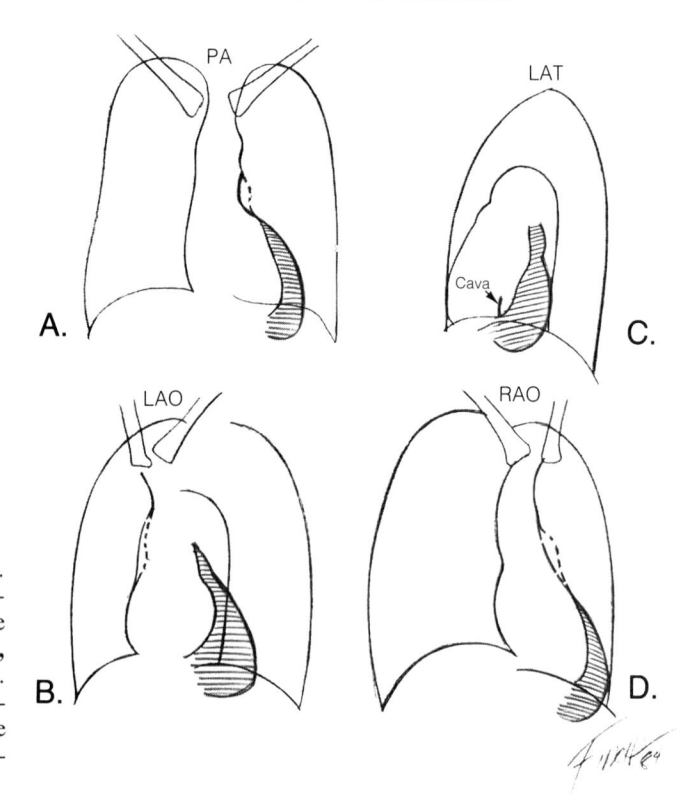

LEFT VENTRICULAR ENLARGEMENT

FIG 5–69.
Diagrams of radiographic signs of left ventricular enlargement. **A,** posteroanterior projection; pulmonary arterial segment concave (counterclockwise rotation of the heart). Left ventricle round and elongated and extends below dome of diaphragm. **B,** steep left anterior oblique projection; left ventricle overlies spine. **C,** lateral projection; left ventricle extends posteriorly to reflection of the inferior vena cava *(arrow)*. **D,** right anterior oblique projection; pulmonary artery segment inconspicuous, left ventricle extends below diaphragm.

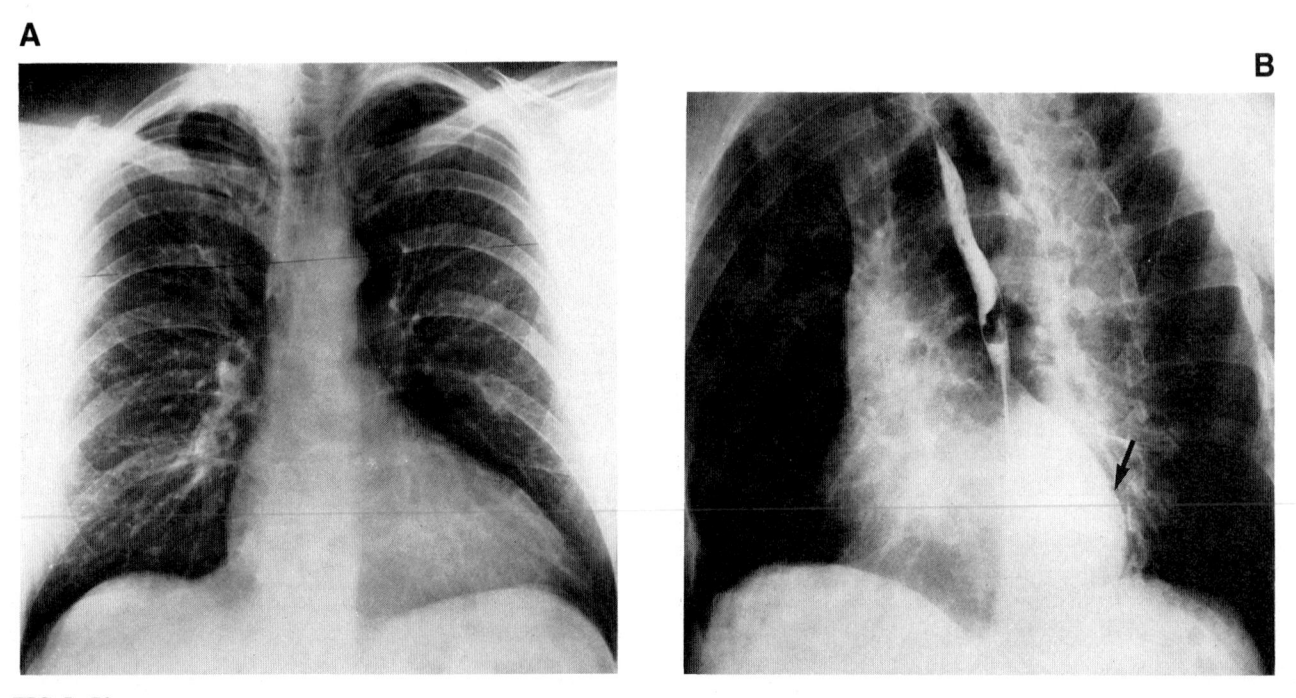

FIG 5–70.
Left ventricular enlargement. **A,** thoracic roentgenogram, pulmonary artery inconspicuous because of counterclockwise rotation. **B,** left anterior oblique projection; left ventricle overlies spine even on his very steep view.

tion (see Fig 5–69) (Check the position of clavicles, because a reversed lordotic view may do the same [see Fig 5–24].)

3. The pulmonary artery segment is concave, and the ascending aorta is more prominent because of counterclockwise rotation of the heart.

4. With a very large left ventricle, the dome of the diaphragm can no longer be seen through the cardiac shadow because the ventricle extends posteriorly. Therefore, the interface of the diaphragm with lung is lost.

5. The left anterior oblique projection is the most diagnostic view, because the left ventricle is rounder (more prominent) and extends lower than normal.

6. When the left ventricle is enlarged, it extends more posteriorly; it extends over the spine on a 60-degree left anterior oblique view. This overlap of the ventricle and the spine varies considerably with the rotation of the chest or the heart and with the shape of the thorax.

7. In a right anterior oblique projection, the pulmonary artery is less prominent because of the counterclockwise rotation from left ventricular enlargement. The cardiac apex extends inferiorly, and the left hemidiaphragm may blend with the cardiac shadow.

8. In the lateral projection, the left ventricle extends posteriorly and inferiorly. Therefore, the density of the supradiaphragmatic portion of the inferior vena cava projects within the cardiac contour.

9. The projections which best show left ventricular enlargement are the posteroanterior and left anterior oblique views (Fig 5–70).

Left Atrial Enlargement

Left atrial size can easily be assessed radiographically because the esophagus lies against the posterior wall. A barium swallow is very helpful. The highest indentation of the esophagus is caused by the aorta, followed (sometimes) by the left mainstem bronchus (Fig 5–71) and the left atrium.

During deep inspiration, the barium-filled esophagus may be indented by a normal-sized left atrium, but it should not be displaced posteriorly (Fig 5–72). However, the esophagus may be displaced posteriorly, giving a false impression of left atrial enlargement, if the view is taken during expiration. Marked right-sided cardiac enlargement may displace the left atrium, and therefore the barium-filled esophagus, posteriorly without the presence of left atrial enlargement (see Fig 5–66).

Left atrial enlargement may not be seen on each of the views because the esophagus may be displaced not only

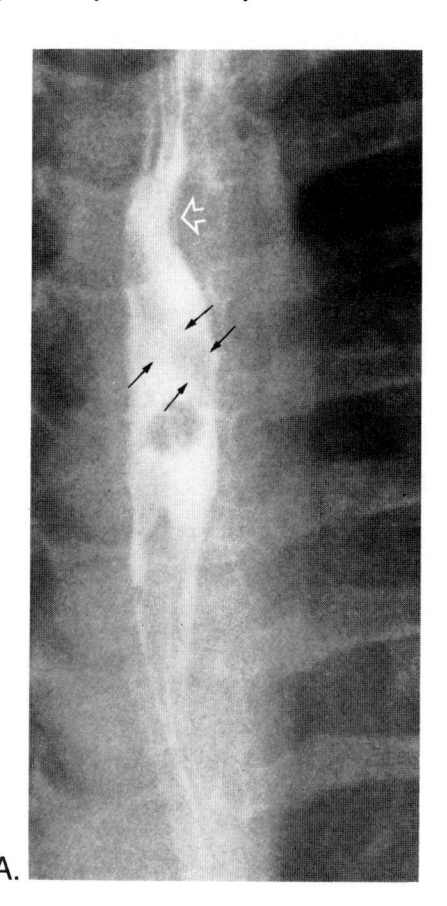

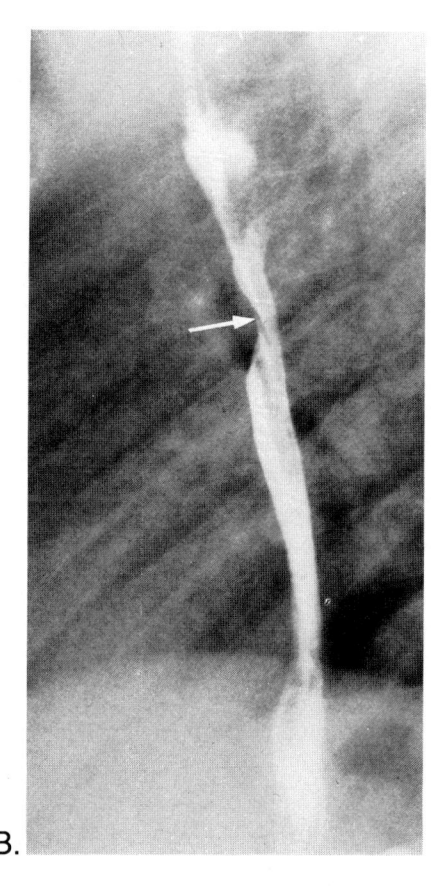

FIG 5–71.
Thoracic roentgenograms. A, anteroposterior projection. Normal identation of the barium-filled esophagus by a left arch *(open arrow)* and the left mainstem bronchus *(black arrows)*. **B,** lateral projection demonstrating indentation of esophagus by left mainstem bronchus *(white arrow)*.

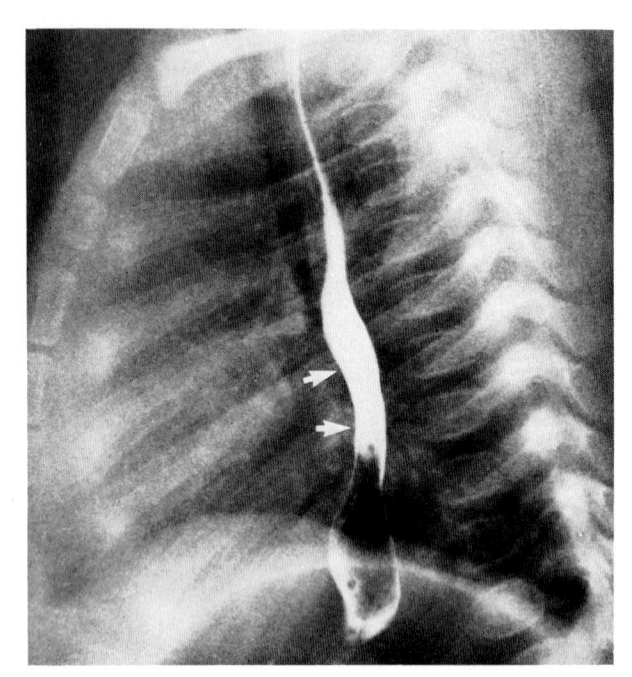

FIG 5–72.
Thoracic roentgenogram, lateral projection with barium swallow in infant with normal heart. Anterior wall of esophagus *(arrows)* indented. This normal finding should not be misdiagnosed as left atrial enlargement.

posteriorly but to either the right or the left. The latter phenomenon has been called esophageal escape. The maximum displacement is seen in the projection in which the x-ray beam passes tangentially to the esophagus (Fig 5–73). Thus, if the esophagus is displaced posteriorly and not laterally, the best view is the lateral projection; if the esophagus is displaced posteriorly and toward the right, maximum displacement is demonstrated on a right anterior oblique projection (see Fig 5–73). In the much rarer situation of displacement toward the left, a left anterior oblique projection is best.

In the elderly, an erroneous diagnosis of left atrial enlargement may be made because the esophagus normally is displaced by a tortuous and elongated thoracic aorta. The esophagus adheres to the descending thoracic aorta, which can be seen on a posteroanterior film as deviation of the esophagus toward the left. This normal deviation should not be confused with displacement by left atrial enlargement on the left anterior oblique projection.

A markedly enlarged left atrium may extend beyond the cardiac silhouette toward either the right or the left. Slight left atrial enlargement may be seen as a double density through the cardiac silhouette. This is abnormal in the adult, indicating left atrial enlargement, but in children younger than 5 years, it may be a normal finding (Fig 5–74). An enlarged confluence of the right pulmonary veins also may create a double density.

The left atrium is anatomically related to the carina. When the chamber enlarges, it expands not only posteriorly but also superiorly, toward the carina, because the heart is firmly supported by the diaphragm. With enlargement, the space between the left mainstem bronchus and left atrium becomes filled in on the left anterior oblique projection, and eventually the angle of the carina becomes splayed. Splaying is more common in adults with acquired

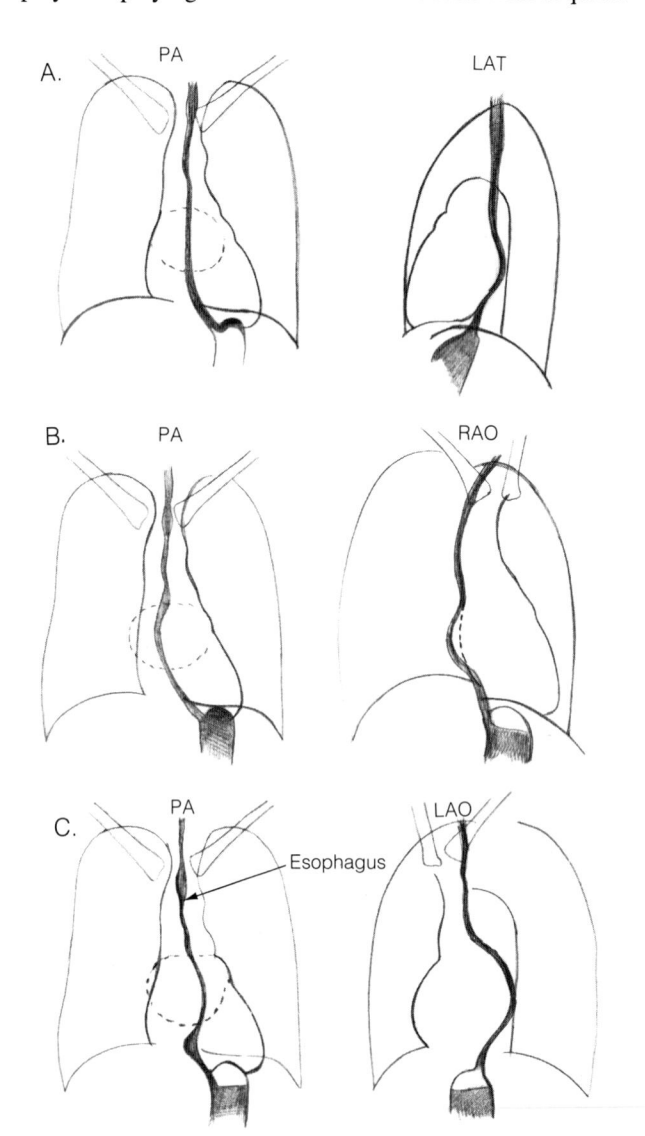

FIG 5–73.
Diagram of left atrial enlargement, with concomitant views that best show the maximum displacement of the barium-filled esophagus. **A,** posterior without lateral displacement; in infants and patients with slight left atrial enlargement. Lateral projection is best view. **B,** displacement posteriorly and toward right; commonly occurs with larger left atria. Right anterior oblique projection is best. **C,** displacement posteriorly and toward the left. Rare occurring only with the large left atria. Left anterior oblique projection is best. Lateral displacement of esophagus has been termed "esophageal escape."

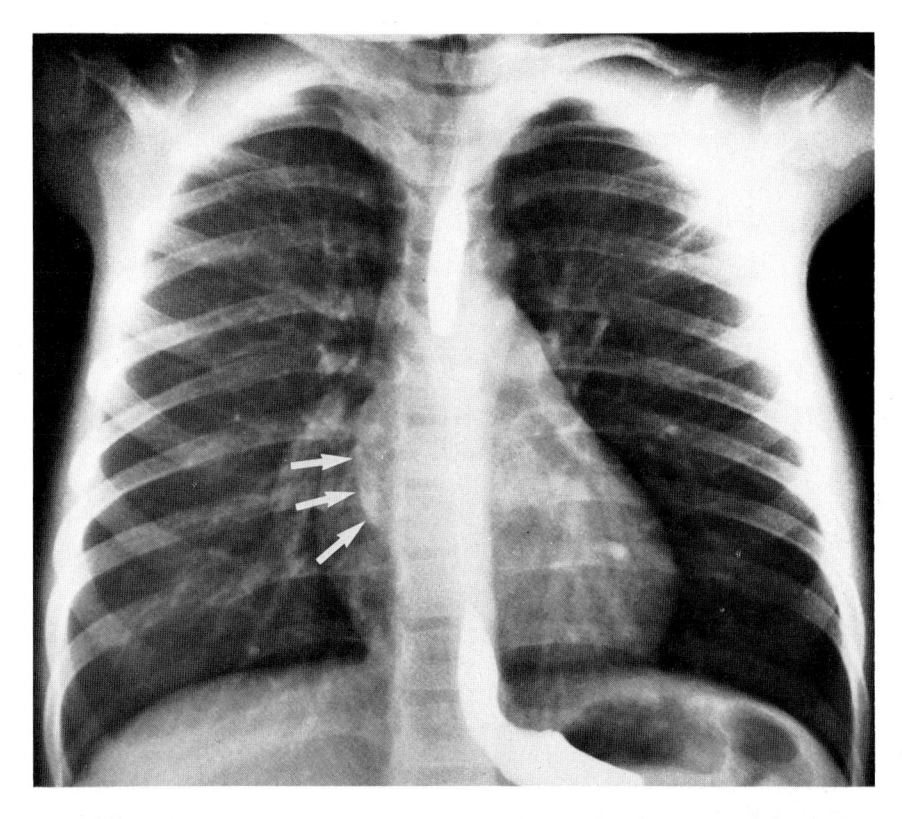

FIG 5–74.
Thoracic roentgenogram, posteroanterior projection in normal child. Left atrium causes double density *(arrows)*, a normal finding in children. In older patients, however, double density indicates left atrial enlargement.

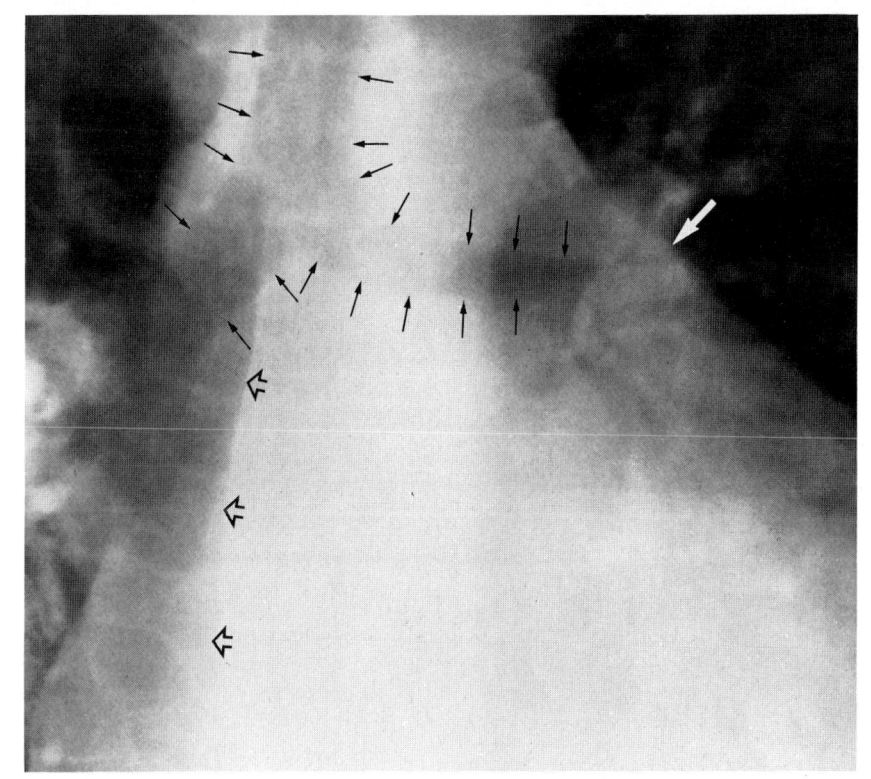

FIG 5–75.
Thoracic roentgenogram, posteroanterior projection, in patient with mitral insufficiency. Huge left atrium; carina (normal angle about 60 degrees) markedly splayed *(arrows)*. Posterior mediastinum *(open arrows)* displaced toward right, simulating a paraspinal mass. Left atrial appendage *(white arrow)* distended, resulting in straight left cardiac border ("mitralization").

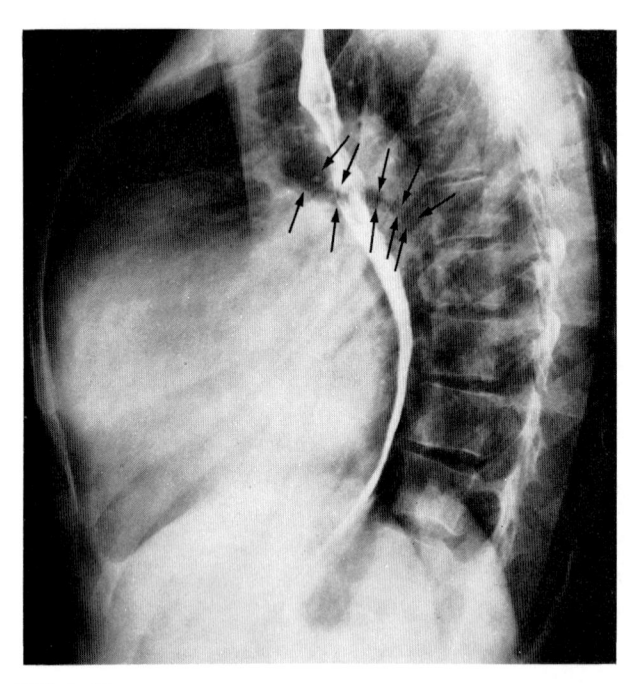

FIG 5–76.
Thoracic roentgenogram, lateral projection shows huge left atrium secondary to mitral disease. Sternum bowed anteriorly. Retrosternal space obliterated, indicating marked right-sided enlargement. Huge left atrium displaces barium-filled esophagus. Left mainstem bronchus elevated, displaced posteriorly, and slightly narrowed *(arrows)*.

mitral disease than in patients with congenital heart disease (Fig 5–75), but it may occur in the latter if the left atrium is very large.

On the left anterior oblique and lateral projections, the left mainstem bronchus is elevated and displaced posteriorly (Fig 5–76). With severe left atrial enlargement, the left main bronchus is narrowed by the pressure exerted by the left atrium below and the left pulmonary artery above. Atelectasis of the left lung may ensue (Fig 5–77).

In mitral valve disease, the left atrial appendage becomes distended and forms a prominent bulge along the left cardiac contour just below the pulmonary arterial segment (see Fig 5–75) ("mitralization" of the cardiac silhouette). After a mitral commissurotomy, the heart may no longer be typically "mitral" because the left atrial appendage has been amputated (see Fig 5–8). Specific distention of the left atrial appendage is rare in congenital heart disease.

CARDIAC FLUOROSCOPY

Previously, fluoroscopy was an integral part of the cardiac examination and performed in addition to the four views of the heart. Because of the high radiation dose—the skin dose to an average patient is about 2,000 mR, whereas a cardiac series is only about 100 mR—the added cost, and the small diagnostic yield, cardiac fluoroscopy is

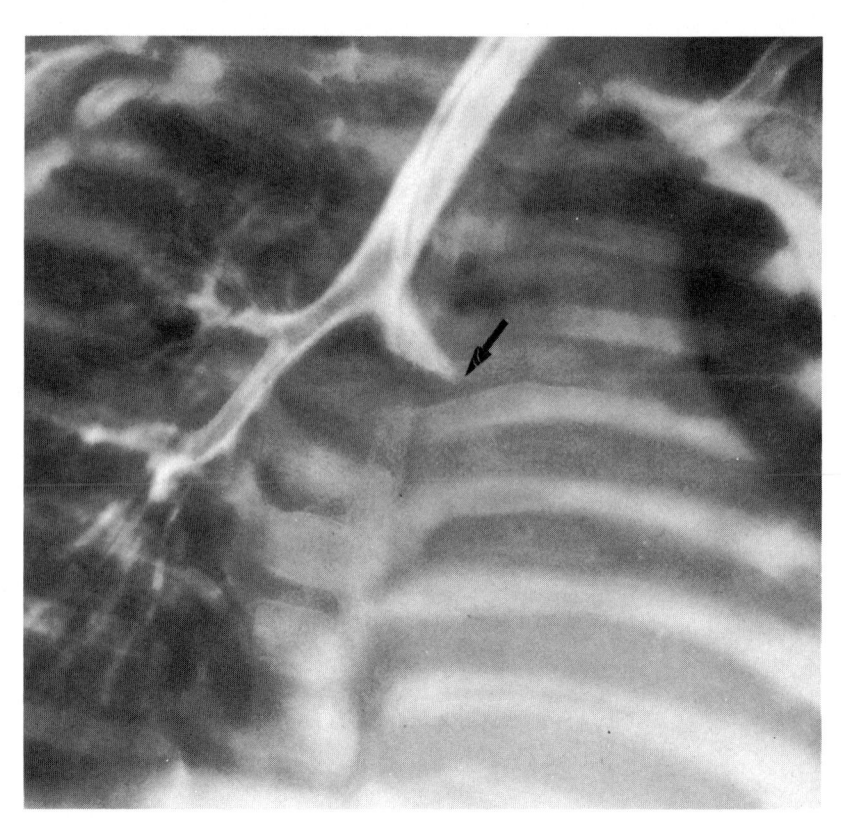

FIG 5–77.
Bronchogram demonstrating atelectasis of the left lung because of compression of the left mainstem bronchus *(arrow)*.

seldom performed now, echocardiography being used to provide similar information. However, fluoroscopy is still a useful tool for differentiating an enlarged thymus from a mediastinal tumor, as well as in emergencies during cardiac catheterization to exclude hemopericardium resulting from vascular performation.

The most useful application of cine fluorography is in the evaluation of artificial cardiac valves. After valve replacement and before discharge from the hospital, the valve is fluoroscoped, and the opening angle of the disk or leaflets is recorded on a cine strip. If valve dysfunction is suspected later, fluoroscopy is repeated for comparison with the baseline cine strip to diagnose valve dysfunction. Fluoroscopy is more reliable than echocardiography in this context. Fluoroscopy is also valuable to study cardiac calcifications, particularly when combined with cine fluorography.

CHAPTER 6

Cardiac Catheterization

Cardiac catheterization is an invasive diagnostic procedure designed to accomplish three functions. First, although most patients have had clinical evaluation and noninvasive studies such as electrocardiography, thoracic roentgenography, and echocardiography, cardiac catheterization may be needed to make a definitive diagnosis. Second, catheterization provides information about the severity of a cardiac lesion, because, through various measurements, the hemodynamics of a given anomaly can be determined. Finally, catheterization may be performed to evaluate the effect of a lesion on the heart and circulation. Some cardiac lesions are well tolerated, whereas others have sufficient effect to alter the response of the myocardium to exercise or even its condition at rest.

In general, catheterization is most often performed before a cardiac operation. The information obtained provides the surgeon with anatomic information to guide operative decisions and provides the cardiologist with insights about the circulation that may assist in the preoperative or postoperative management. Also, cardiac catheterization is often performed postoperatively to determine the success of an operation, to measure changes in the circulation, and to discover any residual abnormalities. Catheterization also may be performed to study the effects of various pharmacologic agents on the heart, either directly or to follow changes during therapy in a patient who has been on medications for some time.

To meet all of these objectives, various types of information are obtained during catheterization, and data are derived from several sources. One is observation of the catheter's course. The passage of a catheter through a communication such as an atrial septal defect, ventricular septal defect, or patent ductus arteriosus can provide important information about the presence of such communications without angiography. However, such a course is only diagnostic if anteroposterior and lateral views are made. Second, pressures can be measured in the various cardiac chambers and great vessels and these values compared with each other and with normal values. Third, blood samples can be obtained from individual cardiac chambers for oxygen measurement to detect shunts and to calculate blood flows. Fourth, angiocardiography usually is performed during routine cardiac catheterization. This technique is used primarily to detect the presence and anatomic form of congenital anomalies and may aid in the assessment of their severity, particularly in the case of insufficient valves. Finally, a variety of specialized diagnostic tests, such as injection of dye, performance of exercise, and administration of vasoactive pharmacologic agents, may be performed to provide additional information.

CATHETER COURSE

The normal catheter course through the right side of the heart and into the pulmonary artery, or through the arterial system into the left side of the heart, is easily recognizable, as are variations. The most common and characteristic catheter positions are diagrammed as seen in the anteroposterior and lateral projections in Figure 6–1, parts 1 to 37. In the presence of communications between the two sides of the heart, such as atrial septal defect (part 19), ventricular septal defect (part 4), or patent ductus arteriosus (part 5), the catheter may go from one side of the heart to the other, frequently following a characteristic course. In addition, the course from a peripheral site to the heart through the inferior vena cava or the descending aorta or from the brachial artery or veins provides information about the course of these vascular structures to the heart. In patients with a left superior vena cava, for instance (part 18), a catheter passed from the left arm will descend on the left side of the mediastinum to enter either the coronary sinus or, less frequently, the left atrium directly. Normally, the inferior vena cava is on the right side of the abdomen and the descending aorta on the left side, both being alongside the spine. If the catheter course is on

116 *General Introduction*

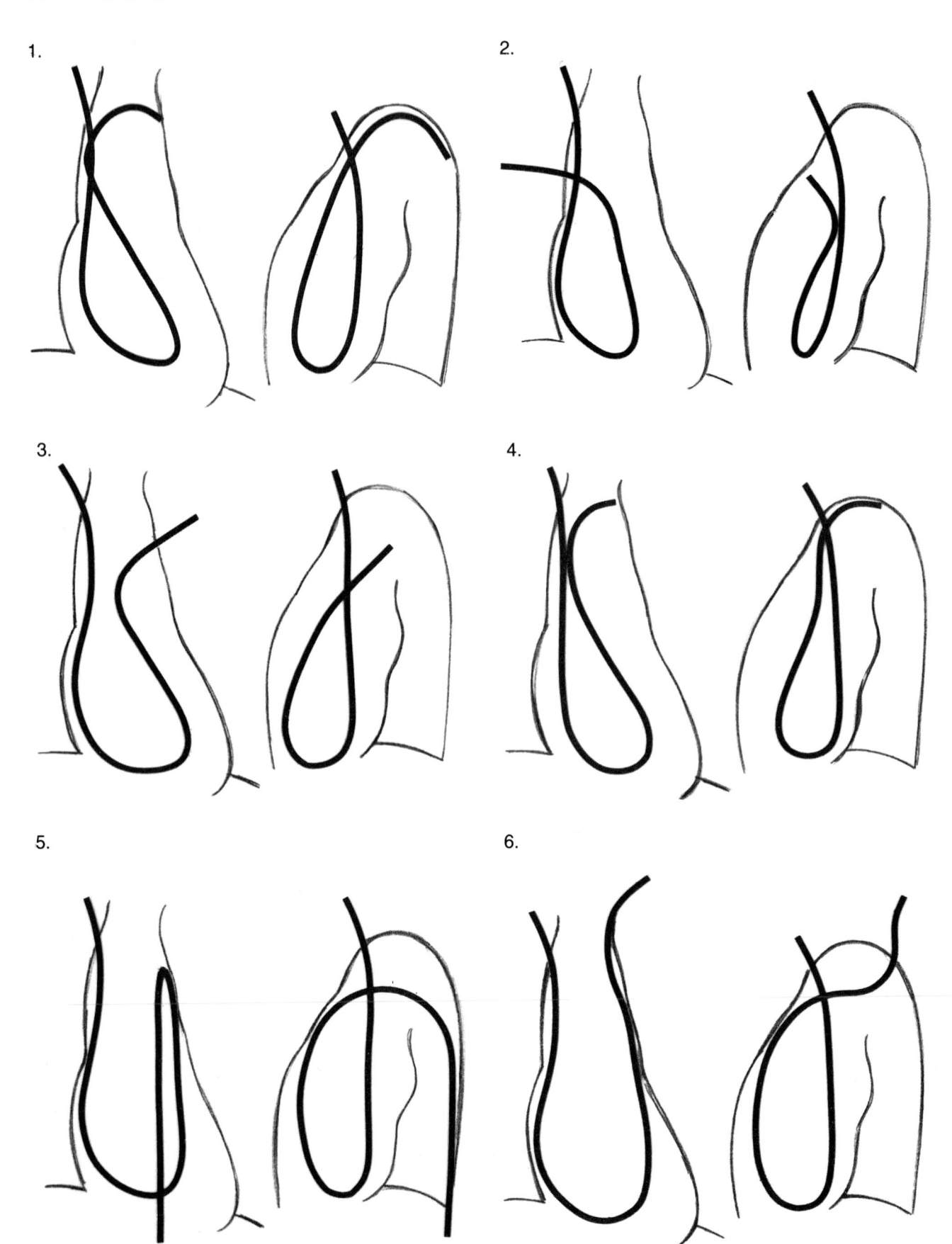

1.

2.

3.

4.

5.

6.

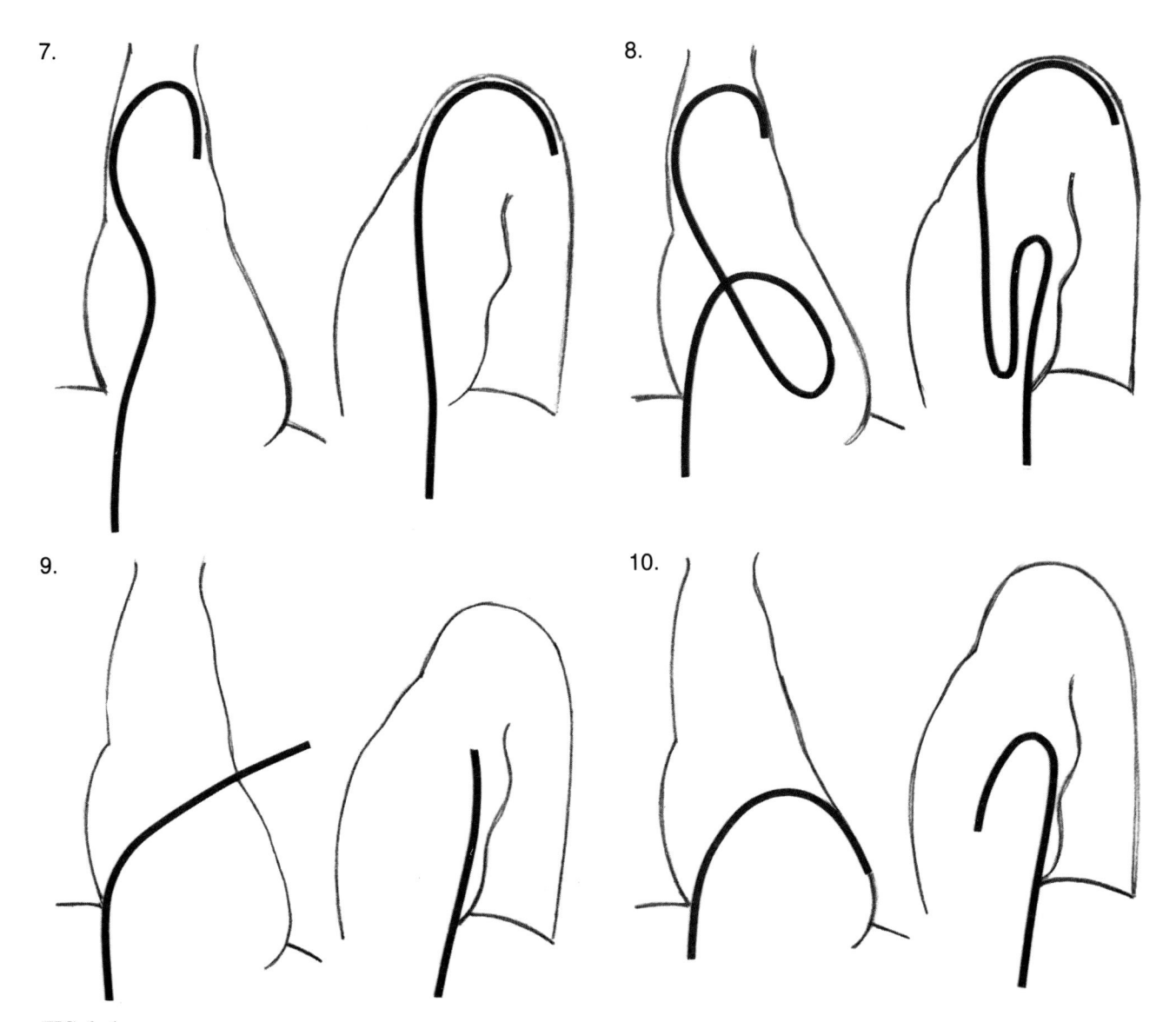

FIG 6–1.
Characteristic catheter positions in the various types of congenital heart disease, showing anteroposterior and lateral views. (Students may find these useful as unknowns for self-testing.) *1.* Complete transposition of great vessels; catheter passes from superior vena cava, through right atrium and ventricle, into aorta, which lies anteriorly and to the right. The view on an anteroposterior projection is identical to that seen with a membranous ventricular septal defect (part *4*). *2.* Congenitally corrected transposition of great vessels; catheter passes from superior vena into right atrium, through inverted left ventricle, into the medially and posteriorly located pulmonary artery and the right pulmonary artery. This is a technically difficult catheter passage because of the tail-shaped inverted ventricle. *3.* Persistent truncus arteriosus; catheter passes from the superior vena cava into the right ventricle, truncus, and left pulmonary artery. The lateral projection excludes congenitally corrected transposition, which may show a similar catheter course on the anteroposterior projection (part *2*). *4.* Membranous ventricular septal defect; catheter passes from superior vena cava through right atrium and medial portion of right ventricle and enters a great vessel (aorta), which is located posteriorly and ascends in normal fashion. The catheter course should not be mistaken for that in complete transposition (part *1*). *5.* Patent ductus arteriosus or Potts anastomosis; catheter passes from superior vena cava through right atrium and ventricle into pulmonary trunk. On lateral projection, posterior direction of passage from pulmonary artery to aorta is evident. The catheter is then advanced below the diaphragm, confirming its location in the aorta. It is this important subdiaphragmatic location of the catheter that rules out the much more common passage into a left pulmonary artery. *6.* Patent ductus arteriosus; unusual course: catheter passes from superior vena cava through right side of heart into pulmonary trunk through a patent ductus into the thoracic aorta and the left subclavian artery. *7.* Membranous ventricular septal defect; catheter enters heart from inferior vena cava, passes through tricuspid valve following typical course close to spine, through ventricular septal defect, into the aortic arch. This course is more common than that demonstrated in part *4*. *8.* Ascending aorta through patent foramen ovale; catheter enters heart from inferior vena cava, passes from right to left atrium through area of foramen ovale, and into left ventricle, where it curves on itself and then shows typical course through ascending aorta and aortic arch. *9.* Left upper pulmonary vein; catheter enters heart from inferior vena cava, passes from right to left atrium, and leaves cardiac silhouette into left midlung field. On lateral projection, however, it is located within cardiac shadow: One view is never diagnostic in determining catheter positions. *10.* Pericardial sac, through left atrial appendage; catheter enters heart from inferior vena cava, passes from right to left atrium, and then follows cardiac border. This course may mimic passage into left lower pulmonary vein, but blood cannot be withdrawn, pressure is negative, and injection of a minute amount of contrast material confirms location.

(Continued.)

11.

12.

13.

14.

15.

16.

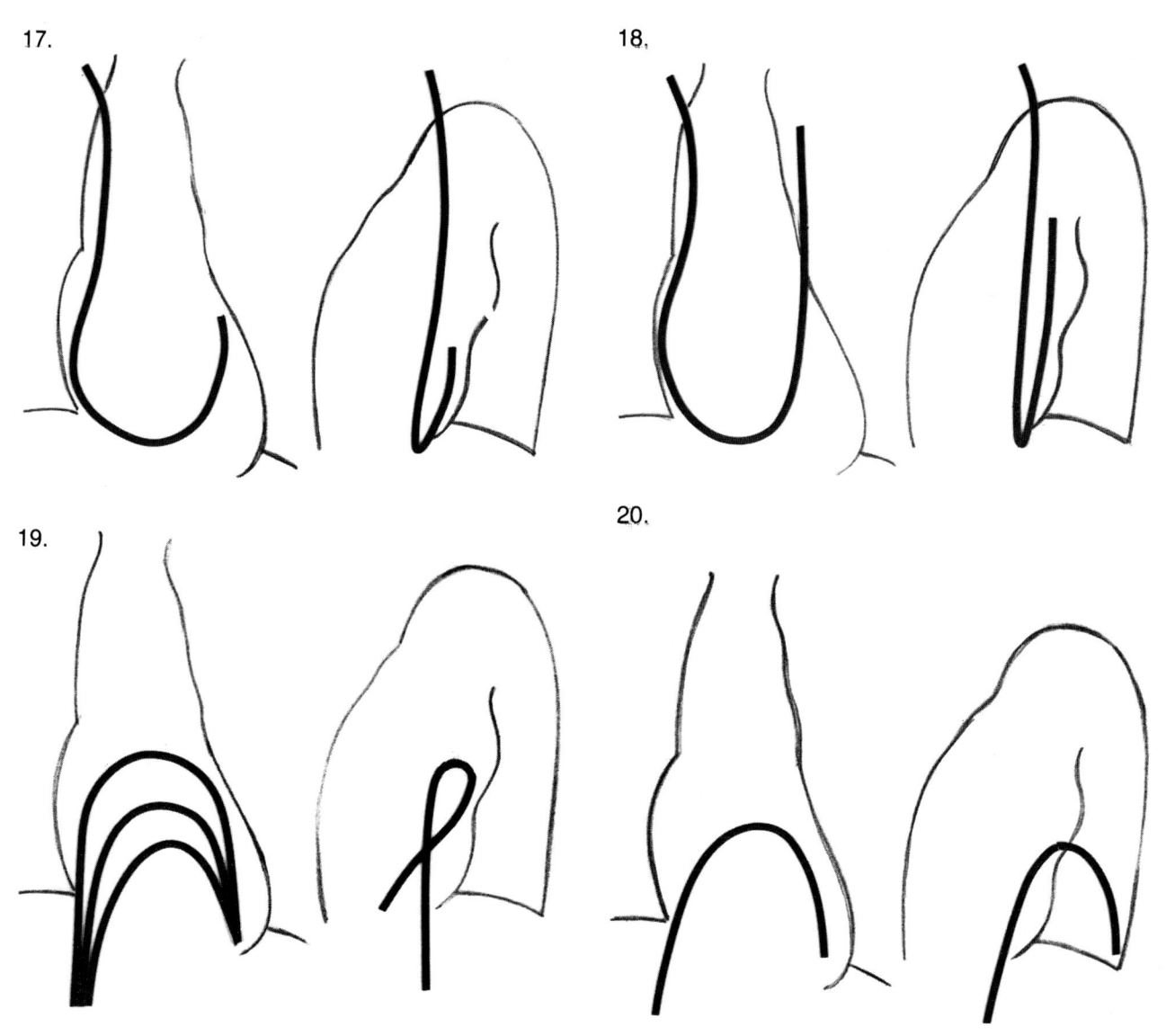

FIG 6–1 (cont.).
11. Interruption of the vena cava with azygous continuation; catheter passed from below. On anteroposterior projection, leading portion of catheter appears within cardiac silhouette, but on lateral projection, it lies behind the heart in azygous vein and passes anteriorly into superior vena cava. Once there, it passes inferiorly into right atrium, and, typically, into apex of right ventricle. *12.* Left lower pulmonary artery; catheter enters heart from superior vena cava and passes through right side of heart into pulmonary artery. Anteroposterior projection resembles that in part *5,* showing catheter through a patent ductus. Here, however, catheter cannot be passed below diaphragm; and on the lateral projection, it extends posteriorly obliquely into lung field two features, excluding patent ductus arteriosus. *13.* Membranous ventricular septal defect (arterial approach); catheter course through aortic arch, across aortic valve, through septal defect, and anteriorly into right ventricle. This course is uncommon with membranous defect and it is suspicious for double-outlet right ventricle or tetralogy of Fallot. *14.* Common atrium (catheter course from superior vena cava); catheter loops from right to left cardiac border and back again at a level above the atrioventricular valves. Catheter outlines the lateral margins of the common atrium. *15.* Hepatic vein; catheter passes from superior vena cava, through right atrium, into right hepatic vein. *16.* Left ventricle through atrial septal defect; catheter passes from superior vena cava, through sinus venosus atrial septal defect, and posteriorly into the left ventricle. *17.* Coronary sinus; catheter passes from superior vena cava into right atrium and then posteriorly and into typical "reverse J" shape. On the anteroposterior projection, catheter position could be mistaken for right ventricle. For the same reason, pacemaker positions have to be determined in two planes. *18.* Left superior vena cava entering coronary sinus; catheter passes from superior vena cava into right atrium. Initial course similar to that in part *17,* but catheter can be advanced superiorly beyond cardiac contour. *19.* Atrial septal defects; catheter passed from inferior vena cava, through various atrial defects. The most superior catheter has passed through a sinus venosus, the lower one through an ostium secundum, the lowest through an ostium primum defect (*see* Chapter 16). *20.* Left lower pulmonary vein; catheter passes from inferior vena cava through right atrium and left atrium into left lower pulmonary vein. (Compare parts *10* and *19:* similar appearance on anteroposterior projection, but lateral projection here shows catheter posteriorly in lung field.) This course is more common with catheterization from the inferior vena cava, because the catheter tip is guided by the limbus of the fossa ovalis.

(Continued.)

21.

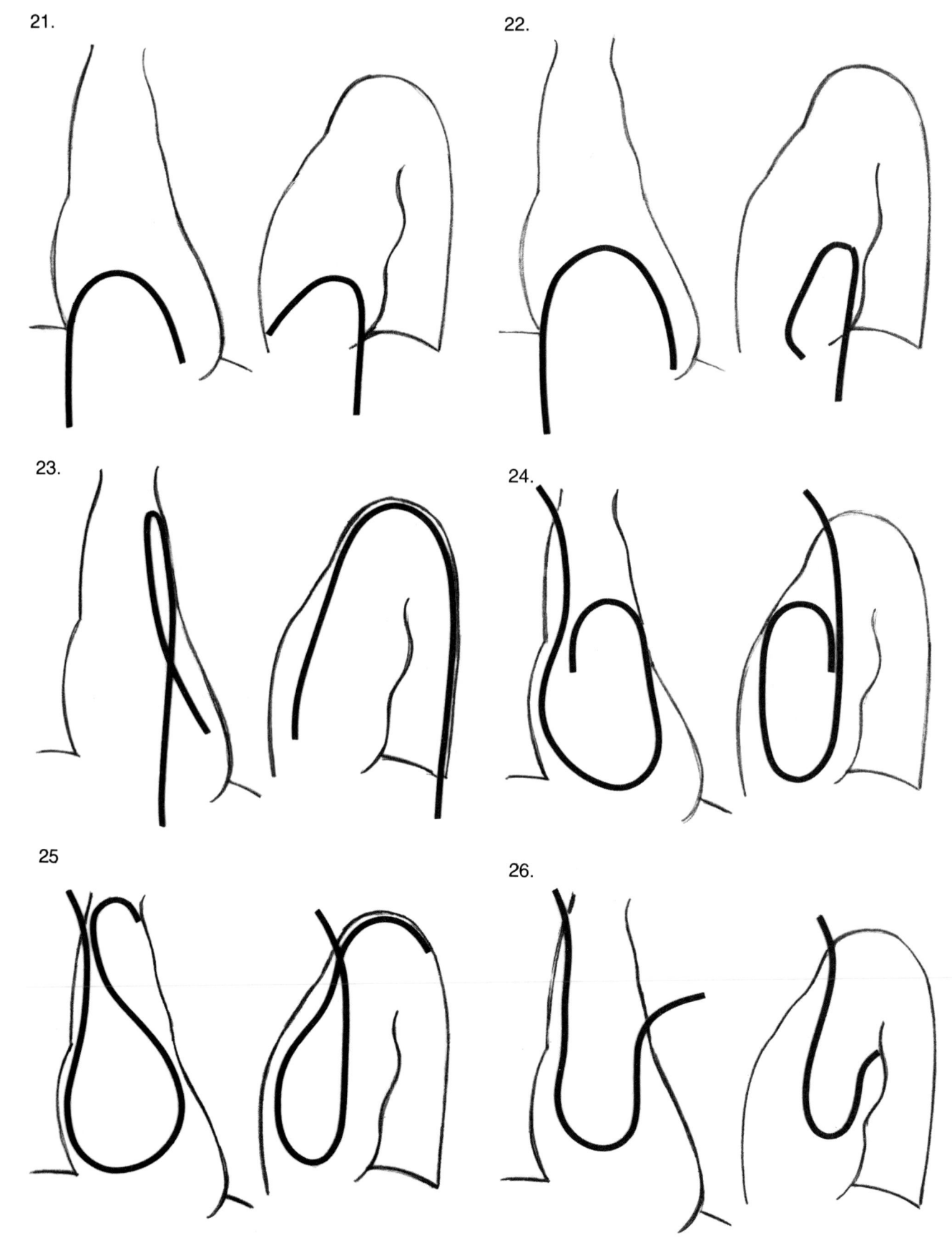

22.

23.

24.

25.

26.

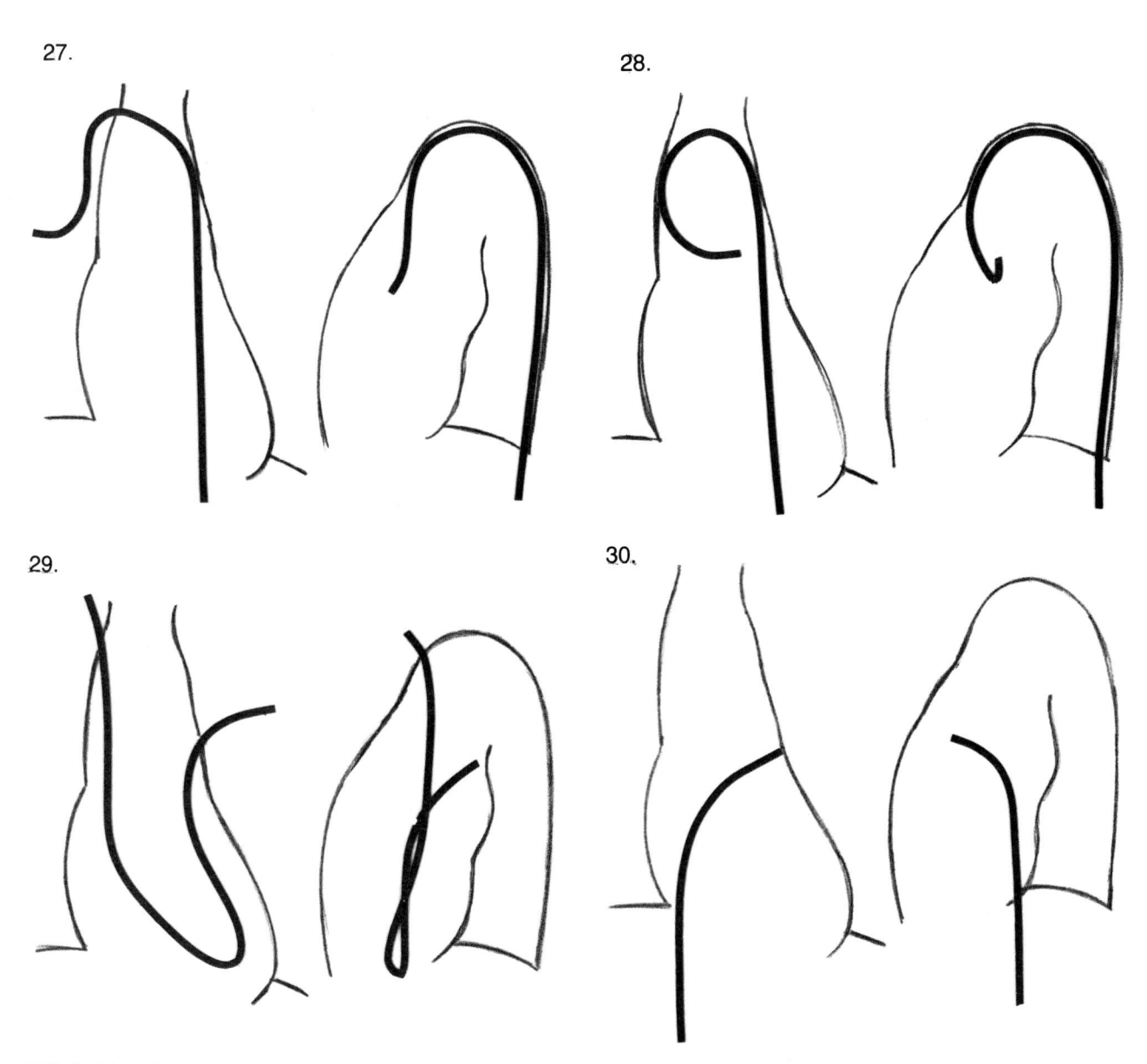

FIG 6–1 (cont.).
21. Right ventricle; catheter passes from inferior vena cava through right atrium anteriorly into right ventricle. *22.* Left ventricle; catheter passes from inferior vena cava across atrial septum, then inferiorly and posteriorly into left ventricle. (Compare parts *10, 19,* and *20.*) *23.* Congenitally corrected transposition (arterial approach); catheter passes through descending aorta and aortic arch. The ascending aorta is located anteriorly and to the left. The catheter enters the systemic ventricle, located anteriorly and to the left (inverted right ventricle). *24.* Aorticopulmonic window; catheter enters heart through superior vena cava and passes through right atrium and right ventricle into pulmonary trunk. It then courses posteriorly and medially to descend in the ascending aorta. Catheter tip lies against the aortic valve. *25.* Aorticopulmonic window; catheter enters heart from superior vena cava and passes through right atrium and ventricle into pulmonary trunk. It then passes through aorticopulmonary window into ascending aorta. (Compare parts *1* and *4*). This is distinguished by being posterior and slightly more lateral on anteroposterior projection. *26.* Left upper pulmonary vein; catheter passes from superior vena cava, from right to left atrium, into left upper pulmonary vein. *27.* Right Blalock-Taussig shunt; catheter passes through aortic arch, into innominate artery, and through shunt into right pulmonary artery. *28.* Waterston shunt; catheter passes through aortic arch. Above aortic valve, catheter passes leftward into proximal left pulmonary artery. *29.* Complete transposition of great vessels, catheter passes through superior vena cava across atrial septum into posteriorly located left ventricle. Catheter then loops on itself to enter posteriorly located pulmonary trunk and left pulmonary artery. *30.* Left atrial appendage; catheter passes from inferior vena cava, through atrial septum, and superiorly and leftward into left atrial appendage. DO NOT PUSH! because catheter course will then become like that in part *10*. The left atrial appendage is preferentially entered after catheter has been passed into left atrium and is a common site of iatrogenic cardiac perforations.

(Continued.)

31.

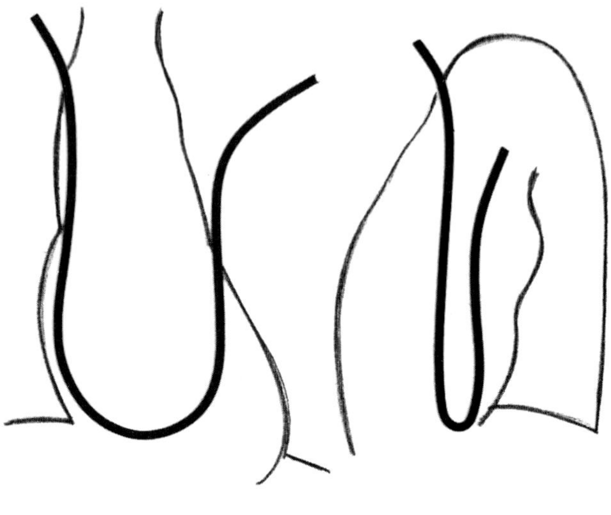

32.

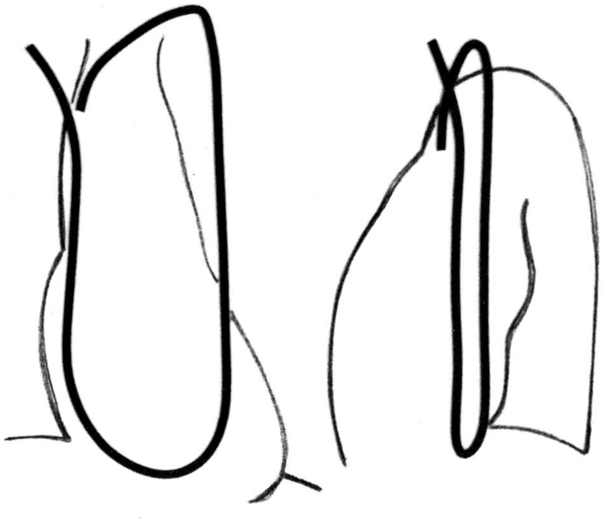

33.

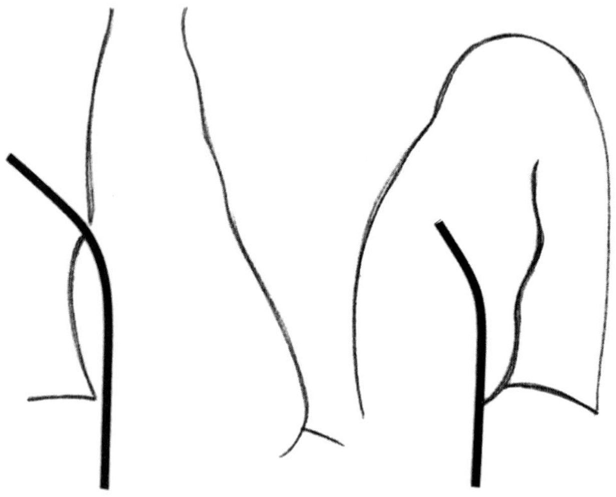

34.

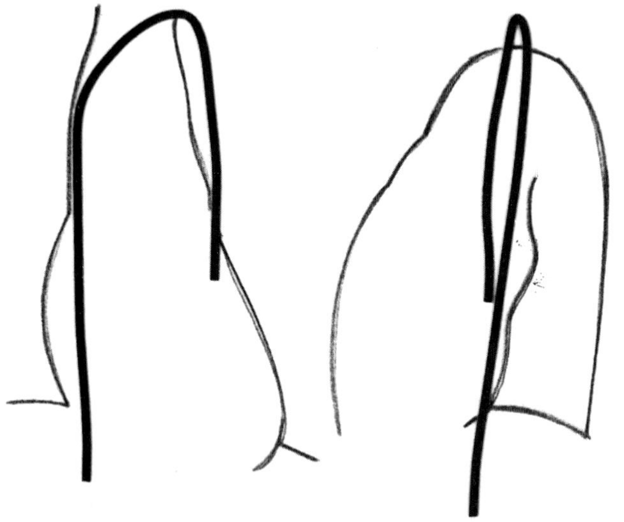

35.

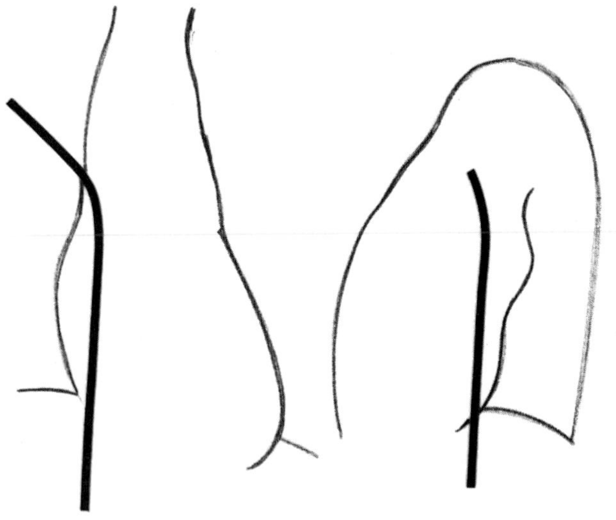

FIG 6–1 (cont.).
31. Anomalous pulmonary venous connections to coronary sinus. (Compare parts *17* and *18.*) Initial part of catheter course similar, but catheter tip passes through left upper pulmonary vein into left upper lung field. *32.* Right superior vena cava; catheter passes from coronary sinus to left superior vena cava, left subclavian vein; and innominate vein. *33.* Right upper pulmonary vein; catheter passes from inferior vena cava through right atrium and ultimately to right upper pulmonary vein. Usually, this course is through a patent foramen ovale. Rarely, it indicates direct connection of pulmonary vein to right atrium. *34.* Left superior vena cava in total anomalous pulmonary venous connection; catheter passes from inferior vena cava to right superior vena cava, left innominate vein, and left superior vena cava. If oxygen saturation is high, partial or total anomalous venous return must be considered. *35.* Partial anomalous pulmonary venous connection of right upper pulmonary vein to superior vena cava; catheter passes from inferior vena cava, through right atrium and proximal superior vena cava, into right upper lung field. (Compare part *33.*) Catheter clearly enters right pulmonry vein from the superior vena cava; in part *33,* catheter does not enter superior vena cava.

(Continued.)

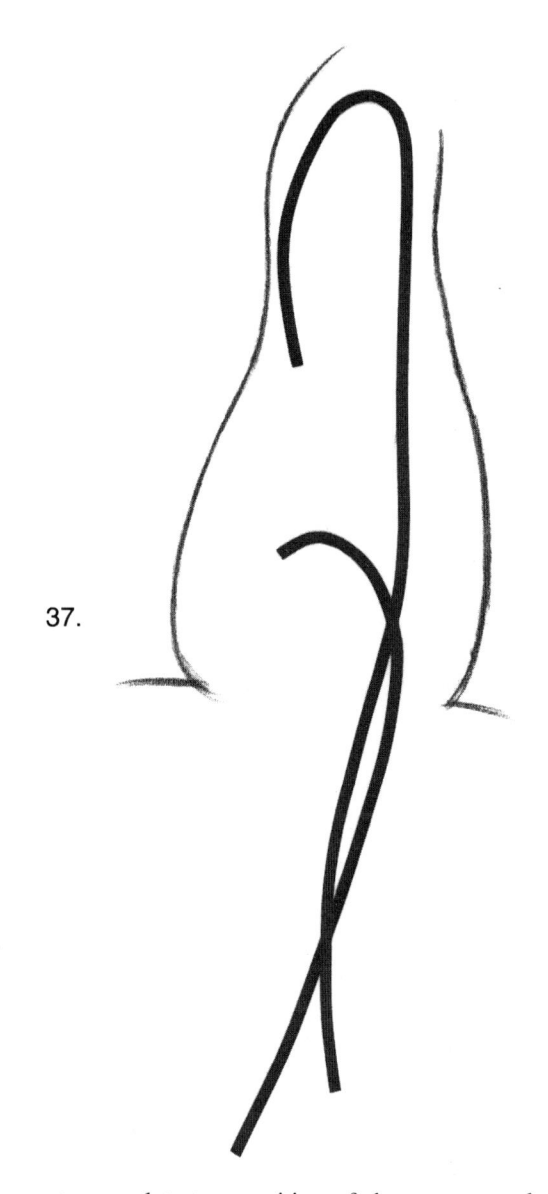

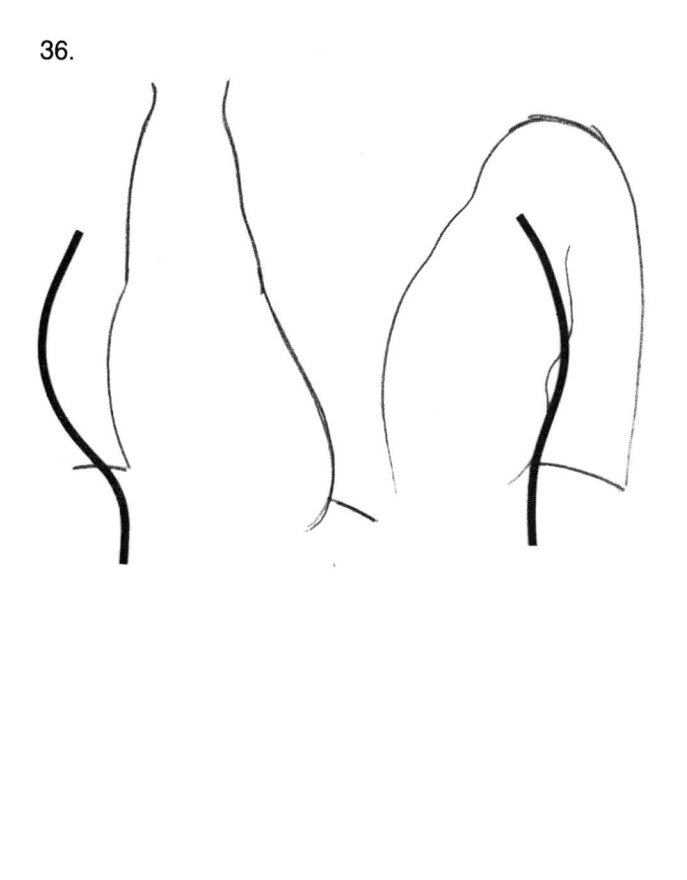

FIG 6–1 (cont.).
36. Scimitar vein; catheter passes from inferior vena cava into right lung. Characteristic curved course is diagnostic of scimitar vein even without a lateral view. *37.* Situs ambiguous (abdominal heterotaxia); both venous and arterial catheters are to left of the spine and cross in abdomen, indicating an indeterminate (ambiguous) situs. (See chapter on cardial malpositions and asplenia.)

the opposite side, it indicates situs inversus. At times, the initial recognition of situs ambiguous, as found in patients with asplenia or polysplenia, is diagnosed by the abnormal relations between the inferior vena cava and the aorta in the abdomen (part *37*). In patients with asplenia, generally the inferior vena cava and aorta lie on the same side of the abdomen. In patients with polysplenia, there is infrahepatic interruption of the inferior vena cava with azygous continuation, so that the catheter passes from the abdomen into the superior vena cava and then down into the right atrium, a very diagnostic course (part *11*).

The catheter course can also be used to recognize malposition of the great vessels. If the catheter can be advanced from the right ventricle to the aorta, this suggests a ventricular septal defect (parts *4* and *7*) if, on a lateral view, the catheter in the aorta is located posteriorly. If, on the other hand, the catheter is located more anteriorly, this suggests complete transposition of the great vessels (part *1*) or persistent truncus arteriosus (part *3*). When the catheter passed from the venous side through a ventricle into the aorta that courses along the upper left cardiac border and is anteriorly located, this indicates either congenitally corrected transposition or single ventricle with inverted infundibulum (part *2*).

An atrial septal defect can be suggested by a catheter course from the right atrium into the left atrium (part *19*). Such a course can also be through a patent foramen ovale. It is much easier to advance the catheter from the right atrium to the left atrium from the inferior vena cava through an ostium secundum–type atrial defect. If the catheter can be passed from the superior vena cava into the left atrium, it suggests either a sinus venosus location of the defect or an ostium primum defect. Characteristically, in an ostium primum defect, the catheter course from the right atrium to the left atrium is low through the atrial septum and well within the cardiac shadow. Generally, catheters can be advanced through a membranous ventricular septal defect and go almost exclusively into the aorta (parts *4* and *7*). It is uncommon to be able to advance the catheter through a ventricular septal defect to other locations or to advance the catheter through a ventricular septal defect into the body of the left ventricle. On the other hand, retrograde passage of a catheter from the aorta into the ventricle almost never occurs through the ventricular septal defect into the right ventricle. If the catheter passes into the right ventricle, a diagnosis of double-outlet right ventricle or tetralogy of Fallot (overriding aorta) should be suspected (part *13*).

From the pulmonary artery, the catheter can be advanced from the proximal left pulmonary artery to the descending aorta through a patent or closing ductus arteriosus (part *5*). It is rare for a catheter to pass from the pulmonary artery through a ductus into the ascending aorta (part *6*); we have encountered only one single case. In a patient with an aorticopulmonary septal defect, the catheter can be advanced from the proximal pulmonary artery into the proximal aorta. Characteristically, the catheter can then be advanced into one of the brachiocephalic vessels, giving a characteristic appearance to this catheter course (parts *24* and *25*).

The catheter can also be advanced into pulmonary veins that are either normally or abnormally connected. In the presence of normally connected veins, frequently, when the catheter is advanced from the right atrium through an atrial defect, it passes readily into the left pulmonary veins (part *26*). The left lower pulmonary vein descends in the left lung and generally appears within the cardiac shadow (part *20*). From the inferior vena cava, the catheter frequently can also be advanced into the right upper pulmonary vein. This course might make the pulmonary vein appear to connect anomalously to the right atrium. It is possible to pass the catheter through the venous system, coronary sinus, or superior vena cava into anomalously connecting veins from either the right superior vena cava or a persistent left superior vena cava (parts *9, 31, 34,* and *35*).

In patients with a surgically created extracardiac shunt, such as a Blalock-Taussig (part *27*) or Waterston (part *28*) shunt or a Gortex graft, the catheter may be advanced through the channel from the aorta into the pulmonary artery.

Thus, considerable information can be obtained by observing the catheter course, and careful attention should be directed to this throughout the catheterization. However, failure to advance a catheter from one chamber to another does not mean that there is an atretic valve or lack of communication between these structures but may merely reflect an inability of the operator to make appropriate maneuvers.

Whenever an unusual or doubtful catheter position is encountered during cardiac catheterization, the location of the catheter tip can be identified in three ways:

1. Pressure measurment
2. Oxygen measurement in a blood sample drawn through the catheter
3. Injection of a small amount of contrast medium

In most cases, pressure measurements and blood sample analysis are adequate for identification. Although the injection of contrast medium is the most definitive technique, it should be used sparingly to limit the cumulative dose of contrast medium.

If the catheter course is unusual, it should always be documented radiographically in both the anteroposterior and lateral projections. Also, even if demonstrated radiographically in two planes, catheter positions are diagnostic only if the pressure and oximetry data confirm the diagnosis.

CARDIAC PRESSURE MEASUREMENTS

Cardiac pressures are measured in each chamber and great vessel that the catheter enters and recorded in millimeters of mercury, whereas venous and portal pressures are usually measured in centimeters of water (saline solution). Conversions can be effected by the formula 1 mm Hg equals 1.36 cm H_2O. In atria and arteries, mean pressures are generally obtained in addition to recordings during systole and diastole.

Right Atrial Pressure

The right atrial pressure, like the left atrial pressure, typically has three wave forms: an *a* wave, occurring with atrial contraction; a *c* wave, occurring shortly after the beginning of systole as the atrioventricular valve is displaced into the atrium; and a *v* wave, occurring at the end of systole and reaching its peak before the onset of diastole (Fig 6–2). The *v* wave represents the continued accumulation of blood in the atrium before the opening of the atrioventricular valve. The normal pressures of the wave forms in the right atrium are $a = 3$ to 7 mm Hg, $c = 2$ to 5 mm Hg, and $v = 2$ to 5 mm Hg, with a mean pressure of 1 to 5 mm Hg. In infants, however, the right atrial pressure is often zero even in the presence of congestive heart failure. This reflects the fact that systemic venous bed is very compliant in the infant and so can accommodate a large volume of blood without an increase in pressure. In older patients, atrial pressures, particularly the *a* wave, may be in-

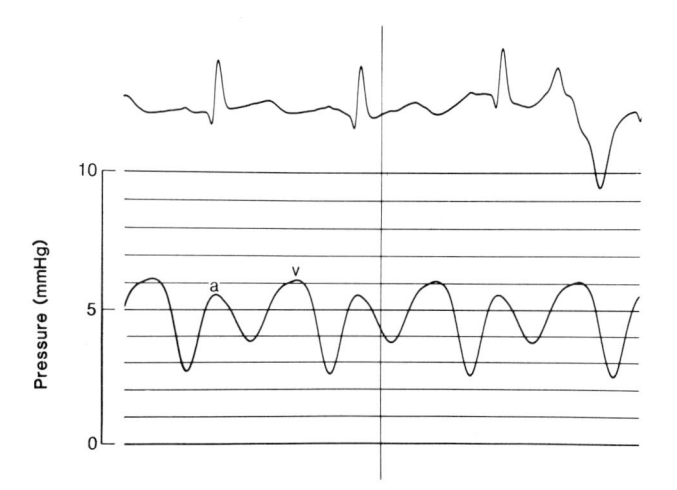

FIG 6–2.
Atrial pressure tracing with simultaneous electrocardiographic tracing. *a* = a wave; *v* = v wave.

creased because of elevated end diastolic pressure in the ventricle or the presence of tricuspid stenosis or atresia. The atrial pressure may also be elevated because of increased volume load, as occurs in an atrial level left-to-right shunt.

Tricuspid insufficiency produces a large *v* wave.

Right Ventricular Pressure

The right ventricular pressure is normally 25/0 to 5 mm Hg (Fig 6–3). Whenever there is a large communication between the ventricles, the right ventricular pressure is elevated, usually to systemic levels. The systolic pressure is elevated in the presence of pulmonary stenosis, pulmonary hypertension, a large ventricular septal defect, or connection of the right ventricle to the aorta, as in complete transposition of the great vessels. In the latter situation or in patients with a large ventricular septal defect, the systolic pressure in the right ventricle is the same as in the aorta, and the pressure curve shows a sharp rise but a rather flat top. This is in contrast to findings in patients with pulmonary hypertension and an intact ventricular septum and those with severe pulmonary stenosis, in whom the right ventricular pressure curves are more peaked and the pressure may exceed the systemic level. The right ventricular end-diastolic pressure may be elevated in patients with increased right ventricular volume, such as those with an atrial septal defect, right ventricular hypertrophy secondary to elevated systemic pressures, as in pulmonary stenosis or large ventricular septal defects, or, rarely, right ventricular cardiomyopathy.

Pulmonary Vascular Pressures

The pulmonary arterial pressure is generally 25/10 mm Hg, with a mean of 15 mm Hg. In patients with congenital heart disease, pulmonary arterial pressure is often elevated, reflecting pulmonary hypertension. This elevation may be related to increased pulmonary vascular resistance, in which both the systolic and diastolic pressures in the pulmonary artery are elevated. It may also be related to an increase in the volume of pulmonary blood flow, in which case the systolic pressure is elevated but the diastolic pressure is only slightly elevated, so that there is a wide pulse pressure in the pulmonary artery. This pattern generally indicates that the pulmonary resistance is fairly normal but that there is a large volume of blood flow. A wide pulse pressure may also be found in the main pulmonary artery proximal to peripheral arterial stenosis, an uncommon condition. The pulmonary arterial pressure may also be widened in patients with pulmonary valvular insufficiency, but in these situations the systolic pressure is rarely greater than 40 mm Hg.

The measurement of the pulmonary capillary, or wedge, pressure is critical in the assessment of patients with congenital heart disease. In this technique, a catheter with an end hole or a balloon catheter is passed through the pulmonary artery until it can be advanced no further into the lung and becomes wedged. Alternatively, a balloon catheter can be used. With successful wedging, the end hole of the catheter measures the pulmonary capillary pressure, since, because of the wedged position, the pulmonary arterial pressure is not transmitted to the catheter tip. Unless there is obstruction in the pulmonary venous system, the pulmonary capillary pressure reflects the left atrial pressure rather closely; it is therefore possible to assess the pressure in that chamber without actually entering it.

A wedge pressure can be verified by three methods.

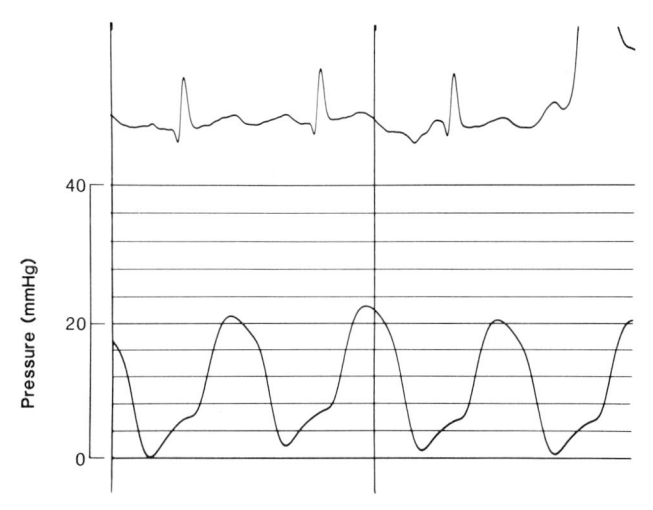

FIG 6–3.
Right ventricular pressure tracing with simultaneous electrocardiogram.

First, fully saturated blood can be withdrawn from this site. Second, the very characteristic wave form, with an *a* wave and a predominant *v* wave, as found in the left atrium, will be noted. Third, a sharp transition between the wedge and the pulmonary arterial pressure will be obtained as the catheter is withdrawn. The mean wedge pressure should not exceed 13 mm Hg; a higher value suggests elevated left atrial pressure.

Left Atrial Pressure

The left atrial pressure, like the right atrial pressure, contains *a, c,* and *v* waves, but in contrast to the finding in the right atrium, the *v* wave is the predominant wave form. The *a* wave is 3 to 7 mm Hg, the *v* wave is 5 to 15 mm Hg, and the mean pressure is 5 to 10 mm Hg. Care should be taken not to measure the pressure from the left atrial appendage, because at this location, an *a* wave is predominant, occurring as the appendage contracts around the catheter (catheter entrapment). In patients with mitral stenosis or other obstructive lesions around the mitral valve, the *a* wave is elevated and is the major wave form. In patients with mitral insufficiency or with a large pulmonary blood flow, as occurs with a communication at the arterial or the ventricular level, the left atrial *v* wave is large.

Left Ventricular Pressure

Left ventricular pressure is normally 120/10 mm Hg in adolescents. In neonates, the systolic pressure may be 70 mm Hg, and this pressure gradually rises as the child grows older. Elevation of left ventricular systolic pressure generally reflects some form of aortic stenosis or systemic hypertension. During diastole when the mitral valve is open, left atrial pressure normally equals the left ventricular diastolic pressure; a gradient indicates mitral stenosis. When the left atrium contracts, it produces a slight increase in pressure, the *a* wave. An identical wave form is also recorded in the left ventricle. Because this occurs at the end of the diastole, the pressure represents the end-diastolic pressure. In atrial fibrillation, the *a* wave is absent, and the pressure does not show a peak at the end of diastole. Elevated left ventricular end-diastolic pressure can indicate a large volume of blood in the left ventricle, as from a left-to-right shunt or valvar regurgitation; hypertrophy secondary to elevated left ventricular systolic pressure; or cardiomyopathies, which preferentially involve the left ventricle.

Aortic Pressure

Aortic pressure also rises during childhood from 70 mm Hg in newborns to 120 or 130 mm Hg in adolescents. The diastolic pressure normally is one third less than the

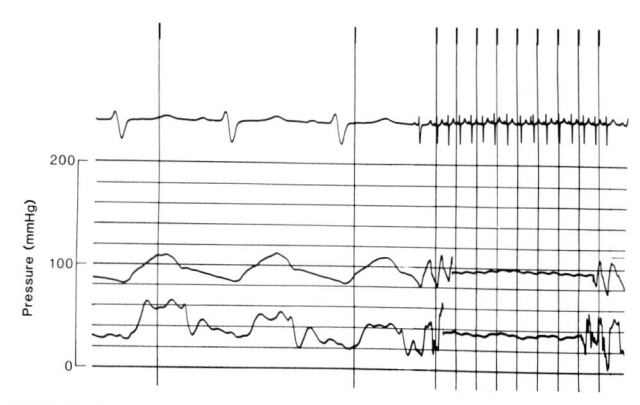

FIG 6–4.
Simultaneous aortic *(upper)* and pulmonary arterial *(lower)* pressure tracings and electrocardiogram.

systolic pressure (Fig 6–4). An elevated systolic pressure in the ascending aorta indicates hypertension or coarctation of the aorta. The diastolic pressure may be lowered because of run-off through an insufficient aortic valve or a shunt from the aorta into the pulmonary arteries, as in patent ductus arteriosus, aorticopulmonary window, or a persistent truncus arteriosus. Systolic pressure may be lowered in patients with decreased myocardial function and low cardiac output.

Withdrawal Pressure

Commonly during cardiac catheterization, pressures are recorded as the catheter is withdrawn from one chamber to another. This is particularly useful in patients with stenotic lesions to determine the site and severity of the obstruction (Fig 6–5). During catheterization, it is helpful to record the location of the pressure change on cine or spot film to verify the position of the catheter tip at the time of a pressure change.

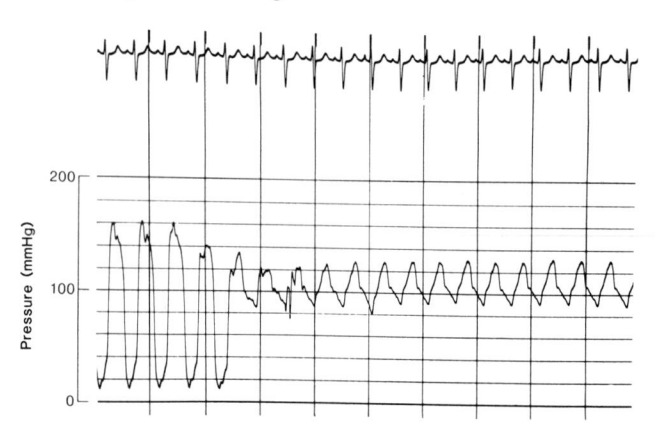

FIG 6–5.
Withdrawal pressure tracing from left ventricle *(left)* to aorta *(right)* and simultaneous electrocardiogram. Pressure gradient indicates left ventricular outflow obstruction.

OXIMETRY DATA

During cardiac catheterization, blood samples are withdrawn from various chambers for blood-gas analysis to determine the presence of either a left-to-right or a right-to-left shunt. In addition, the oxygen data are used to determine the cardiac output by the Fick principle. Usually, serial samples are obtained, and often multiple samples are taken in cardiac chambers to detect small shunts and to take into account mixing of the bloodstreams. The oxygen saturation obtained in various chambers varies considerably, depending on the site at which the blood sample was taken. Mixing of blood improves progressively from the inferior vena cava to the right atrium, right ventricle, and pulmonary artery. Pulmonary arterial samples are considered to best represent "mixed" venous blood.

Normally the superior vena caval oxygen saturation is 65% to 75%. A figure considerably higher than 70% suggests the presence of partial or total anomalous pulmonary venous connection to the superior vena cava or one of its tributaries, an arteriovenous fistula into the superior vena caval system, or high cardiac output. In contrast, low oxygen saturation in the superior vena cava suggests low cardiac output or a cyanotic form of congenital heart disease.

In the inferior vena cava, oxygen saturation is often 80% because this vessel receives a large volume of blood flow from the kidneys and these organs do not extract much oxygen from the arterial blood. It is more difficult to detect the presence of a left-to-right shunt at this site. Because of streaming and consequent incomplete mixing of blood, the inferior vena caval sample is commonly disregarded in shunt calculations. However, when the inferior vena caval saturation is lower than that in the superior vena cava, a reversing ductus arteriosus should be suspected.

Normally the oxygen saturation of blood from the coronary sinus is 30%. A greater figure indicates the presence of a persistent left superior vena cava to the coronary sinus, a form of anomalous pulmonary venous connection to the coronary sinus, or a coronary arteriovenous fistula.

The right atrium receives three significant venous returns, each with a different oxygen saturation: about 30% in the coronary sinus, about 80% in the inferior vena cava, and about 70% in the superior vena cava. Mixing occurs in the right atrium but may be incomplete. Generally the best-mixed blood in the right atrium can be obtained in the middle of the chamber at the lateral wall. To detect the presence of a left-to-right shunt at the atrial level, an increase of >10% oxygen saturation is needed between the superior vena cava and the right atrium. (An increase of only 7% is needed if two oxygen saturation series are performed and averaged.)

Conditions associated with a significant increase in oxygen saturation in the right atrium include atrial septal defect, atrial septal defect associated with a left-sided cardiac condition, endocardial cushion defect, anomalous pulmonary venous connection to the right atrium or coronary sinus, fenestration of the coronary sinus, left ventricular–right atrial communication, ventricular septal defect with tricuspid insufficiency, a ruptured sinus of Valsalva aneurysm into the right atrium, or a coronary arteriovenous fistula.

During blood flow through the right side of the heart, mixing improves, so that a smaller increase in oxygen saturation between the right atrium and right ventricle is considered diagnostic of a left-to-right shunt at the ventricular level. Thus, an increase of 1 ml of O_2/dL or 7% (5% if two oximetry series are obtained), is considered a significant increase, suggesting a left-to-right shunt. Although a ventricular septal defect is the most common cause of left-to-right shunt at the ventricular level, other congenital malformations in which there is a ventricular septal defect or a single ventricle will produce this finding, examples being double-outlet right ventricle or complete transposition of the great vessels.

A 0.5 mL of O_2/dL, or 5%, increase in saturation between the right ventricle and the pulmonary artery is considered significant; if two series are obtained, a 3% increase is considered significant. A patent ductus arteriosus, coronary arteriovenous fistula, truncus arteriosus and systemic pulmonary artery surgical shunts, and aorticopulmonary window are the principal conditions associated with an oxygen increase at the pulmonary arterial level.

Care must be taken in interpreting the oximetry data because of streaming effects. Thus, the presence of a defect and the magnitude of its shunt may be reflected best by the oximetry samples in the chamber immediately downstream of the shunt. Thus, the size of an atrial septal defect may be truly appreciated by right ventricular sampling, and a supracristal ventricular septal defect may be detected by an increase in oxygen saturation in the pulmonary artery.

The oxygen saturation in the pulmonary veins is normally about 96%. A low saturation suggests pulmonary parenchymal disease such as pneumonia, atelectasis, or edema. The oxygen content of pulmonary venous blood may also be reduced by excessive sedation or hypoventilation. Pulmonary arteriovenous fistulas are a rare cause of desaturation.

A 5% decrease in oxygen saturation between the pulmonary veins and the aorta indicates a right-to-left shunt, which may be at the atrial level through a septal defect or the foramen ovale or be the result of such rare conditions as coronary sinus or coronary arterial fenestrations and connections of the left superior vena cava to the left atrium (see Chapter 20). Fenestration between the superior vena cava and left atrium and a connection of the superior or inferior vena cava to the left atrium are rare. If all cardiac and pulmonary right-to-left shunts are ruled out by selective angiography, peripheral angiography should be performed via the left arm to exclude connection of left superior vena cava to left atrium.

Right-to-left shunts may occur at the ventricular level with a ventricular communication or through a communication at the level of the great vessels. Right-to-left shunts at the ventricular level, as in tetralogy of Fallot or truncus arteriosus, may best be detected by sampling from above the aortic valve, because blood from the left ventricle may be fully saturated. This is particularly true if the sample is obtained from the apex of the left ventricle, which is part of the inflow portion and so receives fully saturated blood entering through the mitral valve. The presence of a reversing patent ductus arteriosus is detected by decreased oxygen saturation in the descending aorta and lower extremities and normal saturation in the ascending aorta. If the reversing patent ductus arteriosus is associated with a ventricular septal defect, as in interruption of the aortic arch, the oxygen difference between ascending and descending aorta is minimal.

Occasionally the aortic and pulmonary arterial saturations are identical or nearly so. This occurs in the group of malformations classified as admixture lesions, which includes total anomalous pulmonary venous connection, single atrium, single ventricle, tricuspid atresia, truncus arteriosus, pulmonary atresia, mitral atresia, and tetralogy of Fallot with pulmonary atresia.

DERIVED DATA

The oximetry data can be used to calculate the size of shunts and the volume of systemic and pulmonary blood flows. During catheterization, the patient's oxygen consumption is measured to calculate the cardiac output using the Fick principle. In infants and small children, it may be difficult to measure the oxygen consumption; consequently, a value is assumed, often 150 to 175 mL of O_2/min/m^2 of body surface.

The cardiac output can be determined by the equation:

$$\text{Output} = \frac{\text{Oxygen consumption}}{\text{Arteriovenous oxygen difference}}$$

The principle is simple and is also the basis for the dye dilution technique, which uses, not oxygen, but a green dye as an indicator. If an indicator such as oxygen or green (Wood, Fox) dye is added at a known rate to a flowing stream of liquid, its concentration downstream (dilution) is determined by the flow. From the ratio of the two concentrations of the indicator, blood flow can therefore be calculated. Thus, the Fick principle indicates that the cardiac output can be calculated by measuring the volume of oxygen the patient consumes over a period of time and the difference in oxygen content of blood across the systemic circulation.

Because in congenital heart disease either left-to-right or right-to-left shunts are common, the systemic blood flow and pulmonary blood flow may not be equal. Thus, in these patients, separate blood flows can be calculated for the systemic and pulmonic circulations. The systemic blood flow can be calculated according to the following formula:

$$Qs = \frac{VO_2}{Ao - MV}$$

where Qs = systemic blood flow, VO_2 = oxygen consumption, Ao = aortic oxygen saturation, and MV = mixed venous oxygen saturation.

This formula indicates that the oxygen difference used to calculate systemic blood flow (Qs) is that across the body as represented by the difference between oxygen content in the aorta and that in the blood returning from the body ("mixed venous blood"). Preferably, the sample should be obtained in the pulmonary artery or at a site proximal to a left-to-right shunt. Pulmonary blood flow is calculated by the formula:

$$Qp = \frac{VO_2}{PV - PA}$$

where Qp = pulmonary blood flow, VO_2 = oxygen consumption, PV = pulmonary vein oxygen saturation, and PA = pulmonary artery oxygen saturation. In this formula, the arteriovenous oxygen difference across the lungs (the oxygen content of blood pulmonary venous returning to the heart minus the oxygen concentration in the pulmonary artery) must be measured.

Often the ratio of pulmonary-to-systemic blood flow is used to indicate the size of the left-to-right shunt. This can be calculated by:

$$Qp/Qs = \frac{Ao - MV}{PV - PA}$$

where Ao = aortic oxygen content, MV = mixed venous oxygen content, PV = pulmonary venous content, and PA = pulmonary artery oxygen content.

In addition, the size of shunts may be described as a percentage, determined by the following formulas:

$$\text{L-R shunt (\%)} = \frac{\text{PA} - \text{MV}}{\text{SA} - \text{MV}} \times 100$$

and

$$\text{R-L shunt (\%)} = \frac{\text{PV} - \text{SA}}{\text{SA} - \text{MV}} \times 100$$

where MV = mixed venous oxygen saturation, PV = pulmonary venous saturation, PA = pulmonary arterial saturation, and SA = systemic artery saturation. These three formulas are, of course, modifications of the Fick principle.

Information about cardiac output can be combined with pressure data to determine vascular resistance or, in patients with stenoses, to estimate the orifice area of the valve. Vascular resistance is calculated according to Ohm's law, which states that flow of electricity or a liquid is directly proportional to pressure and inversely proportional to resistance:

$$\text{Resistance} = \frac{\text{Pressure}}{\text{Flow}}$$

The result reflects the resistance to blood flow across a circulatory bed and thus indicates the condition of the arterioles of that bed. With the pressure measurements routinely obtained during cardiac catheterization, both the systemic vascular (SVR) and pulmonary arterial (PAR) resistances can be calculated:

$$\text{SVR} = \frac{\text{Ao} - \text{RA}}{\text{SBF}}$$

and

$$\text{PAR} = \frac{\text{PA} - \text{LA}}{\text{PBF}}$$

where Ao = mean aortic pressure, RA = mean right atrial pressure, PA = mean pulmonary arterial pressure, LA = mean left atrial pressure (all in mm Hg), SBF = systemic blood flow, and PBF = pulmonary blood flow (both in L/min/m^2 of body surface). These formulas calculate resistance using the indexed systemic or pulmonary blood flow. The unit of resistance from these formulas is expressed either as mm Hg/L/min/m^2, or more commonly, as resistance or Woods units. Systemic vascular resistance is normally 10 to 12 units in infants and rises to 14 to 18 units in older children. In contrast, pulmonary vascular resistance is 8 to 10 units at birth and falls to less than 3 units by 8 weeks of age.

Formulas for the size of the orifice of a stenotic semilunar valve express the severity of valvular lesions. These formulas are:

$$\text{AVA} = \frac{\dfrac{\text{Cardiac output}}{\text{Heart rate} \times \text{Systolic ejection period}}}{44.5 \times \sqrt{\text{LVSP} - \text{AO}}}$$

and

$$\text{PVA} = \frac{\dfrac{\text{Cardiac output}}{\text{Heart rate} \times \text{Systolic ejection period}}}{44.5 \times \sqrt{\text{RVSP} - \text{PA}}}$$

where LVSP and RVSP = left and right ventricular systolic pressure, respectively, AO = mean aortic pressure, and PA = mean pulmonary artery pressure, AVA = aortic valve area, PVA = pulmonary valve area. The normal aortic and pulmonary valve orifices are 2 cm^2/m^2.

INDICATOR DILUTION TECHNIQUES

Various indicators have been used to measure cardiac output or to determine patterns of blood flow through the heart. The indicator dilution technique, basically, uses the Fick principle, which was applied to an injected dye by Stewart. A known amount of nonmetabolized dye is added to the bloodstream, and its concentration is measured downstream after complete mixing. The dye is diluted by the degree of flow. The indicator most widely used clinically is Cardio-Green (indocyanine green), which mixes thoroughly with the blood, does not diffuse into blood cells or extravascular spaces, is not metabolized in the lung, and can be measured with a densitometer.

In principle, an indicator dilution technique involves injecting a precisely known amount of dye as a bolus while continuously withdrawing blood downstream past a densitometer, which photoelectrically detects the changing concentrations of the dye and can record it on a strip chart.

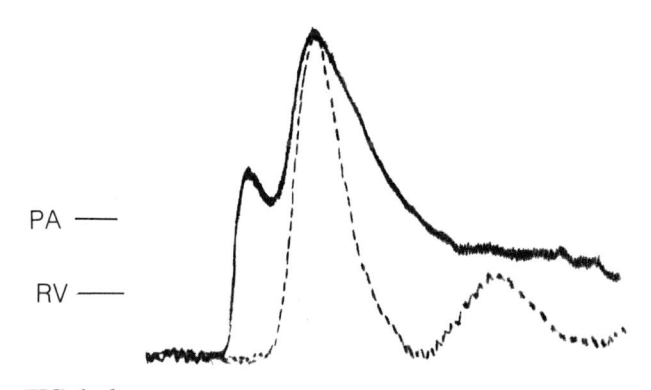

FIG 6-6.
Indicator dilution curves in patient with right-to-left shunt at ventricular level. Curve from right ventricle *(RV)* to systemic artery *(SA)* shows earlier dye appearance than does curve from pulmonary artery *(PA)* to systemic artery *(SA)*.

In the normal circulation, there is a lag between the injection of contrast material on the right side of the heart and the arrival of dye in arteries, because the dye has to pass through the capillary bed to the lungs. Thus, a typical curve has a rather sharp upstroke and a gradual decay, with a small recirculation hump as some of the dye arrives at the sampling site for a second time.

The normal curve can be distorted in several ways. In the presence of a right-to-left shunt, dye appears early after injection into a peripheral venous site (Fig 6–6). In the presence of an insufficient valve, the downslope of the curve is distorted, because the dye is diluted in the dilated chamber by the increased blood flow through the regurgitant valve. A similar distortion of the curve occurs in left-to-right shunts because of early recirculation of dye through the lungs. This distortion may also occur with decreased cardiac output and therefore is not specific for left-to-right shunts. The injection of the dye into the left side of the heart and sampling from the right side is very specific for, and much more sensitive than oximetry in detecting, a left-to-right shunt. It requires the use of two catheters, a disadvantage that can be avoided by using an inhaled indicator (hydrogen, radioactive methyliodide, krypton, xenon). With the advent of selective angiography, however, these techniques have become obsolete.

Without a shunt, dye curves can be used to calculate cardiac output, because the area under the primary curve is related to cardiac output.

More recently, thermal dilution techniques have been used to measure cardiac output using the same principle. Cold saline solution is injected as a bolus, and the temperature is measured downstream of the injection site. The increase in temperature is related to blood flow: the faster the flow, the greater the change in temperature compared with that of the injected saline solution.

CHAPTER 7

Angiographic Equipment

CINE FLUOROSCOPY

Because cine fluorography has become an important imaging method in patients with congenital heart disease, a basic understanding of the equipment is required.[1] Cine recording has several advantages over recording using film changers.

1. Convenience. The patient can easily be positioned under fluoroscopic control, after which the cine camera can immediately be activated by depressing a foot switch.
2. Reliable film density. With proper radiographic equipment, proper coning, and exposure control, the frames should be of uniform density.
3. Good resolution. With modern equipment, acceptable sharpness (resolution) of the film is obtained, approaching the resolution of cut-film radiography. The present resolution of cine radiography is 3.5 line pairs/mm compared with 4 to 5 line pairs/mm with high-speed radiography using rapid film changers.
4. Negligible motion unsharpness. Cardiac structures, such as valves, that move rapidly are better demonstrated by cine recording because of the short exposure time (1–5 msec).
5. High visual sensitivity. Smaller amounts of contrast medium can be injected, because recording at 60 frames/sec (fps) provides many exposures throughout a cardiac cycle. For comparison, rapid film changers operate at only 6 to 12 exposures/sec. Furthermore, the human eye is extremely sensitive to minor temporal density changes on a cine angiogram, allowing recognition of minute shunts or regurgitating jets.
6. Angled projections. Because cine cameras are lightweight, they can be mounted on C or U arms for examination with beam angulation. Proper radiographic exposure can be obtained by the electronic automatic brightness control.

From the recording of the cine frames to their final projection, numerous complex electronic and mechanical manipulations are required. The basic physics and mechanics of various components are discussed briefly, because understanding of them will improve the quality of cine radiography and of trouble-shooting in case of deterioration of the image quality.

THE RADIOGRAPHIC TUBE

Cine radiography places special demands on manufacturers of radiographic x-ray tubes for two reasons:

1. A large amount of heat is created in the target because of the high milliamperage (current flux; mA) necessary to produce a sufficient number of photons (see the section on quantum noise), so the equipment needs a high heat-load capacity. The heat storage capacity of an x-ray tube is measured by heat units. The anode of a modern graphite-backed cine tube may have as much as 2,400,000 heat unit storage capacity. Heat unit (HU) is defined as the product of mA × KV(p) × seconds. Another important number is the tube cooling rate which is expressed by the loss of HU/min. The more meaningful heat storage capacity of the anode should not be confused with the greater heat storage capacity as measured on the x-ray tube housing.
2. A small focal spot, ideally 0.3 or 0.6 mm, is desirable to increase radiographic sharpness.

These factors are antagonistic in that the image becomes sharper the more nearly the source of x-rays (focal spot) resembles a point, yet focusing of electrons to a point would melt the target. Therefore, the focal spot has nominal dimensions, although it should be as small as possible within the limits of the heat capacity of the x-ray tube.

Cine runs of at least 10 seconds should be possible; particularly in younger patients, most events one wishes to observe after the injection of contrast medium do not exceed this span.

The heat-loading capacity of an x-ray tube can be increased by high-speed rotation of a large anode. Modern cine fluorographic x-ray tubes have an anode rotation speed of 10,000 rpm and a diameter of 5 in. (at least 100 mm). The large mass of such anodes and their conductive graphite backing dissipate heat well, thereby allowing longer cine runs at the same current flux.

The instantaneous tube loading capacity of the anode can be increased by a shallow target angle. The length of the actual focal spot is increased, but because of the shallow target angle, the projected (effective) focal spot length remains the same. The instantaneous tube loading capacity thus can be increased without changing the geometry of the effective focal spot. The lower limit on the size of the target angle is the coverage of the input phosphor of the image intensifier: for coverage of a 14 by 14-in. radiographic field, a 12-degree target is required, whereas for cine radiography a 6- to 7-degree target is adequate to cover a 9-in. image intensifier. The instantaneous tube loading capacity with a 6-degree target is obviously much greater than that of a 12-degree target.

To summarize: for effective cine radiography, an x-ray tube must have the following qualities:

1. A large, preferably graphite-backed, anode to allow longer cine recording by improving heat dissipation.
2. The smallest possible target angle to cover the input phosphor of the image-intensifier tube.
3. The smallest possible focal spot, generally 0.6 mm.

Cine tubes are commonly "grid controlled." For cine radiography, intermittent emission of x-rays is required, because the patient should not be irradiated while the camera is transporting the film. An efficient way to produce x-rays intermittently is by intermittent blockage of the current flow; this is accomplished by a grid in the tube, which intermittently is given a negative charge (bias) to stop the electron flux. Therefore, in a grid-controlled x-ray tube, the anode is bombarded rapidly and intermittently, the tube being used as an electronic on-and-off switch. Of course, the bias grid must be charged at exactly the moment the film is in transport in the camera, and the charge has to disappear exactly when the cine film is at rest, ready to be exposed (i.e., the grid and cine camera have to be perfectly synchronized).

Most American manufacturers obtain intermittent emission of x-rays by a grid-controlled tube, whereas some European manufacturers prefer to have electrons produced intermittently in the generator by either a triode or a tetrode. These also are intermittent electron-stopping devices but are located in the generator outside the x-ray tube. Either switching method can be used to produce pulsed x-rays, but the grid-controlled tube is simpler and less expensive.

For biplane recording, each x-ray tube has to be out of phase with the other: If the tubes are fired simultaneously, the secondary radiation would fog the images in each plane. However, if the x-ray tubes are fired intermittently, the film in one camera will be in transit and protected by the shutter during the exposure in the other plane.

The X-Ray Generator

Generally speaking, cine fluorography does not place special demands on the x-ray generator, because current flow is comparatively low and limited by the heat-loading capacity of the x-ray tube. In the United States, standard 12-pulse generators are used, but in Europe, constant-potential generators have been developed that allow a slight increase in the pulse width and slightly improved film blackening. These minimal gains are offset by the increased cost, however.

Cine Fluorography

Shortly after the discovery of x-rays, it became feasible to record the light image on a fluoroscopic screen with a cine camera. However, the dim light output of the screen and the continuous radiation made adequate penetration difficult, and the radiation dose to the patient was excessive. Two major developments made application of this new imaging modality feasible:

1. Intermittent emission of x-rays by a pulsing system (grid-control tube or tetrode), eliminating radiation during film transport.
2. The development of the image intensifier, which increases the light output (brightness).

Basic Principles of Image Intensifiers

As the name suggests, an image intensifier is basically an electronic device for intensifying the brightness of the light image. With this tube, the photon flux can be increased by a factor of many thousands.

To be photographed by a cine camera, the radiographic image must be transformed into a light image, because the radiographic film is relatively insensitive to direct x-ray exposure. The conversion of x-rays to light is accomplished by a phosphor, which glows when struck by x-rays. The image intensifier converts the light image produced by the phosphor into an electron image and then reconverts this electron image to a light image. Thus, the image intensifier tube is basically an energy converter. Because energy conversion is not 100% efficient, some photon energy is lost. How, then, can the image intensifier gain energy and amplify the brightness of the light image? Because electrons have charge and mass, they can be focused by electrostatic lenses and accelerated, and this acceleration in a vacuum allows us to pump energy into the system. Thus, brightness increases despite the basically energy-losing conversion process (Fig 7–1,A).

Light intensification, then, is accomplished by both the acceleration of the electrons and the reduction of the image. Specifically, the brightness gain of an image intensifier is the "minification" gain multiplied by the flux gain. The former follows the inverse-square law: If the input phosphor is 9 in. on each side and the image is reduced to 1 by 1 in., the gain is 81 (9 × 9). The intensification caused by acceleration of the electrons (flux gain) usually is around 50. Therefore, in this example the total brightness gain equals 81 × 50, or a total brightness gain of 4,050.

The components of an image intensifier are shown in Figure 7–1,B. The input phosphor is mounted behind a round curved face of a vacuum tube. In all modern image-intensifying tubes, the input phosphor is made of cesium iodide, which provides the best conversion of x-rays to light and the highest resolution, characteristics that depend largely on the thickness of the input phosphor (about 200 μm). The electrons produced by the photocathode, which is made of a combination of antimony and cesium compounds, are attracted by the anode and accelerated because of a difference in potential. The electrons are focused by a set of electrostatic lenses on the 1-in. output phosphor (usually zinc–cadmium sulfide). Exact electronic focusing is of paramount importance and requires an equal path length for all electrons; this is accomplished by curving the face of the input phosphor. However, despite this curvature and electronic focusing lenses, the electron beam flares toward the periphery, causing some distortion of the image. This imperfection can be demonstrated by imaging a mesh, which will appear slightly distorted and larger around the periphery. The degree of distortion differs from one intensifier to another (Fig 7–2,A and B). In addition to this geometric distortion, resolution and image brightness are lost toward the periphery. This peripheral decrease in brightness is called "vignetting," a term used in photography to describe how the contours of a portrait are shaded off toward the periphery to blend with the background. Thus, the quality of an image is best in the center of the output phosphor.

The output phosphor is coupled with an objective lens

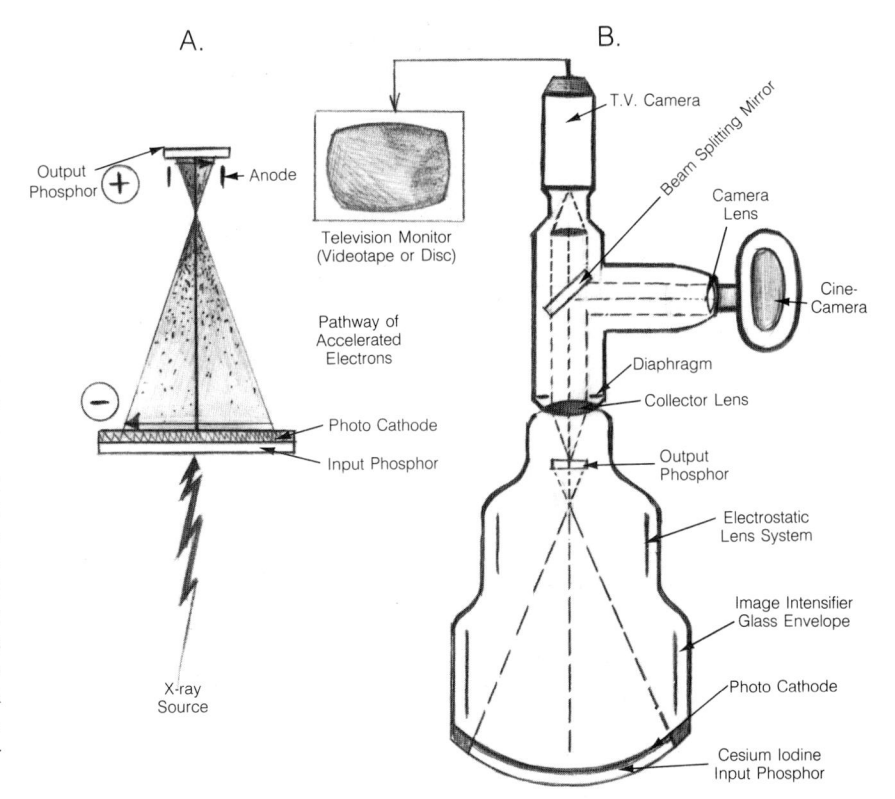

FIG 7–1.
Basic principle of image-intensifying tube. **A,** x-rays are converted into light by the input phosphor, and the light image created by the glow of the phosphor is converted to an electron image by another phosphor (the photocathode) emitting electrons in proportion to the light output of the first phosphor. In a vacuum, a negative charge can be put on the photocathode, and the electrons can be accelerated by a charged anode and focused by electrostatic lenses, which also reduce and invert the image, just as optical lenses do. The image is focused on the smaller output phosphor, which reconverts the electron image into light. Light-intensification is accomplished by the acceleration of the electrons and reduction of the image. **B,** basic structure of an image intensifier–cine-TV system.

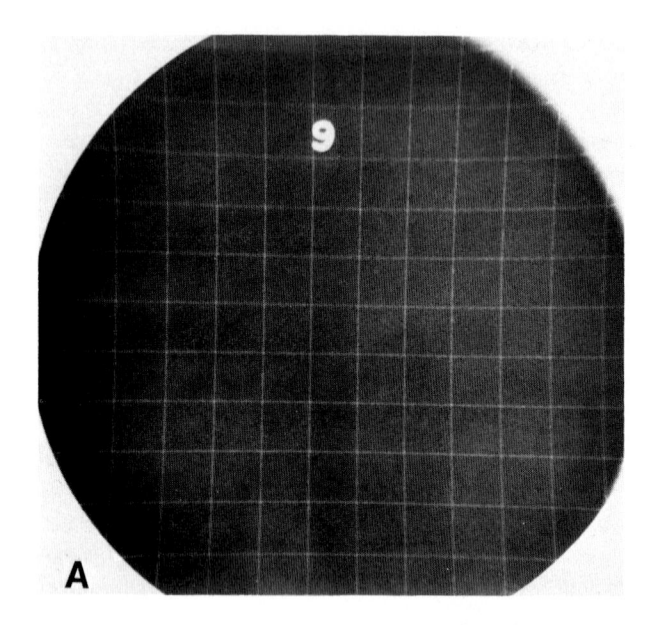

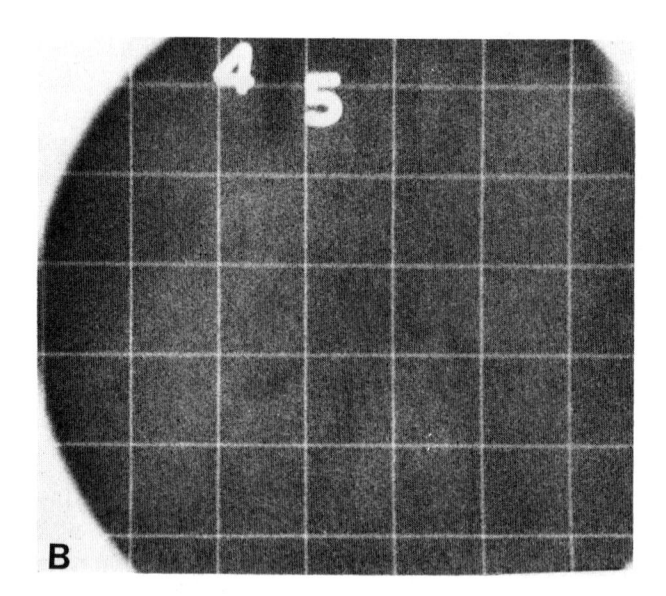

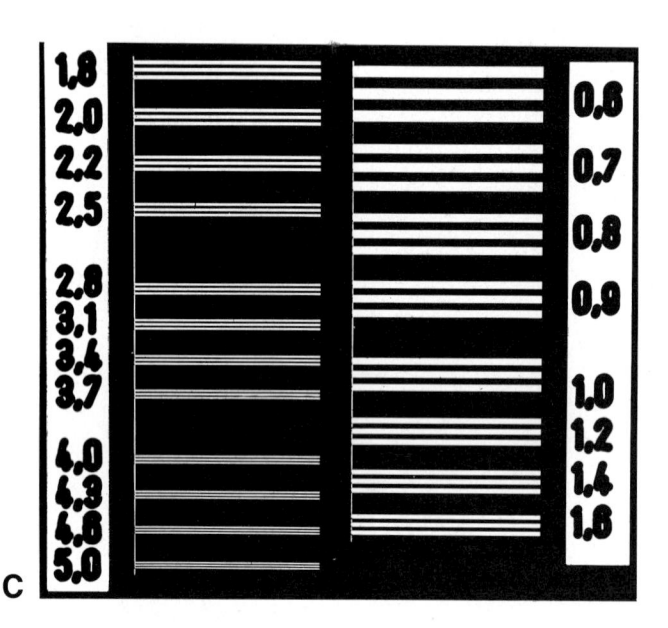

FIG 7–2.
Cine frames of a 1-cm mesh image in the 9-in. mode (**A**) and the 4.5 in. mode (**B**). The distortion of the mesh toward the periphery (more marked in the 9-in. mode) is caused by imperfection in the electronic focusing system ("pincushion effect"). Resolution is increased with the 4.5 in. mode *(grid lines visible)*. Note also the decrease in density at the periphery, particularly the 9-in. mode ("vignetting"). **C,** one of the cine resolution patterns that should be recorded before every angiogram to detect loss of focus of the electronic-optical system. It also serves in focusing the projector. Resolution is indicated as line pairs per millimeter. The mesh must be placed at right angle to the radiographic grid, directly on image intensifier to avoid interference (moiré) patterns. Or, the grid is removed to eliminate moiré artifacts. Moiré (French, meaning watered or wavy), a wavy artifact, is produced by x-ray interference between grid and resolution pattern. Certain fabrics such as silk will produce a wavy moiré pattern.

that projects the image on a partially reflecting, beam-splitting mirror (Fig 7–1,B). Ninety percent of the light output is reflected through the cine objective lens into the camera, and 10% passes through the mirror and is viewed by a standard TV Vidicon or Plumicon camera. The TV image is visible on a standard monitor and can be stored simultaneously on videotape or videodisc.

If one is to preserve optimal resolution, exact focusing of the electronic and optical lens systems is important; and because either system, but especially the electronic, may go out of focus, they should be checked at least every 3 months. Every cine run should start with a cine test pattern, careful observation of which permits early detection of deterioration in focusing (Fig 7–2,C).

For good cine angiography, a rate of 60 fps is desirable; in other words, 1/60 of a second (16 msec) is available per frame. However, because the cine film has to be transported at intervals, only a portion of this time span can be used for exposure: At a rate of 60 fps, the maximum exposure time (pulse width) is usually set at 4 to 5 msec. An exposure of 4 msec is short enough to freeze even rapidly moving cardiac structures, but better results are obtained with an even narrower pulse width, particularly in children.

With a rate of 30 fps, twice as much time is available for each exposure, so the maximum pulse width is usually 8 msec. At this speed, however, fast-moving cardiac structures such as valves may be slightly blurred, so whenever possible, a rate of 60 fps is preferable for angiocardiography. The principal advantage of a 30-fps rate is the increased tube heat-loading capacity. Because only half as many exposures are taken and their exposure time is twice as long, kilovoltage, milliamperage, or both can be decreased to increase the tube loading capacity. Occasionally, very large patients cannot be examined at 60 fps, particularly when the x-ray beam is angulated, because the tube loading capacity will be exceeded; and thus the images will be underexposed. Under such circumstances, a rate of 30 fps with the 8-msec pulse width allows proper exposure (penetration) by staying within the loading capacity. Some manufacturers provide meters or warning lights to indicate when this capacity is exceeded. If this occurs, changing to a slower (30-fps) rate may solve the problem.

Another advantage of an exposure rate of 30 fps is the lower kV(p) level, which increases the contrast; Contrast tends to deteriorate with increasing kilovoltage. However, the longer exposure time increases blurring by motion, particularly in patients with a rapid heart rate and in structures that are markedly active, such as the right coronary artery.

Cine Pulsing System

In cine fluorography, the exposure time (pulse width) is the duration of the x-ray exposure for each frame. The pulse width is determined by the duration of the electron flux in the x-ray tube as regulated by the grid or by tetrodes. With some radiographic systems, the pulse width is variable, whereas in other systems it is fixed. The variable system has the advantage of permitting reduction of the exposure time to 1 to 2 msec for the studies of infants. The maximum pulse width is limited by the time available for exposure of the cine film in the camera, which depends on the frame rate. A pulse width greater than 8 msec results in noticeable blurring.

Automatic Brightness Control

The automatic brightness control is an important part of any modern cine system, which allows the operator to activate a foot switch and obtain a good cine film. However, to achieve the best results, the radiologist must understand it.

The purpose of the control is to keep the density of the cine film constant automatically, regardless of the thickness of the body part or the changing penetration requirements, such as after the injection of contrast medium or during "panning" over various areas of the body. Panning is commonly used in motion-picture photography, as when a mountain range is recorded by continuous motion of the camera, to obtain a panoramic view. In cine fluorography, panning is used when the entire area of interest is too large to be recorded on one frame and is accomplished by moving either the patient or the image intensifier. It is an important part of cine angiography and requires good eye-hand coordination. Panning necessitates continuous changes of penetration, which are compensated for by the automatic brightness control, which therefore assures proper exposure of the film, making cine recording convenient for the operator. The system has limitations, however, that must be recognized to avoid either overexposure or underexposure.

The brightness of the image-intensifier output phosphor can be kept constant either by measuring its optical brightness directly or by measuring the current flow in the image intensifier. If brightness or current flow drop because of the changing penetration requirements, such as during panning or injection of contrast medium, an automatic feedback signal returns this message to the generator, which changes its output to keep the current flow or brightness at a constant level. The feedback system consists of a pick-up signal, a feedback signal, and an answer signal.

The generator can automatically compensate for changing penetration by varying one of the three factors determining the density of the x-ray image.

Variable Kilovoltage.—The potential of the x-ray output can be adjusted automatically by increasing the kV(p) to keep the brightness sensing device at a constant level. Milliamperage and pulse width remain at a constant maximum. The system has a relatively slow response but yields fair results. The principal disadvantage of variable kilovoltage is the deterioration of the image quality for the following reasons:

1. The difference between the x-ray absorption by tissue and contrast medium gradually decreases with increasing kilovoltage. Consequently, the overall contrast of the images decreases.

2. High kilovoltage produces higher-energy secondary radiation that penetrates the antiscatter grid, which

thus becomes less efficient. This causes a further loss of contrast.

3. With higher kilovoltage and energy of the x-ray beam, the number of photons absorbed decreases, resulting in an increased quantum mottle, which may cause a "noisy" grainy image (see the section on quantum mottle).

4. With some generators of European design, the current flow decreases with increasing kV(p) ("falling-load generators"), further decreasing image quality.

Variable Tube Current.—With this system, the pulse width and kV(p) levels can be preselected, and the current flow in the x-ray tube (mA level) is varied according to the electronic brightness-sensing device. The system is relatively slow and requires considerable experience to give satisfactory results, so it is not commonly used in modern equipment.

Variable Exposure Time (Pulse Width).—Basically, the kilovoltage and tube currents are kept constant, whereas the pulse width is changed from 1 to 4 msec at 60 fps. By itself this change of exposure time is inadequate to cover all sizes of patients; therefore, this system is useful only when combined with a system that changes either the tube potential or current flow. Changing the exposure time (pulse width) can be accomplished rapidly, thereby assuring proper exposure of each frame. The greatest versatility and best results are obtained with a combination that allows variation of exposure time, pulse width, and kilovoltage (tube potential) at a maximum permissible tube current (mA). With such a system, it is possible to preselect an ideal kV(p) level, for example, 70 kV(p) in an infant, and the electronic sensing-control system then will automatically select the maximum permissible tube current with a simultaneous decrease in the exposure time. This system gives images with the greatest sharpness and maximum contrast. If the maximum current flow and pulse width (usually 4 msec) are inadequate to penetrate the patient, the electronic control automatically increases the kV(p) level to assure proper cine exposures.

In such a system, if the ideal preselected kV(p) level must be exceeded to maintain proper film density, the operator is warned by an override signal, and the automatically selected kV(p) level will be indicated on a panel. The tube potential can be automatically adjusted only to a certain level (usually 120 kV[p]), above which the system can no longer increase its x-ray output to provide proper penetration. This point may be reached in very heavy patients or in the magnified mode if angled views are used. A warning signal then appears, indicating that maximum pulse width, tube current, and tube potential have been reached and that no further brightness can be delivered.

The operator then has several options to prevent underpenetration.

1. Either the lateral-plane x-ray tube or the anteroposterior image intensifier can be moved as close as possible to the patient (x-ray intensity decreases inversely with the square of the distance).

2. Angulated projections can be changed to less angulation or nonangulated views. Because angulated views are basically transabdominal projections, they require much more penetration than does a straight anteroposterior or lateral projection, which requires only penetration of the tissues of the chest and the air-filled lung.

3. With multiple-field image intensifiers, less magnification can be used. For example, instead of the 4.5-in. mode, a 6- or 9-in. mode can be selected.

4. A 30-fps rate can be selected. At this speed, the maximum pulse width is twice as long as at 60 fps (8–10 msec compared with 4–5 msec), and only one half as many frames per second are taken.

Modern automatic brightness controls work satisfactorily, provided the operator is familiar with their basic construction, limitations, and proper operation. Although the brightness-pickup system can give us an overall brightness level and the feedback system and control system can keep this overall brightness level constant, it cannot guarantee proper exposure of the area of interest. That is, the automatic brightness control system does not "know" that the operator is interested in the heart rather than the lung or the area beneath the diaphragm; it can only produce an average. Therefore, the operator must remove areas of little interest, particularly the lungs, from the image, because they will influence the brightness-sensing device. This can be accomplished in three ways:

1. Proper centering of the field over the area of interest (the heart), with the exclusion of as much lung as possible. Improper positioning, with 50% of the image consisting of "bright" lung, will result in underpenetration of the heart because the automatic brightness control measures the average.

2. Proper coning. Maximum coning not only excludes a large portion of the bright lung but also decreases secondary radiation and increases contrast.

3. Masking. Because most cones are square, the lung cannot be entirely excluded. Therefore, coning may have to be customized. This can be accomplished by placing a lead mask in front of the x-ray tube or by taping a lead-rubber mask over the image intensifier. The image then contains almost no lung, which results in the best penetration of the heart.

These considerations are particularly important if the heart must be penetrated from above or below the diaphragm, as in angled left anterior oblique projections. If too much lung is offered to the automatic brightness-pickup system, the portion of the heart above the diaphragm will be overexposed and the infradiaphragmatic portion will be severely underexposed. Coning is particularly important with image intensifiers of high brightness gain and when using high-contrast rather than latitude cine films (see the section on cine film). The best results are obtained with a semitransparent diaphragm. This wedge filter is motorized and can be conformed to the heart contour (Fig 7–3).

Image Intensifier Size

The sizes of image intensifiers differs, depending on the catheterization laboratory, so image size must be considered carefully. Furthermore, intensifiers are available as single- and multiple-mode tubes.

Single-Mode Image Intensifiers.—Image intensifiers are rated according to the diameter of the round input phosphor, which ranges from 5 to 14 in. whereas the output phosphor is always about 1 in. On a 5-in. image intensifier, therefore, the maximum size of the object that can be recorded is about 5 in. in diameter, provided the object is in contact with the input phosphor. Because the x-rays diverge and the distance between the x-ray tube and the image intensifier is rather short, 20% to 30% magnification occurs. Consequently, the size of the object as seen is not 5 in. but 20% to 30% less. This decrease in field coverage is an important consideration when an image intensifier is selected, although the limitation on field coverage with a 5-in. image intensifier can be overcome to some extent by panning.

Because the input phosphor is electronically focused

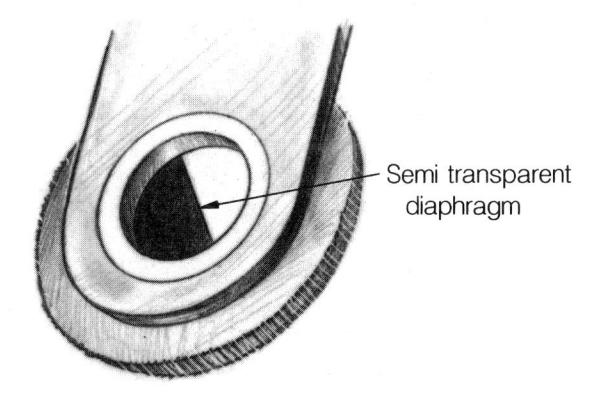

FIG 7–3.
View of a motordriven semitransparent diaphragm, which is a wedge filter providing a gradual contrast change. It can be moved in and out and can be rotated.

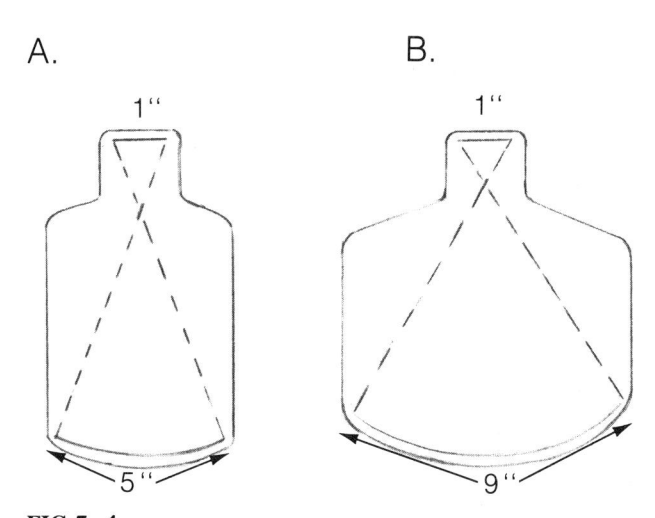

FIG 7–4.
Comparison of 6-in. image intensifier with the 6-in. input phosphor electronically focused to the 1-in. output phosphor (**A**) and 9-in. image intensifier also focused to a 1-in. output phosphor (**B**). The latter image-intensifying tube produces more "minification" (compression of the image).

to fill the 1-in. output phosphor, different-sized image intensifiers provide a different degree of magnification (Fig 7–4). On a 5-in. image intensifier, the input phosphor focuses the electrons on the 1-in. output phosphor (see Fig 7–4,A). In a 9-in. image intensifier, the image from the input phosphor is also reduced to a 1-in. output phosphor (see Fig 7–4,B). Of course, a 5-in. object imaged with a 9-in. image intensifier produces a much smaller image on the output phosphor and will appear smaller than it will with the 5-in. image intensifier. Image intensifiers with a smaller input phosphor therefore have more magnification, and, consequently, the "minification" brightness gain is much less. The loss of minification gain from one intensifier to another is related to the square of the size of the input phosphors. For example, the magnification gain of a 5-in. image intensifier is less than one third that of a 9-in. image intensifier (81 compared with 25). If the electronic gain (flux gain) of a 5- and a 9-in. intensifier are the same, the 5-in. intensifier therefore will require three times the amount of radiation to give the same total brightness. Similarly, the patient receives three times as much radiation, and therefore the smaller image intensifier places a higher demand on the x-ray generator and tube. For large patients, the equipment may "run out of x-rays," so it may not be possible to penetrate heavy patients adequately.

There are, however, several advantages to smaller single-mode image intensifiers:

1. Higher resolution, which is accomplished by the greater degree of magnification and the fact that electronic focusing is easier than it is with a multimode tube.

2. Because the input phosphor is smaller, x-ray tubes

with a shallower target angle and higher tube rating can be used.

3. The higher radiation requirement resulting from the decreased minification brightness gain results in less quantum noise, providing better images.

4. Because it is easier to focus the electrons from a smaller field, there is less vignetting and pincushion effect (i.e., less peripheral brightness loss and distortion).

The smallest possible single-mode image intensifier gives the best result.

Because only structures 20% to 30% smaller than the input phosphor can be demonstrated, it is impossible to see a significantly enlarged left ventricle on a 5-in. image intensifier. On the other hand, the coronary arteries can be ideally imaged by a 5-in. intensifier using panning. One of the solutions to this problem is the selection of an in-between size of 7 in.

This dilemma of field coverage led to the development of the very useful dual- or triple-mode image intensifiers, which have largely replaced the single-mode tube.

Multiple-Mode Image Intensifiers.—The basic principle of multiple-mode image intensifiers is simple, because focusing of the electrons in the image intensifier tube is accomplished by electrostatic lenses: By applying different voltages, one can focus the electrons at a variable distance from the input phosphor and so create a variable degree of magnification (Fig 7–5). A 9-in. image intensifier tube can therefore be converted electronically into a 6- or 5-in. tube. The 9-in./6-in. mode is the most common type of dual-image intensifiers. The triple-field image intensifiers are commonly 4.5, 6, and 9 in.

Dual- and triple-field image intensifiers have several advantages:

1. They provide adequate field coverage even for patients with markedly enlarged hearts.
2. They provide maximum magnification (up to ×4.5), which is highly desirable in children.
3. They allow adequate penetration of even very heavy patients in the 9-in. mode.
4. There is a significant increase in resolution in the 6-in. and, particularly, in the 4.5-in. modes, the images being almost as good as those obtained with a small single-mode image intensifier.

With multiple-mode image intensifier, the maximum possible magnification should be used because of the resulting increased resolution and decreased noise distortion and pincushion effect. However, the radiation dose to the patient is much greater in the magnified mode. To avoid unnecessary exposure of the patient, one must close the

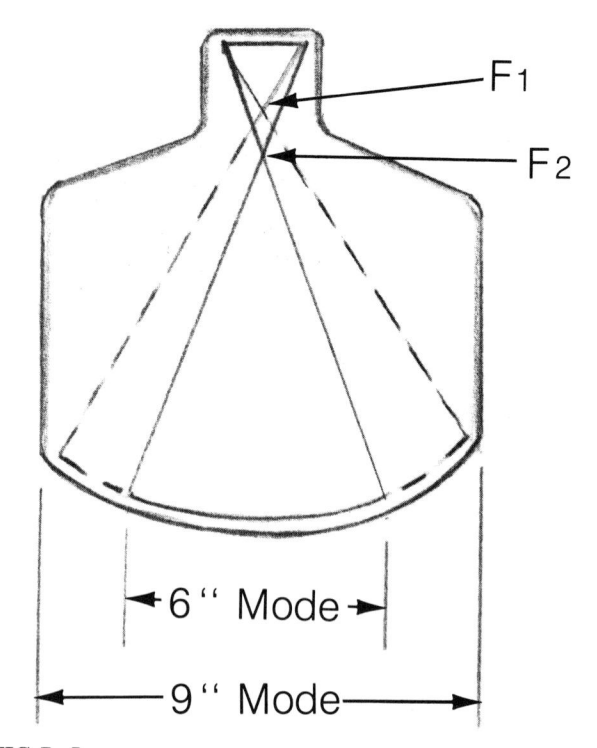

FIG 7–5.
Diagram of a dual-image field (9-in./5-in.) image intensifier. The electrons cross at F1 in the 9-in. mode. Shifting the focus to F2 converts the 9-in. tube to a 5-in. tube. Now only the central, best portion of the input phosphor is used. Unnecesssary exposure of the patient is avoided by an automatic coning system, limiting field size to 5 in.

cones until their image appears in the field; because there is no guarantee that the operator will do this, coning is accomplished automatically as soon as the equipment is switched from the 9- to the 5-in. mode. Coning needs also vary with the distance of the image intensifier, so this distance is sensed automatically by a potentiometer, assuring proper coning without unnecessary radiation to areas that do not appear on the cine frame.

The Optical System

The image from the output phosphor is transmitted to the film in the cine camera by a set of optical lenses. A large collective lens (actually a set of several lenses) "looks" at the output phosphor and projects a parallel bundle of light through an iris diaphragm, the f-stop of which should be about two stops above the maximum. Ninety percent of the light is reflected by the beam-splitting mirror (see Fig 7–1,B) through the smaller objective lens system of the cine camera onto the film, whereas 10% of the light passes through the mirror into the TV camera, allowing simultaneous image monitoring during cine recording. A fast lens system in the cine camera is important to permit the iris to be reduced two f-stops, thus optimizing the performance of the lens. Regardless of film speed or f-stop, the minimum dose per cine frame should not be less than 15 to 20 μR to minimize quantum mottle.

In recent years this dose level has been decreased by increasing the thickness of the input phosphor to 300 μm. This increases the light output and contrast of the phosphor but also decreases resolution.

The entire system must consist of a set of high-quality coated lenses with a higher resolution than the image intensifier, which is the limiting factor in resolution in cine fluorography.

Framing.—The format of 35-mm x-ray cine film is identical to that of commercial film with an 18 by 24-mm^2 field (Fig 7–6). The output phosphor is round, and this causes a mismatch, wasting either part of the information on the output phosphor or part of the available area on the cine frame. The relationship between the size of the output phosphor and the film format is called "framing." Framing is an important part of the cine system, and the degree of overframing must be adjusted to special needs. Underframing is an error, indicating that the output phosphor is less than 18 mm (the smallest dimension of the available film area).

Framing is accomplished by looking at the output phosphor with lenses of focal lengths from 90 to 125 mm. The principle is identical to that of the telephoto lenses used in photography. The degree of framing varies from exact to total overframing, where the entire cine frame is filled and 40% of the available information on the output phosphor is lost (see Fig 7–5). Overframing is an optical means of magnification (see Fig 7–5) using a telephoto system and eliminates the distracting glare around the cine image, but it requires good panning.

Underframing and exact framing are not useful in angiography. Some degree of overframing is recommended but may require panning. A 90- or 100-mm lens is most commonly used for angiocardiography. With overframing, there is always some loss of the image available on the output phosphor. Only a moderate degree of overframing can be used with smaller image intensifiers, because the available area of coverage is small to begin with.

Image-Intensifier Quality Control

The selection of a good image intensifier with an appropriate-sized input phosphor is crucial for satisfactory cine fluorography. The variation in quality between different manufacturers is much less than the variation between image intensifiers, particularly if off-the-shelf tubes are installed. For high-quality cine angiography, a hand-picked image intensifier with either a high gain or high resolution should be purchased; generally, the higher the gain, the lower the resolution. Increased brightness and contrast can usually be achieved by making the input phosphor thicker (200–300 μm). The trade-off is not significant, however, and newer image intensifiers tend to have higher contrast.

Resolution determines the sharpness of the image: The higher the resolution, the sharper the cine image and the smaller the structures that can be seen. Resolution is usually measured using a test pattern containing lead lines (see Fig 7–2,C) that is placed in contact with the input phosphor of the image intensifier. The image on the output phosphor is observed, and the number of lead lines that can still be seen distinctly is recorded. ("Line" actually means one line, and the adjacent interspace. It is more correctly called a "line pair.") The resolution of the entire system can be tested by making a cine recording of the test pattern. Before a cine angiogram is recorded in a patient, a short strip of a cine test pattern should be obtained to test the resolution and the contrast. A careful study of this test

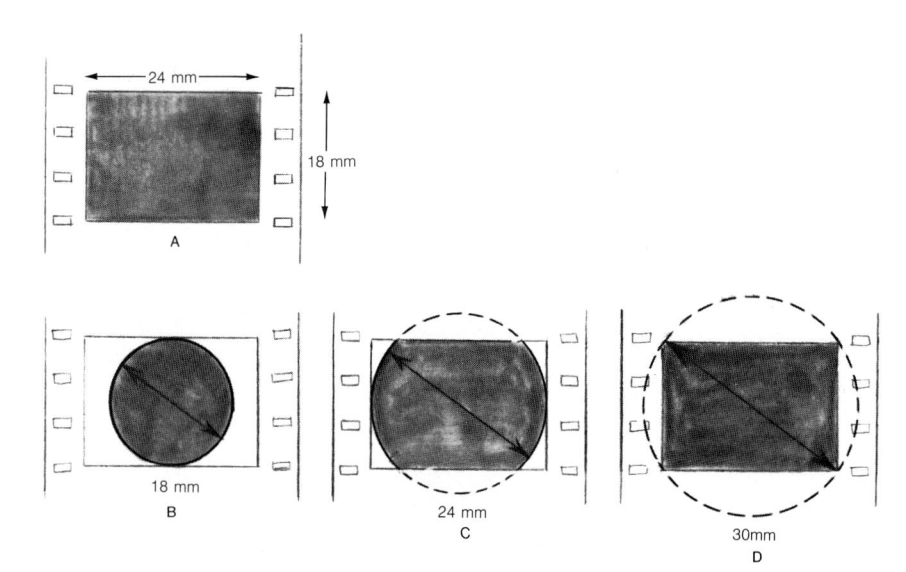

FIG 7–6.
Principle of framing. **A,** cine frame of 35 mm; the available exposure area measures 18 by 24 mm. **B,** exact framing; the size of the image is identical to the height of the frame (18 mm). **C,** partial overframing. **D,** total overframing, with loss of approximately 40% of the available image.

pattern helps in trouble-shooting if the quality of the cine recording deteriorates, as is discussed later.

A modern 5- or 6-in. image intensifier or a multiple-field tube in the 4.5- or 6-in. mode should have a resolution of 4 line pairs/mm; 7- and 9-in. tubes should have a resolution of 2.8 to 3.5 line pairs/mm. A satisfactory modern image intensifier should resolve the lines of an 80 line/in. radiographic grid (see Fig 7–2,B). However, there will be a slight variation from one image intensifier to another, even those from the same manufacturer.

The age of the image tube is another important factor, because brightness and gain tend to decrease with age. After 5 years, even if the image tube is still functional, it should be replaced to maintain high-quality cine radiography.

Radiation Dose per Cine Frame.—For satisfactory cine radiography, each frame must receive an adequate amount of light. Although it is possible to adjust the overall density by opening or stepping down the lens in the cine camera, the output phosphor itself has to produce an adequate amount of light, which, in turn, requires an adequate amount of x-rays. If the radiation dose is less than a certain minimum (16 µR/frame), there is not enough photon flux, and the image on the output phosphor will appear to scintillate. This appearance is also recorded on the cine film, which becomes noisy or grainy. This type of graininess is termed "quantum noise" and should not be confused with *film* graininess, which is negligible (see the section on cine film).

Quantum Noise.—Quantum noise, also called "quantum mottle," is basically the visualization of the statistical fluctuations of the photons striking the phosphor. The impact of these photons is not evenly distributed, and consequently some will partially overlap, whereas spaces will occur between others. Only when enough photons are formed will this statistical fluctuation disappear and the phosphor be evenly illuminated. With an inefficient number of photons striking the phosphor, not only is the image noisy and grainy but the imaged structures appear fuzzy, and resolution and border definition are decreased.

The basic principle can be readily understood if, instead of photons striking a phosphor, paint droplets from a spray gun striking paper are considered. These small droplets, like photons, will have a random distribution and will be seen individually unless the air flow is increased (higher kV[p]) or the area is painted for a longer period of time (mA) to average out the statistical fluctuations of their impact on paper (Fig 7–7).

Translated into cine radiography, photo flux cannot be increased by increasing the exposure time, because this is limited to 4 to 5 msec at a rate of 60 fps. Therefore, a radiation dose 16 to 20 µR/frame can be achieved only with higher mA output, which places great demand on the entire radiographic system.

If the ciné system is calibrated to a dose of at least 16 to 20 µR/frame quantum noise does not occur. The automatic brightness control provides continuous adjustment of KV(p) at MA in order to assure a properly exposed ciné frame. In very obese patients and with extreme angle views in adult coronary angiography the KV(p) and milliamperage limits of the radiographic system may be exceeded, resulting in under penetration.

Some manufacturers have introduced a variable iris for the ciné camera. If the limits of the system are exceeded, the iris will open up automatically, providing more light to the ciné camera. In this way, less dose is needed for proper penetration but the images are grainy due to quantum noise (not enough dose per frame).

The Cine Camera

Cine cameras are standard commercial motion-picture cameras adapted, with minor modifications, for cine angiography. Basically, the cine film from a feed spool (Fig 7–8) is fed continuously through the film gate by a sprocket wheel, which engages the perforations and winds

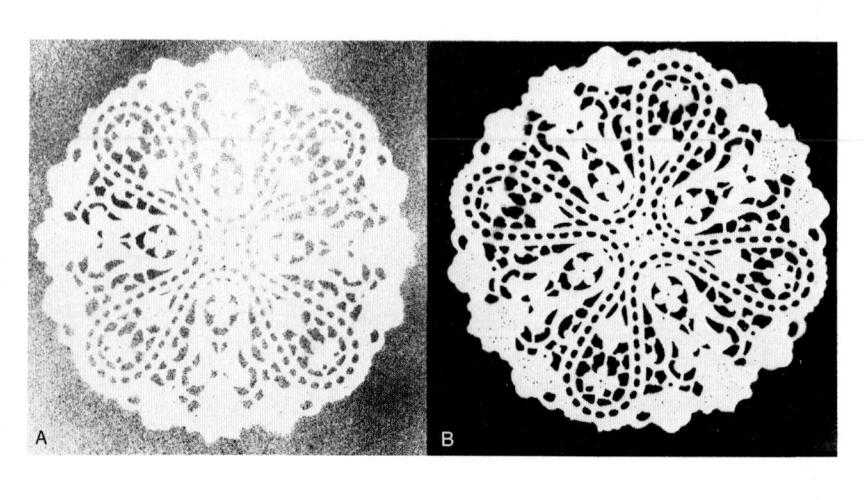

FIG 7–7.
A, spray gun producing an insufficient number of paint droplets; the statistical fluctuation of their impact on paper produces a noisy, fuzzy image (quantum noise). **B,** air flow was increased and now carries many more paint droplets; the paper (phosphor) is uniformly covered, and the grainy image (quantum noise) has disappeared.

A. CINE CAMERA MECHANISM

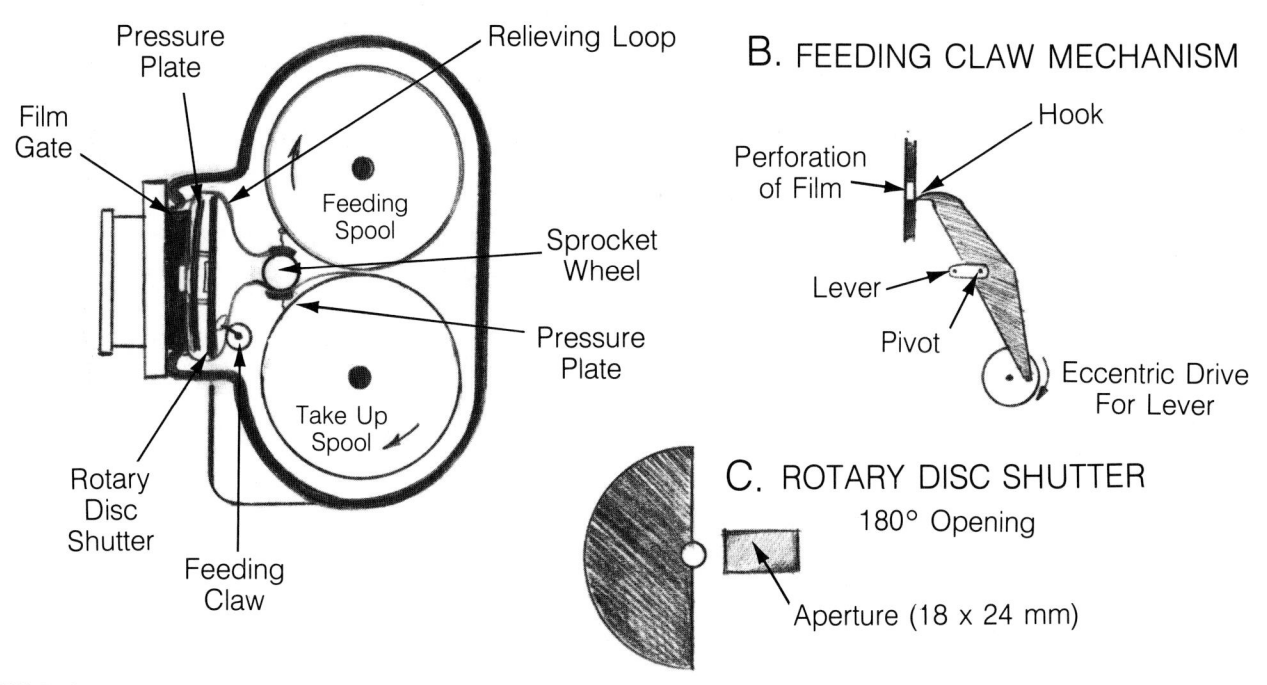

B. FEEDING CLAW MECHANISM

C. ROTARY DISC SHUTTER
180° Opening

FIG 7-8.
Diagrams of a cine camera. **A,** film is fed continuously from a spool by means of a sprocket wheel through the film gate, forming a relieving loop needed because transport is intermittent. The film is held flat by a pressure plate. The film gate is closed intermittently by a rotary-disc shutter. **B,** basic mechanism of intermittent film transport. **C,** rotary-disc shutter with a 180-degree opening covering the aperture intermittently.

the film up on a take-up spool. In the film gate, a pressure plate keeps the film flat so the lens can be precisely focused. Transport through the film gate is accomplished in a jerky (intermittent) motion by an eccentric-lever mechanism (see Fig 7–8,B). The hook of the lever engages the film perforation, resulting in intermittent transport of the film. The film is stationary approximately 50% of the time, although the duty cycle of most cine cameras is about 60/40; in other words, 60% of the time is required for transport, whereas 40% of the time the film is stationary and available for exposure. Transport time with this type mechanism is also called "pull-down time." During film transport, the aperture is covered by a rotary-disk shutter (see Fig 7–8,C). While the film is in motion, light cannot enter the aperture.

Whereas in regular motion-picture photography the exposure time is determined by the time the shutter is open, in cine fluorography, exposure is determined by the pulse width. One could assume that a shutter thus would not be necessary, but there are three reasons shutters are used for cine recording:

1. Although the decay time of the input phosphor (cesium iodide) is in the microsecond range, the decay of the output phosphor is in the millisecond range, and because of this afterglow, the film must be protected while it is in motion.

2. A shutter protects the film in biplane cine radiography, where one plane is exposed while the other camera is transporting. Without the shutter, the film would be exposed by secondary radiation (cross-fogging).

3. Cine cameras are commercial cameras made for light cinematography and thus are always equipped with shutters.

Cine cameras are driven by a synchronous motor similar to that of an electric clock, which rotates exactly according to the line frequency (60 cycles/sec). This is vital, because the pulsing system has to be exactly synchronized with the camera. Because the pulsing system of the generator and the driving mechanism of the cine camera are controlled by the same line frequency, synchronization can be accomplished. The line frequency determines the frame rate, which, in the United States, is 60 fps or some fraction thereof (e.g., 30 or 15). In Europe, standard exposure rates are 50 fps or fractions thereof because of the lower line frequency (50 cycles/sec).

In biplane cine fluorography, the two exposures must

occur out of phase; if they are made simultaneously, the secondary radiation cross-fogs the film. If they are synchronized, however, the quality of biplane cine fluorography is identical to that of single-plane equipment except for some minor drawbacks (see the section on biplane arrangement).

All motors, including the drive mechanism for the cine camera, start at 0 speed. Although the response time of the motor is short, the first few frames may be overexposed because the motor is not at full speed. Consequently, injection of contrast medium should be delayed slightly until the entire mechanical and electronic system is in equilibrium.

BASIC CINE EQUIPMENT

Cine angiograms can be recorded in either a single-plane or a biplane projection. Each technique has advantages and disadvantages.

Single-Plane Cine Angiography

The advantages of this method are as follows:

1. The cost is lower, because only one generator, image intensifier, and cine camera must be purchased.
2. Sharpness is increased, because the image intensifier can always be placed close to the patient.
3. It has quicker and easier handling.
4. It has one half the radiation to patient and personnel as biplane cine angiography.

Biplane Cine Angiography

In biplane cine angiography, two x-ray tubes are fired out of phase at either 60 or 30 fps. Two image intensifiers and cine cameras are required. When the x-ray tube is activated in one plane, the mechanical shutter of the other camera is closed to prevent fogging of the image, so the quality of biplane cine radiography is identical to that of single plane.

The advantages of this method are as follows:

1. With a single injection of contrast medium, two views can be obtained, so fewer injections are required.
2. Because fewer injections are required, the amount of contrast medium per injection can be increased, resulting in better opacification with an acceptable total dose of contrast.

The disadvantages of this method are as follows:

1. Because the patient must be centered over the anteroposterior image intensifier, the lateral image intensifier cannot be moved close because of interference by the table. As a result, the lateral image has greater geometric unsharpness. Whenever possible, the small focal spot should be used to minimize this problem.
2. Biplane equipment is used so routinely that it may be misused when the second plane does not add information. The patient then receives twice the radiation dose unnecessarily.
3. Operating and using biplane equipment is much more cumbersome and time consuming.
4. The cost is almost twice as great as for a single-plane arrangement.

X-Ray Tube Mounting

There are four basic arrangements for tube mountings that are used for angiocardiography: standard biplane, C arm, L/U arm, and parallelogram mounting. The other available arrangements are only variations of these four basic types.

Standard Biplane Technique

One image intensifier is mounted above the patient and the other at a right angle (Fig 7–9). The x-ray tubes and image intensifiers can be attached to either the ceiling or the floor, but suspension from the ceiling is preferable because it allows easier access to the patient, particularly in an emergency.

The principal limitation of this common tube arrangement is the inability to move the lateral image intensifier close to the patient, leading to unsharpness of the lateral image (geometric unsharpness). This can be minimized by using a narrow catheterization table, particularly for pediatric patients. Another limitation is that for doubly angulated views, the patient must be rotated, and this is cumbersome, particularly in heavily sedated children and debilitated adults. In addition, catheters may be dislodged during such positioning.

C-Arm Mounting

C-arm mountings are made in various forms. Basically, the image intensifier and x-ray tube are mounted on a ring (C arm) that can move in an arc around the patient and around a second axis (Fig 7–10). The entire C arm can be raised and lowered, and with some mountings, it can also be moved away, providing excellent access to the patient. C arms are lighter and more mobile and require less floor space than does an L/U arrangement. Also, they

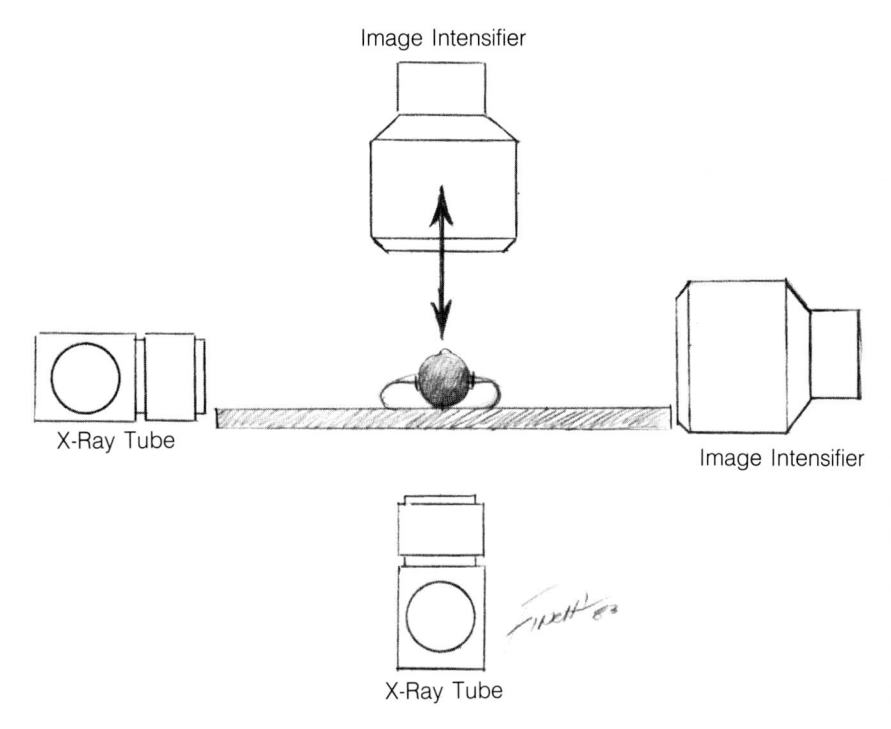

FIG 7-9.
Fixed biplane arrangement of x-ray tube and image intensifiers; only right-angle views can be obtained. Compound biplane angled projections require special positioning of the patient. The anteroposterior image intensifier can be moved close to the patient, but the lateral cannot. However, geometric unsharpness in the lateral projection can be minimized by using the small focal spot and x-ray table.

can be arranged in biplane fashion to allow simultaneous multiangulated projections. However, the light construction and ceiling suspension of standard C arms may not allow vibration-free operation of a cine camera. This drawback led to the construction of a sturdier floor-mounted C arm combined with an L arm (Fig 7-11). The versatility of this equipment is increased when the catheterization table can be raised and lowered.

C arms are designed to rotate around wide catheterization tables, and consequently the source-to-intensifier distance (SID) is large. Because of this, a greater x-ray output is required (inverse-square law). Some of the more sophisticated C-arm systems allow either the image intensifier or the x-ray tube to be raised or lowered, thereby shortening the SID for smaller patients. However, with many designs, the distance is fixed. If arranged in biplane fashion, the axis of both C arms is at the same level. If the heart is positioned at this isocenter (isos is Greek meaning equal), its image will not shift if the system is rotated.

L/U System

Basically, all L/U systems consist of an L arm and a U arm (Fig 7-12) that can be rotated freely in many directions. The catheterization table can be moved, raised, and lowered and can be rotated to obtain access to the patient in an emergency. L/U arms require more floor space and are heavier than C-arm mountings. Recently they have been arranged in biplane fashion.

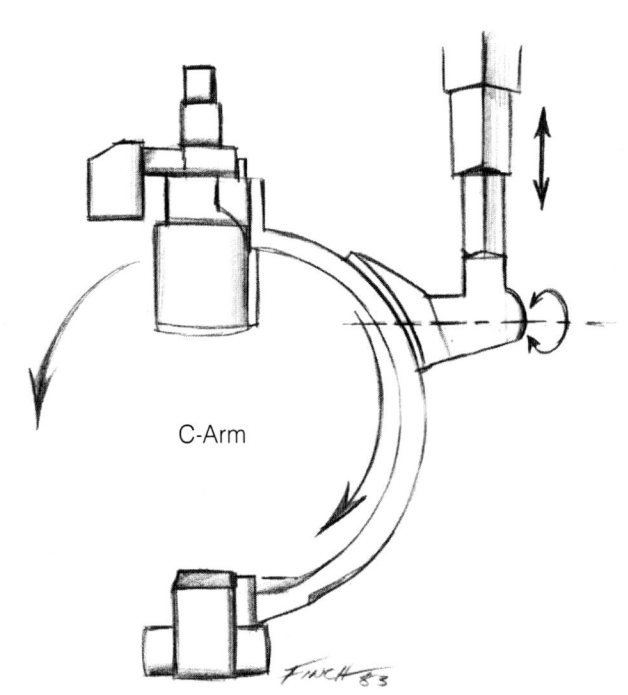

FIG 7-10.
C-arm radiographic unit. X-ray tube and image intensifier are mounted on a C-shaped support, which can be rotated about the patient in direction indicated by large arrows. Rotation *(smaller round arrow)* is possible on a pivot. C-arm units are either mounted on the floor or suspended from the ceiling and can be raised or lowered.

144 *General Introduction*

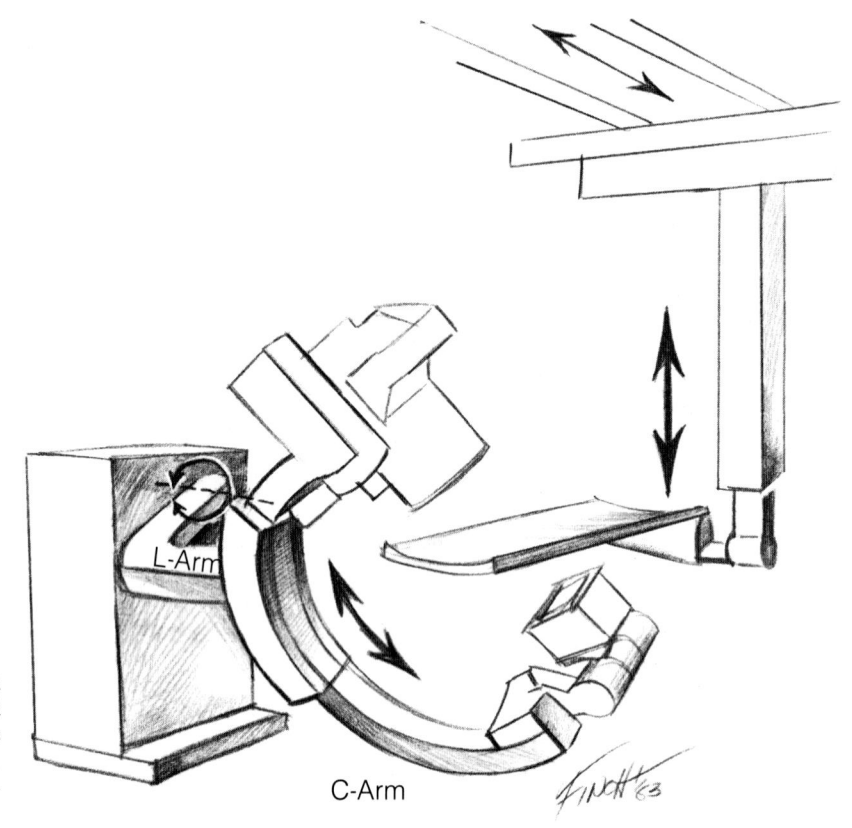

FIG 7–11.
L/C-arm cine unit. A C arm is mounted on an L arm, allowing various motions as indicated by arrows. This combination is more versatile than the standard C arm and is vibration free. A cantilever table is suspended from the ceiling, increasing versatility.

Parallelogram Mounting

Parallelogram mounting is a modified U mount that allows both rotation of the tube assembly around the patient and angulation (Fig 7–13). As with any other U-arm arrangement, the patient rests on a special mobile cantilever table, which can be lowered or raised to the isocenterposition.

ANGIOGRAPHIC POSITIONING

Principles[2]

The aim in positioning the patient for angiography is to demonstrate the anatomic features of cardiac anomalies to their best visual advantage. Ideally, profile views of the important anatomic features should be obtained,

FIG 7–12.
L/U arm radiographic unit. X-ray tube and image intensifier are mounted on an U arm, which rotates around axis (**A**). The U arm is mounted on an L arm, which rotates at its base (**B**). The L arm can be mounted on either the floor or the ceiling. Cantilever x-ray table can be moved in various directions *(arrows)*.

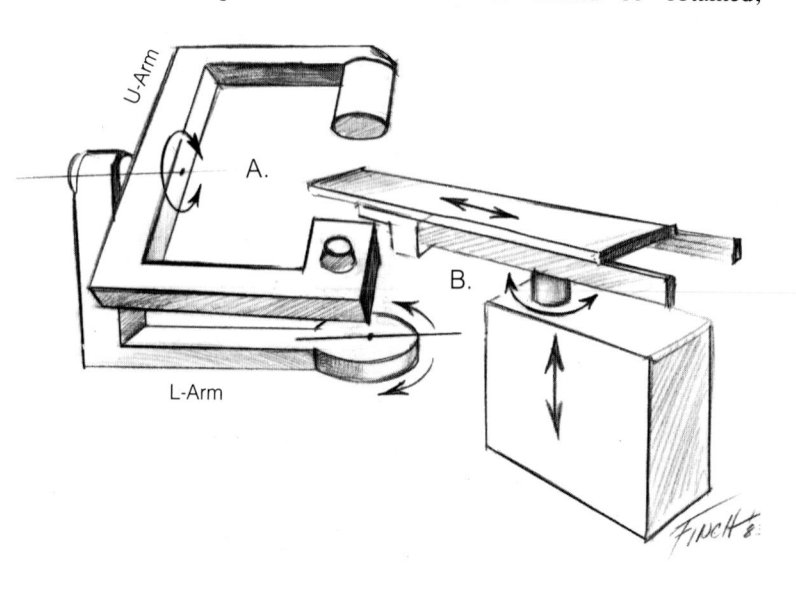

PARALLELOGRAM

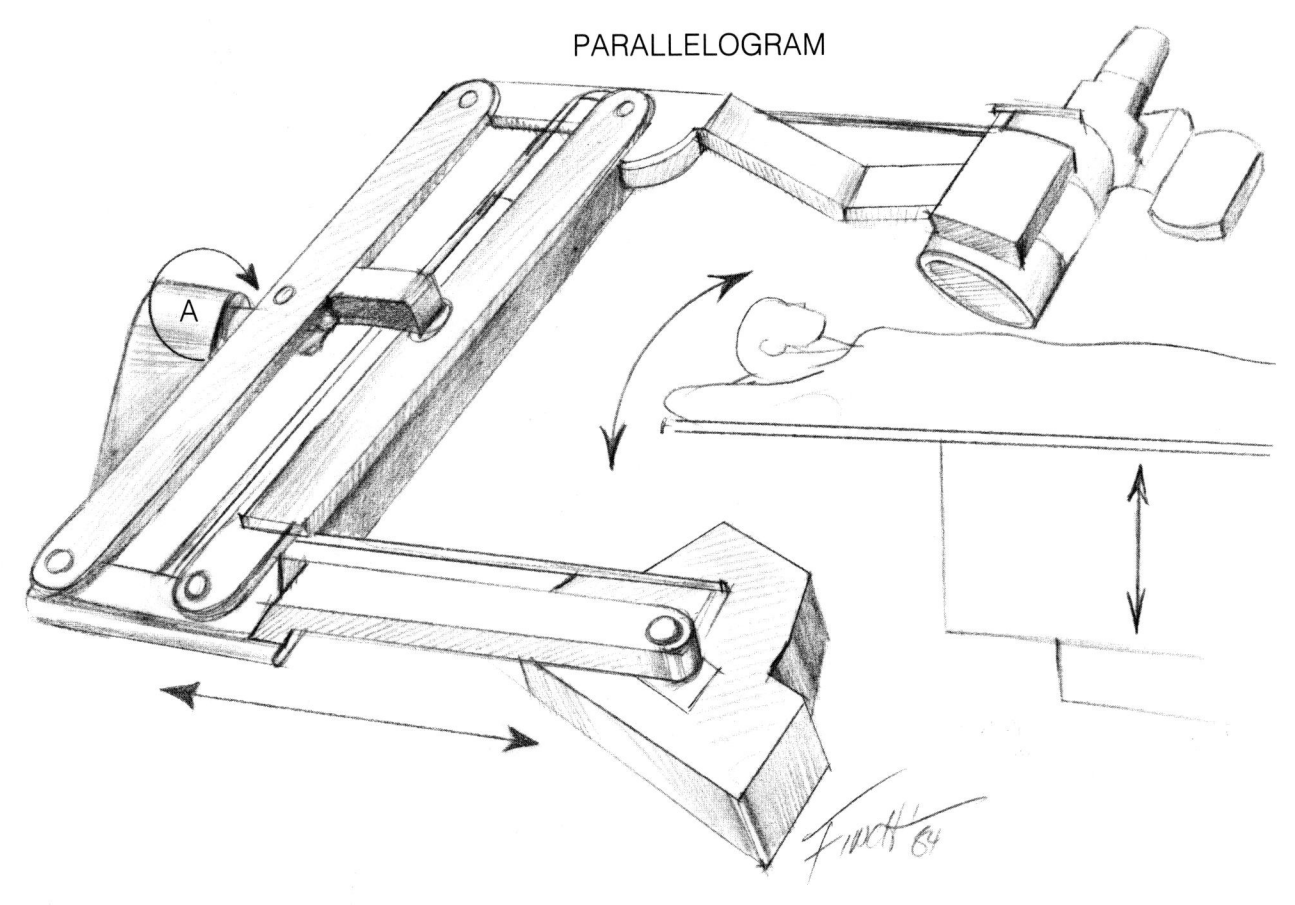

FIG 7–13.
Parallelogram mounting. This is bascially a U-arm mounting, which rotates around axis (**A**). Because of the parallelogram design, the x-ray tube and image intensifier can also be tilted in the direction of the arrows. Cantilever table moves in various directions.

and foreshortening of cardiac structures should be avoided.

The basic principle of positioning is understandable if one has a clear concept of the position of the heart within the thoracic cavity. The long axis of the heart is inclined approximately 45 degrees to each major body plane (Fig 7–14). Therefore, if radiographs are taken in the direction of either the sagittal or the frontal plane of the chest, the image of the heart is markedly foreshortened. For instance, a lateral view of the thorax (Fig 7–15,A) results in a foreshortened projection of the heart, whereas if the lateral view of the heart is taken by positioning the patient obliquely in relation to the x-ray beam (Fig 7–15,B), the heart is depicted without foreshortening. Alternatively, instead of positioning the patient, it is possible to angulate the x-ray beam in relation to the patient. Multidirectional x-ray equipment is available so that the beam can be changed in relation to the long axis of the body. If the x-ray beam enters the body exactly in the midsagittal plane, a straight posteroanterior view is obtained—posteroanterior because the anterior part of the patient is close to the image intensifier and the beam enters the posterior aspect of the body. If the x-ray tube is in front and the image intensifier behind the patient, an anteroposterior view results. Therefore, posteroanterior and anteroposterior are identical projections. If the x-ray beam is angulated in relation to the sagittal plane or the patient is turned, a right anterior oblique or left anterior oblique projection is obtained. Right anterior oblique means that the right anterior part of the chest is close to the image receptor. If the beam is parallel to the table top, a lateral view of the body is obtained (Fig 7–16). A 45-degree left anterior projection of the chest shows an end-on view of the heart (see Fig 7–16), whereas a 45-degree right anterior oblique view shows an en face view of the heart. Posteroanterior and lateral projections are intermediate between these two views.

If the x-ray tube is angulated toward the patient's head, a cranial (Latin: cranium-skull; Greek: cephale head) or cephalad projection is obtained (Fig 7–17); angulation

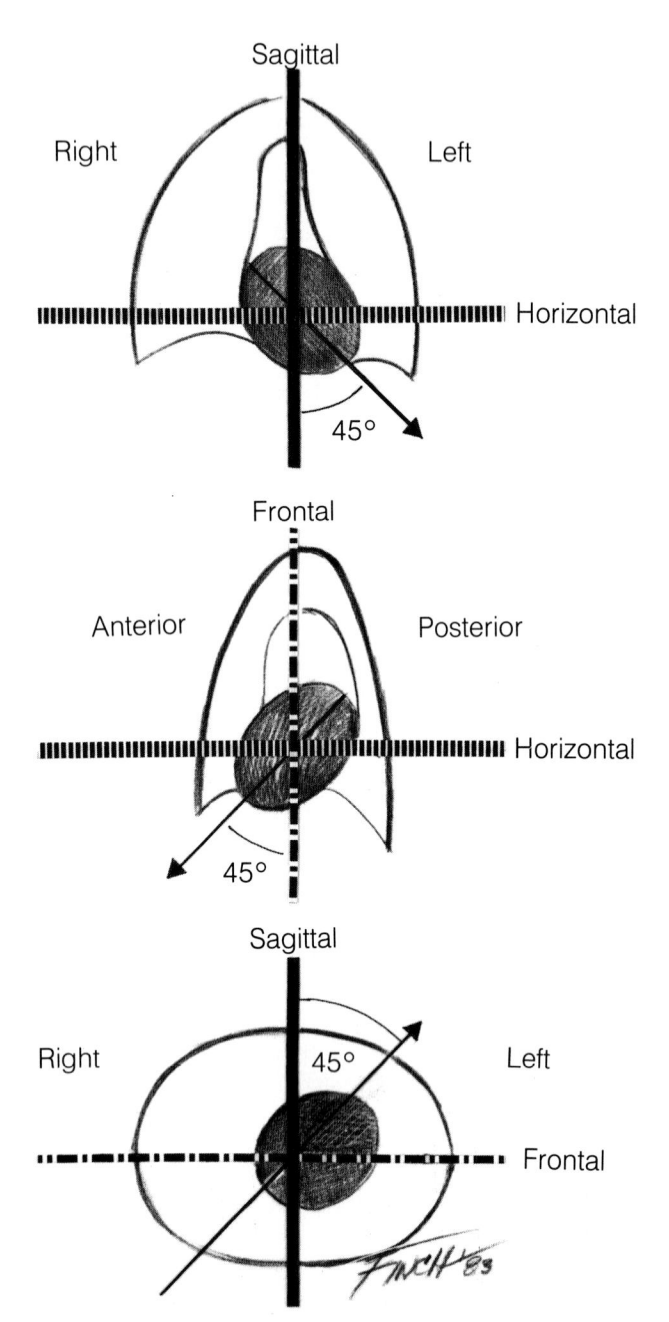

FIG 7–14.
Inclination of long axis of heart to each three major body planes. Inclination is about 45 degrees. If standard views of body are taken, projection of heart is always foreshortened.

of the x-ray beam toward the patient's feet results in the caudal (or caudad) (Latin: cauda-tail) projection. The image on the image tube, however, is the opposite: cranial is looking down toward the feet and caudal is looking up toward the head. Because of the inclined position of the heart within the thorax, the standard posteroanterior projection foreshortens the long axis of the heart and caudad angulation causes even more foreshortening, whereas the cranial angulation eliminates foreshortening as does tilting the body (see Fig 7–15). A 45-degree cranial beam angulation gives a virtually unforeshortened view of the heart. Without multidirectional x-ray equipment, the same result can be obtained by sitting the patient up 40 degrees (see Fig 7–19).

By combining angulations of the x-ray beam in a cranial-caudal direction with a right anterior oblique and left anterior oblique projection, one can obtain compound angles, which are useful for angiocardiography. These views can be made in two ways, depending on the type of equipment available. If the image intensifier is fixed, as in standard biplane equipment, the patient's body must be rotated and elevated to achieve these compound angles. On the other hand, with multidirectional equipment, the patient can lie flat on the table, and compound views are obtained by rotating the x-ray tube and image intensifier about the table. This method is much more convenient for the patient, particularly if heavily sedated. By angulating the x-ray beam along the sagittal plane (i.e., in a cranial-caudad direction) and at a right angle to the sagittal plane in the short axis (horizontal plane) of the body, one can develop a coordinate system about the thorax that provides all compound angles using the multidirectional equipment (Fig 7–18,). Whereas beam angulation in either the right anterior oblique or left anterior oblique direction requires only a slight increase in x-ray penetration, beam angulation in the cranial-caudal direction requires a marked increase in penetration, because the x-ray beam has to pass through the abdomen. Whereas the x-ray beam can be angulated about the short axis of the body in the horizontal plane through an arc of 360 degrees, beam angulation along the long axis of the body (sagittal plane) is limited to 45 degrees, because of the shape of the body and the excessive demands on tube output. A 45-degree beam angulation along the long axis of the body is adequate to eliminate foreshortening of the heart (see Fig 7–14).

With this coordinate system erected over the heart (Fig 7–18,B), it is possible to obtain compound angles with multidirectional equipment without moving the patient. Point B on the coordinate system, for instance, represents a beam angulation of 15-degree cranial and a 15-degree left anterior oblique projection. On the other hand, point A is a 30-degree caudal and 30-degree right anterior oblique projection. These same compound projections can be obtained using standard fixed biplane equipment but only by positioning the patient, which is much more cumbersome.

In situs inversus, tube angulations produce different images of the heart. In situs solitus a right anterior oblique view, for example (Fig 7–19,A), results in an unforeshortened view of the long axis of the heart. In situs inversus (Fig 7–19,B), the same projection results in a foreshort-

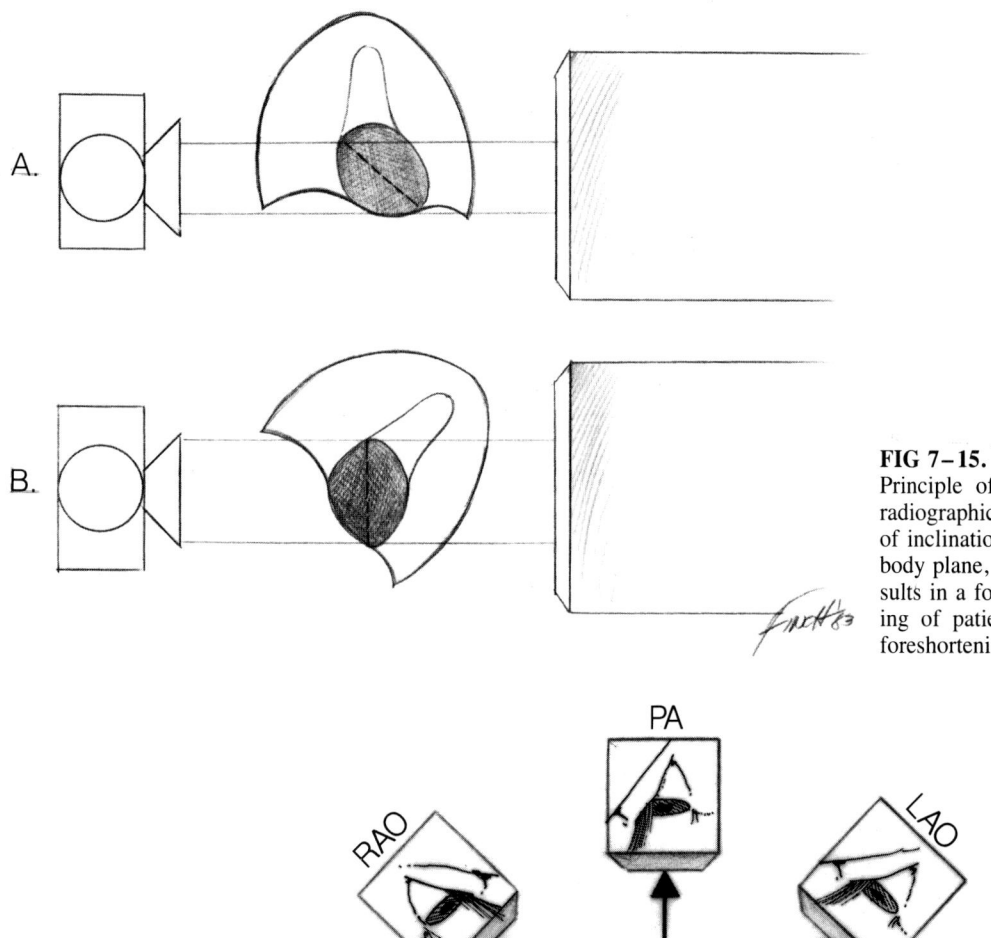

FIG 7–15.
Principle of eliminating foreshortening of radiographic projection of heart. **A,** because of inclination of heart in relation to sagittal body plane, a right-angle view of thorax results in a foreshortened image. **B,** by slanting of patient 45 degrees on x-ray table, foreshortening of long axis is eliminated.

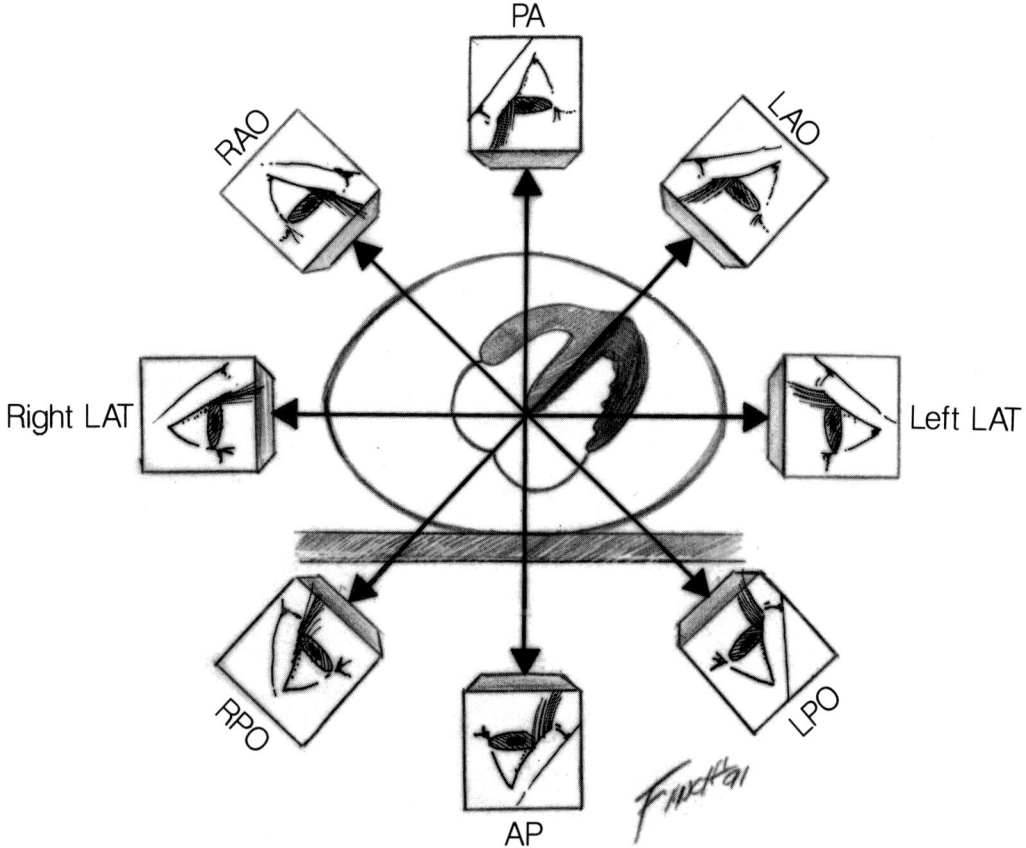

FIG 7–16.
Posteroanterior, lateral, right, and left anterior oblique views of chest, taken with multidirectional equipment. The patient remains supine and the heart can be viewed through a 180-degree arc. Understanding of positioning is facilitated by thinking of the image intensifier as having eyes.

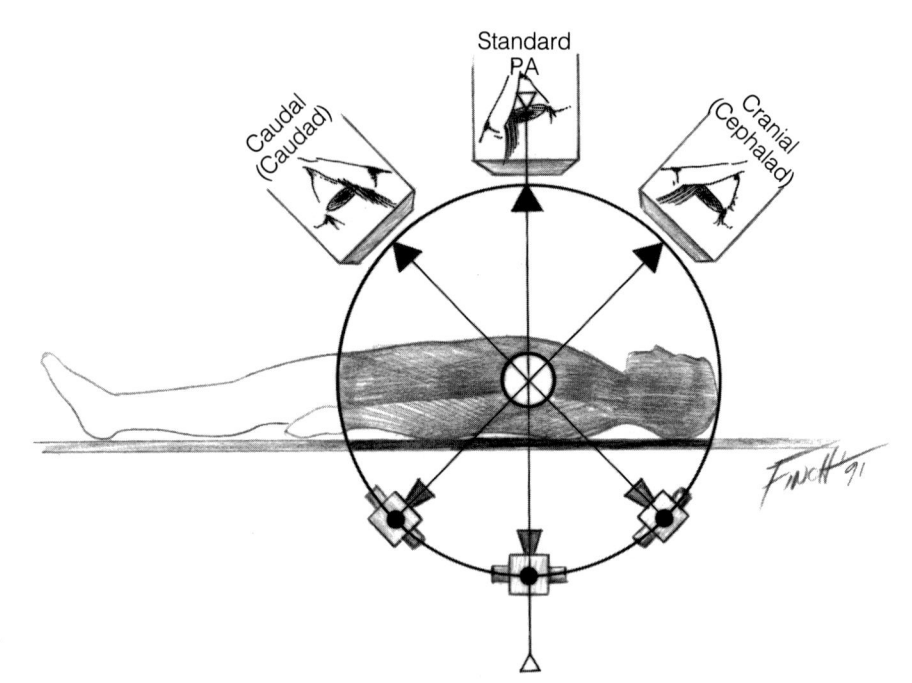

FIG 7–17.
Beam angulation along long axis (sagittal plane) of body. If beam is angulated toward patient's head, projection is cranial or cephalad; if angulated toward feet, it is caudal or caudal. Because the patient's body interferes, angulation is limited to an arc of 90 degrees compared with 180 degrees in short axis of body (see Fig 7–3) with cranial angulation the image intensifier is looking "down" and with caudal angulation it is looking up.

ened view of the heart, which is, in essence, a left anterior oblique projection. To obtain a right anterior oblique view of the heart, one must use the usual left anterior oblique projection.

Similarly, a cranial projection (looking down) in situs solitus (Fig 7–20,A) eliminates the foreshortening of the long axis of the heart. In situs inversus, the same projection (looking down) results in a foreshortening of the ventricles (Fig 7–20,B). To minimize foreshortening, one makes a caudal projection. In summary, in situs inversus all projections have to be reversed except for the true lateral view.

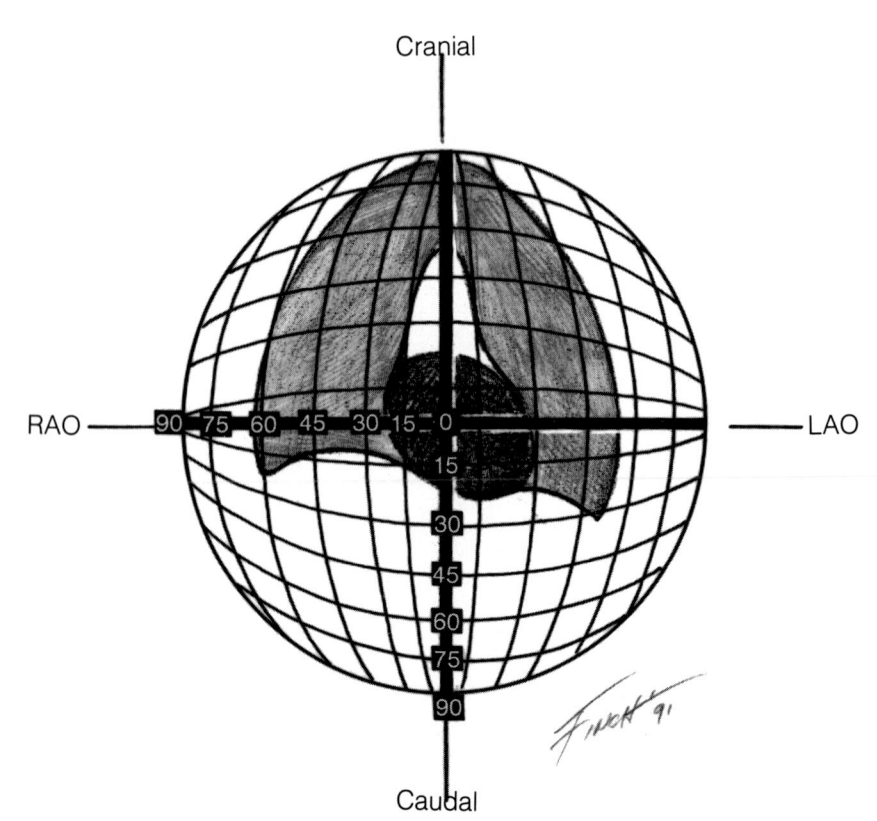

FIG 7–18.
A, combining beam angulation in sagittal and horizontal planes a coordinate system can be erected over the thorax, allowing for determination of compound x-ray beam angulations. Point A, for example, is 30-degree right anterior oblique projection, and 30-degree caudal angulation. Point B is 15-degree left anterior oblique projection and 15-degree cranial view of thorax.

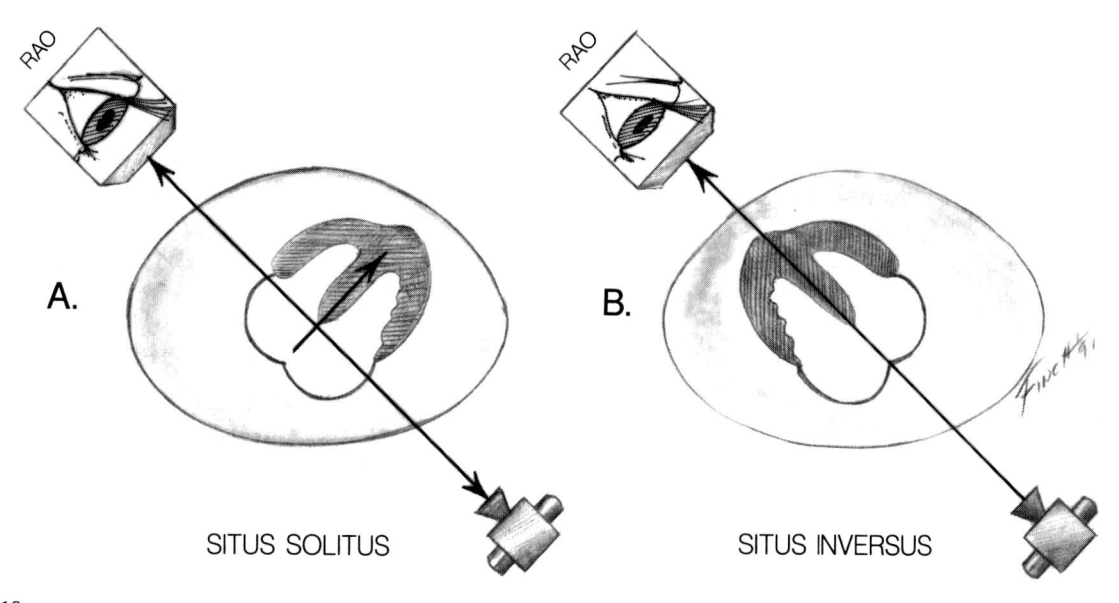

FIG 7–19.
A, situs solitus. Right anterior right projection, which results in an en face view of the heart. **B,** situs inversus. Same right anterior oblique projection results in a end-on view, which is a left anterior oblique projection. In situs inversus, therefore, the projections have to be reversed.

Angiographic Positioning Using Standard Fixed Biplane Equipment

Foreshortening of cardiovascular structures can be eliminated with standard fixed biplane equipment by rotating the patient. Either the anteroposterior or the lateral x-ray tube can be used; the results are the same. Whenever possible, however, the anteroposterior x-ray tube should be used, because the image intensifier can be brought closer to the patient, thereby minimizing geometric unsharpness. Images obtained with the lateral tube are usually of inferior quality, particularly if a small focal spot cannot be used.

On a standard anteroposterior view of the thorax, the right ventricular outflow tract and pulmonary arteries are foreshortened because of their inclination with the horizontal plane (see Chapter 2). A 45-degree cranial tube angulation can be obtained by placing the patient in a semisitting position using a wedged pillow and the anteroposterior x-ray tube system (Fig 7–21). The patient's head must be

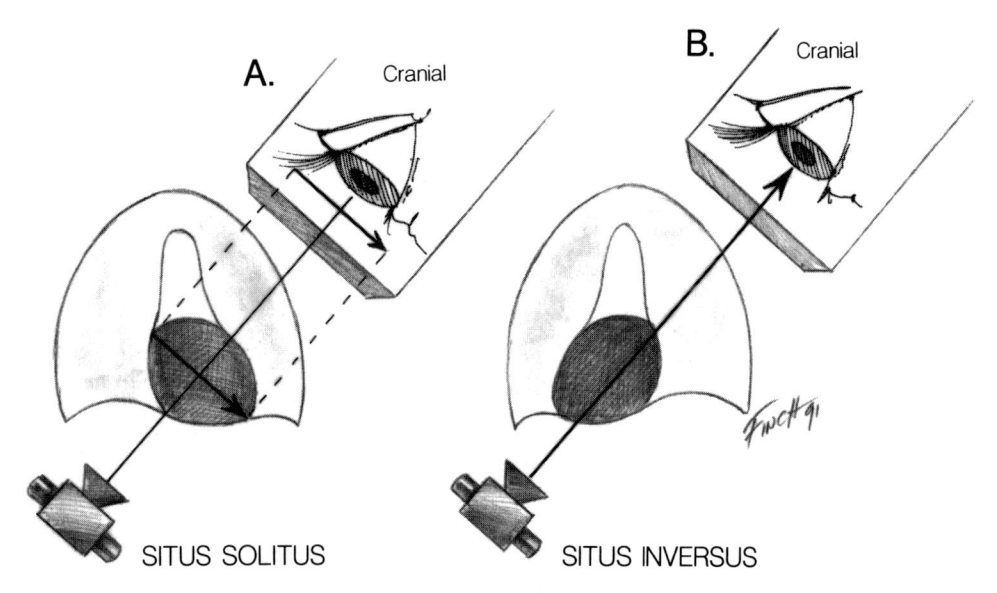

FIG 7–20.
A, situs solitus. Cranial projections result in a elongation of the ventricle. **B,** situs inversus. The same cranial angulation in situs solitus produces a foreshortening of the ventricle. To elongate the long axis of the heart in situs inversus, one must use caudal projections.

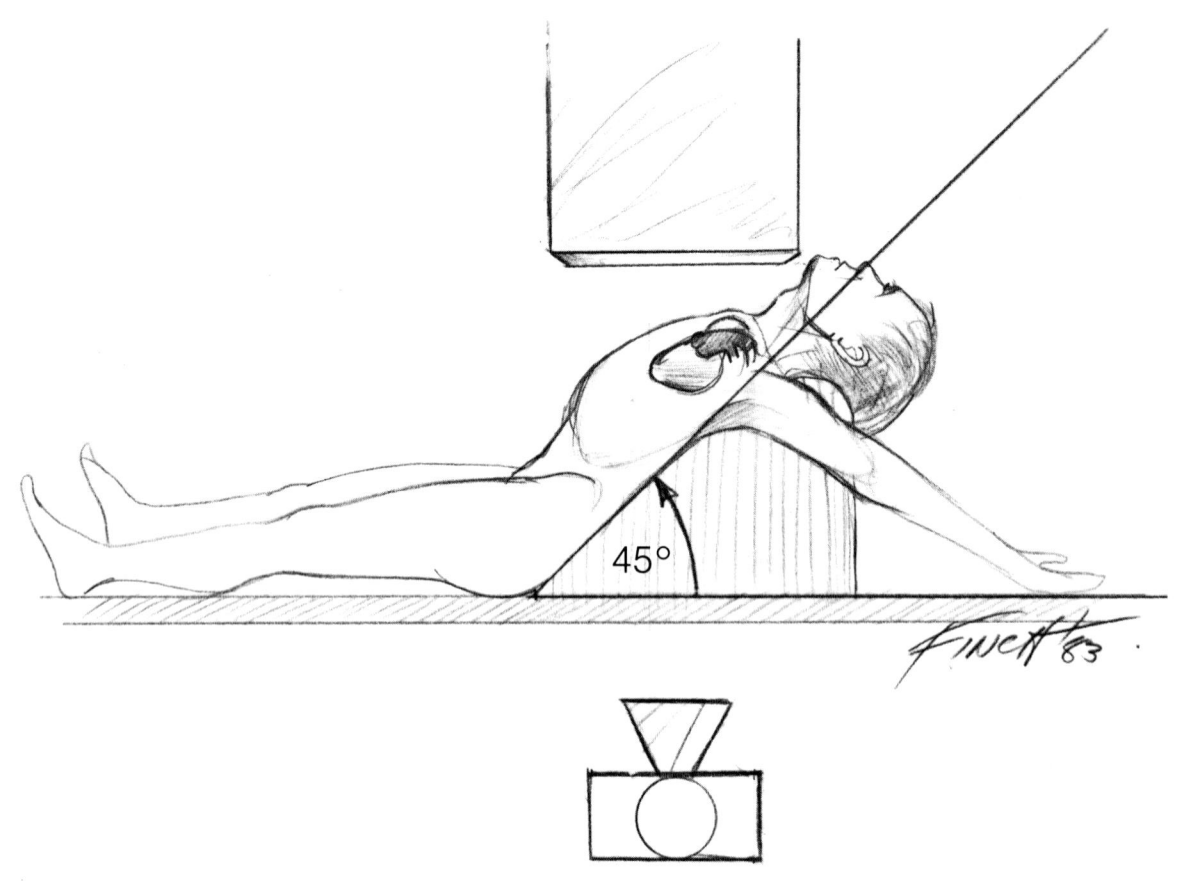

FIG 7–21.
Elimination of foreshortening of right ventricular outflow tract and main pulmonary artery using anteroposterior x-ray tube. By sitting patient up 45 degrees, foreshortening is eliminated. This projection (sitting up projection) is useful for demonstration of right ventricular outflow tract and pulmonary artery.

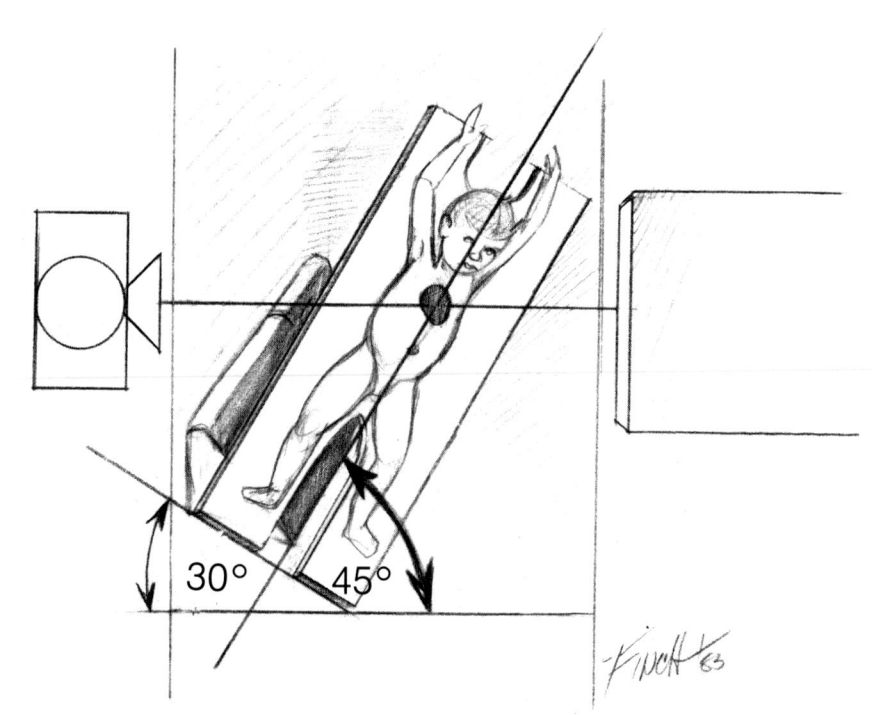

FIG 7–22.
Elimination of foreshortening of long axis of heart using lateral x-ray tube. Patient is slanted 45 degrees across long axis of table and rotated in right anterior oblique position. On the lateral plane, a left anterior oblique projection is obtained. Shallow right anterior oblique position of patient in this long axial oblique projection results in a steep left anterior oblique projection on lateral projection. Both angles add up to 90 degrees.

extended to prevent overlap of the chin, and if films are to be obtained simultaneously with the lateral x-ray tube, the patient's arms must be pulled back. It is difficult to position a patient, particularly a heavily sedated one, in this manner. A similar projection can be obtained by using the lateral x-ray tube; the patient is placed in a lateral decubitus position and slanted 45 degrees across the long axis of the table. However, as noted, images obtained with the lateral tube system are less sharp than those of the anteroposterior system.

Right anterior oblique and left anterior oblique views are common projections and yield an en face and end-on view of the heart, respectively. With fixed biplane equipment, the lateral tube is usually used for the left anterior oblique projection, particularly in infants, who can easily be tilted on the table (Fig 7–22). Slanting the infant 45 degrees across the long axis of the x-ray table can eliminate foreshortening of the heart. Unfortunately, in adult patients, this is impossible because the patient's feet would extend beyond the table top.

If the patient is rotated 30 degrees in a right anterior oblique position (see Fig 7–22), the right-angle view with the lateral tube results in a 60-degree left anterior oblique projection. In other words, a slight right anterior oblique rotation of the patient results in a steep left anterior oblique projection on the lateral tube. Because a 90-degree biplane system is used, the total degrees of right anterior oblique and left anterior oblique views add up to 90 degrees. A 30-degree right anterior oblique rotation of the patient on the x-ray table thus results in a 60-degree left anterior oblique view on the lateral plane (30 + 60 = 90). This degree of obliquity is commonly used for demonstration of membranous ventricular septal defects and has been termed the "long axial oblique" view.

The same views can be obtained by placing the patient properly in relation to the anteroposterior plane, and this produces sharper images because there is less geometric distortion. Foreshortening of the long axis of the heart is eliminated by having the patient sit up 45 degrees (the same as having the patient slanted 45 degrees on the x-ray table and using the lateral tube). In addition, the patient is placed in a left anterior oblique position (Fig 7–23). The left anterior oblique position of the anteroposterior plane results in a right anterior oblique view on the lateral plane. Again, both angles add up to 90 degrees. If the patient is rotated in a 60-degree left anterior oblique position, a 30-degree right anterior oblique view is obtained, as in Figure 7–22. Usually, in this view, a shallow (e.g., 45 degrees) left anterior oblique projection, termed the "four-chamber view," is made. This is a very useful projection for angiographic demonstration of atrioventricular canal and atrial septal defects by rotating the patient in a 45-degree left anterior oblique position. The sharpness of the left anterior oblique image is improved by using the anteroposterior x-ray tube. On the other hand, the degree to which the patient can sit up is limited, and the demands on the x-ray tube are greater. Because the beam enters in the region of the liver and exits near the clavicle, the projection has also been termed the "hepatoclavicular" view.

Thus, angiographic positioning is a simple logical procedure if the position of the heart within the thoracic cavity and the geometry of the x-ray beam are kept in mind. Optimal results can be obtained only if the angiographer has a clear concept of the compound angles that are possi-

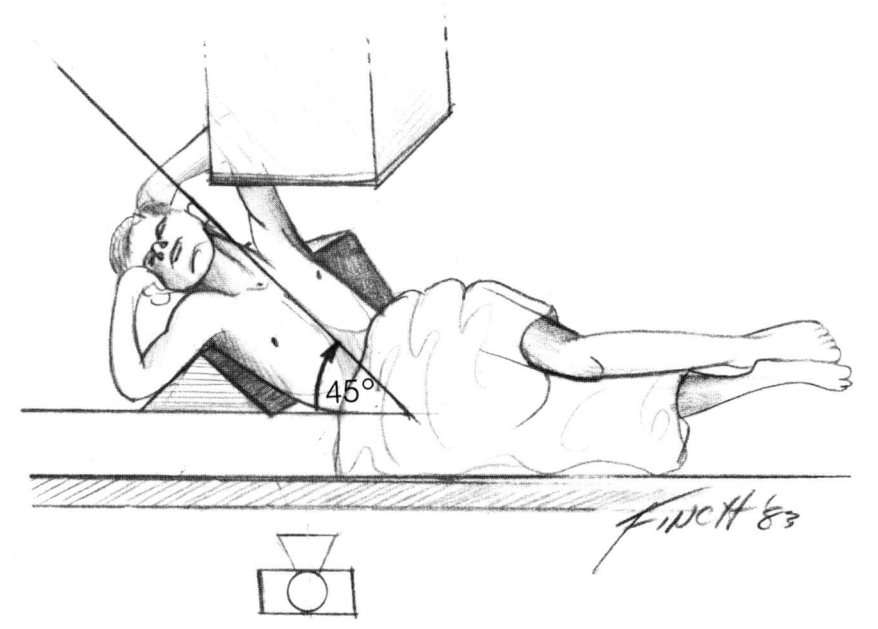

FIG 7–23.
Elimination of foreshortening of heart using the anteroposterior x-ray tube. With fixed biplane equipment, this system has the advantage over the lateral tube technique that geometric unsharpness is minimized because image intensifier can be brought closer to patient. A 45-degree right anterior oblique sitting up projection eliminates foreshortening of long axis of heart and results in 45-degree left anterior oblique projection on lateral plane. This view has been termed "hepatoclavicular," or "four-chamber view." Whether anteroposterior tube or lateral tube is used for demonstration of various cardiac defects depends on size and age of patient, and the anomaly to be demonstrated. With multidirectional equipment, this variable is eliminated.

ble with either multidirectional or fixed biplane equipment. In recent years pluridirectional equipment has largely replaced the fixed biplane arrangement. For both types of equipment, positioning is facilitated if one envisions that the image intensifier has eyes.

CINE FILM

Films used for cine radiography are standard black and white 35 mm with one emulsion and a base of either cellulose acetate or polyester (Mylar).[3] Polyester has an advantage in that the film does not break easily and can be transported with less trouble through cine cameras and projectors. In the case of malfunction, however, polyester films may damage the gear system of the camera.

For cine radiography, a medium-speed film should be selected, because high-speed films have larger silver halide crystals that create a granular image. This type of granularity, referred to as "film grain," is different from quantum mottle, which is unrelated to film quality.

A basic understanding of film characteristics is desirable, because it helps the angiographer judge cine film intelligently. The photographic properties of a cine film can be predicted from the characteristic or H & D (Hurter and Driffield, 1890) curve.[4] The properties of a film are determined by exposing a strip to a series of well-calibrated light sources of increasing intensity to produce a scale of densities (Fig 7–24); the necessary instrument is called a "sensitometer." The density values as measured by a densitometer are plotted against the logarithm of the relative exposure, and this creates the characteristic curve (Fig 7–25). These curves have a fairly long linear portion in the range of densities used in radiography. In the low- and the very high-density areas, the film is insensitive ("toe" and "shoulder" of the H & D curve).

From this curve, the two most important properties of the photographic emulsion, contrast and speed, can be determined so that various films can be compared. If the differences in contrast between various steps on the test strip increase rapidly, the film has "high contrast," and the characteristic curve is steeper (see film A in Fig 7–25). If the increase is less rapid (film B), the film has less contrast or more "latitude." If the angle of the linear portion of the curve is 45 degrees, the film neither enhances nor decreases contrast. All cine films enhance contrast and have an average gradient of more than 1. For good cine radiography, a medium-speed fine-grain latitude (low-contrast) film with an average gradient of 1.2 to 1.5 is most useful. If films with higher contrast are selected, information is lost because of overpenetration of cardiovascular structures.

Film speed also can be determined from the H & D curve. In Figure 7–25, film A not only is higher in con-

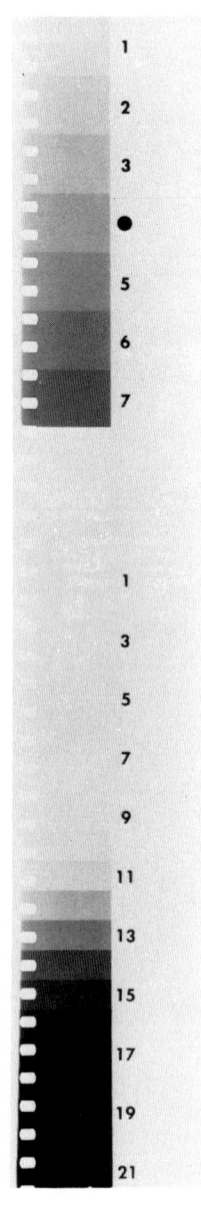

FIG 7–24.
Film strip exposed by a calibrated, accurately repeatable light source of a sensitometer.

trast than B but is more sensitive (has a higher speed) because it takes less exposure to produce the same density. The higher the film speed, the more the curve lies to the left.

Film resolution is relatively unimportant, because the resolving power of the emulsion exceeds by many times the resolving power of the cine system. Film transparency is important, however. Cine films are projected and enlarged for viewing, and the film is adequately illuminated by using high-powered lamps in the projectors. There are limits to the light output of projector lamps because of the difficulty of cooling of the high-power ones, particularly when the film is viewed in the still-frame mode. Conse-

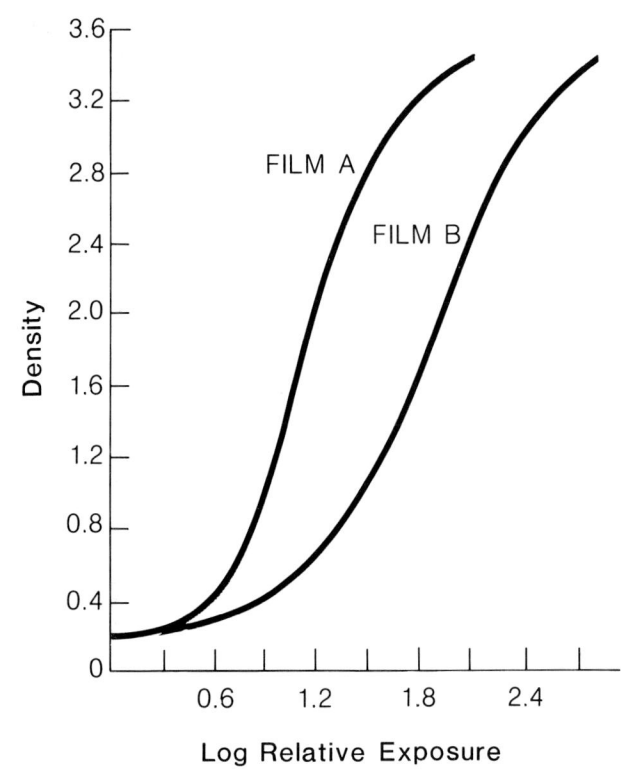

FIG 7–25.
Characteristic (H & D curve) of two different films. The curve of film A lies more to the left; therefore, film A is faster than B. Film A's curve is steeper; therefore film A has more contrast than B. Film B is a slower likely less grainy film that has more "latitude."

quently, it is undesirable for the film base itself to reduce the light output. The base, although of clear plastic, has a certain amount of opacity, or "base density." In addition, the developed-film emulsion (not exposed) produces a slight density called the "film fog." The total opacity of the unexposed but developed film is termed "base + fog" and should be as low as possible. A reading of base + fog should be recorded daily, because it may indicate premature aging, improper storage, or, sometimes, an error in film manufacturing. It is typically about 0.25 for blue base and 0.08 for clear base film.

The base fog on the film comes primarily from exposure to man-made radioactive rays, natural radioactivity, cosmic rays, chemical fumes, improper storage (high temperature, high humidity), and aging of the emulsion. Storage suggestions of film manufacturers and attention to expiration dates thus are important considerations in quality control.

Film Processing and Quality Control

An automatic processor is a critical link in the production of a good cine film, and it is unwise to save money by purchasing an inexpensive but unreliable model. The apparatus also must be installed properly and be supervised by trained technical personnel. X-ray technicians must be well trained in its use and must keep a meticulous record to ensure optimal quality control. The processor must be inspected and cleaned periodically (preventive maintenance) at the time the chemicals are changed.

The automatic processor carries out the basic functions of film processing, namely, development, rinsing, fixing, washing, and drying. The cine film is transported at a constant speed through the various solutions, which are kept at a constant temperature by a thermostatically controlled heating system. The chemicals are replenished automatically to preserve their original strength; this is accomplished by measuring the amount of film transported through the solutions and adjusting the amount of chemicals replaced by the replenishing pump.

The technical details of the apparatus may not be of interest to the angiographer, but a knowledge of the data recorded daily on the control chart is of paramount importance.

Quality Assurance for Automatic Film Processors

Each morning before processing cine angiograms, the technicians perform sensitometry and densitometry to assure proper processing. The film strip is exposed by a sensitometer to produce a density scale (see Fig 7–24). After the solutions have reached the proper temperature, the test strip is passed through the automatic processor, and the densities on the optical step wedge are measured with the densitometer. Although a characteristic curve could be constructed, this is time consuming; and for quality control, it is unnecessary. It is enough to measure the density of one of the intermediate steps (usually step 14), which roughly corresponds to film speed ("speed point"). The density difference of two other steps (usually steps 11 and 15) is also measured, representing contrast. In addition, the density of the unexposed filmstrip is measured, which represents base + fog. Finally, the developer temperature is recorded on a sensitometer control record chart.

This important chart is inspected daily. By connecting various points, trends can be discovered so corrections can be made before points fall outside the upper and lower permissible limits (Fig 7–26). Angiographers should be familiar with this record, because understanding it will facilitate trouble-shooting should cine image quality deteriorate.

CINE PROJECTORS

The projector is an important component of the entire cine process, because inadequate projectors project poor images. Several 35-mm projectors are commercially available, but each is limited in light output and therefore un-

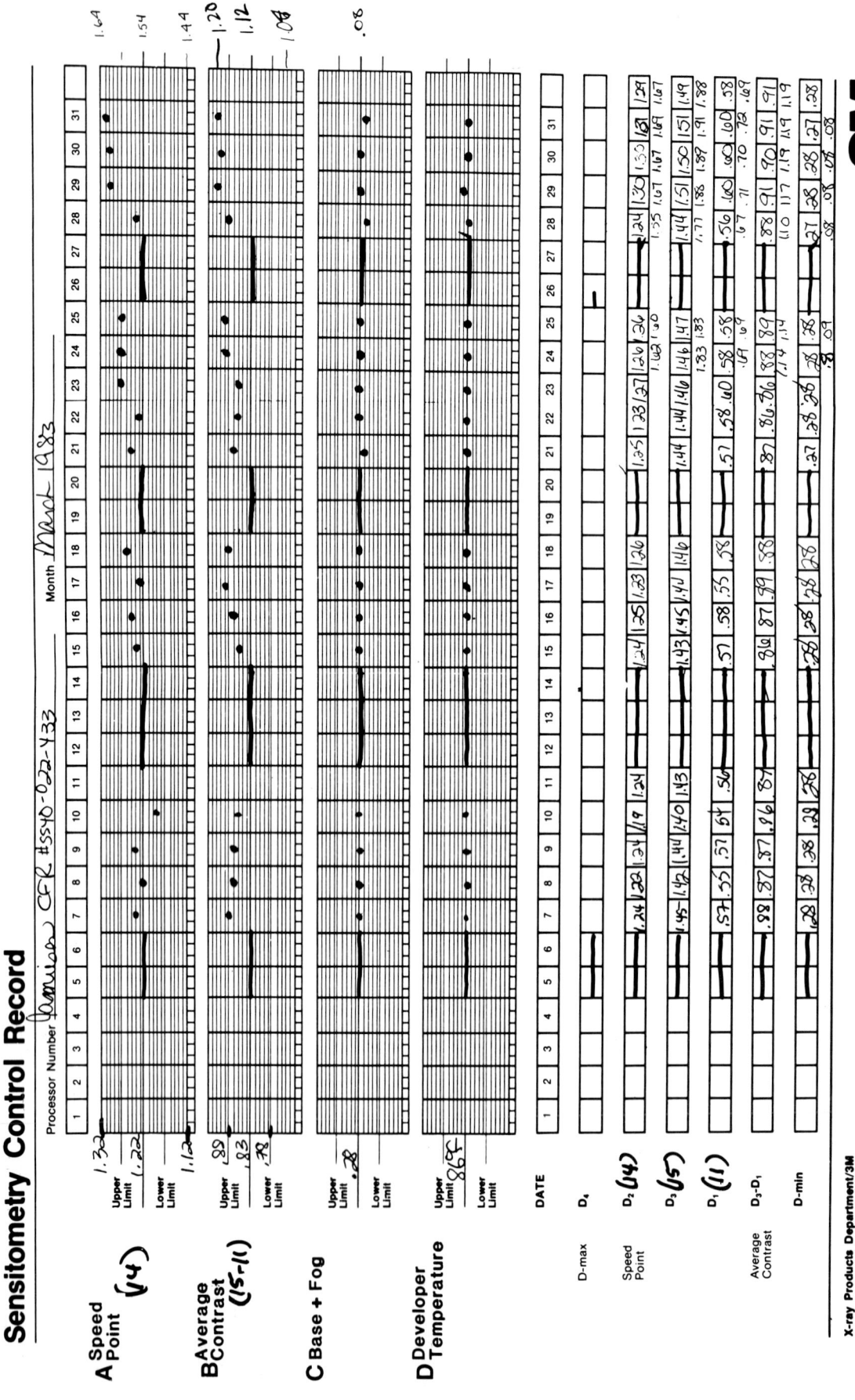

FIG 7–26.
Typical sensitometric control record of an automatic cine processor. **A**, "Speed point" density of step 14 of the sensitometric optical wedge. **B**, "average contrast"; Density difference between step 15 and step 11. **C**, base + fog: Density of developed unexposed portion of the test strip. **D**, "developer temperature". Note that on March 29 and 31, "speed points" and average contrast fall outside the upper permissible limit, indicating problems with the system.

satisfactory for use in a large auditorium. For projection in a large room, cine films should be reduced to 16 mm or a commercial 35-mm movie projector should be used.

Cine projectors transport film either intermittently, at fixed speeds identical to those of a cine camera, or continuously by using rotating prisms. The latter is particularly useful for everyday clinical work, because the projector speed can be varied continuously from single-frame to very fast. In addition, the film is loaded more quickly and easily than in a fixed-speed projector, although the optical sharpness and light output are less. The continuous transport also makes less noise than does the intermittent transport. Older projectors of the prism type have insufficient light output and should be replaced with newer models, which use a higher-wattage lamp. Cine projectors with intermittent film transport provide a slightly sharper image, have a higher light intensity, and so are preferable for use in conference rooms. However, they are somewhat more difficult to load and more likely to jam than are the continuous-transport projectors. Also, their cooling fans and film transport are fairly noisy.

Cine projectors should be inspected and cleaned periodically. The mirror and lens system of the projector become cloudy, particularly if the projector is operated in a smoky room, and this significantly decreases the light output and causes deterioration of the image.

TROUBLE-SHOOTING THE CINE SYSTEM

An understanding of the entire system of cine radiography is essential for effective trouble-shooting, although the angiographer does not need to be familiar with all the minor technical details. He or she should be able to pinpoint the defective link in the chain. After the main fault has been identified, specific checks and tests can be performed to pinpoint the problem. A well-trained staff of repair people and technicians specializing in the various components should be available.

Often, however, an inadequate cine image does not mean equipment failure but either operator error or a large patient. Cine films obtained from heavy patients are always relatively poor:

1. The automatic brightness control of the image intensifier asks for higher kV(p), which decreases contrast.

2. The high kV(p) level required for adequate penetration of the patient causes an increased amount of high-energy scatter, which is inadequately absorbed by the antiscatter grid. This increased amount of secondary radiation further decreases the contrast.

3. The system may not be able to deliver an adequate amount of radiation to penetrate the patient, which results in frank underexposure.

Differentiation of operator error from equipment malfunction is important, because searching for equipment malfunction can be time consuming and expensive. To review what was discussed earlier, the most important and common operator errors are as follows:

1. Improper positioning. If an excessive amount of lung is included in the radiographic image, the area of interest, usually the heart, will be under penetrated. REASON: The automatic brightness control in the image intensifier measures only *average* brightness. Because of the high radiolucency of the lungs, the brightness control automatically decreases the radiation, resulting in underexposure of the heart. The best results are obtained when a lead shield is used to exclude nearly all of the lung from the image.

2. Improper coning. If the shutters are wide open, an unnecessarily large field is exposed. Therefore, the amount of secondary radiation is increased and the contrast is consequently decreased.

3. Improper kV(p) setting. With some equipment, the automatic brightness control allows manual selection of a fixed kV(p). If the operator selects an excessively high kV(p), the mA automatically decreases, causing a grainy, noisy image. Furthermore, excessive high-energy scatter is produced, which decreases the contrast. The kV(p) level chosen should be appropriate for the patient's size.

4. Errors in observing warning signals. If the operator ignores or fails to see the warning signals indicating that the available amount of x-rays is inadequate to produce a good cine image, underpenetration results. This occurs more commonly with the multiple-mode image intensifiers, in which the 4.5- and 6-in. formats require much more radiation. REMEDY: use less magnification or less angulation or change to 30 fps.

5. Error in injection technique. Use of an inadequate amount of contrast medium or a slow delivery rate results in an inadequate angiogram.

6. Use of a large focal spot in infants when the small focus could have been used. The larger focal spot results in more geometric unsharpness, particularly with fixed biplane equipment in the lateral mode.

7. Improper panning. The most common error here is inclusion of too much lung, resulting in underexposure of the heart.

If various operator errors are excluded, the cine image should be carefully analyzed. Four major qualities of the image should be distinguished:

1. Definition. Basically, this is the sharpness of the image. Scientifically, it is expressed as "resolution," which is the ability to distinguish small structures individually. It is measured in line pairs per millimeter. Lack of resolution means a fuzzy image.

2. Contrast. This indicates the degree of difference between the light and dark areas of the film. Lack of contrast results in a grayish or a flat image.

3. Graininess. This denotes the amount of visible grain. Excessive graininess produces a noisy image; a "quiet" image is more pleasing and gives more detail.

4. Improper overall film density. The image can be either too dark or too light.

Unfortunately, most inexperienced angiographers cannot distinguish these qualities and consequently simply classify the image as poor, leaving all the analysis to the service person. The following tests will assist the angiographer in diagnosing an equipment problem.

1. Lack of definition or sharpness makes the image fuzzy. There are two tests to determine the source of a lack of definition:
   a. If the resolution is decreased, the projector must be excluded as a cause. This can be done by using another projector for the film, by review of a previous film known to have good resolution, or by checking the possibly faulty projector with an optical-resolution control strip. All newly purchased projectors should be checked with such a control strip, and those that do not have a uniform resolution should be rejected. Once the projector has been excluded as the cause, the problem will be known to lie with the image-intensifier-cine system.
   b. A careful study of the resolution bar pattern should always precede every cine recording. Of course, the angiographer has to know the resolution limit of the system in various magnification modes. If the resolution test shows unsharpness, the trouble lies in the focusing. Usually (90% of the time) the electronic focus is at fault rather than the optic. Refocusing must be done by an experienced service person, who will observe the image of a resolution test pattern on the output phosphor and make necessary electronic or optical adjustments.
2. The image lacks contrast. The most common cause of this problem is a large patient or an error by the operator, who has selected an unnecessarily high kV(p).

   If these two most common causes are excluded, the sensitometric control strip, particularly the density difference between two optical steps, should be checked. If these contrast measurements are incorrect, the automatic processor has to be serviced and cleaned and the developing solutions changed. If, on the other hand, the automatic developer is functioning properly, check whether the radiographic antiscatter grid is in place. Sometimes grids are removed and not replaced.

   If the entire system is found to operate properly and the cine images are still considered flat, a film with a higher average gradient should be selected.
3. The images are too grainy. The most common cause of noisy film is an excessively high kV(p) and a compensatorily low mA, which results in quantum mottle. This problem can also mean that the dose per cine frame is too low. Check to be certain the dose is as recommended, usually 16 to 20 μR/frame.

   Sometimes, graininess is caused by an excessively fast cine film. This problem can be eliminated by using a slower film, which has a less grainy emulsion.
4. The image is either too dark or too light. The most common cause is operator error, primarily improper positioning or coning. If operator error can be excluded, the sensitometric control chart should be reviewed to ensure that the film is being processed properly. Film storage conditions and expiration dates should also be checked.

   If operator error, film processing, and film characteristics are excluded, the problem may lie in an automatic brightness control that does not "track" properly; this is determined by phantom measurements. If the entire system checks out, proper adjustment should be made by repair people, who will close or open the iris of the cine camera to restore the proper film density.
5. Gradual deterioration of contrast and everything appears to be okay:
   a. A common cause of lack of contrast and light output is a low-wattage lamp or a dirty lens system in the projector, so cleaning the lenses and mirrors may dramatically improve contrast and brightness.
   b. The image tube is losing gain because of age. Ideally, it should not be older than 5 years, but the duration varies from one image tube to another.

REFERENCES

1. Lamel DA, Brown RD, Shaver JW, et al: *The correlated lecture laboratory series in diagnostic radiologic physics,* Washington, DC, Bureau of Radiological Health, Food and Drug Administration, US Public Health Service, Department of Health and Human Services. 1981.
2. Bargaron LM, Elliott LP, Soto B, et al: Axial cine angiography in congenital heart disease, *Circulation* 56:1075–1083, 1977.
3. *The fundamentals of radiology,* Rochester, NY, 1980, Health Sciences Markets Division, Eastman Kodak Co.
4. Hunter F, Driffield VC: *J Soc Chem Ind* 9:455, 1890.

CHAPTER 8

Angiography*

This chapter reviews cardiac catheters, contrast media, and power injectors. In addition, it provides practical hints on angiographic technique.

CARDIAC CATHETERS

Historical Background

Because catheterization of the genitourinary tract was known before the turn of the century, it is not surprising that catheterization of the vascular system was attempted as early as 1907. Two German scientists, Bleichröder[1] and Forssmann,[2,3] using self-experimentation, showed that passage of ureteral catheters into the vascular system was indeed feasible and harmless. Their purpose was to use intravascular catheters for therapy; neither investigator foresaw the impact of his discovery nor imagined that vascular catheterization would be used not only for therapy but also for diagnosis. Indeed, their classic publications suggest that both investigators had doubts about the practical value of their new technique.

Soon, numerous other investigators[4–8] catheterized the right side of the heart using Forssmann's technique and observed the heart and the pulmonary vascular tree after injection of contrast medium. Right-heart catheterization became an accepted procedure after Cournand and Ranges[9] described right atrial catheterization in humans. Those investigators punctured the antecubital vein with a no. 10 Lindeman needle and introduced a no. 8 flexible radiopaque ureteral catheter. Their modified ureteral catheter became known as the Cournand catheter and became the most widely used right-heart catheter. This woven catheter had a shellacked core covered with many x-ray-opaque plastic layers and had a single end hole.

The Cournand catheter was modified by Goodale et al.,[10] who added two side holes (bird's eyes) 2 mm from the catheter tip to facilitate simultaneous flushing of the end hole and side hole to prevent clotting. These authors also recommended soaking the catheters for 1 hour in heparin, the first attempt to apply heparin to catheters to render them nonthrombogenic.

In early selective angiocardiographic studies,[11] Cournand-type catheters and a manually operated injection syringe were used. In the United States, selective angiocardiography gained popularity slowly, because the simpler intravenous technique[12] obviated the introduction of a selective catheter. However, selective injection techniques yielded superior angiographic results, particularly if a power injector and special catheters were used. The forceful jet produced by Cournand catheters was studied in detail,[13] and it was concluded that catheter recoil and cardiac arrhythmias resulted. Therefore, the first catheter designed specifically for angiography had an occluded end and six side holes. The speed of the catheter jets was markedly decreased, because the cross-sectional area of the side holes was ten times that of the catheter. Furthermore, recoil was minimized, because the forces were directed at a right angle to the catheter tip; and because the side holes were arranged circumferentially around the tip, the jets tended to stabilize the catheter during the injection. The subsequently developed NIH catheter was identical except that the holes were round instead of oval. These two types of catheters were the most commonly used for selective angiocardiography.

In 1947, large-bore (12F–14F) catheters were introduced through the jugular vein into the right side of the heart for selective angiocardiography.[14] These catheters were made of rubber, and rapid injections were feasible. In 1949, the use of polyethylene for intravenous catheters was proposed.[15] This nonopaque tubing could be introduced into the venous system through large-bore needles and retained in place for several days for administration of drugs. Helmsworth et al.,[16] recognizing the disadvantages

---

*We are grateful for the diligent help of Mr. James Leslie, who performed the innumerable testing procedures on various catheters described in this chapter.

(namely, slow delivery rates) of woven catheters, also proposed using thin-walled, large-bore polyethylene tubing; Pierce et al.[17] used such tubing for percutaneous femoral aortography. The drawback of Pierce's technique was the need to insert large-bore needles, which was overcome by the Seldinger percutaneous catheterization technique involving a comparatively small needle and guidewire system.[18] Seldinger advocated the use of nonopaque virgin polyethylene tubing.

Percutaneous arterial and venous catheterizations rapidly gained popularity with the introduction of a radiopaque plastic catheter material.[19-23] This material was comparatively smooth and could be easily formed in boiling water, so for the first time, physicians were able to shape their own catheters to conform to the vascular anatomy.[23]

More recently, other plastics have been tried as catheter materials. Teflon is attractive because of its low frictional properties and high tensile strength, which allow high flow rates. Polyurethane is also excellent. For a short time, catheters were produced from polypropylene, but this plastic proved too rigid, so such catheters are no longer manufactured. Silastics are widely used in long-term indwelling catheters for administration of fluids, but because of the limpness of Silastic rubber and its high frictional coefficient, it has not been used for diagnostic catheters. However, Dotter and Straube,[24] realizing the advantage of the softness of Silastic tubing, introduced the concept of flow-guided catheterization, in which the catheter is carried by the bloodstream through the right side of the heart into the pulmonary artery for pressure recording. More recently, Swan et al.[25] have used this concept and improved it by adding a balloon to a limp polyvinyl catheter. The inflated balloon markedly improves the flotation of these flow-guided catheters.

Plastics

Because the characteristics of catheters are governed almost exclusively by the physical properties of the plastic, the angiographer should have a basic understanding of this subject.

Plastics are long-chain organic molecules formed by linkage of small molecules (monomers) by a process referred to as "polymerization." Therefore, plastics are commonly referred to as "polymers" or "resins," the latter term being used because they were originally developed to replace natural resins such as shellac or amber.

Plastics can be divided into two groups depending on their physical change on heating. If the material becomes soft, it is said to be a "thermoplastic." In contrast, thermosetting plastics, or "thermosets," do not soften in response to high temperatures. All materials used for the fabrication of cardiac catheters are thermoplastic and can therefore be deformed and shaped by heat. Deformation of the plastic molecules occurs gradually with heating, and consequently the physical characteristics of catheters at room temperature are not necessarily the same as those at 37°C. Therefore, all tests performed on plastic cardiac catheters should be carried out at body temperature to yield practical results.

Although considerable information is available about the mechanical characteristics of plastics, such data cannot necessarily be applied to catheters made from those plastics, because catheters contain additives such as colorants and radiopaque particles. Nevertheless, the mechanical performance of catheters is governed primarily by its construction and the physical characteristics of the plastic used.

Physical Characteristics of Plastics

Unlike simple molecules such as water, thermoplastics do not have a precise melting point; instead, the material softens gradually until the temperature is reached at which molecules flow freely under minimal stress. These *softening-range* temperatures can be used to give catheters specific shapes. On cooling, the molecules freeze in the new position, so the shape given to the plastic is largely retained.

If the curve of a catheter is straightened and the straightening stress is relieved, the tubing should resume its original shape. This important property is referred to as "plastic memory." With all plastics, however, a certain amount of molecular deformation occurs even at room temperature, referred to as "creep" or "cold flow." As this happens, the catheter loses its given shape. If a stretching stress is applied to most thermoplastic catheters, elongation occurs without recovery. If the plastic returns to its original length after stretching, it is said to be "rubbery" or an "elastomer."

Not all of the desired properties for a cardiac catheter, such as a high flow rate, good memory, high torque, and softness, can be achieved with a single type of fabrication and plastic material. Angiographic catheters are manufactured of particular materials for specific purposes. The few plastics of interest to the angiographer are polyolefins (polyethylene and polypropylene), fluorocarbons (Teflon), vinyls, urethanes, and polyamides (nylons).

Polyolefins.—Polyethylene, the most widely used polyolefin, is of historic interest because it was the material used by Seldinger[18] for his percutaneous catheterization technique. Because a stretch stress readily results in permanent elongation, polyethylene tubing can be tapered by pulling it down over a guidewire. Furthermore, various shapes can be easily given to this tubing by dipping it in boiling water or shaping it with steam. On cooling, shapes are retained that have a good plastic memory. Odman[20] made the nonopaque polyethylene catheters radiopaque by adding lead to the plastic, and these popular catheters are now commercially produced on a large scale.

Polyethylene has the general formula (CH_2) and is essentially a high molecular weight paraffin with excellent resistance to chemicals, including solvents. Polyethylene is a waxlike thermoplastic with a softening range of about 80°C to 120°C, depending on chain length. Depending on molecular structure, polyethylene can be produced as a low-, intermediate-, or high-density polymer. For the fabrication of catheters, the softer, low-density type is preferable. Polyethylene is semitransparent, with a low coefficient of friction. When used as a catheter material, it is usually mixed with a radiopaque substance and a dye to make it red, blue, gray, green or other colors. The ease of stretching, bending, perforating, and shaping has made the material ideal for the fabication of custom-made catheters.

The ability to change the shape of polyethylene or polyurethane catheters for specific angiographic needs is extremely important, because commercially supplied catheters sometimes fail to suit specific situations, such as catheterization of pulmonary artery branches of the truncus arteriosus, bronchial arteries, or a Blalock-Taussig anastomosis. Because the softening temperature of polyethylene is approximately 100°C, these catheters can be reshaped simply with steam from a kettle (Fig 8–1). When heated to 100°C, the curve of the catheter made of polyethylene or polyurethane deforms and thus can be reformed to a specific need. For better retention of the curve, manufacturers apply higher temperatures, as can be obtained by superheated steam, glycerin, or ethylene glycol (antifreeze).

Fluorocarbons.—Fluorine-containing plastics are known by various trade names such as Teflon, Fluon, and Tetraflon. One of these, polytetrafluoroethylene (Teflon), is widely used in industry.

The unique characteristics of this plastic are:

1. High softening point and heat resistance. These qualities make it difficult to shape Teflon, because a temperature of approximately 300°C is required. Therefore, to reshape one of these catheters, a heat gun is desirable. Because Teflon is stiffer than other plastics, vascular perforations are more common. Therefore, Teflon catheters must be manipulated with special care.

2. Very low coefficient of friction. This is desirable because it minimizes irritation of the blood vessels, eliminating spasm. Furthermore, passage of guidewires or Gianturco embolization coils through Teflon catheters is much easier than it is through polyethylene or polyurethane catheters.

3. Considerable cold flow or creep. This property, which causes the catheter to deform, is undesirable.

4. High tensile strength. This allows high injection pressures and high flow rates.

For fabrication of a catheter, Teflon is mixed with a radiopaque filler, usually metallic tungsten powder, and extruded as tubing.

Polyurethane.—Polyurethane plastics encompass a wide range of solid and foamed materials. In the production of catheters, the rubbery polyurethane elastomers are used. These compounds have good resilience, high tensile strength, and tear resistance. The latter property makes polyurethane a very safe catheter material, because breakage is unheard of, provided the catheters are used as recommended by the manufacturer. A low softening point makes it possible to shape these catheters in steam.

An important drawback is that polyurethane ages poorly, so catheters used after their recommended expiration date may break, particularly if they are reused. Another significant drawback of this material is its high coefficient of friction. However, Teflon-coated guidewires facilitate percutaneous introduction.

Other Plastics.—Nylon, because of its excellent mechanical properties, is still used as the inner lining of Rodriguez-Alvarez and NIH catheters. Like Teflon, nylon is relatively stiff, making it difficult to pass the catheter around corners. Therefore, care must be taken to avoid vascular perforations with catheters of either material. In

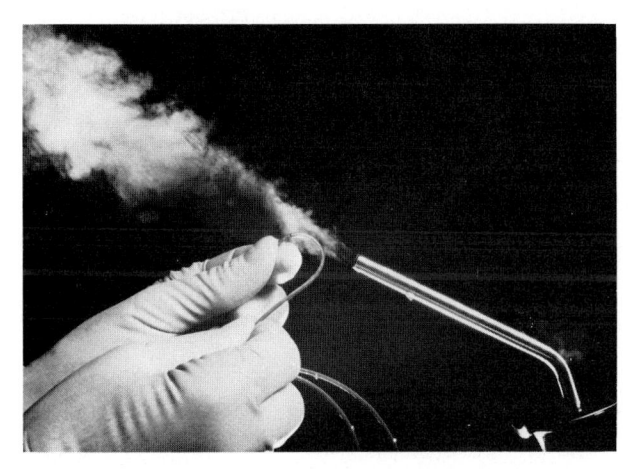

FIG 8–1.
A steam kettle is a simple device for customizing commercially available plastic catheters to meet a specific need. A tip can be given a new shape by holding it for 30 seconds in the stream of steam. This method is particularly valuable for cardiac and peripheral selective catheterization and should be available in every catheterization laboratory.

recent years relatively soft nylons were introduced as catheter materials. These catheters have excellent torque transmission and good memory. Vinyls are used primarily for floppy, flow-guided balloon catheters.

Methods for Making Catheters

Two technologies are used to manufacture catheters: a weaving (more accurately, braiding) and spraying process, and an extrusion process.

Woven Catheters

Woven catheters are widely used for cardiac catheterization. The manufacturing process is complex and largely proprietary to only one company in the United States. Basically, it is the old process used for ureteral catheters, an art originally developed in France. A seamless Dacron tube is woven over a steel mandrel by an ingeniously designed automatic machine, which braids the thread concentrically. (The same braiding technology is used for the manufacture of shoelaces and fire hoses.) By a special arrangement, it is possible to braid side holes directly into the seamless Dacron tube (Fig 8–2). This machine is called the "Maypole braider" and produces a seamless fabric tube; the name derives from the fact that the braiding process is identical to the pattern of ribbons made on a Maypole by dancing girls, a folk custom common in Europe, where this catheter-manufacturing technique was pioneered.

Dacron is braided into cardiac catheters primarily to achieve torque transmission. Because of the design, the torque is the same in both directions, a characteristic that cannot be obtained through a simple weaving process. When a braided catheter is rotated clockwise, the same number of fibers are stretched as when the catheter is rotated counterclockwise. However, the total torque transmitted by a woven cardiac catheter is poor, because the catheter softens markedly when introduced into the body. To overcome this problem, stainless steel wires are used in the braiding. Steel also improves the opacity of the catheter and increases the torque transmission.

The braided fabric core is soaked in a solution of natural resin and dried in an oven. The side holes are pinned with small nylon pins, the mandrel is removed, and the catheter undergoes repeated applications of polyurethane applied by spray guns, which distribute the polymer evenly around the catheter. Each coat is dried and heat cured. Seven to fifteen coats may be required to build the desired wall thickness. The polyurethane contains a radiopaque filler, finely dispersed metallic tin, and because no colors are added, all woven catheters manufactured by U.S. Catheter, Inc. have the dark gray color of the tin powder.

After the polyurethane has been completely cured, the catheters are ground to exact outside dimensions by a centerless grinder. After labeling of the catheter, a final smooth, clear polyurethane layer is applied. The catheters then undergo numerous inspections before they are finally released for sterilization and shipment.

The NIH angiographic and Rodriguez braided catheters are made in similar fashion. Instead of the steel mandrel, however, a permanent nylon tube is used, which gives this catheter increased stiffness and strength and a bursting pressure about 1,500 lb/in.^{2}

The availability of these torque catheters, which are produced in polyurethane and polyethylene under various names, has greatly facilitated selective coronary and peripheral angiography. They are also useful for cardiac angiography in some cases, and therefore the angiographer must be familiar with them.

Extruded Catheters

Several thermoplastics, such as polyethylene, polyurethane, and Teflon, lend themselves readily to a much simpler extrusion process, an industrial technology widely used to manufacture plastic tubing. Plastic pellets are mixed thoroughly with a dye to give the catheter a red, blue, yellow, or other color and with a radiopaque filler such as metallic tin, metallic tungsten (for Teflon cathe-

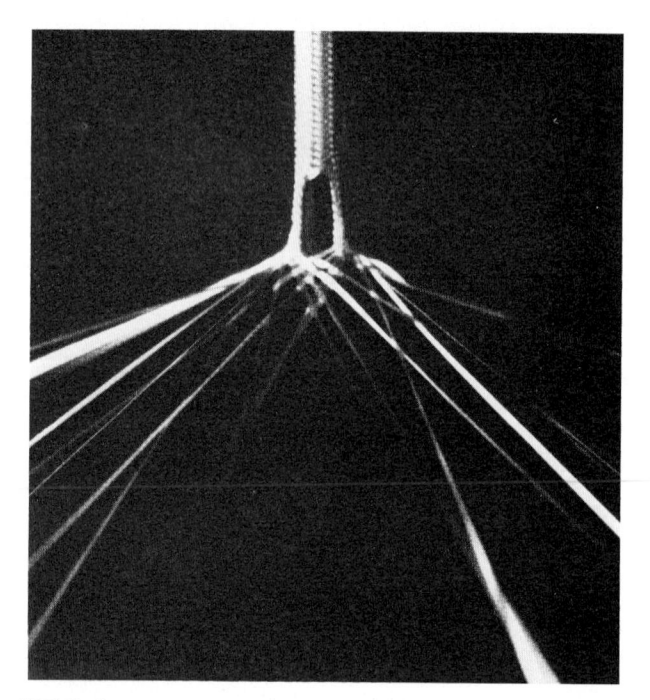

FIG 8–2.
Closeup view of the braiding process of the inner core of a woven catheter. An oval side hole is being formed in the seamless Dacron tube.

ters), bismuth subcarbonate (used mostly for polyurethane catheters), metallic lead, mercuric sulfide, lead oxide, or barium sulfate (commonly used for polyethylene catheters). The plastic pellets containing dye and radiopaque filler are then placed in the hopper of an extruder (Fig 8–3), and a screw transports the mixture through a heating chamber toward the nozzle. At the nozzle of the extruder, a heated die with a center core gives the extrusion its final shape and smooth surface. Extrusions over a plastic or metallic mandrel ensures a constant, precise internal lumen in the tubing.

In the extrusion process for a woven torque catheter, the thin-walled inner catheter tubing is extruded first. Over this tubing, stainless steel wire is braided, as in the production of woven Dacron catheters. Another plastic sleeve is then extruded over this wire mesh so that the catheter shaft contains woven wire inside plastic (Fig 8–4). To this wire-reinforced catheter shaft, a nonbraided catheter tip is welded; side holes can be punched only into this tip. Torque catheters thus have a thicker wall and consequently a decreased flow rate, which is important if hand injections are used. Recently, "high-flow" versions of torque catheters have been introduced that have better flow rates but poorer torque characteristics.

The Soft Tip Catheter

The soft tip catheter is a concept introduced by Dr. Robert Van Tassel, the rationale being stiff catheters may lift off plaques that can result in dissections. In selective, particularly coronary, angiography, torqueability is of paramount importance. Because torque transmission and stiffness are intimately related, selective catheters have to be

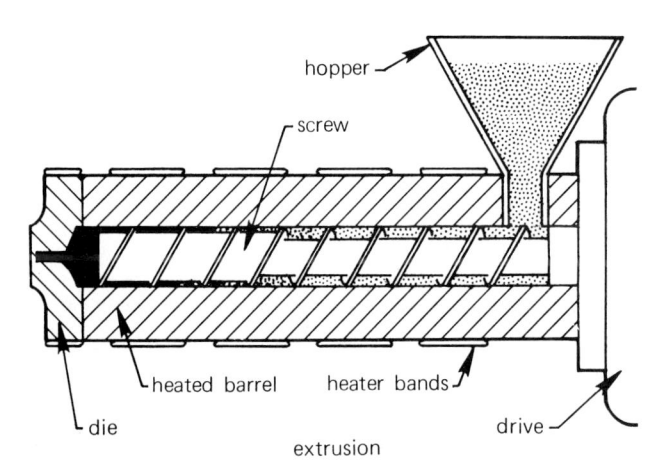

FIG 8–3.
Screw-type extruder used in the manufacture of polyethylene and polyurethane catheters. Hopper contains plastic pellets, dye, and radiopaque filler. The screw, driven by a motor, transports the pellets toward the heated die; during transport, pellets are mixed and heated to the melting point for extrusion.

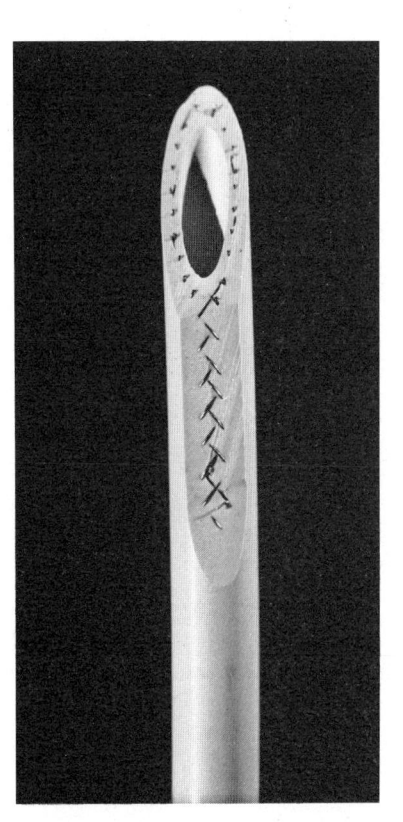

FIG 8–4.
Closeup of wire-reinforced torque catheter; braided-wire mesh is embedded in its wall.

relatively stiff. By attaching a soft tip to a conventional catheter, torqueability remains preserved and intimal damage can be minimized. This is accomplished by so-called insert molding. The catheter shaft is placed over a mandril in the mold, and a soft plastic is injected at the tip and melted together with the shaft.

Catheter Surface

A smooth outer catheter surface is desirable because it decreases friction. Whether it also is important for thrombogenicity is unknown but likely, even though the intima of an artery is not smooth.

Scanning electron microscopic examination of surfaces of catheters from various manufacturers showed wide variation in surface roughness (Fig 8–5). Catheters with a surface coating of polyurethane were the smoothest.

Mechanical Properties of Catheters

The mechanical properties of its plastic material largely determine the handling characteristics of a catheter. Depending on its purpose, a catheter must have a certain stiffness, being neither too stiff nor too flaccid. For example, during selective catheterization, it must be possible to pass the catheter tip into a specific site by manipulating the

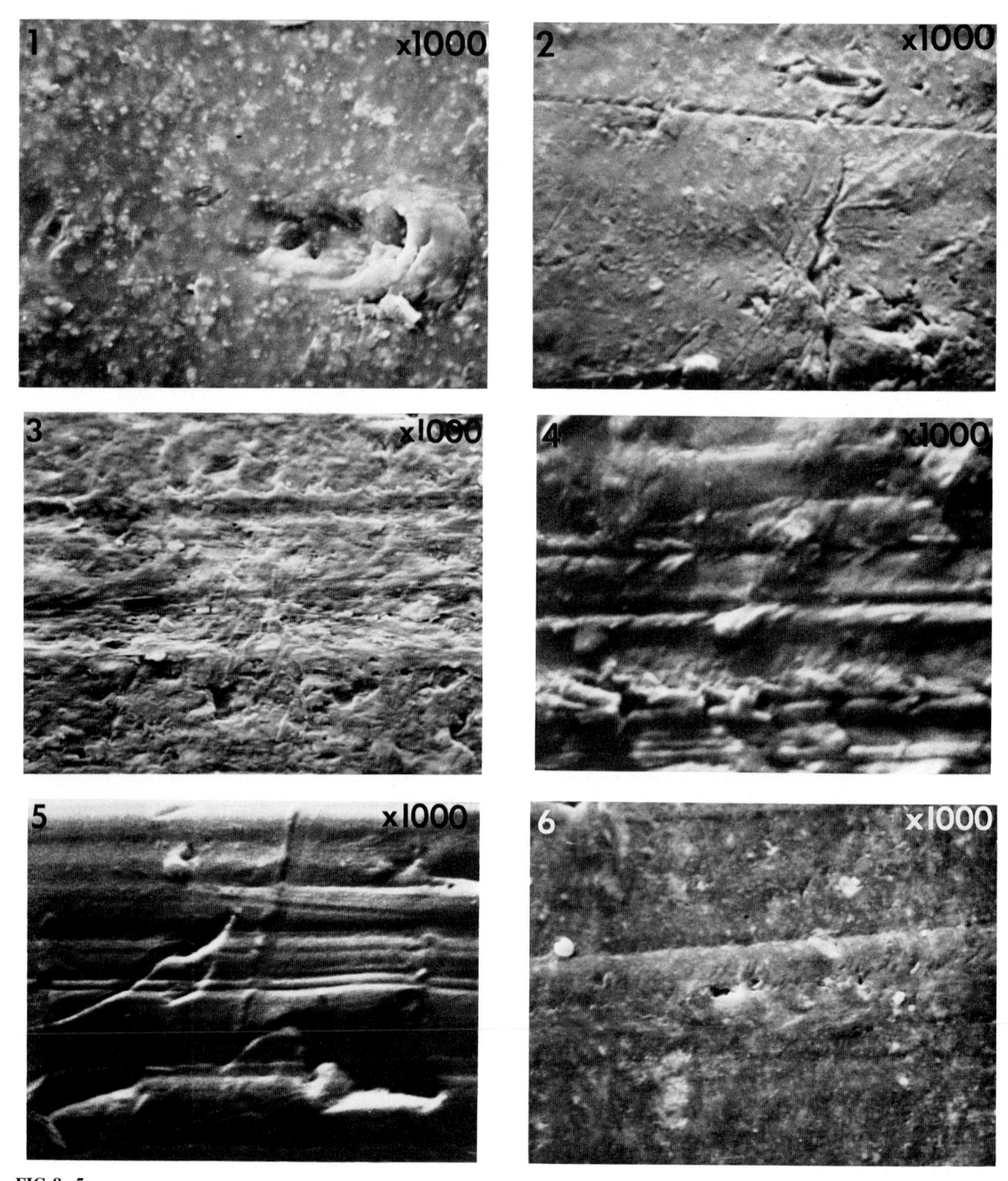

FIG 8–5.
Catheter surfaces examined by scanning electron microscopy. **1–4,** polyethylene catheters from various manufacturers. **5,** extruded Teflon catheter. **6,** polyurethane catheter.
(Continued.)

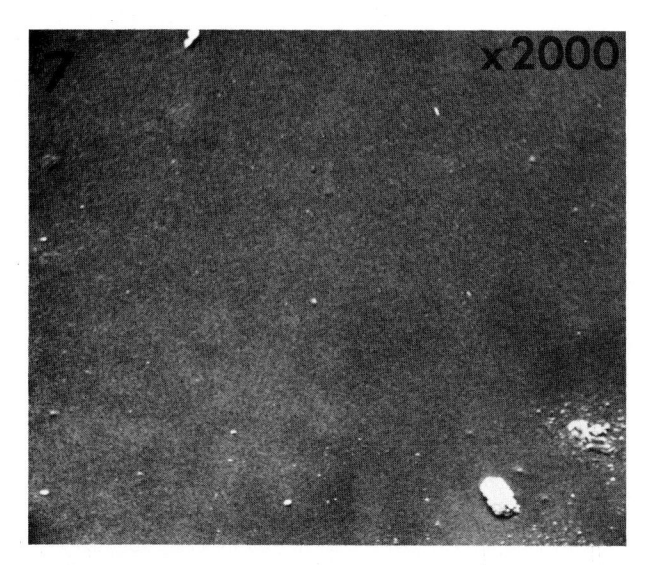

FIG 8–5 (cont.).
7, polyurethane-coated catheter is smooth even at magnification × 2,000.

catheter shaft by axial rotation and to-and-fro motion from an entry point outside the body and as much as 100 cm away from the tip. The mechanical properties of a catheter also depend on the manufacturing process, such as extrusion or weaving, and on the additives, such as radiopaque materials, pigments, and surfactants.

Plastics do not follow the simple behavior patterns of materials such as metals, which obey Hooke's law of elasticity. Rather, under stress, plastics deform in a fashion simultaneously to that of a viscous fluid and an elastic body (viscoelasticity). Consequently, when a catheter is subjected to a force, the deformation that results depends not only on the type of plastic but also on the temperature and on the duration of the stress. This viscoelastic property can be used advantageously during cardiac catheterization to give the tip a different shape while it is in the body. For instance, the catheter can be remolded in the right atrium by curving it against the lateral atrial wall and holding it there for a time.

In practice, certain catheters are said to have good memory, good torque control, or adequate stiffness. Bioengineers can test the stress-strain relations under conditions relevant to angiography.

Plastic Memory

Tests were performed in our laboratory to compare the plastic memory of several commercially available catheters under conditions simulating a clinical catheterization procedure. Test samples were prepared from 8F catheter material, and two samples of each material were preshaped by placing them in a glass tube formed into a coil 3.5 cm in diameter and then heating them to a temperature that allowed plastic deformation. For example, polyethylene and polyurethane samples were placed in boiling water for 5 minutes, whereas Teflon samples were baked in an oven at 200°C for 15 minutes and woven Dacron catheters were baked for 15 minutes at 150°C. After cooling, one of the samples from each pair was stressed by placing it in a straight glass tube and immersing it in a 37°C water bath for 5 minutes. The sample was then removed from the tube, allowed to resume its original shape, and photographed to compare with its unstressed mate (Fig 8–6).

Woven Dacron angiographic catheters retained their curvature best, whereas Teflon showed the poorest plastic memory. Four polyethylene samples from different manufacturers and one sample of polyurethane retained their shape nearly as well as did woven Dacron. There appeared to be no difference between the plastic memories of polyethylene and polyurethane, both being very good.

Torque

If the catheter shaft is rotated during cardiac catheterization, the rotational movement should be transmitted to the tip. Therefore, catheters with good torque characteristics are preferred. The extent of torque control depends largely on the catheter material, the length, and the stiffness: The stiffer the catheter, the better it transmits torque. Therefore, torque also depends on wall thickness, meaning that high-flow catheters, by necessity, have less torque transmission. These facts show why, in clinical practice, knowledge of catheter construction is useful.

We developed a simple apparatus that allows us to measure the torque characteristics of commercially available catheters. In our studies, an exactly measured torque was applied to catheters of identical length, and the twisting force was measured. The results show that nonreinforced catheters of polyethylene, Teflon, and polyurethane have similar torque characteristics, with the exception of polyethylene C, a high-density plastic with greater stiffness (Fig 8–7). The torque transmission of a woven Dacron catheter, particularly a wire-reinforced catheter, is considerably greater, largely because of the increased stiffness imparted by the nylon core.

During angiography, catheters with poor torque transmission must be "overtorqued," which is usually accomplished using a two-handed technique, one hand torquing the catheter shaft while the other fixes the rotated shaft at the skin entry site. Several 360-degree rotations of the shaft may be required to transmit the rotation to the catheter tip. With wire-reinforced catheters, however, overtorquing is neither necessary nor desirable, because the rotation of the catheter shaft is transmitted directly to the tip. Thus, overtorqued catheters will suddenly jump or whip.

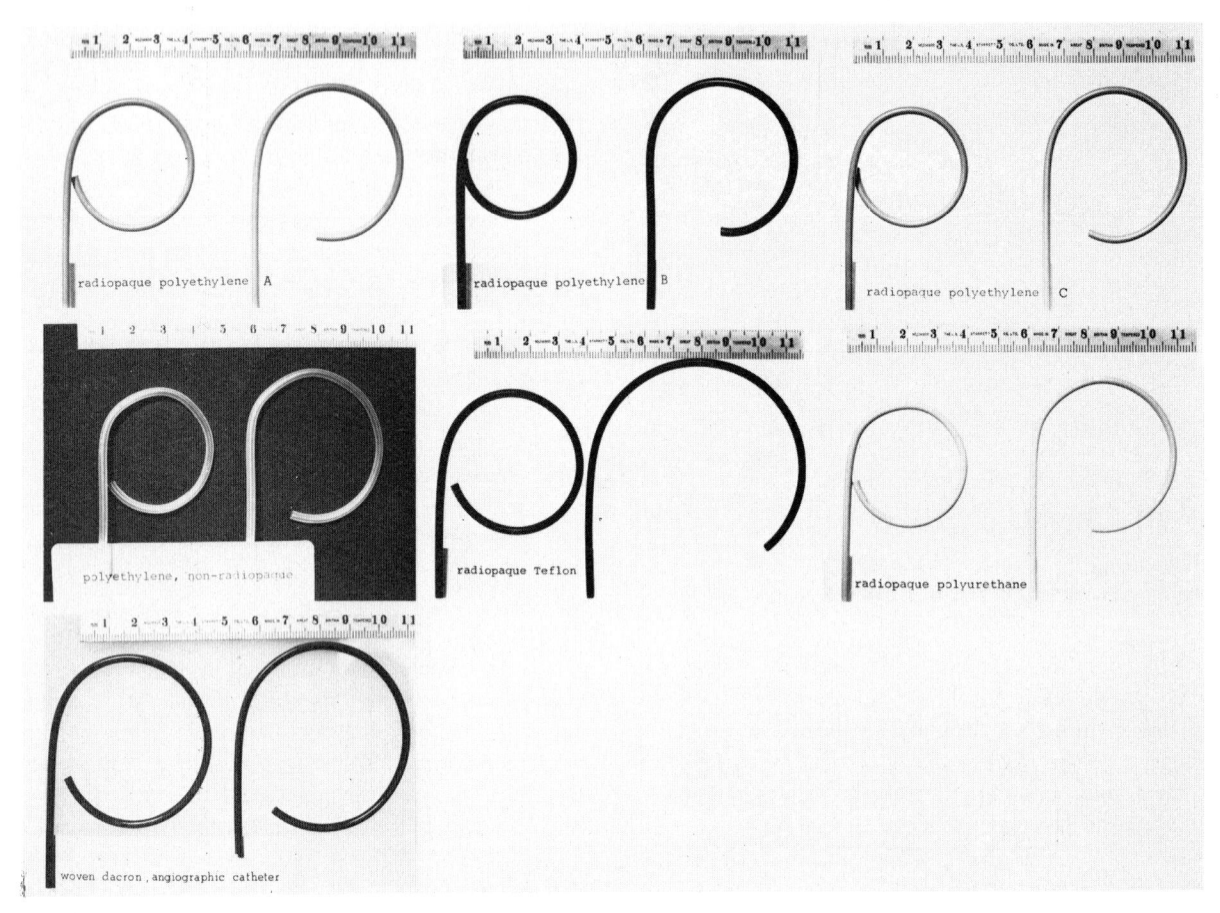

FIG 8–6.
Results of plastic memory tests. In each pair, the catheter on the left shows the preformed curvature; the catheter on the right is the same catheter after straightening procedure. Radiopaque Teflon has the poorest memory. The memory of polyethylene and polyurethane is better and similar.

The rotational motion of the catheter shaft should be combined with to-and-fro motion because:

1. The torque is transmitted better through the skin and subcutaneous tissue to the shaft.
2. The catheter tip is almost never free, usually being braced against either a cardiac or a vascular wall. By imparting a to-and-fro motion simultaneously with the rotational movement, the operator reduces the breakaway friction and therefore minimizes catheter whipping.
3. To-and-fro motion increases the likelihood of passing the catheter tip into the desired anatomic site.

Consequently, the tip of the catheter being manipulated by an experienced angiographer appears to be in constant motion. In contrast, the novice attempts to steer and rotate catheters without moving them, a much less effective maneuver.

Flow Dynamics

The rate of flow of contrast agents through a cardiac catheter is influenced by the injection pressure; the inside diameter of the catheter; catheter length; smoothness of the bore; the number, size, and arrangement of side holes; and the viscosity and density of the contrast medium. Catheter length and diameter are constrained by patient size, whereas all other factors are variable.

The relation between pressure and flow rate for a given catheter and contrast agent must be understood. If a pressure-calibrated injector is used, the angiographer must determine the pressure required to deliver the desired flow rate. If a flow-controlled injector is used, the pressure-flow relations need not be calculated, but the angiographer must know the maximum flow rates tolerated by the catheter. For angiocardiographic catheters, maximum pressures of 1,500 lb/in.^{2} can be used, whereas the bursting pressure of a balloon catheter is much lower. The latter can be determined experimentally as follows. The catheter is

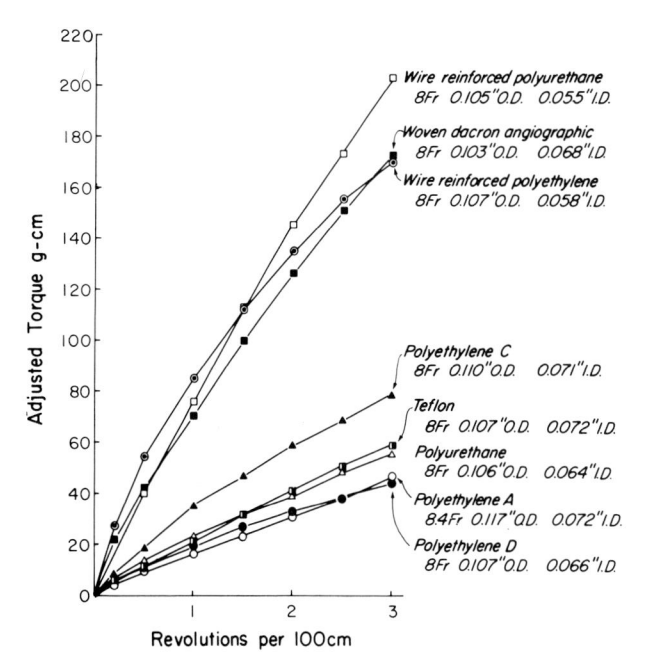

FIG 8–7.
Results of torque transmission studies of commercial catheters; the best torque transmission is achieved with wire-reinforced catheters.

connected to a power syringe loaded with contrast medium, which is injected at increasingly higher flow rates until the catheter bursts. Clinically, a flow rate of 80% to 90% of the bursting rate should not be exceeded, because the variations between catheters mean that some will be more liable to bursting than others. The bursting flow rates also differ for contrast medium with different viscosities.

Pressure drops in a catheter at the inlet, along the length, and at the outlet, and the extent of pressure loss can be calculated for each portion of the catheter. The exact relations between pressure, flow rate, and other factors differ depending on whether the flow is laminar, turbulent, or transitional. Engineers use a dimensionless number, called Reynold's number, to predict whether flow will be laminar or turbulent:

$$N_R = \frac{\rho D \overline{V}}{\eta}$$

where N_R = Reynold's number,

D = inside diameter of catheter,
$\overline{V}$ = mean fluid velocity,
ρ = fluid density, and
η = fluid dynamic viscosity.

If Reynold's number is less than 2,000, laminar flow is expected, whereas when Reynold's number exceeds 3,500, flow is usually turbulent. For intermediate values, flow may be turbulent or laminar or fluctuate between the two (unstable flow).

Under conditions of laminar flow, Poiseuille's law is applicable:

$$Q = \frac{\pi r^4}{8\eta}\Delta P$$

where

Q = flow rate,
L = catheter length (cm),
η = viscosity factor,
r = radius of the catheter, and
ΔP = injector syringe pressure minus patient's intravascular pressure (dynes/cm^2).
(The patient's intravascular pressure usually is negligible compared with the mechanical power of injectors.[26])

Therefore, flow rate through a catheter is inversely related to both catheter length and the fourth power of its radius. Accordingly, torque wire-reinforced catheters, which have slightly thicker walls, offer more resistance to flow and are not useful if high-speed injections are required.

The effects at the ends of the catheter have been neglected in these calculations, and Fischer et al. showed that experimentally neither Poiseuille's law nor the Blasius equation accurately predicts experimental pressure-flow relations.[27] An algorithm for a computer program, which uses Poiseuille's law, a jet equation to account for a tapered tip, and a side hole equation, has been reported by Bove and Gimenez,[28] who found excellent correlation with experimental data. Also, Williamson[29] empirically derived his own equation to determine injection times. Any of these equations is accurate for clinical use, provided it is applied appropriately. For example, Poiseuille's law should be applied only if the calculated Reynold's number is less than 2,000. Side holes and tapered tips must be taken into consideration. All of these calculations are approximations and are no longer needed with flow controlled injectors, which compensate automatically for the various resistance factors.

Side holes are added to catheters for five reasons: (1) to improve mixing of contrast medium and blood; (2) to decrease catheter resistance, thereby increasing the flow rates; (3) to reduce jet velocities; (4) to stabilize the catheter; and (5) to minimize catheter recoil. Studies of multihole catheters showed several significant phenomena.[30]

First, the angle between the axis of the side holes and the axis of the catheter has little effect on the rate of delivery. Second, a distance of 1 to 10 side-hole diameters between the holes has no significant effect on contrast flow. Finally, up to a point, flow rates increase with the number and diameter of side holes, but the addition of more than three side holes does not augment flow rates.

Susman and Diboll[30] applied Bernoulli's equation to data on catheter tips to predict the proportional yield of contrast from side and end holes of various diameters. In their experiments, they drilled three side holes in both tapered and occluded-tip catheters. For holes of equal size, they predicted and confirmed experimentally that each successive side hole toward the catheter tip emitted a larger quantity of contrast medium than did the next most proximal hole, the end hole emitting the greatest quantity of all. This surprising phenomenon can be explained by Bernoulli's law of conservation of energy. With closely spaced side holes, the frictional energy loss between holes may be neglected. Energy conservation requires that any change in kinetic energy (speed) must be replaced by an appropriate change in pressure energy. The linear velocity distal to the first side hole is lower than the proximal velocity, because some of the fluid escapes through the hole. Similarly, there is a further decrease of velocity beyond each subsequent side hole. Bernoulli's law requires that the decrease in velocity be compensated for by an increase in hydrostatic pressure, and this is true for both tapered tip and end-occluded catheters. Consequently, there is a gradual increase in lateral pressure from side hole to the next side hole, so each successive hole emits more fluid.

Of course, the amount of fluid emitted also depends on the size of the side holes, a limiting factor because large side holes weaken the catheter. Oval-shaped side holes can yield the largest cross-sectional area with minimal catheter weakening, and if slits are used instead of side holes, the catheter is weakened to a lesser degree.

Whereas the three large side holes permit maximum total flow, the jet velocity is decreased by additional holes, which is desirable, because high-velocity jets induce cardiac arrhythmias.[13] Recoil forces are decreased by reducing the jet pressure from the end hole, and the radial forces are balanced by arranging the side holes in a symmetric fashion. Side holes can be arranged either opposite each other or in a spiral fashion.

High-pressure injections cause cavitation, and the production of gas bubbles in regions of low pressure. That is, if the catheter jet velocity is high enough to reduce the pressure below the vapor pressure of water, vapor bubbles will form (cavitation). This phenomenon is transient and consequently does not present a clinical problem. In dogs, ultrasonic techniques have been used to prove that cavitation occurs with the injection techniques commonly used clinically.[31]

Catheter rupture is another hazard of high-pressure angiography and occurs with injection pressures or flow rates exceeding the manufacturer's recommended limit.[32] We tested several commercial catheters to determine the sites of rupture. In catheters of nonreinforced plastic and uniform cross section, the rupture consistently occurred within 2 cm of the hub, because the pressure within the catheter decreases linearly toward its tip. Rupture at this location poses little risk, because it occurs outside the patient. If, however, the catheter has a greater wall thickness toward its hub or is wire reinforced, rupture may occur near the tip, inside the patient. Indeed, LePage et al.[32] found that several different wire-reinforced torque catheters consistently rupture near the tip when excessive injection pressures are used. End-occluded angiographic catheters can safely withstand a pressure of 1,500 lb/in.^{2}, whereas nonreinforced polyethylene, vinyl, and woven Dacron catheters rupture at much lower injection pressures. Only nonreinforced Teflon and nylon tubing can withstand high injection pressure. Clearly, the manufacturer's instructions regarding the handling, sterilization, and choice of injection pressures must be followed for each catheter.

Catheter Thrombogenicity

Minor and major complications related to thrombogenicity may follow catheterization. Thrombosis or embolization into catheterized arteries may result in renal, cerebral, or myocardial infarction; fortunately, these emboli are small and subclinical. For many years, embolic complications were believed to result primarily from dislodgement of atherosclerotic plaques, but it now is clear that they are much more often the result of clots.

Nejad et al.[33] showed that fibrin is deposited on the outside of cardiac catheters. In a well-controlled experiment in dogs, these investigators demonstrated fibrin deposits on indwelling plastic catheters of all types and postulated that some embolic complications of catheterization procedures may be caused by the stripping off of thrombi formed on the outside of plastic catheters.[33] The formation of such fibrin deposits has been proved unequivocally in numerous other animal experiments.[31-40] During routine angiography, thrombi are commonly seen on catheters and may become dislodged and embolize. The distribution of such emboli is governed by the distribution of blood flow to various organs. Fortunately, the arteries to the brain have less blood flow than the thoracic aorta; consequently, these small emboli are usually asymptomatic, and strokes are a rather rare complication of catheterization. Because of the potential hazard of embolization, some investigators heparinize patients undergoing cardiac catheterization, but we have not found this necessary.

Thrombi also form on the outside of catheters during human arterial catheterization, as shown by pullout angiography.[41] By this rather insensitive radiographic technique, thrombi could be seen on the outside of the cardiac catheters in 50% of the cases. There was a direct relation between the incidence of thrombi and the duration of catheterization. On removal of an arterial catheter, the fibrin thrombi remain either attached to the arterial wall at the puncture site or embolized into smaller peripheral arterial branches. Very rarely, occlusion of a large vessel, such as the popliteal artery, will occur after the catheter has been removed. In most cases these peripheral embolizations are subclinical.

Because of the clinical importance of thromboembolism during arterial catheterization, an extensive research program was started to develop truly nonthrombogenic surfaces. Much knowledge has accumulated on this subject, but to date no such plastic has been developed. However, thromboembolism can be effectively prevented during cardiac catheterization by systemic anticoagulant therapy or local heparinization of catheters.[42, 43]

Factors Determining Thrombus Formation

Several physical properties of catheters are suspected of increasing thrombogenesis:

1. Catheter material. A systematic evaluation of the relation between catheter material and thrombogenesis was carried out.[36, 37, 40] Teflon was found slightly less thrombogenic in dogs, a finding that contradicts the results of the guidewire studies performed in dogs and humans.[39] All plastic catheters now in use are thrombogenic, although there maybe slight variations in degree.

2. Surface characteristics. Roughness promotes platelet adhesion and thrombosis, so rough catheters may be more thrombogenic than smooth ones. Because of the incorporation of radiopaque materials and the extrusion process, all catheter surfaces are comparatively rough unless they have been coated with clear polyurethane or polyethylene. Whether this coating indeed decreases thrombogenicity has not been determined and may be considered unlikely.

3. Wetability. Nonwetability prolongs the Lee-White clotting time in vitro,[44] apparently because of a delayed thrombocyte action, so it was reasonable to postulate a similar mechanism in vivo. In our laboratory, we applied various vegetable and animal waxes to catheters to increase the nonwetability. Although very hydrophobic and highly polished, the waxes showed no significant effect on thrombogenicity. An animal study was conducted in vivo, applying silicone to stainless-steel guidewires, Teflonized guidewires, and polyethylene catheters, rendering the surface extremely hydrophobic,[36, 37] yet no protection against thrombus formation could be achieved. Apparently, hydrophobic characteristics do not play an important role. Furthermore, all catheter surfaces are inherently hydrophobic yet are uniformly thrombogenic.[17, 36]

4. Surface charge. Because the intima has a negative charge and heparin is strongly electronegative, one might expect that a negative surface charge is important in the prevention of thromboembolism. Also, the extensive work of Sawyer et al.[45-47] emphasized the potential difference across vessel walls and the patency of metallic arterial grafts as a result of a negative charge. Surface charge may be important, but it is not the only crucial factor in thrombogenicity: Even through most plastics and glass have negative surface charges, they are highly thrombogenic.

5. Atherosclerosis. After catheterization, atherosclerosis plays a minor role in arterial thrombosis, provided the lumen of the artery remains large. However, if the diameter of the artery is narrowed by atherosclerotic deposits, the incidence of thrombosis may increase. Furthermore, some of the complications of catheterization may not be the result of fibrin deposits but the result of mechanical depression of an atherosclerotic plaque or subintimal passage of catheters. Whenever blood flow persists around an intra-arterial catheter, postcatheterization thrombosis is rare; but if there is neither flow nor a distal pulse, the incidence of thrombosis is higher (about 0.5%). The incidence of this complication increases with the use of larger catheters and with vascular spasm, particularly in individuals with smaller arteries and in infants.

6. Variation in blood coagulability. This factor is probably important but usually is unknown before catheterization.

In summary, the question of thrombogenicity is complex, because no single factor is responsible for this complication during arterial catheterization. Nevertheless, such complications are preventable in most cases.

Prevention of Thromboembolism

The simplest and most effective protection against thromboembolism is skill in catheter manipulation, which shortens the procedure. Most catheterization procedures, particularly coronary angiography, can be carried out in less than 10 to 15 minutes, which probably is too short a time for formation of clinically significant thrombi.

Systemic or local anticoagulants can be used to minimize thrombus formation. Systemic anticoagulation is commonly used during coronary and cerebral angiography.

168 *General Introduction*

A disadvantage is the risk of bleeding complications such as cardiac tamponade or retroperitoneal hematoma from inadvertent perforation of the cardiovascular system. However, although cardiac perforation as a result of catheterization is fairly commonly observed at postmortem examination, cardiac tamponade is rare in nonheparinized patients.

Another approach to the prevention of thromboembolism is the use of heparinoids such as low molecular weight dextran (Rheomacrodex Dextran 40, Pharmacia Laboratory, Piscataway, N.J.) This artificial plasma expander delays platelet aggregation and increases the LD_{50} of contrast media.[48–53] However, animal experiments with low molecular dextran in our laboratory showed no significant decrease in thrombus formation on the outside of catheters.[42]

Another attractive and simple approach is the use of acetylsalicylic acid and dipyridamole (Persantin), both of which reduce platelet adhesiveness. These drugs are used clinically to prevent thromboembolism in patients with artificial cardiac valves.[54–56] Their usefulness in arterial catheterization has not yet been documented, but our unpublished animal studies demonstrate that these drugs may slightly reduce the size of the thrombi.

Testing for Catheter Thrombogenicity

A reliable simple test for catheter thrombogenicity is needed. The test should expose the catheter to arterial blood flow in vivo under conditions similar to those of a catheterization procedure. Also, formed thrombi should be retrievable without sacrificing the animal.

Because thrombi do not adhere strongly to a slippery catheter surface, we designed a thrombus-retrieval system to collect fibrin deposits. A 5F catheter is inserted percutaneously into the femoral artery of a dog and advanced until the tip just reaches the aorta bifurcation. The catheter is flushed with saline solution and closed with a stopcock. A second catheter may then be introduced into the contralateral femoral artery for simultaneous comparative testing. Fluoroscopy is used to ensure that the catheters do not extend into the aorta, where they could touch each other. After a suitable period, usually 1 hour, the retrieval system is introduced (Fig 8–8). A Teflon dilator is advanced over the test catheter into the artery and followed by a second dilator to which a polyvinyl tubing is attached. The second dilator is sufficiently large to occlude the femoral artery completely, assuring collection of all thrombi.

The test catheter is rapidly removed through a side hole (A in Fig. 8–8) in the polyvinyl tubing, and the blood is allowed to spurt for a moment into an attached filter (B) from a blood infusion set. The thrombus is rinsed and either traded by size on a scale ranging from a trace to 4 (Fig 8–9) or weighed. The test has the following advantages over other thrombogenicity tests:

1. The catheter is introduced percutaneously and thus wetted by tissue thrombokinase, just as in clinical practice.
2. Four to six surfaces can be tested in the same animal.
3. Flow through the iliofemoral system is maintained, so the flow characteristics are not significantly altered.
4. Two surfaces can be tested in the same animal at the same time, thus eliminating variations in the clotting mechanism from one animal to another.

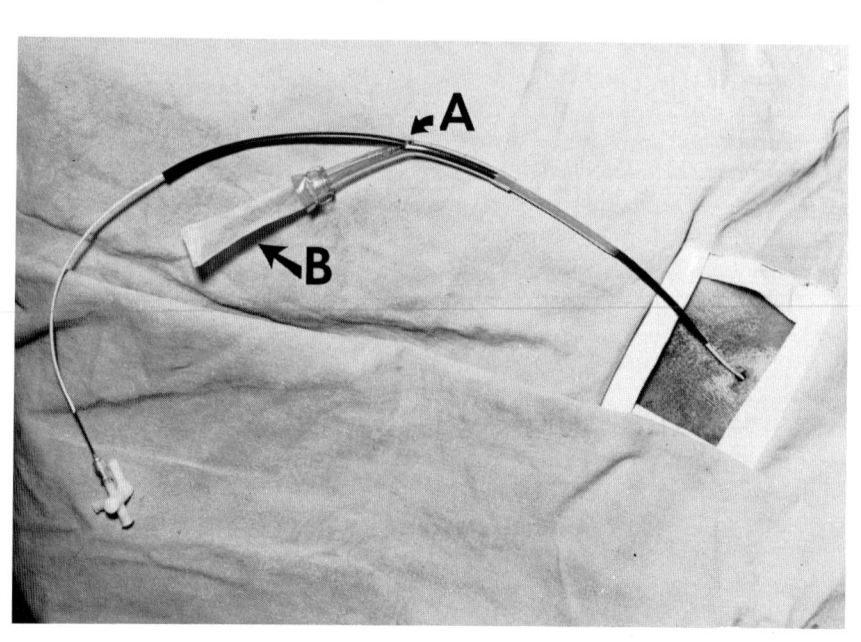

FIG 8–8.
Closeup view of system for retrieving thrombi in thrombogenicity testing. Catheter is withdrawn through the side hole *(A)* of an attached vinyl tube, and thrombi are collected in the filter *(B)*.

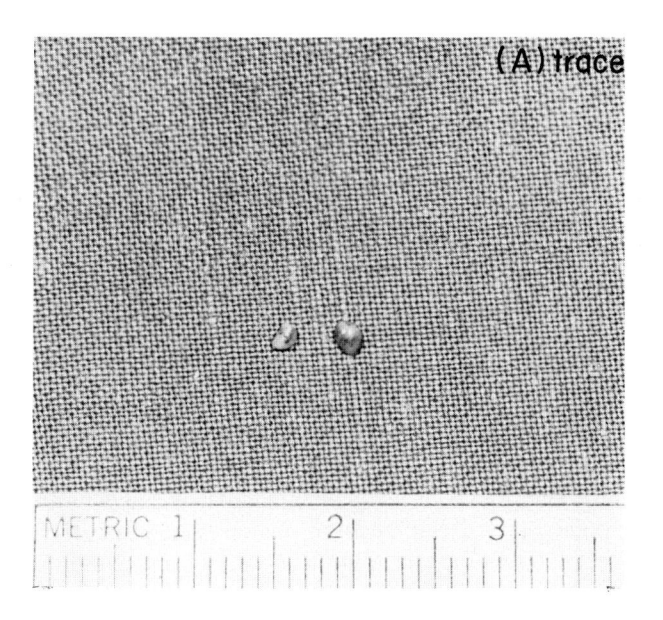

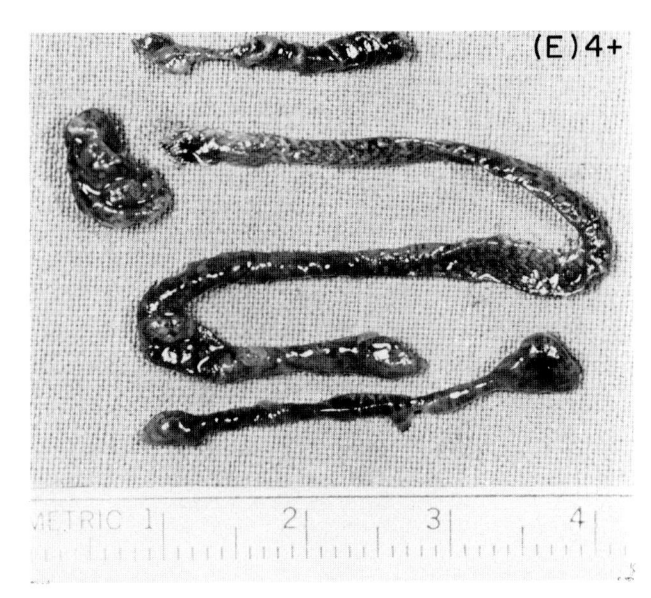

FIG 8–9.
Thrombi collected with retrieval system. **A,** trace thrombus. **B,** 4+ thrombus.

5. The test lasts only 1 hour and is, therefore, comparatively economical, especially because the animals can be used more than once.

A method developed by Lipton et al.,[57] based on nuclear imaging of thrombi in dogs after labeling of platelets with [III]indium-oxine, may permit demonstration of catheter-induced thromboembolic phenomena in humans, but it probably is less sensitive than the direct method.

Guidewire Thrombogenicity

Because of the corrugated construction of guidewires, areas of stasis and turbulence are created and induce early formation of white thrombi. Such thrombotic material may be deposited on guidewires within 90 seconds in dogs and usually within 5 minutes in humans.[39] Contrary to common belief, stainless-steel guidewires are less thrombogenic than the Teflon variety, and guidewires with a thicker Teflon coating show a slightly higher degree of thrombogenicity. After being in a human artery for 10 minutes, all guidewires have considerable fibrin deposits, which could be clinically significant. In dogs, guidewires may become completely encased by fibrin within 20 minutes, creating a huge thrombus (Fig 8–10). Heparinized guidewires are recommended for manipulation in brachiocephalic vessels or across stenotic aortic valves.

The Nonthrombogenic Catheter

Ideally, catheters should be nonthrombogenic, so that thromboembolic complications and the need for systemic heparinization are eliminated, but currently a truly nonthrombogenic plastic catheter is unavailable.

Attempts have been made to render catheters nonthrombogenic by the application of various coatings and adsorption of anticoagulants, particularly heparin, a concept introduced in 1949 by Goodale et al.[10] Gott et al.[58] described a heparin-binding technique using a graphite–benzalkonium treated surface. Local heparinization of catheters and guidewires appears to be the most promising solution, because it provides a powerful, if short-lived, protection from the formation of fibrin. To be useful for angiography, heparin-treated catheters must have the following characteristics:

1. The properties of the catheter, particularly the stiffness, torque, and memory, should not be altered.
2. The treatment should render the catheter clot free with certainty for at least 1 hour.
3. Blood should not clot within the catheter.
4. The duration of vascular compression needed after withdrawal of the catheter should not be significantly prolonged.

Heparinization provides powerful but temporary protection against fibrin formation. There is no significant desorption of heparin from heparinized surfaces in isotonic saline solution, but in plasma, heparin is released rapidly.[58] If the shear rate is increased to the velocity of arterial blood flow, as much as 80% of the heparin is released in 5

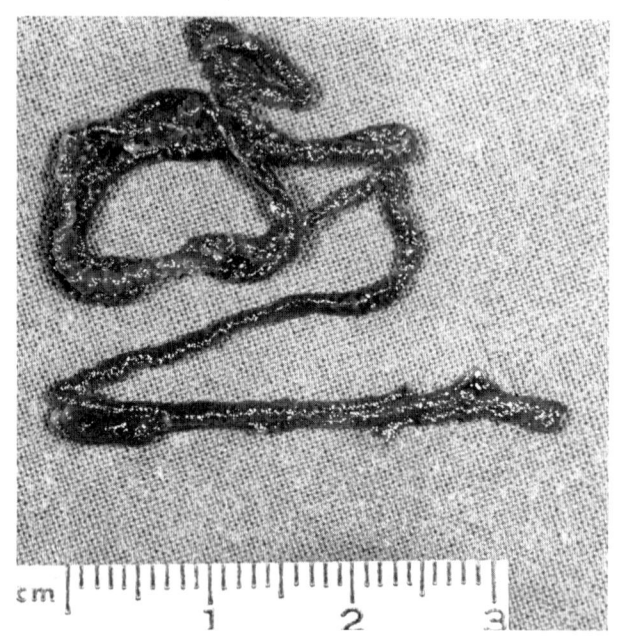

FIG 8–10.
An encasement thrombus on a guidewire retrieved after 20 minutes' exposure in an artery of a dog.

hours. Nevertheless, heparin treatment can make catheters effectively thromboresistant for 1 to 2 hours in dogs and probably longer in humans.

We have developed a coating that can be applied to guidewires and catheters that renders them nonthrombogenic for an adequate period of time for catheterization procedures. However, compression time is increased unless the catheter is introduced with a sheath.

Types of Catheters

Satisfactory diagnostic cardiac catheterization and angiocardiography can be performed using very few different types of catheters. The most commonly used are shown in Figure 8–11.

The Goodale-Lubin Catheter

This catheter represents a modification of the Cournand catheter by the addition of two oval lateral holes, which facilitate blood sampling. This catheter, made of woven Dacron, is useful as a general catheter for both right- and left-sided cardiac catheterization. It is impractical for angiocardiography, as it recoils because of its large end hole and because it bursts at a low pressure.

The NIH Catheter

The NIH catheter has a nylon core, six lateral holes, and an occluded end, which minimizes recoil. The opposing side holes provide an excellent mixing of contrast medium with blood. It is a high-flow angiographic catheter, and in our experience, the catheter has never ruptured, even at maximum flow rates corresponding to an injection pressure of 1,500 lb/in.^{2}

The Pigtail Catheter

This open-end catheter can be introduced percutaneously over a wire guide. The distal end is coiled and has a smaller lumen, which increases resistance, forcing contrast medium through the round or oval side holes. The number of holes varies, but even with 12 side holes, approximately half of the contrast medium is still ejected through the end hole. Increasing the number of side holes decreases the energy of the jets, but the total volume of contrast medium ejected is the same as through three side holes. This catheter is very useful for both ventriculography and aortography. The pigtail configuration minimizes passage of the catheter tip underneath trabeculations, so intramyocardial injections are rare.

During aortography, at higher flow rates, the pigtail portion may straighten partially, and the jet from the end hole then tends to pull the catheter through the aortic valve, producing artificial aortic reflux. The newer high-flow version of this catheter provides less resistance; consequently, the pigtail configuration is preserved even during a rapid injection of contrast medium. Pigtail catheters are available as either torque or nonbraided catheters. The latter have a thinner wall and higher flow.

The Sidewinder Configuration

With this catheter, retrograde catheterization can be performed if direct antegrade catheterization fails. This catheter is useful for catheterization of bronchial and intercostal arteries to obtain pressure measurements and in the truncus arteriosus to exclude associated stenosis of the pulmonary arteries (Fig 8–12). The catheter is made in three tip lengths and can be advanced deep into bronchial arteries beyond areas of stenoses.

Cobra Catheter

This catheter is useful for selective catheterization of the pulmonary arterial tree and is indispensable for embolization procedures. It is wire reinforced and has excellent torque characteristics. A secondary curve of the shaft makes it possible to catheterize upper lobe pulmonary arteries selectively and to advance it deep into bronchial arteries. This is useful in patients with peripheral pulmonary artery stenoses if balloon dilatation is contemplated.

THE MECHANICS OF VENTRICULOGRAPHY

Selective cardiac ventriculography can be performed using an NIH, pigtail, or balloon catheter.

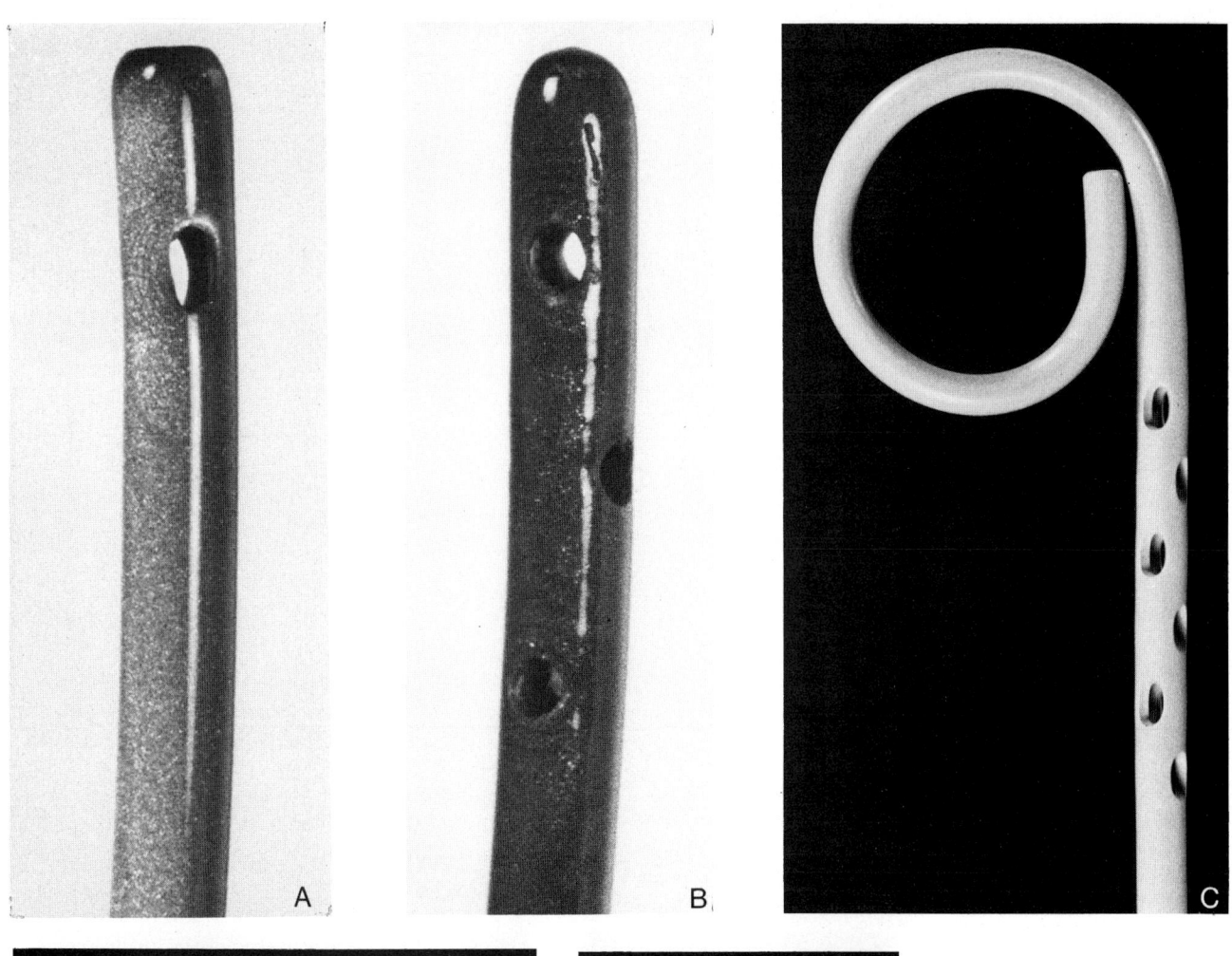

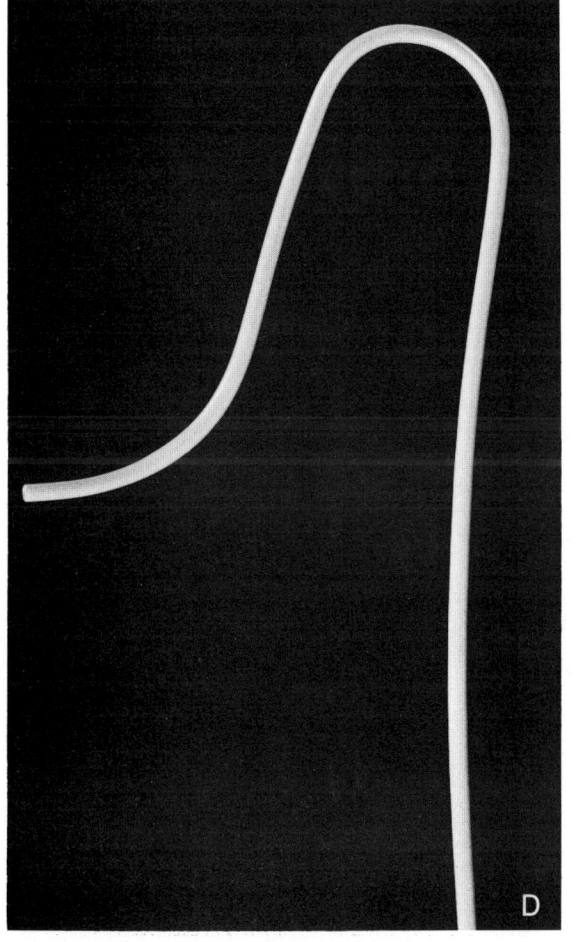

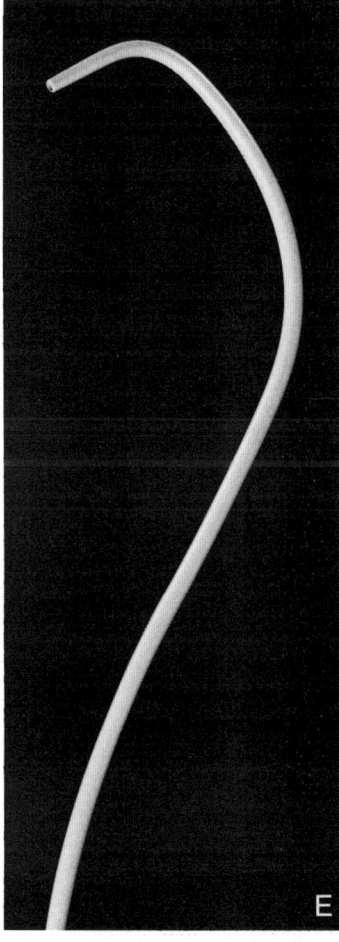

FIG 8–11.
The types of catheters most often used for cardiac catheterization and angiocardiography. **A,** Goodale-Lubin, a useful cardiac catheter. **B,** NIH catheter, useful for high-speed, high-pressure injections. **C,** pigtail catheter, useful for ventriculography. **D,** sidewinder catheter, helpful for catheterization of bronchial arteries, truncus, and shunts. **E,** cobra catheter, practical for catheterization of pulmonary branches, bronchial arteries, system-pulmonary shunts.

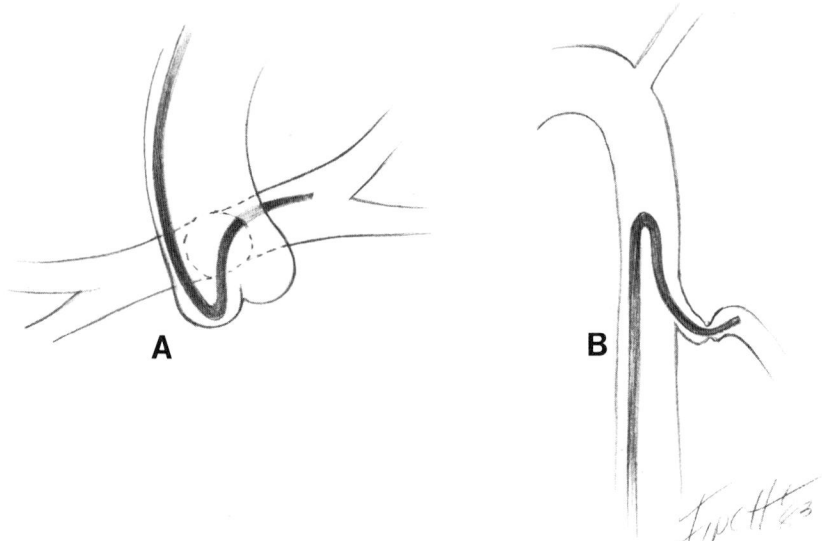

FIG 8–12.
Diagram of retrograde catheterization with a sidewinder catheter. **A,** truncus arteriosus. **B,** stenotic bronchial artery.

With the NIH catheter, it is possible to bury the catheter tip inadvertently in the trabeculations. Also, the side holes of the catheter are in direct contrast with the myocardium, and the energy of the jet of contact medium through the holes is sufficient to deliver the contrast into or even through the myocardium (Fig 8–13,A), particularly if the catheter has been braced against the right atrial wall to prevent recoil. Therefore, with the NIH catheters, care must be taken that the catheter tip lies free within the ventricular cavity, as evidenced by fluoroscopy. A small test injection should be made with the power injector.

With a pigtail catheter (Fig 8–13,B), the trabeculations cannot be entered, but some of the side holes lie close to the myocardium. Subendocardial injections do occur, but intramyocardial injections are rare.

When the balloon of a flow-directed catheter is inflated, the catheter tip is prevented from entering the trabeculations of the ventricle. Also, the balloon has the advantage of increasing the distance between the side holes and the myocardium; consequently, most of the energy of the contrast jets is dissipated by entrainment with blood. Thus, intramyocardial injection almost never occurs with a balloon catheter. Furthermore, because of the increased distance between the side holes and the endocardium, arrhythmias are rare. However, if the catheter is manipulated without the balloon inflated, it may pass under trabeculations and perforate the myocardium, just as any other catheter can (although not as readily as the NIH catheter, which is stiffer). Another problem is that the balloon may be inflated under the epicardium, and a subepicardial injection may occur (Fig 8–14), although this is rare. Thus, even with balloon catheters, small test injections are advisable.

Arrhythmias during angiography are caused by mechanical irritation of the endocardium by either the catheter or the contrast jets. The closer the catheter jets are to the endocardium, the more common the arrhythmias. Consequently, arrhythmias occur much more frequently during injection into small or hypertrophied ventricles (myocardium close to jets) or into the apical portion of a ventricle. To avoid arrhythmias, injection should be made into the inflow portion of a ventricle. Angiography with a large-bore catheter is less likely to induce arrhythmias, because less pressure is required to deliver a given volume of contrast medium, so the jet energy is less. The higher the flow rate, the higher the injection pressure necessary to deliver the contrast medium and the higher the energy of the jets. A slower delivery rate therefore induces fewer arrhythmias than the rapid injection. Delivery at the same rate through a smaller catheter produces more arrhythmias than with a larger catheter (less pressure required, so less energy of the side-hole jets).

Arrhythmias cannot be consistently prevented in spite of careful positioning of the catheter tip.

Balloon Catheters

Balloon catheters have rapidly gained popularity. They are made in two basic configurations: either side holes proximal to the balloon or an end hole distal to the balloon (Fig 8–15). The catheter is made of polyvinyl and has a latex rubber balloon. The chief features of these catheters are as follows:

1. They are safer, because the inflated balloon prevents cardiac perforation or intramyocardial injection.

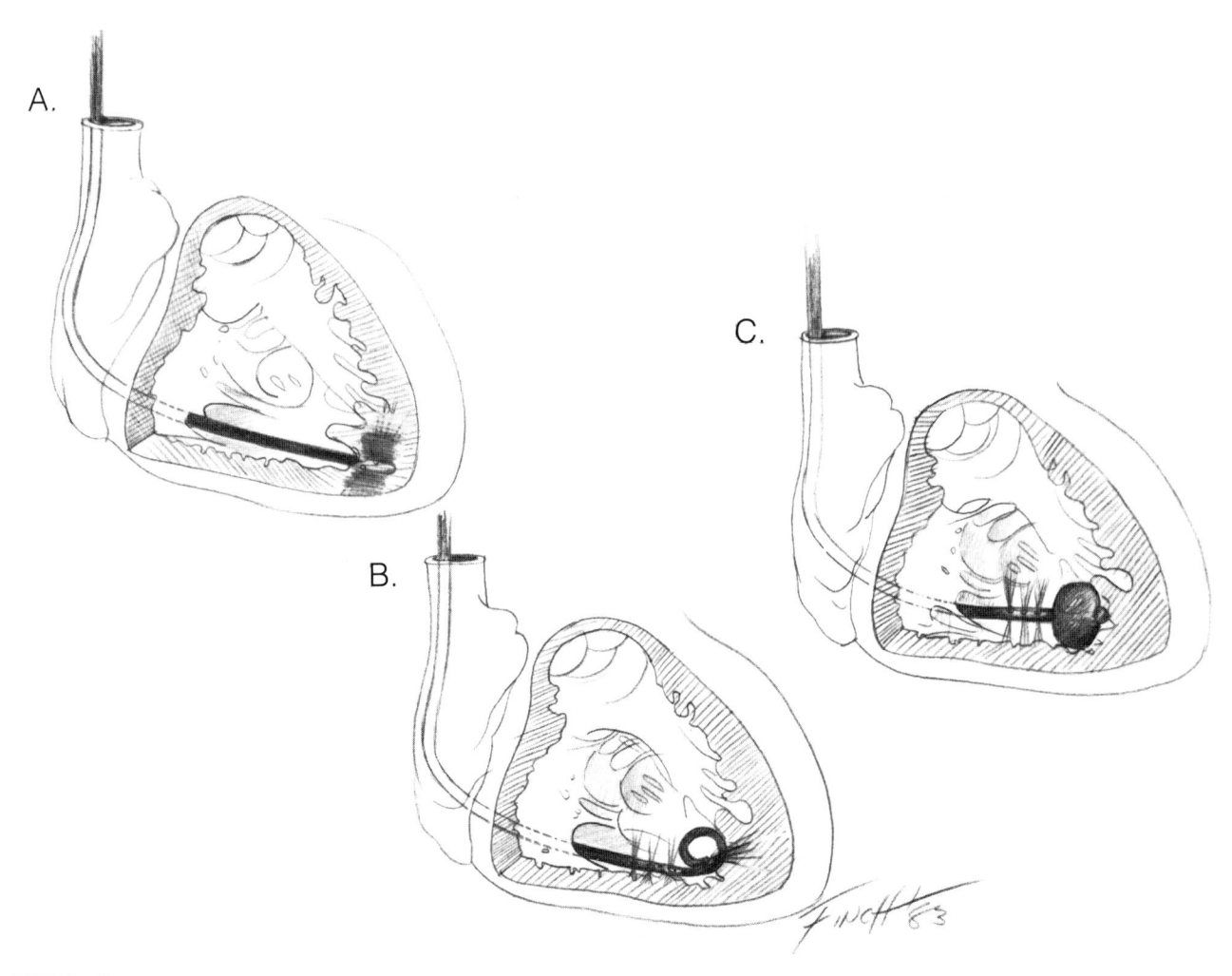

FIG 8–13.
Diagram of the principles of ventriculography with various catheters. **A,** NIH catheter; tip buried in trabeculations of right ventricle and catheter braced against right atrial wall. Recoil cannot occur during injection; therefore, this catheter position may result in intramyocardial and transmyocardial injection. **B,** pigtail catheter; trabeculations cannot be entered; consequently, myocardial injection is much less frequent. Side holes still lie closely to the endocardial surface, and extrasystoles are common. **C,** balloon catheter with balloon inflated; trabeculations cannot be entered. The distance between the side holes and endocardial surface is increased, and energy of the side hole jets is dissipated by blood (entrainment). Therefore, arrhythmias and intramural injection are least common with balloon catheters.

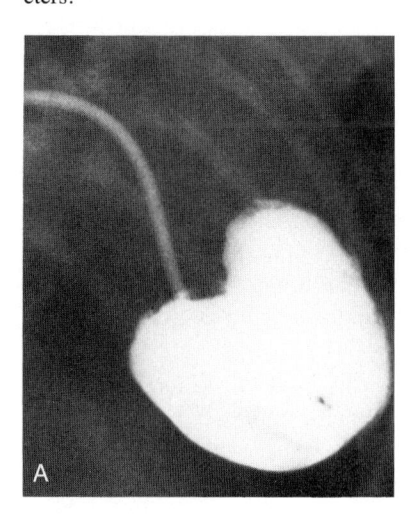

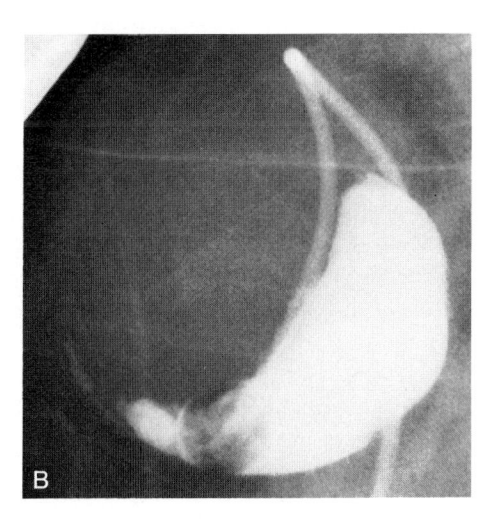

FIG 8–14.
Right ventriculogram in right anterior (**A**) and left anterior (**B**) oblique projections. Balloon catheter, manipulated without balloon inflated, perforated myocardium. No test injection was made; balloon inflated beneath epicardium. Typical subepicardial deposition of contrast medium. No filling of ventricle, pericardial space, or veins. Contrast was aspirated, and patient's clinical course was uneventful.

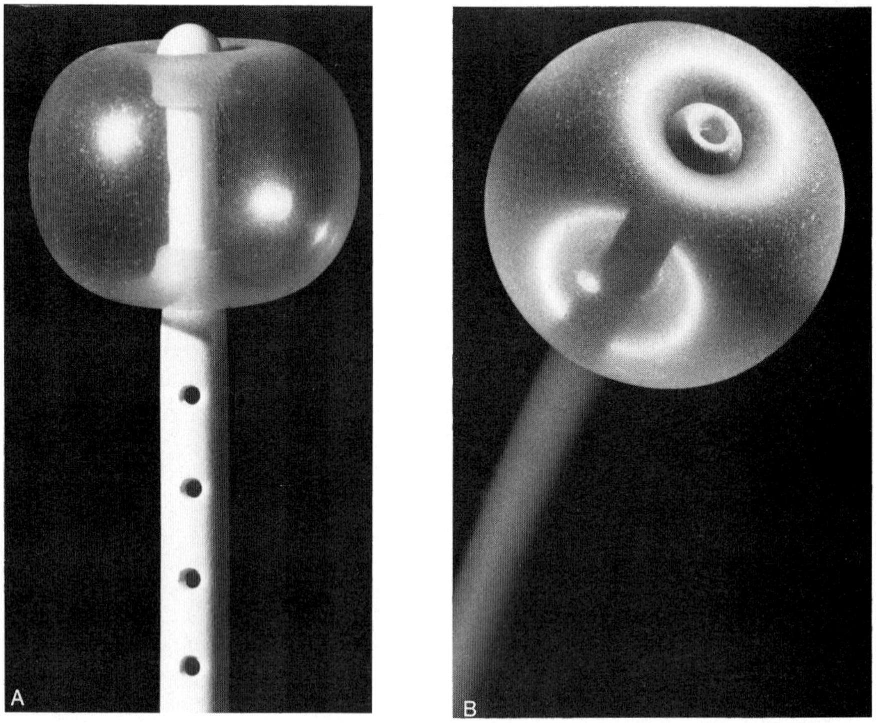

FIG 8–15.
Balloon (Berman) catheter. **A,** side holes proximal to the inflated balloon. **B,** single end hole. This catheter is useful for flow-guided catheterization and safe angiography.

2. They are soft and carried by the bloodstream (flow-guided catheterization).
3. They can be used for pressure recordings, blood sampling, and angiography.
4. Even though they have a double lumen, these catheters allow adequate flow rates for angiography.
5. They can be used for occlusion angiography.

The flow or pressure limits, which have to be determined experimentally, cannot be exceeded without rupturing the catheter.

Balloon Occlusion Angiography

Balloon occlusion angiography is an important technique of selective angiography that markedly improves the quality of the angiograms and conserves contrast medium. Some congenital lesions can be demonstrated only by this technique. The balloon is inflated in a vessel to occlude flow, and contrast injections are made either proximally or distally to the balloon. This technique has several advantages:

1. Because contrast medium is undiluted, less must be injected.
2. The concentration of the contrast medium creates a dense angiogram, which provides excellent anatomic detail.
3. Because flow is occluded, for example, in selectively occluded pulmonary arterial branches, several projections can be examined after a single injection.
4. The direction of blood flow can be reversed. For example, in a reversing patent ductus arteriosus, balloon occlusion angiography allows demonstration of the pulmonary artery and the aortic arch. The need for ascending aortography is thus eliminated.
5. A vessel with very low flow (Fig 8–16) usually cannot be opacified by standard angiography, but with balloon occlusion, the contrast medium is forced into the vessels. For example, standard pulmonary arteriography usually does not opacify stenotic or atretic pulmonary veins well because of low flow rates, whereas pulmonary angiography after balloon occlusion provides excellent opacification by forcing the contrast into the occluded veins and from there into systemic collateral channels (Fig 8–17).
6. Blood flow can be redirected. In patients with a Waterston shunt, after aortography it is common for only the right pulmonary artery to be opacified; thus, it may be impossible to determine continuity between the pulmonary arteries. If the right pulmonary artery is occluded by a balloon and an angiogram performed with injection proximal to the balloon, continuity can be demonstrated.

Balloon catheters can be used to measure the size of atrial septal defects or other communications indirectly. An inflated balloon of known diameter is passed across the defect, and deformation of the balloon is observed fluoro-

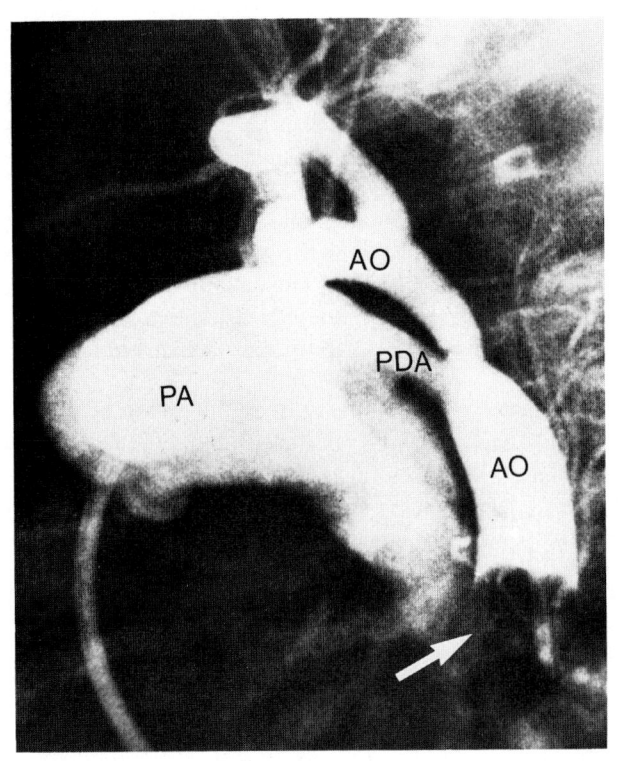

FIG 8–16.
Balloon occlusion angiography in reversing patent ductus arteriosus. Injection made proximally to inflated balloon in descending aorta *(arrow)*. The aortic arch and pulmonary artery are well opacified against the normal direction of blood flow. *AO* = aorta; *PA* = pulmonary artery; *PDA* = patent ductus arteriosus.

scopically. In patients with hypoplastic right ventricles and patent foramen ovale, balloon occlusion can reveal whether the ventricle is of adequate size. At the time of cardiac catheterization, the atrial septal defect is occluded by a balloon, and careful physiologic observations are made to determine if the foramen ovale can be closed safely at operation.

These balloon catheters are of different design than those used for balloon atrial septostomy.

CONTRAST MEDIA

The differential absorption of x-rays by blood and by soft tissues is insufficient to visualize cardiac chambers and blood vessels, so contrast media are needed. The types of contrast media can be divided into two broad groups:

1. Positive contrast media, which absorb more x-rays than do soft tissues. Although these media can be either water soluble or oily, only the aqueous media will be discussed, because oily media are not useful for angiocardiography.

2. Negative contrast media, which absorb less x-rays

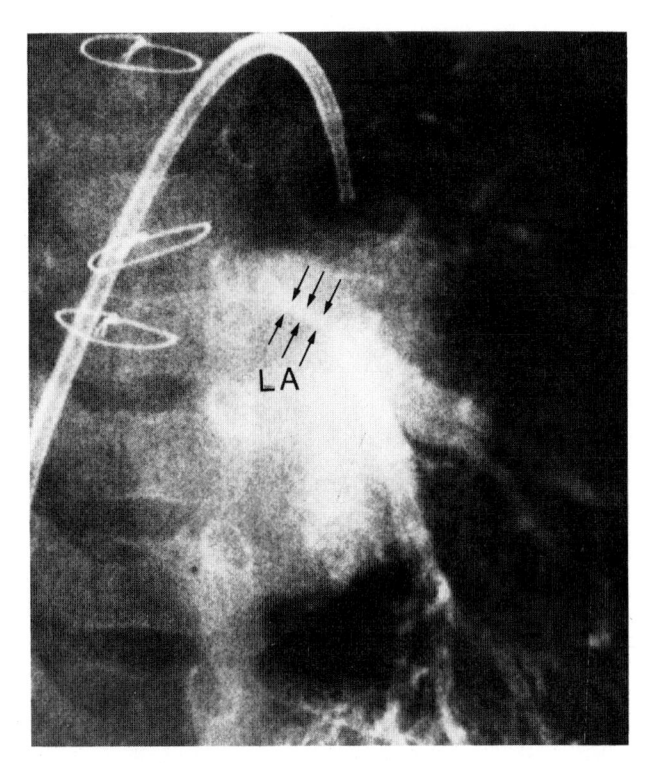

FIG 8–17.
Balloon-occlusion left pulmonary arteriogram, allowing demonstration of stenosis of the individual pulmonary veins *(arrows)*. Jet is from the stenotic veins.

than do soft tissues. Carbon dioxide, a safe negative contrast medium, has previously been used for examination of right atrial wall thickness to diagnose pericardial effusion (Fig 8–18). In this technique, the patient is placed in the left lateral decubitus position and 50 to 100 mL of carbon dioxide is injected into the antecubital vein. One radiograph is adequate to demonstrate the right atrium.

Because gas refluxes into the hepatic veins, the technique is still useful to exclude Budd-Chiari syndrome, but with the advent of ultrasonography, this diagnostic test has otherwise been abandoned. The radiographic detail obtained with negative contrast media is far inferior to that obtained by positive contrast media. Consequently, gases are rarely used for the study of the cardiovascular system.

A detailed description of contrast media, their composition, and their physiologic and toxic effects is beyond the scope of this book; however, a basic understanding is essential to optimize radiographic results and to minimize complications. The injection of contrast media can cause a variety of serious reactions, including death.

Prevention of Contrast Media Reactions

Adverse reactions to the injection of contrast media cannot be completely eliminated, but they can be minimized if certain precautions are taken.

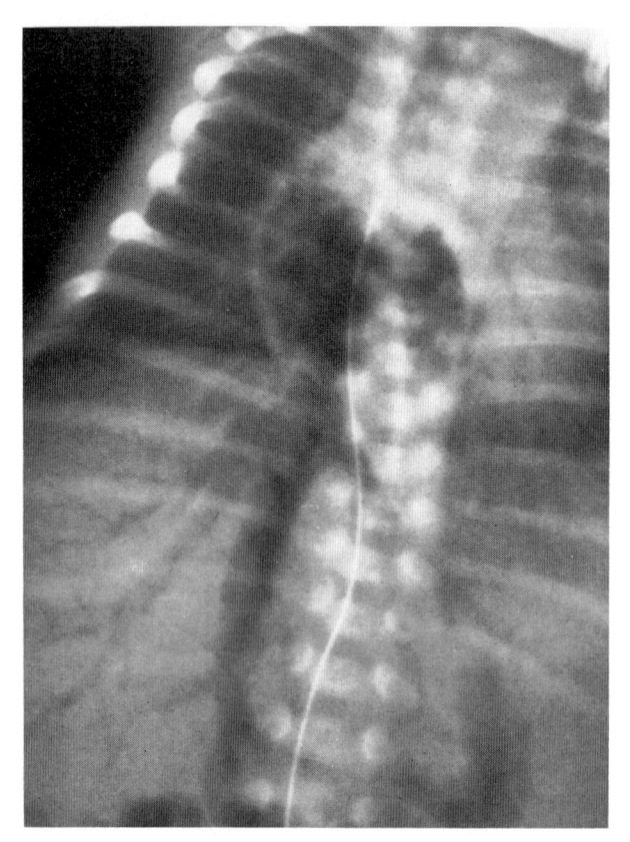

FIG 8-18.
Carbon dioxide injection into right atrium with patient in left lateral decubitus positon; right atrium, its wall, hepatic veins, and inferior vena cava are well outlined. Technique was used to diagnose pericardial effusion and is still useful to exclude Budd-Chiari syndrome.

1. Anesthesia. In most cases, general anesthesia is not indicated for angiography because it represents a risk by itself. However, the quality of angiograms made with the patient under general anesthesia is better because cardiac output is decreased, resulting in a higher concentration of contrast medium because there is less dilution. Sedation with barbiturates and local anesthesia are generally adequate for angiography. Narcotics should be used cautiously, because contrast media themselves have a mildly depressant effect on the respiratory center.

2. Hydration. The nephrotoxic effect of contrast media is dependent not only on the type of medium but also on the concentration reaching the kidneys. Adequate hydration increases renal flow and lowers the concentration of contrast medium in the blood perfusing the renal arterial bed. Adequate hydration is particularly important in patients with compromised renal function, as in diabetes mellitus, hyperuricemia, or multiple myeloma. In the latter group, dehydration predisposes to the precipitation of myeloma protein in the renal tubules. Intravenous fluid should be administered by drip infusion before, during, and after angiography. In very high-risk patients, a diuretic can be given in addition, but there is no evidence that this further increases safety. Contrast media can be used in patients with renal failure because they are also excreted by the mucosa in the stomach, gallbladder, and bowel. Contrast media are hydrolyzable.

3. Sensitivity testing. The intravenous or intradermal injection of a small amount of contrast medium has no predictive value: Severe, even fatal, reactions have occurred with the test dose alone, and patients with a negative sensitivity test result have had serious reactions after full injection.

A history of any allergy or of allergy to iodine-containing compounds does not represent a contraindication to angiography, but certain precautions should be taken. In our experience, the incidence of reactions in this group of patients is only minimally higher, and reactions generally are mild. Patients who had a reaction at the time of intravenous pyelography most commonly have no reaction during angiography; however, the risk is somewhat increased. The risk can be minimized if a nonionic agent is used for repeat examination.

4. Management of patients with an allergic history and previous reaction to contrast medium of intravenous pyelography. First, decide if angiography is absolutely necessary to arrive at the diagnosis; if diagnostic tests that do not require contrast agents are available, angiography should be canceled. If angiography is necessary, we perform it with an experienced anesthetist present to assist in the management of cardiac and respiratory emergencies. Cortisone, antihistamines, epinephrine, and drugs to treat cardiopulmonary emergencies are ready for immediate injection if needed. We do not premedicate our patients with cortisone and antihistamines for 2 to 3 days before angiography because of the increased cost and the absence of sufficient evidence that such medication decreases the risk of allergic reactions.* In our experience, the incidence of reactions has been negligible, and we have had no deaths from anaphylactic reaction over the past 27 years in 36,000 angiocardiograms with ionic agents.

Injections of contrast medium on the venous side of the circulation cause more reactions than those on the arterial side. This difference is believed to be related to histamine release induced by the passage of the contrast medium through the pulmonary circulation.

5. Pheochromocytoma. Patients with suspected pheochromocytoma should be treated with a combination of α- and β-blockers beforehand. Without this precaution, injection of contrast media may induce a life-threatening crisis.

---

*Very recently a large-scale controlled study seemed to prove that the incidence of reactions may be decreased by premedication with corticosteroids. (Personal communication with Dr. Elliot Lasser.)

6. Congestive heart failure. In the presence of congestive heart failure, overhydration should be avoided, because the osmotic load from the contrast medium may aggravate cardiac failure. A nonionic contrast agent or a dimer with lower osmolality should be used.

7. Severe pulmonary hypertension. Acute right-heart failure has been described secondary to angiography in patients with severe pulmonary hypertension because of vasoconstriction. The amount of contrast medium injected should be limited and, if possible, only one lung injected at a time. In our experience, injection of contrast media has been well tolerated by patients with severe pulmonary hypertension, and we have had no fatalities. The use of diluted nonionic agents and digital recording further improves the safety of angiography in pulmonary vascular disease.

8. Electrocardiographic (ECG) monitoring. Because one of the major complications of angiography, particularly ventriculography and coronary angiography, is cardiac arrhythmias, ECG monitoring is imperative. It is usually adequate to observe the ECG on an oscilloscope. A technician or physician should be assigned to observe the tracing continuously.

9. For all angiographic procedures, an intravenous drip infusion of saline, Ringer's lactate, or similar solution should be running to provide access for drugs in case of emergencies.

10. Nonionic agents should be used routinely in neonates and infants.

Contraindications to Angiography

In patients in whom angiography may be the only test that will afford a decisive diagnosis for effective medical or surgical management, there are virtually no contraindications except a life-threatening reaction to a previous injection of contrast medium.

On the other hand, in many patients, angiography is a diagnostic adjunct but not essential. In this latter group, there are relative contraindications to this procedure. Thus, in patients with impaired renal function, a history of allergy, pulmonary hypertension, multiple myeloma, hyperuricemia, uremia, sickle cell anemia, liver failure, cardiac failure, or pheochromocytoma, benefit has to be weighed against risk.

The Choice of Contrast Medium

Currently, there is no evidence that one contrast medium is significantly safer than another. Animal studies in our laboratory showed that the newer nonionic agents and dimers are less nephrotoxic than are ionic media,[59] but human studies are still incomplete.

Because of their lower osmolality, nonionics and dimers cause virtually no pain or heat sensation. Whether the routine use of a nonionic agent for angiocardiography is warranted is uncertain currently.

Ionic Angiographic Contrast Media

Positive contrast agents used for angiocardiography are all water soluble. Their radiopacity is achieved by the incorporation of a heavy metal ion (iodine) into organic molecules. The first iodine-containing contrast medium, sodium iodide, was rapidly replaced by less toxic iodinated organic compounds. Some of the older contrast agents have only two iodine atoms per molecule and are called diiodinated compounds (Iopax, Diotrast, Neo Iopax, Urokon, etc.). These diiodinated media had a high incidence of adverse reactions and consequently are no longer used. All modern contrast media contain three iodine atoms per molecule (triiodinated compounds). Some triiodinated compounds can be coupled into dimers, which have six iodine atoms per molecule.

The subject of contrast media appears confusing because of the endless list of commercially available products, but most of these agents are the same compounds with the same chemical formula. The concentration of the aqueous solution of the generic compound may vary, and, rarely, mixtures of two chemically different compounds are available. The trade names have common suffixes such as "Ray" (from x-ray), "Trast" (from contrast), or "Paque" (from opaque) and prefixes indicating their use, such as "angio," or "cardio." To alleviate the confusion, physicians should use nonproprietary names, particularly in scientific publications.

Diatrizoate.—The diatrizoates (known commercially as Renografin and Hypaque in the United States and by other names elsewhere) are the most commonly used. Renografin and Hypaque have the same chemical formula. They are inexpensive and have been extensively tested. Diatrizoate contrast media are aqueous solutions of either a meglumine or a sodium salt of diatrizoic acid, which is a derivative of benzoic acid. The benzene ring has three iodine atoms, and the compound ionizes in solution, which doubles the osmolality to a level five to eight times that of blood. The sodium salt of diatrizoic acid is less viscous than the meglumine salt, but it has more cardiovascular effects. Pure sodium and meglumine salts of diatrizoic acid are available, but for angiocardiography, a mixture of sodium and meglumine salts is most useful. Particularly for coronary angiography, a balanced sodium concentration is essential, because the incidence of ventricular fibrillation increases significantly when the pure meglumine salt is used.

These contrast agents are available in both 60% and 76% solutions. The former solution is used primarily for peripheral angiography because it causes less discomfort. Its osmolality is 1,420 mOsm/kg of H_2O compared with 1,920 mOsm/kg of H_2O for the 76% solution. A 90% solution was used previously but is no longer commercially available because of its excessive viscosity and tendency to crystallize at room temperature. Early power injectors were always equipped with a heating jacket to dissolve the crystals and decrease the viscosity of the agent.

Iothalamates.—The iothalamates are sodium or methylglucamine salts of iothalamic acid, which is chemically similar to diatrizoic acid except for the side chains on the benzene ring. In the United States, the compounds are commercially available as "Conray," "Conray 400," or "Angioconray." Iothalamates have the same iodine content as the diatrizoates, but their viscosity is lower; consequently, the compound can be injected faster through smaller catheters. Iothalamates are as safe as diatrizoates and have been extensively used for angiocardiography. As with the diatrizoates, the methylglucamine salt is less cardiotoxic than is the sodium salt.

Metrizoates.—The metrizoates are chemically similar to the diatrizoates except for the side chains. The contrast agent, known as "Isopaque," is a mixture of the sodium, meglumine, magnesium, and calcium salts of metrizoic acid. This mixture is ionically better balanced and has the theoretical advantage of being less cardiotoxic, but this is unproved.

Clinical Experience With Diatrizoates

With pure diatrizoate-glucamine, the lack of sodium ions increases the incidence of ventricular fibrillation to about 15% in coronary angiography. When a mixture of the sodium and methylglucamine salts is used, the incidence is less than 1%. Attempts to make a more physiologic contrast medium by using an ionically more balanced sodium and calcium diatrizoate mixture failed because calcium diatrizoate is insoluble. Theoretically, the metrizoates are a more balanced contrast agent, but in practice the incidence of ventricular fibrillation during selective coronary angiography is no lower than with diatrizoates.

Osmolality depends on the number of particles in solution, and because all ionic contrast agents hydrolyze into two particles, their osmolality is high: 1,940 mOsm/kg of H_2O for a 76% solution. Some of the side effects of contrast media are caused by osmotic irritation of the intima and result in hypertension, flushing, pain, hypervolemia, endothelial damage with vascular thrombosis, and erythrocyte aggregation. Therefore, research efforts have been directed toward the development of agents with lower osmolality.

Low Osmolar Agents.—The number of particles formed per triiodinated benzene ring can be reduced in two ways:

1. Creation of a dimer in which two triiodinated benzene rings are linked together, forming a molecule containing six iodine atoms. This new molecule also will form two particles in solution, but now the relation between the numbers of particles and iodine atoms is 2:6 instead of 2:3, as in the monomeric molecule. Thus, dimers with the same concentration of iodine have an osmolality about one half that of the ionic agents.

Dimers of diatrizoic, metrizoic and iothalamic acid have been produced. A well-known agent is a mixture of the sodium and methylglucamine salt of ioxaglic acid, commercially available as Hexabrix. The iodine content of the commercially available solution is similar to that of 76% diatrizoate, but the osmolality is only about 600 mOsm/kg of H_2O; the lethal dose of Hexabrix is about twice that of the monomeric ionic compounds.[60] Hexabrix was proved safe but not necessarily safer than diatrizoates. However, because of the lower osmolality, there is virtually no heat sensation and pain.

2. Use of nonionic substances, which do not dissociate in aqueous solution. That is, nonionic contrast media also contain a triiodinated benzene ring, but because they are not salts, they do not dissociate and consequently form only one particle per benzene ring in solution. Nonionic contrast media are available commercially as Amipaque, Iopamidol, Iohexol, and Iversol, and so on. Each has an osmolality of about 700 mOsm/kg of H_2O. Not only do these agents cause less vasodilation and pain, they are safer for angiocardiography in infants, because the lower osmotic load causes less hypervolemia.

There is experimental evidence[59] that both dimers and nonionic contrast agents are less nephrotoxic than the ionic agents, but clinical confirmation is lacking. The newer agents also cost more. Nonetheless, dimers and nonionic contrast media have replaced the ionic agents for peripheral angiography and also for cardiac angiography in the pediatric age group.

Low osmolar contrast agents have completely replaced the ionic compounds since they produce less or no myocardial depression, less increase of end diastolic pressure and fall in blood pressure due to decreased peripheral resistance.[61]

Adverse Reactions to Contrast Media

Serious reactions, including death, may occur after injection of contrast media, although, fortunately, this is not common.

Death

During our 35 years of angiographic experience at the University of Minnesota, only one death has been directly attributable to angiography with diatrizoate contrast medium. In a newborn with hyaline membrane disease, thought, because of the appearance of the chest film, to have total anomalous pulmonary venous connection below the diaphragm, angiography resulted in immediate pulmonary edema and death. This represents the only lethal complication in 36,000 angiograms.

Minor Side Effects

Ionic contrast media are potent dilators of the peripheral capillary bed, but they increase resistance in the pulmonary arteries. The profound peripheral vasodilatation results in the sensation of heat, pain, and flushing of the skin. The extent of these effects depends on the type of contrast agent used and its concentration in the blood, so they are much more pronounced after selective arterial injections. If the contrast medium is injected on the venous side of the circulation, the concentration reaching the arterial side is so low that heat sensation, burning, and pain are minimal or absent. Nevertheless, the patient should be forewarned.

Pulmonary Complications

Pulmonary complications are rare. Pulmonary embolism is probably the result of dislodgement of fibrin deposits on the catheter rather than of the contrast medium itself. Such emboli are so small that they can be detected only angiographically and do not cause clinical symptoms. The accidental injection of a small amount of air into the lungs is also clinically well tolerated.

If the catheter is in a wedged position, the contrast medium can be injected into the pulmonary parenchyma, which results in extravasation but usually without clinical sequelae.

Angiography carries an additional risk in patients with significantly elevated pulmonary arterial pressure, because contrast media increase pulmonary vascular resistance. Whether this increase in resistance and pressure results from sludging of red blood cells or vasoconstriction is unknown (Fig 8–19). In our experience, pulmonary angiography in patients with arterial or venous pulmonary hypertension has not caused serious complications, although these have been reported by others. The danger of pulmonary angiography in patients with severe pulmonary hypertension can be minimized in four ways:

1. By limiting the amount of contrast medium injected.
2. By injecting only one pulmonary artery and sparing the contralateral lung.
3. By the use of nonionic agents.
4. By diluting the contrast medium and using digital recording.

Balloon occlusion angiography combines these measures, and we use this technique frequently in this clinical situation.

Cheyne-Stokes breathing, respiratory apnea, or respi-

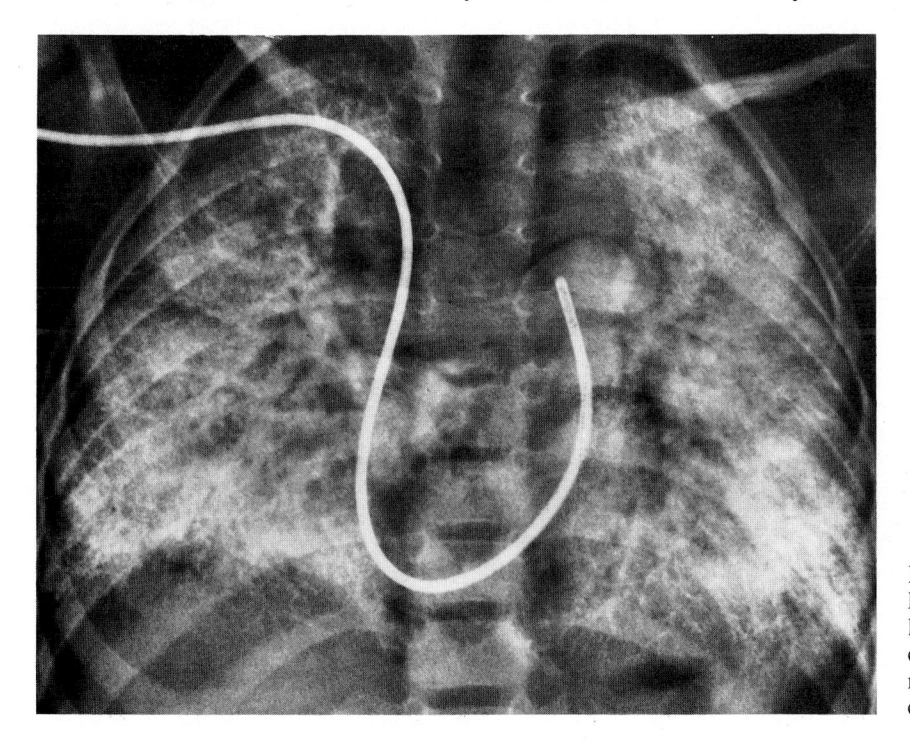

FIG 8–19.
Pulmonary arteriogram; dense stain of both lungs for several seconds, with transient increase in pulmonary artery pressure. The mechanism is probably spasm of pulmonary capillary bed induced by contrast agent.

ratory arrest may occur, but this is exceedingly rare. We have never observed this complication.

Gastrointestinal Complications

Nausea, retching, and vomiting are common after angiography but are self-limited and do not require special treatment. The pathophysiology of these symptoms is not understood. Because of these side effects, patients must fast before angiography. Distracting patients by asking them to breathe deeply and reassuring them are other useful antiemetic measures.

Cardiovascular Complications

Vascular complications of angiography may occur for three reasons.

Embolism.—Embolic phenomena occur primarily from accidental injection of air or from thrombotic or atheromatous material.

Injection of a few air bubbles is well tolerated even when it occurs selectively into the coronary arteries, but injection of a large amount (>40 cc) of air into the left side of the heart results in temporary or permanent stroke (Fig 8–20). In the cerebral circulation, air causes mechanical blockage of the cerebral arteries by a compressible air column. Similarly, if a large amount of air is injected into the venous side of the circulation, the right ventricle compresses the gas during systole (gasses are compressible; fluids are not), and therefore no blood is ejected; the ventricles can expel only noncompressible fluids, such as blood. If accidental injection of air occurs into the venous side of the circulation, the patient should immediately be placed in the left lateral decubitus position. In this position, the air rises through the tricuspid valve into the right atrium, and blood can then enter the right ventricle by gravity. Once the ventricle is filled with blood, cardiac output resumes.

Effects of Contrast Medium on the Coronary Arterial Bed and Myocardium.—As noted earlier, ionic contrast agents are potent peripheral vasodilators, and the diffuse peripheral vasodilatation decreases peripheral resistance and systemic blood pressure. A compensatory increase in stroke volume and tachycardia then occurs; this reflex increases cardiac output and restores the baseline blood pressure. Although normally this decrease in systemic pressure is only transient, in patients with obstructive cardiomyopathy or severe left ventricular outflow tract obstruction, systemic hypotension may persist, causing decreased myocardial perfusion with dysfunction. The result may be death. Consequently, angiocardiography is especially dangerous in patients with left ventricular outflow obstruction and depressed myocardial function.

Contrast media also cause profound vasodilatation of the coronary arterial bed and augment coronary blood flow. This beneficial side effect increases the safety of coronary angiography. Rarely, however, contrast media cause severe coronary arterial spasm, resulting in cessation of blood flow, ECG changes, and severe ischemic pain. A similar paradoxical spastic reaction of other vascular beds may occur, particularly in the pulmonary circulation (see Fig 8–19). The treatment of this complication is intravascular injection of nitroglycerin or papaverine.

When the myocardium is perfused with contrast media, myocardial contractility is immediately depressed, as evidenced by an increased filling pressure (elevation of the end-diastolic pressure). In our experience, the correlation between coronary artery disease and the degree of elevation of the end-diastolic pressure after angiography is of little clinical value. Fortunately, myocardial depression is transient and well tolerated except by patients with severe cardiomyopathy or left ventricular outflow obstruction. Depression of myocardial function is the result of a direct toxic effect of the contrast agent rather than of hypoxia caused by partial replacement of the perfusing blood by

FIG 8–20.
Left ventriculogram with injection of large amount of air. **A,** anteroposterior projection; descending aorta outlined by double contrast *(arrows);* large amount of air in ascending aorta. **B,** lateral projection; air in left ventricle *(white arrow).* Air contrast level with waves *(black arrows)* in ascending aorta. Patient experienced transient bradycardia but did not suffer a stroke.

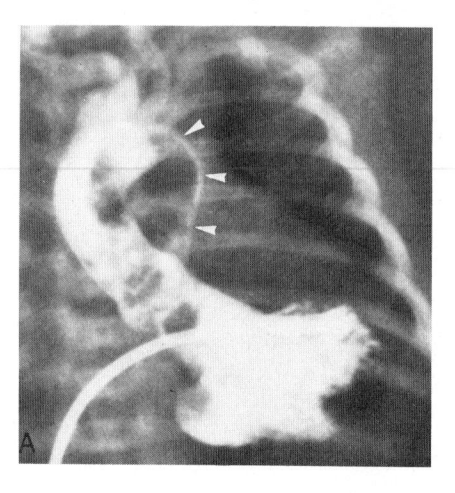

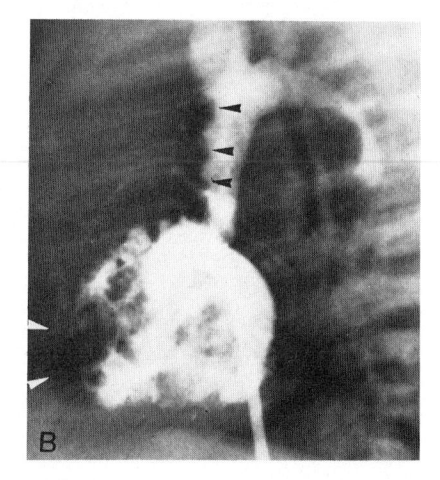

the nonoxygen-carrying contrast medium, because an injection of saline at the same rate does not reduce myocardial function.

Contrast media also have a direct effect on the cardiac conducting system that can lead to cardiac arrhythmias, particularly when the agents are injected selectively into the coronary arteries. Heart block, premature beats, ventricular tachycardia, or ventricular fibrillation may occur. Bradycardia or asystole are the most common arrhythmias during selective coronary angiography, but almost invariably the heart resumes a sinus rhythm after several seconds. This effect is caused by vagal stimulation and can be blocked by premedication with atropine. Severe asystole can be terminated by a blow on the chest, cardiac pacing, or administration of catecholamines. Asystole is almost always self-limited and does not warrant the routine use of a cardiac pacemaker or of having the patient cough. In our experience, all asystoles during coronary angiography are self-limited without having the patient cough, although that may be comforting for the angiographer.

Ventricular fibrillation is a serious arrhythmia that should be treated immediately by electric defibrillation. Ventricular fibrillation occurs in about 0.5% to 1% of patients after selective coronary angiography with 76% diatrizoates but is lower with low osmolar agents. Before coronary angiography the defibrillator should be checked, and the paddles should be prepared with a conductive paste in case they are needed. The best results are obtained with immediate defibrillation before acidosis. After defibrillation, the procedure can be continued, because fibrillation very rarely recurs.

The electrocardiographic changes seen after selective injection of the coronary arteries are identical to those found in myocardial ischemia, but they are caused by a direct effect of the contrast medium on the myocardium rather than by ischemia. Similar electrocardiographic changes cannot be produced if a physiologic solution such as Ringer's lactate solution is injected at the same rate into the coronary arteries.[62]

Depression of the ST segment and either T-wave inversion or development of giant upright T waves regularly occur during coronary angiography using ionic agents. With low osmolar media, ECG changes are minimal. Consequently, they have largely replaced ionics. The specific pattern depends on whether the posterior or the anterior portion of the ventricular septum is perfused predominately by the contrast medium. With coronary obstruction and resultant myocardial perfusion via collaterals, the ECG pattern changes have a characteristic sequential pattern. Another common and harmless ECG change, which is not well understood, is axis shift.

Myocardial infarction is a rare (<0.5%) complication of selective coronary angiography. The exact mechanism is unknown, but it is probably related to embolization rather than to the contrast medium itself, because myocardial infarction is rare unless the contrast medium is injected selectively into coronary arteries.

Allergic Reactions.—Reactions such as skin rashes, angioedema, fever, and anaphylactic shock are clearly allergic and are rare. The exact mechanism is not understood, but it is unlikely that such reactions are caused by antibodies, because contrast media do not contain protein and the incidence of allergic reactions is no higher in patients who have had previous injections of contrast media. However, the incidence is slightly higher in patients with a history of allergy and previous reaction to contrast agents.

Allergic reactions are not dependent on dose, and usually it is not possible to predict their occurrence on the basis of the response to a test dose of contrast medium. Generally the injection on the venous side produces a higher incidence of allergic reaction than does injection on the arterial side, probably because of histamine release when the contrast medium passes through the pulmonary capillary bed. In our experience, patients who give a history of an allergic reaction after intravenous pyleography very rarely have a reaction if an angiogram is performed on the left side of the heart, in spite of the injection of a larger amount of contrast medium. The severity of reaction is decreased with the use of nonionic agents, which should be used in patients with previous allergic reaction to ionic contrast media.

Central Nervous System Complications

Complications, such as cerebrovascular accident and paraplegia, that involve the nervous system are rare. Cerebrovascular accidents are probably related to embolic phenomena rather than to toxicity of the contrast medium unless selective carotid angiography is performed. Paraplegia has been reported after abdominal angiography and selective injection of the bronchial, intercostal, and lumbar arteries.

Convulsions may occur after angiocardiography. The frequency of this complication is related to the dose of contrast medium. We have observed it in one infant after many angiograms for which a total dose of 10 mL/kg had been given. The computed tomography scans revealed contrast medium in the subarachnoid space, indicating a breakdown of the blood-brain barrier. The patient recovered.

Another rare, frightening, and not well understood complication is "cortical blindness," in which the patient is blind but has no other neurologic deficit. Fortunately, normal vision returns without treatment after 24 to 48 hours.

The cause is probably transient ischemia of the visual cortex.

Contrast media do not cross the blood-brain barrier unless administered in either very high concentration or in excessive amounts. Breakdown of the blood-brain barrier may result in neurologic complications caused by cell necrosis. Because neurotoxic complications depend on the amount and concentration of the contrast agent, they are much more common in selective injections into cerebral vessels than with angiocardiography. These complications are expected to be less common with nonionic compounds, which have less neurotoxicity.

Renal Complications

Contrast media are nephrotoxic, although the newer nonionic agents may be less so.[59] Toxic effects follow intravenous, aortic, or renal arterial administration. Renal damage occurs with every angiogram performed with an ionic contrast agent, but because of the large functional reserve of the kidneys, there are no symptoms. Instead, damage may be detectable only by biochemical tests or microscopic examination of the urine. Ten percent to 12% of patients show biochemical evidence of renal impairment after angiography,[62, 63] and in patients with borderline renal function, angiography may cause renal shutdown from acute tubular necrosis.

Because the nephrotoxicity depends on the concentration and dose of the contrast medium, both should be limited in these patients, who also should be forcefully hydrated before the procedure. Alternatively, the more sensitive digital imaging technique, which requires less contrast agent, may be used.

Renal failure is the most common serious complication of angiography and is evidenced by decreased urine output for 24 hours, followed by anuria.[64] Patients with multiple myeloma or diabetes and elderly dehydrated patients are at higher risk. Occurrence of renal failure caused by tubular necrosis can usually be predicted by a very dense nephrogram persisting for hours or days after angiography. Almost invariably, renal function returns to normal, but dialysis may be required temporarily.

POWER INJECTORS

Almost every power injector produces excellent results when properly used, and this requires the operator to be entirely familiar with its operation. Nonetheless, it is the operator's knowledge of hemodynamics and angiocardiographic techniques rather than the mechanical design of the injector that is most important. The various power injectors perform so similarly that there is no detectable difference in the results, although the newer instruments are more convenient and safer.

Manual injection is still widely used in selective coronary angiography because it is more convenient than pressure injection. A larger pressure can be achieved with a syringe, which has a small diameter. If the operator can exert a manual force of 20 lb on a syringe with a 1-in.^{2} piston, an injection pressure of 20 lb/in.^{2} can be delivered. With a smaller syringe, a greater pressure and flow rate can be achieved. For exmple, with a 1-mL tuberculin syringe, 1,000 lb/in.^{2} is attainable with manual injection.

However, larger amounts of contrast medium cannot be delivered quickly enough with manual injection, and this limitation led to the development of mechanical injectors using a lever principle. These injectors represented a significant improvement, since adequate (greater) injection pressures were generated. In addition, the contrast medium could be heated by a circulating water bath, and the film changer could be started any time between the beginning and the end of the injection by adjustable limit switches. With the development of these lever-powered injectors, it became necessary to use stainless-steel syringes that could be autoclaved and reused. The major disadvantage of the lever injector was the uncontrollable delivery rate, which varied largely depending on the force applied by the operator. The lever injectors were subsequently replaced by more sophisticated power injectors, which allowed selection of injection pressure and control of the delivery rate of contrast medium.

Pressure-Controlled Injectors

With pressure-controlled injectors, force is applied by mechanical, pneumatic, or hydraulic power. The delivery rate of contrast medium is determined by the applied force and the resistance, which is, in turn, determined by the internal diameter and length of the catheter and the viscosity of the contrast medium. Because the internal diameters of catheters and the viscosity of various contrast media differ, the delivery rates had to be determined by charts. Pressure-controlled injectors are rarely used now, having been largely replaced by flow-controlled injectors, which automatically adjust flow rates regardless of resistance. However, the results of pressure-controlled and flow-controlled injectors are identical, provided the operator understands the principles of angiography.

Flow-Controlled Injectors

Constant-volume or flow-controlled injectors have largely replaced pressure-controlled injectors because flow charts, nomograms, flow computers, and so on are not required to set the proper pressure to deliver a given volume. The rate of contrast medium delivery is independent of resistance and is adjusted automatically with a pressure range of ≤1,200 or less lb/in.^{2} (Fig 8–21).

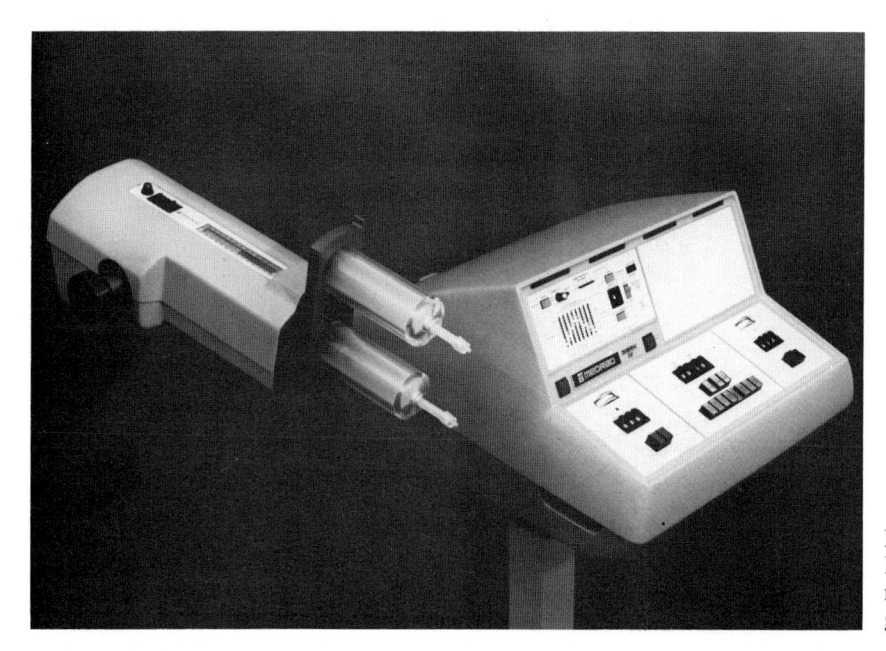

FIG 8–21.
Flow-controlled injector featuring a dual turret-type injector head for more expedient angiography.

Flow-controlled injectors use the rotary motion of an electric motor, converted to linear motion by a ball screw, to propel the plunger of the syringe. The speed of the motor is kept at a selected constant speed regardless of the resistance offered by the viscosity of contrast medium, the diameter of catheters, or other factors. This constant delivery rate is achieved by an electrical feedback system, which compares the selected motor speed with actual motor speed. The electronic loop compares the amplitude of a speed-dependent feedback voltage with the input voltage. When the amplitude of the feedback voltage drops, a higher voltage is applied to accelerate the motor. This injection system added safety and convenience to angiocardiography. Furthermore, these injectors use disposable plastic syringes, thereby minimizing air injection and virtually eliminating the electric shock hazards of a steel syringe.

Flow-controlled injectors are made by various manufacturers and are almost identical in function. Unfortunately, too many buttons are provided that may confuse the inexperienced operator. Consequently, the simplest unit with adequate pressure (at least 1,000 lb/in.^{2}) will yield the best results.

Pressure Limitation

A set of buttons is provided that allows preselection of the force of the motor expressed in pounds per square inch. If a lower injection pressure is selected, the desired flow rate will not be obtained; thus, the injector should always operate at maximal pressure. If the selected flow rate is too high, some of the catheters such as the soft balloon catheters will burst. Consequently, the operator has to determine bursting pressure for various flow rates. A chart of maximal tolerated flow rates should be made for each angiographic catheter and posted in the catheterization laboratory.

Rise Time

Rise time is an attempt of the manufacturer to provide a more gradual onset of injection. It is true that the motor will be up to full speed in a few milliseconds, but all injections have a very gradual onset because of the compliance of the plastic syringe, which expands, and the compression of the rubber piston. This is particularly pronounced with large syringes, which should not be used in pediatric angiography. The compliance factor also prolongs delivery of contrast medium after the motor has stopped, which is clearly visible on all angiograms. Because of the gradual onset and gradual termination of the injection, the rise time should always be zero, because a square wave injection cannot be obtained.

Phasic Dye Injection

The phasic delivery of contrast medium was first used at the University of Minnesota by Richards and Thal[70] for coronary angiography and later was used by others.[71, 72] The ECG controls the injection syringe, starting the injection during diastole and stopping it at the beginning of systole. Recently, multiple intermittent injections have been advocated, with cine recording as the patient is slowly rotated in a cradle.[73] There is no value in phasic dye injection for clinical angiography, and the purchase of an ECG module is unnecessary except for investigational purposes.

Complications Associated With Power Injection of Contrast Media

Many hazards, and some fatal mishaps, accompany the use of power injectors. The operator must be entirely familiar with these hazards, because they are avoidable; in the hands of a careful operator, the power syringe is a reliable and safe instrument.

Breakage of power cords, corrosion of leads, and consequent lack of electric or ground contact are malfunctions that can be eliminated only by preventive maintenance. Damaged power cords and plugs must be replaced, and ground connections have to be checked periodically. Human errors, as in setting dials, can be minimized but not eliminated by a thorough knowledge of the instrument and by elimination of all unnecessary switches and buttons.

Other complications and their prevention are as follows:

1. Injection of air. The injection of small air bubbles usually causes no clinical problems, but it may be serious during cerebral angiography. We demonstrated that small air emboli cause transient obstruction of capillaries. They become elastic cushions, which are compressed intermittently during systole and produce transient ischemia. Slowly they pass through the capillaries into the venous side of the circulation, and immediately afterward there is a markedly increased blood flow through the capillary bed because of reactive hyperemia. Ischemic changes because of the injection of small air bubbles are therefore only transient and not evident clinically.

   On the other hand, injection of a large amount of air has disastrous consequences. In one patient, 50 cc of air was injected into the ascending aorta, resulting in transient stroke. A technician had loaded the syringe with air instead of contrast medium, and the physician, unaware of the mistake, performed an ascending aortogram.

   In most modern power injectors, filling of the syringe is accomplished by activating either a toggle or a rocker switch into the "fill" position, allowing either contrast medium or, inadvertently, air, to be aspirated. If these switches are activated mistakenly, a large amount of air can be aspirated and subsequently injected.

   The inadvertent aspiration of air into a partially filled syringe is possible but rare. Unfortunately, the more common serious incidents occur when the technician places an empty syringe in the injector, having forgotten the entire loading procedure. The catheter is then connected to the empty syringe, and the entire volume of the air-filled syringe is injected, resulting in stroke or even death. Such serious complications can be prevented by:

   a. Adding a small amount of dye (e.g., green dye) to the contrast medium, making it easy to verify its presence in the injection syringe. (It would be more convenient if the manufacturers of contrast media would supply these agents as colored solution.)
   b. By connecting the injection syringe to transparent pressure tubing, which, in turn, is connected to the catheter. Before the catheter is connected to the pressure tubing, the syringe and tubing are purged of air, virtually eliminating the possibility of having the syringe loaded with air.
   c. By aspirating a small amount of blood into the syringe after the catheter has been connected. Because of its specific gravity, blood floats on top of the contrast medium.
   d. By using an air detection device. The development of a device to detect air bubbles is feasible but poses a major engineering problem and has been investigated only theoretically. If such a device were not sensitive enough, injection of a small amount of air would not be prevented, yet this amount would be significant in cerebral angiography. If the device were too sensitive, it could complicate angiography by shutdown of the injection. Furthermore, such sophisticated devices may fail while giving the operator a false sense of security.

   In most catheterization laboratories, the technician is responsible for both the loading and the injection procedures. However, the ultimate responsibility rests with the physician, who must check the injection syringe and injector settings before making an injection.

   The major error in construction of commercially available injectors is the loading of the syringe after it is in the injector. Although slightly less convenient, it is safer to load the syringe separately and place the loaded syringe in the injector.

2. Injection of an excessive amount of contrast medium. Modern contrast injectors use either a 100- or 130-mL syringe, and the entire volume may be injected because of human error or failure of the volume-control mechanism. The injection of such a large amount of contrast material into an infant may be fatal. This danger can be eliminated by not loading a dangerous volume of contrast medium, particularly for angiocardiography in infants. The volume loaded into a single syringe should not exceed 9 mL/kg of body weight of the patient. It is also advisable to use smaller syringes, as we have done in our injector.

   The volume control of the amount of contrast medium to be injected is achieved by various means: (1) mechanical stop; (2) electrical limits switches, which deenergize the motor or the solenoid valves; (3) a potentiometer and electronic circuit that sense the position of the plunger; and (4) a photoelectric chopper wheel that counts the rotation of the driving motor photoelectrically. Because electrical or electronic devices are more prone to failure than the mechanical stop, the latter is preferred. The injection of an excessive amount of contrast medium may still occur, however, because of human error.

ELECTRIC SHOCK HAZARDS IN THE CATHETERIZATION LABORATORY

With the introduction of a catheter or pacemaker into the heart, a conductive lead is created to the endocardium. Because a very small current may induce ventricular fibrillation (microshock), a basic understanding of this hazard is helpful in avoiding electrical accidents.

Basic Principles of Electrocution

When an alternating current is conducted through the heart, ventricular fibrillation may occur. The low frequency, 60 cycles/sec, is particularly dangerous to the heart.

The danger of producing ventricular fibrillation is directly related to *current flow,* which, in turn, is directly proportional to voltage and indirectly proportional to resistance. When electric current is applied to the outside of the body, current flow is largely limited by the skin resistance, which varies with moisture and electrolyte content but is approximately 500 Ω. Electrocution by the application of a current to the skin is referred to as macroshock. The danger of macroshock in the catheterization laboratory exists and is the same as the risk involved with the everyday use of electrical household appliances. Furthermore, because of the large cross-sectional area of the body and, consequently, the low current density, a comparatively large current flow (in the milliampere range) is required before ventricular fibrillation is induced. However, the "safe" current levels are unknown, because the available data are derived from animal experiments. There is undoubtedly a wide variation in the susceptibility to ventricular fibrillation induced by electric currents. The diseased human heart may be extremely sensitive to current flow and may even fibrillate spontaneously. With the new regulations regarding grounding, injuries from macroshock have been virtually eliminated.

When conductors such as saline-filled angiographic catheters and pacemakers are introduced into the heart, a low resistance path is created from the outside of the body and a danger of microshock results. Because of the small cross-sectional area of the conductor, the current density is high, and ventricular fibrillation may be induced in dogs with currents ranging from 20 to 160 μA.[74, 75] More recent information derived from human subjects indicates a higher threshold for ventricular fibrillation, perhaps justifying the present safety standard of 100 μA as permissible stray current.

An improperly grounded power injector may induce ventricular fibrillation, because it is an alternating current apparatus and is connected directly to a conductor (catheter) leading to the heart.

Prevention of Electric Shock Hazards

Safety can be achieved by proper grounding and by double insulation of the injector; the grounding approach has been more popular in the United States, whereas double insulation has been more common in Europe. Because of the excellent safety record of insulation achieved over the past 25 years in Europe, there is now a trend toward this approach in the United States as well.[76, 77]

A satisfactory ground from a three-pronged plug of the new safety design offers excellent protection against stray current. Grounding is particularly vulnerable to failure because of either corrosion or breakage of ground wires. A safe grounding system may also be negated by a negligent operator who uses "cheater" plugs. To make the grounding system more reliable, redundant grounding (an additional, separate ground wire connected to ground) may be used.

Various instruments in the catheterization laboratory are not always attached to the same ground. In modern design of catheterization laboratories, particular care is taken to assure a *common* ground, preventing potential differences from developing between various pieces of equipment. Older catheterization laboratories have been upgraded to fulfill this safety requirement.

Dangerous leakage of alternating current to ground can also be detected or interrupted by electronic devices (ground fault detectors and ground fault interrupters). This approach has been used in some injectors, but ground-fault alarms are triggered at a current flow above microshock levels.

The best protection can be achieved by an isolation transformer and double insulation, namely, insulating the electrical component and its housing. A major improvement in electric safety of power injectors was insulation by the use of disposable plastic syringes.

The quality of angiography does not depend on the type of injection equipment used, and the development of flow-control injectors has not improved angiography. However, flow-controlled injectors are more convenient and safer and have largely replaced pressure-controlled devices. An injector of the simplest design with a minimal number of modules is the most useful, because it tends to minimize human error, which increases with the number of unnecessary options. In spite of the improved control of

186   General Introduction

electrical shock hazards, power cords should be periodically inspected.

Hazards From Hydraulic Forces

Power injectors develop enormous pressures (800–1,500 lb/in.^{2}), which may damage vascular structures. With a delivery rate of 50 mL/sec, the contrast medium is discharged through a no. 8 catheter with a linear velocity of 13 m/sec. If such high-velocity jets are directed against vessel walls, the hydraulic forces may cause rupture, which may be fatal. The positive force of the jet decreases rapidly with distance because of mixing with the surrounding blood, so the damage depends not only on the force of injection but also on the distance between the catheter tip and the area of impact. Transmural injections, therefore, occur almost invariably when the catheter is in a wedged position and cannot recoil. The angiographer must understand this phenomenon.

What is the pressure at the catheter tip with high-power injections? This question is commonly asked, but it cannot be answered intelligently unless one specifies at what angle the pressure is measured. Pressure is defined as force applied per unit area (lb/in.^{2} or kg/cm^2). All forces, being vectors, have not only magnitude but also direction. If a catheter is connected to a power syringe that delivers a certain pressure (indicated in the diagram in Fig 8–22 as hydrostatic pressure), and if there is no flow, the lateral pressures in the attached catheter will be identical to the hydrostatic pressure. Of course, the same pressure relation is present at the catheter tip (see Fig 8–22,A). The high pressure from the injector is transmitted to the catheter tip if it is held firmly against a vascular structure, eliminating flow and resulting in vascular perforation. The addition of side holes decreases these forces and increases safety. A catheter tip with side holes may be entrapped between trabeculations, which is also dangerous. A small test injection should be made before injecting the entire volume of contrast material.

In a flowing system, the lateral pressure in the catheter gradually decreases toward the top, where all pressure energy has been converted to kinetic energy (Fig 8–22,B). Consequently, the lateral pressure at the catheter tip is zero. The lateral pressures indicated in the diagram also explains why a catheter tends to burst near its hub, safely outside the body, although with wire mesh–reinforced catheters, rupture may occur inside the body at a distal site where there is no wire enforcement.

At the tip of the catheter, the high-velocity jet carries great kinetic energy, which is rapidly dissipated with distance by interaction of the jet with the surrounding blood (jet entrainment). The forces in the jet may vary from markedly positive to markedly negative. If pressures are measured in the direction of the jet, kinetic energy is being converted into static pressure, and a positive pressure is recorded by a manometer (Fig 8–22,C). If the pressure is measured at a right angle to the jet, it is markedly negative. The sum of all these forces is zero (the law of preservation of energy).

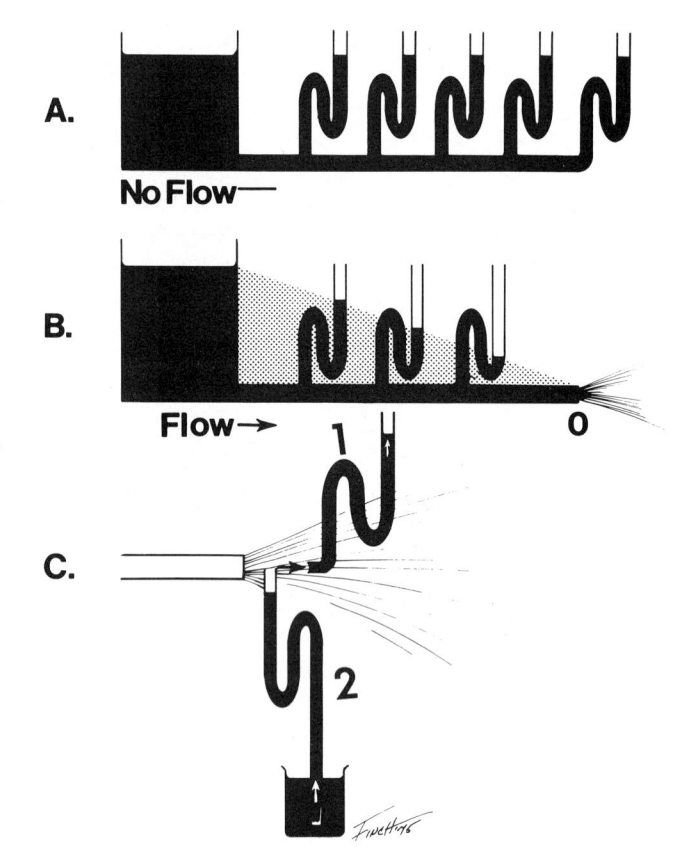

FIG 8–22.
Diagram showing pressure relations of a catheter during power injection. **A,** with no flow in the catheter, pressure is transmitted from the reservoir to the catheter tip as indicated by equal levels in the manometers along catheter course. **B,** when flow occurs through the catheter, lateral pressure gradually decreases along the catheter course to a level of zero at the catheter tip. **C,** pressures in catheter jet; manometer *(1)* against the jet records a positive pressure; monometer *(2)* at right angle to the jet, a markedly negative pressure.

Damage may occur from either the positive or the negative forces of jets.

If the catheter lies freely in the vascular system, it can recoil and move away from the vascular wall. On the other hand, if recoil is prevented for some reason (wedge injection), the catheter jet cuts through the vessel wall and results in extravasation. In angiography, such situations may occur under the following circumstances:

1. Wedging of side-hole catheters in arteries or veins (coronary sinus, peripheral pulmonary artery, my-

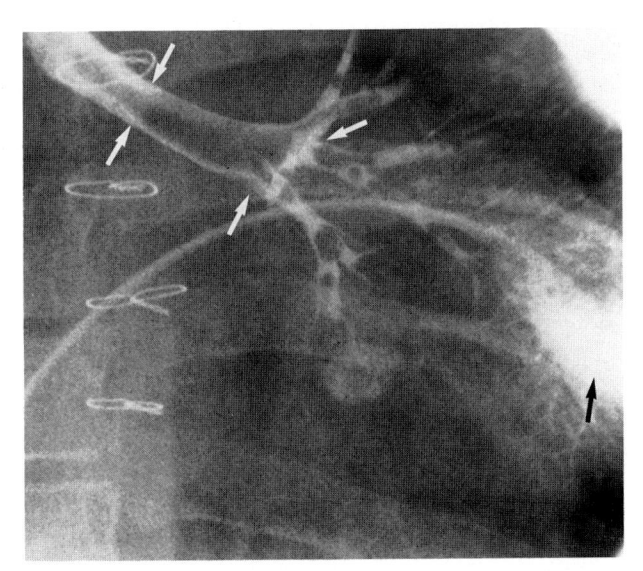

FIG 8–23.
Pulmonary venogram with catheter wedged; rupture of pulmonary parenchyma *(black arrow)* and filling of bronchial tree *(white arrows)*. No clinical sequelae.

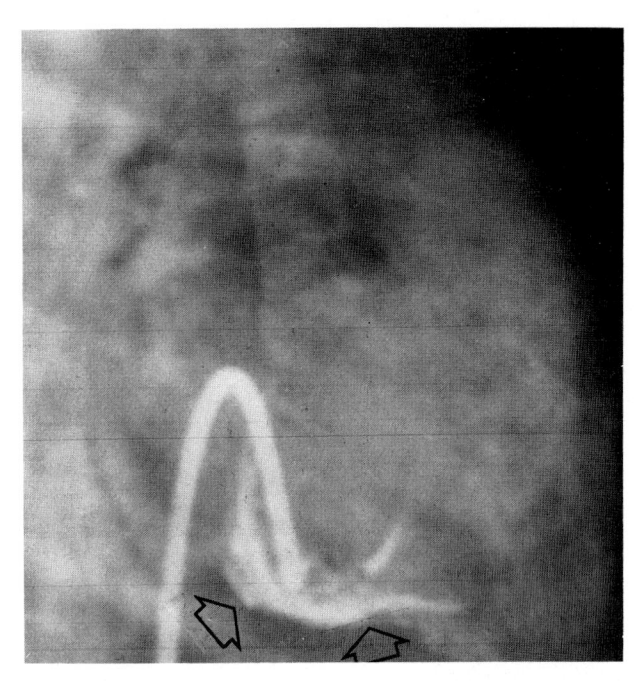

FIG 8–24.
Left ventriculogram in lateral projection showing persistent stain in the left ventricle *(arrows)* characteristic of subendocardial deposition of contrast medium. The incidence has decreased with use of balloon catheters.

ocardium, etc.). In spite of numerous side holes, disruption of the vascular structure may occur by the positive forces of the jets.
2. Entrapment of side-hole catheters in trabeculations of the ventricle and bracing of the catheter against the heart to prevent its recoil.
3. End-hole catheters, needles, or cannulas held firmly at a right angle to vascular walls.
4. Wedging of catheters in the pulmonary veins (Fig 8–23).

Such vascular complications are evidenced angiographically as subintimal, or, more commonly, subadventitial, staining with contrast medium. Occasionally the staining will be perivascular, indicating complete disruption of the intima and media. Within the heart, contrast medium may be deposited in various layers, resulting in characteristic angiographic findings. Subendocardial deposition of contrast medium is the most common, usually resulting from the jets from one or two of the side holes. Such a complication is usually not clinically significant and is evidenced angiographically as an irregular "stain" (Fig 8–24). Intramyocardial injections of contrast medium are recognizable by the larger "stain" and immediate filling of cardiac veins. Opacification of the coronary sinus always occurs (Fig 8–25). Usually this complication is well tolerated, but in very sick infants, it may be fatal.

The catheter jet may traverse the myocardium, not filling cardiac veins, and create a subepicardial deposition. Radiographically, the contrast deposit is a smooth collection outlining the myocardium (Fig 8–26). At postmortem examination, blood can be found subepipericardially, giving the appearance of a "bruise." Sometimes, endocardial, myocardial, and epicardial injection occur simultaneously.

The contrast jets may traverse the endocardium, myocardium, and epicardium and opacify only the pericardial space. This complication is easily recognized angiographically (Fig 8–27) and may cause cardiac tamponade. With intrapericardial injections, a further increase in fluid may occur because of the high osmotic pressure of the contrast medium. Patients with this complication should be carefully watched, and pericardiocentesis should not be delayed if tamponade develops. Particularly in patients with aortic stenosis, acute pericardial effusion is not well tolerated. Transmural injection may also occur through the ventricular septum and mimic a ventricular septal defect, with which it must not be confused. Such a transseptal injection usually causes no clinical problems.

The catheter itself may cause perforations. At postmortem examinations, perforations of cardiac chambers sometimes are found after cardiac catheterization. Perforation of a semilunar valve is rare, most often occurring when guidewires are advanced through a catheter that is firmly braced against the aortic valve (Fig 8–28). As the guidewire exits from the catheter tip, it acts as a stylet, causing valve perforation, and the catheter is then advanced through the hole. Angiographically this complica-

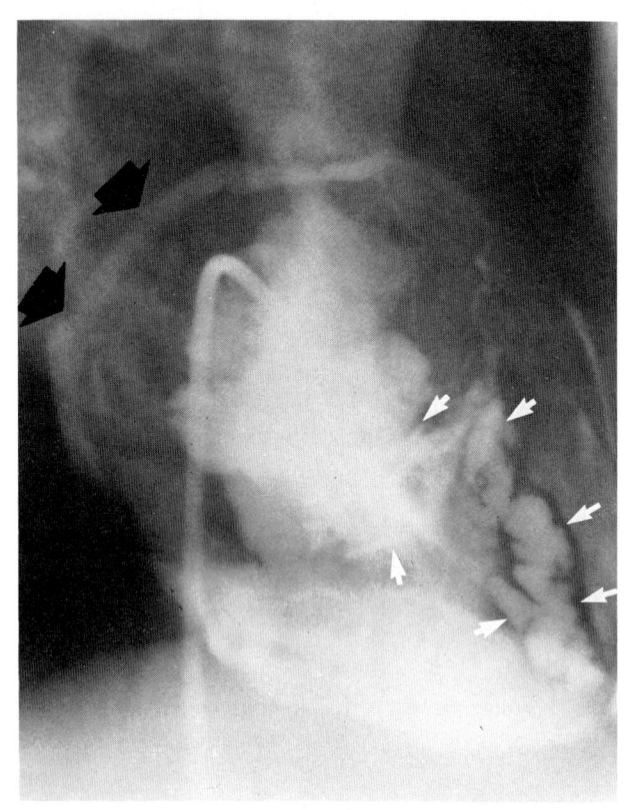

FIG 8–25.
Left ventriculogram in lateral projection showing intramyocardial injection of contrast medium. Large intramyocardial stain *(white arrows),* immediate filling of cardiac veins, and opacification of coronary sinus *(black arrows).*

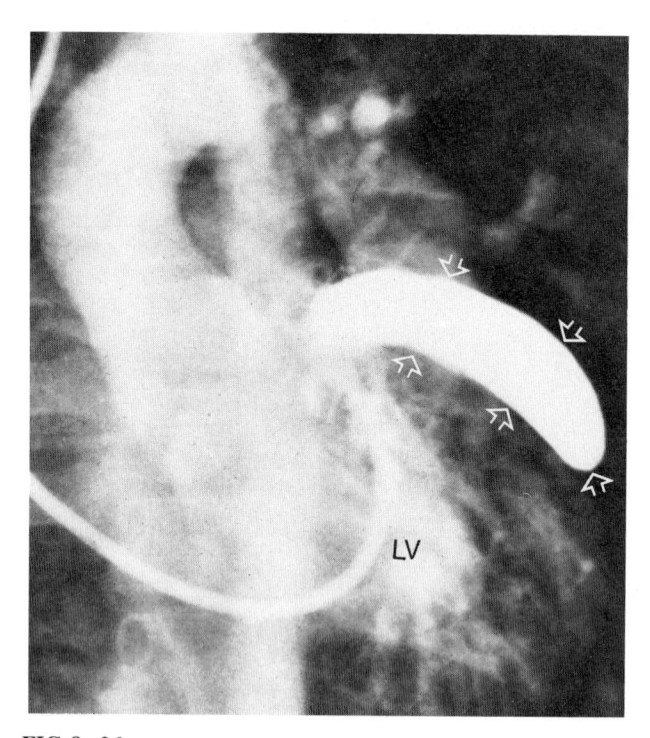

FIG 8–26.
Left ventriculogram showing typical subepicardial deposition of contrast medium *(arrows).* Epicardium is stripped from myocardium. Smooth pocket of contrast medium is formed. It is usually possible to aspirate the contrast from subepicardial collections if the catheter tip lies in subepicardial position. (see also Fig 8–14).

tion is recognizable by a regurgitating round jet (in both projections) at the base of the aortic cusp (see Fig 8–28).

Another type of vascular injury is caused by the negative force of the jet. It occurs whenever a forceful injection is made through a needle, cannula, or open-end catheter through an artery or a vein. This complication can be seen when contrast medium is injected through a plastic sheath in retrograde fashion through the femoral arteries or the brachial arteries, as in retrograde brachial angiography (Fig 8–29). It is most commonly encountered in children because their arteries are more collapsible. It occurs whenever very high injection pressures or flow rates corresponding to 1,000 lb/in.^{2} are used.

The mechanism of this injury has been termed jet collapse.[78] The jet coming from a needle or open-end catheter produces a negative force that pulls the vessel wall into the jet (Fig 8–30). As soon as the vascular wall is pulled into the jet, which can be seen angiographically as narrowing (Fig 8–31), it is pushed away by the positive forces. As soon as it is pushed away, it is pulled into the jet again. This to-and-fro motion of the vascular wall is fast, so that the wall flutters. If the injection force is very high, the jet cuts through the vessel wall when it is pulled into the jet, and extravasation of blood occurs. The jet becomes a "hydraulic knife," making a longitudinal cut in the intima and media. Subadventitial extravasation of contrast medium occurs (Fig 8–32).

Vascular jet collapse can occur in the tubelike vessels such as the iliac artery, aorta, and vena cava. During digital angiography, which requires injection into the superior vena cava, rupture and extravasation has occurred because of jet collapse using open-end catheters. Pigtail catheters, which mimimize the jet effect from the end hole, eliminate such complications. However, in newborns, aortography is usually performed through an end-hole umbilical catheter, and if high flow rates are used, the collapsible abdominal aorta may be pulled into the jet. Extravasation may result (see Fig 8–32).

Because of these considerable positive and negative forces of catheter jets, end-hole catheters should not be used unless they have a pigtail configuration and additional side holes. The catheter tip should always move freely in the heart before injection of contrast medium, because trabecular entrapment of an end-occluded catheter with side holes may also cause extravasation. Balloon catheters cannot readily become entrapped in trabeculations, eliminat-

Angiography 189

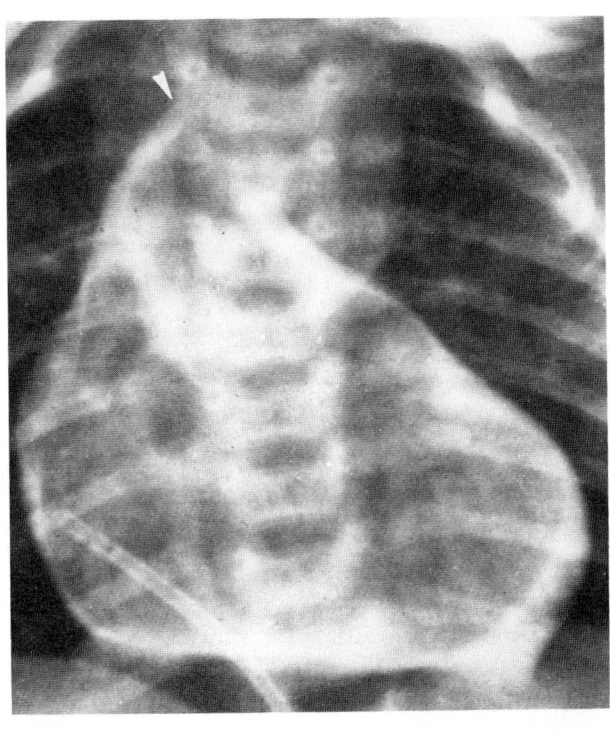

FIG 8–27.
Transventricular injection of contrast medium into pericardial space in anteroposterior projection. Note the high attachment of the pericardial sac at the level of the innominate artery *(arrow)*.

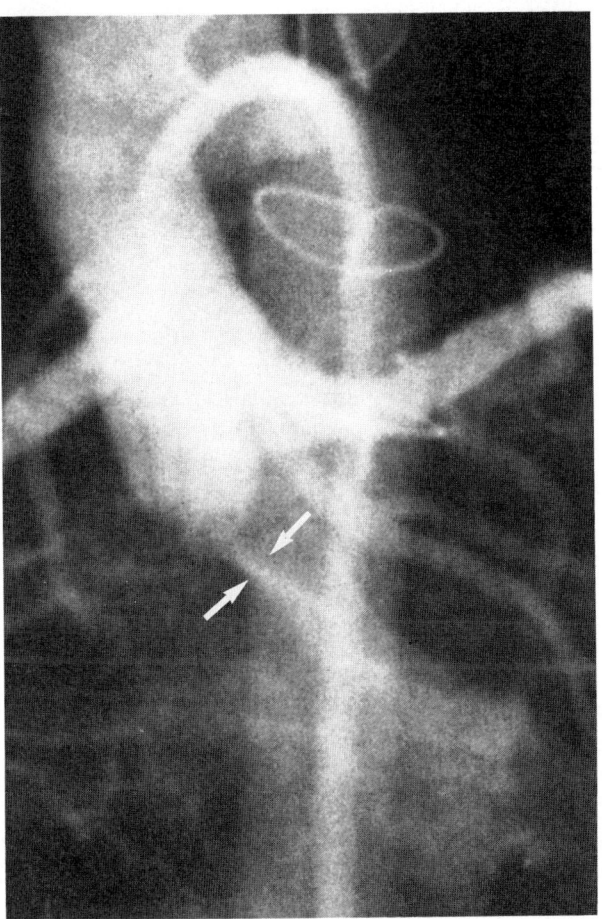

A. B.

FIG 8–28.
Perforation by catheter. **A,** aortogram in anteroposterior projection shows narrow round regurgitating jet; regurgitation occurs in the nonappositional portion at base of right aortic cusp. This appearance is characteristic of catheter perforation. **B,** postmortem specimen of same patient; perforation in the right cusp exactly the size of catheter.

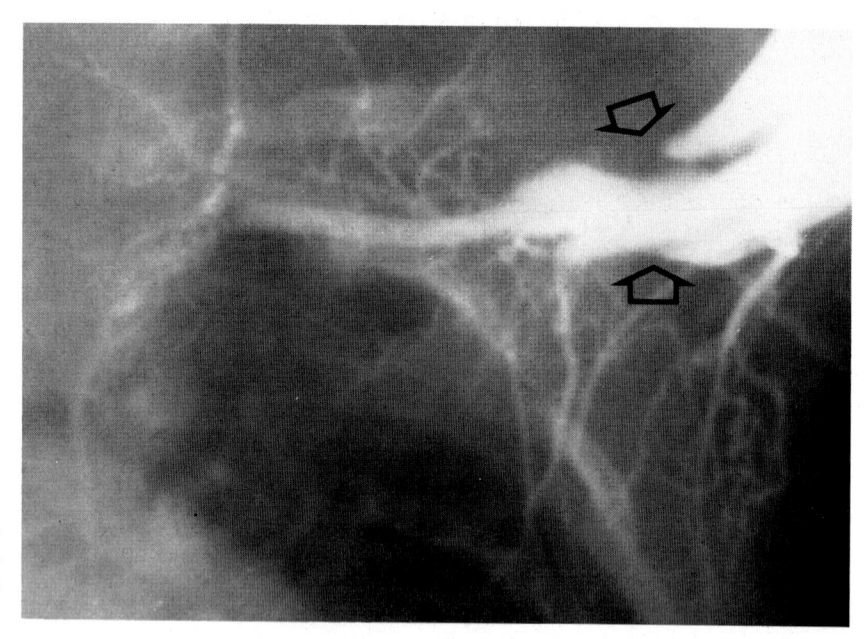

FIG 8–29.
Retrograde brachial angiogram in anteroposterior projection shows extensive paravascular extravasation as a result of jet collapse and rupture *(arrows)* of the axillary artery.

ing this complication. However, if used uninflated, they too may perforate the heart (see the earlier section on catheters).

Catheter whip does not result in vascular damage. In air, with high-power injections, catheters whip considerably, but in blood, the whipping motion is markedly dampened, so the forces are minimal.

PRACTICAL HINTS

Because angiocardiography is generally performed to evaluate the anatomy rather than the physiology of cardiac disease, dense opacification of cardiac chambers and great vessels is required. Angiographic density depends largely on the delivery rate of contrast medium and on the extent of dilution by blood flow: The greater the delivery rate, the denser the angiogram, and the higher the blood flow, the poorer the opacification. To perform adequate angiocardiography, the angiographer must have a knowledge of the physiology, particularly the speed of blood flow. Patients with a high cardiac output and tachycardia require a faster rate of injection than do patients with a low cardiac output.

The size of the chamber or vessel to be opacified needs to be considered also, since the radiographic density also depends on size: The larger the opacified structure, the higher the radiographic density. Conversely, a very high concentration of contrast medium is necessary to see smaller arteries, such as the coronary arteries. Under those circumstances, the contrast medium is better delivered selectively into the artery rather than into the aorta, where it is diluted.

Radiographic density depends also on the amount of contrast medium injected. When cardiac chambers and great vessels are opacified, the injected opaque medium is diluted by the blood in the chamber. Because cardiac chambers and ventricles do not empty completely during systole, residual contrast remains, so there is an increase in concentration if the contrast is injected over several cardiac cycles. Another reason to extend the injection over several cycles is the convenience of viewing cine angiograms.

The amount of contrast medium required is also determined by the size of the chamber to be opacified. Dilated ventricles and great arteries contain more blood; consequently, more contrast medium is necessary to counteract the effects of dilution. Small hypoplastic chambers can be opacified with only a few milliliters of opaque medium.

The rapid delivery of contrast media into ventricles usually causes premature ventricular contractions. The mechanical irritation of the endocardium by contrast jets causes these arrhythmias, which are beneficial angiographically because during this time there is virtually no cardiac output and dilution is thus minimized. On the other hand, no hemodynamic conclusions can be made, because the physiology has been disturbed. For physiological studies, the contrast agent should be injected into the atria, where arrhythmias are not induced. Generally, physiologic conclusions reached from angiography are inferior to those of careful cardiac catheterization because of the vasodilatory and myocardial depressive effect of the contrast medium. Hemodynamic data should therefore always be obtained before angiography.

Currently, angiography is the best technique to evalu-

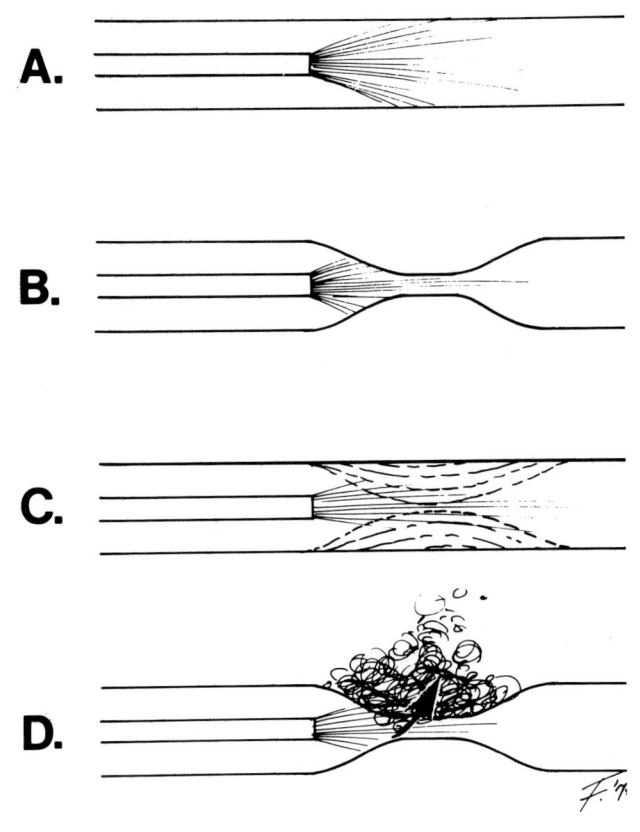

FIG 8–30.
Diagram of mechanism of vascular jet collapse. **A,** jet of contrast medium injected. **B,** the jet causes the vessel wall to collapse because of the negative forces. **C,** the intermittent negative and positive forces result in flutter of arterial wall. **D,** the high-velocity jet may cause disruption of the vessel and extravasation.

ate atrioventricular valve insufficiency. For this purpose, the catheter must be positioned in a "quiet" area in the ventricle, and the injection must be made slowly to minimize the jet irritation of the myocardium. Unfortunately, extrasystoles cannot always be avoided, but nevertheless, approximations of the degree of regurgitation can be obtained.

The Dose of Contrast Medium

Generally, infants have a higher blood volume than older children and adolescents, and consequently the volume of contrast injected per unit of body weight can be higher. The dose of contrast medium is usually calculated in milliliters per kilogram. Manufacturers invariably recommend a dose that is inadequate for satisfactory cardioangiography. In our experience with 36,000 angiocardiograms, an injection of 2 mL/kg delivered approximately over 1 second almost invariably results in excellent opacification of cardiac chambers and great vessels in

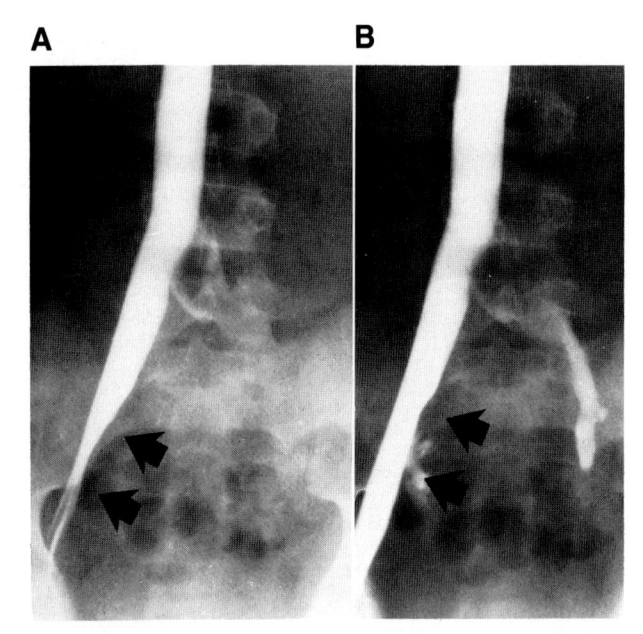

FIG 8–31.
A, injection of contrast medium into the femoral vein through a plastic sheath. Marked narrowing *(arrows)* of femoral vein from jet collapse. **B,** after termination of the injection, the vein *(arrows)* resumes its normal size.

infants. Previously, only 1 to 1.5 mL/kg was used, and this gave less satisfactory results. In spite of this increase in dose, the mortality rate in infants in the cardiac catheterization laboratory decreased from 3.4% to less than 0.5%. A total dose of 7 mL/kg is commonly reached in our patients, which is well tolerated. Our average dose is 5.5 mL/kg. There was only 1 death in 36,000 angiograms that could be attributed to the contrast agent itself; however, this death was not related to an overdose of the agent.

These are only general guidelines for infants. Older children and adults are less tolerant of contrast media, and such a large dose not only is unnecessary but may cause complications. In older children, 1.5 mL/kg and, in adults, 1 mL/kg yields adequate results. The safe dose is unknown but probably significantly lower than in infants.

The amount of contrast medium and injection speed are governed by many factors, such as speed of blood flow, chamber size, condition of the patient, renal status, and number of injections contemplated. One should not compromise the diagnostic yield of angiography by not using an adequate amount of contrast medium. On the other hand, in many cases, a diagnosis can be made with very small injections. Angiographic injections should not be carried out in rapid succession and angiography is said to be much more risky in cyanotic patients, but this has not been our experience. Optimal results and safety are ac-

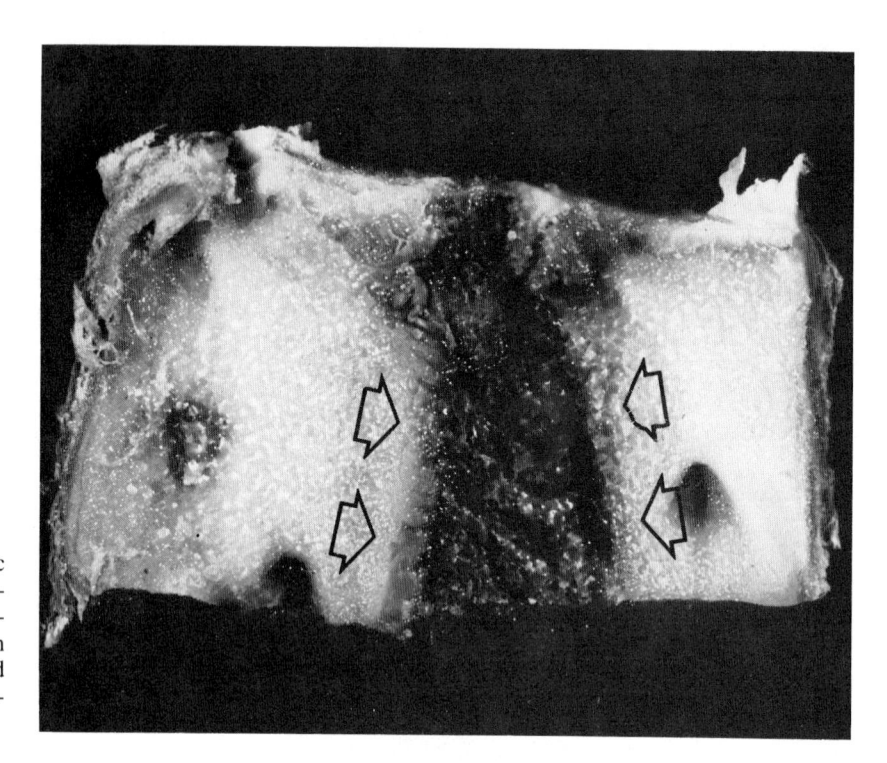

FIG 8–32.
Postmortem specimen of an infantile thoracic aorta after angiography with an open-end umbilical catheter. Extravasation of contrast medium occurred. Microscopically, a section in this area showed disruption of the intima and media. Open arrows point to vascular disruption.

complished if an experienced radiologist assists the cardiologist in the catheterization laboratory.

CONCLUSION

Angiography is the most invasive definitive test performed before cardiac operations. Because of its potential hazard, it should be carried out only by an experienced team. The radiologist should be largely responsible for the angiographic aspects of cardiac catheterization.

During angiocardiography, fluids should be given to expedite the excretion of contrast media and minimize renal damage, which is rare in the pediatric age group. It is wise to perform a small test injection, which will also give an idea about the expected flow and possible recoil of the

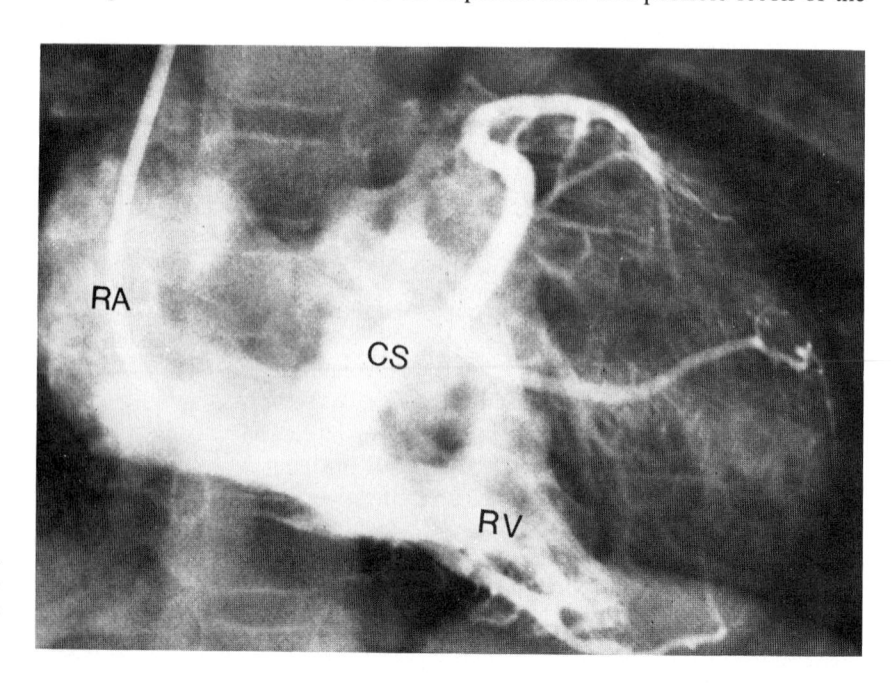

FIG 8–33.
Right ventriculogram. Catheter recoiled during the injection and entered coronary sinus *(CS)*. This represents an unavoidable complication.

catheter. Nevertheless, sometimes, complications cannot be avoided even with a test injection, because the catheter may become dislodged during the injection. (Fig 8–33)

REFERENCES

1. Bleichröder F: Intra-Arterielle Therapie, *Klin Wschr* 49:1503, 1912.
2. Forssmann W: Die Sondierung des rechten Herzens, *Klin Wschr* 8:2085, 1929.
3. Forssmann W: Uber Kontrastdarstellung der Höhlen des lebenden rechten Herzens und der Lungenschlagader, *Münch Med Wschr* 78:489, 1931.
4. Moniz E: Angiopneumographie, *Presse Med* 39:996, 1931.
5. Heuser C: Arteriografia directa aortografia por impregnacion del reticuloendotelium, vasos grafias del pulmon por medio del sondeo de la Auricula Derecha, *Rev Assoc Argent Microbiol* 46:1119, 1932.
6. Conte E, Costa A: Angiopneumography, *Radiology* 21:461, 1933.
7. Ravina A: L'exploration radiologique des vaisseaux pulmonaires par l'injection de substances de contraste, *Progres Med* 1701, 1934.
8. Ameuille P, Ronneaux G, Hinault V, et al: Remarques sur quelques cas d'arteriographie pulmonaire chez l'homme vivant, *Bull Mém Soc Med Hôp Paris* 52:729, 1936.
9. Cournand A, Ranges HA: Catheterization of the right auricle in man, *Proc Soc Exp Biol Med* 46:462, 1941.
10. Goodale WT, Lubin M, Banfield WG, et al: Catheterization of the coronary sinus, right heart, and other viscera with a modified venous catheter, *Science* 109:117, 1949.
11. Jonsson G, Broden B, Karnell J: Selective angiocardiography, *Acta Radiol* 32:486, 1949.
12. Robb GP, Steinberg I: A practical method of visualization of the chambers of the heart, the pulmonary circulation, and the great blood vessels in man, *J Clin Invest* 17:507, 1938.
13. Rodriguez-Alvarez A, Martinez de Rodriguez G: Studies in angiocardiography: the problems involved in the rapid, selective, and safe injections of radiopaque materials: development of a special catheter for selective angiography, *Am Heart J* 53:841, 1957.
14. Chavez I, Dorbecker N, Celis A: Direct intracardiac angiography: its diagnostic value, *Am Heart J* 33:560, 1947.
15. Duffy BJ Jr: The clinical use of polyethylene tubing for intravenous therapy: a report of seventy-two cases, *Ann Surg* 130:929, 1949.
16. Helmsworth JA, McGuire J, Felson B: Arteriography of the aorta and its branches by means of the polyethylene catheter, *Am J Roentgenol Radium Ther Nucl Med* 64:196, 1950.
17. Pierce EC: Percutaneous femoral artery catheterization in man with special reference to aortography, *Surg Gynecol Obstet* 93:56, 1951.
18. Seldinger SI: Visualization of aortic and arterial occlusion by percutaneous puncture or catheterization of peripheral arteries, *Angiology* 8:73, 1957.
19. Arner O, Edholm P, Odman P: Percutaneous selective angiography of the internal mammary artery, *Acta Radiol* 51:433, 1959.
20. Odman P: Thoracic aortography by means of a radiopaque polythene catheter inserted percutaneously, *Acta Radiol* 45:117, 1956.
21. Odman P: Percutaneous selective angiography of the main branches of the aorta: preliminary report, *Acta Radiol* 45:1, 1956.
22. Odman P: Percutaneous selective angiography of the superior mesenteric artery, *Acta Radiol* 51:25, 1959.
23. Odman P: The radiopaque polythene catheter, *Acta Radiol* 52:52, 1959.
24. Dotter CT, Straube KR: Flow guided catheterization, *Am J Roentgenol Radium Ther Nucl Med* 88:27, 1962.
25. Swan HJC, Ganz W, Forrester J, et al: Catheterization of the heart in man with use of a flow-directed balloon-tipped catheter, *N Engl J Med* 283:447, 1970.
26. Gonzales LL, Lewis CM, Wiot JF: A study of factors influencing delivery rates of contrast media during arteriography: preliminary observations of a new contrast medium, *Angiology* 15:283, 1964.
27. Fischer HW, Roller G, Hubbard PG: An analysis of several factors influencing injection rates in angiography, *Radiology* 83:396, 1964.
28. Bove AA, Gimenez JL: Computer analysis of flow characteristics of injection catheters, *Invest Radiol* 3:427, 1968.
29. Williamson DE: Experimental determination of flow equation of catheters for cardiology, *Am J Roentgenol Radium Ther Nucl Med* 94:704, 1965.
30. Susman N, Diboll WB Jr: Fluid dynamics in the tip of the multiholed angiographic catheter. *Radiology* 92:843, 1969.
31. Bove AA, Ziskin MC, Mulchin WL: Ultrasonic detection of in-vivo cavitation and pressure effects of high-speed injections through catheters. *Invest. Radiol* 4:236, 1969.
32. LePage JR, Pratt AD Jr, Sorondo E: Intravascular catheter rupture, *Angiology* 24:62, 1973.
33. Nejad MS, Klaper MA, Steggerda FR, et al: Clotting on the outer surfaces of vascular catheters, *Radiology* 91:248, 1968.
34. Amplatz K: A simple non-thrombogenic coating, *Invest Radiol* 6:280, 1971.
35. Amplatz K, Amplatz C, Johnson BS, et al: A new simple test for thrombogenicity, *Radiology* 120: 53–55, 1976.
36. Durst S, Johnson BS, Amplatz K: The effect of silicone coatings on thrombogenicity, *Am J Roentgenol Radium Ther Nucl Med* 120:904, 1974.
37. Durst S, Leslie J, Moore R, et al: A comparison of the thrombogenicity of commercially available catheters, *Radiology* 113:599, 1974.
38. Glancy JJ, Fishbone G, Heinz ER: Nonthrombogenic arterial catheters, *Am J Roentgenol Radium Ther Nucl Med* 111:43, 1970.
39. Ovitt TW, Durst S, Moore R, et al: Guide wire thrombogenicity and its reduction, *Radiology* 111:43, 1974.

40. Schlossman D: Thrombogenic properties of vascular catheter materials in vivo: the differences between materials, *Acta Radiol* 14:186, 1973.
41. Formanek G, Frech RS, Amplatz K: Arterial thrombus formation during clinical percutaneous catheterization, *Circulation* 41:833, 1970.
42. Cramer R: A simple nonthrombogenic coating: experimental and clinical studies, Thesis, Saint Paul, Minn, 1972, University of Minnesota.
43. Cramer R, Moore R, Amplatz K: Reduction of the surgical complication rate by the use of hypothrombogenic catheter coating, *Radiology* 109:585, 1973.
44. Lewis RC, Glueck HI: A micromethod for determining clotting time using capillary blood and siliconized tubes, *J Lab Clin Med* 52:299, 1958.
45. Sawyer PN, Brattain WH, Boddy PJ: Electrochemical precipitation of human blood cells and its possible relation to intravascular thrombosis, *Proc Natl Acad Sci USA* 51:428, 1964.
46. Sawyer PN, Wu KT, Wesolowski SA, et al: Electrochemical precipitation of blood cells on metal electrodes: an aid in the selection of vascular prostheses, *Proc Natl Acad Sci USA* 53:294, 1965.
47. Sawyer PN: The electrochemical metabolism of the blood vessel wall: its possible role in myocardial infarction. Reprinted from the Henry Ford Hospital International Symposium: *The etiology of myocardial infarction,* Boston, 1968, Little, Brown.
48. Bernstein EF, Evans RL: Low-molecular-weight dextran, *JAMA* 174:1417, 1960.
49. Dean RE, Andrew JH, Read RC: The red cell factor in renal damage from angiographic media: perfusion studies of the in situ canine kidney with cellular and acellular perfusates, *JAMA* 187:27, 1964.
50. Lindgren P et al: Intravascular erythrocyte aggregation after intravenous injection of contrast media, *Acta Radiol* 2:334, 1964.
51. Sessions RT, Killan DA, Foster JH: Low molecular weight dextran as a protective agent against the toxic effects of Urokon, *Am Surg* 28:455, 1962.
52. Whetsell WO Jr, Lockard I: Responses to intracarotid hypaque in rabbits with and without low molecular weight dextran, *J Neuropathol Exp Neurol* 25:283, 1966.
53. Wiedeman MP: Influence of low molecular weight dextran on vascular and intravascular responses to contrast media, *Am J Roentgenol Radium Ther Nucl Med* 92:682, 1964.
54. Emmons PR, Harrison MJG, Honour AJ, et al: Effect of dipyridamole on human platelet behaviour, *Lancet* 2:603, 1965.
55. Smythe HA, Ogryzlo MA, Murphy EA, et al: The effect of sulfinpyrazone (Antruran) on platelet economy and blood coagulation in man, *Can Med Assoc J* 92:818, 1965.
56. Weiss HJ, Aledort LM, Kochwa S: The effect of salicylates on the hemostatic properties of platelets in man, *J Clin Invest* 47:2169, 1968.
57. Lipton MJ, Doherty P, et al: [111]Indium-oxine labelled platelets for diagnosing vascular thrombus in patients, *Radiology* 129:363, 1978.
58. Gott VL, Whiffen JD, Dutton RC: Heparin binding on colloidal graphite surfaces, *Science* 142:1297, 1963.
59. Lund G, Einzin S, Rysavy JA, et al: The role of ischemia in contrast induced renal damage: an experimental study, *Circulation* 69(4):783–789, 1984.
60. Grainger RG: Formulation and clinical introduction of low osmolality contrast media, *Radiology* 21:261, 1981.
61. Higgins C, Sovak M, Schmidt W, et al: *Invest Radiol* 15:39–46, 1980.
62. Ovitt T, Rizk G, Frech RS, et al: Electrocardiographic changes in selective coronary arteriography: the importance of ions, *Radiology* 104:705, 1972.
63. Oler R, Miller J, Jackson D, et al: Angiographically induced renal failure and its radiographic detection, *Am J Radiol* 126:1039, 1976.
64. Schwartz RD, Rubin JE, Leeming BW, et al: Renal failure following major angiography, *Am J Med* 65:31, 1978.
65. Shipps FC: An automatic injector for angiography, *Am J Roentgenol Radium Ther Nucl Med* 80:982, 1962.
66. Shipps FC: Physical aspects of high pressure angiography, *Am J Roentgenol Radium Ther Nucl Med* 88:93, 1962.
67. Amplatz K: A vascular injector with program selector, *Radiology* 75:955, 1960.
68. Amplatz K: Automatic injection syringe and cassette changer for cerebral angiography, *JAMA* 183:430, 1963.
69. Viamonte M Jr, Hobbs J: Automatic electric injector: development to prevent electromechanical hazards of selective angiocardiography, *Invest Radiol* 2:262, 1967.
70. Richards LS, Thal AP: Phasic dye injection control system for coronary arteriography in human, *Surg Gynecol Obstet* 107:739, 1958.
71. Hettler MG: Angiographic problems and possibilities: III, controlled cardiac phase angiography as a basis of exact morphological and functional blood vessel diagnosis, *Fortschr Röntgenstr* 92:420, 1960.
72. Olin T: *Studies in angiographic technique,* Stockholm, 1963, Lund, Sweden, 1963, Hakon Ohlssons Boktryckerei.
73. Schad N, McKnight R, Kunz H, et al: Superselective left atrial cineangiocardiography, *Invest Radiol* 9:133, 1974.
74. Starmer CF, Whalen RE, McIntosh HD: Hazards of electric shock in cardiology, *Am J Cardiol* 14:537, 1964.
75. Starmer CF, Whalen RE, McIntosh HD: Determination of leakage currents in medical equipment, *Am J Cardiol* 17:437, 1966.
76. Danziel CF: Electric shock hazard, *IEEE Spectrum* 9:41, 1972.
77. Dalziel CF, Lee WR: Reevaluation of lethal electric currents, *IEEE Trans Ind Gen Appl* 4:467, 676, 1968.
78. Doumanian HO, Amplatz K: Vascular jet collapse in selective angiocardiography, *Am J Roentgenol Radium Ther Nucl Med* 100:344, 1967.

CHAPTER 9

Cardiac Ultrasound

G. Wayne Moore, B.Sc., M.B.A.

Steven C. Cassidy, M.D.

Wayne H. Franklin, M.D.

Hugh D. Allen, M.D.

Cardiac ultrasound has become an important method of imaging the heart and major blood vessels to determine structure and function. In this chapter two major aspects of cardiac ultrasound are described. First the physical principles of ultrasound are presented, and then the techniques of performing cardiac ultrasound to assess cardiac malformation are described. Details of ultrasound findings of individual cardiac anomalies are not described in this chapter but in the chapters that follow.

PHYSICAL PRINCIPLES OF ULTRASOUND

The ultrasound spectrum of frequencies is defined as sound beyond human perception and begins at 20 kHz (2×10^3 Hz or cycles per second) (Fig 9–1). For diagnostic ultrasound applications, frequencies ranging from 2 MHz (2×10^6 Hz) up to 30 MHz are used. An inverse relationship between frequency and depth of penetration exists. This inverse relationship defines the appropriate frequency to use for a given clinical application. Higher frequencies provide better spatial resolution than lower frequencies as demonstrated in the equation:

$$\lambda = \frac{c}{f}$$

where λ = wavelength,
c = speed of sound in the medium (in soft tissue about 1,540 m/sec), and
f = the frequency.
The higher the operating frequency, the smaller the wavelength, and, consequently, the better the imaging resolution. Therefore, in diagnostic imaging applications such as pediatric echocardiography, frequencies as high as 7.5 MHz are often used, whereas in adult echocardiographic applications where greater penetration is needed, frequencies as low as 2.0 MHz are used.

An ultrasound wave is created by electronically stimulating a piezoelectric crystal, which is usually made from a synthetic ceramic material such as lead zirconate titanate or barium titanate. This piezoelectric (from the Greek, meaning pressure/electric) material has the property of generating an acoustic pressure wavefront when excited by an electronic pulse. Conversely, when it is strained by a pressure pulse, it will generate a small electrical signal (Fig 9–2). The wavefront is a series of compressions and rarefactions similar in nature to the audible sound pulses created by a speaker transmitting music. When a strong bass note is applied to a speaker, its cone moves toward the listener and the note is "pushed," or compressed, toward the listener. As the note is lowered in intensity or removed, the speaker cone retracts and the acoustic wavefront becomes a rarefaction (minimal compression). The physical principle of the piezoelectric crystal is known as "transduction." From the transduction process, we have the term "transducer," which is applied to a multitude of ultrasound probes. These probes or transducers can consist of either a single continuous aperture piezoelectric crystal or an array of small crystals (also known as "elements"), which form a sampled aperture, connected electronically.

When the piezoelectric crystal is pulsed electronically, it exhibits the same basic characteristics as a bell being struck by a hammer. As a bell is struck, it rings and con-

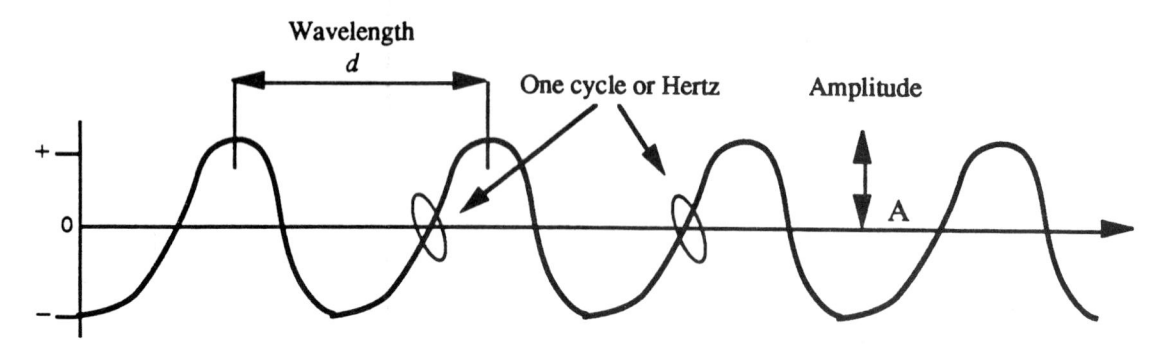

FIG 9–1.
Various components of a periodic wave. A = amplitude; d = wavelength.

tinues to ring for a period of time after being struck. This "ring-down" time is an undesirable condition when ultrasound is used for diagnostic purposes. Therefore, when a transducer is constructed, a backing material is placed behind the crystals to lessen the ring-down time. This controls pulse length. Short pulse length improves axial resolution, which is discussed later. In addition, during transducer construction, an epoxy-based material that has the same basic acoustic properties as soft tissue is adhered to the front of the piezoelectric crystals. This covering protects the delicate crystals from damage, provides electrical isolation between elements and patient, and, in some transducer configurations, provides a means of altering the focal characteristics of the transmitted acoustic beam. The section of the transducer through which the ultrasound beam passes and through which echoes are received is known as the "transducer aperture." In most echocardiographic applications, the transducer aperture is less than 21 mm in diameter because of limited acoustic access between ribs. The diameter of the active aperture dictates the depth of field or the depth over which the ultrasound beam remains in focus; the larger the diameter, the better the depth of field.

Once the transducer is pulsed electronically, an ultrasound wave passes through the aperture and enters the patient. As the acoustic wave propagates through the patient's body, a resulting series of alternating conditions of compressions and rarefactions takes place (Fig 9–3). The ultrasound wave, mechanical energy, travels through media (blood, soft tissue) as longitudinal waves in a generally straight direction. When the acoustic wave strikes an interface between two media of differing acoustic impedances, a portion of the mechanical energy is returned to the transducer as an echo. Acoustic impedance is described by the equation:

$$Z = pv$$

where Z = acoustic impedance,
p = density of media, and
v = sound velocity.

For example, a blood–soft tissue interface causes an echo to return to the transducer. If molecular bonding is tight, the medium has a high density; the denser the media, the faster the ultrasound wave passes through it. For example, the speed of ultrasound through blood is approximately 1,570 m/sec, whereas the speed of ultrasound through bone, obviously a much denser media, is 3,380 m/sec. All diagnostic ultrasound systems used in echocardiographic applications are calibrated at 1,540 m/sec, which is roughly the velocity of sound through soft tissue. The velocity component of the ultrasonic wave through a medium is critical in determining the distance between the transducer aperture and the echo interface. The ability of an ul-

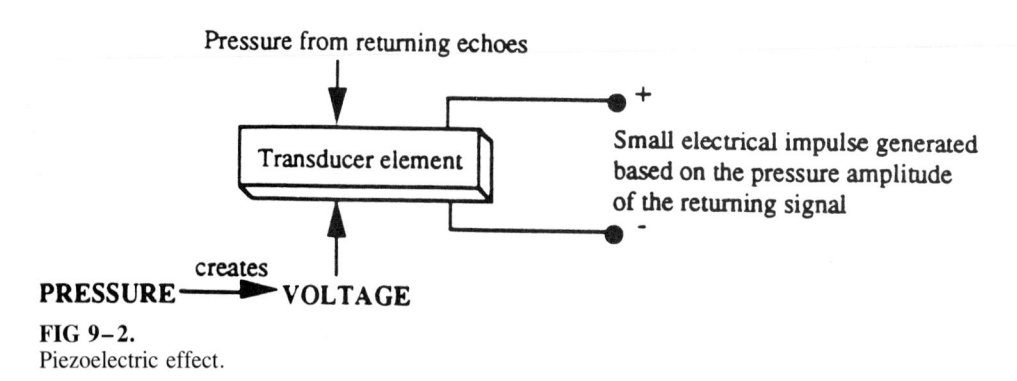

FIG 9–2.
Piezoelectric effect.

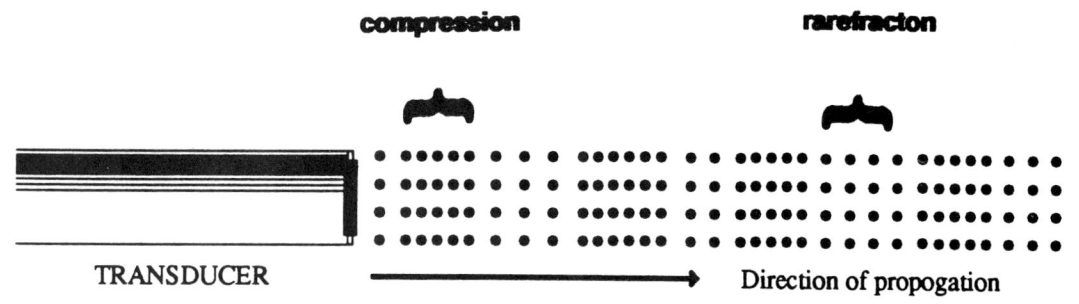

FIG 9-3.
Accoustic wavefront compression and rarefaction.

trasound system to accurately display a target's depth (location) is known as its "tissue registration accuracy."

If the tissue target is larger than the wavelength of the transducer frequency being used, it is known as a "specular reflector." A specular reflector is an angle-dependent reflector. An angle-dependent reflector is a reflector in which the ultrasound beam returns from the target at an angle that equals the angle of incidence. The amount of mechanical energy returned to the transducer aperture as an echo will, in this case, be a function of the angle of incidence between the transmitted acoustic beam and the target interface (Fig 9-4). Therefore, in the case of a specular reflector, the highest returned energy level occurs when the target is exactly perpendicular to the transducer.

As the ultrasound beam propagates into soft tissue media, acoustic energy is attenuated in a rather linear fashion, expressed by a rule of thumb equation:

$$\text{Attenuation} = 1 \text{ dB/cm/MHz}$$

This means that the ultrasound waves from higher-frequency transducers, which supply excellent spatial resolution, will not penetrate as deeply as those from lower-frequency transducers. Most energy attenuation is a function of absorption where the energy is converted to heat as it passes through the medium's molecular matrix. Maximum depth of penetration for any given frequency transducer is ensured by focusing the acoustic beam into a small area as deeply as possible. In diagnostic ultrasound applications, the ability to maintain beam collimation is restricted in part by the size of the transducer aperture. In clinical applications with virtually unrestricted acoustic access (e.g., abdominal imaging), a large-diameter transducer can be used. Therefore, beam collimation can be maintained for a greater depth, whereas cardiac applications require small apertures and collimation is sacrificed.

The echoes returning from the targets encountered by the transmitted ultrasound beam are translated by the transducer into electrical pulses of an amplitude equal to those of the various intensity levels of the returning echoes. These electrical pulses are processed by the ultrasound system into various shades of gray, mapped into exact pixel (picture elements that comprise the display monitor) locations, and are displayed as real-time two-dimensional images on the system's television monitor. With this in mind, the distribution of the reflected intensities of the ultrasound wave as a function of the time from a transducer may be looked at as a map of tissue discontinuities along the scanning axis direction.

A key aspect of two-dimensional ultrasound imaging is resolution. One form of resolution to be considered is spatial resolution. Spatial resolution is that property that allows for the differentiation as distinct targets of two or more targets that lie in close proximity to one another. There are two measures of this type of imaging resolution: axial and lateral. Axial resolution, which is resolution in depth, is a function of two performance parameters: the transducer frequency and the transmit pulse length (again determined in part by the degree of damping done on the

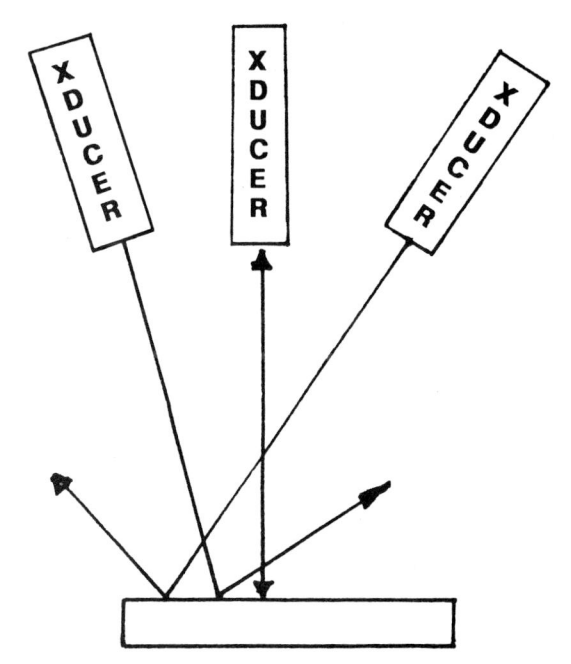

FIG 9-4.
Angle-dependent and specular reflectors. *xducer* = transducer

piezoelectric crystals in the transducer). A higher transducer frequency has a shorter wavelength and, consequently, better axial resolution. Shorter transmit pulse length also has better axial resolution. In no case, however, can the axial resolution be better than the transducer wavelength. Axial resolution in ultrasound systems is always much better than lateral resolution. Lateral resolution is a measure of the ultrasound system's ability to distinguish between two or more targets that lie in a line perpendicular to the axis of the ultrasound beam. This quality of imaging resolution is typically a function of beam width. The more collimated the beam (i.e., the narrower the beam), the better the resultant lateral resolution. Advances in large-aperture, linear-phased array and annular array transducers employing a technique known as "dynamic focusing" have greatly improved the lateral resolution qualities in modern ultrasound systems.

Two other measures of ultrasound imaging resolution include temporal resolution and contrast resolution. Temporal resolution is a measure of the ability of an ultrasound system to accurately track and display the changing loci of a moving target with respect to time. An example is a system's ability to accurately represent the movement of the anterior leaflet of the mitral valve during the various phases of diastole. Basically, systems that have faster imaging frame rates (a frame is a single complete two-dimensional image; frame rate is the number of frames acquired and displayed per second) have better temporal resolution. Some current ultrasound systems have the ability to acquire data at frame rates in excess of 160 frames/sec. Data acquired at this frame rate can then be reviewed in slow motion via a cine loop format.

One other measure of resolution is contrast resolution. Contrast resolution is a measure of the system's ability to accurately display two echo signals that are only slightly different in amplitude as two distinct echoes with different gray scale levels (e.g., the epicardial-pericardial interface). When gray scale is used to represent the various echoes in a two-dimensional image, the strong intensity echoes receive the brightest gray shade (white) and the weakest returning echoes are assigned the darkest (black). The intensity levels between these two extremes represent more than 70 dB of dynamic range that modern systems can detect in soft tissue. As an example, the range of echo signal strength in adult cardiac applications ranges from nearly 1 V in magnitude (e.g., the reflection to the transducer aperture from the patient's chest wall) to roughly 10 μV (or 1×10^{-6}), as is present in the reflection from the epicardial-pericardial interface.

The wide dynamic range of returning echoes received by the ultrasound system through the transducer requires an electronic normalization of the echoes to provide a uniform gray scale presentation of the display monitor. This process is known by a variety of names; two of the most common are time gain compensation (TGC) and depth gain compensation (DGC). This process provides the system operator with the ability to dampen the echoes returning from targets close to the transducer, such as the chest wall, and to provide additional system gain (amplification) to those echoes returning from targets farthest away from the transducer, such as the epicardial-pericardial interface. Other analog processing techniques such as signal detection are also done in the receiver section of the ultrasound system.

Once the echo signals pass through the transducer and the receiver portion of the ultrasound system, they are usually converted from the analog to the digital domain for further processing. This is accomplished in a circuit known as an "analog-to-digital converter" (A/D). These digital data are generally sent to a scan converter, where the echo data, which were acquired along radial sector scan lines (typically one per degree of sector), are converted into a rectangular format for video display. Echo data can be processed relatively easily in the digital domain. The types of processing used are extremely varied and beyond the scope of this discussion. The accuracy and precision of the digital scan conversion process are typically expressed by the write rate of the scan converter and the number of bits used to represent a given echo amplitude, again displayed as a shade of gray. For example, a scan converter's precision is often expressed in the format $512 \times 512 \times 8$. These numbers mean that on the display monitor there are 512 vertical pixels and 512 horizontal pixels being illuminated in the display field, comprised of both alphanumeric data (such as this date) and the echo information contained within the imaging sector. The last number, 8, means there are 8 bits of data for each echo interpretation, or 256 levels of gray scale analyzed ($2^8 = 256$). The higher the number of bits, the more precise the resultant displayed echo. Most modern echocardiographic systems have a minimum of 6-bit (64 levels of gray) precision.

One digital processing issue is that of interpolation. To understand the need for interpolation, observe Figure 9–5. When the sector format for the display of two-dimensional echo data is used, the lines that make up the sector are very close together at the apex of the sector but diverge at depth. To display a smooth contiguous two-dimensional image, the system must have a means to fill the pixels with shades of gray that are not covered or interrogated by an acoustic scan line. Most echo systems use at least one acoustic scan line per degree of the sector; some use more. The interpolation process in echo systems takes the true echo information from two adjacent scan lines and calculates a linear transition between them. The pixels between those two adjacent scan lines then receive a gray scale level that is somewhat lighter (less intense) than the two real data points but bright enough so that a smooth-

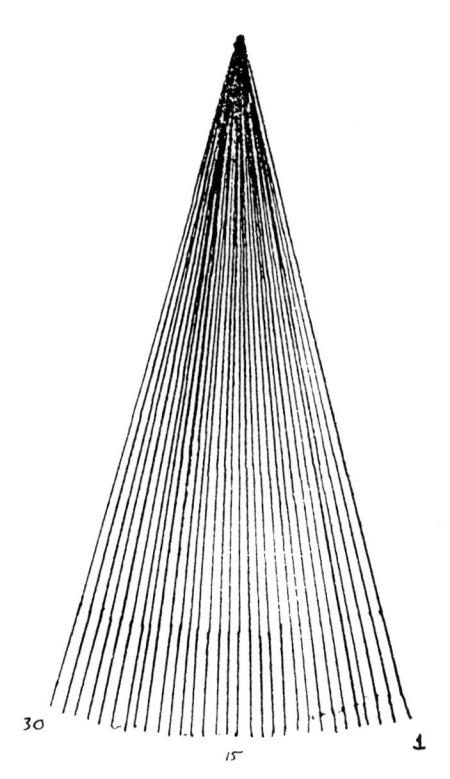

FIG 9–5.
Thirty lines comprising a 30-degree echo sector. Interpolation techniques fill in missing data points.

appearing transition is displayed. Interpolation algorithms are also used, with various degrees of success, in color flow mapping modality to fill in missing data points in the color flow matrix. There are no industry standards with regard to interpolation or other digital processing issues, so the degree of processing and techniques used can vary dramatically from manufacturer to manufacturer.

Recent advances in the ability of ultrasound systems to process a wider dynamic range of two-dimensional echoes have given rise to new methods of echo information presentation. The most dramatic of these new techniques is the so-called B-color mode (Color Plate 1). B-color displays the two-dimensional image in various color schemes rather than in a traditional gray scale format (Fig 9–6). Because the human eye can discern a greater bandwidth of colors than gray scale, these new B-color formats are better at displaying low-intensity echoes, such as those developed when the sound beam passes through a newly formed clot. These types of image processing display algorithms may develop into a means of quantitatively displaying various tissue signatures (tissue characterization). B-color is not limited to two-dimensional image display but can also be used in time axis modalities such as pulsed wave Doppler (Color Plate 2). It may be that when color is used to display a spectral waveform, as in Color Plate 2, the mean velocity of the Doppler envelope may be more readily discernable.

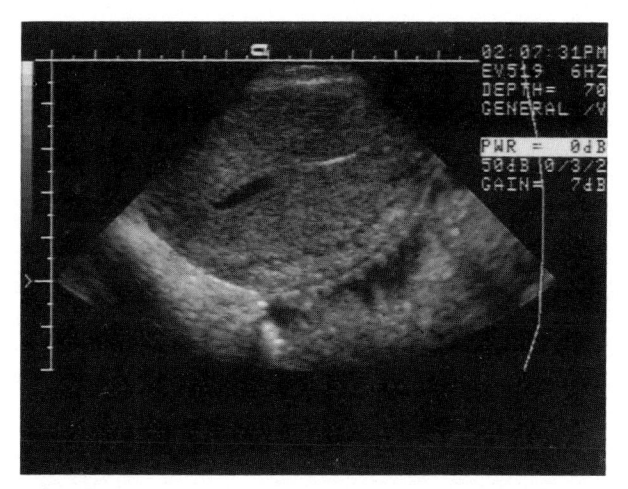

FIG 9–6.
Traditional gray scale two-dimensional image. (Courtesy of Accuson Corp.)

In addition to identification of changes in morphology with the two-dimensional image, data relative to the physiologic processes can also be acquired. In noninvasive diagnostic ultrasound, physiologic data is obtained using the Doppler technique. The Doppler phenomenon, first described by Christian Johann Doppler in the mid-19th century, is the change in the observed frequency of a sound wave caused by movement of a target toward or away from a stationary source. In clinical ultrasound, a Doppler shift is usually the result of the detected movement of red blood cell (RBC) clusters as they move either toward or away from the transducer; the greater the number of blood cells observed, the more intense the backscatter data received by the transducer. Because individual RBCs are so much smaller than the wavelength of the interrogating Doppler frequency (usually the transducer frequency) they cannot be individually resolved by the Doppler system. Red blood cells are classified as diffuse reflectors (equal intensity scattering in all directions, i.e., non–angle dependent reflector) rather that specular reflectors (angle-dependent reflectors). The echoes received by the system from moving RBCs has been likened to the manner in which light is reflected from a fog bank or a heavy mist. In this analogy, individual vapor droplets are smaller than the wavelength of light and therefore do not individually reflect light; however, because they are in such close proximity to other vapor droplets, their aggregate effect produces a light reflection.

The fundamental Doppler formula is:

$$\Delta f = \frac{2 f_o \cdot v \cdot \cos \theta}{c}$$

where f_o = the transmitted frequency (sometimes, but not always, the transducer frequency),

Δf = the frequency shift (the difference between the transmitted frequency, the received frequency)
v = velocity
c = the velocity of sound in soft tissue (about 1,540 m/sec), and
cos θ = angle of incidence between the sound beam and the target motion, and (Fig 9–7). With some basic algebraic manipulation, the ultrasound system converts frequency shift information into a more clinical useful format, velocity information. Velocity is calculated from the detected frequency shift by the equation:

$$V = \frac{c \cdot \Delta f}{2f_o \cdot \cos \theta}$$

One can observe from the velocity formula that as the transducer frequency (f_o) decreases, the system's ability to resolve higher velocities is increased. Therefore, whereas the highest frequency transducer practical is used to achieve better axial resolution, in the Doppler mode, the lowest frequency transducer is used. Because this angle of incidence (cosine of angle θ) is in the denominator in the velocity formula to observe maximum Doppler velocities, the transducer (the transmitted acoustic pulse) is placed parallel with blood flow. Whereas the best imaging of echoes is achieved with the transducer perpendicular to the target, the best Doppler signals are achieved parallel to flow. Therefore, a complete ultrasound examination of the heart often requires compromises between various angles of interrogation.

There are currently four types of clinical Doppler modalities: (1) pulsed-wave Doppler (PWD); (2) continuous-wave Doppler (CWD); (3) high pulse repetition–frequency Doppler (HPRF), and (4) the most recently developed Doppler display modality, color flow Doppler. Color flow Doppler is known by a number of other names such as color flow mapping, color flow imaging, 2D Doppler, and color Doppler. In this discussion, it is referred to as color flow imaging (CFI).

Pulsed-wave Doppler is created by periodically pulsing the transducer with a relatively short-duration pulse, typically a four-cycle bipolar electrical pulse. The frequency of excitation is a function of the depth the interrogation site is from the transducer aperture. The time delay between transducer excitations is known as the "pulse repetition frequency" (PRF). By a process known as "range gating," the operator can place a Doppler sample cell (Fig 9–8) at a discrete area within the two-dimensional imaging sector and obtain Doppler data from that specific site. This is known as "range resolution." Because pulsed Doppler is a sampled technique, there is a limitation to its ability to resolve velocities. The Nyquist sampling theorem dictates that for a sample system to unambiguously resolve a moving target, the frequency of sampling must be at a level twice the velocity of the target. In general, the Nyquist limit in PWD is approximately the PRF/2. A more useful equation for determining the maximum velocity one could hope to resolve using PWD is the range-velocity product:

$$V_m = \frac{c^2}{8f_o R}$$

where V_m = the maximum resolvable velocity,
c = the speed of sound through soft tissue,
f_o = the Doppler transmit frequency, and
R = depth of the PWD sample cell.

If the velocity exceeds the Nyquist limit, the ability of the system to display accurately the velocity and direction of the flow is lost. The result is known as "aliasing" (Fig 9–9). Once aliasing occurs, and if the clinician wishes to

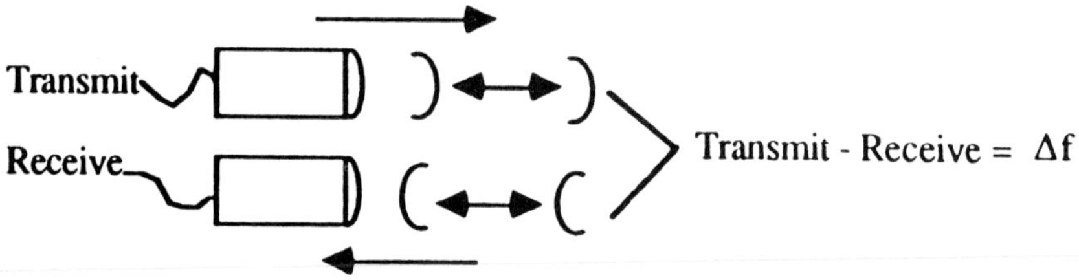

$$\Delta f = \frac{(2fo)(v)(\cos\Theta)}{C} \quad \text{OR} \quad V = \frac{(c)(\Delta f)}{(2fo)(\cos\Theta)}$$

WHERE:
Δf = the difference between transmitted and received frequency
fo = the frequency of the transmitter (e.g. transducer frequency)
v = the velocity of the target
c = the velocity of sound in the medium
cosΘ = angle of incidence between souce of transmission and target

FIG 9–7.
Calculation of frequency shift velocity.

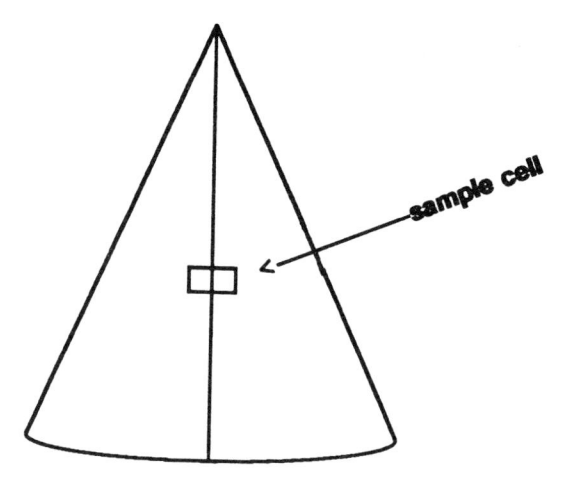

FIG 9-8.
Range gating. Within a two-dimensional imaging section, Doppler data can be obtained from a specific site.

resolve the velocity and direction of flow, a different technique of Doppler acquisition must be used. To resolve higher-velocity flows, one must use either an HPRF Doppler or a CWD.

The HPRF Doppler is similar to the PWD in that there are sample cells located along a radial line cursor located within the two-dimensional imaging sector (Fig 9-10). The HPRF Doppler takes advantage of a phenomenon known as "range ambiguity." As in standard PWD, HPRF Doppler pulses the transducer with a short duration burst of electrical energy. Unlike PWD, the PRF in the HPRF Doppler is determined by the location of the first sample cell location of perhaps four sample cells rather than the depth of a single sample cell from the transducer. Because the PRF is so much higher in HPRF Doppler than regular PWD, higher velocities may be resolved.

For all practical purposes in clinical ultrasound, CWD does not have a PRF, so it is not a sampled technique. Therefore, CWD is not bounded by the Nyquist limit and does not alias. Continuous-wave Doppler does not have range resolution, however, because all velocities along the line of interrogation are processed and displayed. Because CWD allows sampling of all velocities within the range seen in normal and abnormal clinical states, it has a major advantage of allowing prediction of maximal instantaneou pressure drops across short segment stenoses. This is achieved by using the modified Bernoulli equation:

$$\text{Gradient} = 4\,(V_{2-V_1})$$

where V_2 = the maximal velocity distal to an obstruction, and
V_1 = the maximal velocity proximal to an obstruction.

Pulsed-wave Doppler, HPRF, and CWD are all-time axis Doppler techniques and are generally displayed as spectral waveforms. These Doppler data are typically analyzed using a fast Fourier transform (FFT) algorithm, which converts Doppler information from the time domain to the frequency domain. This allows the system to display the velocity and power content of the frequency shifts encountered by the Doppler transmit pulse. This velocity and power information is usually displayed as a gray scale contour. Advances in technology allow for the display of spectral waveforms in various color formats. Color display of these data allows the operator to discern the mean velocity content with greater ease. Also, the operator may be able to visualize the various velocity components that comprise a CWD waveform, whereas range resolution data are not directly observed.

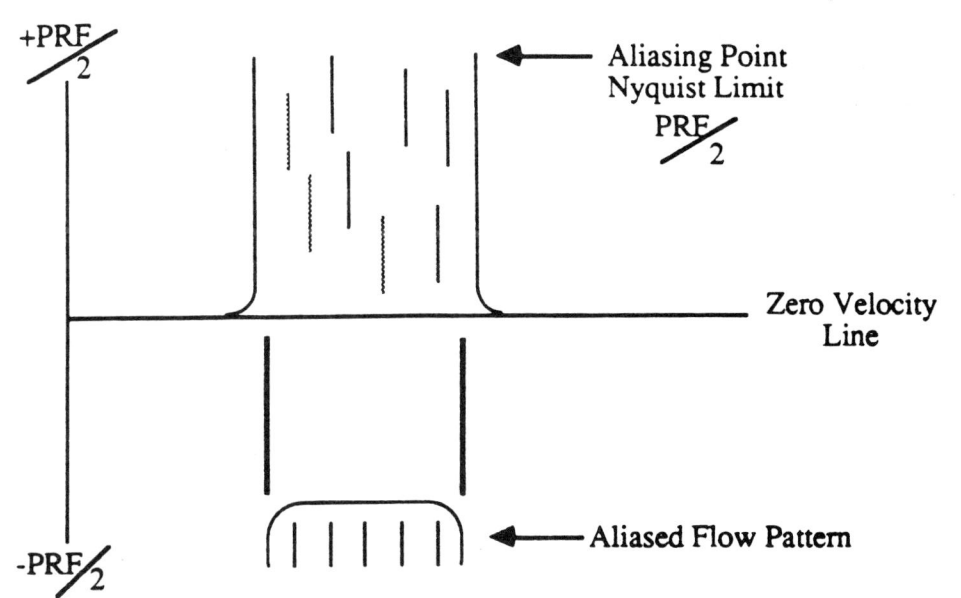

FIG 9-9.
Time axis Doppler aliasing. *PRF* = pulse repetition frequency.

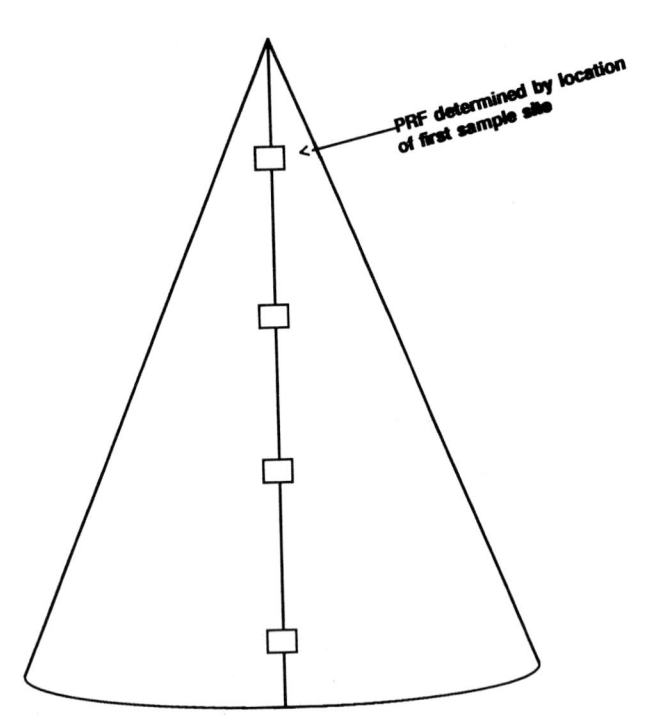

FIG 9–10.
High pulse repetition–frequency Doppler allows multiple sampling sites along a radius within a two-dimensional imaging section.

Color flow imaging is an extension of the PWD technique. It provides the operator with a global hemodynamic perspective of flow by rapidly acquiring Doppler-derived mean velocities along each of the radial lines that comprise the CFI sector, displaying those data in a color flow matrix with, and synchronous with, the two-dimensional gray scale image (Color Plate 3). This information about mean velocity is then displayed by using one of the several color "maps" available to the operator. The three most common color maps are (1) velocity, (2) velocity/variance, and (3) the power or intensity mode. These maps display, with various degrees of accuracy, the mean velocities, flow direction, variance components, and the energy contained within the Doppler backscatter. The most frequently used color map in echocardiographic applications is the velocity/variance display. Conventional echocardiographic applications display flow toward the transducer in red and flow away from the transducer in blue. Variance, the calculated deviation from the mean velocity, is displayed by mixing green with red for turbulent flow toward the transducer and blue for turbulent flow away from the transducer. As with any sampled system, CFI also has a Nyquist limit above which it will alias, and both velocity and directional coherence are lost. In CFI, aliasing is displayed by the sudden shift from a primary color (Fig 9–11). As with standard PWD, CFI aliasing occurs approximately at the PRF/2. The PRF in CFI is often determined by the depth of the image and certainly by the depth of the last CFI sample cell (Fig 9–12). The equation used to derive the CFI velocity (V) content is:

$$V = \frac{\Lambda\theta}{\frac{4\pi f}{c} \times \frac{1}{PRF}}$$

where f = the transmitted frequency,
c = sound speed through soft tissue,
$\Lambda\theta$ = phase shift (determined by a mathematical technique known as auto correlation),
and PRF = pulse repetition frequency.

Although extremely useful for visualizing the flow in a two-dimensional format, CFI-displayed velocities are not as accurate as the more computationally intensive PWD

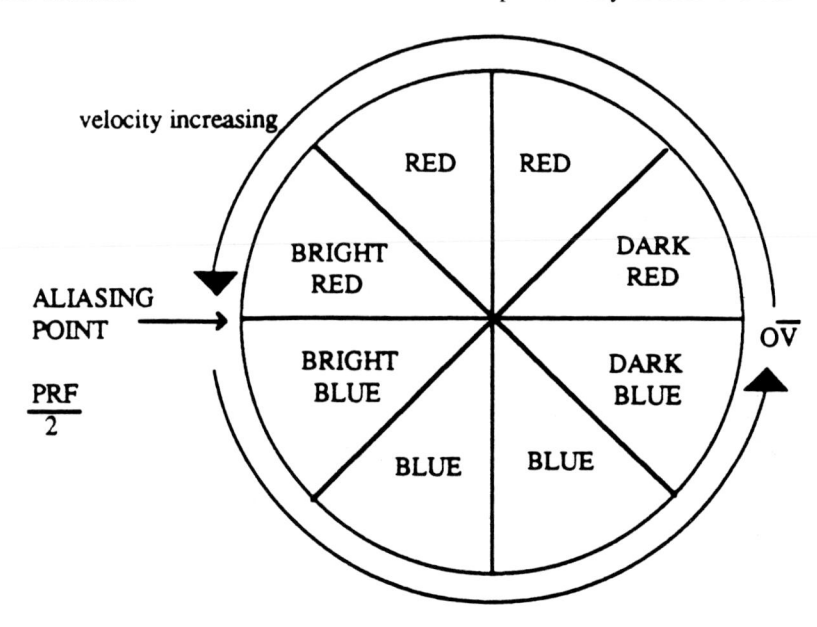

FIG 9–11.
Color flow imaging. Aliasing displayed by sudden shift of primary color. *PRF* = pulse repetition frequency.

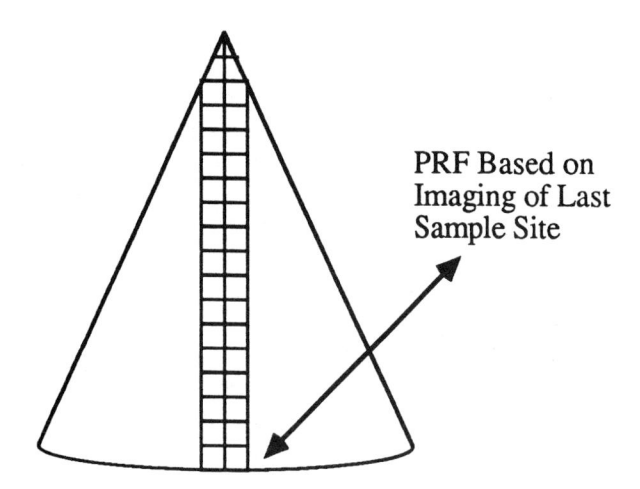

FIG 9–12.
Color flow imaging. Pulse repetition frequency *(PRF)* determined by depth of image and depth of last sampling site.

and CWD spectral displays. Therefore, CFI is viewed as a complimentary modality to PWD and CWD. As shown in Figure 9–13, each of the current ultrasound modalities contributes to the overall evaluation.

TECHNIQUES OF CARDIAC ULTRASOUND

Many clinical decisions can be made primarily on the basis of integrating the results of an echo-Doppler examination with information provided by history, physical examination, electrocardiography, and chest x-ray film. Alternatively, an inadequate ultrasound examination can provide misleading information that could cause harm. To perform ultrasound for cardiac anomalies, the examiner should be completely familiar with the anatomy and physiology of cardiac malformations. Ultrasound technicians are usually excellent, but physician supervision is necessary. The physician often is present during the examination and even performs it, especially when the anatomy is confusing.

Most patients can be evaluated on an examination table, hospital bed, or isolette, but occasionally cooperation is best achieved if the child is held on the parent's lap. Some phases of the evaluation are uncomfortable, especially the suprasternal and subcostal portions. These can disturb, especially infants and younger patients. Thus, sedation is often administered as in preparation for magnetic resonance imaging studies. Although chloral hydrate sedation has commonly been used, many patients achieve smoother sedation with intranasal midazolam sedation.[1] If any form of sedation is used, the patient should be both monitored and observed until he or she has returned to fully conscious state. Guidelines for conscious sedation have been published[2] and should be followed in any laboratory that deals with children.

An electrocardiogram should be recorded during each examination. A standard lead II is displayed if the electrodes and leads are consistently mounted and connected. This allows the examiner to monitor the sedated and very young patient during the examination and provides a timing cross-reference for later evaluation of echo and Doppler data. Liberal amounts of ultrasonic transmission contact gel should be applied to the transducer-skin interface. This excludes air between the transducer and the skin and allows a cleaner image. If the patient has had a recent operation, avoid contact with the wound. We use an antibiotic gel as the contact medium to minimize the risk of wound infection.

Some patients with overexpanded lungs, obesity, or thoracic wall deformities cannot be evaluated. Most patients, however, can be evaluated if the examiner is skilled and if the patient is properly prepared.

Every attempt should be made to obtain a complete

COMPLIMENTARY MODALITIES

Mode	Application
M-Mode	Measurement of Dimensions
2D Echo	Definition of Anatomy & Morphology
PW Doppler	Localization of Hemodynamic Flow
CW Doppler	Measurement of Flow Velocities
CFM	Global Hemodynamic Blood Flow
M-Mode CFM	Precise Timing of Flow

FIG 9–13.
Current ultrasound methods. Each method can provide information to understanding cardiac structures and features.

examination on each patient. A two-dimensional echo study should be performed long enough to obtain a thorough understanding of cardiac structures. Then M-mode echo tracings are derived for measurement purposes from a cursor placed in the proper area of interest. Finally, CFD interrogation is performed. When the color flow Doppler shows an area of flow disturbance, that area should be evaluated quantitatively with PWD, CWD, or both. The color M-mode Doppler should be used to obtain on-line depth and timing information regarding flows in various areas. The combined imaging and color flow Doppler should serve as a guide to the best areas for obtaining normal physiologic information from pulsed Doppler tracings regarding intracardiac and great-vessel flows. A complete study is accomplished by sweeping the beam through the entire heart and by systematically combining various modalities in each imaging location. When each aspect of the evaluation has been completed, the ultrasonographer moves to the next location. If an abnormality is detected, it should be evaluated thoroughly and its characteristics defined. Random jumping from location to location during a routine examination should be avoided.

ECHOCARDIOGRAPHIC LOCATIONS

The following sections describe the usual examination locations and emphasize the important findings in each. From each of the locations different planes through the heart and great vessels can be obtained.

Subcostal Location

The subcostal location is the most important site for examination of cardiac malformations. Nearly every cardiac and great-vessel structure can be imaged from this location because little lung tissue interferes with the passage of the ultrasound beam. Unfortunately, transducer placement under the ribs during the subcostal examination causes patient discomfort. Several manufacturers have transducers that fit this area well. The laboratory choosing equipment for use on children should consider this factor before purchasing equipment.

If possible, the echo-Doppler examination should start subcostally. The imaging sector is set on the screen so that the apex of the sector triangle is at the bottom. This displays the images anatomically correctly. The subcostal examination consists of three planes and an additional static view. The imaging of each plane proceeds as a sweep from one side of the heart to the opposite side and then returns to the point of origin. The sweeps are first performed with two-dimensional imaging alone to optimize anatomic detail. The sweeps are then repeated with color Doppler to screen for abnormal flow patterns. The transducer is placed so that the plane of the ultrasonic beam gives a cross-section of the abdomen with the spine in the center of the transducer. This allows the situs of the patient to be determined by noting the position of the abdominal aorta, the inferior vena cava (or lack of an inferior vena cava), the position of the liver, hepatic veins, and stomach (Fig 9–14). After situs is determined, the inferior vena cava is followed as it enters the right atrium. All of the sweeps begin and end at the inferior vena caval–right atrial junction. Doing this adds consistency for comparing patient studies and allows the ultrasonographer to obtain pattern recognition for detection of subtle abnormalities.

Four planes are observed from a subcostal location: (1) frontal, (2) long axial oblique, (3) sagittal, and (4) right anterior oblique.

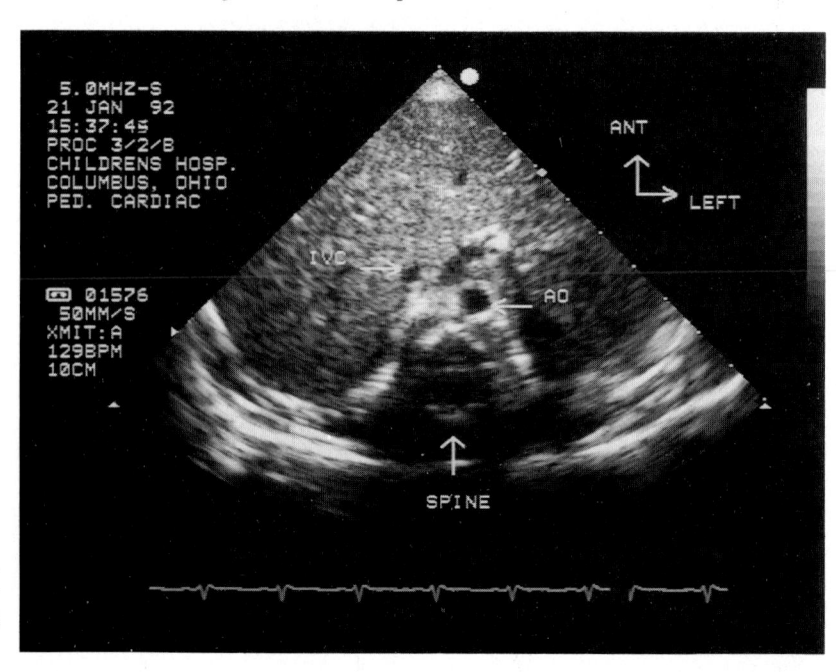

FIG 9–14.
Subcostal cross-sectional plane of abdomen. This view is used to examine situs of abdominal great vessels and viscera. *Ant* = anterior; *AO* = aorta, *IVC* = inferior vena cava.

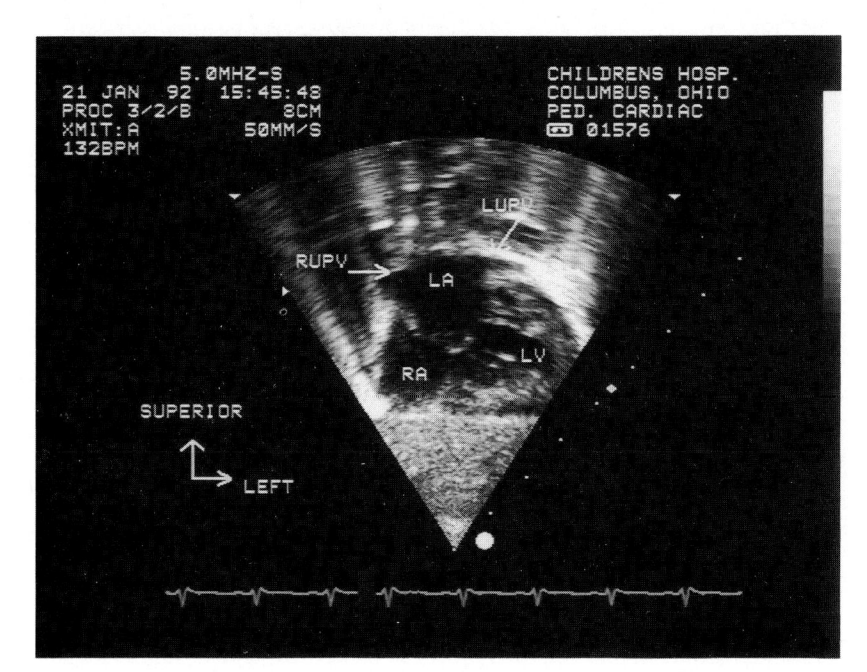

FIG 9–15.
Subcostal frontal plane of heart used to examine atrial size, location of pulmonary veins, and atrial septum. *LA* = left atrium; *LUPV* = left upper pulmonary vein; *LV* = left ventricle; *RA* = right atrium; *RUPV* = right upper pulmonary vein.

Frontal Plane

The sector fan of the ultrasonic beam is first directed in a frontal plane, with the sector parallel to the patient's back. The sweep starts at the junction of the inferior vena cava and the right atrium, and the transducer is slowly flattened with respect to the patient's abdomen so that its face gradually is directed anteriorly. As this is done, the coronary sinus, pulmonary veins, and left atrium come into view (Fig 9–15). Directing more anteriorly allows visualization of the ventricular septum, right ventricle, and finally the pulmonary valve (Fig 9–16). The transducer is slowly directed posteriorly to complete the sweep back to the inferior vena caval–right atrial junction.

Long Axial Oblique Plane

The second sweep, obtaining a long axial oblique plane, is performed with the transducer rotated 30 degrees clockwise from the frontal plane. The transducer is directed with its face tilting from the direction of the patient's right hip and slowly sweeping toward the direction of the patient's left shoulder. This allows both the atrial and ventricular septa to be positioned perpendicular to the ultrasound beam (Fig 9–17) and flow across defects to be

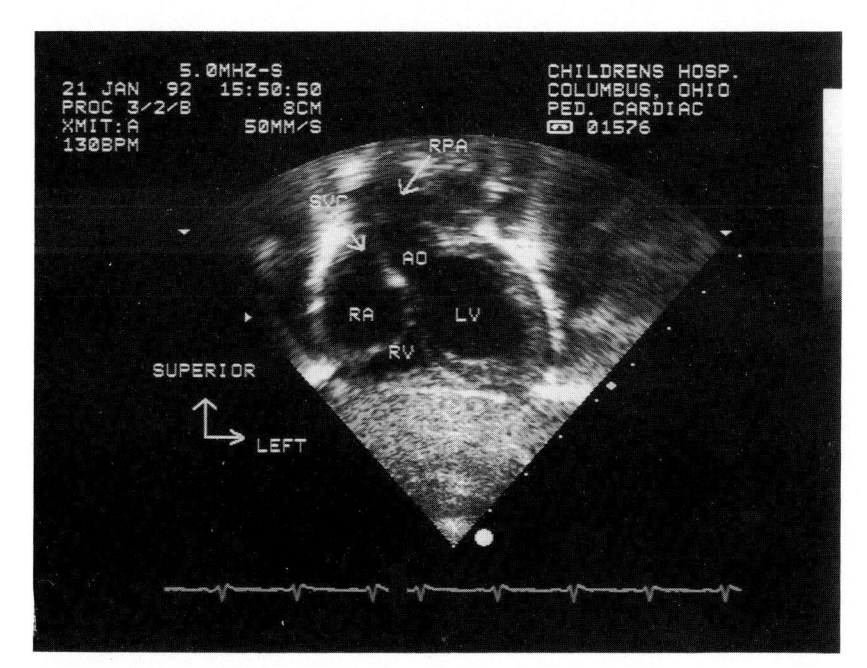

FIG 9–16.
Subcostal frontal plane of heart angled more anteriorly to examine left ventricle and aorta. *AO* = aorta; *LV* = left ventricle; *RA* = right atrium; *RPA* = right pulmonary artery; *RV* = right ventricle; *SVC* = superior vena cava.

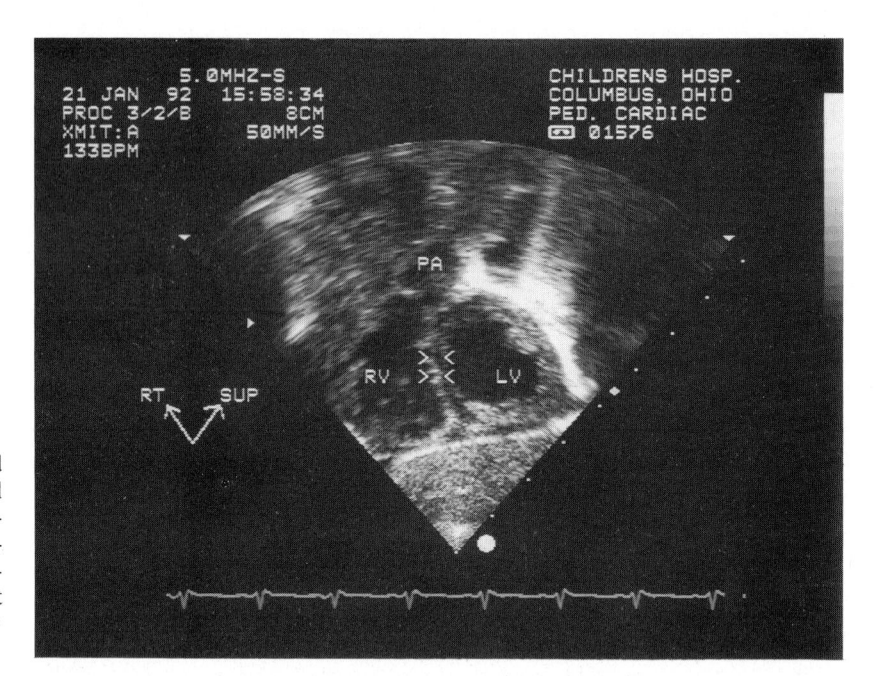

FIG 9–17.
Subcostal long axial oblique view, obtained by rotating 30 degrees clockwise from coronal plane. This view is used to examine ventricles, interventricular septum, and atrioventricular valves in short axis. Interventricular septum lies between the arrowheads. *LV* = left ventricle; *PA* = pulmonary artery; *RT* = right; *RV* = right ventricle; *SUP* = superior.

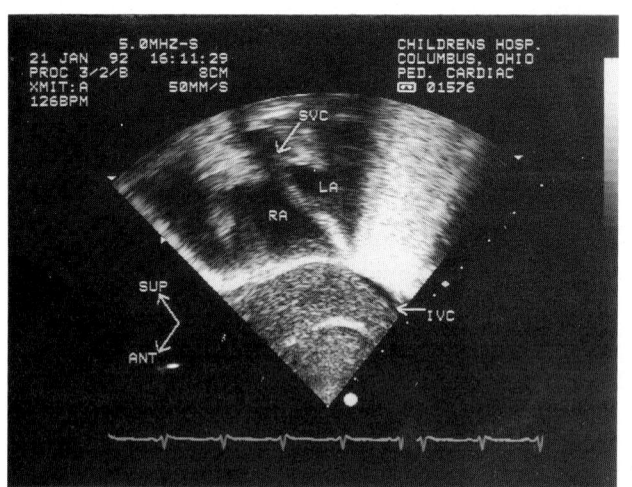

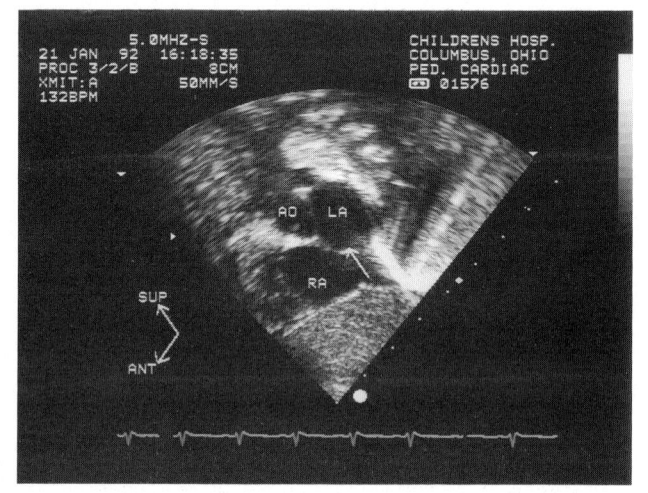

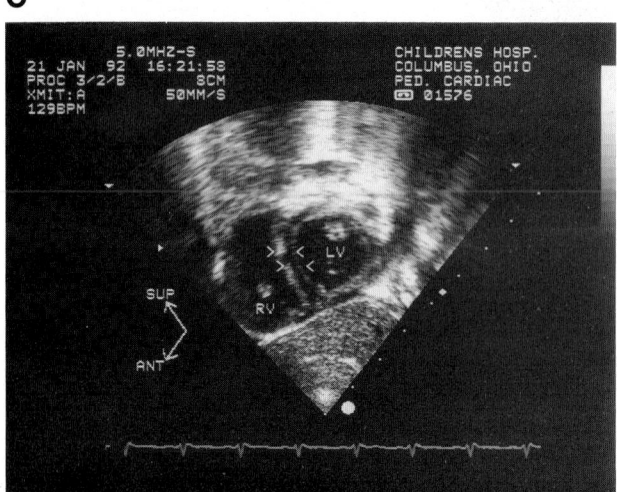

FIG 9–18.
Subcostal sagittal plane. **A,** sagittal view of atria and vena cava. **B,** sagittal view of atria and interatrial septum *(arrow)*. **C,** sagittal view of ventricles and intraventricular septum *(arrowheads)*. *ANT* = anterior; *AO* = aorta; *IVC* = inferior vena cava; *LA* = left atrium; *LV* = left ventricle; *RA* = right atrium; *RV* = right ventricle; *SUP* = superior; *SVC* = superior vena cava.

parallel to the beam. The descending aorta is visualized at the level of the diaphragm.

Sagittal Plane

The third sweep obtains the sagittal plane. The transducer is rotated 90 degrees clockwise from the frontal plane position. This view is equivalent to a lateral chest x-ray film. This sweep starts with both the superior and inferior vena cavae entering the right atrium (Fig 9–18,A). The transducer is slowly directed to the patient's left. The left atrium and atrial septum are then visualized (Fig 9–18,B). The tricuspid valve, right ventricle, and right ventricular outflow tracts are next visualized after the ventricular septum and the mitral valve apparatus (Fig 9–18,C). This sweep gives a cross-sectional view of the atrioventricular valves and is particularly helpful in patients with an atrioventricular septal defect. The sweep proceeds to the apex of the heart and is slowly returned to the point of origin of the sweep.

Right Anterior Oblique Plane

The final view from the subcostal window is a "static" view. It is termed the right anterior oblique plane because it correlates with the right anterior oblique view of angiography. The transducer is rotated 20 to 30 degrees counterclockwise from the frontal plane, with the transducer virtually flat on the child's abdomen. This shows the inferior vena cava, right atrium, tricuspid valve, right ventricular outflow tract, pulmonary valve, and main and right pulmonary arteries in one view (Fig 9–19). Abnormalities of the infundibular septum such as occur in tetralogy of Fallot can be visualized well in this plane.

Precordial Location

From a precordial location both a long-axis and a short-axis plane can be obtained from a parasternal location.

Parasternal Long-Axis Plane

The imaging sector is set on the screen so that the apex of the sector triangle is located at the top. The transducer is placed in the left third or fourth intercostal space, with the front of the sector directed toward the patient's right shoulder. Most examinations are facilitated by having the patient lie on his or her left side to displace the overlying lung, which could interfere. Sometimes asking the patient to exhale helps. Occasionally (to achieve a clear image) the patient's position must be changed to nearly a supine face-down location.

The image is adjusted until the right ventricle, ventricular septum, any aorta, left ventricle, and left atrium are imaged (Fig 9–20). Angling the transducer slightly rightward demonstrates the right atrium, tricuspid valve, and perimembranous septal area; angling it slightly leftward demonstrates the right ventricular outflow tract. Once the imaging is completed, the plane through the chordal-mitral apparatus is used to derive M-mode echo tracings for measurement purposes (Fig 9–21). After this is completed, the Doppler analysis is performed. Pulmonary venous and transmitral flows are directed toward the transducer, and aortic flows are directed away from it (Color Plate 4). Ventricular septal defects, if present, are associated with flow toward the transducer, whereas mitral regurgitant flows are directed away from it. Because it is commonly

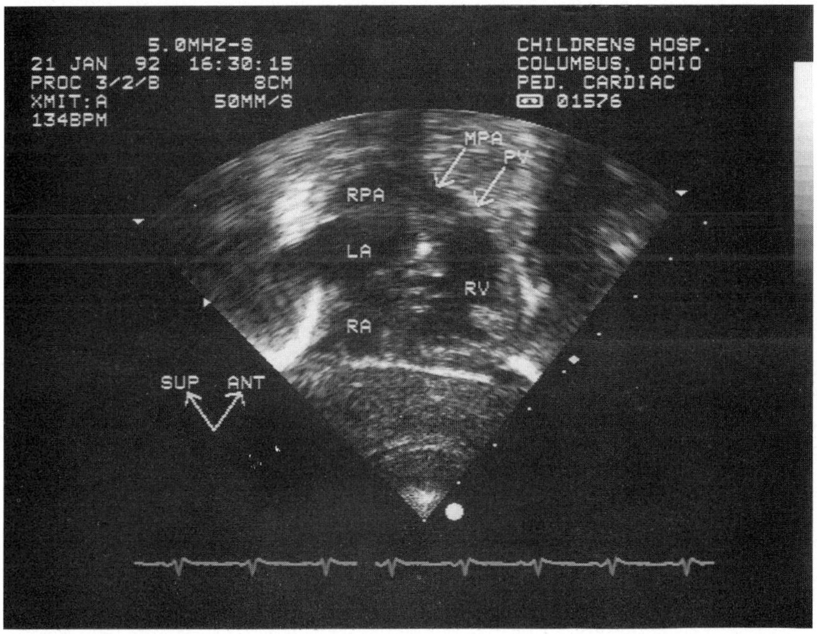

FIG 9–19.
Subcostal right anterior oblique plane obtained by rotating 30 to 45 degrees counterclockwise from coronal plane. It is used to examine entire right ventricle and pulmonary artery. *ANT* = anterior; *LA* = left atrium; *MPA* = main pulmonary artery; *PV* = pulmonic valve; *RA* = right atrium; *RPA* = right pulmonary artery; *RV* = right ventricle; *SUP* = superior.

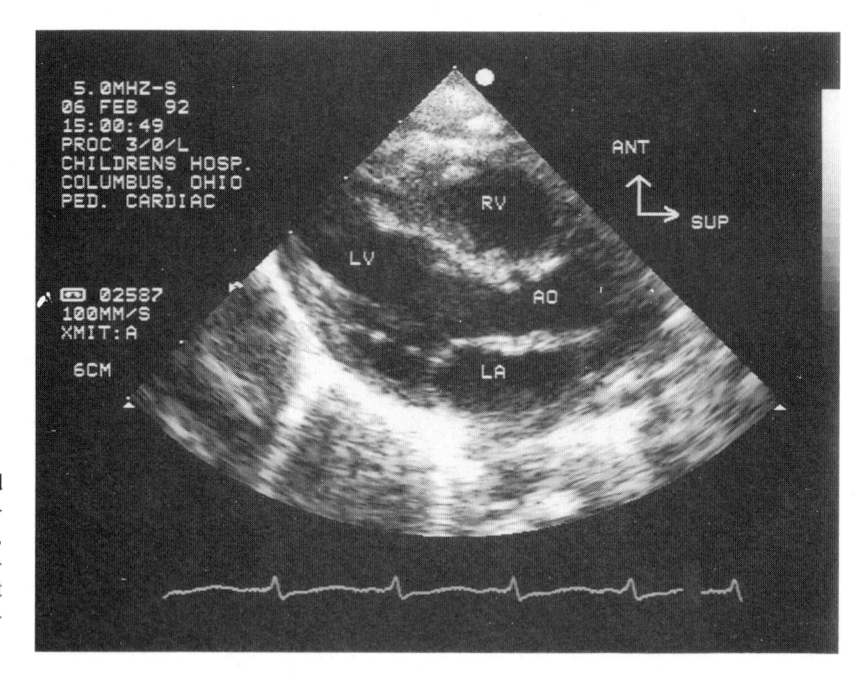

FIG 9-20.
Parasternal long-axis plane. This view is used to examine left ventricular size and wall motion, aortic and mitral valves, left atrial size, and proximal ascending aorta. *ANT* = anterior; *AO* = aorta; *LA* = left atrium; *LV* = left ventricle; *RV* = right ventricle; *SUP* = superior.

detectable on the color examination, mitral backflow without a murmur should be considered a normal physiologic event.[3]

Parasternal Short-Axis Plane

The same precordial transducer position is used as for the long-axis examination, but the front of the sector is directed leftward and perpendicularly to the long-axis plane. The transducer is then tilted so that the sector plane is at the apex. Cross-sectional slices of the heart are obtained from planes at the apex, the chordae tendineae, the anterior and posterior mitral valve leaflets, and the aorta (Fig 9-22). The transducer is then angulated slightly more leftward to allow clear visualization of the pulmonary artery and its bifurcation (Fig 9-23). The short-axis plane is useful for assessment of left ventricular geometry and areas of dyskinesis and of abnormal tricuspid morphology. The plane also allows identification of the location of ventricular septal defects, perimembranous defects (located beneath the tricuspid valve at a 10 o'clock position), muscular defects (at a 12 o'clock position), and subpulmonic defects (at a 2 o'clock position). It is the preferred view for demonstration of right

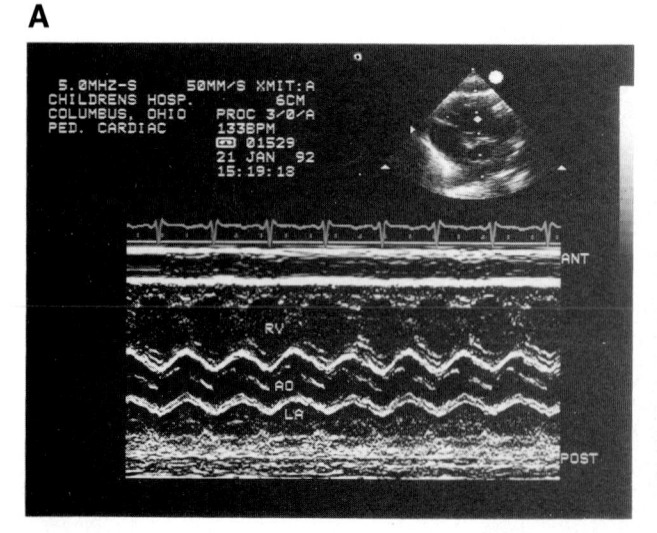

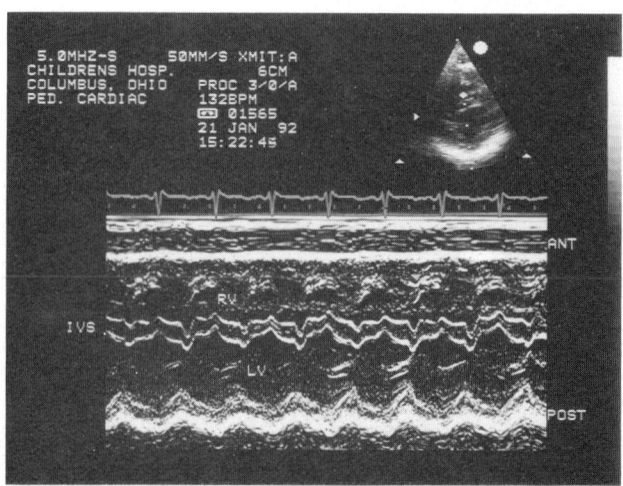

FIG 9-21.
Parasternal M-mode recording. **A,** M-mode of aortic valve. Closed aortic cusps are seen centrally in aortic root during diastole and against anterior and posterior aortic walls during systole. This view is used for standardized measurements of aortic valve. **B,** M-mode recording through ventricles. This view is used for standardized measurements of the left ventricle and interventricular septum. *ANT* = anterior; *AO* = aorta; *IVS* = interventricular septum; *LA* = left atrium; *LV* = left ventricle; *POST* = posterior; *RV* = right ventricle.

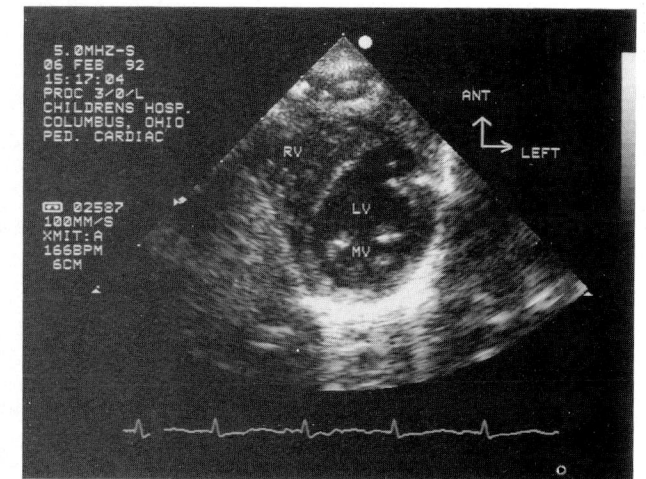

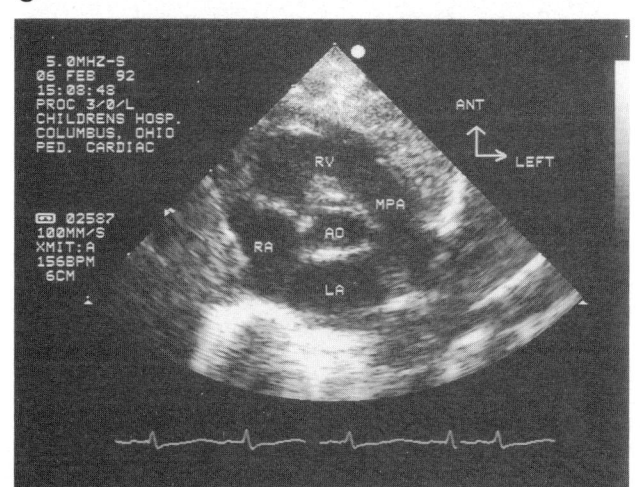

FIG 9–22.
Parasternal short-axis plane. **A,** short-axis view of ventricles and interventricular septum, imaged between arrowheads. **B,** short-axis view at left of mitral valve. **C,** short-axis view at level of aortic root. *ANT* = anterior; *AO* = aorta; *LA* = left atrium; *LV* = left ventricle; *MPA* = main pulmonary artery; *MV* = mitral valve; *RA* = right atrium; *RV* right ventricle.

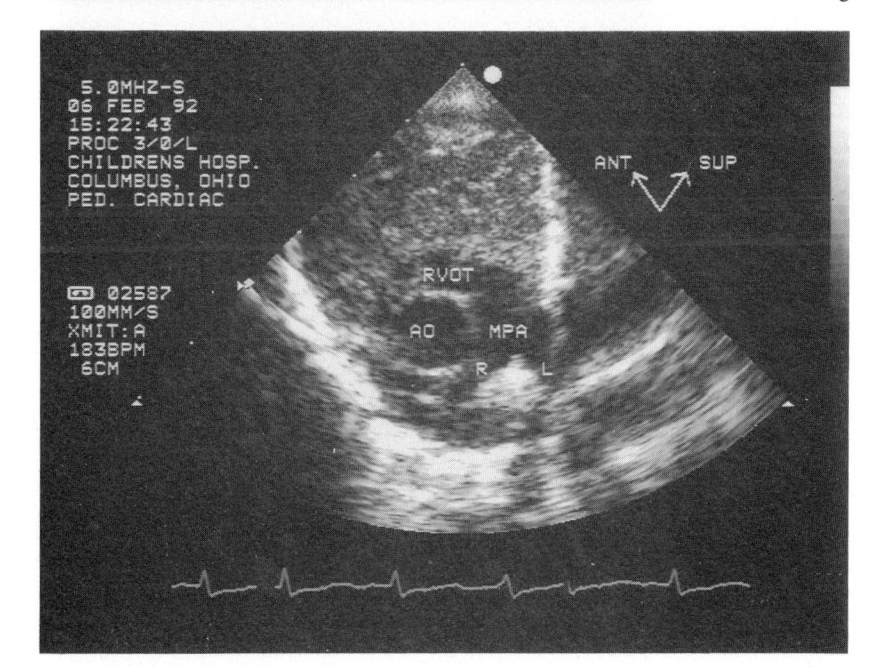

FIG 9–23.
High parasternal short-axis plane. This view is used to demonstrate pulmonary artery anatomy and to examine for patency of ductus arteriosus. Bifurcation of the pulmonary artery is seen. *ANT* = anterior; *AO* = aorta; *L* = left pulmonary artery; *MPA* = main pulmonary artery; *R* = right pulmonary artery; *RVOT* = right ventricular outflow tract; *SUP* = superior.

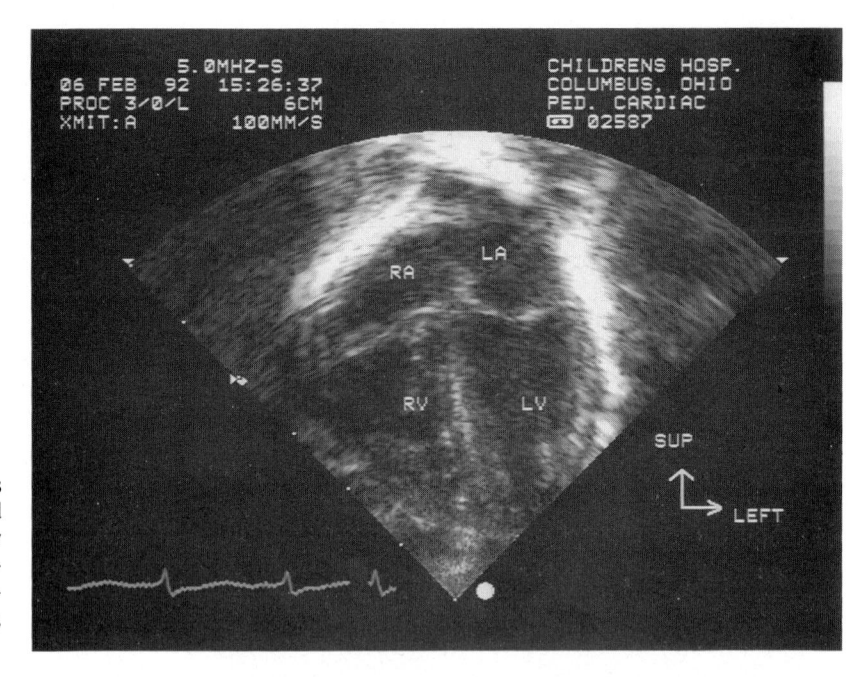

FIG 9–24.
Apical four-chamber plane. This demonstrates relative size of cardiac chambers and tricuspid and mitral valve motion and is an ideal view for Doppler interrogation of the atrioventricular valves. *LA* = left atrium; *LV* = left ventricle; *RA* = right atrium; *RV* = right ventricle; *SUP* = superior.

ventricular outflow obstructions, coronary abnormalities near the aortic root, aortic valve morphology, and the presence of a patent ductus arteriosus. Often atrial septal abnormalities are detected in this plane as well.

Precordial Apical Location

From the cardiac apex a four-chamber plane, aortic outflow plane, and two-chamber plane can be obtained.

Four-Chamber Plane

The transducer is placed at the point of maximal impulse (the cardiac apex). The anterior sector is oriented in the same direction as used in the short-axis examination. The apex of the sector should be displayed at the bottom of the video screen so that structures are displayed anatomically correctly. The scan includes both atrioventricular valves, the ventricles, and the atria. In this slightly posterior plane, the superior posterior pulmonary veins, atrial septum, mitral and tricuspid valves, and ventricular septum can be evaluated (Fig 9–24). After the imaging examination is completed, the color sector is slowly swept from one side to the other so that abnormalities such as anomalous pulmonary venous connection, atrial septal defect, mitral or tricuspid regurgitation, and ventricular septal defect can be detected. The color examination is followed

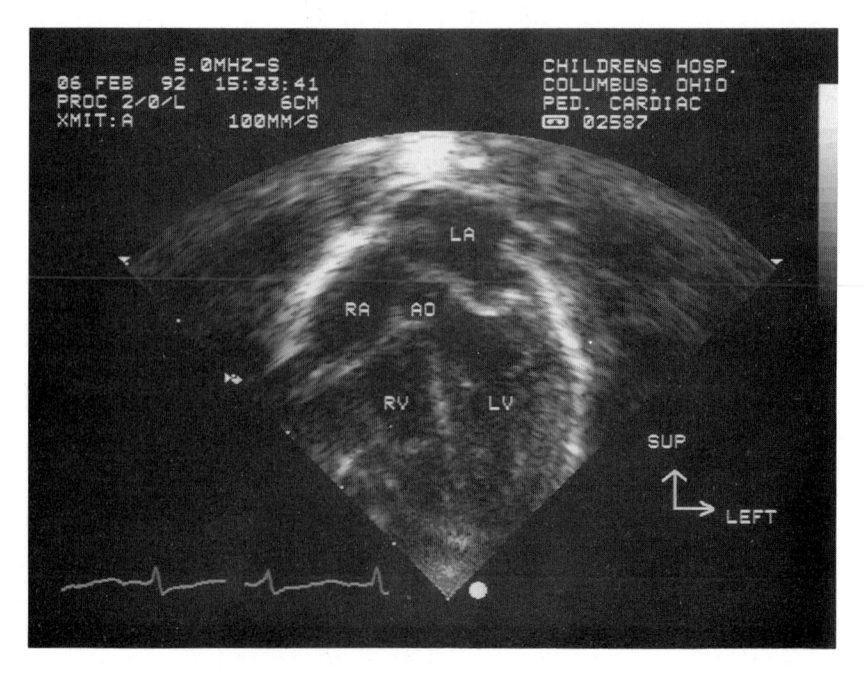

FIG 9–25.
Apical four-chamber plane, including the aorta. This view is obtained by tipping the transducer back from the four-chamber view to examine the more anteriorly located aortic valve. *AO* = aorta; *LA* = left atrium; *LV* = left ventricle; *RA* = right atrium; *RV* = right ventricle; *SUP* = superior.

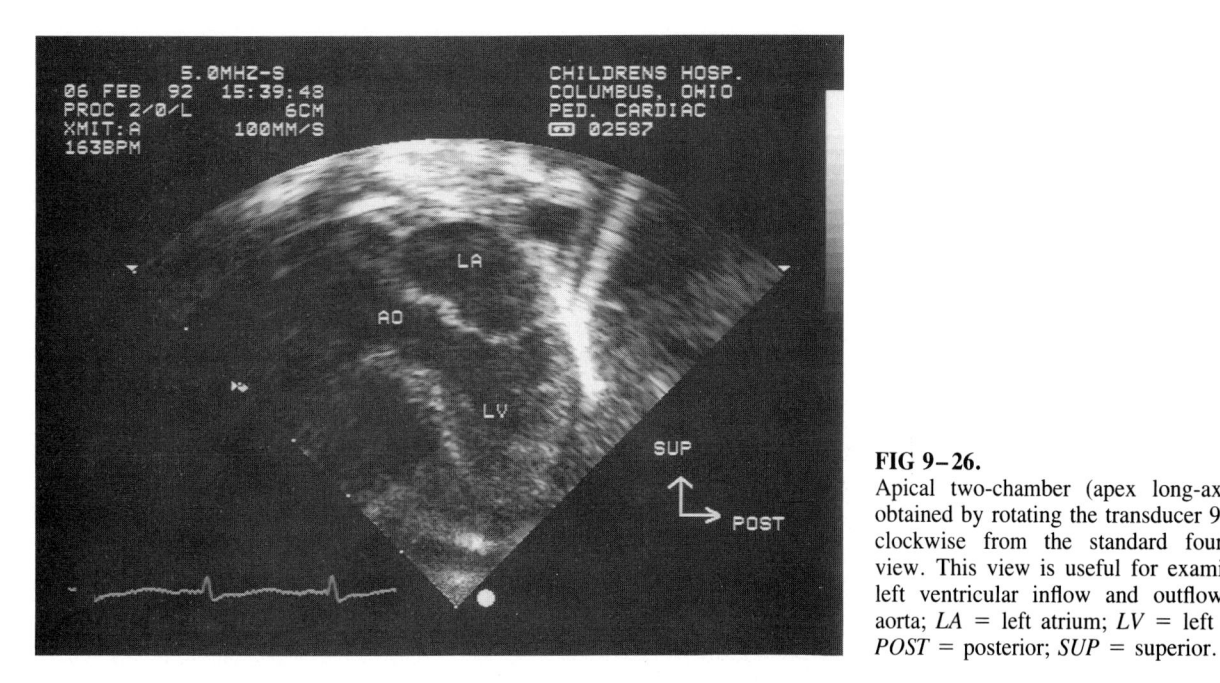

FIG 9–26.
Apical two-chamber (apex long-axis) plane obtained by rotating the transducer 90 degrees clockwise from the standard four-chamber view. This view is useful for examination of left ventricular inflow and outflow. *AO* = aorta; *LA* = left atrium; *LV* = left ventricle; *POST* = posterior; *SUP* = superior.

with quantitative PWD and CWD evaluation on both sides of the valves. If anomalous pulmonary venous connection is suspected, the transducer is aimed even more posteriorly, behind and superior to the left atrium to detect a venous confluence.

Aortic Outflow Plane

After the apical four-chamber examination is completed, the sector is moved anteriorly and the left ventricular outflow tract and aorta are visualized (Fig 9–25). The orifice and proximal segments of the coronary arteries can be evaluated. Again, the color sector is swept from side to side to detect left ventricular outflow tract abnormalities, anteriorly located ventricular septal defects, and atrial septal defects.

Apical Two-Chamber Plane

Turning the transducer 90 degrees counterclockwise so that the anterior sector is again in the long axis plane allows imaging of the left ventricular inflow and outflow (Fig 9–26). This is often called the apical two-chamber view and is especially useful for evaluation of the left ventricular outflow tract in adults in whom left ventricular aneurysms are suspected. Color flow analysis in this plane

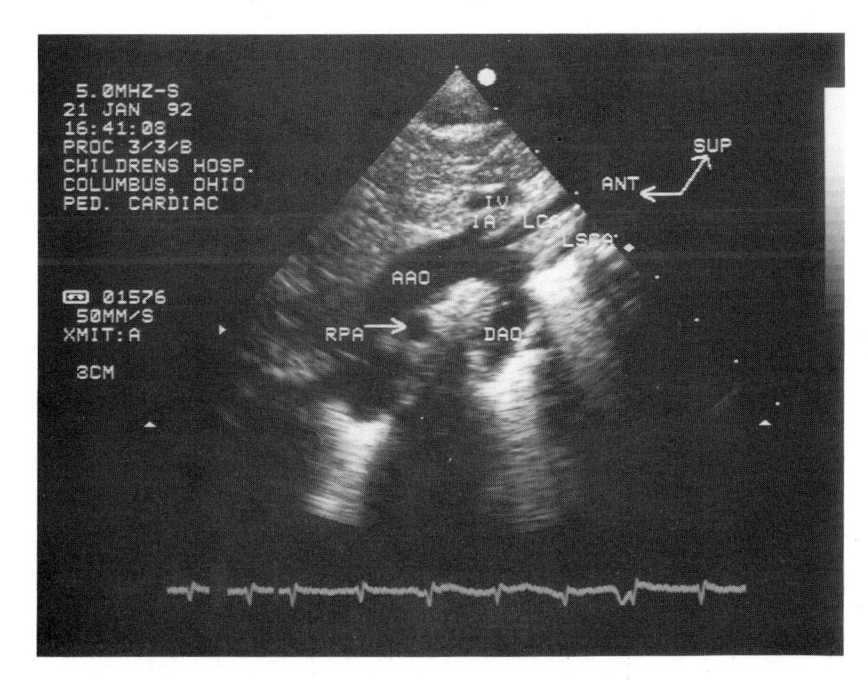

FIG 9–27.
Suprasternal notch view of the aorta. The transducer is placed in the suprasternal notch with the neck slightly extended. The plane of image is rotated clockwise from the sagittal plane into the plane of the aortic arch. This view is used to examine the aortic arch and the anatomy of the head and neck arteries. *AAO* = ascending aorta; *ANT* = anterior; *DAO* = descending aorta; *IA* = innominate artery; *IV* = innominate vein; *LCA* = left carotid artery; *LSCA* = left subclavian artery; *RPA* = right pulmonary artery; *SUP* = superior.

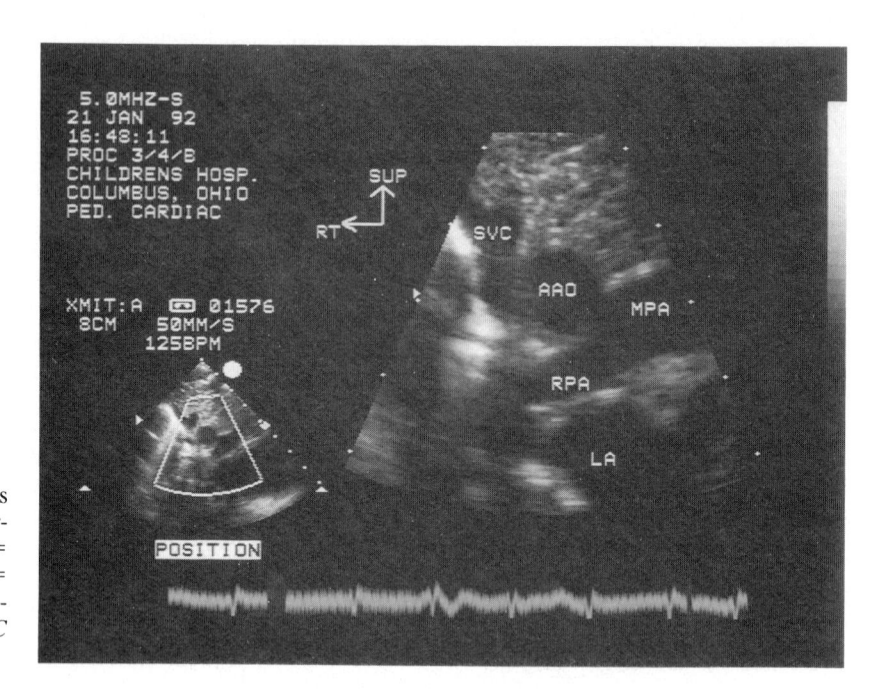

FIG 9–28.
Suprasternal notch coronal plane. This view is used to examine the anatomy of the great arteries and veins of the head and neck. *AAO* = ascending aorta; *LA* = left atrium; *MPA* = main pulmonary artery; *RPA* = right pulmonary artery; *RT* = right; *SUP* = superior; *SVC* = superior vena cava.

Division of Cardiology Columbus Children's Hospital
ECHOCARDIOGRAM DATA SHEET

Patient's Name:_____   Tape #:_____
Referring Physician:_____
Medical Record #:_____
Date of Study:_____
Date of Birth/Age:_____
Equipment:_____

MEASUREMENTS   PREVIOUS: _____

LVEDD: _____   _____
LVESD: _____   _____
RVEDD: _____   _____
LVPW: _____   _____
IVS: _____   _____
AoR: _____   _____
LA: _____   _____
FS: _____   _____

COMMENTS:
                                 Ht: _____
                                 Wt: _____
                                 BSA: _____

Initials:_____

FIG 9–29.
Data worksheet used in echocardiographic laboratory.

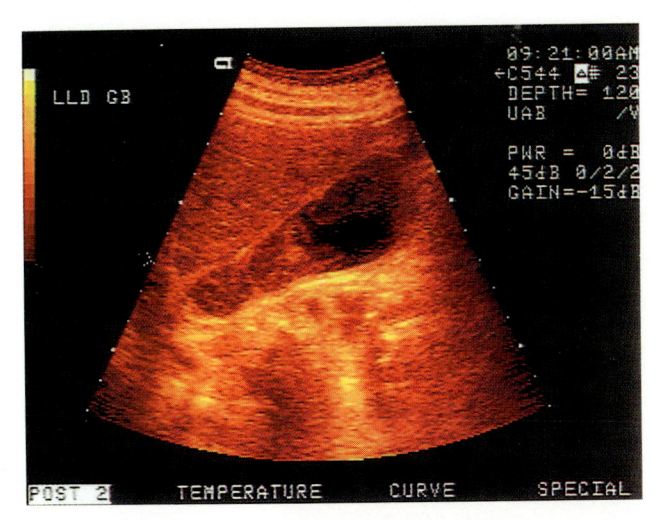

COLOR PLATE 1.
B-color two-dimensional imaging mode. Gallbladder and its contents. (Courtesy of Accuson Corp.)

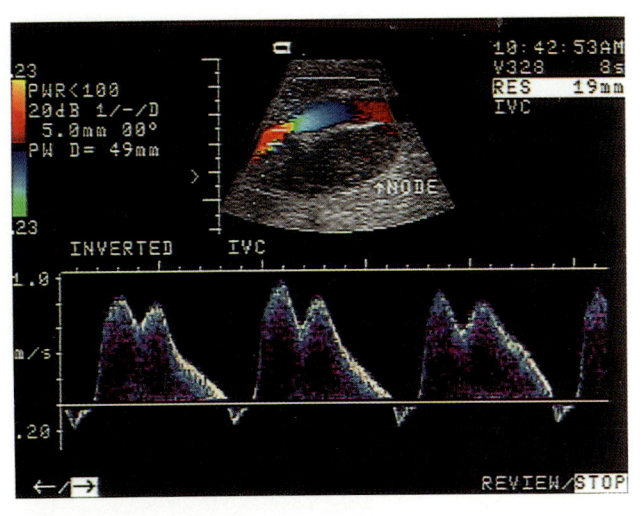

COLOR PLATE 2.
Color Spectra Doppler display. (Courtesy of Accuson Corp.)

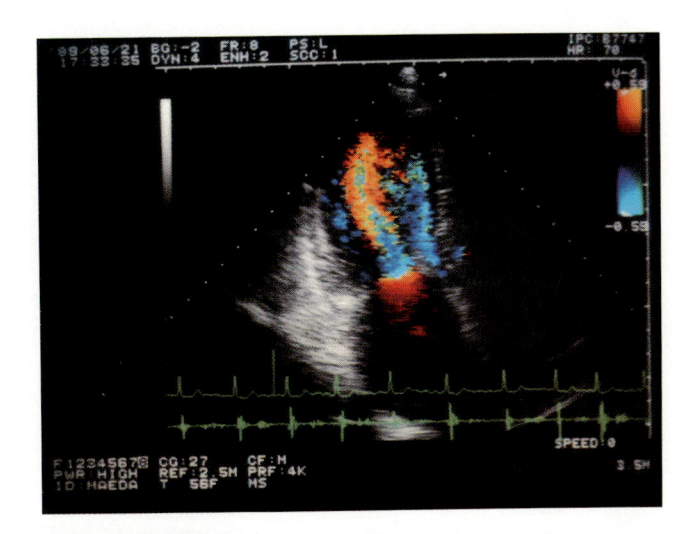

COLOR PLATE 3.
Color flow imaging. Simultaneous recording of color flow matrix and two-dimensional gray scale image.

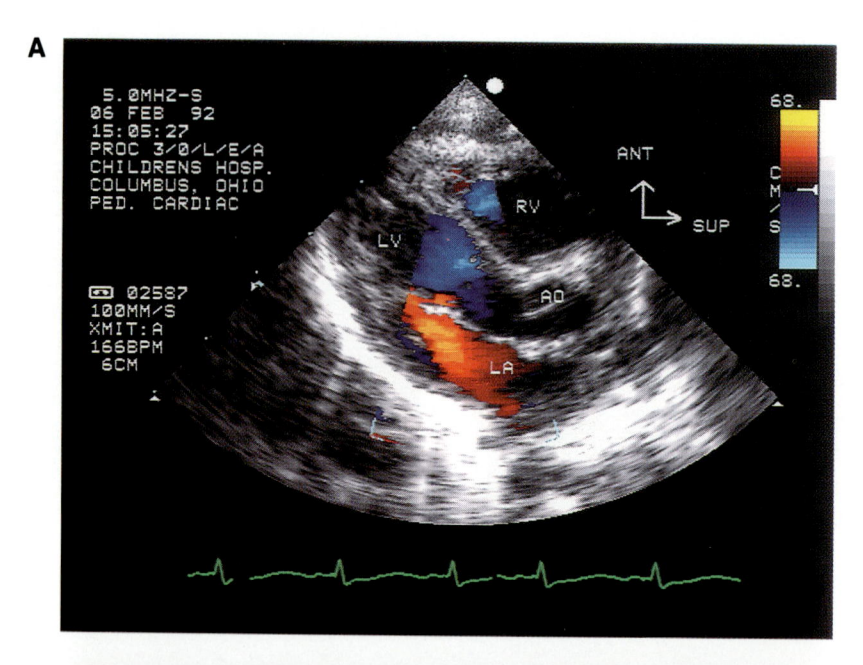

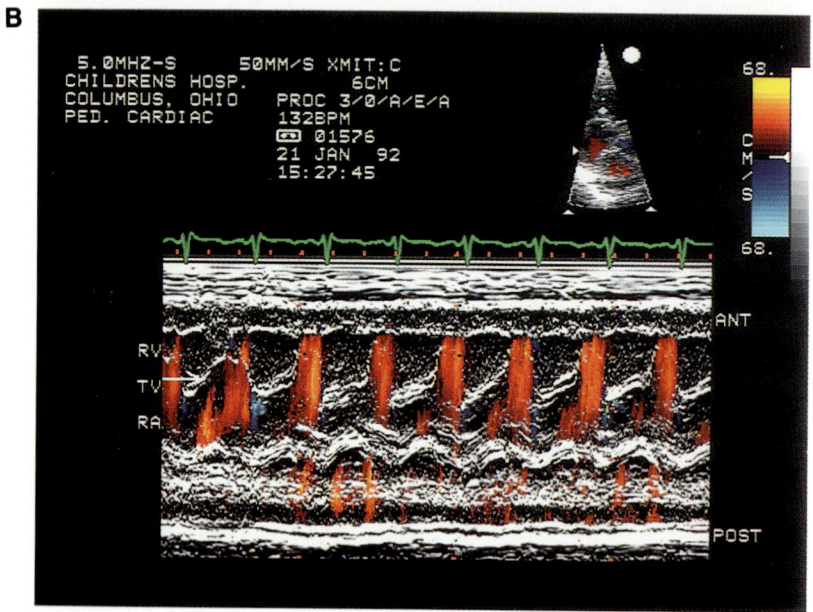

COLOR PLATE 4.
Parasternal color Doppler flow velocity mapping. **A,** color Doppler flow map in long axis view showing direction and velocity of flow *(red-orange color map)* through mitral valve. **B,** color M-mode analysis of tricuspid valve flow. Trivial amount of tricuspid valve regurgitation *(blue color map)* on right atrial side of valve in early systole during some cycles. *Ant* = anterior; *AO* = aorta; *LA* = left atrium; *LV* = left ventricle; *POST* = posterior; *RA* = right atrium; *RV* = right ventricle; *SUP* = superior; *TV* = tricuspid valve.

allows a composite evaluation of mitral inflow and aortic outflow and is especially helpful if the patient has abnormalities of either valve or combined valve abnormalities.

Precordial Right Upper Sternal Border Location

The precordial right upper sternal border location is used primarily for Doppler interrogation of the ascending aorta, particularly for patients with aortic valve stenosis, especially when the poststenotic jet is directed toward the patient's right. It is useful in some patients to image the aortic arch when the suprasternal notch locations cannot be used.

Suprasternal Notch Location

From the suprasternal notch, both a sagittal and coronal plane can be obtained.

Sagittal Plane

The transducer is placed in the notch between the clavicles without placing undue pressure on the trachea or underlying structures. The head is hyperextended and rotated slightly, and liberal amounts of contact gel are applied. The transducer is oriented so that the anterior sector plane is in the same general direction as used for the short-axis precordial examination. The transducer is gently manipulated until the entire ascending aorta arch and proximal descending aorta are seen (Fig 9–27). Immediately underlying the aorta is the proximal right pulmonary artery and below that the left atrium. The superior vena cava lies adjacent to the ascending aorta and connects superiorly to the transverse innominate vein. The great arteries should be visualized arising from the ascending aorta. The first vessel, the innominate artery, should be directed rightward. The sweep of the aorta should be leftward. The color flow and pulsed Doppler examination involves interrogation of each structure in this plane for flow patterns. This view is particularly useful in patients with either aortic stenosis or coarctation of aorta.

Coronal Plane

After the structures in the sagittal plane are evaluated, the transducer is rotated slightly so that the top of the sector is oriented toward the patient's left. The aorta is seen in cross-section in the coronal plane (Fig 9–28). This allows evaluation of the entire caval system, including a left superior vena cava, if present. In addition, the right pulmonary artery can be followed from its origin to the first bifurcation. The left atrium can be evaluated from anterior to posterior, and the pulmonary venous connection can be interrogated in this plane as well.

In our institution, after the examination is completed, M-mode measurements and calculations are made, appropriate Doppler measurements and gradients are calculated, and the technician and physician record their impressions on a worksheet (Fig 9–29). This is used in conjunction with playback review, sometimes frame-by-frame analysis, of the videotape recording of the examination. A final procedural report is then dictated.

BIBLIOGRAPHY

Committee on Drugs, Section on Anesthesiology, American Academy of Pediatric Dentistry: Guidelines for the elective use of conscious sedation, deep sedation, and general anesthesia in pediatric patients, *Pediatrics* 76:317–321, 1985.

Latson LA, Cheatham JP, Gumbiner CH, et al: Midazolam nose drops for outpatient echocardiography sedation in infants, *Am Heart J* 121:209–210, 1991.

Yoshida K, Yoshikawa J, Shakudo M, et al: Color Doppler evaluation of valvular regurgitation in normal subjects, *Circulation* 78:840–847, 1988.

CHAPTER 10

Isotope Scanning

Robert J. Boudreau, Ph.D., M.D.

Claudia M. Engeler, M.D.

Nuclear medicine differs from the other imaging modalities in that it provides functional rather than anatomic information and cannot provide the exquisite anatomical detail available from magnetic resonance imaging (MRI), computed tomography (CT), ultrasound, or angiography. Furthermore, the techniques of nuclear medicine require expensive and cumbersome equipment and are lengthy procedures. Although the doses of radioactive materials are quite safe, consideration has to be given in children to the fact that MRI and ultrasound do not use ionizing radiation. Therefore, what is the role of nuclear medicine in the evaluation of cardiac malformations? Nuclear techniques can provide accurate quantitative measures of blood flow and function of the heart and lungs. For example, nuclear medicine can noninvasively provide a left ventricular ejection fraction with a typical error of four ejection fraction (EF) units. In contrast, left ventricular EF can only be estimated by echocardiographic techniques, and it is extremely expensive to use MRI for this application. In the evaluation of cardiac malformations, quantitative lung scans can easily and accurately determine the relative blood flow to each lung.

In the sections that follow, we review the indications, methodology, and results for several types of nuclear techniques as they relate to cardiac malformations. The underlying principle of each technique is the same: short-lived radionuclides are used as tracers. These are chemically attached to radiopharmaceuticals that track a biochemical or physiologic process. The injected or inhaled radionuclide is imaged with a gamma camera that forms an image of γ-rays. The count density of the image is transferred to a computer for quantitative analysis. Any anatomic information obtained is usually secondary to the physiologic or biochemical information sought.

GATED BLOOD POOL IMAGING OF THE HEART

Equilibrium radionuclide angiocardiography is a frequently used nuclear medicine technique. By synchronizing cardiac contraction with scintillation detection, images of the cardiac blood pool are formed that allow evaluation of ventricular function. The most widely used isotope for this technique is technetium 99m, which is readily available from a molybdenum generator. It has a 6-hour half-life, and its main photopeak is 140 keV, which is ideal for the presently used gamma cameras.

Radiopharmaceuticals used for gated blood pool imaging include ^{99m}Tc human serum albumin (HSA) and red blood cells (RBCs) labeled with ^{99m}Tc. Human serum albumin is a macromolecular radiopharmaceutical that has the advantage of being supplied as a ready-to-use kit. It is given as a single intravenous injection, with the usual dose being 200 μCi/kg and the maximum dose being 25 mCi. Patient preparation is not required, and unlike RBCs, medication does not interfere with the labeling. A disadvantage is the slow leakage of the tracer from the vascular space, which decreases target/background ratio. Part of the tracer is excreted by the kidneys, whereas the remainder accumulates in the liver and extravascular space. The effective half-life in the blood is 4 hours. The target organ is the blood, which receives an estimated dose of 0.063 rad/mCi.[1, 2]

Erythrocytes labeled with ^{99m}Tc are the most commonly used radiopharmaceuticals for gated blood pool imaging. They allow higher target/background ratios than HSA but frequently require two injections. The process involves treating erythrocytes with cold stannous pyrophosphate, a reducing agent. Then ^{99m}Tc pertechnetate is administered. It enters the erythrocyte, is reduced, and binds to the β-chain of hemoglobin. Various medications, including heparin, doxorubicin, hydralazine, prazosin, phenylalanine, penicillin, quinidine, iodinated contrast, and proteins,[3, 4] can interfere with the uptake of stannous chloride into erythrocytes, thereby reducing labeling efficiency.

Three different labeling techniques exist. First is *in vivo labeling,* in which cold stannous chloride and then 20 minutes later ^{99m}Tc pertechnetate are injected intravenously; labeling occurs within the intravascular space.[5] Labeling efficiency is between 80% and 90%. Second is *in vitro labeling,*[6] in which erythrocytes are withdrawn, labeled, and then injected. This time-consuming method is the least frequently used. It achieves, however, the highest labeling efficiency (> 95%). Third is *modified in vivo labeling,*[6] in which after cold stannous pyrophosphate administration, blood is withdrawn into a syringe containing ^{99m}Tc pertechnetate with sodium citrate as an anticoagulant. Heparin should not be used, because it interferes with the labeling process. The syringe is then gently agitated and incubated for 5 to 10 minutes, and the labeled RBCs are reinjected. The usual dose is 200 μCi/kg, with a minimum of 2 to 3 mCi and a maximum of 30 mCi administered. The target organ is the heart wall, with 0.054 rad/mCi and 0.015 rad/mCi total body dose.[7] Labeling efficiency exceeds 90%.

Once the vascular pool is labeled, a computerized gamma camera is used to obtain data. An electrocardiogram (ECG) is connected to the patient and the computer. The R wave triggers the beginning of data acquisition. The R-R interval is divided into at least 16 frames, and data of consecutive cycles are recorded for either a preset time or for the number of counts per frame. In Figure 10–1, schematic time correlation of image sequence, ECG, and volume curve are shown. Each R wave triggers the beginning of the data acquisition, with the cardiac cycle being divided into segments. Counts are consecutively added into the appropriate time segment for a fixed period of time or counts. Typical framing rates are 35 to 50 msec/frame. Data acquisition is done in either a frame mode or, more frequently, in dual buffered list mode, which needs larger memory capacity but allows for more adequate arrhythmia correction. For accurate assessment of regional wall motion, a minimum matrix size of 64 by 64 is needed.

Typically, anterior, 45-degree left anterior oblique, and left lateral views are obtained. This allows optimal

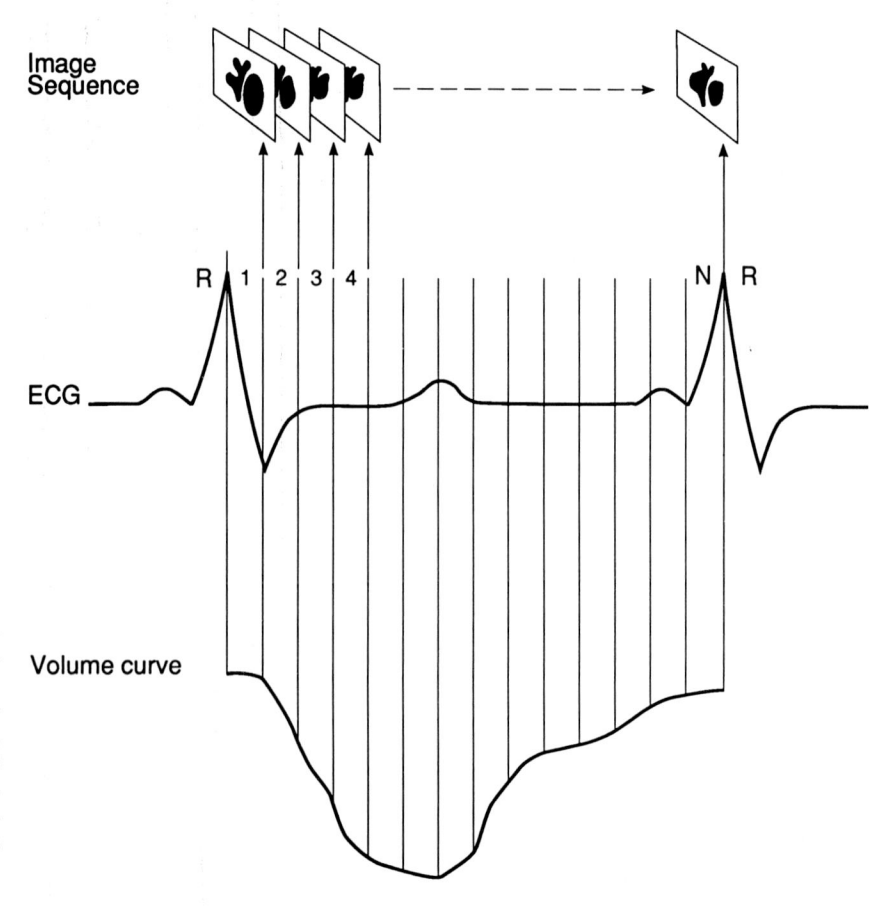

FIG 10–1.
Diagram of gated blood pool imaging. Following detection of R wave, computer begins acquiring data for short-time intervals. This procedure is repeated over many cardiac cycles, typically 10 minutes or until each one of the frames contains 250,000 counts. Then left ventricular region of interest is analyzed for each frame, and subsequent time activity curves of ventricle are generated.

separation of the right and left ventricles. The ventricular ejection fraction is computed as follows:

$$EF = (ED\ counts - ES\ counts)/(ED\ counts - BG)$$

where ED = end diastolic,

ES = end systolic, and

BG = background.

Although the technique can be applied to either the left or right ventricle, because of poor separation of the right atrium from the right ventricle, the calculation of right ventricular ejection fraction (RVEF) is less accurate than calculation of the left ventricular ejection fraction (LVEF). In Figure 10–2,A, a 45-degree left anterior oblique view of a normal resting gated blood pool image is shown. The LVEF is in the normal range, and the time activity curve (lower left) has a normal appearance. The end diastolic and end systolic frames are also shown in the upper left and right images, respectively. The image in the right lower corner represents the end diastolic (dotted line) and end systolic (straight line) contours of the left ventricle.

Functional image analysis from time activity curves of individual pixels is available and useful in the interpretation of the cine display.[8] Both phase and amplitude images can be studied, considering the properties of continuous and periodic (wavelike) mathematical functions. The amplitude image represents the counts ejected (or stroke volume) throughout the cycle. The phase image refers to the point when the peak of contraction occurs, in other words, the timing of the contraction of each pixel in relation to the R wave (ventricular and atrial pixels are about 180 degrees out of phase) (Fig 10–2,B). The image is computed by plotting the location where 25% of the maximum activity in the left ventricle is for frames 1 through 12, starting from end diastolic frame and proceeding to end systole. A crude but useful method of edge detection and wall motion display is by computing the 25% isocontour image of the LVEF (Fig 10–3,A). Segmental EFs can be calculated for any given radian, as well as for the entire ventricle (Fig 10–3,B).

The radionuclide EF determination from gated blood pool imaging has high reproducibility and accuracy.[9] Consideration of tracer labeling, patient motion, positioning, and proper background selection all are important for correct data analysis (Fig 10–4). Normal values of LVEF using equilibrium radionuclide angiocardiography are unavailable for children. First-pass measurements of LVEF are available for children using ^{99m}Tc MDP or Meckel's scanning with ^{99m}Tc pertechnetate.[10] The mean RVEF was

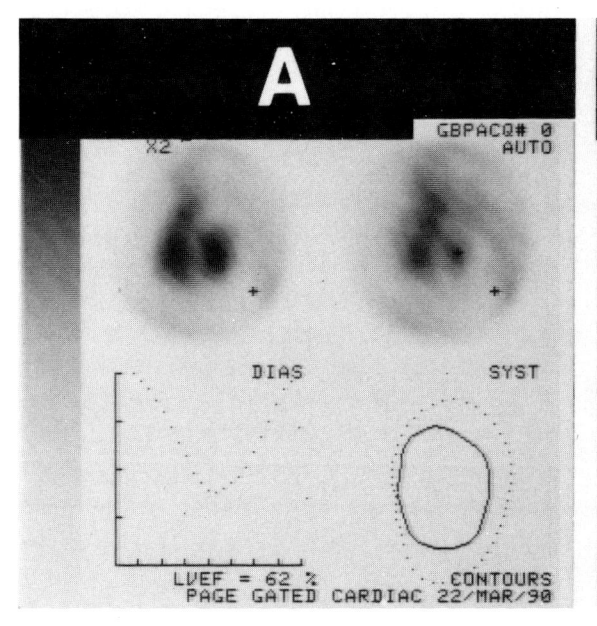

FIG 10–2.
Typical output data. Gated blood pool study. Left ventricle. **A,** end diastolic and end systolic frames. Time activity curve. Left ventricular ejection fraction equals 62%. **B,** phase and amplitude functional images of the heart. *Upper right panel,* left anterior oblique 45-degree end diastolic image. Ventricles separated by interventricular septum. *Lower right panel,* phase image that gray-scales timing of contraction of pixels in entire image. Right and left ventricles contract in synchrony; in other words, they are the same intensity of gray. In contrast, atria and great vessels are 180 degrees out of phase and show as black in this image. *Upper left image;* amplitude of contraction, which is typically more intense in the ventricular region than in the right.

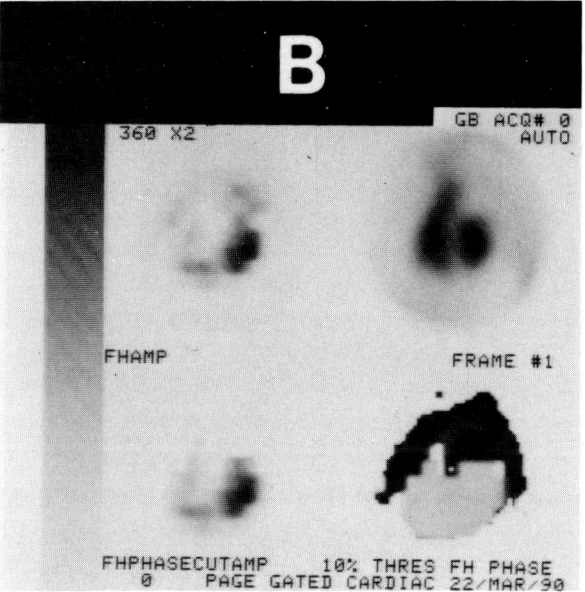

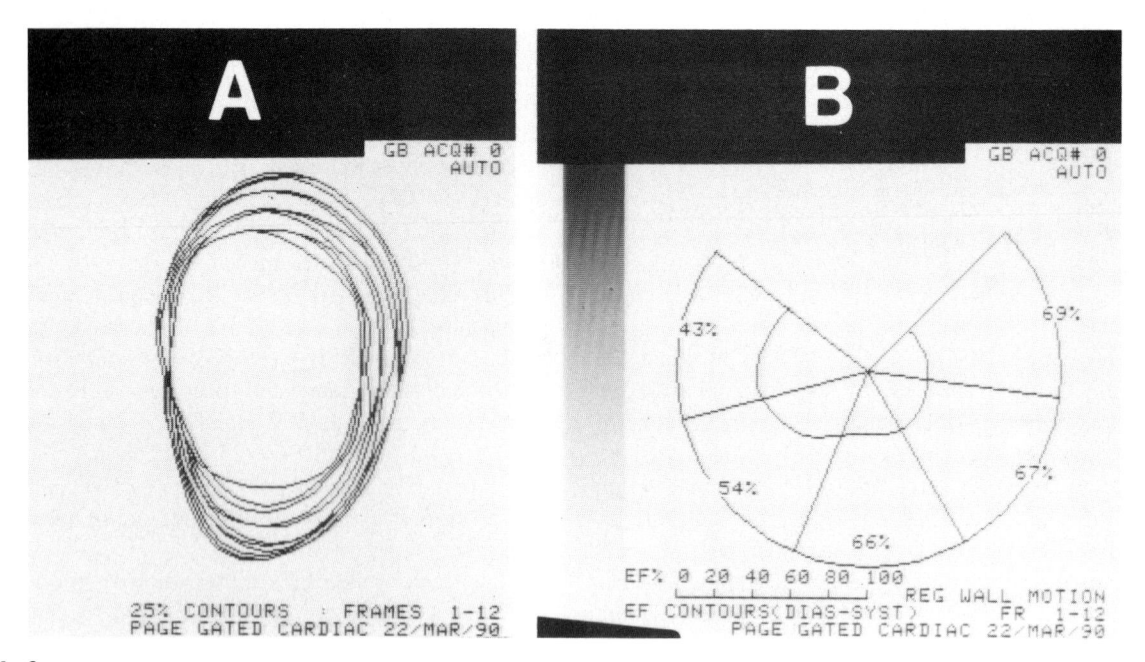

FIG 10–3.
Typical normal gated blood pool output. **A,** 25% isocontours show uniform contraction of left ventricle from end diastole to end systole. **B,** regional ejection fractions of left ventricle.

0.53 ± 0.06, and the mean LVEF was 0.68 ± 0.09.[10]

Equilibrium radionuclide angiocardiography is commonly used to assess ventricular function in patients with cardiomyopathy[11, 12] or a cardiac malformation.[13] Examples are shown in Figures 10–5 and 10–6.

Monitoring of ventricular function in patients with valvar heart disease can assist in medical management.[14]

Attempts to quantitate the amount of valvar regurgitation[15, 16] have a sensitivity 60%–78% but cannot differentiate between degrees of regurgitation.[17] Furthermore, impaired ventricular function significantly interferes with accurate calculations of the regurgitation index.[18]

Ventricular function can be evaluated during exercise testing (Fig 10–7). Normally, LVEF increases by 5 points during exercise. Focal abnormalities of ventricular wall

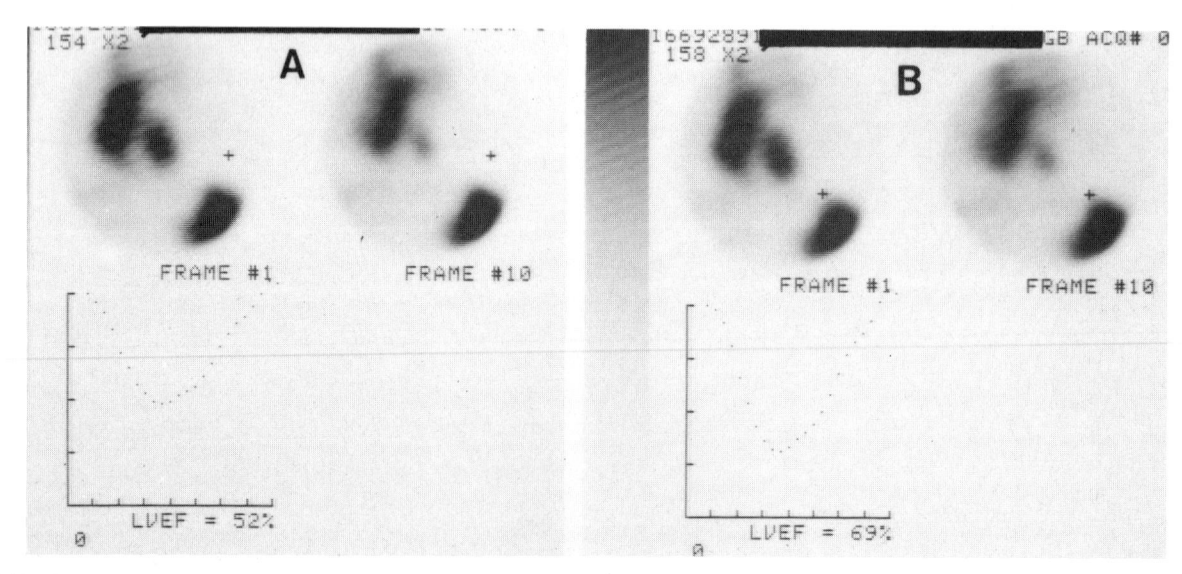

FIG 10–4.
Effect of background position on left ventricular ejection fraction calculation. **A,** cross hair marks background location which is appropriately placed. Calculated left ventricular ejection fraction is 52%. **B,** background deliberately moved too close to spleen. Resulting increase in background results in ejection fraction of 69%. This case illustrates importance of careful quality control.

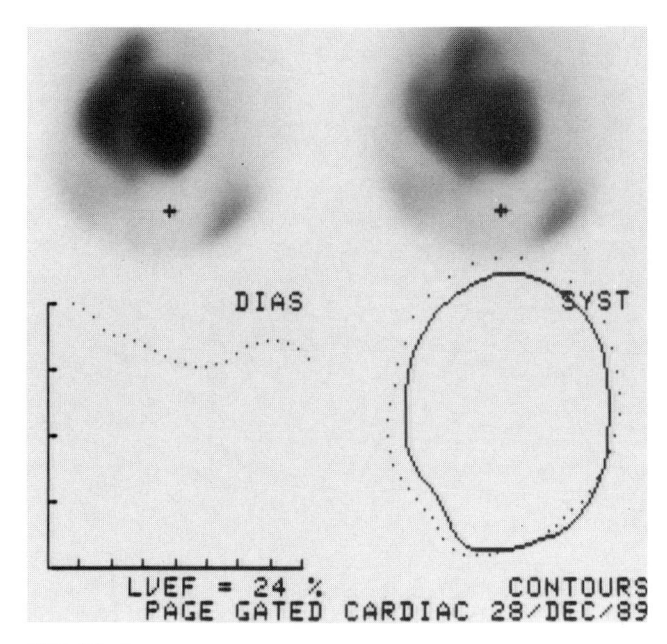

FIG 10–5.
Idiopathic cardiomyopathy. Gated blood pool study. Forty-five-degree left anterior oblique view. Left ventricle massively dilated and hypokinetic. Ejection fraction is very low (24%).

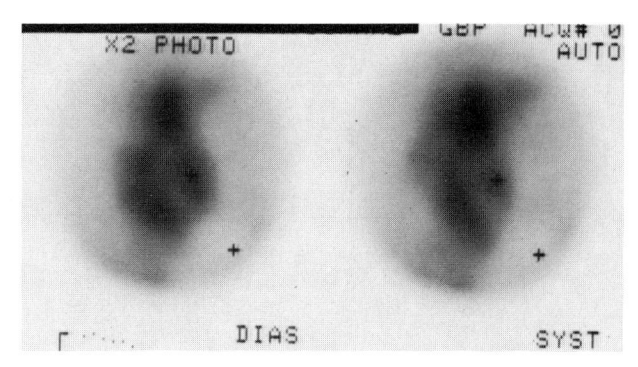

FIG 10–6.
Atrial septal defect and Eisenmenger's syndrome. Gated blood pool study. Forty-five-degree left anterior oblique view. Enlarged and hypokinetic right ventricle. Normal left ventricle.

motion are evident on blood pool imaging in patients with various conditions such as anomalous left coronary artery, thalassemia, mucocutaneous lymph node syndrome, and cardiac tumors.

Attempts have been made to measure ventricular volumes using the labeled erythrocyte techniques. Although good correlation between angiographically measured volumes and radionuclide-based volumes have been reported in children,[19] the mean absolute error is high. Although absolute measurements vary, serial measurements in the same patient are helpful.

FIRST-PASS IMAGING OF THE HEART

Although the gated blood pool technique has been used to obtain an RVEF, the first-pass method is an alternative. This technique can separate temporarily a bolus of radioactive tracer as it travels from the right to the left side of the heart.[20] Furthermore, by correct positioning of the patient, the right atrial counts can be eliminated from the right ventricular activity. Unfortunately, counting statistics are a problem unless a multicrystal detector is used. Although the multicrystal detector is extremely sensitive, these devices have not been available commercially for some time. The spatial resolution of this detector is limited, however. Therefore, its use is confined to the first-pass analysis of VEF and relationship between pulmonary and systemic blood flows (Qp/Qs). If a standard gamma camera is used instead of a multicrystal detector for a first-pass study, disappointing counting statistics are obtained. Because the error of any radioactive measurement is proportional to the square root of the counts, the error of the calculated EFs can become significant.

The counting statistics of the first-pass technique using a conventional gamma camera, have been increased by gating the bolus as it transits the heart.[21] By adding several successive heartbeats (typically 3–8), in a matter analogous to the equilibrium method, the counting statistics are improved. This technique, gated first-pass study, is a reasonable alternative to the multicrystal camera but requires appropriate software for data acquisition and analysis.

To perform satisfactory first-pass imaging, one must have a highly sensitive gamma camera and a bolus injection of radioactivity. The injection may be made through a centrally placed catheter. Complete mixing of the bolus of radioactivity with nonradioactive blood from the inferior vena cava is assumed. The processing of a first-pass study with current clinically available software is lengthy.

The first-pass imaging technique has been used to study both ventricles.[22,23] Because the left ventricle is usually well separated from the other cardiac chambers, the use of this cumbersome technique for this purpose is not as justifiable. The accuracy of determination of RVEF is less than the LVEF with both techniques. A typical normal first-pass study of the heart is shown in Figures 10–8 and 10–9.

The first-pass technique could theoretically be performed using any ^{99m}Tc based radiopharmaceutical except macroaggregated albumin. Usually tracers such as glucoheptonate or diethylenetriaminepentaacetic acid (DTPA) that are rapidly cleared by the kidney are used, so radiation exposure to the patient is reduced and repetitive studies can be performed. As with the gated technique, first-pass EFs can be obtained either at rest or with stress. The first-pass technique is limited in the number of studies that

220 General Introduction

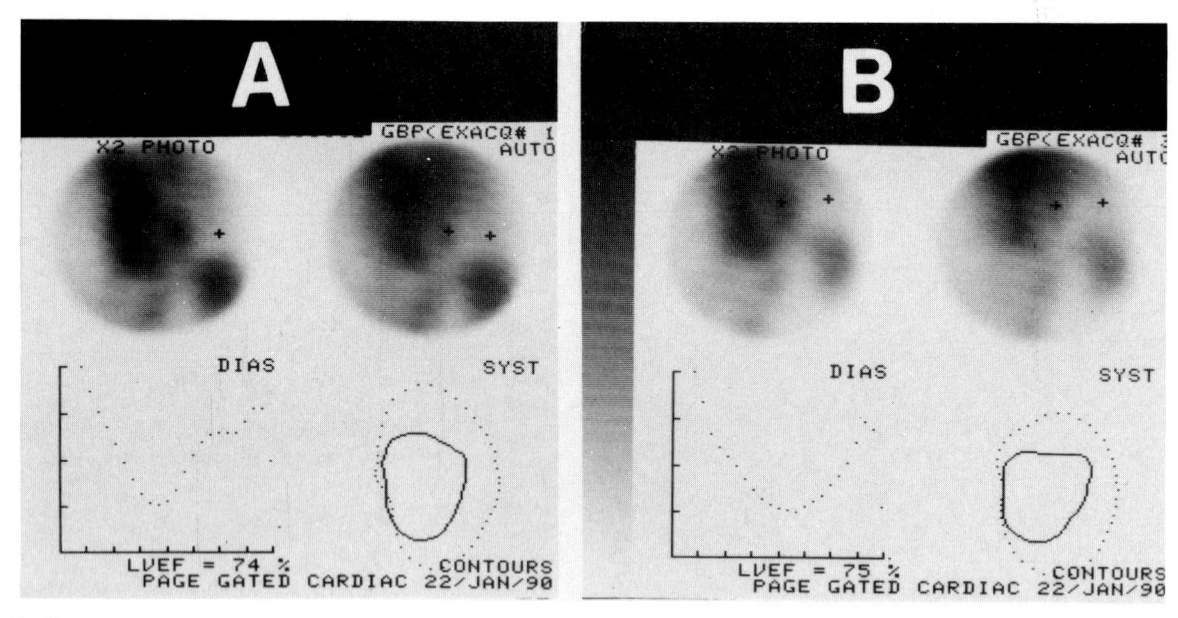

FIG 10–7.
Atrial septal defect. Gated blood pool study. Lateral anterior oblique view. **A**, rest and, **B**, maximum exercise. Left ventricular ejection fraction 74% at rest and 75% with exercise. Failure to increase the injection fraction is abnormal. The right ventricle is enlarged.

can be performed, because each study requires an injection of a radiopharmaceutical. With each study, both the patient dose and the background activity are increased. The clinical indications for first-pass determinations of right or left ventricular function are identical to those of the gated technique.

The first-pass technique has a unique capability. It can measure the QP/QS, an indicator of the degree of left-to-right shunt.[24,25] The patient is positioned in an anterior projection with the lung fields, not just the heart, in the field of view. A bolus of tracer is injected, and data are acquired in a first-pass study. The areas of the right lung and superior vena cava are scanned. The time activity curve of the right lung region is recorded in a computer and displayed.

A normal study shows an increase in activity after the injection, which is followed by a decrease as the bolus passes through the lung. The activity continues to decline until the systemic recirculation returns radioactivity to the lungs. If a left-to-right shunt is present, early pulmonary recirculation is noted as a second hump on the downsloping part of the lung time activity curves (Fig 10–10, solid line). Computer analysis is necessary to separate the pulmonary flow, which is represented by the area under the initial bolus (A1), from the early recirculation activity, which is represented by the area under the second curve (A2). Typically a γ-variate fit, an exponential curve-fitting operation, is applied to the activity curves. The fit begins when the counts are 10% above background on the upslope and terminates when the activity returns to 70% of maximal on the downslope. The remainder of the activity is extrapolated from the γ-variate fit to this small portion of the curve. The dashed line in Figure 10–10 represents this extrapolation. The area under this first curve (A1) is subtracted from the total time activity curve, which results in the recirculation curve (cross-hatched line in Fig 10–10). Another γ-variate is used to determine the extra-

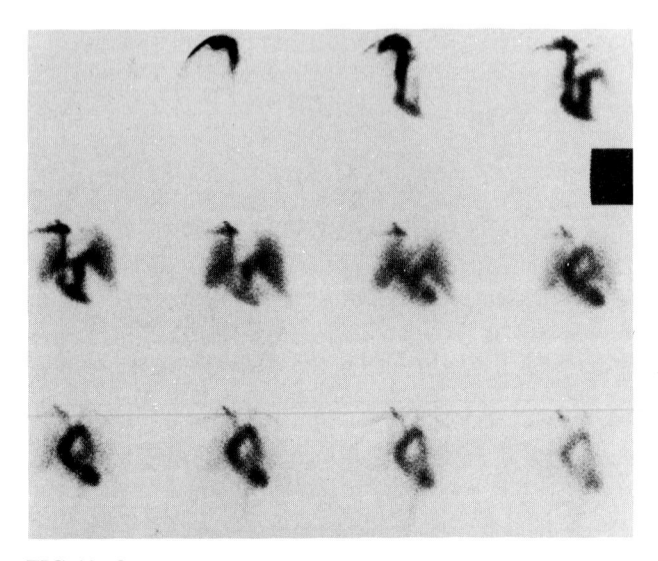

FIG 10–8.
First-pass study of the heart. Two-second sequential images. Left to right, top to bottom. *Upper panel* (sequentially), superior vena cava, right atrium, right ventricle and pulmonary outflow tract. *Middle panel,* lung activity, and by the third image, left ventricle *(third image).* Aorta and great vessels *(fourth image.)*

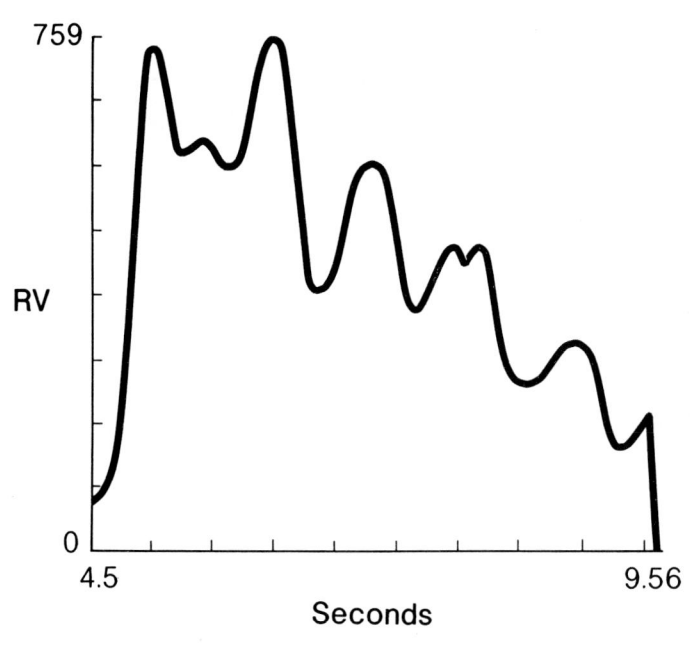

FIG 10-9.
First-pass-time-activity curve of right ventricular region of interest. Right ventricular counts against time. Peaks and valleys represent end diastole and end systole, respectively. Right ventricular ejection fraction 48% (normal).

polated area under this curve (A2). The ratio of pulmonic to systemic flow can then be calculated from the equation:

$$QP/QS = A1/(A1 - A2)$$

Although this technique has been applied successfully in many clinical situations with increased pulmonary blood flow, there are several potential problems. First, an inadequate bolus can adversely affect the accuracy of the study. Second, tricuspid regurgitation or a bidirectional shunt results in erroneous results. Third, it may be difficult to obtain an adequate number of data points on the downslope of the curve to extrapolate the remainder of the curve. In this case, reprocessing the data can then result in fluctuations in the calculated value of the QP/QS that are problematic, especially if the value is of borderline clinical significance (1.5:1). The theoretical normal QP/QS ratio should be 1, but values less than 1.2 are considered normal using this technique. QP/QS measurements may be useful in patients where a variation in volume of pulmonary blood flow is presented or suspected.

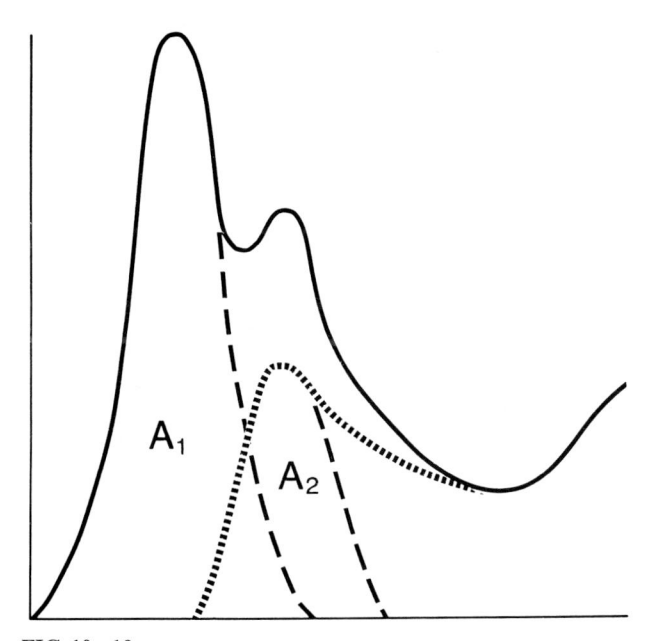

MYOCARDIAL PERFUSION IMAGING

Thallium 201 is currently the most widely used radioactive agent used to study myocardial perfusion in children. As a monovalent cation, similar to potassium, thallium concentrates in the myocardium by the energy requiring sodium-potassium–adenosine triphosphatase (ATPase) mechanisms.[26] Thallium 201 is produced by a cyclotron and has a half-life of 73 hours. It has a low-energy principle emission of 68 to 80 keV (98% abundance). Two γ-photons, with energies of 135 and 167 keV are also emitted, but these have only a 10% abundance.[26] The minimum dose administered is 150 μCi, and maximum dose is 5 mCi, although some states limit the dose to 3 mCi. Regional myocardial uptake of ^{201}Tl is proportional to myocardial blood flow (Fig 10–11). It has a high extraction efficiency (85%), and about 4% of the injected dose localizes in the myocardium. Maximal uptake occurs at 10 to 30 minutes in the resting state, and at 5 to 10 minutes with exercise. The radionuclide then has a half-life of 4 to 6 hours in the myocardium.

FIG 10-10.
Diagram of first-pass QP/QS study. Solid line plots counts over right lung vs. time. Left-to-right shunt. For details, see text.

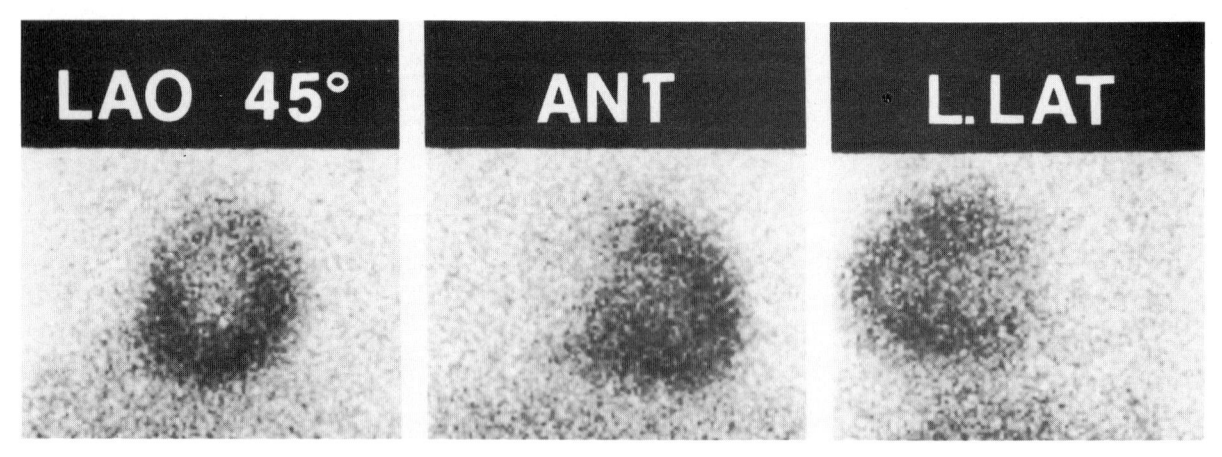

FIG 10–11.
Resting thallium 201 scan. Mucopolysaccharidosis. Left anterior oblique 45-degree view, moving counterclockwise, interventricular septum, inferoapical region, and postlateral wall of heart. Anterior view, moving clockwise, anterolateral wall, apex, and inferior wall of left ventricle. Left lateral view, moving counterclockwise, anterior wall, apex, and inferoposterior regions of left ventricle. Normal study.

The change of the myocardial ^{201}Tl activity with time is called "redistribution." The rate of redistribution is affected by the presence of ischemia (slower washout) (Figs 10–12 and 10–13),[27] level of exercise at the time of injection (accelerated loss with high levels of exercise) (Fig 10–14),[28] and plasma insulin levels (increased loss from ischemic and normal tissue with glucose, potassium, and insulin administration).[29]

A gamma camera with ¼-in. thick crystal usually achieves optimal resolution for the low-energy photons of ^{201}Tl. Anterior, 45-degree left anterior oblique, 70-degree left anterior oblique, and optionally 45-degree right anterior oblique projections should be obtained, each projection containing a total of 150,000 to 500,000 counts. Projections are recorded on either film or the computer. Computer image enhancement with background subtraction, smoothing, and interpolation are helpful. Tomographic reconstruction may increase the sensitivity for detection of abnormalities.[30] A radionuclide angiogram may be added in complex cardiac malformations.

Under resting conditions, the image acquisition is started 20 to 30 minutes after injection. In patients with congestive cardiac failure and therefore increased pulmonary uptake, imaging at 4 to 6 hours improves the target/background ratio.

For studies during exercise, 60 to 90 seconds before termination of the exercise, thallium is injected. The patient must continue to exercise for the remaining time, maintaining maximum stress. Accuracy of the result depends on the maximum exercise level achieved. Imaging begins within 10 minutes of the thallium injection to avoid the effects of early redistribution. Delayed imaging is also performed 2 to 4 hours after injection.

Thallium perfusion studies require strict adherence to technical details, including appropriate background subtraction, identical patient positioning after exercise and at rest (best accomplished with a laser positioner), avoidance of extravasation at the injection site, adequate exercise level, and proper patient preparation.

Although ^{201}Tl studies are performed commonly in

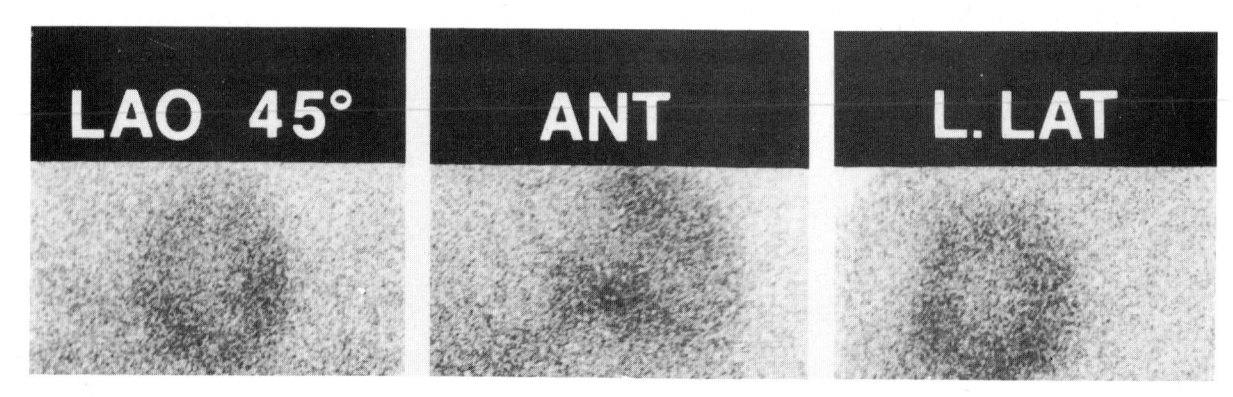

FIG 10–12.
Abnormal resting thallium 201 image. Mucopolysaccharidosis. Reduced thallium accumulation in septum, anterolateral wall, and apex.

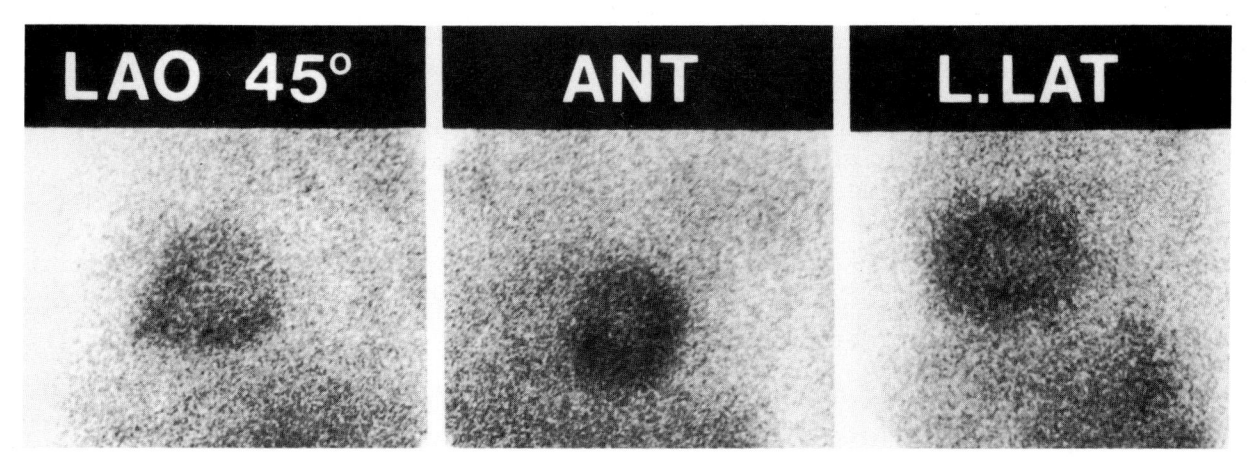

FIG 10–13.
Thallium 201 scan, Hurler's syndrome. Left anterior oblique 45-degree view. Nonhomogeneous perfusion of left ventricle, particularly septal region. Patient has narrowing of left anterior descending coronary artery.

adults to diagnose coronary artery disease, the study is also helpful in children with congenital coronary abnormalities,[31] Kawasaki disease,[34] mucopolysaccharidosis (see Figs 10–12 and 10–13),[31, 35] and to assess myocardial perfusion before and after surgical intervention.[32, 33]

An area of infarction shows decreased uptake during both rest and exercise, whereas areas of ishemia demonstrate decreased tracer accumulation during exercise.

Dipyridamole-enhanced thallium imaging has been helpful in patients who cannot be exercised. Dipyridamole

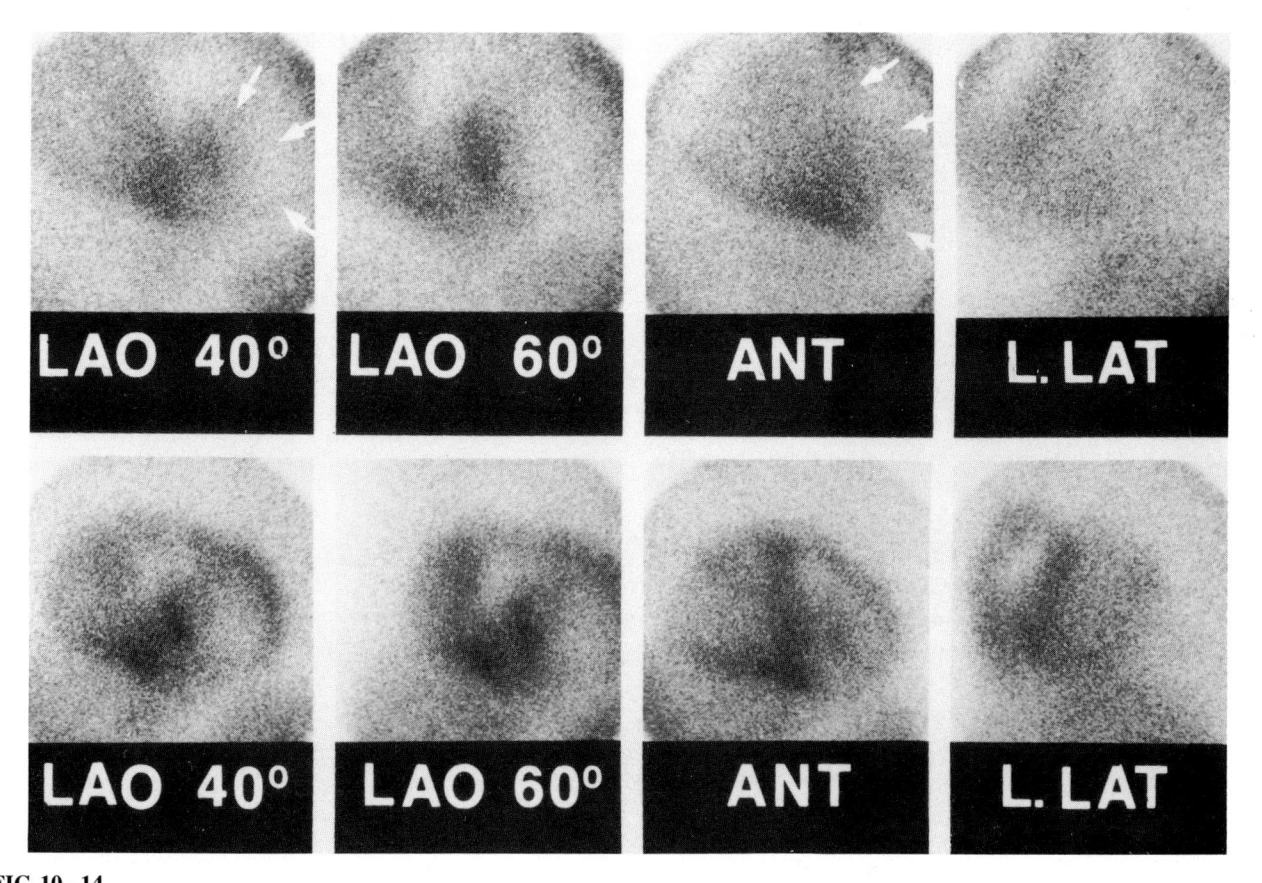

FIG 10–14.
Stress *(upper)* and delayed *(lower)* thallium scans. Tetralogy of Fallot. Large area of reversibly ischemic myocardium *(arrowheads)*. This area, which is not visualized at stress, fills on delayed images *(lower)*. Inferior wall shows fixed defect. Right ventricular hypertrophy and abnormal-appearing septum.

vasodilates normal but not diseased coronary arteries; therefore, ^{201}Tl activity is reduced in the distribution of the diseased artery.

Soon radiopharmaceuticals labeled with ^{99m}Tc will be approved for use in the United States. These agents will expand the role of perfusion imaging in cardiac malformations because of the high count rates that can be obtained at rest. Also first-pass and perfusion studies can be performed using the same agent.

QUANTITATIVE LUNG PERFUSION STUDIES

Macroaggregates of albumin (MAA) labeled with ^{99m}Tc are used for quantitative lung perfusion studies. *U.S. Pharmacopeial* (USP) requirements state that at least 90% of the MAA particles have a diameter between 10 and 90 μm, and none of the particles has a diameter greater than 150 μm. Once injected, ^{99m}Tc MAA is cleared from the lung with a half-life of 2 to 4 hours.[37, 38] After intravenous injection, the particles lodge in the pulmonary arterioles in a distribution directly proportional to blood flow. Because pulmonary blood flow depends on both gravity and the depth of respiration, the particles are administered while the patient is breathing moderately deeply and is in a supine position.

At least 60,000 particles should be injected to obtain sufficient numbers of particles and produce accurate statistical results.[39] Typically, 200,000 to 500,000 particles are injected for a routine adult study. This dose is safe because only 0.1% of the pulmonary arterioles and capillaries are blocked by this number of particles, and the occlusion is only temporary. Albumin microspheres are an alternative but less commonly used radiopharmaceutical, because they have a much longer residence time in the lungs and are not used for cardiac malformations with a right-to-left shunt.

In malformations with a right-to-left shunt, particles are shunted into the systemic circulation. Toxicity of MAA for cerebral embolism[40] shows a margin of safety exceeding 2,000-fold, even with a 50% right-to-left shunt. We routinely study patients with a right-to-left shunt and have not encountered cerebral complications. In such patients, the number of administered particles should be kept to a minimum by preparing fresh MAA and injecting between 50,000 and 100,000 particles. Because deaths have occurred after the administration of MAA in patients with severe pulmonary hypertension, a minimum number of particles should also be used in this situation. Idiosyncratic reactions to MAA have been reported; they should not be administered to patients with hypersensitivity to products containing HSA.

Quantitative lung perfusion studies are useful in patients with cardiac conditions with reduced or segmental pulmonary blood flow to evaluate the distribution caused by stenosis or atresia of the pulmonary arterial branches and after palliative shunt procedures between the systemic and pulmonary circulations.

A quantitative lung perfusion scan is performed by injecting MAA labeled with ^{99m}Tc and imaging both anterior and posterior projections. The counts are averaged for both lungs and the percentage contribution of each lung calculated. In normals, the distribution is 45% to the left lung and 55% to the right lung (Fig 10–15).

The percentage of right-to-left shunting can be estimated by two methods. In one, the counts over the lungs and over the head on the posterior views are determined. Then the counts in the head are expressed as a percentage of counts over the lungs (Fig 10–16). This calculation is not an absolute quantification of the right-to-left shunt but is a useful indicator of the size of the shunt and can be used for serial observations. A second and more sophisticated method determines the total body counts from a gamma camera capable of performing a digital total body scan. Regions of interest over the lungs are drawn, and then the shunt is calculated as (total body counts − total lung counts)/total body counts × 100%.

Quantitative lung scans can be used to assess treatment (Fig 10–17) and to evaluate patients after heart-lung and lung transplants (Fig 10–18). The scans provide useful information concerning the relative severity of disease in each lung preoperatively and also can be used to follow the patients postoperatively.

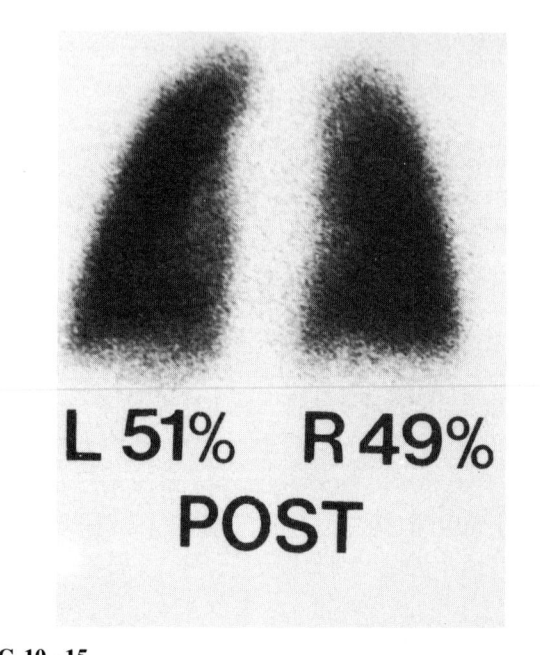

FIG 10–15.
Quantitative lung perfusion scan. Symmetric distribution of tracer and homogenous lung perfusion bilaterally.

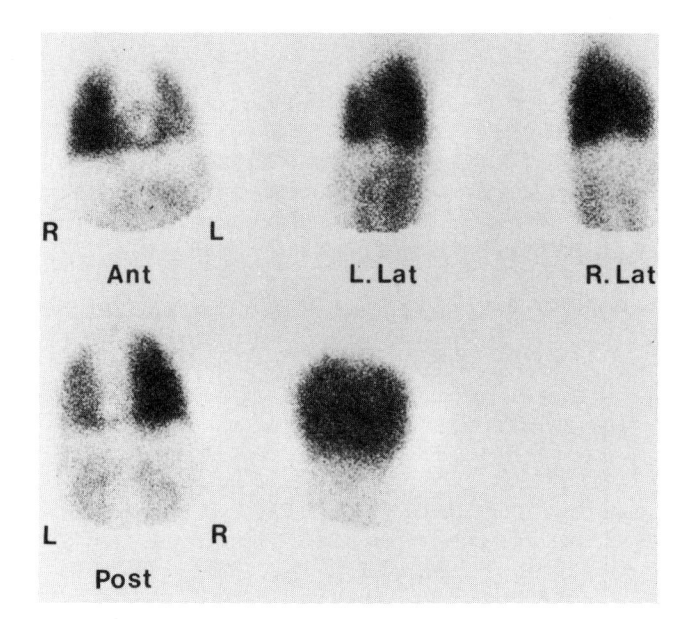

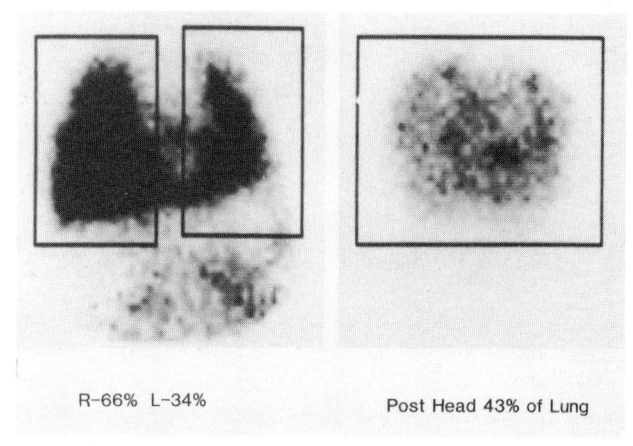

FIG 10–16.
Quantitative lung perfusion study. Patient with very large right-to-left shunt. **A,** five views of head, kidneys, and myocardium. **B,** relative distribution of pulmonary perfusion. Right lung = 66%, left lung = 34%, head = 43% of pulmonary activity.

Scans using ^{99m}Tc MAA are helpful in the evaluation of systemic-pulmonary arterial shunts.[41] These surgical procedures can dramatically alter the distribution of MAA injected intravenously. The appearance of the lung scan can differ from patient to patient because of differing hemodynamic states. Therefore, a study before surgical placement of a shunt is extremely helpful in the evaluation of these patients. Systemic-to-pulmonary arterial shunts all produce a similar pattern of MAA imaging. Because the systemic blood contains less radioactive material than the venous blood, a patent shunt dilutes the radioactivity in the pulmonary region supplied by the systemic-to-pulmonary

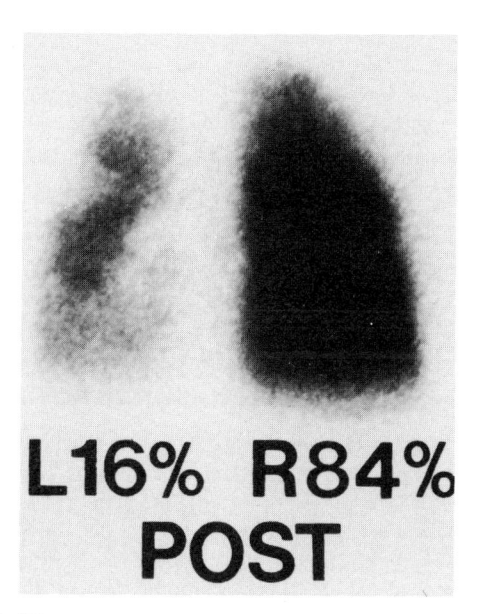

FIG 10–17.
Left pulmonary artery stenosis. Before balloon dilatation, the left lung = 30% pulmonary blood flow. After balloon dilatation the left lung = 16%. Segmental defects in left lung raise possibility of pulmonary embolic disease.

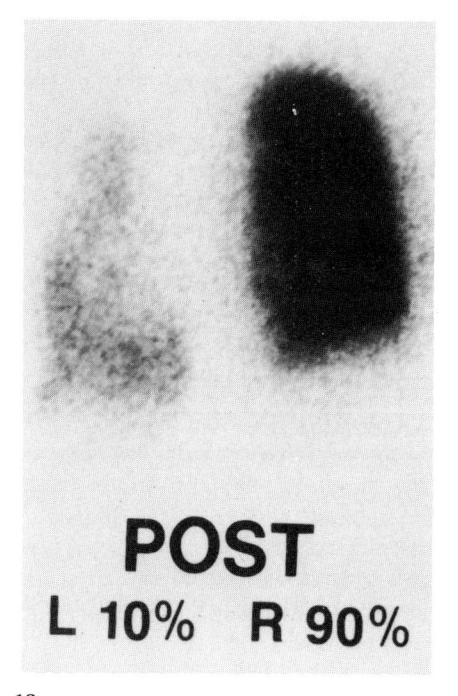

FIG 10–18.
Successful single right lung transplant. Macroaggregates of albumin scan. Transplanted right lung receives 90% of pulmonary blood flow. Homogenous distribution of flow.

shunt. Radioactivity appears preferentially diverted to the nonshunted lung regions. The pattern varies according to the type of shunt. In severe stenosis or atresia of the right ventricular outflow tract, all of the RV blood (and radioactivity) is directed to the systemic circulation. Therefore, the MAA is preferentially directed toward the lung region supplied by the shunt. Thus, knowledge of the patient's hemodynamics and baseline studies is essential to interpret the studies. The pattern of a successful shunt can vary between reduced or augmented radioactivity.

A final application of MAA imaging is in patients with anomalous origin of the left coronary artery. Because the left coronary artery originates from the pulmonary artery rather than the aorta, visualization of the myocardium on a ^{99m}Tc perfusion scan in the absence of a very large right-to-left shunt is diagnostic of anomalous origin of the left coronary artery. Unlike thallium imaging, however, this study does not provide information concerning the relative ischemia of the ventricles.

REFERENCES

1. Harbert JC, Pollina R: Absorbed dose estimates from radionuclides. *Clin Nucl Med* 9:210–221, 1984.
2. Gottschalk A, Hoffer PB, Potchen EJ: Diagnostic nuclear medicine. In *Golden's diagnostic radiology,* Baltimore, Williams and Wilkins, 1988, pp 196–205.
3. Dewanjee MK: The chemistry of Tc-99m labelled radiopharmaceuticals, *Semin Nucl Med* 20:1–98, 1990.
4. duCret RP, Boudreau RJ, Larson T, et al: Suboptimal red blood cell labeling with Tc-99m, *Semin Nucl Med* 18:74–75, 1988.
5. Hegge FN, Hamilton GW, Larson SM, et al: Cardiac chamber imaging: a comparison of red blood cells labeled with Tc-99m in vitro and in vivo, *J Nucl Med* 19:129–134, 1978.
6. Srivastava SC, Chervu LR: Radionuclide labelled red blood cells: current status and future prospects, *Semin Nucl Med* 14:68–82, 1984.
7. Atkins HL, Thomas SR, Buddemeyer U, et al: MIRD dose estimate report no. 14: radiation absorbed dose from technetium 99m labeled red blood cells, *J Nucl Med* 31:378–380, 1990.
8. Boudreau RJ, Loken MK: Functional imaging of the heart, *Semin Nucl Med* 17:28–38, 1987.
9. Pfisterer ME, Ricci DR, Schuler G, et al: Validity of left ventricular ejection fractions measured at rest and peak exercise by equilibrium radionuclide angiography using short acquisition times, *J Nucl Med* 20:484–490, 1979.
10. Hurwitz RA, Treves S, Kuruc A: Right ventricular and left ventricular ejection fraction in pediatric patients with normal hearts: first pass radionuclide angiocardiography, *Am Heart J* 107:727–732, 1984.
11. Pohost GM, Fallon JT, Strauss HW: Radionuclide techniques in cardiomyopathy. In Strauss HW, Pitt B, editors: *Cardiovascular nuclear medicine,* ed 2, St Louis, 1979, Mosby–Year Book, pp 326–342.
12. Alexander J, Dainiak N, Berger HJ, et al: Serial assessment of doxorubicin cardiotoxicity with quantitative radionuclide angiocardiography, *N Engl J Med* 300:278–283, 1979.
13. Parrish MD, Graham TP Jr, Born ML, et al: Radionuclide evaluation of right and left ventricular function in children: validation of methodology, *Am J Cardiol* 49:1241–1247, 1982.
14. Dilsizian V, Rocco TP, Bonow RO, et al: Cardiac blood pool imaging: II, applications in noncoronary heart disease. *J Nucl Med* 31:10–22, 1990.
15. Hurwitz RA, Treves S, Freed M, et al: Quantitation of aortic and mitral regurgitation in the pediatric population: evaluation of radionuclide angiography, *Am J Cardiol* 51:252–255, 1983.
16. Rigo P, Alderson PO, Robertson RM, et al: Measurement of aortic and mitral regurgitation by gated cardiac blood pool scans, *Circulation* 60:306–312, 1979.
17. Nicod P, Corbett JR, Firth BG, et al: Radionuclide techniques for valvular regurgitant index: comparison in patients with normal and depressed ventricular function, *J Nucl Med* 23:763–769, 1982.
18. Lam W, Pavel D, Byron E, et al: Radionuclide regurgitant index: value and limitations, *Am J Cardiol* 47:292–298, 1981.
19. Parrish MD, Graham TP Jr, Born ML, et al: Radionuclide ventriculography for assessment of absolute right and left ventricular volumes in children, *Circulation* 66:811–819, 1982.
20. Berger HJ, Matthay RA, Pytlik LM, et al: First-pass radionuclide assessment of right and left ventricular performance in patients with cardiac and pulmonary disease, *Semin Nucl Med* 9:275–295, 1979.
21. Harolds JA, Grove RB, Bowen RD, et al: Right-ventricular function as assessed by two radionuclide techniques: concise communication, *J Nucl Med* 22:113–115, 1981.
22. Holman BL, Wynne J, Zielonka JS, et al: A simplified technique for measuring right ventricular ejection fraction using the equilibrium radionuclide angiocardiogram and the slant-hole collimator, *Radiology* 138:429–435, 1981.
23. Legrand V, Chevigne M, Foulon J, et al: Evaluation of right-ventricular function by gated blood-pool scintigraphy, *J Nucl Med* 24:886–893, 1983.
24. Maltz DL, Treves S: Quantative radionuclide angiocardiography: determination of QP/QS in children, *Circulation* 47:1049–1056, 1973.
25. Alderson PO: Basic principles of shunt quantitation by radionuclide angiocardiography, *Appl Radiol* 9:162–170, 1980.
26. Lebowitz E, Green MW, Fairchild R, et al: Thallium-201 for medical use: I, *J Nucl Med* 16:151–155, 1975.
27. Pohost GM, Alpert NM, Ingwall JS, et al: Thallium redistribution mechanism and clinical utility, *Semin Nucl Med* 10:70–93, 1980.
28. Kaul S, Chesler DA, Pohost GM, et al: Influence of peak exercise heart rate on normal thallium myocardial clearance, *J Nucl Med* 27:26–30, 1986.
29. Wilson RA, Okada RD, Strauss HW, et al: Effect of

30. glucose-insulin potassium infusion on thallium clearance, *Circulation* 68:203–209, 1983.
30. Treves S, Hill TC, VanPraagh R, et al: Computed tomography of the heart using thallium 201 in children, *Radiology* 132:707, 1979.
31. Anderson RH, Macartney FJ, Shinebourne EA, et al: *Pediatric Cardiology,* New York, 1987, Churchill Livingstone, vol. 2.
32. Finley JP, Howman-Giles RB, Gilday DL, et al: Thallium-201 myocardial imaging in anomalous left coronary artery arising from the pulmonary artery: application before and after medical and surgical treatment, *Am J Cardiol* 42:675, 1978.
33. Gutgesell HP, Pinskey WW, DePuey EG: Tl-201 myocardial perfusion imaging in infants and children: value in distinguishing anomalous left coronary artery from congestive cardiomyopathy, *Circulation* 61:596, 1980.
34. Kato H, Ichinose E, Yoohioka F, et al: Fate of coronary aneurysms in Kawasaki disease; serial coronary angiography and long term follow up study, *Am J Cardiol* 49:1758, 1982.
35. Hudson REB: The cardiomyopathies: order from chaos, *Am J Cardiol* 25:70–77, 1970.
36. Khaja F, Alam M, Goldstein S, et al: Diagnostic value of visualization of the right ventricle using thallium 201 myocardial imaging, *Circulation* 59:182, 1979.
37. Robbins PJ, Feller PA, Nishiyama H: Evaluation and dosimetry of a Tc99m Sn-MAA lung imaging agent in humans, *Health Physics* 30:173, 1976.
38. Malone LA, Malone JF, Ennis JT: Kinetics of technetium 99m labelled macroaggregated albumin in humans, *Br J Radiol* 56:109, 1983.
39. Heck LL, Duley JW: Statistical considerations in lung imaging with Tc-99m albumin particles, *Radiology* 113:675, 1974.
40. Taplin GV, MacDonald NS: Radiochemistry of macroaggregated albumin and newer lung scanning agents, *Semin Nucl Med* 1:132, 1971.
41. Rosenthal A: Care of the postoperative child and adolescent with congenital heart disease. In Barness LA, et al, editors: *Advances in pediatrics,* Chicago, 1983, Mosby–Year Book, vol 30, pp 131–167.

CHAPTER 11

Magnetic Resonance Imaging

Antoinette S. Gomes, M.D.

Gustav Formanek, M.D.

During the first half of the 1980s, the new imaging modality magnetic resonance imaging (MRI) was developed.

Of all the currently available noninvasive imaging techniques, magnetic resonance (MR) imaging is unique in its ability to depict cardiac structures. It affords visualization of the entire heart in multiple projections in both a static and dynamic format. Several characteristics of MR make it particularly suitable for imaging the heart. These include the absence of ionizing radiation, the high natural contrast between flowing blood and soft tissue, the wide field of view obtained, and the ability to image the heart in multiple standard and compound oblique projections. In a short time, MRI has become an important cardiac imaging tool. It is an important noninvasive complement to echocardiography and in many instances affords information similar to angiocardiography.

MRI has been found useful in the evaluation of the folllowing: (1) complex cardiac malformations in which the visceroatrial situs and spatial relationships of the heart must be clearly identified; (2) anomalies of the aortic arch, including aortic interruption, coarctation of the aorta, vascular rings, and acquired conditions such as Marfan's syndrome and aortic dissection; (3) anomalies of the central pulmonary arterial tree; (4) cardiac masses; (5) postoperative evaluation, particularly in complex lesions or for assessment of shunt patency; and (6) conditions for which angiography is contraindicated. It also offers the potential for assessment of wall motion and determination of regurgitant and shunt fraction.

MRI PHYSICAL PRINCIPLES

The images obtained with MRI resemble those of computer tomography (CT) in that organs are distinguished by their contrast on a black-white scale. The underlying principles of image formation are different, however. In CT, contrast depends on differences in the x-ray attenuation, whereas in MRI, tissue contrast is dependent on difference in tissue behavior when placed in an external magnetic field and exposed to radiofrequency radiation. Magnetic resonance imaging is based on the nuclear magnetic properties of tissues. Imaging depends on the characteristic resonance of the atomic nucleus. After exposure to a magnetic field and absorption of an appropriate radiofrequency pulse, resonance is induced and nuclei continue to resonate and emit radiofrequency electromagnetic waves until they return to their original state of equilibrium. These waves can be detected and converted into images. The two principal components of exponential decay of the nuclear resonance are characterized as T1 (longitudinal) and T2 (transverse) relaxation times. The T1 and T2 values of tissues vary with the molecular structure and physical state of the material. Of all the isotopes in the body the hydrogen atom is the most abundant and produces the highest signal strength. Because the hydrogen atom has a single proton in the nucleus, proton density indicates the distribution of the resonating nuclei of hydrogen within the imaging sample. The sensitivity and abundance of hydrogen atoms serve as the basis for MRI.

It is beyond the scope of this book to analyze MRI technique in detail (for the fundamental principles of MRI see references 1–4). In MRI, there is high natural contrast between flowing blood and soft tissues. Currently, most cardiac imaging is performed using spin-echo and gradient-echo pulse sequences. Spin-echo (SE) pulse sequences used are static imaging. Within the physiologic range, on SE images moving blood does not produce a signal. Therefore, it appears black (signal void) and creates excellent contrast to signals emitted by the myocardium of the heart or from walls of the vascular tree. This technique uses a 90° pulse followed by a 180° refocusing pulse. Flowing blood that leaves the imaging slice before receiv-

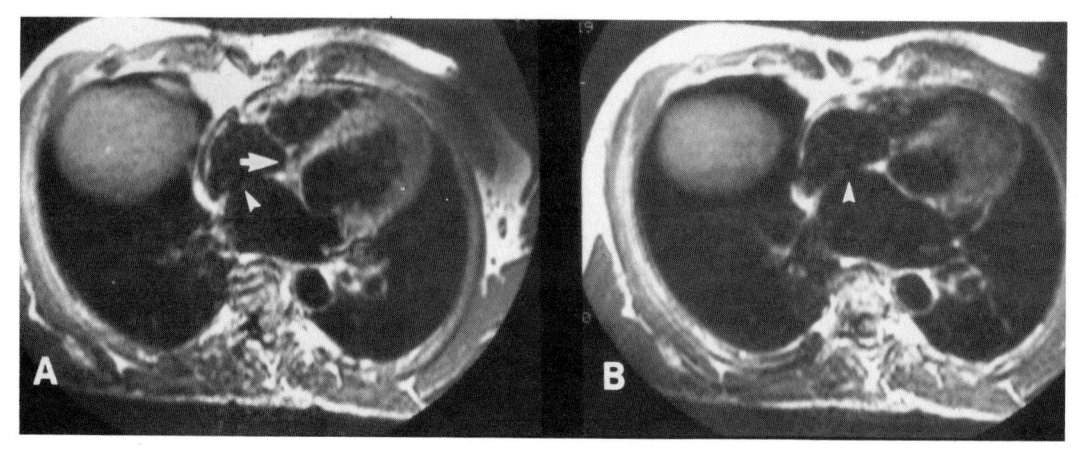

FIG 11-1.
Magnetic resonance images. Axial plane. Caudocranial sequence. Spin-echo protocol. Flowing blood rveals signal void, is imaged black, and creates contrast with signal-emitting tissues. **A,** characteristic anterior insertion of septal leaflet of tricuspid valve *(arrow),* an important hallmark for identification of right ventricle. **B,** thinning of atrial septum *(arrowhead)* at foramen ovale. Spatial relationship of individual cardiac chambers and proximal vessels is shown.

ing the second RF pulse is not excited and therefore produces no echo signal (Fig 11–1). The second technique used for cardiovascular imaging is gradient-echo imaging sometimes displayed as "cine MR".[5-7]

In this pulse sequence, a selective RF pulse excites the spins, but the spins are not tipped a full 90° and instead of the 180° refocusing pulse, a nonselective RF refocusing-gradient pulse is applied a short time after the initial RF pulse, producing a gradient echo. Because heart muscle is relatively stationary in the slice being imaged, it is contin-

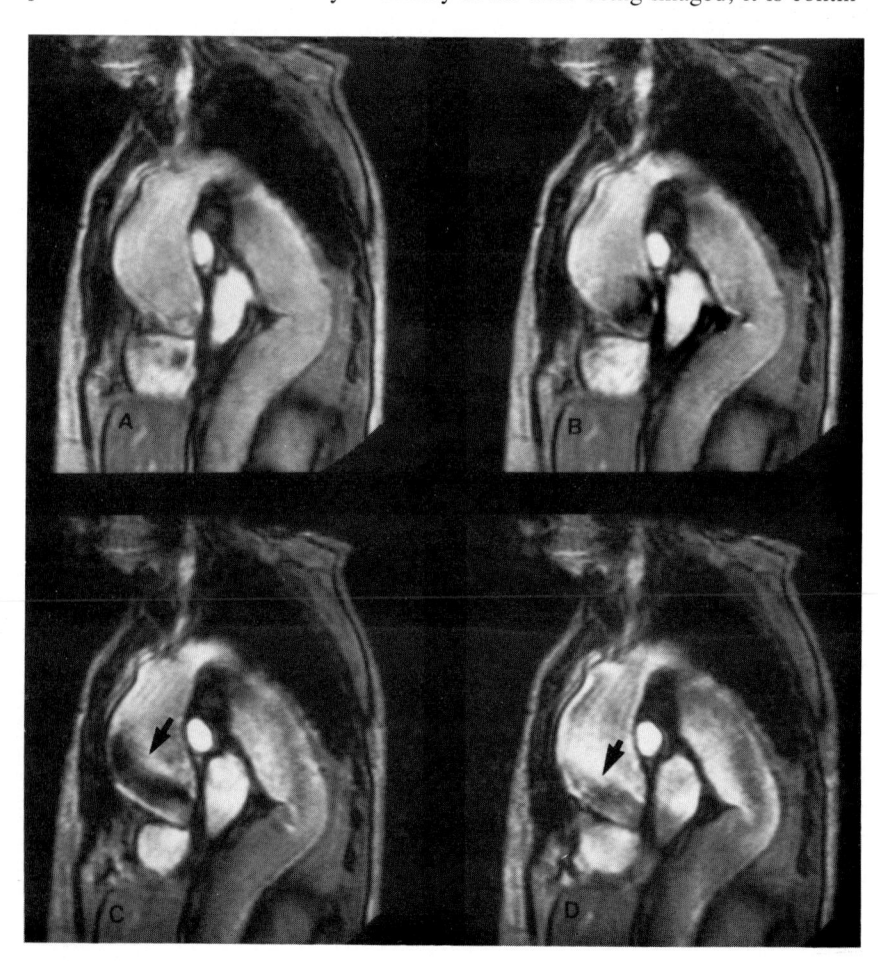

FIG 11-2.
Magnetic resonance images. Thoracic aorta with bicuspid aortic valve. Left anterior oblique plane. Gradient echo sequence. Bicuspid aortic valve. Different phases of cardiac cycle. **A,** diastole. **B–D,** various stages of systole. Normally flowing blood emits high-intensity signals *(white),* turbulent flow with high-velocity moving blood *(black).* Turbulent flow at site of eccentric jet *(arrows)* are seen on **C** and **D.**

uously re-excited by the rapid RF pulses. As the spins do not have time to recover between successive excitations, they become saturated and return little signal. Rapidly moving blood, however, has not been exposed to any of the previous RF pulses, is not saturated, and returns a very strong signal. Flowing blood, therefore, appears as bright signal relative to myocardium. (Fig 11-2)

The full potential of MR techniques in the assessment of the functional status of the heart has yet to be realized. The dynamic display of cardiac function provided by cine MR represents only the first stage of development. The phase data acquired during the formation of MR images (magnitude data) has the potential to provide information on blood flow and velocity, and newer MR techniques offer the potential to image the heart in very short periods of time, on the order of seconds.[8]

ADVANTAGES

The low energy of radiofrequency radiation of MRI is harmless to humans. MR cardiac imaging is done with ECG gating or ECG triggering. Electronic angulation is used to obtain images in multiple obliquities and imaging planes.[9]

With current MRI techniques, certain patients should not undergo MRI. These include patients with pacemakers, as the changing magnetic fields may reset the pacemaker.[10] In addition, patients with intracerebral aneurysm clips or metallic foreign body in the eye should not undergo MRI. Prosthetic heart valves are not a contraindication to MRI unless the valve is partially dehisced.[11,12] Sternal wires and cardiac surgical clips may produce artifact in some imaging planes, but are not a contraindication to imaging with current imaging systems. When imaging children, sedation is necessary, as motion artifacts seriously degrade images.

MRI: CARDIAC APPLICATIONS

Although MRI is still evolving, MRI is used routinely in the evaluation of a variety of congenital lesions. With MRI, the configuration and size of the atrial and ventricu-

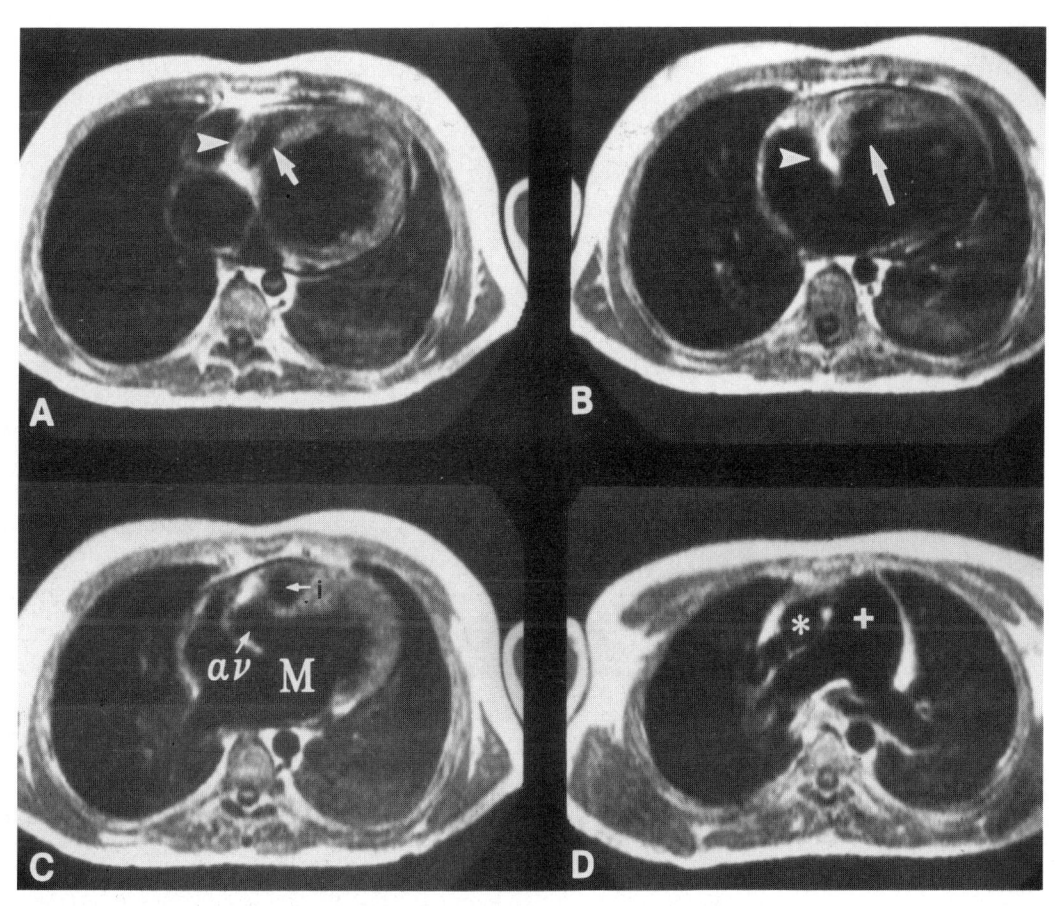

FIG 11-3.
Magnetic resonance images. Axial plane. **A-D,** caudocranial sequence. Tricuspid atresia. At site of tricuspid valve a membrane with medium intensity present *(arrowhead)*. **C,** large mitral valve *(M)*. Hypoplastic right ventricle *(small arrow)*, bulboventricular foramen *(large arrow)*. Large pulmonary artery (+) from widely opened infundibulum *(i)*. Ascending aorta (*). Aortic valve *(av)*.

232 General Introduction

lar chambers is readily identified, as is the number and location of AV valves and the relationship of the great vessels (Fig 11-3). The anatomy and drainage of the systemic veins is clearly delineated. These factors make MRI useful in the identification of abnormalities of situs.

VISCEROATRIAL SITUS

While displaying the structures of the heart within the particular imaging slice, the spatial relationship is not distorted, and the visceroatrial situs and ventriculoarterial connections can be readily identified (Fig 11-4). Because the intrinsic details of the heart are not obscured by contrast medium, the segmental anatomy is clearly seen, with better spatial resolution than echocardiography.[13,14] For instance, identification of the moderator band and the septal leaflet of the right ventricle make it possible to identify the bulboventricular loop (see Fig 11-1).[15] Of the imaging modalities currently available, MRI gives the most detailed images of cardiac anatomy.[16]

The following examples illustrate the advantage of MRI compared to angiocardiography in the determination of visceroatrial situs. The first patient underwent angiography in infancy, and the diagnosis of dextrocardia and single ventricle with right aortic arch was made. At age 15 years, coronal and sagittal magnetic resonance images (Fig 11-5) contributed to the final diagnosis: dextrocardia with abdominal heterotaxia, left-sided azygous continuation of the inferior vena cava, cor biloculare with morphologic right ventricle, anterior aorta with right arch, pulmonary atresia with absent main pulmonary artery, and large single collateral from the proximal descending aorta to both good-sized right and left pulmonary arteries, which are not interconnected. Unfortunately, axial scans, which would have given information about the pulmonary venous return and the status of the systemic veins, were not performed.

In the second patient the diagnosis was ventricular septal defect and coarctation. The chest radiograph showed dextrocardia. With the help of axial MRI scans, the type of dextrocardia was determined as a d-cardiac loop (Fig 11-6). This assessment was based on the identification of the morphologic right ventricle as a right-sided cardiac structure. The excellent portrayal of intrinsic cardiac anatomy, including connections and spatial relations, by MRI obviates the need for angiocardiographic studies and supplies more detailed information.

Knowledge of the anatomic details of systemic veins that can be shown by MRI in certain forms of complex cardiac malformations is important preoperatively because of the high incidence of associated systemic venous anom-

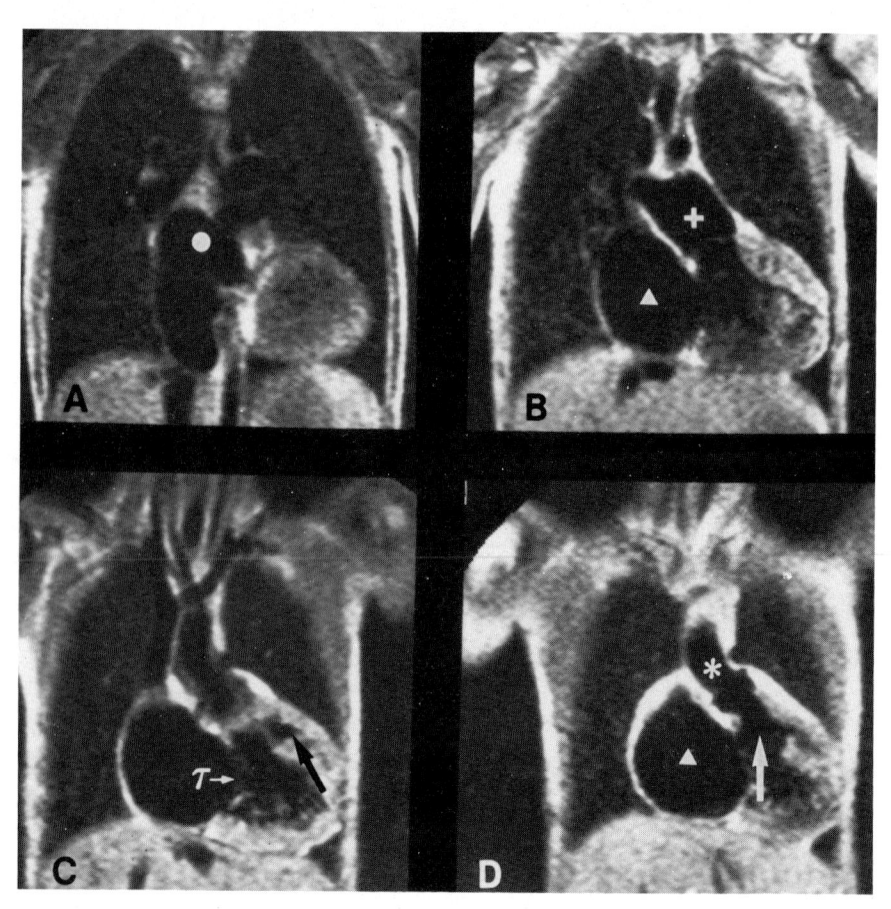

FIG 11-4.
Magnetic resonance images. Posteroanterior plane. Coronal scan. Mitral atresia and rudimentary subaortic chamber. Small left (○), large right (△) atrium. Only right (tricuspid, T) atrioventricular valve is demonstrated. Large pulmonary artery (+) posterior to small descending aorta (*). Bulboventricular foramen and subaortic chamber (arrow).

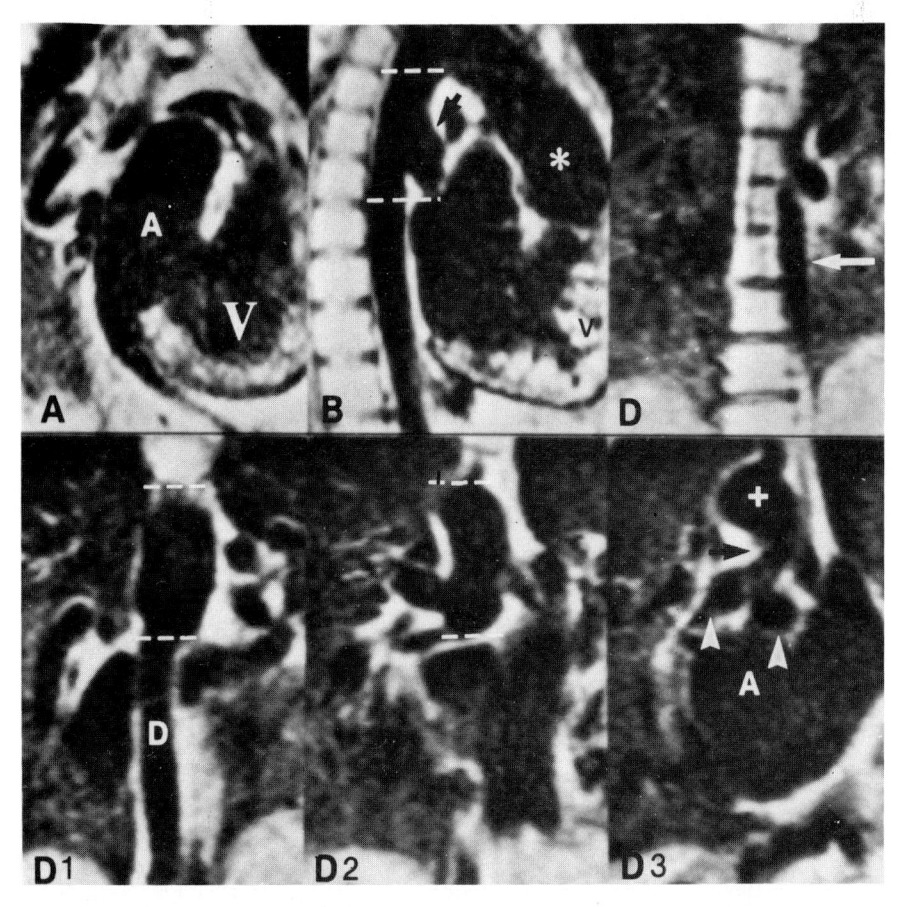

FIG 11–5.
Magnetic resonance images. Posteroanterior sequence. **A** and **B** sagittal; **D** coronal. Hemiazygous continuation of left inferior vena cava *(white arrow)*, single atrium *(A)* and single trabeculated ventricle *(V)*, anterior aorta (*), with right arch (+) and right descending aorta *(D)*. Pulmonary artery absent, large systemic collateral *(black arrows)* connected to central pulmonary artery branches *(arrowheads)*. Portion of aorta between the lines of **B** corresponds to the marked part on *D1* and *D2* frames.

alies.[17] In one series, magnetic resonance imaging accurately identified 98% of the systemic veins and 95% of the pulmonary veins.[18]

It is uncommon that MRI is employed to evaluate simple congenital lesions, such as an atrial septal defect or ventricular septal defect, as they can usually be identified with echocardiography. Because these lesions are usually constituents of complex congenital heart disease, it is important to appreciate their appearance on MRI. Atrial septal defects are identified on spin-echo images as defects in the interatrial septum.[19] With selection of the appropriate projection, their type can be determined. There is a tendency to overcall ostium secundum–type defects with spin-echo MR imaging, as signal dropout may occur in the region of the fossa ovalis, where the interatrial septum is normally thinner (see Fig 11–1,B). Ventricular septal de-

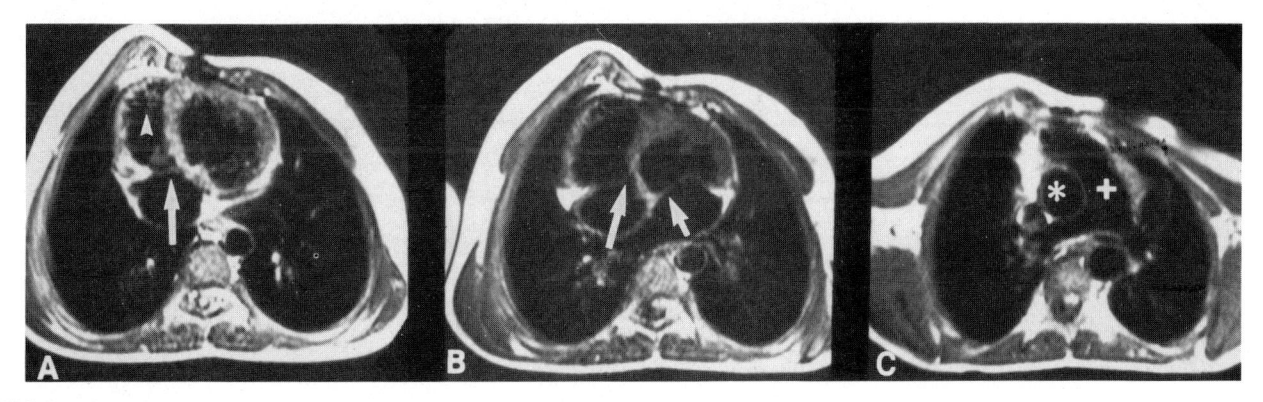

FIG 11–6.
Magnetic resonance images. Axial plane. **A–C,** caudocranial sequence. Dextroversion. Moderator band *(arrowhead)* and tricuspid valve *(arrow)* identified by characteristic more apical insertion of septal leaflet *(arrow)* as opposed to **B** mitral valve *(small arrow)*. Therefore, right-sided ventricle is the morphologic right ventricle. Normally related aorta (*) and pulmonary artery (+). The pulmonary veins drain into the left-sided atrium.

fects, if large, can be readily identified (Fig 11–7,A), and their location and relationship to the great vessels identified.[20] Small defects may be missed, and it is important to note that muscular defects are usually not seen with spin-echo techniques. In general, the presence of atrial or ventricular shunts is more readily identified on gradient-echo images as the bright signal of the shunted blood is seen traversing the defect (Fig 11–7,B).

Complex congenital lesions, such as single ventricle and double-outlet right ventricle, can also be diagnosed with MR imaging. There have been no large series describing the applicability of MRI in the evaluation of patients with these lesions; however, the type of double-outlet right ventricle and relationship of the ventricular septal defect to the great vessels can be determined.[21] Single ventricle anatomy can also be determined.

Congenital abnormalities of the great Vessels

On spin-echo transverse images, the anteroposterior relationship of the aorta and pulmonary artery is readily identified. The thoracic aorta may not be seen in its entirety on sagittal views, as it may buckle in and out of plane. In these cases, it is necessary to synthesize the entire aorta from multiple views or to perform image reconstruction.

Truncus arteriosus, patent ductus arteriosus, and aorticopulmonary window have all been diagnosed with MRI. MRI studies are frequently performed to evaluate suspected vascular rings[22] and tracheal compression. Double aortic arch has a characteristic appearance on MRI, as both limbs of the arch can be identified (Fig 11–8).

MRI is used both preoperatively and postoperatively to evaluate coarctation of the aorta (Fig 11–9). Estimation

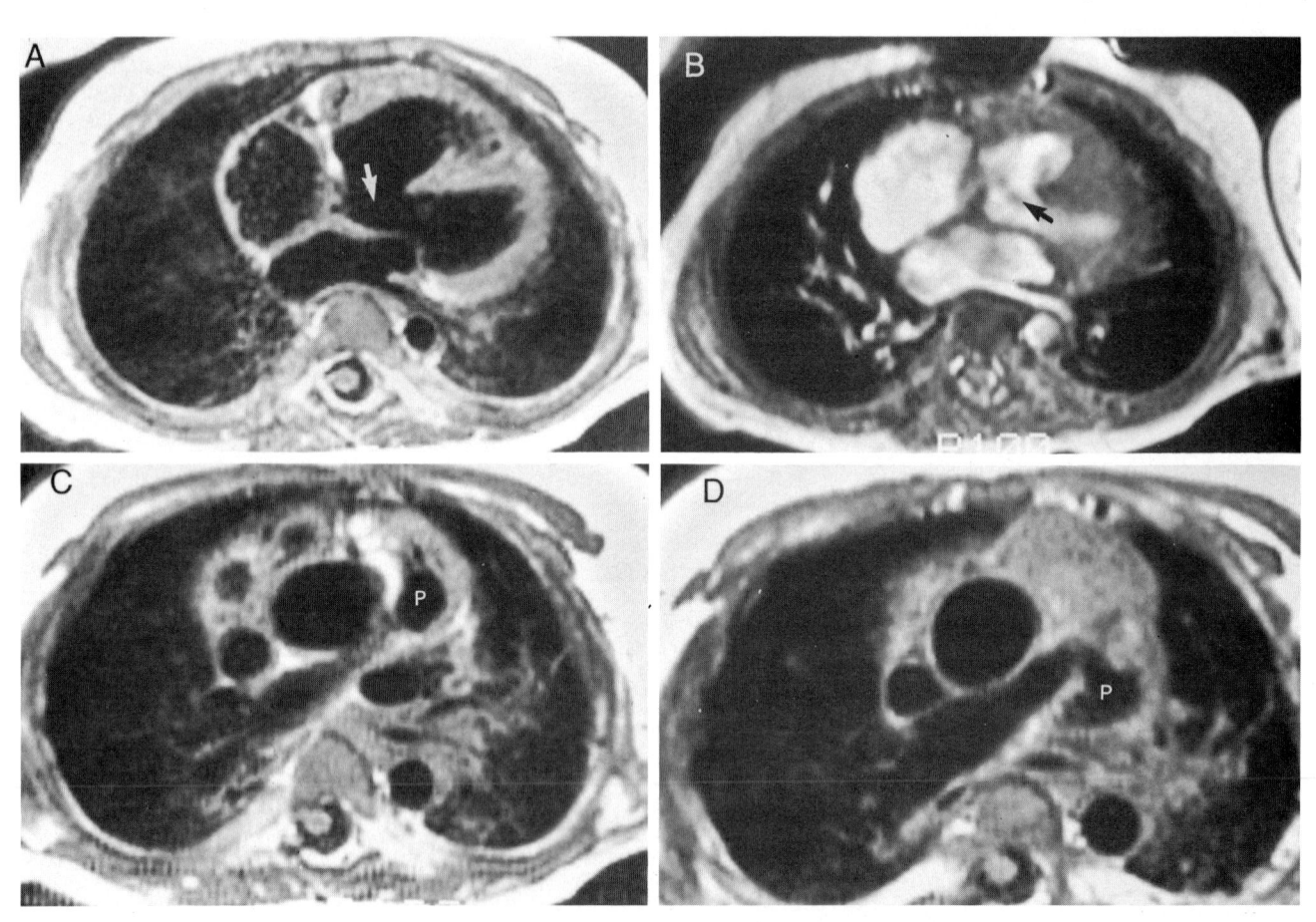

FIG 11–7.
Magnetic resonance imaging. Tetralogy of Fallot with pulmonary atresia. **A,** spin-echo section, axial plane through ventricles shows right ventricular hypertrophy and a VSD (*arrow*). **B,** gradient-echo axial section shows shunting across the ventricualr septal defect (*arrow*). **C,** axial section at base of heart shows small pulmonary outflow tract (*p*). **D** higher section shows large right pulmonary artery with dilated midportion at site of insertion of modified right Blalock-Taussig shunt. The pulmonary arteries are confluent, but the left pulmonary artery (*p*) ends in a small aneurysmal sac and is occluded distally. The obstruction occurred postoperatively.

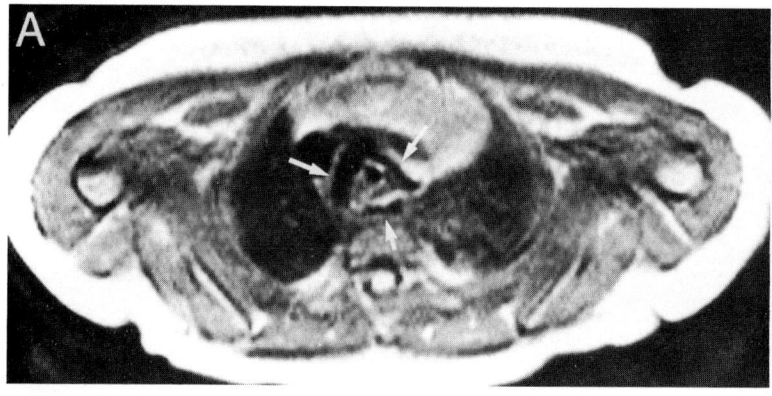

FIG 11-8.
Magnetic resonance images. Double aortic arch. **A,** axial section. Spin-echo images. The right and left limbs of the double aortic arch are seen as a "V"-like region of signal void passing along each side of the airway (*arrows*). Posteriorly, the two limbs are seen before they join the descending aorta (*small arrow*). **B,** sagittal section shows the left arch and a small portion of the right arch (*arrow*).

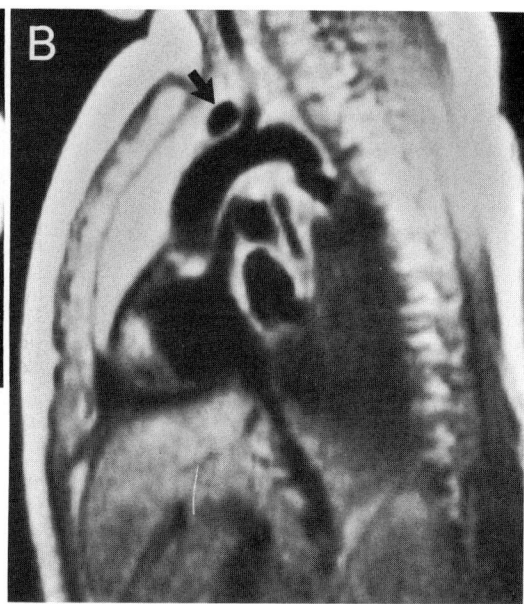

of the degree of stenosis at the site of coarctation may be difficult, and it may be necessary to obtain oblique sections through the coarcted segment in order to assess orifice size. The pressure or absence of collaterals can also be determined. On gradient-echo images, signal loss at site of coarctation is often seen. Efforts at quantifying the degree of stenosis or regurgitation from assessment of the region of signal loss have met with mixed success.[23] Newer techniques such as "phase mapping" may allow this capability with greater accuracy.

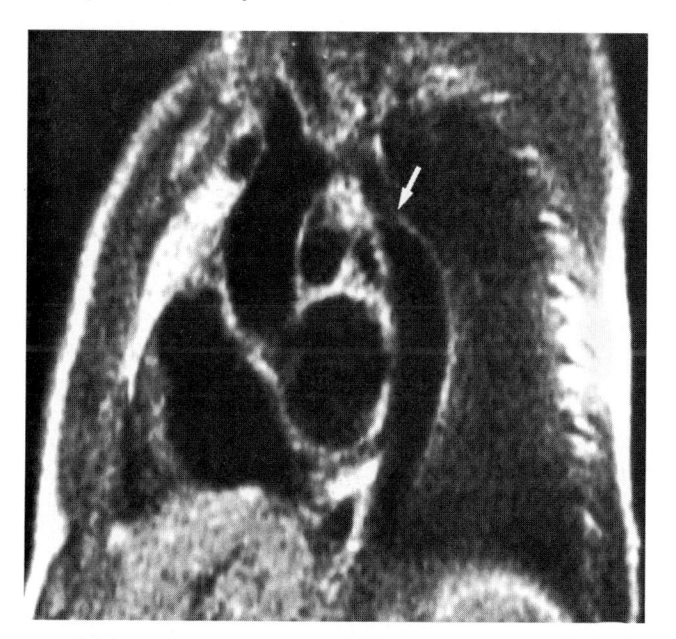

FIG 11-9.
Magnetic resonance images. Sagittal oblique projection. Coarcatation (*arrow*) of the aorta. Mild hypoplasia of the aortic isthmus is also present.

MRI imaging has now become the noninvasive imaging procedure of choice for monitoring changes in the aortic root width in patients with Marfan's and Turner's syndrome. Echocardiography is also used; however, the echocardiographic findings may be misleading when the dilation is above the level of the aortic valve. Gradient-echo techniques permit detection of concomitant aortic insufficiency.

Aneurysms of the sinus of Valsalva may also be detected with MRI and present a characteristic appearance seen best on axial and sagittal oblique views.

Abnormalities of the pulmonary vessels

MRI has been of particular value in the evaluation of the main and branch pulmonary arteries.[24-27] The pulmonary arteries are seen best on axial sections at the base of the heart and can be followed to the outer mediastinum. Small central arterial branches, the pulmonary arterial confluence, and systemic pulmonary collaterals can be seen (see Fig 11-7,C and D). The pulmonary arteries are not well seen beyond their hilar portions on axial scans, but in some instances pulmonary branches may be identified on thin-section coronal studies. Nonetheless, for determining the distribution of collateral flow or the size of the lobar or segmental pulmonary artery branches, selective angiography is better.[27,28]

MRI is frequently used in the evaluation of right ventricular outflow tract obstruction and pulmonary stenosis or atresia. The decision to perform a one-stage total surgical correction or a preliminary palliative surgical shunt to promote pulmonary artery growth in patients with these lesions is based largely on the size of the pulmonary arteries and the presence or absence of a pulmonary artery confluence.[29] Further, pulmonary artery growth following placement of a systemic-to-pulmonary-artery shunt is unpredictable. In neonates, two-dimensional Doppler echocardiography is usually successful in identifying the presence of pulmonary arteries and determining their confluence.[30] In older children and adults, however, the main pulmonary artery and right pulmonary artery are often seen on echocardiography, but the left pulmonary artery is seen only 65% of the time.[31] With CT scanning, the pulmonary confluence may not be seen, and it is difficult to detect stenosis at the origin of the left pulmonary artery or to detect peripheral stenosis within branch pulmonary arteries. CT also requires contrast infusion and has not been widely used in children. MRI provides a simple noninvasive method for serial monitoring the pulmonary arteries (Fig 11–10).

Abnormalities of pulmonary veins can also be identified with MR imaging. Partial and total anomalous pulmonary venous connections can be identified with spin-echo MR imaging (Fig 11–11). The location of superior vena cava can also be ascertained.

POSTOPERATIVE EVALUATION

The noninvasive nature of MRI and the excellent anatomic detail it provides suggests it can replace angiography for evaluation of operative results.

Postoperative anatomy is usually clearly seen on MRI (Figs 11–12 and 11–13). Systemic to pulmonary shunts, including Blalock-Taussig shunts, Glenn anastomoses, and Waterston and Potts anastomoses, can be identified on

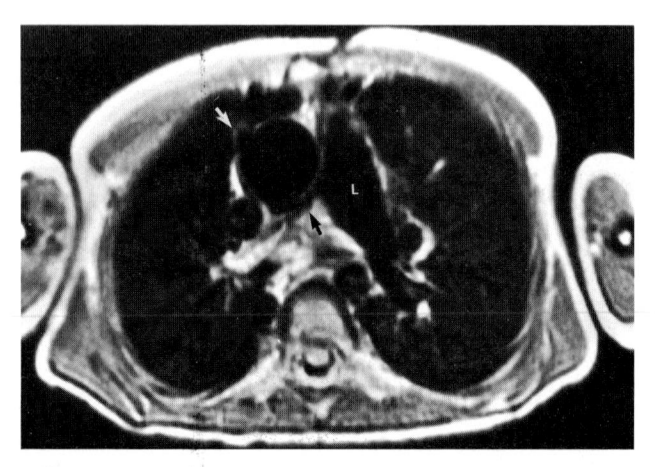

FIG 11–10.
Magnetic resonance images. Tetralogy of Fallot and pulmonary atresia. Axial sections. Spin-echo images. The main pulmonary artery which is anastomosed to a Rastelli conduit, is patent. The left pulmonary artery (L) is dilated. The right pulmonary artery is hypoplastic (black arrow). The stump of an occluded shunt from the aorta to the right pulmonary artery is seen (white arrow).

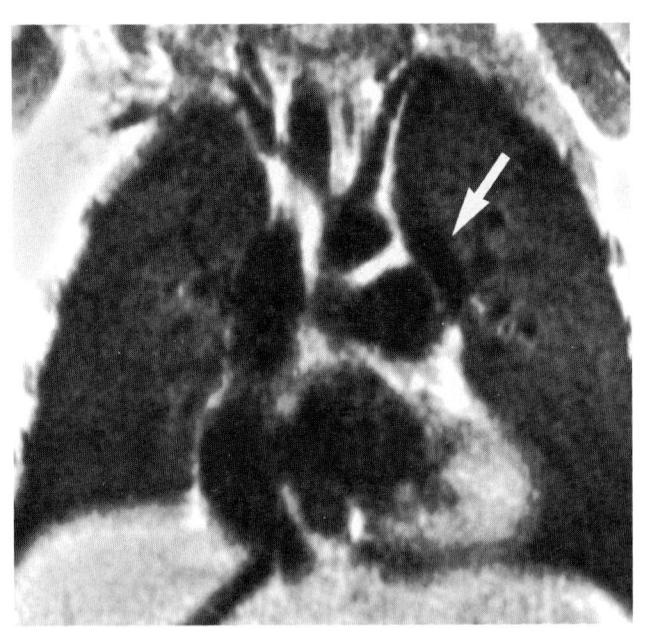

FIG 11–11.
Magnetic resonance images. Anomalous pulmonary venous connection. Coronal spin-echo image. This patient had undergone prior operation for total anomalous pulmonary venous connection to the left vertical vein in infancy. The left upper lobe could not be connected to the left atrium at time of surgery. On this new preoperative study, the left upper pulmonary vein is seen to drain into the left vertical vein (arrow). (From Casarella WJ, editor: *ARRS Categorical Course Syllabus: Cardiovascular imaging.* Baltimore 1990, American Roentgen Ray Society. Used with permission.)

MRI, although focal stenoses in the shunt usually are not reliably seen with current techniques[32] (Fig 11–14). Conduits such as those placed in Fontan or Rastelli repairs also can be readily identified (Fig 11–15). Postoperative results in complex repairs, such as the Mustard and Senning atrial baffle procedures, may be shown better with MRI than angiography as the angiographic appearance in these baffles may be similar.[33] Perigraft and pericardial collections can be clearly detected.

CINE MRI TECHNIQUES

Gradient-echo cine MRI techniques are used as an adjunct to spin-echo imaging in order to obtain functional information. With gradient-echo techniques, flowing blood is seen as high signal. Areas of turbulence are seen as regions of signal void due to spin dephasing. Nonturbulent shunt flow can often be seen as high signal passing across the defect. In general, shunts are more readily appreciated on cine MRI. Ventricular volumes, ejection fraction, and stroke volume can be calculated. Preliminary studies have suggested that under normal conditions, right ventricular

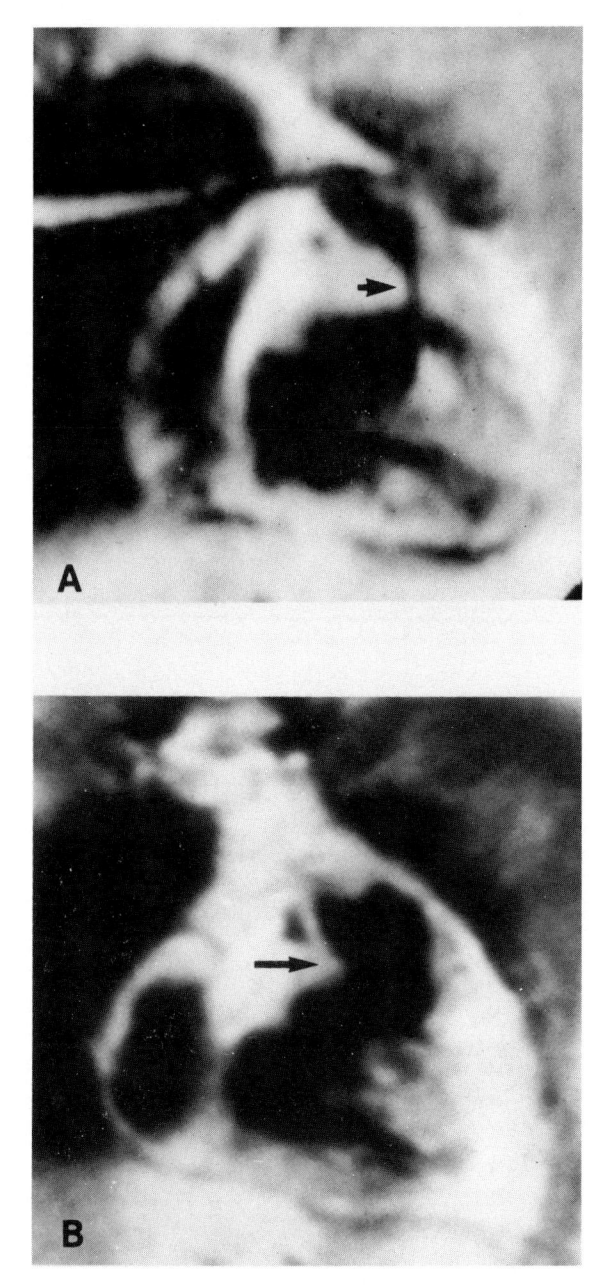

FIG 11–12.
Magnetic resonance images. Coronal plane. Tetralogy of Fallot. **A,** preoperative severe infundibular stenosis *(arrow)*. **B,** six days after operation, relief of infundibular stenosis *(large arrow)*.

and left ventricular stroke volumes are approximately equal.[34] The potential to determine shunt fraction by comparing right and left ventricular stroke volumes has been proposed, but awaits validation.

Valvar regurgitation is seen as signal void on gradient-echo sequences. Attempts at quantification of the regurgitant volume have met with mixed success to date. The apparent size of the regurgitant jet varies with the TE used, and shorter TEs result in apparently larger areas of turbulence. Newer approaches to measurement of blood flow with MR involve the use of phase imaging. Spins passing through an applied magnetic gradient field undergo a motion-induced phase shift that is proportional to the component of velocity coincident with the direction of the gradient. Phase imaging utilizes a computer-generated image in which pixel intensity is proportional to the amount of phase shift within its voxel. Phase imaging has the potential to allow accurate measurements of blood flow and other derived measurements, such as cardiac ouput. These newer applications of MR imaging offer great promise for future noninvasive determinations of cardiac function. Fast imaging techniques are also under development that will permit real-time acquisition of cardiac images.

Magnetic resonance imaging has drawbacks. The equipment is expensive and unavailable in many medical centers. With current MR systems, sedation is required in

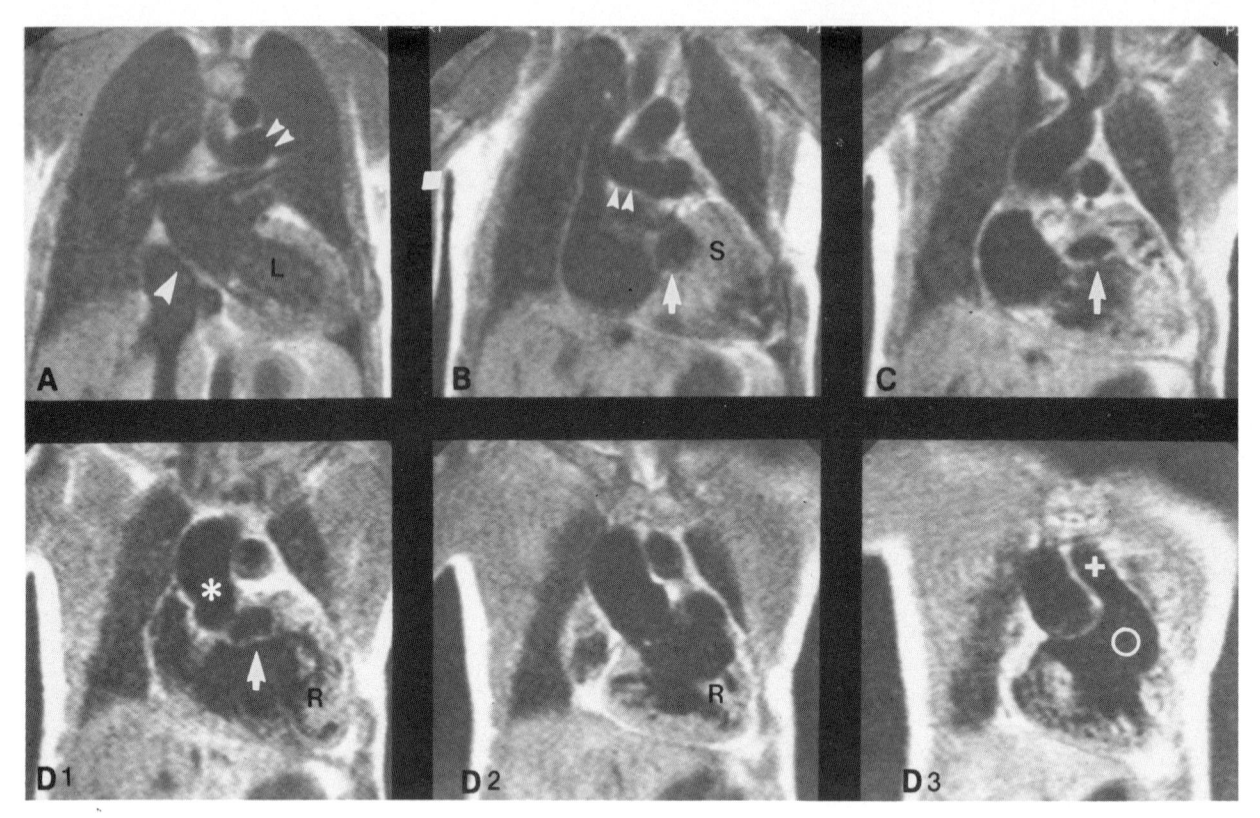

FIG 11-13.
D, Magnetic resonance images. Coronal scans. Posteroanterior plane. **A-C,** complete transposition with large ventricular septal defect and severe infundibular and valvular pulmonary stenosis. **D,** after operation. Surgically created tunnel *(small arrows)* from left ventricle through septal defect toward aorta (*). **D3,** patent right ventricular outflow tract (○). Graft (+) to distal pulmonary artery. Interventricular septum *(S)*. Interatrial septum *(large arrowhead)*. Right and left pulmonary artery *(double small arrowheads)*. *Small arrows* indicate infundibular and valvar stenosis in **B, C,** and **D.**

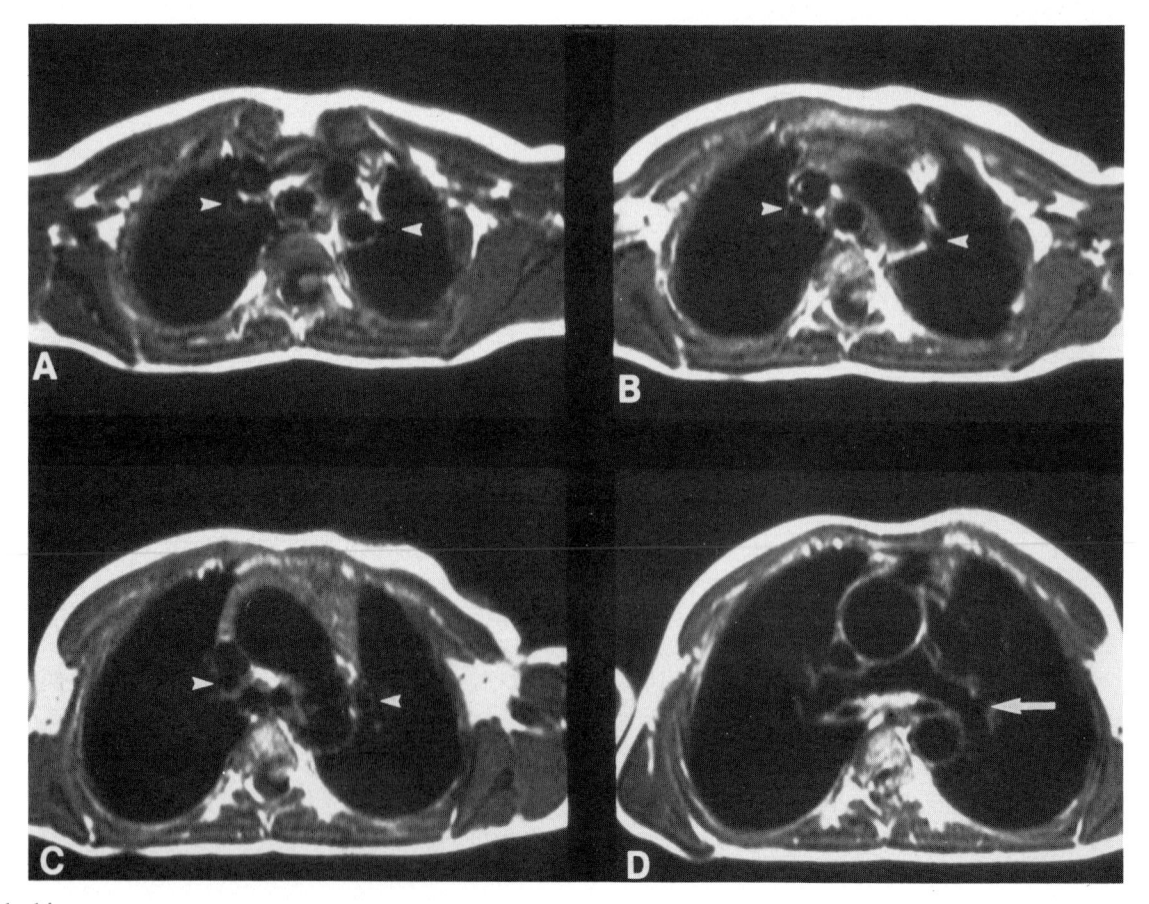

FIG 11-14.
Magnetic resonance images. Axial plane. Spin-echo protocol. **A-D,** craniocaudal sequence. Pulmonary atresia and bilateral modified Blalock-Taussig shunts. Patency of shunts *(arrowheads)* is evident by signal void. **D,** Anastomosis with branch of left pulmonary artery (arrow). Continuity of central pulmonary arterial branches is present.

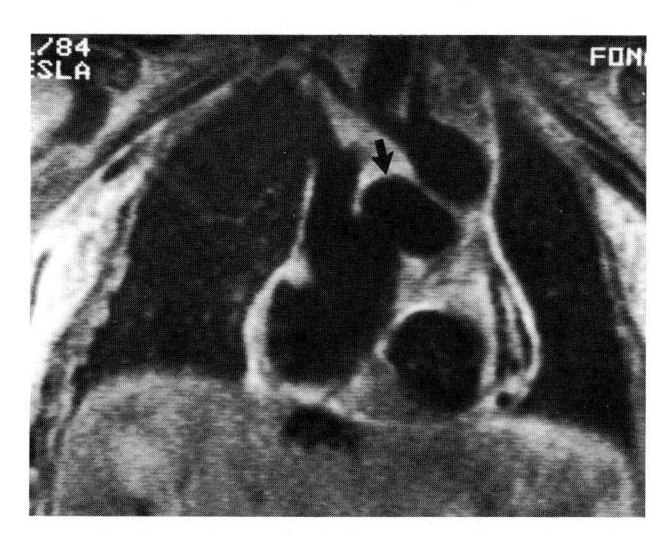

FIG 11–15.
Magnetic resonance image. Fontan procedure. Coronal plane, spin-echo image. The Fontan conduit is clearly identified connecting the right atrium and the pulmonary artery (*arrow*). (From Casarella WJ, editor: *ARRS Categorical Course Syllabus: Cardiovascular imaging*. Baltimore, 1990, American Roentgen Ray Society. Used with permission.)

patients who are incapable of holding still during the study, such as infants and claustrophobic patients, and image quality is degraded in patients with an irregular heart rate.

Despite these limitations, the anatomic and functional information provided by MRI has made it a useful noninvasive imaging technique in the evaluation of cardiac disease. It is a useful adjunct to echocardiography in those instances in which the echocardiographic findings are uncertain or when additional noninvasive corroboration of echocardiographic findings is needed. In some instances it can replace angiography, and in other instances reduce the need for repeat angiography.

SUMMARY

MR imaging is a noninvasive imaging modality that takes advantage of the safe interaction that occurs between the nuclei of certain atoms and radiofrequency waves in the presence of a magnetic field. The technique affords high-quality images in the heart and great vessels and has great promise as a technique for providing information regarding both anatomy and function of the heart in patients with cardiac disease.

REFERENCES

1. Bushong SC: *Magnetic resonance imaging: physical and biological principles*. St. Louis, 1988, Mosby–Year Book.
2. Fullerton GD: Basic concepts for nuclear magnetic resonance imaging. *Magn Reson Imaging* 1:39–55, 1982.
3. Smith MA: The technology of magnetic resonance imaging. *Clin Radiol* 36:553–559, 1985.
4. Stark D, Bradley WG: *Magnetic resonance imaging*. St Louis, 1988, Mosby–Year Book.
5. Haase A, Frahm J, Matthaei D, et al: FLASH imaging: rapid NMR imaging using low flip-angle pulses. *J Magn Reson* 67:258–266, 1986.
6. Glover GH, Pelc NJ: A rapid-gated cine MRI technique. In Kressel HK, editor: *Magnetic resonance annual*. Raven Press, 1988, New York, 1988;299-333.
7. Sechtm U, Pflugfelder PW, White RD, Gould RG, et al. Cine MR imaging: potential for the evaluation of cardiovascular function. *AJR* pp 239–246.
8. Matthaei D, Haase A, Henrich D, et al: Cardiac and vascular imaging with an MR snapshot technique. *Radiology* 177:527, 1990.
9. Dinsmore RE, Wismer GL, Levine RA, et al: Magnetic resonance imaging of the heart: positioning and gradient angle selection for optimal imaging planes. *AJR* 143:1135–1142, 1984.
10. Pavlicek WA, Geisinger M, Castle L, et al: Effects of nuclear magnetic resonance on patients with cardiac pacemakers. *Radiology* 147:149–153, 1983.
11. Soulen RL: Magnetic resonance imaging of prosthetic heart valves. *Radiology* 154:705–707, 1985.
12. Shellock FG: MR imaging of metallic implants and materials: a compilation of the literature. *AJR* 151:811–814, 1985.
13. Fisher MR, Lipton MJ, Higgins CB: Magnetic resonance imaging and computed tomography in congenital heart disease. *Semin Roentgenol* 3:272–282, 1985.
14. Didier D, Higgins CB, Fisher MR, et al: Congenital heart disease: gated MR imaging in 72 patients. *Radiology* 158:227–235, 1986.
15. Guit GL, Bluemm R, Rohmer J, et al: Levotransposition of the aorta: identification of segmental cardiac anatomy using MR imaging. *Radiology* 161:673–679, 1986.
16. Higgins CB: Overview of MR of the heart—1986. *AJR* 146:907–918, 1986.
17. Humes RA, Feldt RH, Porter CJ, et al: The modified Fontan operation for asplenia and polysplenia syndromes. *J Thorac Cardiovasc Surg* 96:212–218, 1988.
18. Julsrud PR, Ehman RL, Hagler DJ, et al: Extracardiac vasculature in candidates for Fontan surgery: MR imaging. *Radiology* 173:503–506, 1989.
19. Dinsmore RE, Wismer GL, Guyer D, et al: Magnetic resonance imaging of the interatrial septum and atrial septal defects. *AJR* 145:697–703, 1985.
20. Didier D, Higgins CB: Identification and localization of ventricular septal defect by gated magnetic resonance imaging. *Am J Cardiol* 57:1363–1368, 1986.
21. Akins EW, Martin TD, James AA, et al: MR imaging of double-outlet right ventricle: Case report. *AJR* 152:128–130, 1989.
22. Bisset GS, Strife JL, Kirks DR, et al: Vascular rings: MR imaging. *AJR* 149:251–256, 1987.

23. Wagner S, Auffermann W, Buser P, et al: Diagnostic accuracy and estimation of the severity of valvular regurgitation from signal void on cine MRI. *Am Heart J* 118:760–767, 1989.
24. Rees RSO, Somerville J, Underwood SR, et al: Magnetic resonance imaging of the pulmonary arteries and their systemic connections in pulmonary atresia: comparison with angiographic and surgical findings. *Br Heart J* 58:621–626, 1987.
25. Mirowitz SA, Gutierrez FR, Canter CE, et al: Tetralogy of Fallot: MR findings. *Radiology* 171:207–212, 1989.
26. Canter CE, Gutierrez FR, Mirowitz SA, et al: Evaluation of pulmonary arterial morphology in cyanotic congenital heart disease by magnetic resonance imaging. *Am Heart J* 118:347–354, 1989.
27. Gomes AS, Lois JF, Williams RG: Pulmonary arteries: MR imaging in patients with congenital obstruction of the right ventricular outflow tract. *Radiology* 174:51–57, 1990.
28. Canter CE, Gutierrez FR, Mirowitz SA, et al: Evaluation of pulmonary arterial morphology in cyanotic congenital heart disease by magnetic resonance imaging. *Am Heart J* 118:347–354, 1989.
29. Edwards JE, McGoon DC: Absence of anatomic origin from heart of pulmonary arterial supply. *Circulation* 47:393, 1973.
30. Gutgesell HP, Huhta JC, Cohen MH, et al: Two dimensional echocardiographic assessment of pulmonary artery and aortic arch anatomy in cyanotic infants. *J Am Coll Cardiol* 4:1242, 1984.
31. Huhta JC, Piehler JM, Tajik AJ, et al: Two dimensional echocardiographic detection and measurement of the right pulmonary artery in pulmonary atresia-ventricular septal defect: angiographic and surgical correlation. *Am J Cardiol* 49:1235, 1982.
32. Jacobstein MD, Fletcher BD, Nelson AD, et al: Magnetic resonance imaging: evaluation of palliative systemic-pulmonary artery shunts. *Circulation* 70:650–656, 1984.
33. Soulen RL, Donner RM, Capitanio M: Postoperative evaluation of complex congenital heart disease by magnetic resonance imaging. *RadioGraphis* 7:975–1000, 1987.
34. Sechtum U, Pflugfelder PW, Gould RG, et al: Measurement of right and left ventricular volumes in healthy individuals with cine MR imaging. *Radiology* 163:697–702, 1987.

PART TWO

Cardiac Conditions Associated With a Left-to-Right Shunt

The cardiac conditions associated with left-to-right shunting of blood represent at least half of all instances of congenital heart disease, and indeed one, ventricular septal defect, represents one-fourth of all cases. Many patients with these conditions are asymptomatic, and the cardiac disease is recognized only by the presence of a murmur. Ventricular septal defect represents a typical example. In two thirds of the cases of this anomaly, the defect is small and does not require treatment, either medically or surgically. On the other hand, anomalies of a moderate size may be associated with symptoms such as easy fatigability, delayed growth, perhaps a tendency to respiratory infections, whereas in those patients with a large communication the major symptoms are related to development of congestive cardiac failure. In the latter group of patients, pneumonia and serious respiratory infections are frequent.

Pulmonary vascular disease may develop in patients with large communications between the left and right sides of the heart. The pulmonary vascular changes increase pulmonary vascular resistance, which, when it exceeds systemic vascular resistance, causes the shunt to become right-to-left. In this modern surgical era of early recognition and diagnosis of congenital heart disease, such a complication is unusual. Yet there are patients in whom this complication occurs, and in those instances these patients have to be considered in the differential diagnosis of patients with cyanosis and increased pulmonary vascular markings.

The left-to-right shunt may occur at any level of the heart: at the level of the great veins, in the form of partial anomalous pulmonary venous connection, at the artrial level as various types of atrial defects, at the ventricular level such as in ventricular septal defect, or between the great vessels as in patent ductus arteriosus.

Three general hemodynamic principles govern blood flow among the cardiac conditions associated with a left-to-right shunt:

1. Relative resistance to blood flow, as in shunts at either the ventricular or great vessel level.
2. Relative ventricular compliance as in shunts at the atrial level.
3. An obligatory mechanism in which a high-pressure chamber is in free association with a low-pressure chamber during some portion of the cardiac cycle. Examples of this hemodynamic principle are left ventricular-right atrial shunt, coronary arteriovenous fistula, and ruptured sinus of Valsalva aneurysm.

In the chapters that follow, the congenital cardiac anomalies associated with a left-to-right shunt are presented on basically an anatomic and hemodynamic order.

Chapters 12 to 15 present ventricular septal defect and variations of ventricular septal defect, such as coexistent ventricular septal defect and aortic insufficiency, of left ventricular-right artrial shunt. Chapters 16 to 18 present shunt conditions with a communication between the aorta and pulmonary arteries, examples being patent ductus arteriosus, aorticopulmonary window, and aortic origin of pulmonary artery. The shunts that occur at the atrial level are discussed, including atrial septal defect, endocardial cushion defect, partial anomalous pulmonary venous connection and its variations. Finally, two examples of obligatory shunts are discussed, namely, ruptured sinus of Valsalva aneurysm and coronary arteriovenous fistula.

CHAPTER 12

Ventricular Septal Defect

Isolated ventricular septal defect (VSD) is the most common congenital cardiac malformation, accounting for 20% of all instances of congenital heart disease. In 2%, there is more than one VSD, with the frequency being higher in symptomatic infants. In 5% of patients with congenital heart disease, VSD coexists with other major cardiac anomalies, particularly coarctation of the aorta and patent ductus arteriosus, and the septal defect plays a dominant role in the hemodynamics and clinical features. Ventricular septal defect is present in 2 per 1,000 live births overall, with a higher incidence in premature infants[1] and a slightly higher incidence in girls. Ventricular defects in a supracristal location occur more commonly in patients of Asian descent.

In another 25% of patients with congenital heart disease, VSD is a component and a hemodynamic factor, such as tetralogy of Fallot, persistent truncus arteriosus, single ventricle, tricuspid atresia, double-outlet right ventricle, and interruption of the aortic arch. In this group, the flow through the ventricular communication is similar to that in isolated VSD, but the clinical picture is influenced significantly by the other components of the malformation and thus usually differs greatly from that of isolated VSD. These conditions are therefore discussed individually elsewhere in this work.

ANATOMY

The size of the defect varies considerably—from 1 mm to 2.5 cm in diameter—and is one of the major determinants of the hemodynamics. Defects greater than 1 cm^2/m^2 or 75% of the diameter of the aorta are considered large. About 5% of VSD are of such size.

Ventricular septal defects can be located in various positions in the septum. The location is generally described relative to landmarks in the right ventricle, but we also describe the left ventricle location of each.

The subaortic area of the left ventricle passes obliquely behind the infundibulum of the right ventricle (Fig 12–1). Therefore, a VSD located immediately below the aortic valve may emerge at different sites in the right ventricle, depending on its location about the circumference of the subaortic area.

Normal Anatomy

The right and the anterior half of the noncoronary aortic cusp are related to the ventricular septum (Fig 12–2). Between the right and posterior cusps, there is a small translucent fibrous area termed the "membranous septum." Because the membranous septum is small, so-called membranous VSDs are larger and include adjacent muscular tissue (perimembranous VSD). Some subaortic VSDs are located more anteriorly and do not involve the membranous septum; these also are called "perimembranous defects." The anterior leaflet of the mitral valve is in continuity with the posterior half of the noncoronary cusp, whereas the left aortic cusp has no anatomic relation to the ventricular septum. A defect confined to the membranous ventricular septum is rare.

In the right ventricle, an important anatomic landmark is the papillary muscle of the conus (Lancisi or Luschka Lancisi, 17th century physician, Luschka, 19th century German anatomist), which gives rise to chordae tendineae extending toward the adjacent halves of the septal and anterior leaflets of the tricuspid valve. The crista supraventricularis with its septal and parietal limbs divides the right

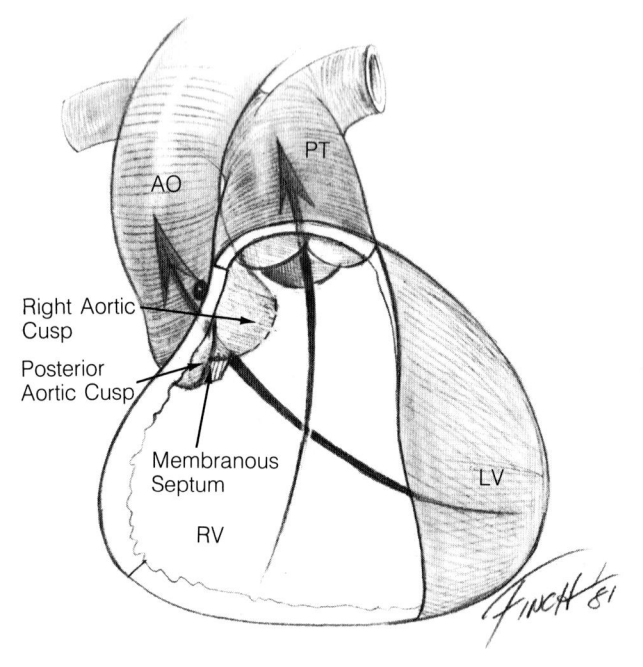

FIG 12–1.
Diagram of heart with anterior wall of right ventricle removed. Right *(RV)* and left ventricular *(LV)* outflow tracts cross. Because of the tilt of the aortic valve, membranous and perimembranous defects emerge at different levels in the right ventricle. The membranous septum *(cross-hatched area)* lies between the posterior and right aortic cusps.

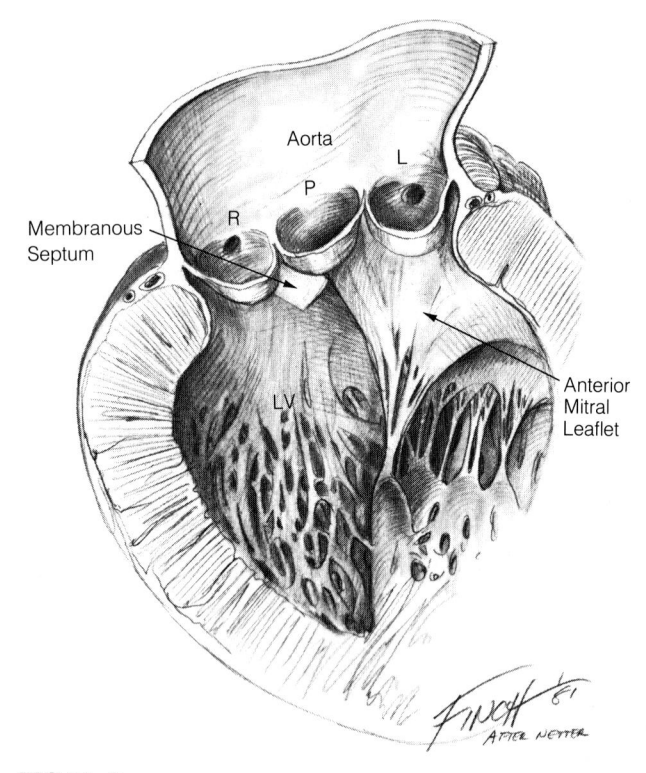

FIG 12–2.
Diagram of left ventricular aspect of interventricular septum. Membranous septum located between right *(R)* and posterior *(P)* aortic cusps. *(L)* = left aortic cusp.

ventricle into an inflow (sinus) and outflow (infundibular) portion.

Classification of Ventricular Septal Defect[2]

1. Supracristal VSD (5% of the total) located beneath the pulmonary valve (Fig 12–3). The upper border of these defects lies beneath the right coronary cusp of the aortic valve, so they are remote from the membranous septum. Often the pulmonary and aortic cusps are contiguous through the defect.
2. Defect inferior to the crista supraventricularis (80%). This, the most common type of VSD, has two subtypes:
   a. Membranous VSD. This involves the true membranous septum and the adjacent muscular septum. In the right ventricle, the defect lies beneath the crista supraventricularis, posterior to the papillary muscle of the conus, and is at least partially covered by the septal leaflet of the tricuspid valve. On the left side, it lies in the commissure between the posterior (noncoronary) and right aortic cusps (see Fig 12–2) and immediately anterior to the anterior leaflet of the mitral valve.
   b. A defect between the papillary muscle of the conus and the crista supraventricularis. These defects lie more anteriorly in the left ventricle and extend below the right cusp of the aortic valve.
3. Defects in the inflow portion of the septum (5%). This is the VSD of the atrioventricular (AV)–canal type. In the right ventricle, this defect involves the posterior ventricular septum and extends to the tricuspid anulus. In the left ventricle, it passes from the posteromedial commissure of the mitral valve toward the left ventricular outflow area. This defect may be associated with left-axis deviation on the electrocardiogram (ECG).
4. Defects in the midportion of the septum (10%). These defects may be isolated or multiple and may appear anywhere in the muscular ventricular septum. Commonly they are hidden in the coarse trabeculations of the right ventricle and are more easily seen from the left ventricle because the septum is less trabeculated.

In general, the posterior (AV canal–type) defects and infracristal communications are large and single. Muscular defects, in contrast, tend to be small and multiple,[3] occasionally giving the ventricular septum a Swiss cheese appearance. Systolic blood flow through a muscular VSD is diminished by the contraction of the ventricular septum, which decreases the size of the communication. Sometimes, however, a muscular septal defect is large and causes a hemodynamically significant left-to-right shunt.

Associated Abnormalities

In membranous VSD, the conduction system passes along the posteroinferior margin of the defect. One of the complications of the operative closure of such defects is complete heart block caused by the injury of the bundle of His. In muscular and supracristal VSDs, the conduction system is remote from the defect.

The changes in the pulmonary vasculature may be significant. In a small VSD, the left-to-right shunt is limited, and consequently the right ventricular systolic pressure is normal or slightly elevated. In these patients, the vascular bed matures in normal or near-normal fashion, and pulmonary vascular disease rarely develops. In contrast, because of the large pulmonary blood flow and the increased pulmonary arterial pressure in patients with a large VSD, histologic changes develop in the pulmonary arterioles, and maturation of the pulmonary arterial tree is delayed (Fig 12–4). Medial hypertrophy of the muscular pulmonary arteries develops. Eventually, fibrous thickening of the intima may almost completely occlude the pulmonary arteries. Subsequently, a mass of endothelial cells may intrude into the vascular lumen, causing mechanical obstruction. Called a "plexiform lesion," it is present in patients with severe pulmonary hypertension and a bidirectional or right-to-left shunt. Distal to the plexiform lesion, dilatation and thinning of the arteries may occur.

VENTRICULAR SEPTAL DEFECTS
(Viewed from Right Ventricle)

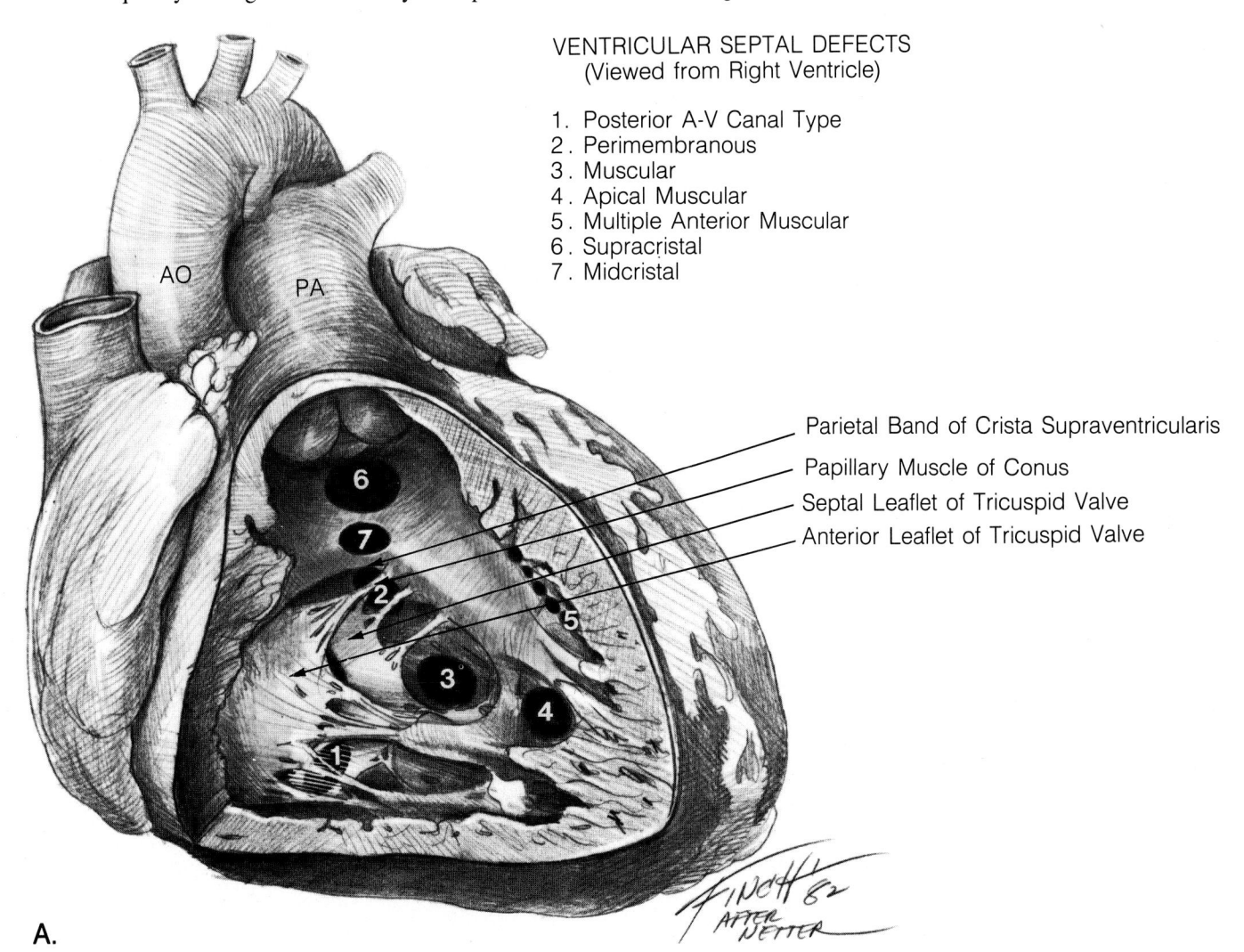

1. Posterior A-V Canal Type
2. Perimembranous
3. Muscular
4. Apical Muscular
5. Multiple Anterior Muscular
6. Supracristal
7. Midcristal

FIG 12–3.
Diagram of right ventricular (**A**) and left ventricular (**B**) views of ventricular septum, with relative position of five types of ventricular septal defects shown on each side of the septum. *AO* = aorta; *PT* = pulmonary trunk; *L* = left; *P* = posterior; *R* = right aortic valve cusps.
(Continued.)

VENTRICULAR SEPTAL DEFECTS
(Viewed From Left Ventricle)

1. Posterior A-V Canal Type
2. Perimembranous
3. Muscular
4. Apical Muscular
5. Multiple Anterior Muscular
6. Supracristal

B.

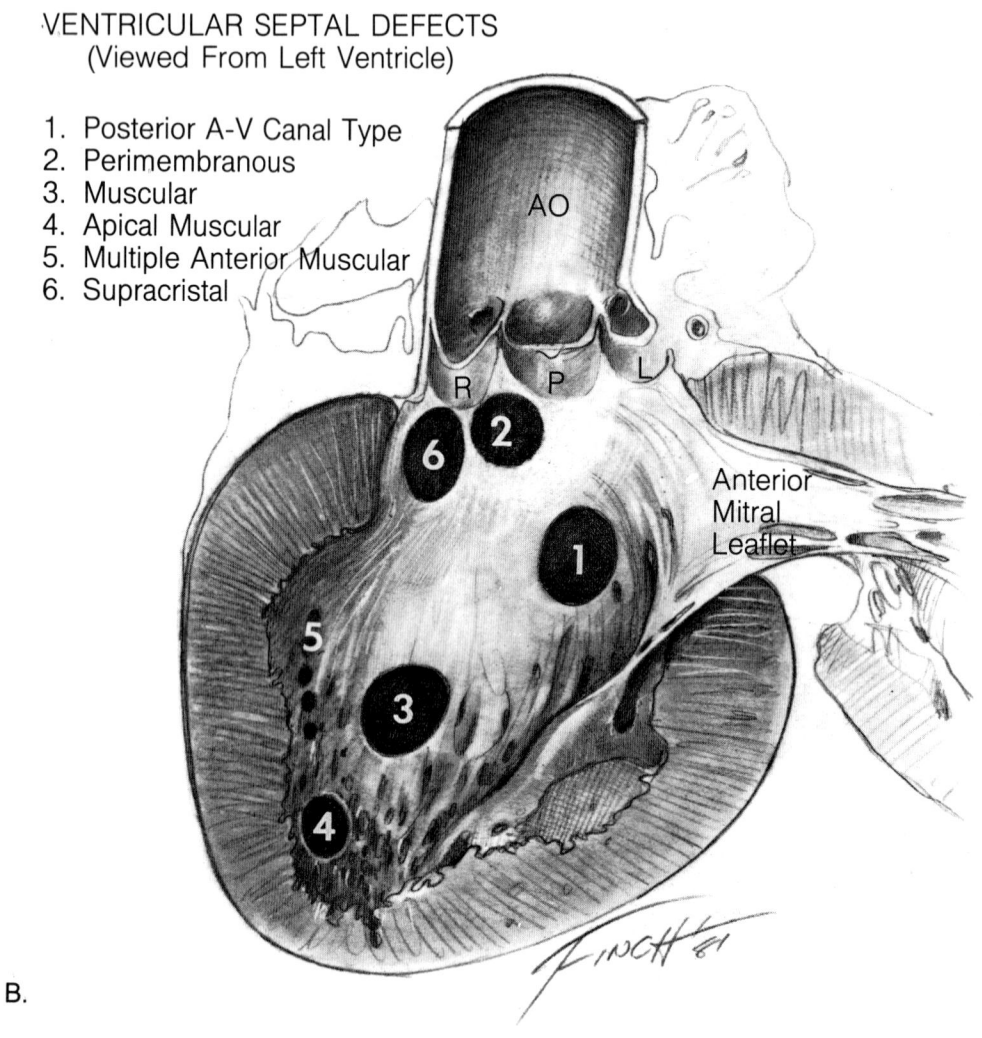

FIG 12–3 (cont'd.).

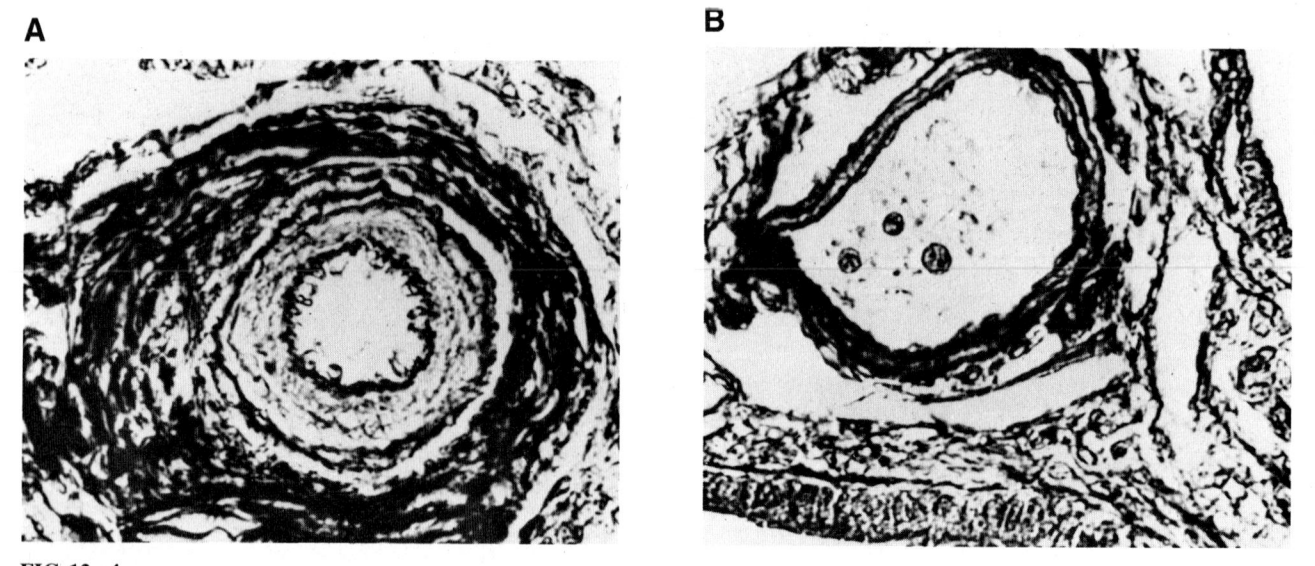

FIG 12–4.
Maturation of muscular pulmonary arteries; normal lung × 65. **A**, at birth. **B**, at 9 months.

Secondary Anatomic Changes

1. Long-standing pulmonary hypertension. In this circumstance, the pulmonary trunk becomes dilated, and intimal atherosclerotic lesions develop that are identical to those found in the aorta of older persons. The atherosclerotic plaques may calcify and become visible on a thoracic roentgenogram; this indicates severe, long-standing pulmonary vascular disease.

2. In the right ventricle opposite the VSD, a jet lesion may develop. This fibrotic thickened patch of endocardium is caused by the trauma of the high-velocity jet through the defect. Jet lesions occur more commonly with small defects than with large ones, because the jet has a high velocity from the high left ventricular–right ventricular pressure gradient.

3. Bacterial endocarditis. Jet lesions in the right ventricle, the rim of the septal defect, or the mitral valve (rare) may be the site of bacterial infection.

4. Partial obstruction of the left mainstem bronchus (rare). Increased blood flow through the left side of the heart causes enlargement of both the left atrium and the left ventricle. As the left atrium enlarges, it elevates the left mainstem bronchus, which may be compressed between the enlarged hypertensive left pulmonary artery and the enlarged left atrium ("hemodynamic vise") (Fig 12–5). As a result, either emphysema or atelectasis may occur in the left lung.

Other Associated Conditions

1. Left ventricular–right atrial communications. Left ventricular–right atrial shunts (see Chapter 15) are rare but most often are associated with a VSD. The shunt is caused by adherence of the septal leaflet of the tricuspid valve to the defect, with an associated perforation or cleft in the tricuspid valve. Isolated left ventricular–right atrial shunt without a ventricular component is rare.

2. Atrial septal defect or patent foramen ovale. A left-to-right shunt is common in infants with a large VSD, but it subsequently disappears. In most instances, the shunt occurs through a foramen ovale stretched open by left atrial dilatation.

3. Patent ductus arteriosus. In 10% of patients with a large VSD, there is a patent ductus arteriosus. Because large septal defects invariably lead to pulmonary hypertension so that the pressures in the pulmonary artery and aorta are equal, the patent ductus arteriosus is not heard, being obscured by the loud murmur of the septal defect.[4, 5] This state, "silent ductus arteriosus," must be excluded by angiography before operation, because its presence makes extracorporeal circulation hazardous.

4. Mitral insufficiency. Insufficiency because of a cleft in the mitral valve may occur without the association of an ostium primum defect. In other patients, mitral insufficiency results from accessory chordae tendineae or abnormally located papillary muscles. Malfunction of the mitral valve follows.

5. Tricuspid insufficiency. Associated tricuspid reflux may rarely occur from fibrotic changes secondary to the jet of blood through the VSD striking the valve leaflets.

6. Valvar pulmonary stenosis. Ventricular septal defect may be associated with valvular pulmonary stenosis, usually from a bicuspid pulmonary valve.

7. Infundibular pulmonary stenosis. Obstruction of the right ventricular outflow tract at the infundibular level

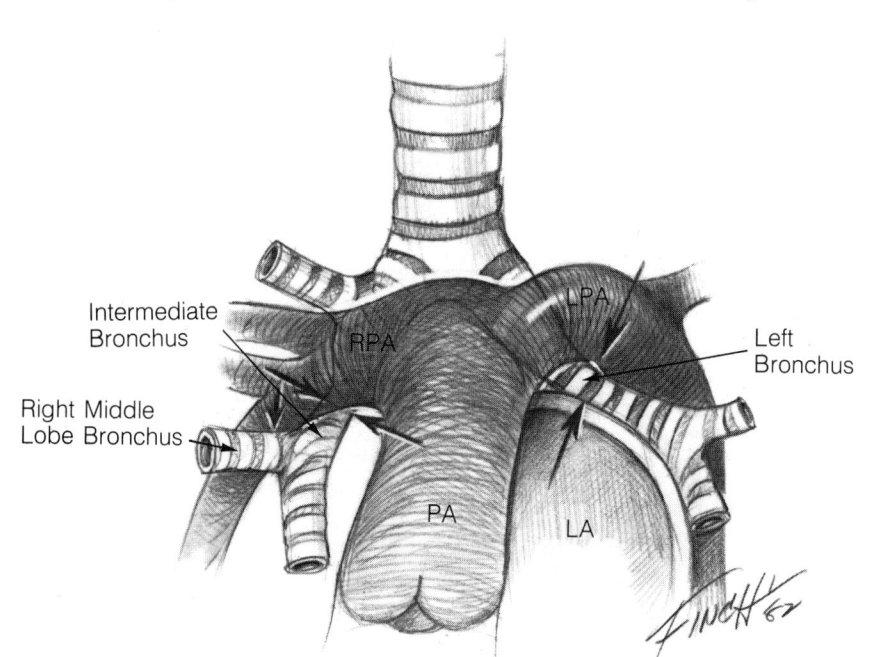

FIG 12–5.
The left mainstem bronchus compresses by left atrium *(LA)* below *(arrow)* and left pulmonary artery *(LPA)* above. Both structures are enlarged in patients with a large ventricular septal defect (VSD). *RPA* = right pulmonary artery. Left mainstem bronchus and right intermediate bronchus are most commonly compressed by an enlarged pulmonary artery.

may occur in association with VSD. In infants, associated infundibular pulmonary stenosis may be masked by pulmonary hypertension, and a minimal or no pressure gradient is found. As the child grows, the infundibular stenosis becomes more severe, and pulmonary artery pressure falls. When the stenosis is mild, a left-to-right shunt is present. This condition is referred to as "acyanotic tetralogy of Fallot," or "pink tetralogy." If the infundibular stenosis increases and a right-to-left shunt develops, the clinical picture resembles that of typical tetralogy of Fallot.

8. Anomalous muscle bundles. Another obstructive lesion, these bundles occur in the inflow portion of the right ventricle (Fig 12–6). When the anomalous muscle bundle lies proximal to the VSD, a left-to-right shunt occurs through the defect; if the muscle bundles lie beyond the defect, a right-to-left shunt may occur. Muscle bundles may be either obstructive or nonobstructive and are best diagnosed by angiography.

9. Subaortic stenosis. This condition may not be diagnosed unless careful pressure measurements and left ventricular angiography are carried out. Subaortic stenosis may be either muscular or membranous and the VSD located either proximal or distal to the stenosis. If the defect is proximal to the stenosis (Fig 12–7,A), the right and left ventricular systolic pressures are equal, but a gradient is recorded across the subaortic area. This combination of defects is commonly associated with obstruction in the aortic arch, such as coarctation or interruption of the aorta, and produces a characteristic angiographic picture. If the VSD is located distal to the subaortic stenosis, the aorta and right ventricular systolic pressures are equal, but a gradient is recorded within the left ventricle (Fig 12–7,B). A third type of obstruction results from a subaortic membrane (Fig 12–7,C) coexisting with a small VSD between the aortic valve and the membrane.

10. Aneurysm of the membranous septum. The pathologic details of aneurysm of the membranous septum are unclear. A VSD may be associated with either a true aneurysm or an aneurysm formed by adherence of the septal leaflet of the tricuspid valve to the edge of the septal defect being the most common. Ventricular septal defects associated with aneurysm of the membranous septum tend to close. Often the angiographic appearance is of a bulging, partially adherent septal leaflet of the tricuspid valve, particularly if there is a left ventricular–right atrial shunt. Differentiation between a true aneurysm of the membranous septum and a closing VSD by adherence of the septal leaflet of the tricuspid valve cannot be made even at postmortem examination (see Chapter 14).

HEMODYNAMICS

The hemodynamics of a VSD are determined by the size of the defect and the status of the pulmonary vasculature.[6, 7]

In the normal newborn infant, pulmonary vascular resistance is elevated. It decreases in the immediate neonatal period because of the rise in oxygen tension in the arterial bed (Fig 12–8). The neonatal expansion of the lungs results in a negative intrathoracic pressure, which also lowers pulmonary vascular resistance. The pulmonary vascular bed does not fully mature until about 4 years of age, probably because of a further decrease in pulmonary resistance caused by an increase in the cross-sectional area of the total pulmonary vascular bed resulting from growth of the lungs.

In the presence of a large VSD (> 1 cm^2/m^2), pulmonary vascular resistance declines at a slower than normal

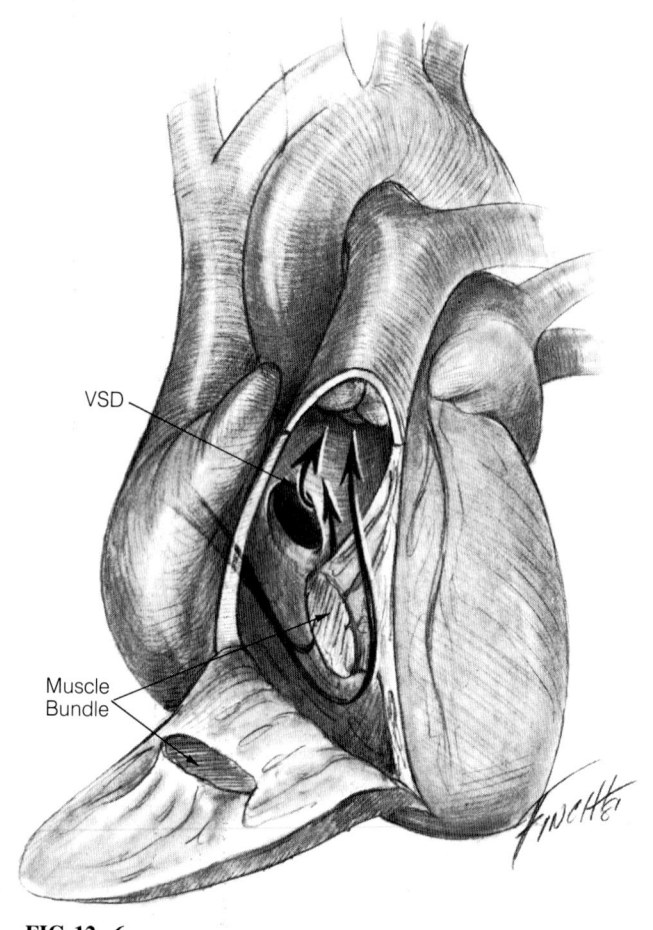

FIG 12–6.
Diagram of VSD and anomalous muscle bundle in right ventricle; right ventricular anterior wall removed. Large circular anomalous muscle bundle dividing right ventricular inflow portion *(arrows)*. Large septal defect *(VSD)* with left-to-right shunt; three pathways are now present *(arrows)*. The anatomy may even be more confusing to the operating surgeon if there is more than one muscle bundle.

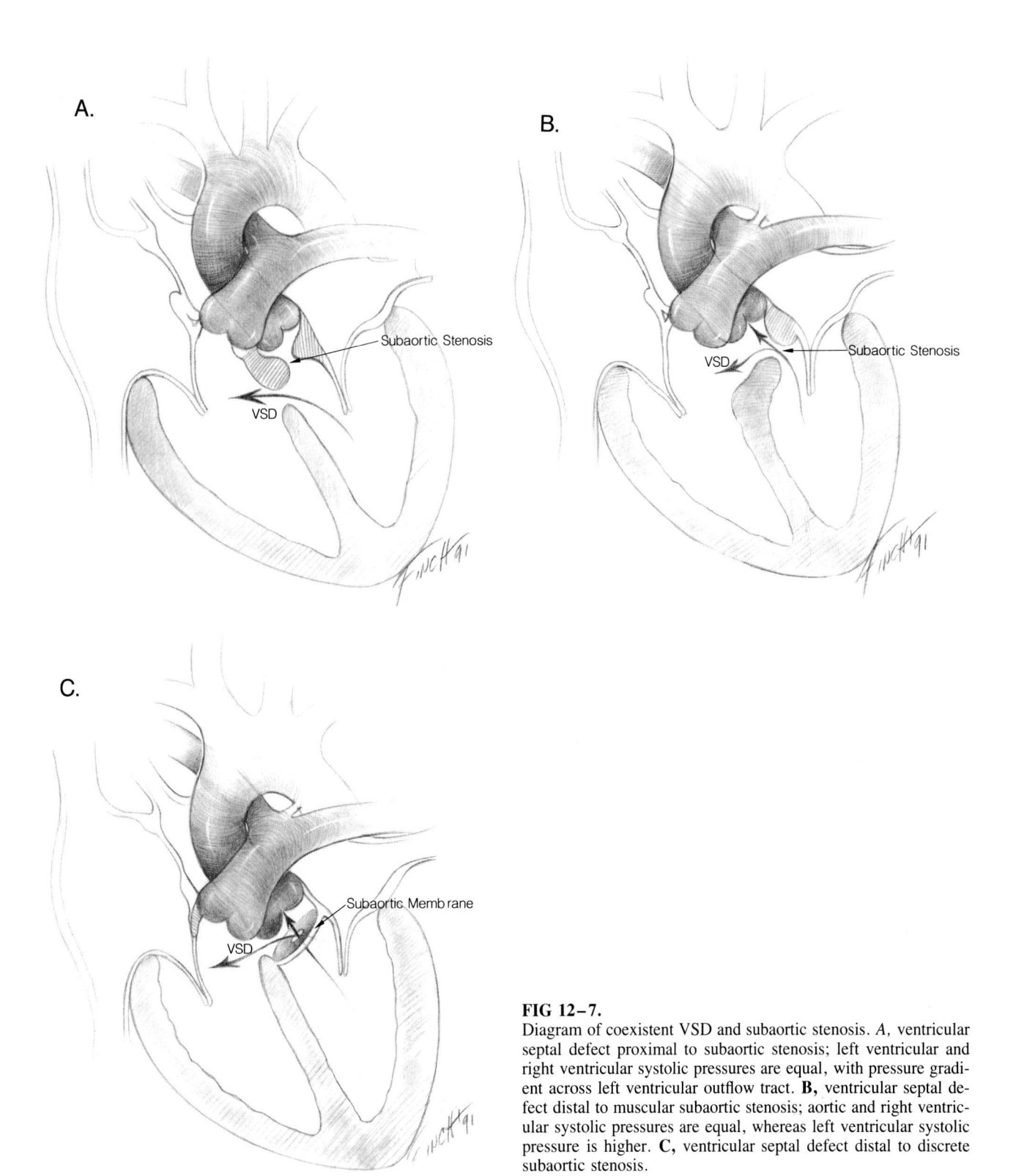

FIG 12–7.
Diagram of coexistent VSD and subaortic stenosis. *A,* ventricular septal defect proximal to subaortic stenosis; left ventricular and right ventricular systolic pressures are equal, with pressure gradient across left ventricular outflow tract. **B,** ventricular septal defect distal to muscular subaortic stenosis; aortic and right ventricular systolic pressures are equal, whereas left ventricular systolic pressure is higher. **C,** ventricular septal defect distal to discrete subaortic stenosis.

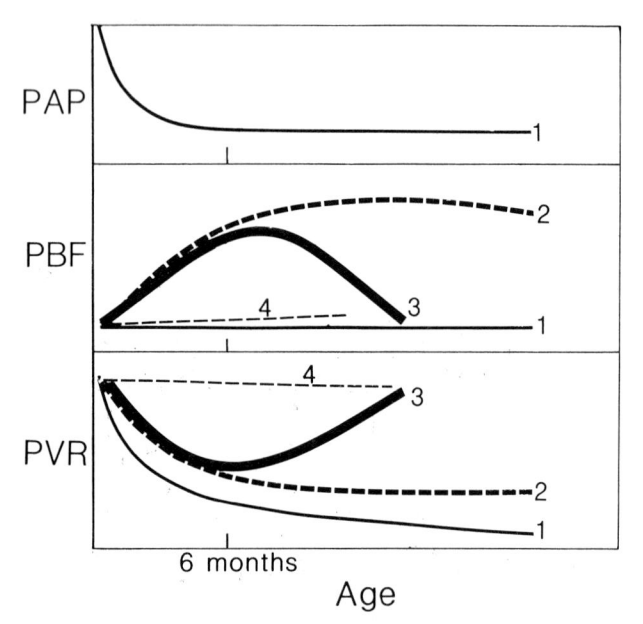

FIG 12–8.
Comparison of pulmonary arterial pressure *(PAP)*, pulmonary blood flow *(PBF)*, and pulmonary vascular resistance *(PVR)* in normal patients *(1)* and patients with VSDs *(2–4)*. In most patients with a large defect *(2)*, PVR falls, but along a higher than normal curve. In other patients, pulmonary vascular disease may develop *(3)*, while in an occasional patient *(4)*, the pulmonary vasculature does not mature postnatally, and the PVR remains elevated.

rate (see Fig 12–8). One factor maintaining elevated pulmonary resistance is distention of the left atrium by increased pulmonary blood flow. This increased left atrial pressure probably causes pulmonary vasoconstriction by a reflex mechanism. In these patients, the pulmonary arterial pressure equals the aortic pressure because the ventricles are in free communication through the large defect. Blood flow across the defect, either right-to-left or left-to-right, is governed by the relative pulmonary and systemic vascular resistances (Fig 12–9,B). If the resistances are equal, as at birth, there is no significant blood flow across the defect. In infancy, flow is left to right through the defect because of the decrease in pulmonary vascular resistance.

As the volume of pulmonary blood flow increases, the amount of blood returning to the left atrium and left ventricle is also increased. This elevates the pulmonary venous pressure, dilates the left atrium and left ventricle, and leads to an increase in left ventricular mass as a compensatory mechanism.

With progressive decrease in the pulmonary vascular resistance, the volume load on the left ventricle may exceed the compensatory mechanism of hypertrophy, the Frank-Starling mechanism, and catecholamine stimulation. Congestive cardiac failure thus typically develops at about 2 to 3 months of age.

The clinical course and hemodynamics are different in patients with a small VSD. When the ventricles communicate through a small defect, the left ventricular pressure is only partially transmitted to the right ventricle, so there is a pressure gradient across the defect (pressure-limiting VSD). The blood flow is always left to right through the defect, the amount being determined primarily by the size of the defect and the pressure differential between the ventricles (Fig 12–9,A). If the right ventricular systolic pressure is less than the left, the defect must be small.

In patients with a small VSD, the decline in the pulmonary vascular resistance usually follows a normal curve or is only slightly retarded. Various degrees of right ventricular hypertrophy are found, depending on the right ventricular systolic pressure. In a very small VSD with normal right-sided pressure, the right ventricle is of normal thickness. With a larger VSD and pulmonary hypertension, the thickness of the right ventricular wall equals that of the left ventricle.

Although the greatest volume load is placed on the left ventricle, studies of the right ventricle show a modest increase in right ventricular volume from diastolic shunting.[8] The major flow through the ventricular septal defect occurs during systole, when the pressure differential between the ventricles is the greatest. The right ventricle is more distensible (compliant), particularly in patients with only a minor degree of right ventricular hypertrophy, and this favors blood flow across the defect during diastole. During systole, right ventricular volume is not increased by the left-to-right shunt, because the blood is ejected directly through the defect into the right ventricular infundibulum, which merely acts as a conduit.

NATURAL HISTORY OF VENTRICULAR SEPTAL DEFECT

In patients with a VSD, three events may occur naturally.[9–15] (1) the defect may close spontaneously, (2) pulmonary vascular disease may develop, or (3) infundibular pulmonary stenosis may develop. Small defects with only slightly elevated right ventricular pressure do not lead to pulmonary vascular disease.

1. Spontaneous closure.[16–19] Spontaneous closure of VSD may occur by several mechanisms
   a. The septal leaflet of tricuspid valve may adhere to a membranous defect.
   b. A muscular VSD may be sealed by hypertrophy of muscle bundles.
   c. The margins of defects may undergo fibrotic changes, which finally close the defect.

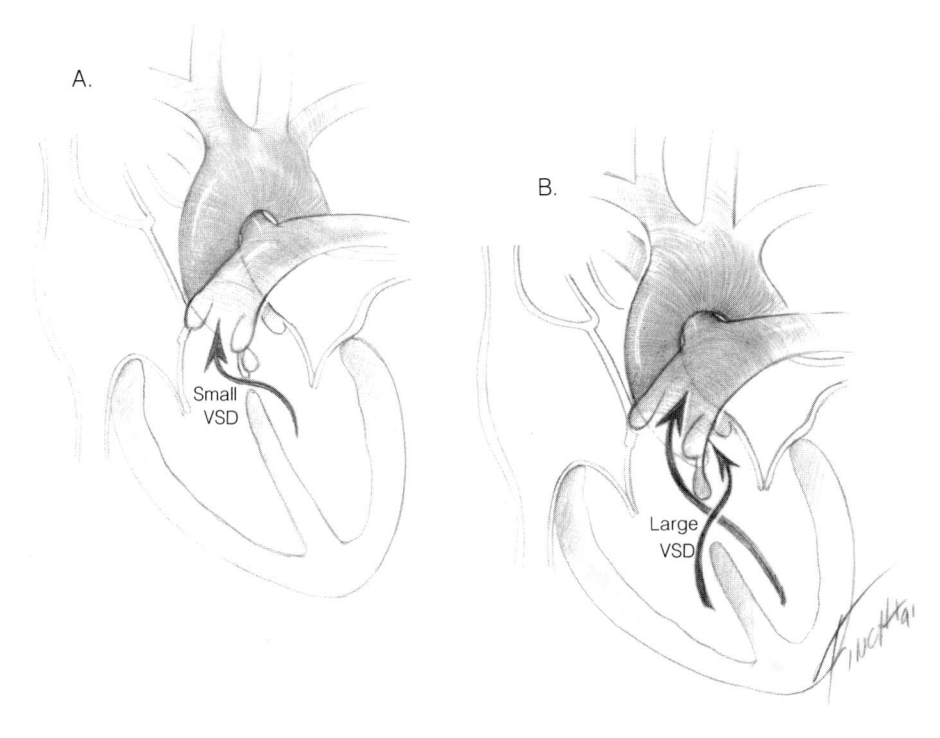

FIG 12–9.
Central circulation of a ventricular septal defect *(VSD)*. **A,** small VSD; volume of flow through the defect depends on the relative systolic pressures in the ventricles. **B,** large VSD; direction and magnitude of flow depend on relative systemic and pulmonary vascular resistances.

    d. The defect may become sealed by vegetations of subacute bacterial endocarditis.

The exact number of VSDs that close is unknown. In routine autopsy data, anatomic evidence for a spontaneously closed defect is found in 1 of 225 cases; this figure is greater than the incidence of clinically recognizable VSD. At least 25% of small defects close spontaneously before adulthood, many in the first 3 years of life; although we have had one patient between the ages of 22 and 26 years in whom a defect closed.

Muscular VSDs are more likely to close spontaneously, as are defects in females. The incidence of moderate-sized or large defects closing is less than that in small defects, but perhaps 5% to 10% of large defects also undergo spontaneous closure. Even if spontaneous closure does not occur, the defect becomes smaller in 70% of patients, again more commonly in those with a small defect. The defect does not grow in proportion to cardiac size, and because cardiac output increases with growth, the defect and shunt flow become relatively smaller.

If an aneurysm of the membranous septum is demonstrable angiographically, the defect is much more likely to close.[17] Many defects with an aneurysm of the membranous septum are actually closing membranous defects with partial adherence to the septal defect of the tricuspid valve.

2. Development of infundibular pulmonary stenosis. In patients with a VSD, infundibular stenosis, in the form of anomalous muscle bundles or infundibular hypertrophy, may develop. Eventually the stenosis may become severe enough to cause a right-to-left shunt.[21] Stenosis is much more common in patients with a right aortic arch.[22]

3. Development of pulmonary vascular disease. In patients with a large VSD and long-standing pulmonary hypertension, progressive medial thickening and, subsequently, intimal proliferation can occur in the pulmonary arterioles, increasing the resistance to blood flow.[14, 23] These changes rarely occur during childhood, but, rather, appear in the teenage years or early adulthood. By the age of 20 years, perhaps 10% of patients with VSDs have markedly elevated pulmonary vascular resistance. The mechanism of these pathologic changes is unknown.

The pulmonary vascular resistance may eventually exceed the systemic vascular resistance, and the shunt through the defect becomes right to left. Cyanosis then develops (see Fig 12–8). As the pulmonary vascular resistance rises, the volume of pulmonary blood flow falls, thereby reducing the volume load on the left ventricle. Thus, congestive cardiac failure disappears, the heart becomes smaller, and left atrial enlargement disappears. Some patients with a VSD retain their high fetal resistance and never develop a large left-to-right shunt.

It is rare for a patient with a VSD and normal or slightly elevated pulmonary artery pressure to develop pulmonary vascular disease for the same reason it is rare for those with atrial septal defects to become cyanotic.

CLINICAL FEATURES

The presence of a VSD is usually evidenced by a murmur, which generally is not heard in the neonatal period but appears at age 4 to 6 weeks. At this age, the pulmonary vascular resistance has fallen sufficiently to allow a large enough left-to-right shunt to create the murmur. However, in a patient with a small VSD, a murmur may be heard in the neonatal period because of the high velocity of the jet.

Patients with a small VSD remain asymptomatic throughout childhood. If the VSD is large, symptoms develop between 1 and 6 months of age. Infants with a large left-to-right shunt develop congestive heart failure during this interval, because the pulmonary vascular resistance has fallen sufficiently to allow a large shunt and increase the left ventricular volume. Dyspnea and recurrent respiratory tract infections are common in those with a large left-to-right shunt, probably from reduced pulmonary compliance, secondary to elevated pulmonary venous pressure. One manifestation of dyspnea on exertion is fatigue while feeding. This factor, plus the increased metabolic demands, retard growth.

Many symptomatic infants, if not treated surgically, show improvement of symptoms between 12 and 24 months, which may be caused by one of three factors:

1. Reduction in size or closure of the VSD
2. Development of infundibular stenosis
3. Development of increased pulmonary vascular resistance

The physician must carefully evaluate the clinical and laboratory data to determine which of these natural events is occurring; in doubtful cases, cardiac catheterization is indicated.

Physical Examination

The appearance of children with small VSDs is normal, whereas those with large defects may be thin and show retarded growth. Blood pressure is normal. If the defect is large, there is a precordial bulge because of right ventricular enlargement.

The most diagnostic feature is a systolic murmur best heard along the left sternal border in the third and fourth interspaces.[24] The loudness of the murmur varies and does not correlate with the size of the defect. In a small muscular VSD, the murmur is soft, squirting, and not pansystolic. In most other VSDs with a left-to-right shunt, the murmur is grade 3 to 4/6, pansystolic, harsh, and well heard throughout the precordium. In patients with severe pulmonary vascular disease and little or no left-to-right shunt, there is no systolic murmur. If the murmur is grade 5/6, an anomalous muscle bundle may coexist or the defect may be supracristal.[25]

The other findings include:

1. First heart sound. In patients with a large left-to-right shunt, the first heart sound is loud at the apex, because left ventricular filling is prolonged, and the mitral valve has a longer excursion as it closes.
2. Second heart sound. The aortic component is normal, but the intensity of the pulmonic component may be increased because P_2 reflects the pulmonary arterial pressure. As pulmonary vascular resistance increases, the degree of splitting narrows, because the pressure contours of the left and right ventricles are nearly identical.
3. Middiastolic murmur. When the volume of pulmonary blood flow exceeds twice the normal amount, the volume of flow across the mitral valve causes turbulence, leading to an apical middiastolic murmur (relative mitral stenosis). This accurately reflects the volume of pulmonary blood flow. The murmur is usually grade 1 to 2/6 and low pitched.
4. Early diastolic murmur. In patients with pulmonary hypertension and markedly elevated pulmonary vascular resistance, an early diastolic murmur of pulmonary insufficiency develops. This murmur results from dilatation of the pulmonary trunk and elevated pulmonary artery diastolic pressure.

Electrocardiographic Features

The ECG reflects the hemodynamics of the VSD. Basically, two abnormal workloads can be placed on the ventricles: an increased left ventricular volume, which leads to a pattern of left ventricular hypertrophy, and increased right ventricular systolic pressure, which leads to a pattern of right ventricular hypertrophy.

Four patterns of ventricular hypertrophy may be found among patients with a VSD:

1. Normal. This indicates a small defect, with a nearly normal pulmonary artery pressure and a small (< 2:1) left-to-right shunt.
2. Left ventricular hypertrophy. This indicates a moderate-sized defect, with a 2:1 or 3:1 left-to-right shunt, low pulmonary vascular resistance, and normal or slightly increased pulmonary vascular resistance.
3. Combined ventricular hypertrophy. This indicates a large defect, with large pulmonary blood flow, pulmonary hypertension, and normal or slightly increased pulmonary vascular resistance.
4. Right ventricular hypertrophy. This indicates a large defect and pulmonary vascular disease. Because of

the severe pulmonary hypertension and the increased pulmonary vascular resistance, the volume of pulmonary blood flow is limited.

The QRS axis is variable. With increasing pulmonary vascular resistance, the QRS axis shifts toward the right. Left-axis deviation up to −30° may be found and is not indicative of a defect of the AV-canal type. The P waves are usually normal. The T waves may be tall in the left precordial leads of patients with a large pulmonary blood flow.

Echocardiographic Features

The echocardiogram is most useful in the identification of unexpected coexistent conditions, and therefore we perform echocardiography before cardiac catheterization. The clinical diagnosis of VSD is usually evident, and an echocardiogram is unnecessary for the diagnosis in most cases.

With the development of cross-sectional echocardiograms, it has been possible to identify the location of some of the defects. In one study, most large defects were identified, but defects less than 4 mm in diameter were not demonstrated.[26]

CHEST RADIOGRAPHY

The radiographic appearance of a VSD is not uniform, but in most patients, the correct diagnosis can be made when clinical information is also considered. The chest radiograph is consistent with the hemodynamics, which range from small defects with small shunts and normal pulmonary artery pressure to large defects with large pulmonary blood flow and pulmonary hypertension or with pulmonary vascular disease.

1. In patients with small or medium-sized defects:
   a. Cardiac size is usually normal or slightly increased.
   b. The pulmonary arterial segment and pulmonary vasculature appear normal or at the upper limits of normal.
   c. The left atrium is not enlarged. REASON: The pulmonary blood flow is not large enough to distend the left atrium.
   d. A left-to-right shunt of 50% may be present and associated with minimal or borderline radiographic findings (Fig 12–10).
2. In patients with a large defect and large pulmonary blood flow without increased pulmonary resistance:
   a. The cardiac size is moderately to severely increased. REASON: The large volume of pulmonary blood flow enlarges the left ventricle; this may be complicated by congestive cardiac failure.
   b. The pulmonary arterial segment is enlarged. The pulmonary vasculature is markedly increased and has a fluffy appearance similar to that in atrial septal defect (Fig 12–11,A). REASON: Arteries and veins are diffusely distended by flow. Pulmonary vascular disease is not present, which causes diminution of pulmonary blood flow and tortuosity of the pulmonary arteries.
   c. Enlargement of the left ventricle can be seen on a left anterior oblique view (Fig 12–11,B). This view is helpful in the differentiation of VSD from atrial septal defect, which causes right atrial enlargement and an elevated small left ventricle (see Chapter 19).
   d. Left atrial enlargement is also evident on the left anterior oblique or lateral views (Fig 12–11,C). REASON: The markedly increased blood flow through the pulmonary circulation distends not only the pulmonary veins but also the left atrium. Enlargement of the left atrium indicates that the pulmonary blood flow is large. There is a fair correlation between left atrial size and the mitral diastolic-flow murmur. It is usually evident in infancy, but the shunt flow invariably decreases later in life.

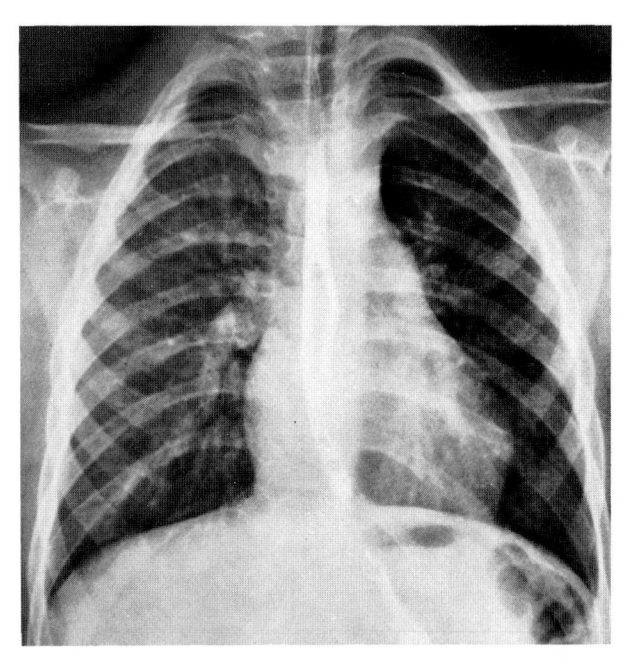

FIG 12–10.
Thoracic roentgenogram in posteroanterior projection of VSD with 40% left-to-right shunt and normal pulmonary arterial pressure. Normal cardiac size. Pulmonary vasculature and pulmonary arterial segment at upper limits of normal. Diagnosis of a left-to-right shunt cannot be made radiographically.

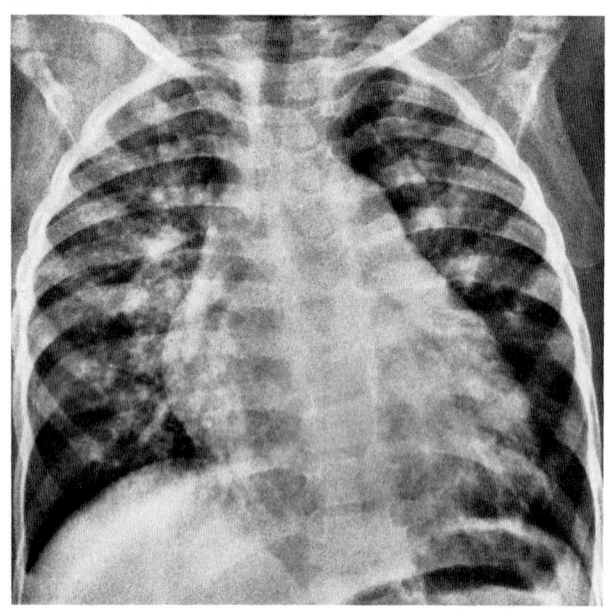

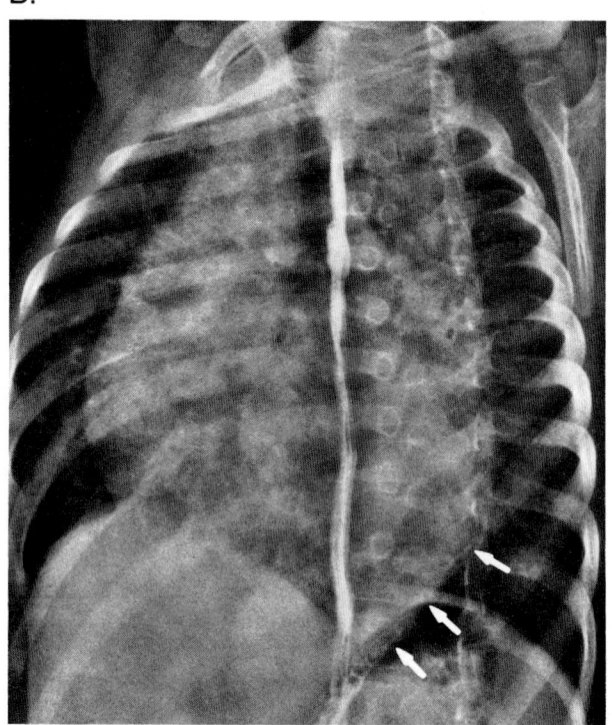

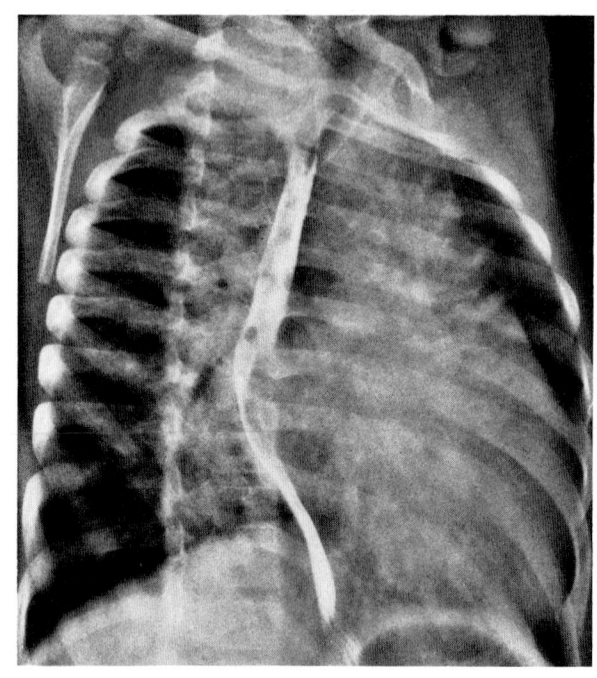

FIG 12–11.
Thoracic roentgenogram of large VSD with normal pulmonary vascular resistance. **A,** posteroanterior projection shows marked cardiomegaly and markedly enlarged main pulmonary arterial segment. Pulmonary vasculature diffusely accentuated but with indistinct fluffy appearance. Aortic knob inconspicuous because aortic flow is normal. **B,** left anterior oblique projection shows left ventricular enlargement *(arrows)* from large volume of pulmonary blood flow. **C,** right anterior oblique projection shows left atrial enlargement proportional to volume of pulmonary blood flow.

Cardiac size, pulmonary vasculature, and degree of left atrial enlargement correlate well. Left atrial size is a reliable indicator of the volume of pulmonary blood flow. If the degree of left atrial enlargement appears disproportionate to the pulmonary vasculature and the degree of cardiomegaly, associated mitral disease should be suspected.

In spite of the increased blood flow through the left atrium and elevation of the left atrial pressure, Kerley B lines are never seen unless there is associated mitral disease, a rare situation. Mitral reflux is more common than mitral stenosis.

3. In patients with a large VSD and pulmonary vascular disease:
   a. The pulmonary vasculature is better defined.
   REASON: The pulmonary arteries are enlarged and have become tortuous because of long-standing pulmonary hypertension.
   b. Pneumonitis and pneumonic residues are common.
   REASON: These patients are particularly likely to develop pneumonitis, probably because of the decreased pulmonary compliance as a result of the elevated pulmonary venous pressure.
   c. Left atrial enlargement may be present or absent, depending on the degree of left-to-right shunt.
   d. Rarely, atelectasis of the left lung develops (Fig 12–12). The left mainstem bronchus is narrowed between the enlarged left pulmonary artery above and the enlarged left atrium below (see Fig 12–5).
4. In patients with VSD with severe pulmonary vascular disease (Eisenmenger's syndrome*), as the pulmonary vascular disease worsens, the left-to-right shunt disappears, and the following x-ray features are noted:
   a. Left atrial enlargement disappears.
   b. Cardiac size decreases.
   c. The central pulmonary arteries remain enlarged and tortuous.
   d. The peripheral pulmonary arteries become constricted (peripheral pruning), suggesting pulmonary vascular disease (Fig 12–13).
   e. Calcification may be observed in the main and left pulmonary arterial branches, because the atherosclerotic plaques that develop secondary to long-standing pulmonary hypertension calcify.
   f. The pulmonary valve also may calcify (Fig 12–14). (The pulmonary valve may calcify in valvular pulmonary stenosis, also.)

*Eisenmenger's syndrome is named after Victor Eisenmenger, a German physician who described in 1897 a patient who was cyanotic from birth and who had a ventricular septal defect, hypertrophy of the right ventricle, and an overriding aorta (Eisenmenger complex). Today "Eisenmenger's syndrome" or "reaction" is used to describe the development of pulmonary vascular disease secondary to a left-to-right shunt.

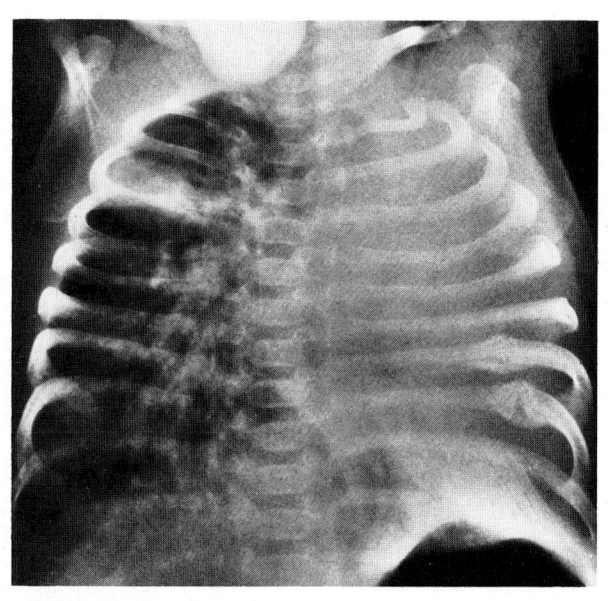

FIG 12–12.
Thoracic roentgenogram in posteroanterior projection of VSD and pulmonary vascular disease. Markedly increased vasculature in right lung; branch arteries are tortuous. Pneumonitis in right upper lobe, a common finding in patients with a large defect. Marked mediastinal shift to left from atelectasis of left lung. At necropsy, left mainstem bronchus was found to be compressed between enlarged left atrium and left pulmonary artery. Incidental fracture of left eighth and ninth ribs.

In a few patients with VSD and severe pulmonary vascular disease, another radiographic appearance is encountered. This happens in patients whose pulmonary vasculature does not mature and who never developed a significant left-to-right shunt. In these patients, the radiographic appearance is close to normal (Fig 12–15). The cardiac size and pulmonary vasculature are normal, and the pulmonary artery segment is normal or slightly prominent. Radiographically its appearance is more consistent with valvar pulmonary stenosis than with VSD.

5. Generally the diminution of the left-to-right shunt as the patients become older is evidenced radiographically by the following:
   a. Cardiac size decreases.
   b. Left atrial enlargement diminishes and finally disappears.
   c. The pulmonary vasculature decreases, particularly in the periphery of the lung fields, indicating a decrease in pulmonary flow.

This change can be caused by the following events, which are better diagnosed by clinical than by radiographic means:
   a. The defect may become smaller or close.
   b. Infundibular pulmonary stenosis may develop.

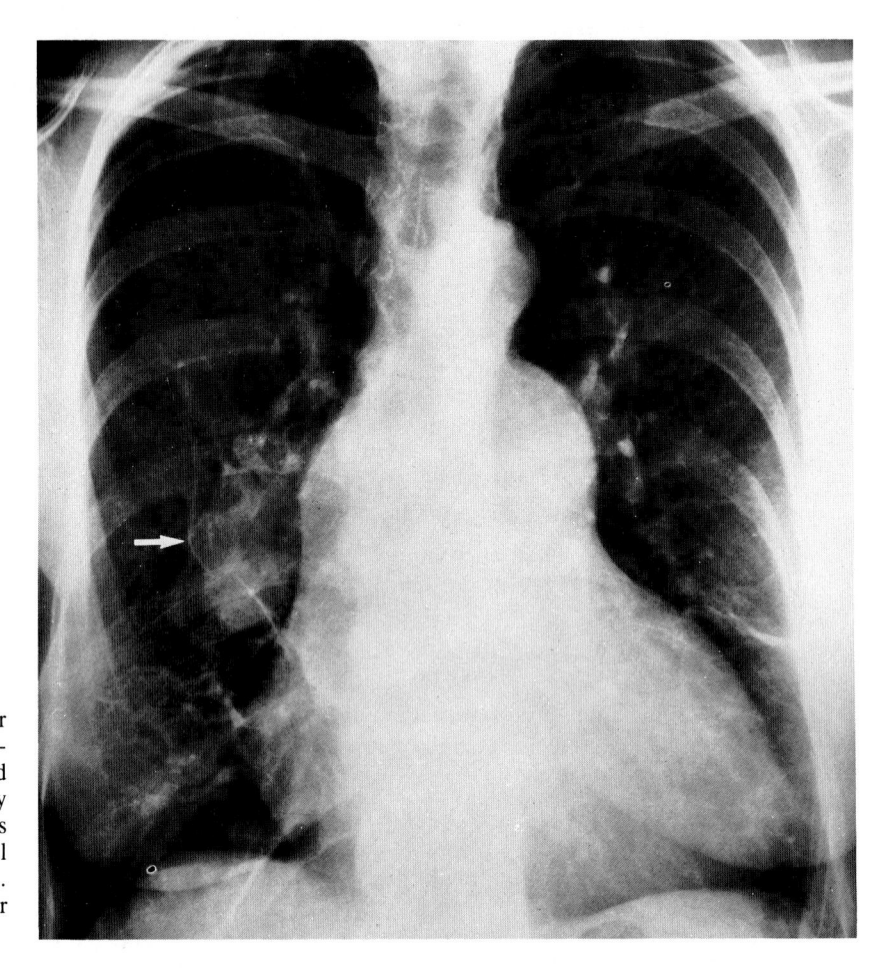

FIG 12–13.
Thoracic roentgenogram in posteroanterior projection of VSD, severe pulmonary vascular disease, and right-to-left shunt. Enlarged main pulmonary artery and central pulmonary arteries; sparse peripheral pulmonary arteries (pruning). Calcium flecks (arrow) in small pulmonary arteries indicate atherosclerosis. Increased cardiac size from right ventricular enlargement.

    c. Anomalous muscle bundles may become more significant hemodynamically.
    d. Pulmonary vascular disease may appear.

Radiographically, the differentiation among these events is difficult. A VSD without a prominent pulmonary artery segment suggests the presence of infundibular stenosis (pink tetrad).

If the patient has a right aortic arch and a left-to-right shunt, the most likely diagnosis is VSD. A right arch without an aortic diverticulum strongly suggests associated pulmonary stenosis.

6. After pulmonary arterial banding, chest radiographic changes are identical to those in other conditions that decrease the left-to-right shunt (Fig 12–16). REASON: The tight band creates a pressure gradient across the pulmonary valve and limits the shunt flow. If the band is properly placed, the shunt decreases in both lungs equally. Serial roentgenograms should be examined carefully to detect any unilateral decrease of pulmonary flow, which suggests displacement of the band and compression of one of the pulmonary arteries. Compression of the right pulmonary artery is more common (Fig 12–17). REASON: The left pulmonary artery is a continuation of the main pulmonary artery and is not as readily compressed by distal displacement of the band. Exceptions occur, however.

7. In patients with a VSD and anomalous muscle bundle, the chest radiographic findings depend on the degree of obstruction and range from a pattern of left-to-right shunt to a pattern of right-to-left shunt:
    a. The cardiac silhouette may be enlarged, the pulmonary vasculature increased, and the left atrium enlarged when the muscle bundle causes a minor degree of obstruction or the VSD is located distal to the anomalous muscle bundle.
    b. The cardiac size may be normal, and the pulmonary vasculature may be within normal limits when the muscle bundle causes a moderate degree of obstruction and results in a "balanced" shunt, indicating a small left-to-right, right-to-left, or bidirectional shunt.
    c. The cardiac size may be normal, and the

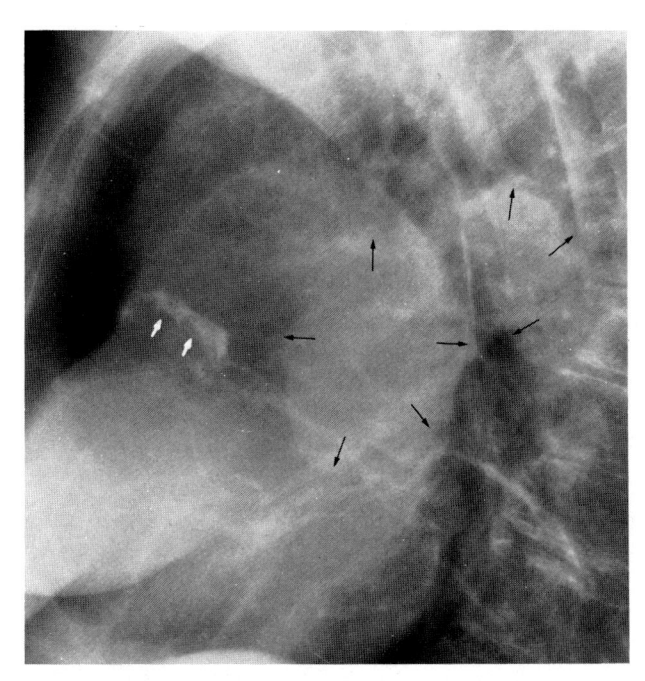

FIG 12-14.
Thoracic roentgenogram in lateral projection of VSD, pulmonary vascular disease, and right-to-left shunt. Calcification of pulmonary valve *(arrows)*. Right and left pulmonary arteries are huge *(black arrows)*.

pulmonary vasculature decreased when the muscle bundle is severely obstructive and there is a right-to-left shunt at the ventricular level. In these patients, the hemodynamics resemble those of tetralogy of Fallot, and the obstructing muscle bundle is distal to the VSD.

8. In patients with a VSD and aortic stenosis:
   a. Subaortic stenosis complicating VSD cannot be suspected from thoracic roentgenograms.
   b. The radiographic findings are usually normal when subaortic stenosis proximal to the VSD limits the left-to-right shunt.

CARDIAC CATHETERIZATION

The purposes of cardiac catheterization in patients with a VSD are to:

1. Establish the diagnosis.
2. Measure the pulmonary blood flow and pulmonary artery pressure to calculate pulmonary vascular resistance.
3. Identify any coexisting conditions.
4. Determine the location of the VSD.
5. Exclude coexisting muscular VSDs.

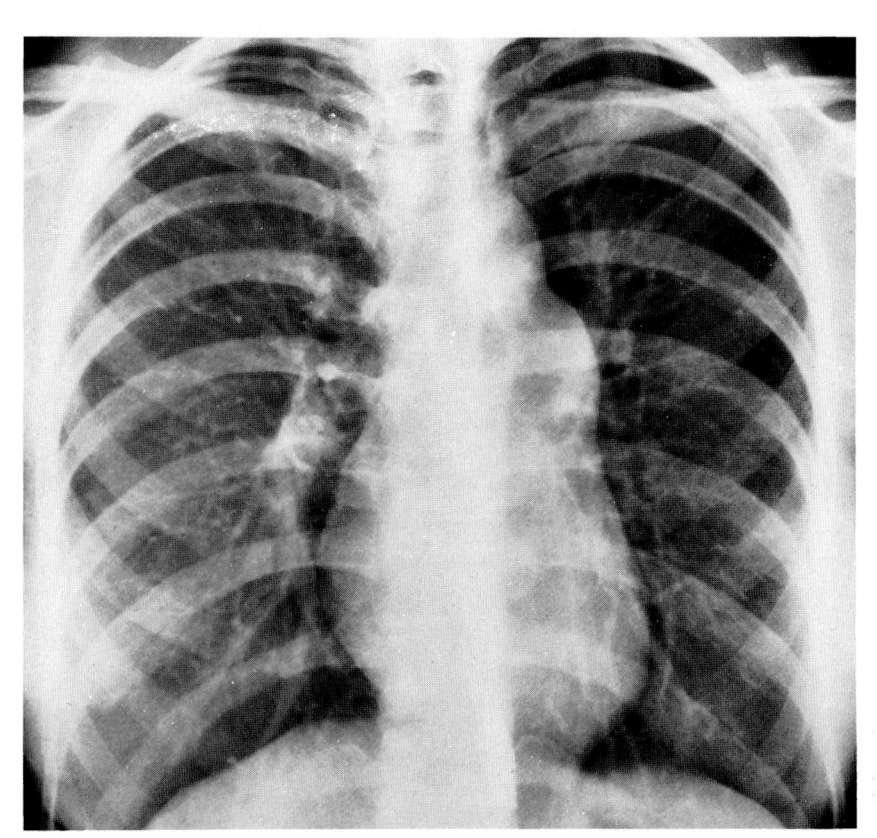

FIG 12-15.
Thoracic roentgenogram in posteroanterior projection of VSD and pulmonary vascular disease. Normal cardiac size and pulmonary vasculature; slightly prominent main pulmonary arterial segment. Radiographic appearance resembles that of pulmonary stenosis.

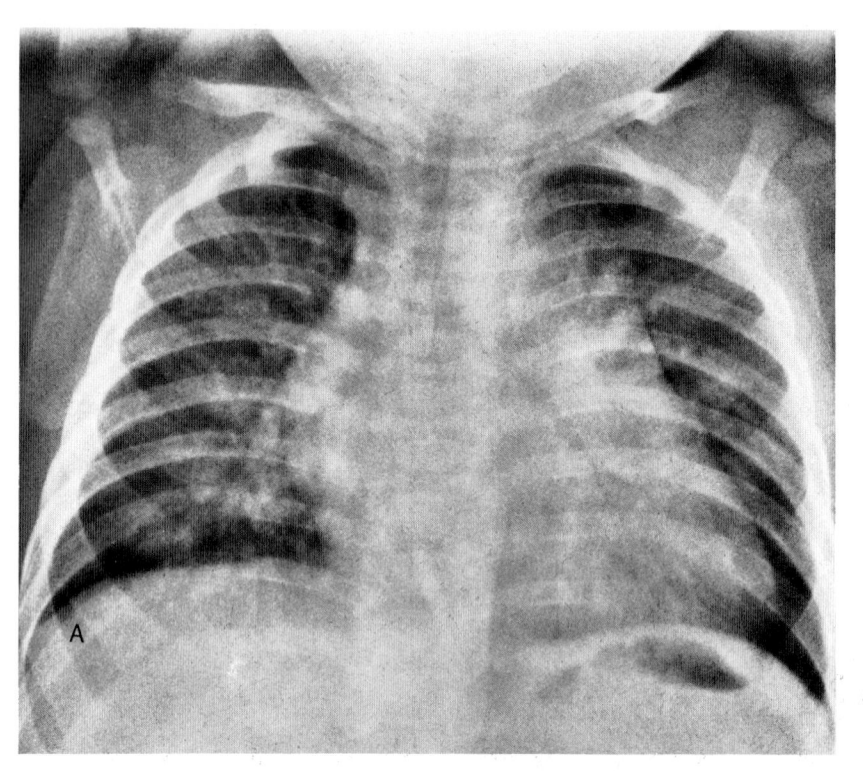

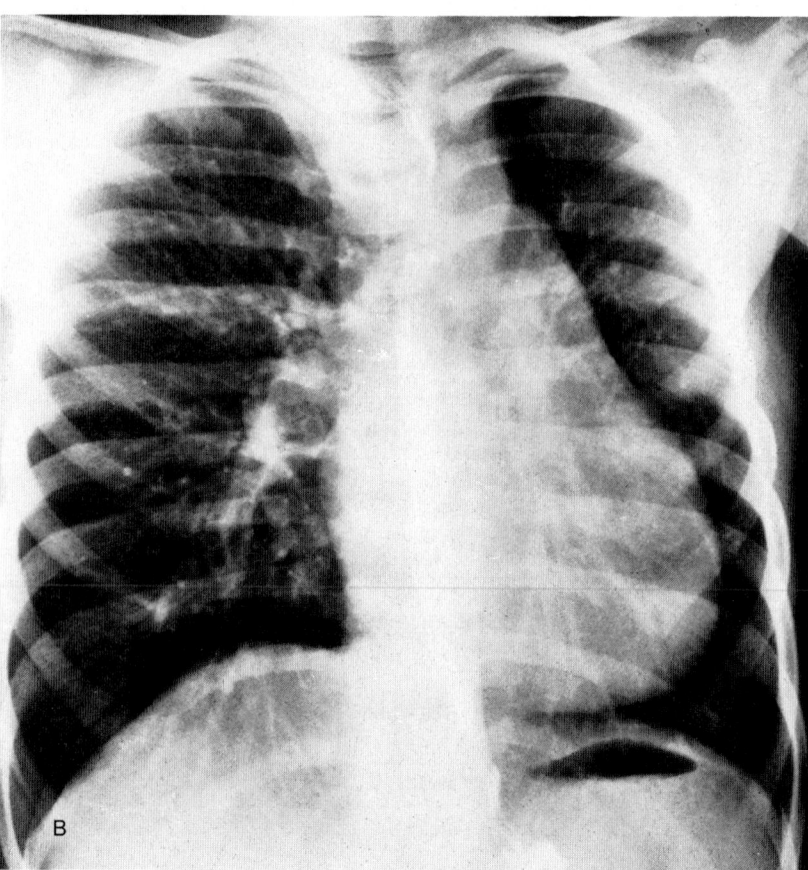

FIG 12–16.
Thoracic roentgenogram in posteroanterior projection of large VSD and large pulmonary blood flow before **(A)** and 2 years after **(B)** pulmonary arterial banding. Decreased cardiac size and pulmonary vasculature. Vasculature in left lung is sparse, suggesting obstruction of left pulmonary artery by band. This is less common than obstruction of the right pulmonary artery.

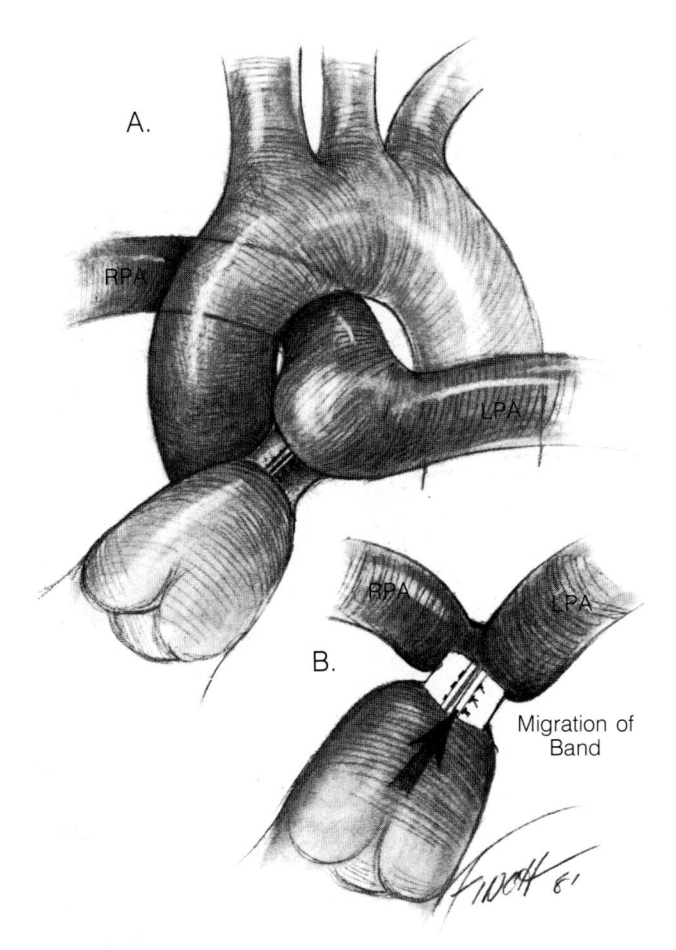

FIG 12–17.
Diagram of banding of main pulmonary artery; proper position of band. If the band slips *(arrow)*, right pulmonary artery *(RPA)* is more likely to be occluded than the left *(LPA)*, because the latter is a continuation of main pulmonary artery.

The indications for cardiac catheterization are:

1. In infants, a VSD and congestive heart failure.
2. All children with a VSD in whom operation is contemplated.
3. Children with evidence of increasing pulmonary vascular resistance.

The approach is generally through the femoral vein. In infants, the catheter can often be passed from the right to the left atrium through a patent foramen ovale. From the left atrium, the left ventricle can be entered; this is the most convenient approach for left ventriculography in infants. The catheter may be passed through a membranous VSD into the ascending aorta, and this is the preferred route for measuring aortic pressures and carrying out aortography. The catheter course is characteristic. It is generally difficult to pass a catheter through a VSD into the body of the left ventricle. When the catheter is in the pulmonary artery of infants with pulmonary hypertension, attempts should be made to pass it across the ductus arteriosus.

The pulmonary arterial wedge or left atrial pressure should be measured. In patients with a large left-to-right shunt, these pressures may be slightly elevated. Withdrawal pressures from the pulmonary artery through the right ventricle should be recorded to exclude right ventricular obstruction. If right-sided pressures are elevated, pressure should be measured simultaneously in the aorta or a systemic artery to determine vascular resistance.

A careful oximetry series should be obtained through the right side of the heart, and aortic oxygen saturation should be determined to calculate both the systemic and the pulmonary blood flows. Diagnosis of a ventricular septal defect by oximetry requires at least a 1 vol% increase in oxygen content between the right atrium and ventricle. In many infants, a small shunt is detectable at the atrial level as well. Left-to-right shunts of less than 20% cannot be detected by oximetry.

Angiography—General Remarks

Exact angiographic location of the VSD is important for the surgeon, because the surgical approach depends on the location, and a proper approach makes the operation more expedient. For example, if the defect is supracristal, it cannot be closed through a right atrial approach; rather, a right ventriculotomy over the infundibulum is required. Also, multiple muscular VSDs are difficult to identify at operation. Closure of such defects may require a left ventriculotomy, or corrective surgery may be deferred until patients are older, because these defects have a tendency to close spontaneously. An isolated posterior VSD (AV-canal type) may require a left ventriculotomy for repair and may be overlooked at surgery unless an exact diagnosis has been established preoperatively.

Knowledge of the anatomy of the ventricular septum is essential for the angiographic demonstration of these defects. The left ventricular surface of the septum is concave and the right ventricular surface convex (Fig 12–18). Angiographic demonstration of a VSD depends on observation of the contrast jet through the defect without superimposition of an opacified ventricle. Therefore, the x-ray beam must be directed tangentially to the defect. Because the septum is also curved in spiral fashion, a single left anterior oblique view is inadequate to demonstrate all VSDs.

Because of the tilt of the aortic valve plane and the crossing of the right and left ventricular outflow tracts (indicated by arrows in Fig 12–1), membranous and perimembranous defects, which comprise 80% of all VSDs, emerge in the right ventricle at various locations. True membranous defects emerge relatively low in the right

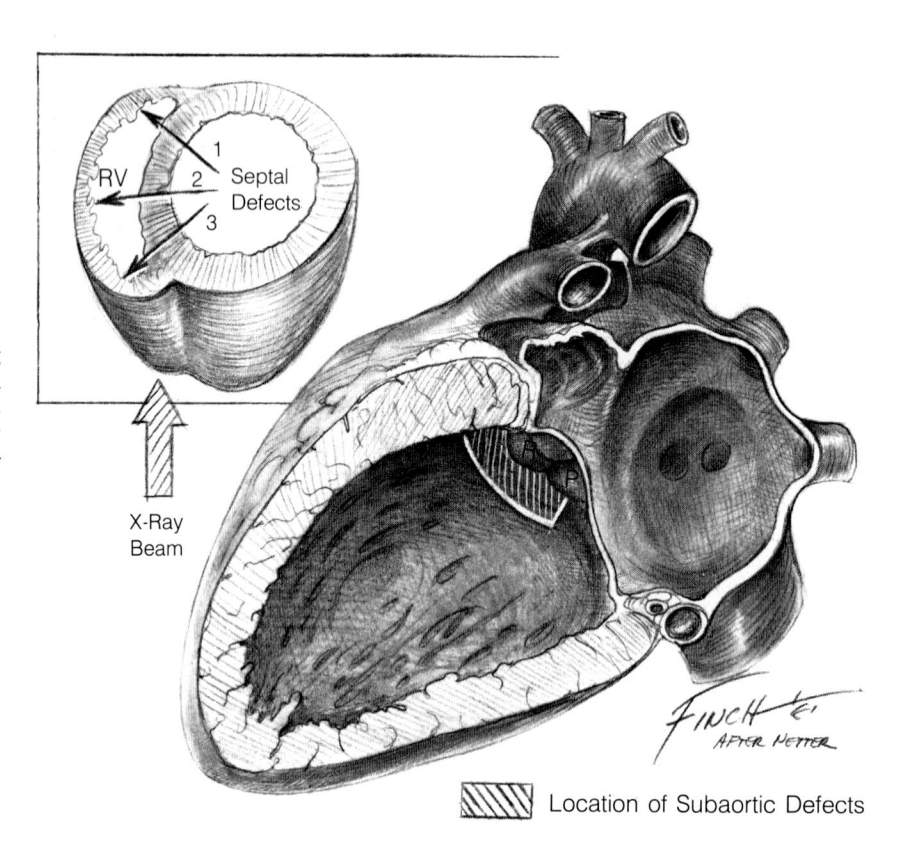

260 Cardiac Conditions Associated With a Left-to-Right Shunt

FIG 12–18.
Diagram of left ventricle, demonstrating concavity of ventricular septum. Location of the membranous and perimembranous defects indicated by the hatched area below the right and anterior half of the posterior aortic cusps. The membranous septum occupies a small area between the right *(R)* and posterior *(P)* aortic cusps. *Insert,* cross-section through ventricles, showing curved ventricular septum. Location of three VSDs shown by arrows *(1, 2,* and *3).* If the hatched arrow indicates direction of x-ray beams, it will be apparent that the patient must be rotated in different obliquities so that the defect is seen in profile. A different degree of rotation would be required for each of the three defects indicated. *RV* = right ventricle

ventricle, whereas defects beneath the right aortic cusp are located higher in the right ventricle, being infrapulmonary (supracristal).

On a standard left anterior oblique view, the septum is foreshortened, and this causes superimposition of various defects (Fig 12–19). This foreshortening of the septum can be avoided by using a left anterior oblique projection with angulation of the x-ray beam or by having the patient partially sit up.

Generally speaking, the higher and the more anterior

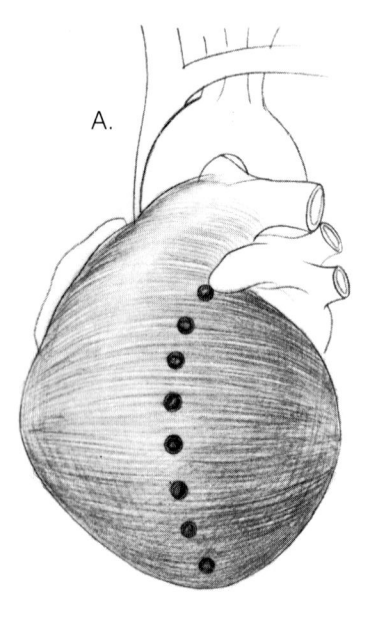

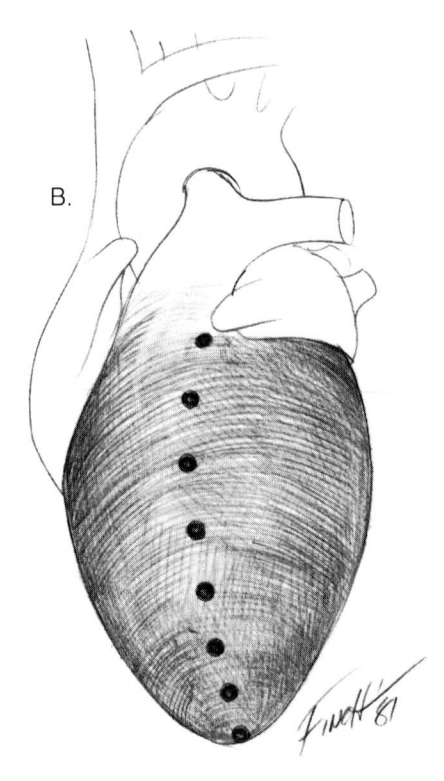

FIG 12–19.
Diagram of left anterior oblique view of heart; edge of the ventricular septum outlined by beads. **A,** patient in supine position; interventricular septum foreshortened. Therefore, multiple VSDs may be superimposed. **B,** by angling the x-ray beam cranially (looking down) or having the patient sit up, foreshortening of the ventricular septum is minimized. Ventricular septum is not straight but is slightly curved.

Ventricular Septal Defect **261**

VENTRICULAR SEPTAL DEFECTS
(Viewed from Right Ventricle)

1. Posterior A-V Canal Type
2. Perimembranous
3. Muscular
4. Apical Muscular
5. Multiple Anterior Muscular
6. Supracristal

FIG 12–20.
Cutaway view of the right ventricle, demonstrting four zones in which a VSD may be located. The zones require increasingly steeper left anterior oblique projections from *zone 1* to *zone 4* to demonstrate the defect in profile. *AO* = aorta; *PA* = pulmonary artery.

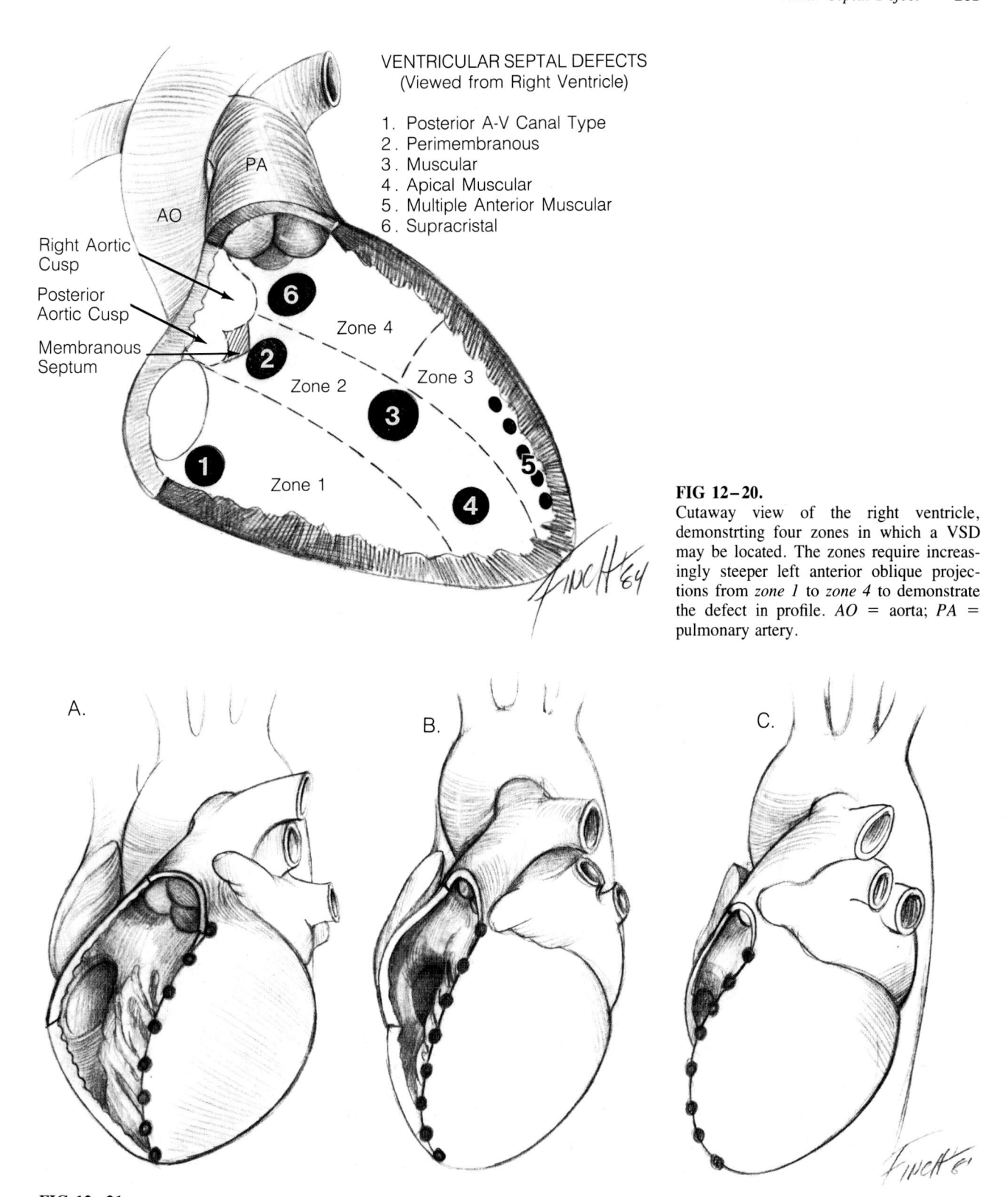

FIG 12–21.
Diagram of ventricular septum and exposed right ventricle, indicating the different degrees of obliquity required to demonstrate VSDs in various loctions. **A,** shallow (about 45 degrees) left anterior oblique view; posterior muscular defects near the tricuspid valve, such as VSD of the AV-canal type, are demonstrated. **B,** steeper (about 60 degrees) left anterior oblique projection; defects of anterior ventricular septum and the area of the membranous septum are demonstrated. **C,** steep left anterior oblique projection (lateral view); infrapulmonary (supracristal) defects demonstrated. Rarely, a right anterior oblique projection is required to demonstrate supracristal defects.

the defect, the more obliquity is required for its demonstration. The right ventricular surface can therefore be divided in four zones, which require increasingly steeper left anterior oblique projections to demonstrate communications in profile (Fig 12–20). Because of the spiral contour of the ventricular septum, these obliquities are necessary (Fig 12–21).

The degree of rotation of the chest required for visualization of a VSD also varies with the rotation of the heart. In patients with nonrotated hearts, the angle of the left anterior oblique projections varies from 40 degrees for zone 1 to 90 degrees for zone 4. Hearts with clockwise rotation as, for example, in patients with atrial septal defects or tetralogy of Fallot require steeper left anterior oblique projections.

Angiographic Appearance

1. The angiographic technique of choice to demonstrate a VSD is left ventriculography in the left anterior oblique position, with either tube or patient angulation to eliminate foreshortening of the ventricular septum (Fig 12–22).

2. The angled projection is better than a standard left anterior oblique projection, which does not allow distinction of defects in various locations. For example, without angulation, the two ventricular septal defects in Figure 12–23 would have been superimposed.

3. The correct degree of left anterior oblique projection should be used to observe the defect in profile.

4. The appropriate degree of the left anterior oblique projection is not constant, differing with rotation of the heart. The heart may be rotated by thoracic cage deformities, cardiac malposition, and other congenital anomalies.

5. If the heart is already rotated in counterclockwise fashion as seen from below, the degree of left anterior obliquity required to observe the septum is less. In hearts with clockwise rotation, as in atrial septal defect, a lateral projection may be required to show the membranous septum in profile.

6. Ventricular septal defects in the posterior septum (septal defects of the AV-canal type) and defects in the inflow portion of the muscular septum require the least obliquity (about 45 degrees). If such a defect is suspected clinically on the basis of left-axis deviation of the ECG, a shallow left anterior oblique view should be obtained as the initial projection.

7. Defects in the true membranous septum (between the commissure of the posterior and right aortic cusps) and left ventricular–right atrial shunts require a steeper left anterior oblique projection (about 60 degrees) (Fig 12–23).

8. In the right anterior oblique view the defects are

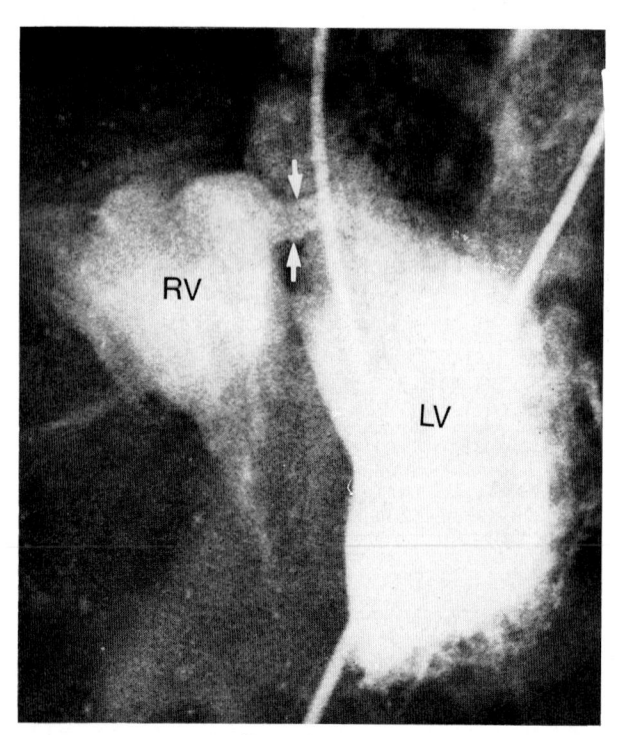

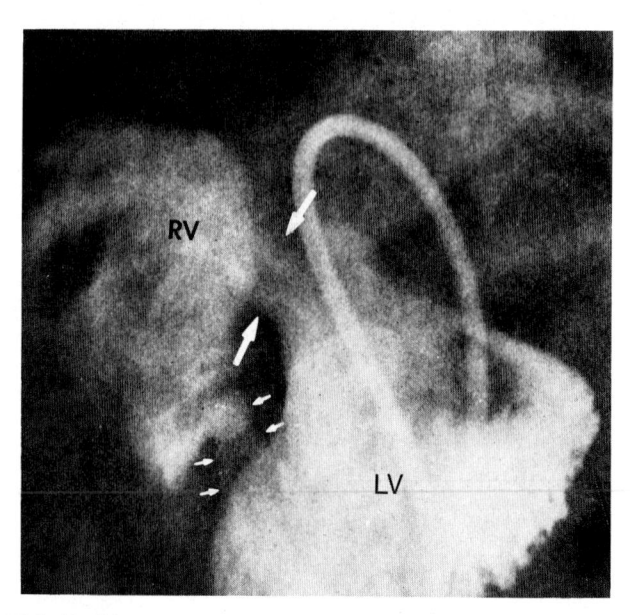

FIG 12–22.
Left ventriculogram *(LV)* in steeply angled (60 degrees) left anterior oblique projection; true membranous VSD *(arrow)* located immediately below aortic valve. No additional defects evident. *RV* = right ventricle.

FIG 12–23.
Left ventriculogram *(LV)* in about 60-degree left anterior oblique projection; large membranous VSD *(large arrows)* seen in profile. Additional muscular defect *(small arrows)* more anterior in the ventricular septum and therefore not demonstrated in profile, although well seen. The latter defect would require a steeper left anterior oblique projection, because of the spiral shape of the septum. *LV* = left ventricle; *RV* = right ventricle.

usually not seen. By the degree of left anterior oblique projection, which demonstrates the defect in profile, one can predict the location of the defect in the muscular septum. The more obliquity, the more anterior in location (Fig 12–24).

9. Demonstration of the location and number of muscular defects is of great practical importance to the surgeon, because multiple defects in the trabecular portion of the septum require a left ventriculotomy for repair. REASON: Defects are difficult to identify from the right ventricular side because of trabeculation. On left ventriculography, trabeculations in the right ventricle form numerous contrast jets simulating multiple defects (Swiss cheese appearance) (Fig 12–25,A). However, on right ventriculography, a single muscular defect can be demonstrated.

10. Ventricular septal defects lying underneath the right aortic cusp require more obliquity for their demonstration, because they exit high in the right ventricle (zone 4 in Fig 12–20). If the heart has a normal position within the chest, this area is seen in profile on a very steep left anterior oblique view, about 80 degrees to 90 degrees (lateral view).

11. Observation of supracristal VSDs requires a lateral or right anterior oblique projection (see Fig 12–26). Supracristal defects shunt directly into the infundibulum and fail to opacify the inflow portion of the right ventricle. REASON: The infundibular portion of the ventricular septum is inclined posteriorly, directing the jet upward through the defect (Figs 12–26 and 12–27). Because the shunt occurs primarily during systole, the rapid blood flow through the infundibulum directs the contrast medium into the pulmonary trunk, and the inflow portion does not opacify, although there are exceptions (see Fig 12–27).

12. Ventricular septal defects in the membranous septum are closely related to the septal leaflet of the tricuspid valve. Therefore, after left ventriculography, there is some opacification of the body of the right ventricle. Dense opacification of the apex of the right ventricle suggests a muscular defect.

13. To allow a shunt proximal to the crista supraventricularis, the aortic valve must be relatively high in relation to the crista (see Fig 12–27).

14. Ventricular septal defects can also be demonstrated on the levophase of a pulmonary arteriogram. In patients with a left-to-right shunt of less than 50% who will not undergo operation, the diagnosis can be established by this technique. Left-heart catheterization can thereby be avoided, but pulmonary arteriography is much less sensitive.

15. When an anomalous muscle bundle coexists with a VSD, it causes a characteristic round filling defect on an anteroposterior projection (Fig 12–28,A), and a bar-shaped filling defect extending across the ventricular outflow tract on the lateral view (Fig 12–28,B).

16. Subaortic stenosis may coexist with VSD and may be readily identified by left ventriculography. Subaortic stenosis distal to the VSD increases the left-to-right shunt (Fig 12–29). This type of subaortic obstruction is commonly associated with coarctation or interruption of the aortic arch. The ventricular defect is slightly lower, and the stenosis is caused by a characteristic muscular spur (see Fig 12–29). In discrete subaortic stenosis, a small VSD may be visible immediately below the aortic valve and above the membrane. It is important to make this diagnosis, because this defect may be difficult to see during operation (Fig 12–30).

17. Aortography is an integral part of catheterization, because patent ductus arteriosus has to be excluded. With a systemic level of pressure in the pulmonary artery, the ductus cannot be heard (silent ductus). The catheter can be passed through a membranous defect from the right ventricle into the aorta, following a characteristic course (see Fig 6–1).

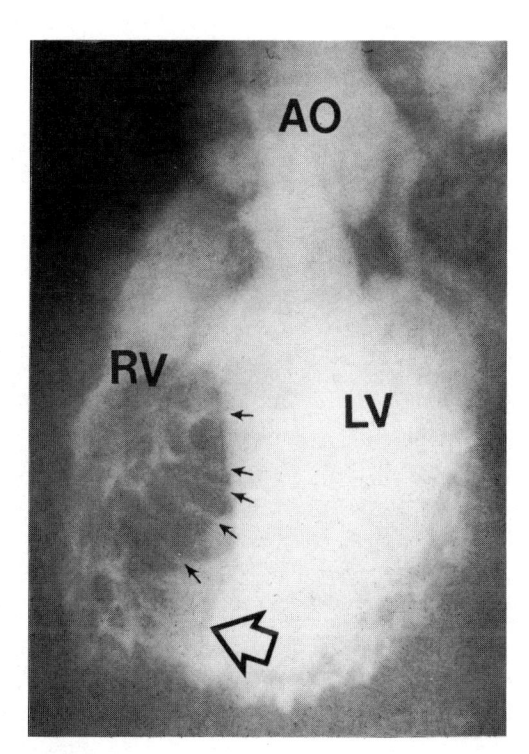

FIG 12–24.
Very steep left anterior oblique view of a left ventriculogram demonstrating numerous muscular defects in profile *(arrows)*. Because almost a lateral view was required for their demonstration, they must be located in the apical and anterior septum (Swiss cheese septum). For each defect there is a separate orifice in the left ventricular septum (see also Fig 12–28). At the apex there is a large muscular defect *(open arrow)*. In this location these defects are notoriously difficult to find through a right-sided surgical approach.

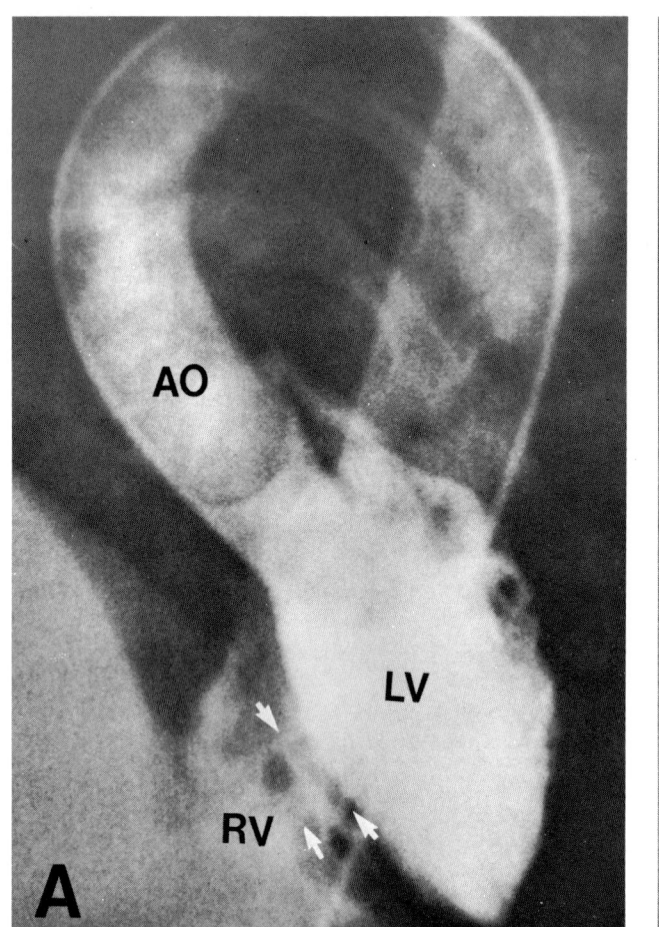

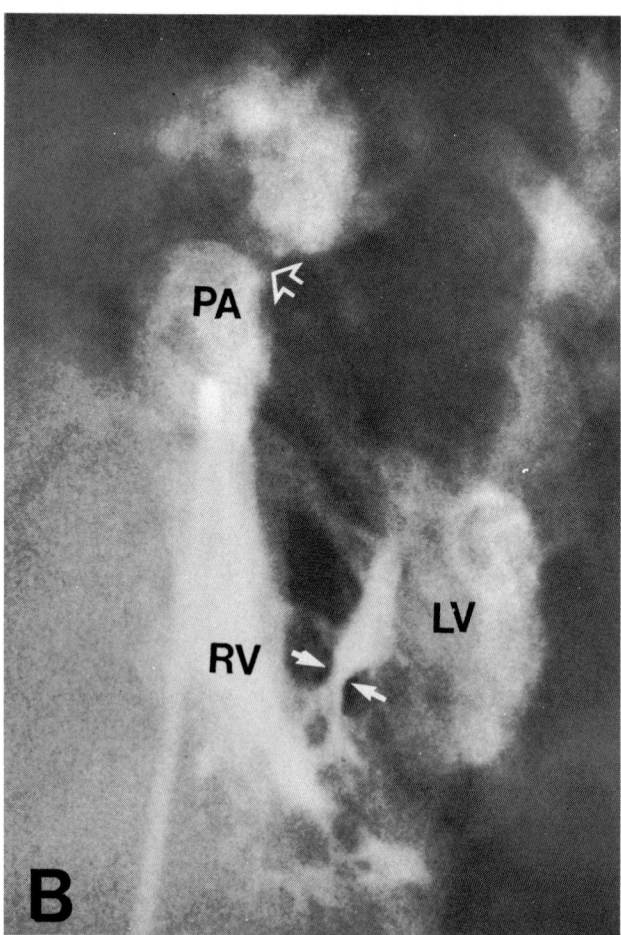

FIG 12–25.
A, left anterior oblique left ventriculogram with cranial beam angulation demonstrates what appears to be numerous muscular septal defects *(arrows)* simulated by trabeculations in the right ventricle. **B,** same patient; right ventriculogram shows only a single defect on the left ventricular side *(arrows)*. Pulmonary band well seen *(open arrow)*.

FIG 12–26.
Left ventriculogram *(LV)* in lateral projection showing supracristal VSD *(white arrow)*. The shunt occurs directly into the infundibulum above the crista supraventricularis. The defect lies immediately beneath the pulmonary valve. Because of the inclination of the infundibular septum, the jet of contrast medium is directed superiorly toward the pulmonary valve. *AO* = aorta; *PA* = pulmonary artery.

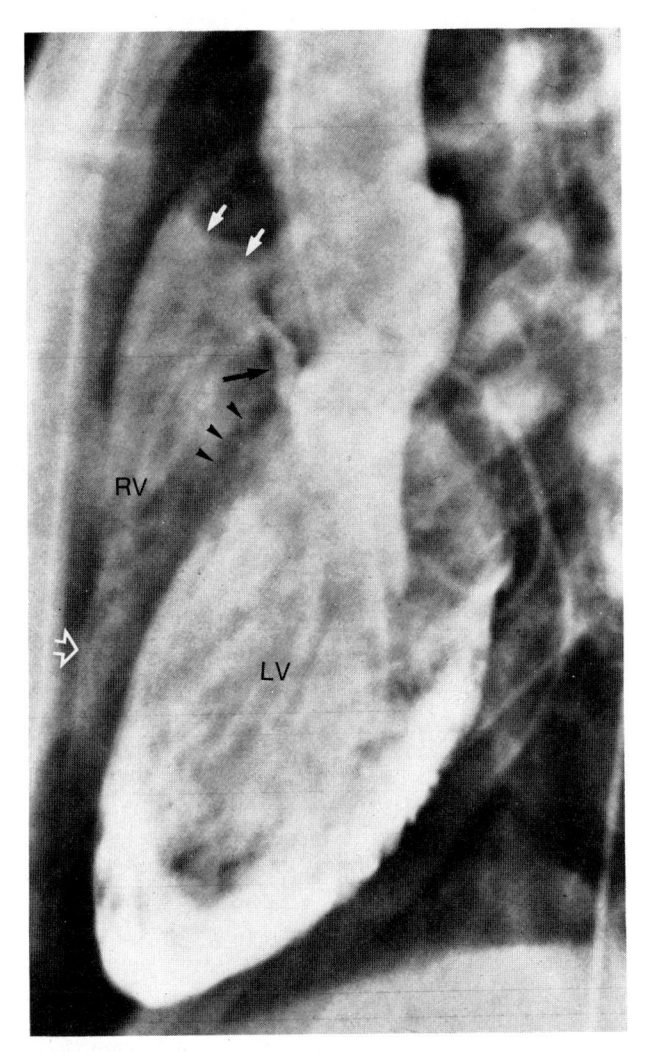

FIG 12–27.
Left ventriculogram *(LV)* in lateral projection showing VSD *(large arrow)* immediately beneath the right aortic cusp. The location is supracristal (infrapulmonary), and the area of the crista supraventricularis *(small black arrows)* is clearly seen. The contrast jet is directed cephalad toward the pulmonary valve *(white arrows)*, but some opacification of the inflow portion of the right ventricle *(open arrow)* is visible. The aortic valve is unusually high in relation to the pulmonary valve, allowing a supracristal shunt. *RV* = right ventricle.

18. Membranous defects may close spontaneously by adherence of the septal leaflet of the tricuspid valve, forming a membranous septal aneurysm (Fig 12–31,A). Muscular defects close by muscle growth and fibrointimal reaction (Fig 12–31,B and C).

MANAGEMENT

The management of children with VSDs varies according to the size of the defect and the level of pulmonary vascular resistance.

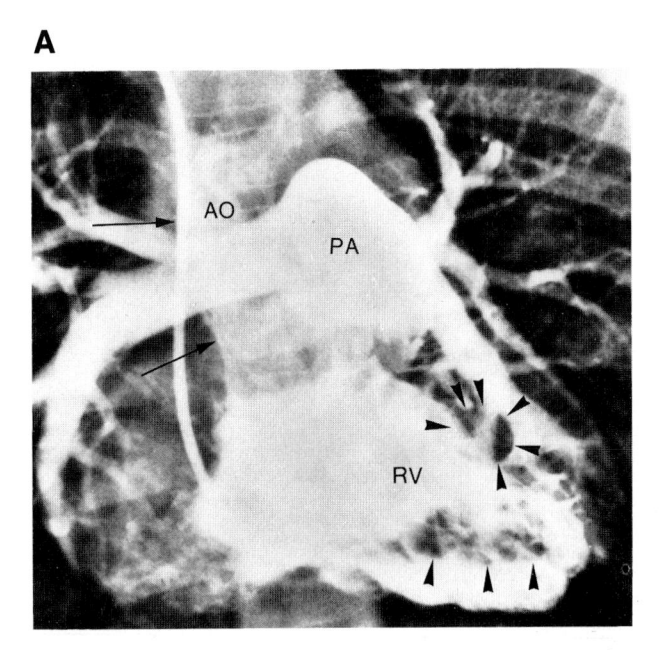

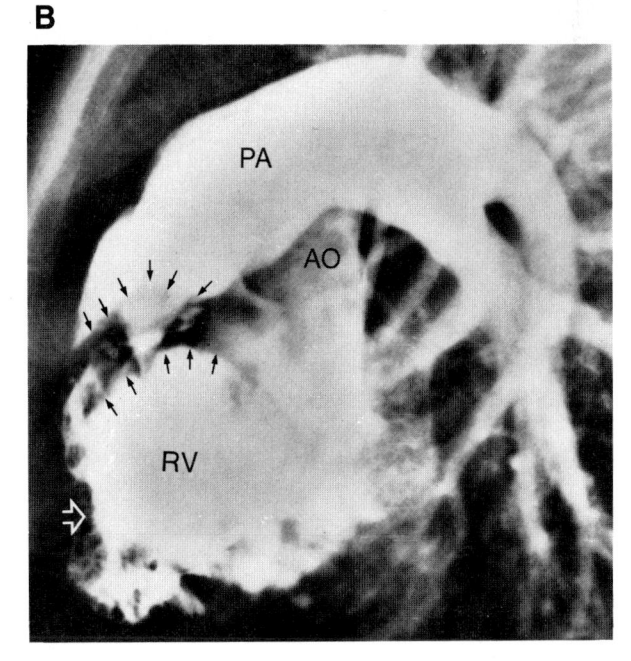

FIG 12–28.
Right ventriculogram. **A,** anteroposterior projection; filling defect of an anomalous muscle bundle in the right ventricular outflow tract and at the inflow portion, which is a hypertrophied moderator band *(arrow)*. The muscle bundle was partially obstructive and results in a balanced shunt with faint opacification of the aorta. Long arrows indicate aorta. **B,** lateral projection; anomalous muscle bundle *(small arrows)* extends from the anterior surface of the right ventricle contrast material extends into the right ventricle *(black arrows)* and right atrium *(white arrows)*. This angiogram is characteristic of malformation shown in Figure 12–1,C. *AO* = aortic; *LV* = left ventricle; *RA* = right atrium; *RV* = right ventricle.

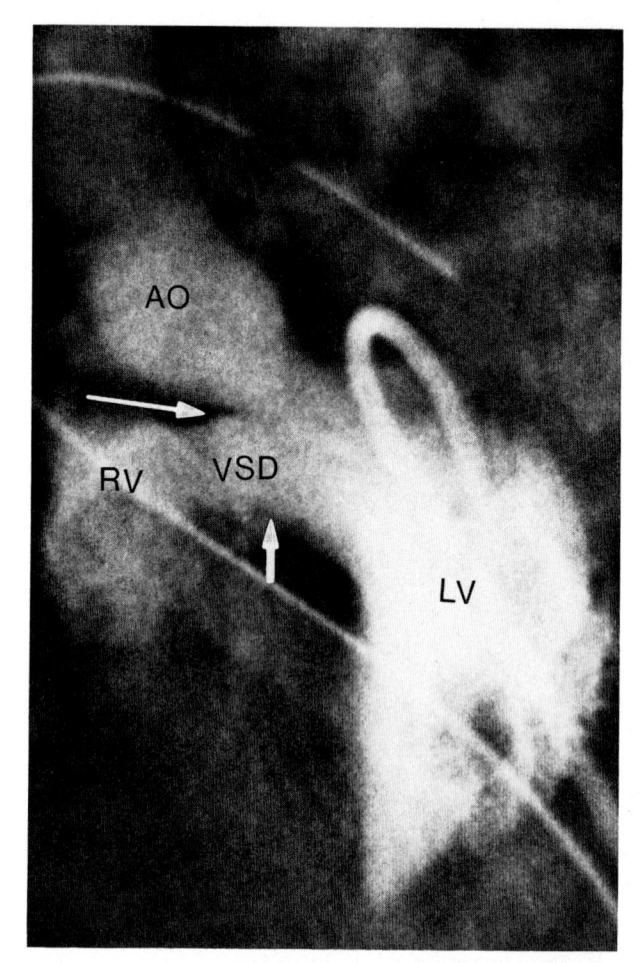

FIG 12–29.
Left ventriculogram in left anterior oblique projection showing VSD *(short white arow)* and subaortic stenosis. Subaortic stenosis caused by a spurlike protrusion of septum *(long arrow);* this type of VSD with subaortic stenosis is common in patients with interruption of the aortic arch. *AO* = aorta; *LV* = left ventricle; *RV* = right ventricle.

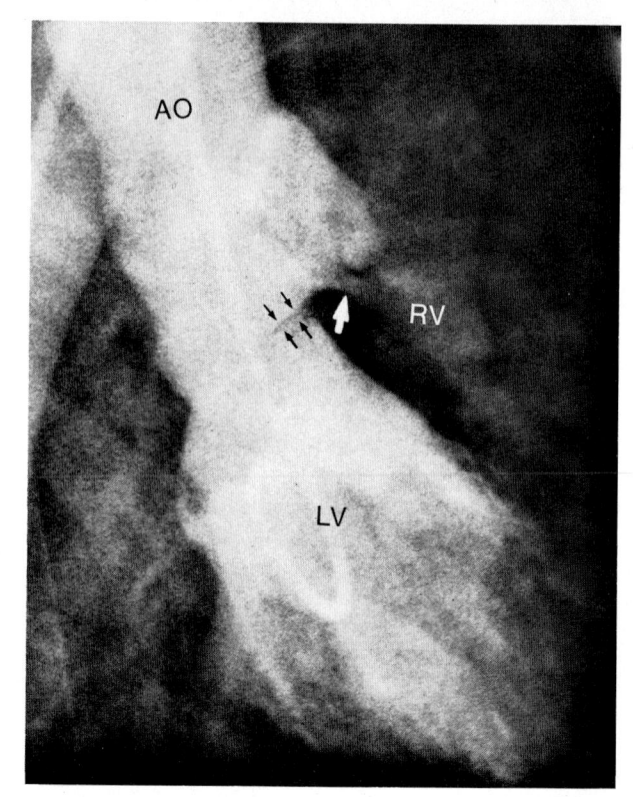

FIG 12–30.
Left ventriculogram in right anterior oblique projection showing discrete subaortic membrane *(black arrows)* and small VSD *(white arrow)* imediately beneath the right aortic cusp, which is slightly deformed because of prolapse through the defect (see also Chapter 10). Prolapse of the right aortic cusp causes partial obliteration of the ventricular septal defect resulting in a narrow jet *(white arrow)*. *RV* = right ventricle; *LV* = left ventricle.

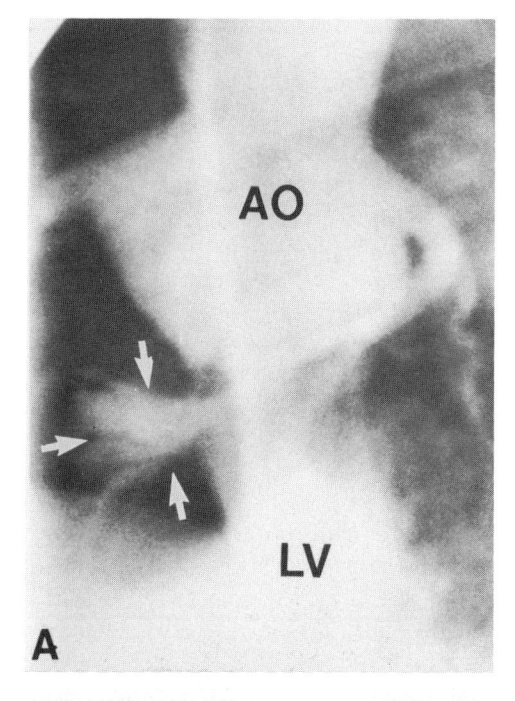

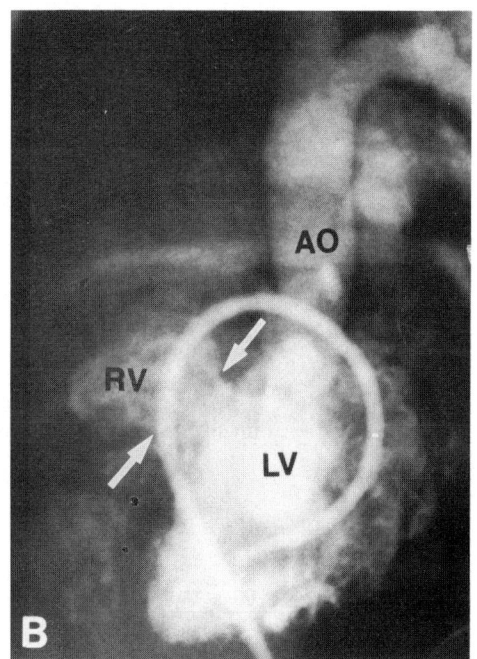

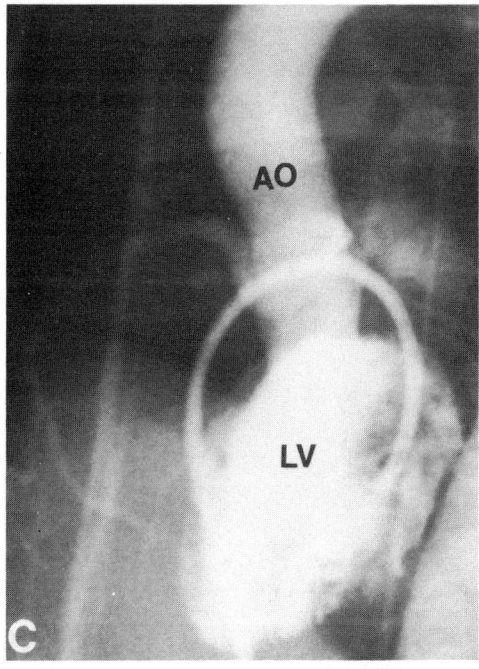

FIG 12–31.
A, lateral anterior oblique left ventriculogram showing closure of a previously demonstrated membranous septal defect. The septal leaflet of the tricuspid valve is circumferentially adherent to the defect, forming an aneurysm of the membranous septum *(arrow).* **B,** patient with large muscular septal defect *(arrows).* Lateral anterior oblique left ventriculogram. **C,** same patient repeat angiogram 1 year later demonstrates spontaneous closure. (Courtesy of Dr. R. Stone.)

For the infant with a large defect who develops congestive cardiac failure, digitalis and diuretics are administered. Most infants do not respond and retain some features of cardiac failure. Cardiac catheterization is then performed. If the VSD is membranous or supracristal, our choice is a corrective operation. If the defect is muscular or multiple, thus requiring a right or left ventriculotomy for repair, we recommend a pulmonary artery band, with closure of the VSD and removal of the band at 18 months of age. We perform cardiac catheterization before the second operation.

Patients who do not develop cardiac failure and in whom clinical data do not suggest pulmonary hypertension are followed until the age of 4 years. We believe that many VSDs will become smaller or close spontaneously during this time, and the likelihood of the child developing pulmonary vascular disease is small. However, if there are striking ECG or x-ray abnormalities, cardiac catheterization is performed. If the shunt is greater than 2:1 or the pulmonary artery pressure is elevated, corrective surgery is recommended. If, at 4 years clinical evidence indicates normal pulmonary artery pressure and a small (≤ 50%) left-to-right shunt, we do not catheterize and continue to follow the child clinically.

In the patient with a large VSD and pulmonary vascular disease with a ratio between the systemic and pulmonary vascular resistances of 0.7, we do not recommend operation.

Operation

Corrective surgery is carried out in infancy with cardio-pulmonary bypass or deep hypothermia and circulatory arrest. Ventricular septal defects are closed by a Dacron patch or, if the defect is small, direct suturing. Angiographic location of the defect preoperatively helps the surgeon select the operative approach.

A membranous ventricular septal defect is exposed through either a right ventriculotomy (Fig 12–32) or more often, by a right atrial approach. In patients with pulmonary hypertension, a right atrial approach is preferred. Through the right atrium, the defect is usually readily visible and can be repaired by retracting the papillary muscle of the conus and its chordae tendineae. Rarely, the septal leaflet of the tricuspid valve has to be detached to reach the defect. Supracristal (infrapulmonary) defects require a small right ventriculotomy because they cannot be repaired by a right atrial approach.

Muscular defects, particularly of the AV-canal type, which are located posteriorly and usually hidden by the septal leaflet of the tricuspid valve, are difficult to repair. Because of their location, they may be overlooked at the time of surgery. Muscular defects located more anteriorly in the septum are also difficult to repair. They are commonly multiple, small, and hidden within the trabeculations of the septum. These defects can usually be closed more easily through a left ventriculotomy performed near the cardiac apex, with a large patch used to close all the defects rather than closing each defect individually.

There is evidence that when a VSD is repaired in a child younger than 2 years, the pulmonary vascular resistance is more likely to fall, whereas after that age, it usually remains constant.[27–30] However, in an occasional patient, it rises after successful closure. Furthermore, ven-

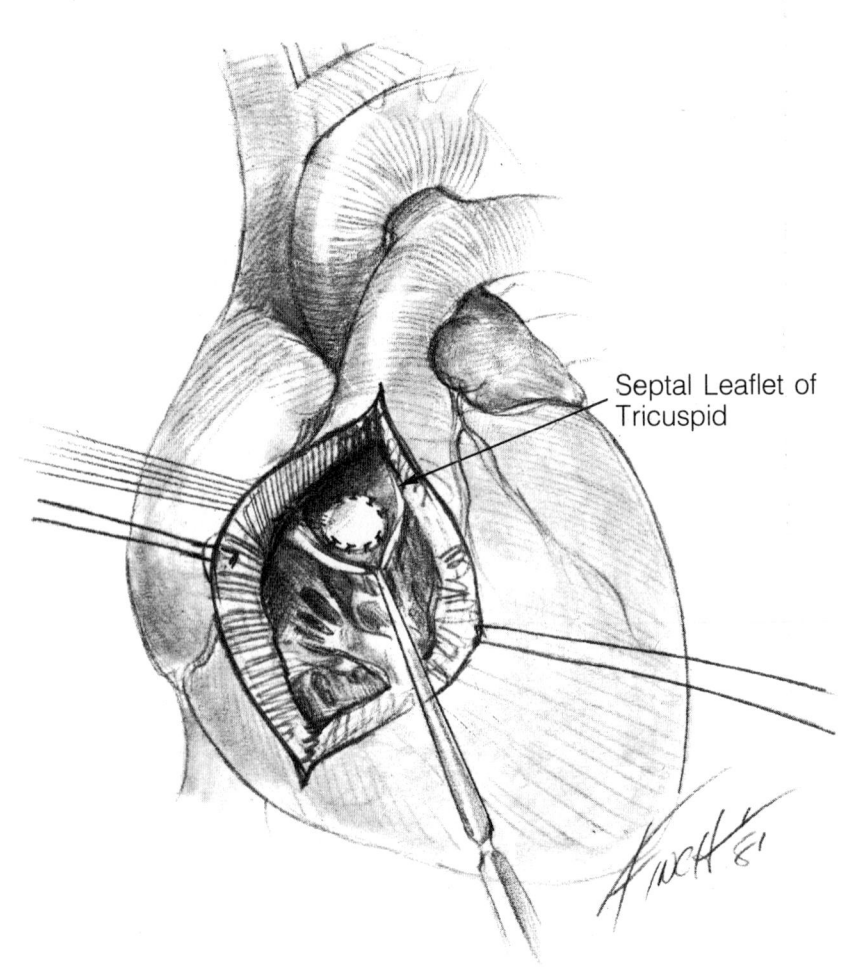

FIG 12–32.
Diagram of closure of membranous VSD by a transventricular approach. A longitudinal ventriculotomy has been made; some surgeons prefer a transverse incision.

tricular volume studies show more normal left ventricular function after early operation.[31, 32]

Pulmonary Artery Banding

In some infants with either multiple or muscular VSDs a constricting band of Dacron is placed around the main pulmonary artery (see Fig 12–17) through a small left anterior thoracotomy. The pulmonary arterial band offers resistance to right ventricular outflow, reducing the volume of pulmonary blood flow and thereby reducing the congestive cardiac failure. When the infant is older, often around 18 months of age, the band is removed and the VSD closed.

Postoperative Chest Film Features

1. The amount of decrease of the pulmonary vasculature and cardiac size after corrective operation depends largely on the preoperative hemodynamics. In patients with a large pulmonary blood flow and low pulmonary resistance, striking improvement follows defect closure.

2. Because most large VSDs are associated with slightly or moderately increased pulmonary resistance and pulmonary hypertension, postoperative improvement is not as striking and is usually gradual. Cardiac size becomes relatively smaller as the child grows, reaching normal in a few years.

3. Persistent cardiomegaly (Fig 12–33) may result from partial closure of the defect or tricuspid insufficiency from damage to the valve during operative closure of the defect. REASON: Many defects lie close to the septal leaflet of the tricuspid valve, which may have to be incised or detached during the operation. Currently, however, tricuspid insufficiency is an uncommon complication of surgery.

4. If there is increasing cardiac size and a persistent murmur, left ventriculography should be performed to search for a residual defect or an additional anomaly overlooked at the time of operation.

5. The patch over the defect may calcify (see Fig 12–33). This has no clinical significance.

6. After placement of an adequate pulmonary arterial band, cardiac size and pulmonary vasculature gradually decrease.

7. If the pulmonary band is placed too close to the pulmonary valve, thickening of the valvular leaflets may occur because of the mechanical impact (Fig 12–34). This thickening is of no clinical consequence.

8. After placement of a pulmonary arterial band, decrease of the pulmonary vasculature may be greater in one lung than the other, suggesting either migration of the band or an improperly placed band. Migration of the band most commonly causes partial or complete occlusion of

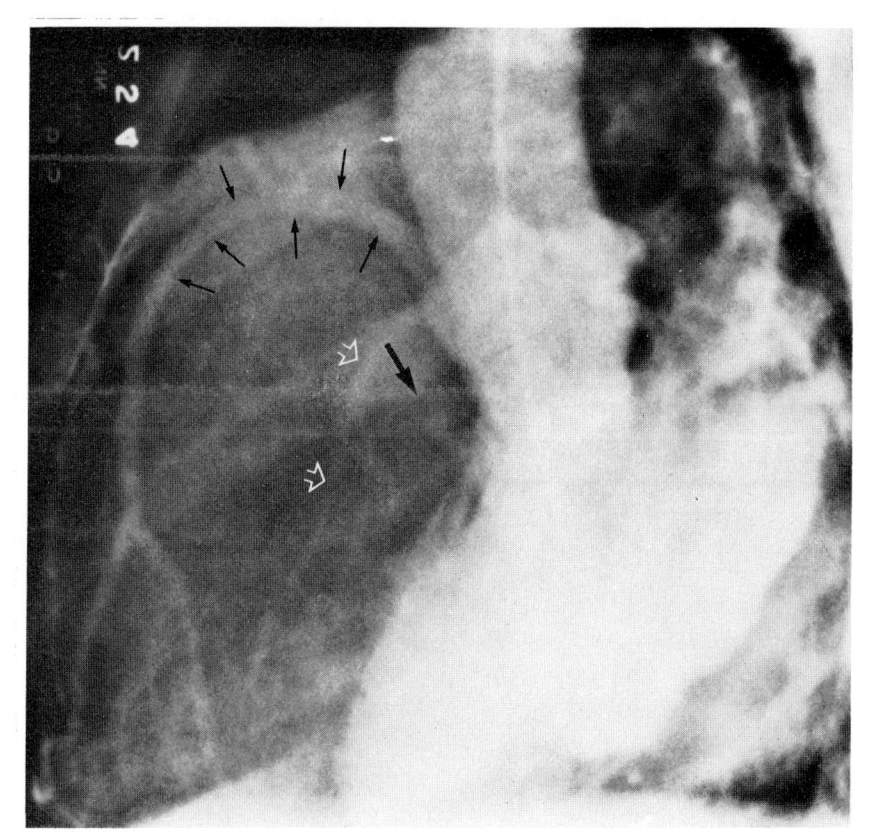

FIG 12–33.
Left ventriculogram in lateral projection showing postoperative VSD. Persistent cardiomegaly and systolic murmur of tricuspid regurgitation. Left ventricle displaced posteriorly by marked enlarged right ventricle, evidenced by the sweeping course of the right coronary artery *(small black arrows)*. Because the right coronary artery lies in the right atrioventricular groove, it conforms to the shape of the right ventricle. Marked right ventricular enlargement has caused clockwise rotation of the heart, displacing the left anterior descending coronary artery *(small white arrows)* posteriorly. Calcified patch *(large black arrow)*.

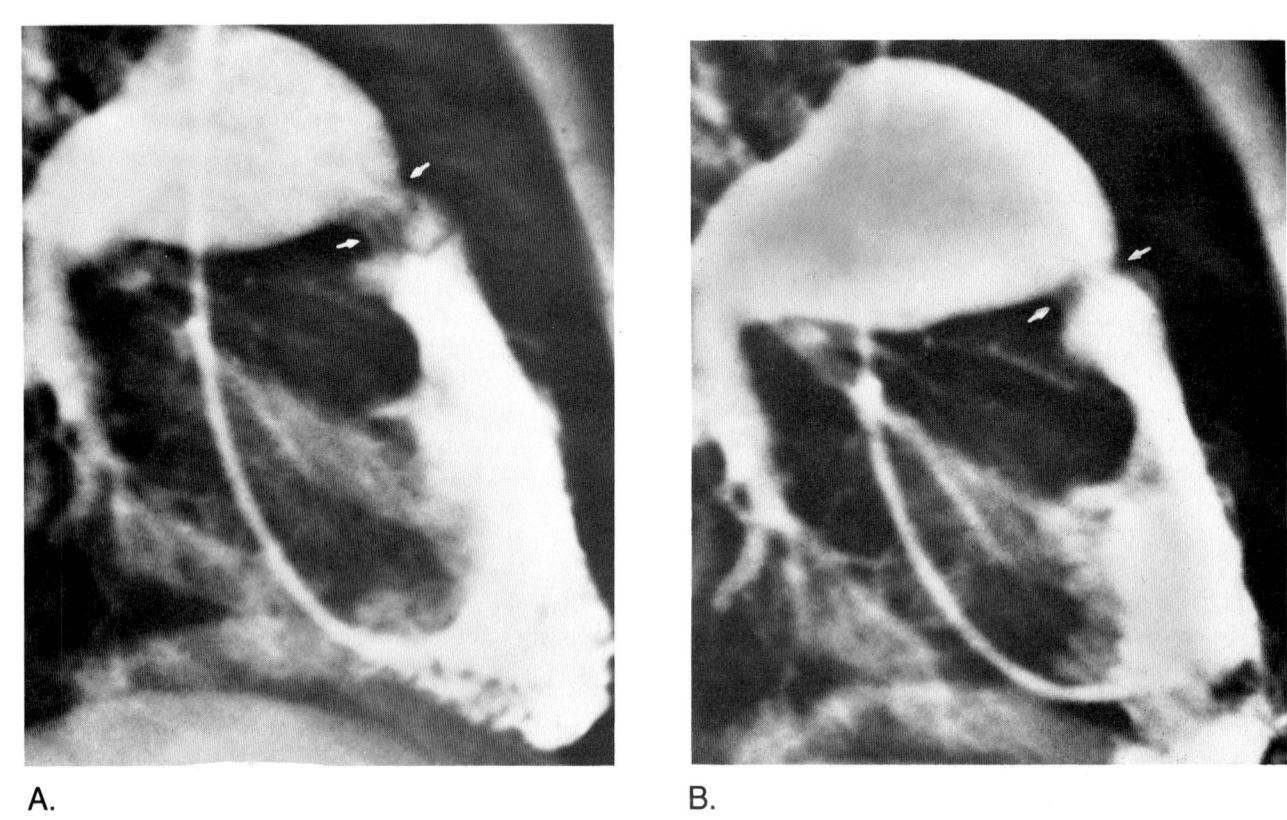

270 *Cardiac Conditions Associated With a Left-to-Right Shunt*

FIG 12–34.
Right ventriculogram in lateral projection of pulmonary banding. **A,** diastole; pulmonary arterial band placed close to pulmonary valve *(arrows)*. **B,** systole; pulmonary valve markedly thickened and shows "pseudodoming" *(white arrows)*. The angiographic appearance is similar to that of valvular pulmonary stenosis.

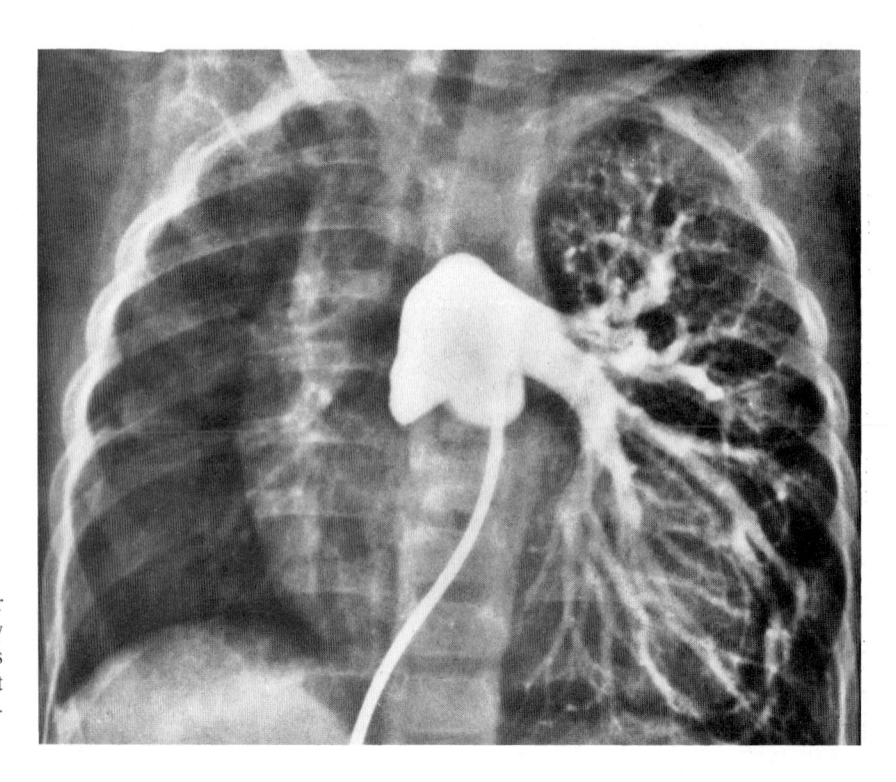

FIG 12–35.
Pulmonary arteriogram in anteroposterior projection after banding. Right pulmonary artery occluded by slippage of band; this is the most common event, because the right pulmonary artery arises almost at a right angle from main pulmonary artery.

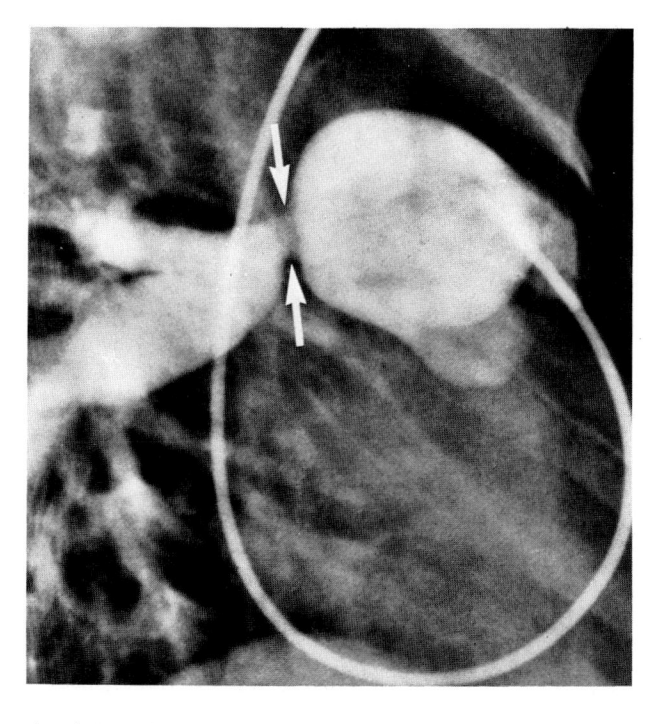

FIG 12–36.
Right anterior oblique pulmonary arteriogram after banding. Left pulmonary artery is occluded (uncommon), and right pulmonary artery is severely stenotic.

the right pulmonary artery (Fig 12–35). REASON: The right pulmonary artery originates acutely from the main pulmonary artery (see Fig 2–31).

9. The origin of both pulmonary arteries may be narrowed; rarely, only the left pulmonary artery is obstructed (Fig 12–36).

10. Despite obstruction, the pulmonary artery remains patent. The obstructed artery is supplied by collateral blood flow through the bronchial arteries. If the pleural space is obliterated by adhesions, collateral flow from intercostal arteries provides a major blood source to the occluded pulmonary artery (Fig 12–37). If the pleural space has not been entered surgically and there are no adhesions, collateral blood flow occurs primarily via bronchi inflow.

REFERENCES

1. Mitchell SC, Berendes HW, Clark WM Jr: The normal closure of the ventricular septum, *Am Heart J* 73:334, 1967.
2. Edwards JE: The pathology of ventricular septal defect, *Semin Roentgenol* 1:2, 1966.
3. Wenink ACG, Openheimer-Dekker A, Moulaert AJ: Muscular ventricular septal defects: a reappraisal of the anatomy *Am J Cardiol* 43:259, 1979.
4. Elliott LP, Ernst RW, Anderson RC, et al: Silent patent ductus arteriosus in association with ventricular septal defect: clinical, hemodynamic, pathologic and surgical observations in forty patients, *Am J Cardiol* 10:475, 1962.
5. Sasahara AA, Nadas AS, Rudolph AM, et al: Ventricular septal defect with patent ductus arteriosus: a clinical and hemodynamic study, *Circulation* 22:254, 1960.
6. Kidd L, Rose V, Collins G, et al: The hemodynamics in ventricular septal defect in childhood, *Am Heart J* 70:732, 1965.
7. Rose V, Collins G, Kidd L, et al: Clinico-hemodynamic correlations in ventricular septal defect in childhood, *J Pediatr* 69:359, 1966.
8. Graham TP Jr, Atwood GF, Boucek RJ Jr, et al: Right ven-

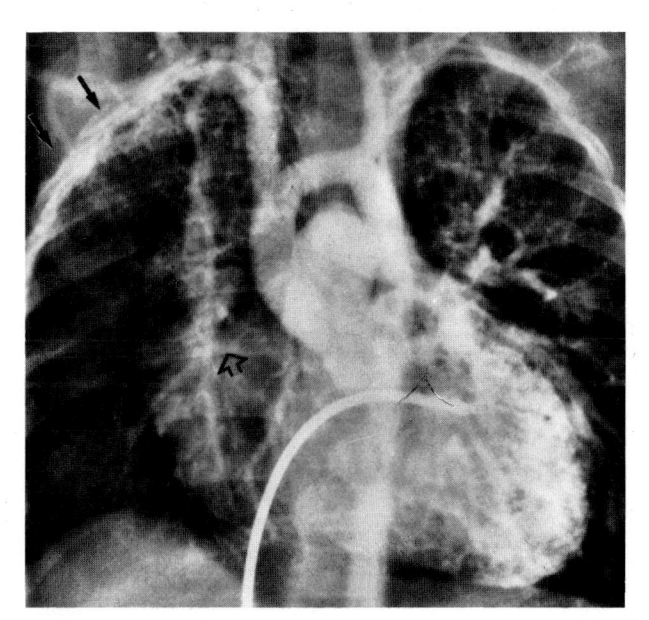

FIG 12–37.
Left ventriculogram in anteroposterior projection after pulmonary banding for VSD. Only left pulmonary artery is patent. Extensive transpleural collaterals *(arrows)* faintly fill the right pulmonary artery *(open arrow)* via intercostal collaterals.

tricular volume characteristics in ventricular septal defect, *Circulation* 54:800, 1976.
9. Hoffman JIE: Natural history of congenital heart disease: problems in its assessment with special reference to ventricular septal defects, *Circulation* 37:97, 1968.
10. Corone P, Doyon F, Gaudeau S, et al: Natural history of ventricular septal defect: a study involving 790 cases, *Circulation* 55:908, 1977.
11. Ritter DG, Feldt RH, Weidman WH, et al: Ventricular septal defect, *Circulation* 31 and 32(suppl III):42, 1965.
12. Weidman WH, Blount SG Jr, DuShane JW, et al: Clinical course in ventricular septal defect, *Circulation* 56(suppl I):56, 1977.
13. Bloomfield DK: The natural history of ventricular septal defect in patients surviving infancy, *Circulation* 29:914, 1964.
14. Lucas RV Jr, Adams P Jr, Anderson RC, et al: The natural history of isolated ventricular septal defect: a serial physiologic study, *Circulation* 24:1372, 1961.
15. Arcilla RA, Agustsson MH, Bicoff JP, et al: Further observations on the natural history of isolated ventricular septal defects in infancy and childhood: serial cardiac catheterization studies in 75 patients, *Circulation* 28:560, 1963.
16. Agustsson MH, Arcilla RA, Bicoff JP, et al: Spontaneous functional closure of ventricular septal defects in fourteen children demonstrated by serial cardiac catheterizations and angiocardiography, *Pediatrics* 31:958, 1963.
17. Varghese PJ, Izukawa T, Celermajer J, et al: Aneurysm of the membranous ventricular septum: a method of spontaneous closure of small ventricular septal defect, *Am J Cardiol* 24:531, 1969.
18. Moore D, Vlad P, Lambert EC: Spontaneous closure of ventricular septal defect following cardiac failure in infancy, *J Pediatr* 66:712, 1965.
19. Simmons RL, Moller JH, Edwards JE: Anatomic evidence for spontaneous closure of ventricular septal defect, *Circulation* 34:38, 1966.
20. Alpert BS, Mellits ED, Rowe RD: Spontaneous closure of small ventricular septal defects, *Am J Dis Child* 125:194, 1973.
21. Gasul BM, Dillon RF, Vrla V, et al: Ventricular septal defects: their natural transformation into those with infundibular stenosis or into the cyanotic or noncyanotic type of tetralogy of Fallot, *JAMA* 184:847, 1957.
22. Varghese PJ, Allen JR, Rosenquist GC, et al: Natural history of ventricular septal defect with right-sided aortic arch, *Br Heart J* 32:537, 1970.
23. Weidman WH, DuShane JW, Kincaid OW: Observations concerning progressive pulmonary vascular obstruction in children with ventricular septal defects, *Am Heart J* 65:148, 1963.
24. Leatham A, Segal B: Auscultatory and phonocardiographic signs of ventricular septal defect with left-to-right shunt, *Circulation* 25:318, 1962.
25. Steinfeld L, Dimich I, Park SC, et al: Clinical diagnosis of isolated subpulmonic (supracristal) ventricular septal defect, *Am J Cardiol* 30:19, 1972.
26. Cheatham JP, Latson LA, Gutgesell HP: Ventricular septal defect in infancy: detection with two dimensional echocardiography, *Am J Cardiol* 47:85, 1981.
27. Sigmann JM, Perry BL, Behrendt DM, et al: Ventricular septal defect: results after repair in infancy, *Am J Cardiol* 39:66, 1977.
28. Allen HD, Anderson RC, Noren GR, et al: Postoperative follow-up of patients with ventricular septal defect, *Circulation* 50:465, 1974.
29. Hallidie-Smith KA, Wilson RSE, et al: Functional status of patients with large ventricular septal defect and pulmonary vascular disease 6 to 16 years after surgical closure of their defect in childhood, *Br Heart J* 39:1093, 1977.
30. Maron BJ, Redwood DR, Hirshfeld JW Jr, et al: Postoperative assessment of patients with ventricular septal defect and pulmonary hypertension: response to intense upright exercise, *Circulation* 48:864, 1973.
31. Jarmakani JMM, Graham TP Jr, Canent RV Jr, et al: The effect of corrective surgery on left heart volume and mass in children with ventricular septal defect, *Am J Cardiol* 27:254, 1971.
32. Cordell D, Graham TP Jr, Atwood GF, et al: Left heart volume characteristics following ventricular septal defect in infancy, *Circulation* 54:294, 1976.

CHAPTER 13

Ventricular Septal Defect With Aortic Insufficiency or Aortic Stenosis

In 2% to 5% of patients with a ventricular septal defect (VSD), aortic insufficiency coexists. Aortic regurgitation is rarely present in infancy but develops with age because of prolapse of an aortic cusp. The associated aortic insufficiency occurs more commonly in males.

PATHOLOGY

In hearts with coexisting VSD and aortic insufficiency, the septal defect is adjacent to the aortic anulus, in other words, immediately below the valve cusps and with no tissue separating the defect from the anulus. The defect lies either under the right cusp or between the right and noncoronary cusps (Fig 13–1), so on the right side of the heart the VSD is either supracristal or infracristal, respectively. Infracristal VSD is most common in patients in the United States, whereas supracristal defects are more common in Japan. In some instances, infundibular stenosis coexists. This has led to the following classification:[1,2]

1. Type I: Supracristal VSD with aortic insufficiency
   a. Without aortic cusp herniation
   b. With aortic cusp herniation and conal muscle rim below the pulmonary valve
   c. With aortic cusp herniation and without conal muscle rim below the pulmonary valve
2. Type II: Infracristal VSD with aortic insufficiency
   a. Without aortic cusp herniation
   b. With aortic cusp herniation
3. Type III: Infracristal VSD with aortic insufficiency and infundibular pulmonary stenosis
4. Type IV: Supracristal VSD with aortic insufficiency and infundibular pulmonary stenosis

This classification is used by some surgeons as a guide to operative decisions.

The involved aortic cusp is dilated and forms a pouch, which may project into or through the VSD. Because the cusp prolapses into the defect, the effective size of the defect is reduced. The free margin of the cusp is thickened (Fig 13–2). The left ventricle is dilated because of the aortic regurgitation. The right ventricle may be hypertrophied but not greatly, because the pulmonary arterial pressure is usually normal or only slightly elevated. This malformation has been thought to be caused by two factors:[3] lack of support of the aortic cusp because of the VSD and the left-to-right shunt exerting force on the prolapsed cusp, resulting in a distortion of the valve leaflets and causing further aortic insufficiency (Venturi effect).

Although in many patients with VSD, the defect is located adjacent the aortic anulus, aortic reflux does not always develop. Therefore, the location of the defect is not the only factor leading to aortic regurgitation. The aortic valve loses the support of the anulus because of a deficiency of the conal musculature and tissue of the sinus of Valsalva. The aortic valve may be further damaged by the left-to-right shunt through the defect, which causes further sagging of the cusp, which may bulge into the right ventricular outflow tract (Fig 13–3).

Herniation is most pronounced during systole because of the Venturi effect. Eventually, the aortic cusp separates from the adjacent cusps during diastole, and aortic incompetence results. Prolapse of the cusp and aortic regurgitation may disappear after a simple closure of the VSD. Aortic insufficiency in patients with supracristal VSDs results from deficiency of the conal musculature, which normally supports the anulus of the aortic valve. In infracris-

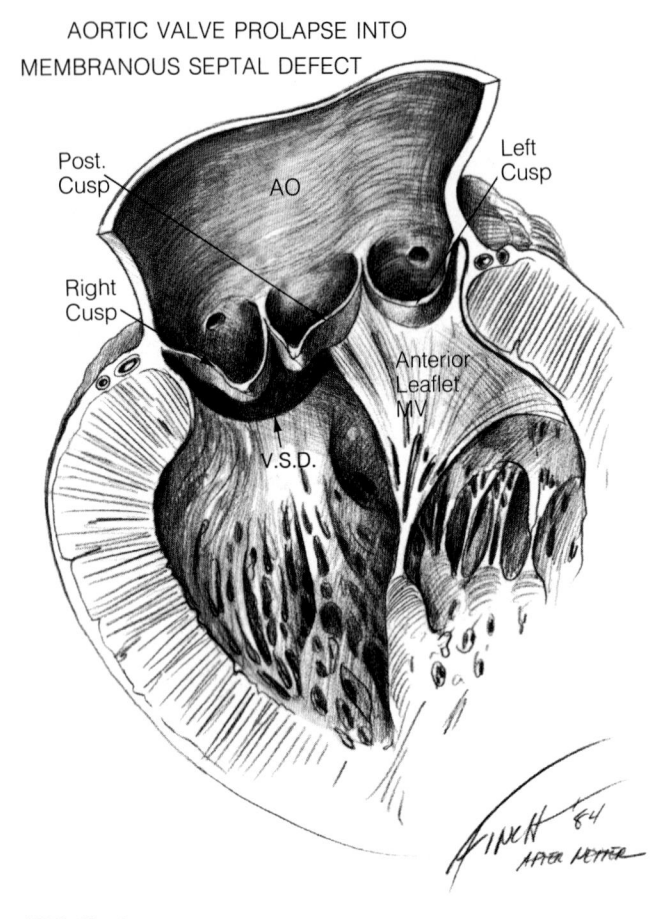

FIG 13-1.
Diagram of left side of ventricular septum, showing defect *(VSD)* immediately beneath right and noncoronary cusps of the aortic valve. *AO* = aorta; *MV* = mitral valve.

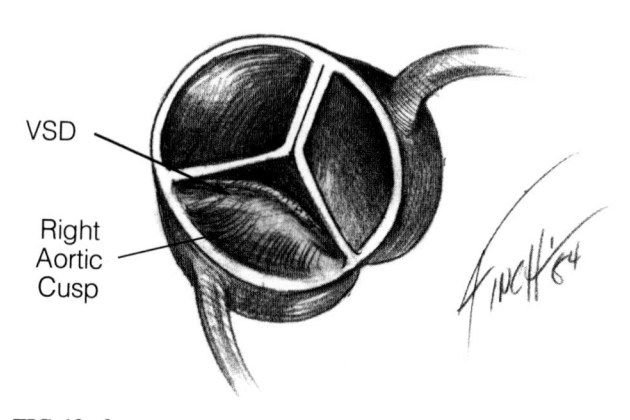

FIG 13-2.
Diagram of prolapse right aortic valve cusp into ventricular septal defect *(VSD)*. Aorta opened, and aortic valve cusps viewed from above. In this case, only the right cusp is pulled down into the defect.

tal VSD, aortic insufficiency may also result from underdevelopment of the aortic valvar commissures or from endocarditis.

CLINICAL FEATURES

The clinical features[4-7] indicate that the murmur of aortic insufficiency is rarely heard in the first year of life. The patient is initially diagnosed as having a VSD because of a pansystolic murmur. The left-to-right shunt is rarely large enough to cause heart failure or other symptoms. The diastolic murmur of the aortic insufficiency usually appears in the early school years. Aortic regurgitation may increase to cause cardiac failure but usually not until later childhood.

Physical Examination

If there is considerable aortic regurgitation, a wide pulse pressure and sharp peripheral arterial pulses are found. There is a grade 3 to 4/6 harsh pansystolic murmur and thrill along the left sternal border. If infundibular pulmonary stenosis is present, the murmur has ejection qualities in the pulmonary area. A grade 1 to 3/6 early diastolic murmur of aortic regurgitation is found in the third and fourth left intercostal spaces. In some patients, even those with a small shunt, an apical middiastolic murmur is present,[4-7] presumably representing an Austin-Flint murmur (flutter of the anterior leaflet of the mitral valve caused by the regurgitation of blood through the aortic valve).

It is difficult to evaluate the components of the second heart sound, because they are obscured by the prominent murmurs.

Electrocardiographic Features

The QRS axis is usually normal but may show the variation generally found among patients with VSDs. Left ventricular hypertrophy (tall R in lead V6) is present in most patients. Associated ST depression and T-wave inversion in the left precordial leads[4] suggest left ventricular strain. Occasionally right ventricular hypertrophy coexists if the right ventricular systolic pressure is increased by pulmonary hypertension or infundibular pulmonary stenosis.

Echocardiographic Features

One study using scanning identified supracristal VSDs by a deficiency of echoes in the subaortic region.[8] The affected aortic cusp prolapsed during early systole, stabilized in midsystole, and prolapsed more in early diastole be-

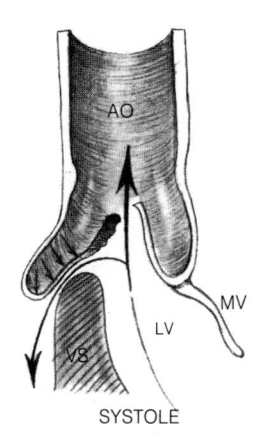

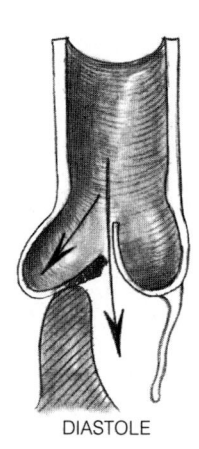

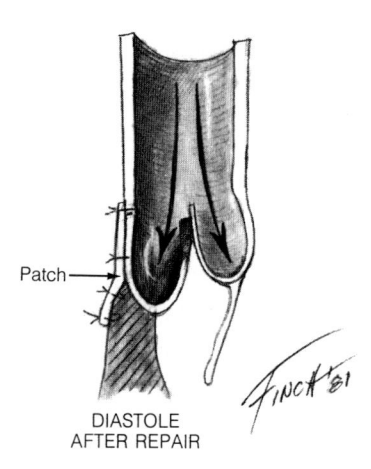

FIG 13-3.
Diagram of prolapsed aortic cusp and VSD. *Left,* during systole, left-to-right shunt through defect creates a Venturi (suction) effect. *Middle,* during diastole, septal defect is occluded by prolapsed cusp. Aortic regurgitation occurs. *Right,* during diastole, after repair of defect; prolapsed cusp buttressed and rendered competent by patch closure of VSD. *AO* = aorta; *LV* = left ventricle; *MV* = mitral valve; *VS* = interventricular septum.

cause of the regurgitation. The prolapsed aortic cusp is apparent as anterior motion of an anomalous echo through the defect.

RADIOGRAPHIC FEATURES

The radiographic appearance is not uniform and depends largely on the degree of aortic regurgitation and the size of the septal defect. With marked aortic reflux, the radiographic findings resemble those of aortic insufficiency, with prominence of the ascending aorta and, occasionally, left atrial enlargement secondary to left ventricular failure. When the right aortic cusp prolapses, usually there are no radiographic signs of a left-to-right shunt. REASON: Although the defect is large, the prolapsing cusp partially occludes it, reducing the left-to-right shunt. The shunt may not even be demonstrable by indicator dye dilution techniques or angiography.

CARDIAC CATHETERIZATION

Cardiac catheterization combined with aortography should be performed in any patient with a VSD when a murmur of aortic insufficiency is discovered so that the diagnosis can be established and treatment initiated promptly.

The oximetry data show a left-to-right shunt, which is rarely larger than 2:1. The shunt becomes smaller with time because increasing aortic cusp prolapse reduces the size of the defect. The pulmonary arterial systolic pressure is usually normal or slightly elevated and is seldom more than 35 mm Hg, although occasionally it exceeds 60 mm Hg.

In about one third of the cases, a gradient is present between the pulmonary artery and the body of the right ventricle, in which case the right ventricular systolic pressure may reach systemic levels. The pressure tracing from the aorta shows elevated systolic and lowered diastolic pressures. The wedge pressure is usually normal.[5, 6]

Angiographic Appearance

The VSD may not be demonstrable by angiography or dye dilution curves because it is entirely occluded by the prolapsing aortic cusp or because of elevated right ventricular systolic pressure. Typically, a previous angiogram shows a VSD with no or mild aortic regurgitation, whereas the most recent angiogram usually shows significant aortic reflux and no ventricular communication. REASON: The aortic cusp is being progressively pulled down, increasing the aortic reflux but occluding the septal defect. Aortic regurgitation is usually into the left ventricle but may be directed primarily into the right ventricle, as demonstrated by angiography.

The main differential diagnosis lies with a ruptured or unruptured sinus of Valsalva's aneurysm, which also forms a baglike extension below the level of the aortic valve. With a prolapsed cusp, the configuration varies considerably during systole and diastole, because part of the deformity is formed by the valve leaflet. A sinus of Valsalva's aneurysm, on the other hand, lies below the freely moving valve leaflet and thus does not change significantly during the cardiac cycle.

Angiographic Indications and Findings

1. Aortography and right ventriculography are indicated in patients with a VSD and clinical signs of aortic regurgitation.

2. Angiography allows the differentiation between prolapse of the aortic cusp and other causes of aortic regurgitation, such as sinus of Valsalva aneurysm or aneurysm of the membranous septum. In the former, the prolapsed aortic cusp varies considerably between systole and diastole, in contrast to an aneurysm of the sinus of Valsalva.

3. If aortic regurgitation is marked, a large catheter will be needed for rapid delivery of an adequate amount of contrast medium.

4. When the aortic cusp herniates, marked deformity of the aortic valve is clearly seen. The cusp protrudes anteriorly and downward through the defect into the right ventricle (see Fig 13–4).

5. Differentiation from a sinus of Valsalva aneurysm may be difficult. With a prolapsed aortic valve, the valve leaflet can be clearly observed during systole and diastole as it prolapses through the defect anteriorly (see Fig 13–5).

6. Another differential consideration is an aortico–left ventricular tunnel (see Chapter 27), which also is an aortic run-off lesion. However, a tunnel originates above the level of the right coronary artery.

7. Because a prolapsed aortic cusp may cause right ventricular outflow tract obstruction and murmur, right ventriculography is indicated. It will reveal a round filling defect (Fig 13–5), which corresponds to the prolapsed aortic cusp demonstrated by aortography (Fig 13–4).

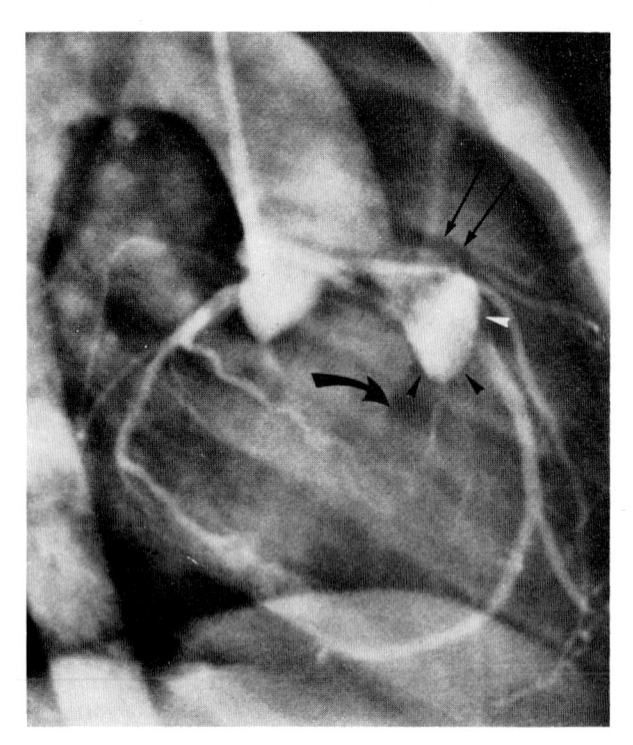

FIG 13–4.
Aortogram; lateral view of herniated right aortic cusp prolapsing through a VSD into the right ventricular outflow tract. The right cusp is pulled down and almost completely obilerates the defect *(small arrows)*. A small amount of contrast medium is seen in the right ventricular outflow tract, outlining the wall, which is seen as a radiolucent band *(large arrows)*. The edge of the ventricular septum is seen because of aortic regurgitation *(curved arrow)*, which is mild in this case.

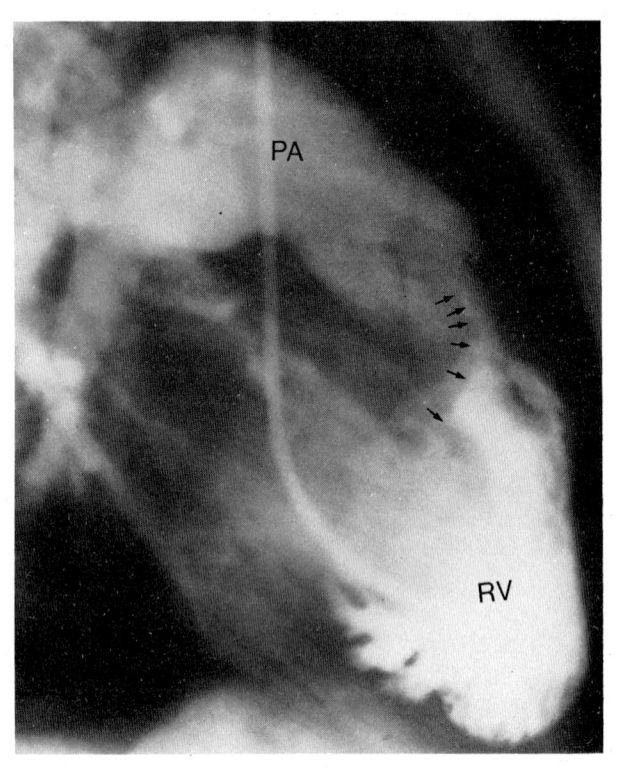

FIG 13–5.
Right ventriculogram, lateral view (same patient as in Fig 13–4). Prolapsed right aortic cusp causes large filling defect *(arrows)* in the right ventricular outflow tract, which resulted in a pressure gradient. The right aortic cusp has herniated through a supracristal defect into the outflow tract of the right ventricle.

OPERATION

The operative indications and approach to a VSD with aortic insufficiency are controversial, and each medical center probably has established its own approach. Nonetheless, certain guidelines are generally accepted:

1. The principal hemodynamic feature in most candidates is the aortic regurgitation, not the left-to-right shunt or right ventricular outflow tract obstruction.

2. Patients undergoing closure of a VSD without aortic valve repair have the best results if the defect is in the supracristal position.[1, 9]

3. Patients with minimal aortic regurgitation of short duration or with minimal or no exercise limitation benefit from early closure of the defect.[1]

4. Moderate aortic regurgitation remains relatively stable over a long period of time. Progression is more likely in subpulmonary VSDs.[9]

Long-term results of closing the defect to prevent worsening of aortic regurgitation have not been reported.

Various operative procedures on the aortic valve, such as replacement and plication, have been combined with closure of the VSD. Because the defect is immediately beneath the aortic valve, it is possible to close it through the aorta. Care must be taken not to place stitches in the valve leaflet and to use the patch to support the prolapsed cusp (see Fig 13–3) We prefer to operate early, when the aortic regurgitation is mild, and avoid operating on the aortic valve if possible.

VENTRICULAR SEPTAL DEFECT WITH AORTIC STENOSIS

Thoracic roentgenographic findings in these patients are:

1. Subaortic stenosis complicating VSD cannot be suspected from thoracic roentgenograms, because the findings are usually normal. REASON: Subaortic stenosis proximal to the VSD limits the left-to-right shunt.
2. Subaortic stenosis distal to the defect increases the left-to-right shunt (see Fig 12–29). This type of subaortic obstruction is commonly associated with coarctation or interruption of the aortic arch.
3. Ventricular septal defect with valvular aortic stenosis can be readily identified at the time of left ventriculography.
4. In discrete subaortic stenosis, a small VSD may be found immediately below the aortic valve and above the stenosis. Angiographic observation is important, because this defect may be difficult to see during the operation (see Fig 12–30).

REFERENCES

1. Kawashima Y, Danno M, Shimizu Y, et al: Ventricular septal defect associated with aortic insufficiency: anatomic classification and method of operation, *Circulation* 47:1057, 1973.
2. VanPraagh R, McNamara JJ: Anatomic types of ventricular septal defect with aortic insufficiency, *Am Heart J* 75:604, 1968.
3. Tatsuno K, Konno S, Ando M, et al: Pathogenetic mechanisms of prolapsing aortic valve and aortic regurgitation associated with ventricular septal defect: anatomical, angiographic, and surgical considerations, *Circulation* 48:1028, 1973.
4. Sommerville J, Brandao A, Ross DN: Aortic regurgitation with ventricular septal defect: surgical management and clinical features, *Circulation* 41:317, 1970.
5. Keck EWO, Ongley PA, Kincaid OW, et al: Ventricular septal defect with aortic insufficiency: a clinical and hemodynamic study of 18 proved cases, *Circulation* 27:203, 1963.
6. Nadas AS, Thilenius OG, LaFarge CG, et al: Ventricular septal defect with aortic regurgitation: medical and pathologic aspects, *Circulation* 29:862, 1964.
7. Halloran KH, Talner NS, Browne MJ: A study of ventricular septal defect associated with aortic insufficiency, *Am Heart J* 69:320, 1965.
8. Aziz KU, Cole RB, Paul MH: Echocardiographic features of supracristal ventricular septal defect with prolapsed aortic valve leaflet, *Am J Cardiol* 43:854, 1979.
9. Keane JF, Plauth WH Jr, Nadas AS: Ventricular septal defect with aortic regurgitation, *Circulation* 56 (suppl I):72, 1977.

CHAPTER 14

Aneurysm of the Membranous Ventricular Septum

Aneurysms of the membranous ventricular septum may be either congenital or acquired, and the two types cannot be distinguished angiographically or anatomically. Acquired aneurysms are usually the result of bacterial endocarditis of the aortic valve or secondary erosion of the ventricular septum. Rarely, congenital aneurysms of the ventricular septum become secondarily infected, and under those circumstances, differentiation between acquired and congenital aneurysms is virtually impossible.

Congenital aneurysm of the membranous septum is the more common type. The aneurysm is a fibrous sac arising from the ventricular portion of the membranous septum and protruding into the right ventricle beneath the septal leaflet of the tricuspid valve. The aneurysm may be intact, or there may be a perforation, which results in a left ventricular–right atrial shunt (see Chapter 15).

Some aneurysms considered congenital subsequently rupture, resulting in a left-to-right shunt at the ventricular level. However, there is evidence that aneurysms of the membranous septum may develop in conjunction with a ventricular septal defect (VSD). For example, aneurysms are rarely seen angiographically before the age of 2 years but are commonly found with VSDs in older children.[1,2] The frequent association of a small VSD and an aneurysm of the membranous septum strongly suggests that under these circumstances, the aneurysm is acquired. In patients with large VSDs demonstrated before the age of 2 years, the defect often becomes smaller, and subsequent angiograms show an aneurysm of the membranous septum. The decreasing size of the left-to-right shunt and the formation of the aneurysm may result from adherence of the septal leaflet of the tricuspid valve to the ventricular septum, partially or completely sealing the ventricular communication (Fig 14–1). Adherence of the septal leaflet of the tricuspid valve is a major mechanism of spontaneous closure of VSDs.

Rarely, an aneurysm develops in the muscular portion of the ventricular septum when the septal leaflet of the tricuspid valve adheres to the septum over a muscular VSD. A similar aneurysmal structure results from a VSD and a pouchlike malformation of the tricuspid valve.[3] This is usually associated with a large VSD in contrast to aneurysms of the ventricular septum, in which the defect is small.

COMPLICATIONS

Unruptured aneurysms of the membranous septum cause no hemodynamic alteration and therefore escape clinical recognition. Hence, the incidence of aneurysms of the ventricular septum is difficult to determine, but it appears to be small. Complications occur occasionally in patients with an aneurysm of the membranous septum.

Although most aneurysms are small, measuring 1 to 3 cm in diameter, rarely they are large enough to cause right ventricular outflow obstruction (see Chapter 29). When an aneurysm occurs in patients with complete transposition of the great arteries and other cardiac anomalies in which the right ventricular systolic pressure is greater than the left ventricular systolic pressure, the aneurysm bulges into the left ventricle and may cause obstruction, either subaortic

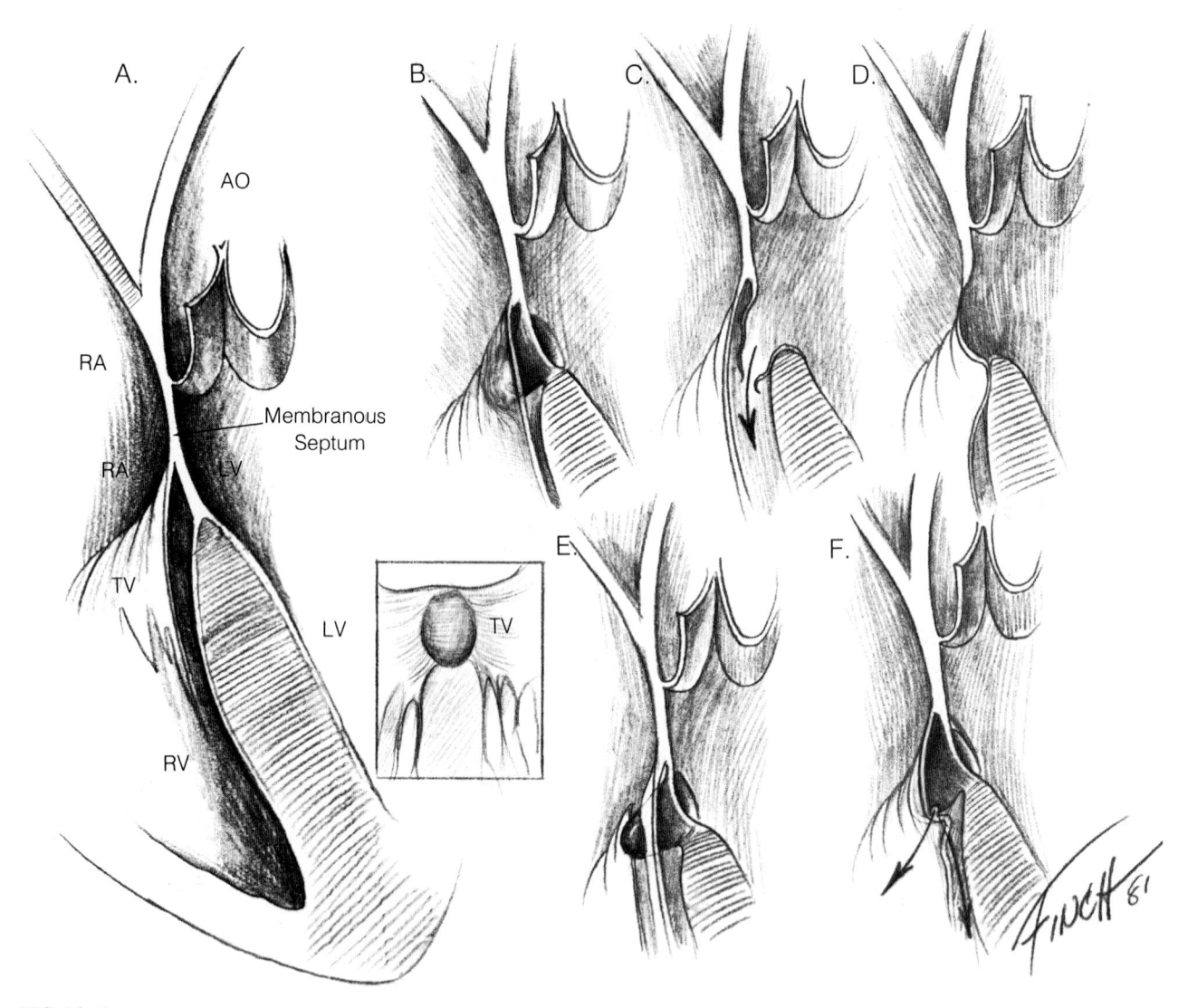

FIG 14–1.
Aneurysm of membranous septum. **A,** normal anatomic relations of membranous septum. **B,** unruptured aneurysm of membranous septum projecting beneath septal leaflet of the tricuspid valve. **C,** rupture of aneurysm of membranous septum into right ventricle, associated with left-to-right shunt at ventricular level. **D,** adherence of septal leaflet of tricuspid valve to interventricular septum, sealing a membranous VSD. **E,** projection of aneurysm of membranous septum through cleft of tricuspid valve. **F,** adherence of tricuspid valve to ruptured aneurysm of membranous septum, with left-to-right shunts into both right atrium and ventricle. *Insert,* view of septal leaflet of tricuspid valve with aneurysm of membranous septum projecting beneath it. *AO* = aorta; *LV* = left ventricle; *RA* = right atrium; *RV* = right ventricle; *TV* = tricuspid valve.

or subpulmonary, depending on the great vessel originating from the left ventricle.

Rarely, a thrombus in an aneurysm of the membranous septum is the source of systemic emboli.

Cardiac arrhythmias have been described with aneurysms, probably because of the proximity of the bundle of His.

Tricuspid insufficiency is an uncommon complication, resulting from the bulging aneurysm's interference with tricuspid valvular function.

When the aneurysm of the membranous septum lies beneath a normal septal leaflet of the tricuspid valve, rupture of the aneurysm results in a ventricular level shunt. When the aneurysm is attached to a cleft in the tricuspid valve, rupture leads to a left ventricular–right atrial shunt and frequently to a ventricular shunt as well (see Chapter 15) (see Fig 14–1).

Thus, an aneurysm of the membranous septum is usually an isolated, asymptomatic abnormality. However, it may coexist with other congenital cardiac malformations, particularly small VSDs and, less frequently, coarctation of the aorta, aortic insufficiency, or subaortic stenosis.

CLINICAL AND LABORATORY FINDINGS

In patients with a VSD, the presence of an aneurysm of the membranous septum may be suspected on the basis of an early systolic clicky sound along the lower left sternal border.[4] There are no other distinctive clinical features.[2]

Echocardiography is useful for diagnosing an aneurysm of the membranous septum, which has a variable echocardiographic appearance. The echoes from the aneurysm may appear as abnormal segments in the tricuspid valve and are better seen during diastole.[5]

RADIOGRAPHIC FEATURES

1. Most aneurysms of the membranous septum are associated with a VSD or with a left ventricular–right atrial shunt. Usually the left-to-right shunt is small, so chest radiographic findings are normal.

2. An aneurysm without an interventricular communication cannot be suspected from plain films. REASON: The aneurysm is an intracardiac structure, outlined by blood on both sides and therefore does not cast a radiographic density unless contrast medium is injected.

ANGIOGRAPHIC APPEARANCE

1. An aneurysm of the membranous septum is best observed by left ventriculography using either a steep left anterior oblique or a lateral projection. Beam angulation is helpful.

2. The aneurysm is a berry-shaped outpouching of the ventricular septum immediately below the aortic valve in the region of the membranous septum. During both systole and diastole, the aneurysm bulges into the right ventricle. REASON: Left ventricular pressure is greater than the right ventricular pressure throughout systole and diastole.

3. The aneurysm is larger and more prominent during ventricular systole. REASON: The pressure differential between the ventricles is greater in this phase of the cardiac cycle. (Fig 14–2).

4. There may be a small communication with the right ventricle (Fig 14–3).

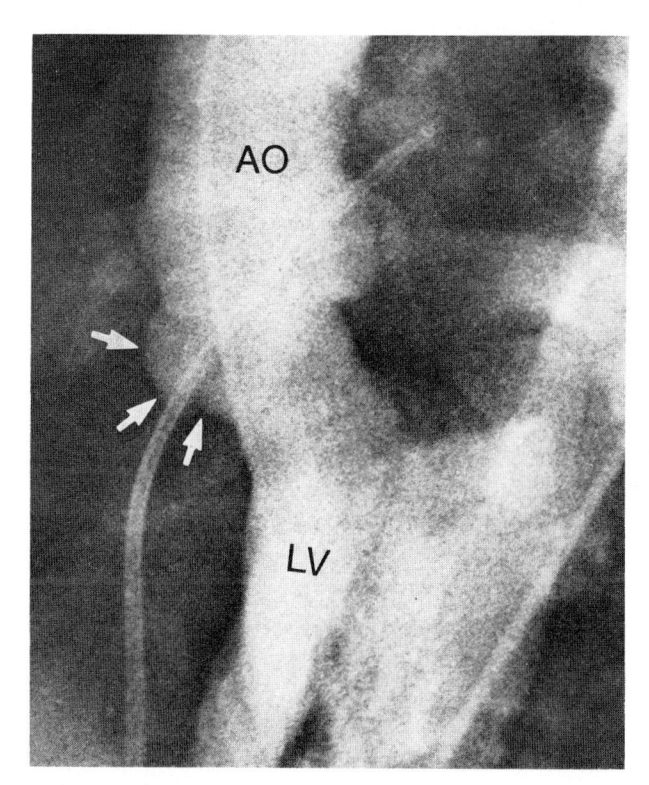

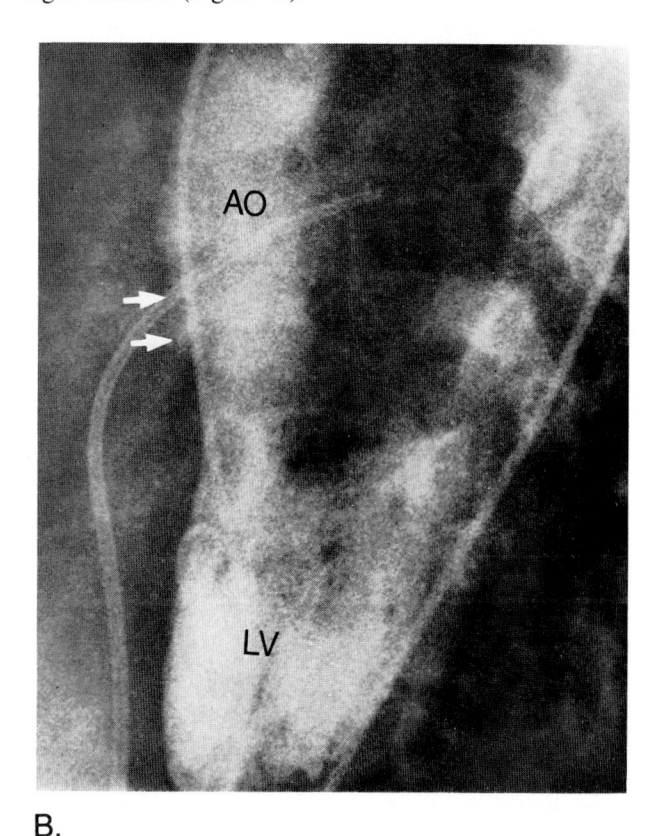

FIG 14–2.
Change in prominence of aneurysm during cardiac cycle. **A,** left ventriculogram in left anterior oblique projection during systole shows smooth aneurysm of the membranous septum without VSD *(arrows)*. Probably congenital. **B,** during diastole, aneurysm disappears, suggesting that the diastolic pressure in both ventricles is similar. *AO* = aorta; *LV* = left ventricle.

5. The aneurysm may be smooth (Fig 14–3) or lobulated (Fig 14–4). The latter appearance is more suggestive of a closing VSD and adherence of the septal leaflet, creating a pouch. The presence of a jet along the edge of an aneurysm also suggests a closing VSD. A true aneurysm of membranous septum that ruptures into the right ventricle should have a jet arising from the dome of the aneurysm (Fig 14–2).

6. Demonstration of an aneurysm of the membranous septum with a small VSD strongly suggests that the defect will close spontaneously.

7. An aneurysm of the membranous septum can be suspected from an anteroposterior or right anterior oblique view of a left ventriculogram. Characteristically, a double density is seen beneath the junction of the right and posterior aortic cusps, the location of the true membranous septum (Fig 14–5).

8. On right ventriculography, an aneurysm may appear as a filling defect in the right ventricular outflow area (see Chapter 26).

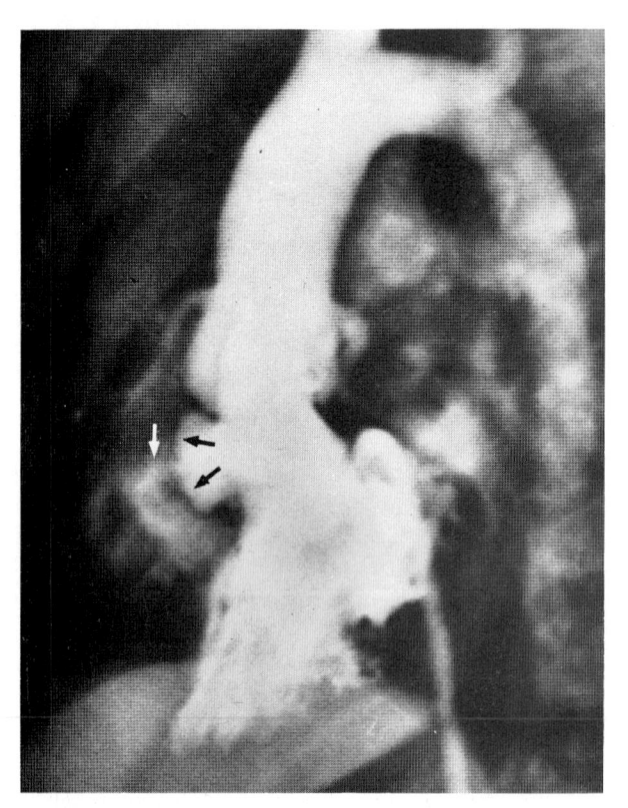

FIG 14–4.
Left ventriculogram in left anterior oblique projection showing huge, irregular, lobulated aneurysm of membranous septum without VSD. Irregular contour suggests closure of a previous septal defect with adherence of tricuspid leaflet and formation of a large pouch of septal leaflet of tricuspid valve.

FIG 14–3.
Left ventriculogram, lateral view, showing large aneurysm of the membranous septum. The aneurysm forms a large bulge beneath the aortic valve in the region of the true membranous septum *(small black arrows)*. It is intracristal. The aneurysm bulges during systole. A central small communication results in a left-to-right shunt *(white arrow)* and faint opacification of the right ventricle. The smooth appearance of the aneurysm and its central opening suggest a congenital aneurysm of the ventricular septum with a small ventricular communication. *LV* = left ventricle.

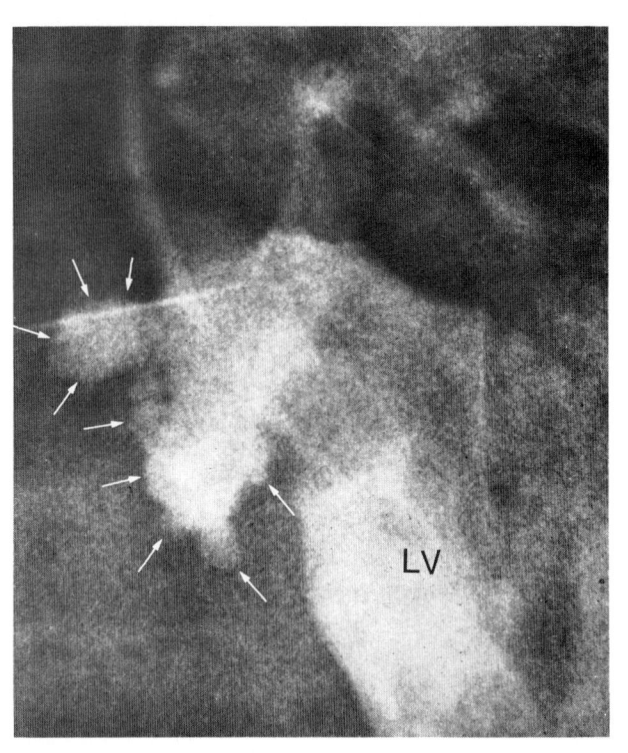

9. Aneurysms are usually not large enough to cause significant obstruction in the right ventricle, but rarely a right ventricular systolic pressure gradient may be created (see Chapter 26).

10. If the right ventricular systolic pressure exceeds the left ventricular systolic pressure, the aneurysm bulges into the left ventricular outflow area.

11. Rarely, the tricuspid valve adheres to a VSD, forming a pouch that is indistinguishable angiographically from a true congenital aneurysm of the membranous septum (see Fig 12–13,A).[3]

12. It is likely that the majority of aneurysms of the membranous septum are caused by closure of a membranous ventricular defect by the septal leaflet of the tricuspid valve.

13. An aneurysm of the membranous septum can be confused with either a prolapsing aortic cusp or an aneurysm of the sinus of Valsalva with rupture into the right ventricle. The sinus of Valsalva's aneurysm, however, arises from the aortic cusp, and the left-to-right shunt is predominant during diastole, particularly if the right ventricular pressure is elevated. A prolapsing aortic cusp changes its angiographic appearance dramatically between systole and diastole because of motion of the leaflet.

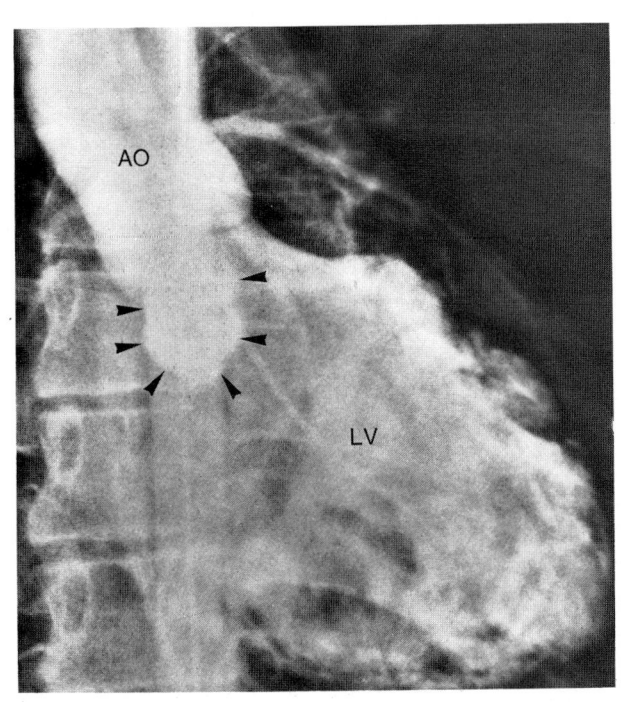

FIG 14-5.
Clues to the presence of aneurysm of membranous septum. **A,** left ventriculogram in anteroposterior projection. Double density *(arrows)* in area of membranous septum. **B,** lateral projection showing irregular aneurysm with tiny left-to-right shunt *(white arrows).* Anatomic nature of aneurysm uncertain. Jet appears to originate at edge of aneurysm, suggesting adherence of septal leaflet to a VSD rather than a congenital aneurysm. *AO* = aorta; *LV* = left ventricle.

OPERATIVE CONSIDERATIONS

Because complications of unruptured aneurysms of the membranous septum are so uncommon, operation is not indicated. If an aneurysm is associated with a VSD, the defect is usually small and the left-to-right shunt less than 40%. It decreases with time. Therefore, closure of the septal defect and repair of the aneurysm are not indicated in most instances.

REFERENCES

1. Nugent EW, Freedom RM, Rowe RD, et al: Aneurysm of the membranous septum in ventricular septal defect, *Circulation* 56(suppl I):82, 1977.
2. Freedom RM, White RD, Pieroni DR, et al: The natural history of the so-called aneurysm of the membranous ventricular septum in childhood, *Circulation* 49:375, 1974.
3. Tandon R, Edwards JE: Aneurysm-like formations in relation to membranous ventricular septum *Circulation* 47:1089, 1973.
4. Pieroni P, Bell BB, Krovetz LJ, et al: Auscultatory recognition of aneurysm of the membranous ventricular septum associated with small ventricular septal defect, *Circulation* 44:733, 1971.
5. Sapire DW, Black IFS: Echocardiographic detection of aneurysms of the interventricular septum associated with ventricular septal defect: a method of noninvasive diagnosis and follow-up, *Am J Cardiol* 36:797, 1975.

CHAPTER 15

Left Ventricular–Right Atrial Communication

This uncommon anomaly results from several anatomic arrangements that permit shunting of blood directly from the left ventricle to the right atrium. Characteristically, the clinical findings suggest a ventricular septal defect, but at catheterization, a left-to-right shunt is found at the atrial level.

PATHOLOGIC ANATOMY

Normally the membranous portion of the ventricular septum faces both the right ventricle and the right atrium. The septal leaflet of the tricuspid valve divides the membranous septum into a larger right atrial and a smaller right ventricular portion (Fig 15–1). Left ventricular–right atrial communication occurs through the membranous portion of the ventricular septum.

In one third of patients with a left ventricular–right atrial communication, the defect lies above the tricuspid valve (atrial portion of membranous septum), although it may extend to the attachment of the valve, resulting in a direct communication between the left ventricle and right atrium. In the other two thirds of patients, the defect is located below the tricuspid valve in the ventricular portion of the membranous septum. Therefore, a ventricular septal defect is present, which is associated with an abnormality of the tricuspid valve. The septal defect allows passage of blood from the left ventricle into the right ventricle; and through the abnormality of the tricuspid valve, blood flows into the right atrium. The latter type of left ventricular–right atrial communication has several anatomic varieties[1]:

1. Adherence of a cleft in septal leaflet of the tricuspid valve to edges of membranous ventricular septal defect.
2. Ventricular septal defect and accessory orifice of tricuspid valve.
3. Ruptured aneurysm of membranous septum through tricuspid valve.
4. Ventricular septal defect with adherent tricuspid valve.
5. Isolated ventricular septal defect of the atrioventricular-canal type and tricuspid valvular abnormality.

Associated cardiac malformations are present in one third of patients with left ventricular–right atrial communication:

1. Atrial septal defect (most common).
2. Subaortic stenosis, coarctation of aorta, patent ductus arteriosus, bicuspid aortic valve, and pulmonary stenosis (less frequent).
3. Transposition of the great vessels, tetralogy of Fallot, and pulmonary atresia with intact septum (a few reported cases).

Each of the cardiac chambers in left ventricular–right atrial communication is dilated, because each carries blood involved in the shunt.

NATURAL HISTORY, SIGNS, AND SYMPTOMS

Cardiac disease is often recognized in the neonatal period because of the presence of a murmur.[2] A shunt is present through the communication from birth because of the large pressure difference between the left ventricle and

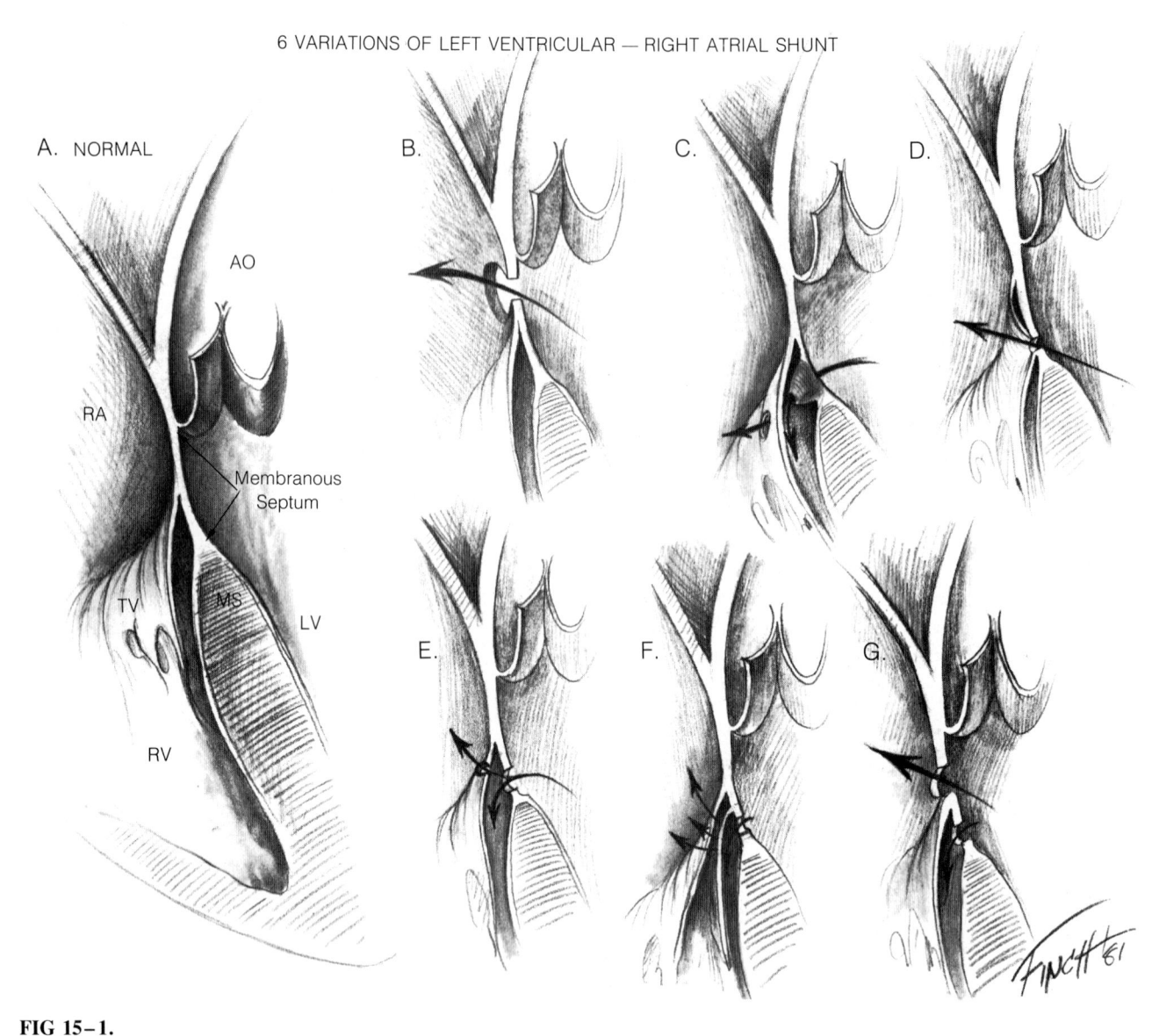

286 *Cardiac Conditions Associated With a Left-to-Right Shunt*

FIG 15–1.
Diagram of varieties of left ventricular–right atrial communication. **A,** normal anatomic relation of membranous septum, largest portion of which separates left ventricle and right atrium. Septal leaflet of tricuspid valve inserts across septum, and small portion of septum lies below attachment of tricuspid valve. **B,** isolated left ventricular–right atrial communication. Defect in membranous septum above septal leaflet of tricuspid valve. **C,** ruptured aneurysm of membranous septum, with defect of septal leaflet of tricuspid valve. **D,** defect in interventricular portion of membranous septum, with adherence of septal leaflet of tricuspid valve and perforation of the leaflet. **E,** defect in interventricular portion of membranous septum, with fenestration in septal leaflet of tricuspid valve. **F,** defect in interventricular portion of membranous septum and cleft in septal leaflet of tricuspid valve. **G,** coexistent defects in both portions of membranous septum. *AO* = aorta; *LV* = left ventricle; *MS* = muscular septum; *RA* = right atrium; *RV* = right ventricle; *TV* = tricuspid valve.

the right atrium. This is in contrast to instances of isolated ventricular septal defect, where the magnitude of left-to-right shunt depends on the pulmonary vascular resistance so the murmur usually is not heard until vascular resistance has begun to decrease.

Many patients are asymptomatic, but others have frequent respiratory infections and tire easily. Approximately 25% develop congestive cardiac failure because of the left ventricular volume overload. Symptoms may appear as early as 1 month of age.

PHYSICAL EXAMINATION

The prominent finding is a loud, harsh pansystolic murmur, often associated with a thrill along the left sternal border.[2] The murmur is usually interpreted as a ventricular septal defect, and its loudness masks the murmur of the flow across the right ventricular outflow tract. Because of the increased volume ejected by the right ventricle, the second heart sound is more widely split than normal. It varies normally with respiration, because there is no atrial communication. This is in distinction to atrial septal defects, which cause wide, fixed splitting.

An apical middiastolic murmur, related to the increased blood flow and turbulence across the mitral valve, is present in patients with moderate or large shunts. Less frequently, a tricuspid middiastolic murmur is heard as well.

ELECTROCARDIOGRAPHIC FEATURES

No consistent pattern is found, perhaps because of the variations in the size of the shunt. Typically the electrocardiogram would be expected to show right atrial enlargement, incomplete right bundle-branch block (right ventricular enlargement), and left ventricular hypertrophy because of the dilatation and hypertrophy of each of these chambers. In the rare instance in which a left ventricular–right atrial shunt occurs as a part of an endocardial cushion defect, left-axis deviation is usually found.

ECHOCARDIOGRAPHIC FEATURES

On M-mode echocardiography, each cardiac chamber is dilated, its size being proportional to the magnitude of the shunt. In those patients in whom the shunt occurs through the ventricular septal defect, a high-frequency, low-amplitude flutter of the tricuspid valve occurs during systole but not in diastole.[3]

RADIOGRAPHIC FEATURES

Because of the many anatomic variations among left ventricular–right atrial shunt, the hemodynamics and radiographic picture are not uniform.[4]

1. X-ray findings may be normal. REASON: In many patients, the left-to-right shunt through the left ventricular–right atrial communication is small.

2. The pulmonary vasculature is increased when the left-to-right shunt is large and resembles that of an atrial septal defect. REASON: In the uncommon, isolated left ventricular–right atrial shunt, the pulmonary artery pressure is normal, as in atrial septal defect.

3. Large left-to-right shunts through a concomitant ventricular communication may lead to radiographic signs of pulmonary hypertension. REASON: The ventricular component transmits left ventricular systolic pressure directly to the right ventricle, causing pulmonary hypertension

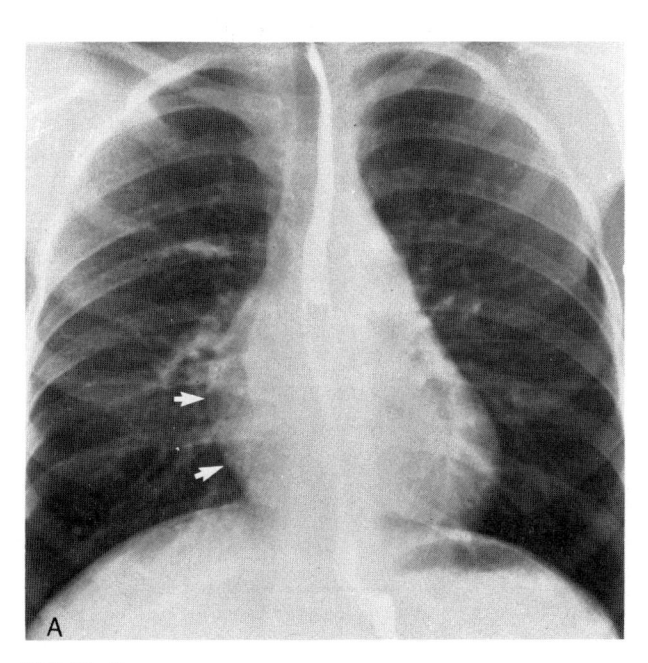

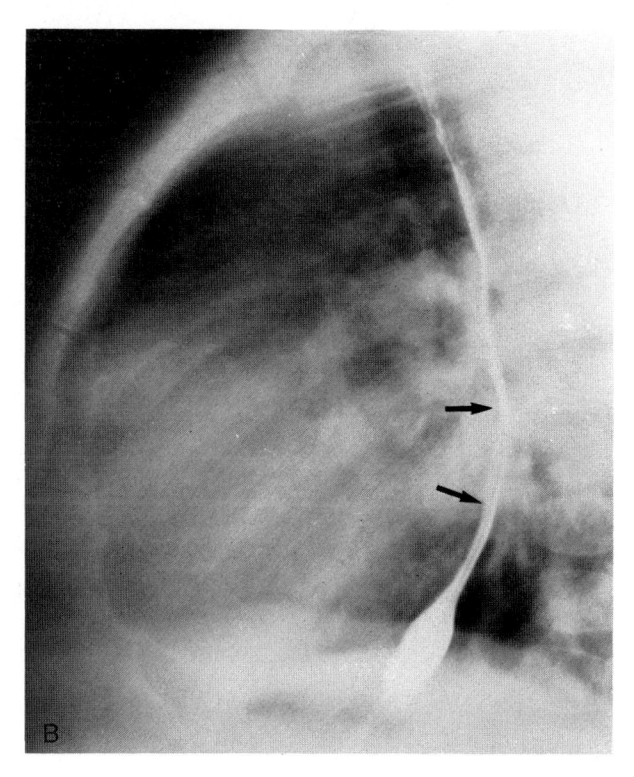

FIG 15–2.
Thoracic roentgenogram of isolated left ventricular–right atrial shunt. **A**, posteroanterior projection shows normal pulmonary vasculature and slight prominence of right atrium *(arrows)*. The radiographic findings are normal, as is commonly observed in instances of small left ventricular–right atrial communication. **B**, lateral projection shows enlargement of the heart and displacement of the esophagus by an enlarged left atrium. This is in contrast to the picture in atrial septal defect, which does not cause left atrial enlargement.

identical to that seen with a large ventricular septal defect.

4. The right atrial border may be prominent (Fig 15–2,A). REASON: As in atrial septal defect, the blood flow through the right atrium is increased, so the chamber is distended.

5. The left atrium and left ventricle are dilated (Fig 15–2,B). REASON: The blood flow through the left side of the heart is increased because of the left-to-right shunt. In contrast to what happens in atrial septal defect, the left atrium cannot decompress itself, because there is no atrial shunt. Therefore, left atrial distention occurs.

6. Radiographic findings of a large left ventricular–right atrial shunt are identical to those of a ventricular septal defect except for enlargement of the right atrium. The latter is the only helpful radiographic finding, but it is difficult to determine radiographically. Thus, the diagnosis is virtually never made from chest radiographs.

CARDIAC CATHETERIZATION

The catheter course is normal. In fact, the inability to advance a catheter from the femoral vein across the atrial septum in the presence of an atrial level left-to-right shunt should suggest this diagnosis.

Oximetry data show increased oxygen saturation at the right atrial level. An additional increase may occur at the ventricular level, depending on the size of the concomitant ventricular communication. However, because of streaming, any ventricular component is difficult to detect. Angiography is essential.

ANGIOGRAPHIC APPEARANCE

The diagnosis can be established by left ventriculography with anteroposterior and lateral projections or, preferably, angled left anterior oblique and right anterior oblique views. The diagnosis is usually missed if only a lateral or

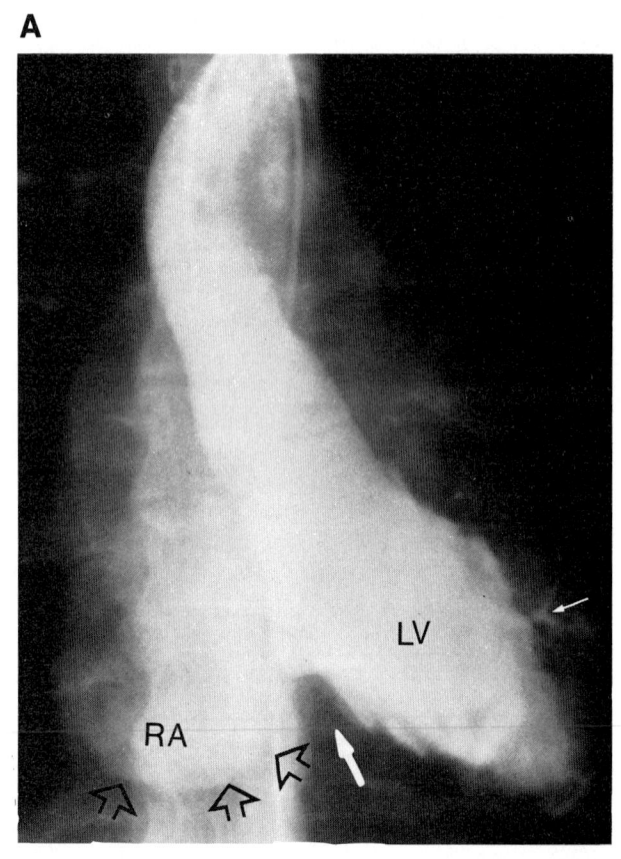

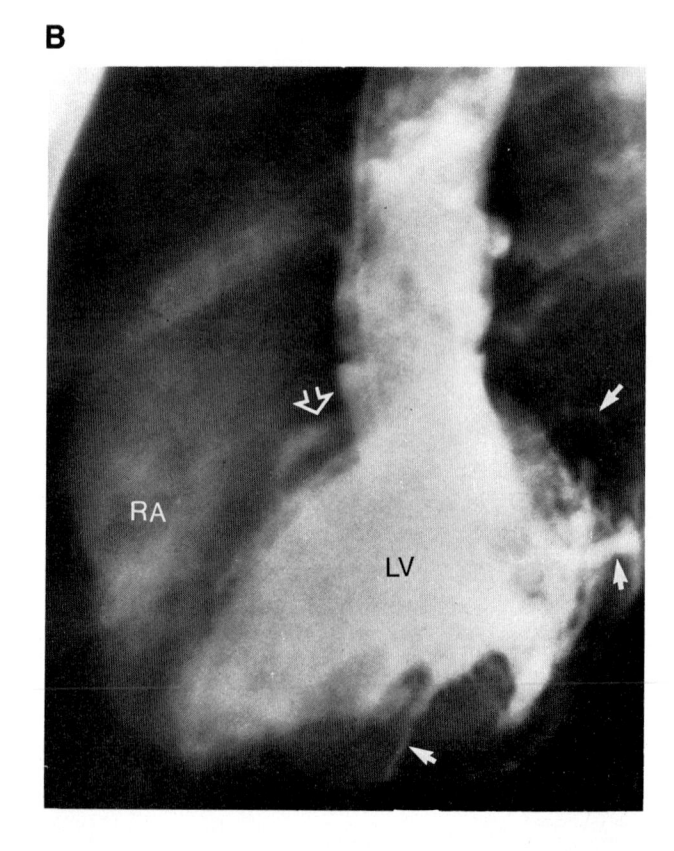

FIG 15–3.
Left ventriculogram of isolated left ventricular–right atrial communication above tricuspid valve. **A,** anteroposterior projection shows dense opacification of the right atrium *(open arrows)*. The inflow portion of the right ventricle is unopacified, as indicated by clear space *(white arrow)* between the opacified left ventricle and right atrium. **B,** lateral projection with opacification of the right atrium. The jet of contrast medium is clearly visible *(open arrow)*. Simultaneous opacification of right atrium and right ventricle could not be excluded on the basis of the lateral projection alone. Note intramyocardial injection, with filling of coronary veins *(small white arrows)*. LV = left ventricle; RA = right atrium.

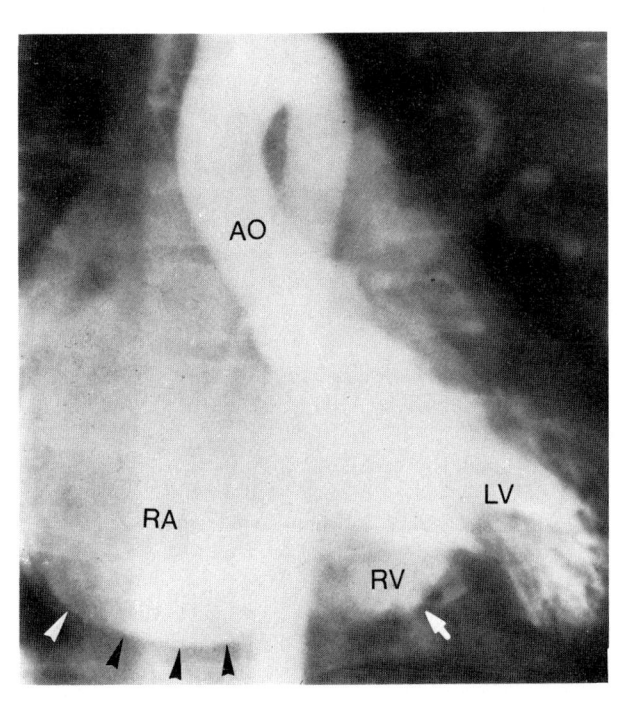

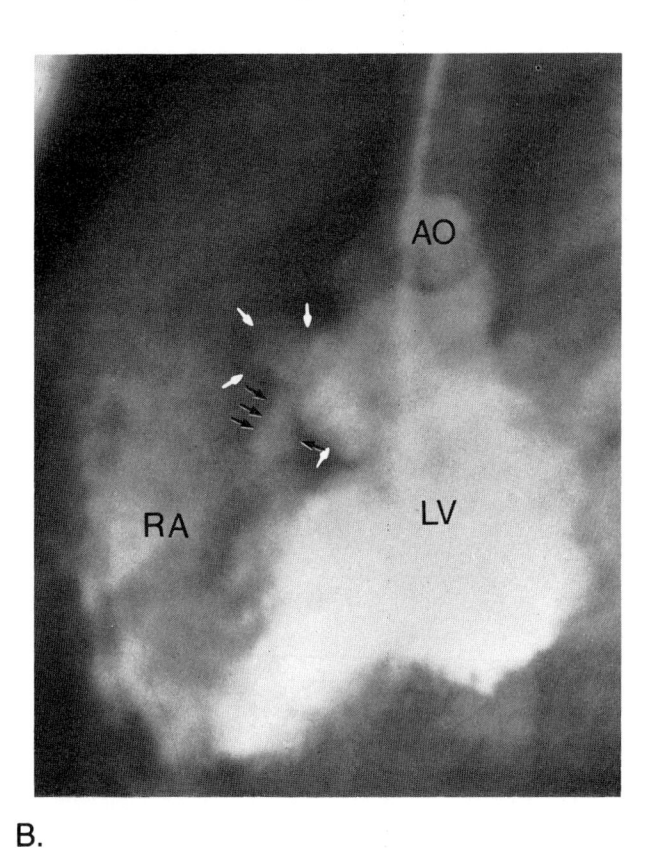

FIG 15–4.
Left ventriculogram of large left ventricular–right atrial communication. **A,** anteroposterior projection; dilated right atrium is densely opacified *(black arrows).* Simultaneous dense opacification of the inflow portion of the right ventricle *(white arrow).* **B,** lateral projections; large aneurysm of the membranous septum *(white arrows).* A fan-shaped jet of contrast material extends into the right ventricle *(black arrows)* and right atrium *(white arrows).* This angiogram is characteristic of malformation shown in Figure 15–1, **C.** *AO* = aorta; *LV* = left ventricle; *RA* = right atrium; *RV* = right ventricle.

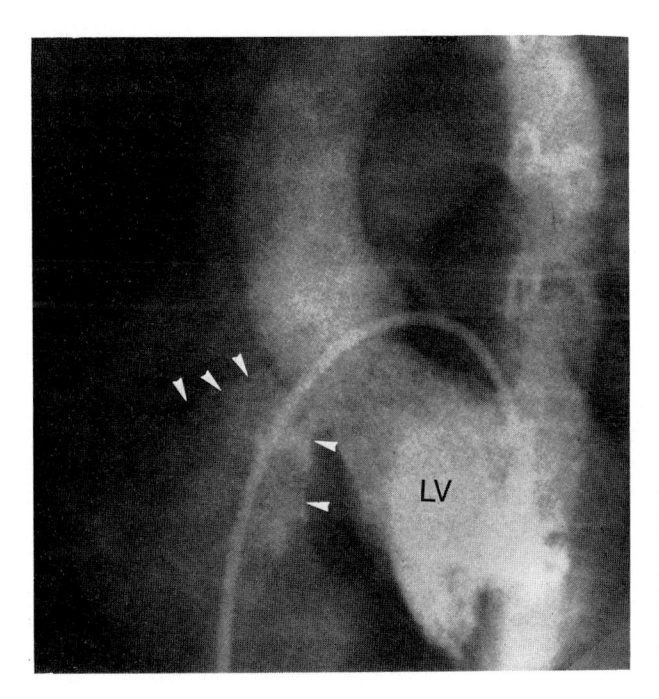

FIG 15–5.
Long axial oblique left ventriculogram via transatrial catheterization shows simultaneous opacification of right ventricle and right atrium. In this projection, the chambers are superimposed and cannot be distinguished. The fan-shaped jet *(arrows)* suggests a cleft in the tricuspid valve, although the exact anatomy cannot be discerned. *LV* = left ventricle.

left anterior oblique projection is made. REASON: The right ventricle and right atrium are then superimposed.

1. In a true left ventricular–right atrial shunt with an isolated communication in the atrial portion of the membranous septum, early films after left ventricular injection show opacification of the right atrium but not the right ventricle (Fig 15–3,A). The opacified right atrial border is separated from the opacified left ventricle by a clear space, which represents the unopacified inflow portion of the right ventricle (see Fig 15–3,A). This is best seen on an anteroposterior or right anterior oblique projection.

2. On a lateral view, the opacified right atrium may be confused with the right ventricle (Fig 15–3,B).

3. Most left ventricular–right atrial shunts occur through ventricular septal defects and are associated with some type of tricuspid valvular abnormality (see Fig 15–3,C and G); in such cases, the right atrium and right ventricle opacify simultaneously after left ventricular injection.

4. The association of a left ventricular–right atrial shunt with a ventricular communication and an aneurysm of the membranous septum is common (Fig 15–4), indicating adherence of the tricuspid valve to the defect.

5. A fan-shaped jet (Fig 15–5) suggests a cleft in the tricuspid valve with a ventricular septal defect (see Fig 15–1,F). The exact anatomy cannot always be predicted.

MANAGEMENT

Left ventricular–right atrial communications do not close spontaneously, and the incidence of bacterial endocarditis is probably higher than in isolated ventricular septal defect. Therefore, all such communications should be operatively repaired. Those defects located above the tricuspid valve may be closed by direct suture; those located below the level of the valve should be closed by a patch, which may necessitate mobilization of a portion of the valve.[5] Care must be taken during the operation, because of the proximity of the conduction system, not to cause postoperative heart block.

REFERENCES

1. Perry EL, Burchell HB, Edwards JE: Congenital communications between the left ventricle and the right atrium: coexisting ventricular septal defect and double tricuspid orifice, *Mayo Clin Proc* 24:198, 1949.
2. Riemenschneider TA, Moss AJ: Left ventricular–right atrial communication, *Am J Cardiol* 19:710, 1967.
3. Nanda NC, Gramiak R, Manning JA: Echocardiography of the tricuspid valve in congenital left ventricular–right atrial communication, *Circulation* 51:268, 1975.
4. Elliott LP, Gedgaudas E, Levy MJ, et al: The roentgenologic findings in left ventricular–right atrial communication, *AJR* 93:304, 1965.
5. Levy M, Lillehei CW: Left ventricular–right atrial canal: ten cases treated surgically, *Am J Cardiol* 10:623, 1962.

CHAPTER 16

Patent Ductus Arteriosus

Patent ductus arteriosus (PDA) is the best known of all congenital cardiac anomalies because of its presence in fetal life, its early conquest by the surgeon, and its glamorous murmur.

The ductus arteriosus represents persistence of the distal part of the primitive sixth aortic arch, which, although a bilateral structure, usually regresses on the right early in fetal life (see Chapter 1). Therefore, most instances of PDA are on the left side, and because the ductus connects the aorta and the left pulmonary artery, there is a shunt, which is usually in a left-to-right direction.

INCIDENCE

The incidence of PDA is difficult to determine, because it is an essential component of the fetal circulation. In full-term infants beyond the immediate neonatal period, PDA represents about 8% of all congenital heart disease. It occurs twice as frequently in females as in males. The incidence is considerably higher in prematurely born infants, particularly those with the respiratory distress syndrome.[1,2] The incidence in these infants correlates with birth weight, being 75% in those weighing less than 1,200 g and 50% in those weighing less than 1,750 g.[3] The incidence is also higher in populations living at high altitudes, especially above 10,000 ft.[4]

ETIOLOGY

In a few families, PDA occurs in more than one member or generation.[5] Maternal rubella during the first trimester of pregnancy causes a well-recognized triad of deafness, congenital cataracts, and congenital heart disease, the heart disease almost always being either PDA or peripheral pulmonary arterial stenosis.[6] However, the histologic appearance of a PDA in these children is different from that in non-rubella-associated ductus, with a lesser amount of smooth muscle tissue. The angiographic appearance is also different.

Oxygen is important in the normal closure of the ductus arteriosus, but the exact mechanisms are not fully understood. Evidence for the role of oxygen includes the increased incidence of PDA in populations living at high altitudes.[4] This effect apparently is mediated through a reduced arterial Po_2. Studies by Moss and others of normal neonates showed that when an infant is placed in an environment of 100% oxygen, the ductus closes, whereas an environment of 12% oxygen leads to opening of the ductus. This responsiveness depends on the concentration of oxygen in the blood traversing the ductus arteriosus. Unfortunately, however, in many neonates with cyanotic forms of cardiac disease, such as pulmonary atresia, who depend on the ductus as the primary or sole source of pulmonary blood flow, the lifesaving ductus closes despite severe hypoxia.

In premature infants, a PDA often closes spontaneously at the time the child normally would have been born.[8] What factors determine this spontaneous closure are unknown. Perhaps prostaglandin E_1 plays an important role because it is a potent dilator of the ductus arteriosus.[9-11] Indomethacin administered to neonates is associated with ductal closure.[12]

PATHOLOGY AND ANATOMY

The ductus arteriosus connects the proximal portion of the left pulmonary artery with the proximal descending aorta immediately below the entrance of the left subclavian artery. In its course from the left pulmonary artery, the ductus passes posteriorly and inferiorly to the descending aorta, forming an arch. If there is a right-sided arch and right-sided ductus arteriosus, the relations are the same, only on the other side. If there is a ductus arteriosus arising opposite the aortic arch, as in right aortic arch and left PDA, the ductus courses between the ipsilateral subclavian artery and the pulmonary artery.

The size and shape of the PDA vary, ranging from long, narrow, and tortuous to short and wide.

The histologic appearance of ductus arteriosus differs considerably from that of the adjacent aorta and pulmonary artery, whose walls are composed principally of elastic tissue. In utero the ductus has a thick intimal layer, a media with a single elastic lamina, spiral muscle, and mucoid material.[13, 14] A patent ductus shows a marked reduction in muscular tissue and, perhaps, more elastic tissue.

There usually are secondary changes in the heart, depending on the volume of pulmonary blood flow and the pulmonary arterial pressure. With a large shunt, the left atrium, left ventricle, ascending aorta, aortic arch, and pulmonary artery are dilated. Right ventricular hypertrophy is found in patients with pulmonary hypertension.

The recurrent laryngeal nerve passes around the ductus arteriosus whether left- or right-sided; this relation allows definite differentiation between a bronchial artery and a PDA at postmortem examination. It also has important surgical implications.

HEMODYNAMICS

Because the ductus arteriosus is a normal component of the fetal circulation, we will review its function because of the information it provides about the hemodynamics of PDA.

The lumen of the fetal ductus is large and offers no impediment to flow, so that the pulmonary arterial pressure equals the aortic pressure. The direction and magnitude of flow through the ductus depend on the relative pulmonary vascular and systemic vascular resistances. Pulmonary resistance is determined by the pulmonary arterioles, which are constricted by the normal prenatal hypoxia, whereas the systemic resistance is determined primarily by the large, low-resistance placenta. At birth, two events happen that significantly alter this relationship. First, pulmonary vascular resistance decreases because of inflation of the lungs and improvement of oxygenation. Second, systemic vascular resistance increases because of the elimination of the placenta from the circulation. The ductus shunt becomes bidirectional for the first 6 hours and then left to right, with the ductus closing functionally in most normal neonates by 18 to 24 hours.[15]

In fetal ductus arteriosus, intimal cushions develop that are associated with medial hypertrophy at their bases. After birth, the spiral musculature of the ductus contracts. The intimal cushions from longitudinal ridges further narrow the lumen and eventually fuse. The muscle in the media is separated by mucoid material. Cytolytic necrosis occurs, the central channel of the ductus shrinks, and the muscle tissue disappears, ultimately forming a fibrous ligament. Anatomic closure is usually complete by 1 month. In the neonatal period, it may be possible to pass a catheter through a ductus arteriosus that cannot be demonstrated angiographically or by oximetry measurements.

Like the ventricular septal defect, PDA can be divided into two groups according to size. When the ductus arteriosus is large, approaching the size of the aorta, the direction and flow depend on the relative vascular resistances. Normally, as the pulmonary vascular resistance decreases, the volume of pulmonary blood flow increases, leading eventually to congestive cardiac failure from left ventricular volume overload. Ultimately, some of these patients have pulmonary vascular disease if they are not operated on. Eventually, pulmonary vascular resistance may exceed systemic vascular resistance, and the shunt then becomes right to left. Occasionally the pulmonary vasculature fails to mature, and the pulmonary vascular resistance remains elevated from birth.

In most patients, however, the caliber of the ductus is less than that of the aorta, and the narrowed ductal lumen offers resistance to flow. The pulmonary vascular resistance usually declines normally, and pulmonary vascular disease is rare in this group. The pulmonary arterial pressure may be normal or elevated, although rarely to systemic levels, and the level of pressure depends on the volume of pulmonary blood flow. Cardiac failure may occur in this group if the shunt flow is great.

The hemodynamics of a PDA in a premature infant are considerably different, principally because left ventricular compliance is reduced in these infants by edema of the ventricular myocardium and disorganization of the myocardial fibers. Thus, the increased left ventricular volume from the ductus causes a marked increase in the left atrial and pulmonary venous pressures.[16] The systemic output is often inadequate. As a result, systemic arterial pressures are low, and inadequate peripheral organ perfusion leads to inadequate renal blood flow or necrotizing enterocolitis. Furthermore, the lower diastolic pressure decreases the coronary perfusion pressure, which may lead to subendocardial ischemia and consequent reduction of left ventricular function.[17]

Another significant hemodynamic effect of PDA resembles that of any aortic runoff lesion, with widening of the pulse pressure. The systolic pressure increases because of the large left ventricular stroke volume into the aorta, and the diastolic pressure is lower because of the flow through the ductus arteriosus during diastole ("aortic runoff").

CLINICAL FEATURES

The clinical course of a premature infant with a PDA differs from that of full-term infants or children. The premature infant develops respiratory distress from hyaline membrane disease within hours of birth. The infant is supported, usually by a respirator, and the respiratory condition improves within days. Respiratory difficulties then reappear, which may necessitate reinstitution of ventilatory support or an increase in the level of support. The respiratory distress is caused by pulmonary congestion secondary to decreased left ventricular compliance. This is associated with increased precordial activity, bounding peripheral arterial pulses, and, often, the characteristic murmur of a PDA over the upper sternum or beneath the left clavicle.[8] The murmur can be variable because of changing levels of pulmonary and systemic vascular resistances.

Except for prematurely born infants, most patients with PDA are asymptomatic. A few, those with large left-to-right shunts, develop congestive cardiac failure, usually by age 3 months. Cardiac disease is usually diagnosed by the discovery of a murmur. A typical continuous murmur may be found in a neonate, and some of these murmurs disappear spontaneously. More commonly, the murmur is found on a examination later during infancy. The height and weight may be low.

In most patients, the physical findings are diagnostic. The pulse pressure is widened, and there are increased peripheral pulses. In neonates, these may be manifested by a palmar pulse. The heart may be enlarged. Prominent pulsations and, occasionally, a thrill are found in the suprasternal notch. The characteristic murmur is located over the area of the ductus, namely, under the left clavicle. It is continuous, beginning with the first heart sound, reaching a peak about the second heart sound, then tailing off into diastole. The loudness varies from grade 1 to 4/6 depending on the size and flow through the ductus. In neonates and infants, the murmur of a PDA is heard in the same area but is primarily systolic, perhaps extending briefly into diastole. It has a hollow quality.

The pulmonary component of the second heart sound is accentuated if pulmonary hypertension is present, but it may be obscured by the murmur.

With a large volume of pulmonary blood flow, an apical middiastolic murmur is heard.

In the patient with pulmonary vascular disease and right-to-left flow through the ductus, there is no murmur ("silent ductus"), a markedly accentuated P_2, and differential cyanosis (cyanosis of the legs but not of the arms).

ELECTROCARDIOGRAPHIC FEATURES

The electrocardiographic findings resemble those of ventricular septal defect and vary considerably depending on the hemodynamics. The QRS axis and P wave are usually normal. Four QRS patterns are found:

1. Normal, suggesting a small ductus arteriosus.
2. Isolated left ventricular hypertrophy, suggesting a moderate-sized PDA with nearly normal pulmonary arterial pressure and a moderate increase in pulmonary blood flow.
3. Biventricular hypertrophy, suggesting a large PDA with elevated pulmonary arterial pressure and blood flow but nearly normal pulmonary vascular resistance.
4. Isolated right ventricular hypertrophy, indicating a large PDA with pulmonary hypertension secondary to severe pulmonary vascular disease.

In premature infants, the only abnormality of a symptomatic PDA may be ST-segment depression and T-wave inversion in the left precordial leads.

In our experience, the q wave in lead V_6 is often deeper than in a ventricular septal defect with similar hemodynamics, and abnormalities of ST and T waves are more often found in the left precordial leads, perhaps suggesting myocardial ischemia secondary to lowered coronary arterial perfusion pressure.

ECHOCARDIOGRAPHIC FEATURES

There has been considerable interest in the ability of the echocardiogram to predict the hemodynamics of PDA, particularly in premature infants.[18, 19] The dimension of the aorta and left atrium have been compared, on the assumption that left atrial size would increase with a large volume of pulmonary blood flow. Unfortunately, the left atrial dimension or any ratio involving this measurement correlates poorly with the volume of pulmonary blood flow, even in older children. In premature infants, shifts of fluids and the effects of the respirator interfere with measurement of left atrial dimension even further. Serial measurements in an individual infant may, however, help in determining changes in hemodynamics, particularly when combined with other clinical data.

Cross-sectional echocardiography, especially from the suprasternal notch, has been useful in identifying PDA.

RADIOGRAPHIC FEATURES

The radiographic manifestations of PDA vary greatly, depending on the hemodynamic state.

1. Commonly, the radiographic findings are normal. REASON: In many patients, the shunt is small. In addition, its length creates further resistance to flow.
2. Calcification of the ductus arteriosus commonly occurs in infancy following normal closure. The calcified ductus can be seen radiographically as a tiny area of in-

FIG 16–1.
Thoracic roentgenogram in posteroanterior projection of asymptomatic patient. Characteristic density *(arrow)* of calcified closed ductus arteriosus (calcified ductus ligament). This appearance indicates closure of ductus. (Courtesy of Dr. Ken Fellows.)

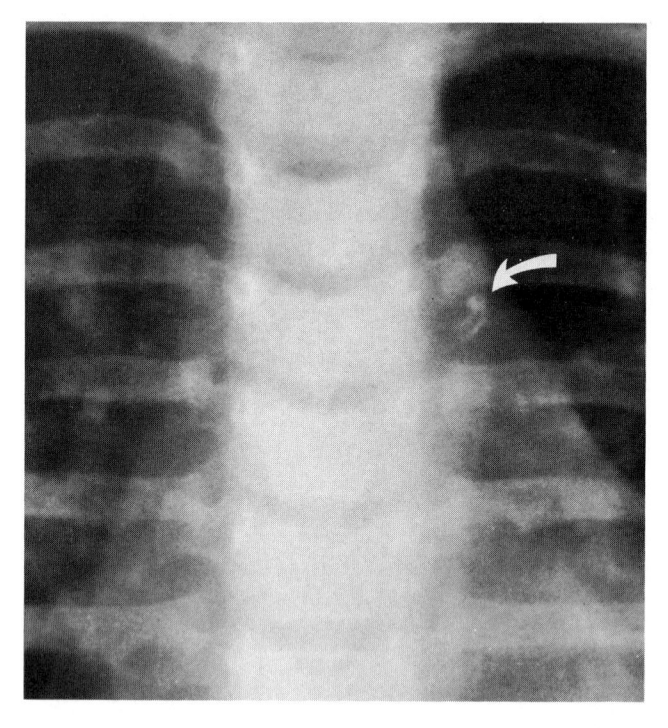

creased density on a posteroanterior projection. This fairly common radiographic finding in children is rare in adults, because calcifications of the ductus ligament tend to disappear later in life. The radiographic finding of a calcified ductus ligament rules out patency (Fig 16–1).

3. In a large PDA with normal pulmonary vascular resistance, enormous volumes of blood flow through the left side of the heart. REASON: Shunt during systole and diastole. This causes a marked increase in pulmonary vascularity, as well as left atrial and left ventricular enlarge-

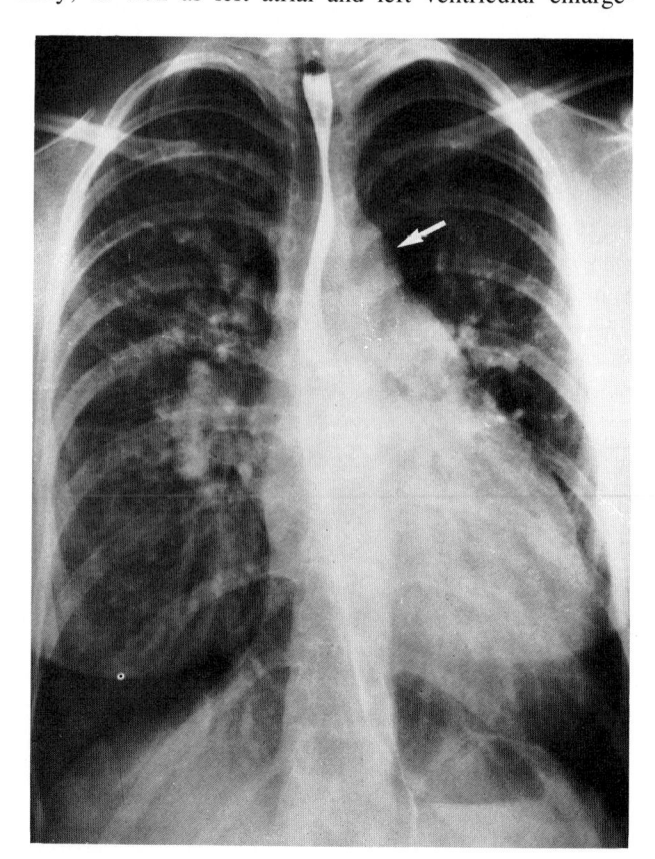

FIG 16–2.
Thoracic roentgenogram in posteroanterior projection of patients with large patent ductus arteriosus (PDA). Increased pulmonary vasculature except in left upper lobe. Prominent main pulmonary artery segment; prominent left ventricle; normal right cardiac border. Features identical to those of ventricular septal defect except that aortic knob *(arrow)* is prominent. REASON: Blood flowing through the ascending aorta consists of the cardiac output plus the volume shunted through the patent ductus. Hypovascularity of left upper lobe is more consistent with PDA than with ventricular septal defect.

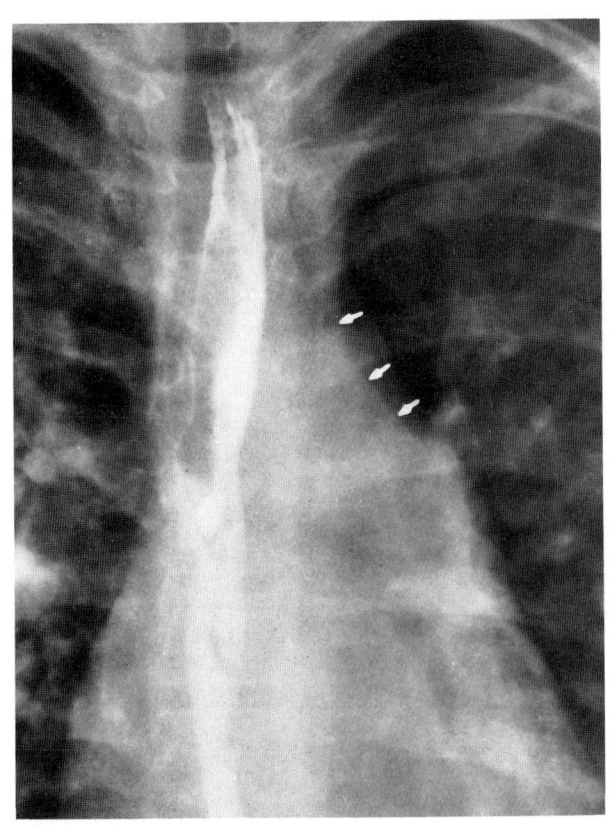

FIG 16–3.
Thoracic roentgenogram in posteroanterior projection of patients with moderate-sized PDA. Minimal cardiomegaly; increased pulmonary vascularity except in left upper lobe. Double density *(arrows)* seen through the pulmonary artery segment is caused by the patent ductus but is sometimes also seen in normal individuals; therefore, it is not diagnostic.

ment, as in patients with a large ventricular septal defect with low pulmonary vascular resistance.

4. In many patients, the radiographic appearance cannot be differentiated from that of a large ventricular septal defect. Patients with a large PDA, however, tend to have a prominent aortic knob (Fig 16–2). REASON: The blood flow through the ascending aorta and aortic arch up to the level of the ductus arteriosus is increased, because it represents the cardiac output plus the volume of blood shunted through the ductus.

5. The aortic pulsations are increased, which can be seen fluoroscopically. REASON: Patent ductus arteriosus is a diastolic runoff lesion that lowers aortic diastolic pressure. The pulse pressure is widened, and the peripheral pulses are "snappy."

6. If pulmonary vascular disease develops, the shunt flow decreases, and left atrial and left ventricular enlargement gradually disappear.

7. The increased pulmonary vascular resistance causes right ventricular hypertrophy and, subsequently, right ventricular enlargement.

8. The PDA may be visible on thoracic radiographs as a faint additional density that is seen through the pulmonary arterial segment or, in the case of a large lesion, as part of the upper left cardiac border (Fig 16–3).

9. Either a PDA or a ductus diverticulum of the aorta may cause a mass density (Fig 16–4). A ductus diverticulum is a funnel-shaped widening of the aortic origin of a ductus, which may not be patent. Closure of the ductus from the pulmonary arterial end to the aortic end of the ductus is incomplete. The density may be mistaken for a mediastinal mass, and aortography (see Fig 16–4,C) is required to establish a diagnosis and obviate surgical exploration or needle biopsy. The ductus diverticulum may persist into adulthood, when needle biopsy of such a "mass" may result in life-threatening or fatal hemorrhage.

10. Incomplete closure of the pulmonary end of the ductus results into a pulmonary ductus diverticulum (see Chapter 30).

11. The ductus arteriosus may calcify. This does not indicate the state of patency, because a ductus ligament also may calcify. However, if the calcification has a ring-like configuration, the ductus arteriosus is probably patent (Fig 16–5). A pointlike calcification is diagnostic of a calcified ductus ligament (see Fig 16–1).

12. In patients with a large PDA and pulmonary hypertension, calcifications may occur in the intima of the ductus (atherosclerosis). Under those circumstances, a posteroanterior projection shows a ring density rather than a solid calcification (see Fig 16–5).

13. The distribution of pulmonary blood flow is commonly unequal, with less blood flow through the left lung, particularly the upper lobe. This causes a difference in the appearance of the vasculature in the two lungs (see Figs 16–2, 16–3, and 16–5). PROBABLE REASON: The patent ductus attaches to the left pulmonary artery, and the jet

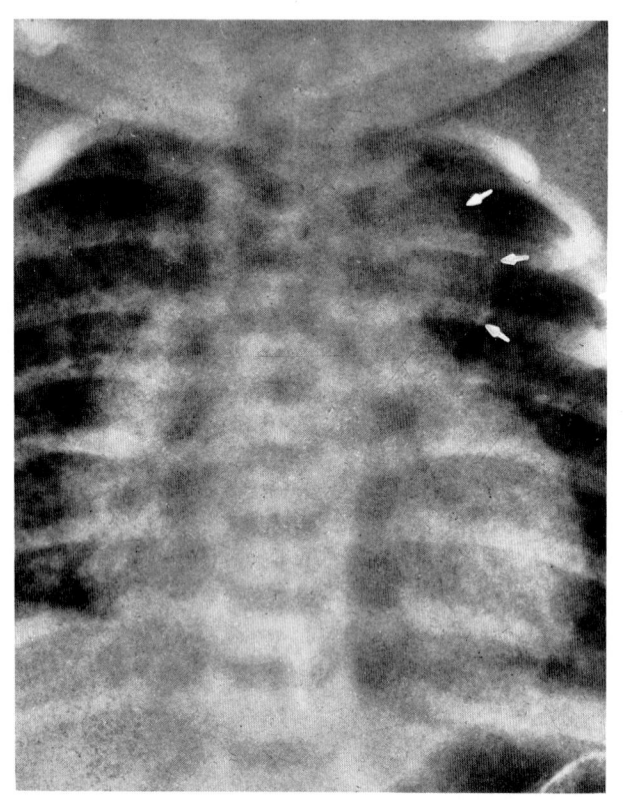

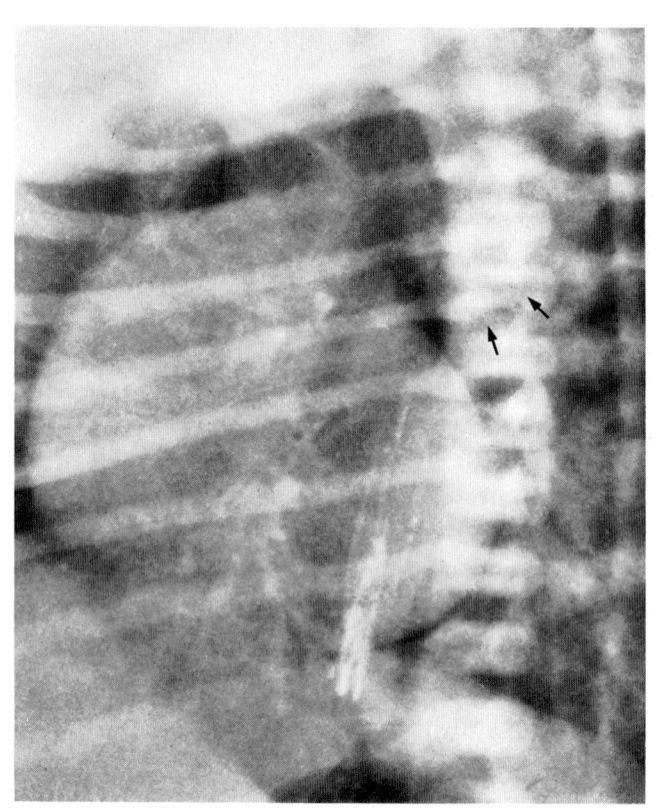

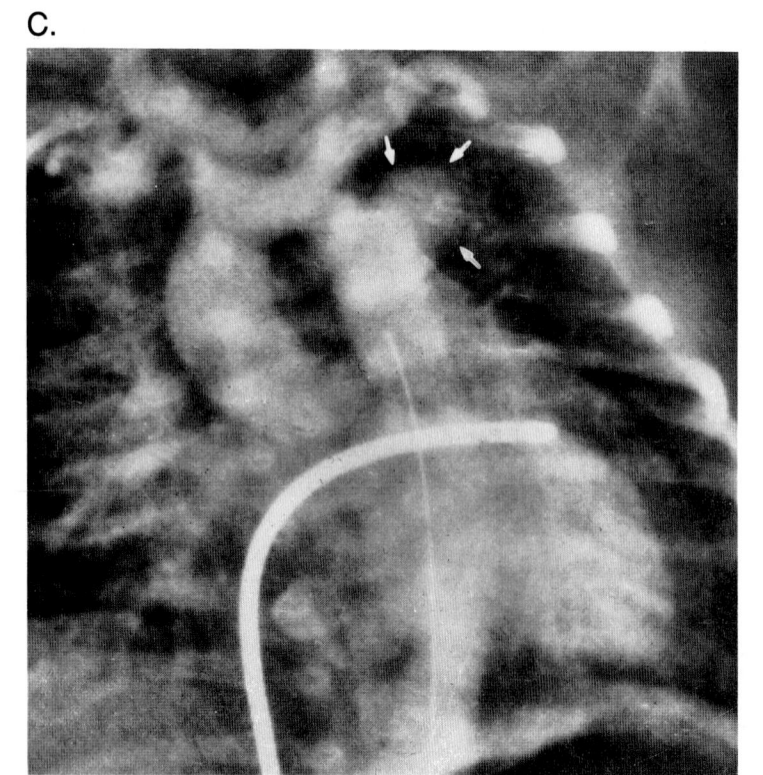

296 Cardiac Conditions Associated With a Left-to-Right Shunt

FIG 16–4.
Thoracic roentgenogram of asymptomatic patient with ductus diverticulum; posteroanterior (**A**) and left anterior oblique (**B**) projections. Large mass *(arrows)* in left upper mediastinum (**A**) and in the region of the posterior aortic arch (**B**). Right ventriculogram, late phase in anteroposterior (**C**) projection. Large aortic ductus diverticulum *(arrows);* the ductus arteriosus is not patent.

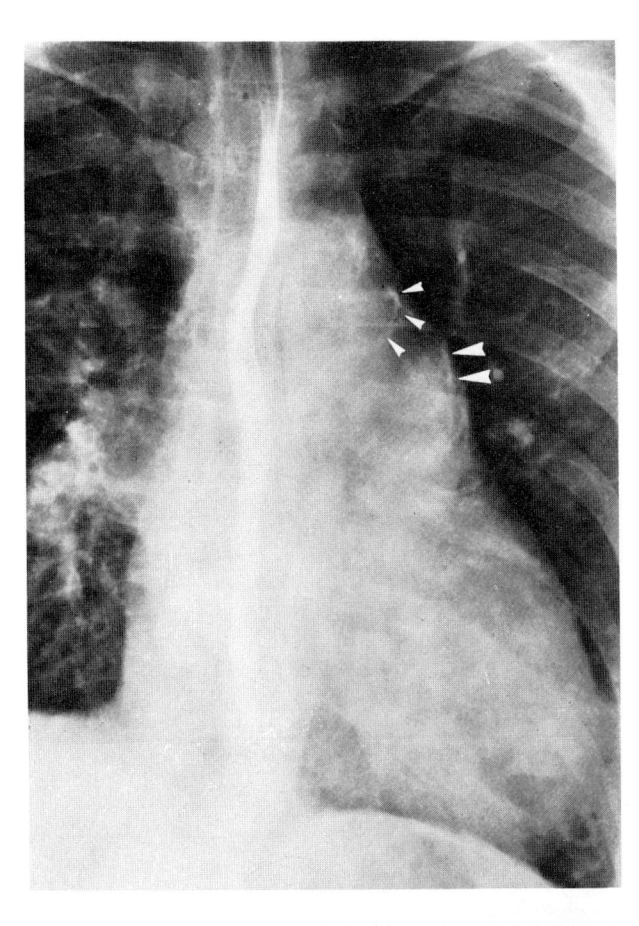

FIG 16–5.
Thoracic roentgenogram, posteroanterior projection of PDA in adult. Ringlike calcium deposits *(small arrows)* in the wall of the ductus. Calcifications *(large arrows)* in the main pulmonary artery indicate pulmonary atherosclerosis caused by long-standing pulmonary hypertension. The left upper lobe is hypovascular.

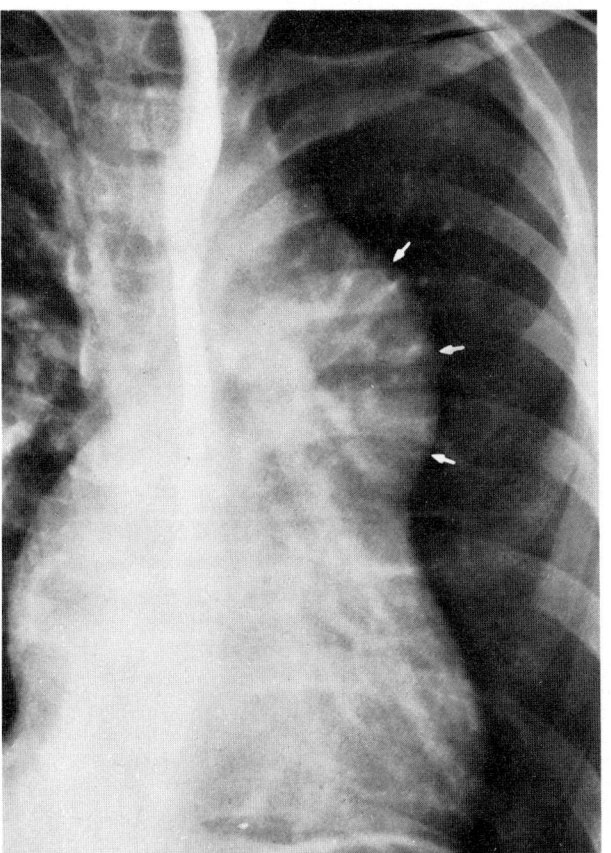

FIG 16–6.
Thoracic roentgenogram, posteroanterior projection of patient with PDA, pulmonary vascular disease, and right-to-left shunt. Aneurysmal dilatation of the main pulmonary artery segment; this occurs most commonly in reversing patent ductus (reason unknown). The right pulmonary artery and peripheral pulmonary arteries appear normal. Sparsity of blood flow throughout the left lung. Radiographically, the appearance resembles that of valvular pulmonary stenosis or idiopathic dilatation of the pulmonary artery, but most patients with valvular pulmonary stenosis also have poststenotic dilatation of the left pulmonary artery. This does not occur in reversing ductus arteriosus.

through the ductus is directed against the direction of blood flow in the left pulmonary artery. Blood flow into the left pulmonary artery decreases, particularly during diastole, because of inflow of blood from the ductus in the opposite direction (entrainment of the surrounding blood by the jet).

14. Patent ductus arteriosus with a right-to-left shunt commonly causes enormous enlargement of the pulmonary artery, which may grow to aneurysmal proportions (Fig 16–6). The cause of this enlargement is unknown but probably is the combination of increased pulmonary arterial pressure and increased flow through the reversing ductus. (Blood flows predominately into the descending aorta from the main pulmonary artery and the PDA; Fig 16–7.)

15. Although cardiomegaly and radiographic signs of pulmonary hypertension usually are found in patients with a reversing PDA, there are exceptions. As in ventricular septal defect with pulmonary vascular disease, cardiac size and the pulmonary vasculature may appear normal (Fig 16–8). These patients probably maintain their high fetal pulmonary vascular resistance and never develop a left-to-right shunt. For some unknown reason, the thick-walled pulmonary arteries do not dilate.

16. In prematurely born infants, the radiographic findings of a large PDA are different. In this age group, the ductus is usually complicated by the respiratory distress syndrome. The lung fields show a diffuse reticular-alveolar pattern, which is typical for respiratory syndrome but may also reflect some degree of pulmonary edema (Fig 16–9).

CARDIAC CATHETERIZATION

Because the diagnosis of PDA usually can be made clinically, the value of cardiac catheterization data is not as great as in many other conditions.

The diagnosis can be suspected from the characteristic

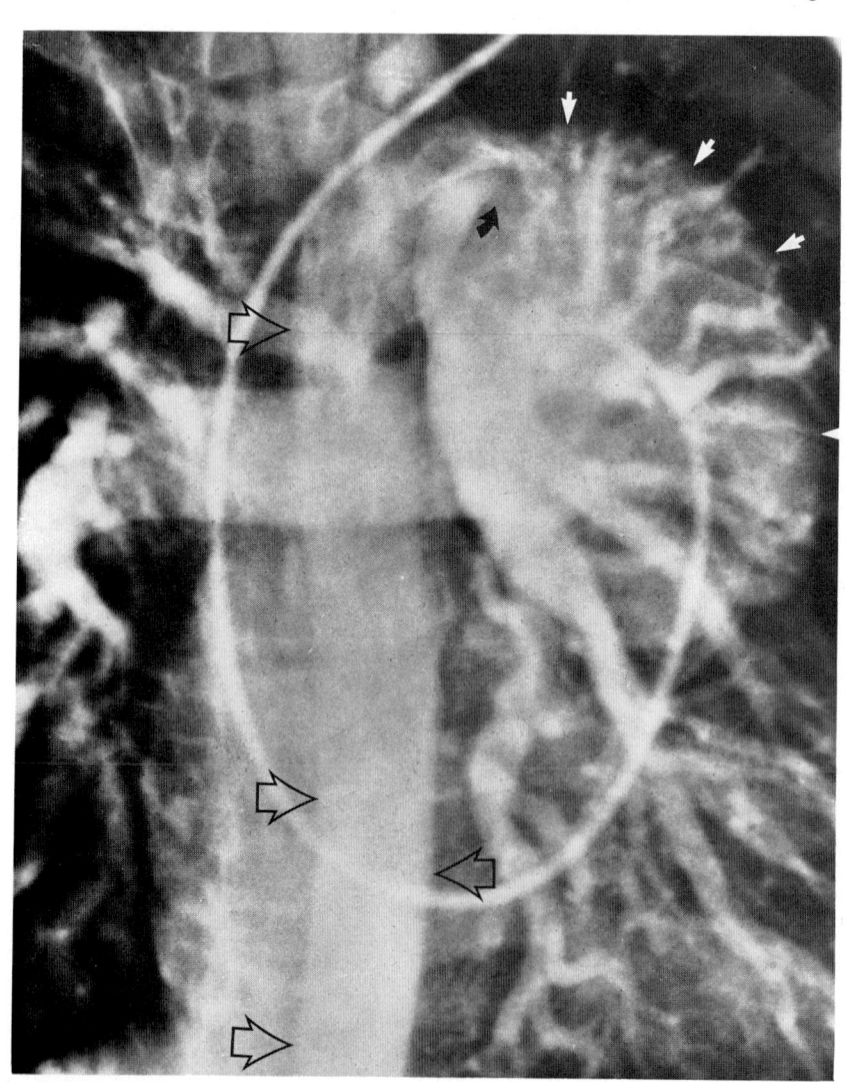

FIG 16–7.
Pulmonary arteriogram, anteroposterior projection of patients with reversing patent ductus with huge, aneurysmal main pulmonary artery *(white arrows)*. The peripheral pulmonary arteries are normal in size but tortuous, a radiographic sign of pulmonary vascular disease. The descending aorta is well opacified *(open arrows)* through the reversing patent ductus *(curved black arrow)*. Very likely, the increased flow and pressure cause the aneurysmal dilatation of the pulmonary artery.

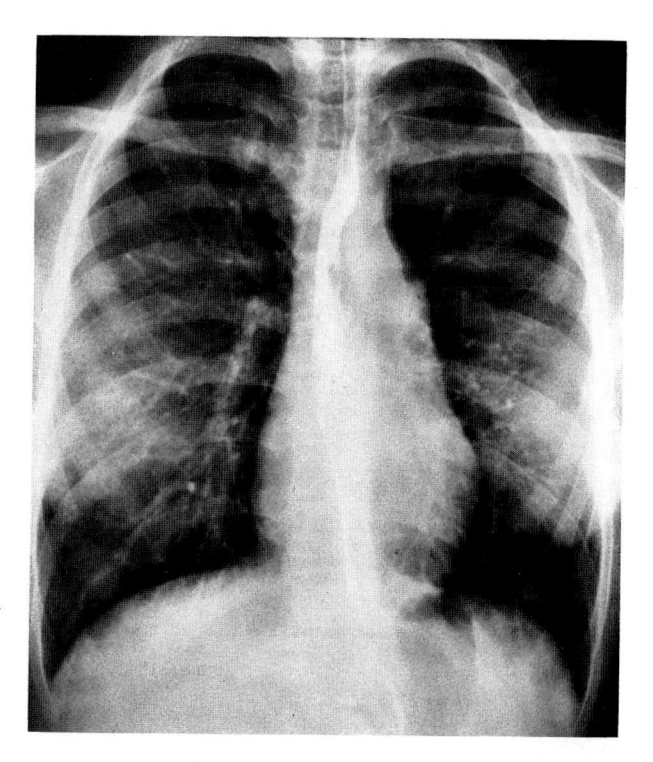

FIG 16–8.
Thoracic roentgenogram, posteroanterior projection of patient with PDA, severe pulmonary vascular disease, and right-to-left shunt. Normal cardiac size. Pulmonary vasculature appears at lower range of normal, with no radiographic signs of disease. Nonetheless, severe pulmonary hypertension may be present without radiographic evidence, similar to instances of ventricular septal defect (Eisenmenger's syndrome and pulmonary vascular disease).

catheter course into the descending aorta (see Fig 6–1). The presence of a ductus can be verified by always passing the catheter below the diaphragm to rule out passage into the left pulmonary artery. On very rare occasions, the catheter passes upward into the aortic arch. Passage of the catheter through a ductus does not necessarily mean patency, particularly in neonates.

Oximetry data show an increase in oxygen saturation in the pulmonary artery, particularly the left pulmonary artery. Because of streaming effects, it is difficult to determine the volume of the shunt from oximetry data. It is impossible to obtain a representative sample from the pulmonary artery. An increase in oxygen saturation between the right ventricle and the pulmonary artery of at least 5% is required for the diagnosis of a significant left-to-right shunt. When a ventricular septal defect and PDA coexist, it is usually impossible to detect the ductus arteriosus by oximetry data.[20] When a right-to-left shunt occurs through a ductus, oxygen saturation in the descending aorta is lower than the ascending aorta.

The pulmonary arterial and right ventricular systolic pressures range from normal to systemic levels. The aortic and pulmonary arterial pulse pressures are wide in most patients. As pulmonary vascular disease develops, the

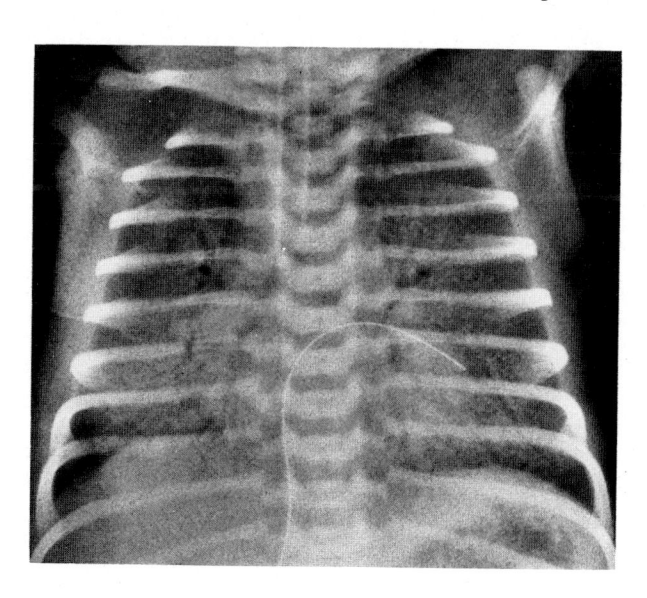

FIG 16–9.
Thoracic roentgenogram, posteroanterior projection of premature infant with respiratory distress syndrome and PDA. Air bronchogram indicates lung disease. Diagnosis of associated PDA can be made only by aortography.

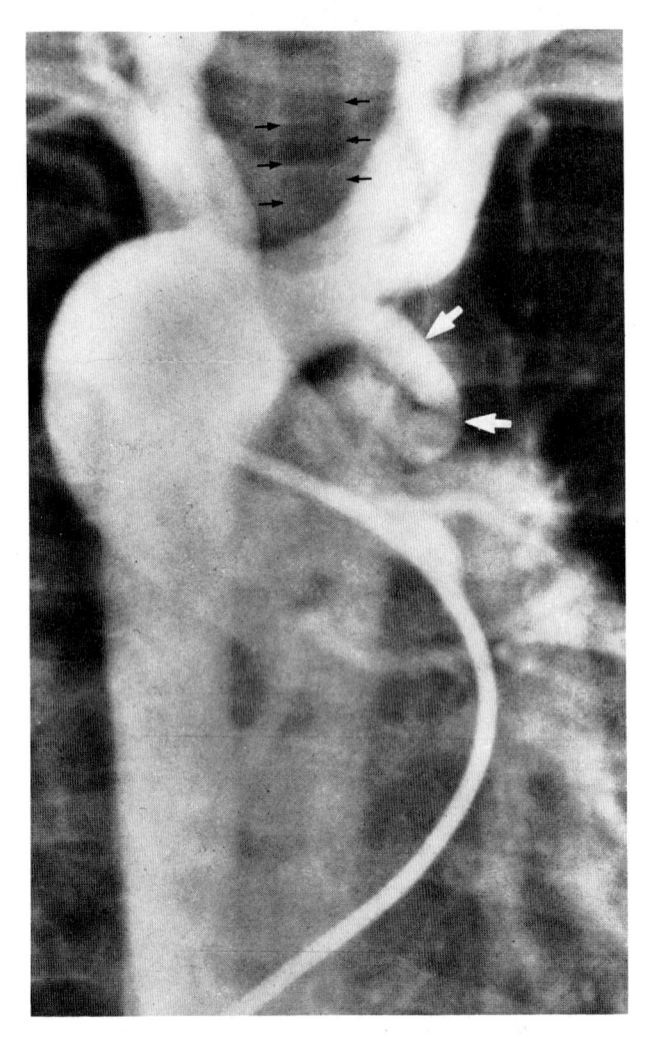

FIG 16–10.
Aortogram, anteroposterior projection of patients with coexisting ventricular septal defect and PDA. Catheter passed through the ventricular septal defect into the ascending aorta. Right aortic arch, passing to right of the trachea *(small black arrows)*. A long, tortuous, left-sided patent ductus *(small white arrows)* arises from the left subclavian artery. (A ductus opposite the aortic arch always arises from the subclavian artery). The trachea is not shifted, because the aorta and ductus form a vascular ring that prevents it.

1. The most sensitive technique for demonstrating a PDA with a left-to-right shunt is aortography performed through a catheter, which can be introduced via the brachial, umbilical, or femoral route and advanced to the ascending aorta. However, a ductus can also be demonstrated by retrograde brachial angiography, which does not require a catheter. Contrast medium is injected through a cannula into the brachial artery, which serves as the catheter. If the left arm was used, the contrast medium opacifies the ductus, which lies just opposite the left subclavian artery.
   If there is an associated ventricular septal defect, the catheter can usually be passed through the defect into the ascending aorta during right-heart catheterization and an aortogram performed at that site (Fig 16–10).
2. In patients with a PDA and a left-to-right shunt, pulmonary angiography usually does not opacify the ductus. Unopacified blood coming through the patent ductus causes a well-defined radiolucency on the superior aspect of the opacified pulmonary artery (Fig 16–11).

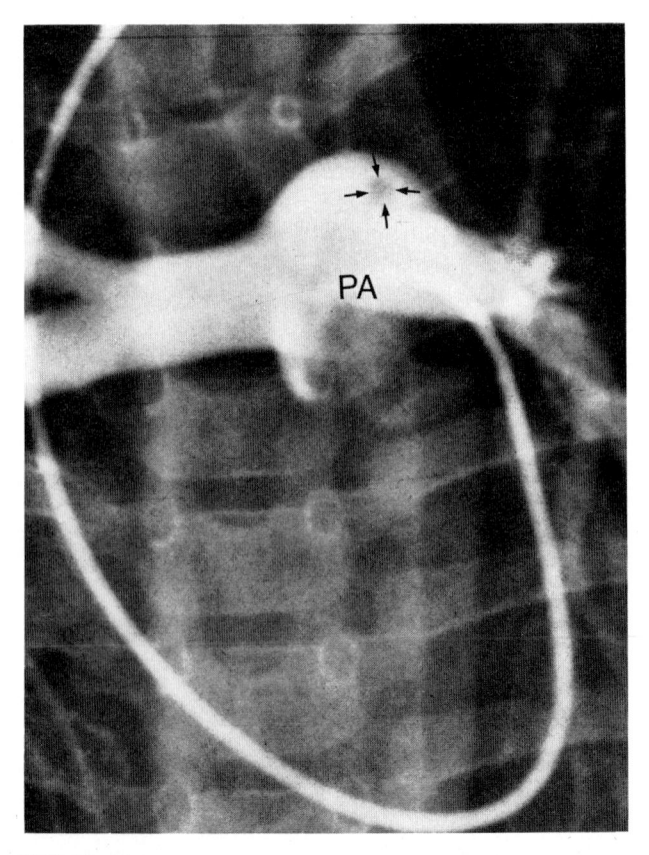

FIG 16–11.
Pulmonary angiogram *(PA)*, anteroposterior projection of patient with small PDA, evidenced by a small round filling defect *(arrow)*. REASON: Jet of unopacified blood through the patent ductus dilutes the contrast medium.

pulse pressure in both great vessels narrows, and the murmur disappears (silent ductus).

ANGIOGRAPHIC APPEARANCE

Various angiographic techniques have been used to demonstrate a PDA. Because of the great variability in size and direction of blood flow (left to right, right to left, or little flow; usually referred to as "balanced ductus"), the techniques vary in their usefulness in observing a patent ductus:

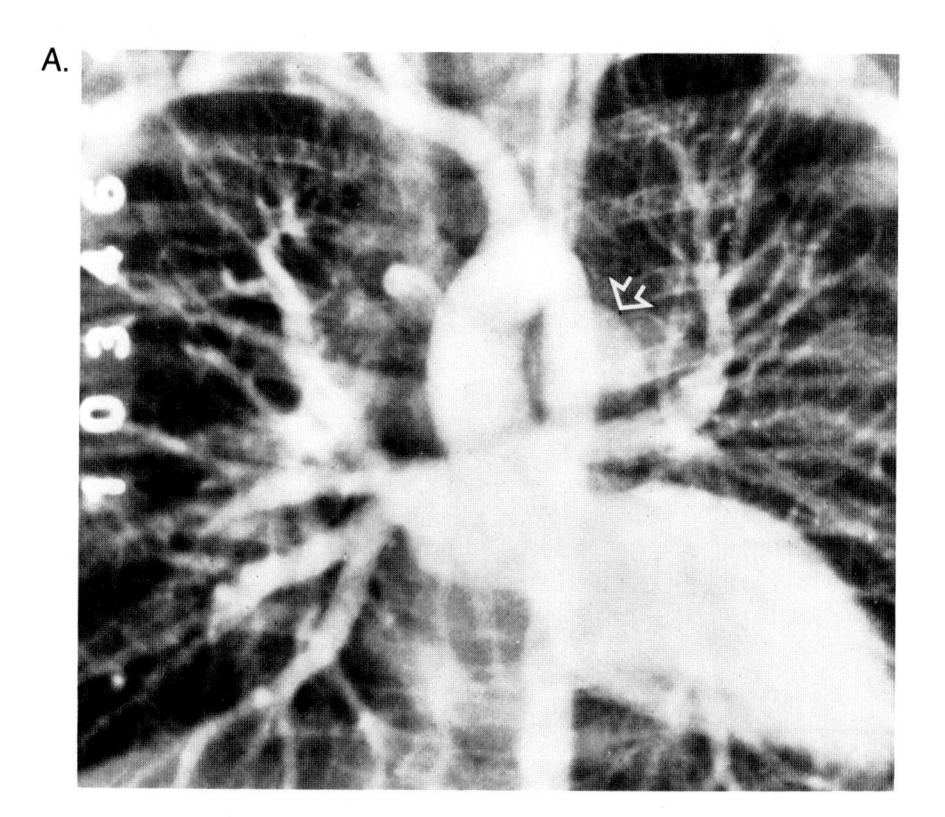

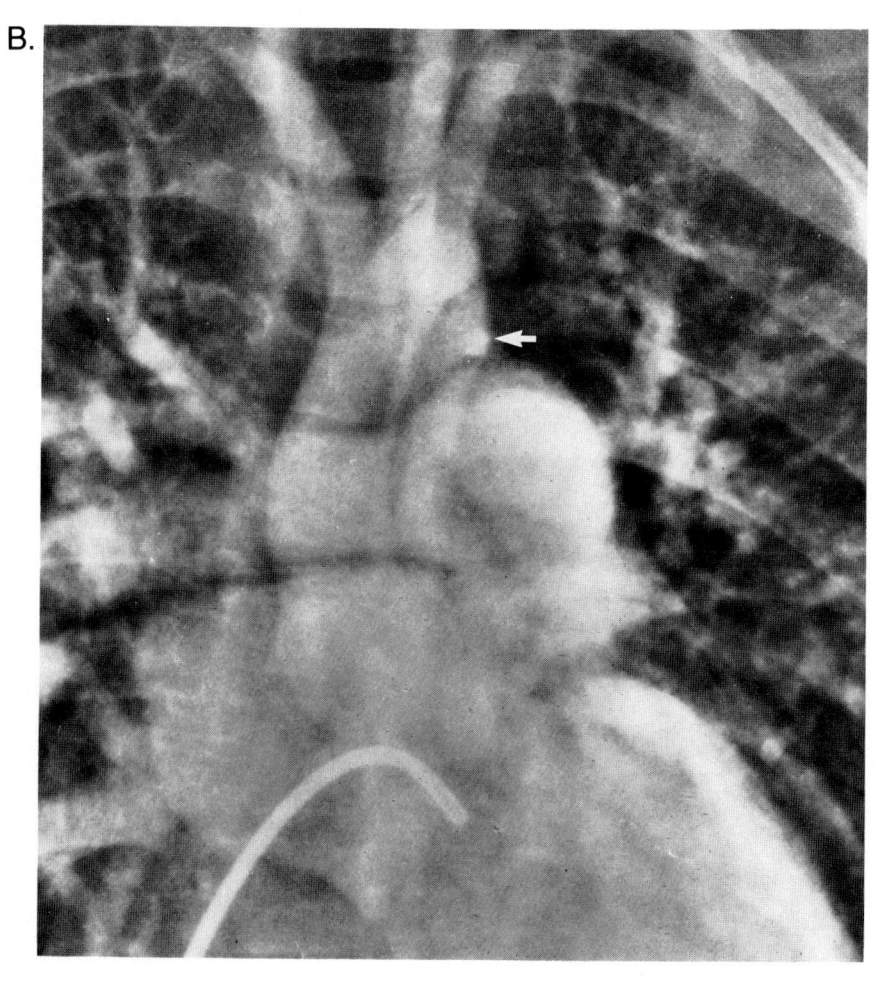

FIG 16–12.
Patent ductus arteriosus. **A,** venous angiogram, anteroposterior projection; reopacification of the pulmonary artery *(open arrow)*. This technique is successful only in young patients without additional shunts. **B,** right ventriculogram, anteroposterior projection late phase. Reopacification of the pulmonary artery. Small PDA visible as round density *(arrow)*. REASON: The ductus is filled with contrast medium and seen on end in the anteroposterior projection.

3. On the levophase of an injection of contrast medium into the right ventricle or pulmonary artery, reopacification of the pulmonary artery occurs. A PDA is usually seen as an added density in the area of the pulmonary artery on an anteroposterior projection (Fig 16–12). This technique is the least sensitive for diagnosis of PDA.
4. It is more difficult to demonstrate a PDA with a right-to-left shunt by aortography unless balloon occlusion is used (see Chapter 8). It can usually be seen on aortography as a filling defect by dilution.
   REASON: Unopacified blood flows through the PDA and enters the opacified descending aorta (Fig 16–13).
5. Patent ductus arteriosus with a right-to-left shunt can best be demonstrated by pulmonary arteriography. Whenever there is a right-to-left shunt through a ductus arteriosus, an aortic obstruction, either coarctation or interruption of the aortic arch proximal to the ductus, must be excluded. Pulmonary arteriography with a right-to-left shunt does not opacify the distal portion of the aortic arch. This drawback can usually be overcome by balloon occlusion aortography (Fig 16–14).
6. Patent ductus secondary to rubella infection can be angiographically recognized because of the characteristic abnormalities of the pulmonary artery and valve (Fig 16–15):
   a. A short main pulmonary artery with a normal caliber.
   b. A vertical position of the pulmonary valve.
   c. Thickening of the pulmonary valve.
   d. Pulmonary insufficiency.
      Not all features are present in an individual patient.
7. Occasionally the distinction between a PDA, a systemic origin of a pulmonary artery, or origin of the pulmonary artery from the ascending aorta may be impossible angiographically (Figs 16–16 and 16–17). In these circumstances, only surgery postmortem examination allows the identification of a PDA, by finding of the recurrent nerve passing around the ductus.
8. A right-sided PDA with a right descending aorta may compress the right bronchus and result in lobar emphysema (Fig 16–18). In the reconstruction of an interrupted right aortic arch with a graft, this compression must be relieved.
9. The catheter course through a right-sided PDA and right aortic arch is characteristic.

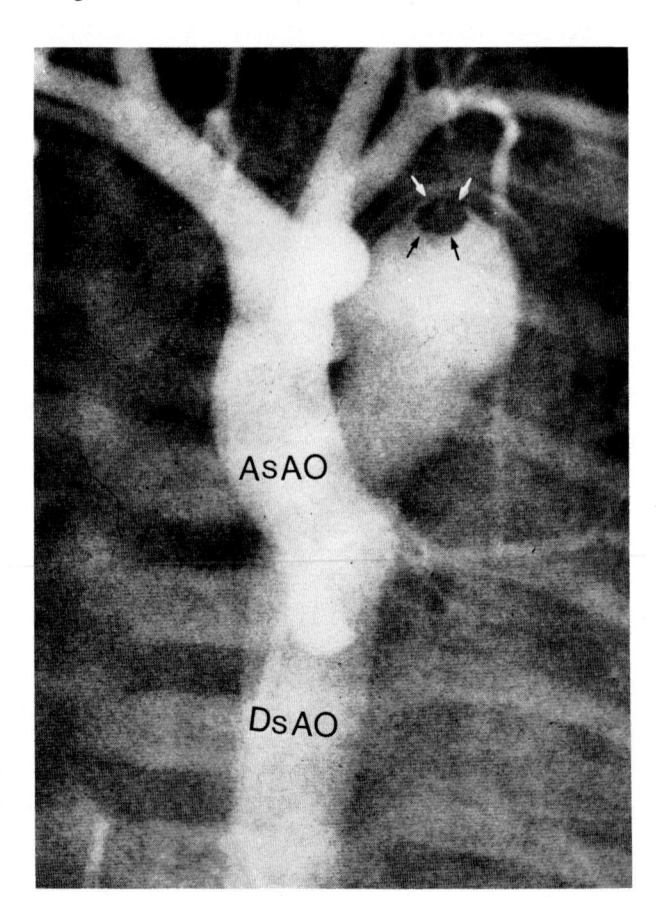

FIG 16–13.
Aortogram, in patient with reversing PDA. The ductus appears as a round filling defect *(white arrows)* in the opacified decending aorta. Descending aorta is larger than the ascending aorta, a common finding in reversing patent ductus. Dilution of contrast medium in the descending aorta from inflow of unopacified blood through the reversing patent ductus. *AsAO* = ascending aorta; *DsAO* = descending aorta.

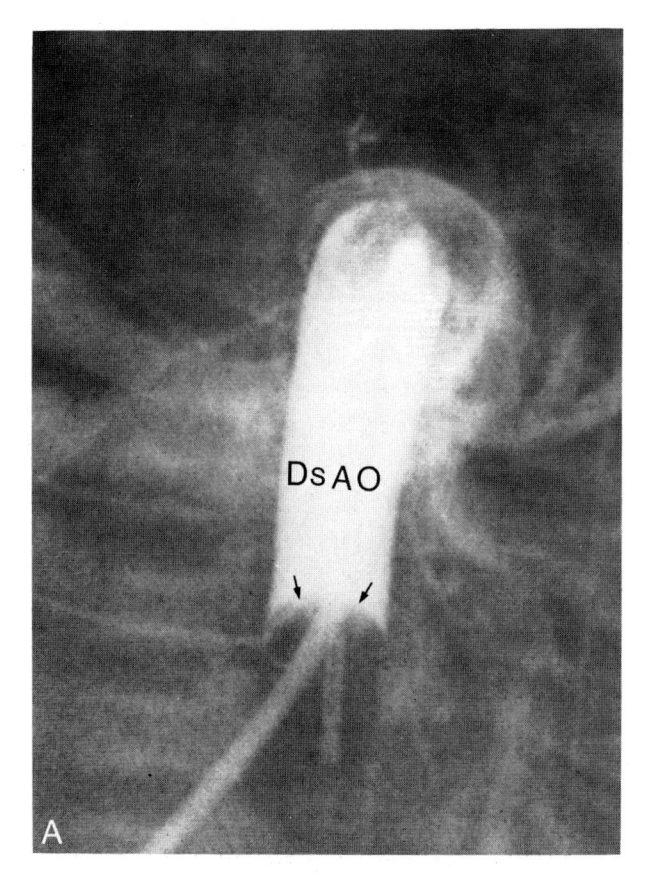

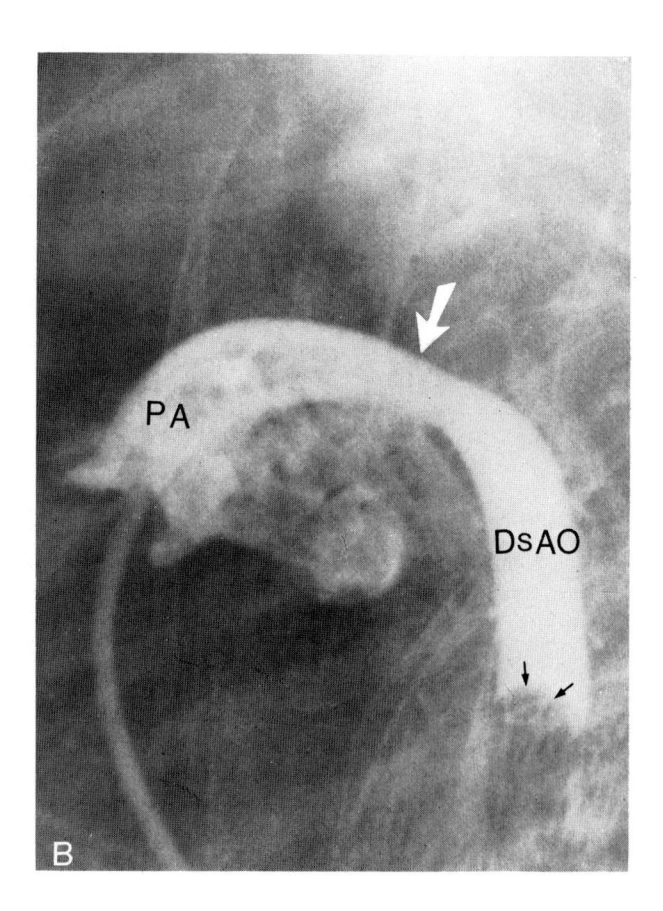

FIG 16-14.
Aortogram with balloon occlusion in anteroposterior **(A)** and lateral **(B)** projections. Catheter passed through the pulmonary artery and ductus arteriosus into the descending aorta. The inflated balloon *(small black arrows)* obstructs the descending aorta; contrast medium has been injected through the proximally located holes of the catheter. Large PDA visible *(white arrow)*. The distal aortic arch is not opacified, indicating an interruption. Descending aortography or selective pulmonary angiography without balloon occlusion commonly results in inadequate anatomic demonstration of the ductus and distal aortic arch. Exact demonstration of the anatomy, particularly of coarctation, is of great practical importance, and balloon occlusion aortography, although unphysiological, provides the best anatomic information. *DsAO* = descending aorta; *PA* = pulmonary artery.

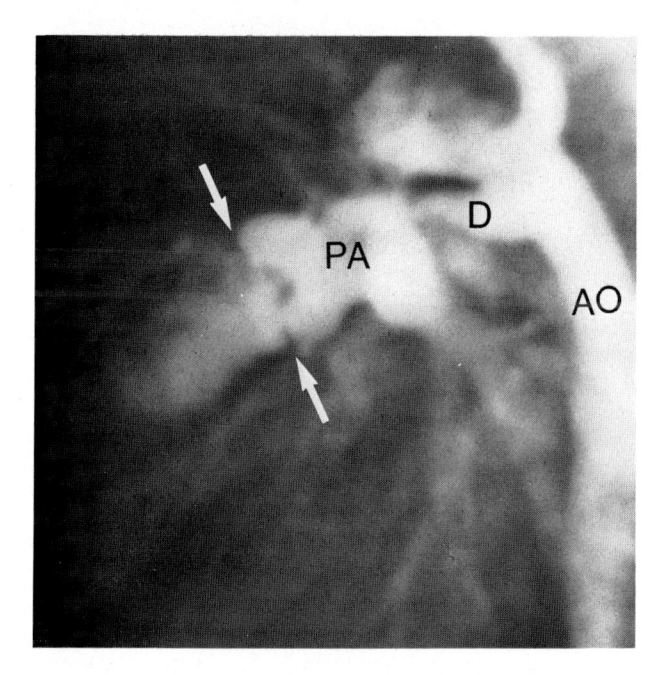

FIG 16-15.
Aortogram, lateral projection shows characteristic angiographic features associated with a ductus arteriosus *(D)* in rubella syndrome. The main pulmonary artery *(PA)* is of normal diameter. Plane of thickened pulmonary valve oriented more vertically. Main pulmonary artery *(PA)* is short, with considerable pulmonary insufficiency. Pulmonary artery is not enlarged in spite of patent ductus. *AO* = aorta.

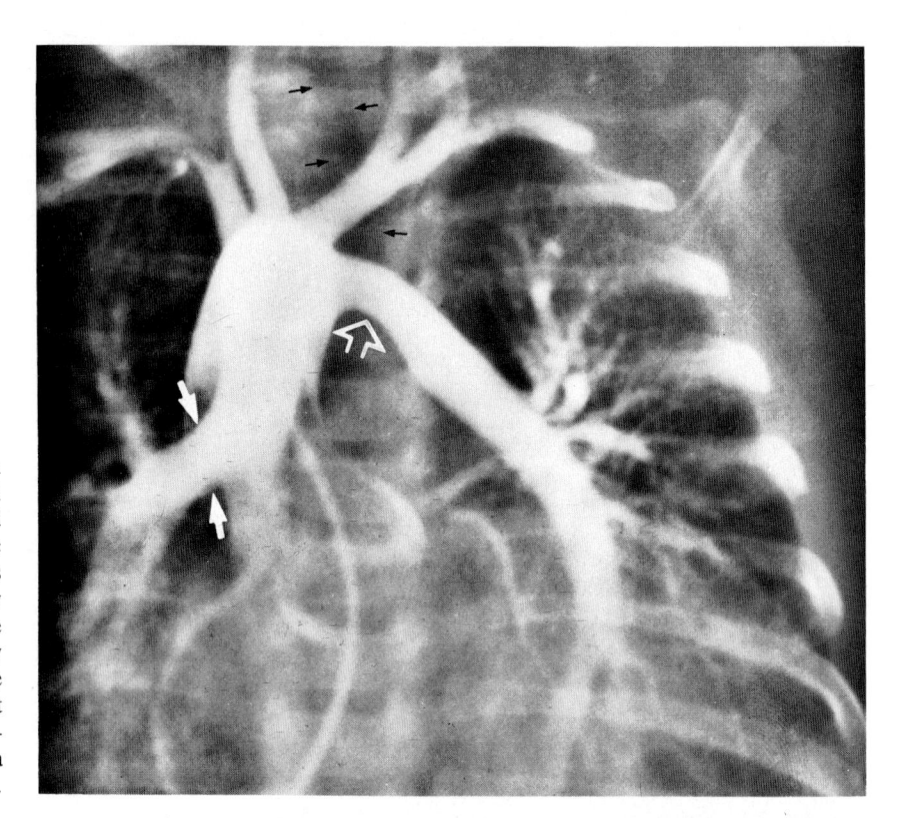

FIG 16–16.
Aortogram, anteroposterior projection with catheter passed through a ventricular septal defect into the ascending aorta. Associated pulmonary atresia and right-sided aortic arch. Trachea *(small black arrows)* passes to the left of the arch. The right pulmonary artery *(small white arrows)* arises from the descending aorta. Left pulmonary artery *(open arrow)* arises atypically high from the aortic arch; this could represent a PDA, but it should arise from the left subclavian artery. More likely, the finding represents a systemic origin of the left pulmonary artery.

10. Not only may the aortic side of the ductus remain open and form a ductus diverticulum, but so may the pulmonary arterial end of the ductus. This pulmonary ductus diverticulum (Fig 16–19) cannot be seen on thoracic roentgenograms because it lies within the mediastinum. Its presence interferes with the angiographic demonstration of the pulmonary artery bifurcation.

Rarely are cardiac catheterization and angiocardiography required before operation. In most patients, the diagnosis can be made accurately without these methods, being based principally on the finding of a continuous murmur. However, it is essential to identify patients with conditions associated with pulmonary atresia or severe pulmonary stenosis, when the ductus may be patent and create a continuous murmur, because in these cases, ligation would be lethal. Differentiation of PDA from an aorticopulmonary window may be difficult by auscultation alone.

MANAGEMENT

With the discovery of the vasoactive prostaglandins, therapy of PDA in the neonate has changed considerably. Prostaglandin E_1 is a potent dilator of the ductus,[9–11] and indeed is now widely used to maintain ductal patency in neonates with ductus-dependent lesions. If prostaglandin synthesis could be inhibited, then perhaps the ductus would close. Indomethacin, a prostaglandin synthetase inhibitor, thus has been given to premature infants to effect

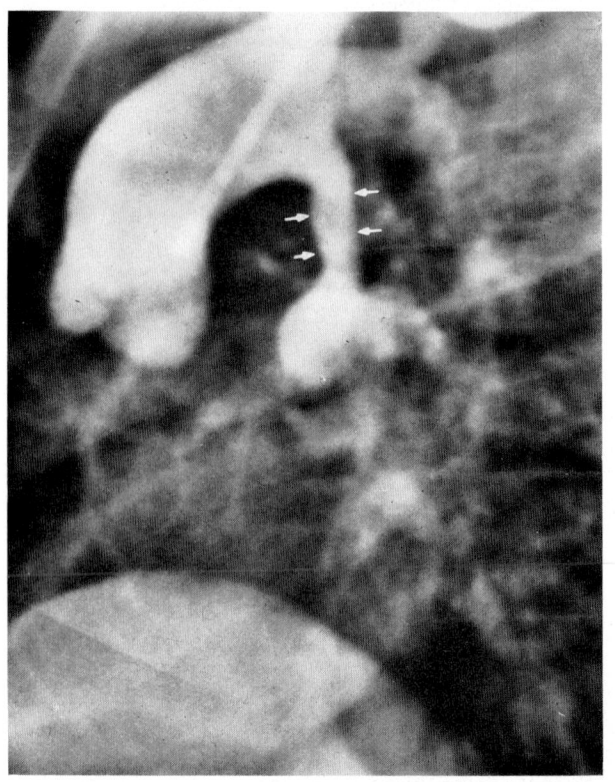

FIG 16–17.
Aortogram, lateral projection in patient with asplenia and pulmonary atresia. Ductuslike structure *(arrows)* arises high in the aortic arch supplying the pulmonary artery. The location is atypical for a PDA but most commonly seen in pulmonary atresia and intact septum.

closure of a patent ductus.[21-23] This treatment is most effective in the more premature infant and during the first week of life; in these groups, perhaps one half of the ductus lesions close or shrink, although it is difficult to determine the exact incidence because of the natural occurrence of spontaneous closure. Medical management of a premature infant with a PDA also includes restriction of fluid intake (to reduce pulmonary edema), use of a respirator, maintenance of hemoglobin concentration, and digitalis administration.

Operation remains the mainstay of management. Ligation of PDA was first accomplished by Robert Gross in 1938, and although some modifications have been made, his remains the standard technique. The procedure is carried out without extracorporeal circulation through a left lateral thoracotomy. Previously, single ligation of patent ductus led to a high recurrence rate, probably because of inadequate exposure and the use of silk sutures. Now most surgeons prefer to divide the ductus, although in infants, single, double, or triple ligation is usually carried out (Fig

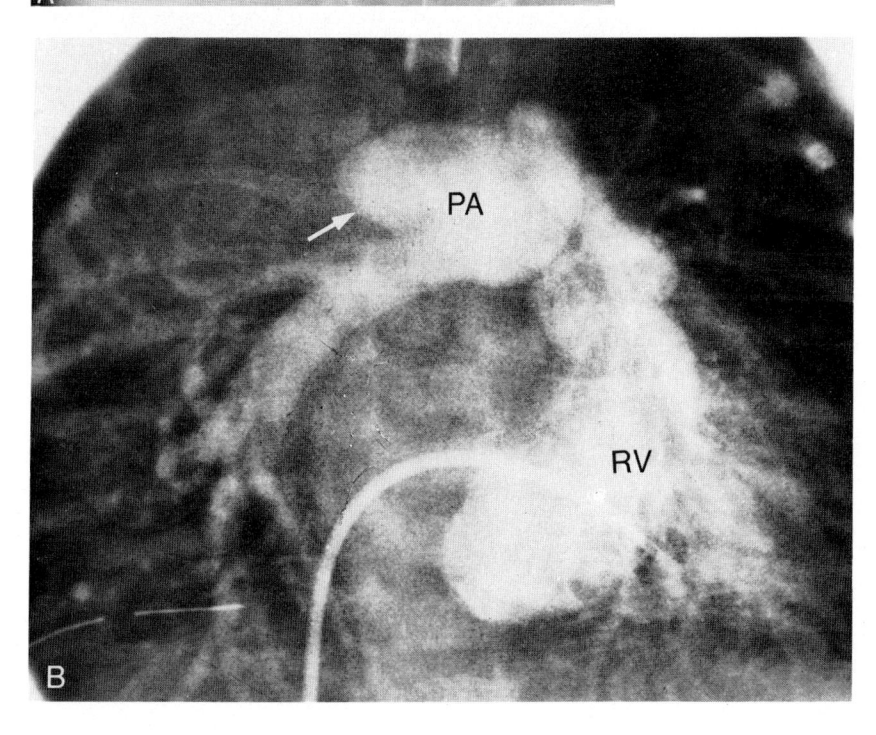

FIG 16–18.
Neonate with respiratory distress syndrome; right aortic arch and large right-sided ductus arteriosus compresses the right mainstem bronchus. **A,** thoracic roentgenogram, posteroanterior projection shows lobar emphysema of entire right lung. Marked mediastinal shift to left, depression of right hemidiaphragm, and herniation of mediastinum toward left *(arrows)*. **B,** right ventriculogram, anteroposterior projection shows right-sided aortic arch. Large right-sided ductus diverticulum *(arrows)* causes compression with atelectasis of right upper lobe.

C. BRONCHIAL COMPRESSION BY RIGHT SIDED P.D.A.

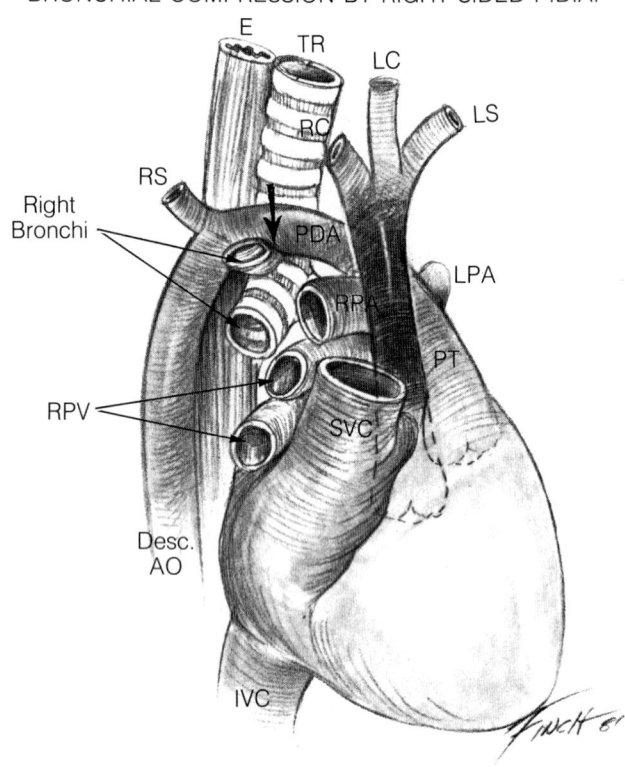

FIG 16–18 (cont'd.).
C, diagram of heart viewed from right; right-sided aortic arch is interrupted. Descending aorta supplied by right-sided PDA, which compresses right upper lobe bronchus, leading to emphysema. IVC = inferior vena cava; SVC = superior vena cava; RPA = right pulmonary artery; LPA = left pulmonary artery; PDA = patent ductus arteriosus; RS = right subclavian artery; RC = right carotid artery; TR = trachea; LC = left carotid artery; LS = left subclavian artery; PT = pulmonary trunk.

16–20). If the ductus is an incidental lesion, as in a patient with a ventricular septal defect, it is ligated through a midline sternotomy. Proper ligation of the ductus arteriosus with modern suture material does not result in a significant recurrence rate.

Preoperative radiographic demonstration of calcium within the ductus of older patients is important to the surgeon, because it may necessitate a more difficult and complicated surgical repair.[24–27]

The operative risk is extremely low in children after the age of 6 months, but the risk is higher in older adults or infants less than 6 months. The operative risk in premature infants is surprisingly low; in one study, no different than for medical management.

The principal problem encountered in the operation is proper identification of the ductus arteriosus: The aortic arch, left pulmonary artery, left subclavian artery, or left mainstem bronchus may be ligated inadvertently. This

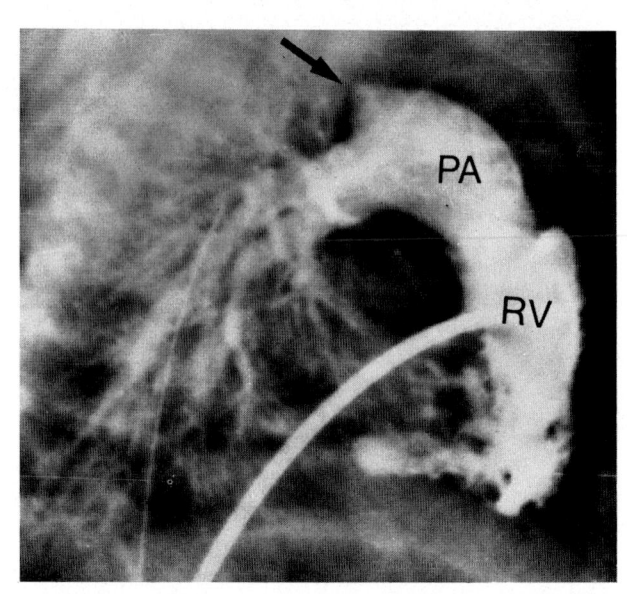

FIG 16–19.
Right ventriculogram, lateral projection showing ductus diverticulum of the pulmonary artery *(arrow)* that is not clinically significant. Unlike a ductus diverticulum of the aorta, this type of ductus diverticulum cannot be seen on thoracic roentgenograms because it is not outlined by air. It may interfere with angiographic demonstration of origins of right and left pulmonary arteries from pulmonary trunk.

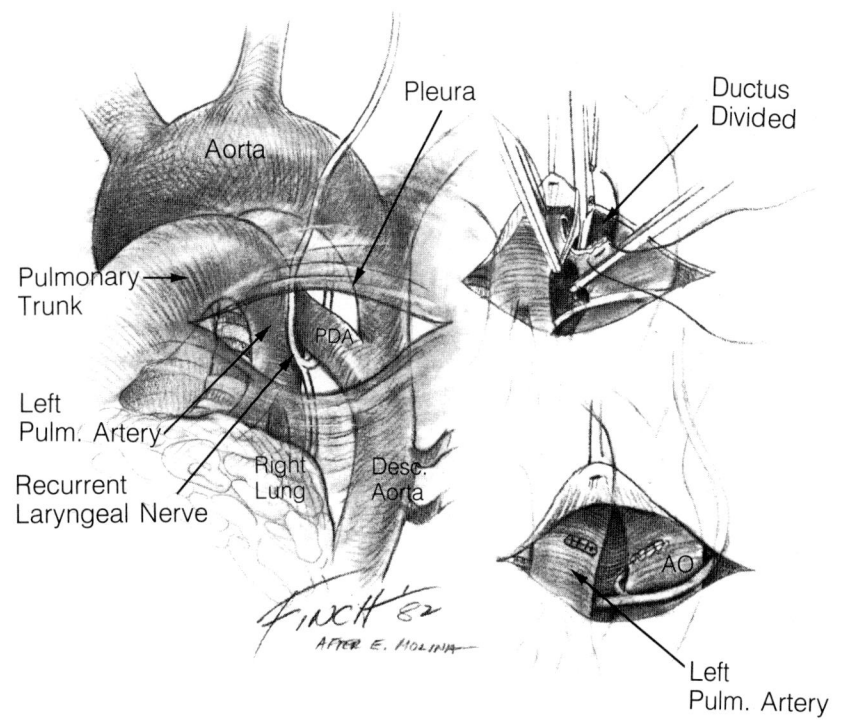

FIG 16–20.
Drawing of division of patent ductus (PDA) through left thoracotomy. Pleura has been incised, and ductus is identified on the basis of its relation to left recurrent nerve. Ductus is divided and closed by sutures. In infants, a ductus is commonly ligated two or three times rather than divided.

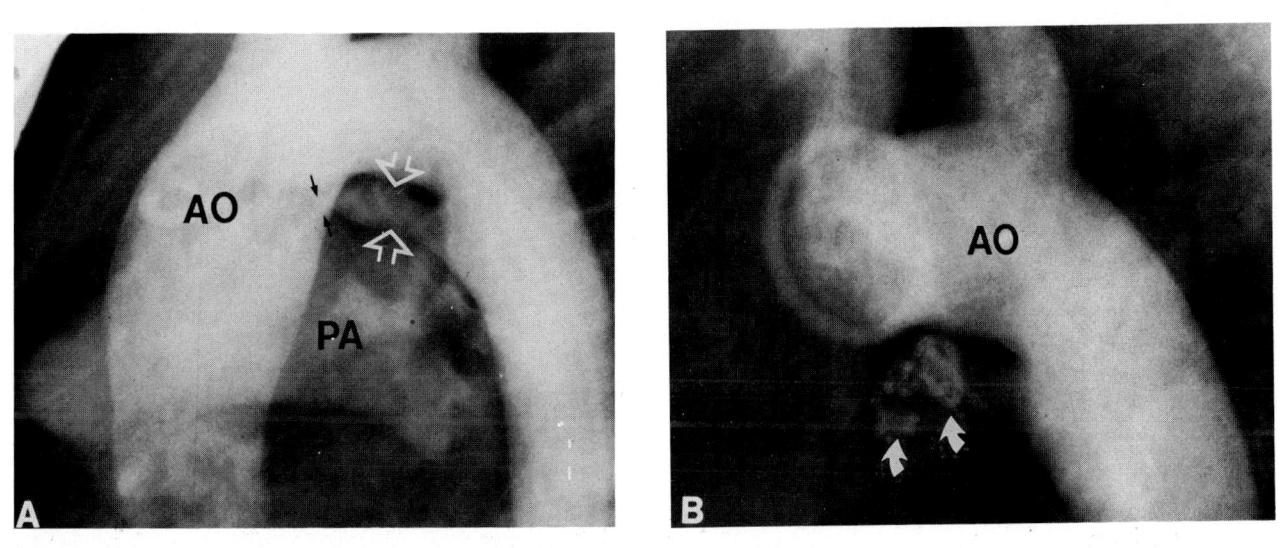

FIG 16–21.
A, lateral thoracic aortogram showing a large patent ductus *(open arrow)* with a small neck at the junction with the pulmonary artery *(small arrow)*. Because of its length and narrow pulmonary junction coil occlusion was safely carried out. **B,** successful occlusion of patent ductus by coils *(arrow)*.

usually results from incomplete exposure of the ductus, distal aortic arch, and proximal descending aorta. Most commonly, the ductus itself is mistaken for the aortic arch, particularly by the novice surgeon. Therefore, at the time of operation, the recurrent nerve, which always passes around the ductus arteriosus, must be identified.

Nonsurgical techniques for closing a patent ductus using cardiac catheterization have been developed, but so far they are technically difficult and limited to small long ductus with a neck at the pulmonary end (Fig 16–21).

POSTOPERATIVE RADIOGRAPHIC FEATURES

As in other conditions with a large left-to-right shunt, the division of a PDA causes a striking decrease in cardiac size and pulmonary vasculature (see Fig 16–21).

REFERENCES

1. Danilowicz D, Rudolph AM, Hoffman JIE: Delayed closure of the ductus arteriosus in premature infants, *Pediatrics* 37:74, 1966.
2. Thibeault DW, Emmanouilides GC, Nelson RJ, et al: Patent ductus arteriosus complicating the respiratory distress syndrome in preterm infants, *J Pediatr* 86:120, 1975.
3. Emmanouilides GC: Persistent patency of the ductus arteriosus in premature infants: incidence, perinatal factors, and natural history. In: Heymann MA, Rudolph AM, editors: *The Ductus Arteriosus,* Report of the Seventy-Fifth Ross Conference on Pediatric Research. Ross Laboratories, Columbus Ohio, pp. 63–68, 1978.
4. Alzamora-Castro V, Battilana G, Abugattas R, et al: Patent ductus arteriosus and high altitude, *Am J Cardiol* 5:761, 1960.
5. Anderson RC: Causative factors underlying congenital heart malformations: patent ductus arteriosus, *Pediatrics* 14:143, 1954.
6. Hastreiter AR, Joorabachi B, Pujatti G, et al: Cardiovascular lesions associated with congenital rubella, *J Pediatr* 71:59, 1967.
7. Moss AJ, Emmanouilides GC, Adams FH, et al: Response of ductus arteriosus and pulmonary and systemic arterial pressure to changes in oxygen environment in newborn infants, *Pediatrics* 33:937, 1964.
8. Neal WA, Bessinger FB Jr, Hunt CE, et al: Patent ductus arteriosus complicating respiratory distress syndrome, *J Pediatr* 86:127, 1975.
9. Coceani F, Olley PM: The response of the ductus arteriosus to prostaglandin, *Can J Physiol Pharmacol* 51:220, 1973.
10. Elliott RB, Starling MB, Neutze JM: Medical manipulations of the ductus arteriosus, *Lancet* 1:140, 1975.
11. Coceani F, Olley PM, Bodach E: Prostaglandins: a possible regulator of muscle tone in the ductus arteriosus, *Adv Prostagland Thrombox Res* 1:417, 1976.
12. McCarthy JS, Zies LG, Gelband H: Age-dependent closure of the patent ductus arteriosus by indomethacin, *Pediatrics* 62:706, 1978.
13. Gittenberger–de Groot AC, van Ertgruggen I, Moulaert AJMG, et al: The ductus arteriosus in the preterm infant: histologic and clinical observations, *J Pediatr* 96:88, 1980.
14. Gittenberger–de Groot AC: Persistent ductus arteriosus: most probably a primary congenital malformation, *Br Heart J* 39:610, 1977.
15. Moss A, Emmanouilides G, Duffie E: Closure of the ductus arteriosus in the newborn infant, *Pediatrics* 32:25, 1963.
16. Friedman WF, Pool, PE, Jacobowitz D, et al: Sympathetic innervation of the developing rabbit heart: biochemical and histochemical comparisons of fetal, neonatal, and adult myocardium, *Cir Res* 23:25, 1968.
17. Hoffman JIE, Buckberg GD: The myocardial supply: demand ratio—a critical review, *Am J Cardiol* 41:327, 1978.
18. Baylen BG, Meyer RA, Kaplan S, et al: The critically ill premature infant with patent ductus arteriosus and pulmonary disease: an echocardiographic assessment, *J Pediatr* 86:423, 1975.
19. Silverman NH, Lewis AB, Heymann MA, et al: Echocardiographic assessment of ductus arteriosus shunt in premature infants, *Circulation* 50:821, 1974.
20. Elliott LP, Ernst RW, Anderson RC, et al: Silent patent ductus arteriosus in association with ventricular septal defect: clinical, hemodynamic, pathological and surgical observations in forty patients, *Am J Cardiol* 10:475, 1962.
21. Yeh TF, Luken JA, Thalji A, et al: Intravenous indomethacin therapy in premature infants with persistent ductus arteriosus: a double-blind controlled study, *J Pediatr* 98:137, 1981.
22. Cifuentes RF, Olley PM, Balfe JW, et al: Indomethacin and renal function in premature infants with persistent patent ductus arteriosus, *J Pediatr* 95:583, 1979.
23. Merritt TA, White CL, Jacob J, et al: Patent ductus arteriosus treated with ligation or indomethacin: a follow-up study, *J Pediatr* 95:588, 1979.
24. Currarino G, Jackson J: Calcification of the ductus arteriosus and ligamentum botalli, *Radiology* 94:139, 1970.
25. Childe AE, Mackenzie E: Calcification in the ductus arteriosus. *Am J Roentgenol Radium Ther* 54:370, 1945.
26. Morrow AG, Clark WD: Closure of the calcified patent ductus: a new operative method utilizing cardiopulmonary bypass, *J Thorac Cardiovasc Surg* 51:534, 1966.
27. Ruskin H, Samuel E: Calcification in the patent ductus arteriosus, *Br J Radiol* 23:710, 1950.

CHAPTER 17

Aorticopulmonary Septal Defect (Window)

In aorticopulmonary septal defect (APSD), a communication exists between the proximal ascending aorta and the pulmonary artery. This location differs from that of patent ductus arteriosus, in which the proximal descending aorta and the left pulmonary artery communicate. Aorticopulmonary septal defect must be considered in the differential diagnosis of either large patent ductus arteriosus or ventricular septal defect with pulmonary hypertension. The condition is rare and occurs slightly more frequently in males.

EMBRYOLOGY

Aorticopulmonary septal defect results from incomplete fusion of the truncal ridges, which, as they develop, separate the aorta from the pulmonary trunk. Because of this incomplete fusion, a communication exists between the great arteries. The embryogenesis of this condition thus resembles that of truncus arteriosus, with an abnormal formation of the truncal ridges.

PATHOLOGIC ANATOMY

Aorticopulmonary septal defect is a fenestration between adjacent portions of the ascending aorta and pulmonary trunk or right pulmonary artery. In contrast to truncus arteriosus, both semilunar valves are present, and almost invariably, the ventricular septum is intact. The defect is usually large, ranging from 1 to 6 cm in diameter. Typically the defect lies about 1.5 cm above the level of the coronary arteries, but occasionally it is either higher in the aorta or below the level of the coronary arteries.

The anatomic forms of APSD have been classified in two ways.[1,2] In both classifications, a type I defect, the most common form, lies between the right wall of the pulmonary trunk and the left wall of the ascending aorta (Fig 17–1). Type II defects lie on the posterior wall of the ascending aorta and the proximal right pulmonary artery at its junction with the pulmonary trunk. In one classification,[2] a type III defect is defined as one involving both areas, whereas in the other classification,[1] a type III defect is defined as anomalous origin of the right pulmonary artery from the ascending aorta. We have discussed the latter as a separate condition (see Chapter 18), although the embryogenesis is probably similar.

Rarely, two APSDs coexist.[3] Usually the defect is merely a fenestration, having no length, but it may have a tiny channel.

ASSOCIATED ANOMALIES

Other cardiac anomalies coexist in 25% of patients. The most prevalent conditions are:

1. Patent ductus arteriosus.
2. Coarctation of aorta.
3. Ventricular septal defect.[4]
4. Interruption of aortic arch.[5]
5. Right aortic arch.

HEMODYNAMICS

Because in most patients the APSD is large, the aortic and pulmonary arterial pressures are equal. Thus, as in a large patent ductus arteriosus, the direction and magnitude of the shunt through the defect vary with the relative systemic and pulmonary vascular resistances. In most patients, there is a large left-to-right shunt, which causes cardiac failure because of the excessive left ventricular volume load. As in all types of large ventricular or great-

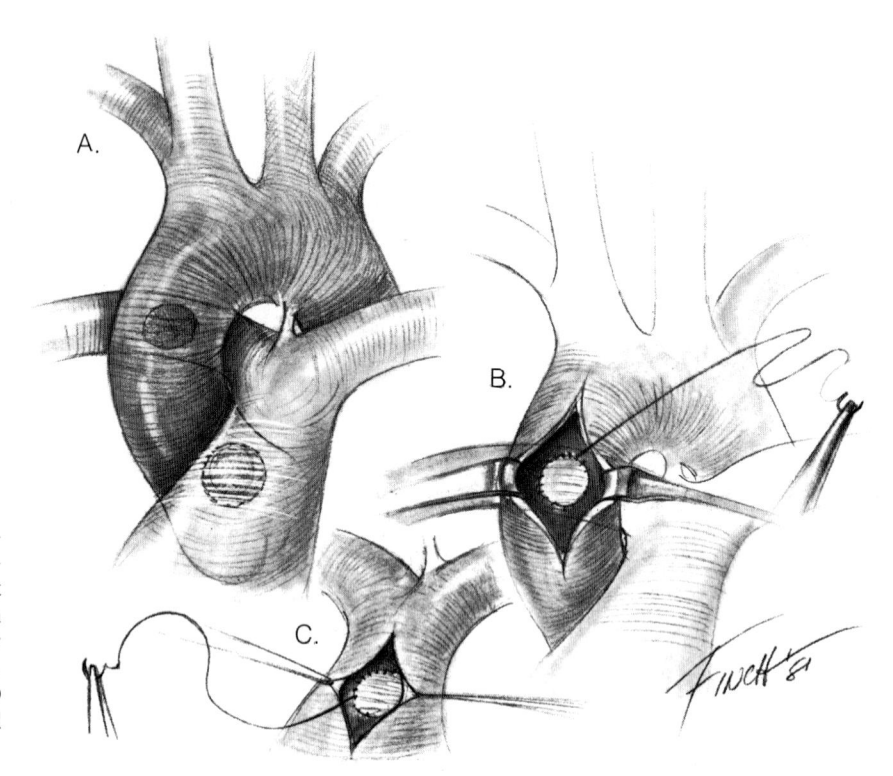

FIG 17–1.
Diagram of common locations of aortico-pulmonary septal defects (APSDs). **A,** between ascending aorta and proximal right pulmonary artery (distal type) and between ascending aorta and main pulmonary artery (proximal type), both defects may coexist. **B,** operative repair of distal type of APSD through ascending aorta and **(C)** proximal type through main pulmonary artery.

vessel communications, pulmonary vascular disease may develop, and eventually the shunt becomes right to left (Eisenmenger's Syndrome).

Rarely, the defect is small, and the pulmonary artery pressure remains below the systemic pressure.

CLINICAL FEATURES

Most patients are identified by the appearance of congestive cardiac failure and recurrent respiratory tract infections.[6] Occasionally, in patients with a small defect, cardiac disease is first recognized by the presence of a murmur. The pulse pressure may be increased, as in other aortic "runoff" lesions.

Auscultatory findings include:

1. A normal first heart sound.
2. Accentuated pulmonary component of the second heart sound, because of pulmonary hypertension.
3. Occasionally, a pulmonary systolic ejection click if the pulmonary trunk is dilated.
4. A loud systolic ejection murmur along the upper left sternal border, caused by blood flow through the defect.
5. Rarely, an early diastolic murmur of pulmonary regurgitation if pulmonary vascular disease develops.
6. An apical middiastolic murmur, caused by increased flow across the mitral valve because of large volume of pulmonary blood flow.
7. Rarely, a continuous murmur in patients with a small defect.

ELECTROCARDIOGRAPHIC FEATURES

The electrocardiogram varies and reflects the pulmonary arterial pressure, the pulmonary vascular resistance, and the volume of pulmonary blood flow. Typically, biventricular hypertrophy is present, but in infants and in patients with marked elevation of pulmonary vascular resistance, isolated right ventricular hypertrophy is found. The QRS axis varies widely. P waves are usually normal.

ECHOCARDIOGRAPHIC FEATURES

M-mode echocardiography shows dilatation of the left atrium and left ventricle and hypertrophy of the right ventricle. The structure and anatomic relations within the heart are normal. On cross-sectional echocardiography, echoes may drop out between the great vessels, suggesting the diagnosis.

RADIOGRAPHIC FEATURES

The specific diagnosis of an APSD cannot be made from a chest roentgenogram, because the radiographic

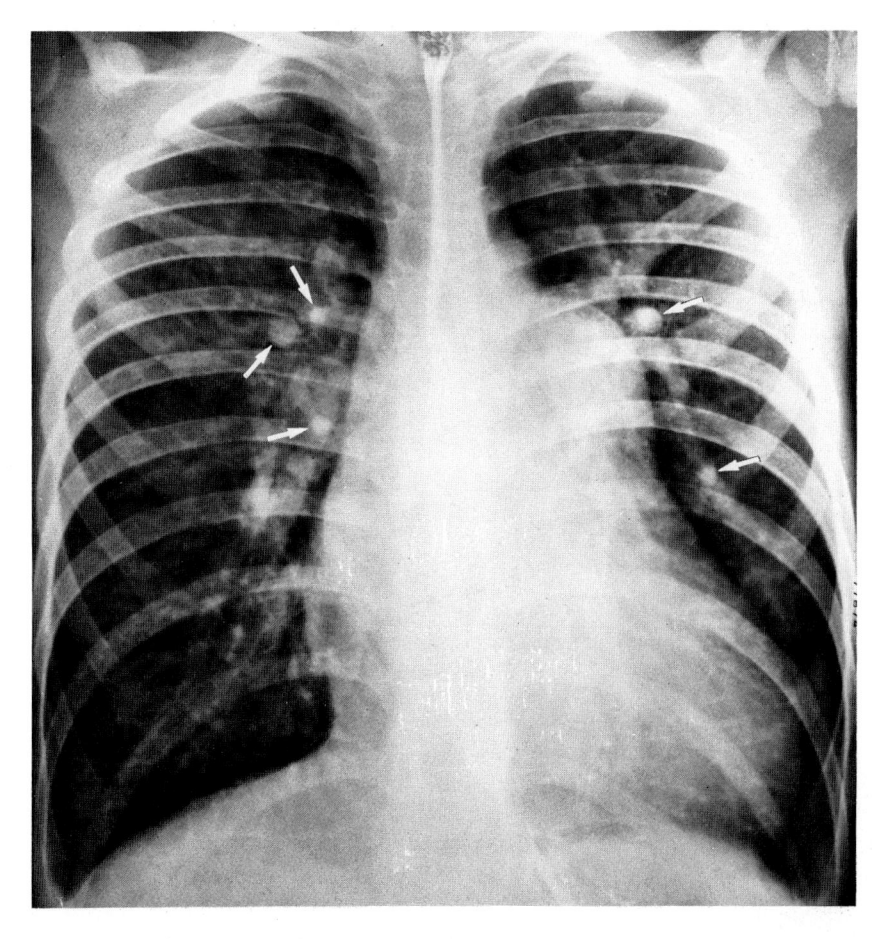

FIG 17–2.
Thoracic roentgenogram, posteroanterior projection of patient with APSD shows cardiomegaly. Enlargment of main pulmonary artery and well-defined, enlarged peripheral pulmonary arteries suggest pulmonary hypertension. Many pulmonary arterial branches are seen on-end because pulmonary hypertension causes tortuosity of the pulmonary arteries *(arrows)*. Minimal prominence of ascending aorta and knob. Radiographic findings identical to those of ventricular septal defect or patent ductus; correct diagnosis is not suggested by this film.

findings are identical to those of ventricular septal defect or patent ductus arteriosus:

1. Cardiac size and the pulmonary vasculature are usually markedly increased. REASON: Most APSDs are large and create a large left-to-right shunt. Patent ductus arteriosus, on the other hand, differs considerably in diameter and length, factors that increase the resistance to flow and decrease the left-to-right shunt.

2. The left atrium is enlarged in patients with low pulmonary resistance and a large volume of pulmonary blood flow. REASON: The increased blood flow through the left side of the heart causes left atrial and left ventricular enlargement.

3. If pulmonary resistance increases because of pulmonary vascular disease, radiographic signs of pulmonary hypertension become apparent. Cardiac size and left atrial enlargement decrease, as in instances of ventricular septal defect or patent ductus arteriosus with pulmonary vascular disease (Eisenmenger's syndrome).

4. The ascending aorta and aortic arch are either not prominent or only slightly enlarged. REASON: The blood flow through the ascending aorta is increased only to the level of the defect. Because these communications are located immediately above the aortic valve, the aortic knob is of normal size. In contrast, in patent ductus arteriosus, blood flow through the aortic arch is increased to the level of the ductus arteriosus. However, because APSDs result in a shunt during both systole and diastole, there is retrograde blood flow through the aortic arch during diastole. This may cause some prominence of the aortic knob, as in aortic insufficiency (Fig 17–2).

CARDIAC CATHETERIZATION

Cardiac catheterization and angiocardiography are usually needed to establish the diagnosis, because most patients with aortic pulmonic window cannot be differentiated from ventricular septal defect or an atypical patent ductus arteriosus. At time of catheterization, other cardiac conditions must be excluded as well.

The catheter course may be diagnostic (Fig 17–3). From the pulmonary trunk, it may be possible to advance the catheter into either the root of the aorta or the innominate artery. In a patent ductus arteriosus, with rare exceptions, the catheter tip would pass only into the descending aorta.

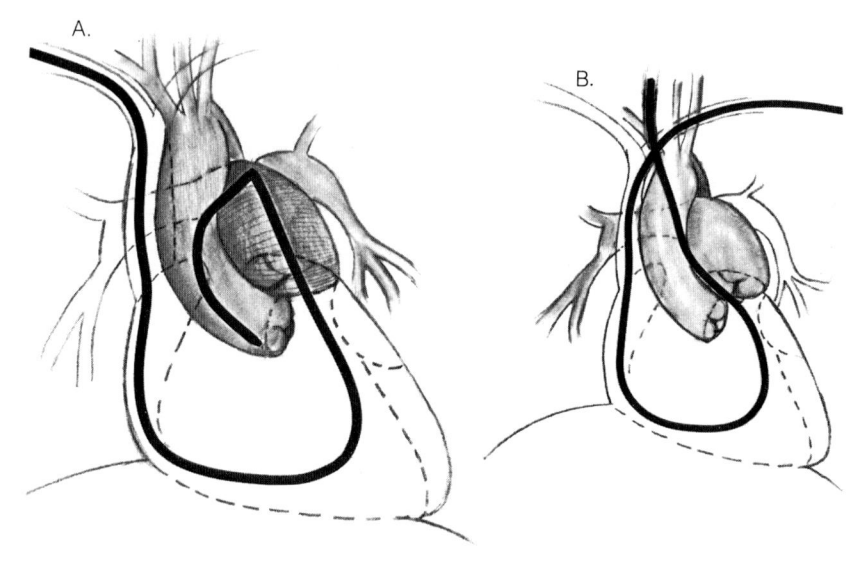

312 Cardiac Conditions Associated With a Left-to-Right Shunt

FIG 17–3.
Cardiac catheterization in APSD. **A,** diagram of catheter course; venous catheter passed through right-sided cardiac chambers into pulmonary trunk and through defect into ascending aorta. Catheter course virtually diagnostic for aortic pulmonic window. **B,** catheter tip advanced into right carotid artery; this catheter course is indistinguishable from the much more common passage through a high ventricular septal defect.

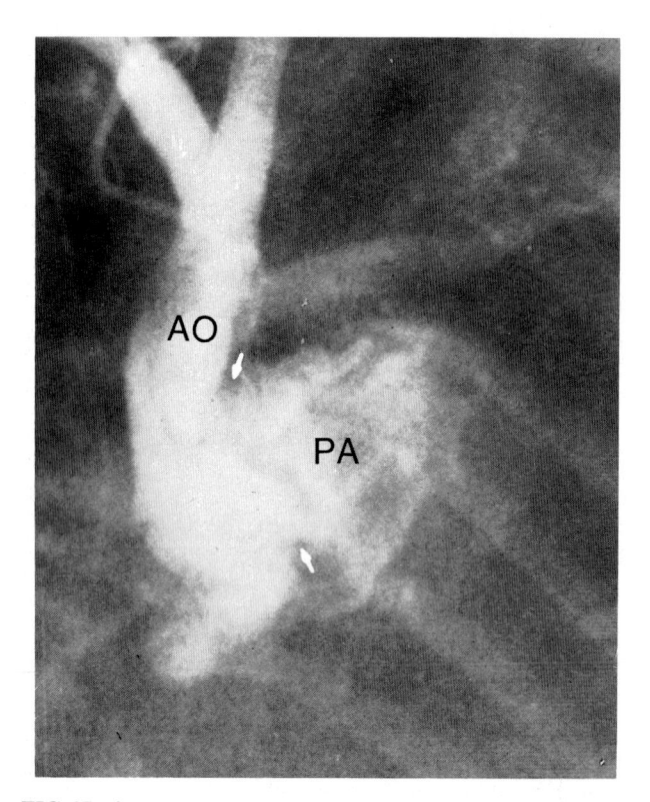

FIG 17–4.
Retrograde aortogram, anteroposterior projection shows opacification of ascending aorta *(AO)* and pulmonary artery *(PA)* through an unusually large aorticopulmonary window *(arrows)*. Normally, ascending aora does not opacify on retrograde aortography.

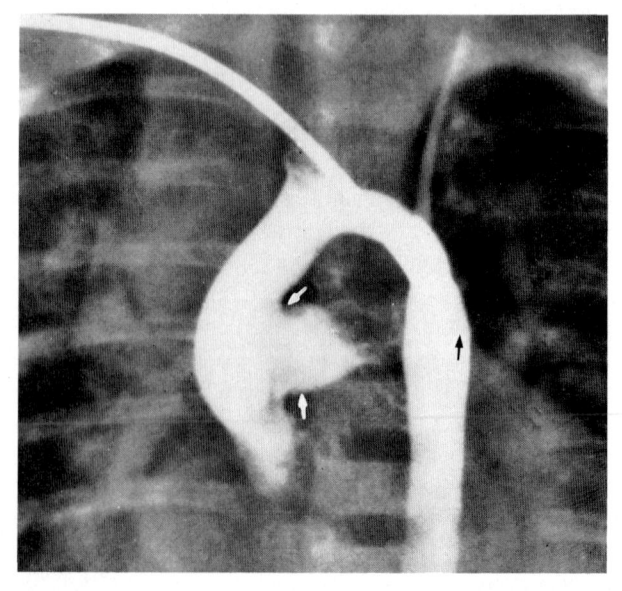

FIG 17–5.
Aortogram from descending aorta, anteroposterior projection. The stiff catheter could not be passed into the ascending aorta; because of diastolic back flow there is satisfactory demonstration of large proximal aorticopulmonary window *(white arrows)*.

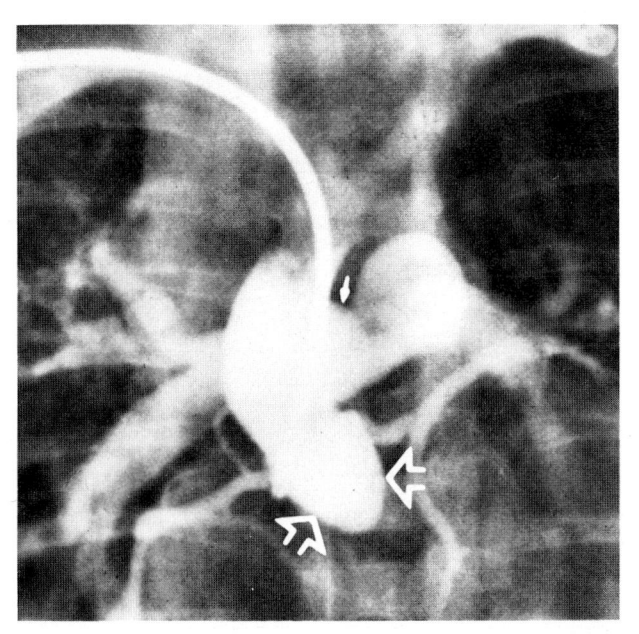

FIG 17-6.
Ascending aortogram, anteroposterior view shows APSD with a short "neck" *(white arrow)*. The aortic and pulmonary valves are distinctly demonstrated, excluding a truncus arteriosus. Patient also has a bicuspid aortic valve *(open arrows)*.

Oximetry data show a large increase in oxygen saturation at the level of the pulmonary trunk. Rarely, aortic desaturation is found, indicating pulmonary vascular disease.

Pulmonary arterial and right ventricular systolic pressures are elevated, usually to systemic levels.

ANGIOGRAPHIC APPEARANCE

Satisfactory angiographic demonstration of the APSD is important, because the operative approach differs according to the type of defect and the associated conditions (see Fig 17-1). Ventriculography should be performed to exclude an associated ventricular septal defect. If such a defect is present, distinct and separate aortic and pulmonary valves must be identified to exclude truncus arteriosus. Truncus arteriosus is always associated with a ventricular septal defect, APSD rarely.

1. In contrast to the findings in patent ductus arteriosus, aortography from the descending aorta or the brachial artery opacifies the ascending aorta because of the enormous diastolic backflow (Fig 17-4).

2. The diastolic backflow can be used advantageously if the catheter cannot be passed into the ascending aorta. Even descending aortography may result in demonstration of the aorticopulmonary window (Fig 17-5).

3. The best technique for demonstrating an APSD is a very rapid injection of contrast medium into the ascending aorta via a catheter (Fig 17-6).

4. After right ventriculography or pulmonary arteriography, contrast medium is diluted in the pulmonary artery by the left-to-right shunt. The site of dilution allows differentiation between a proximal and distal septal defect. The APSD with low pulmonary vascular resistance allows a large left-to-right shunt during both systole and diastole. Unopacified blood enters either the main pulmonary artery

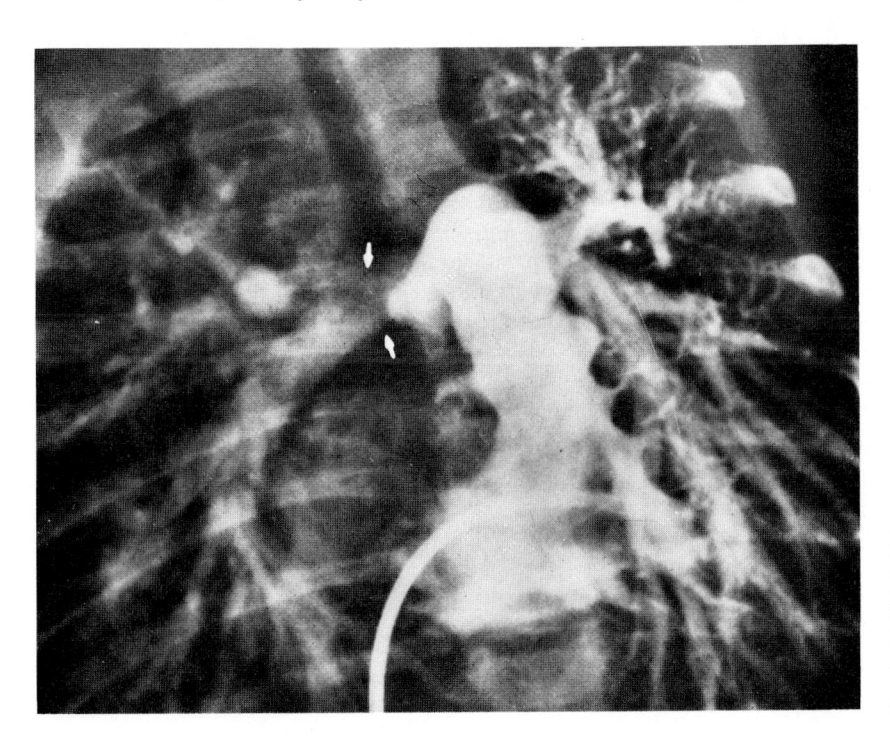

FIG 17-7.
Right ventriculogram, anteroposterior projection shows right ventricular hypertrophy as a result of pulmonary hypertension. Dilution of contrast material *(white arrows)* in the right pulmonary artery from a distal-type aorticopulmonary window.

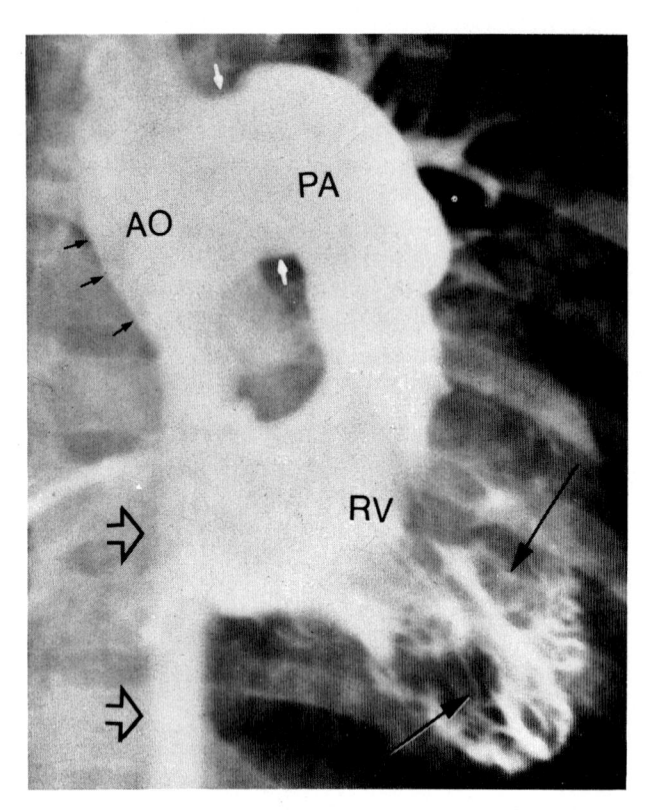

FIG 17–8.
Right ventriculogram, anteroposterior projection of patients with APSD, severe pulmonary disease, and interruption of aortic arch. Long-standing pulmonary hypertension has resulted in right ventricular hypertrophy and increased trabeculation *(black arrows)*. Because of elevated pulmonary vascular resistance, the ascending aorta *(small black arrows)* opacifies through a huge proximal APSD *(small white arrows)*. Aortic opacification usually does not occur in APSD with low pulmonary vascular resistance (see Fig 17–9). Descending aorta *(open black arrows)* is well demonstrated. *AO* = aorta; *PA* = pulmonary artery; *RV* = right ventricle.

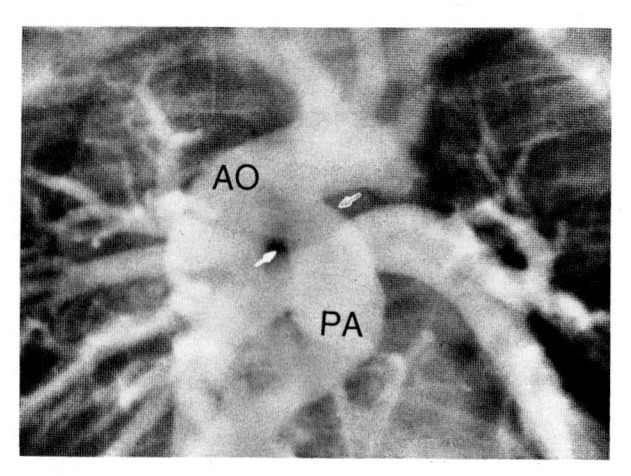

FIG 17–9.
Aortogram. Slight left anterior oblique projection. Distal aorticopulmonary septal defect *(arrows)*. Defect located posteriorly and higher on aorta than in usual aorticopulmonary septal defect.

(proximal aorticopulmonary defect) or the right pulmonary artery (distal defect) (Fig 17–7).

5. In patients with severe pulmonary vascular disease, after right ventriculography, the ascending aorta is opacified through a right-to-left shunt (Fig 17–8).

6. Aorticopulmonary septal defects located in the proximal aorta are easily seen on anteroposterior projections (see Figs 17–5, 17–6, and 17–8).

7. Aorticopulmonary septal defects to the right pulmonary artery are higher and located on the posterior wall of the aorta. Therefore, a slight left anterior oblique projection is required for adequate demonstration (Fig 17–9).

OPERATIVE CONSIDERATIONS

Previously, attempts were made to repair this condition without cardiopulmonary bypass by ligation of the defect, similar to the operation used for ductus arteriosus. This proved difficult in most patients, because of the diameter and short length of the defect. Currently APSDs are corrected with the patient on cardiopulmonary bypass. Depending on the location of the defect, it is approached through either the pulmonary trunk or the aorta, and a patch is applied (see Fig 17–1).

REFERENCES

1. Richardson JV, Doty DB, Rossi NP, et al: The spectrum of anomalies of aortopulmonary septation, *J Thorac Cardiovasc Surg* 78:21, 1979.
2. Mori K, Ando M, Takao A, et al: Distal type of aortopulmonary window: report of 4 cases, *Br Heart J* 40:681, 1978.
3. Baronofsky ID, Gordon AJ, Grishman A, et al: Aorticopulmonary septal defect, *Am J Cardiol* 5:273, 1960.
4. Tandon R, DaSilva CL, Moller JH, et al: Aorticopulmonary septal defect coexisting with ventricular septal defect, *Circulation* 50:188, 1974.
5. Moller JH, Edwards JE: Interruption of the aortic arch: anatomic patterns and associated malformations, *Am J Roentgenol Radium Ther Nucl Med* 95:557, 1965.
6. Blieden LC, Moller JH: Aorticopulmonary septal defect: an experience with 17 patients, *Br Heart J* 36:630, 1974.

CHAPTER 18

Origin of Pulmonary Artery From Ascending Aorta (Hemitruncus)

Origin of a pulmonary artery from the ascending aorta, a rare condition that occurs with equal frequency in males and females, has also been called hemitruncus arteriosus. It has three features:

1. Absence of one pulmonary artery arising from the pulmonary trunk.
2. A single large artery arising from the ascending aorta and entering the hilus of the involved lung, which is most commonly the right.
3. Normal size and structure of involved lung.

ANATOMY AND PATHOLOGY

A large arterial vessel originates from the ascending aorta, usually on the posterior wall, enters the pulmonary hilus, and joins the pulmonary artery, so blood follows the normal distribution in the lung (Fig 18–1). The orifice of this artery from the aorta is usually large. The involved pulmonary artery almost always arises opposite the side of the aortic arch; therefore, the right pulmonary artery is usually the one that arises anomalously. Origin of the left pulmonary artery may occur, but almost exclusively in tetralogy of Fallot, and in these instances, the arch may be either left or right sided.[1,2] Ventricular septal defect and patent ductus arteriosus frequently coexist.

The pulmonary trunk arising from the right ventricle gives rise to only one pulmonary artery. Right ventricular hypertrophy may be present, because pulmonary arterial pressure is usually elevated.

There are conflicting views about the status of the pulmonary arterioles. One or both lungs may show intimal proliferation and medial hypertrophy. These changes are expected in the involved lung, because it is perfused at systemic pressure, resulting in pulmonary vascular disease.[3,4] Pulmonary vascular disease may also develop in the opposite lung, probably because it is perfused with twice the normal volume of blood, which retards the normal neonatal decrease in pulmonary vascular resistance.

The left atrium and ventricle are dilated because of the increased volume of blood flow through the lungs.

ASSOCIATED CONDITIONS

The most commonly associated cardiac anomaly is patent ductus arteriosus connecting to the normally arising pulmonary artery. Ventricular septal defect, either with or without pulmonary stenosis, is much less common.

EMBRYOLOGY

One embryologic explanation for this condition is unequal division of the primitive truncus arteriosus, from which the right and left pulmonary arteries originate in the proximal segments of the respective sixth aortic arches. Partition of the primitive truncus arteriosus occurs by fusion of the conotruncal ridges, which arise opposite each other.[5] If the truncal ridges do not arise opposite each other and one of the ridges emerges more from a dorsal position, the proximal sixth aortic arch becomes incorporated into the ascending aorta (see Fig 45–1,B). As a result, a pulmonary artery arises from the dorsal aspect of the ascending aorta. Embryologic development thus resembles that of the distal type of aorticopulmonary window.

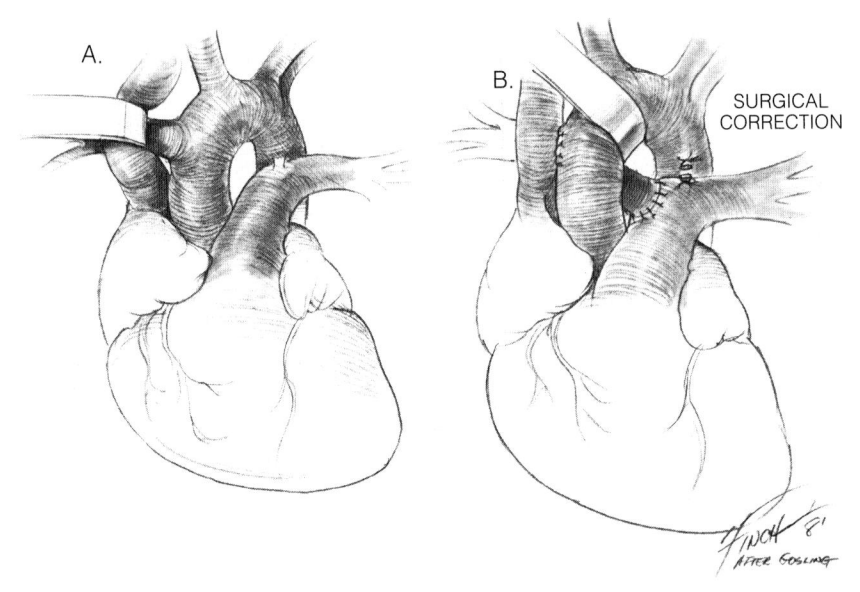

FIG 18–1.
Diagram of origin of right pulmonary artery from ascending aorta. **A,** right pulmonary artery arises from ascending aorta; pulmonary trunk gives rise only to the left pulmonary artery. **B,** operative repair; right pulmonary artery has been disconnected from aorta and sutured directly to the side of the pulmonary trunk. A coincidental ductus has been ligated and divided.

HEMODYNAMICS

The blood flow through the normally connected lung is twice normal because it is perfused by the entire systemic venous return (cardiac output). This large volume of pulmonary blood flow delays the normal postnatal decrease in pulmonary vascular resistance in this lung.[6] Therefore, the pulmonary arterial and right ventricular systolic pressures are elevated from birth in most patients. This is in contrast to the effect of pneumonectomy in older patients, in which the pulmonary arterial pressure is normal, although blood flow through the remaining lung is also twice normal.

Blood flows from the ascending aorta into the opposite lung, the volume depending on the pulmonary vascular resistance. As the pulmonary resistance declines postnatally in this lung, the volume of blood flow increases. Pulmonary vascular disease may develop in this lung, eventually reducing the volume of blood flow.

CLINICAL FEATURES

The clinical picture resembles that of a large left-to-right shunt with pulmonary hypertension.[6, 7] Poor weight gain and symptoms of respiratory distress and congestive cardiac failure develop in the second or third months of life. Mild cyanosis has been described and results from pulmonary disease rather than from an intracardiac right-to-left shunt.

Because of aortic runoff into the pulmonary artery, the pulse pressure is wide, and the peripheral pulses are snappy. The first and second heart sounds are prominent. There is a moderately loud systolic murmur along the left sternal border. In patients with a large volume of pulmonary blood flow, an apical diastolic murmur is heard because of turbulent flow across the mitral valve.

ELECTROCARDIOGRAPHIC FEATURES

The electrocardiogram is indistinguishable from that of a large patent ductus arteriosus. Usually there is biventricular hypertrophy, although if pulmonary vascular disease develops, only right ventricular hypertrophy is found.

ECHOCARDIOGRAPHIC FEATURES

The echocardiogram shows a dilated left atrium and ventricle secondary to the increased pulmonary blood flow. Right ventricular hypertrophy related to pulmonary hypertension is also present.

With two-dimensional echocardiography, it is impossible to demonstrate continuity between the pulmonary trunk and the involved pulmonary artery. The usual pattern of the bifurcation of the pulmonary artery is not present. It may be possible to demonstrate the origin of the involved pulmonary artery from the aorta.

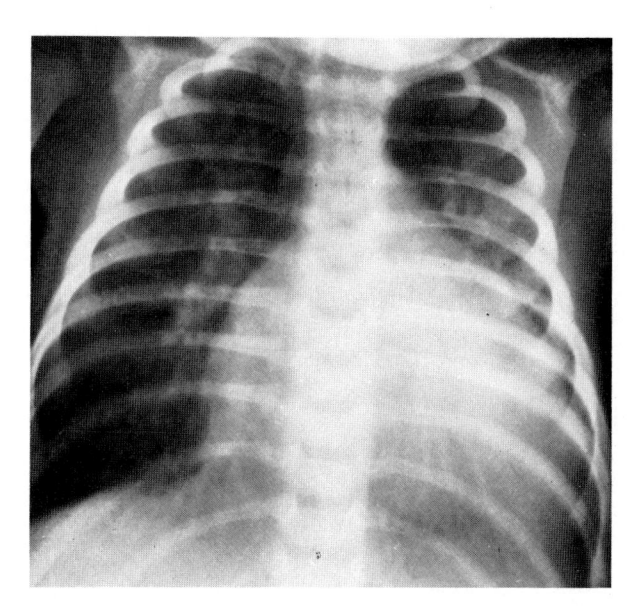

FIG 18–2.
Thoracic roentgenogram, posteroanterior projection of patient with origin of right pulmonary artery from ascending aorta. Marked cardiomegaly; pulmonary vasculature increased bilaterally. Correct diagnosis can be suggested.

RADIOGRAPHIC FEATURES

1. The cardiac silhouette is usually enlarged. REASON: Origin of pulmonary artery from the ascending aorta causes a serious hemodynamic abnormality from the increased blood flow through the anomalously arising pulmonary artery. Furthermore, pulmonary hypertension occurs in the anomalously connected and often the normally connected lung.

2. The diagnosis could be suggested by increased vascularity in one lung (usually the right lung), but the difference in the radiographic appearance is minimal (Fig 18–2). REASON: Origin of the pulmonary artery from the ascending aorta almost invariably occurs opposite the aortic arch. Left aortic arch is much more common than right aortic arch; therefore, this condition usually involves the right lung.

3. The pulmonary vasculature in the normally connected lung is usually normal, although blood flow through this lung is increased, because it receives the total systemic venous return.

4. The diagnosis can be confirmed by an intravenous injection of radionuclides. This study shows no perfusion of one lung during the early phase.

5. If a large patent ductus arteriosus joins the normally connected pulmonary artery, both lung fields show hypervascularity. In these cases, the diagnosis cannot be suspected from thoracic roentgenogram. The left atrium is enlarged. REASON: Increased pulmonary blood flow: total systemic output through one lung plus the aortic runoff to either lung. With the development of pulmonary vascular disease, however, pulmonary flow and left atrial enlargement disappear.

CARDIAC CATHETERIZATION

During cardiac catheterization, the catheter cannot be advanced from the pulmonary trunk into both pulmonary arteries. The involved pulmonary artery, however, may be catheterized from the ascending aorta.

Pressures in the anomalously arising pulmonary artery are usually at systemic levels. The pulmonary arterial pressure in the opposite lung may be normal but is usually elevated. The pulse pressure in the aorta is increased (aortic runoff lesion).

Oximetry data through the right side of the heart are normal, unless there is a coexisting intracardiac shunt or patent ductus arteriosus.

The oxygen saturation in the artery to the involved lung is increased because of the shunt from aorta to the pulmonary artery.

ANGIOGRAPHIC APPEARANCE

The diagnosis can be established by either the intravenous or the selective injection of contrast medium into the right ventricle (Fig 18–3).

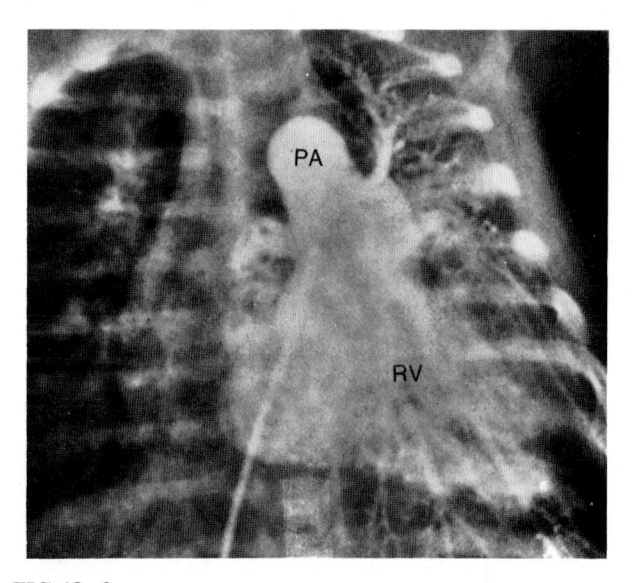

FIG 18–3.
Right ventriculogram, anteroposterior projection of origin of right pulmonary artery from ascending aorta. Opacification of right ventricle, pulmonary trunk, and only the left pulmonary artery.

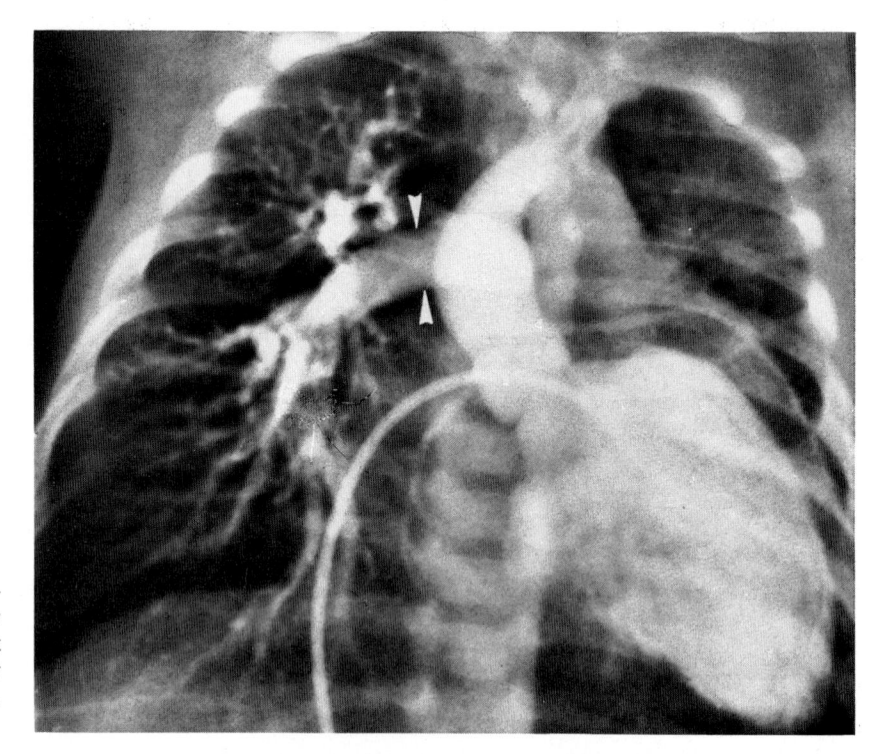

318 *Cardiac Conditions Associated With a Left-to-Right Shunt*

FIG 18–4.
Left ventriculogram, anteroposterior projection of origin of right pulmonary artery from ascending aorta. Opacification of left ventricle and aortic arch. Right pulmonary artery *(arrows)* arises from ascending aorta. Intact ventricular septum.

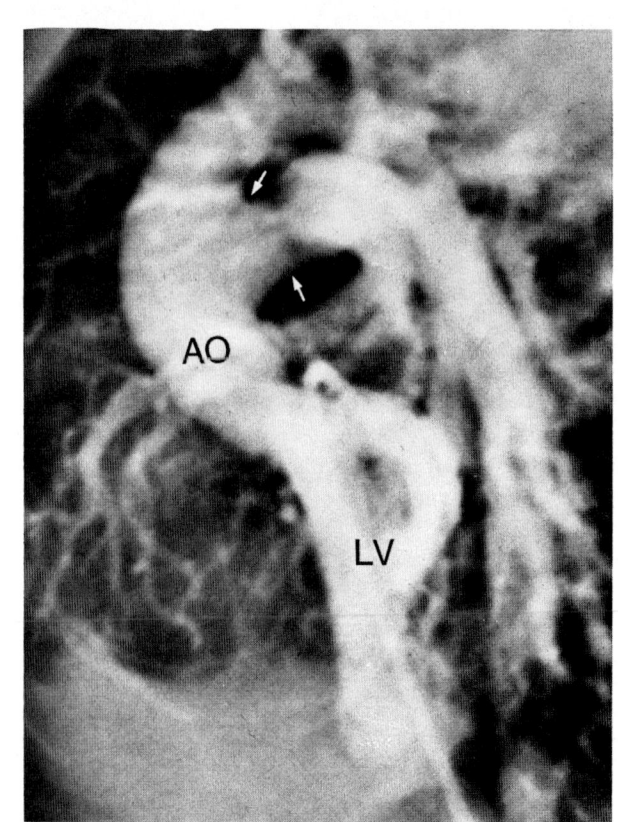

FIG 18–5.
Left ventriculogram *(LV)*, left anterior oblique projection of origin of right pulmonary artery from ascending aorta. Intact ventricular septum; posterior displacement of left ventricle because of dilatation of the right ventricle. Right pulmonary artery *(arrows)* arises from posterior aspect of ascending aorta *(AO)*.

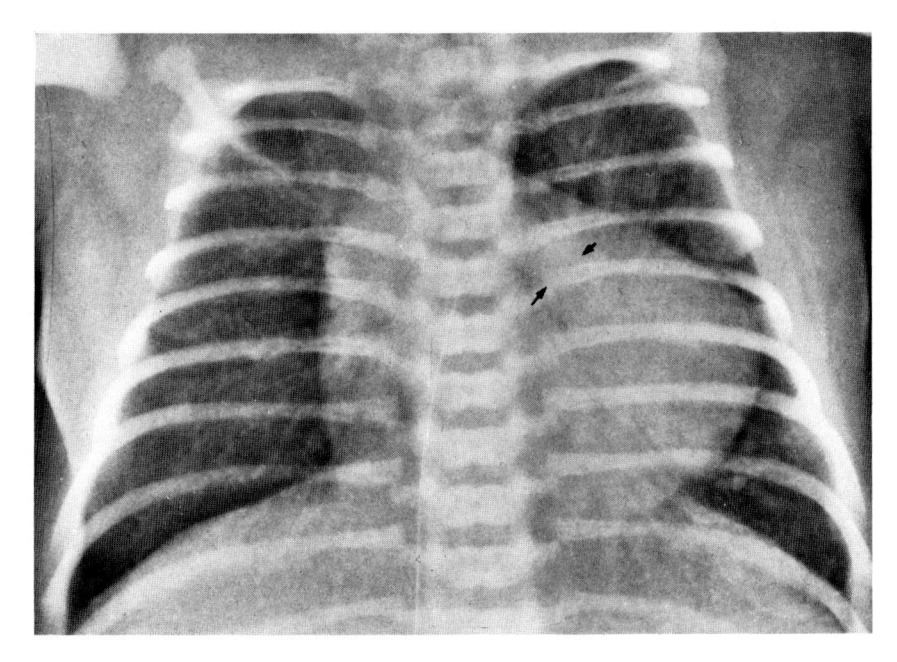

FIG 18-6.
Thoracic roentgenogram, posteroanterior projection ventricular defect and pulmonary atresia, origin of the left pulmonary artery from the ascending aorta. Discrepancy of the vascularity in right and left lung. A large left pulmonary artery *(arrows)* is seen through the heart shadow. Right aortic arch is difficult to see.

1. After injection of a large volume of contrast medium, the anomalous origin of the pulmonary artery from the aorta can be observed on the levophase of the study.
2. The condition is best seen by either left ventriculography or aortography (Fig 18-4).
3. The involved pulmonary artery arises from the aorta on either the posterior or lateral aspect (Fig 18-5). Because of right ventricular enlargement, the left ventricle may be displaced posteriorly.
4. Systemic origin of the pulmonary artery may be part of the tetralogy of Fallot with or without pulmonary atresia.
5. Usually the systemic pulmonary artery arises opposite the aortic arch; in tetralogy or pulmonary atresia with ventricular septal defect, it may arise from the ipsilateral or contralateral side of the aortic arch.
6. Because of pulmonary stenosis, the discrepancy in pulmonary vasculature between the lung fields may be obvious (Figs 18-6 and 18-7).

MANAGEMENT

Without operation, this condition is frequently associated with death in infancy.[7] Depending on the site of origin from the aorta, operative repair is accomplished by ei-

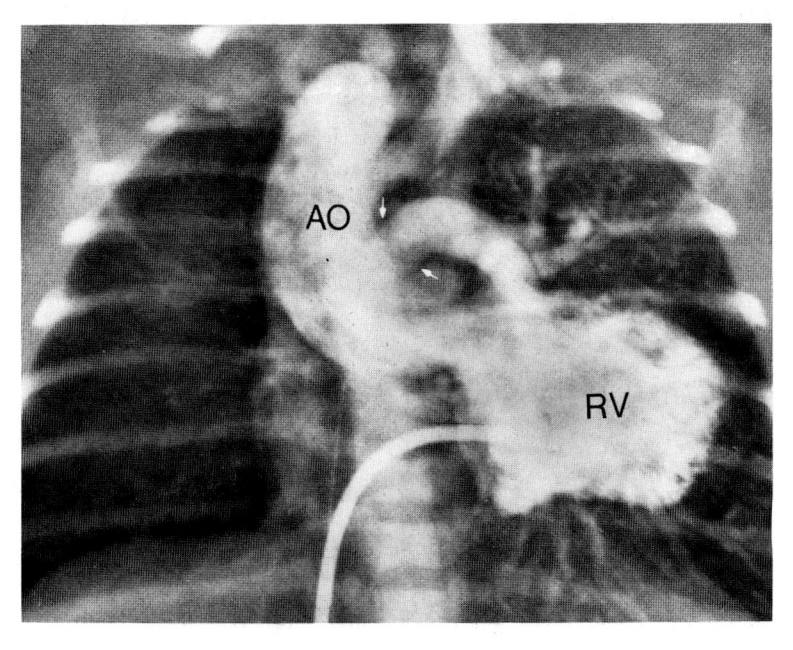

FIG 18-7.
Right ventriculography *(RV)* in anteroposterior projection of patient in Figure 18-6. Filling of the aorta *(AO)* through ventricular septal defect. There is pulmonary atresia and the left pulmonary artery arises from the ascending aorta *(arrows).* Vascular supply of the right lung occurred via bronchial and systemic collaterals. The systemic origin of the left pulmonary artery is opposite the right-sided aortic arch although in tetralogy of Fallot and its variants, the systemic pulmonary artery may arise from either the same or opposite side as aortic arch.

ther direct anastomosis behind the aorta or a graft anastomosis to the pulmonary trunk (see Fig 18–1). Operation should be performed early to prevent the development of pulmonary vascular disease.[7]

REFERENCES

1. Robin E, Silberberg B, Ganguly SN, et al: Aortic origin of the left pulmonary artery: variant of tetralogy of Fallot, *Am J Cardiol* 35:324, 1975.
2. Morgan JR: Left pulmonary artery from ascending aorta in tetralogy of Fallot, *Circulation* 45:653, 1972.
3. Rosenberg HS, Hallman GL, Wolfe RR, et al: Origin of the right pulmonary artery from the aorta, *Am Heart J* 72:106, 1966.
4. Griffiths SP, Levine OR, Anderson DH: Aortic origin of the right pulmonary artery, *Circulation* 25:73, 1962.
5. Cucci CE, Doyle EF, Lewis EW Jr: Absence of a primary division of the pulmonary trunk: An ontogenetic theory, *Circulation* 29:124, 1964.
6. Cumming GR, Ferguson CC, Sanchez J: Aortic origin of the right pulmonary artery, *Am J Cardiol* 30:674, 1972.
7. Keane JF, Maltz D, Bernhard WF, et al: Anomalous origin of one pulmonary artery from the ascending aorta: diagnostic, physiological and surgical considerations, *Circulation* 50:588, 1974.

CHAPTER 19

Atrial Septal Defect

Atrial septal defect (ASD) is the fifth most common form of congenital heart disease and is the type most commonly seen in adults, because the life span may be 50 years. The location of ASDs varies, and in this chapter, we do not discuss one form, the ostium primum defect, because that condition is reviewed in Chapter 23.

INCIDENCE

Atrial septal defect accounts for 10% of congenital heart disease, with a 3:2 female/male ratio. It sometimes occurs in families, and, interestingly, in these patients the PR interval tends to be prolonged. Atrial septal defect has also been described as a portion of the Holt-Oram syndrome, an autosomal dominant condition that also includes anomalies of the digits of the hands, such as absent or fingerlike thumbs.

PATHOLOGY

Edwards[1] has classified defects of the atrial septum according to location (Fig 19-1):

1. At the fossa ovalis (ostium secundum defect).
2. In the superior portion of atrial septum (sinus venosus defect), usually associated with partial anomalous pulmonary venous connection of right upper lobe pulmonary veins.
3. In the lowermost portion of atrial septum (ostium primum defect).
4. Posterior to the fossa ovalis.
5. In the region of the ostium of the coronary sinus, which is associated with absence of the coronary sinus and with left superior vena cava connection directly to the left atrium (Raghib-type ASD).[2]
6. At the junction of the inferior vena cava with the right atrium.
7. Multiple perforations and coalescence of defects, leading to an almost complete absence of the atrial septum (single atrium).

Atrial septal defects are usually large, often 2 to 4 cm in diameter, and permit free communication between the left and right atria.

Because of the proximity of the right pulmonary veins to the atrial defects, particularly in the sinus venosus type, the blood from the right pulmonary veins usually flows preferentially through the atrial defect (anomalous venous drainage), whereas the blood from the left pulmonary veins flows predominantly into the left atrium and through the mitral valve into the left ventricle. This has been termed "anomalous pulmonary venous drainage with normal pulmonary venous connection."

In patients with an ASD adjacent to the inferior vena cava, a small right-to-left shunt may occur through the defect. In infants with defects at the fossa ovalis, a right-to-left shunt may occur, because the upper rim of the defect may straddle the inferior vena cava and divert vena caval blood into the left atrium. This represents a residue of the fetal circulation.

Because, in most patients, there is a large left-to-right shunt through the defect, the right atrium, ventricle, and pulmonary trunk are dilated. However, the right ventricle is not hypertrophied unless pulmonary hypertension develops. The left ventricle may be slightly smaller than normal.

ASSOCIATED CONDITIONS

1. Persistent left superior vena cava to the coronary sinus (10% of cases).
2. Partial anomalous pulmonary venous connection to right atrium or superior vena cava (10% of cases).
3. Mitral valve prolapse (an incidence as high as 30% has been reported).[3, 4]

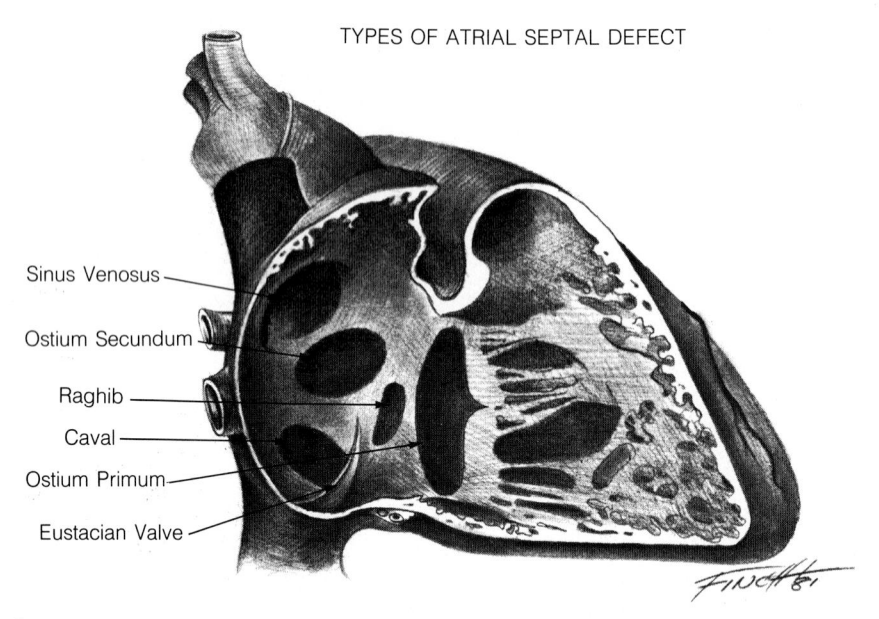

TYPES OF ATRIAL SEPTAL DEFECT

Sinus Venosus
Ostium Secundum
Raghib
Caval
Ostium Primum
Eustacian Valve

FIG 19–1.
Diagram of right atrium and right ventricle, showing location of various types of atrial septal defect (ASD).

HEMODYNAMICS AND PATHOPHYSIOLOGY

In the presence of a large atrial septal communication, the right and left atrial pressures and the end-diastolic pressures in the two ventricles are equal.[5] All four chambers are connected by nonrestrictive pathways (the atria through the ASD and the ventricles through the atrioventricular valves). Therefore, pressure is not the predominant factor influencing the direction and magnitude of the shunt. Rather, ventricular distensibility or compliance is the primary factor. Because the right ventricular wall is thinner than the left ventricular wall, the right ventricle is more compliant or distensible; and at equal filling pressures, more blood flows into the right ventricle (Fig 19–2). The difference in ventricular wall thickness and therefore in compliance is the result of differences between the pulmonary and systemic arterial resistances and pressures.

Because during diastole all four cardiac chambers are in free communication, a large amount of blood flows through the ASD into the more distensible right ventricle (Fig 19–3). In addition to the diastolic shunt, there is also a smaller left-to-right shunt at the atrial level during systole. Reason: during systole when the atrioventricular valves are closed, the normal-sized left atrium cannot accommodate the increased venous return from the lungs. Blood flow therefore occurs into the more distensible (compliant) right atrium, which becomes enlarged. A very large diastolic and systolic left-to-right shunt occurs similar to a patent ductus arteriosus (see Chapter 16). With a large defect, the flow into the left ventricle may be diminished because left atrial pressure is lower than normal and only as high as the right atrial pressure.

In newborns, the right and left ventricular wall thicknesses are the same, favoring a balanced or right-to-left shunt. As pulmonary vascular resistance falls after birth, pulmonary arterial pressure drops, right ventricular compliance increases, and the left-to-right shunt increases. Because the pulmonary and systemic vascular resistances are similar in most people, the difference in ventricular compliance between individuals is also fairly constant. Therefore, in most patients with an ASD, the size of left-to-right shunt is similar, about 65%. The systemic cardiac output is normal at rest.

The right atrium, particularly because it receives the

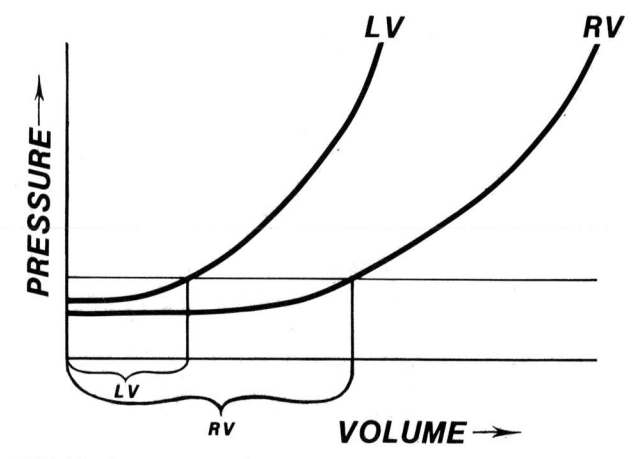

FIG 19–2.
Graph illustrating principle of ventricular compliance and effect on blood flow in ASD; at any filling pressure, a larger volume of blood flows into the right *(RV)* than into the left ventricle *(LV)*.

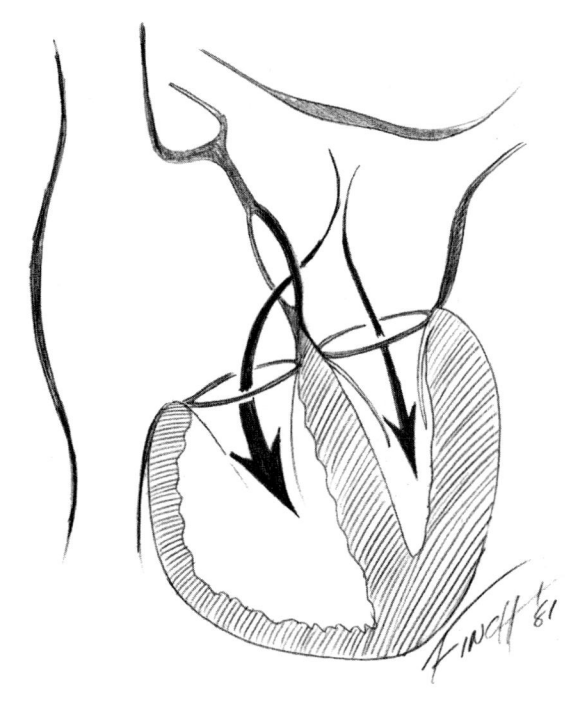

FIG 19-3.
Diagram of heart during diastole; all four chambers are in free communication and pressures are equal. Blood flows preferentially into thinner, more distensible (compliant) right ventricle, resulting in a large blood flow through atrial communication (left-to-right shunt).

venae cavae, is more distensible than the left atrium, and this difference also favors a left-to-right shunt. The volume load placed on the right ventricle by the shunt is well tolerated, and cardiac failure rarely occurs during childhood.

With each decade after the age of 30 years, the incidence of pulmonary vascular disease becomes higher, with an incidence of 15% between the ages of 20 and 40 years.[6] The incidence at higher altitudes is significantly greater.[7] However, some patients reach old age with only slight pulmonary hypertension. The life span of patients with ASD averages 50 years, with adults developing tricuspid insufficiency, atrial fibrillation, and, subsequently, cyanosis and a potential for paradoxical emboli.[8, 9]

With the elevation of the pulmonary arterial pressure, right ventricular hypertrophy develops and compliance drops, and the shunt may become right to left.

CLINICAL FEATURES

Most patients are asymptomatic and remain so until the second or third decade of life. During childhood, there may be slight exercise intolerance and an increased susceptibility to respiratory infections or pneumonia. Cardiac failure is rare in childhood but has been reported in infancy.[10-13] If cardiac failure develops, a coexisting condition such as cardiomyopathy or an obstructive lesion about the mitral valve should be suspected. In the adult, rheumatic mitral valve disease may complicate ASD; this combination has been called "Lutenbacher's syndrome." In adults, congestive cardiac failure and cyanosis may develop.[8, 9] Atrial fibrillation also can occur because of right atrial dilatation.

The usual initial manifestation a murmur discovered in an asymptomatic child, often found during the preschool examination.

PHYSICAL EXAMINATION

The children are usually normal in height and weight for their age. There is no cyanosis except in those with a coronary sinus ASD (Raghib's syndrome), where it is mild. A precordial bulge is present because of the dilated right ventricle, and precordial cardiac activity is increased because of the large stroke volume of the right ventricle.

The auscultatory findings are diagnostic:

1. Loud first heart sound in the tricuspid area.[14] Because of the large volume of blood flow across the tricuspid valve, the leaflets have a longer excursion, so closure of the valve at the beginning of systole is louder.

2. Pulmonary systolic ejection murmur. This murmur originates from the large volume of blood flowing across the right ventricular outflow area. It is soft (grade 1 to 3/6) and therefore is rarely associated with a thrill.

3. Wide, fixed splitting of the second heart sound.[15, 16] Wide splitting comes from delayed pulmonary valve closure, presumably from the prolonged right ventricular ejection because of the large stroke volume. Fixed splitting, meaning that the splitting of the components of the second heart sound does not vary with the phases of breathing as in normal persons, is found in the presence of an atrial communication.

4. Soft middiastolic murmur in the tricuspid area. It is caused by the turbulence of the large volume of blood flowing across the tricuspid valve.

In children, the pulmonary component of the second heart sound has a normal intensity, but in adults, it may be accentuated when pulmonary hypertension is present.

ELECTROCARDIOGRAPHIC FEATURES

In most patients, the electrocardiogram (ECG) is typical:

1. The QRS axis shows right-axis deviation between +90 and +150 degrees. Fewer than 2% of patients have

left-axis deviation in contrast to patients with ostium primum defect.

2. The P waves are tall and peaked in 25% and indicate right atrial enlargement.

3. The PR interval is prolonged in 10% of patients,[17] particularly those with a familial history of this lesion.

4. The QRS complexes show a precordial lead pattern of incomplete right bundle-branch block[18] (80% of cases). Leads V_4R or V_1 show an rSR' pattern, and the terminal part of the QRS complex is delayed. This pattern has been called incomplete right bundle–branch block.

ECHOCARDIOGRAPHIC FEATURES

M-mode echocardiography shows the features of right ventricular volume overload[19]:

1. Increased right ventricular internal diameter.
2. Paradoxical septal motion (i.e., during diastole, the ventricular septum moves away from the anterior chest wall).
3. Right ventricular free wall, which is of normal thickness.

On two-dimensional or cross-sectional echocardiography, the atrial septum can be seen, and the location of the septal defect is apparent.[20]

RADIOGRAPHIC FEATURES

In most instances, the roentgenographic appearance is characteristic. Together with the echocardiographic and clinical findings, it permits a diagnosis with a sufficiently high degree of accuracy that cardiac catheterization is not necessary.

1. Unlike ventricular septal defects, which differ in size, ASDs are usually large, and pulmonary hypertension is uncommon before the age of 30 years. Because the shunt is determined by the compliance of the ventricles which is fairly constant between patients, the size of the shunt is large and similar between patients.

2. The pulmonary arterial vasculature is increased; and the main, central, and peripheral pulmonary arteries are markedly enlarged. REASON: A large left-to-right shunt distends the pulmonary arteries, even with a normal pulmonary artery pressure, and the pulmonary arteries actually grow, adapting to the increased blood flow.

3. The pulmonary arteries in both lung fields are less distinct than in other types of large left-to-right shunt. REASON: Most large left-to-right shunts not located at the atrial level result in pulmonary hypertension. Pulmonary hypertension causes an increased tortuosity of the pulmonary arteries, so that many pulmonary arteries are seen "on end." In ASD and normal pulmonary artery pressure, the pulmonary vasculature tends to be more fluffy appearing (Fig 19–4), although exceptions are seen.

4. Because the pulmonary arteries in the hilar areas may be obscured by cardiomegaly, the size of the right pulmonary artery should be observed on the lateral view. If enlarged, it is a helpful sign for detecting the large shunt (Fig 19–5). The left atrium is not enlarged. Although blood flow through it is markedly increased, it is decompressed by the atrial communication. The retrosternal space is obliterated by right atrial and right ventricular enlargement (Fig 19–5).

5. Although the right atrium is enlarged on the posteroanterior roentgenograms, the right atrium does not necessarily extend farther to the right side of the spine than normal. REASON: As the right ventricle enlarges against the sternum, the heart rotates clockwise, and this minimizes the bulge of the chamber toward the right. This rotation also makes the superior vena cava and ascending aorta in-

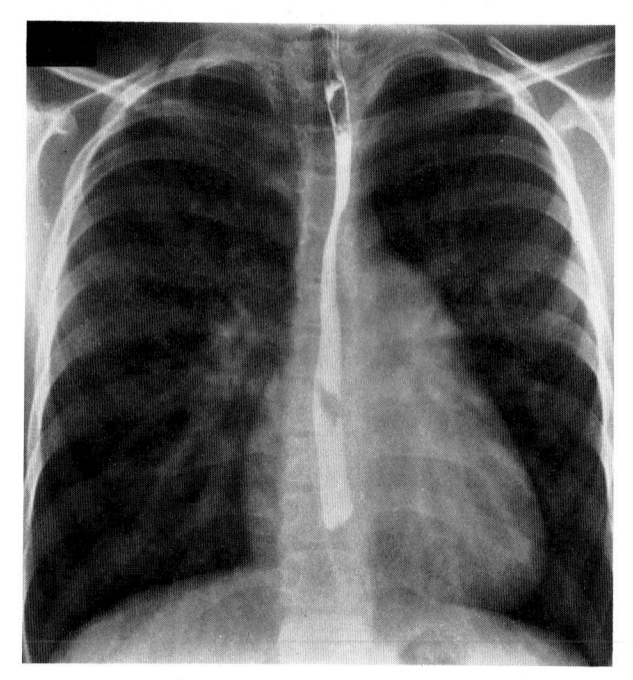

FIG 19–4.
Thoracic roentgenogram, posteroanterior projection of patient with typical ASD. Cardiomegaly. Pulmonary vasculature is diffusely increased and "fluffy"; main pulmonary arterial segment is enlarged. Ascending aorta and aortic arch are inconspicuous. Esophagus is not displaced. Right atrial border is slightly prominent but does not extend significantly beyond right side of spine because of clockwise rotation of heart. Cardiac apex is slightly elevated above diaphragm. Superior vena cava and ascending aorta are not seen because of clockwise rotation of heart.

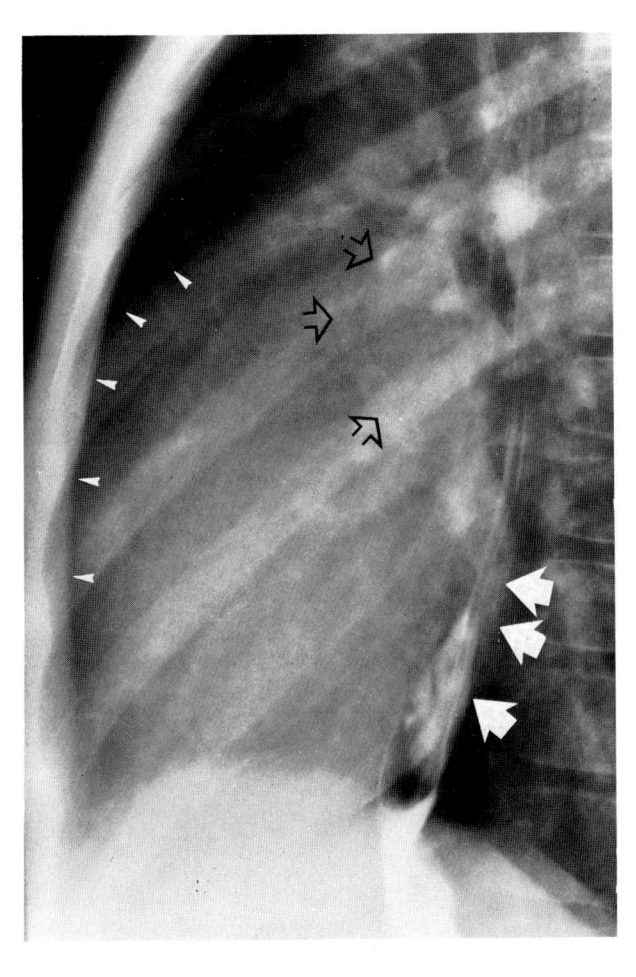

FIG 19-5.
Thoracic roentgenogram, lateral projection of patient with typical ASD. Anteroposterior dimension of heart is markedly increased. Enlarged right ventricle and right ventricular outflow tract make a long area of contact with sternum *(small white arrows)*, which is slightly bowed anteriorly. Enlarged right ventricle pushes left ventricle posteriorly, so that it projects behind esophagus *(large white arrows)*. Left ventricle does not project downward, as in instances of left ventricular enlargement, but is lifted off the diaphragm. Enlargement of right pulmonary artery is well demonstrated *(open black arrows)*.

conspicuous (Fig 19–6). Enlargement of the right atrium is indicated on a posteroanterior projection as a large diameter arc along the right cardiac border. This is better seen on a left anterior oblique projection (Fig 19–7).

6. The cardiac contour on the posteroanterior roentgenogram may mimic that of left ventricular enlargement (see Fig 19–4). REASON: With the clockwise rotation of the heart, the dilated right ventricle forms the left cardiac border, causing a contour similar to that of left ventricular enlargement. However, the apex of the heart, because it is formed by the right ventricle, tends to be elevated (Fig 19–4).

7. The left ventricle is rotated posteriorly and is elevated by the enlarged right ventricle. The left ventricle is best seen on left anterior oblique and lateral projections (see Figs 19–5 and 19–6). This appearance is helpful in excluding left ventricular enlargement.

8. The huge right ventricle displaces the left ventricle posteriorly. Consequently, the left ventricle may extend beyond the esophagus on a lateral view (see Fig 19–5) and project beyond the spine on a left anterior oblique projection (see Fig 19–7).

9. Left atrial enlargement is absent. REASON: In spite of the markedly increased blood volume returning to the left atrium, that chamber decompresses itself through the septal defect directly into the right atrium and through the mitral valve into the left ventricle (see Fig 19–3). The left atrial and right atrial pressures are equal.

10. In some patients, the left atrium indents or displaces the barium-filled esophagus. REASON: A markedly enlarged right ventricle causes a generalized posterior displacement of the heart. The normal-sized left atrium is displaced posteriorly against the esophagus, mimicking left atrial enlargement (Fig 19–8). The indentation on the esophagus is small, suggesting a normal-sized left atrium (pseudo left atrial enlargement).

11. The right ventricle enlarges anteriorly against the sternum, causing an increased area of contact between the heart and sternum (see Fig 19–5). Clinically, anterior bowing of the sternum (precordial bulge) may be observed.

12. The right ventricular outflow tract is enlarged and is best seen on the right anterior oblique view (see Fig 19–8).

13. The aortic knob is inconspicuous. REASON: The large pulmonary artery overshadows the aortic knob. How-

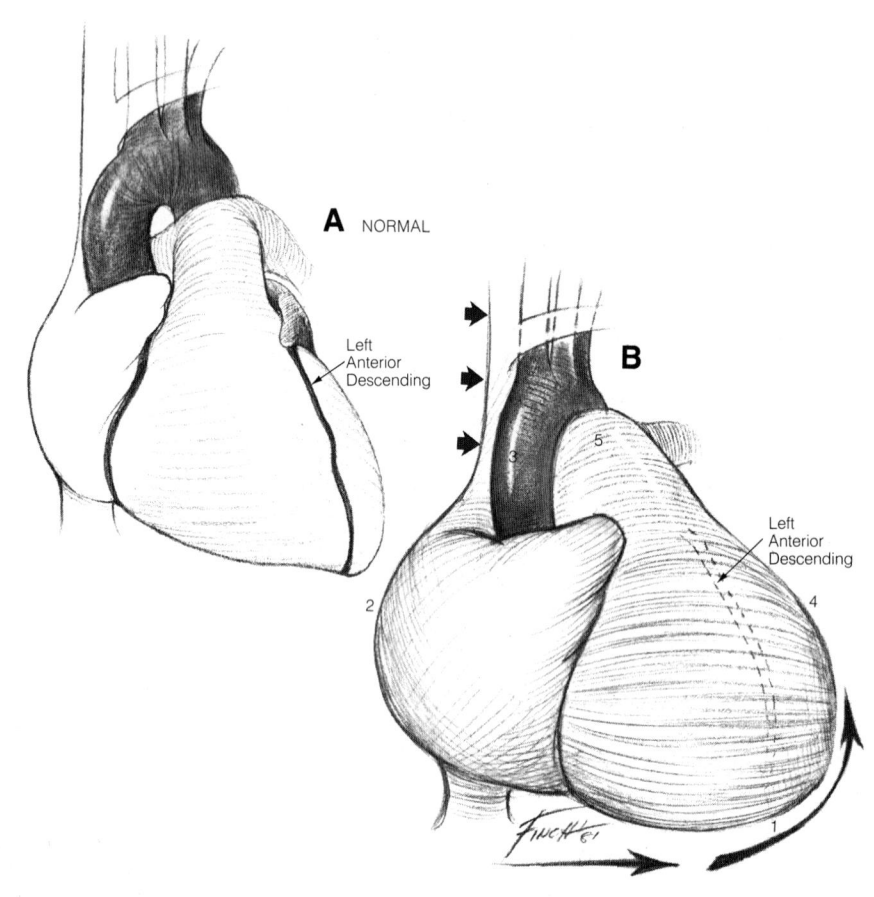

FIG 19-6.
Diagram of change of cardiac silhouette caused by right ventricular enlargement in ASD. **A,** normal heart. **B,** Atrial septal defect and right ventricular dilatation. Because right ventricle can enlarge anteriorly only against the sternum, enlargement causes a clockwise rotation *(arrow)* of heart. Cardiac apex, normally formed by left ventricle, is now formed by right ventricle. As a result, cardiac apex *(1)* is elevated off diaphragm. Right atrium *(2),* although markedly enlarged, does not extend significantly beyond right side of the spine because of clockwise rotation. "Arc" formed by lateral wall of right atrium may, however, be enlarged. Ascending aorta *(3)* and superior vena cava are in a more medial position and are therefore inconspicuous. Left cardiac border is formed by enlarged right ventricle and dilated right ventricular outflow tract *(4),* sometimes resulting in a continuous arc with the dilated pulmonary artery, simulating the contour of corrected transposition. Enlarged main pulmonary artery partially overshadows the aorta, resulting in an inconspicuous aortic knob *(5).* **C,** magnetic resonance image of heart in patient with atrial septal defect. Enlargement of right ventricle against the anterior rib cage and clockwise rotation of the heart *(arrows)* are well demonstrated. Left ventricle displaced posteriorly.

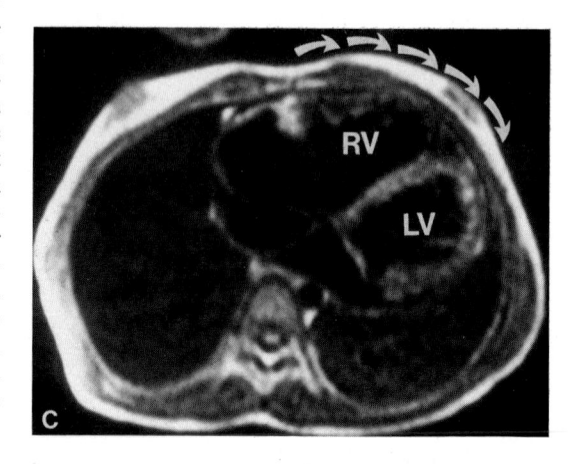

ever, the aorta is of normal size, because these patients have a normal cardiac output. The aorta also appears small compared with the pulmonary artery.

14. The ascending aorta is not prominent and sometimes is not seen. REASON: The clockwise rotation of the heart causes a more medial position of the aorta, minimizing the aortic prominence along the right cardiac border (see Figs 19–4 and 19–6).

15. A faint density along the left superior mediastinum suggests a persistent left superior vena cava (Fig 19–9), which occurs in 10% of patients with ASD. Therefore, cardiac catheterization is best performed from the right antecubital or a femoral vein, because it is difficult to pass the catheter into the pulmonary artery if it enters the heart from a persistent left superior vena cava.

16. Partial anomalous pulmonary venous connection, which is common with a sinus venosus–type ASD, can be suspected from an anomalous course of the right upper

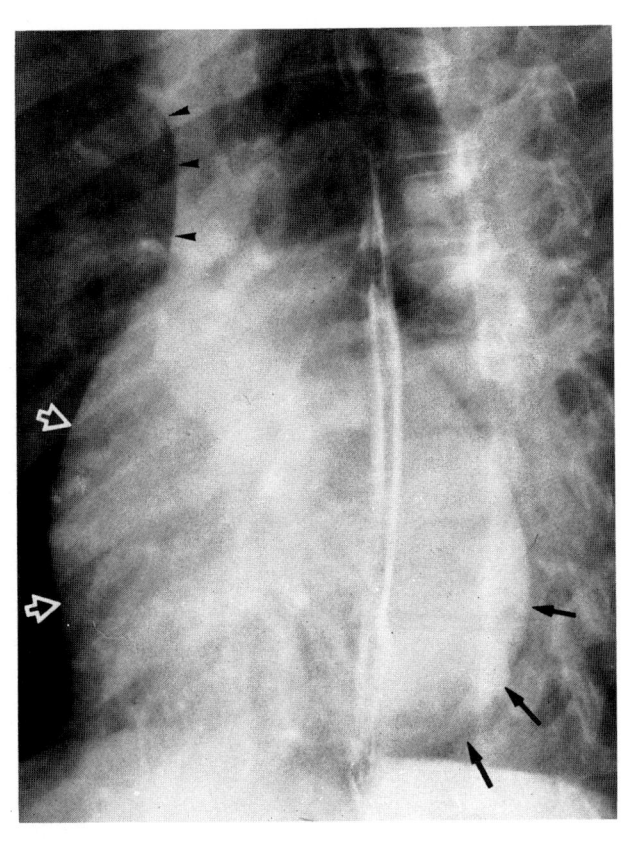

FIG 19–7.
Thoracic roentgenogram, left anterior oblique projection of patient with typical ASD. Cardiac apex is elevated above diaphragm *(black arrows)* and extends beyond spine because of marked right ventricular enlargement and clockwise rotation of heart. Increased diameter of the right atrium *(white open arrows)* is evident and indicates enlargement. Ascending aorta and superior vena cava are inconspicuous because of clockwise rotation of heart. In this roentgenogram, superior vena cava *(small black arrows)* rather than ascending aorta is seen along upper mediastinum.

pulmonary vein. The specific location of the defect cannot be suspected from plain film findings, but sinus venosus defects tend to have a smaller left-to-right shunt than do the ostium secundum type.

17. Some adult patients with ASDs develop pulmonary vascular disease, which can be seen radiographically as "pruning" of the peripheral pulmonary arteries (Fig 19–10). A similar appearance may be present in some patients without pulmonary hypertension. Therefore, it is difficult to predict the pulmonary arterial pressure radiographically, nor can the pulmonary hypertension secondary to ASD be differentiated from that from other causes.

18. Fluoroscopic observations demonstrate an actively pulsating right ventricle and increased pulsations of the pulmonary arteries ("hilar dance"). This is not specific for ASD but may occur in any form of left-to-right shunt because of the increased blood flow through the pulmonary arteries. It is, however, most common in ASD and once was an important fluoroscopic sign. The increased pulsations can be recorded by kymography (Fig 19–11).

19. Rarely, the increased pulsations of the pulmonary arteries are the only radiographic finding, because the pulmonary arteries and the heart size may be normal radiographically (Fig 19–12). The reason some patients with large ASD have normal chest roentgenograms is unknown. A normal chest x-ray film therefore does not exclude an ASD with large left to right shunt.

CARDIAC CATHETERIZATION

We believe that the diagnosis of ASD can be made with a high degree of accuracy on clinical grounds alone and so do not routinely perform cardiac catheterization on

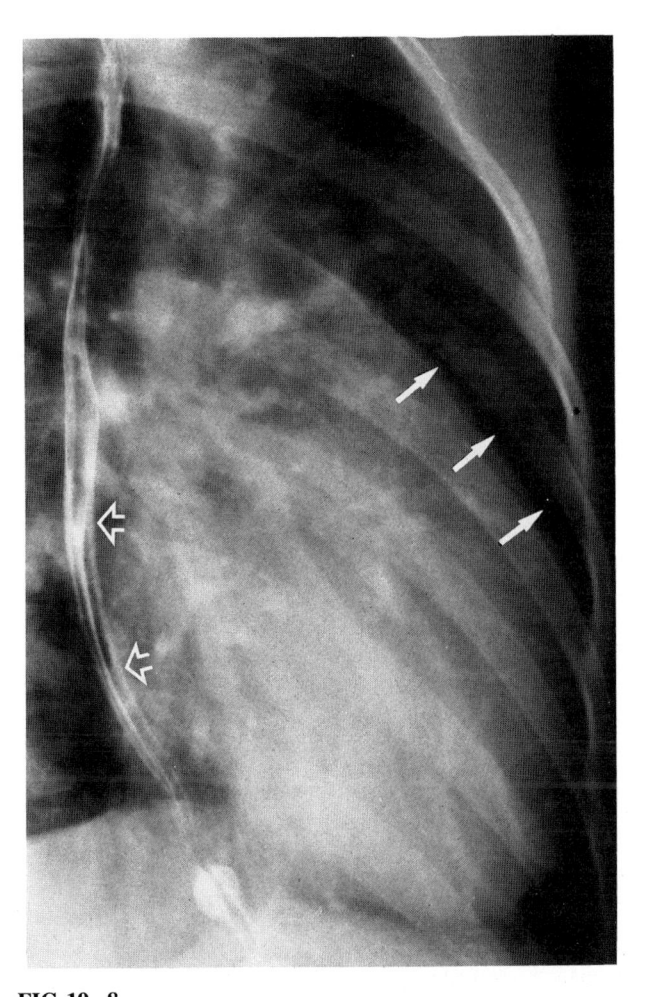

FIG 19–8.
Thoracic roentgenogram, right anterior oblique projection of patient with typical ASD. Enlarged right ventricular outflow tract *(solid arrows)* is best seen in this projection. Barium-filled esophagus is slightly indented and displaced (pseudo left atrial enlargement) *(open arrows)*.

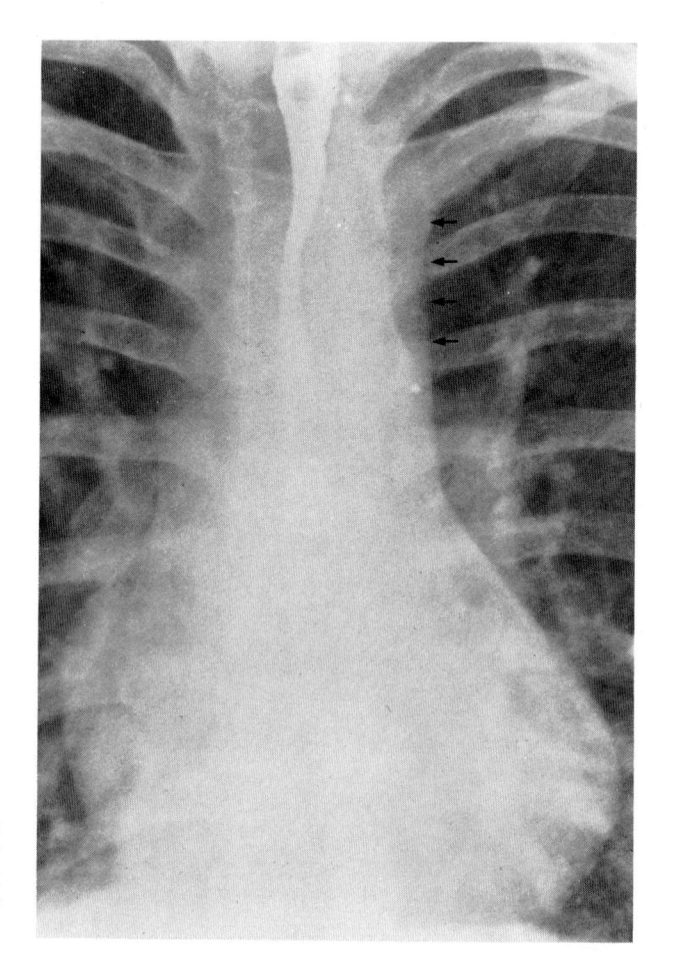

FIG 19–9.
Thoracic roentgenogram, posteroanterior projection of patient with ASD. The right atrial border is slightly prominent. The pulmonary vasculature is increased, but a pulmonary artery segment is not prominent, which is atypical. Faint density along the left superior mediastinum *(arrows)* indicates a persistent left superior vena cava.

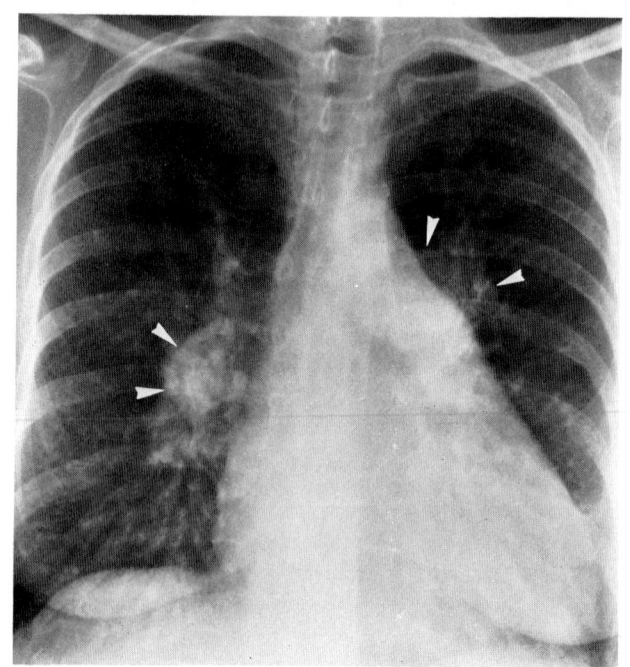

FIG 19–10.
Thoracic roentgenogram, posteroanterior projection of patient with ASD and pulmonary vascular disease. Marked cardiomegaly. Central pulmonary arteries *(arrows)* are enlarged, whereas peripheral pulmonary vasculature is normal (pruning). Appearance of pulmonary vasculature is suggestive of only pulmonary hypertension because it may be present in patients with ASD and normal pulmonary artery pressure.

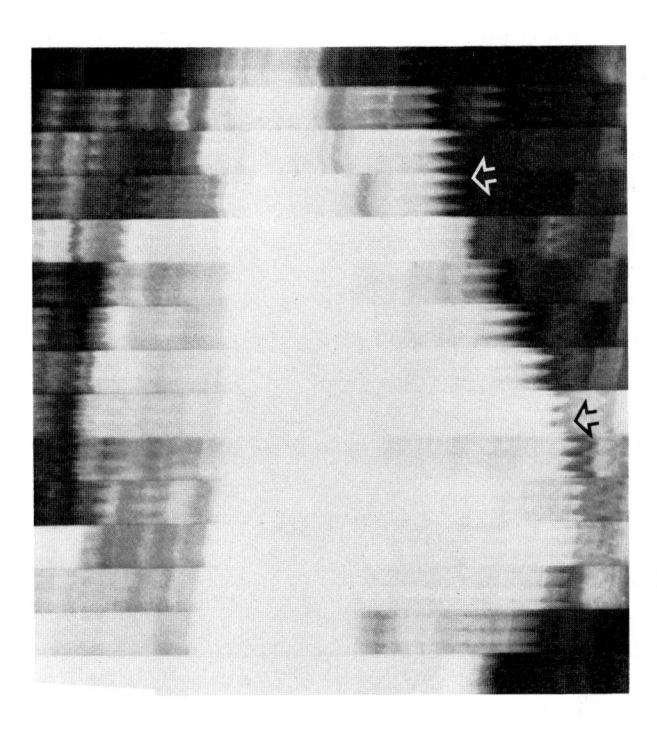

FIG 19–11.
Kymogram, posteroanterior projection in patient with ASD. Increased pulsations of the pulmonary arteries (hilar dance; *white arrow*). Increase pulsation of right ventricle *(black arrow)* because of increased stroke volume.

children with suspected ASD unless the clinical or laboratory findings are atypical.[21] As a result, we currently catheterize less than 10% of our patients with ASD who are to undergo operation.

The catheter tip may be passed through the septal defect, particularly if catheterization is performed through the femoral vein. The passage of the catheter usually suggests the location of the defect. Thus, passage into the left atrium in the center usually indicates a secundum defect (Fig 19–13). It is possible, however, to pass a catheter through a patent foramen ovale, so the catheter course is not totally diagnostic of the position or presence of an ASD. A high passage strongly suggests a sinus venosus location, and a low passage suggests an ostium primum or a low caval defect. Commonly, the catheter enters a right pulmonary vein (Fig 19–14). In the posteroanterior projection, it may appear that the catheter has passed directly from the right atrium into a pulmonary vein. This does not

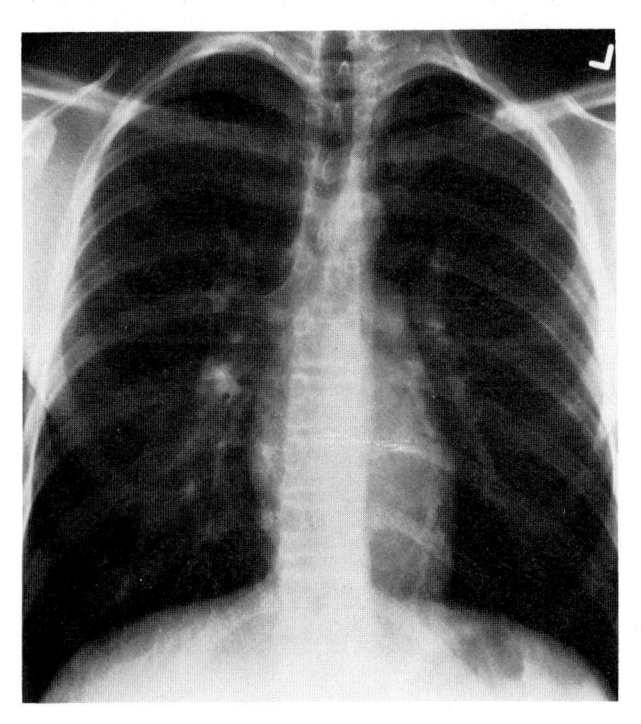

FIG 19–12.
Thoracic roentgenogram, posteroanterior projection of patient with 76% left-to-right shunt. Normal cardiac size and pulmonary vasculature; the reason for such a normal radiograph is not known. A normal chest roentgenogram does not exclude ASD with a large left-to-right shunt.

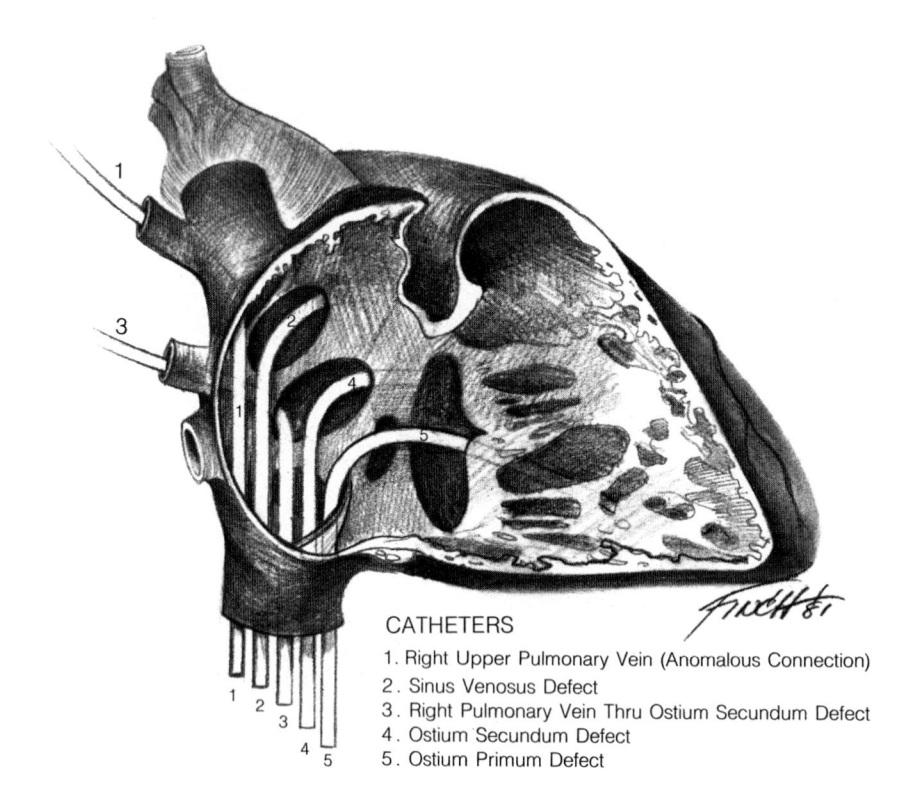

FIG 19–13.
Diagram of catheter course through various types of ASDs. *1*, catheter passed into right lung field outside right atrium, indicating anomalous connection of right upper pulmonary vein to right atrium. *2*, high catheter course, suggesting sinus venosus defect. *3* and *4*, catheter course in center of right atrium, suggesting a secundum defect. *5*, low catheter course, suggesting ostium primum defect.

CATHETERS
1. Right Upper Pulmonary Vein (Anomalous Connection)
2. Sinus Venosus Defect
3. Right Pulmonary Vein Thru Ostium Secundum Defect
4. Ostium Secundum Defect
5. Ostium Primum Defect

necessarily indicate an anomalous pulmonary connection to the right atrium. In most cases, the catheter has passed first through the septal defect and then into the normally connecting pulmonary vein (see Chapter 6).

The catheter can be passed more easily across the septal defect from the left arm than from the right arm. However, because 10% of patients have a persistent left superior vena cava, the left arm is not the preferred route for cardiac catheterization of a patient with ASD.

Pressure tracings show equal pressures in the atria, the left atrial pressure being lower than normal. Pulmonary arterial pressures are normal or slightly elevated, but in children pulmonary vascular resistance is lower than normal. There may be a gradient as large as 30 mm Hg across the right ventricular outflow area without any form of obstruction. This gradient is caused by turbulent flow through the right ventricular outflow tract.

The oximetry data show a large increase in oxygen saturation at the atrial level, usually with a 65% left-to-right shunt. The saturation in the inferior vena cava may be slightly higher than normal because of reflux of fully saturated blood from the right atrium. There may be a slight additional increase in oxygen saturation in the right ventricle, because during diastole fully saturated blood from the left atrium flows through the open tricuspid valve directly into the right ventricle. In the rare condition of ASD associated with a persistent left superior vena cava connecting directly to the left atrium, arterial desaturation is found (see Chapter 20).

A careful oximetry series should be performed throughout the right atrium and superior vena cava to detect anomalous pulmonary venous connection.

ANGIOGRAPHIC APPEARANCE

Angiographic demonstration of the atrial septal defect usually is not indicated, although it can be accomplished by a very rapid injection of contrast medium into the left atrium while filming a 45-degree angulated left anterior oblique projection angulated cranially (see Chapter 8). In some patients with a persistent right-to-left shunt after surgical repair of pulmonary stenosis, angiographic demonstration of the defect may be indicated. In these patients, a fast right atrial injection is made (Fig 19–15) in an angled 45-degree left anterior oblique projection.

1. The size of the atrial septal defect can easily be gauged by a balloon catheter,[22] the dimension of which has been calibrated by injection of a known amount of

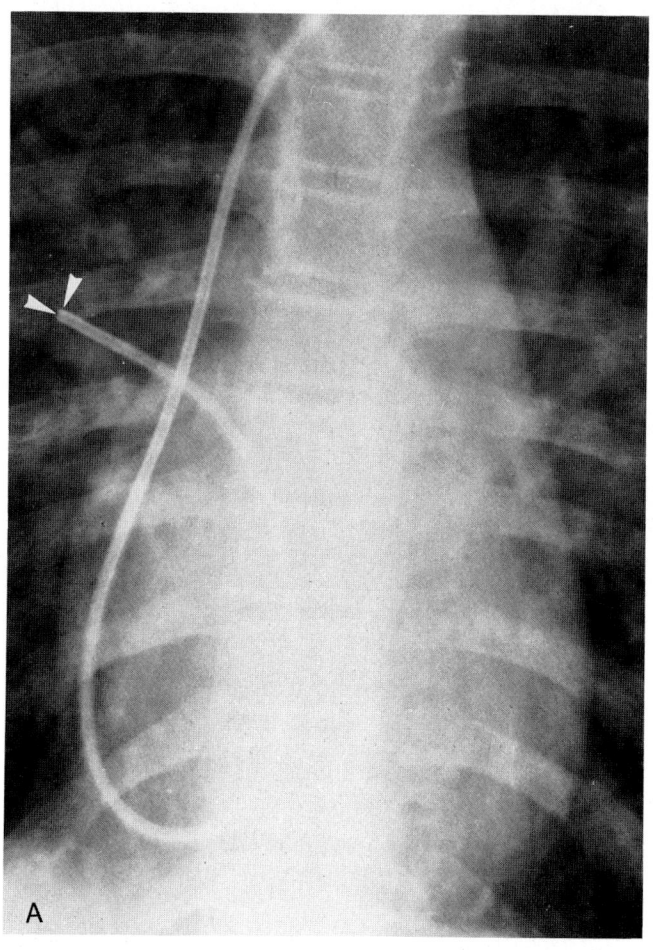

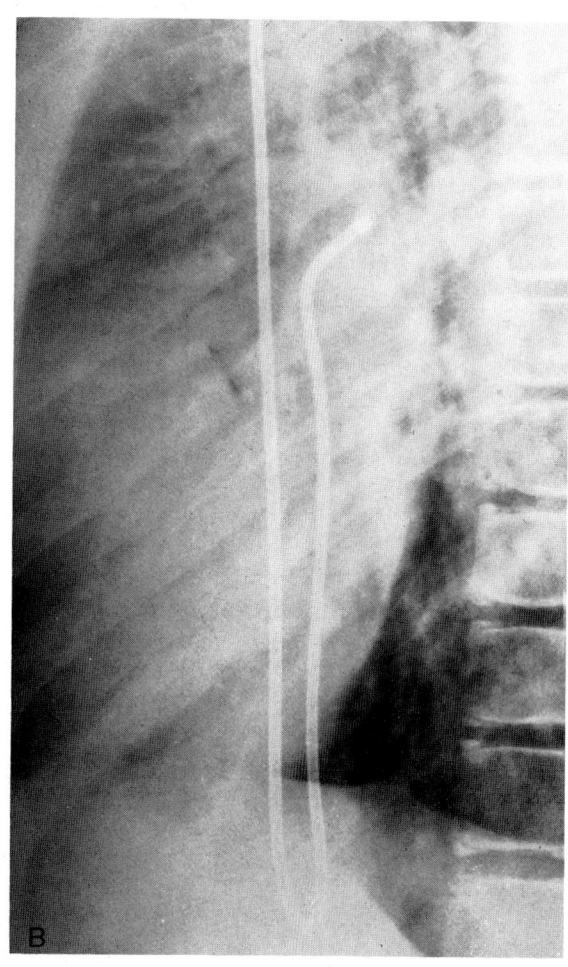

FIG 19–14.
Thoracic roentgenograms of patient with ASD. **A,** anteroposterior projection; catheter tip *(arrows)* outside cardiac silhouette in right pulmonary vein. **B,** lateral projection; catheter course posterior, suggesting passage through an atrial communication from right to left atrium and then into right upper pulmonary vein. This catheter position is commonly misinterpreted as showing anomalous connection of right upper pulmonary vein to right atrium.

contrast medium. The catheter is passed from the left atrium through the defect into the right atrium, and the size of the defect is measured by withdrawing the inflated balloon through the defect and observing its deformation fluoroscopically.

2. Pulmonary angiography demonstrates the increased pulsation of the pulmonary arteries (hilar dance) (Fig 19–16). REASON: The stroke volume of the right ventricle is markedly increased; therefore, the difference in systolic and diastolic calibers is more marked than in patients without left-to-right shunts. Pulmonary angiography must be performed by injecting a very large amount of contrast medium very rapidly. REASON: The pulmonary blood flow is markedly increased, so the contrast material tends to be diluted.

3. Pulmonary angiography is indicated to observe coexisting anomalous connecting pulmonary veins, which are recognized by the anomalous course of a pulmonary vein (Fig 19–17) and opacification of either the right or the left superior vena cava. PITFALL: Slight opacification of the right superior vena cava may occur without anomalous pulmonary venous connection because of the normal reflux of blood from the right atrium.

4. The late phase of a satisfactory pulmonary arteriogram accurately demonstrates the left-to-right shunt through the septal defect (Fig 19–18).

5. Right ventriculography is not indicated unless tricuspid insufficiency is suspected (uncommon), or there is a significant pressure gradient between the right ventricle and the pulmonary artery. Most commonly, the gradient is caused by turbulent blood flow through the right ventricular outflow tract (systolic murmur). However, on occasion, pulmonary valvular stenosis and ASD coexist.

6. If tricuspid insufficiency is suspected, a right ven-

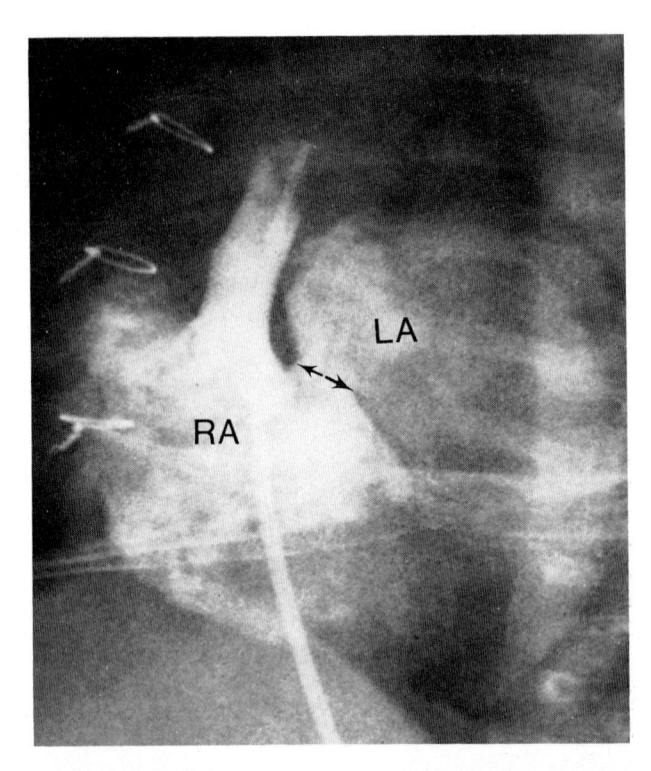

332 *Cardiac Conditions Associated With a Left-to-Right Shunt*

FIG 19–15.
Right atriogram; 45-degree left anterior oblique projection with cranial beam angulation. Atrial right-to-left shunt after repair of pulmonary artery stenosis. After injection into the right atrium, contrast material passes through the foramen ovale into left atrium. The diameter of the defect *(small arrows)* can be measured.

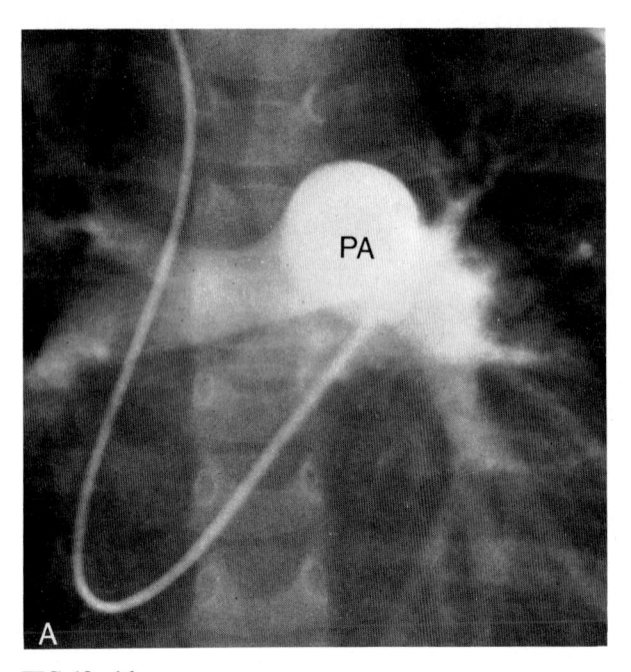

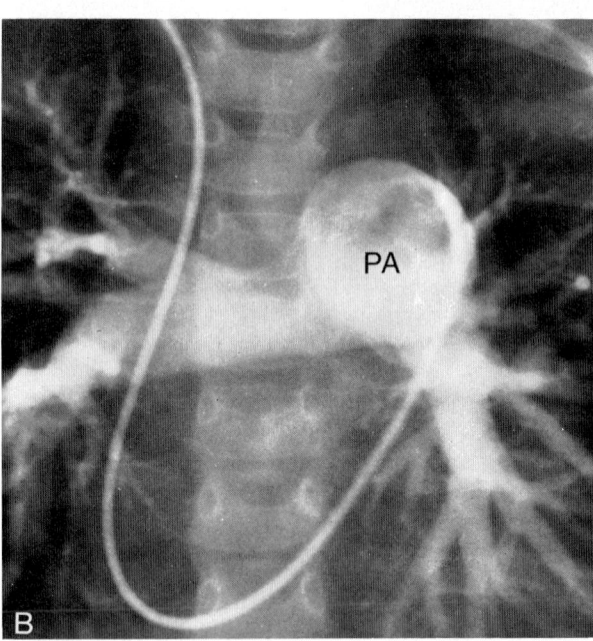

FIG 19–16.
Pulmonary arteriogram, anteroposterior projection of patient with ASD during systole **(B)** and diastole **(A)**. Marked expansion of the pulmonary arteries in systole; smaller caliber in diastole. This is the angiographic demonstration of the hilar dance caused by massively increased stroke volume of right ventricle.

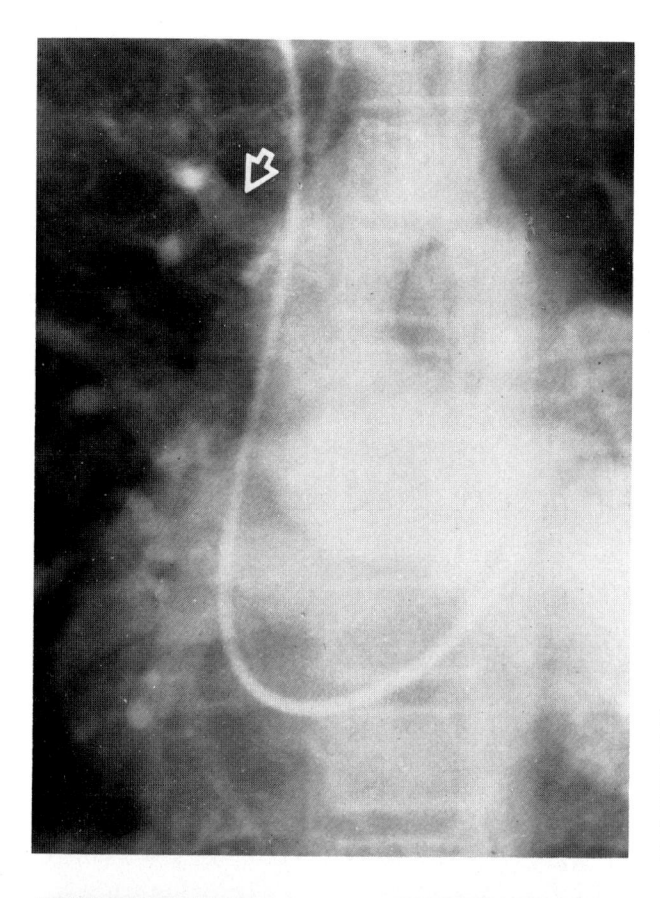

FIG 19–17.
Levophase of pulmonary arteriogram, anteroposterior projection in patient with partial anomalous pulmonary venous connection. An anomalous pulmonary vein *(arrow)* joins the superior vena cava. No shunt is present at the atrial level. The anomalous vein is identified by its abnormal, high course.

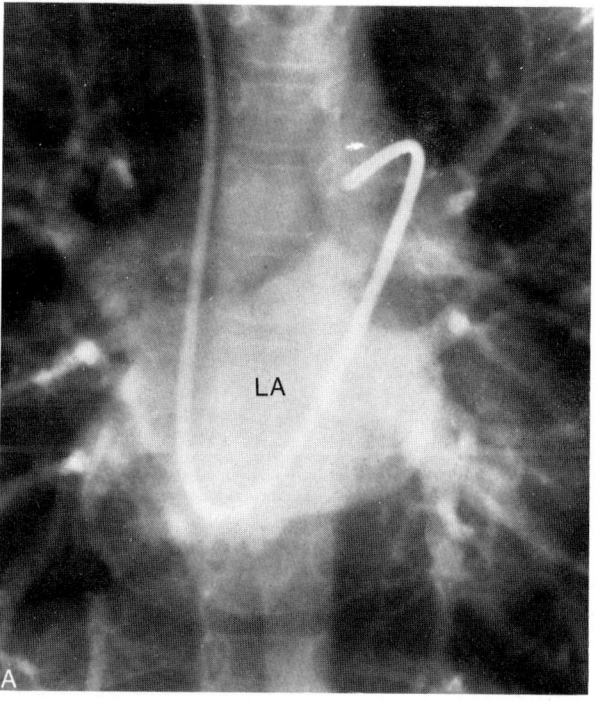

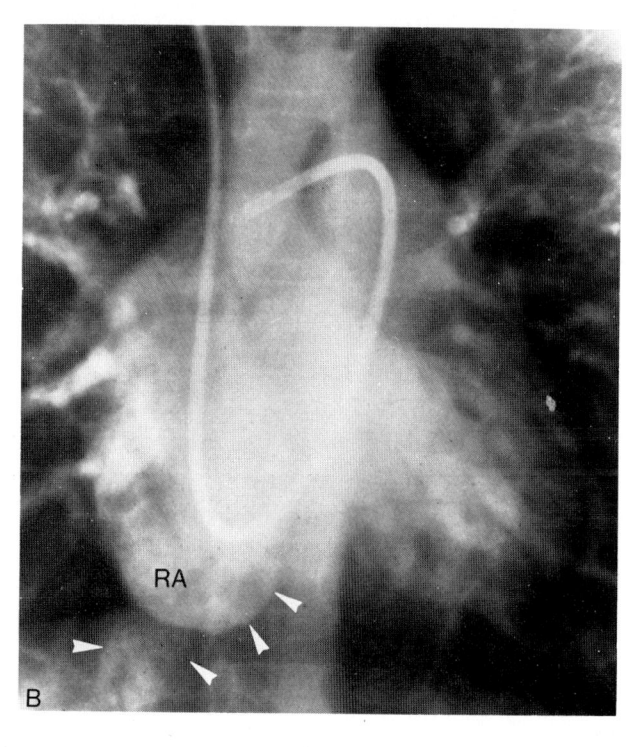

FIG 19–18.
Late phase of pulmonary arteriogram, anteroposterior projection in patient with ASD. **A,** left atrium *(LA)* and moderately enlarged pulmonary veins visible. **B,** subsequent film shows opacification of the right atrium *(RA)* and inferior vena cava *(arrows)* from atrial left-to-right shunt.

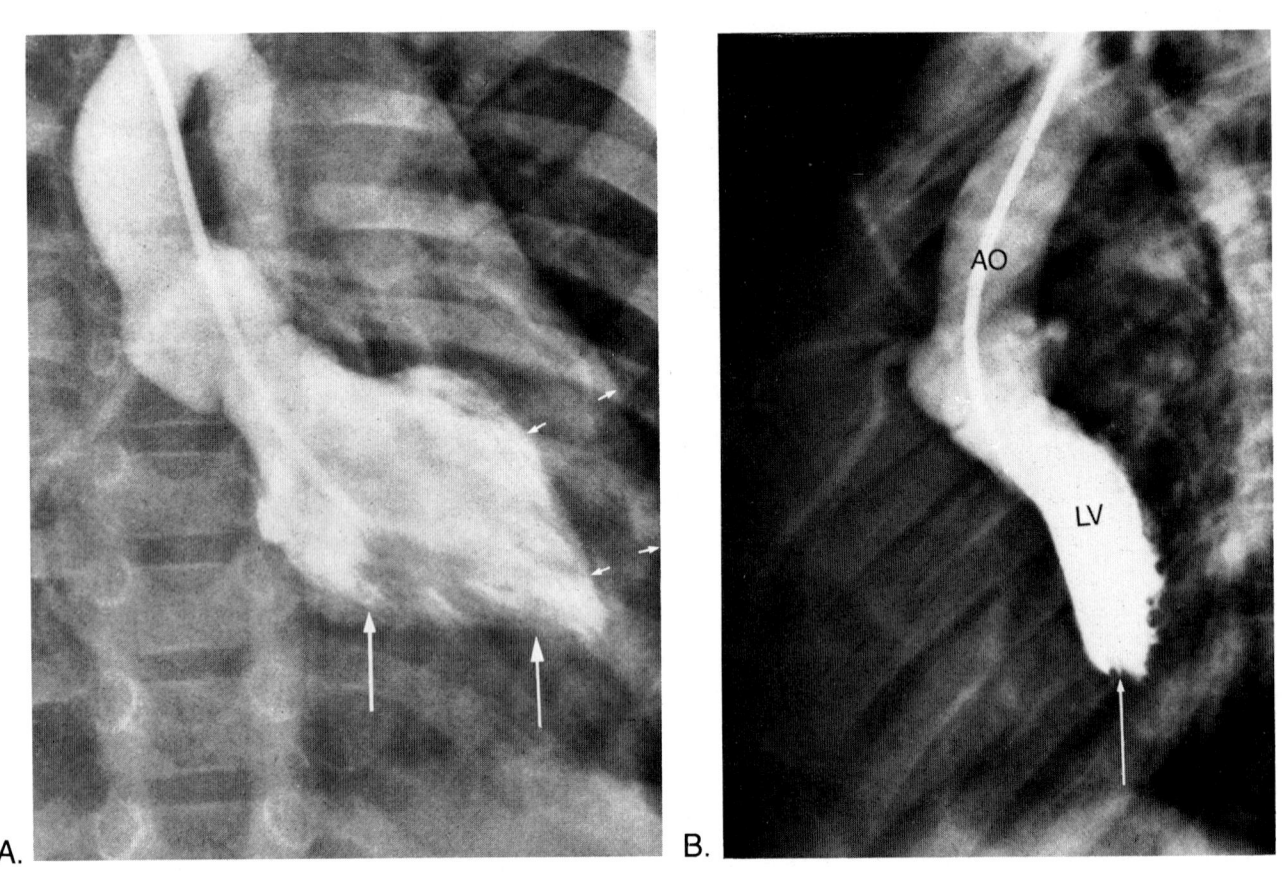

334 Cardiac Conditions Associated With a Left-to-Right Shunt

FIG 19–19.
Left ventriculogram, anteroposterior projection in patient with ASD. **A,** left ventricle is comparatively small and elevated *(long arrows).* Left ventricular wall appears thick *(small arrows),* but left cardiac border is now formed by enlarged right ventricle from clockwise rotation (pseudo left ventricular hypertrophy). This should not be mistaken for true left ventricular hypertrophy. **B,** lateral projection. Left ventricle is displaced posteriorly and elevated *(arrow)* by huge right ventricle AO = aorta; LV = left ventricle.

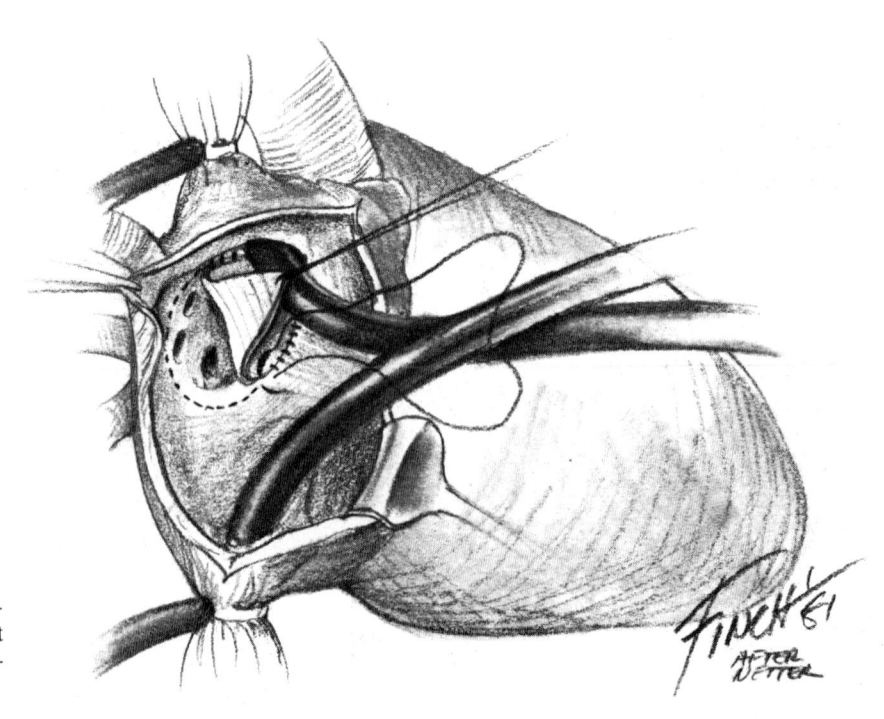

FIG 19–20.
Diagram of patch closure of ostium secundum type defect. Lateral wall of right atrium opened; cannulas in superior and inferior venae cavae.

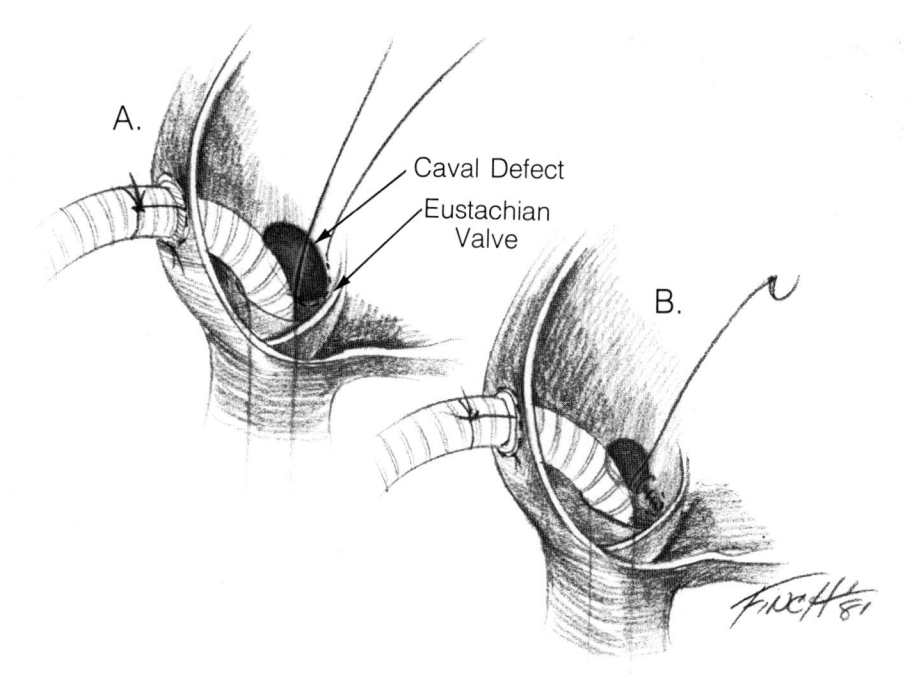

FIG 19–21.
Diagram of suture closure of inferior vena caval type of ASD. Initial sutures placed in inferior rim of defect. Cannula in inferior vena cava facilitates orientation; the defect, caval orifice, and eustachian valve may present a confusing anatomy.

triculogram should be performed. If right-sided pressure measurements are normal and clinical signs of tricuspid regurgitation are absent, right ventriculography is not indicated.

Left ventriculography should be performed to exclude the commonly associated mitral valve prolapse (15%–20%), to diagnose an associated ventricular septal defect or a left ventricular–right atrial shunt, which cannot be demonstrated by pulmonary arteriography.

1. The left ventricle is displaced posteriorly and appears to be elevated (Fig 19–19). REASON: Enlargement of the right ventricle causes clockwise rotation (see Fig 19–6), displacing the ventricle posteriorly.
2. The left ventricle appears small in comparison with the overall cardiac size.
3. On the lateral view, the septum is seen more on end. REASON: Clockwise rotation of the heart.
4. The thickness of the left ventricular wall may appear to be increased (Fig 19–19). REASON: With the clockwise rotation of the heart, the cardiac border may be formed by the enlarged right ventricle. Therefore, the distance between the opacified left ventricle and the free margin of the heart does not represent the true thickness of the left ventricular wall, as it does in the normal heart.

OPERATIVE CONSIDERATIONS

Operation is indicated in all children with an ASD and left-to-right shunt more than 50%.[23] It should be performed on an elective basis about the age of 5 years, because pulmonary vascular disease does not develop before that age. Atrial septal defects should not be closed before the age of 1 year, because perhaps 50% of these defects

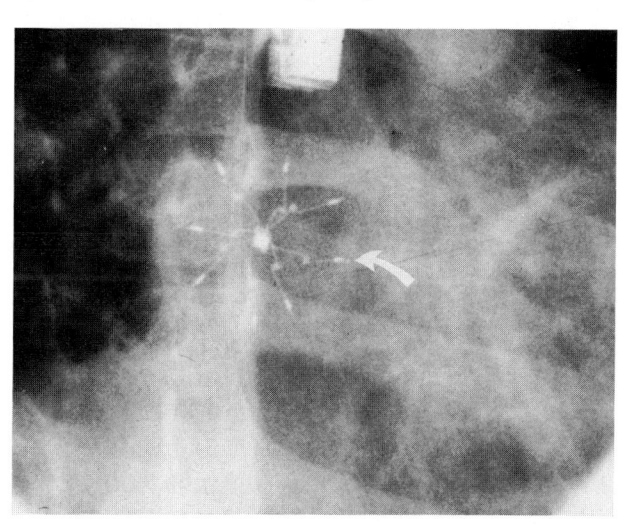

FIG 19–22.
Patient with small atrial septal defect and repeated peripheral emboli who had closure of his defect *(arrow)* by transcatheter technique.

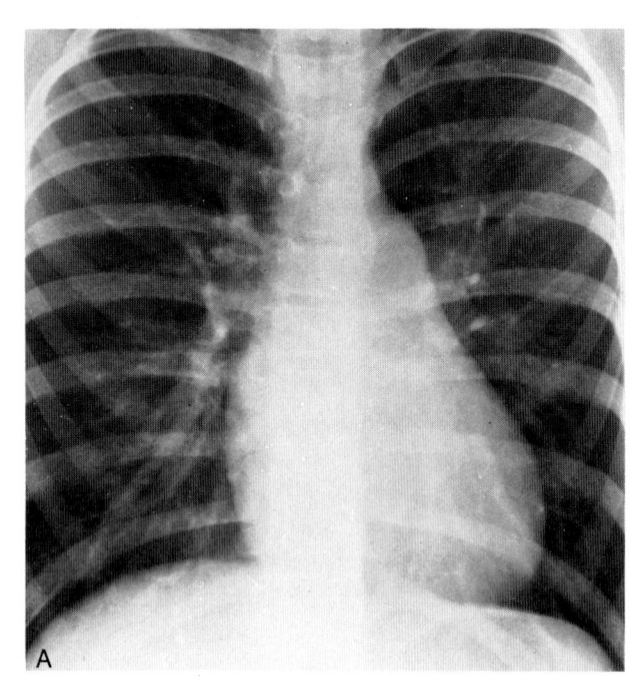

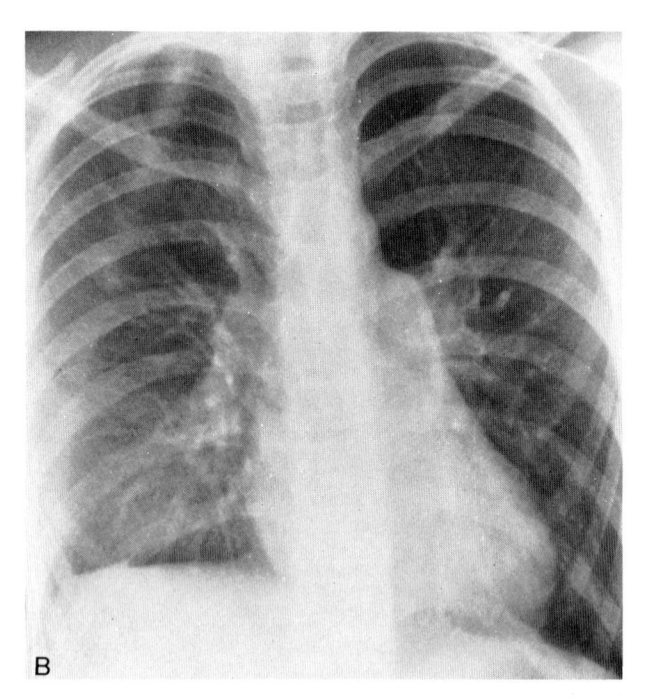

FIG 19–23.
Thoracic roentengenograms, posteroanterior projection of patient with ASD. **A,** preoperative film. **B,** week after closure of ASD; marked reduction in cardiac size and pulmonary blood flow.

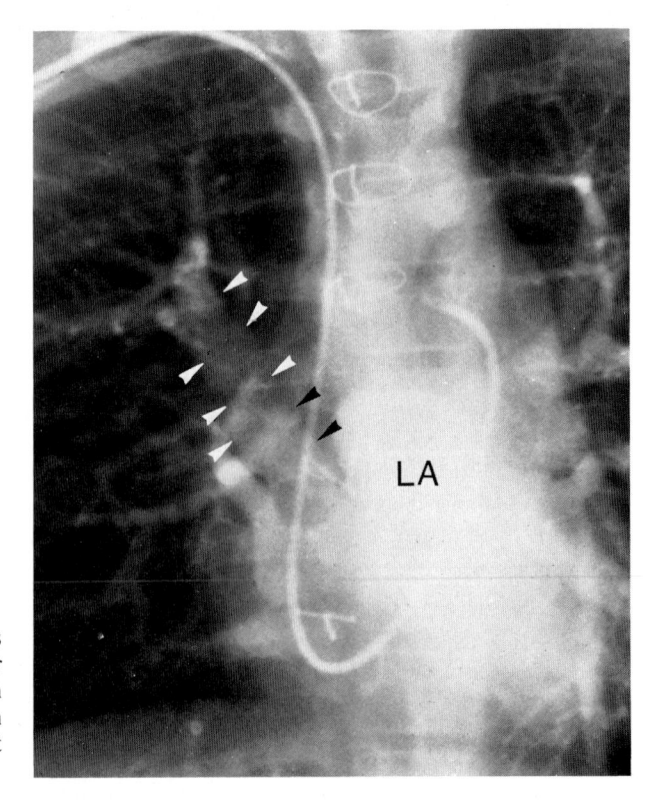

FIG 19–24.
Levophase of a pulmonary angiogram in patient with sinus venosus defect and anomalous pulmonary venous connection of right upper lobe vein. Atrial septal defect was closed, and patch was sewn in such a fashion that the anomalous right upper lobe pulmonary vein *(arrows)* now drains normally into left atrium *(LA)*. Left-to-right shunt has been completely corrected.

close spontaneously.[24-26] Operative closure is also indicated in adults except in those with severe pulmonary vascular disease. Closure usually does not reverse pulmonary hypertension.

Operation is performed using cardiopulmonary bypass. The defect is closed either by direct suture or by suturing a patch of Dacron or pericardium over the defect (Fig 19–20). Care must be taken in repairing the low cavaltype of defect. The initial sutures should be placed in the inferior aspect of the defect and continued superiorly; if the order of suturing is reversed, it is possible to close the defect in such a way that the inferior vena cava empties into the left atrium (Fig 19–21).

The operative mortality in children is less than 1% and slightly higher in adults.

Smaller defects can be closed with prosthetic devices during cardiac catheterization (Fig 19–22).

POSTOPERATIVE STATUS

The patient should be given prophylactic penicillin for dental procedures for 6 months postoperatively, but after that, the risk of bacterial endocarditis is nonexistent.

In children, auscultatory, ECG, and radiographic findings return to normal postoperatively, but in adolescents or adults, ECG or radiographic findings may remain abnormal.[27-29] An occasional child, and perhaps 10% of adults, have an atrial arrhythmia postoperatively. Our postoperative catheterization studies have shown an incidence of residual shunt of less than 1%. Children have a normal exercise response.

Other points:

1. Shortly after closure of an atrial septal defect, there is a decrease in cardiac size and pulmonary flow (Fig 19–23).
2. Operative correction of anomalous pulmonary venous connection and ASD can be accomplished by extending the patch obliquely over the entry site of the anomalous pulmonary veins (Fig 19–24).
3. When the eustachian valve is sutured to the edges of a low-lying caval defect, the vena cava may be incorporated accidentally into the left atrium, resulting in a right-to-left shunt (Fig 19–25).

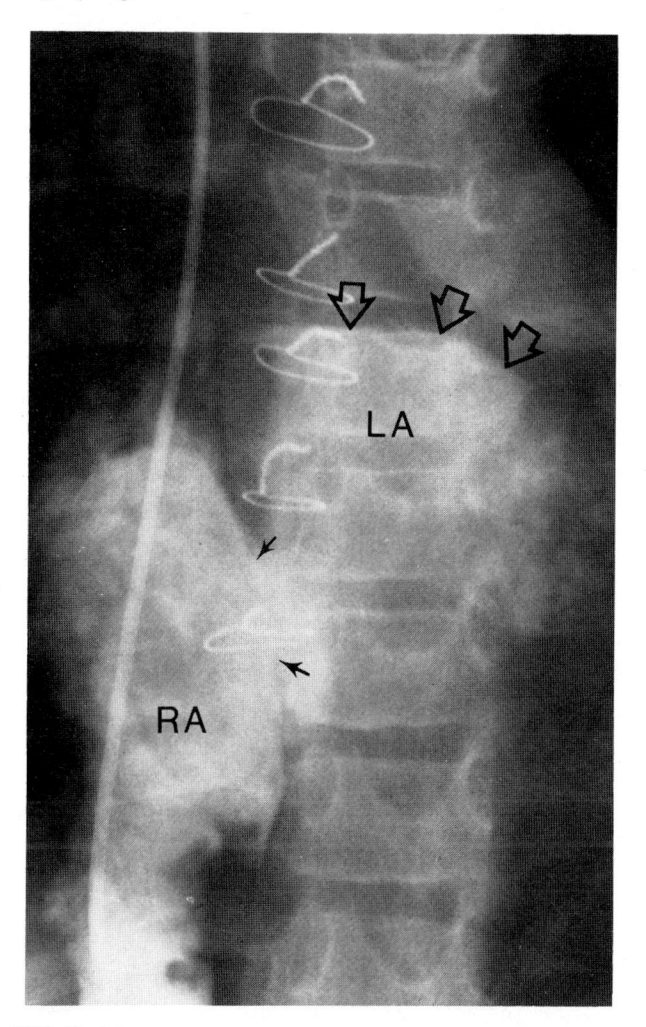

FIG 19–25.
Inferior vena cavogram, anteroposterior projection of patient who became cyanotic after repair of an inferior vena cava–type ASD. A right-to-left shunt through defect *(small arrows)* is demonstrated. Opacification of left atrium *(LA) (large arrows)*. This shunt accounted for the postoperative cyanosis. RA = right atrium.

REFERENCES

1. Edwards JE: The pathology of atrial septal defect, *Semin Roentgenol* 1:24, 1966.
2. Raghib G, Ruttenberg HD, Anderson RC, et al: Termination of left superior vena cava in left atrium, atrial septal defect, and absence of coronary sinus: a developmental complex, *Circulation* 31:906, 1965.
3. Hynes KM, Frye RL, Brandenburg RO, et al: Atrial septal defect (secundum) associated with mitral regurgitation, *Am J Cardiol* 34:333, 1974.
4. Victorica BE, Elliott LP, Gessner IH: Ostium secundum atrial septal defect associated with balloon mitral valve in children, *Am J Cardiol* 33:668, 1974.
5. Levin AR, Spach MS, Boineau JP, et al: Atrial pressure-flow dynamics in atrial septal defects (secundum type), *Circulation* 37:476, 1968.
6. Craig RJ, Selzer A: Natural history and prognosis of atrial septal defect, *Circulation* 37:805, 1968.
7. Khoury GH, Hawes CR: Atrial septal defect associated with pulmonary hypertension in children living at high altitude, *J Pediatr* 70:432, 1967.
8. Saksena FB, Aldridge HE: Atrial septal defect in the older

patient: a clinical and hemodynamic study in patients operated on after age 35, *Circulation* 42:1009, 1979.
9. Gault JH, Morrow AG, Gay WA Jr, et al: Atrial septal defect in patients over the age of forty years: clinical and hemodynamic studies and the effects of operation, *Circulation* 37:261, 1968.
10. Hastreiter AR, Wennemark JR, Miller RA, et al: Secundum atrial septal defects with congestive heart failure during infancy and early childhood, *Am Heart J* 64:467, 1962.
11. Hunt CE, Lucas RV Jr: Symptomatic atrial septal defect in infancy, *Circulation* 47:1042, 1973.
12. Hoffman JIE, Rudolph AM, Danilowicz D: Left to right atrial shunts in infants, *Am J Cardiol* 30:868, 1972.
13. Nakamura FF, Hauck AJ, Nadas AS: Atrial septal defect in infants, *Pediatrics* 34:101, 1964.
14. Lopez JF, Linn H, Shaffer AB: The apical first heart sound as an aid in the diagnosis of atrial septal defect, *Circulation* 26:1296, 1962.
15. O'Toole JD, Reddy PS, Curtiss EI, et al: The mechanism of splitting of the second heart sound in atrial septal defect, *Circulation* 56:1047, 1977.
16. Kumar S, Luisada AA: The second heart sound in atrial septal defect, *Am J Cardiol* 28:168, 1971.
17. Anderson PAW, Rogers MC, Canent RV Jr, et al: Atrioventricular conduction in secundum atrial septal defects, *Circulation* 48:27, 1973.
18. Boineau JP, Spach MS, Ayers CR: Genesis of the electrocardiogram in atrial septal defect, *Am Heart J* 68:637, 1964.
19. Diamond MA, Dillon JC, Haine CL, et al: Echocardiographic features of atrial septal defect, *Circulation* 43:129, 1971.
20. Lieppe W, Scallion R, Behar VS, et al: Two-dimensional echocardiographic findings in atrial septal defect, *Circulation* 56:447, 1977.
21. Neal WA, Moller JH, Varco RL, et al: Operative repair of atrial septal defect without cardiac catheterization, *J Pediatr* 86:189, 1975.
22. King TD, Thompson SL, Mills NL: Measurement of atrial septal defect during cardiac catheterization: experimental and clinical results, *Am J Cardiol* 41:537, 1978.
23. Moss AJ, Siassi B: The small atrial septal defect—operate or procrastinate? *J Pediatr* 79:854, 1971.
24. Cumming GR: Functional closure of atrial septal defects, *Am J Cardiol* 22:888, 1968.
25. Mody MR: Serial hemodynamic observations in secundum atrial septal defect with special reference to spontaneous closure, *Am J Cardiol* 32:978, 1973.
26. Cayler GC: Spontaneous functional closure of symptomatic atrial septal defects, *N Engl J Med* 276:65, 1967.
27. Liberthson RR, Boucher CA, Strauss HW, et al: Right ventricular function in adult atrial septal defect: preoperative and postoperative assessment and clinical implications, *Am J Cardiol* 47:56, 1961.
28. Dave KS, Pakrashi BC, Wooler GH, et al: Atrial septal defect in adults: clinical and hemodynamic results of surgery, *Am J Cardiol* 31:7, 1973.
29. Nasrallah AT, Hall RJ, Garcia E, et al: Surgical repair of atrial septal defect in patients over 60 years of age: long-term results, *Circulation* 53:329, 1976.

CHAPTER 20

Raghib Syndrome and Other Coronary Sinus Anomalies Allowing Intracardiac Shunts

In 1965, Raghib et al.[1] described a developmental complex of termination of left superior vena cava in the left atrium, atrial septal defect, and absence of the coronary sinus. This is an uncommon cardiac anomaly, which has unique clinical and angiographic findings.

PATHOLOGIC ANATOMY

The left jugular venous system and left subclavian vein join to form the left superior vena cava, which passes anteriorly to the aortic arch and left pulmonary artery to join the left atrium between the left pulmonary veins posteriorly and the base of the left atrial appendage anteriorly (Fig 20–1). In most cases, a small bridging vein connects the left superior vena cava to the right superior vena cava. The coronary sinus is absent, and the cardiac veins drain directly into the atria.

An atrial septal defect is present at the normal site of the coronary sinus, posteroinferiorly to the fossa ovalis, medial to the entrance of the inferior vena cava, and above the septal leaflet of the tricuspid valve (see Chapter 19). In the left atrium, the defect is located near the posterior atrial wall and above the posteromedial commissure of the mitral valve.

There may also be an endocardial cushion defect. In such cases, the atrial septal defect extends the atrial component of the endocardial cushion defect more posteriorly.

EMBRYOLOGIC DEVELOPMENT

Raghib syndrome results from abnormal development in the sinoatrial portion of the heart (Fig 20–2). At an early stage, the right and left common cardinal veins join the sinus venosus, which has a broad communication with the common atrium. Subsequently, two processes begin simultaneously: the initial development of the septum primum, which starts the process of division of the common atrium, and development of a fold between the common cardinal vein and the common atrium. This fold deepens progressively, directing the left common cardinal vein into the right atrium, while the septum primum is completing the division of the common atrium. Normally the branches of the left anterior cardinal vein involute, but the coronary sinus remains.

If this infolding process is arrested, the coronary sinus is not formed; the left superior vena cava, representing a remnant of the left anterior cardinal vein, connects directly with the left atrium; and there is an atrial septal defect in the location of the coronary sinus. Because the septum primum is also developing at this time, ostium primum defects may coexist.

HEMODYNAMICS

The hemodynamics are those of an atrial septal defect, but there is a small right-to-left shunt because the left superior vena cava connects directly to the left atrium.

CLINICAL FEATURES

The clinical findings are those of atrial septal defect or of a form of endocardial cushion defect. The history of cyanosis or its presence on physical examination of a patient with an atrial left-to-right shunt should alert the clinician

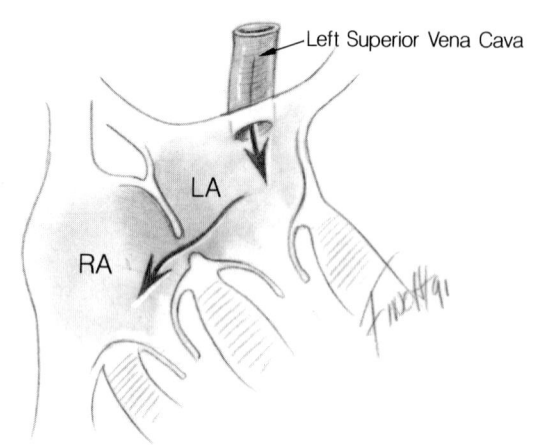

340 *Cardiac Conditions Associated With a Left-to-Right Shunt*

FIG 20–1.
Diagram of pathologic anatomy of Raghib syndrome. Left superior vena cava terminates in left atrium; coronary sinus is absent. Atrial communication at location of the normally encountered coronary sinus ostium. *LA* = left atrium; *LV* = left ventricle; *RA* = right atrium; *RV* = right ventricle.

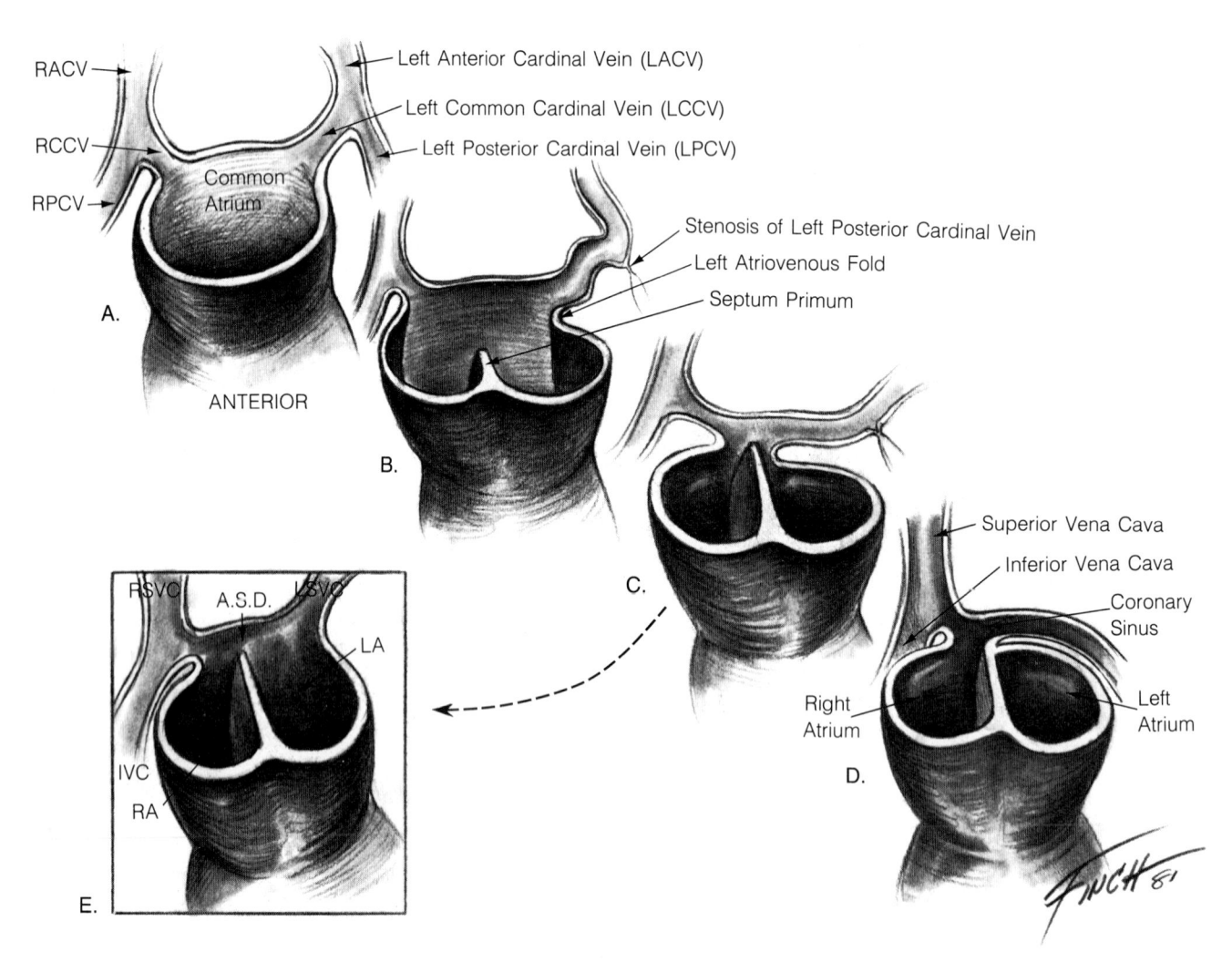

FIG 20–2.
Diagram of development of coronary sinus; superior view of sinoatrial region of embryo from above. **A,** common cardinal veins join respective sides of atrium. **B,** left posterior cardinal vein has involuted. Beginning of formation of atrial septum. **C,** continued formation of atrial septum. Evagination in posterior wall of left atrium separating the coronary sinus. **D,** atrial septum fused; coronary sinus completely formed. **E,** abnormality in Raghib syndrome: left superior vena cava *(LSVC)* to left atrium *(LA),* absence of coronary sinus, posterior atrial septal defect *(ASD).* *IVC* = inferior vena cava; *RA* = right atrium; *RSVC* = right superior vena cava.

to this condition. The auscultatory findings are those of an atrial septal defect.

ELECTROCARDIOGRAPHIC FEATURES

The electrocardiogram resembles that of either an ostium secundum atrial septal defect or an endocardial cushion defect but has no distinctive features.

RADIOGRAPHIC FEATURES

1. In isolated Raghib syndrome, the chest roentgenograms resemble those seen in atrial septal defect (see Chapter 19).
2. When another congenital malformation coexists, the chest roentgenogram is not altered by Raghib syndrome.
3. Careful examination of the posteroanterior roentgenogram may demonstrate a faint density along the left superior mediastinum, suggesting a persistent left vena cava (see Chapter 19). In patients with systemic arterial desaturation, this subtle radiographic finding may suggest the diagnosis of Raghib syndrome.

CARDIAC CATHETERIZATION

The correct diagnosis can be made before cardiac catheterization by echocardiography.

The basic hemodynamics are those of an atrial septal defect, or those of an endocardial cushion defect, if it is coexistent. Therefore, Raghib syndrome must be considered in any patient with an atrial level shunt. The unique clue is the presence of mild systemic arterial desaturation, which may be from 83% to 93%, because the left superior vena cava, carrying desaturated blood, joins the left atrium directly. Passage of the catheter through a very low-lying defect should suggest the diagnosis: Whereas this low passage is to be expected in patients with complete atrioventricular canal, it is unexpected in ostium secundum defect.

ANGIOGRAPHIC APPEARANCE

The angiograms are diagnostic. However, angiographic recognition of the anomaly can be difficult unless one is aware of this malformation and the contrast medium is injected into the left superior vena cava.

1. If the catheter is passed from the right atrium into a persistent left superior vena cava, a small volume of contrast medium should be introduced with a power injector to determine the site of termination of the superior vena cava.

2. In cases of Raghib syndrome, contrast medium flows from the left superior vena cava directly into the left atrium rather than through the coronary sinus into the right atrium (Fig 20–3).

3. If suspected, the diagnosis of Raghib syndrome can be made by a peripheral injection of contrast medium into the left arm, whereby contrast medium flows from the left superior vena cava into the left atrium (Fig 20–4). However, several variants of Raghib syndrome can be excluded only by selective injections. This anomaly can also be excluded after the catheterization by an ultrasonic "bubblegram."

4. In contrast to circumstances when the left superior

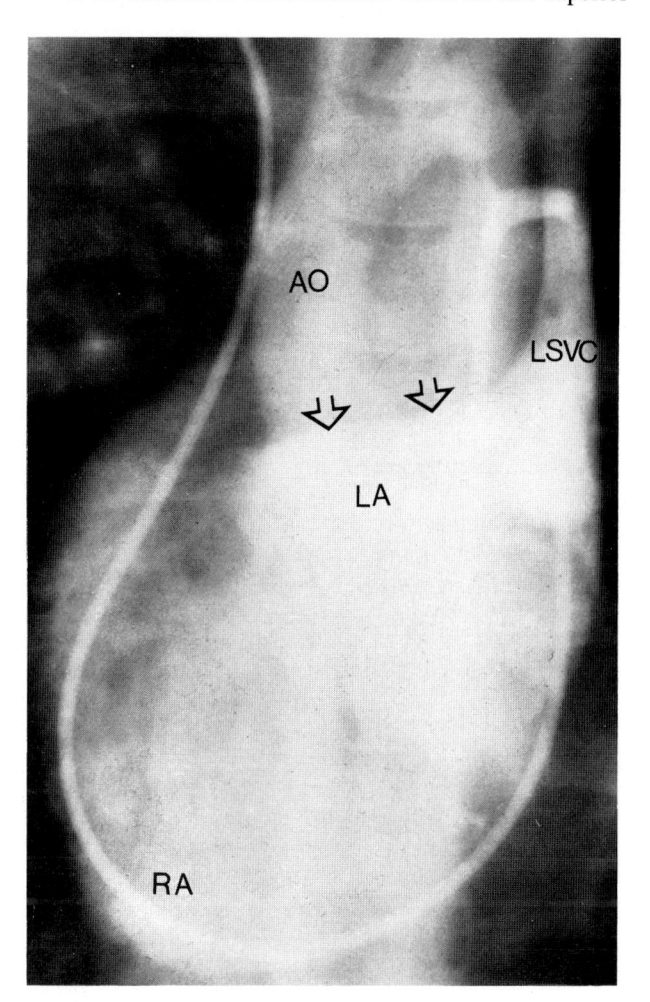

FIG 20–3.
Venous catheter passed from right atrium *(RA)* into left superior vena cava; course is typical for coronary sinus passage. Injection of contrast medium demonstrates a left superior vena cava *(LSVC)*, and there is immediate opacification of the left atrium *(LA) (arrows)*. Left superior vena cava terminates directly in left atrium. Coronary sinus is not opacified. Dense opacification of right atrium from left-to-right shunt through atrial septal defect. Opacification of aorta *(AO)* also confirms connection of left superior vena cava with left atrium; aorta does not immediately opacify if left superior vena cava connects with coronary sinus.

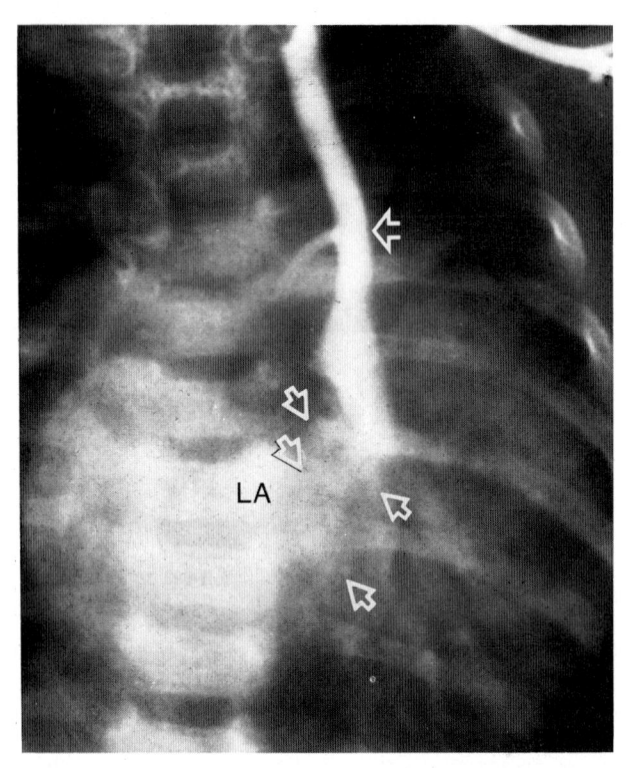

FIG 20-4.
Injection of contrast medium into left antecubital vein, posteroanterior projection. Persistent left superior vena cava *(white arrow)* connecting directly with the left atrium *(LA)*. Immediate dilution of contrast medium by blood in left atrium *(open arrows)*.

vena cava terminates in the coronary sinus, the contrast medium is diluted immediately at the junction of the left superior vena cava with the left atrium.

OPERATIVE CONSIDERATIONS

The atrial defect is closed with a patch as in simple atrial septal defect. If an endocardial cushion defect coexists, it is corrected in the usual manner (see Chapter 23). If there are bilateral superior venae cavae, the left superior vena cava can often be ligated, because the bridging innominate and jugular veins provide adequate collateral flow. An alternative to ligation is rerouting the left superior vena cava to the right atrium.

VARIANTS OF RAGHIB SYNDROME (CORONARY SINUS–LEFT ATRIAL WINDOW)

In some patients, the wall of the coronary sinus is partially formed, resulting in one or more fenestrations between the coronary sinus and the left atrium. As in Raghib syndrome, a persistent left superior vena cava may be present. These variants are often associated with atresia or stenosis of one of the atrioventricular valves.[2]

Hemodynamics

Because the left atrial pressure exceeds the right atrial pressure, a left-to-right shunt usually occurs, with blood passing from the left atrium through the fenestration into the coronary sinus and thence to the right atrium. Because the pressure differential between the atria is low, a small right-to-left shunt may be present as well (Fig 20–5).

In one variant (Fig 20–6,A), there is associated tricuspid atresia. If the foramen ovale is closed, the only egress of blood from the right atrium is through the coronary sinus and through the fenestrations into the left atrium. In another variant (Fig 20–6,B), with mitral atresia and coronary sinus ostial stenosis, blood leaves the left atrium through the coronary sinus and passes to the left superior vena cava, forming a left-to-right shunt.

In these situations with atrioventricular valve atresia, the left atrial–coronary sinus window represents the only pathway for regress of blood and creates an obligatory right-to-left or left-to-right shunt.

A very rare form of a left-to-right shunt is atresia of the coronary sinus and fenestration with persistent left superior vena cava.

RADIOGRAPHIC AND CLINICAL FEATURES

1. The chest roentgenogram. The coronary sinus–left atrial window is commonly associated with complex congenital heart disease and provides an obligatory shunt that is necessary to sustain life. A correct diagnosis can be made only by angiography.

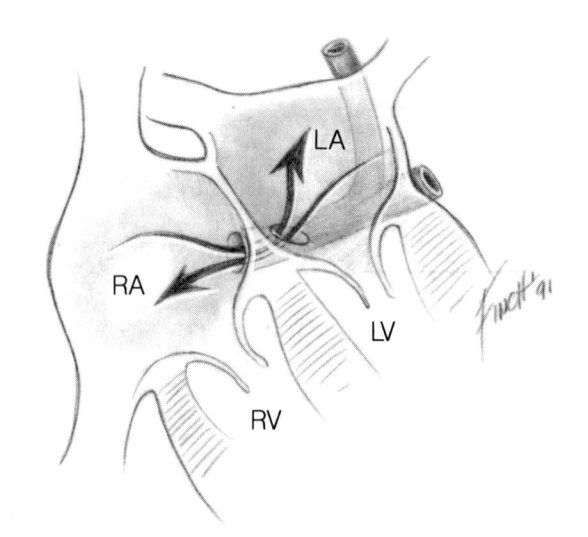

FIG 20-5.
Diagram of pathologic anatomy of coronary sinus fenestration. Because of low pressure difference between right *(RA)* and left atrium *(LA)*, bidirectional shunt is present.

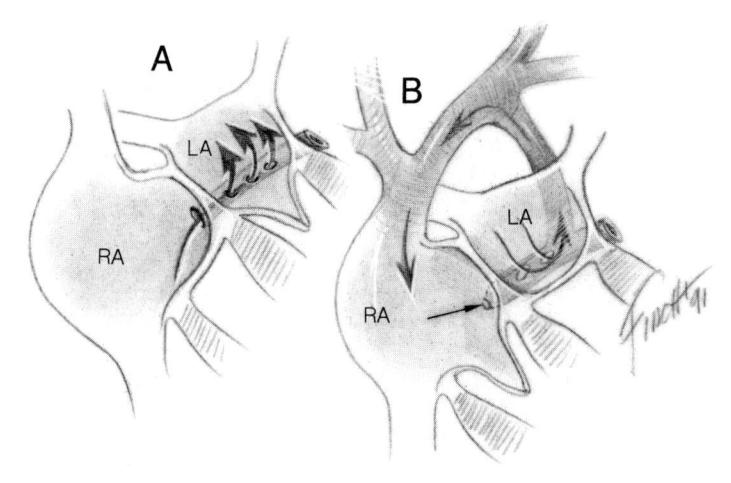

FIG 20–6.
Coronary sinus fenestration and atrioventricular valve atresia. **A,** tricuspid atresia and intact atrial septum; obligatory right-to-left shunt occurs through coronary sinus and coronary sinus fenestrations *(arrows)*. **B,** mitral atresia and intact atrial septum. Obligatory left-to-right shunt occurs through coronary sinus fenestration in the direction indicated by arrows. Associated stenosis of coronary ostium *(straight arrow)*. *LA* = left atrium; *RA* = right atrium.

There are no distinctive clinical or laboratory findings. These rare anomalies are suspected only during cardiac catheterization or angiography.

CARDIAC CATHETERIZATION AND ANGIOGRAPHY

1. In addition to the results of careful oxygen sampling at time of cardiac catheterization, coronary sinus–left atrial windows can be diagnosed on the basis of the course of the catheter. Characteristically, the catheter is passed into the coronary sinus and then through a fenestration (window) into the left atrium (Fig 20–7).

2. In most cases, coronary sinus–left atrial window causes a left-to-right shunt, which can be demonstrated by angiography (Fig 20–7).

3. In spite of the predominant left-to-right shunt through most coronary sinus–left atrial windows, left superior cavography usually demonstrates the fenestration by slight opacification of the left atrium because the shunt is

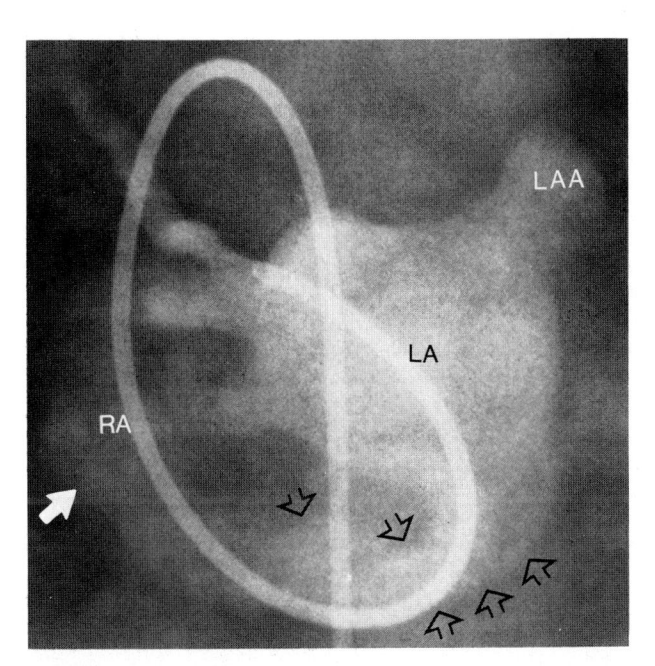

FIG 20–7.
Left atriogram, anteroposterior projection of coronary sinus–left atrial window. Interruption of hepatic segment of the inferior vena cava. Catheter course is from azygous vein to right superior vena cava, right atrium, coronary sinus, and finally through window into left atrium *(LA)*. Contrast medium flows into coronary sinus *(open arrows)* and right atrium *(RA)*. Right atrium *(white arrow)* is clearly opacified because of left-to-right shunt. *LAA* = left atrial appendage.

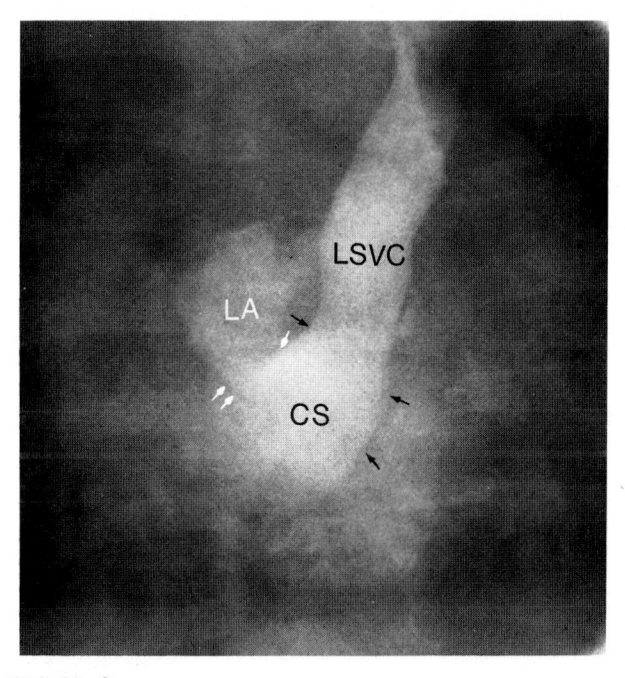

FIG 20–8.
Left superior vena cavogram, anteroposterior projection. Dilated left superior vena cava *(LSVC)* terminates in coronary sinus *(CS)* *(small black arrows)*. Left superior vena cava is dilated because of predominant left-to-right shunt. However, left atrium *(LA)* also opacifies through coronary sinus–left atrial window *(white arrows)* because of bidirectional shunt.

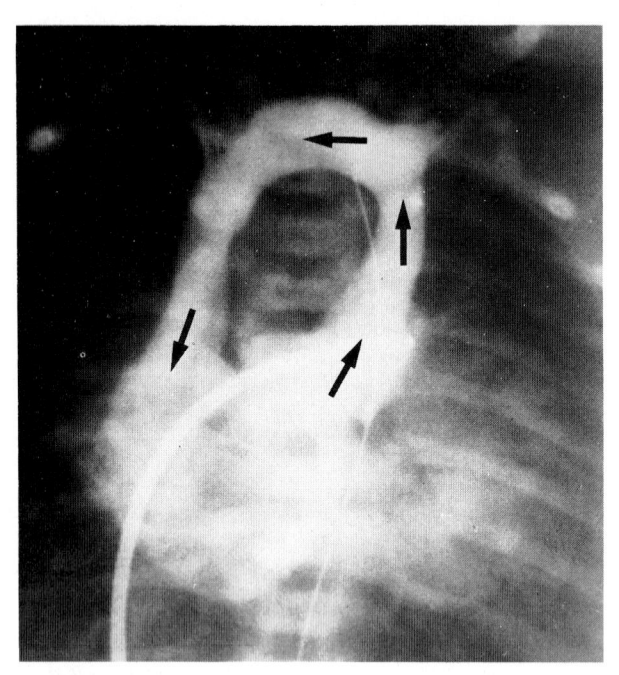

FIG 20–9.
Left atriogram, anteroposterior projection in mitral atresia, coronary sinus–left atrial window, and left superior vena cava connecting to left atrium. Contrast flows from left atrium into left superior vena cava, innominate vein, right superior vena cava, and right atrium *(arrows)*. In this patient, the foramen ovale was sealed, and obligatory left-to-right shunt could not occur through atrial defect.

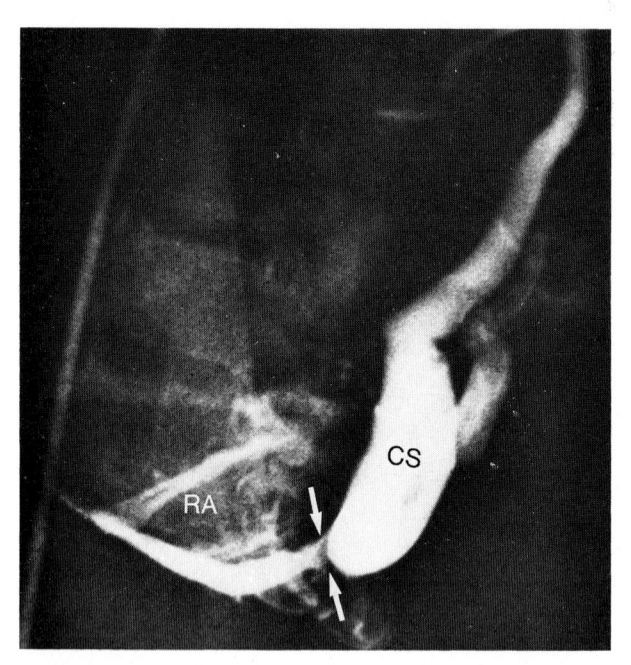

FIG 20–10.
Coronary sinus angiogram, anteroposterior projection in stenosis of coronary ostium. Catheter passed through persistent left superior vena cava into coronary sinus *(CS)*. Oxygen saturation in coronary sinus was low, indicating absence of fenestration. Severe stenosis of coronary ostium *(arrows)*; slight opacification of right atrium *(RA)*.

bidirectional (Fig 20–8). Unlike the findings in Raghib syndrome, the coronary sinus is clearly visible.

    4. In cases of atresia of the mitral valve or atresia of the coronary sinus ostium, blood flow through the left superior vena cava is reversed: Blood flows into the innominate vein, and then into the right superior vena cava (Fig 20–9). This is a very rare form of a left-to-right shunt.

    5. Similarly, in patients with tricuspid atresia, Raghib syndrome or coronary sinus–left atrial windows may allow an obligatory right-to-left shunt in patients with a competent foramen ovale (see Fig 20–6,A).

    6. Coronary sinus stenosis or atresia may occur without fenestration. It is usually of no hemodynamic significance (Fig 20–10).

SUMMARY

Coronary sinus abnormalities are important in the explanation of the peripheral desaturation without a murmur and left-to-right shunts at the atrial level without atrial septal defects or anomalous veins. They may provide egress of blood in patients with mitral or tricuspid atresia and no atrial communication.

    The coronary sinus may be completely absent (Raghib syndrome) or partially absent (fenestration). The coronary sinus ostium may be stenotic or atretic. If no other defect is present, egress of coronary venous blood occurs via enlarged thebesian veins into the atria. Rarely, a fistula between coronary sinus and left ventricle or coronary artery occurs.

REFERENCES

1. Raghib G, Ruttenberg HD, Anderson RC, et al: Termination of left superior vena cava in left atrium, atrial septal defect, and absence of coronary sinus: a developmental complex, *Circulation* 31:906, 1965.
2. Nath PH, Delaney DJ, Zollikofer C, et al: Coronary sinus–left atrial window, *Radiology* 135:319, 1980.

CHAPTER 21

Partial Anomalous Pulmonary Venous Connection

In partial anomalous pulmonary venous connection (PAPVC), one or more—but not all—pulmonary veins do not connect with the left atrium but with the right atrium or a systemic venous channel. Partial anomalous pulmonary venous connection results in an isolated left-to-right shunt. This is in contrast to total anomalous pulmonary venous connection, in which an obligatory right-to-left shunt is present, resulting in cyanosis (see Chapter 46).

INCIDENCE

In necropsy studies, an incidence of 0.6% to 0.7% has been reported for PAPVC. This is considerably greater than the incidence recognized clinically, indicating that PAPVC, particularly when unassociated with other cardiac anomalies, is not always diagnosed. Most cases discovered during life coexist with atrial septal defect, because PAPVC occurs in 10% of such patients.

ANATOMIC PATHOLOGY

Partial anomalous pulmonary venous connection affects the right lung more commonly than the left lung. Generally, the anomalous pulmonary venous connection is to the derivatives of the right or left cardinal venous system.

Regardless of the site of connection, the hemodynamic effects are the same. Because of the left-to-right shunt, the right atrium and the right ventricle are dilated. The left side of the heart is normal.

Several anatomic types of partial anomalous pulmonary venous connection have been described (Fig 21-1) and are listed according to site of the connecting pulmonary veins.

1. Right superior pulmonary vein connecting with the right superior vena cava or right atrium. This is the most common form of PAPVC (Fig 21-1,A) and is usually associated with a sinus venosus–type atrial septal defect. Sometimes, pulmonary veins from both the right upper lobe and the right middle lobe enter the superior vena cava (Fig 21-1,B). The pulmonary vein from the right lower lobe usually connects normally with the left atrium.
2. Right pulmonary veins with the inferior vena cava immediately below the diaphragm. This may be an isolated anomaly or a part of the scimitar syndrome (Fig 21-1,C).
3. Right superior pulmonary vein connecting with the azygous vein (rare) (Fig 21-1,D).
4. All of the right pulmonary veins directly with the right atrium. This type of anomalous pulmonary venous connection is almost invariably associated with an atrial septal defect and the polysplenia syndrome (Fig 21-2,A).
5. Right pulmonary veins with the coronary sinus (Fig 21-2,B).
6. Connection with the ductus venosus or portal vein (very rare) (Fig 21-2,C); much more commonly associated with total anomalous pulmonary venous connection.
7. Left pulmonary veins with the left innominate vein (Fig 21-3,A).

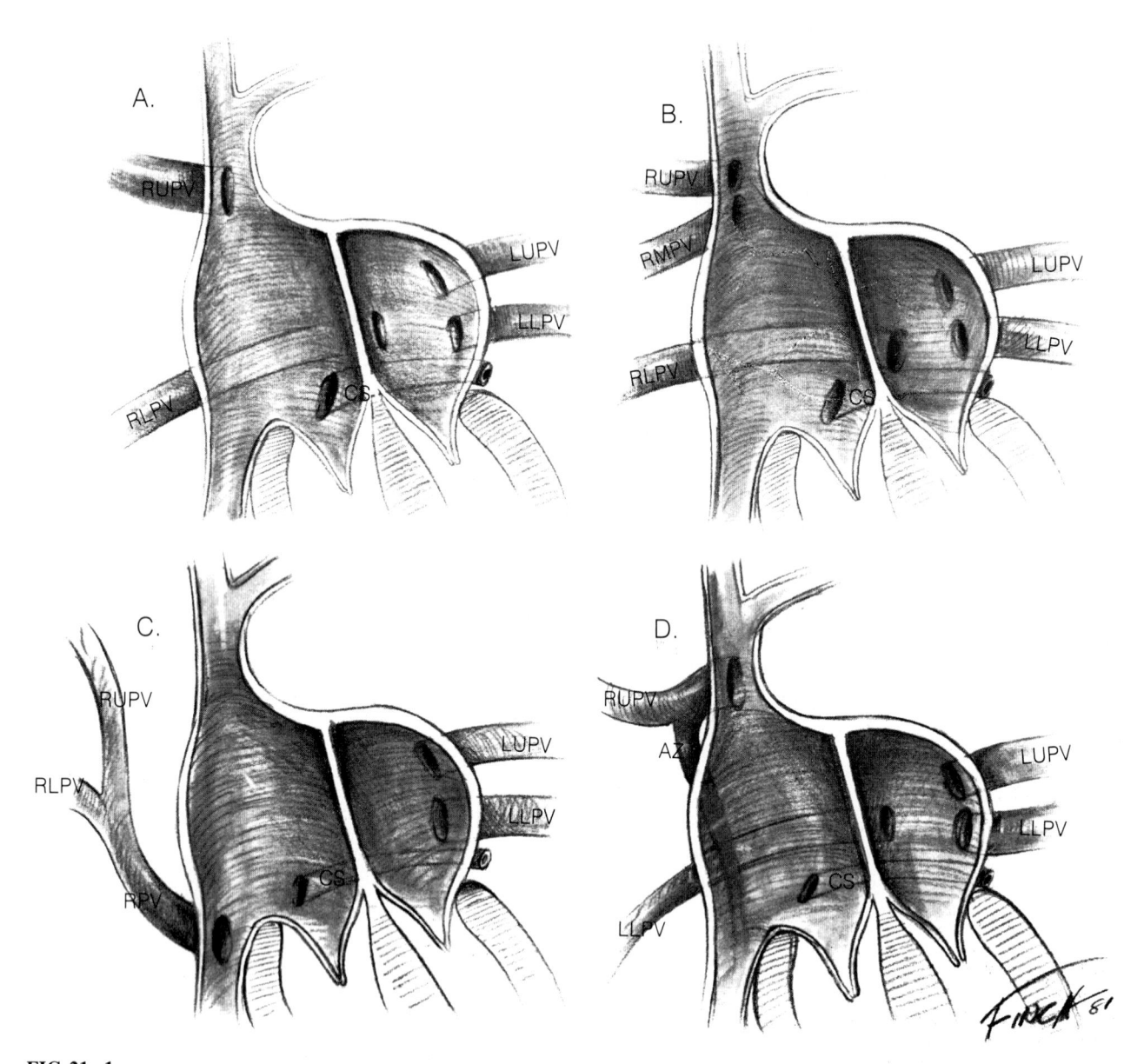

FIG 21–1.
Diagram of various anatomic forms of partial anomalous pulmonary venous connection (PAPVC). **A,** right upper pulmonary vein connecting anomalously with superior vena cava. **B,** right upper and middle pulmonary vein connecting with superior vena cava. **C,** right upper and right lower pulmonary vein connecting with inferior vena cava. **D,** right upper pulmonary vein connecting with azygous vein and from there with superior vena cava. *RUPV* = right upper pulmonary vein; *RLPV* = right lower pulmonary vein; *LUPV* = left upper pulmonary vein; *LLPV* = left lower pulmonary vein; *AZ* = azygous vein; *CS* = coronary sinus.

8. Left pulmonary veins with a persistent left superior vena cava (fairly common).
9. Left pulmonary veins with the left subclavian vein.
10. Left pulmonary veins with the coronary sinus (Fig 21–3,B).
11. Left pulmonary veins with the supradiaphragmatic portion of the inferior vena cava; this is a very rare type of anomalous pulmonary venous connection, being the mirror image of the scimitar syndrome (Fig 21–3,C).

HEMODYNAMICS

In the presence of an atrial septal defect, the coexisting PAPVC does not alter the hemodynamics. When the atrial septum is intact, the hemodynamics are affected by:

1. The number of pulmonary veins connecting anomalously.
2. The resistance to flow through the lung with nor-

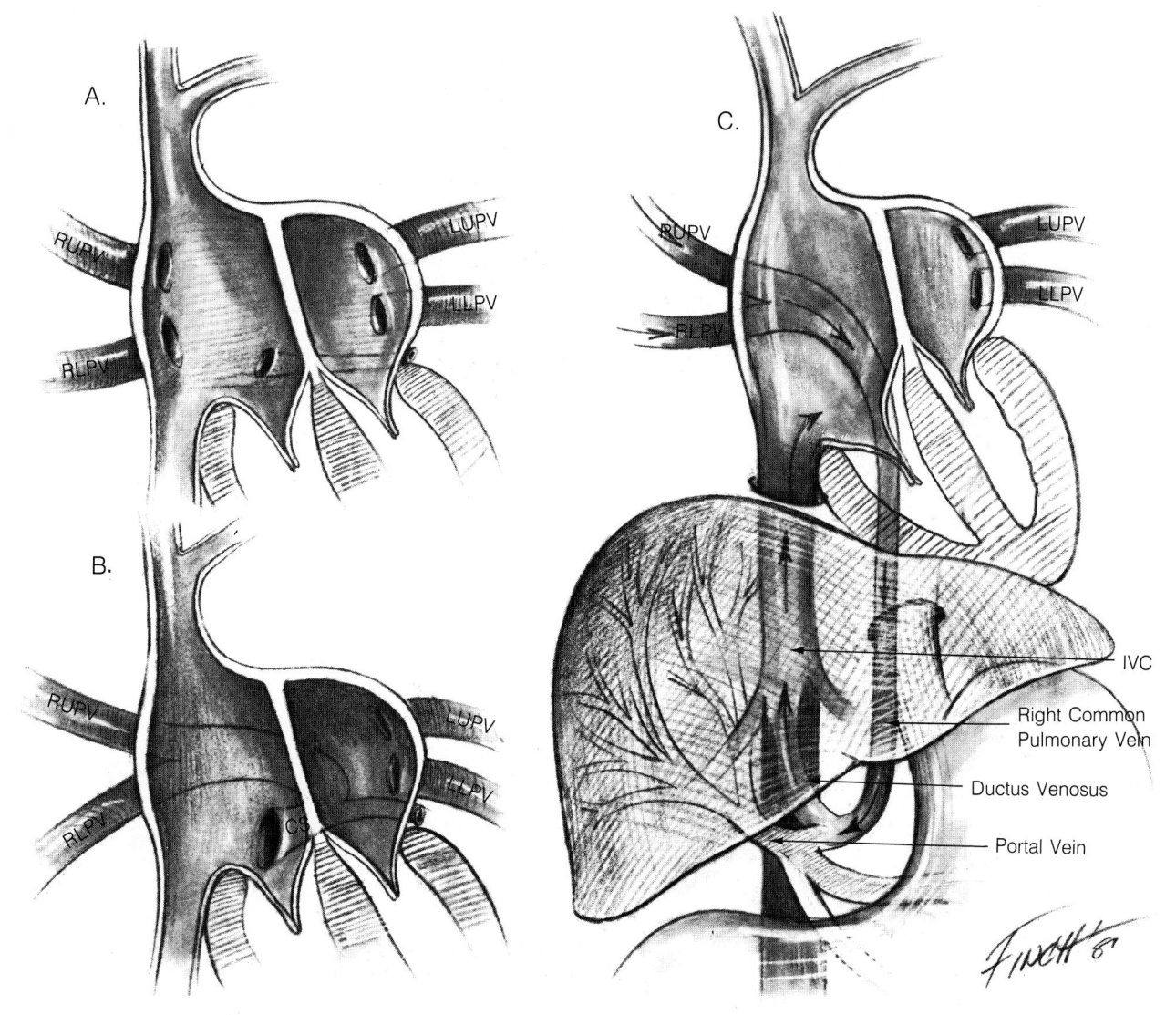

FIG 21-2.
Diagram of forms of PAPVC (cont.) **A,** both right pulmonary veins connecting with right atrium; almost invariably associated with the polysplenia syndrome. **B,** right pulmonary veins connecting anomalously with coronary sinus. **C,** right pulmonary veins connecting with the ductus venosus or portal vein.

mal (and through the lung with abnormal) pulmonary venous connection.
  3. The relative compliances of the right and left atria.

If more than one pulmonary vein connects anomalously, the hemodynamics resemble those of atrial septal defect.

Because the amount of blood flow through each pulmonary vein is approximately 25% of the total pulmonary blood flow in patients with PAPVC and an intact atrial septum, the left-to-right shunt is usually less than 50%. Left-to-right shunts greater than 65% occurring at the atrial level are usually caused by atrial septal defect or PAPVC coexisting with atrial septal defect.

The volume of blood flowing through an anomalously connecting pulmonary vein is slightly greater than normal. REASON: Right atrial pressure is lower than left atrial pressure; therefore, a larger pressure difference exists between the pulmonary artery and the anomalously connecting pulmonary vein than between the pulmonary artery and a normally connecting pulmonary vein.

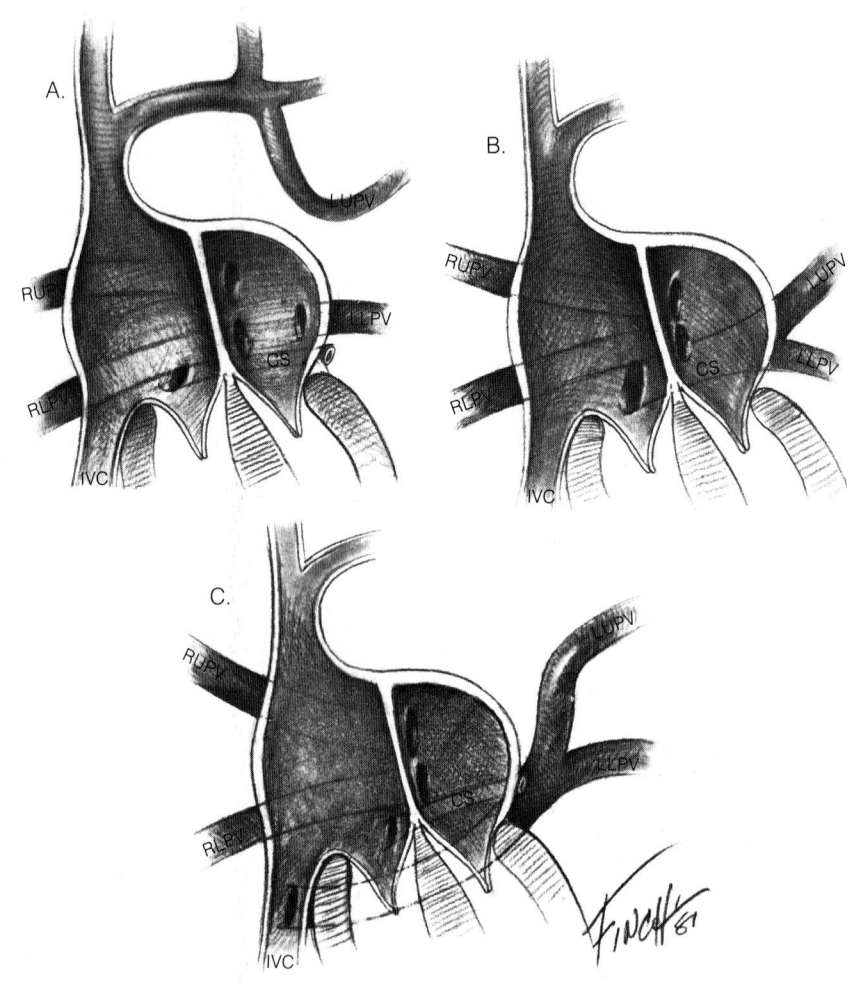

FIG 21-3.
Diagram of forms of PAPVC (cont.) **A,** left upper pulmonary vein connecting with left innominate vein. **B,** left pulmonary veins connecting with coronary sinus. **C,** left pulmonary veins connecting with the inferior vena cava.

CLINICAL FEATURES

In most patients, only one pulmonary vein connects anomalously. Therefore, the patient is asymptomatic and the findings on physical examination and electrocardiogram (ECG), are normal.

In patients with more than one anomalously connecting pulmonary vein, the findings resemble those in atrial septal defect.[1] There may be slow growth and an increased number of respiratory infections. Auscultation shows:

1. Loud first heart sound in the tricuspid area. Because of the large volume of flow into the right ventricle, the excursion of the tricuspid valve at the onset of systole is longer, and valve closure is more forceful.
2. Pulmonary systolic ejection murmur as a result of the increased volume of blood flowing over the right ventricular outflow tract.
3. Middiastolic murmur in the tricuspid area caused by the increased volume of flow across the tricuspid valve.
4. Wide, but *variable*, splitting of the second heart sound. Wide splitting results from delayed pulmonary valve closure secondary to prolonged right ventricular ejection. Unlike the findings in atrial septal defect, the second heart sound is variably split. In atrial septal defect, the volume of flow into the ventricle depends on the relative ventricular compliances; therefore, regardless of the volume of flow into the atria, the amount of blood entering the right and left ventricle is relatively constant.

When the atrial septum is intact, the volume of flow into the right ventricle depends on the volume of flow into the right atrium. Thus, the right atrium receives a constant volume of pulmonary venous return but a variable systemic venous return, depending on the phase of breathing.

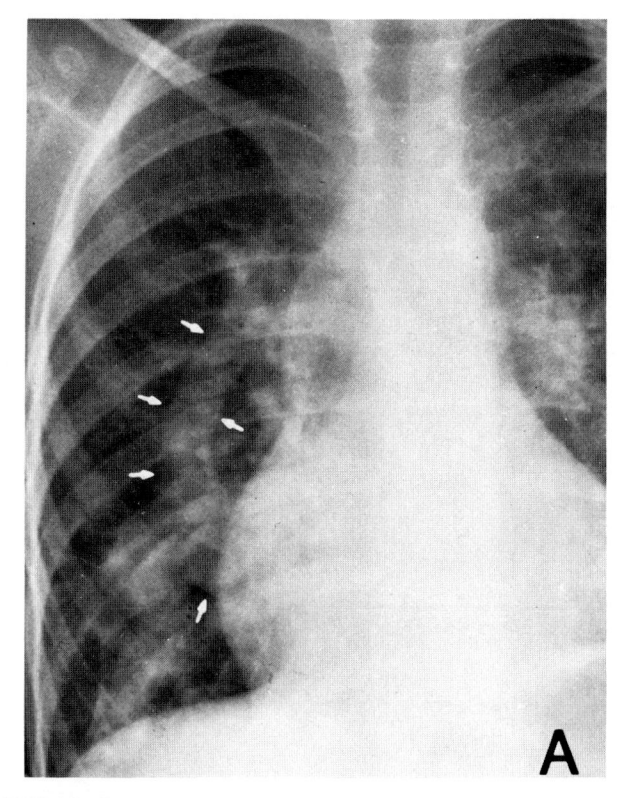

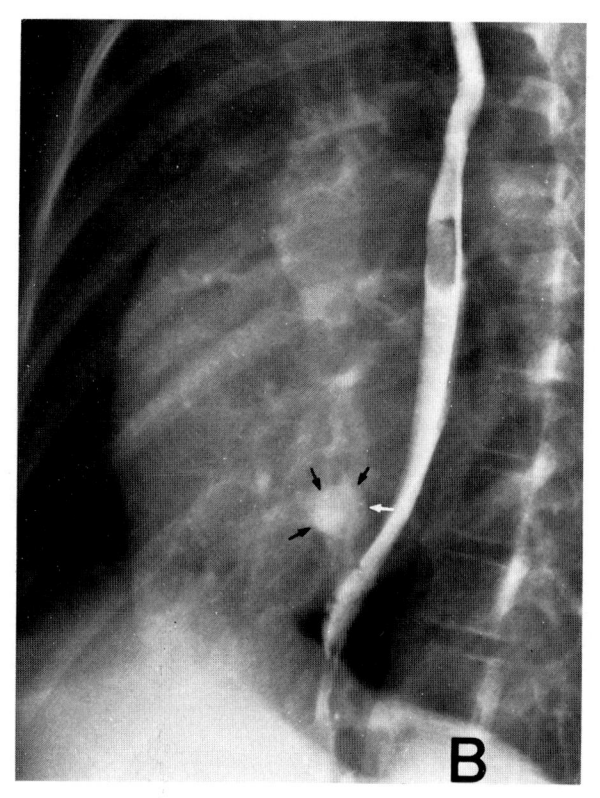

FIG 21–4.
Partial anomalous pulmonary venous connection of right lung with supradiaphragmatic portion of inferior vena cava. **A,** posteroanterior projection; the connecting venous channel *(white arrows)* clearly recognizable by its anomalous course. **B,** lateral projection; connecting vein *(black arrows)* appears as a masslike density seen on end.

Therefore, the right ventricular inflow increases in inspiration and decreases on expiration, resulting in variable splitting of the second heart sound.

ELECTROCARDIOGRAPHIC FEATURES

The ECG resembles that in atrial septal defect and reflects the increased volume of blood flow through the right side of the heart:

1. Mild right-axis deviation.
2. Right atrial enlargement.
3. An RSR' pattern in lead V_4R or V_1.

ECHOCARDIOGRAPHIC FEATURES

When more than one pulmonary vein connects anomalously, the findings resemble those of atrial septal defect:

1. Increased right ventricular diameter.
2. Paradoxical movement of the ventricular septum.

RADIOGRAPHIC FEATURES

1. In most patients, the anomalous pulmonary vein cannot be seen on a thoracic roentgenogram, particularly if only a posteroanterior projection is obtained.
2. Occasionally the anomalous pulmonary vein can be recognized on posteroanterior and lateral chest films by identification of an anomalous course of a pulmonary vein (Fig 21–4). This is particularly obvious if an entire lung drains anomalously, because the anomalous venous channel is large.
3. If only a portion of a lung drains anomalously, the involved pulmonary vein is usually too small to be visible on the posteroanterior roentgenogram. Because the right lower lobe pulmonary vein normally has a fairly horizontal course, an anomalous connection of this vein cannot be diagnosed from a posteroanterior roentgenogram.
4. Although an anomalous course of a pulmonary vein is highly suspicious for anomalous pulmonary venous connection, a pulmonary vein with an anomalous course may connect normally with the left atrium (Fig 21–5).
5. An anomalously connecting pulmonary vein from the right lower lobe is so similar in course to a normally

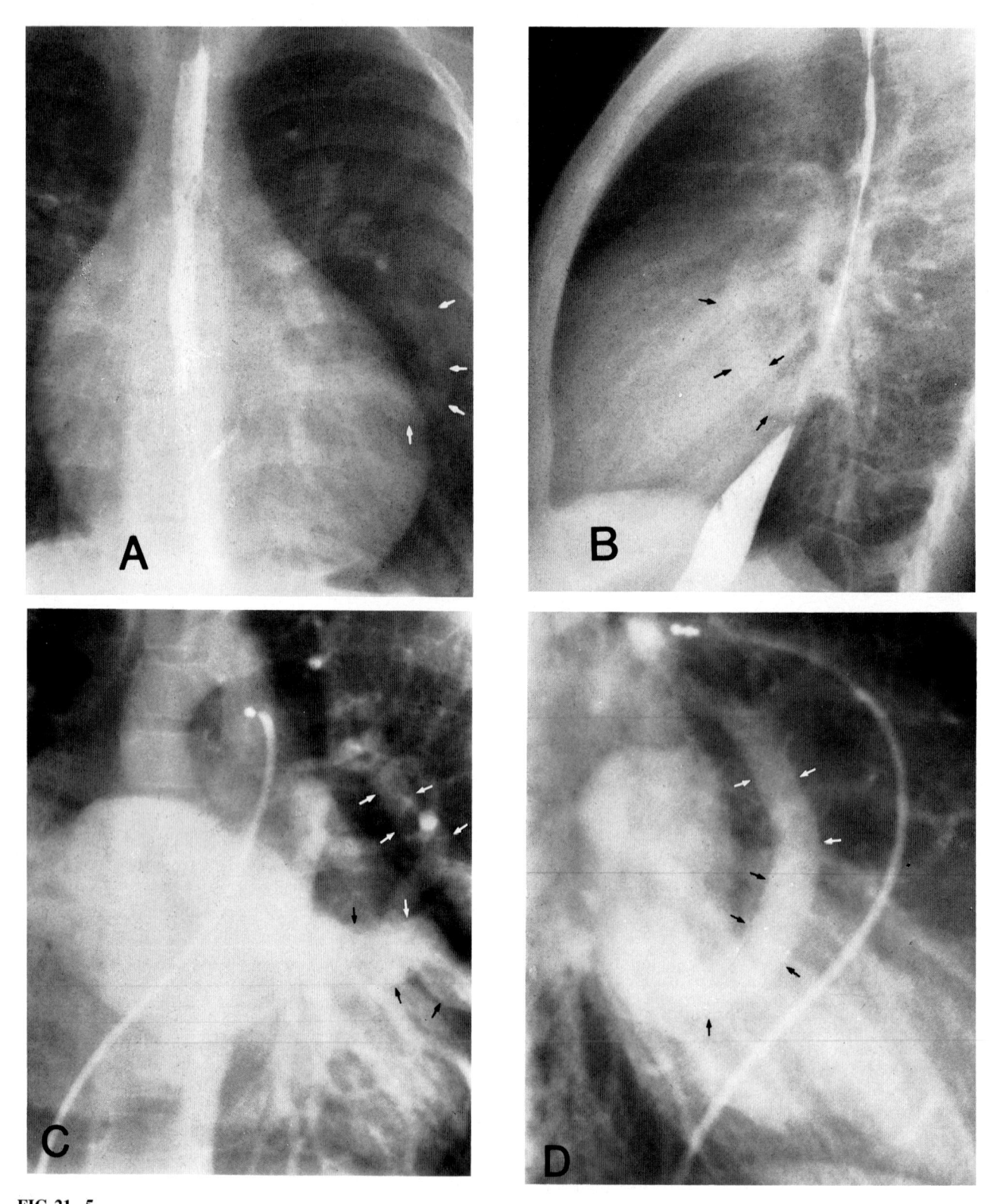

FIG 21-5.
Anomalous course of left pulmonary vein to left atrium. **A,** posteroanterior projection; anomalous course on left pulmonary vein *(white arrows)*. **B,** lateral projection; anomalous course of left pulmonary vein *(black arrows)*. Pulmonary angiogram, late phase; anteroposterior **(C)** and lateral **(D)** projections; the anomalous vein indicated by arrows. An anomalous course of a pulmonary vein is highly suggestive but not diagnostic of anomalous connection.

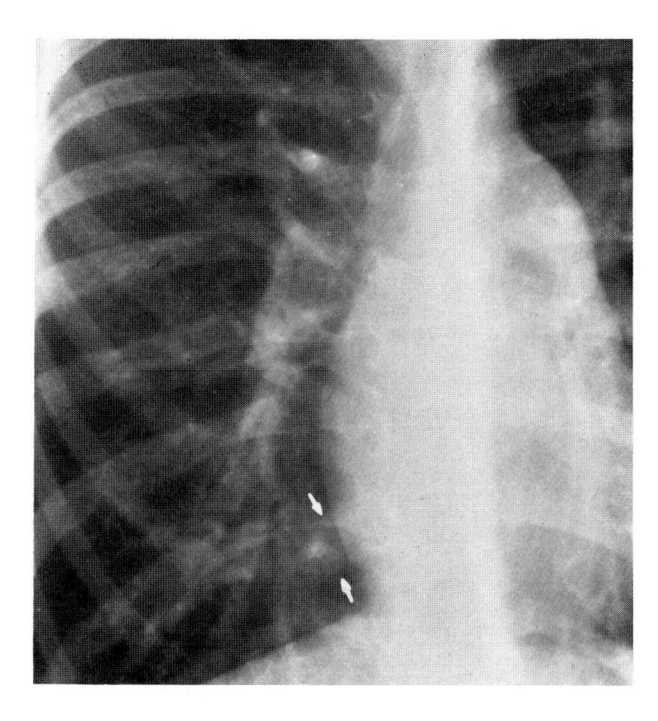

FIG 21–6.
Partial anomalous pulmonary venous connection of right lower lobe to right atrium; posteroanterior projection. The course of the right lower lobe pulmonary vein *(white arrows)* is slightly lower, but still normal. Consequently, the specific diagnosis was not made.

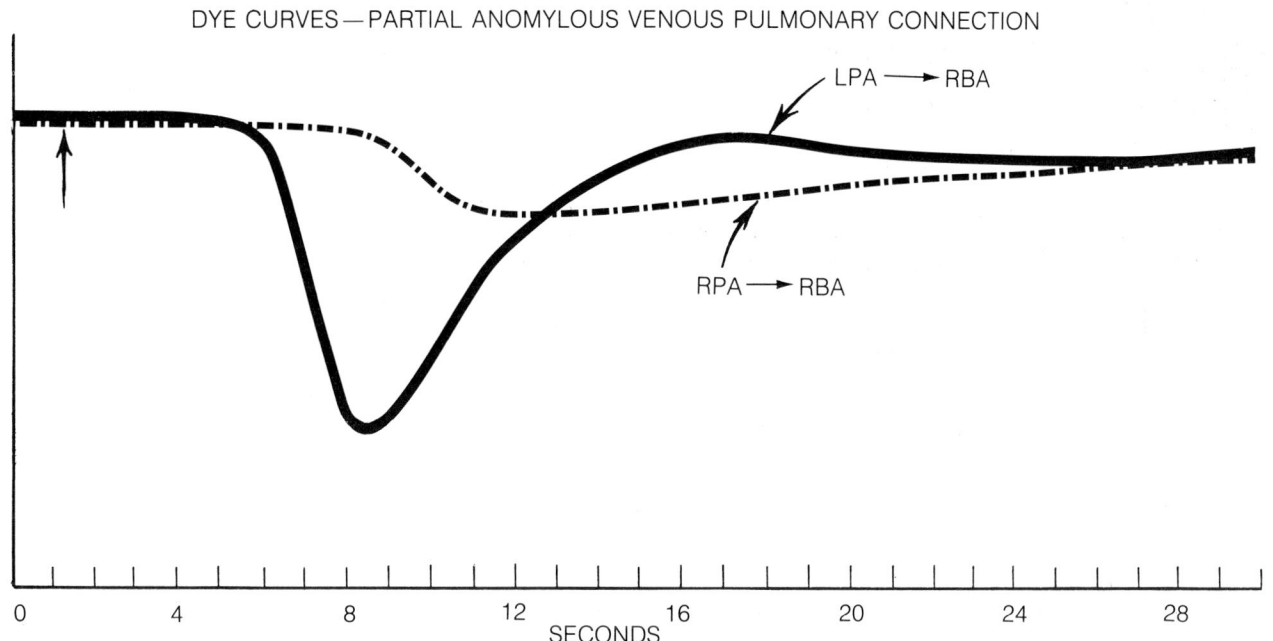

DYE CURVES—PARTIAL ANOMYLOUS VENOUS PULMONARY CONNECTION

LPA ⟶ RBA

RPA ⟶ RBA

FIG 21–7.
Partial anomalous pulmonary venous connection of right pulmonary veins with right atrium and with intact atrial septum. Indicator dilution curves. Injection into left pulmonary artery *(LPA)* and sampling from right brachial artery *(RBA)*; appearance time = 4.5 seconds. Injection into the right pulmonary artery *(RPA)* and sampling from right brachial artery *(RBA)*; appearance time = 8.0 seconds.

FIG 21–8.
Partial anomalous pulmonary venous connection to right superior vena cava; pulmonary arteriogram, late phase, anteroposterior projection. A large anomalous pulmonary vein *(open arrows)* connects with superior vena cava *(solid arrows),* which is clearly opacified.

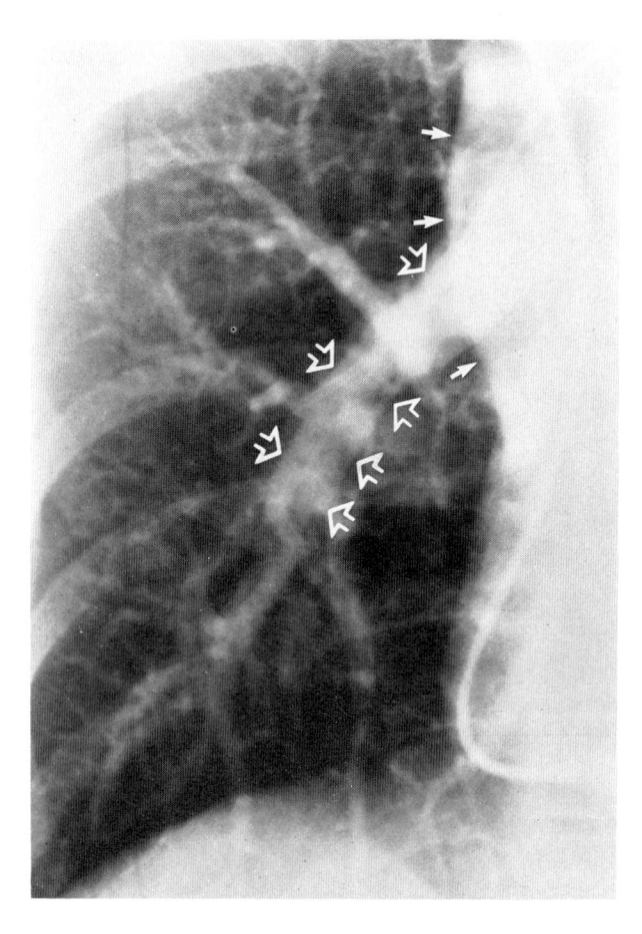

connecting right lower lobe pulmonary vein that the diagnosis cannot be suggested on plain film (Fig 21–6).

CARDIAC CATHETERIZATION

In many patients with PAPVC associated with atrial septal defect, the anomalous pulmonary venous connection may be difficult to diagnose. Repeated oximetry series may reveal the entrance of an anomalous vein into the superior vena cava, coronary sinus, innominate vein, or inferior vena cava by a distinct increase in oxygen saturation at that site.

If the atrial septum is intact, the pulmonary arterial wedge pressure is different between the normally and abnormally connecting lobes. In the lobes with normally connecting veins, the wedge pressure is higher, because it reflects the left atrial pressure. The wedge pressure of the lobe with the abnormally connecting pulmonary vein is lower, because right atrial pressure is lower.

The catheter course may be diagnostic, showing passage into the lung field at an abnormal site.

When the atrial septum is intact, indicator dilution curves are helpful. With selective injection into the pulmonary artery with normally connecting veins and sampling from a peripheral artery, the indicator dilution curve has a normal appearance time (Fig 21–7).

In contrast, injection into pulmonary arterial segments of the anomalously connected lung shows a delayed appearance time (see Fig 21–7), because the dye, on its first passage through the lung, returns to the right atrium. It then passes into the pulmonary trunk, with some passing through normally connecting pulmonary veins, which return to the left side of the heart and eventually reach the peripheral arterial sampling site.

ANGIOGRAPHIC APPEARANCE

Angiography is the best technique for observing anomalously connecting pulmonary veins.

1. If an anomalously connecting pulmonary vein is suspected on the basis of an abnormal catheter course, contrast medium should be injected directly into the pulmonary vein. During injection, the tip of the catheter should be free to prevent wedge injections with retrograde filling of the pulmonary artery. A power injector should be used because the blood flow through pulmonary veins is rapid. An inadequate amount of contrast medium is usu-

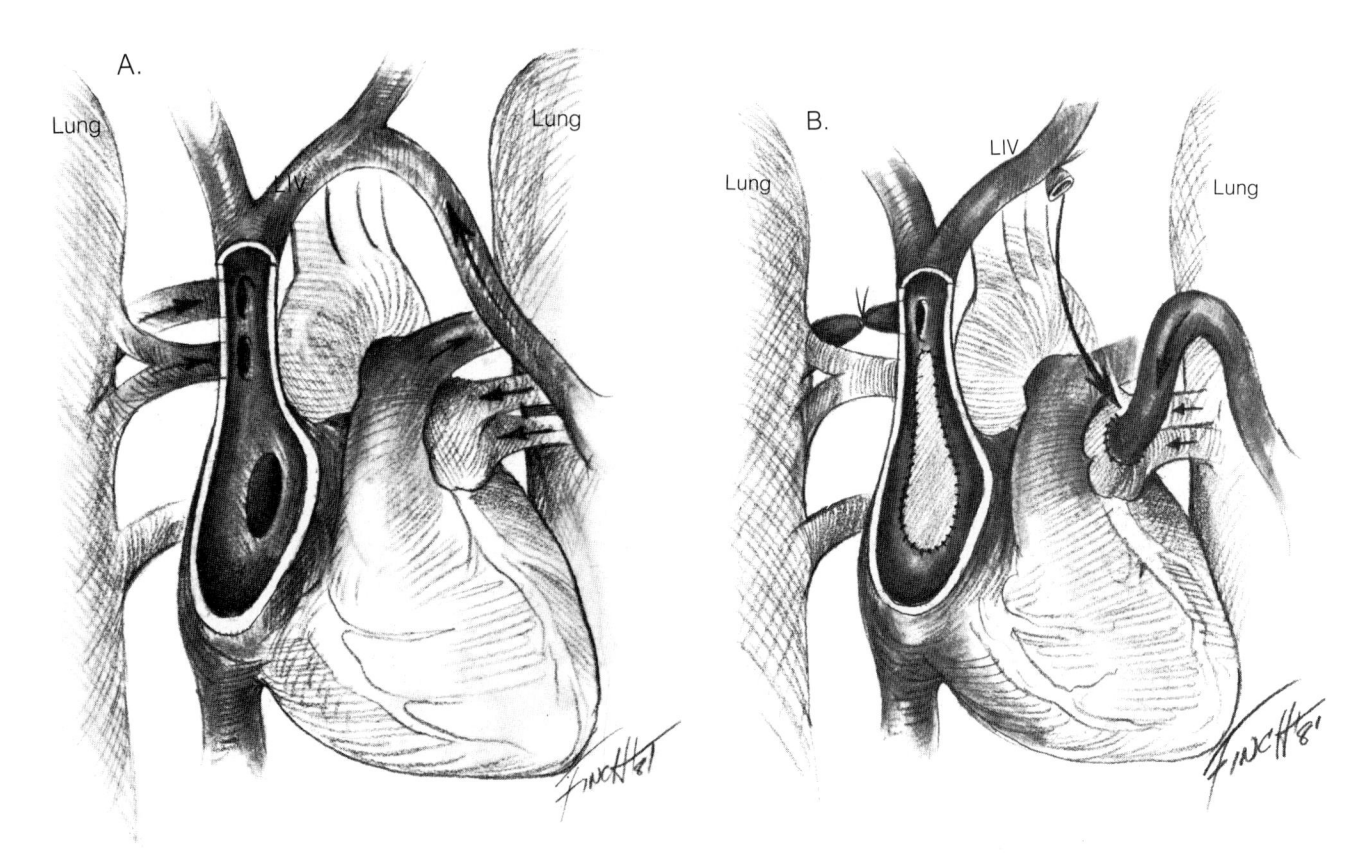

FIG 21–9.
Diagram of operations for PAPVC. **A,** three anomalous pulmonary venous connections are present. Two pulmonary veins from right lung connect with superior vena cava; one vein from left lung connects with innominate vein. An atrial septal defect coexists. **B,** right upper pulmonary vein has been ligated, because there are interpulmonary venous connections with other pulmonary veins from right upper lobe. A patch has been placed in superior vena cava and right atrium to divert blood from other right upper pulmonary vein through the atrial septal defect into left atrium. The anomalously connecting left pulmonary vein has been connected directly with left atrium. *LIV* = left innominate vein.

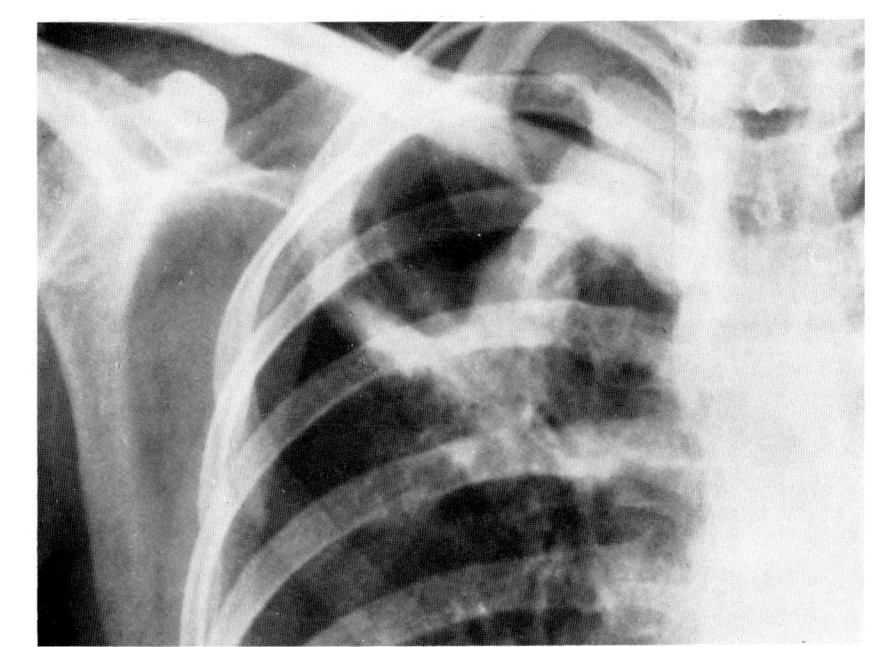

FIG 21–10.
Thoracic roentgenogram, posteroanterior projection of right upper lung field in PAPVC of right upper lobe pulmonary vein to superior vena cava and atrial septal defect. Anomalously connecting pulmonary vein was ligated. Immediately after the operation, patient developed consolidation of right upper lobe, which was followed by cavitation.

ally delivered by manual injection through the small-bore catheters frequently used for cardiac catheterization.

2. A technically satisfactory selective right or left pulmonary arteriogram allows recognition of anomalous pulmonary venous connection. On the pulmonary venous phase, the abnormal course of pulmonary veins is seen, and subsequent opacification of right-sided cardiac structures occurs (Fig 21–8).

OPERATIVE CONSIDERATIONS

Operation is indicated only when a large left-to-right shunt exists through the anomalously connecting pulmonary vein or an atrial septal defect coexists. A single anomalously connected pulmonary vein, draining only one lobe of the lung, is compatible with a normal life span, so operation is not indicated.

The operative correction of anomalously connecting pulmonary veins is more complicated than closure of an atrial septal defect.[1–4] Basically, three techniques can be used:

1. Ligation of the anomalously connecting pulmonary vein (Fig 21–9). This has been advocated for right upper lobe pulmonary veins that join the high superior vena cava because of the difficulty in surgical exposure of the vein. However, on very rare occasions ligation may result in pulmonary infarction and abscess formation, as occurred

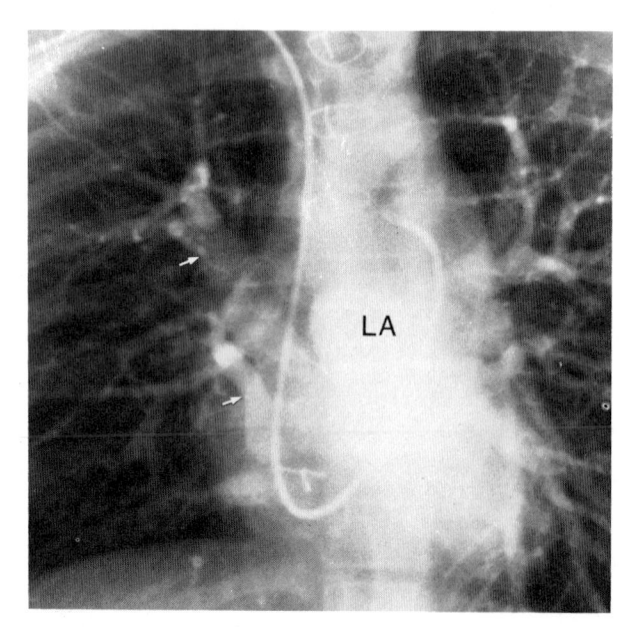

FIG 21–11.
Levophase of postoperative pulmonary arteriogram, anteroposterior projection of PAPVC of right lung with right atrium. Anomalous course of right pulmonary veins, which connect normally with the left atrium *(arrows)*. Contour of left atrium *(LA)* altered by operation. Right atrium no longer opacified.

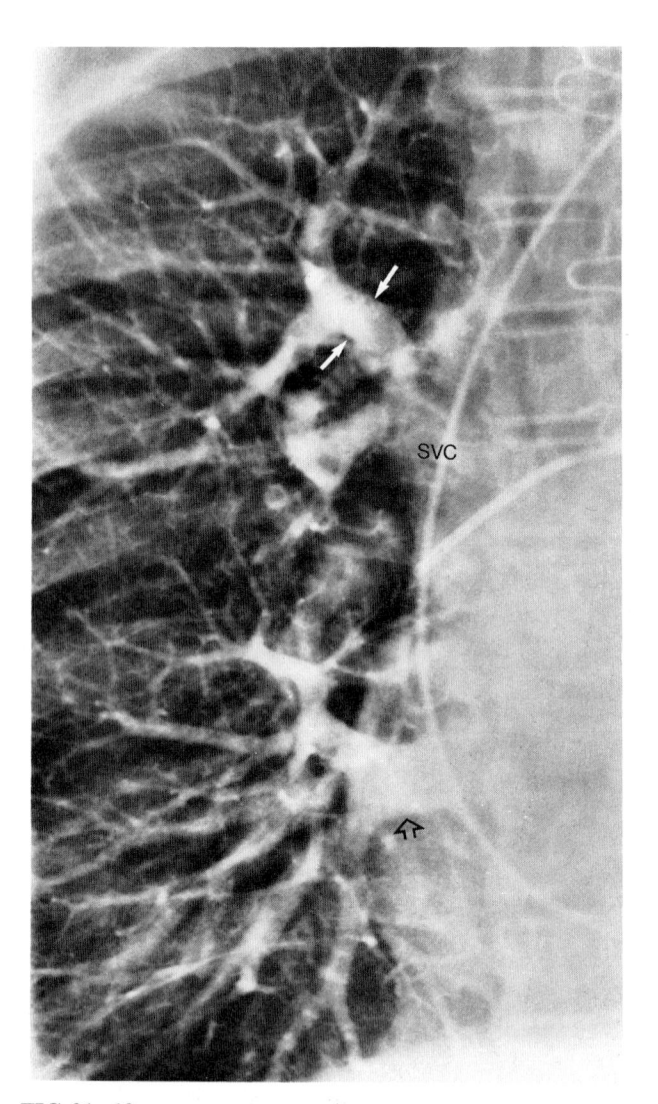

FIG 21–12.
Pulmonary arteriogram, anteroposterior projection of PAPVC of right upper lobe with superior vena cava after closure of atrial septal defect. Right upper pulmonary vein *(white arrows)* connects with superior vena cava *(SVC)*; right lower pulmonary vein joins left atrium *(open arrow)*.

in one of our patients (Fig 21–10). Consequently, one should not attempt to correct a single right pulmonary vein anomalously connecting with the high superior vena cava.

2. Longitudinal partitioning procedures (Fig 21–9). When an anomalously draining vein connects with the right superior vena cava immediately above the right atrium, it can be corrected by a patch sewn into the superior vena cava to direct the blood flow through an atrial septal defect into the left atrium. A patch of either pericardium or fabric may be used, because such partitioning may narrow the superior vena cava, causing superior vena caval syndrome. Many surgeons simultaneously perform a patchplasty of the superior vena cava, thus enlarging its lumen.

3. Ligation and reimplantation (Fig 21–9). The

anomalously connected pulmonary vein is ligated and reimplanted into the left atrium. Although feasible only if the anomalous vein is long enough, this technique yields excellent results.

POSTOPERATIVE FEATURES

The postoperative chest roentgenographic findings are identical to those of correction of atrial septal defect (see Chapter 19).

Pulmonary angiography demonstrates normal flow of contrast medium from the pulmonary vein into the left atrium (Fig 21–11). In the levophase of pulmonary arteriograms in patients with anomalous drainage of the entire right lung to the right atrium, the anomalous course of the pulmonary veins is still demonstrable, but the drainage is now normal into the left side of the heart. The shape of the left atrium is altered by the surgical procedure. When the right upper pulmonary vein enters the superior vena cava at some distance above the right atrium, it usually is left in place. Therefore, postoperative pulmonary angiograms show this persistent anomalous connection and opacification of the right side of the heart (Fig 21–12).

REFERENCES

1. Kalke BR, Carlson RG, Ferlic RM, et al: Partial anomalous pulmonary venous connections, *Am J Cardiol* 20:91, 1967.
2. Ellis FH Jr, Callahan JA, DuShane JW, et al: Partial anomalous pulmonary venous connections involving both lungs with interatrial communication: a report of two cases treated surgically, *Staff Meet Mayo Clin* 33:65, 1958.
3. Neptune WB, Bailey CP, Goldberg H: The surgical correction of atrial septal defects associated with transposition of the pulmonary veins, *J Thorac Surg* 25:263, 1953.
4. Friedli B, Guerin R, Davignon A, et al: Surgical treatment of partial anomalous pulmonary venous drainage: a long-term follow-up study, *Circulation* 45:159, 1972.

CHAPTER 22

Scimitar Syndrome

The scimitar syndrome is a rare anomaly that has four features:

1. Hypoplasia of right lung with dextroposition of heart.
2. Hypoplasia of right pulmonary artery.
3. Anomalous arterial supply of right lower lobe from abdominal aorta.
4. Anomalous pulmonary venous connection of right lung to inferior vena cava.

Not all features are present in every case. Approximately 80 cases have been reported in the literature, two-thirds of them in females.

The scimitar syndrome is recognized by characteristic roentgen findings, and the diagnosis must be considered in the differential diagnosis of dextrocardia and of partial anomalous pulmonary venous connection.

PATHOLOGIC ANATOMY[1, 2]

The right lung is smaller than the left and has from one to three lobes. The right upper and middle lobes are usually absent or hypoplastic, but the lower lobe is invariably present. The right lung may consist of two lobes, suggesting isomerism of the left lung, but the bronchial configuration is an imperfect mirror image of the left lung. One instance of "horseshoe" lung has been described, in which there was fusion of the right and left lungs.[3]

The right bronchial tree is abnormal. The exact bronchial anatomy, especially of the upper and middle lobes, may be difficult to determine. There may be absence or hypoplasia of bronchi and compression and displacement of the right lower lobe bronchus. Diverticula or cystic changes of the bronchi of the lower lobe have been described. Because of the bronchial anomalies, superimposed infection may occur and cause further bronchial changes. Pulmonary sequestration has not been described.

There are three sources of blood supply to the right lung[4]:

1. The right pulmonary artery that is hypoplastic or occasionally absent. The volume of blood flow to the right lung is usually 30% to 50% of normal.
2. Systemic arteries. The right lung, particularly the right lower lobe, is supplied by a single, or, commonly, multiple and small systemic arteries. These arteries originate from the abdominal aorta, pierce the right hemidiaphragm, and enter the right lower lobe. It is not known whether they enter the bronchial or pulmonary arterial system.
3. Systemic arteries. Uncommonly, arteries arise from the thoracic aorta and enter the right lung.

The anomalous pulmonary venous connection is through the characteristic scimitar vein, which receives pulmonary veins from one, two, or three of the lobes of the right lung. This connection is shaped like a scimitar (a sword with a curved blade used in Turkey), curves parallel to the right cardiac border, and enlarges as it descends. The scimitar vein connects with the inferior vena cava either above or, more commonly, below the diaphragm.

A single case of a left scimitar syndrome with drainage of the left lung through a scimitar vein to the infradiaphragmatic portion of the inferior vena cava has been described (see Fig 21–3,C).

Abnormalities of the right hemidiaphragm are common. The lateral attachment of the diaphragm may be higher in the thorax than normal. The right hepatic lobe occasionally herniates through the Bochdalek foramen.

The atrial septum is usually intact.

ASSOCIATED ANOMALIES

Scimitar syndrome may coexist with other congenital cardiac anomalies, but only coarctation of the aorta has a higher than expected incidence (20% of cases). Scimitar syndrome has been described in association with tetralogy of Fallot, pulmonary atresia, ventricular septal defect, patent ductus arteriosus, bicuspid aortic valve, and atrial septal defect.

HEMODYNAMICS

The hemodynamics may be dominated by the coexisting cardiac anomaly. The anomalously connecting pulmonary vein creates a left-to-right shunt, but the volume of shunt is usually small because of the hypoplasia of the right lung and right pulmonary artery. In patients with a larger shunt, the right atrium and ventricle are dilated. Pulmonary hypertension may be present when there is a coexisting cardiac anomaly causing a left-to-right shunt.

CLINICAL FEATURES

The symptoms vary considerably, depending on the degree of pulmonary hypoplasia.[1, 2] If the lung is slightly hypoplastic, the patient is asymptomatic, and the scimitar syndrome is an incidental finding on a thoracic roentgenogram. With more extreme pulmonary hypoplasia and major bronchial abnormalities, there may be recurrent pulmonary infections, pneumonia, and dyspnea.

Physical examination may reveal a small right hemithorax and displacement of the cardiac apex toward the right. There may be auscultatory findings of the coexisting cardiac anomalies. Even in patients without other cardiac anomalies, significant murmurs may be present, representing increased blood flow through the right side of the heart. As in partial anomalous pulmonary venous connection, wide but variable splitting of the second heart sound is found. The pulmonary component of the second heart

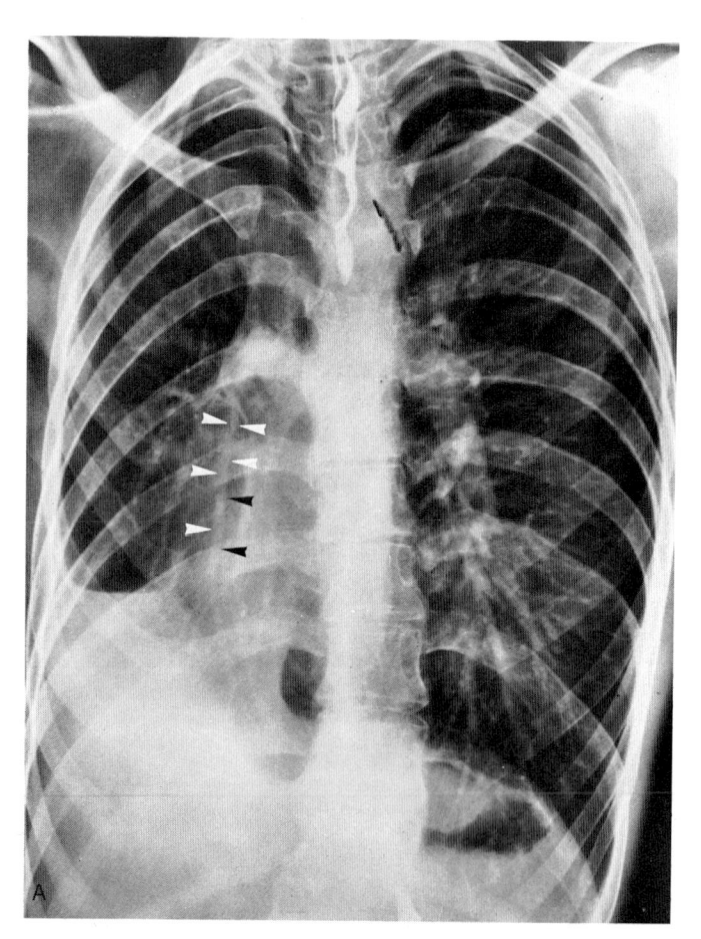

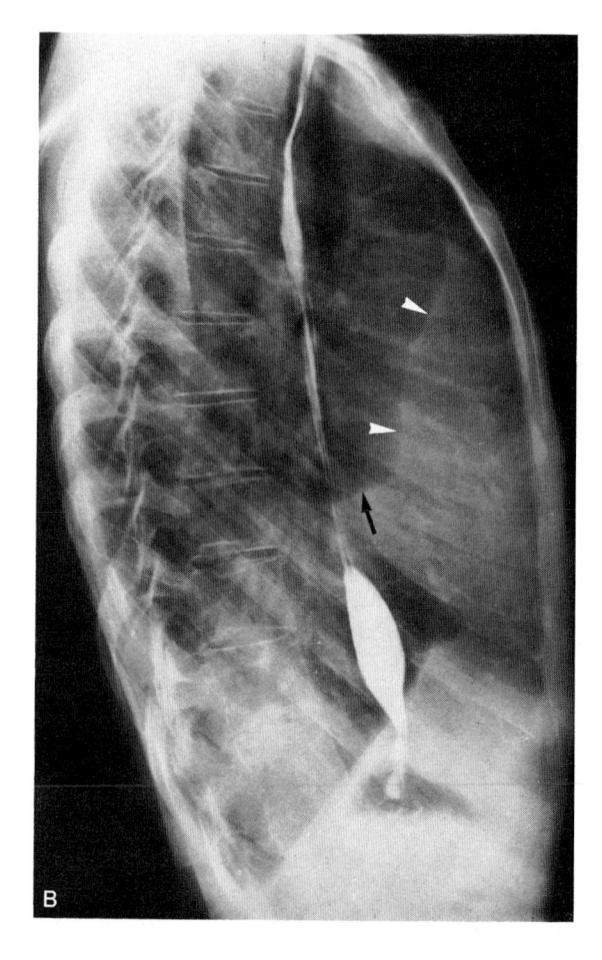

FIG 22–1.
Thoracic roentgenograms in scimitar syndrome. **A,** posteroanterior projection shows marked hypoplasia of the right hemithorax and mediastinal shift to right. High attachment of the lateral border of the right hemidiaphragm, simulating pleural changes. Indistinct right cardiac border. Prominence of the left pulmonary artery; hypoplasia of the right pulmonary artery *(small arrows)*. Scimitar vein not seen, being overshadowed by the cardiac silhouette. **B,** lateral projection shows elevation of the right hemidiaphragm *(black arrow)*. Characteristic mediastinal density probably caused by compensatory overgrowth of fat *(white arrows)* and the smaller right hemithorax.

sound is accentuated in patients with pulmonary hypertension.

ELECTROCARDIOGRAPHIC FEATURES

The electrocardiogram may be normal in patients with mild degrees of hypoplasia. In distinction to dextrocardia secondary to situs inversus, the P-wave axis is normal. Right ventricular hypertrophy, often with rSR' in the right precordial leads, is found. This pattern reflects the left-to-right shunt and increased right ventricular volume.

ECHOCARDIOGRAPHIC FEATURES

If the left-to-right shunt is small, the echocardiogram is normal. When the shunt is larger, the findings resemble those of atrial septal defect, namely:

1. Increased right ventricular diameter.
2. Paradoxical motion of the ventricular septum.

RADIOGRAPHIC FEATURES

The thoracic roentgenographic findings are usually diagnostic.[5] In most cases, no additional radiographic studies are required to establish a diagnosis, but if the characteristic scimitar vein is not seen, laminography may be in-

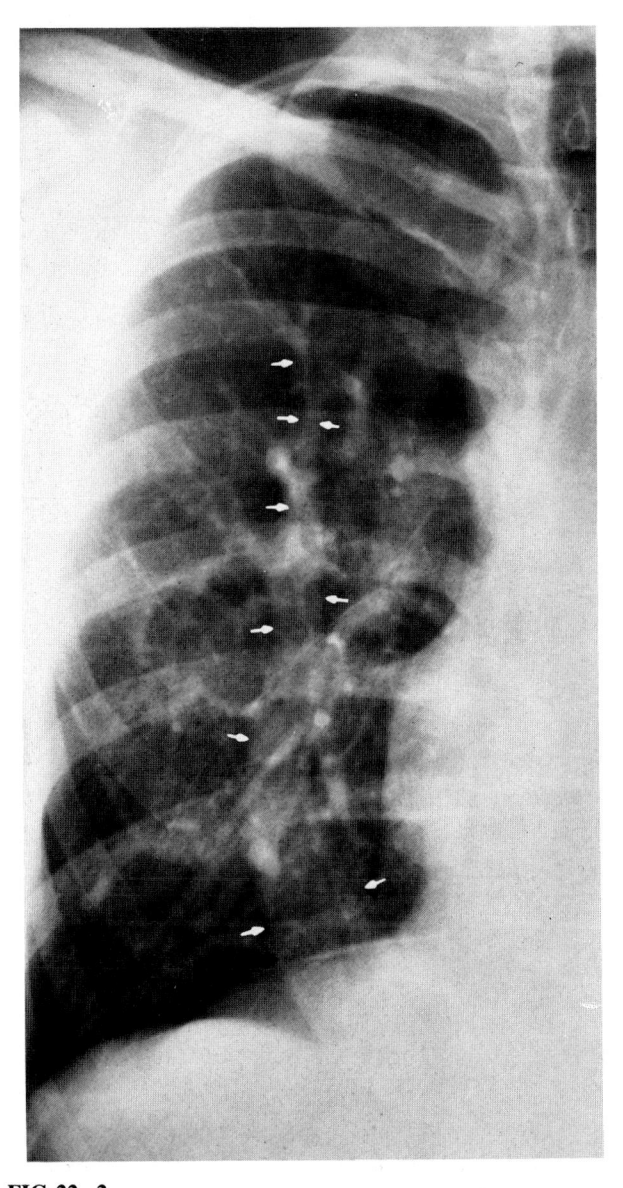

FIG 22–2.
Thoracic roentgenogram, posteroanterior projection of right lung in scimitar syndrome shows minor mediastinal shift. Large, typical scimitar vein *(white arrows)* drains the entire right lung.

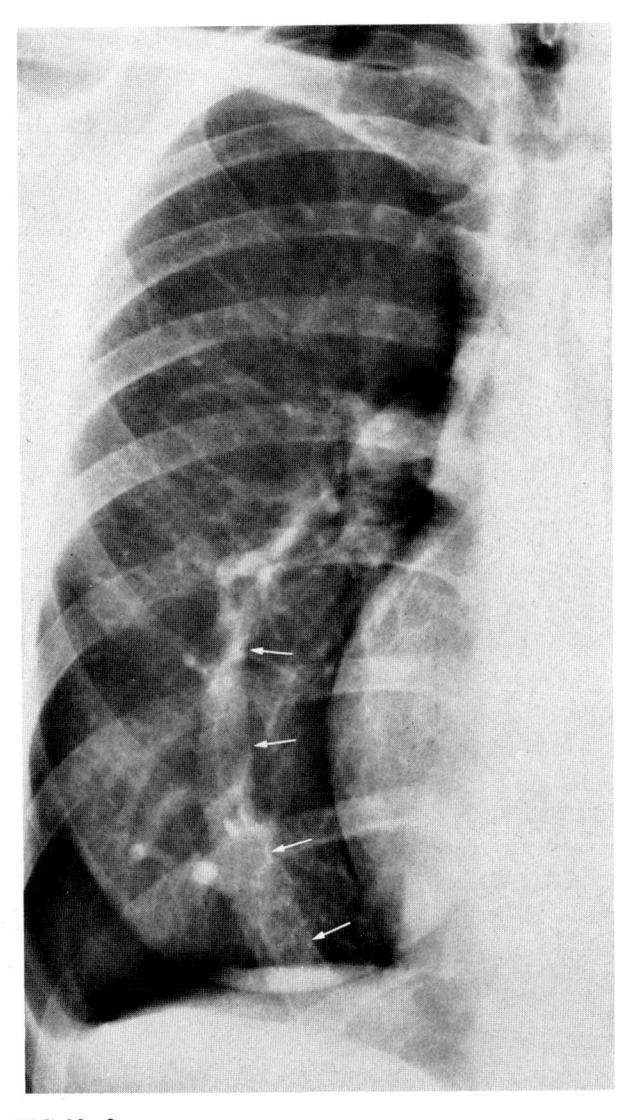

FIG 22–3.
Thoracic roentgenogram, posteroanterior projection of right lung shows scimitar vein draining only the right lower lobe.

dicated. In patients with repeated pulmonary infections, bronchography is useful for delineation of bronchial diverticula or cysts. During cardiac catheterization, pulmonary angiography is the best method for opacifying the scimitar vein.

1. The right hemithorax is smaller than the left, and the mediastinum is usually shifted toward the right (Fig 22–1,A). REASON: The right lung is hypoplastic.

2. In any patient with unexplained shift of the mediastinum toward the right, the right lung should be examined carefully for a scimitar vein.

3. In a patient with minimal hypoplasia of the right lung, the mediastinum is not displaced and is midline.

4. The right hemidiaphragm is usually higher than normal, and the right costophrenic sinus may be obliterated. REASON: The elevated lateral attachment of the right hemidiaphragm occurs secondary to hypoplasia of the right lung (see Fig 22–1,A).

5. The right cardiac border may be indistinct, giving the appearance of pleural changes. At postmortem examination, however, the pleura is usually normal. These changes probably result from an overgrowth of fatty tissue secondary to pulmonary hypoplasia.

6. The overgrowth of fatty tissue may cause a characteristic density on the lateral view (Fig 22–1,B).

7. The left pulmonary artery may appear prominent. REASON: The blood flow through the left lung is greater than normal, and the left hilum is more apparent because of the mediastinal shift (see Fig 22–1,A).

8. The right pulmonary artery shows a variable degree of hypoplasia (see Fig 22–1,A).

9. The scimitar vein is not always seen (see Fig 22–1,A).

10. A scimitar vein forms a characteristic comma-shaped curved density, which widens as it descends toward the right hemidiaphragm (Figs 22–2 and 22–3).

11. The size of the scimitar vein varies depending on whether the entire lung (see Fig 22–2) or only the right lower lobe is drained anomalously into the inferior vena cava (see Fig 22–3).

12. The density cast by the scimitar vein may be subtle (Fig 22–4,A), and in patients with marked mediastinal shift (see Fig 22–1,A) the scimitar vein may not be visible.

13. Under the latter circumstances, the diagnosis can be made by laminography (Fig 22–4,B).

14. Rarely, a scimitar-like vein drains normally into the left atrium (Fig 22–5).[6, 7]

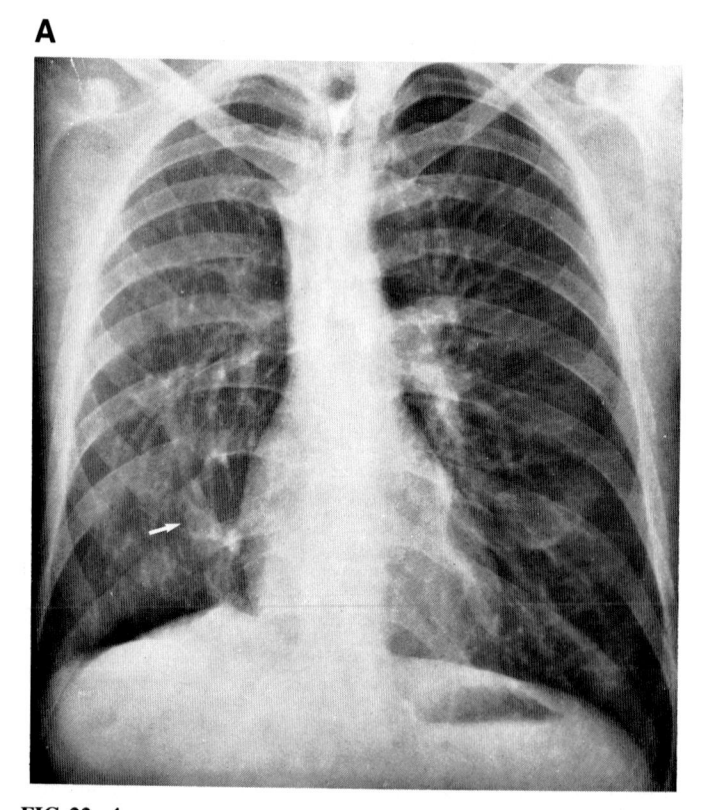

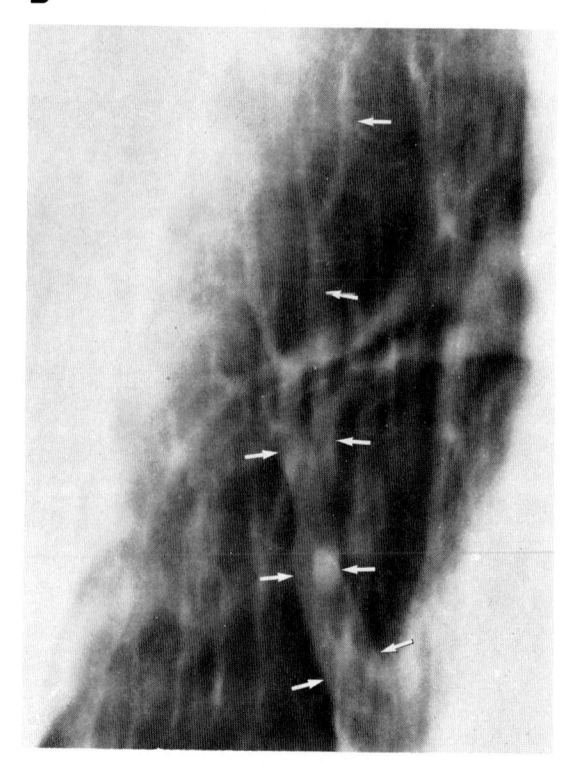

FIG 22–4.
Scimitar syndrome. **A,** thoracic roentgenogram, posteroanterior projection shows mild hypoplasia of the right hemithorax and marked hypoplasia of right pulmonary artery. Prominent left pulmonary artery. Minimal mediastinal shift. Density *(arrow)* cast by the scimitar vein is subtle. **B,** laminography; the scimitar vein is easily visible *(arrows)*.

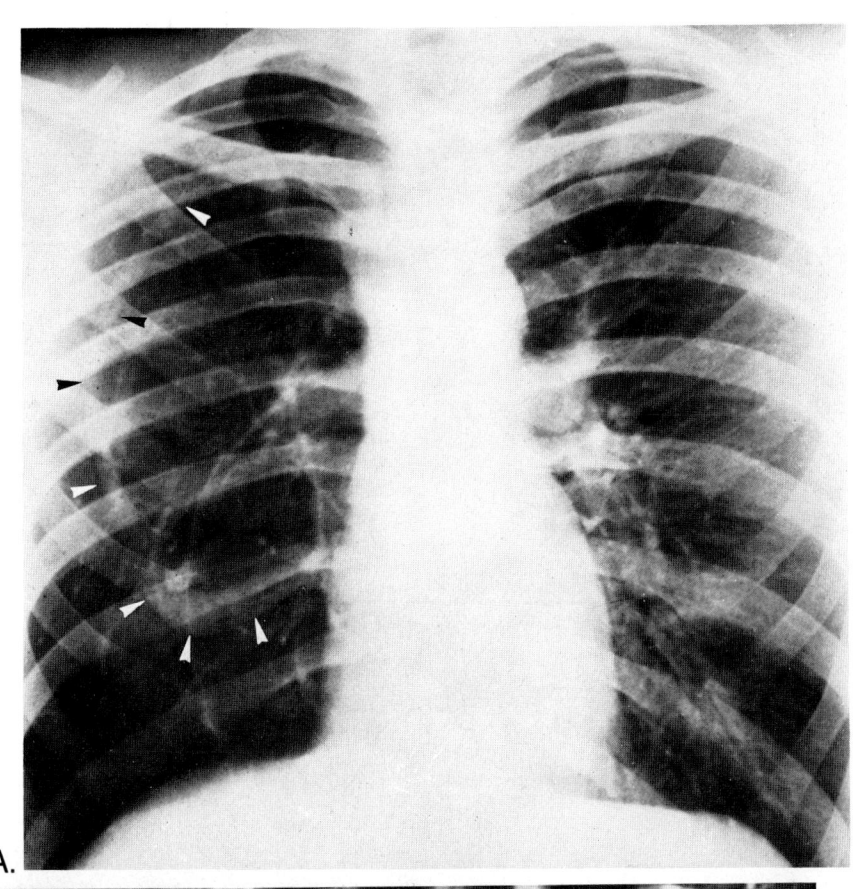

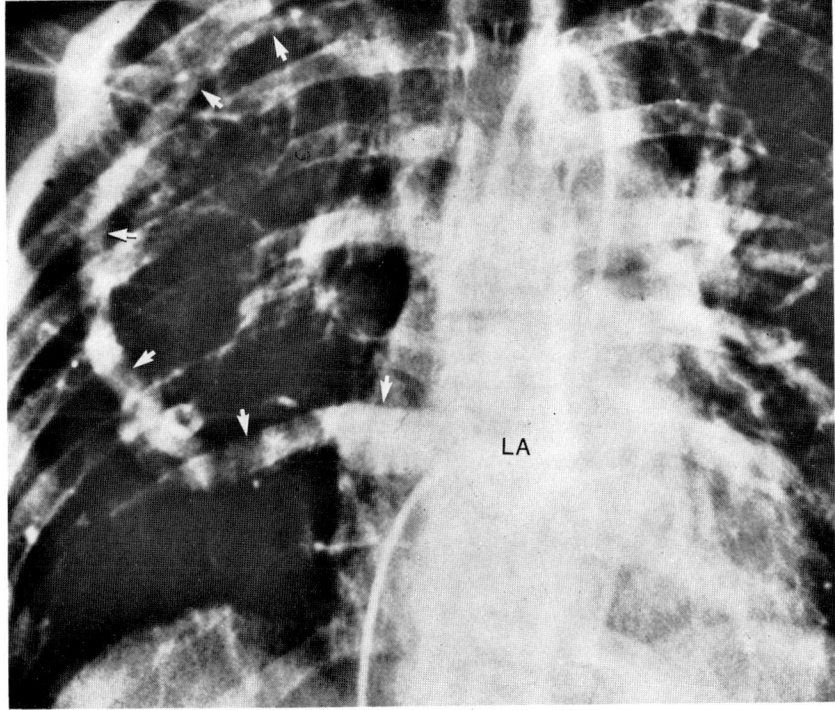

FIG 22–5.
Scimitar-like vein connecting normally with the left atrium. **A,** thoracic roentgenogram, posteroanterior projection shows hypoplasia of right lung, right pulmonary artery, and a curvilinear abnormal vein *(arrows),* strongly suggesting scimitar syndrome. **B,** pulmonary arteriogram, anteroposterior projection in late phase. Scimitar-like vein drains normally into left atrium *(LA).* Probably this is a variation of scimitar syndrome.

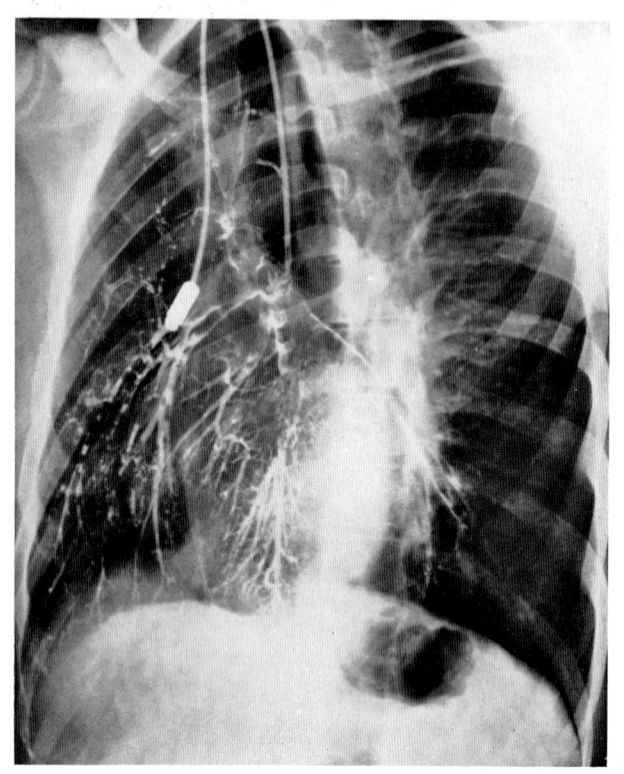

FIG 22-6.
Bronchography, left anterior oblique projection of right lung. Overexpansion of the lung, as demonstrated by spreading of bronchial radicals. Exact bronchial anatomy is difficult to determine. No bronchial cysts.

BRONCHOGRAPHIC FEATURES

In patients with repeated respiratory tract infections, bronchography is indicated to delineate bronchial abnormalities. Interpretation of the bronchogram in scimitar syndrome is difficult and confusing because of variations in anatomic form. The right lower lobe is invariably present.

1. The bronchogram usually demonstrates fewer branches than normal (Fig 22-6). REASON: The right upper and right middle lobe are commonly absent or hypoplastic.
2. The bronchi appear to be spread apart. REASON: The right upper and right middle lobe are absent, so the right lower lobe fills the entire right thoracic cavity.
3. Bronchial cysts and diverticula may be seen.

CARDIAC CATHETERIZATION

The catheter may be advanced from the inferior vena cava into the scimitar vein. The right atrial and ventricular pressures may be normal or elevated, and the right ventricular and pulmonary arterial pressures may reach systemic levels.

An increased oxygen saturation may be found in the inferior vena cava, but it is often small.

ANGIOGRAPHIC FEATURES

At the time of cardiac catheterization, angiography is indicated for the following reasons:

1. Not all scimitar-like veins drain into the right side of the heart (see Fig 22-5).
2. Demonstration of a supradiaphragmatic or infradiaphragmatic entry site into the inferior vena cava.
3. Delineation of the anatomy of the right pulmonary veins, particularly at the level of the diaphragm, is helpful for the surgeon (Fig 22-7).
4. Demonstration of the arterial supply from the aorta.

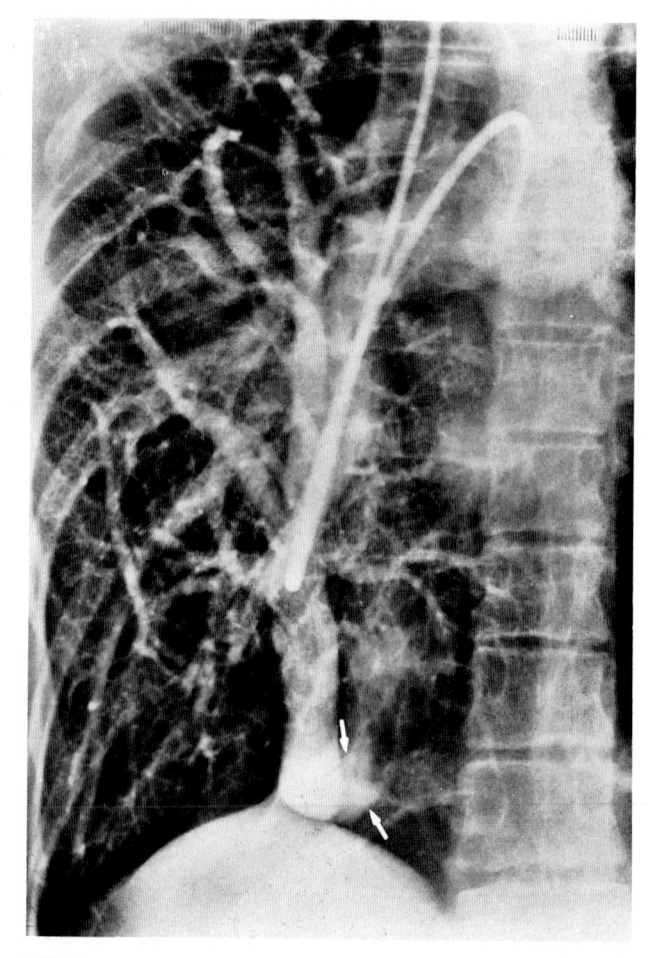

FIG 22-7.
Pulmonary arteriogram, anteroposterior projection in late phase. Right scimitar vein drains entire right lung. The vein does not pierce the diaphragm and enters the supradiaphragmatic portion of the inferior vena cava (arrows). Catheter course in main pulmonary artery shows displacement to the right due to mediastinal shift.

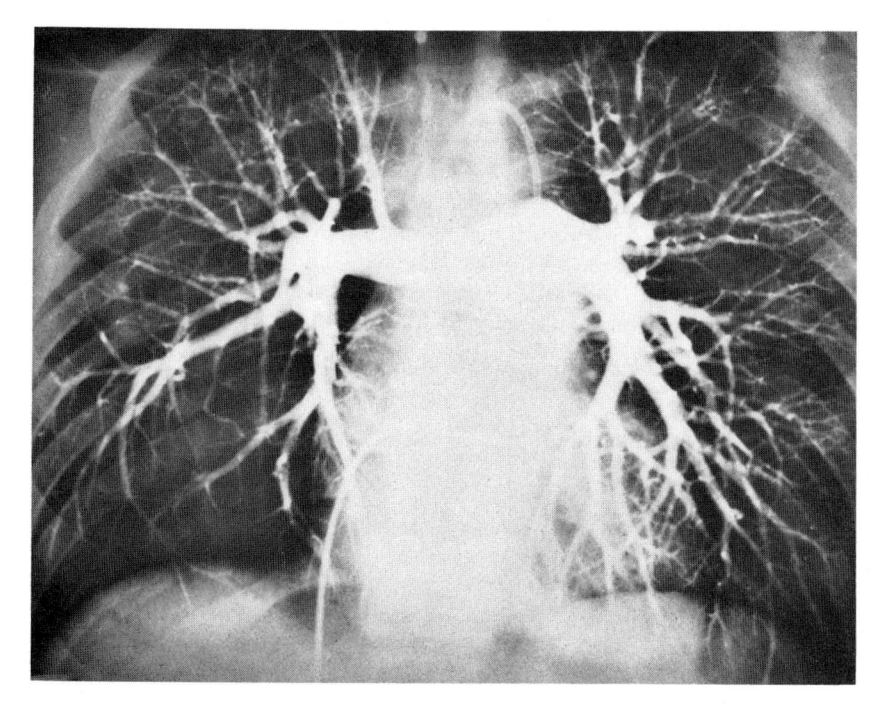

FIG 22–8.
Pulmonary arteriogram, anteroposterior projection shows mediastinal shift to the right. Hypoplasia of the right pulmonary artery with fewer vascular branches than on the left; hypoplasia of the right lung is mild in this case.

If the vein is accidentally entered during cardiac catheterization, injection of contrast medium can demonstrate its course. The vein also can be opacified by rapid injection of a large amount of contrast medium into the right pulmonary artery. Pulmonary arteriography demonstrates the degree of pulmonary hypoplasia (Fig 22–8), and the late phase allows demonstration of all pulmonary veins.

Aortography should be performed to demonstrate the arteries that pass from the aorta to the right lung (Fig 22–9). This information is of great value to the surgeon.

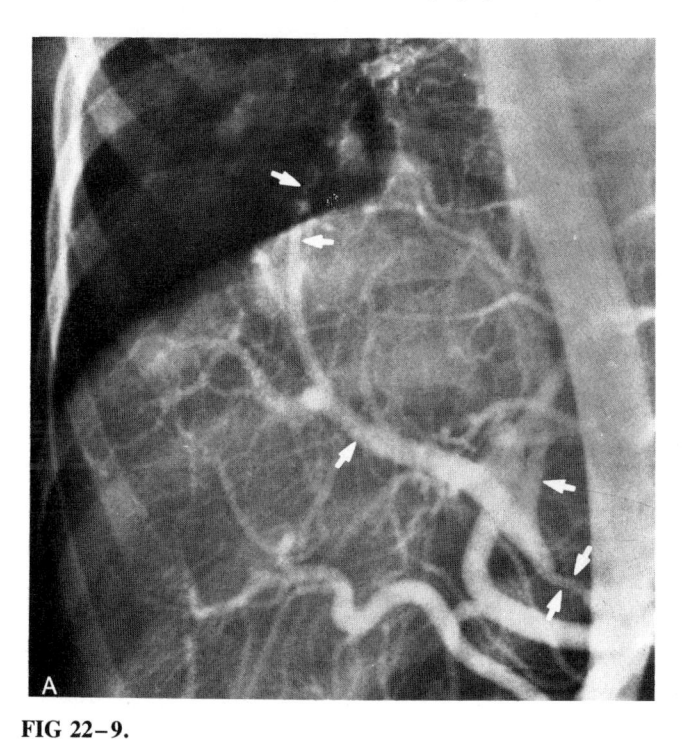

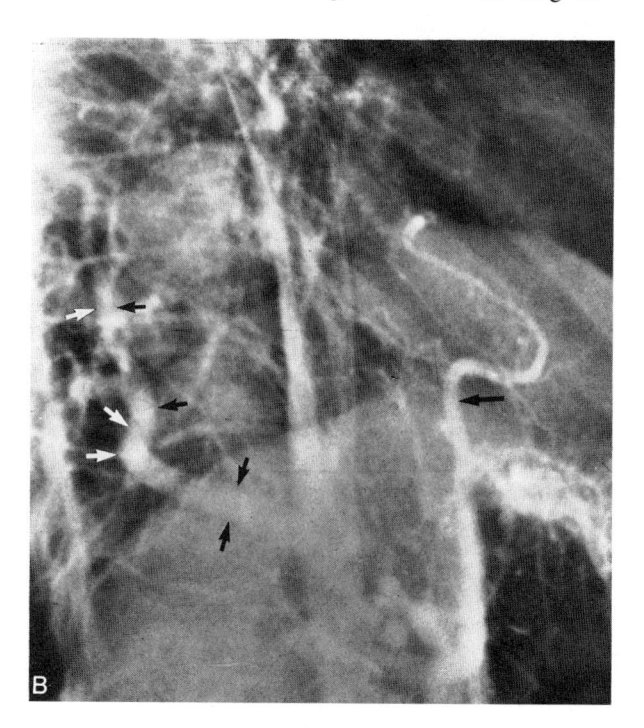

FIG 22–9.
Abdominal aortogram. **A,** anteroposterior projection shows stenotic aberrant systemic artery with two branches *(arrows)* to right lower lobe. **B,** lateral projection shows two systemic arterial branches *(short and long arrows)* to the right lower lobe. Both branches pierce the diaphragm and supply right lower lobe.

OPERATIVE CONSIDERATIONS

Surgery is indicated when there are symptoms secondary to the pulmonary abnormalities. Isolated drainage of a hypoplastic right lobe into the inferior vena cava, by itself, does not warrant operative correction, because the left-to-right shunt is not large and is well tolerated. Pulmonary hypertension usually does not result from scimitar syndrome unless there are coexistent congenital cardiac anomalies associated with increased pulmonary blood flow.

The preferred operative procedure is reimplantation of the scimitar vein into the left atrium. This usually is not possible, because the vein is short; thus, a graft may be required. If scimitar syndrome is associated with an atrial septal defect, the scimitar vein can be attached to the right atrium and a patch placed as in cases with sinus venosus defect. If the atrial septum is intact, the vein can be implanted into the right atrium, and a patch can be sewn to an operatively created atrial communication.

Patients with marked pulmonary hypoplasia, a large systemic blood supply to the right lung, severe pulmonary infections, and bronchial abnormalities may require pneumonectomy.

REFERENCES

1. Jue KL, Amplatz K, Adams P Jr, et al: Anomalies of great vessels associated with lung hypoplasia: the scimitar syndrome, *Am J Dis Child* 111:35, 1966.
2. Kiely B, Filler J, Stone S, et al: Syndrome of anomalous venous drainage of the right lung to the inferior vena cava: a review of 67 reported cases and three new cases in children, *Am J Cardiol* 20:102, 1967.
3. Dische MR, Teixeira ML, Winchester PH, et al: Horseshoe lung associated with a variant of the 'scimitar' syndrome, *Br Heart J* 36:617, 1974.
4. Halasz NA, Halloran KH, Liebow AA: Bronchial and arterial anomalies with drainage of the right lung into the inferior vena cava, *Circulation* 14:826, 1956.
5. Roehm JOF Jr, Jue KL, Amplatz K: Radiographic features of the scimitar syndrome, *Radiology* 86:856, 1966.
6. Valdez-Davila O, Avila-Varguez J, Castaneda-Zuniga WR, et al: A variation of scimitar syndrome, *Röfo* 128:271, 1978.
7. Morgan JR, Forker AD: Syndrome of hypoplasia of the right lung and dextroposition of the heart: "scimitar sign" with normal pulmonary venous drainage, *Circulation* 43:27, 1971.

CHAPTER 23

Endocardial Cushion Defect

Endocardial cushion defect (ECD) is a term that describes a spectrum of cardiac anomalies that are the result of abnormalities in the development of the embryonic endocardial cushion tissues. Endocardial cushion defects account for 4% of cases of congenital heart disease, with an equal sex incidence. This is the most common cardiac malformation in patients with Down syndrome.

EMBRYOLOGY

To understand the origin and anatomic forms of ECD, it is helpful to review the role of the endocardial cushion tissue in the formation of the heart.[1] This important tissue forms four components of the heart:

1. The lower portion of the atrial septum.
2. The upper portion of the ventricular septum.
3. The septal leaflet of the mitral valve.
4. The septal leaflet of the tricuspid valve.

Early in the embryo, a channel (the atrioventricular canal) connects the primitive left atrium and left ventricle (Fig 23–1). Gradually the channel shifts toward the midline, so that a communication also exists between the right atrium and right ventricle. Soon, the atrioventricular canal begins to be separated into a left and right channel by the development of two masses of tissue, the endocardial cushions, one located dorsally and the other ventrally (Figs 23–2 and 23–3). These grow into the atrioventricular canal, meeting initially on the right side and fusing to form the atrioventricular septum. As a result, separate tricuspid and mitral channels are formed.

While the endocardial cushions are forming, the common atrium is being divided by a septum (septum primum), which arises from the dorsal and cephalic atrial wall (Figs 23–3 and 23–4). The crescent-shape leading edge of the septum primum grows toward the atrioventricular septum. Below the free margin of the septum primum and above the atrioventricular septum, there is a communication (the ostium primum) between the primitive right and left atria. The ostium primum gradually closes as the septum primum joins the atrioventricular septum. The ostium secundum then develops in the superior portion of the septum primum, after which the septum secundum develops to the right of the septum primum from the superior portion of the right atrium.

As it develops, the lower portion of the atrioventricular septum becomes concave, with a convexity directed toward the atria (see Fig 23–1). The right limb of the atrioventricular septum fuses with ventricular septum, closing the interventricular foramen. Portions of the atrioventricular septum continue to differentiate into fibrous tissue, so that eventually the two limbs of this septum form the septal leaflets of the tricuspid and mitral valves, respectively.

Endocardial cushion defects result from interruption of the normal development of the endocardial cushion tissue at some stage. In all instances of this anomaly, there is some degree of failure of fusion of the endocardial cushion tissue. As a result of the interrupted development, although the free margin of the septum primum forms normally, there is no atrioventricular septum to which it can attach. This leads to an interatrial communication below the free margin of the septum primum. Failure of normal endocardial cushion development causes a low position of the midportions of the septal leaflets of the mitral and tricuspid valves. The crest of the ventricular septum beneath the atrioventricular valve is scooped out and forms the lower margin of a septal defect involving adjacent portions of atrial and ventricular septa.

Depending on the stage at which development is interrupted, the status of the atrioventricular valves differs, particularly that of the septal leaflet of the mitral valve. If the endocardial cushions fuse but incompletely, a cleft in the mitral valve results. If they fail to fuse, a common atrioventricular valve orifice is formed, with continuous com-

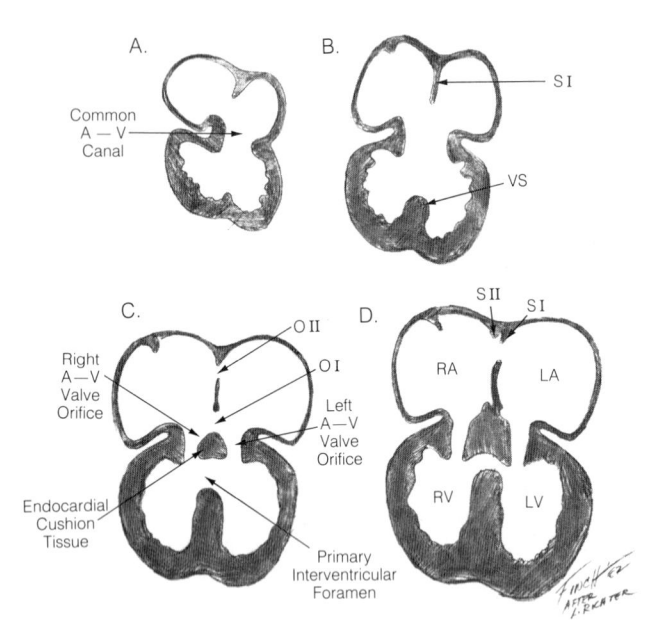

FIG 23–1.
Development of the heart, anterior projection. **A,** complete atrioventricular canal connects primitive left atrium and left ventricle. **B,** complete atrioventricular canal shifts, permitting communication between primitive right atrium and ventricle also. Septum primum *(SI)* and ventricular septum are developing. **C,** endocardial cushions have fused to divide common atrioventricular canal into separate right and left atrioventricular *(A-V)* orifices. The septum primum has completed its growth, sealing the ostium primum *(OI)*. Ostium secundum *(OII)* has developed in septum primum. **D,** ventricular septum and atrial septum are nearing completion. Septum secundum *(SII)* is developing. *LA* = left atrium; *LV* = left ventricle; *RA* = right atrium; *RV* = right ventricle.

mon atrioventricular valve leaflets passing through the septal defect from one ventricle to the other.

PATHOLOGIC ANATOMY

The anatomy of ECD represents a spectrum of malformations, which have been classified as follows[2]:

I. Complete atrioventricular canal
   A. With divided septally attached anterior common leaflet
   B. With divided septally unattached anterior common leaflet
   C. With undivided septally unattached anterior common leaflet
II. Incomplete atrioventricular canal
   A. Without ventricular communication
      1. Partial form (ostium primum atrial defect and cleft mitral valve)
      2. Common atrium with atrioventricular valve deformity
      3. Isolated ostium primum defect
      4. Isolated cleft of anterior leaflet of mitral valve
      5. Isolated cleft of anterior leaflet of tricuspid valve
   B. With interventricular communication
      1. Ventricular septal defect of atrioventricular-canal type, normal atrioventricular valves
      2. Ventricular septal defect of atrioventricular-canal type, abnormal atrioventricular valves

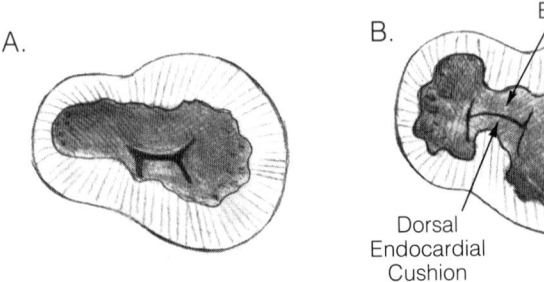

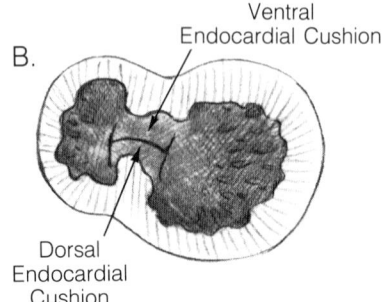

FIG 23–2.
Development of the heart; view from cardiac apex. Stages similar to those in Figure 23–1. **A,** common atrioventricular canal, with single valve orifice entering a common ventricle. **B,** endocardial cushions developing. **C,** continued development of cushion tissue, with differentiation to form to atrioventricular valvular tissue. **D,** complete formation of endocardial cushions, resulting in separate mitral and tricuspid orifices. Interventricular septum *(IVS)* developing. *LV* = left ventricle; *RV* = right ventricle.

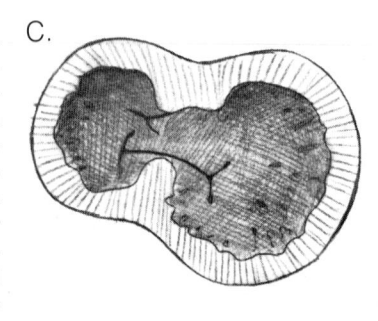

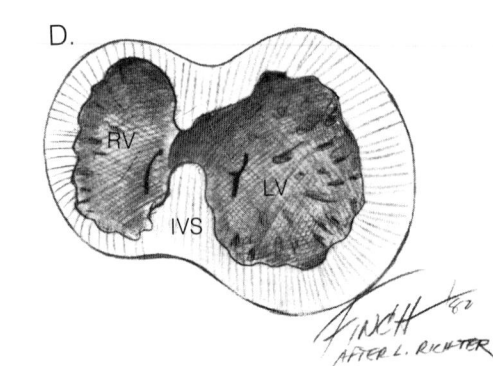

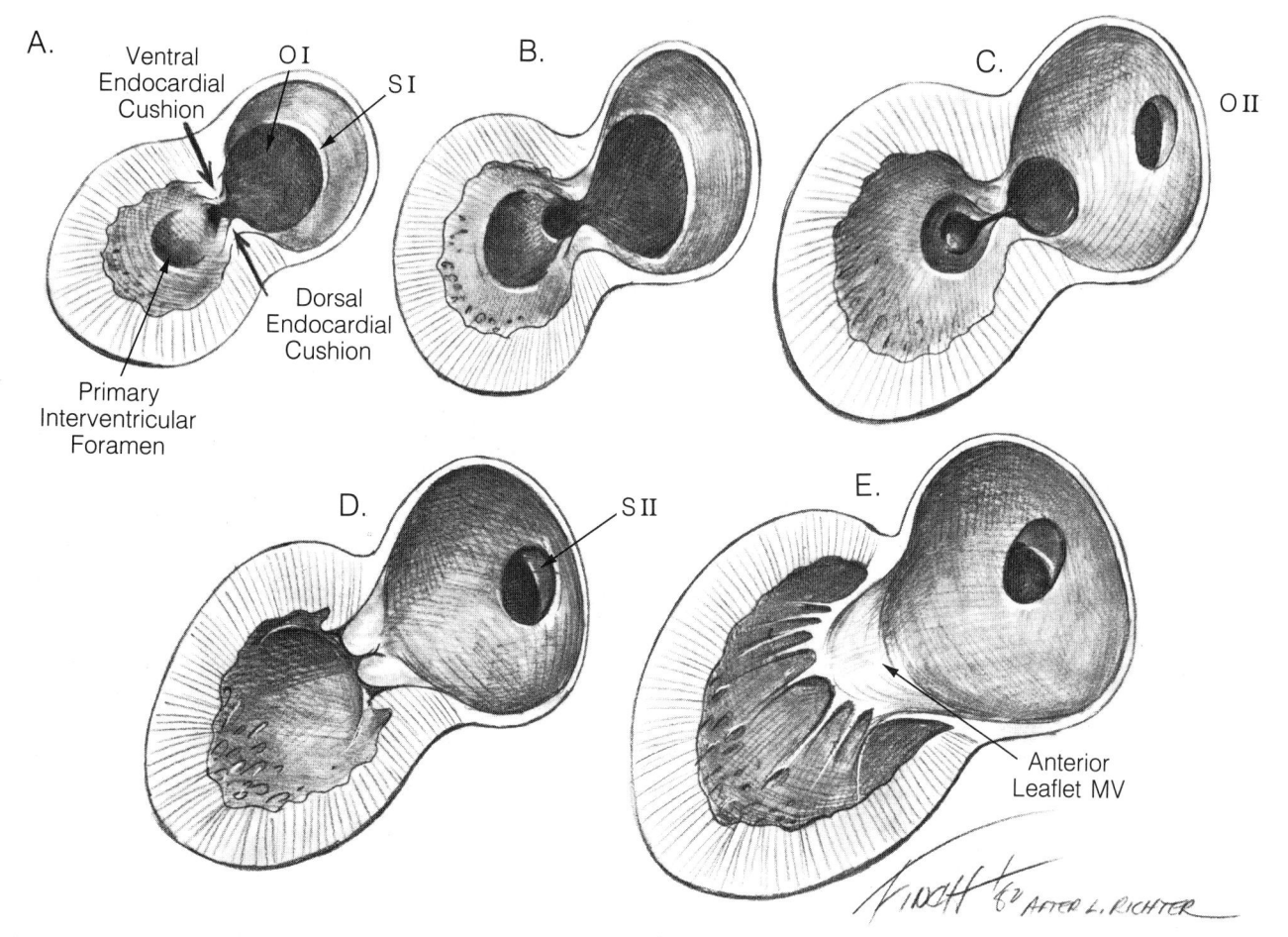

FIG 23-3.
Development of the heart; left lateral projection. **A,** endocardial cushions forming and beginning separation of the common atrioventricular canal. Septum primum *(SI)* forming. *OI* = ostium primum. **B,** continued growth of endocardial cushions. **C,** endocardial cushions nearly formed, and size of ostium primum and interventricular communication diminishing. Ostium secundum *(OII)* forming in the septum primum. **D,** endocardial cushions fused, and septal leaflet of mitral valve differentiating. Septum secundum *(SII)* visible through ostium secundum. **E,** development complete.

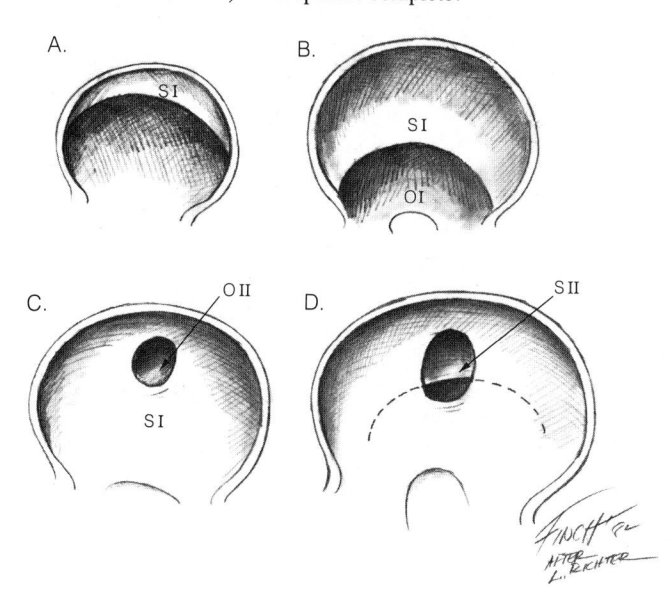

FIG 23-4.
Development of atrial septum, left lateral projection. **A,** septum primum developing from cephalic portion of atrium. **B,** septum primum *(SI)* has partially divided atrium, but communication between left and right atrium exists through the ostium primum *(OI)*. **C,** septum primum has fused to endocardial cushion, and ostium secundum *(OII)* has developed. **D,** septum secundum *(SII)* developing in the right atrium and visible through ostium secundum.

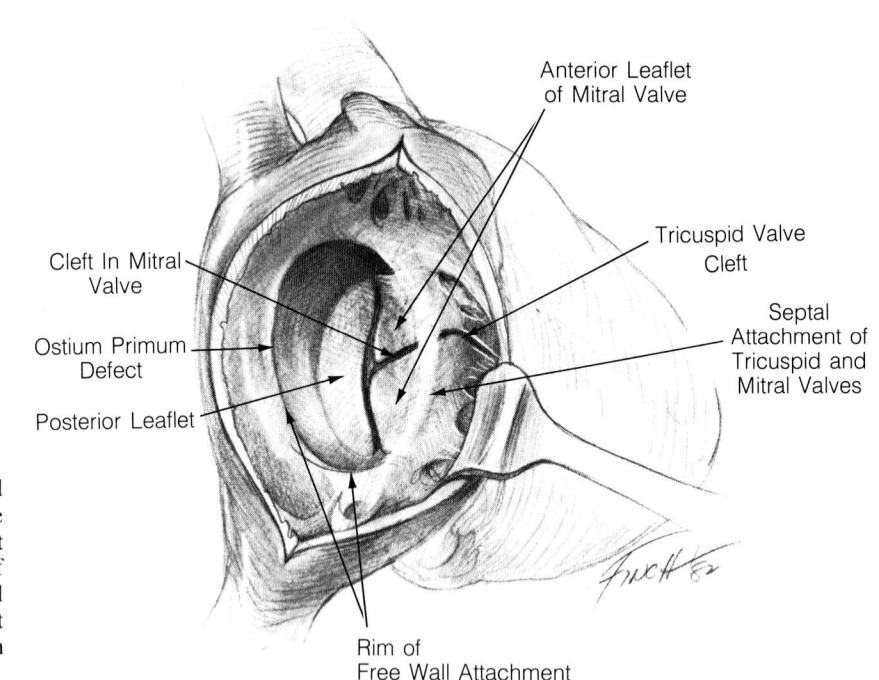

FIG 23-5.
Ostium primum defect and cleft mitral valve viewed through right atriotomy. The ostium primum defect located in lower part of atrial septum and extends to upper part of ventricular septum. Septal leaflets of mitral and tricuspid valves firmly attached to crest of ventricular septum. Adjacent clefts in mitral and tricuspid valve.

In almost all forms of ECD, there is a deficiency of the upper portion of the ventricular septum, giving it a scooped-out, or concave, appearance. The principal difference between complete and incomplete forms relates to the characteristics of the atrioventricular valves and their method of attachment to the crest of the ventricular septum. In partial atrioventricular canal, the atrioventricular valves are attached firmly to the ventricular septum, preventing an interventricular communication (Fig 23-5). In complete atrioventricular canal, there is a single continuous defect involving the lower portion of the atrial septum and an adjacent portion of the ventricular septum underly-

FIG 23-6.
Complete atrioventricular canal and variations of common anterior leaflet. **A,** type A; common atrioventricular canal. Atrial defect continuous with area of deficiency of the upper portion of the ventricular septum. Common posterior leaflet and common anterior leaflet, split into two portions, the medial margins being attached to crest of interventricular septum. **B,** type B; common atrioventricular canal. Chordae tendineae from midportion of common anterior leaflet attached to papillary muscle in right ventricle. **C,** type C; common atrioventricular canal. Midportion of common anterior leaflet unattached.

In each type, because common leaflets are not attached directly to crest of interventricular septum, an interventricular communication exists beneath the atrioventricular valve.

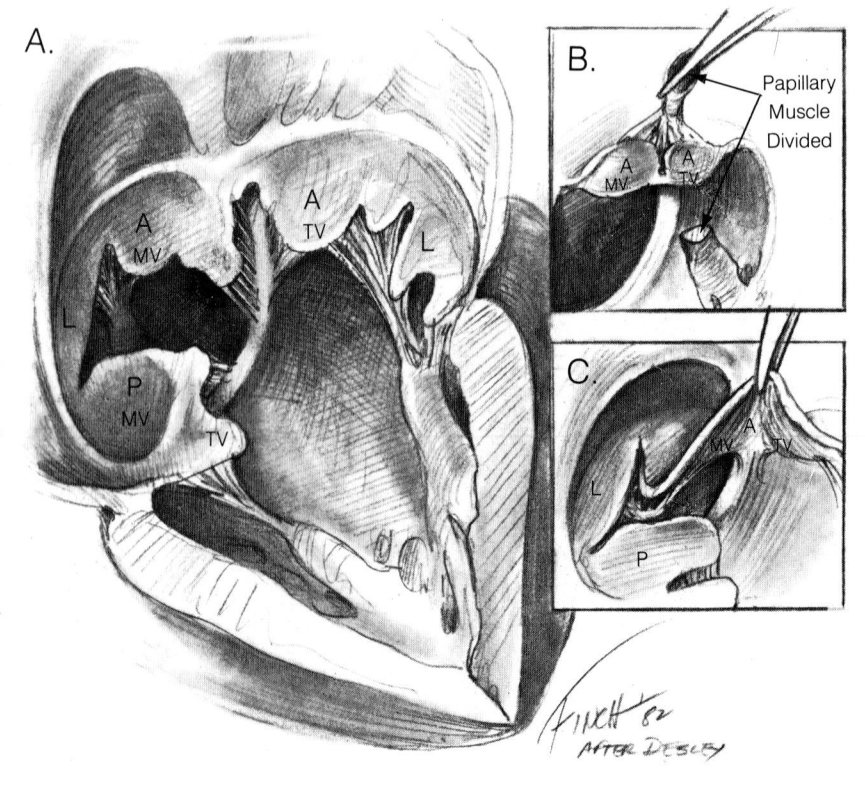

ing the atrioventricular anulus (Fig 23–6). Portions of the atrioventricular valves are abnormal. There is a common anterior and a common posterior atrioventricular leaflet, each of which crosses through the septal defect, extending from one ventricle to the other. These common leaflets represent fusions of portions of the septal leaflets of the mitral and tricuspid valves. The common posterior leaflet is usually rudimentary, whereas the anterior common leaflet is well formed. Chordae tendineae may pass from portions of the valve into either ventricle. In addition, the midportion of the common leaflets may attach by short chordae tendineae to the crest of the ventricular septum.

Complete atrioventricular canal can be divided into three categories, depending on the status of the common anterior leaflet, which represents fusion of the anterior halves of the septal leaflets of the mitral and tricuspid valves (Fig 23–6). In the first category, type A, the anterior leaflet is divided into two equal portions: one related to the left ventricle and the other to the right ventricle (Fig 23–6,A). The medial aspects of these two portions of the anterior leaflet are attached to the crest of the ventricular septum by multiple short chordae tendineae. In type B, the anterior leaflet is also divided into two portions, but these do not attach to the crest of the ventricular septum (Fig 23–6,B). There are, however, chordae tendineae from the medial aspect of each portion which attach to a papillary muscle in the right ventricle. In type C, there is a common undivided anterior leaflet, which has no attachment to either the crest of the ventricular septum or a papillary muscle (Fig 23–6,C). In each type, the lateral aspects of the common anterior leaflet are attached appropriately to chordae tendineae.

In complete atrioventricular canal, the common anterior and posterior atrioventricular valve leaflets are positioned above the crest of the ventricular septum. Thus, an interventricular communication exists above the ventricular septum and beneath the atrioventricular valve leaflets.

In all forms of ECD, there are several common features. First, the posterior leaflets of the mitral and tricuspid valves are normal. Second, because of the deficiency of the ventricular septum, and attachment of portions of the mitral valve to the crest of the ventricular septum, the left ventricular outflow tract may be narrowed and elongated. Third, because of the deficiency in the ventricular septum, the septal portions of the atrioventricular anulus are displaced downward toward the cardiac apex. This reduces the length of the posterior interventricular septum and reduces the base-apex dimension of the left ventricle.

Ostium primum defect and cleft mitral valve is the most common form of incomplete atrioventricular canal. The anterior leaflet of the valve is divided (cleft) into two equal portions. The cleft varies in length and width. Chordae tendineae pass from the margins of the cleft to the ventricular septum and limit the excursion of this leaflet. The anterior leaflet of the valve is in continuity with equivalent portions of the septal leaflet of the tricuspid valve through the defect.

Rare forms of incomplete atrioventricular canal are isolated forms of ostium primum defect, cleft anterior leaflet of the mitral valve, cleft septal leaflet of tricuspid valve, or ventricular septal defect of atrioventricular-canal type.[2-5]

ASSOCIATED CONDITIONS

The cardiac anomaly most often associated with ECD is persistent left superior vena cava.[2] Hypoplasia of the aortic arch may be present in neonates with severe mitral regurgitation in utero; presumably, this develops from reduced antegrade flow into the ascending aorta. Pulmonary stenosis occasionally coexists, in which case the clinical picture resembles a "tetrad variant." Complete atrioventricular canal is common among patients with the asplenia syndrome and ostium primum defect in polysplenia. Ostium secundum defect coexists in 1% of instances of ECD.

HEMODYNAMICS

The hemodynamics are extremely variable and depend on the type and severity of the components of the ECD present. There are four potential hemodynamic problems:

1. Shunt at the atrial level.
2. Shunt at the ventricular level.
3. Mitral regurgitation.
4. Pulmonary hypertension.

The incomplete form of ECD with ostium primum defect and cleft mitral valve results in an atrial level shunt and mitral regurgitation. The direction and magnitude of the atrial shunt depends on the relative compliances of the left and right ventricles. Thus, in most patients the shunt is large and left to right, because the right ventricle is more compliant than the left. The degree of mitral regurgitation varies considerably, depending on the extent of the mitral valvular anomaly; it ranges from minimal to severe. Proportional increases occur in left ventricular volume with increasing severity of mitral regurgitation. Because the cleft is located at the base of the ostium primum defect, the regurgitant flow is predominantly from left ventricle to the right atrium. Because of this relation and the left-to-right shunt, left atrial enlargement is minimal. Pulmonary hypertension is uncommon in patients with ostium primum defect.

In complete atrioventricular canal, in addition to the

atrial level shunt and mitral regurgitation, there is an additional shunt at the ventricular level. The direction and magnitude of this shunt depend on the relative systemic and pulmonary vascular resistances. Usually, the shunt is left to right and large because the pulmonary vascular resistance is low, but the magnitude of the shunt decreases if pulmonary vascular disease develops. In most patients with complete atrioventricular canal, pulmonary hypertension is present, usually at systemic levels. The left ventricle is dilated in proportion to the size of the left-to-right shunt and the degree of mitral regurgitation. Right ventricular hypertrophy is present because of the elevated pulmonary arterial pressure. Right ventricular hypertrophy decreases the compliance of the ventricle, and this decreases the left-to-right shunt at the atrial level. Among patients with complete atrioventricular canal, the hemodynamics vary, depending on the relative magnitude of the shunt through the ventricular communication and the degree of mitral insufficiency.

CLINICAL FEATURES

The clinical features differ according to the form and severity of the ECD and the presence of coexisting conditions. Among patients with partial atrioventricular canal (ostium primum defect), the age of onset and severity of symptoms depend principally on the degree of mitral regurgitation. In most instances, the presence of cardiac disease is recognized by the discovery of a murmur in an asymptomatic child, but in patients with severe mitral regurgitation, congestive cardiac failure develops, sometimes in early infancy. Frequent respiratory infections, growth retardation, and easy fatigability are more common than in patients with atrial septal defect.

There usually is a left precordial bulge caused by the cardiomegaly. The auscultatory findings resemble those of atrial septal defect and mitral insufficiency. The former is evidenced by a soft pulmonary ejection systolic murmur, tricuspid middiastolic murmur, and wide fixed splitting of the second heart sound. An apical pansystolic murmur is heard, its loudness reflecting the degree of mitral regurgitation. In patients with moderate or severe regurgitation, an apical middiastolic murmur is heard, reflecting the increased antegrade flow across the mitral valve. The systolic murmur of mitral regurgitation may be associated with a thrill.

Patients with complete atrioventricular canal present significant symptoms within the first year of life, often within the first month. These symptoms include congestive cardiac failure, failure to thrive, and frequent respiratory infections. Cardiac failure results from the increased left ventricular volume generated by mitral regurgitation and the ventricular septal defect. If mitral regurgitation is the primary hemodynamic condition, severe cardiac failure may develop in the neonatal period. In contrast, if the ventricular septal defect is predominant and mitral regurgitation is minimal, cardiac failure does not develop until 6 weeks to 3 months, as in patients with isolated ventricular septal defect, when the pulmonary vascular resistance has declined.

The infant with a complete atrioventricular canal is usually small and shows tachypnea, tachycardia, and a prominent precordial bulge. The second heart sound is accentuated and narrowly split because of the pulmonary hypertension. A loud pansystolic murmur of the ventricular septal defect is heard diffusely throughout the precordium and may be associated with a thrill. It may be difficult to identify a separate systolic murmur of mitral regurgitation, but when the systolic murmur is heard well at the apex and on the left side of the back, mitral regurgitation should be strongly suspected. An apical middiastolic murmur from the increased flow across the mitral valve secondary to the left-to-right ventricular shunt or mitral insufficiency is heard. A middiastolic murmur is often heard in the tricuspid area from the atrial shunt, and this finding distinguishes complete atrioventricular canal from isolated ventricular septal defect. A pulmonary ejection murmur from the atrial level shunt is not heard, because it is masked by the loud pansystolic murmur.

ELECTROCARDIOGRAPHIC FEATURES

The electrocardiogram (ECG) is diagnostic of ECD and results from both the abnormality of the cardiac conduction system and the hemodynamics. Because of the position of the ventricular component of the cushion defect, the bundle of His is displaced and passes posteriorly and inferiorly around the cushion defect.[6] The atrioventricular node is also displaced posteriorly in relation to the coronary sinus. Other abnormalities of the cardiac conduction system have also been described: early origin of fibers to the left bundle, displacement of the distal left bundle-branch fascicles to the posterior aspect of the interventricular septum, and hypoplasia of the anterior fascicle of the left bundle. These abnormalities result in early depolarization of the posterior aspect of the ventricular septum.[6] From this site, ventricular depolarization generally proceeds from right and inferior to left and superior.[7] This leads to the characteristic finding of left-axis deviation. Indeed, so constant is left-axis deviation that it is difficult to make a diagnosis of ECD without its presence. Patients with complete atrioventricular canal tend to show a greater degree of left-axis deviation (>90 degrees) than do those with partial atrioventricular canal, probably because of the associated right ventricular hypertrophy in the former.[8]

The PR interval is usually prolonged. The reason is unknown. Right atrial enlargement is present in one third of patients and reflects the left-to-right shunt at the atrial level.

In at least three fourths of patients, lead V_4R or V_1 shows either an rsR' or rR' complex. The height of the R' correlates roughly with the level of pulmonary arterial pressure.[8] Left ventricular hypertrophy is common, also reflecting the left ventricular dilatation that results from either ventricular septal defect or mitral regurgitation. It is difficult to assess the degree of mitral regurgitation from the ECG, presumably because left ventricular hypertrophy may be masked by coexisting right ventricular hypertrophy.

ECHOCARDIOGRAPHIC FEATURES

Endocardial cushion defect is associated with characteristic M-mode and two-dimensional echocardiographic findings. In partial atrioventricular canal, these features are found: paradoxical septal motion from the increased right ventricular diameter and abnormalities of the mitral valvular echoes, including anterior displacement of anterior mitral valve leaflet into the left ventricular outflow tract and apparent diastolic movement of the anterior mitral valve leaflet across the ventricular septum.[9, 10]

In complete atrioventricular canal, the echocardiogram shows little ventricular septum. The atrioventricular valvular motion is exaggerated, completely crossing the interventricular septum and appearing as a single atrioventricular valve. Paradoxical septal motion is not found because of the presence of pulmonary hypertension.

Two-dimensional echocardiography clearly outlines the defect involving the atrial and adjacent portions of the interventricular septum and its extent.[11] The characteristics of the atrioventricular valves can be outlined in sufficient detail that the three types of complete atrioventricular canal can be distinguished.

RADIOGRAPHIC FEATURES

Thoracic radiographic findings of atrioventricular canal are not uniform because of the variation in hemodynamics among patients. In complete atrioventricular canal, atrial and ventricular left-to-right shunt and atrioventricular valve insufficiency may coexist, and the magnitude of the shunts and the degree of mitral regurgitation vary, causing a range of radiographic appearances. In the incomplete form of ECD without significant mitral regurgitation, the radiographic findings are indistinguishable from those of a secundum atrial septal defect. However, a normal radiograph, as present in medium-sized ostium secundum atrial septal defects, is uncommon because the atrial communication in ECD is usually large.

Partial Atrioventricular Canal (Ostium Primum Defect)

1. Among patients with ostium primum defect but with little or no mitral regurgitation, the cardiac silhouette is almost always enlarged, because the defect tends to be large and is associated with a large left-to-right shunt (Fig 23–7).

2. Left atrial enlargement is absent. Although blood flow through the left atrium is markedly increased because of the left-to-right shunt, the left atrium is decompressed through the ostium primum atrial defect. Left and right atrial pressures are equal.

3. As in ostium secundum atrial septal defect, increased pulmonary vasculature, prominence of the main pulmonary arterial segment, right ventricular enlargement, and right atrial prominence are present (see Fig 23–7). The hemodynamic alterations of an ostium primum defect without atrioventricular valvar insufficiency are identical

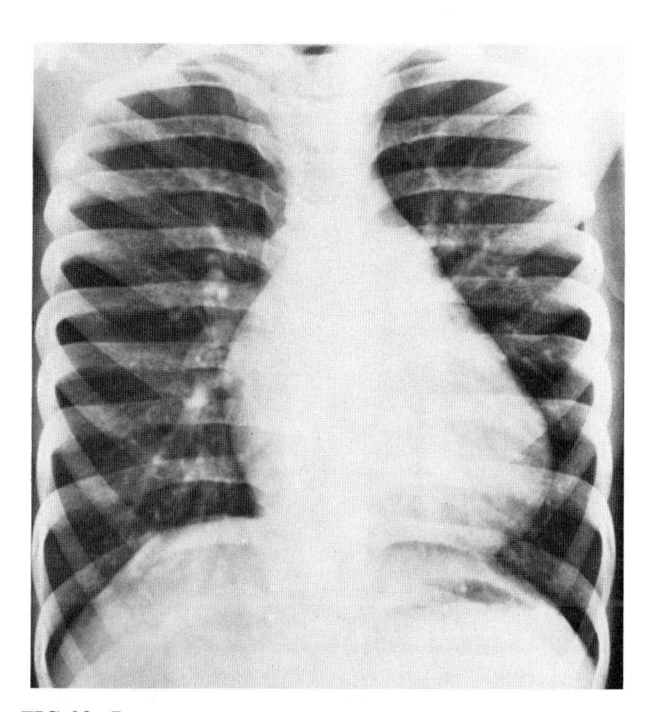

FIG 23–7.
Thoracic roentgenogram, posteroanterior projection of patient with partial atrioventricular canal. Cardiomegaly. Increased pulmonary vasculature with prominent main pulmonary artery segment. Inconspicuous aortic knob. Superior vena cava and ascending aorta inconspicuous due to clockwise rotation of the heart. Large diameter of right atrial border suggests right atrial enlargement; left atrial enlargement absent. Findings indistinguishable from those of ostium secundum type atrial septal defect, which causes identical hemodynamic alterations.

Partial Atrioventricular Canal With Mitral Regurgitation

1. The chest roentgenogram is different in patients with ostium primum defect and moderate or severe mitral regurgitation (Fig 23–8). The cardiac silhouette is markedly enlarged. REASON: In addition to the large left-to-right shunt at the atrial level, which causes right ventricular enlargement, there is volume load on the left ventricle because of mitral regurgitation.
2. The pulmonary arterial vasculature is accentuated, but cardiac size appears out of proportion to the increase of the pulmonary vascularity (Fig 23–8). Whereas an ostium primum defect causes right ventricular enlargement, partial atrioventricular canal with mitral regurgitation results in biventricular enlargement.
3. The combination of the left-to-right shunt and significant mitral regurgitation can cause congestive cardiac failure. Therefore, pulmonary venous distention from associated cardiac failure results in pulmonary vasculature with a fluffy and indistinct appearance (see Fig 23–8).
4. Depending on the degree of mitral regurgitation, the pulmonary vasculature ranges from a pattern consistent with a left-to-right shunt to one with pulmonary venous distension, as found in cardiac failure and mitral reflux.
5. Left atrial enlargement is uncommon (see Fig 23–8), as the chamber is decompressed through the large atrial septal defect. However, the left atrium may appear enlarged on the chest film for one of three reasons:
   a. "Pseudo left atrial enlargement." If the right ventricle is markedly enlarged, it can displace a normal-sized left atrium posteriorly against the barium-filled esophagus, causing posterior displacement and indentation (see Chapter 19).
   b. Rarely, the atrial communication is small (Fig 23–9). Therefore, the left atrium is not decompressed through the pressure-limiting atrial communication, and the left atrium is enlarged because of the mitral regurgitation.
   c. If left ventricular failure develops, left ventricular filling pressure increases, elevating the left atrial pressure. This may also dilate the left atrium.

Complete Atrioventricular Canal

The thoracic roentgenographic findings in the complete form of atrioventricular canal are indistinguishable

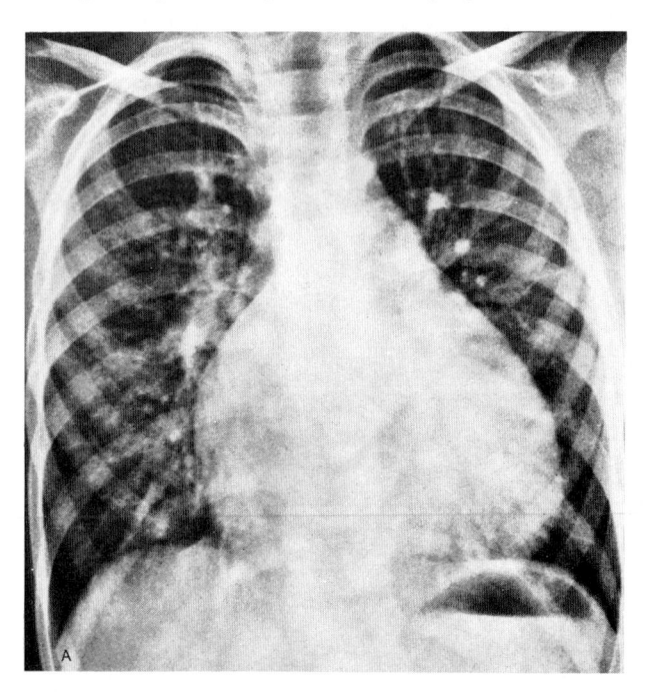

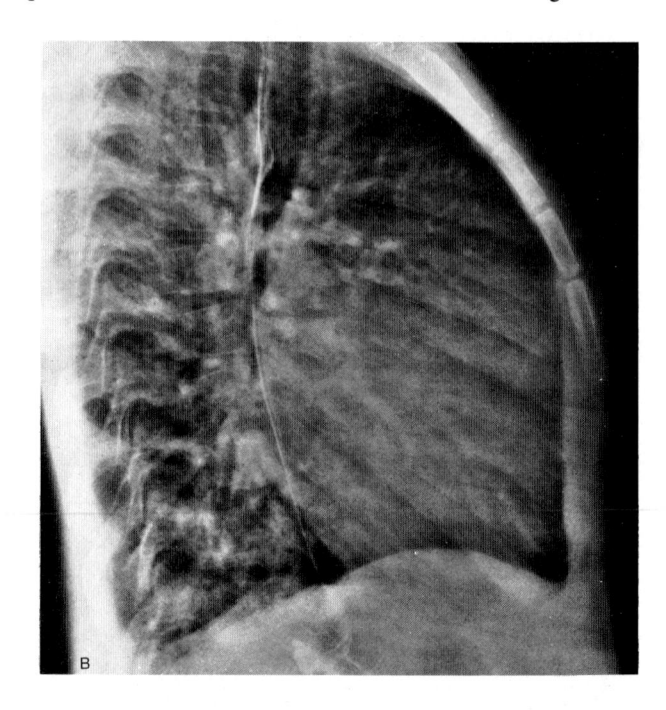

FIG 23–8.
Thoracic roentgenogram, posteroanterior projection of patient with partial atrioventricular canal with significant mitral regurgitation. **A,** marked cardiomegaly. Pulmonary vasculature diffusely increased, with pattern of venous distention. Cardiac image is larger than expected for degree of accentuation of pulmonary arterial vasculature. This is a common radiographic appearance of atrioventricular canal with mitral regurgitation, but a specific radiographic diagnosis often is impossible because the picture is similar to that of cardiomyopathy with congestive cardiac failure or atrial septal defect. **B,** lateral projection. Bowing of lower sternum from right ventricular enlargement. No left atrial enlargement despite severe mitral reflux because left atrium is decompressed via atrial communication.

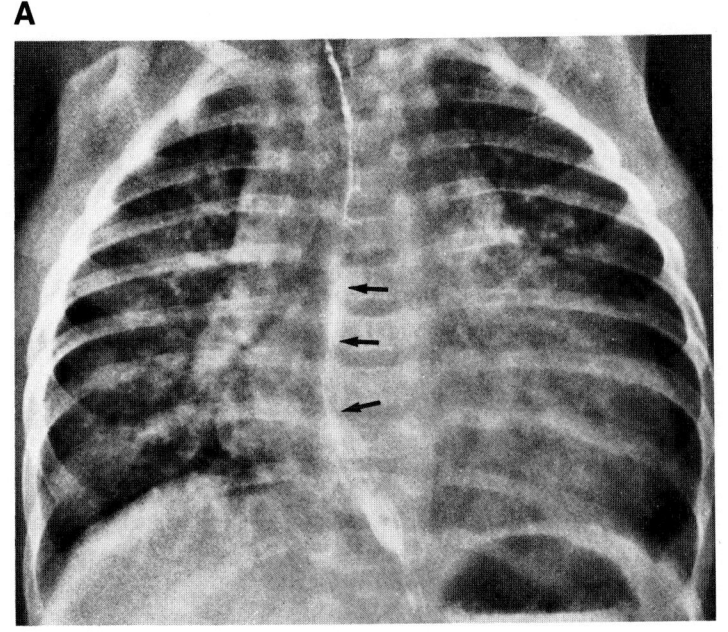

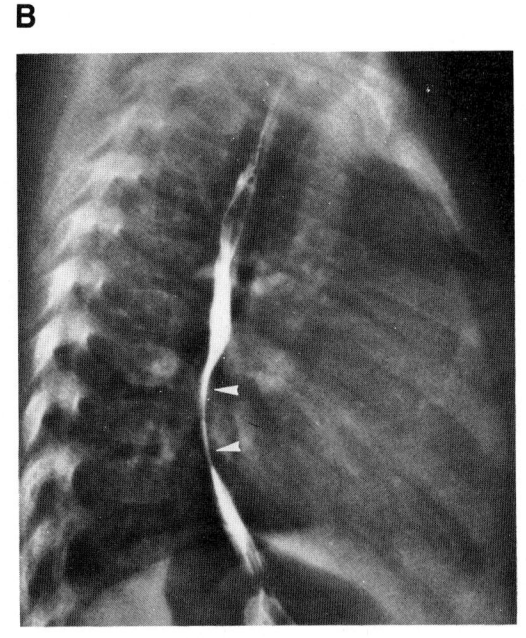

FIG 23-9.
Thoracic roentgenograms of patient with partial atrioventricular canal, considerable mitral regurgitation, and small atrial communication. **A**, posteroanterior projection. Marked cardiomegaly. Pulmonary vasculature diffusely increased and indistinct. Esophagus pushed to right by enlarged left atrium. **B**, lateral projection. Left atrial enlargement *(white arrows)* caused by mitral regurgitation and small atrial communication.

from those of partial atrioventricular canal with mitral regurgitation, but the cardiac image is even larger, especially when compared with the degree of increase in the pulmonary arterial vasculature.

CARDIAC CATHETERIZATION

Cardiac catheterization and angiocardiography are performed to assess the magnitude of shunt, the pulmonary arterial pressure, and the degree of mitral regurgitation; to detect the presence of a ventricular septal defect; and to exclude coexisting anomalies.

The course of the catheter as it passes from the right to the left atrium is characteristic, because it crosses low in the septum through the ostium primum defect. Therefore, the catheter course has a low position within the cardiac silhouette (see Chapter 19). Also, it is easier to advance the catheter from the right atrium into the left ventricle than it is in instances of secundum atrial septal defect because of the location of the ostium primum defect immediately adjacent to the mitral valve. It may be possible to advance the catheter from the right ventricle through the ventricular septal defect into the aorta.

Oximetry data show an increase in oxygen saturation in the right atrium, and the increase is usually large.[12] The left-to-right atrial shunt in partial atrioventricular canal is usually about 65%, similar to that in ostium secundum atrial septal defect. A small right-to-left shunt may also be present at the atrial level. Even in the absence of a ventricular septal defect, there may be an additional, but smaller, increase in oxygen saturation in the right ventricle because of streaming. It is usually difficult to detect a separate ventricular septal defect or coexisting patent ductus arteriosus from the oximetry data.

Atrial pressures are equal and usually normal. The degree of mitral regurgitation cannot be assessed from atrial pressure tracings, because the atria are in free communication. In partial atrioventricular canal, the pulmonary arterial pressure rarely exceeds 60% of the systemic pressure. Rarely is the elevated pressure caused by pulmonary vascular disease; rather, it is caused by the large volume of pulmonary blood flow. In contrast, among patients with complete atrioventricular canal, pulmonary arterial pressures are usually at systemic levels; and elevated pulmonary vascular resistance is common, especially in older patients and those with Down syndrome. Pulmonary vascular disease often develops early (before age 5 years) in patients with complete atrioventricular canal.

ANGIOGRAPHIC APPEARANCE

Angiography is the most important diagnostic test in the evaluation of patients with ECDs. In most patients, left ventriculography allows distinction between ostium primum defect and complete atrioventricular canal.[13] When it is present, the ventricular communication and mitral regur-

FIG 23–10.
Diagram of complete atrioventricular canal. Ventricular and atrial septa are deficient, resulting in an ostium primum defect and deficiency of the adjacent interventricular septum. Anterior leaflet of mitral valve is divided into two segments by cleft. Septal leaflets of mitral and tricuspid valves are continuous across ventricular septum but attach firmly to septum. Anterior half of anterior leaflet of mitral valve and adjacent portion of tricuspid valve are usually called the common anterior leaflet. Posterior half and portions of tricuspid valve form common posterior leaflet. Posterior leaflet of the mitral valve and anterior and posterior leaflets of tricuspid valve are normal. Space beneath leaflets and crest of ventricular septum forms ventricular communication (ventricular septal defect). **A,** leaflets have short chordal attachments. **B,** anomalous chordal attachments to contralateral papillary muscle. **C,** leaflets are free floating. A = anterior leaflet; PMV = posterior mitral valve leaflet; ATV = anterior tricuspid valve leaflet; PTV = posterior tricuspid valve leaflet; P = posterior leaflet.

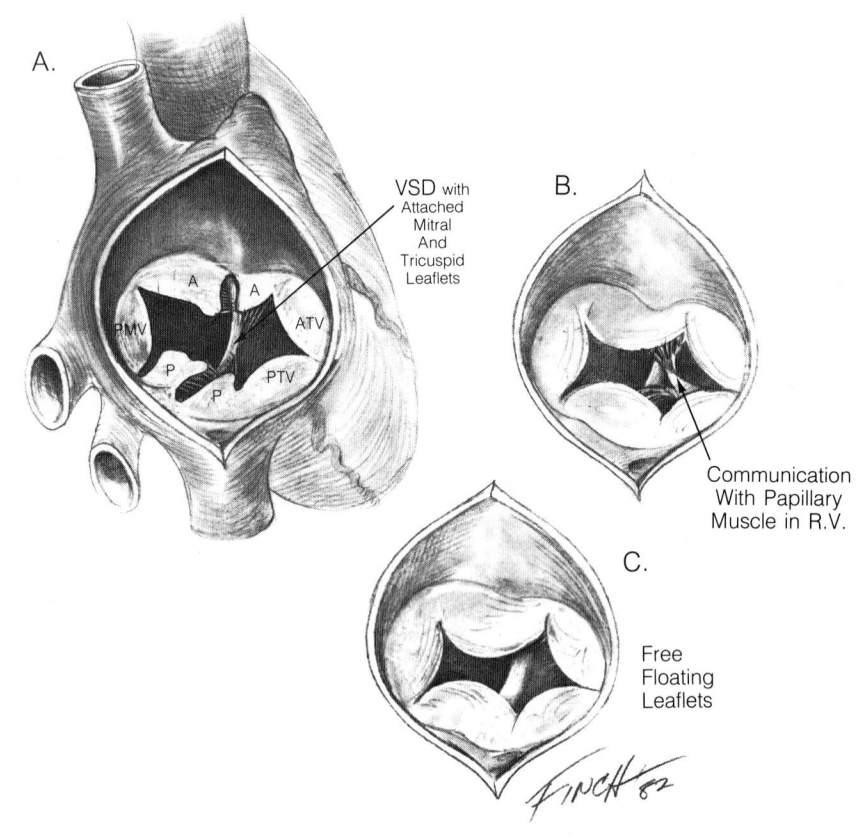

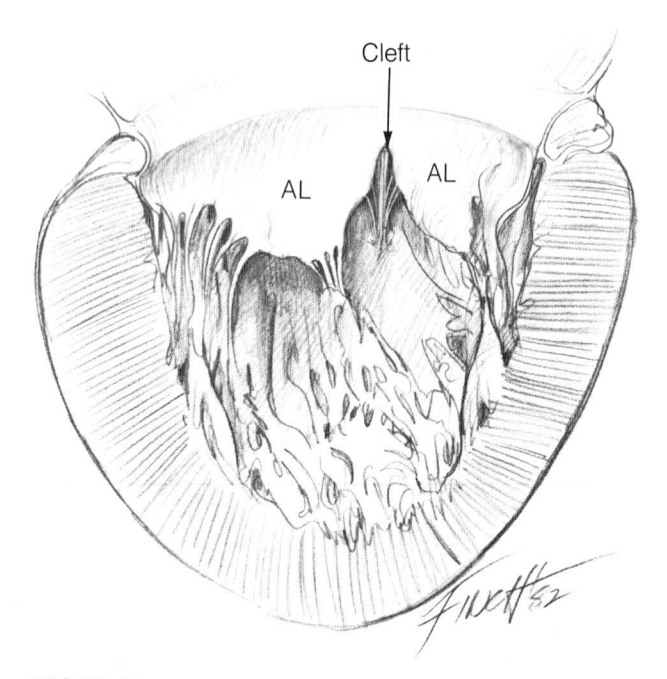

FIG 23–11.
View of anterior leaflet of mitral valve *(AL),* which is attached to ventricular septum (incomplete atrioventricular canal). Anterior leaflet is divided in half by cleft, which has additional chordal attachments.

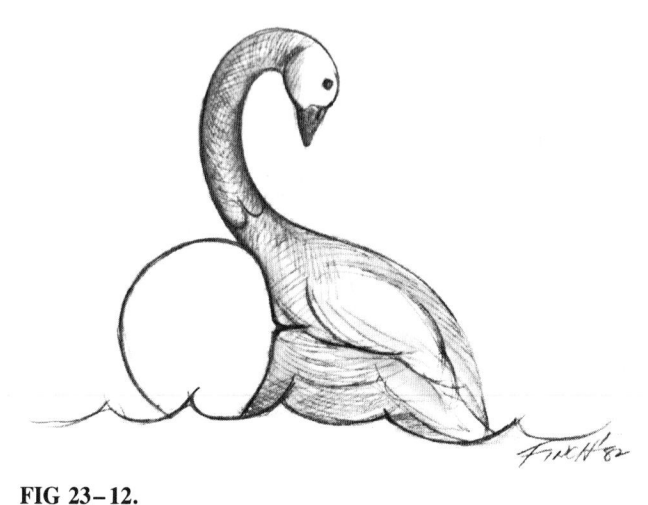

FIG 23–12.
Drawing of a swimming goose, depicting gooseneck deformity observed on left ventriculogram in patients with endocardial cushion defect. Scooped-out appearance of medial margin of left ventricle and elongation and narrowing of left ventricular outflow tract cause gooseneck deformity present in an anteroposterior projection. Goose rests on an egg, which represents ostium primum defect, lying immediately above deficient portion of interventricular septum.

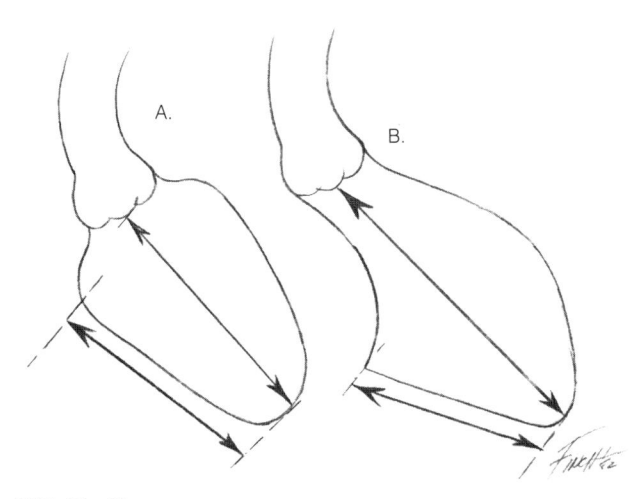

FIG 23–13.
Diagrams of left ventriculograms, anteroposterior projection during systole. **A,** normal heart; inferior margin of interventricular septum slightly shorter than distance from cardiac apex to aortic valve. **B,** endocardial cushion defect; inferior margin of interventricular septum considerably shorter than normal. Distance between cardiac apex and aortic valve is greater than normal.

gitation can be identified in most patients, but the precise anatomic details of the mitral valve cannot always be determined. The assessment of the degree of mitral regurgitation and the demonstration of a common atrioventricular valve is of practical importance, because they each complicate surgical repair and increase the risk of operation. The observation of a ventricular septal defect is important if pulmonary banding is being considered, because in patients with ostium primum defect or complete atrioventricular canal and significant mitral regurgitation, pulmonary artery banding is contraindicated.

To help one understand the angiographic findings of the various features of endocardial cushion defect, we have included a section on radiographic anatomy of these anomalies.[14]

Radiographic Anatomy

1. The underlying anatomic anomaly in atrioventricular canal is a deficiency of the ventricular septum beneath the mitral anulus and a shortened posterior length of the interventricular septum, giving it a scooped-out appearance.

2. The mitral and tricuspid valves are always in continuity across the interventricular septum (Fig 23–10,A).

3. The attachment of the anterior leaflet of the mitral valve varies. It may be firmly attached to the crest of the septum, as in ostium primum defect (see Figs 23–5 and 23–35).

4. In complete atrioventricular canal, the mitral valve may be attached by short chordae tendineae to the crest of the interventricular septum (see Fig 23–10) or chordae tendineae to a contralateral papillary muscle (Fig 23–10,B), or it may be free floating (Fig 23–10,C). The space beneath the valve leaflets and the crest of the scooped-out interventricular septum forms the ventricular communication (see Fig 23–10), and it does not have the usual well-defined round appearance of a ventricular septal defect.

5. The anterior leaflet of the mitral valve is divided into equal segments by the cleft, a superior (anterior) and an inferior (posterior) segment (Fig 23–11). The anterior segment is continuous with the septal leaflet of the tricuspid valve, forming a common anterior leaflet. The posterior segment is also continuous with the tricuspid leaflet, forming a common posterior leaflet.

6. The attachment of the posterior leaflet of the mitral valve to the free wall of the ventricle is normal and appears uninvolved in the development complex of ECD.

Left Ventriculogram: Anteroposterior Projection

1. The scooped-out appearance of the ventricular septum below the mitral valve results in a characteristic defor-

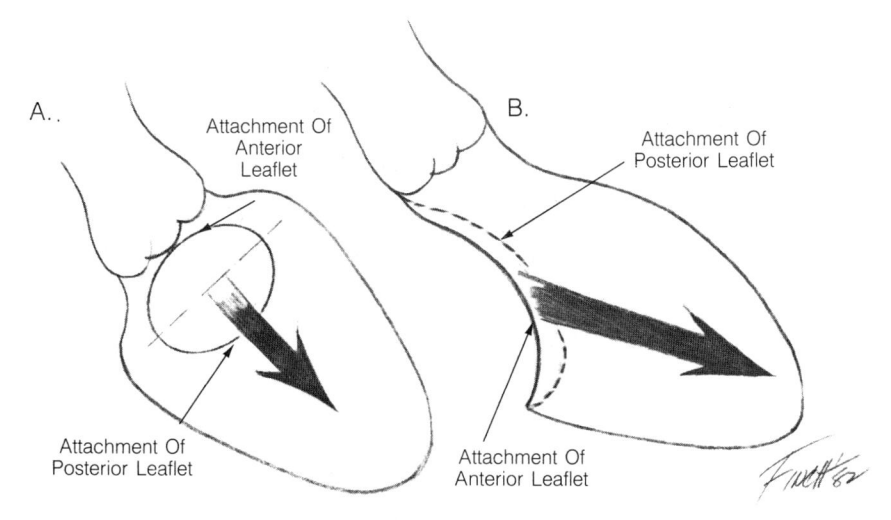

FIG 23–14.
Diagrams of left ventriculograms, anteroposterior projections during diastole. **A,** normal heart; mitral anulus forms an oval radiolucency. Mitral valve is oriented anteriorly. **B,** endocardial cushion defect; anterior (septal) and posterior (free wall) attachments of mitral valve are almost superimposed. Mitral valve is oriented toward the left.

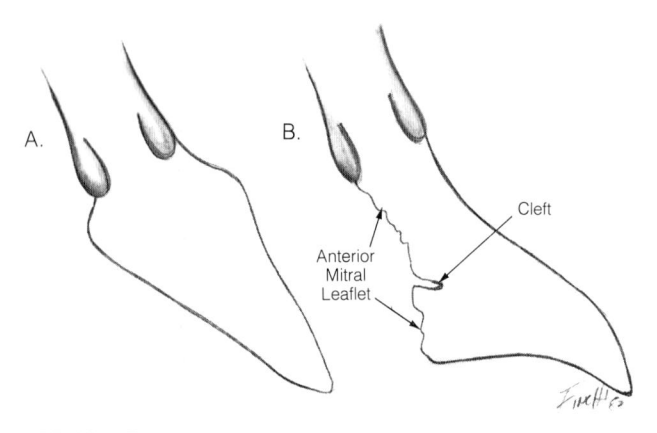

FIG 23–15.
Diagrams of left ventriculograms, anteroposterior projections during systole. **A,** normal; mitral valve is closed and not visible. **B,** endocardial cushion defect; anterior mitral valve leaflet seen as a small filling defect in profile and has a scalloped appearance. Cleft in anterior leaflet seen in midportion of mitral valve.

mity of the left ventricle that has been compared with a sitting goose (Fig 23–12).

2. The gooseneck deformity of ECD is caused by a deficiency of both the conal and the sinus portions of the ventricular septum and causes a narrowing of the left ventricular outflow tract.

3. The inferior margin of the ventricular septum is shortened because of the deficiency of the inflow portion. In addition, the distance between the apex of the left ventricle and the aortic valve is greater than normal, because the aortic valve commonly occupies an abnormally high position (Fig 23–13).

4. Because of the attachment of the anterior leaflet of the mitral valve to the crest of the interventricular septum, the mitral valvular anulus is abnormally located (Fig 23–14).

5. In an anteroposterior projection, the attachments of the anterior and posterior leaflets of the mitral valve are almost superimposed, and both have a similar scooped-out or concave appearance. The gooseneck deformity can be seen during both systole and diastole. The abnormal orientation of the mitral valve (see Fig 23–14) is caused partially by right ventricular enlargement secondary to the left-to-right shunt at the atrial level.

6. Because of its abnormal orientation, the anterior leaflet of the mitral valve can be seen in systole, when the approximated edges of the cleft form a characteristic filling defect (Fig 23–15,B).

7. Because of the attachment of the anterior leaflet of the mitral valve to the crest of the interventricular septum either by direct attachment, as in ostium primum defect, or by unfused shortened chordae tendineae, as in complete atrioventricular canal, the valve balloons into the left atrium during systole and has an irregular, puckered appearance (Figs 23–15,B and 23–16).

8. During diastole, the mitral valve opens, and the posterior anulus of the valve becomes visible, having a smooth appearance (Fig 23–17,A). Contrast medium is trapped behind the open leaflets, although that beneath the

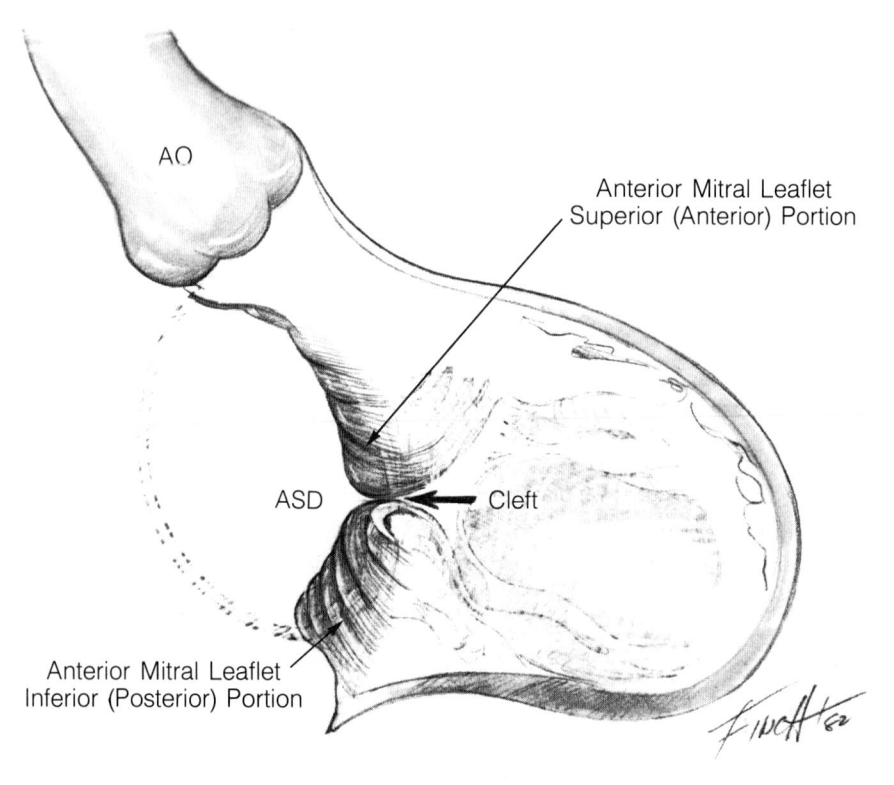

FIG 23–16.
Diagram of ostium primum defect in systole. Anterior leaflet of mitral valve, attached to ventricular septum, balloons into atrium and is outlined by contrast medium beneath leaflet. Leaflet appears scalloped. Edges of leaflets along cleft are slightly thickened and form a linear filling defect.

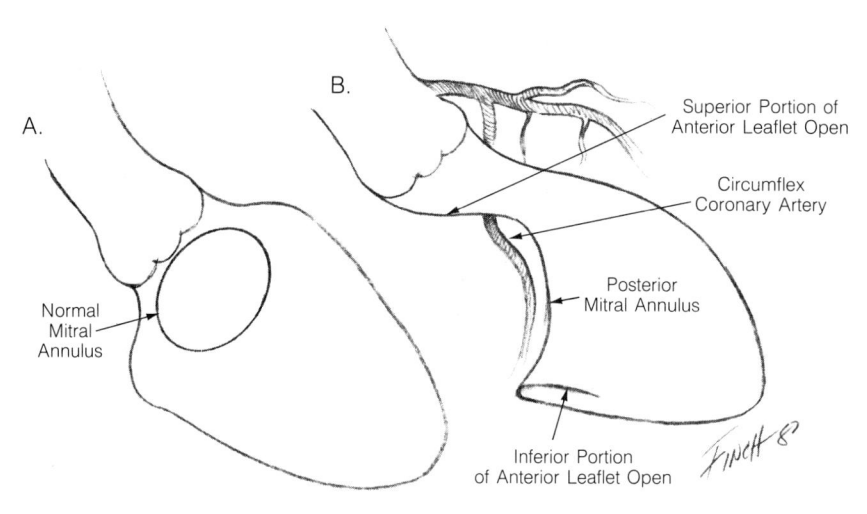

FIG 23-17.
Diagram of left ventriculograms, anteroposterior projection during diastole. **A,** normal heart; unopacified blood crossing mitral valve; contrast medium trapped behind valve leaflets outlines mitral anulus, which in this projection has an oval outline. **B,** endocardial cushion defect; anterior leaflet of mitral valve forms upper portion of gooseneck deformity, and lower portion is formed by free wall attachment of posterior leaflet of mitral valve. Thus, gooseneck in diastole has a smooth appearance. Circumflex branch of left coronary artery parallels posterior anulus.

anterior leaflet may be invisible or only faintly visible. Contrast medium trapped behind the posterior leaflet outlines the smooth free wall attachment of this leaflet to the mitral anulus, creating the gooseneck deformity during diastole (Fig 23–17,B).

9. During diastole, the open anterior leaflet causes further narrowing of the left ventricular outflow tract. The gooseneck deformity during diastole is more marked than that of systole (see Fig 23–17,B).

10. The free wall attachment of the mitral anulus is closely paralleled by the circumflex coronary artery, which lies in the atrioventricular groove. Its course is also abnormal because of the deficiency of the ventricular septum (see Figs 23–17,B and 23–30).

11. When the septal leaflets of the mitral and tricuspid leaflets attach to the crest of the interventricular septum, the anulus of each valve is distinctly visible during diastole provided the right ventricle is also opacified. If the septal leaflets are not firmly attached, as in some forms of atrioventricular canal (free-floating leaflets), only the posterior attachments of the valve to the free walls is visible. Therefore, only one atrioventricular anulus (a common anulus for both the tricuspid and mitral valves) is seen (Fig 23–18).

12. The radiographic appearance of the right anterior oblique projection of a left ventriculogram is similar to the anteroposterior projection. Depending on the degree of obliquity, however, the septal attachment of the mitral valve may no longer be seen in profile; and the free wall attachment of the mitral valve may form the medial border of the opacified left ventricle. In this projection, the gooseneck deformity is less obvious, but the distance between the cardiac apex and the mitral valve remains shortened (Fig 23–19).

13. In both the anteroposterior and the right anterior oblique projections, the presence of mitral regurgitation can be distinguished from the presence of a ventricular left-to-right shunt. The left anterior oblique projection with beam angulation is helpful in patients with complete atrioventricular canal to see both the characteristic location of the ventricular septal communication underneath the atrioventricular valves and any coexisting muscular ventricular septal defects.

Left Ventriculogram: Left Anterior Oblique Projection—Diastole

1. During diastole, contrast medium is trapped behind the open mitral valve leaflets and outlines the anulus.

2. The abnormal orientation of the mitral valve is also apparent (Fig 23–20).

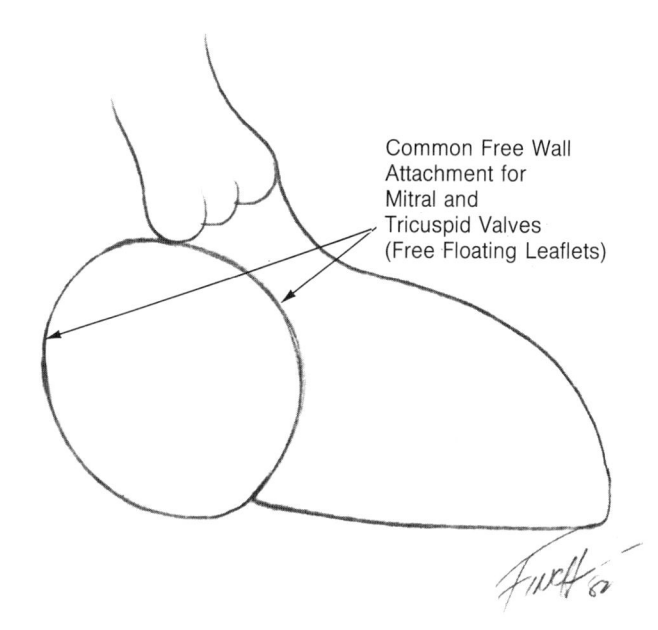

FIG 23-18.
Diagram of left ventriculogram, anteroposterior projection. Complete atrioventricular canal with unattached common anterior atrioventricular valve. Septal portions of mitral and tricuspid valve are not attached to crest of interventricular septum. Valve leaflets are attached only to free walls of ventricles, thus forming a common anulus.

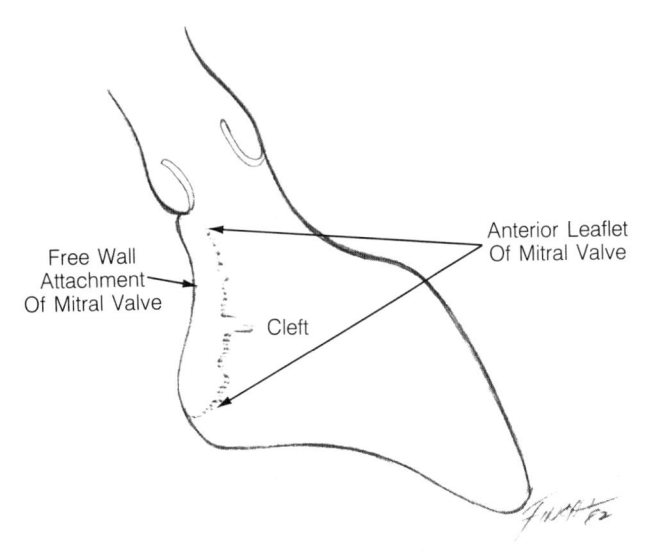

FIG 23–19.
Diagram of left ventriculogram, right anterior oblique projection during systole. Anterior leaflet of mitral valve no longer forms medial margin of left ventricle. Gooseneck deformity is less obvious.

3. When the anterior leaflet of the mitral valve is attached to the crest of the interventricular septum, as in ostium primum defect and some forms of complete atrioventricular canal, a distinct anulus for both the mitral and the tricuspid valve is seen.

4. In complete atrioventricular canal without attachment of the common leaflets to the crest of the interventricular septum (free-floating leaflets), only the attachment of the leaflets to the free walls is seen, forming a common anulus for the tricuspid and mitral valves (Fig 23–21).

5. The right ventricle is opacified because of the ventricular communication.

6. The ventricles communicate through the space between the common atrioventricular valve leaflets and the crest of the interventricular septum (see Fig 23–21).

Left Ventriculogram: Left Anterior Oblique Projection—Systole

1. Unlike the findings in a normal heart (Fig 23–22,A), the anterior leaflet of the mitral valve is seen in profile along the anterior margin of the left ventricle (Fig 23–22,B).

2. Even with the firm attachment of the anterior leaflets to the crest of the ventricular septum, as in ostium primum defect, the contrast medium beneath the valve causes an irregular and scalloped appearance.

3. The mitral valve leaflet balloons into the atrial septal defect; this should not be confused with an aneurysm of the interventricular septum.

4. A jet of contrast medium through the ventricular

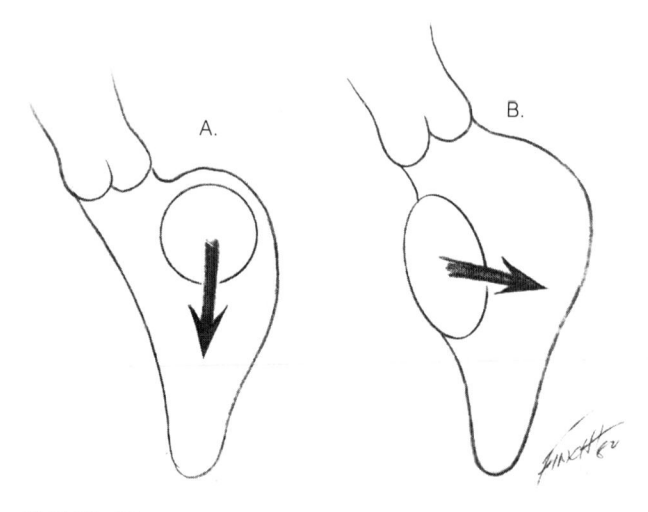

FIG 23–20.
Diagram of left ventriculograms, left anterior oblique projection with beam angulation. **A,** normal heart; arrow indicates direction of blood flow into left ventricle. **B,** endocardial cushion defect; blood flow into the left ventricle is directed toward left. Mitral valve anulus is seen along medial border, indicating attachment to interventricular septum.

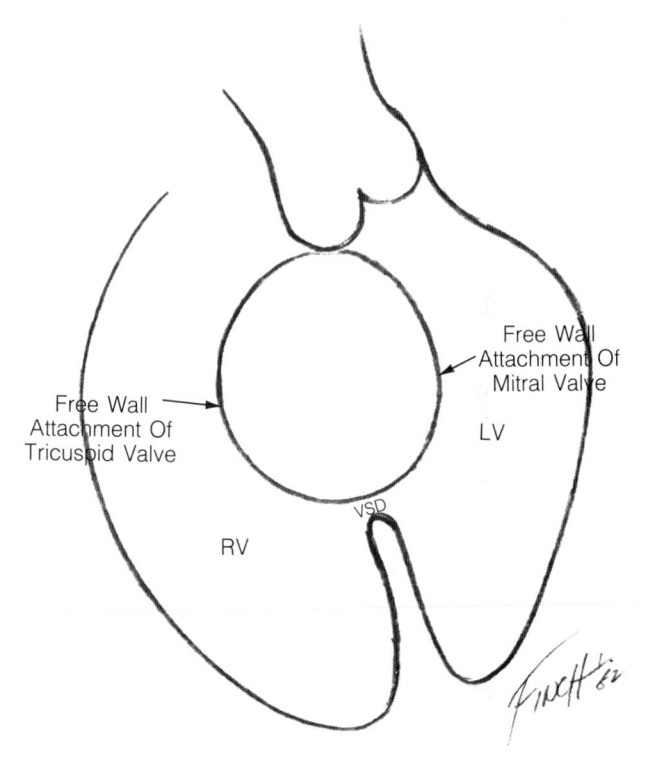

FIG 23–21.
Diagram of left ventriculogram, left anterior oblique projection. Complete atrioventricular canal without attachment of common atrioventricular valve leaflets to ventricular septum. Mural (free wall) attachment of entire atrioventricular valve forms a single anulus. Ventricular septal communication lies beneath common leaflets and crest of interventricular septum.

Endocardial Cushion Defect   379

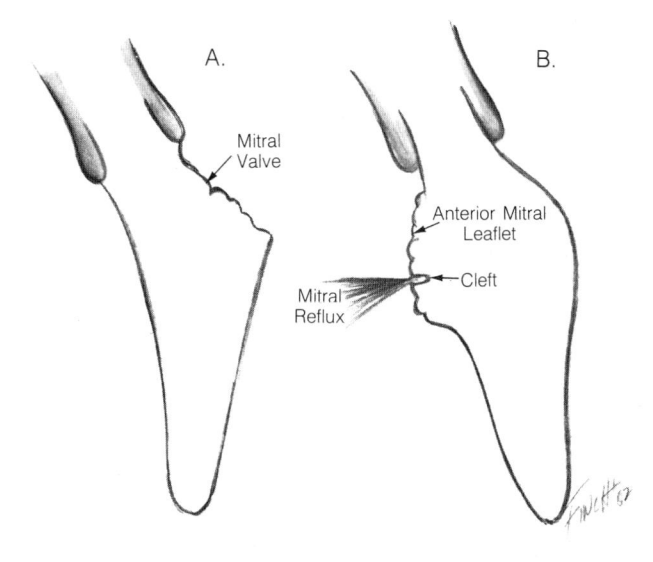

FIG 23–22.
Diagram of left ventriculograms, left anterior oblique projection with cranial beam angulation during systole. **A,** normal heart; mitral valve is closed and not well seen. **B,** endocardial cushion defect; mitral valve seen in profile, has a scalloped appearance, and balloons into atrium. Cleft in anterior leaflet well seen. Mitral regurgitation occurs directly through ostium primum defect into right atrium.

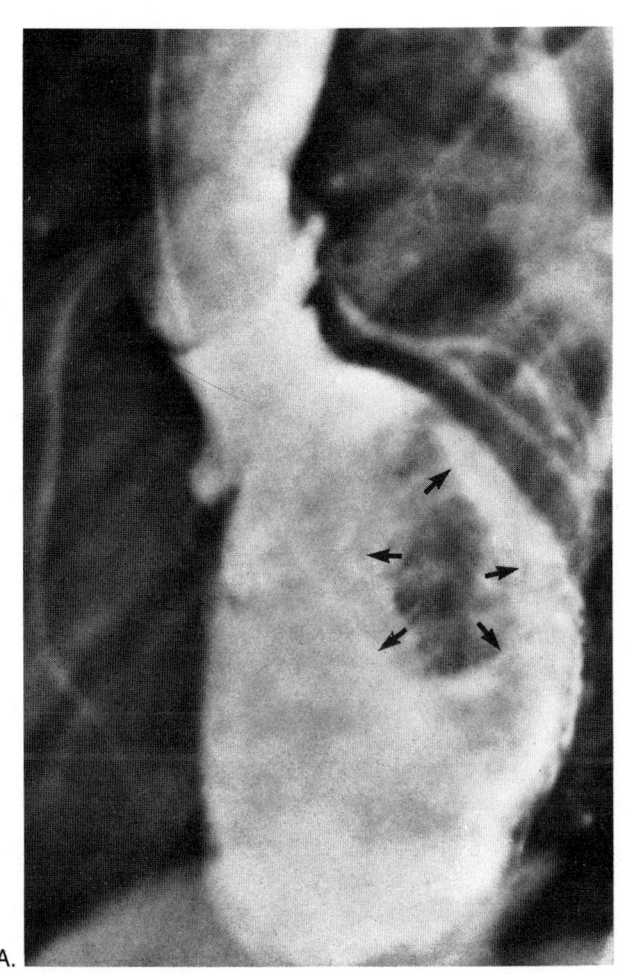

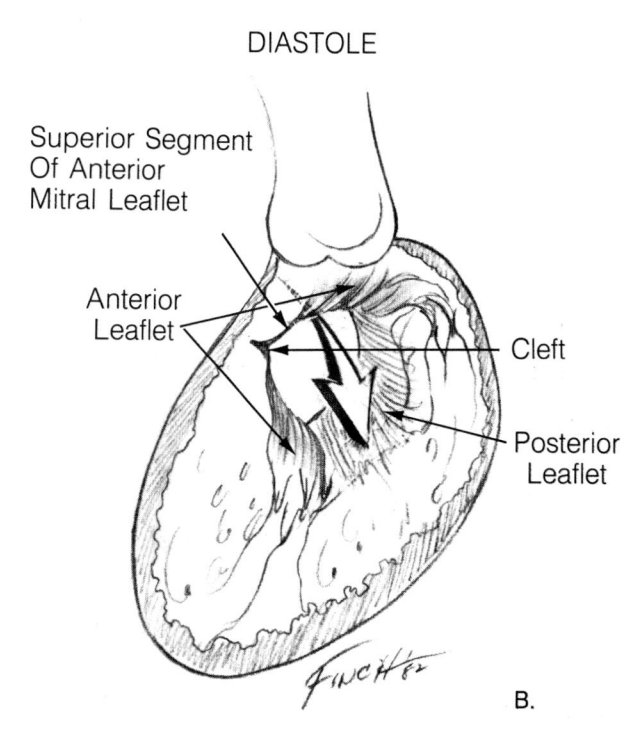

FIG 23–23.
A, ventriculogram in lateral projection in diastole. Mitral anulus *(arrows)* seen more en face than normally. **B,** explanatory diagram.

communication is wide and ill defined compared with a regular ventricular septal defect. The ventricular communication is not round but a moon-shaped space between the common mitral-tricuspid anterior leaflets and the crest of the septum.

5. The coapted and slightly thickened edges of the cleft of the anterior leaflet can be seen on this projection.

6. Because of the abnormal orientation of the mitral valve, the regurgitating jet usually is directed through the ostium primum defect directly into the right atrium. Rarely, the jet is directed into the left atrium.

7. The jet from mitral regurgitation originates from the area of the mitral cleft. Thus, it is located higher than a jet through a communication in the ventricular septum. The latter is present below the anterior leaflet of the mitral valve.

Left Ventriculogram: Lateral Projection—Diastole

1. Unopacified blood passing through the mitral valve outlines the mitral anulus.

2. In a normal heart, the mitral anulus is observed posteriorly as an oval filling defect, whereas in atrioventricular canal, the mitral anulus is seen more anteriorly and on end (Fig 23–23,A and B) as a result of the abnormal orientation of the mitral valve because of the deficiency of the septum.

3. The lateral projection provides an en face view of the mitral valve. Therefore, this is the least useful projection for demonstrating anatomic details of ECD.

4. The left ventricle is displaced posteriorly by the enlarged right ventricle.

Angiographic Techniques and Findings

Mitral Anatomy

The ventricular communication and the degree of mitral reflux are best assessed by a 30-degree right anterior oblique and 45-degree left anterior oblique projection. The left anterior oblique view is made with cranial ("looking down") beam angulation. In the right anterior oblique view mitral reflux can be separated from a left-to-right shunt through a ventricular communication. The foreshortened septum and mitral cleft are clearly seen during systole and

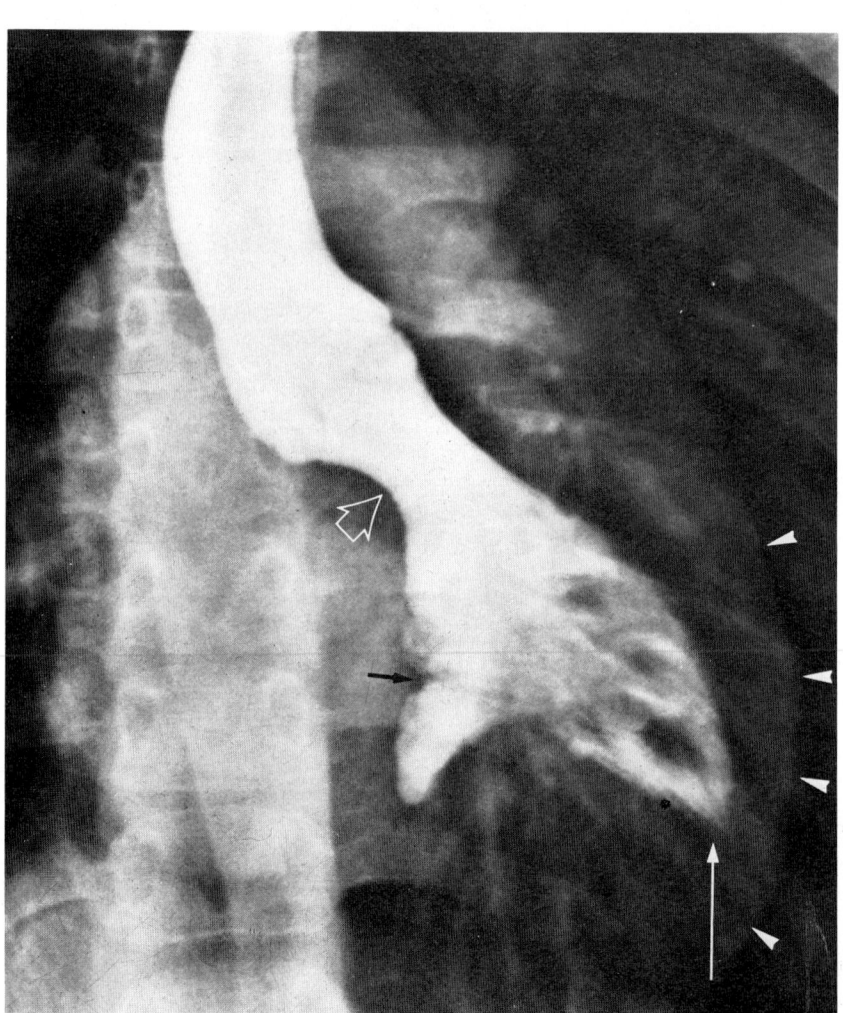

FIG 23–24.
Left ventriculogram, anteroposterior projection during systole. Ostium primum defect without mitral regurgitation. Left ventricle is normal sized, elevated, and displaced posteriorly by huge right ventricle induced by the large left-to-right atrial level shunt *(long white arrow)*. Enlarged right ventricle forms left cardiac border *(small white arrows)*, giving false impression of thickened left ventricular wall. Inferior margin of left ventricle is foreshortened. Left ventricular outlow tract scooped-out and elongated *(open white arrow)*, forming gooseneck deformity. Anterior leaflet of mitral valve, seen in profile, is slightly scalloped. Prominent notch *(black arrow)* corresponds to cleft in anterior leaflet.

diastole. The left anterior oblique view demonstrates mitral anatomy, left-to-right ventricular shunt, and occasional muscular defects.

Anteroposterior and Right Anterior Oblique Projections: Systolic Appearance

1. The left ventricular chamber is elevated by the enlarged right ventricle (Fig 23–24). The left cardiac border is formed by the left ventricle, giving the wrong impression of a thick-walled left ventricle.

2. Because of the clockwise rotation of the heart, a left ventriculogram performed in an anteroposterior projection is actually a right anterior oblique view compared with the normal left ventricle.

3. The inflow portion of the left ventricle is shorter than normal because of foreshortening of the interventricular septum along the diaphragmatic left ventricular wall. This results from absence of the membranous septum and a part of the inflow portion of the muscular septum. In addition, the left ventricular outflow tract is elongated, and the aortic valve is located in a relatively high position (Fig 23–25,A).

4. The scooped-out appearance of the mitral valvular area and the narrowing and elongation of the left ventricular outflow tract is commonly termed "gooseneck deformity." Together with the foreshortened diaphragmatic length of the left ventricle, the appearance is similar to that of a sitting goose (see Fig 23–12).

5. The gooseneck deformity is present in both partial and complete forms of atrioventricular canal and common atrium. REASON: Each of the three forms of ECD has a similar deficiency of the inflow and outflow portions of the interventricular septum. The angiographic appearance may vary depending on the degree of septal deficiency.

6. The appearance of the mitral valve and the outflow tract changes considerably between systole and diastole.

7. The scooped-out deficiency of the interventricular

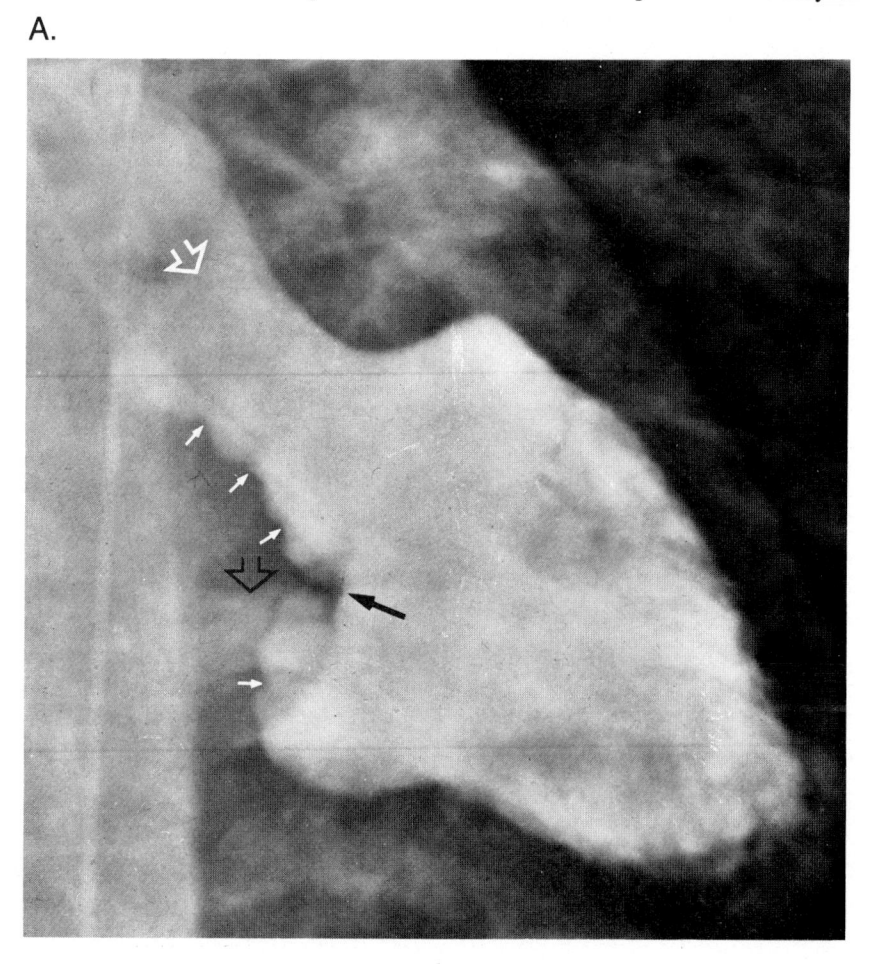

FIG 23–25.
Left ventriculogram, anteroposterior projection in patient with ostium primum defect. **A,** systole; anterior leaflet of mitral valve, attached to crest of interventricular septum, forms gooseneck deformity, which is not marked in this case. Leaflet has a scalloped appearance *(white arrows)* because of attachment by short chordae tendineae to the edge of septum. Prominent notch *(black arrow)* corresponds to cleft in anterior leaflet. Trace of mitral regurgitation *(open black arrow).* Aortic valve located higher than normal *(open white arrow).*
(Continued.)

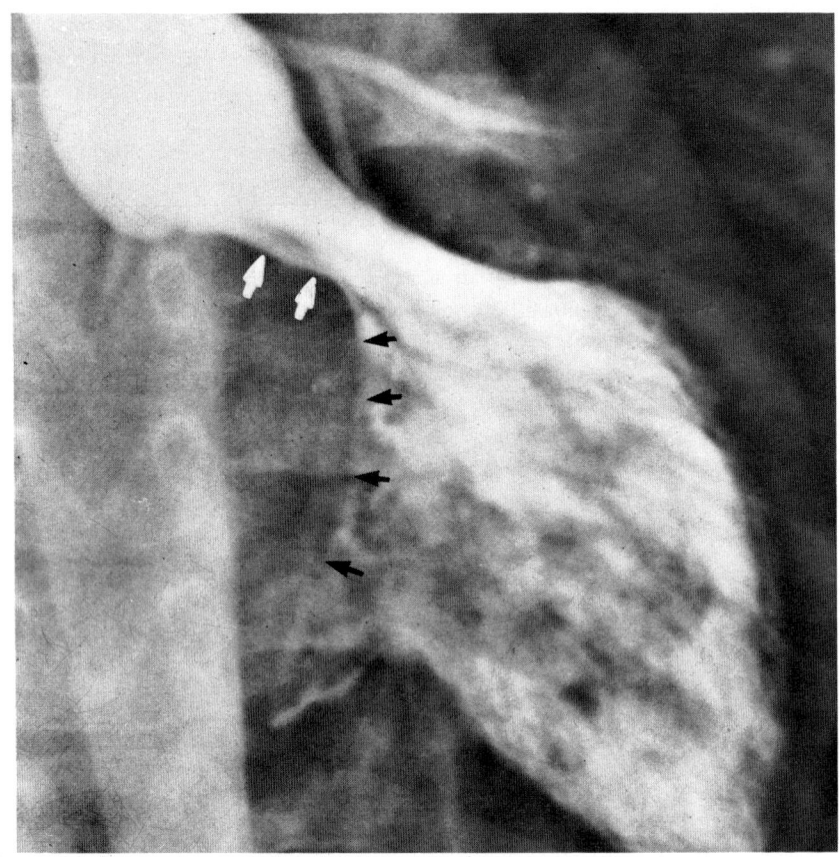

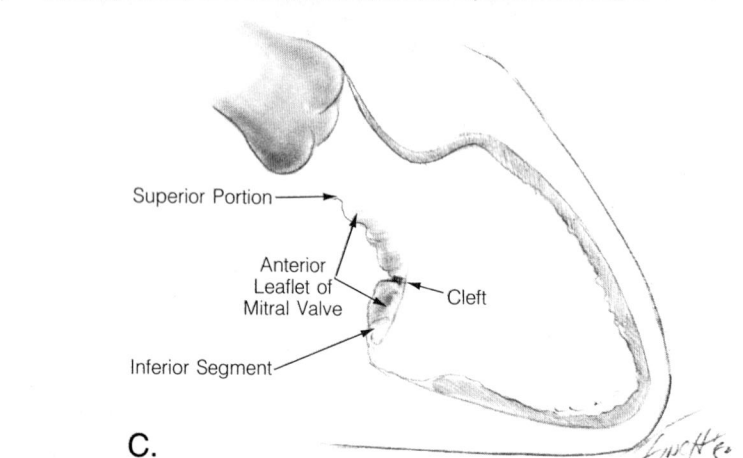

382 Cardiac Conditions Associated With a Left-to-Right Shunt

FIG 23–25 (cont.).
B, diastole. The superior (anterior) half of the split anterior mitral leaflet is seen in profile *(white arrows)* accentuating the gooseneck deformity. This is the most consistent finding in atrioventricular canal. Contrast medium is trapped underneath normal posterior leaflet *(black arrows)*. Circumflex coronary artery closely parallels posterior free wall attachment of mitral valve. **C,** drawing of angiographic systolic appearance.

septum is outlined by contrast medium beneath the anterior mitral valve leaflet (Fig 23–25,A). REASON: The anterior leaflet of the mitral valve is either directly attached or attached by numerous short chordae tendineae to the crest of the interventricular septum. During systole, the gooseneck is formed by the anterior leaflet of the mitral valve, which usually has a serrated, scalloped appearance (see Figs 23–24 and 23–25,A). REASON: The attachment of the anterior mitral valve leaflet to the crest of the ventricular septum occurs by fused or unfused chordae tendineae and permits irregular ballooning pouches of the leaflet during systole.

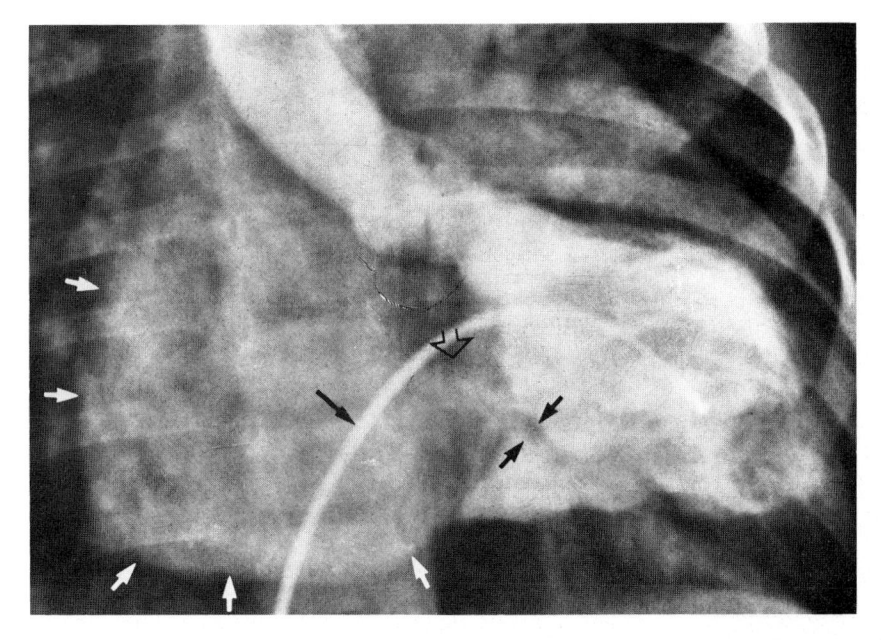

FIG 23–26.
Left ventriculogram, anteroposterior projection in patient with ostium primum defect. Characteristic catheter course *(black arrow)* through ostium primum defect and mitral valve into left ventricle. Fan-shaped jet *(open arrow)* of contrast medium regurgitating through mitral valve is directed toward right atrium *(white arrows)*. Jet originates at site of mitral cleft *(small black arrows)*. Pulmonary artery is unopacified, thereby excluding a major left-to-right shunt at ventricular level.

8. A notchlike filling defect corresponding to the coapted edges of the cleft of the anterior leaflet of the mitral valve is seen along the midportion of the scooped-out area (see Figs 23–24 and 23–25).

9. During systole, the anterior leaflet of the mitral valve bulges and forms the medial margin of the opacified left ventricle (see Fig 23–25). REASON: The anterior leaflet of the mitral valve attaches to the scooped-out ventricular septum and therefore has an abnormal orientation (see Fig 23–14).

10. During diastole the superior (anterior) half of the split mitral leaflet is seen in profile outlined by contrast medium above and unopacified blood from below (see Fig 23–25,B). Sometimes also the inferior (posterior) half of the split valve leaflet can be seen. The profile view of the split leaflet is the most constant and characteristic angiographic finding because incoming blood through the normal mitral valve results in diffuse mixing with contrast medium (see Fig 23–25,A).

11. Mitral regurgitation is evident as a well-defined jet of contrast medium originating in the region of the mitral cleft. It usually passes directly into the right atrium through the ostium primum defect and does not opacify the left atrium (Fig 23–26), although exceptions exist. REASON: In ECDs, the mitral valve has an abnormal orientation, being displaced toward the apex and anteriorly. Therefore, the direction of the regurgitant jet is to the right, into the right atrium. Because the ostium primum defect lies immediately above the mitral valve, the jet passes directly into the right atrium.

12. A ventricular septal defect in complete atrioventricular canal is suggested by immediate opacification of the right ventricular outflow tract and pulmonary artery during the first systolic contraction (Fig 23–27). Diagnosis of a complete atrioventricular canal from an anteroposterior projection may be difficult, and a slow and careful review of the cine angiogram is important. A left anterior oblique projection with cranial angulation is essential for demonstration of the ventricular septal communication.

13. Pouches of accessory mitral valve tissue may project into the left ventricular outflow tract during systole and cause subaortic obstruction (Fig 23–28). This mechanism of obstruction is similar to that on the right side of the heart caused by a windsock of the tricuspid valve (see Chapter 29).

14. Rarely, ECD and a cleft in the anterior leaflet of the mitral valve are an isolated cause of mitral regurgitation.

Anteroposterior and Right Anterior Oblique Projections: Diastolic Appearance

1. During diastole, unopacified blood enters the left ventricle, and the open mitral valve is seen on these projections. During diastole, both segments of the cleft anterior mitral leaflet open, and the superior segment is usually seen well in profile, causing a further apparent narrowing of the left outflow tract. The inferior portion of the anterior mitral leaflet is not as well seen. The gooseneck deformity is usually more pronounced in diastole than in systole (Fig 23–29).

2. The posterior anulus of the mitral valve is visible. REASON: Contrast medium trapped between the left ventricular wall and the open posterior leaflet outlines the mitral anulus, as in the normal heart.

3. The attachment of the posterior leaflet of the mitral

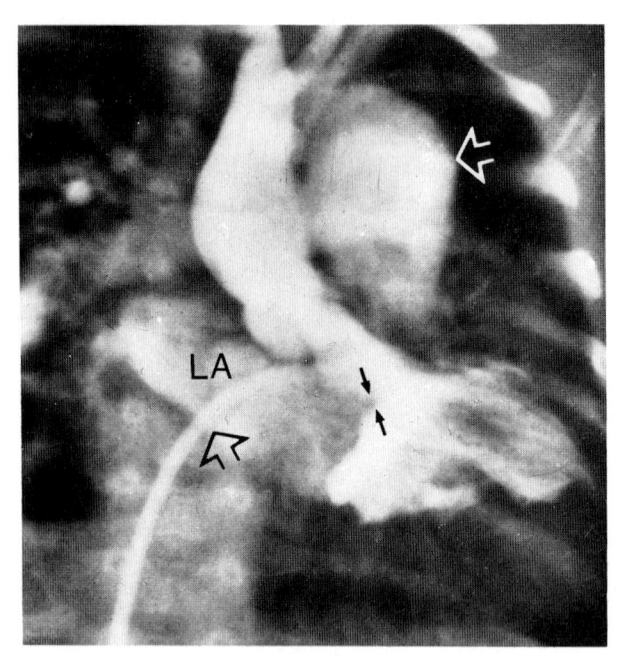

FIG 23-27.
Left ventriculogram, anteroposterior projection in patient with complete atrioventricular canal and mitral regurgitation into left atrium. Gooseneck deformity and cleft *(small black arrows)* in mitral valve. Catheter *(open black arrows)* has been passed through ostium primum defect into the left ventricle. Catheter may also pass through patent foramen ovale. During first systole, pulmonary artery *(open white arrow)* is densely opacified, indicating a significant left-to-right shunt at ventricular level. In this patient, regurgitating jet originating at cleft is directed into left atrium *(LA)*.

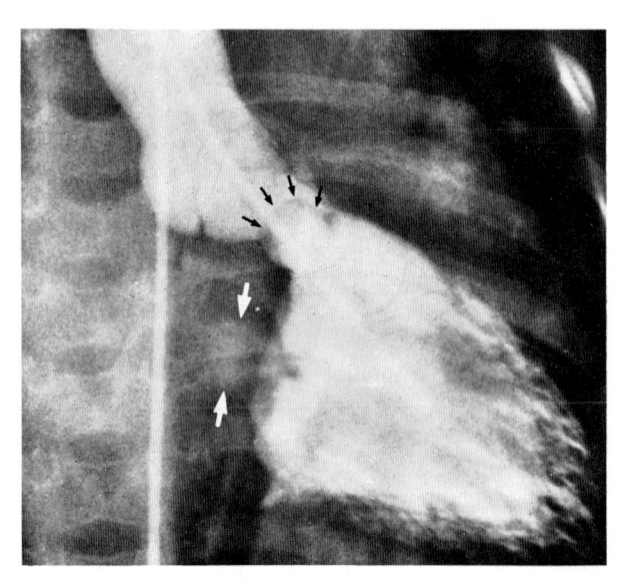

FIG 23-28.
Left ventriculogram, anteroposterior projection in patient with ostium primum defect. Outpouching *(small black arrows)* of mitral valve gives a windsock appearance in left ventricular outflow tract. Cleft in anterior leaflet of mitral valve, associated with trace of mitral regurgitation *(white arrows)*. Pulmonary artery unopacified, indicating no ventricular level shunt.

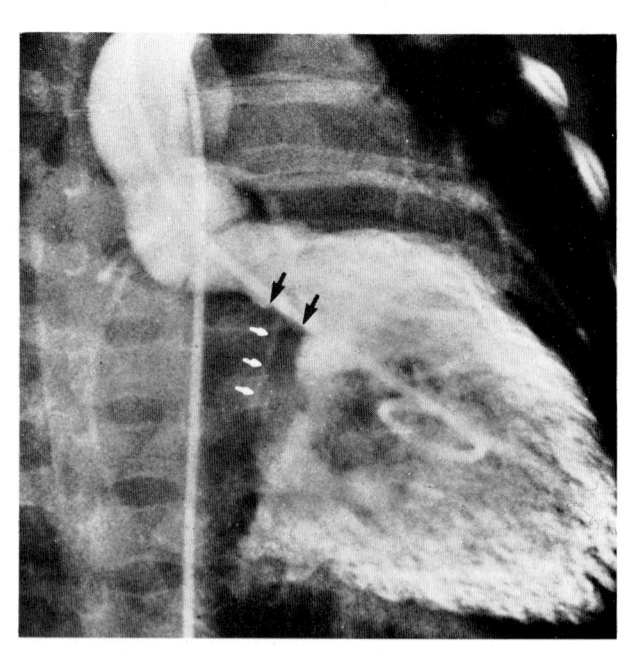

FIG 23-29.
Left ventriculogram, anteroposterior projection during diastole. Anterior leaflet of open mitral valve *(black arrows)* forms a right-angle junction with free wall attachment of mitral valve. Circumflex branch of left coronary artery *(white arrows)* parallels free wall attachment and has an abnormal course because of deficiency of interventricular septum.

valve to the free wall of the left ventricle can be identified by the course of the circumflex coronary artery, which always parallels the free wall attachment; in other words, it has a different course than normal (Fig 23-29). REASON: Deficiency of the muscular septum and foreshortening of the base of the left ventricle cause an altered course of the coronary sinus and circumflex coronary artery (Fig 23-30).

Left Anterior Oblique Projection: Systolic and Diastolic Appearance

1. In an angled left anterior oblique projection, the mitral valve bulges anteriorly through the ostium primum defect during systole. The mitral valve has a puckered appearance, and the cleft can be identified as in either the anteroposterior or right anterior oblique projections (Fig 23-31).

2. Mitral regurgitation usually occurs directly into the right atrium; consequently, the regurgitating jet passes anteriorly. Rarely, the regurgitating jet is directed into the left atrium itself (see Fig 23-27).

3. Because the right ventricle and right atrium are superimposed in this view, it may be difficult to distinguish mitral regurgitation from an interventricular communication. During diastole, the interventricular communication is clearly delineated by contrast medium observed above

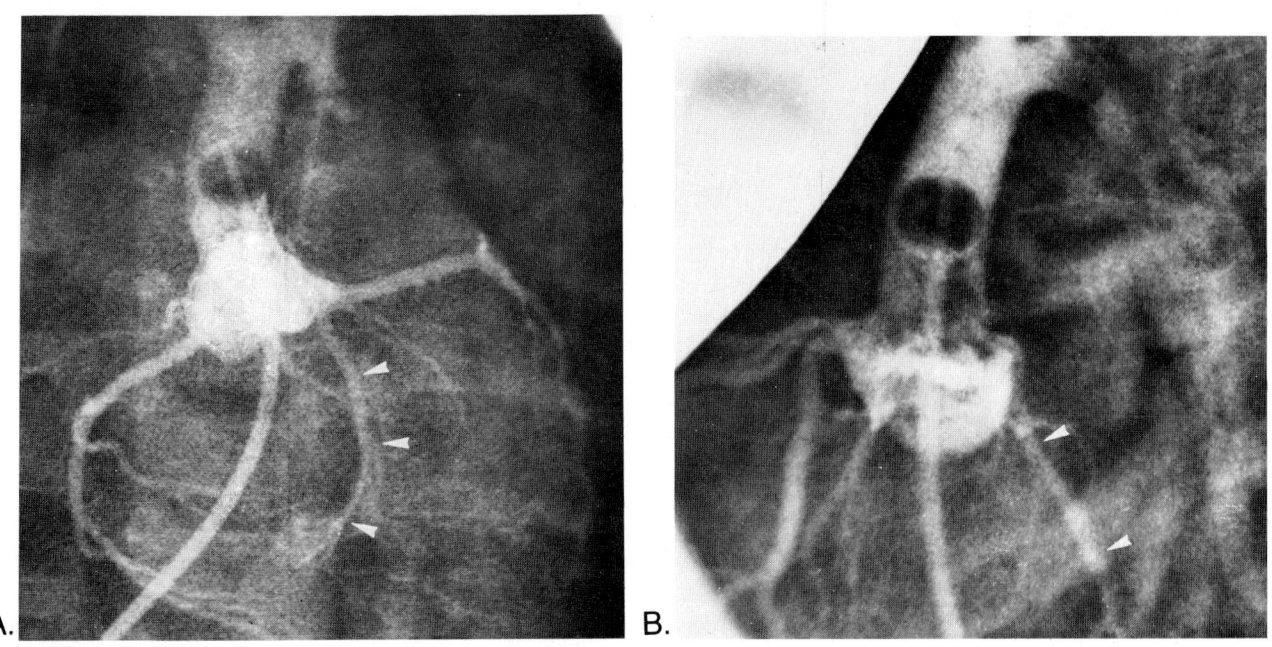

FIG 23–30.
Aortogram, anteroposterior (**A**) and lateral (**B**) projection in patient with complete atrioventricular canal. Circumflex coronary artery *(arrowheads)* has an altered and more vertical course because of deficiency of ventricular septum and foreshortening of base of left ventricle. The atrioventricular groove is also outlined by the right coronary artery and has a more vertical course than normal.

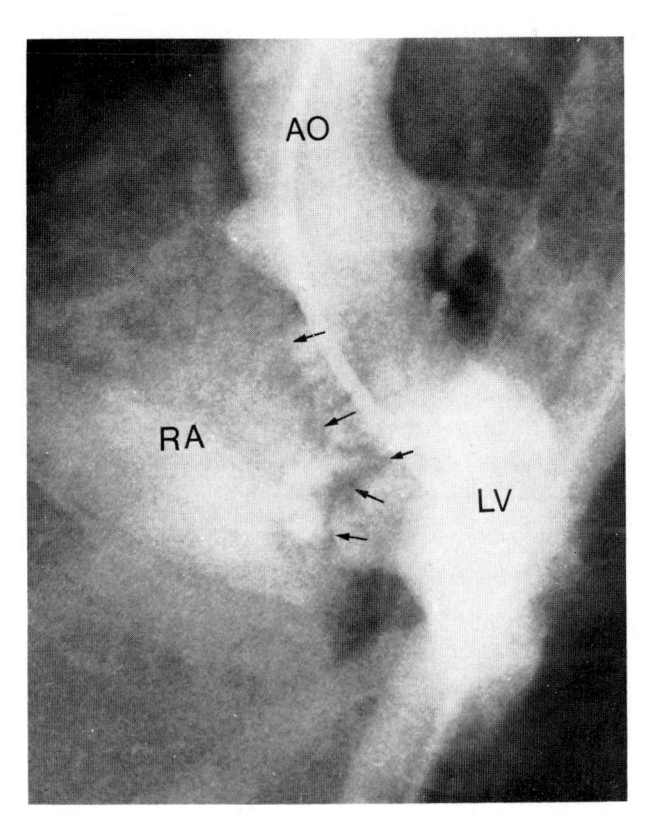

FIG 23–31.
Left ventriculogram, left anterior oblique projection with beam angulation during systole. Anterior leaflet of the mitral valve bulges into ostium primum defect and has a cleft and scalloped appearance. Mitral regurgitation occurs directly into right atrium. Ventricular septum is intact. Ballooning of scalloped anterior leaflet is commonly seen in atrioventricular canal and should not be confused with an aneurysm of the membranous septum. *AO* = aorta; *LV* = left ventricle; *RA* = right atrium.

the crest of the interventricular septum and below the anterior leaflet of the mitral valve (Fig 23–32).

4. If the anterior leaflet of the mitral valve is attached by chordae tendineae to the crest of the ventricular septum, separate mitral and tricuspid anuli can be identified in diastole (see Fig 23–32).

5. The ventricular communication is located much lower than in a membranous ventricular septal defect.

6. During systole, a jet through the ventricular communication is not well defined. REASON: The communication is not a circumscribed defect in the septum, and shunting occurs beneath the entire anterior leaflet of the mitral valve. Sometimes, several jets are produced because of the chordal attachments of the mitral valve to the crest of the ventricular septum.

7. The attachment of the common leaflet to the crest of the septum usually occurs by short chordae tendineae. Therefore, the space beneath the leaflet (ventricular communication) usually appears small. With longer chordal attachment, or if the midportion of the valve is unattached (see Fig 23–6, C), the defect beneath the common valve may be large (Fig 23–33).

8. If the leaflet is unattached to the ventricular septum (free-floating common leaflet), contrast medium is trapped behind the free wall attachment of mitral and tricuspid valves and outlines a common anulus (Figs 23–34 and 23–21).

Quantification of the Degree of Mitral Regurgitation

Estimation of the degree of mitral regurgitation is determined most reliably by left ventriculography and is of

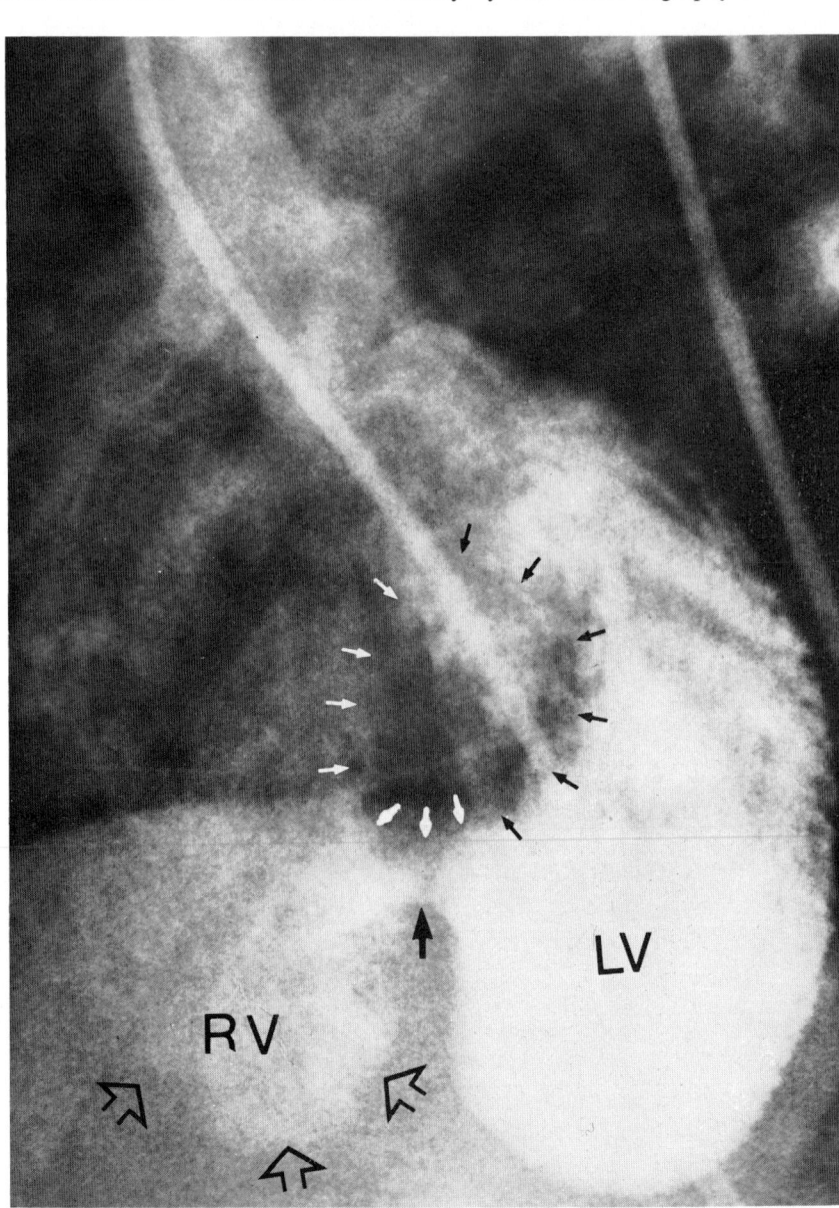

FIG 23–32.
Left ventriculogram *(LV)*, left anterior oblique projection with beam angulation in patient with complete atrioventricular canal. Crest *(black arrow)* of interventricular septum outlined by contrast medium beneath common atrioventricular valve *(arrows)*. Common leaflets attached by chordae tendineae to crest of interventricular septum. Therefore, a separate mitral anulus *(small black arrows)* is demonstrated. Inflow portion of the right ventricle *(RV)* *(open black arrows)* is opacified.

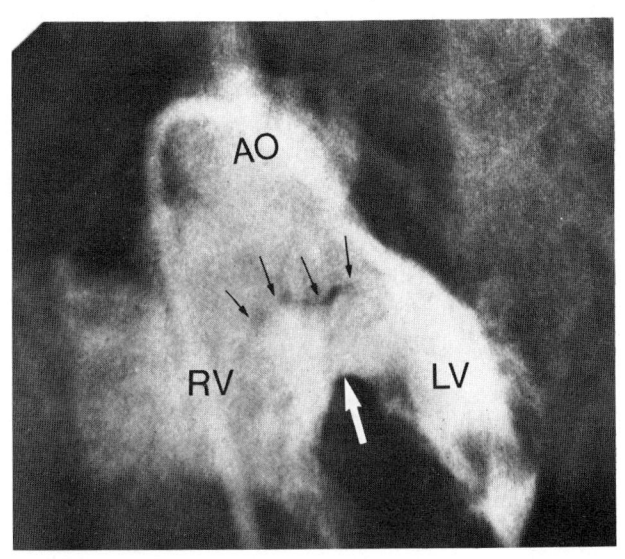

FIG 23–33.
Left ventriculogram *(LV)*, left anterior oblique projection. Large ventricular communication *(small black arrows)* between crest of ventricular septum *(white arrow)* and common valve. Either chordal attachment is longer or midportion of the valve is unattached. Additional information may be gained by echocardiography. *AO* = aorta; *RV* = right ventricle.

practical and prognostic importance. Operative repair of ECDs without or with only a minor degree of mitral regurgitation carries a low risk and yields excellent hemodynamic results. In contrast, complete atrioventricular canal with marked mitral regurgitation requires a more complex operation, which usually does not result in complete elimination of hemodynamic abnormalities.

When mitral regurgitation occurs in patients with an intact atrial septum, the degree can be estimated with considerable accuracy, but it is difficult to assess in atrioventricular canal. REASON: When the atrial septum is intact, the regurgitating contrast medium remains in the left atrium and is diluted only by the pulmonary venous return. Therefore, during the injection of contrast medium, the left atrium becomes increasingly dense. On the other hand, among patients with ECD and mitral regurgitation, the regurgitating contrast medium is directed principally into the right atrium, and the contrast medium is markedly diluted by the large amount of blood shunted left to right through the atrial communication and also by the systemic venous return through the venae cavae. This marked dilution of contrast medium causes only weak opacification of the right-sided cardiac chambers and pulmonary artery, particularly if a slow injection of contrast medium is made to avoid extrasystoles. Thus, the degree of mitral incompetence may be underestimated.

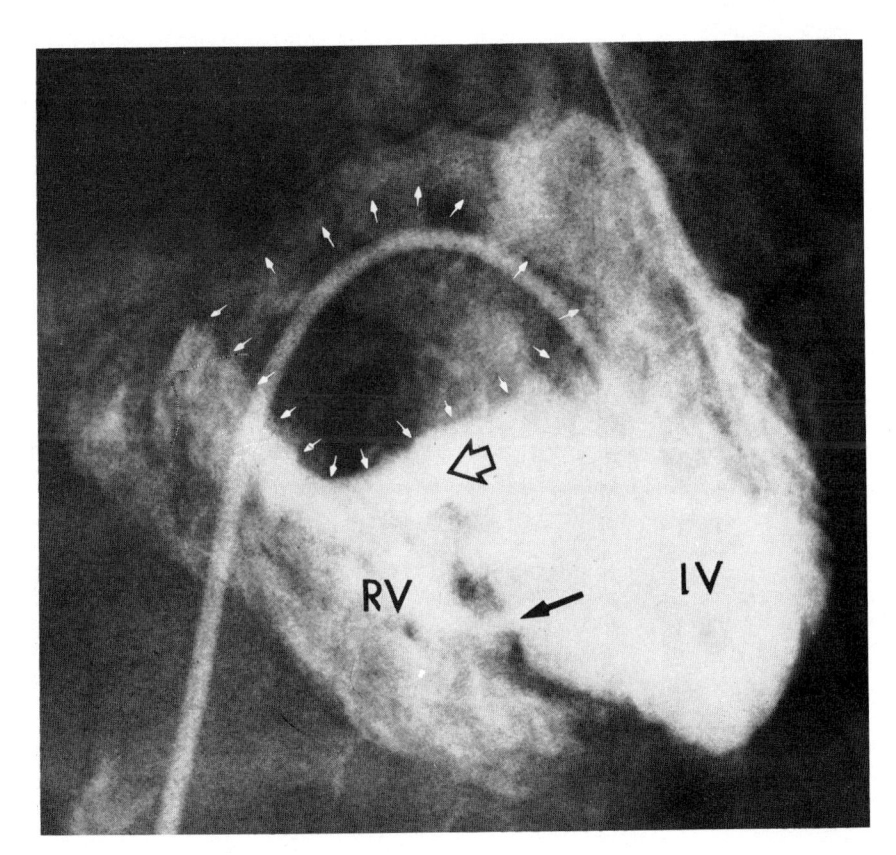

FIG 23–34.
Left ventriculogram, left anterior oblique projection with beam angulation during diastole. Complete atrioventricular canal with common leaflets unattached to crest of interventricular septum (free-floating leaflet). A single common atrioventricular orifice is outlined *(white arrows)*. After injection into left ventricle *(LV)*, right ventricle *(RV)* opacifies through ventricular communication *(open arrows)*. Coexisting muscular ventricular septal defect *(black arrow)*.

Operative Considerations

Partial atrioventricular canal (ostium primum defect and cleft mitral valve) is repaired through a right atrial approach (Fig 23–35). In most instances, the mitral valve is repaired by suturing together the adjacent portions of the mitral valve cleft, unless the degree of mitral regurgitation is minimal or alignment of the edges of the cleft seems impossible. The ostium primum defect is then closed using a knitted prosthesis. During the operation, care must be taken to avoid damage to the bundle of His, which lies in the superficial tissue along the posteroinferior margin of the ventricular portion of the septal defect. The operative mortality is low (< 5%), and the hemodynamic results are good.[15] Often a soft murmur of mitral regurgitation is present postoperatively.

In an occasional patient, subsequent operation may be needed for significant residual mitral regurgitation, which may require valve replacement. It is difficult to assess the degree of mitral regurgitation preoperatively by clinical or laboratory means, so the effect of the degree of mitral regurgitation on operative mortality or postoperative results is difficult to assess.

Operation for ostium primum defect and cleft mitral valve is generally deferred until age 5 years, unless there is deterioration of the patient's condition, which would usually occur from significant mitral regurgitation.

Despite the specific anatomic form of the common atrioventricular valve leaflets in complete atrioventricular canal, the operation is basically the same (Fig 23–36).[16] The mitral portions of the common anterior and posterior leaflets are sutured together, much as in repair of a cleft in the mitral valve. If the common valve leaflets are of the undivided type, they are surgically divided in the midline into separate mitral and tricuspid portions (see Fig 23–36,B). A knitted patch is then sutured to the right side of the ventricular septum (to avoid damage to the conduction system) around the inferior rim of the ECD (see Fig 23–36,D). The mitral portions of the common valves are sutured to the left side of the prosthetic septum at the level of the normal mitral anulus. The corresponding portions of the tricuspid aspect of the common leaflets are then sutured to the right side of the prosthetic septum (see Fig 23–36,E), and the remainder of the patch is sutured to close the ostium primum defect.

Because most patients with complete atrioventricular canal develop symptoms in infancy, operation is usually required early in life. The operative risk is high for corrective operations in infants younger than 6 months of age but less in older children.[17] The operative risk is also higher in patients with pulmonary vascular disease. In some infants who do not respond to medical treatment and have a large left-to-right ventricular shunt and minimal mitral regurgitation, we have used pulmonary arterial banding.[18, 19] Subsequently, at age 18 months, the band is removed and the atrioventricular canal repaired.

POSTOPERATIVE APPEARANCE

1. Closure of an ostium primum defect is usually successful and results in a rapid decrease in cardiac size and pulmonary flow, as seen after closure of an ostium secundum defect.

2. In complete atrioventricular canal without signifi-

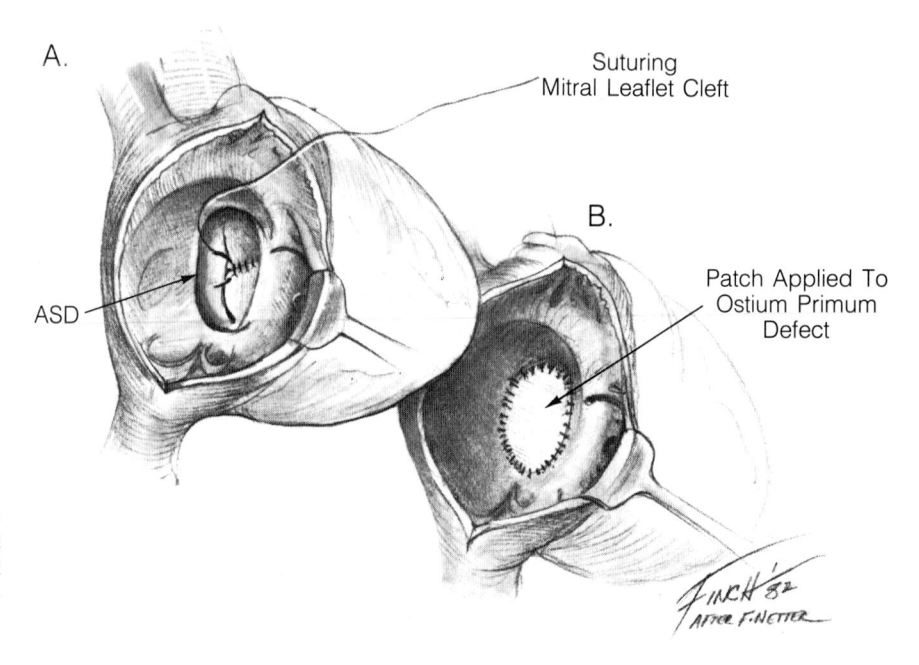

FIG 23–35.
Diagram of repair of ostium primum defect and cleft mitral valve through a right atriotomy. **A,** sutures placed through cleft in anterior leaflet of mitral valve. **B,** ostium primum closed with patch.

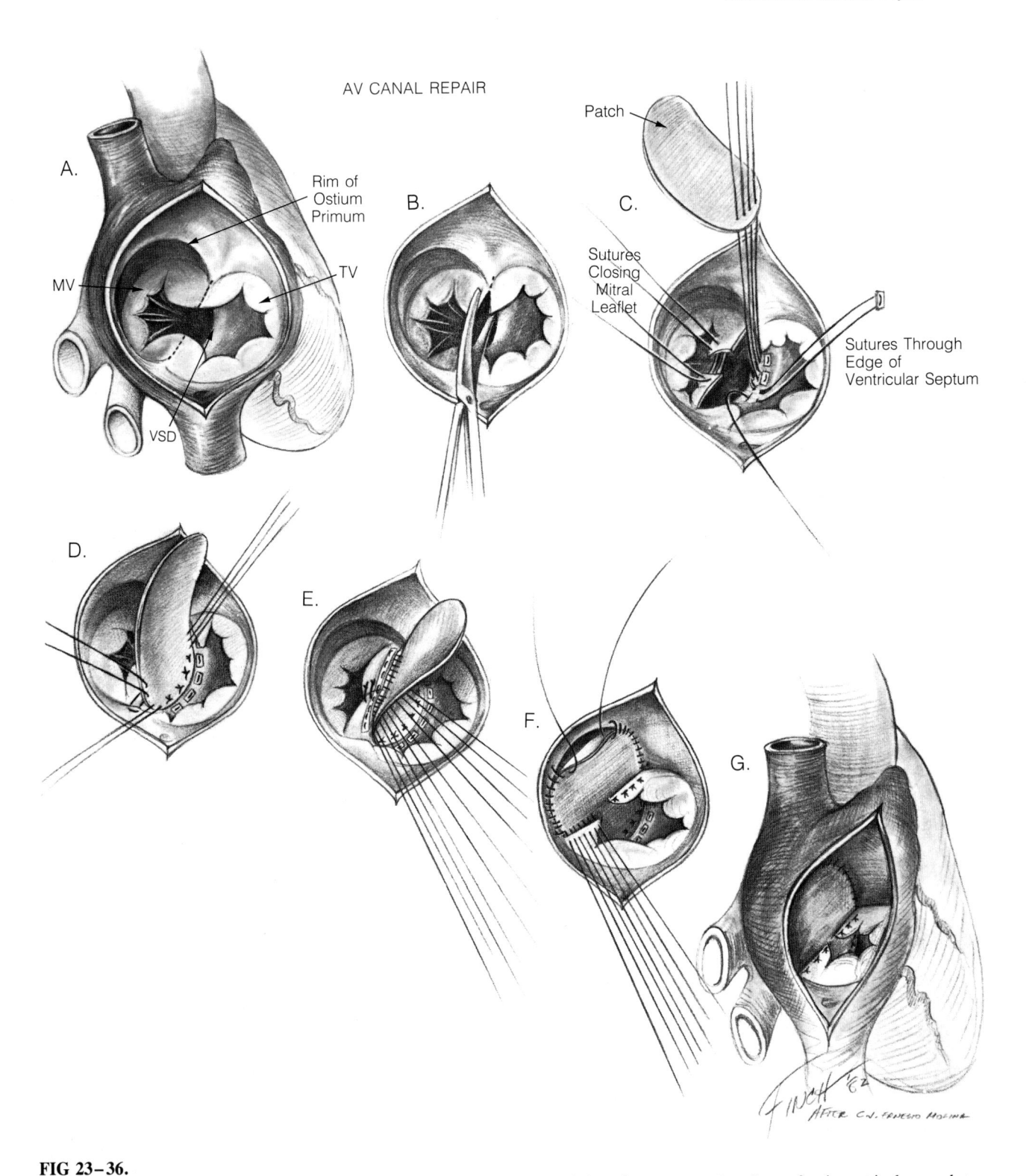

FIG 23-36.
Diagram of repair of complete atrioventricular canal type C. **A,** through a right atriotomy, complete form of atrioventricular canal, type C (Rastelli) viewed. **B,** common anterior and posterior atrioventricular valvular leaflets are divided, separating into separate mitral and tricuspid components. **C,** anterior and posterior halves of mitral valve leaflet are sutured together, creating a single leaflet. Stitches in right side of ventricular septum placed and threaded through inferior border of a Teflon patch. **D,** stitches placed in ventricular septum are tied, and patch is lowered into position. **E,** septal border of sutured septal leaflet of mitral valve is stitched to patch, using a reinforcing strip of Dacron to prevent tearing of leaflet. **F,** septal portions of tricuspid leaflet are sutured to patch at same level as mitral, using same sutures used to attach mitral valve. **G,** repair completed. The atrial septal defect is closed. *ASD* = atrial septal defect; *MV* = mitral valve; *RA* = right atrium; *RV* = right ventricle; *TV* = tricuspid valve; *VSD* = ventricular septal defect.

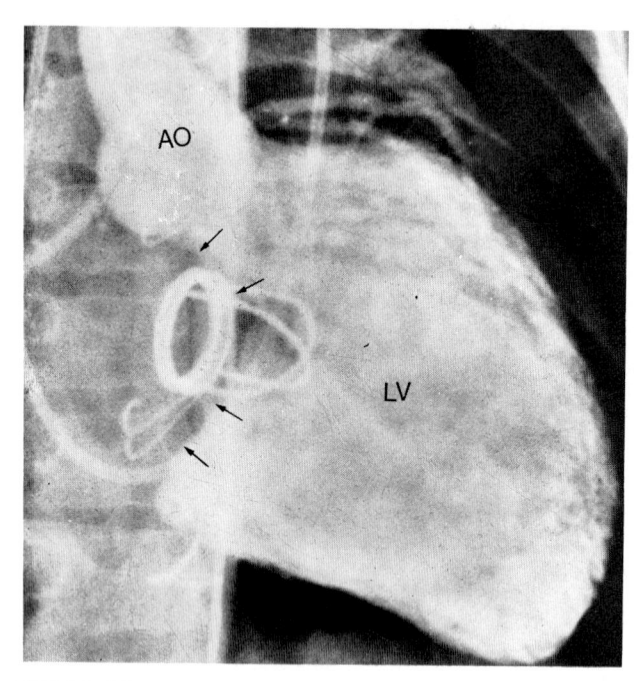

FIG 23–37.
Left ventriculogram *(LV)*, anteroposterior projection after repair of complete atrioventricular canal, using a Starr-Edwards prosthetic mitral valve; gooseneck deformity persists. No other residual abnormality. *AO* = aorta.

commonly incomplete because of residual mitral regurgitation.

4. After placement of a prosthetic mitral valve, the gooseneck deformity persists because of foreshortening of the inferior margin of the ventricular septum (Fig 23–37).

5. Because of the abnormal position of the mitral anulus, the surgeon may incorrectly suture the prosthetic valve directly into the left atrium rather than at the level of the valvular anulus (Fig 23–38).

6. In two of our patients with complete atrioventricular canal, a subaortic membrane developed after insertion of a prosthetic mitral valve (Fig 23–39).

CLEFT MITRAL VALVE

Isolated cleft of the anterior leaflet of the mitral valve is the mildest form of ECD. In this rare condition, the endocardial cushion tissue closes the interatrial and interventricular septa, but fusion of the dorsal and ventral cushions on the left side is incomplete in the formation of the anterior leaflet of the mitral valve, so it is cleft.

Anatomy

A cleft is present in the midportion of the anterior leaflet of the mitral valve, as in other forms of ECD. From the edges of the cleft, chordae tendineae pass either to the papillary muscles or abnormally to the ventricular septum (Fig 23–40). In contrast to other types of ECD, the ventricular septum is not deficient.

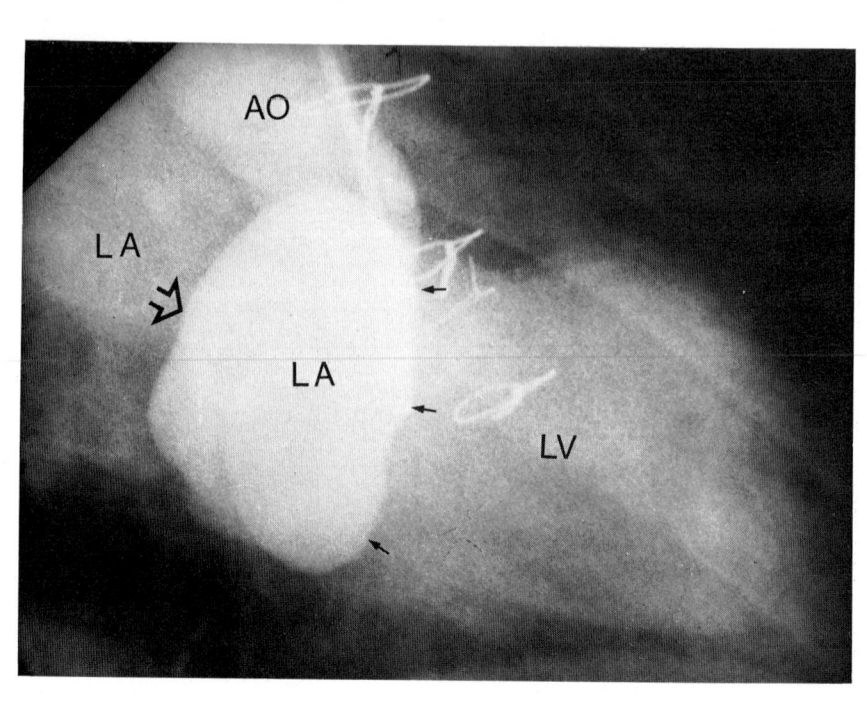

cant mitral regurgitation, closure of the atrial and ventricular communications is usually successful. Marked hemodynamic improvement results.

3. After surgical correction of complete atrioventricular canal with significant mitral regurgitation, repair is

FIG 23–38.
Left ventriculogram *(LV)*, anteroposterior projection after repair of complete atrioventricular canal using a low-profile prosthetic mitral valve *(open arrow)*. Valve inserted above mitral anulus *(black arrows)*. Marked residual mitral reflux into left atrium *(LA)*. The ventricularized portion of the left atrium lies between mitral anulus and prosthetic mitral valve. *AO* = aorta.

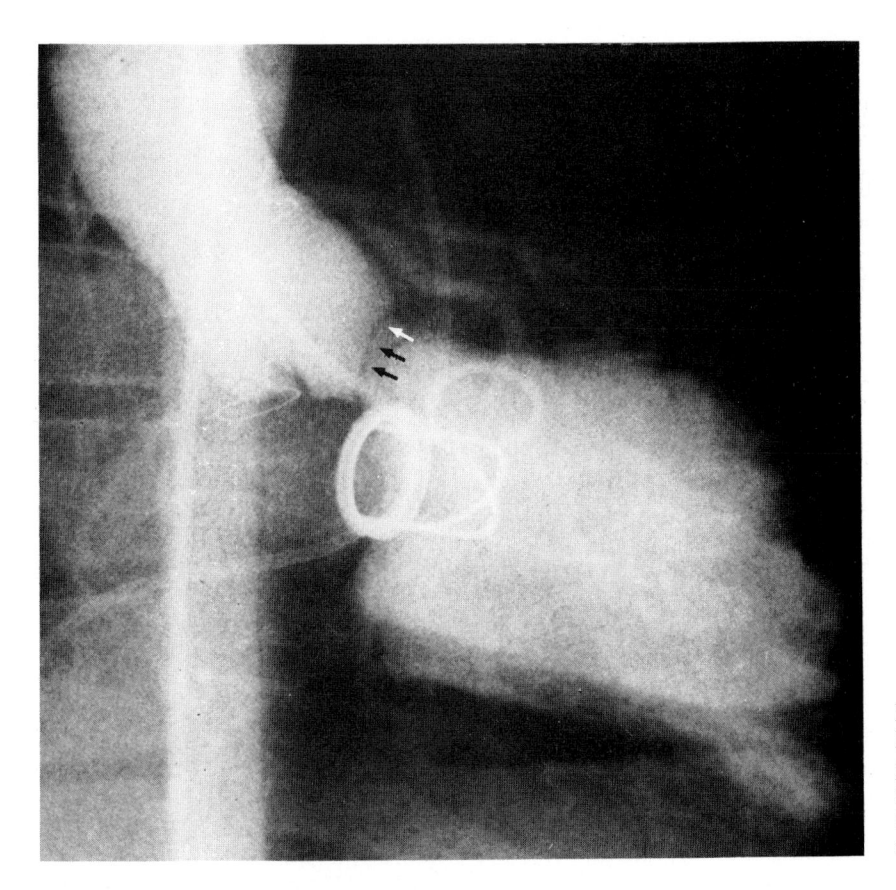

FIG 23–39.
Left ventriculogram, right anterior oblique projection after repair of a complete atrioventricular canal with prosthetic mitral valve. Subaortic membrane *(arrows)*, which was not seen preoperatively, now visible.

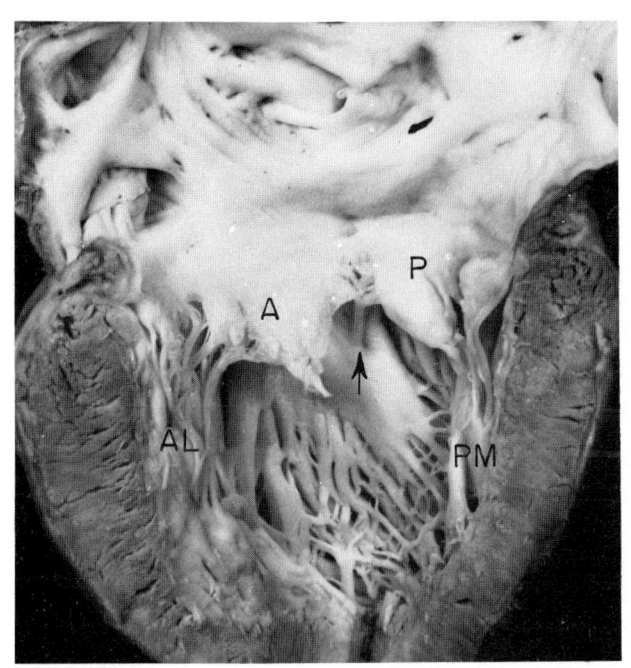

FIG 23–40.
Specimen with isolated cleft in anterior leaflet of mitral valve *(arrow)*. Edges of cleft are slightly thickened and are attached by short chordae tendineae to ventricular septum. Appearance is identical to that of atrioventricular canal, but there is no ostium primum or ventricular septal defect. A = anterior portion of anterior leaflet of mitral valve; AL = anterolateral; P = posterior; PM = posteromedial papillary muscles.

Hemodynamics

The cleft in the mitral valve permits mitral regurgitation, which may be severe. As a consequence, both the left atrium and left ventricle are dilated. Left atrial enlargement occurs, in contrast to other forms of ECD, in which the atrial septal defect allows decompression of the left atrium.

Clinical Features

Depending on the degree of mitral regurgitation, the patient may be asymptomatic or have the features of congestive cardiac failure.

Cleft mitral valve must be considered in the differential diagnosis of mitral regurgitation. There is an apical pansystolic murmur, which may be associated with a thrill, and a prominent third heart sound. Middiastolic murmurs are found in patients with larger amounts of mitral regurgitation.

In contrast to other forms of ECD, left-axis deviation is rare. Left ventricular hypertrophy and left atrial enlargement are found among patients with moderate or severe regurgitation.

Echocardiographic Features

The diagnosis can usually be made on a two-dimensional echocardiographic tracing performed from a subcostal view. In this view, the mitral valve leaflets can be seen, and as they open and close, the anterior leaflet of the mitral valve separates in its midportion.

The left atrial and left ventricular internal dimensions are increased.

Radiographic Features

1. Cardiac size is usually markedly increased.
2. The left atrium and left atrial appendage are enlarged.
3. The pulmonary vasculature is either normal or increased. Increased pulmonary arterial vasculature is not present, because the atrial and ventricular septa are intact.

Cardiac Catheterization

Oximetry data do not show a shunt. Intracardiac pressures may be normal in patients with minimal regurgitation, whereas with more severe degrees of regurgitation, left ventricular end-diastolic pressure and therefore, the left atrial and wedge pressures are elevated. Modest elevation of pulmonary arterial pressure may occur as a consequence.

Angiographic Appearance

1. Left ventriculograms demonstrate an enlarged, actively contracting left ventricle. REASON: The stroke volume of the left ventricle is increased because of the mitral regurgitation.
2. After injection into the left ventricle, there is prompt opacification of the left atrium only.
3. The anterior leaflet of the mitral valve may show a

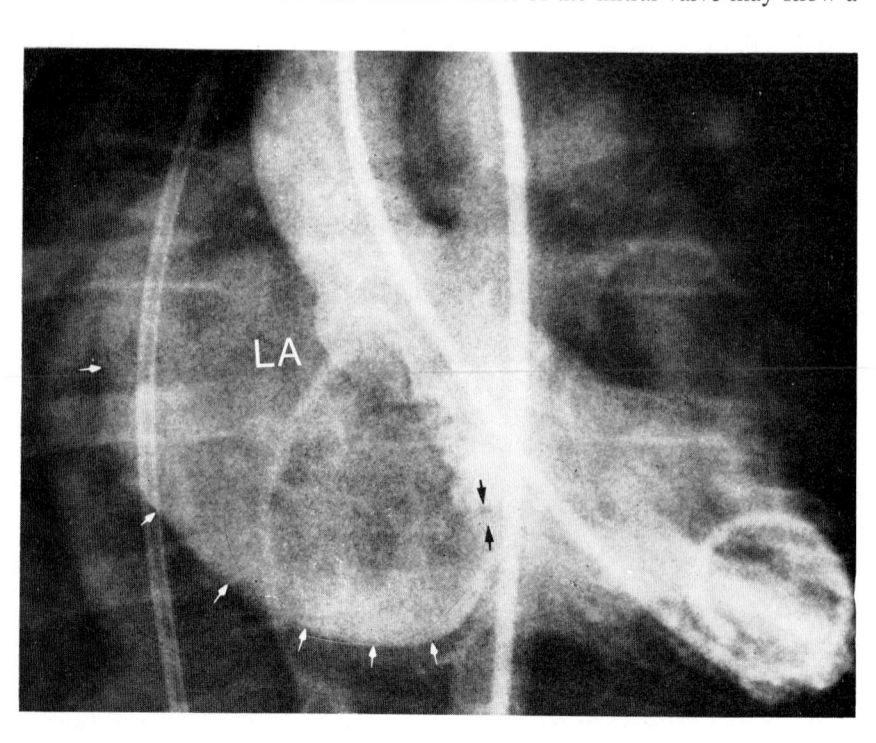

FIG 23–41.
Left ventriculogram, anteroposterior projection of mitral regurgitation secondary to isolated cleft *(black arrows)* in anterior leaflet of mitral valve. Anterior leaflet scalloped, but no gooseneck deformity of left ventricular outflow tract. Left atrium *(LA) (white arrows)* opacified and enlarged, but right atrium is not opacified, indicating an intact atrial septum.

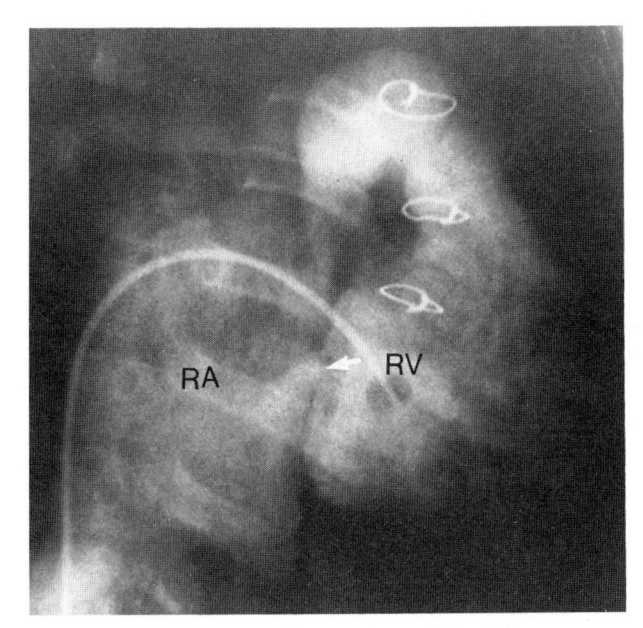

FIG 23-42.
Right ventriculogram *(RV)*, right anterior oblique projection of patient who underwent repair of complete atrioventricular canal. Cleft in tricuspid leaflet was not repaired, and there is marked tricuspid reflux *(arrow)*. RA = right atrium.

scalloped appearance. REASON: The cleft is attached by short chordae tendineae to the ventricular septum.

4. Angiographically, the cleft cannot be consistently identified (Fig 23-41).

5. The typical deficiency of the interventricular septum forming the gooseneck deformity is not present. REASON: The interventricular septum is not deficient, and the mitral valve is attached at the normal location. As a result, angiographic diagnosis is difficult.

Management

In patients with symptoms, cardiomegaly, and elevated left ventricular end-diastolic pressure, operation is recommended. Usually, the cleft can be closed by suturing. Rarely, mitral valve replacement is required.

CLEFT TRICUSPID VALVE

A cleft in the septal leaflet of the tricuspid valve is usually present in complete atrioventricular valve and may cause considerable tricuspid insufficiency (Fig 23-42). As an isolated lesion, it is rare.

REFERENCES

1. Van Mierop LHS, Alley RD, Kausel HW, et al: The anatomy and embryology of endocardial cushion defects, *J Thorac Cardiovasc Surg* 43:71, 1962.
2. Titus JL, Rastelli GC: Anatomic features of persistent common atrioventricular canal. In Feldt RH, editor, *Atrioventricular canal defects,* Philadelphia, 1976, pp 13-35.
3. Goor D, Lillehei CW, Edwards JE: Further observations on the pathology of the atrioventricular canal malformation, *Ann Surg* 97:954, 1968.
4. Baron MG: Abnormalities of the mitral valve in endocardial cushion defects, *Circulation* 45:672, 1972.
5. Wakai CS, Edwards JE: Pathologic study of persistent common atrioventricular canal, *Am Heart J* 56:779, 1958.
6. Feldt RH, DuShane JW, Titus JL: The atrioventricular conduction system in persistent common atrioventricular canal defect: correlations with electrocardiogram, *Circulation* 42:437, 1970.
7. Spach MS, Boincau JP, Long EC, et al: Genesis of the vectorcardiogram (electrocardiogram) in endocardial cushion defects. In Hoffman I, Taynor RC, editors: *Vectorcardiography,* 1966, Elsevier North-Holland, pp 307-326. New York,
8. Ongley PA, Pongpanich B, Spangler JG, et al: The electrocardiogram in atrioventricular canal. In Felt RH, editor: *Atrioventricular canal defects,* Philadelphia, 1976, Saunders, pp 51-75.
9. Hagler DJ: Echocardiographic findings in atrioventricular canal defect, Hoffman I, Taynor RC, editors: *Vectorcardiography,* New York, 1966, Elsevier North-Holland, pp 87-109.
10. Bass JL, Bessinger FB Jr, Lawrence C: Echocardiographic differentiation of partial and complete atrioventricular canal, *Circulation* 57:1144, 1978.
11. Hagler DJ, Tajik AJ, Seward JB, et al: Real-time wide-angle sector echocardiography: atrioventricular canal defects, *Circulation* 59:140, 1979.
12. Park JM, Ritter DG, Mair DD: Cardiac catheterization findings in persistent common atrioventricular canal. In Feldt RH, editor: *Atrioventricular canal defects,* Philadelphia, 1976, Saunders, pp 76-86.
13. Macartney FJ, Rees PG, Daly K, et al: Angiocardiographic appearance of atrioventricular defects with particular reference to distinction of ostium primum atrial septal defect from common atrioventricular orifice, *Br Heart J* 42:640, 1979.
14. Towbin R, Schwartz D: Endocardial cushion defects: embryology, anatomy, and angiography, *AJR* 136:157, 1981.
15. Losay J, Rosenthal A, Castaneda AR, et al: Repair of atrial septal defect primum: results, course, and prognosis, *J Thorac Cardiovasc Surg* 75:248, 1978.
16. McGoon DC, McMullan MH, Mair DD, et al: Correction of complete atrioventricular canal in infants, *Mayo Clin Proc* 48:769, 1973.
17. Berger TJ, Blackstone EH, Kirklin JW, et al: Survival and probability of cure without and with operation in complete atrioventricular canal, *Ann Thorac Surg* 27:104, 1979.
18. Newfeld EA, Sher M, Paul MH, et al: Pulmonary vascular disease in complete atrioventricular canal defect, *Am J Cardiol* 39:721, 1977.
19. Epstein ML, Moller JH, Amplatz K, et al: Pulmonary artery banding in infants with complete atrioventricular canal, *J Thorac Cardiovasc Surg* 78:28, 1979.

CHAPTER 24

Sinus of Valsalva Aneurysm

Aneurysms of the sinus of Valsalva of the aortic valve are uncommon (<1% of congenital heart disease) and affect males more often than females. Any of several clinical pictures may be seen. An unruptured sinus of Valsalva aneurysm may be an incidental finding at aortography. In most clinically recognized cases, the aneurysm has ruptured and created a left-to-right shunt and aortic run off.

PATHOLOGIC ANATOMY[1]

A review of the normal anatomy of the aortic sinuses is required to understand the clinical and laboratory findings in this condition.

The sinuses of Valsalva are bulbous swellings at the root of the aorta below the level of the aortic cusps. They are surrounded by other cardiac structures, and thus, depending on the portion and the sinus involved, the aneurysm may be related to different structures. Most aneurysms of the sinus of Valsalva are congenital and are caused by a separation between the aortic media and the heart.[2] This separation occurs at the anulus fibrosus of the aortic valve, so the aneurysm is located below the level of the valve (Fig 24–1). Because of the separation of the aortic wall, an aneurysm develops gradually and may eventrate into the adjacent cardiac chamber. An aneurysm of the posterior (noncoronary) sinus ruptures into the right atrium, and those of the right sinus rupture into the right ventricle or, rarely, the right atrium, depending on the site of attachment of the tricuspid valve, which is variable. (Figs 24–2 and 24–3). Rupture of the right sinus is more frequent than the posterior sinus. Aneurysms of the left sinus are exceedingly rare. They appear in the epicardium, may compress coronary branches, and rupture into the pericardial sac.

Bacterial endocarditis may affect the aortic valve and erode into adjacent structures, causing anatomic and hemodynamic features similar to those of a congenital aneurysm of the sinus of Valsalva. To further complicate matters, congenital aneurysms of the sinuses of Valsalva may become infected and rupture. Thus, differentiation between congenital and acquired aneurysms may be impossible, even at postmortem examination. The huge sinuses of Valsalva seen in Marfan syndrome and similar connective tissue disorders have also been termed aneurysms, but because the anatomic, histologic features, and clinical findings differ, they are discussed separately.

Aneurysms may form in any of the aortic sinuses. Those of the right sinus are the most common (70%). The posterior sinus is involved less frequently (29%) and the left sinus rarely (1%). The aneurysms may be either unruptured or ruptured, the latter being more common. Aneurysms are rarely detected in neonates or infants and tend to enlarge gradually with age.

Depending on their location, size, and state, the aneurysms may result in:

1. Right ventricular outflow tract obstruction.
2. Tricuspid insufficiency.
3. Conduction abnormalities.
4. A left-to-right shunt.
5. Aortic insufficiency.

If unruptured, aneurysms of the right anterior sinus may protrude into the right ventricular outflow area and

FIG 24–1.
Aneurysm of sinus of Valsalva. Diagram of cross-sectional view through heart, ascending aorta, and an aneurysm of sinus of Valsalva. Aneurysm results from disruption of aortic media, forming a bulge into adjacent cardiac chamber. *LV* = left ventricle; *RA* = right atrium; *RV* = right ventricle; *TV* = tricuspid valve.

cause obstruction or interfere with tricuspid valve closure, producing tricuspid insufficiency. When an aneurysm of the posterior sinus ruptures into the right atrium, a left-to-right shunt occurs (Fig 24–4,A and B). Because attachment of the septal leaflet of the tricuspid valve is variable, rupture of an aneurysm of the posterior sinus occasionally occurs into the right ventricle. Rupture of an aneurysm of the right anterior sinus occurs into the right ventricle, resulting in a left-to-right ventricular level shunt. Aneurysms of the right anterior sinus may be associated with a ventricular septal defect.

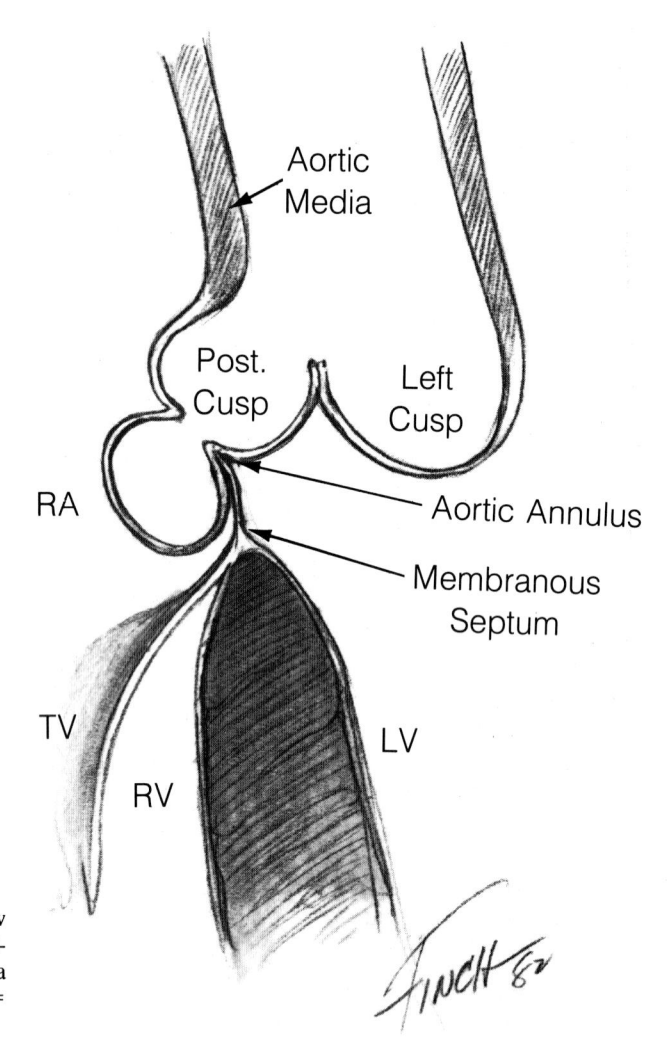

Aneurysms of the left sinus of Valsalva are rare and even more rarely rupture. When they do, a left-to-right shunt does not occur, because the sinus is unrelated to right-sided cardiac chambers. Rupture occurs into the left atrium or ventricle or the pericardial space.

Multiple aneurysms of the sinuses of Valsalva of the aortic valve and aneurysms of the sinuses of the pulmonary valve are rare.

CLINICAL FEATURES

The clinical features vary. Rarely the lesion is discovered at birth; more commonly, it is found later in childhood or in adulthood. The average age of rupture in one series was 32 years.[3]

Unruptured sinuses of Valsalva are usually asymptomatic and cause no abnormal findings, although if they project into the right ventricular outflow tract, they cause a pulmonary systolic ejection murmur.[4] Aneurysms of the posterior sinus may interfere with tricuspid valve closure and cause tricuspid regurgitation. A systolic murmur is present along the lower sternal border in these patients.

Complete heart block and junctional rhythm have been described in patients with aneurysms of the sinus of Valsalva, perhaps by injury or pressure on the bundles of His. This complication may cause sudden death. Sudden death has also been described from obstruction of the ostium of

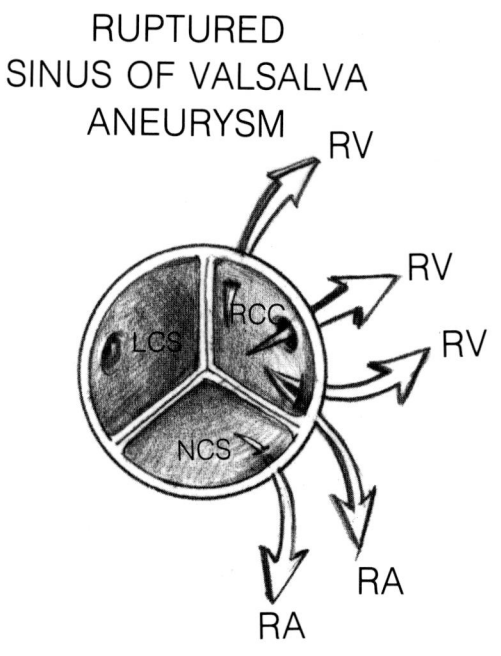

FIG 24–2.
Diagram of aortic valve and sinuses of Valsalva viewed from above, with arrows indicating caridac chambers into which aneurysms from the respective sinuses might rupture. *LCS* = left coronary sinus; *NCS* = non-coronary sinus; *RCS* = right coronary sinus, *RA* = right atrium; *RV* = right ventricle.

the right coronary artery by a thrombus in the right sinus of Valsalva.[4]

When an aneurysm of the sinus of Valsalva ruptures, there may be sudden onset of chest pain and congestive cardiac failure, but more commonly, symptoms of easy fatigability and congestive cardiac failure develop gradually.[3, 5]

Most patients have both a loud systolic and a loud diastolic murmur, each associated with a thrill. The murmurs are loudest along the left sternal border from the second to the fourth intercostal spaces, but they radiate widely. The systolic murmur is of an ejection type and related to the increased volume of blood being ejected across both the aorta and the pulmonary outflow areas. The diastolic murmur is high pitched, starts early in diastole, and has features of aortic insufficiency. At times, the murmurs appear continuous, resembling the murmur of patent ductus arteriosus.[6]

The pulse pressure is increased.

ELECTROCARDIOGRAPHIC FINDINGS

There is no distinctive electrocardiographic finding. Patterns of left, right, or combined ventricular hypertrophy may be present, and these reflect the hemodynamics. Abnormalities of atrioventricular nodal conduction or right bundle-branch block occur.[3, 5]

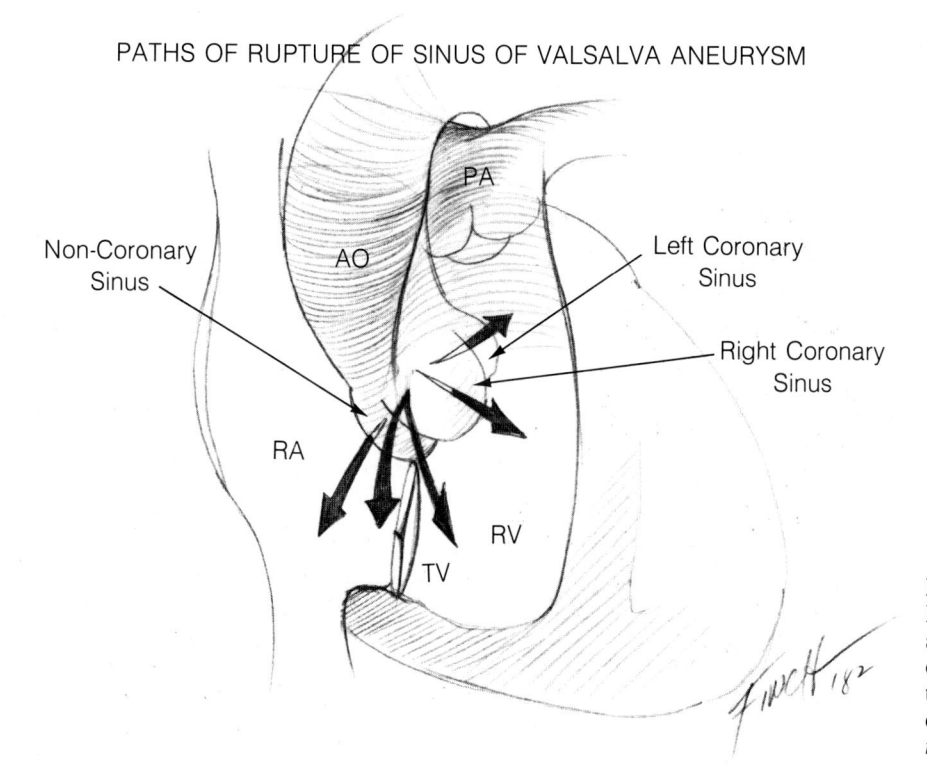

FIG 24–3.
Diagram of anteroposterior projection of aorta *(AO)* and pulmonary artery *(PA)* and opened right atrium *(RA)* showing relations of aortic sinuses to surrounding cardiac structures and sites of rupture *(arrows)*. *TV* = tricuspid valve.

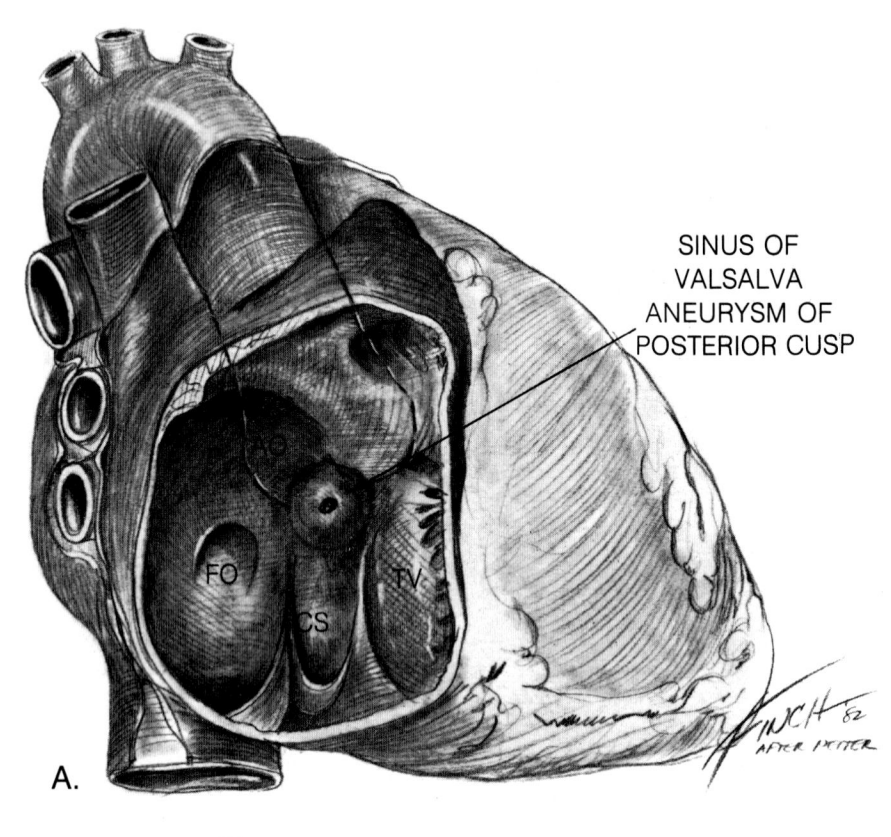

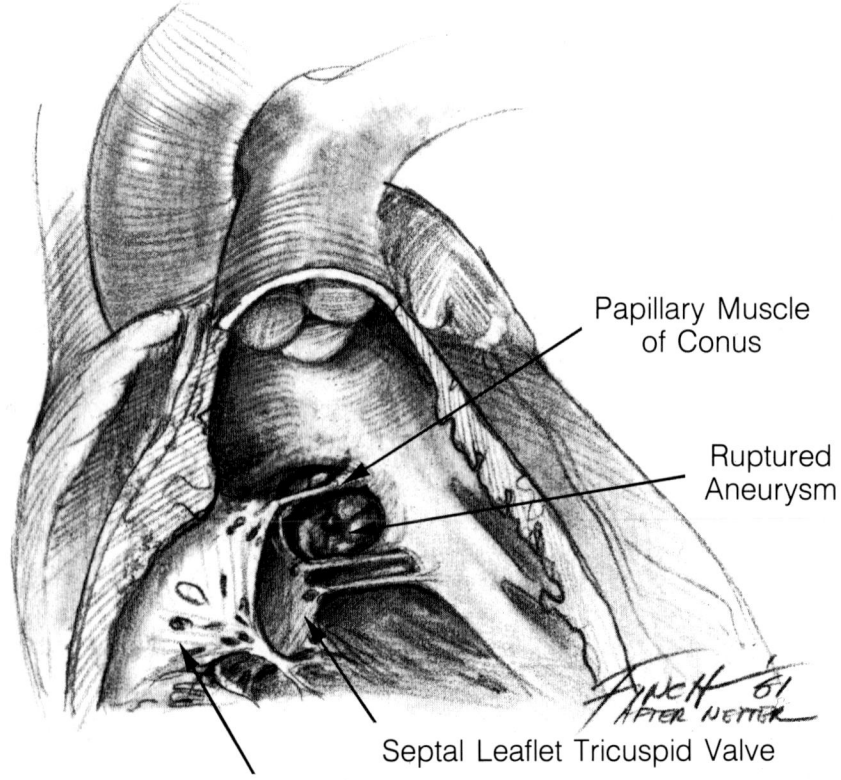

398 Cardiac Conditions Associated With a Left-to-Right Shunt

FIG 24–4.
A, diagram of opened right atrium, showing aneurysm of the posterior sinus of Valsalva projecting above the tricuspid valve *(TV)*. **B,** diagram of ruptured sinus of Valsalva aneurysm immediately behind the papillary muscle of the conus (Lancisi) and the septal leaflet producing tricuspid reflux. *CS* = coronary sinus; *FO* = foramen ovale: *TV* = tricuspid valve.

ECHOCARDIOGRAPHIC FEATURES

Several reports have described both M-mode and cross-sectional echocardiographic findings.[7-10] The echocardiographic findings resemble those of the angiogram. An unruptured aneurysm may appear as a dense echoproducing mass, similar to a tumor. This abnormal structure originates from the aortic root and extends into a cardiac chamber. The discontinuity of the proximal aorta may be identified, but care must be used to distinguish this from technically produced dropout of echo.

When the aneurysm is viewed on two-dimensional echocardiograms, rupture is suggested when there is discontinuity of the echoes from the wall of the aneurysm.

If the aneurysm ruptures near the tricuspid valve, flutter of that valve may be identified.

RADIOGRAPHIC FEATURES

The radiographic findings of the thorax differ, depending on the size and site of rupture of the sinus of Valsalva aneurysm. The aneurysm itself is not evident, because it is an intracardiac structure and does not form a border of the cardiac silhouette. Rarely, an aneurysm of the sinus of Valsalva, usually those involving the left cusp, may calcify and become visible on chest films.

1. Cardiac size and pulmonary vasculature are normal in patients with unruptured sinus of Valsalva aneurysm. REASON: An unruptured aneurysm usually has no hemodynamic consequence.

2. Rarely, an unruptured sinus of Valsalva aneurysm causes right ventricular outflow tract obstruction, giving a picture similar to that of infundibular pulmonary stenosis.

3. The sudden or gradual development of cardiomegaly and increased pulmonary vasculature, and the appearance of a diastolic murmur, are almost pathognomonic of rupture of a sinus of Valsalva aneurysm (Fig 24–5). If the rupture is secondary to endocarditis, a history of fever is present.

4. Depending on the size of the rupture, the heart is enlarged and the pulmonary vasculature is increased. REASON: Rupture of a sinus of Valsalva aneurysm into the right-sided cardiac chambers causes a left-to-right shunt.

5. Rupture into right-sided cardiac chambers results in left atrial enlargement. REASON: Blood flow through the lungs and left atrium is increased, distending the left atrium and enlarging the left ventricle. The left atrium

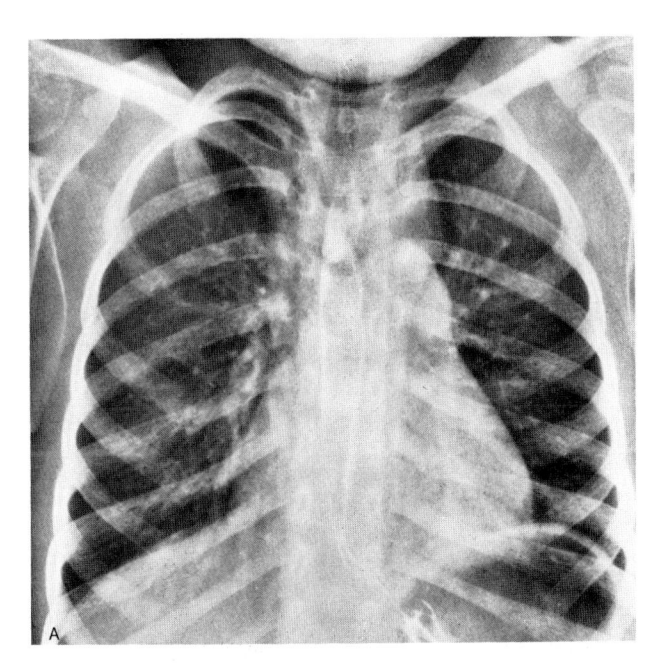

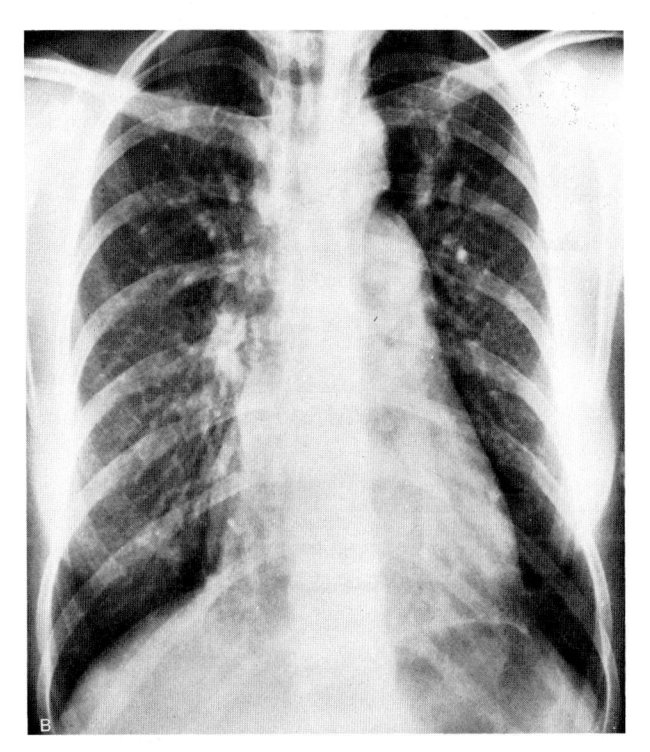

FIG 24–5.
Thoracic roentgenograms, posteroanterior projection in patient with sinus of Valsalva aneurysm. **A,** aneurysm unruptured. Normal pulmonary vasculature and cardiac size. The aorta is slightly prominent for unknown reasons. **B,** after rupture of sinus of Valsalva aneurysm. Significant cardiomegaly, prominent pulmonary arterial segment, and increased pulmonary vasculature. The radiographic findings of a left-to right shunt with the history of the development of a murmur of aortic regurgitation strongly suggests ruptured sinus of Valsalva aneurysm into a right-sided cardiac chamber.

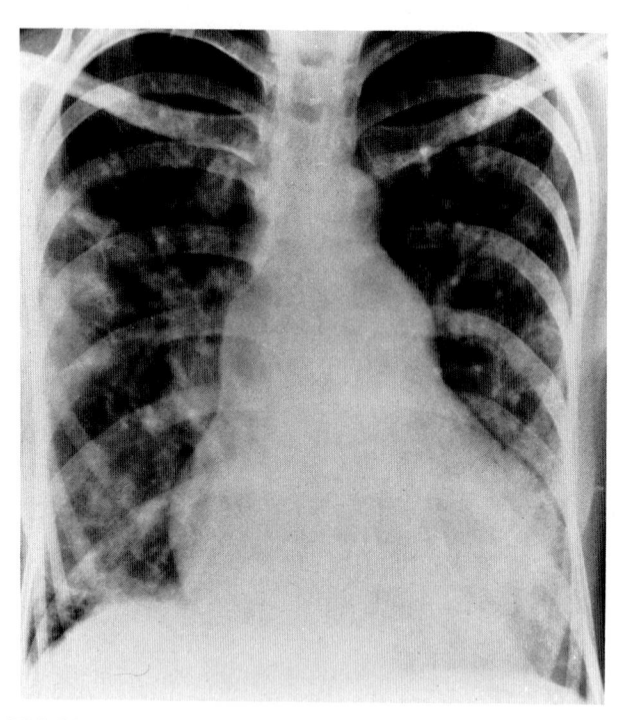

400 Cardiac Conditions Associated With a Left-to-Right Shunt

FIG 24–6.
Thoracic roentgenogram, posteroanterior projection in patient with long-standing rupture of a large sinus of Valsalva aneurysm. Increased pulmonary vasculature and chronic infiltrates from repeated episodes of pneumonia, as is commonly observed in patients with a left-to-right shunt and pulmonary hypertension (see Chapter 12). Marked cardiomegaly, prominent pulmonary artery segment, and prominence of the aorta. The radiographic findings are indistinguishable from those of an extracardiac left-to-right shunt, as in patent ductus arteriosus and associated pulmonary hypertension.

cannot decompress itself, as it can with atrial septal defect.

6. The aorta tends to be prominent. REASON: Ruptured sinus of Valsalva is an aortic runoff lesion. Blood flow in the ascending aorta is increased because of the diastolic backflow through the ruptured aneurysm into the right-sided cardiac chambers. The increased flow into the aorta gradually widens it, as in aortic regurgitation (Fig 24–6). The radiographic appearance is therefore identical to that of patent ductus arteriosus.

7. In most patients, the correct diagnosis can be suggested only radiographically in light of the information that a patient has developed a diastolic murmur of aortic regurgitation.

8. Definitive diagnosis can be made only by angiography.

CARDIAC CATHETERIZATION

In unruptured aneurysm, there may be no abnormal hemodynamic findings, except in the occasional patient in whom it causes obstruction in the right ventricular outflow tract. In such cases, a gradient may be identified, but the gradient is usually not large.

When rupture occurs into a right-sided cardiac chamber (Fig 24–7), an increase in oxygen saturation is found in the chamber receiving the aneurysm. In our experience,[5] the shunt has always been more than 30% and sometimes as large as 75%. Pulmonary arterial pressures are usually normal, although if a ventricular septal defect

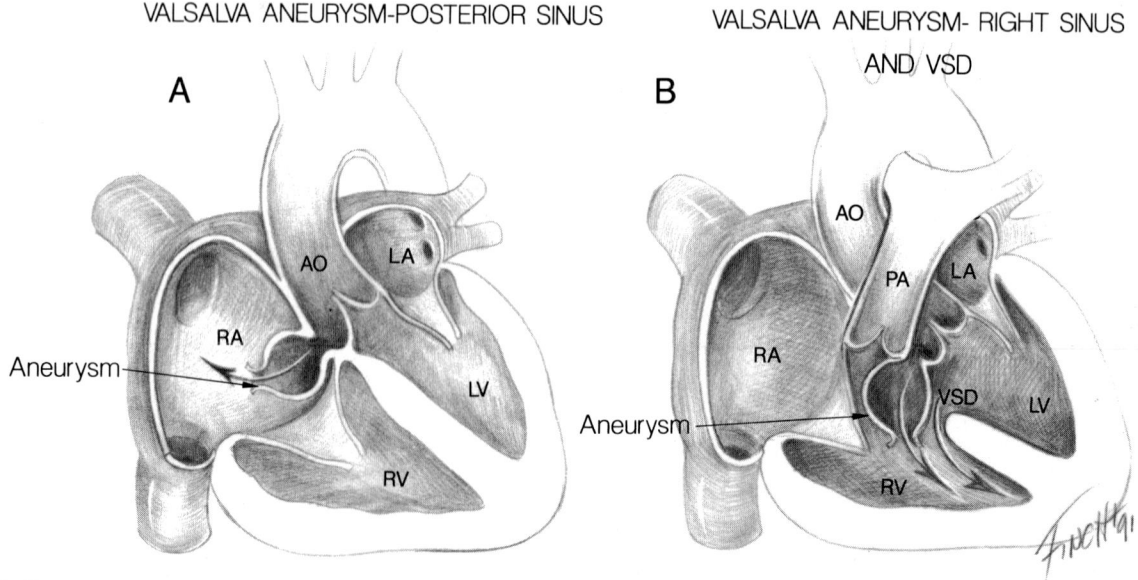

FIG 24–7.
A, diagram of central circulation of aneurysm of the posterior sinus of Valsalva with rupture into the right atrium resulting in an atrial level left-to-right shunt. **B,** ruptured right sinus of Valsalva aneurysm (more common) with ventricular septal defect, resulting in a systolic and diastolic left-to-right shunt at the ventricular level. *AO* = aorta; *LA* = left atrium; *LV* = left ventricle; *PA* = pulmonary artery; *RA* = right atrium; *RV* = right ventricle.

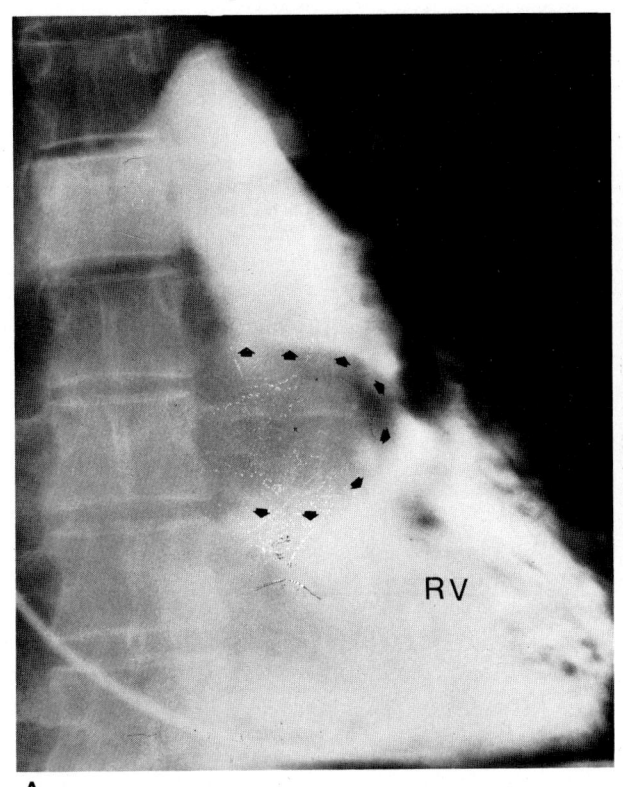

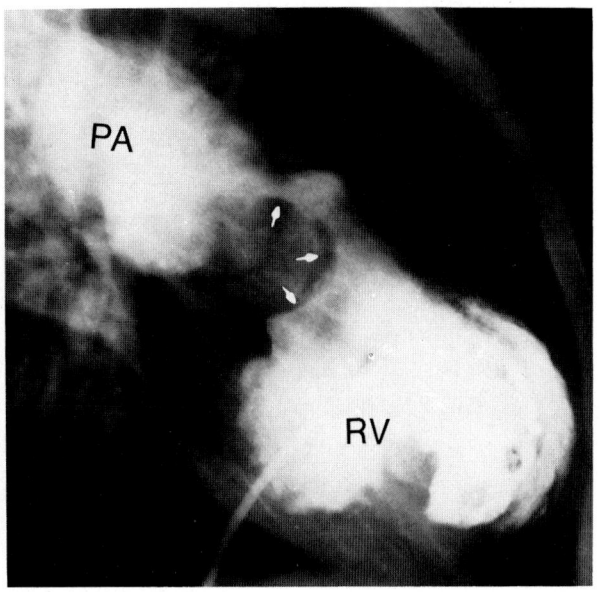

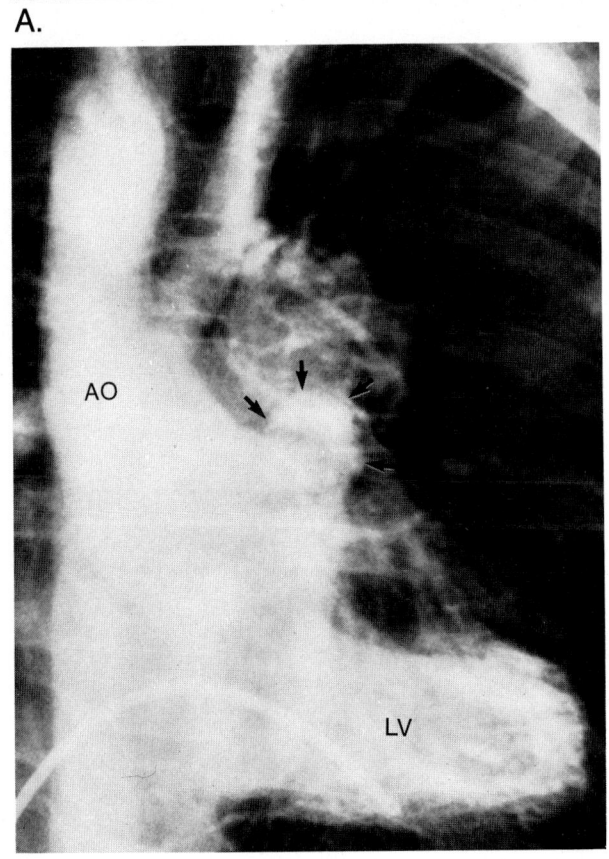

FIG 24–8.
Sinus of Valsalva aneurysm. **A,** right ventriculogram, anteroposterior projection of unruptured aneurysm; large round filling defect *(arrows),* causing severe obstruction in the right ventricular *(RV)* outflow tract. **B,** right ventriculogram, lateral projection; large posterior obstructing filling defect *(white arrows)* in right ventricular outflow tract. Degree of obstruction is unusually severe. **C,** left ventriculogram *(LV);* large sinus of Valsalva aneurysm *(arrows)* of right cusp in area of filling defect in right ventricular outflow tract.

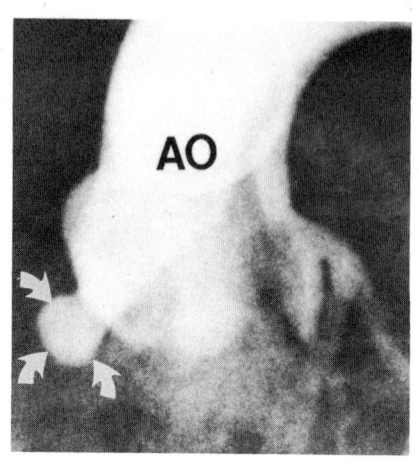

FIG 24–9.
Aortogram left anterior oblique projection demonstrating a typical small unruptured sinus of Valsalva aneurysm of the right sinus *(arrows)*. *AO* = aorta.

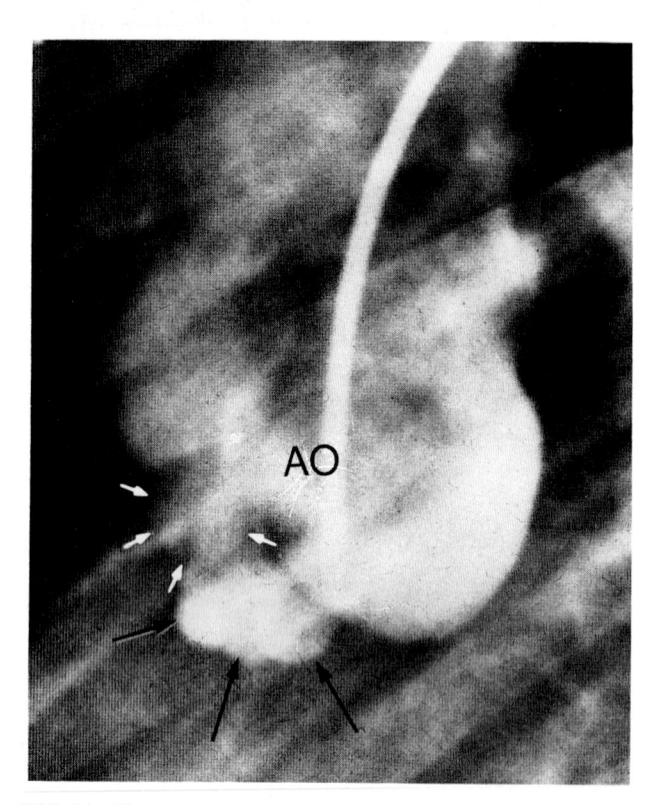

FIG 24–10.
Aortogram *(AO)* lateral projection of multiple unruptured sinus of Valsalva aneurysms. Larger lobulated aneurysm *(black arrows)* arises from posterior cusp, and smaller aneurysm *(white arrows)* originates from right aortic cusp.

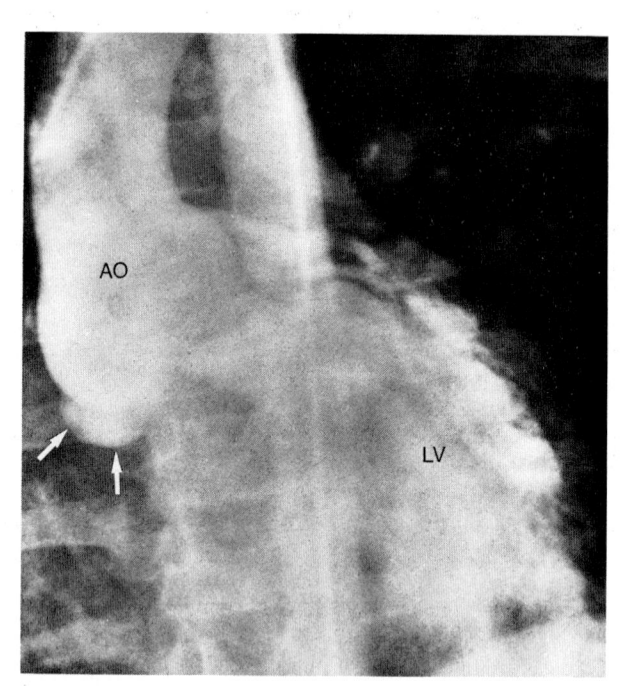

FIG 24–11.
Aortogram, anteroposterior projection of large unruptured aneurysm *(arrows)* of sinus of Valsalva arising from right aortic cusp. Marked aortic insufficiency, with opacification of left ventricle *(LV)*. *AO* = aorta.

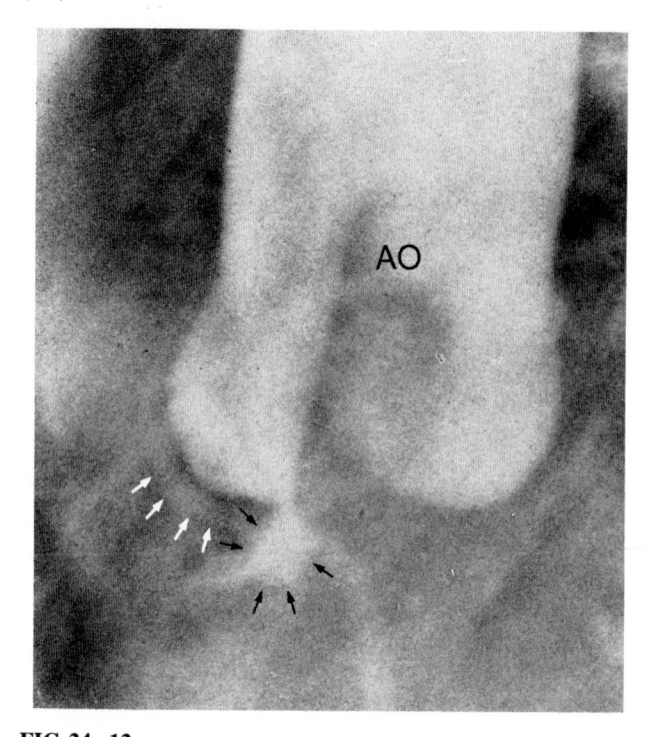

FIG 24–12.
Aortogram, lateral projection of tiny sinus of Valsalva aneurysm *(small black arrows)* arising from right aortic cusp. Aneurysm is distinctly separated from open right aortic valve leaflet, distinguishing if from a prolapsing aortic cusp. Aneurysm has ruptured into right ventricle, as is indicated by a minute jet of contrast medium *(white arrows)* immediately beneath aortic valve. *AO* = aorta.

coexists, pulmonary arterial pressure may be (see Fig 24-7) increased.

When rupture occurs into a left-sided cardiac chamber, there is no left-to-right shunt; but there is regurgitation from the aorta into a cardiac chamber either the left ventricle or left atrium. Systolic pressure is increased because of a large stroke volume, and diastolic pressure is lower because of aortic runoff.

ANGIOGRAPHY

Aortography and selective right and left ventriculography should be performed for complete assessment of a patient with a sinus of Valsalva aneurysm. REASON: Aortography is the most definitive diagnostic technique for demonstrating this lesion. Aortography is also useful to

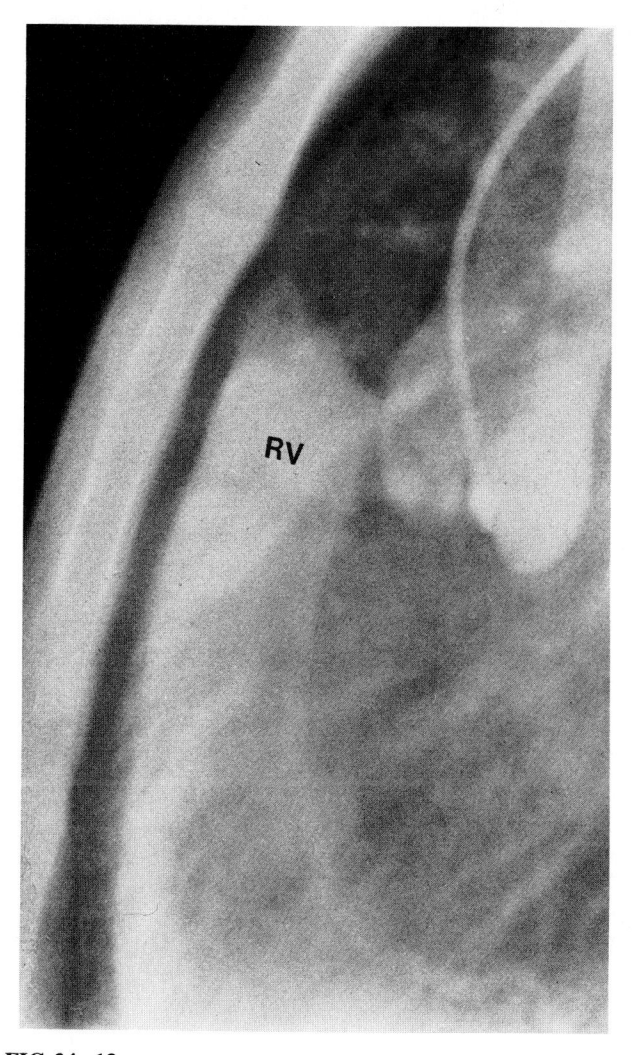

FIG 24-13.
Aortogram, lateral projection of rupture of sinus of Valsalva aneurysm into right ventricular *(RV)* outflow tract. Large shunt, but aneurysm itself is not seen.

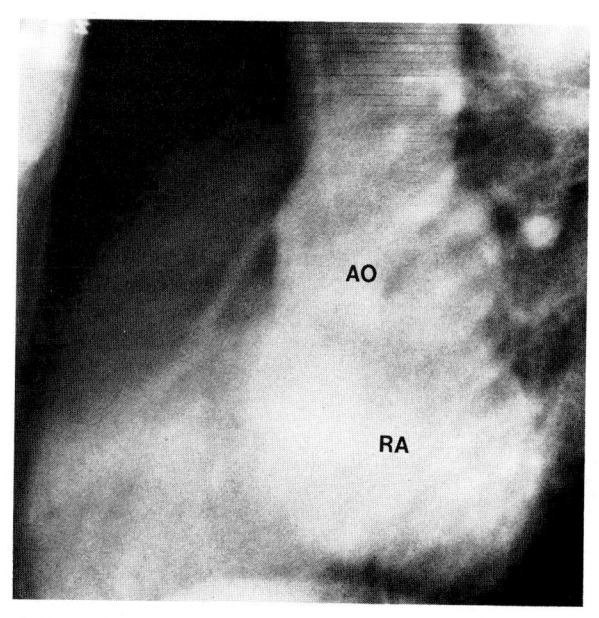

FIG 24-14.
Aortogram, lateral projection of rupture of aneurysm of sinus of Valsalva, with large communication with right atrium *(RA)*. Dense opacification of right atrium. Aneurysm cannot be seen because of the large shunt and, probably, because of its small size. *AO* = aorta.

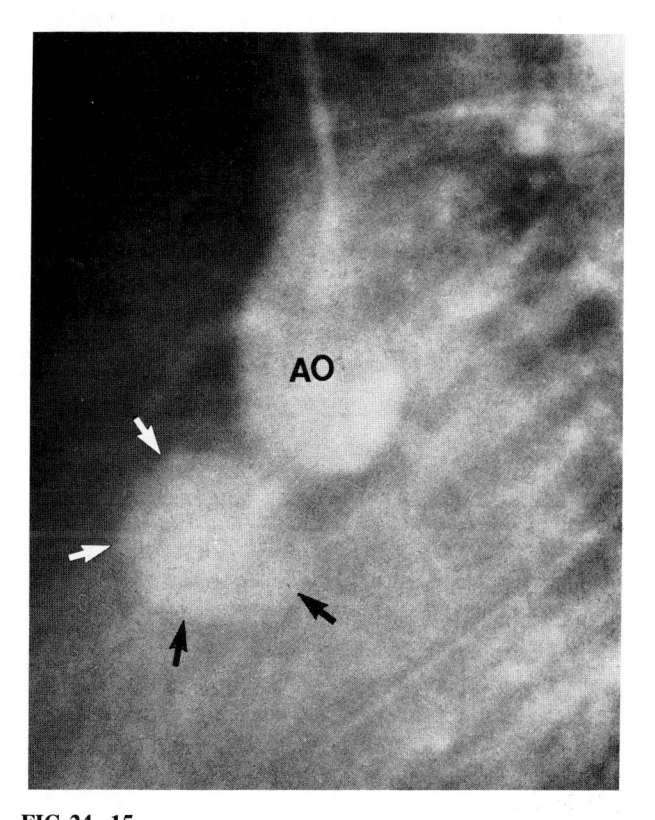

FIG 24-15.
Aortogram, lateral projection of huge sinus of Valsalva aneurysm *(arrows)* (right cusp), which has not ruptured.

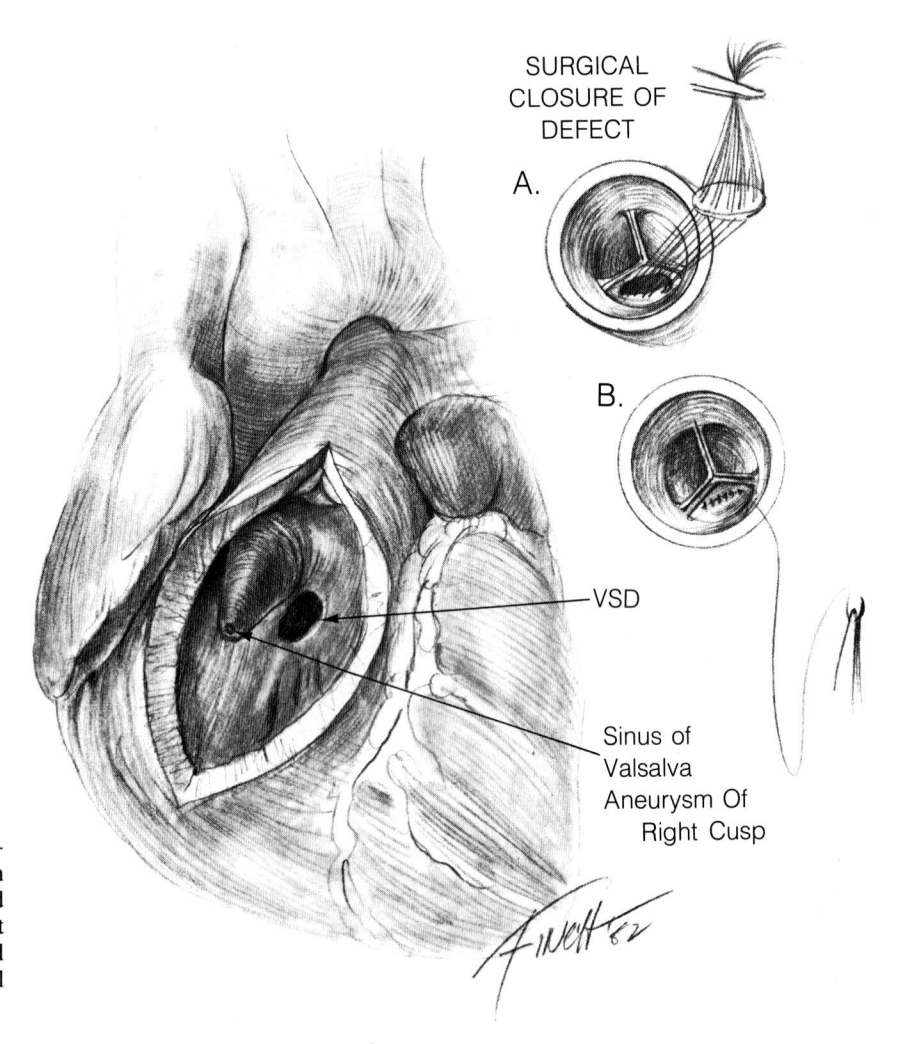

FIG 24–16.
Diagram of operative repair of sinus of Valsalva aneurysm. Aortic valve viewed from above. Aneurysm may be either patched **(A)** or directly sutured closed **(B)**. Right ventricle is opened also, and aneurysmal sac excised and associated ventricular septal defect *(VSD)* closed.

distinguish sinus of Valsalva aneurysm from aneurysm of the membranous ventricular septum, prolapsing aortic cusp, and aortico–left ventricular tunnel (Chapters 13, 14, and 27). Left ventriculography is indicated to exclude a commonly associated ventricular septal defect. Right ventriculography is indicated because large sinus of Valsalva aneurysms may bulge into the right ventricular outflow tract, causing right-sided obstruction (Fig 24–8).

1. A sinus of Valsalva aneurysm is discovered on aortography as a round collection of contrast material below the sinus and the coronary arterial orifice. This is in contrast to the finding in aortico–left ventricular tunnel, which arises above the coronary arterial ostia.

2. Unruptured sinus of Valsalva aneurysm is usually an incidental finding of aortography, when a round pocket slightly above the level of the aortic anulus but distinctly below the level of the coronary ostia is seen (Fig 24–9). There is no significant change in the size of a sinus of Valsalva aneurysm between systole and diastole, unlike a prolapsing aortic cusp, which is larger during diastole. The motion of the valve leaflet is visible on cine aortography.

3. In patients with an aneurysm of the membranous septum or adherence of the septal leaflet of the tricuspid valve to a membranous ventricular septal defect (see Chapter 14), the angiographic appearance of a left ventriculogram is similar to that in sinus of Valsalva aneurysm. However, an aneurysm of the membranous septum is not demonstrated by aortography.

4. More than one unruptured aneurysm may be present in a given patient and arise from either one or several aortic valve cusps (Fig 24–10).

5. Unruptured sinus of Valsalva aneurysm may be large (Fig 24–11) and present as right ventricular outflow tract obstruction (Fig 24–8). Sudden rupture of a large aneurysm usually creates a large left-to-right shunt, but clinical symptoms develop gradually, suggesting that the rupture is initially small and enlarges with time.

6. Even tiny aneurysms may rupture (Fig 24–12).

7. A small aneurysm may be difficult to identify after

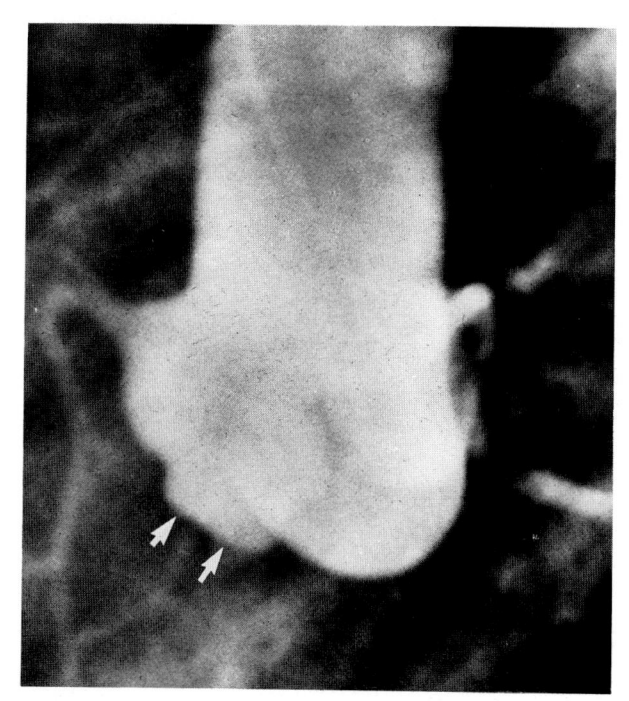

FIG 24–17.
Aortogram, anteroposterior projection after repair of a large ruptured sinus of Valsalva aneurysm arising from right aortic cusp. Mouth of aneurysm *(arrows)* is visible. Opacification of a cardiac chamber does not occur.

rupture. Opacification of the right ventricle (Fig 24–13) or the right atrium (Fig 24–14) after aortography is virtually pathognomonic of rupture of either congenital aneurysms or an acquired aneurysm secondary to subacute endocarditis. It may be difficult to distinguish congenital from acquired aneurysm even at postmortem examination, but a history of a prolonged febrile episode suggests a bacterial origin.

8. Contrary to the findings of atherosclerotic aneurysms of the aorta, the relation between size and time of rupture is not clear. Very large aneurysms may be present without rupture (Fig 24–15), and a tiny aneurysm can rupture early, producing a large shunt.

SURGICAL APPROACH

We recommend that all ruptured aneurysms of the sinus of Valsalva be repaired and that at operation, coexisting conditions be corrected.[5]

At operation, the chamber that receives the aneurysm is opened and the aneurysm resected (Fig 24–16). The ascending aorta is also opened to repair the orifice of the aneurysm. This transaortic approach allows selection of firmer tissue for placement of sutures and reduces the possibility of distortion of the aortic valve cusp, which may lead to aortic incompetence.

The operation can be performed with little risk except in patients with a coexisting condition, when the operative mortality is higher. This additional mortality is perhaps related to the fact that many patients undergoing the operation are adults. The postoperative clinical status and cardiac catheterization data in most patients are excellent.

POSTOPERATIVE RADIOGRAPHIC APPEARANCE

The postoperative radiographic changes of a chest film resemble those seen after correction of other conditions with a large left-to-right shunt or aortic runoff. That is, cardiac size and pulmonary vasculature decrease rapidly. The mouth of the aneurysm may still be demonstrable after aortography, but the shunt is obliterated (Fig 24–17).

REFERENCES

1. Sakakibara S, Konno S: Congenital aneurysm of the sinus of Valsalva: anatomy and classification, *Am Heart J* 63:405, 1962.
2. Edwards JE, Burchell HB: The pathological anatomy of deficiencies between the aortic root and the heart, including aortic sinus aneurysms, *Thorax* 12:125, 1957.
3. Sakakibara S, Konno S: Congenital aneurysms of sinus of Valsalva: a clinical study, *Am Heart J* 63:708, 1962.
4. Buckley BH, Hutchins GM, Ross RS: Aortic sinus of Valsalva aneurysms simulating primary right-sided valvular heart disease, *Circulation* 52:696, 1975.
5. Howard RJ, Moller J, Castaneda AR, et al: Surgical correction of sinus of Valsalva aneurysm, *J Thorac Cardiovasc Surg* 66:420, 1973.
6. Magidson O, Kay JH: Ruptured aortic sinus aneurysms: clinical and surgical aspects of seven cases, *Am Heart J* 65:597, 1963.
7. Nishimura K, Hibi N, Kato T, et al: Real-time observation of ruptured sinus of Valsalva aneurysm by high speed ultrasono-cardiotomography: report of a case, *Circulation* 53:732, 1976.
8. Matsumoto M, Matsuo H, Beppu S, et al: Echocardiographic diagnosis of ruptured aneurysm of sinus of Valsalva: report of two cases, *Circulation* 53:382, 1976.
9. Rothbaum DA, Dillon JC, Chang S, et al: Echocardiographic manifestation of right sinus of Valsalva aneurysm, *Circulation* 49:768, 1974.
10. Weyman AE, Dillon JC, Feigenbaum H, et al: Premature pulmonic valve opening following sinus of Valsalva aneurysm rupture into the right atrium, *Circulation* 51:556, 1975.

CHAPTER 25

Coronary Artery Fistula

Coronary artery fistula is a rare condition in which a communication exists between a coronary artery and a cardiac chamber or systemic vein. It causes an obligatory shunt from the high-pressure coronary artery to a lower-pressure cardiac chamber.

PATHOLOGIC ANATOMY

The fistula more commonly terminates in the right side of the heart and may be to the superior vena cava, right atrium, coronary sinus, right ventricle, or pulmonary artery (Fig 25–1). However, it may terminate in the left side of the heart, either to the left atrium or the left ventricle. Communications to either peripheral pulmonary artery branches, pulmonary veins or mediastinal veins are extremely rare. Either the right or the left coronary artery may be involved in the fistula, and it may terminate in any of the cardiac chambers.

Because of increased blood flow, the involved coronary artery is dilated and tortuous. In some instances the left-to-right shunt through the fistula may be small, but the afferent coronary arteries may be greatly dilated. Focal saccular aneurysms may develop, which eventually calcify. Because of these aneurysms, the condition has also been called coronary aneurysm or congenital coronary aneurysm. These terms are misleading, because they do not describe the basic abnormality.

Because the fistula allows increased blood flow from the aorta into cardiac chambers, the involved chambers may be dilated in proportion to the volume of shunt.

HEMODYNAMICS

Coronary artery fistula resembles other aortic runoff lesions in that blood leaves the aorta through the fistula during diastole, in this instance entering one of the cardiac chambers. This anomaly causes an obligatory shunt, because it connects the high-pressure aorta with a lower-pressure cardiac chamber. When the shunt is into a right-sided cardiac chamber, the hemodynamics resemble those of an extracardiac left-to-right shunt. Shunt flow occurs during systole and diastole except with fistulas to the left ventricle, which have largely diastolic flow. When the connection is to a left-sided cardiac chamber, the hemodynamics mimic those of aortic insufficiency.

Usually the volume of blood through the fistula is small, but it may be as large as twice the cardiac output. When it is large, a wide aortic pulse pressure is found. Myocardial perfusion may be diminished for that portion of the myocardium supplied by the abnormally connecting coronary artery (hemodynamic steal phenomenon). There are conflicting data on whether the coronary artery fistula and shunt increase with age.[1,2] Spontaneous closure of a fistula has been reported, but is exceedingly rare.[3]

CLINICAL FEATURES

Most children with this condition are eventually recognized by the appearance of a murmur. It rarely causes symptoms, other than angina in an adult. Congestive cardiac failure is rare.

On physical examination, there may be evidence of cardiac enlargement and increased cardiac activity. The first and second heart sounds may be normal or slightly increased if the flow through the heart is moderately increased.

The typical finding is a continuous murmur, which may be loud. It can be distinguished from the murmur of a patent ductus arteriosus, because it sounds more superficial and usually is heard best in an area other than below the left clavicle. In most patients, the murmur is heard along either the left or the right lower sternal borders. When the fistula enters the pulmonary trunk or outflow tract, the murmur is localized along the upper left sternal border. Usually, the systolic portion of this murmur is louder,

TERMINATIONS OF CORONARY ARTERY FISTULAE

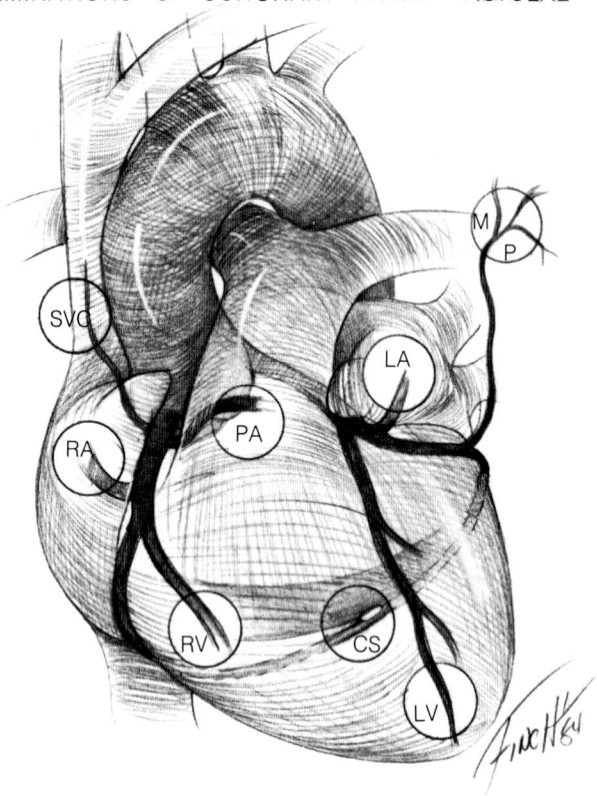

FIG 25-1.
Diagram of external surface of heart and major coronary arterial branches. Sites of termination of coronary artery fistula shown. LA = left atrium; LV = left ventricle; PA = pulmonary artery; RA = right atrium; RV = right ventricle; SVC = superior vena cava; M = mediastinal arteries; P = pulmonary arterial branches, CS = Coronary sinus.

since the pressure difference is greater during that portion of the cardiac cycle, except in connection to the left ventricle, when only a diastolic murmur is heard.

A middiastolic murmur may be present at the apex in patients with considerable left-to-right shunt.

ELECTROCARDIOGRAPHIC FEATURES

The electrocardiogram is usually normal, but in patients with considerable flow, it may show patterns of ventricular hypertrophy. Biventricular hypertrophy develops with a large shunt into the right side of the heart, and left ventricular hypertrophy develops when the fistula involves either the left atrium or left ventricle.

ECHOCARDIOGRAPHIC FEATURES

Cardiac chamber enlargement may be found. The origin of the involved coronary artery is dilated. The fistula may be visible on two-dimensional echocardiography.[4]

RADIOGRAPHIC FEATURES

1. The appearance of the heart and pulmonary vasculature is not uniform. Although the coronary artery fistula is an aortic runoff lesion, the hemodynamic consequences are variable. A fistula into the right side of the heart represents a left-to-right shunt and a fistula into the left-sided cardiac chambers represents an aortic runoff lesion similar to aortic regurgitation.

2. The thoracic roentgenogram may be entirely normal. REASON: A coronary artery fistula is commonly small, sometimes representing only an incidental finding during selective coronary arteriography and not causing significant hemodynamic alterations. The most common small coronary fistula is a communication between the conal branches and the main pulmonary artery.

3. The radiographic appearance of a large coronary artery fistula to the right side of the heart resembles an intracardiac left-to-right shunt, showing cardiomegaly, increased pulmonary vasculature, prominent pulmonary arterial vasculature, and, at times, left atrial enlargement.

4. The heart is enlarged out of proportion to the vol-

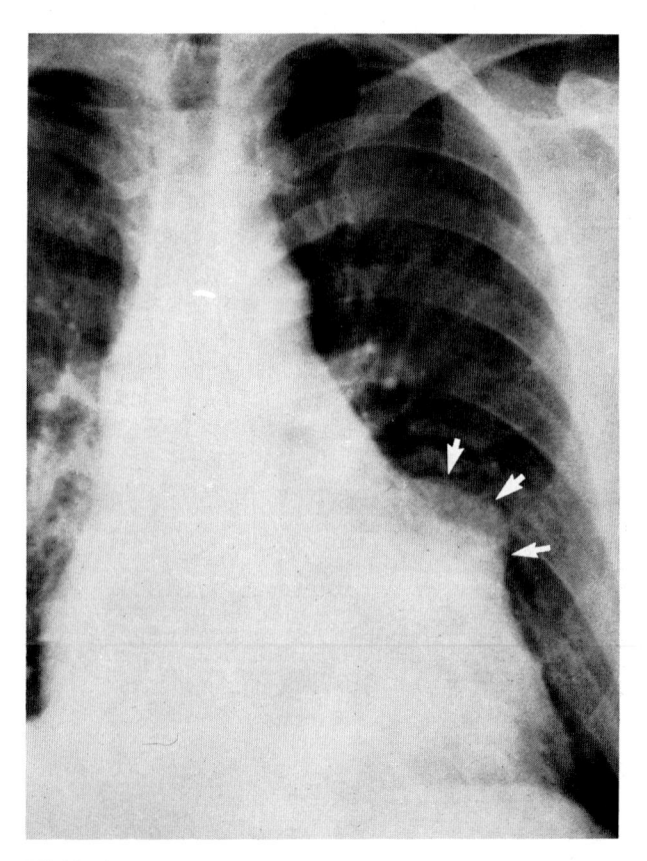

FIG 25-2.
Thoracic roentgenogram, posteroanterior projection in patient with coronary artery fistula. The description of the murmur and the radiographic observation of a small hump *(arrows)* along cardiac border suggested the diagnosis of coronary artery fistula.

ume of left-to-right shunt. REASON: In addition to the hemodynamic effect of the shunt, there is cardiac enlargement from the development of cardiac failure.

5. In most patients, the radiographic diagnosis cannot be made from thoracic roentgenograms unless a saccular aneurysm causes an additional "bump" along the left heart contour (Fig 25–2) or an aneurysm calcifies. Calcification in the fistula provides a valuable radiographic clue but it is very rare, particularly in childhood.

6. Thoracic roentgenographic findings in patients with a left-sided communication are usually normal. REASON: The volume of blood flow through such communication is usually minimal and causes minor hemodynamic change.

CARDIAC CATHETERIZATION

If the fistula is small, the shunt cannot be detected by oximetry sampling in the right side of the heart. With a large shunt, an increase in oxygen saturation will be found in the right side of the heart, being detected in the chamber where the fistula terminates. When the fistula is to a left-sided cardiac chamber, it cannot be detected by oximetry.

Pulmonary arterial and right ventricular pressures are usually normal. When they are elevated, rarely is it to more than half the systemic level.

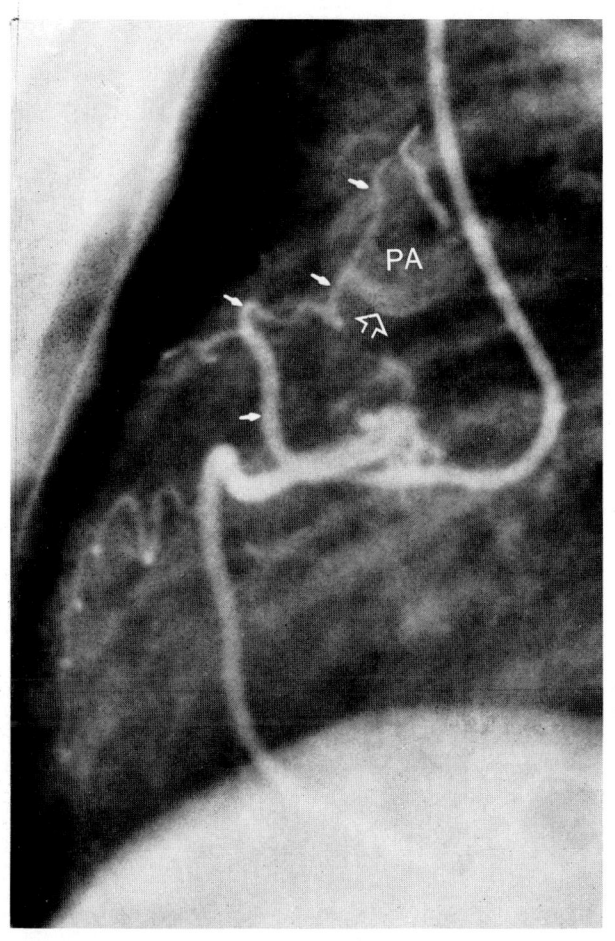

FIG 25–3.
Selective right coronary arteriogram; diastolic frame with pulmonary valve closed *(open arrow)*. Enlarged right conal branch *(arrows)* in patient with chest pain; probably unrelated to fistulous communication with pulmonary artery. Right conal branch is enlarged *(small arrows)*, and there is opacification of pulmonary artery *(PA)*.

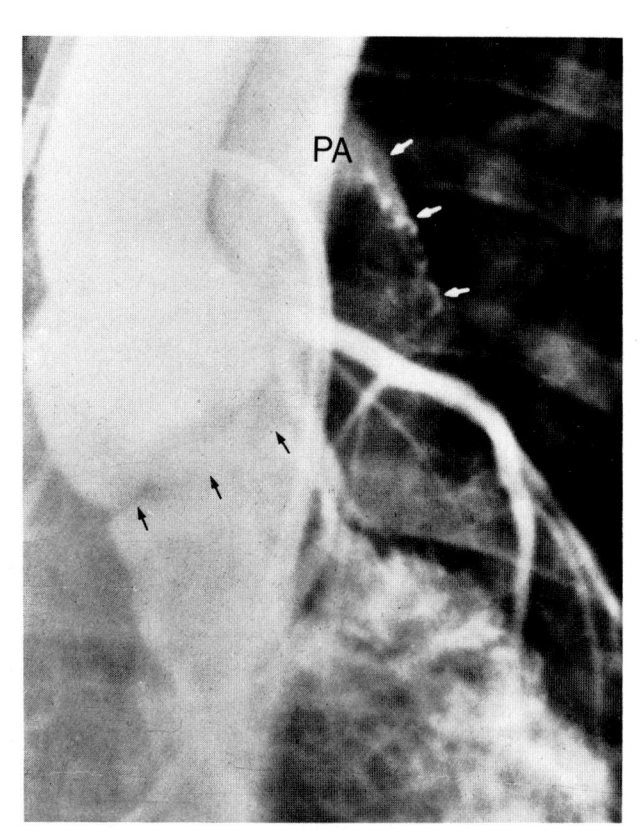

FIG 25–4.
Left ventriculogram; anteroposterior projection in patient with membranous subaortic stenosis *(small black arrows)*. Incidental coronary artery fistula *(white arrows)* from the left conal branch to the pulmonary artery *(PA)* is faintly opacified. The fistula is probably of no clinical importance. In our experience, fistulas of right or left conal branches to pulmonary artery are the most common. Their clincial significance is uncertain.

ANGIOGRAPHIC APPEARANCE

Selective coronary arteriography is essential for exact delineation of the fistula. Aortography can provide the diagnosis in patients with a large fistula and provide guidance for subsequent selective coronary arteriography.

1. A small fistula results in only minor coronary arterial dilatation and very faint filling of the receiving chamber.

2. Small fistulas are frequently found from the conal arteries to the pulmonary artery (Fig 25–3). Such lesions

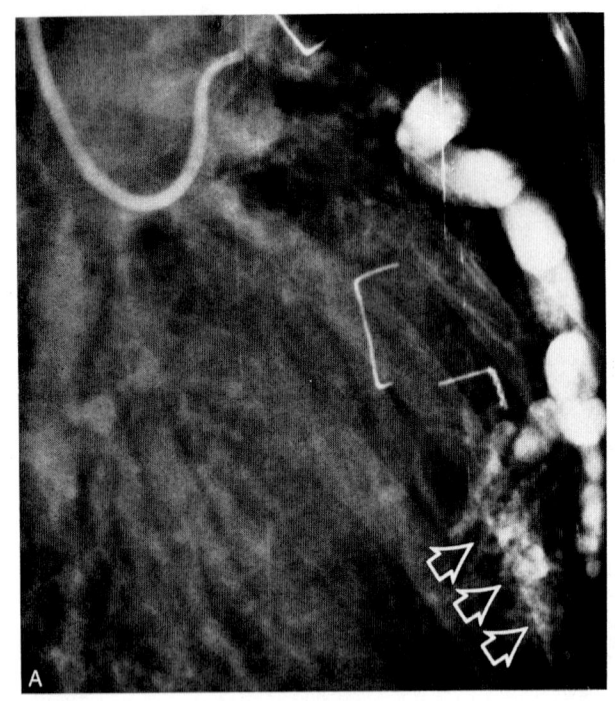

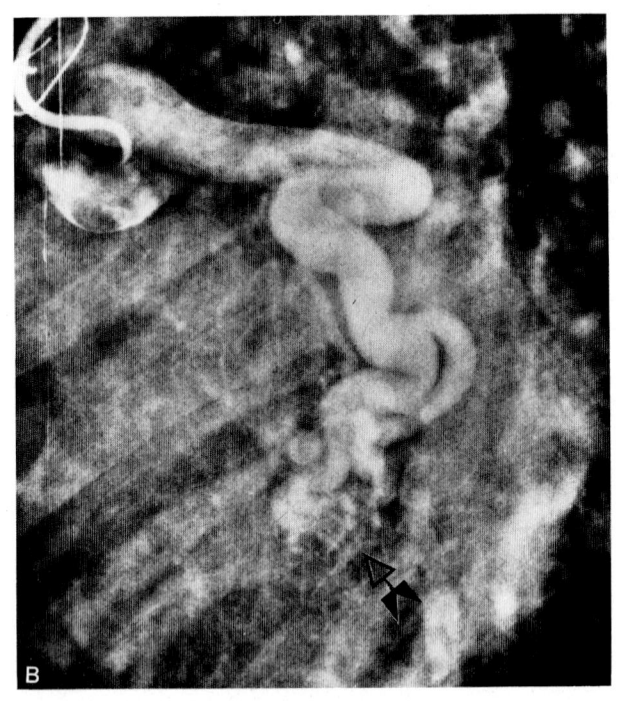

FIG 25–5.
Selective left coronary arteriogram in patient with transposition of the great arteries. **A,** right anterior oblique projection; left anterior descending coronary artery arises from posterior cusp and forms a fistula with left ventricle *(arrows)*. Marked dilatation and tortuosity of left anterior descending coronary artery indicates large blood flow. **B,** left anterior oblique projection; large left anterior descending coronary artery. Numerous tiny communications *(arrows)* within the septum and left ventricle *(arrow)*. Involvement of ventricular septum and diffuse nature of fistula rule out surgical correction.

are commonly identified as an incidental finding during cardiac catheterization for another condition (Fig 25–4) or at time of coronary arteriography.

3. Small communications between the left coronary artery and left ventricle are a common incidental finding of coronary angiography. A small blush of contrast medium can be seen entering the left ventricular cavity during diastole. Communication probably occurs through a normal connection between the myocardium and the left ventricular cavity and is of no clinical importance. To the best of our knowledge, this communication does not enlarge with time. These same communications provide egress of blood from the ventricle into the coronary arteries (sinusoids) in pulmonary atresia.

4. Blood flow through a large anomalously connecting coronary artery is markedly increased. REASON: Normally, the coronary blood flow represents only about 10% of the cardiac output because of the relatively high resistance in the myocardium. With an arteriovenous malformation, resistance to flow is decreased, and therefore the coronary blood flow is markedly increased. Selective coronary angiography must be performed by injecting a large amount of contrast medium rapidly. Best results are obtained if a large (8F) catheter is used.

5. Opacification of the right-sided receiving cardiac chamber occurs throughout the cardiac cycle, because the

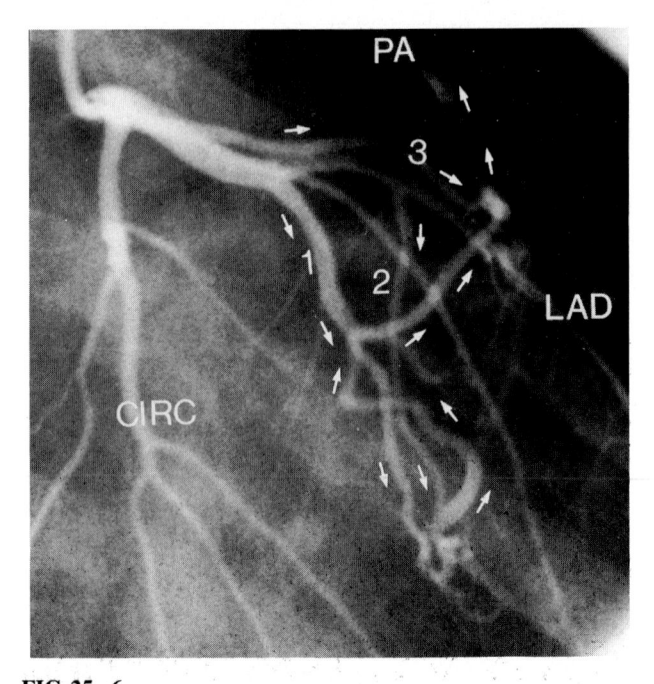

FIG 25–6.
Selective left coronary arteriogram demonstrating a coronary fistula with the pulmonary artery. Feeders come from the first *(1)*, second *(2)*, and a diagonal branch *(3)*. In spite of multiple inflow, the patient can be surgically cured by oversewing the single entry to the pulmonary artery.

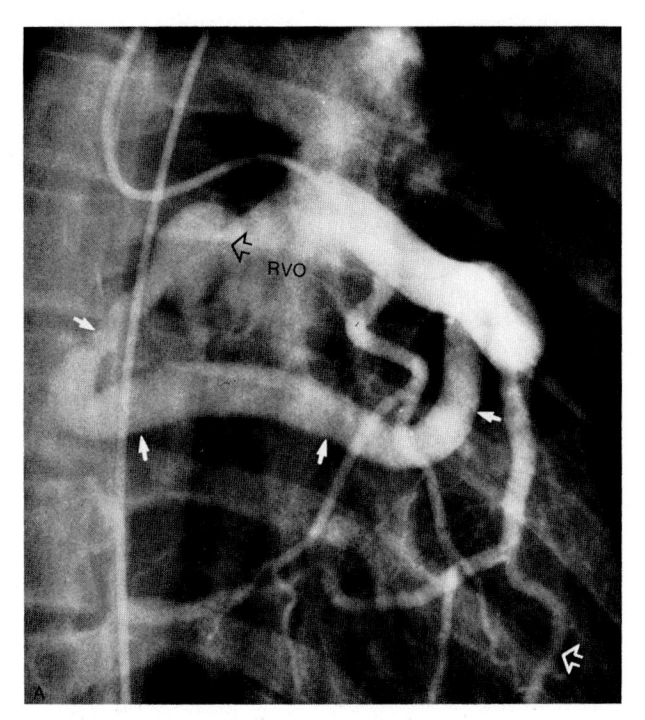

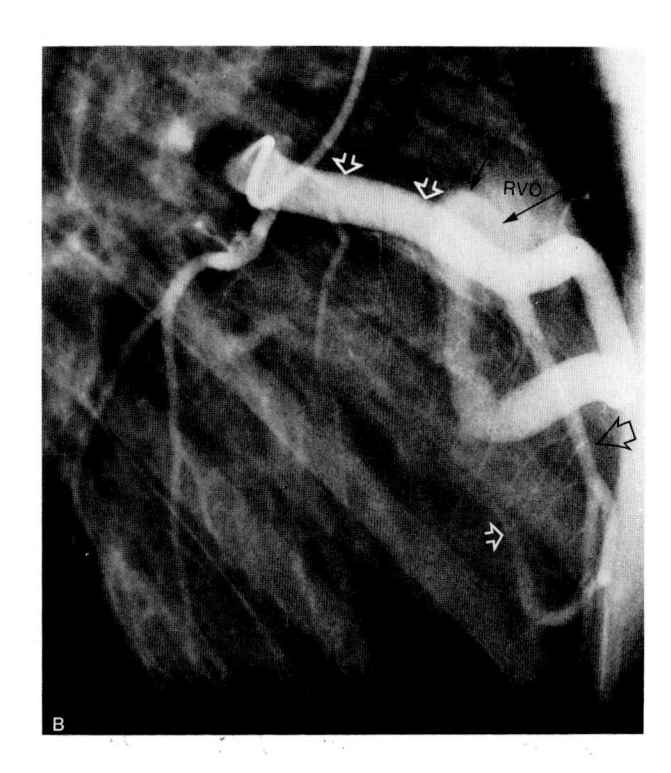

FIG 25-7.
Selective coronary arteriogram in patient with coronary artery fistula. **A,** anteroposterior projection; large single coronary artery fistula with the right ventricular outflow tract *(RVO)*. At the communication, the afferent artery forms an aneurysm *(open black arrow)*. Fistula is supplied by a single branch from left anterior descending coronary artery, being a low left conal branch *(white arrows)*. Left anterior descending coronary artery distal to the fistula appears of normal size but shows delayed opacification *(white open arrow)* because of hemodynamic runoff. **B,** lateral projection. Marked enlargement of left anterior descending coronary artery to level of origin of feeding branch *(open white arrows)*. Distal left anterior descending coronary artery is of normal caliber *(open black arrows)*, but opacification is delayed because of runoff into right ventricle. Right ventricular outflow tract is densely opacified by fistula *(RVO)*. Aneurysm is visible *(black arrow)*.

systolic and diastolic pressures in the aorta are higher than in the cardiac chamber. The speed of flow varies during the cardiac cycle. This is best observed in the main pulmonary artery so even very small amounts of contrast media can be seen. Cine coronary angiography therefore is a very sensitive means of detecting even a tiny fistula.

6. Both coronary arteries and even the mediastinal vessels may be involved in the fistula.

7. The fistula may be single, multiple, or have an angiomatous appearance (Fig 25-5).

8. Coronary artery fistulas usually have numerous feeders (Fig 25-6), obviating surgical ligation or embolization. Surgical cure can be accomplished by oversewing the communications to the ventricular chambers or pulmonary artery.

9. Only the portion of the coronary artery proximal to the fistula is enlarged. The distal segment of the coronary artery is of normal size but may show delayed and decreased opacification because of the effect of the fistula on distal flow (hemodynamic steal) (Fig 25-7).

10. With a large fistula, the involved coronary artery is markedly dilated, and saccular aneurysms may be observed (Fig 25-8).

11. Rarely, the coronary artery fistula occurs to the coronary sinus (see Fig 25-8,B) or left atrium (Fig 25-9).

OPERATIVE CONSIDERATIONS

Whether chest pain can be caused by small coronary artery fistulas is uncertain. Larger communications represent a hemodynamic burden and may cause myocardial ischemia. Almost all coronary artery fistulas can be repaired by surgery except the diffuse angiomatous communications, as in Figure 25-5.

Surgical treatment should be performed in midchildhood and can be carried out with low risk. Selective angiography is essential to demonstrate the number of feeding branches. If a single nonessential branch is involved, it can be ligated. In many cases, it is preferable to open the cardiac chamber or pulmonary artery and repair the mouth of the fistula from the inside either by direct stitches or a patch. By doing so, most coronary artery fistulas can be eliminated. The fistula is divided at the entrance to the cardiac chamber. Rarely do signs of ischemia develop after

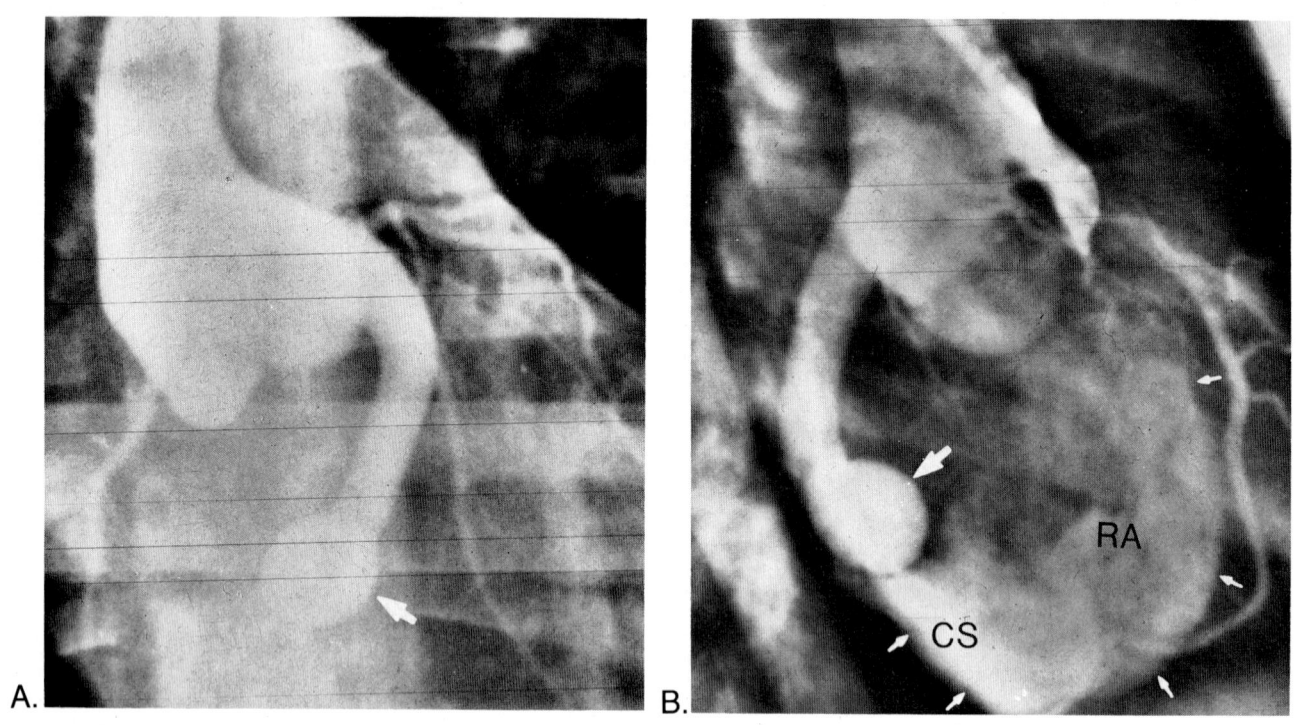

FIG 25–8.
Aortogram in anteroposterior (**A**) and lateral (**B**) projections. Huge circumflex coronary artery with fistulous communication to coronary sinus *(CS)*. At site of communication, there is a saccular aneurysm *(large arrow)*. Branches not involved in fistula appear of normal size. Dense opacification of right atrium *(RA) (small white arrows)* on lateral projection indicates a large shunt. This fistula was closed by operation.

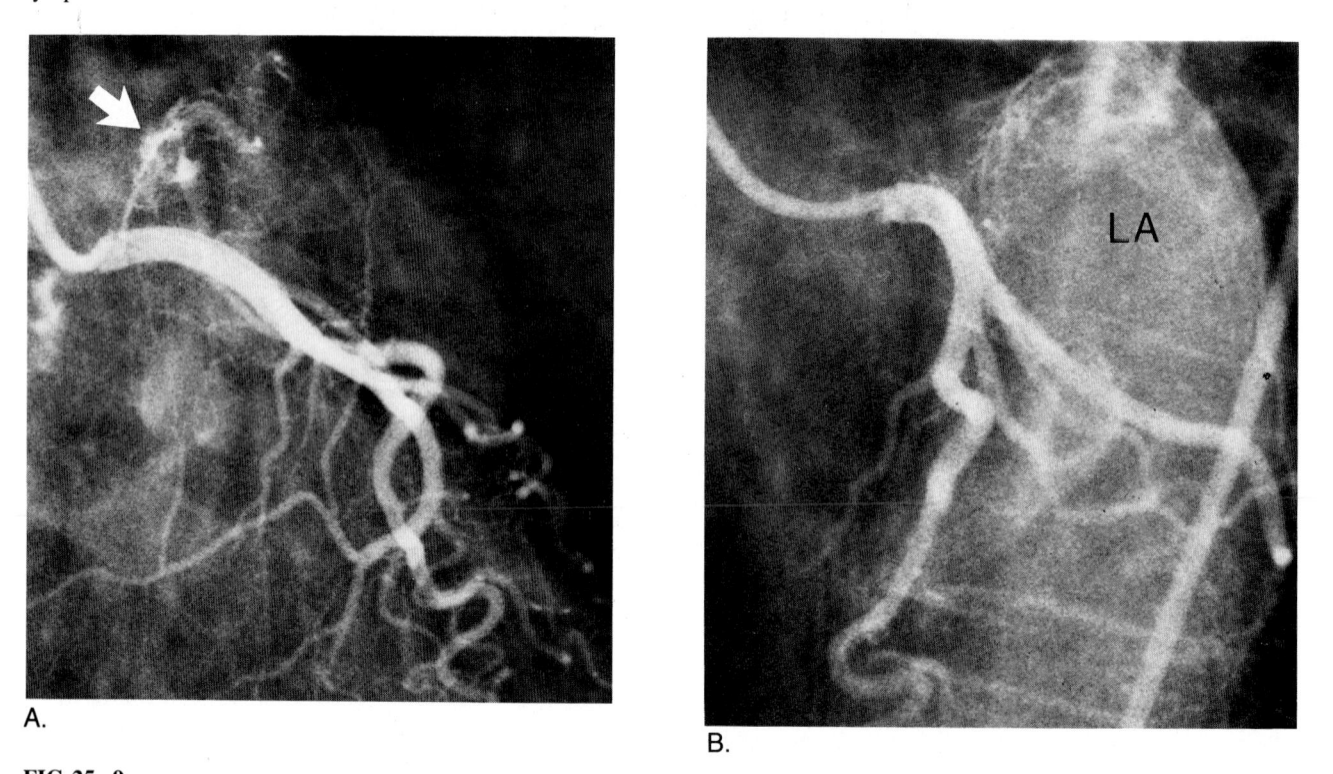

FIG 25–9.
Selective left coronary arteriogram. **A**, several small feeding arteries *(arrows)* are seen to feed a fistula with the left atrium. **B**, left anterior oblique projection shows fistula and faint opacification of the left atrium.

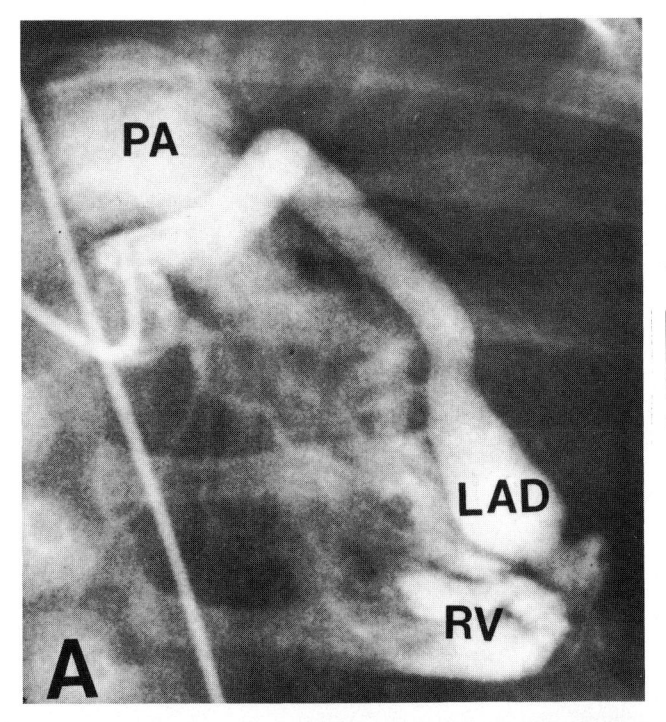

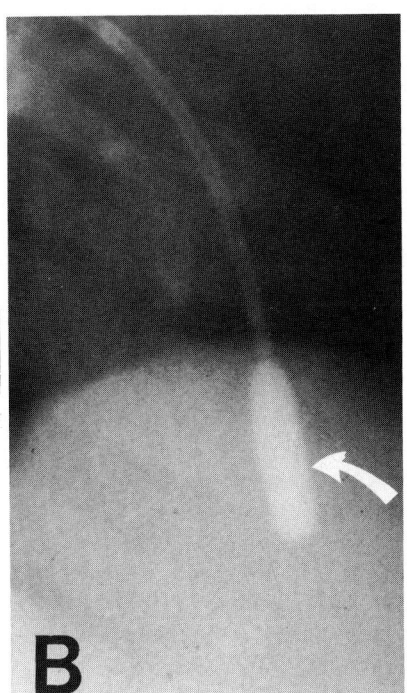

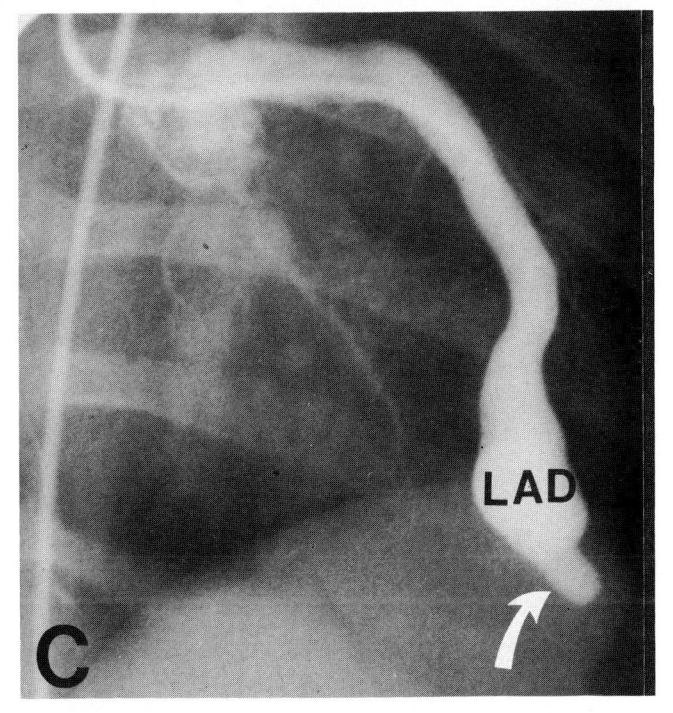

ligation. Anerurysmectomy is not required. Fistulas that have single inflow and are peripheral can be closed by detachable balloons or coils (Fig 25–10).

POSTOPERATIVE APPEARANCE

After closure of a large coronary fistula, heart size returns rapidly toward normal. REASON: The hemodynamic burden of the left-to-right shunt and the hemodynamic steal phenomenon are eliminated, providing adequate myocardial perfusion.

FIG 25–10.
A, right anterior oblique selective left coronary arteriogram demonstrating a huge left anterior descending artery *(LAD)* communicating at the apex with the right ventricle *(RV)*. The pulmonary artery is opacified *(PA)*. No branches of the left anterior descending artery are opacified, consistent with a hemodynamic steal. **B,** same projection during placement of detachable balloon, which is seen injected with contrast medium *(arrow)*. **C,** repeat injection demonstrates the balloon in good position *(arrow)*, and there is complete occlusion of the fistulas. Side branches of the left anterior descending artery are now better opacified.

REFERENCES

1. Liberthson RR, Sagar K, Berkoben JP, et al: Congenital coronary arteriovenous fistula: report of 13 patients, review of

the literature and delineation of management, *Circulation* 59:849, 1979.
2. Jaffe RB, Glancy DL, Epstein SE, et al: Coronary arterial–right heart fistulae: long-term observations in seven patients, *Circulation* 47:133, 1973.
3. Mühler E, Keutel J, von Bernuth G: Spontanverschluβ einer angeborenen Koronararterienfistel, *Z Kardiol* 73:538–540, 1984.
4. Reeder GS, Tajik AJ, Smith HC: Visualization of coronary artery fistula by two-dimensional echocardiography, *Mayo Clin Proc* 55:185, 1980.
5. Edis AJ, Schattenberg TT, Feldt RH, et al: Congenital coronary artery fistula: surgical considerations and results of operation, *Mayo Clin Proc* 47:567, 1972.
6. Gasul BM, Arcilla RA, Fell EH, et al: Congenital coronary arteriovenous fistula: clinical, phonocardiographic, angiocardiographic and hemodynamic studies in five patients, *Pediatrics* 25:531, 1960.

PART THREE

Introduction to Outflow Obstructive Lesions

The conditions that cause obstruction to ventricular outflow represent about 25% of all instances of congenital heart disease. These conditions may occur in the outflow tract of the right ventricle, in the outflow tract of the left ventricle, or within the aorta. The anatomic form of the obstructive lesion may vary considerably. They increase the pressure proximal to the obstruction, to a degree proportional to the severity of obstruction and the volume of cardiac output. Provided the myocardium is normal, the primary ventricular response to the obstruction is ventricular hypertrophy. Dilatation of the involved ventricle can occur in neonates or in older children who develop myocardial abnormalities over a period of time, secondary to the sustained pressure elevation. In addition, turbulent blood flow through the stenotic area causes a murmur and often poststenotic dilatation, which has distinctive radiographic findings.

Although many patients with obstructive lesions are asymptomatic during childhood, in perhaps 10% of the cases the obstruction is severe enough to cause congestive heart failure in the neonatal period. In neonates or infants with severe pulmonary stenosis, cyanosis may occur because elevated right atrial pressure stretches the foramen ovale and permits a right-to-left atrial shunt. Thus, severe pulmonary stenosis with right-to-left atrial shunt must be considered in the differential diagnosis of patients with cyanosis and decreased pulmonary vasculature.

Most of the patients with obstructive lesions can be operated on or treated by balloon dilatation. The operative mortality is low. Although in patients with aortic stenosis or coarctation of the aorta, residual abnormalities frequently persist after the procedures. The radiographic diagnosis of the major obstructive lesions can be made with a high degree of accuracy.

CHAPTER 26

Aortic Stenosis

Obstruction to left ventricular outflow may occur at one of several sites. In most instances, it occurs at the level of the aortic valve in the form of either a bicuspid or, less commonly, a unicuspid unicommissural aortic valve. Less common forms of aortic stenosis are supravalvar aortic stenosis and subaortic stenosis. In this section, we discuss:

1. Valvar aortic stenosis.
2. Discrete membranous subaortic stenosis.
3. Supravalvar aortic stenosis.
4. Muscular subaortic stenosis.

Aortic valvar atresia and aortic stenosis with hypoplastic left ventricle are not discussed subsequently, because the clinical picture is that of pulmonary venous obstruction, and cyanosis is present.

GENERAL CONSIDERATIONS

Although there are unique hemodynamic, clinical, and laboratory features of each of the four major forms of aortic stenosis, there are common hemodynamic consequences of the aortic obstruction, regardless of its site. The primary effect of the obstruction can be understood by the formula

$$AVA \cong \frac{\text{Cardiac output}}{\sqrt{\text{LVSP} - \text{AO}}}$$

where AVA = aortic valve area, LVSP = left ventricular systolic pressure, and AO = aortic pressure. This indicates the relation between the size of the stenotic aortic valve orifice, the cardiac output, and the gradient across the valve.[1]

In most children with aortic stenosis, the cardiac output is normal, and despite the stenosis, the aortic systolic pressure is normal or only slightly reduced. Therefore, the major change in gradient occurs because of an increase in left ventricular systolic pressure.

From the formula, it is apparent that:

1. With more severe stenosis (i.e., reduced AVA), the left ventricular systolic pressure increases to maintain a normal cardiac output.
2. An increased cardiac output, as during exercise, is accomplished through elevation of the left ventricular systolic pressure.

Left ventricular hypertrophy develops in response to elevated left ventricular systolic pressure. Left ventricular dilatation is a late finding, at the time the left ventricle decompensates.

Subendocardial myocardial ischemia[2–4] occurs in infants and some children with more severe aortic stenosis and may be associated with clinical manifestations of ST-T wave changes on the electrocardiogram (ECG), anginal chest pain, and syncope. Two mechanisms may explain the ischemia: (1) the elevated left ventricular systolic pressure, which may compress the subendocardial myocardium; and (2) an imbalance between the myocardial oxygen supply and the increased demand caused by elevated left ventricular systolic pressure, heart rate, and myocardial mass. Eventually, myocardial fibrosis results. If it is extensive, left ventricular dilatation occurs and eventually congestive cardiac failure develops.

In all forms of aortic stenosis, the symptoms vary according to the degree of obstruction. Mild obstruction causes no symptoms, whereas severe forms lead to heart failure in infancy. Unicuspid aortic valves cause more severe obstruction than do bicuspid aortic valves. An infant with severe symptomatic aortic stenosis, therefore, almost invariably has a unicuspid aortic valve.[5]

VALVAR AORTIC STENOSIS

Valvar aortic stenosis may occur as an isolated condition or coexist with coarctation of the aorta or hypoplasia of the left ventricle.

Clinical Features

Aortic stenosis is usually recognized by finding a murmur at birth or in infancy.[6, 7] Most patients grow and develop normally, but in 13% of our patients with valvar aortic stenosis who were catheterized, congestive cardiac failure had developed during the first year of life. After the first year of life, cardiac failure rarely occurs during childhood.

Most patients are asymptomatic throughout childhood but may have mild complaints of fatigue or dyspnea. Two symptoms are important and indicate severe stenosis:

1. Anginal chest pain, which indicates myocardial ischemia and, generally, a left ventricular systolic pressure greater than 200 mm Hg. It may be associated with ST segment depression in lead V_5 and V_6 on a resting ECG. Sudden death may occur in such patients.
2. Syncope, the exact mechanism of which is unknown. It may be related to a reflex mechanism or occur as a complication of myocardial ischemia with decrease of cardiac output. Syncope usually occurs on exercise and may be fatal.

Physical Examination

Most children with valvar aortic stenosis appear robust and healthy. The blood pressure is normal, or occasionally there is a narrowed pulse pressure. On palpation of the thorax, the cardiac apex is normally located, but there may be an apical left ventricular heave from left ventricular hypertrophy. A thrill is present in the suprasternal notch and often below the right clavicle.

Auscultation is characteristic. The first heart sound is normal and followed by an apical systolic ejection click from the poststenotic dilatation of the ascending aorta. A systolic ejection murmur, usually grade 3 to 4/6, follows the click and is heard maximally in the aortic area and less well along the midleft sternal border. The murmur radiates to the neck, particularly the right side.

In one half of school-aged children with aortic stenosis from bicuspid aortic valve, a soft (grade 1–2/6) high-pitched early diastolic murmur of aortic insufficiency is present along the midleft sternal border.

Electrocardiographic Features

Although there are rough correlations between the ECG tracings and the severity of aortic stenosis, they are not specific enough to be uniformly predictive of the left ventricular systolic pressure.

In patients with mild stenosis, the ECG is normal. Among patients with moderate or severe stenosis, a pattern of left ventricular hypertrophy is usually present. The pattern of hypertrophy often shows deep S waves in lead V_1 and a normal R in lead V_6. The depth of the q wave is reduced in lead V_6.

In severe stenosis, ST segment depression, reduction in amplitude, and then inversion of the T wave in left precordial leads indicate myocardial ischemia.

The ECG is more helpful than the chest roentgenogram in monitoring a patient with valvar aortic stenosis.

Echocardiographic Features

Because, in a bicuspid aortic valve, the aortic cusps are of unequal size, the echocardiogram shows an eccentric diastolic echo of the valve within the aorta (Fig 26–1). There are usually multiple diastolic echoes from the aortic valve because the leaflets are thickened.[8]

The left ventricular posterior wall and the interventricular septum are thickened, and various methods of measurements of these structures have been used to determine the severity of the stenosis.[9–11]

If aortic regurgitation is present, flutter of the anterior leaflet of the mitral valve is found.

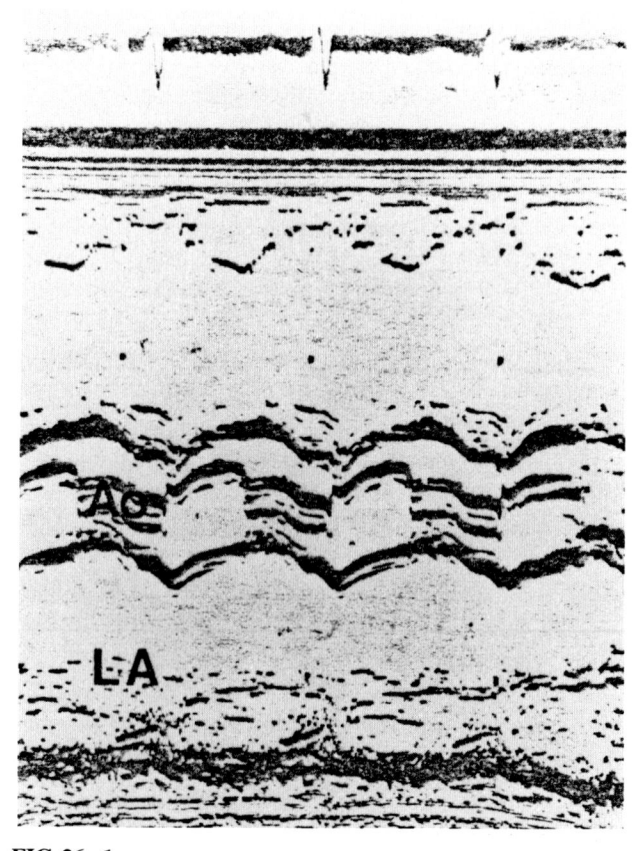

FIG 26–1.
Echocardiogram in patient with valvar aortic stenosis. Aorta *(Ao)* and left atrium *(LA)* seen. Multiple diastolic echoes of aortic valve.

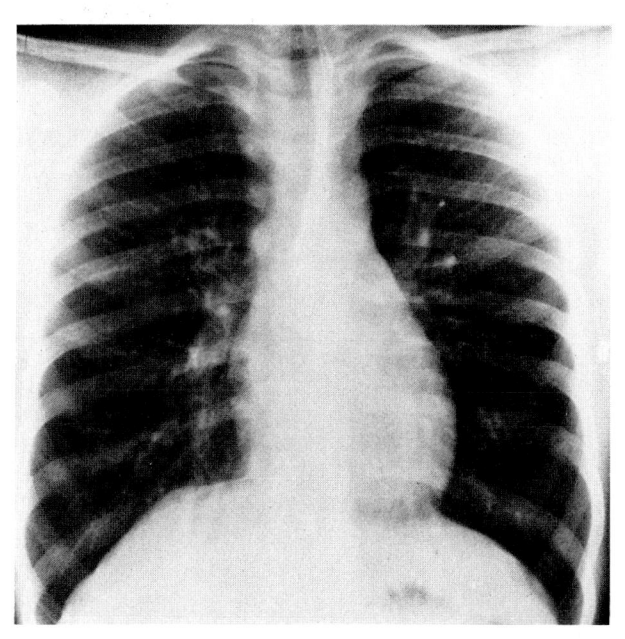

FIG 26–2.
Thoracic roentgenogram in patients with severe valvar aortic stenosis may be entirely normal as long as the left ventricle remains compensated. Left ventricular hypertrophy may not be visible on thoracic radiograph. Murmur, ECG, and echocardiogram are the most helpful diagnostic findings. Normal thoracic roentgenogram, therefore, cannot exclude severe aortic stenosis; this patient had a 100 mm Hg pressure gradient across aortic valve.

Radiographic Features

1. Normal cardiac silhouette and vasculature are seen in most compensated cases (Fig 26–2).
2. The ascending aorta is prominent. This is best seen on a left anterior oblique projection (Fig 26–3). In most patients, however, the ascending aorta tends to be within normal range. Interpretation of the films therefore must be carried out in light of the clinical findings (ECG and murmur of aortic stenosis) and the patient's age (Fig 26–4).
3. Left ventricular enlargement indicates decompensation or associated aortic reflux (Fig 26–5).
4. In infancy, decompensation results in severe generalized cardiomegaly and left atrial enlargement (Fig 26–6).
5. Decompensation may also be evident by cephalization and Kerley B lines, but these are not found in infancy (Fig 26–7).
6. Poststenotic dilatation may be severe, causing a radiographic mediastinal mass density (Fig 26–8,A and B).

Later in life (30–50 years), the aortic valve calcifies, and the gradient increases. There also is a gradual increase in poststenotic dilatation. Isolated aortic valvar stenosis in a man could be either acquired or congenital; if there is marked poststenotic dilatation, the stenosis probably is

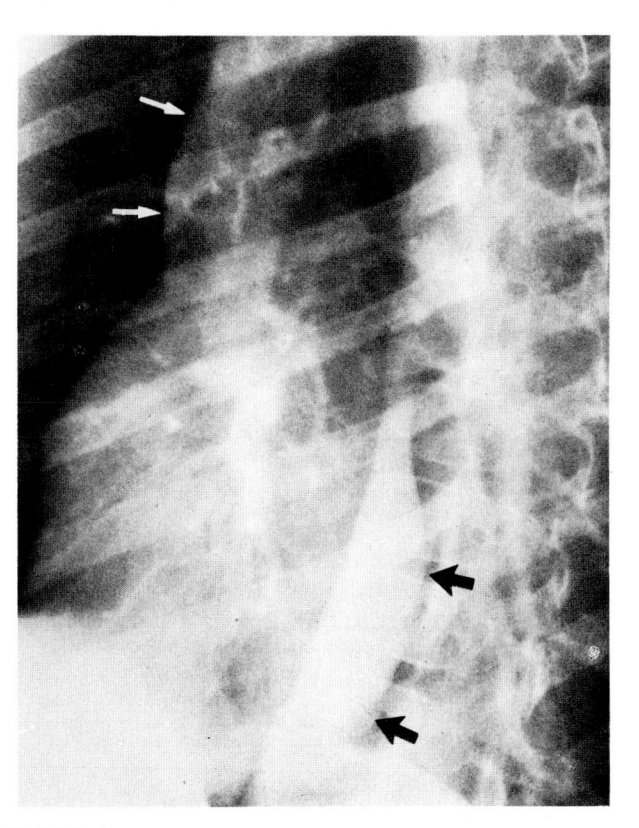

FIG 26–3.
Left anterior oblique projection in patient with valvar aortic stenosis, showing prominence of the ascending aorta caused by poststenotic dilation *(white arrows)*. Left ventricular enlargement *(black arrows)* indicates left ventricular decompensation or associated aortic reflux.

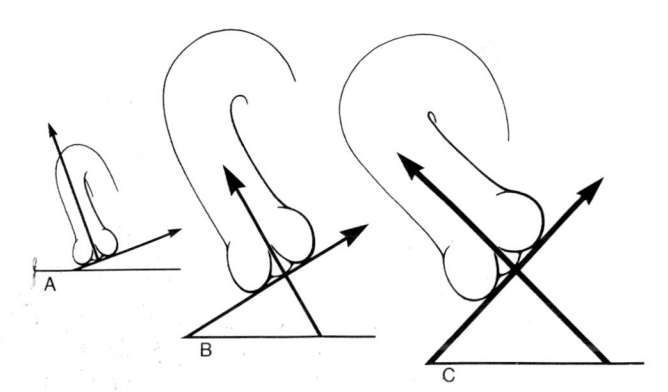

FIG 26–4.
Appearance of normal aorta on posteroanterior projection of thoracic roentgenogram. **A,** infant. Aorta has a more vertical course, not seen because of large thymus. **B,** adolescent. Normal aorta or superior vena cava may form superior right cardiac border. **C,** adult. Right cardiac border is formed by ascending aorta. REASON: Atherosclerosis with elongation of aorta, resulting in "uncoiling." With increasing age, aortic valve plane becomes more vertical *(arrows)*. Two important considerations for judging aortic prominence are the age of the patient and the rotation of the chest film. The posteroanterior projection must be obtained perfectly straight, because slight left anterior oblique rotation results in false prominence of the ascending aorta.

420 Outflow Obstructive Lesions

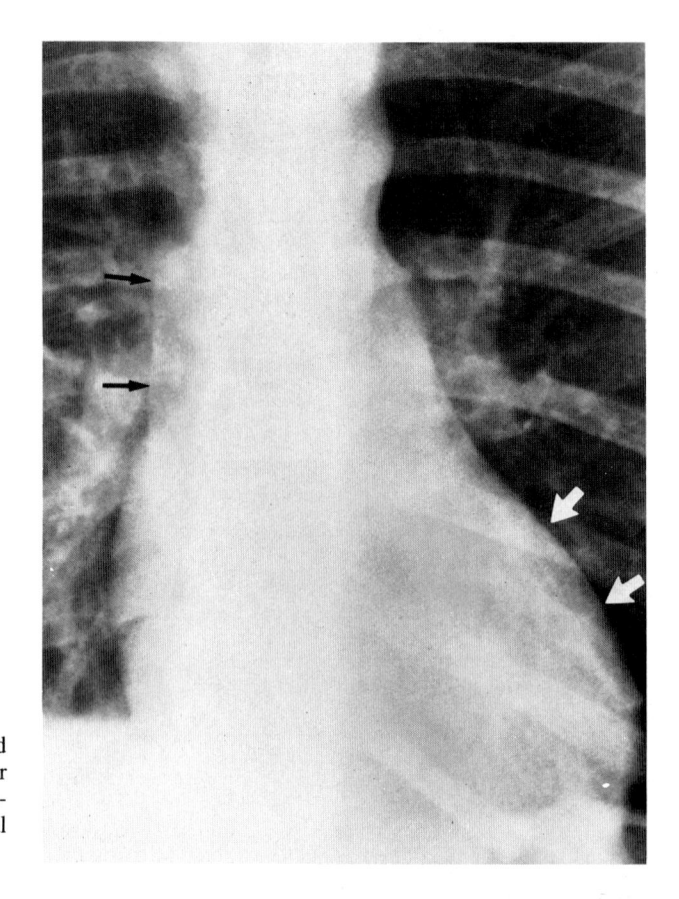

FIG 26–5.
Congential aortic stenosis with left ventricular decompensation and left ventricular enlargement *(white arrows)*. Isolated left ventricular hypertrophy may be difficult to detect by roentgen examination. Ascending aorta *(black arrows)* slightly prominent but within normal range.

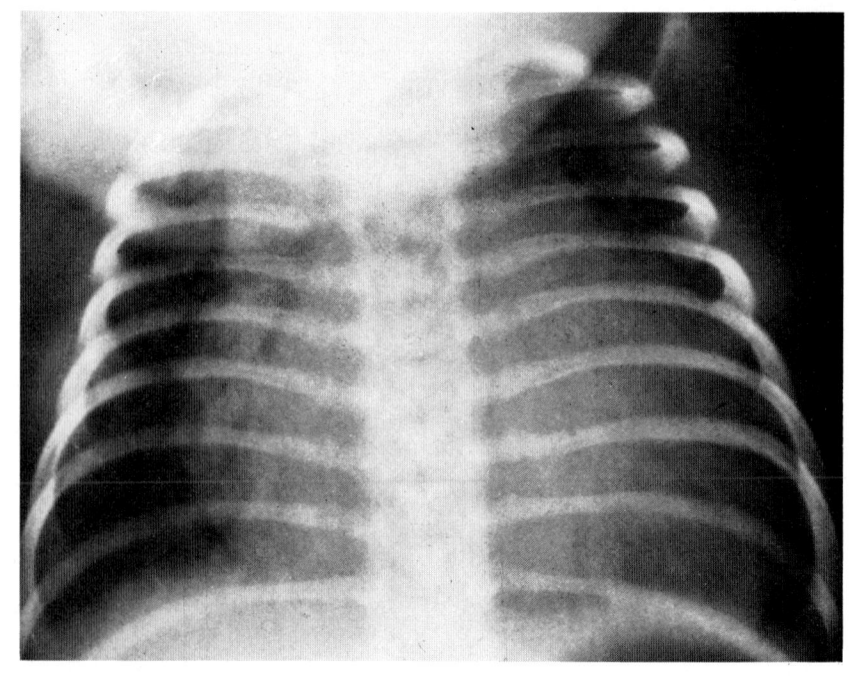

FIG 26–6.
Thoracic roentgenogram, posteroanterior projection in patient with decompensated aortic stenosis. Diffuse generalized cardiomegaly. Congestive pulmonary vasculature is not seen because both hila are overshadowed by cardiac silhouette. Pleural effusion does not occur. Left atrial enlargement present from increased end-diastolic pressure in left ventricle. Radiographic findings are nonspecific but consistent with decompensated aortic stenosis. Older patients with aortic stenosis usually do not have left atrial enlargement until decompensation occurs.

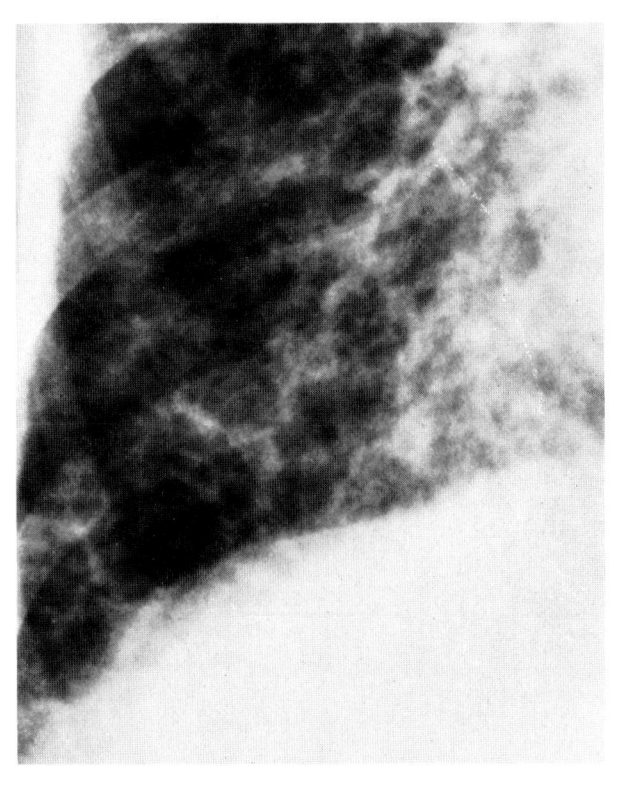

FIG 26–7.
Thoracic roentgenogram, posteroanterior projection of decompensated aortic stenosis in a 6-year-old patient. Pulmonary congestion and Kerley B lines. Rare radiographic manifestation of increased venous pressure as a result of left ventricular decompensation. Pleural effusion almost never observed in infancy and childhood. Kerley B lines are rarely present in left ventricular decompensation occuring in children. If they do occur, as in this patient, they are not as typical as in mitral obstructive disease.

congenital. In a woman, isolated calcific aortic stenosis is virtually always pathognomonic of a congenital lesion (Fig 26–8,C). REASON: In women, rheumatic fever manifests itself predominantly in mitral valvar disease.

Cardiac Catheterization

Cardiac catheterization is performed to:

1. Determine the location of aortic outflow obstruction.
2. Determine the severity of aortic outflow obstruction.
3. Identify coexisting cardiac malformations. However, these are rare. Aortic insufficiency is present in 50% of patients. An occasional infant shows mitral insufficiency, in part from infarction of papillary muscles.[2] An association between aortic stenosis and angiodysplasia of the cecum has been demonstrated. If a patient with aortic stenosis presents with lower gastrointestinal bleeding, angiodysplasia is the most likely diagnosis.[12, 13]

Indications for cardiac catheterization are as follows:

1. Any infant or child with valvar aortic stenosis and congestive cardiac failure.
2. Any infant or child with signs or symptoms suggesting myocardial ischemia or severe aortic stenosis.
3. As an elective procedure in an asymptomatic child to measure gradient and perform balloon valvuloplasty.

At cardiac catheterization, the oximetry data and right-sided cardiac pressures are normal, except in the infant with cardiac failure, in whom the wedge pressure is elevated. The left ventricular end-diastolic pressure rises, causing an increase in left atrial and, subsequently, wedge pressure.

A systolic pressure gradient is found across the aortic valve (Fig 26–9). Left ventricular end-diastolic pressure is usually normal but may be elevated in patients with a markedly hypertrophied left ventricle or with left ventricular failure.

Pathology and Angiographic Anatomy

1. The normal aortic valve consists of three independent cusps (Fig 26–10,1-A).
2. The free margin of all three valves equals three diameters of the aortic circumference, allowing unrestricted movement.
3. Consequently, during systole, the normal aortic valve leaflets approximate the aortic wall (Fig 26–10,1-B) and look straight angiographically (Fig 26–10,1-C).
4. Three types of aortic valvar stenosis occur:
    a. Unicommissural or unicuspid valve (Fig 26–10,2-A).
    b. Bicuspid aortic valve (Fig 26–10,3-A).
    c. Tricuspid valve with fused commissures (extremely rare).
5. In unicommissural aortic valve, two of the commissures either are fused or do not develop.[14] The free margin of the aortic valve leaflets of the orifice equals, at most, one diameter of the aortic anulus. Consequently, during systole, the aortic orifice is constricted and the valve domes (Fig 26–10,2-C).
6. In a bicuspid valve, one of the commissures is fused or does not develop.[15] The free margin of the aortic orifice equals two diameters. Therefore, during systole, the aortic orifice is restricted and the valve domes (Fig 26–10,3-C). One of the cusps is oversized, and the other partially divided by a small raphae (Fig 26–10,3-A and 3-B).
7. Because the free margin of the bicuspid valve is greater than the free margin of a unicuspid valve, the stenosis is usually more severe with unicuspid valve, and the

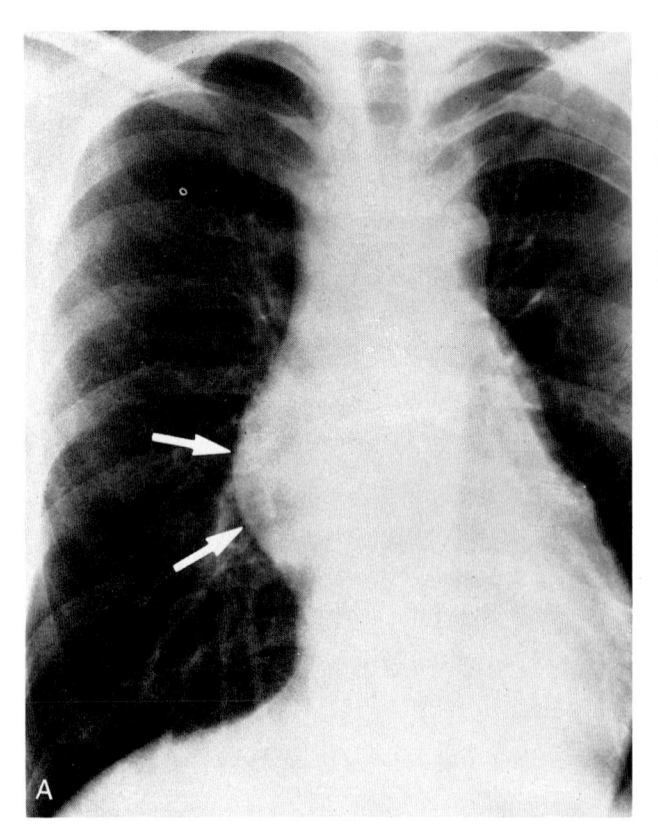

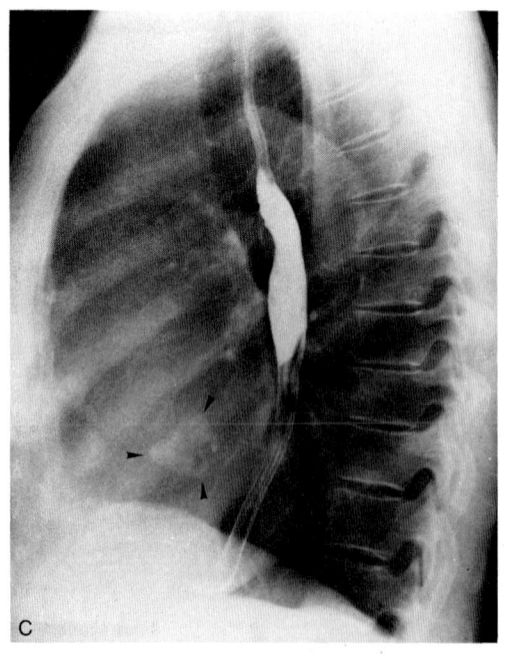

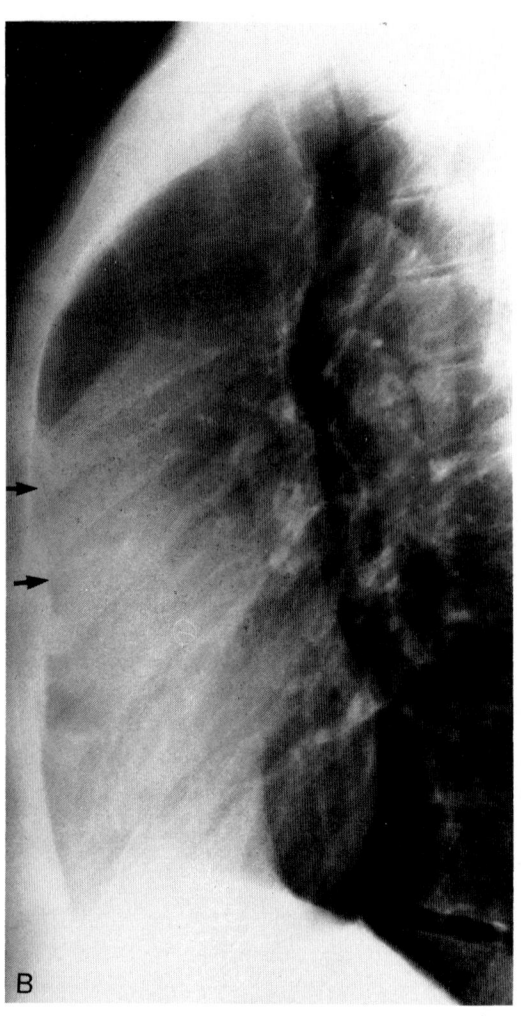

FIG 26–8.
Aortic stenosis as seen on thoracic roentgenogram. **A,** posteroanterior projection; severe poststenotic dilation of the ascending aorta that could be mistaken for a mediastinal mass. **B,** lateral projection; retrosternal space is obliterated by enormously dilated ascending aorta *(black arrows)*. Fluoroscopy may be helpful in demonstrating a calcified aortic valve, which is almost always present in adult patients with congenital aortic stenosis. **C,** lateral projection; densely calcified aortic stenosis. Marked poststenotic dilation (filled-in retrosternal space) is virtually diagnostic of congenital aortic stenosis.

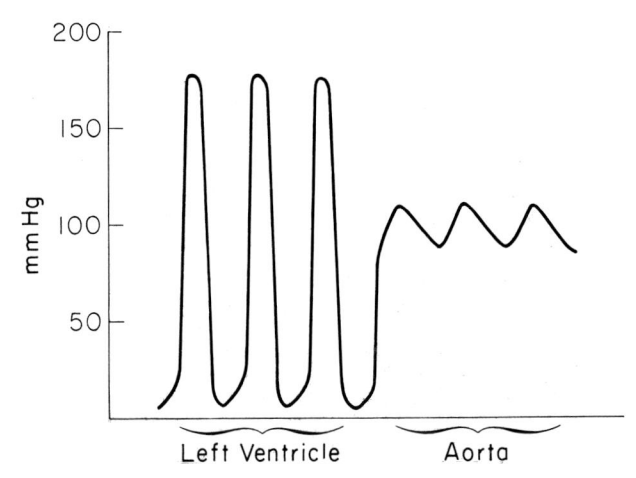

FIG 26–9.
Diagram of pressure tracing of patient with valvar aortic stenosis; abrupt pressure gradient is recorded at level of aortic valve.

symptoms appear earlier. Symptomatic children with aortic valve stenosis younger than 1 year almost always have a unicuspid rather than bicuspid aortic valve.

8. Even with a bicuspid or unicuspid valve, there are three sinuses of Valsalva, because the raphae divide the fused cusp forming rudimentary sinuses. Therefore, the angiographic demonstration of three sinuses during diastole does not exclude either a unicommissural or a bicuspid aortic valve.

Angiographic Appearance

1. Left ventriculography shows the following abnormalities:
   a. Doming of the aortic valve.
   b. Narrow positive jet (Fig 26–11).
   c. Left ventricular hypertrophy (Fig 26–12).
   d. Prominent papillary muscles.
   e. Small left ventricular end-systolic volume.
   f. Poststenotic dilatation of aorta (see Fig 26–12, arrow).
2. Aortography shows the following abnormalities:
   a. Doming of the aortic valve.
   b. Negative jet (Fig 26–13).
   c. Poststenotic dilatation at the point of impact of the jet with the aortic wall, usually at the anterior lateral portion of the ascending aorta.
   d. A central jet causes poststenotic dilatation of the brachiocephalic vessels (Fig 26–14,A).
   e. Marked poststenotic dilatation of the aorta is an excellent sign of congenital origin of the stenosis; because acquired aortic stenosis develops later in life, the less pliable aorta shows little or no poststenotic dilatation.
   f. Poststenotic dilatation may be severe, making the

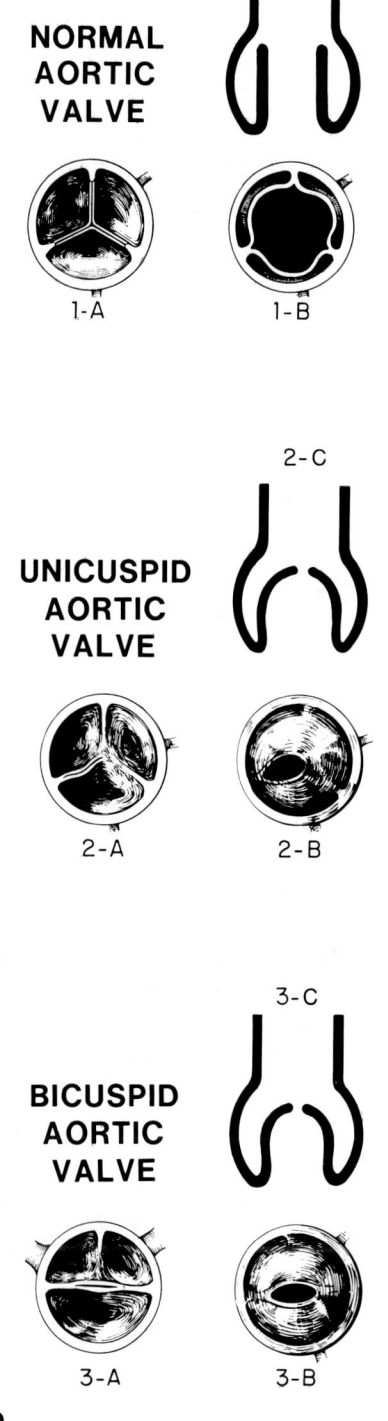

FIG 26–10.
Diagrams of normal and stenotic valves. Normal aortic valve during diastole (**1-A**), during systole (**1-B**), and angiographic systolic appearance (**1-C**). Unicuspid aortic valve during diastole (**2-A**), during systole (**2-B**), and angiographic systolic appearance (**2-C**) showing doming. Bicuspid aortic valve during diastole (**3-A**), during systole (**3-B**), and angiographic systolic appearance (**3-C**).

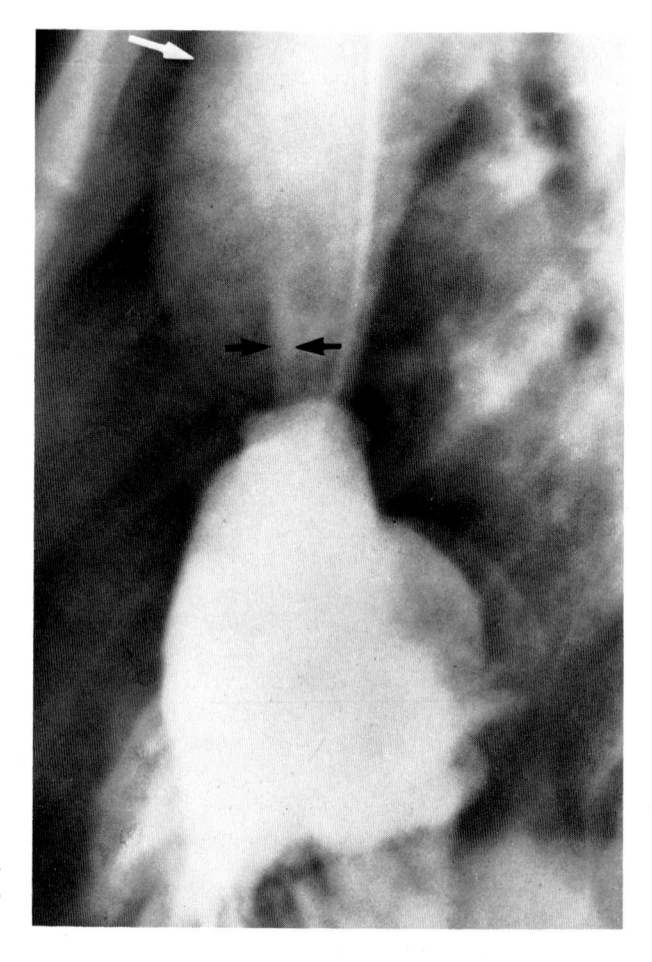

FIG 26–11.
Left ventriculogram, anteroposterior projection showing narrow positive jet through a doming aortic valve *(black arrows)*. Poststenotic dilation occurs at level of impact of jet on aortic wall *(white arrow)*.

differential diagnosis of poststenotic dilatation and cystic medial necrosis difficult. When in doubt, the surgeon should be advised to replace the ascending aorta by a graft.

g. There is a higher incidence of cystic medial necrosis in patients with congenital aortic stenosis which may result in dissecting aneurysms (Fig 26–14,B).

h. During diastole, an oversized aortic cusp is visualized (Fig 26–15) on the lateral projection.

3. Angiographic demonstration of three sinuses during diastole does not exclude a unicommissural or

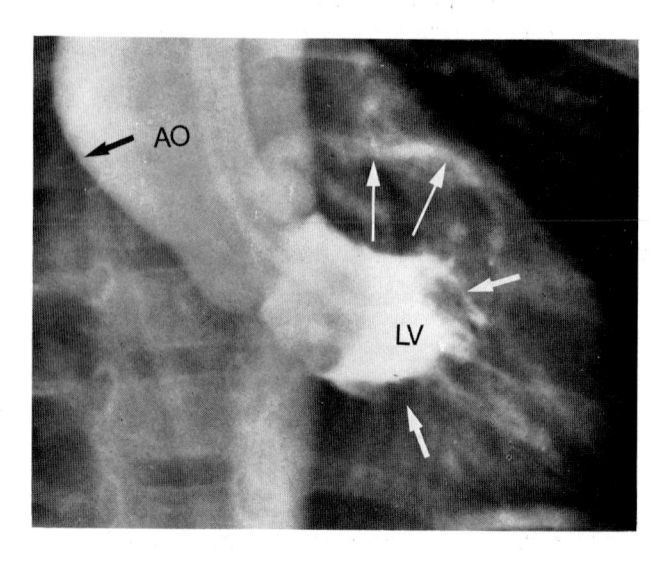

FIG 26–12.
Left ventriculogram, anteroposterior projection showing valvular aortic stenosis. Very small end-systolic volume. Papillary muscles *(short white arrows)* are left coronary artery *(long white arrows)* is increased, indicating left ventricular hypertrophy. Poststenotic dilation of ascending aorta *(black arrow)*.

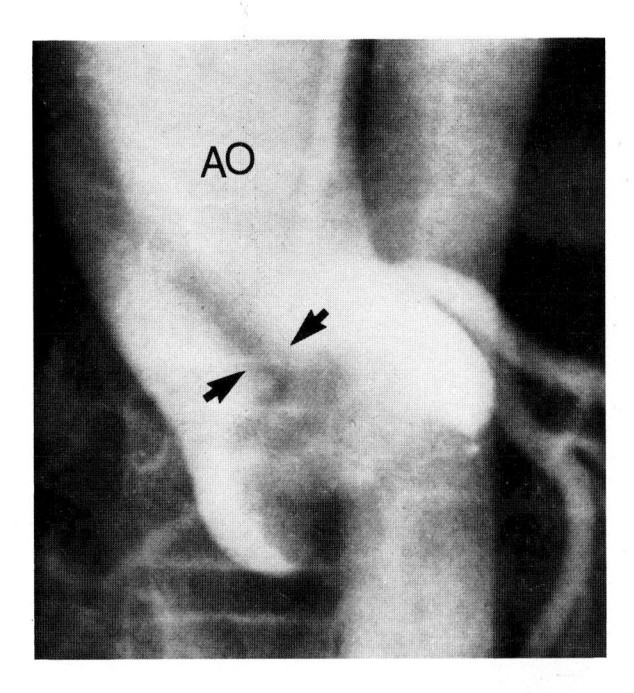

FIG 26–13.
Aortogram *(Ao)*; anteroposterior projection of congenital aortic stenosis. Doming of aortic valve and negative jet *(arrows)*. Appearance has been compared with Prussian helmet. Doming occurs in both bicuspid and unicuspid valves.

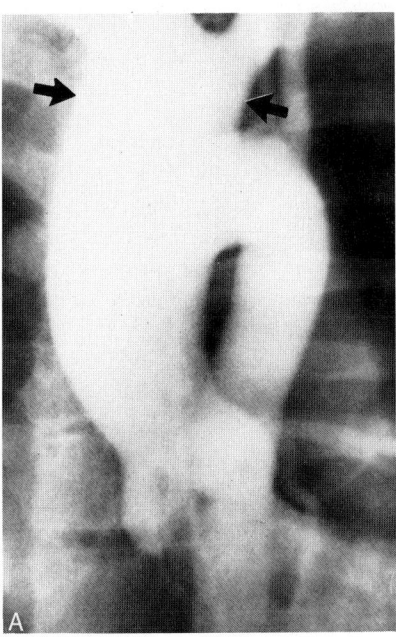

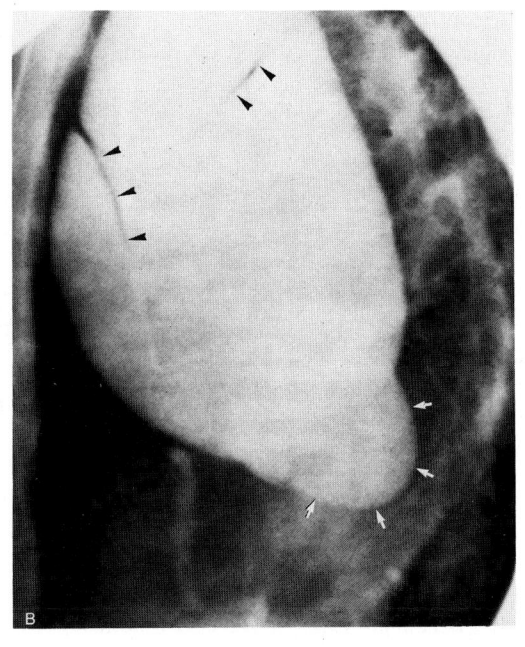

FIG 26–14.
Aortogram. **A,** posteroanterior projection; marked poststenotic dilatation of origin of brachiocephalic vessels *(arrows)*. Impact of centrally located jet on aortic wall occurred high in ascending aorta, resulting in dilatation of origin of brachiocephalic vessels. Anterolateral aspect of ascending aorta not dilated. **B,** aortogram, lateral projection; bicuspid aortic valve with oversized posterior cusp *(white arrows)*. Severe dilatation of ascending aorta from cystic medial necrosis. Dissection *(black arrows)* demonstrated. Increased incidence of cystic medial necrosis in congenital aortic stenosis. Without dissection, it may be impossible to decide if aortic dilatation is poststenotic or the result of medial cystic necrosis.

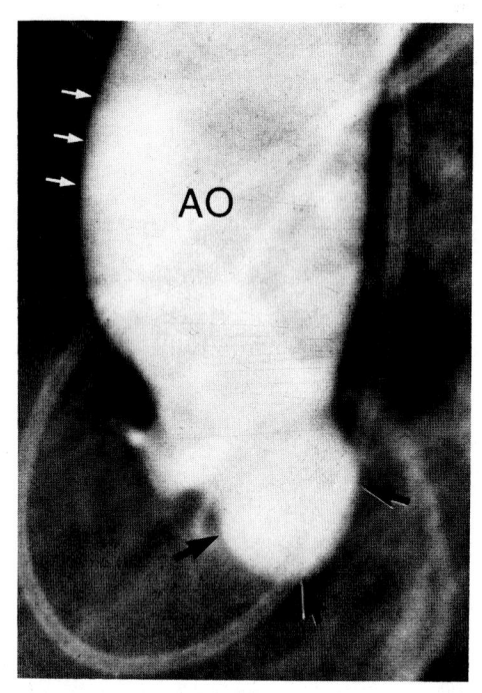

FIG 26–15.
Aortogram *(Ao);* anteroposterior projection during diastole in congenital bicuspid aortic stenosis. One cusp is oversized *(black arrows).* Marked poststenotic dilatation *(white arrows)* along anterolateral aspect of ascending aorta (the most common site).

  bicuspid aortic valve (Fig 26–16). Angiographically, three sinuses are usually seen.
  4. Angiographic distinction between a unicommissural and a bicuspid aortic valve is not possible.
  5. Aortic insufficiency. If it occurs, in most patients it is minor.
  6. If severe aortic regurgitation is present in infancy, the most likely diagnosis is aortico–left ventricular tunnel (Chapter 27).

Operative Considerations

The indications for operation are as follows:

  1. Congestive cardiac failure, in which case the operation is carried out as an urgent procedure.
  2. Signs or symptoms of myocardial ischemia or syncope.
  3. On an elective basis in asymptomatic children.

The exact criteria for selection of such patients differ among institutions. In asymptomatic children, we recommend operation if there is a peak systolic gradient greater than 40 mm Hg or an aortic valve area less than 0.7 cm^2/m^2.

The operation is carried out under cardiopulmonary bypass, and through an incision in the ascending aorta,

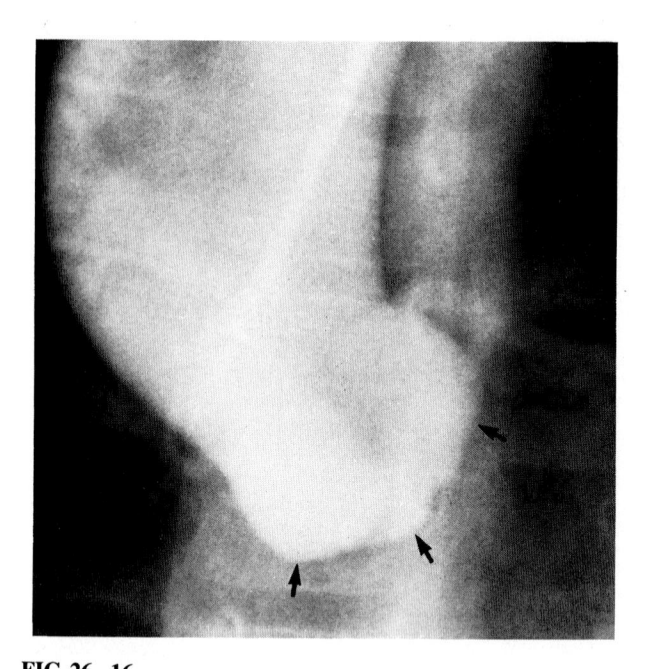

FIG 26–16.
Aortogram, anteroposterior projection during diastole in aortic stenosis. Three distinct sinuses *(arrows).* This finding does not exclude either bicuspid or unicommissural aortic valve, because three sinuses are formed by rudimentary commissures or raphaes.

the commissures of the aortic valve are incised (Fig 26–17).[16–18] Beyond infancy, the operative mortality is low and the results are good. Most patients have satisfactory relief of the obstruction, although there may be an increase in the degree of aortic insufficiency.[16, 19]

In an occasional child, the aortic valve must be replaced.

A balloon valvuloplasty can be performed as a pallia-

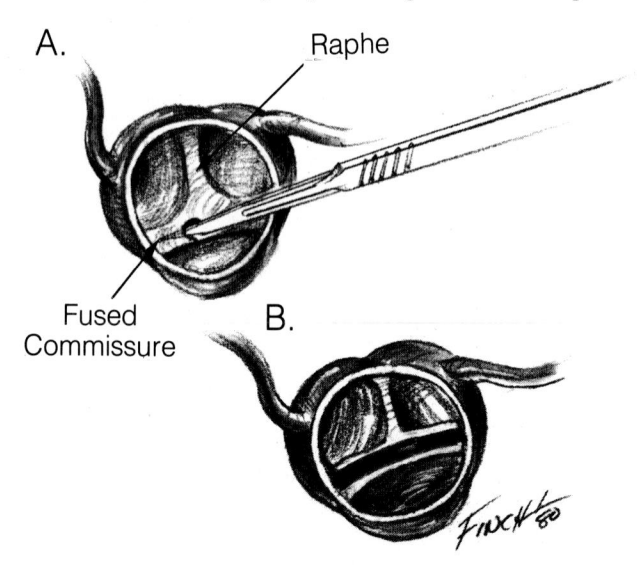

FIG 26–17.
Diagram of aortic valvotomy. Through aortotomy, fused commissures of bicuspid valve are incised to anulus.

tive procedure (see Fig 26–18). In most patients the gradient can be significantly reduced without causing aortic regurgitation, although exceptions exist.

Complications of Valvar Aortic Stenosis

The severity of aortic stenosis increases with age because of fibrosis and, ultimately, calcification of the valve.[20-23] Calcification is rarely found before the age of 20 years. Because of this progression, aortic stenosis caused by a bicuspid aortic valve may be discovered later in childhood or during adulthood.

The bicuspid or stenotic aortic valve is one of the most common sites for bacterial endocarditis, which leads to an increase in aortic insufficiency.

The aortic jet lesion may calcify and also may be a site of endocarditis.

Postoperative Radiographic and Angiographic Appearance

1. In patients with left ventricular decompensation and successful aortic valvotomy, cardiac size returns toward normal and signs of pulmonary congestion disappear.
2. In patients with normal cardiac size preoperatively, there is no change postoperatively.
3. Cardiac size may increase because of aortic insufficiency.
4. Poststenotic dilatation does not change.
5. In spite of incision of the aortic valve, the valve shows persistent doming angiographically (Fig 26–19).

DISCRETE MEMBRANOUS SUBAORTIC STENOSIS

Discrete membranous subaortic stenosis accounts for 10% of aortic stenosis occurring in children and is more likely than valvar aortic stenosis to coexist with other congenital cardiac anomalies.[24, 25]

Anatomic and Hemodynamic Considerations

A discrete, well-circumscribed, thin membrane with a central orifice is present in the left ventricular outflow tract, usually within 0.5 cm of the aortic valve. The hemodynamic consequences are similar to those of valvar aortic stenosis, with elevation of the left ventricular systolic pressure and the development of left ventricular hypertrophy.

The left ventricular output passes at high velocity through the orifice of the membrane. The resultant forceful jet strikes the aortic valve cusps opposite the orifice. This causes thickening of the cusps and asymmetric opening. This feature may be observed echocardiographically and angiographically.

The jet may cause poststenotic dilatation of the ascending aorta, particularly if the obstruction is close to the

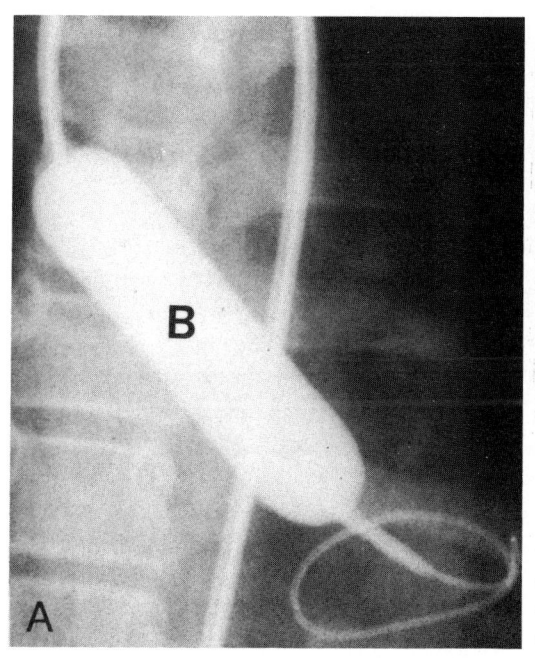

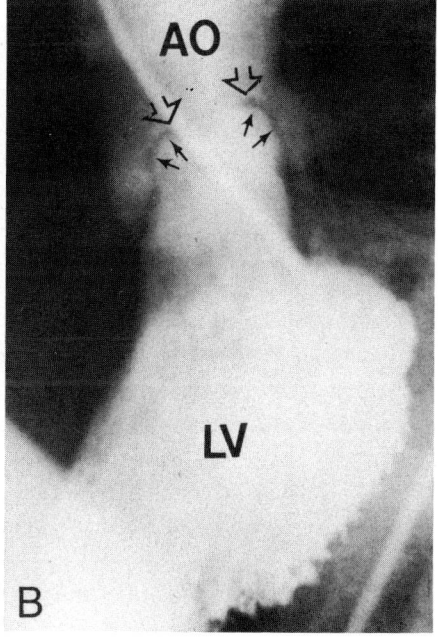

FIG 26–18.
A, severe congenital aortic stenosis. Balloon valvuloplasty. Balloon *(B)* inflated. Waist has disappeared, indicting successful rupture of stenotic valve. In older patients, two balloons may have to be used. **B,** after valvuloplasty. Left ventriculogram. Aortic opening is wide *(open arrows)*, but doming persists *(solid black arrows)*. Left ventricular systolic pressure decreased from 120 to 65 mm Hg.

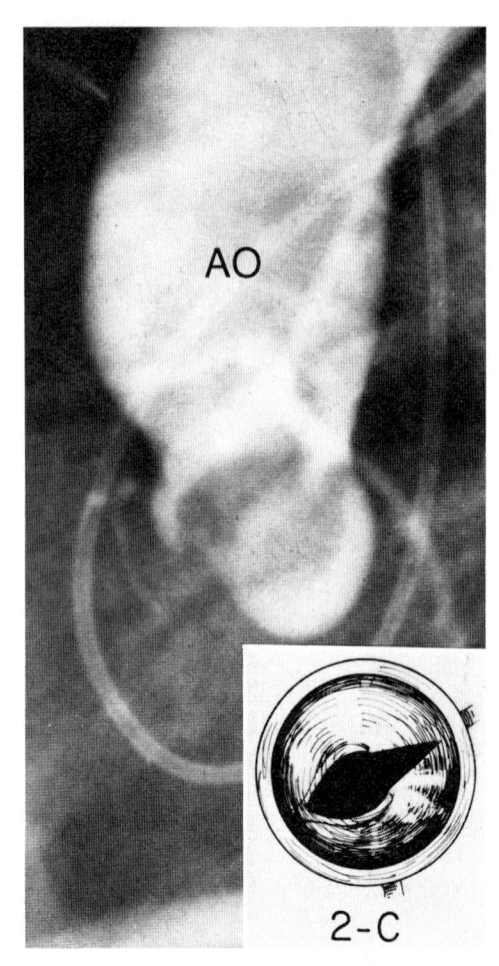

FIG 26–19.
Postoperative aortogram *(Ao)*; lateral projection in valvar aortic stenosis. Persistent doming of aortic valve. Angiographic appearance similar to preoperative aortogram, but aortic jet is larger. *Insert,* systolic view of aortic valve that has been incised by surgeon: doming occurs during systole. Because of persistent bicuspid configuration of valve, length of free margin of valve leaflets is inadequate, and doming occurs (see Fig. 26–10, **2-C**).

aortic valve. Generally, poststenotic dilatation is less marked than in patients with valvar aortic stenosis. Low-lying membranes may cause no aortic dilatation, probably because the energy of the jet is largely dissipated before it strikes the aortic wall.

Clinical Features

The clinical findings resemble those of valvar aortic stenosis, although congestive cardiac failure is rare and few patients have symptoms of myocardial ischemia.

Physical Examination

The patients appear healthy. The blood pressure is normal, as is cardiac size. As in valvular aortic stenosis, a left ventricular heave may be found. A suprasternal notch thrill is rare, but there may be a thrill along the midleft sternal border.

Auscultation helps to distinguish discrete membranous subaortic stenosis from valvular aortic stenosis. Unlike the findings in the latter, an ejection click is rare, because poststenotic dilatation is either mild or absent. A grade 3 to 4/6 systolic ejection murmur is present but is heard maximally along the left sternal border rather than over the aortic area.

A soft early diastolic murmur develops with age.

Electrocardiographic Features

In 90% of patients, the ECG findings are identical to those with valvar aortic stenosis, showing variable degrees of left ventricular hypertrophy and occasionally ST-segment and T-wave changes in the left precordial leads.

In the remaining 10%, lead V_1 shows an rSR' pattern or a deeper than normal S wave in lead V_6. The reason for this pattern is unknown.

Echocardiographic Features[26, 27]

The echocardiographic tracings are diagnostic of discrete membranous subaortic stenosis. There may be fine, high-intensity echoes below the aortic valve. Early systolic closure of the aortic valve is common, probably from the subvalvar jet striking the aortic valve, preventing complete opening of all cusps. Flutter of the valve is common from a Venturi effect caused by the high-velocity jet. The negative pressure in the jet pulls the valve leaflet into the jet, yet once the leaflet has been pulled into the jet, the positive force returns the leaflet to its original position outside the jet. The cycle repeats itself at a high flutter frequency. If we blow over a piece of paper, the negative pressure in the air jet causes the paper to rise and to flutter identically to the valve leaflet (Fig 26–20). The negative pressure in the jet is directly related to its speed, so the normal aortic valve shows little or no flutter. However, if it is struck by a high-velocity jet created from a subaortic diaphragm, flutter is invariably seen. A similar flutter of the anterior mitral valve is seen in aortic regurgitation. Left ventricular posterior wall and ventricular septal hypertrophy, proportional to the degree of stenosis, is found.

Radiographic Features

1. Normal cardiac size and configuration are present in compensated cases (Fig 26–21).
2. The pulmonary vasculature is normal.
3. Marked poststenotic dilatation is rare (Fig 26–22).
4. Fifty percent of patients show some degree of poststenotic dilatation, because the energy of the jet through a

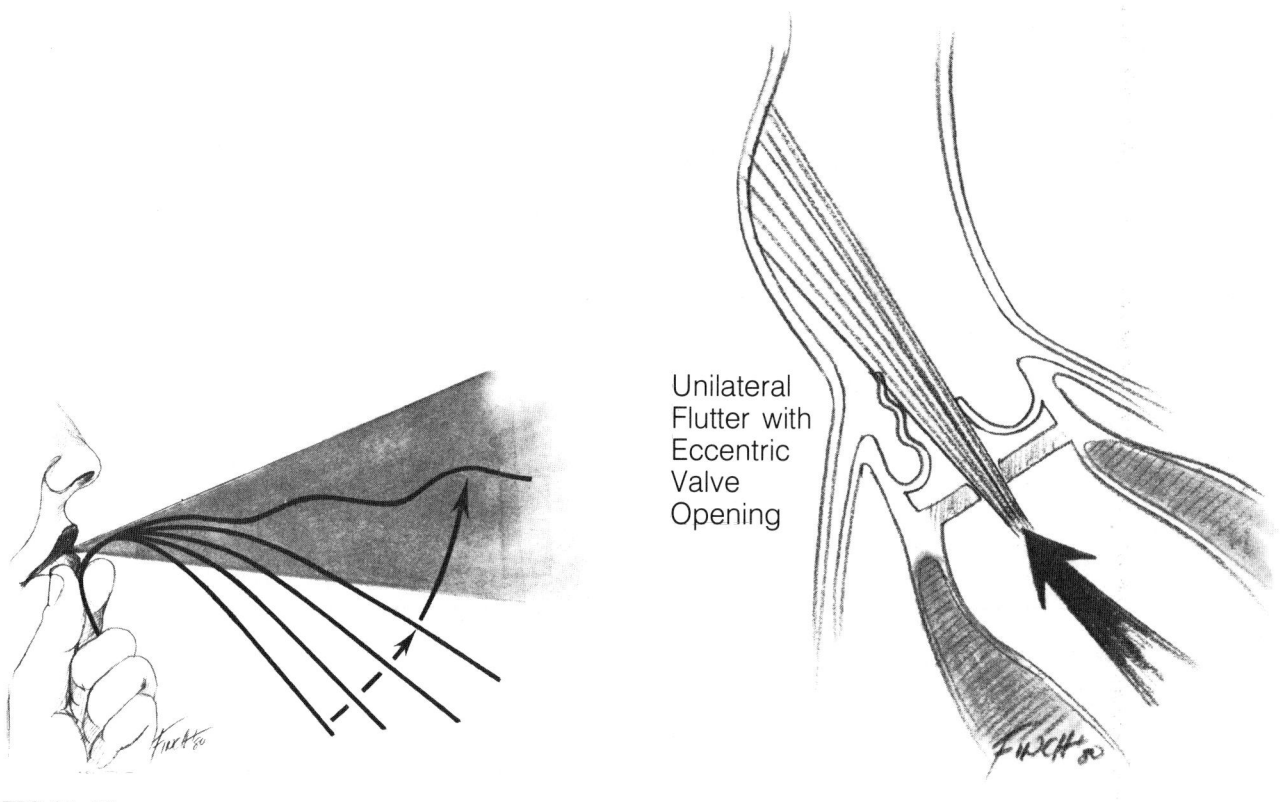

FIG 26–20.
Diagram of Venturi effect. **A,** blowing across a piece of paper results in a flutter by the negative pressure in jet. Similarly, aortic valve leaflet is pulled into jet, which produces a coarse flutter of leaflet. **B,** ultimately, the leaflets become thickened, and aortic insufficiency results.

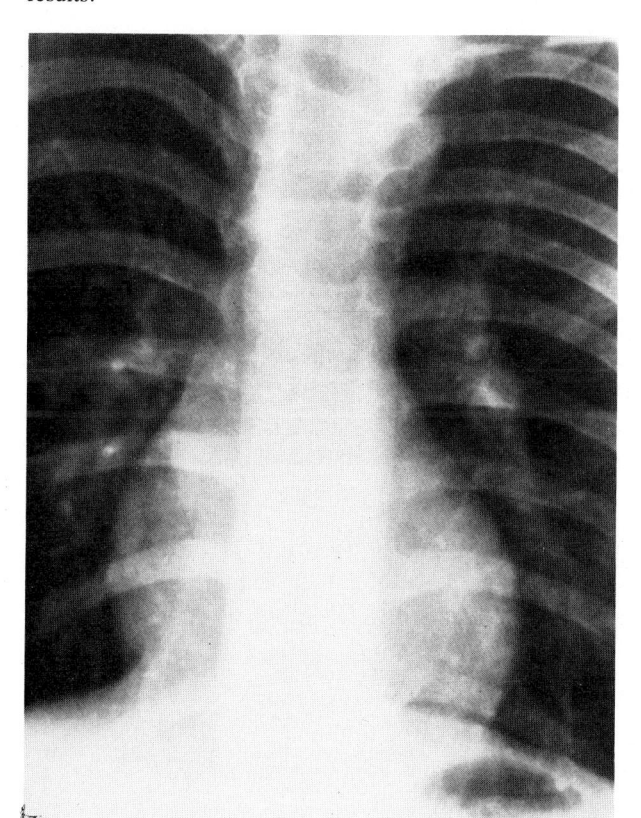

FIG 26–21.
Thoracic roentgenogram, posteroanterior projection in discrete subvalvar aortic stenosis. Normal cardiac configuration; normal pulmonary vasculature. No poststenotic dilatation of aorta. Location of subaortic membrane correlates with presence of poststenotic dilatation: membranes immediately beneath aortic valve have a higher incidence. REASON: Impact of subvalvular jet is more forceful because of short distance. In valvar stenosis, distance between jet and the aortic wall is even shorter, so poststenotic dilatation is more marked. With a low-lying subaortic membrane, energy of jet is largely dissipated before it strikes aortic wall.

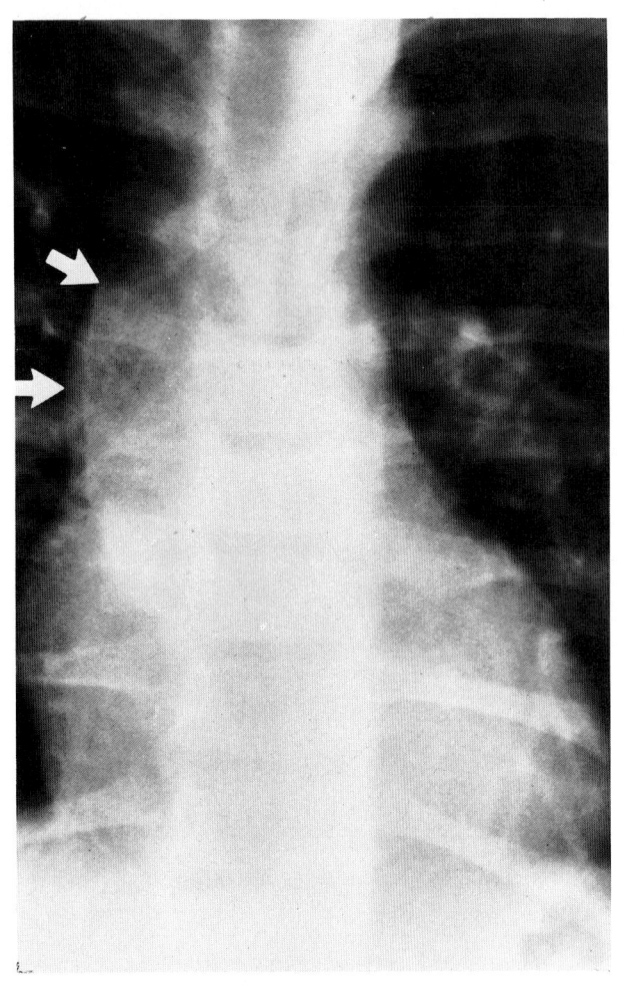

FIG 26–22.
Thoracic roentgenogram, anteroposterior projection of subaortic membrane. Marked poststenotic dilatation *(arrows)*. This unusual finding suggests a very high-lying membrane with jet directed obliquely against aortic wall.

low-lying membrane is dissipated before it strikes the aortic wall.

5. Left ventricular enlargement is rare; when present it indicates left ventricular decompensation or associated mitral reflux.

Cardiac Catheterization

The indications and purposes of cardiac catheterization in patients with discrete membranous subaortic stenosis are similar to those in valvar aortic stenosis. Most patients undergo catheterization on an elective basis, but there is a higher frequency of coexisting cardiac conditions. In our experience, the principal coexisting conditions are: aortic insufficiency (70%); ventricular septal defect (20%); coarctation of the aorta (16%); and mitral insufficiency (8%).

Pressure data from the left side of the heart are characteristic. A systolic pressure is found within the left ventricle, usually immediately below the aortic valve (Fig 26–23). The end-diastolic pressure is normal.

During cardiac catheterization, a pressure tracing should be recorded around the aortic arch to the descending aorta to identify coexistant coarctation of the aorta.

Angiographic Appearance

Angiographic demonstration of a subvalvar membrane may be a challenge, but careful analysis of the anatomic orientation of the aortic cusps allows observation of a subaortic diaphragm with a high degree of accuracy.

A subaortic membrane can be demonstrated only when the x-ray beam passes parallel to the membrane. With such a projection, the membrane appears as a fine line of radiolucency best seen in the anteroposterior or either the right anterior oblique or the left anterior oblique projection. If the x-ray beam transverses a membrane obliquely, the membrane is usually not visible. A tangential view is essential for identification of these thin membranes.

Subvalvar membranes almost invariably lie in a plane parallel with the three aortic cusps in diastole (Fig 26–24,A). The aortic cusps can be readily identified angiographically on left ventriculography or aortography. If all three cusps are at the same level, as is commonly the case in infants and children (see Fig 26–24), angulation of the x-ray beam is not necessary. Superimposition of the descending aorta is avoided by a slight right or left anterior oblique projection.

Commonly, the aortic valve plane is tilted anteriorly in the anteroposterior and, particularly, the slightly right anterior oblique projection, and therefore the right aortic cusp lies lower than the left and posterior cusps (see Fig

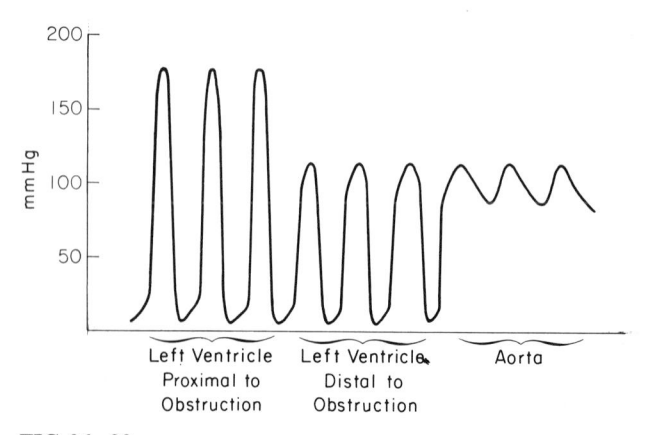

FIG 26–23.
Diagram of pressure tracing in discrete membranous subaortic stenosis; abrupt change in systolic pressure found in left ventricle.

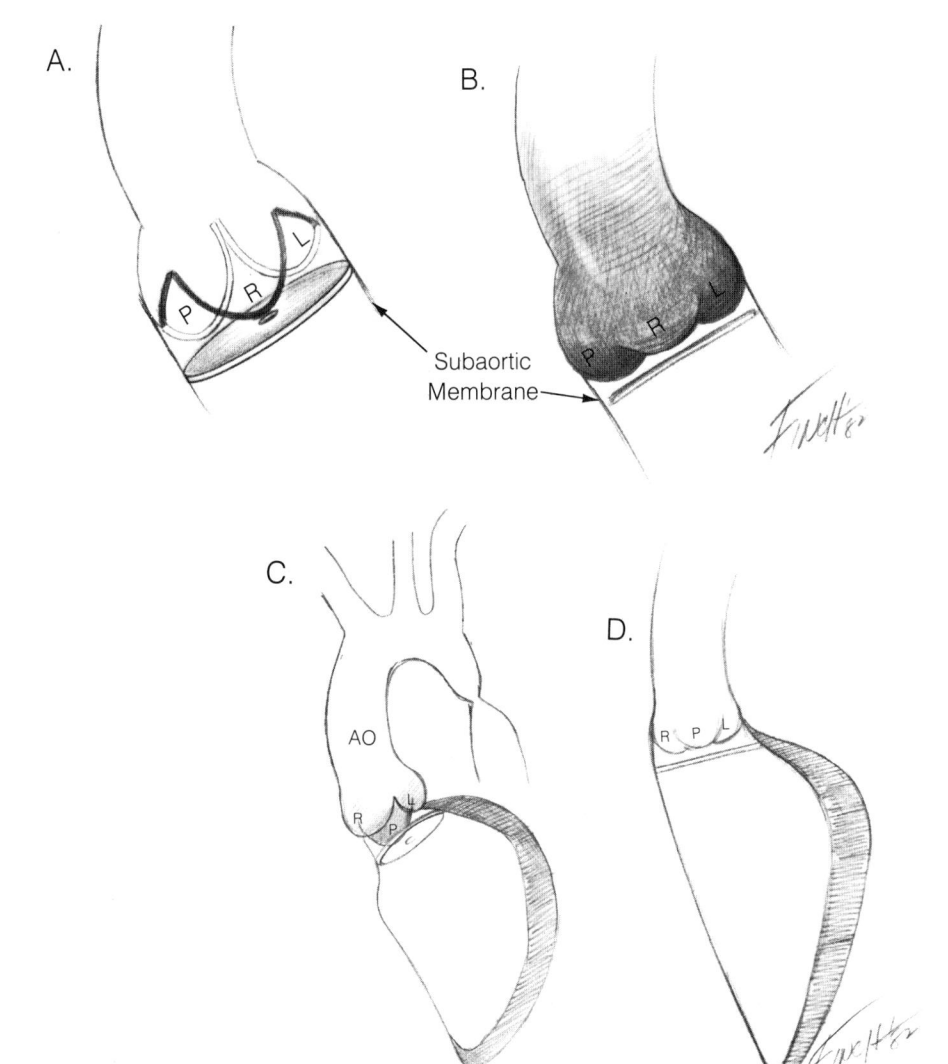

Aortic Stenosis **431**

FIG 26–24.
Diagram of angiographic demonstration of subaortic diaphragm according to projection of aortic valve cusps, which parallel diaphragm. **A,** common appearance on slight right anterior oblique projection and anteroposterior projection; diaphragm projected as a disk and not seen angiographically. **B,** caudad beam angulation restores a true tangential view, demonstrating diaphragm. If right cusp (R) projects higher, cranial angulation has to be used. **C,** left anterior oblique projection; projects diaphragm as a nonvisible disk. **D,** cranial beam angulation (long axial oblique); diaphragm seen on end, allowing observation. *AO* = aorta; *L* = left aortic cusp; *P* = posterior aortic cusp.

26–24). Now the membrane projects as a disk and is no longer visible angiographically. Therefore, the anatomic relation seen in Figure 26–24,B must be established to see the membrane. This can be accomplished either by caudad angulation of the x-ray beam or by elevating the patient's hips and using a straight beam.

In the left anterior oblique projection (Fig 26–24,C), the aortic valve plane is invariably tilted, and the subaortic membrane projects as a disk and is invisible angiographically. The anatomic relation shown in Figure 26–24,D must be present for successful demonstration in the left anterior oblique projection. The projection is identical to that for demonstration of a ventricular septal defect (see Chapter 12), but maximal cranial tube angulation has to be used. Angulation can be increased by placing the patient obliquely on the x-ray table.

Membranes can be demonstrated by left ventriculography and aortography, but their demonstration may be a challenge to the angiographer.

1. Subaortic membrane
   a. Left ventriculography shows a radiolucent thin line parallel to the plane of the aortic valve, differing in thickness. Very thin membranes can be easily overlooked (Fig 26–25).
   b. Two membranes may be present (rare).
   c. Membranes are usually not seen on lateral or angulated left anterior oblique left ventriculograms (Fig 26–26). REASON: The plane of the membrane is oblique to the direction of the x-ray beam. The membrane can be demonstrated on left anterior oblique or lateral projections only with marked cranial beam angulation (Figs 26–24 and 26–27).
   d. Visibility is further improved by placing the catheter tip immediately below the membrane and injecting less contrast medium at a slower rate (see Fig 26–27,B). A very dense ventriculogram may obscure the membrane.
2. Subaortic jet. The subvalvar jet is an important

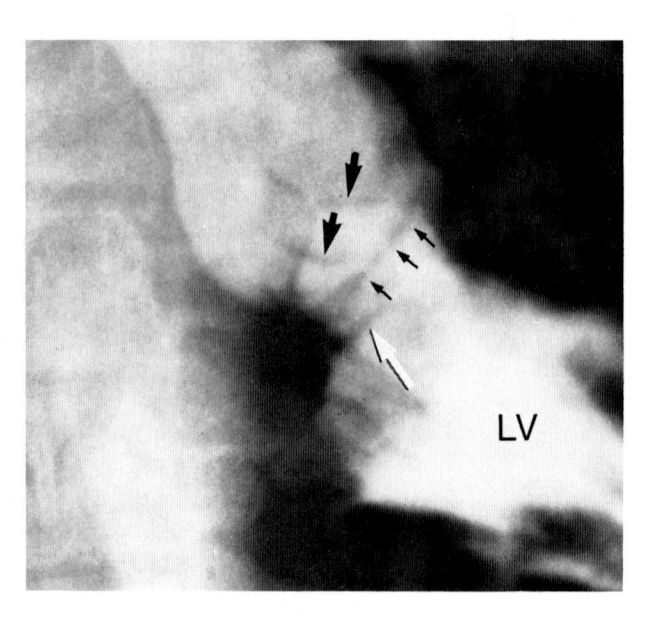

432 Outflow Obstructive Lesions

FIG 26–25.
Left ventriculogram *(LV)*, slight right anterior oblique projection of well-defined subaortic membrane *(small black arrows)* immediately beneath aortic valve. Aortic valve distinctly seen *(larger black arrows)* and slightly thickened from damage of subvalvar jet. Because subaortic membrane touches aortic valve leaflets in diastole, it can easily be confused with the aortic valve itself. Systolic views are most helpful in diagnosis, because aorta valve opens during systole, whereas the subaortic membrane remains visible during diastole and systole. A small distinct second membrane *(white arrow)* is demonstrated. This is very rare.

finding, because it may be the only angiographic evidence of a subaortic membrane. It will confirm an echocardiographic diagnosis.

a. Subaortic jet causes incomplete opening of aortic valve[28] (Figs 26–20 and 26–28). REASON: The jet strikes only one or two aortic valve leaflets, and the remaining leaflet remains closed during systole.

b. The aortic valve is usually thickened and insufficient (Fig 26–29). REASON: The subaortic jet striking the valve cusp induces fibrotic thickening.

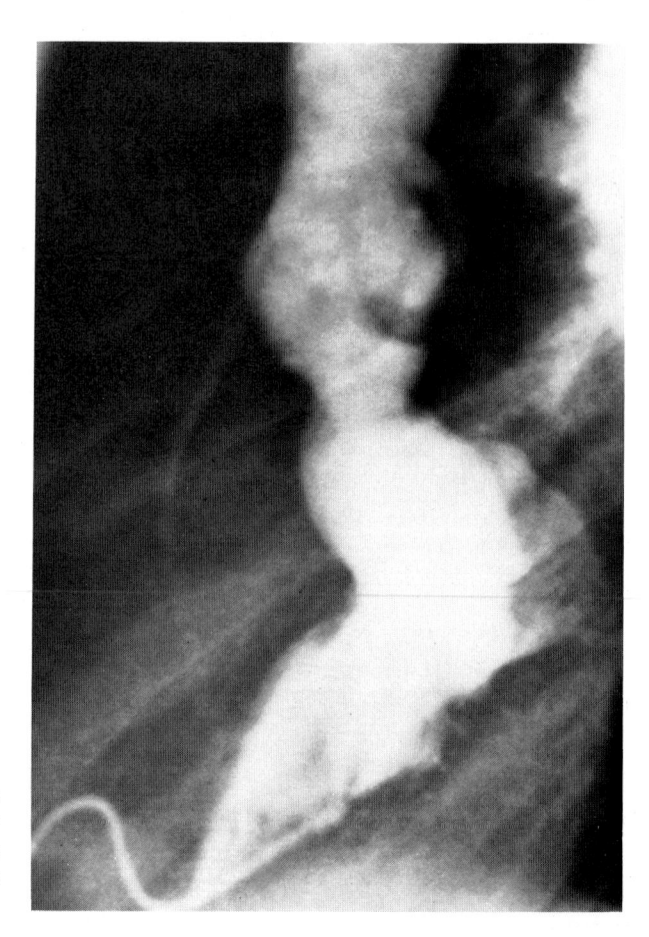

FIG 26–26.
Left ventriculogram, lateral projection of transapical catheterization in patient with proved subaortic stenosis. Angiogram does not show the membrane clearly. REASON: The membrane lies obliquely to the direction of the x-ray beam and is therefore not seen on end because insufficient cranial angulation was used.

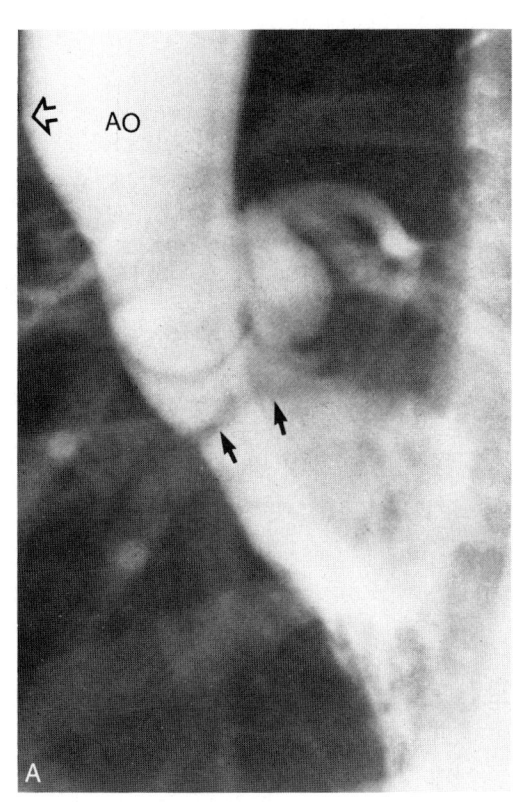

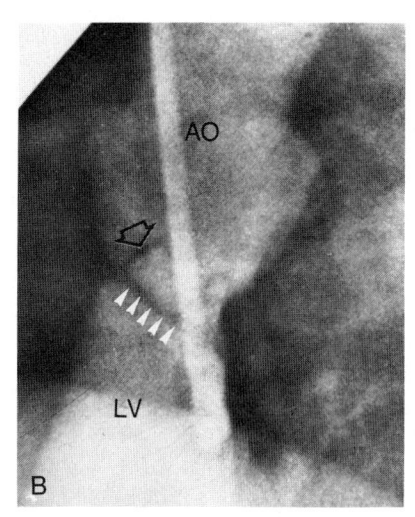

FIG 26–27.
Subaortic membrane. **A,** left ventriculogram, left anterior oblique projection; cranial beam angulation shows subaortic membrane *(black arrows)*. Aortic valve thickened by subvalvar jet. Poststenotic dilatation of the aorta *(open arrows)*. **B,** excellent demonstration of subaortic membrane in left anterior oblique projection. side holes of catheter placed at level of membrane, and contrast medium injected. Thick membrane *(small white arrows)*; thickened right aortic cusp *(open arrow)*. *AO* = aorta; *LV* = left ventricle.

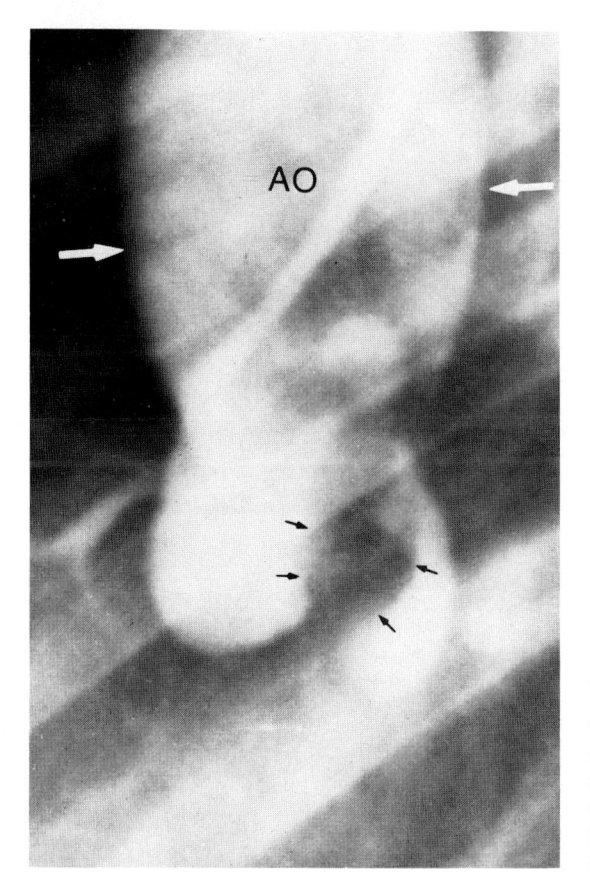

FIG 26–28.
Aortogram *(Ao)*: anteroposterior projection in subaortic membrane. Eccentric opening of aortic valve *(arrows)*; subaortic jet strikes only one or two cusps. The third aortic cusp is not struck by the jet (in this case the right cusp) remains closed during systole. Aortic leaflets, struck by the jet, flutter (Venturi effect). This case is unusual in that the subvalvar jet is directed posteriorly. Distinct poststenotic dilatation of the aorta is present *(white arrows)*, also involving the posterior wall of the aorta (impact of jet).

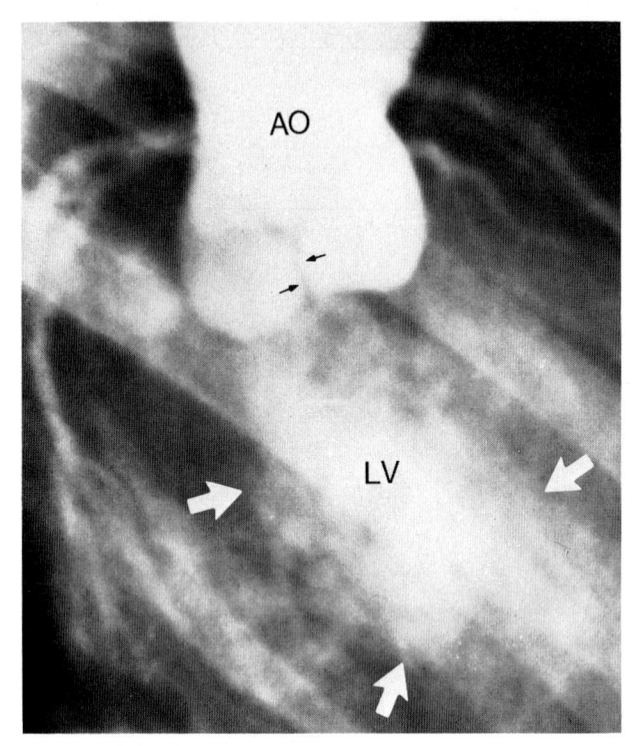

FIG 26–29.
Aortogram *(Ao)*, lateral projection in subaortic stenosis. Distinct thickening of aortic valve *(black arrows)*. REASON: Damage to valve leaflet by subvalvar jet induces fibrotic thickening. Mild aortic reflux *(white arrows)*. LV = left ventricle.

   c. The subaortic membrane may be best seen on aortography when aortic insufficiency is present. Only the superior aspect of the membrane is delineated, and contrast medium may regurgitate through the orifice of the membrane into the left ventricle (Fig 26–30).
   d. The subaortic membrane occasionally is more than 0.5 cm below the aortic valve and therefore involves the mobile portion of the anterior leaflet of the mitral valve (Fig 26–31).
   e. For the best demonstration of subaortic membranes by either left ventriculography or aortography, it is advantageous to project the area of the aortic valve off the spine by using a slight right anterior oblique projection (Fig 26–32).
   f. The membrane may not be parallel with the aortic valve plane (rare) (see Fig 26–30).
   g. The aortic leaflets struck by the high speed jet are seen to flutter (Venturi effect; see Fig 26–20).
3. Subaortic membranes may be associated with other cardiac malformations[29] and are easily overlooked (Fig 26–32). A membrane that is unusually thick is commonly referred to as a fibromuscular ridge (Fig 26–33).
4. Fibromuscular narrowing of the outflow tract may also occur without a ridge. The rigid circumferential tubular narrowing of the left ventricular outflow tract is very rare and is known as "fibromuscular tunnel."
5. Subaortic stenosis may occur in interruption of the aortic arch with ventricular septal defect by a characteristic muscular "spur" (see Chapter 62).

Operative Considerations and Procedure

The indications for resection of a subaortic membrane are similar to those in valvar aortic stenosis. We recommend operation on an elective basis for a smaller gradient than in valvar aortic stenosis, because the operation does not cause aortic insufficiency as it does in valvar aortic stenosis. Complete resection of the membrane eliminates the damaging effect of the subaortic jet on the aortic valve.

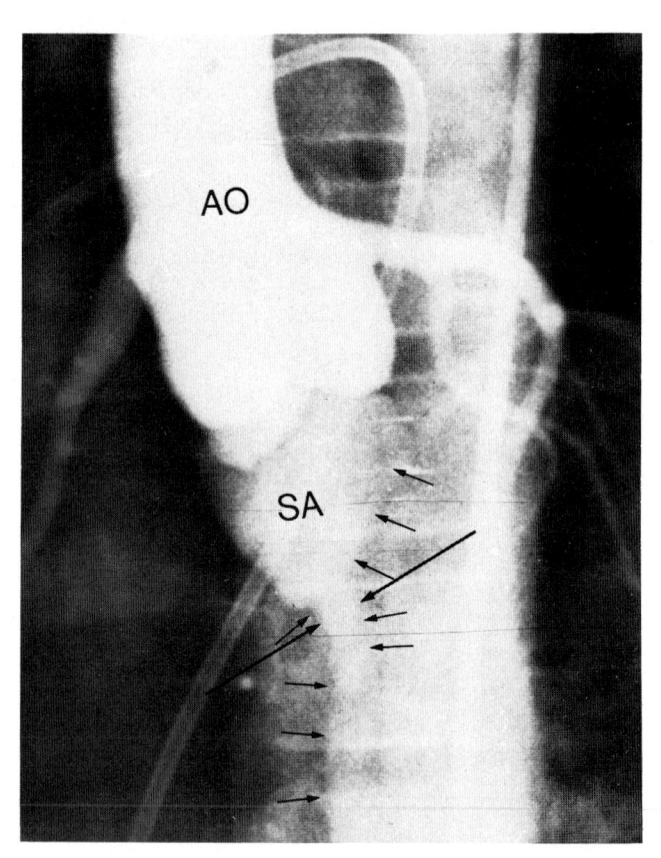

FIG 26–30.
Aortogram *(Ao):* anteroposterior projection showing slight thickening of aortic valve. Aortic regurgitation into subaortic chamber *(SA)* oulining a low-lying subaortic membrane *(small black arrows)*. Jet formed by regurgitation of contrast medium through narrow orifice in membrane *(long black arrows)* into left ventricle. This represents an example of an eccentric orifice in a subaortic membrane. Membrane located very low (1.5 cm below level of aortic valve). The membrane does not parallel the aortic valve plane.

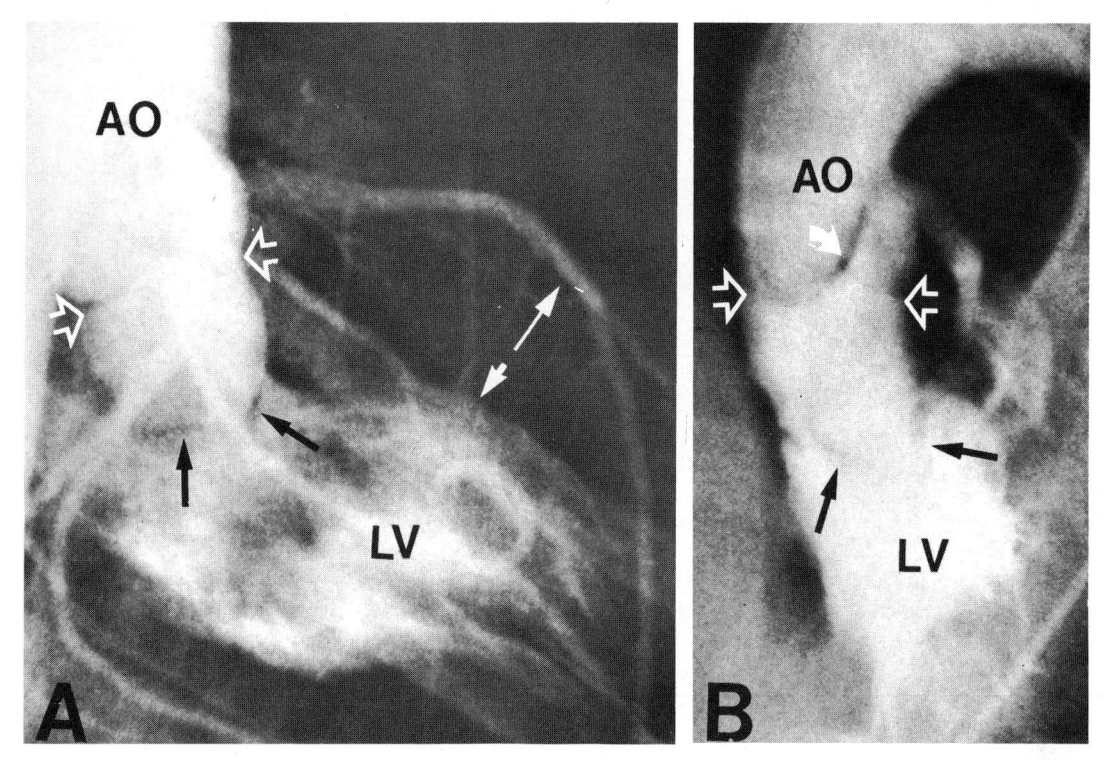

FIG 26–31.
A, discrete subaortic stenosis. Left ventriculogram. Right anterior oblique projection with caudal beam angulation. Subaortic membrane *(small arrows)* 2 cm below aortic valve plane *(open arrows)*. Severe left ventricular hypertrophy *(double arrow)*. **B,** same patient. Left ventriculogram. Marked cranial beam angulation. Subaortic membrane *(arrows)* at least 2 cm below aortic valve plane *(open arrows)*. Marked thickening of one of aortic valve leaflets *(curved white arrow)*.

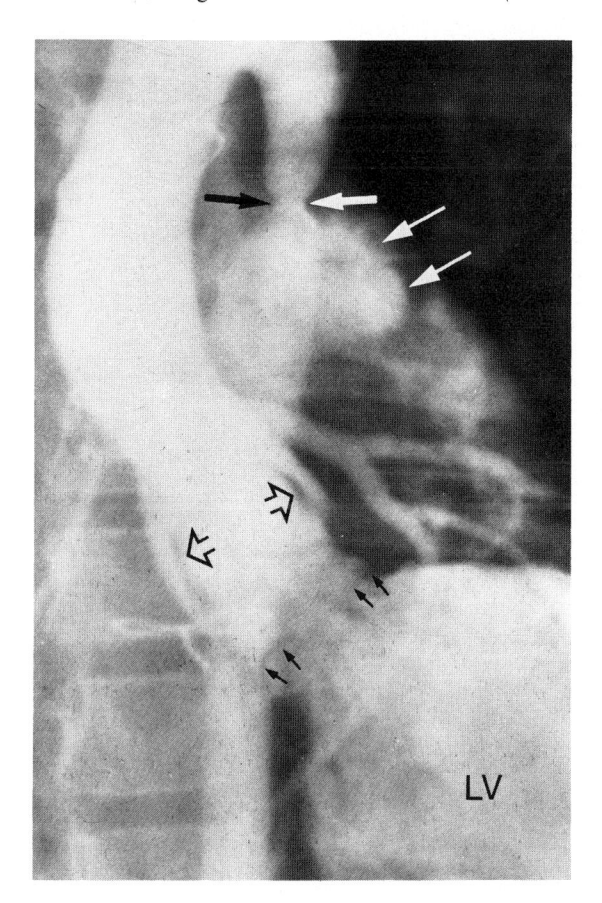

FIG 26–32.
Left ventriculogram *(LV)*, anteroposterior projection in subaortic membrane with coexisting congenital cardiac anomalies. Very thin subaortic membrane *(small black arrows)* visible during systole. Thickened, domed aortic valve *(open black arrows)* after surgery for aortic stenosis. Coarctation of aorta *(fat black arrow)*. Patent ductus arteriosus *(white arrows)*. A subaortic membrane is likely to be missed when it coexists with other cardiac malformations. Subaortic membrane associated with valvar aortic stenosis is difficult to diagnose by catheterization and angiography. Subaortic area should always be inspected at surgery for subaortic stenosis.

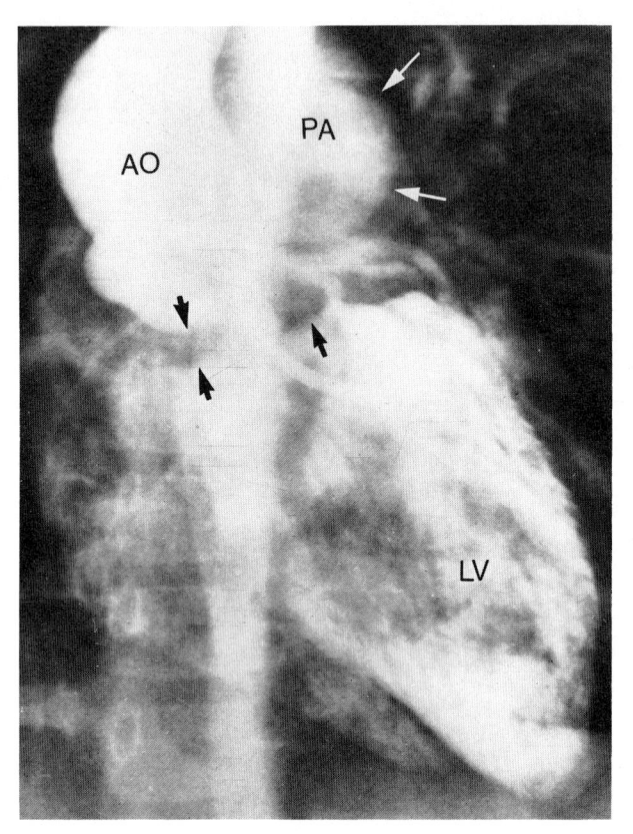

FIG 26–33.
Left ventriculogram, anteroposterior projection shows large bar-like filling defect *(black arrows)* immediately beneath aortic valve. This represents an unusually thick membrane, referred to as a "fibromuscular ridge." Angiographic findings should not be confused with "kissing" mitral valve found in muscular subaortic stenosis, which projects lower into left ventricular outflow area and changes during the cardiac cycle. Small ventricular septal defect indicated by opacification of pulmonary artery *(white arrows)*. Such defects are commonly small and located immediately above aortic membrane. *AO* = aorta; *PA* = pulmonary artery.

After years significant subaortic stenosis may recur because of regrowth of the membrane. The fact that subaortic membranes have not been observed in neonates suggests that they may develop during life.

Under cardiopulmonary bypass, an aortotomy is performed. The aortic valve leaflets are retracted, and the membrane is excised (Fig 26–34). Care must be taken when that portion of the membrane attached to the anterior leaflet of the mitral valve is excised. Too vigorous excision in this region may damage the valve and result in mitral insufficiency. To prevent this, resection of the membrane may be incomplete, and a small residual gradient is commonly found at postoperative cardiac catheterization. Even with successful relief of the gradient, remnants of the subaortic membrane are commonly seen on a left ventriculogram performed postoperatively (Fig 26–35).

Balloon dilatation of a subaortic membrane has been performed and may decrease the gradient. The damaging subaortic jet remains, however, and consequently the procedure is controversial.

RARE CAUSES OF SUBAORTIC STENOSIS

Rarely, obstruction occurs in the left ventricle from conditions other than discrete membranous subaortic stenosis or muscular subaortic stenosis.

1. Accessory mitral valve tissue may bulge into the left ventricular outflow area. This obstructive mechanism is more commonly found in complete transposition of the great vessels (see Chapter 38).

2. In patients with an isolated cleft in the anterior leaflet of the mitral valve, chordae tendineae from the margin of the cleft may insert into the ventricular septum, immobilizing the leaflet and thus obstructing the left ventricular outflow area (see Chapter 23).

3. Subaortic stenosis may occur as a component of complete atrioventricular canal because of deficiency of the ventricular septum and displacement of the atrioven-

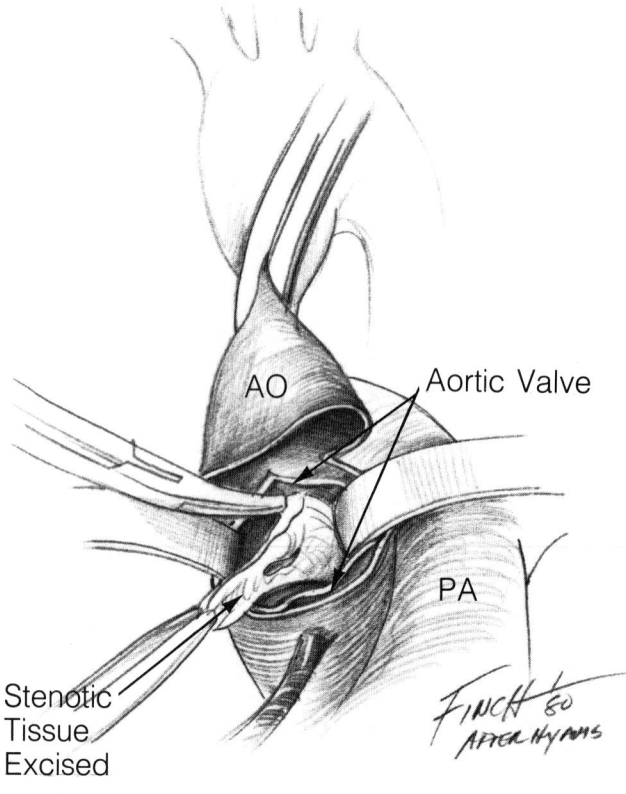

FIG 26–34.
Diagram of operation for discrete membranous subaortic stenosis. *AO* = aorta; *PA* = pulmonary artery.

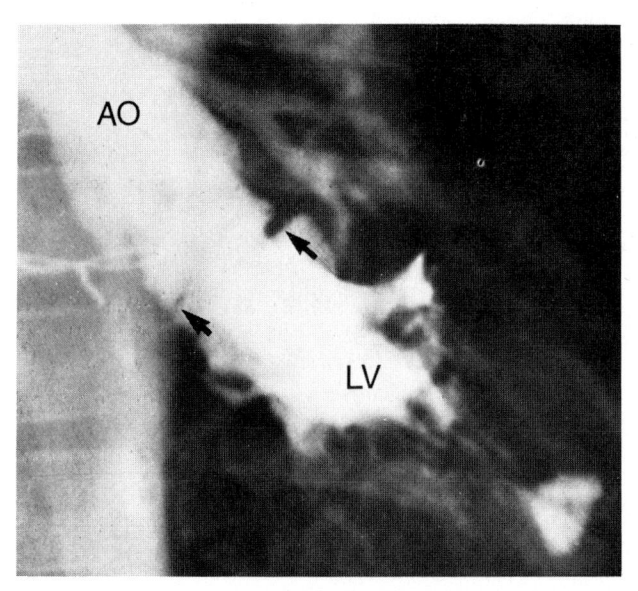

FIG 26–35.
Left ventriculogram after resection of subaortic membrane. Residues of membrane *(arrows)* remain. Complete excision of low-lying membranes may be difficult because of risk of partial excision of mitral valve. Some surgeons are therefore cautious and prefer to leave remnants behind, resulting in a residual pressure gradient. Angiographically, such residual aortic membranes are commonly demonstrated. Complete excision has been rare in our experience. *AO* = aorta.

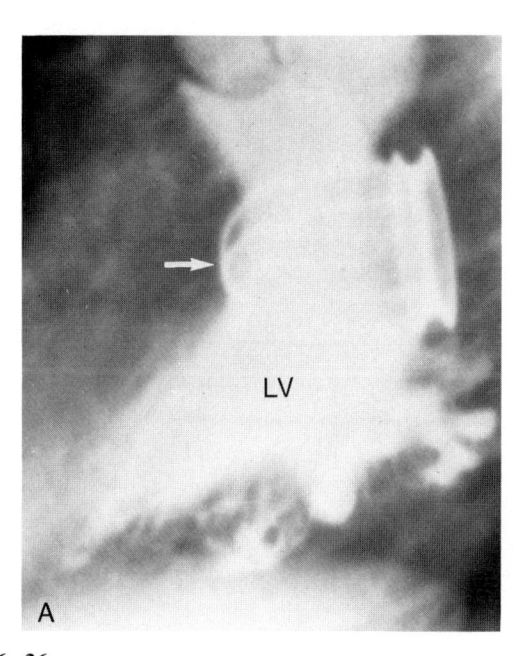

tricular valve into the ventricle and encroachment on the left ventricular outflow area.

4. In patients in whom the mitral valve has been replaced by a prosthetic ball valve, the bulk of the prosthesis may obstruct left ventricular outflow (Fig 26–36). This is much less common with low-profile or tissue prostheses.

5. Cardiac tumors are a rare cause of subaortic stenosis. Rhabdomyoma is the most frequent cardiac tumor of children and can manifest as an obstructive lesion (Figs 26–37 and 26–38).

SUPRAVALVAR AORTIC STENOSIS

Supravalvar aortic stenosis is the least frequently occurring form of aortic stenosis. Three anatomic types of this anomaly have been described[30]:

1. Hourglass deformity of ascending aorta (see Fig 26–39,A).
2. Diffuse hypoplasia of the ascending aorta (see Fig 26–39,B).
3. Narrow membrane at or immediately above the sinus of Valsalva (rare) (see Fig 26–39,C).

The first two forms reflect different degrees of the same condition, causing generalized involvement of the aortic wall, that probably represents a more generalized arterial disease, because the brachiocephalic vessels are commonly narrowed, as, on occasion, are the renal arter-

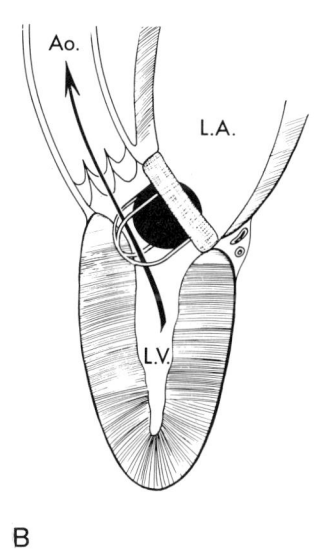

FIG 26–36.
Obstruction by prosthetic valve. **A,** left ventriculogram *(LV)*, lateral projection of prosthetic ball valve *(arrow)* partially obstructing left ventricular outflow area. Impingement of metallic cage on left ventricular septum. **B,** Diagram of obstructive mechanism. *AO* = aorta; *LA* = left atrium.

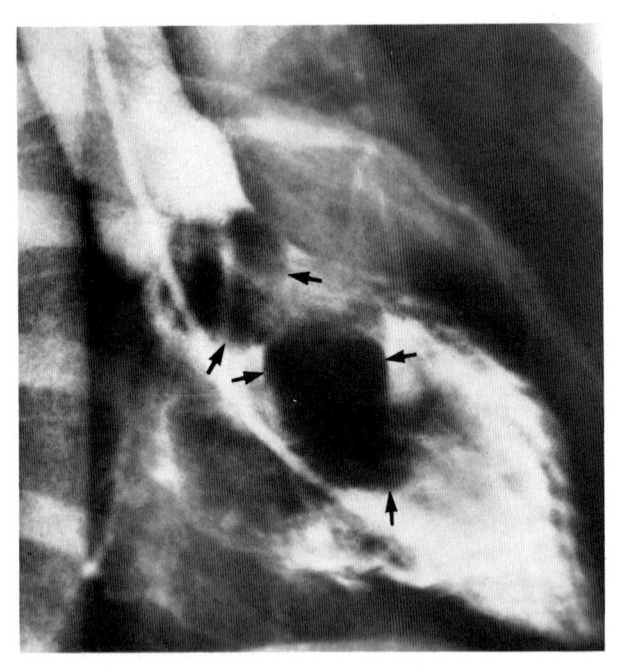

FIG 26–37.
Left ventriculogram, anteroposterior projection during diastole rhabdomyoma left ventricle. Large pedunculated filling defect in left ventricle *(black arrows)* is clearly demonstrated.

ies. Peripheral pulmonary arterial stenosis frequently coexists, supporting the view that this malformation is a generalized arterial disease. The histologic appearance of the ascending aorta and other involved arteries shows disorganization of the media, with focal interruptions of medial fibers and replacement with fibrous tissue. In some areas, the media shows a mosaic pattern, representing the irregular orientation of medial fibers.

Although coexisting congenital cardiac anomalies are rare, other arterial problems may be present. These include peripheral pulmonary arterial stenosis; stenosis of brachiocephalic arteries; coronary arterial anomalies, including stenosis of the coronary ostia; premature coronary atherosclerosis; and acquired aortic valvar anomalies, such as thickening of the cusps and adherence of the free margin of aortic cusps to the aortic wall.

Anatomic and Hemodynamic Considerations

The primary effect of supravalvar stenosis is an increase in systolic pressure proximal to the obstruction. The systolic pressure is elevated not only in the left ventricle, which leads to left ventricular hypertrophy, but also in the aorta proximal to the obstruction, which leads to dilatation, tortuosity, and premature atherosclerosis of the coronary arteries. The coronary blood flow may be compromised by an associated stenosis of the coronary ostia or adherence of an aortic valve cusp to the aortic wall.

Hemodynamically, supravalvar aortic stenosis progresses with age.[31] REASON: Lack of normal growth of the stenosis. The peripheral pulmonary artery stenosis improves hemodynamically in most patients (about 80%).[31] REASON: Increase in the systolic distensibility of the pulmonary arteries.

Clinical Features

Most patients are asymptomatic, and congestive cardiac failure is rare. Symptoms of angina may occur because of the coronary arterial abnormalities.

The history may suggest an etiologic factor for the supravalvar aortic stenosis. There may be a positive family history of supravalvar aortic stenosis,[31] and, indeed, we have seen a family in which all of the six children were affected. Many of the children have signs and symptoms resembling those idiopathic hypercalcemia of infancy,[33, 34] such as irritability and constipation in the first year of life, along with slow growth and mild mental retardation.

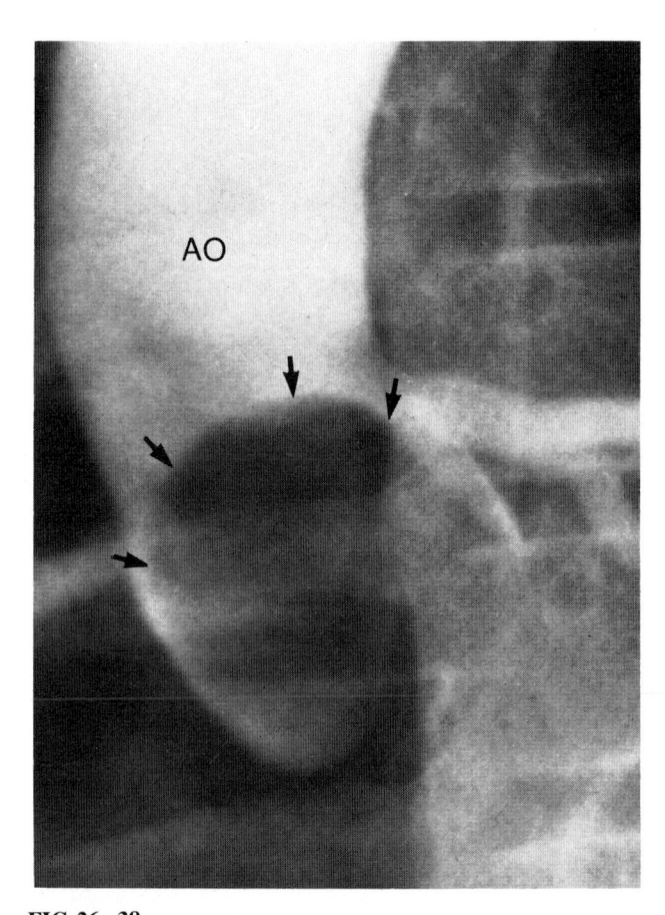

FIG 26–38.
Aortogram delineating prolapsing tumor *(arrows)*. Angiographic appearance similar to doming aortic valve, but no well-defined jet.

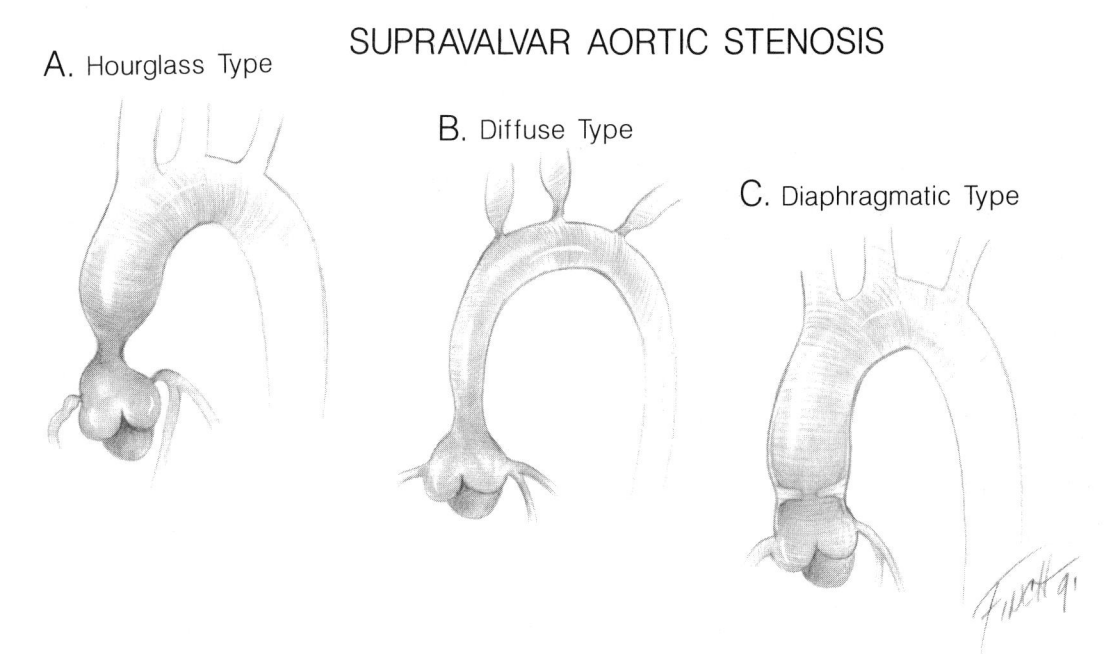

FIG 26–39.
Supravalvar aortic stenosis. Diagram of three types. **A,** hourglass deformity (most common). **B,** diffuse hypoplastic type. **C,** diaphragmatic type (least common). Each type may be associated with stenoses of other arteries (pulmonary artery, coronary arteries, brachiocephalic vessels, renal arteries, etc.). Stenoses of coronary arteries are caused by (1) fibrous changes in media, (2) fusion of aortic valve with area above valve cusps, and (3) atherosclerosis.

Physical Examination

The facies in most patients are typical and highly suggestive of the diagnosis. These have been described as "elfin"[33] or elflike, with periorbital fullness, prominent epicanthal folds, and anteverted nares (Fig 26–40). These patients are very loquacious and may be small in stature.

Commonly, a blood pressure difference is recorded between the arms, the right usually being significantly higher than the left. This is caused by the jet stream that is directly directed into the orifice of the innominate artery. Slowing of the jet causes conversion of kinetic energy into pressure energy, thus increasing the pressure in the right arm. Similar pressure differences between the right and left arm have also been observed in valvar aortic stenosis but to a much lesser degree because the distance between the stenotic aortic valve orifice and the innominate artery is much larger. Consequently, the energy of the jet is largely dissipated by distance.

The preservation of energy of the jet extending into the innominate artery is explained by the Coanda effect (named after Henri Coanda, a Romanian aeronautic engineer who worked in Paris). Coanda discovered that a jet stream tends to adhere to a wall, thus preserving its energy. Because the ascending aorta is curved, the jet adheres to its greater curvature. It is propagated without energy loss and deviated into the innominate artery, where its kinetic energy is converted to pressure energy resulting in an elevated blood pressure.

Cardiac size is normal, although there may be a left ventricular heave. In most patients, a suprasternal notch thrill is found. A systolic ejection murmur is present beneath the right clavicle, which radiates well to the neck. Systolic ejection clicks are not present because there is no poststenotic dilatation. Rarely, a murmur of aortic insufficiency is found. There may be an additional murmur of peripheral pulmonary arterial stenosis.

Electrocardiographic Features

In most instances, the ECG findings resemble those of valvar aortic stenosis. ST-segment and T-wave abnormalities occur more commonly because of coronary artery involvement. Patients with significant coexisting peripheral pulmonary arterial stenosis may show associated right ventricular hypertrophy.

Echocardiographic Features

Echocardiographic tracings show narrowing of the ascending aorta when the stenosis is located immediately above the sinus of Valsalva. Depending on the degree of stenosis, increased thickness of the left ventricular posterior wall and septum may be found, indicating left ventricular hypertrophy.[35, 36]

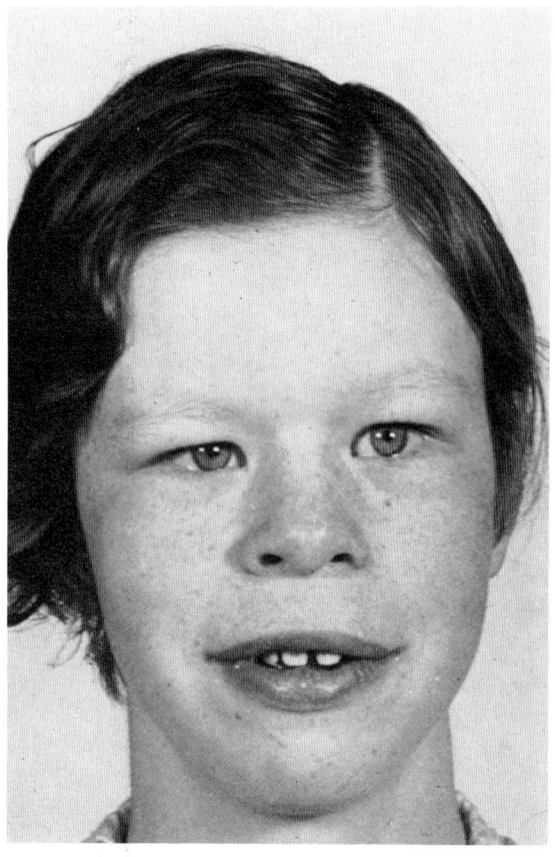

440 Outflow Obstructive Lesions

FIG 26–40.
Facies of patient with supravalvar aortic stenosis.

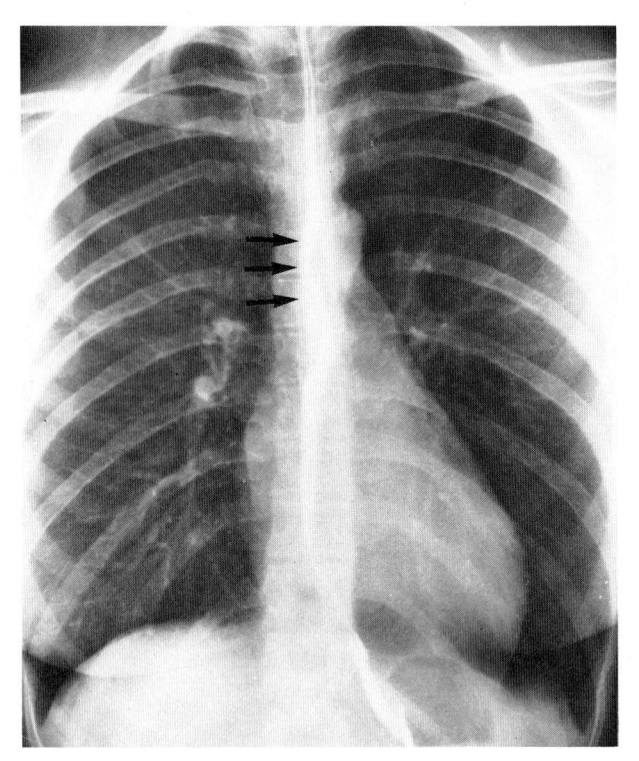

FIG 26–41.
Thoracic roentgenogram, posteroanterior projection in supravalvar aortic stenosis. Normal cardiac size; normal pulmonary vasculature. Left ventricular configuration. With clinical information of aortic systolic ejection murmur and left ventricular hypertrophy, possibility of muscular subaortic or supravalvar aortic stenosis may be suggested. On the basis of absent ascending aortic shadow *(arrows)* and comparatively small aortic knob, supravalvar aortic stenosis should be considered. Absent ascending aortic shadow could also be caused by clockwise cardiac rotation.

Radiographic Features

1. Cardiac silhouette and pulmonary vasculature are normal.
2. Sometimes a diagnosis of supravalvar aortic stenosis will be suggested by the clinical findings of aortic stenosis in a patient with an inconspicuous ascending aorta and a small aortic arch (Fig 26–41). However, muscular subaortic stenosis and, in some patients, subaortic membranes also do not lead to poststenotic dilatation of the ascending aorta; therefore, no specific diagnosis can be made from plain films in most cases.

Cardiac Catheterization

The oximetry data are normal. Pressure tracings from the pulmonary arteries may indicate the presence of peripheral pulmonary arterial stenosis.

Pressure tracings should be obtained on withdrawal of the catheter from the left ventricle through the aortic arch to the descending aorta. Such tracings are diagnostic and characteristically show a systolic gradient within the aorta, with the systolic pressures being identical in the left ventricle and in the aorta proximal to the stenosis. Beyond the obstruction, the systolic pressure is normal. Another characteristic feature is the widened pulse pressure proximal to the obstruction (Fig 26–42). This finding is explained by the fact that during systole, the aorta proximal to the stenosis is merely an extension of the left ventricle, and the systolic portion of the aortic pressure curve is identical to that in the left ventricle. The diastolic pressures on either side of the supravalvar stenosis are identical, because the aorta is in free communication and isolated from the left ventricle by the closed aortic valve. During diastole, there is only coronary flow in the aorta proximal to the obstruction, and this small aortic backflow does not produce a diastolic gradient across the stenosis.

Angiographic Appearance

1. The types of supravalvular aortic stenosis are well demonstrated angiographically.
   a. Hourglass deformity (Fig 26–43), a localized narrowing immediately above the sinuses of Valsalva.

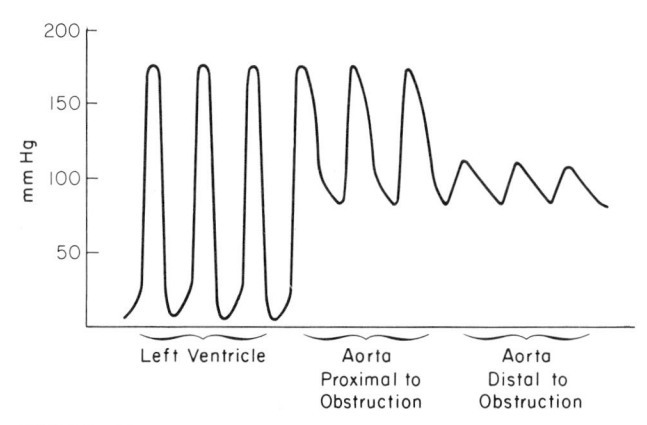

FIG 26-42.
Diagram of pressure tracing of supravalvar stenosis; systolic gradient in aorta.

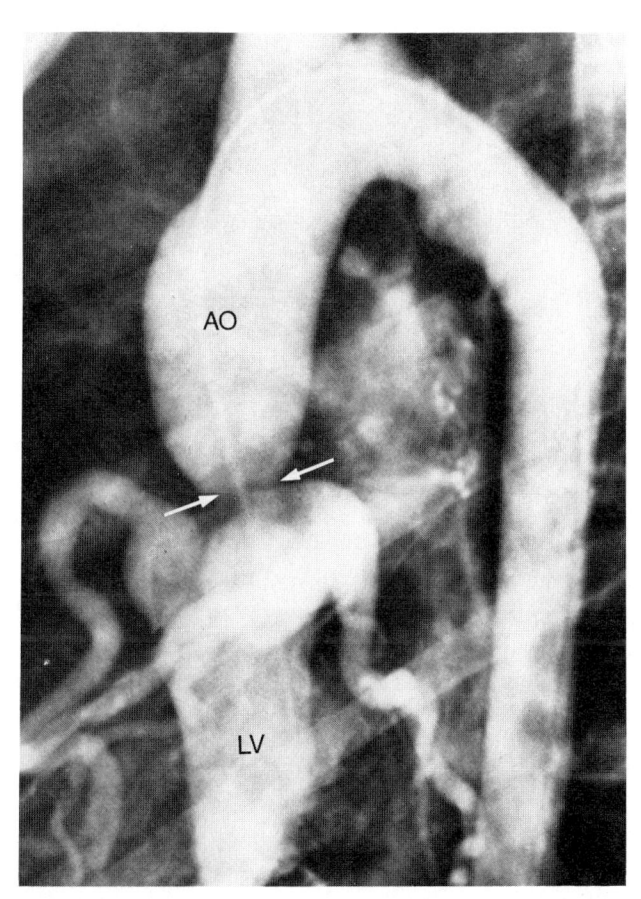

FIG 26-43.
A left ventriculogram (LV) of supravalvar aortic stenosis of hourglass type (arrows). Localized narrowing above sinuses of Valsalva. Enlarged coronary arteries. Aortic valve shows pseudodoming and thickened leaflets. Mild poststenotic dilation of ascending aorta.

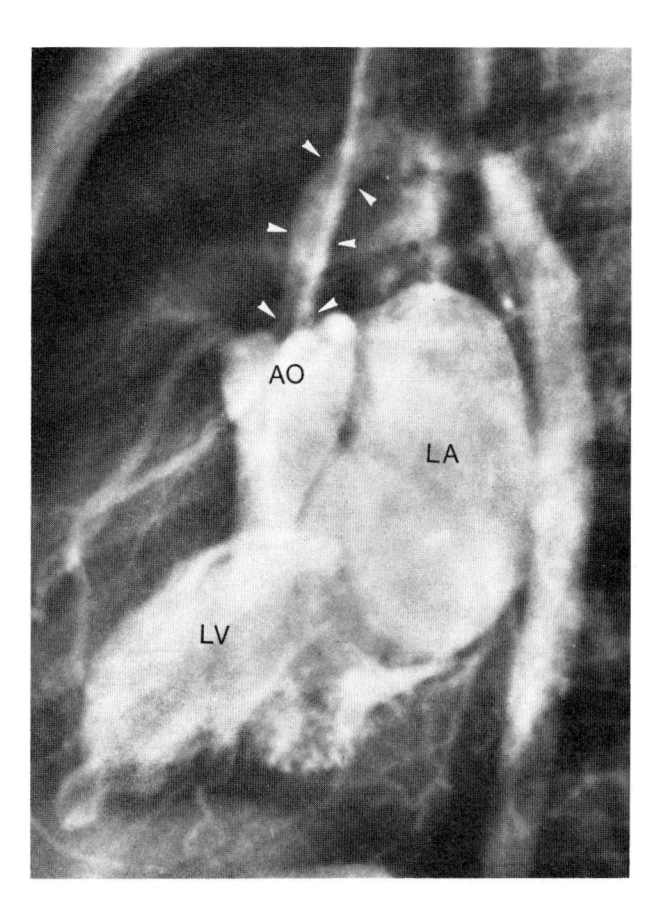

FIG 26-44.
Left ventriculogram (LV) of supravalvar aortic stenosis of diffuse hypoplastic type (arrows). Marked narrowing of entire ascending aorta (AO) and aortic arch; stenosis of brachiocephalic vessels and extension of stenotic process beyond aortic arch into descending aorta. Marked mitral reflux. LA = left atrium.

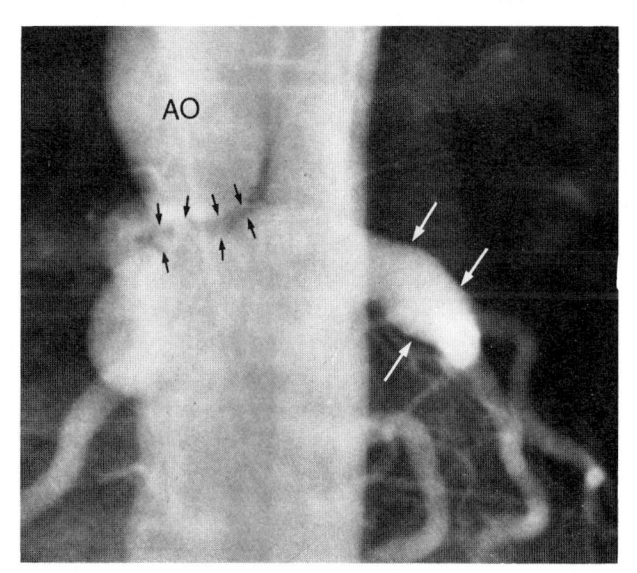

FIG 26-45.
Supravalvar aortic stenosis of discrete supravalvar membrane type (arrows). Enlarged coronary arteries. Aneurysm of left coronary artery (white arrows), suggesting diffuse arterial disease. AO = aorta.

FIG 26–46.
Left ventriculogram *(LV)* of supravalvar aortic stenosis of diffuse hypoplastic type. Left ventricular enlargement. Aortic valve distinctly thickened and domed *(small arrows)*. Pseudodoming because of narrowed supravalvar area—aortic valve leaflets cannot straighten out during systole. This appearance should not be confused with true doming seen in valvar aortic stenosis. Thickening of aortic valve explained by constant impact of aortic valve leaflets on supravalvar narrowing.

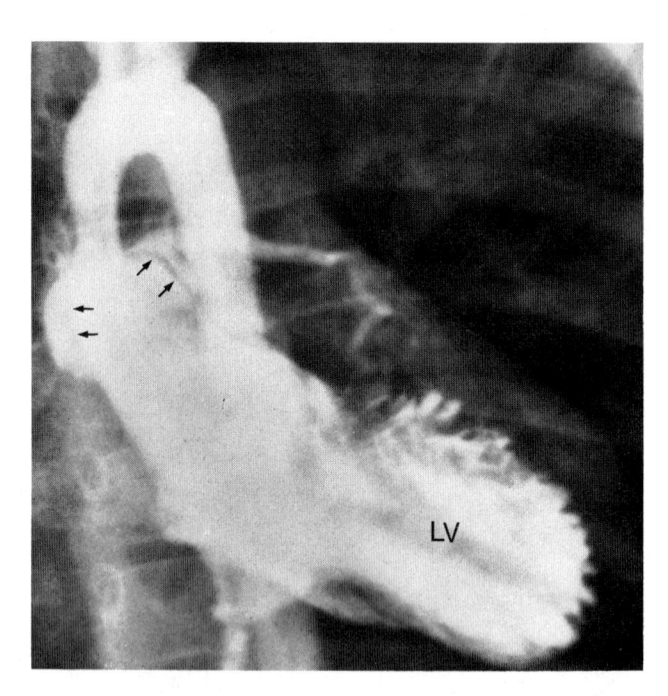

FIG 26–47.
Aortogram, lateral projection of supravalvar aortic stenosis. Marked aortic reflux. Aortic valve is distinctly thickened *(small black arrows)*. Stenosis of right coronary ostium *(small white arrows)*. Pathologic process of supravalvar aortic stenosis may involve aortic valve leaflets, causing secondary aortic insufficiency, as well as the coronary ostial orifice, resulting in stenosis or atresia. *LV* = left ventricle.

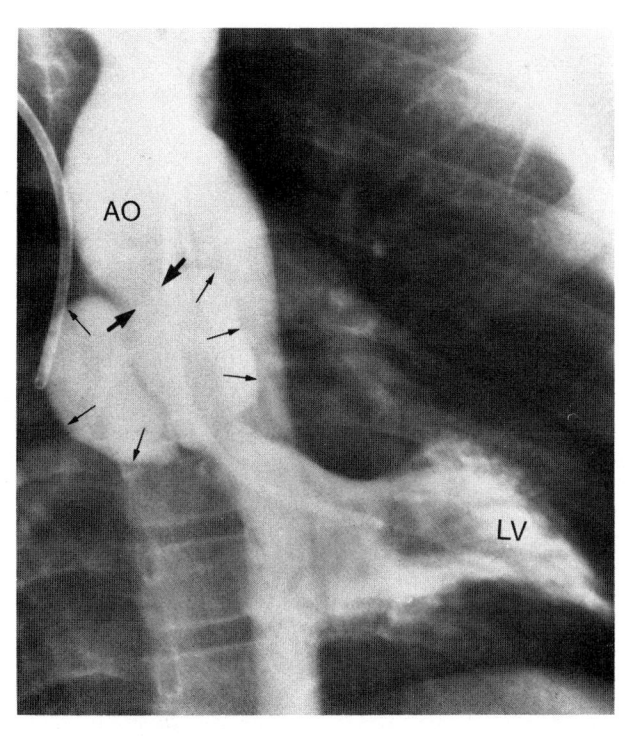

FIG 26-48.
Left ventriculogram *(LV)*, anteroposterior projection in supravalvar aortic stenosis of hourglass type *(large black arrows)*. Left ventricular hypertrophy. Sinuses of Valsalva aneurysmally dilated *(small black arrows)*; this should not be confused with congenital sinus of Valsalva aneurysm. *AO* = aorta.

b. Diffuse narrowing of ascending aorta (Fig 26-44) extending into the descending aorta.
c. Localized supravalvular membrane (Fig 26-45), a discrete membrane immediately above the sinuses of Valsalva.

2. Thickening of aortic valve occurs. REASON: The impact and limited excursion of aortic valve leaflets with supra-aortic narrowing during systole damages the valve leaflets, inducing fibrotic thickening. A similar thickening of the pulmonary valve is seen in

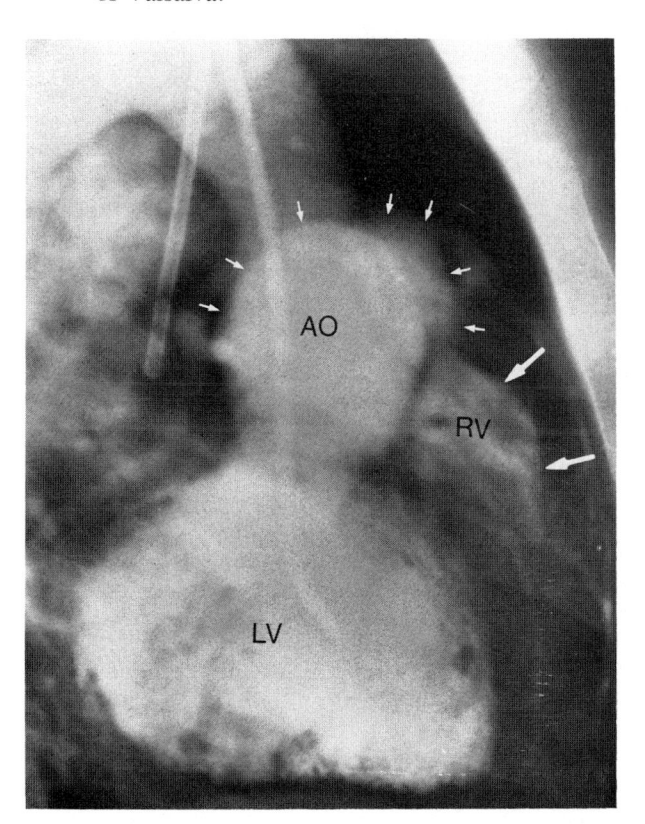

FIG 26-49.
Left ventriculogram *(LV)*, lateral projection in mild supravalvar stenosis of hourglass type. Aneurysmal of sinuses of Valsalva, particularly the right *(small white arrows)*. Opacification of infundibulum of right ventricle *(RV) (white arrows)* through small supracristal ventricular septal defect. *AO* = aorta.

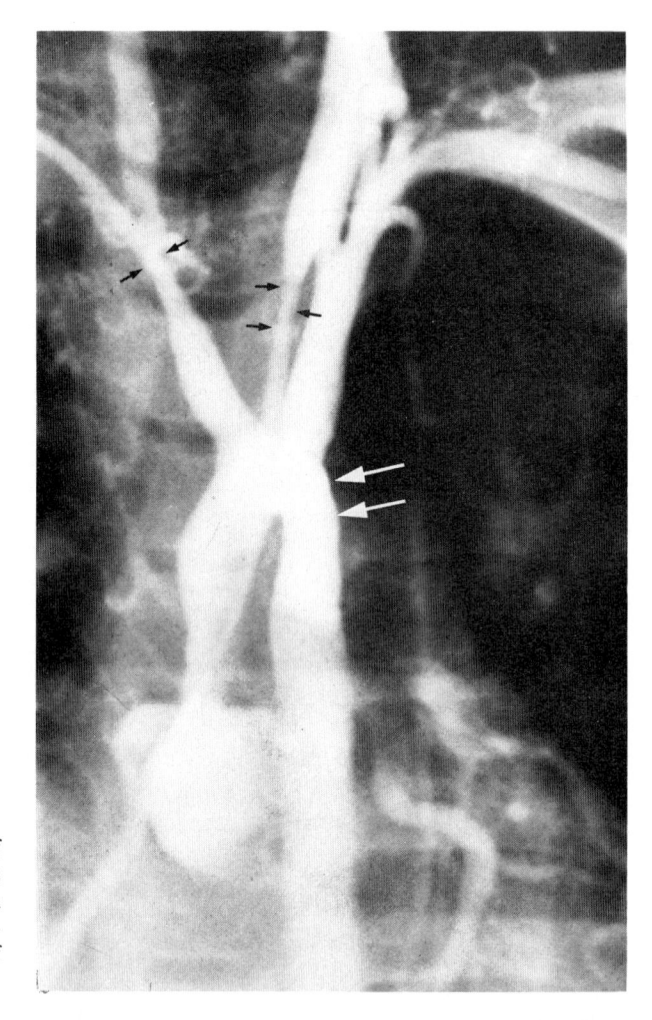

FIG 26–50.
Diffuse hypoplastic type of supravalvar aortic stenosis. Extension of stenotic process *(white arrows)* beyond aortic arch. At surgery, this type of supravalvar stenosis may not be as impressive, because of a very thick inner lining of aortic wall. Origin of brachiocephalic vessels commonly involved *(small black arrows)* with the diffuse type of supravalvar stenosis.

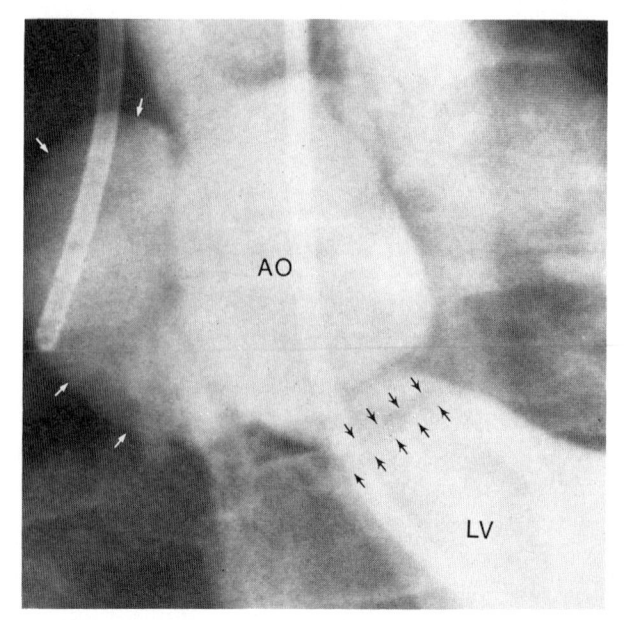

FIG 26–51.
Supravalvar aortic stenosis of the hourglass type *(open white arrows)*. Aneurysmal dilatation of sinuses of Valsalva *(small white arrows)*. Beneath slightly thickened aortic valve, a distinct, discrete, thick subvalvar diaphragm is present *(small black arrows)*. Rare association presents a diagnostic challenge to radiologist and cardiologist. *AO* = aorta; *LV* = left ventricle.

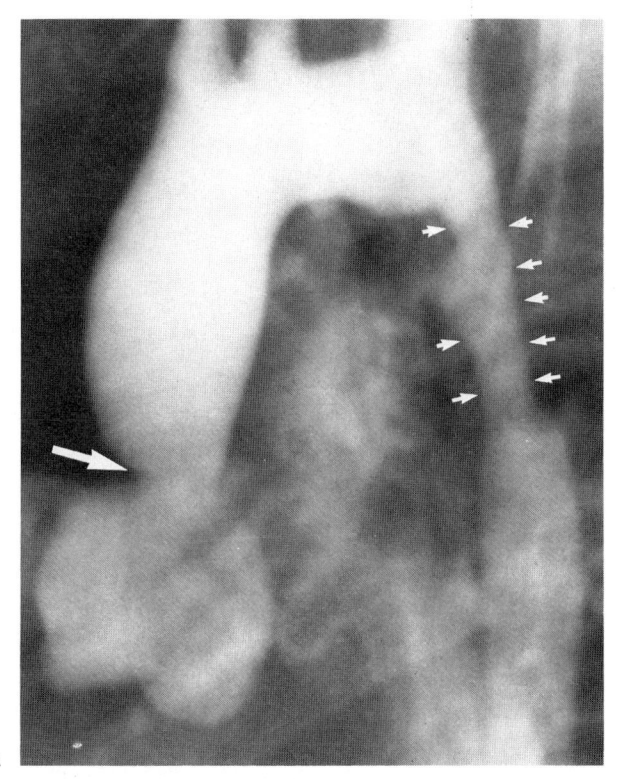

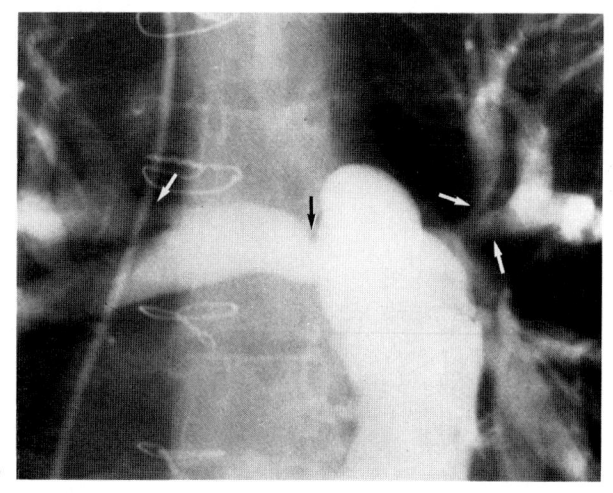

FIG 26–52.
Supravalvar aortic stenosis with diffuse involvement of descending aorta. **A,** lateral aortogram showing typical findings of stenosis *(large arrow)* and distal aortic involvement *(small arrows)*. **B,** pulmonary arteriogram showing numerous areas of peripheral pulmonary artery stenosis.

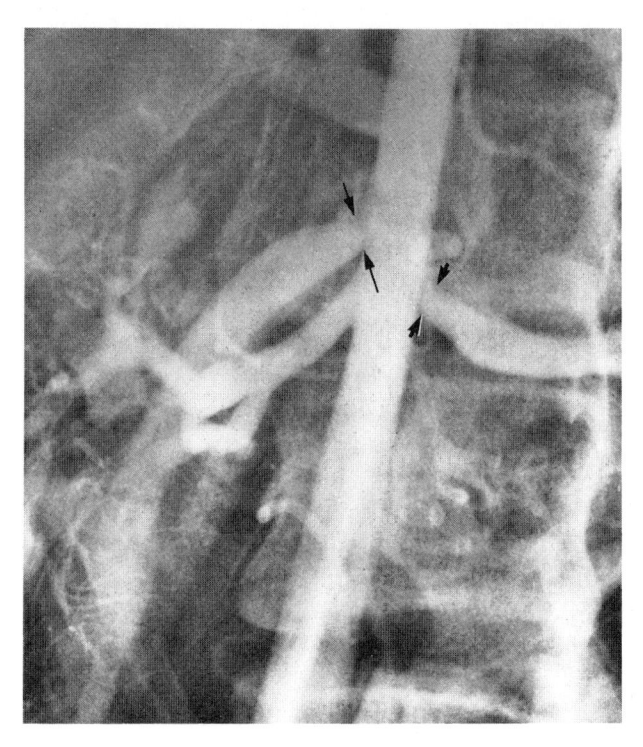

FIG 26–53.
Supravalvar aortic stenosis and diffuse mild narrowing of abdominal aorta (abdominal coarctation). Stenosis of origin of both renal arteries *(short arrows)* is common and may cause systemic hypertension. Stenosis of superior mesenteric artery, with marked poststenotic dilatation *(long arrows)*.

pulmonary banding (pseudodoming) (see Chapter 12).
3. Pseudodoming of the aortic valve is seen. REASON: Aortic valve opening is limited by supravalvar stenosis during systole (Fig 26–46). An identical finding of the pulmonary valve occurs with pulmonary banding.
4. Aortic insufficiency may be found (Fig 26–47). REASON: Thickening of the valve cusps and, sometimes, adherence of a cusp to aortic wall.
5. Aneurysmal dilatation of the sinuses of Valsalva is found occasionally (Fig 26–48). REASON: Probably increased pressure.
6. Dilatation and increased tortuosity of coronary arteries with premature atherosclerosis are common. REASON: Coronary arteries are submitted to high level of systolic pressure.
7. Coronary ostial stenosis (Figs 26–46 and 26–49) or atresia (see Fig 26–57) may be visualized.
8. Associated lesions may be present, including:
    a. Aortic insufficiency (Fig 26–47).
    b. Mitral insufficiency (see Fig 26–44).
    c. Dilation of the sinuses of Valsalva (Figs 26–48 and 26–51).
    d. Ventricular septal defect (Fig 26–49).
    e. Stenosis of brachiocephalic vessels (Fig 26–50).
    f. Subaortic stenosis (Fig 26–51).
    g. Peripheral pulmonary arterial stenosis (Fig 26–52).
    h. Abdominal coarctation and renal artery stenosis (Fig 26–53).
    i. Stenosis of visceral arteries (Fig 26–54).

Operative Considerations[37, 38]

Because of the anatomic features of supravalvar stenosis, the possible associated narrowing of brachiocephalic vessels, and involvement of coronary arteries, the operative risk is greater, and the results may be less satisfactory than with correction of valvar aortic stenosis. Therefore, operation is undertaken with stricter criteria. A surgical procedure is carried out if there are symptoms from the outflow obstruction, a significant gradient is present, or angina pectoris occurs.

Patients with an hourglass deformity are more amenable to operation than those with more diffuse hypoplasia of the aorta.

Under cardiopulmonary bypass, a longitudinal incision is made across the area of stenosis, and a patch is inserted to widen the area (Fig 26–55). It may be necessary to extend the patch around the arch or into brachiocephalic vessels in patients with a long stenotic area (Fig 26–56). Coronary bypass may be carried out in patients with coronary ostial stenosis or atresia (Figs 26–57 and 26–58).

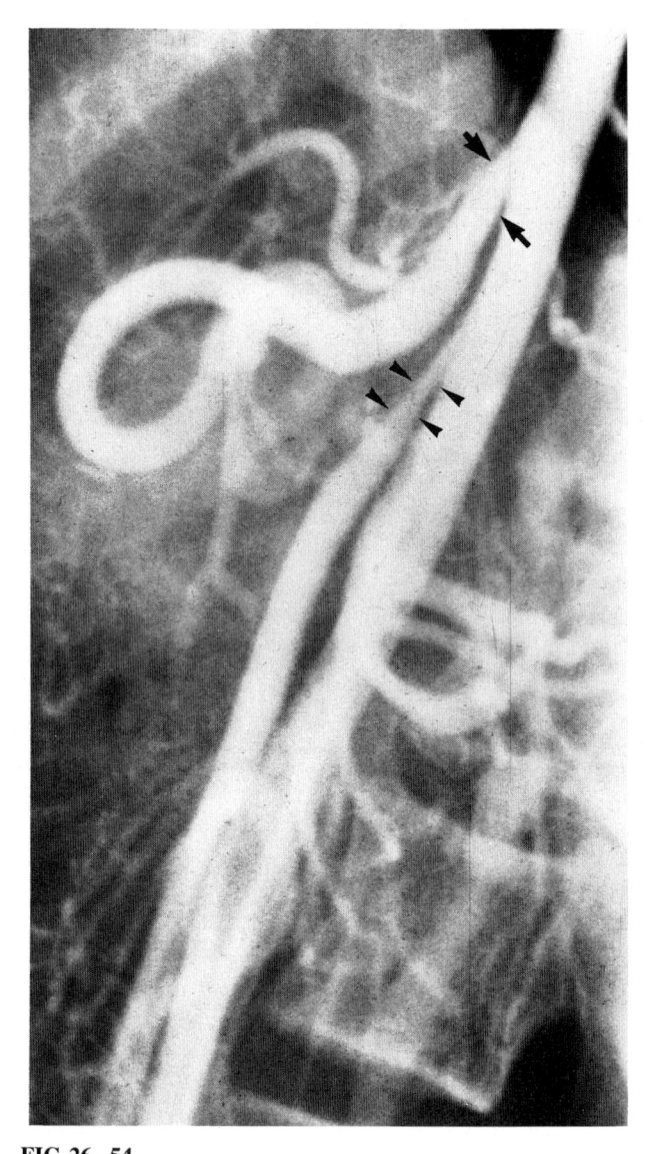

FIG 26–54.
Aortogram, lateral projection in supravalvar aortic stenosis and involvement of the abdominal aorta. Stenosis of superior mesenteric artery and celiac axis (*small and large black arrows*, respectively).

MUSCULAR SUBAORTIC STENOSIS

Muscular subaortic stenosis is known by a number of names, including asymmetric septal hypertrophy, idiopathic hypertrophic subaortic stenosis, and hypertrophic cardiomyopathy. With the advent of echocardiography, the ability to diagnose this condition has been markedly improved. Many patients with asymmetric septal hypertrophy have no hemodynamic obstruction and are without symptoms. In this section, we emphasize the clinical and radiologic features of patients with obstruction.

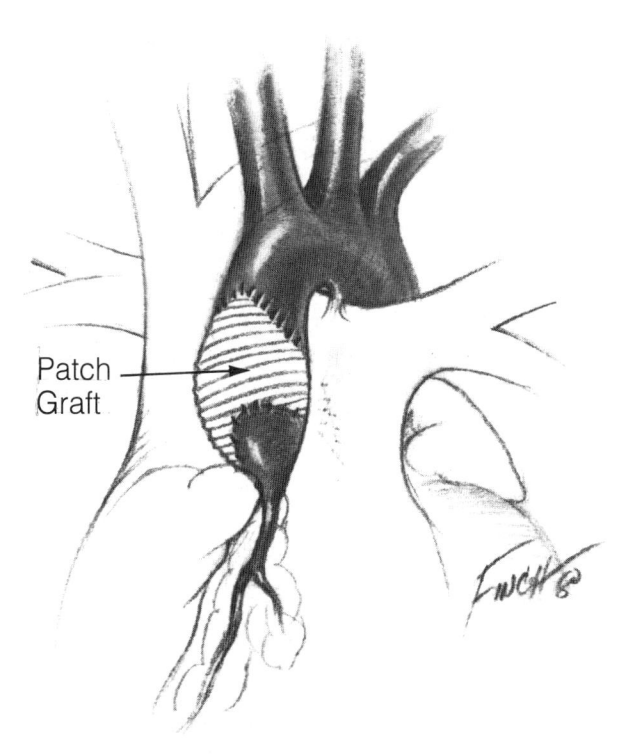

FIG 26–55.
Diagram of operative correction of supravalvar aortic stenosis. Longitudinal incision made in ascending aorta and patch inserted to widen lumen.

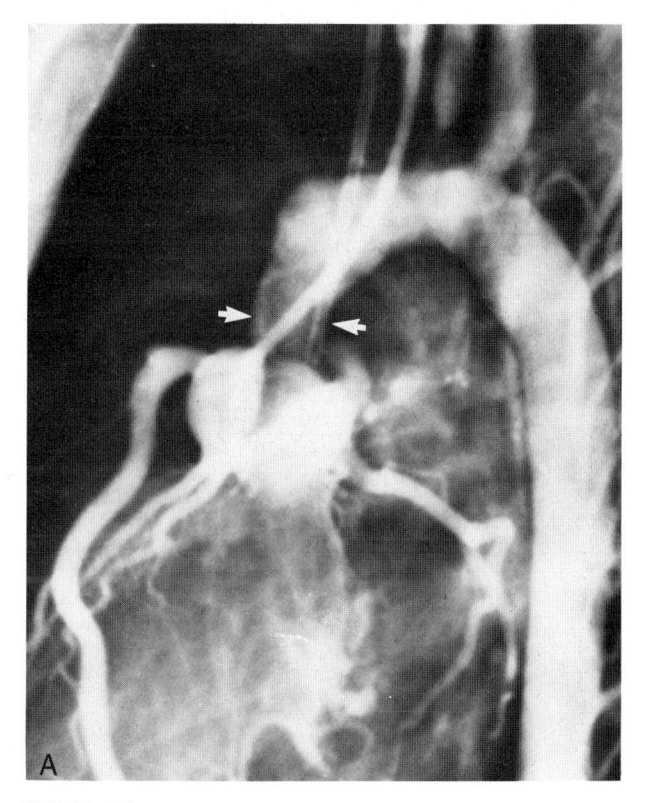

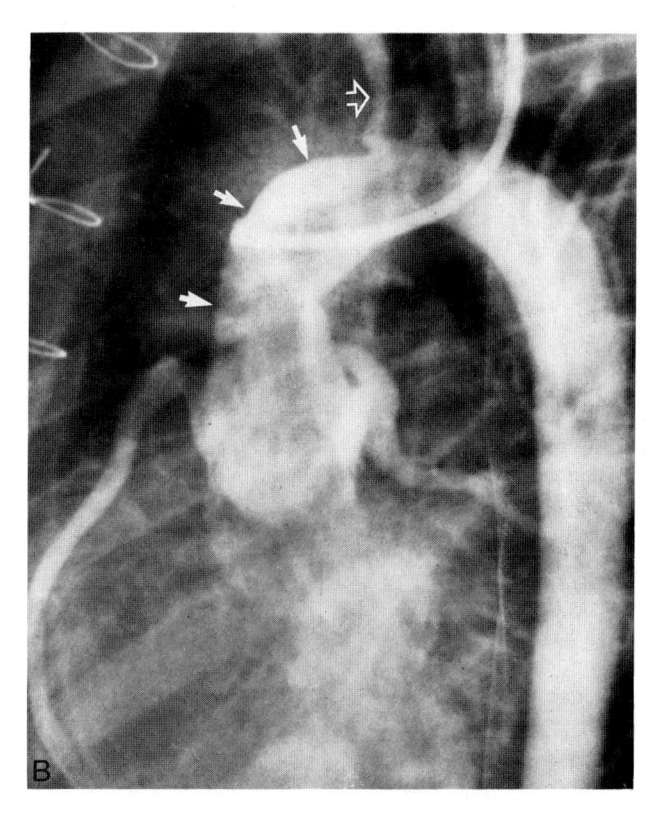

FIG 26–56.
A, Hypoplastic type of supravalvar aortic stenosis *(white arrows)*. Marked involvement of brachiocephalic vessels. **B,** Postoperative aortogram; successful repair of stenosis by patch *(arrows)*. Extension of patch into innominate artery was attempted. Residual stenosis present *(open arrow)*.

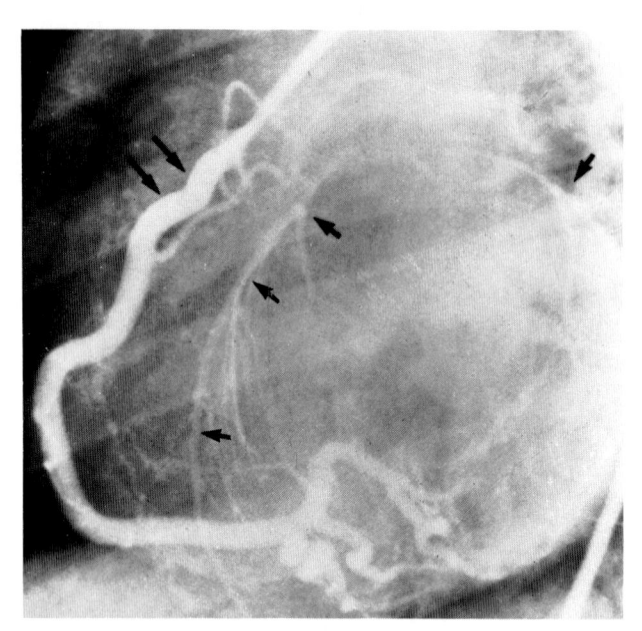

FIG 26–57.
Selective right coronary arteriogram, lateral projection in supravalvar aortic stenosis. Enlarged right coronary artery *(long arrows)*. Atresia of left coronary ostium *(short arrows)*: left coronary artery fills via collaterals.

Pathologic Features

The principal feature is hypertrophy of the ventricular septum and the free wall of the left ventricle. The septum is particularly thickened and encroaches on the subaortic and, occasionally, the subpulmonary area. The subaortic stenosis occurs from apposition of the anterior leaflet of the mitral valve against the septum during systole, and as a result of this contact, the free edge of the mitral valve is thickened. Left atrial enlargement may be present because of commonly associated mitral insufficiency. The latter probably results from abnormal insertion of papillary muscles and angulation of the left ventricle.

Some patients with muscular subaortic stenosis have severe left ventricular hypertrophy with little or no pressure gradient.[39] Subaortic stenosis is probably a myocardial abnormality, which is the cause, not a consequence, of left ventricular outflow tract obstruction. The etiology of the myocardial abnormality is unknown. The hemodynamic obstruction probably is caused by the mitral valve, which is pulled anteriorly against the septum during systole.[40, 41] Sometimes, the pressure gradient is found lower in the body of the left ventricle, probably at the level of the hypertrophied papillary muscles. As a result of the contact with the septum, the mitral valve leaflets become thickened, and there may be a fibrous ridge on the ventricular septum at the contact site of the mitral valve.

Histologic examination of the myocardium shows a characteristic disarray of myofibrils and myofilaments and abnormally shaped and arranged myocardial cells.[42–44]

Hemodynamic Considerations

Regardless of the degree of myocardial hypertrophy, the pressure gradient in a given case is quite variable.[45] Determinants of the gradient are as follows:

1. The state of myocardial contractility.
2. Left ventricular stroke volume.
3. Peripheral resistance.

In general, a decrease of the left ventricular stroke volume, a decrease in contractility, or an increase in left ventricular afterload reduces the gradient. The gradient is increased by increased contractility of the myocardium, a reduced afterload, or increased left ventricular stroke volume.

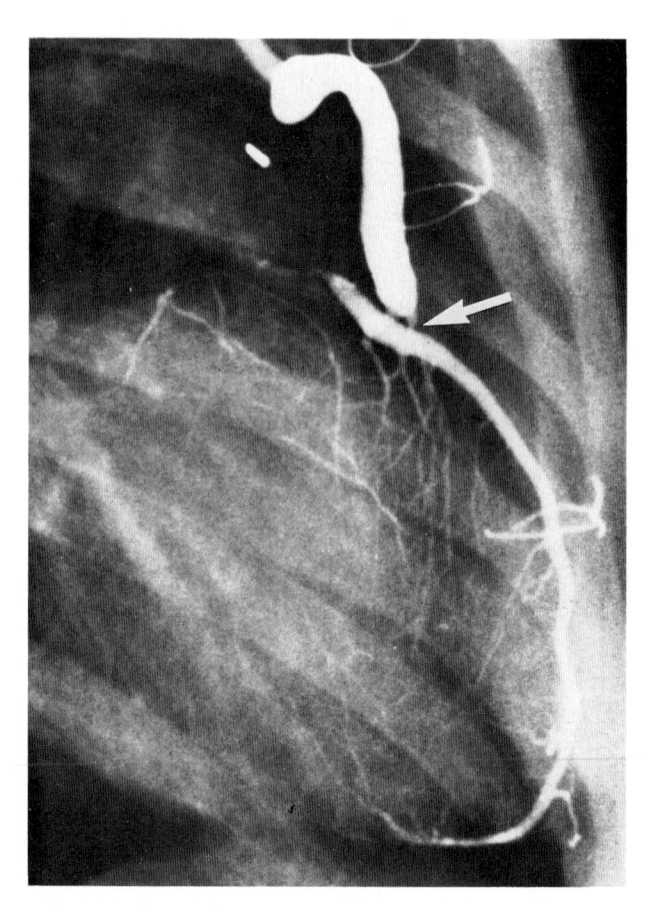

FIG 26–58.
Atresia of left coronary ostium with injection of a saphenous bypass, seen in lateral projection. Graft connected to small diagonal branch of left anterior descending coronary artery. Increased profusion pressure resulted in marked enlargement of left anterior descending branch compared with preoperative angiogram.

Drugs that alter these variables, as well as exercise, can be used to diagnose asymmetric septal hypertrophy. Drugs that decrease myocardial contractility are the basis for the medical treatment.[46, 47]

Clinical Features

Most patients are asymptomatic.[48] A few patients have symptoms of easy fatigability, angina, dizziness, or syncope.

Physical Examination[48]

The patients appear healthy, although occasionally there are features of Leopard syndrome (see Chapter 29). Unlike the findings in other forms of aortic stenosis, the peripheral pulses are brisk and have a double systolic beat. A large portion of the stroke volume is ejected early during systole while there is little gradient. As systole progresses, the gradient increases, and ejection slows considerably. As the stenosis relaxes, there is ejection again and the second part of the pulse beat.

Cardiac size may be either normal or increased. The apical impulse is prominent and may have two impulses. One of these is the normally expected apical impulse that occurs with ventricular systole; the second is presystolic

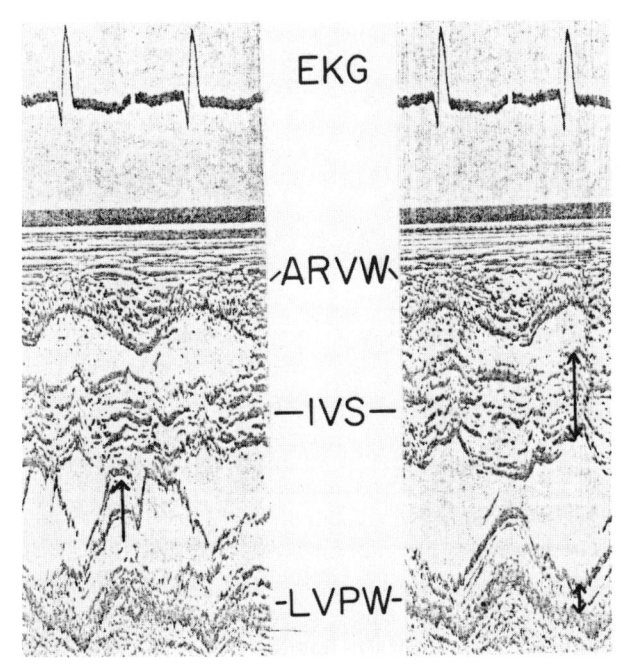

FIG 26–59.
Echocardiogram in muscular aortic stenosis. Thickening of interventricular septum *(IVS)* is out of proportion to size of left ventricular posterior wall *(LVPW) (double arrows)*. Characteristic systolic anterior motion of anterior leaflet of mitral valve (SAM) *(single arrow)*. ARVW = anterior right ventricular wall.

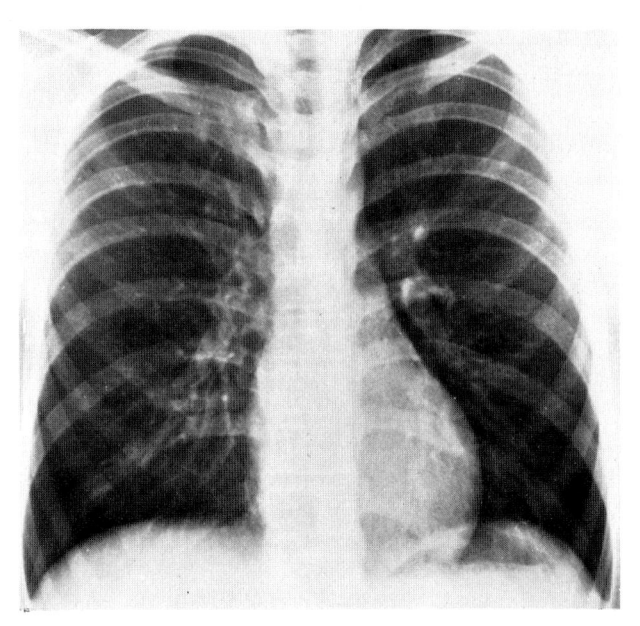

FIG 26–60.
Thoracic roentgenogram, posteroanterior projection of muscular subaortic stenosis in patient with highly abnormal ECG and 100 mm Hg pressure gradient. Normal radiograph. Ascending aorta not evident. With clinical information of systolic ejection murmur, left ventricular hypertrophy on the ECG, and absence of poststenotic dilatation on radiograph, possibility of supravalvar, muscular subaortic, or discrete membranous subaortic stenosis should be considered, rather than valvar aortic stenosis.

and occurs from forceful atrial contraction because of the diminished ventricular compliance. A thrill is found along the left sternal border in one half of the patients. The heart sounds are normal, although a fourth heart sound may be heard. Systolic ejection clicks are rare, because poststenotic dilatation of the aorta is absent.

A systolic ejection murmur is present and is best heard between the lower left sternal border and the apex. A soft high-pitched murmur may be heard at the apex in patients who develop mitral insufficiency. A soft middiastolic murmur is found at the apex in one fourth of patients. The origin of this murmur is not understood. The systolic murmur characteristically decreases in loudness when the patient squats and increases on standing, because the systemic vascular resistance is elevated in the former position and decreased in the latter.

Electrocardiographic Features[49]

The QRS axis is normal. Most patients show left ventricular hypertrophy, and about one third develop ST-segment depression and reduced or inverted T waves in the left precordial leads. An occasional patient shows a Wolff-Parkinson-White syndrome. Deep Q waves are found in the left precordial leads in about 20% of patients and are believed related to septal hypertrophy.

Echocardiographic Features[50-53]

Echocardiography is the most helpful noninvasive diagnostic test for detecting muscular subaortic stenosis. The ratio of the ventricular septal to left ventricular posterior wall thickness exceeds 1.3:1 (the upper limit of normal).

The most pathognomonic finding is systolic anterior motion of the mitral valve (Fig 26–59). Closure of the aortic valve occurs during midsystole because aortic flow is very low during this period of maximum obstruction. This midsystolic closure of the aortic valve occurs because of the high initial velocity of the left ventricular ejection of blood and the relatively small amount of flow in midsystole as a result of systolic anterior motion.

Radiographic Features

1. Radiographs may be entirely normal despite severe destruction and a markedly abnormal ECG (Fig 26–60).
2. Most patients show some degree of cardiac enlargement and signs of left ventricular hypertrophy (Fig 26–61).
3. Rarely, cardiac enlargement is severe (Fig 26–62); the pulmonary vasculature remains normal.

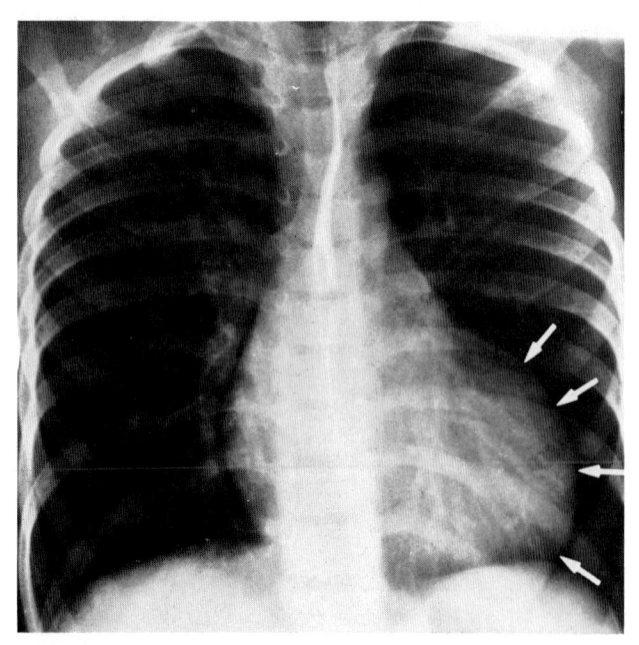

FIG 26–61.
Thoracic roentgenogram, posteroanterior projection of muscular subaortic stenosis. Rounded left ventricular contour *(arrows)*, indicating left ventricular hypertrophy. Slightly enlarged heart. Normal pulmonary vasculature. No aortic dilatation. Nonvalvar left ventricular outflow tract obstruction should be considered.

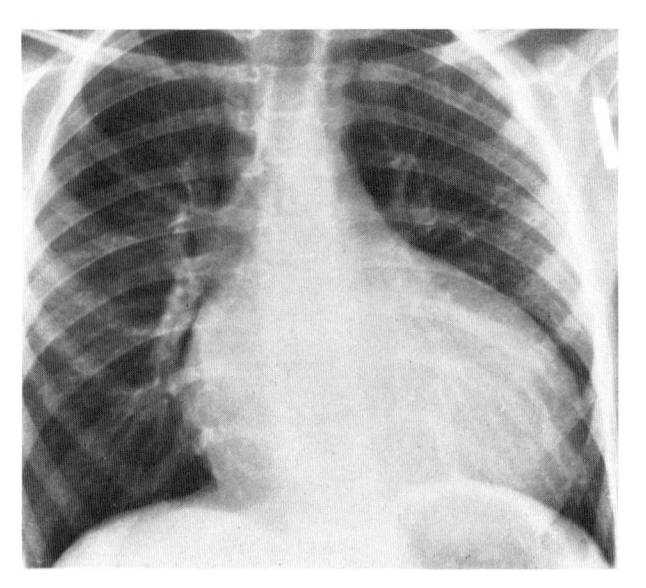

FIG 26–62.
Thoracic roentgenogram, posteroanterior projection in muscular subaortic stenosis. Severe cardiomegaly. Rounded cardiac apex. Congestive changes or pleural effusion and cephalization not present. No correlation between degree of cardiomegaly and left ventricular gradient; this patient had only a small gradient.

4. Radiographic findings of decompensation are rare.
5. The ascending aorta is normal (poststenotic dilatation absent).
6. Left atrial enlargement may be present because of mitral insufficiency, which is commonly found in muscular subaortic stenosis.

Cardiac Catheterization

The oximetry data are normal.

The major abnormalities are found in pressure recordings. A pressure gradient is found within the left ventricle at a lower level than in discrete membranous subaortic stenosis. Characteristically, the left ventricular pressure curve shows a notch at the point where the aortic valve opens (Fig 26–63). Occasionally, no pressure gradient is found at rest, but one can be provoked by exercise or ionotropic drugs, such as isoproterenol or digitalis.

The aortic pressure tracing shows a very rapid upstroke because of the rapid left ventricular ejection during the first portion of systole. The aortic pressure also shows a characteristic feature on a postextrasystolic beat[54]. In contrast to normal, after a postextrasystolic pause, when the pulse pressure increases, the pulse pressure is reduced. The subaortic obstruction increases because of postextrasystolic potentiation of myocardial contractility by the prolonged filling of the left ventricle during a compensatory pause.

On occasion, a systolic gradient is found in the right ventricle because of encroachment on the right ventricular

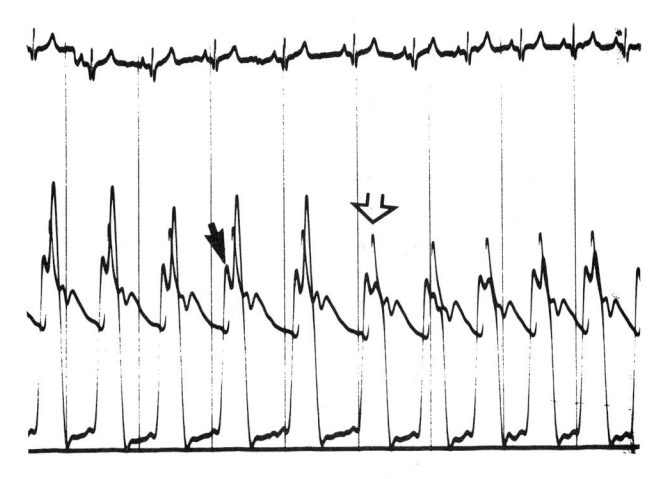

FIG 26-63.
Pressure tracing with simultaneous recording of aortic and left ventricular pressures in muscular subaortic stenosis. Typical notch in ventricular tracing *(solid arrow)* and systolic pressure gradient *(open black arrow).*

outflow area by the hypertrophied septum (Bernheim phenomenon).

Angiographic Appearance[55, 56]

1. There is hypertrophy of the ventricular septum, which is best seen by simultaneous left and right ventricular injections (Fig 26–64).
2. The free wall of the left ventricle may also be thickened (Fig 26–65).
3. End-systolic volume is decreased (Fig 26–65), as with other types of aortic stenosis.
4. During diastole, the space between the anterior leaflet of the mitral valve and the ventricular septum is narrowed (Fig 26–66), creating pseudonarrowing of left ventricular outflow tract.
5. Systolic anterior motion of the mitral valve (Fig 26–67) may be difficult to see angiographically. The best view is an angulated left anterior oblique projection, but the motion can also be seen on the lateral projection.
6. Peculiar angulation of the left ventricle and abnormal orientation of the anterior papillary muscle are found (Fig 26–68) in many cases.
7. Abnormal angulation of left ventricle is also found on lateral projection (Fig 26–69).
8. An hourglass deformity of left ventricle as a result

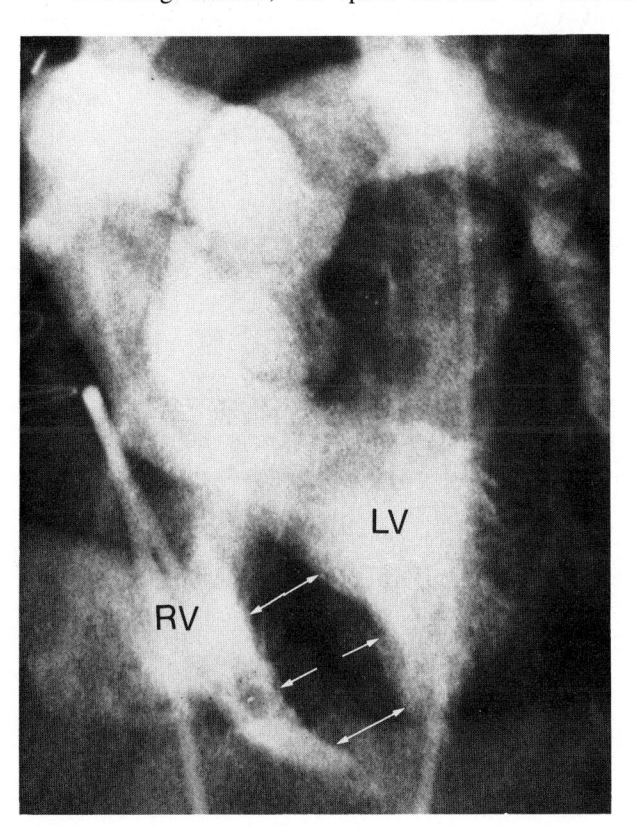

FIG 26-64.
Left ventriculogram *(LV)*, left anterior oblique projection in muscular subaortic stenosis. Simultaneous injection of left and right ventricles *(RV)* reveals enormously thickened ventricular septum *(small arrows).*

452 Outflow Obstructive Lesions

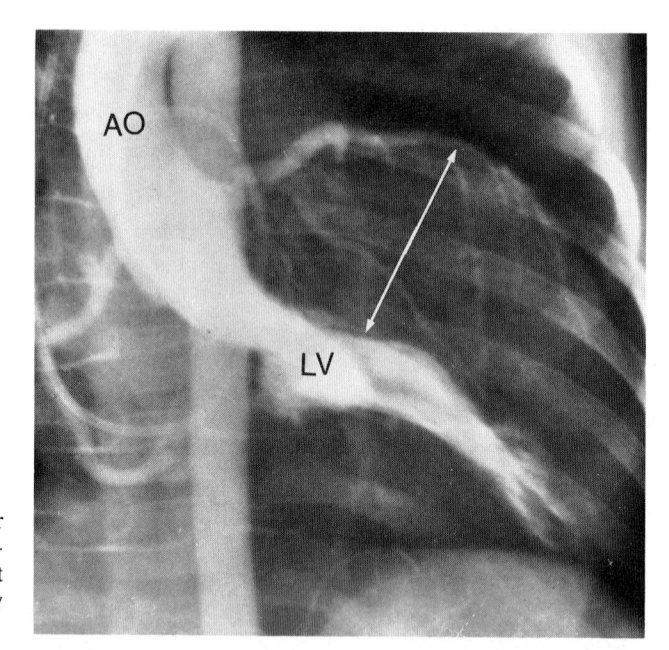

FIG 26–65.
Left ventriculogram *(LV)*, anteroposterior projection in muscular subaortic stenosis. Decreased end-systolic volume. Severe thickening of myocardium, evidenced by increased distance between left ventricular cavity and coronary arteries *(arrows)*. Large coronary arteries are commonly present in this condition. *AO* = aorta.

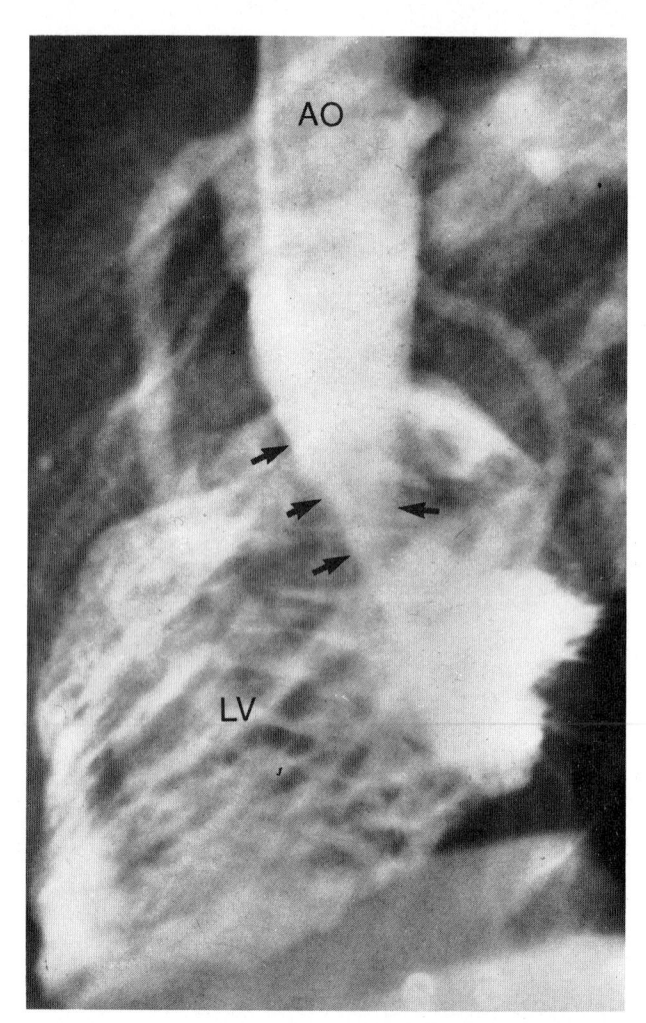

FIG 26–66.
Left ventriculogram *(LV)*, lateral projection during diastole in muscular subaortic stenosis. Encroachment of anterior leaflet of mitral valve and hypertrophied septum *(arrows)*, with characteristic cone-shaped appearance of left ventricular outflow area. Previously, this appearance was thought to be angiographic demonstration of obstruction, until it was realized that narrowing occurs during diastole and consequently is not responsible for the systolic gradient. Only after systolic anterior motion of mitral valve was demonstrated by echocardiography could it also be seen by angiography. *AO* = aorta.

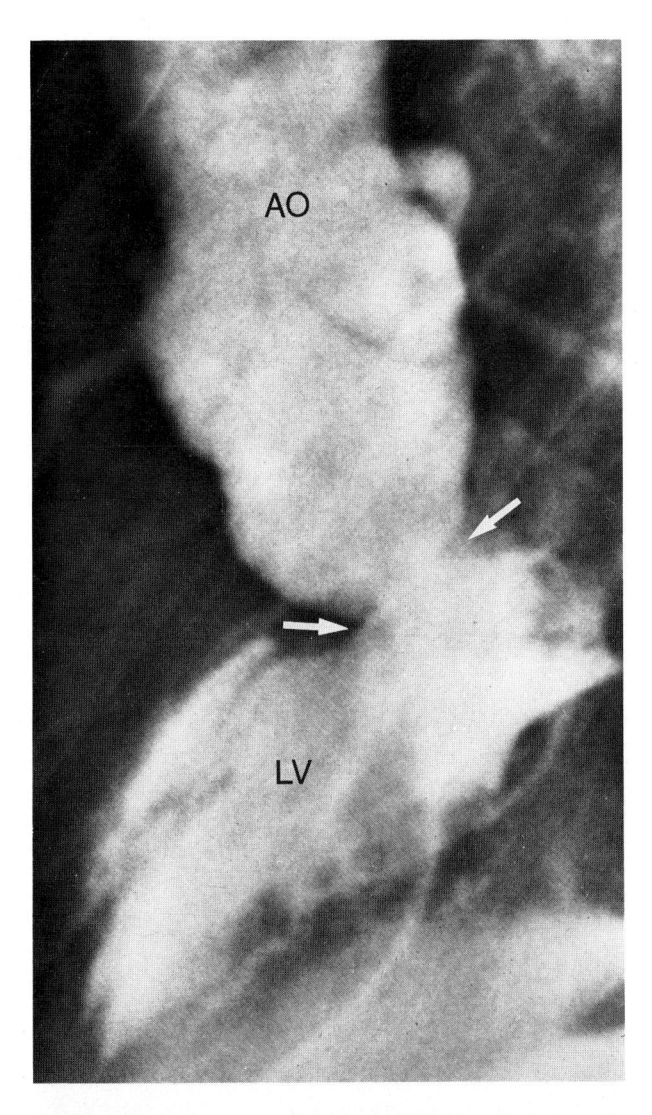

Aortic Stenosis 453

FIG 26–67.
Left ventriculogram, lateral projection in muscular subaortic stenosis in systole. Marked encroachment of outflow area by hypertrophied septum *(white arrow)*. Encroachment posteriorly *(arrow)* from anterior leaflet of mitral valve. This appearance is caused by systolic anterior motion of mitral valve. Left ventricular cavity shows unusual angulation and abnormal direction of papillary muscles and chordae tendineae, believed to cause abnormal valve motion and possibly mitral insufficiency. *AO* = aorta.

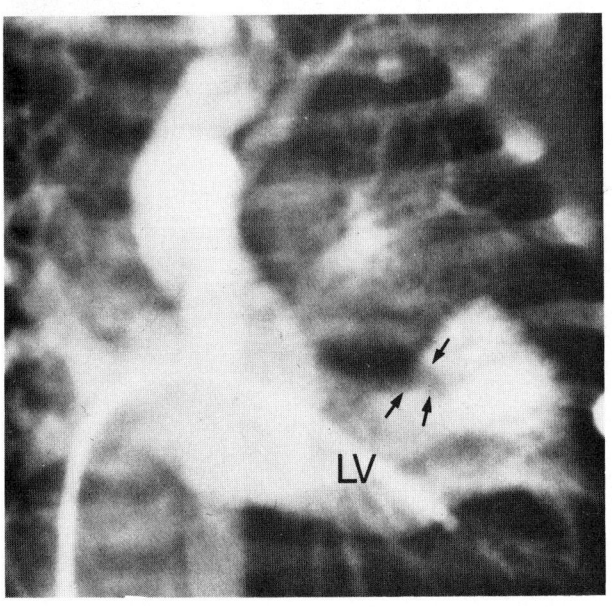

FIG 26–68.
Left ventriculogram *(LV)*, anteroposterior projection in muscular subaortic stenosis. Marked angulation of left ventricular cavity also seen on lateral projection (see also Figures 26–70 and 26–73). Hypertrophied papillary muscles *(black arrows)*. Because of angulation of left ventricular cavity, direction of papillary muscles and chordae tendineae is altered. During systole, anterior leaflet of mitral valve moves anteriorly and may be held open, leading to mitral regurgitation.

454 Outflow Obstructive Lesions

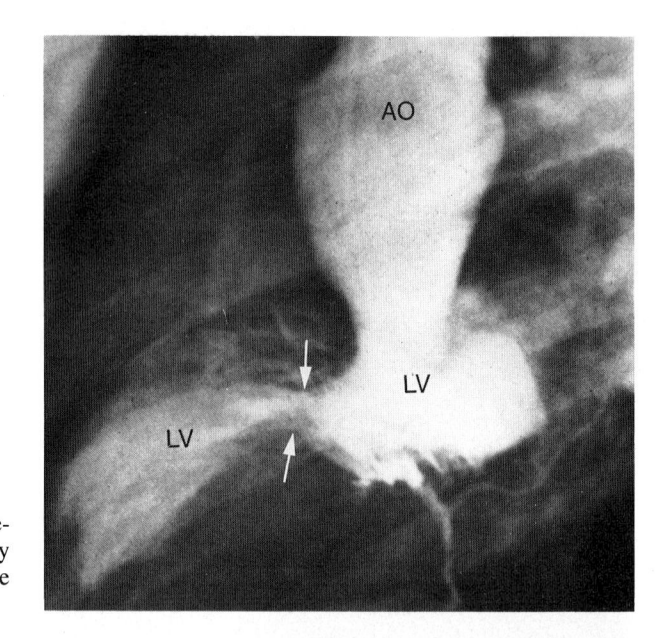

FIG 26–69.
Left ventriculogram *(LV)*, lateral projection in muscular subaortic stenosis. Abnormal angulation of left ventricle. Hourglass deformity *(white arrows)* caused by hypertrophied papillary muscles. Pressure gradient may be recorded at this level. *AO* = aorta.

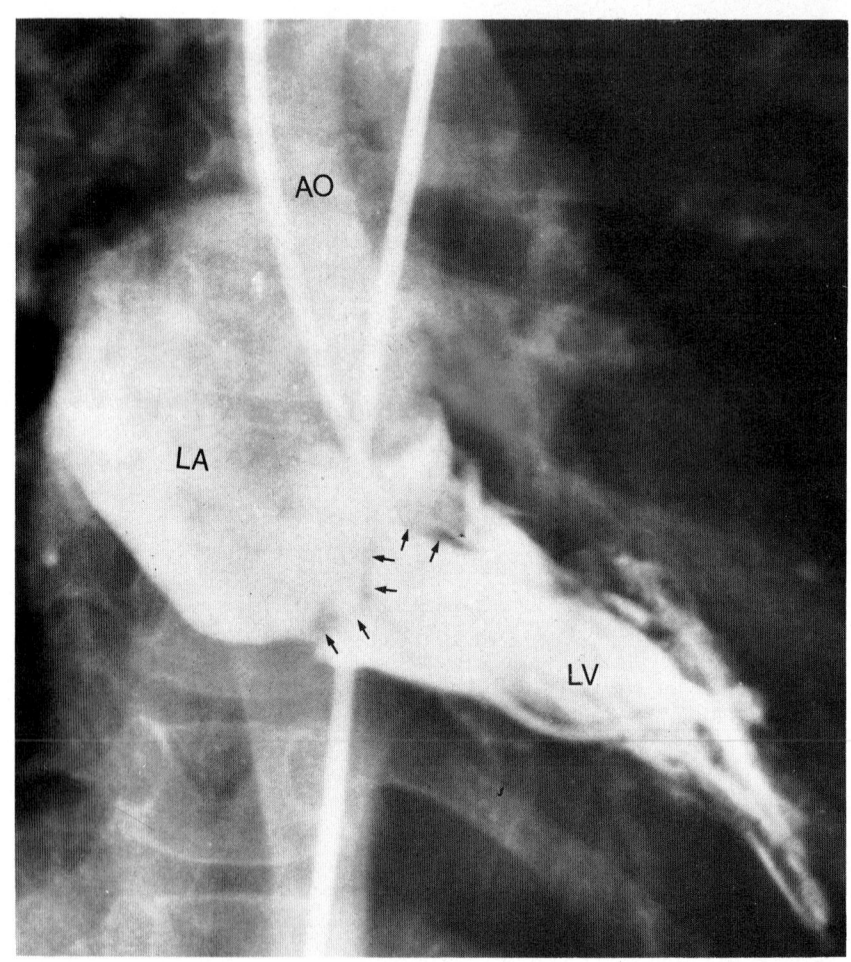

FIG 26–70.
Left ventriculogram, anteroposterior projection in muscular subaortic stenosis. Characteristic V-shaped filling defect in left ventricular outflow area caused by contact of mitral valve with the ventricular septum; there is mitral reflux. Marked left ventricular hypertrophy. Angulation of left ventricle not present. *AO* = aorta; *LA* = left atrium; *LV* = left ventricle.

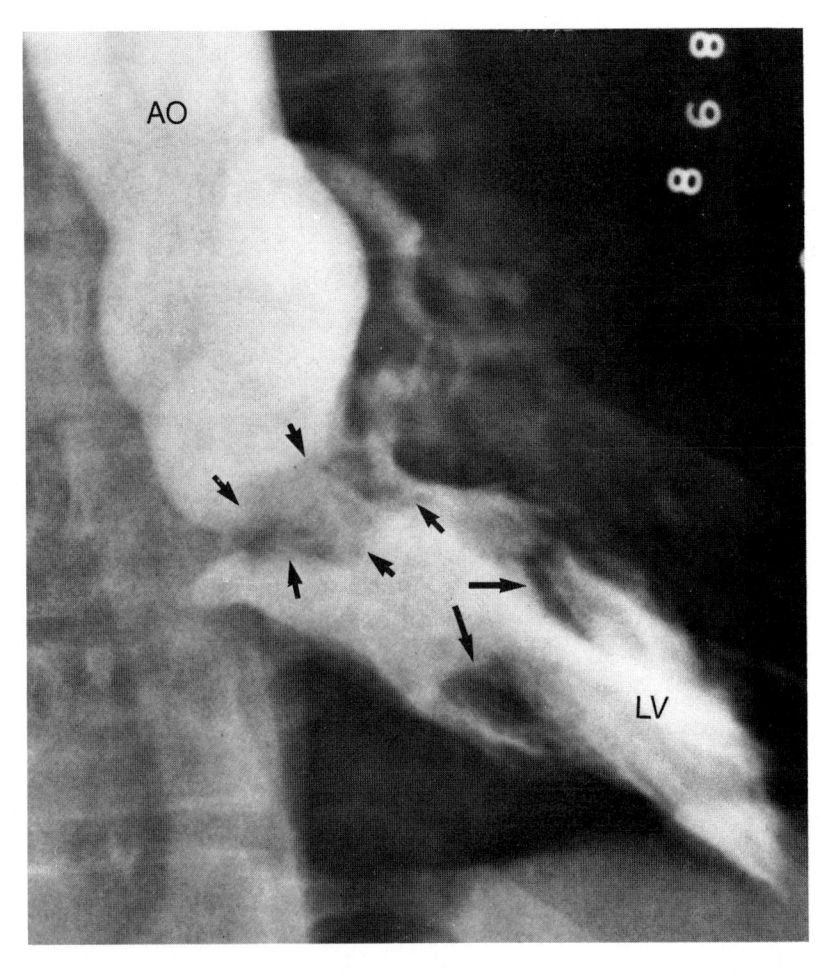

FIG 26–71.
Filling defect in left ventricular outflow tract caused by contact of markedly thickened anterior leaflet of mitral valve with septum during anterior motion of valve *(small arrows)*. Hypertrophied papillary muscles *(larger arrows)*. Angiographic appearance could be confused with fibromuscular ridge of discrete subaortic stenosis. The filling defect disappears during diastole in muscular subaortic stenosis and changes during cardiac cycle, whereas fibromuscular ridge persists throughout cardiac cycle. *AO* = aorta; *LV* = left ventricle.

of hypertrophied papillary muscle may be observed angiographically. A pressure gradient may be found at this level.

9. On the anteroposterior or right anterior oblique projection, systolic V-shaped radiolucency in the left ventricular outflow tract is caused by contact ("kissing") of anterior leaflet with ventricular septum; it results from anterior motion of the anterior leaflet of the mitral valve and hypertrophy of ventricular septum (Fig 26–70). A fibrous thickening may be found at the area of impact on the ventricular septum.

10. Markedly thickened mitral valve may cause a prominent radiolucency in left ventricular outflow tract (Fig 26–71) during systole from the anterior motion of mitral valve.

11. The hypertrophied septum may encroach on the right ventricle (Fig 26–72; Bernheim phenomenon) and cause right ventricular outflow obstruction and a subvalvar jet (Fig 26–73).

12. Coronary arteries may enlarge. REASON: Increased left ventricular mass (Fig 26–74), requiring more blood flow.

Biventriculography may be helpful in demonstrating the thickened interventricular septum.[57]

Treatment (Including Operation)

Both medical and surgical forms of therapy are available for patients with muscular subaortic stenosis. The indications and long-term results of each form of treatment are not well known.

In asymptomatic patients, regardless of the level of gradient, we give no treatment. Propranolol, a β-adrenergic blocker that decreases myocardial contractility, has been used in symptomatic patients with relief of symptoms,[58–60] but tolerance to the drug may develop. Thus, although during cardiac catheterization propranolol can reduce the gradient, prolonged oral administration may be associated with return of the gradient.

The indications for operation are debatable. Patients with significant mitral insufficiency, syncope, or angina are candidates for surgery. Patients with a large pressure gradient and no symptoms are not operated on, because there is no uniformly successful surgical procedure.

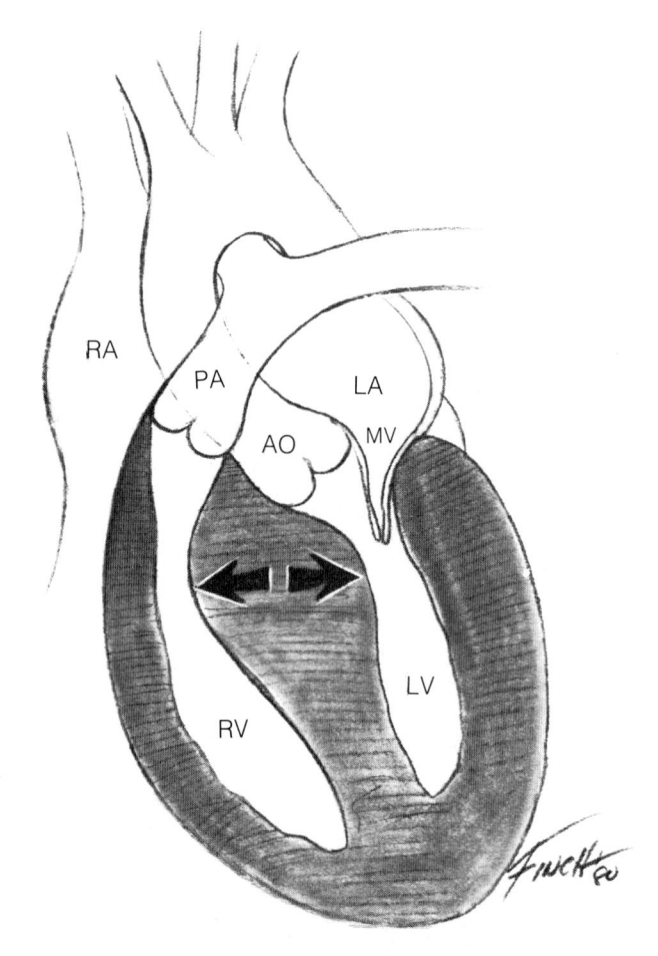

456 Outflow Obstructive Lesions

FIG 26–72.
Diagram of muscular subaortic stenosis with enormous thickening of ventricular septum. Outflow obstruction, mostly in left ventricular hypertrophied septum may cause severe right ventricular outflow obstruction (Bernheim phenomenon). *AO* = aorta; *LA* = left atrium; *LV* = left ventricle; *MV* = mitral valve; *PA* = pulmonary artery; *RA* = right atrium; *RV* = right ventricle.

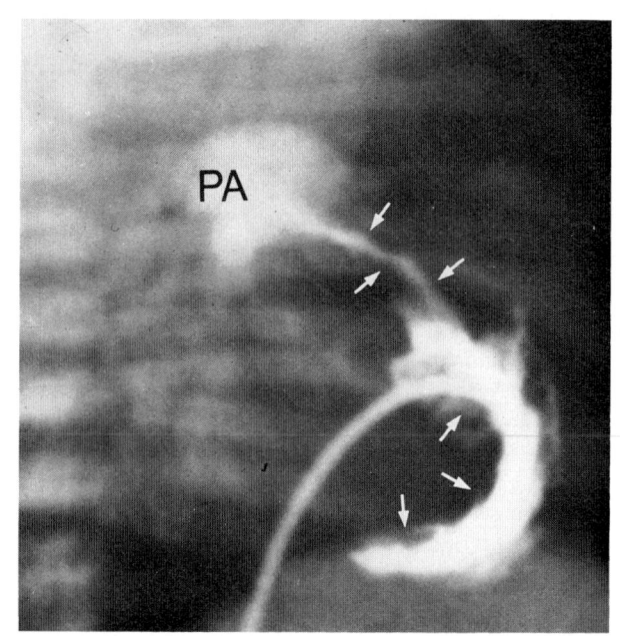

FIG 26–73.
Right ventriculogram, lateral projection in muscular subaortic stenosis. Bernheim phenomenon: marked encroachment on right ventricular cavity by enormously thickened septum *(arrows)*. Narrow jet of contrast medium extends into pulmonary artery and originates from infundibulum *(small arrows)*. Subvalvar jet, because pulmonary valve does not dome; this was misinterpreted as valvular pulmonary stenosis, and patient was operated on. A normal pulmonary valve was found.

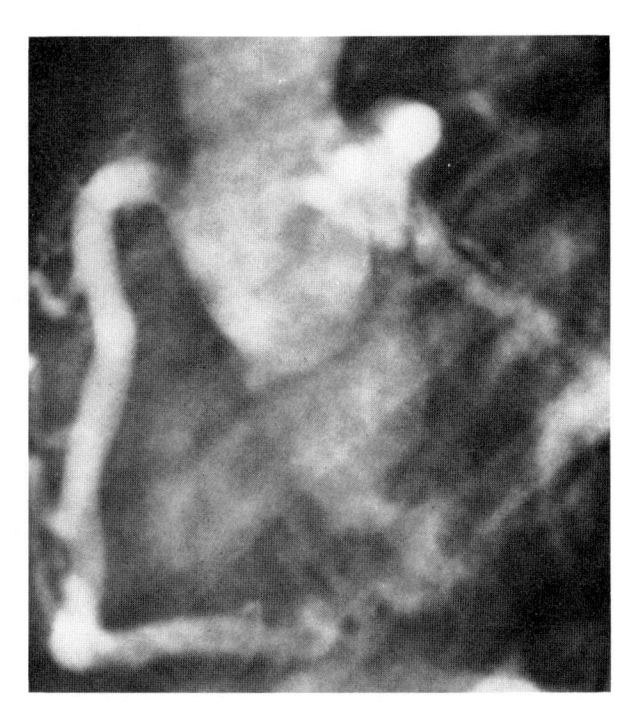

FIG 26-74.
Aortogram in muscular subaortic stenosis. Huge coronary arteries. Markedly increased left ventricular mass, requiring more blood than in normal heart.

Several operative approaches have been advocated. Replacement of the mitral valve by a prosthesis has been used to eliminate the obstructive mechanism that might be caused by systolic anterior motion of the mitral valve.[61] In another approach, a left ventricular myotomy and myectomy have been used to remove hypertrophied septal tissue.[62-64] Muscle can be removed from the left and the right ventricular sides of the septum. Although this technique can eliminate the gradient, the underlying myocardial process is still present. Whether operation affects the long-term course of the disease is unknown; it does not eliminate the chance of sudden death.[64, 65]

REFERENCES

1. Gorlin R, Gorlin SG: Hydraulic formula for calculation of the area of the stenotic mitral valve, other cardiac valves, and central circulatory shunts, *Am Heart J* 41:1, 1951.
2. Moller JH, Nakib A, Edwards JE: Infarction of papillary muscles and mitral insufficiency associated with congenital aortic stenosis, *Circulation* 34:87, 1966.
3. Krovetz LJ, Kurlinski JP: Subendocardial blood flow in children with congenital aortic stenosis, *Circulation* 54:961, 1976.
4. Vincent WR, Buckberg GD, Hoffman JIE: Left ventricular subendocardial ischemia in severe valvar and supravalvar aortic stenosis: a common mechanism, *Circulation* 49:326, 1974.
5. Moller JH, Nakib A, Eliot RS, et al: Symptomatic congenital aortic stenosis in the first year of life, *J Pediatr* 69:728, 1966.
6. Braunwald E, Goldblatt A, Aygen MM, et al: Congenital aortic stenosis: clinical and hemodynamic findings in 100 patients, *Circulation* 27:426, 1963.
7. Hohn AR, Van Praagh S, Moore AAD, et al: Aortic stenosis, *Circulation* 31,32(suppl. III):4, 1965.
8. Nanda NC, Gramiak R, Manning J, et al: Echocardiographic recognition of the congenital bicuspid aortic valve, *Circulation* 49:870, 1974.
9. Gewitz MH, Werner JC, Kleinman CS, et al: Role of echocardiography in aortic stenosis: pre- and postoperative studies, *Am J Cardiol* 43:67, 1979.
10. Bass JL, Einzig S, Hong CY et al: Echocardiographic screening to assess the severity of congenital aortic valve stenosis in children, *Am J Cardiol* 44:82, 1979.
11. Aziz KU, van Grondelle A, Paul MH, et al: Echocardiographic assessment of the relation between left ventricular wall and cavity dimensions and peak systolic pressure in children with aortic stenosis, *Am J Cardiol* 40:775, 1977.
12. Athanasoulis CA, Galdabini JJ, Waltman AC, et al: Angiodysplasia of the colon: a cause of rectal bleeding, *Cardiovasc Radiol* 1:3, 1978.
13. Galloway SJ, Casarella WJ, Shimkin PM: Vascular malformations of the right colon as a cause of bleeding in patients with aortic stenosis, *Radiology* 113:11, 1974.
14. Edwards JE: Pathology of left ventricular outflow tract obstruction, *Circulation* 31:586, 1965.
15. Waller BF, Carter JB, Williams HJ Jr, et al: Bicuspid aortic valve: comparison of congenital and acquired types, *Circulation* 48:1140, 1973.
16. Morrow AG, Goldblatt A, Braunwald E: Congenital aortic stenosis: II, surgical treatment and the results of operation, *Circulation* 27:426, 1963.
17. Keane JF, Berhard WF, Nadas AS: Aortic stenosis surgery in infancy, *Circulation* 52:1138, 1975.
18. McGoon DC, Geha AS, Scofield EL, et al: Surgical treatment of congenital aortic stenosis, *Dis Chest* 55:388, 1969.
19. Jack WD II, Kelly DT: Long-term follow-up of valvulotomy for congenital aortic stenosis, *Am J Cardiol* 38:231, 1976.
20. Friedman WF, Modlinger J, Morgan JR: Serial hemodynamic observations in asymptomatic children with valvar aortic stenosis, *Circulation* 43:91, 1971.
21. Cohen LS, Friedman WF, Braunwald E: Natural history of mild congenital aortic stenosis elucidated by serial hemodynamic studies, *Am J Cardiol* 30:1, 1972.
22. Hurwitz RA: Valvar aortic stenosis in childhood: clinical and hemodynamic history, *J Pediatr* 82:228, 1973.
23. Lakier JB, Lewis AB, Heymann MA, et al: Isolated aortic stenosis in the neonate: natural history and hemodynamic considerations, *Circulation* 50:801, 1974.
24. Newfeld EA, Muster AJ, Paul MH, et al: Discrete subvalvular aortic stenosis in childhood: study of 51 patients, *Am J Cardiol* 38:53, 1976.
25. Katz NM, Buckley MJ, Liberthson RR: Discrete membranous subaortic stenosis: report of 31 patients, review of the

literature, and delineation of management, *Circulation* 56:1034, 1977.
26. Popp RL, Silverman JF, French JW, et al: Echocardiographic findings in discrete subvalvular aortic stenosis, *Circulation* 49:226, 1974.
27. Davis RH, Feigenbaum H, Chang S, et al: Echocardiographic manifestations of discrete subaortic stenosis, *Am J Cardiol* 33:277, 1974.
28. Lundquist CB, Amplatz K: The subvalvar aortic jet, *Radiology* 85:635, 1965.
29. Baltaxe HA, Moller JH, Amplatz K: Membranous subaortic stenosis and its associated malformations, *Radiology* 95:287, 1970.
30. Peterson TA, Todd DB, Edwards JE: Supravalvular aortic stenosis, *J Thorac Cardiovasc Surg* 50:734, 1965.
31. Giddins NG, Finley JP, Nanton MA, et al: The natural course of supravalvar aortic stenosis and peripheral pulmonary artery stenosis in Williams's syndrome, *Br Heart J* 62:315, 1989.
32. Underhill WL, Tredway JB, D'Angelo GJ, et al: Familial supravalvular aortic stenosis: comments on the mechanisms of angina pectoris, *Am J Cardiol* 27:560, 1971.
33. Antia AU, Wiltse HE, Rowe RD, et al: Pathogenesis of the supravalvular aortic stenosis syndrome, *J Pediatr* 71:431, 1967.
34. Jones KL, Smith DW: The Williams elfin facies syndrome: a new perspective, *J Pediatr* 86:718, 1975.
35. Nasrallah AT, Nihill M: Supravalvular aortic stenosis: echocardiographic features, *Br Heart J* 37:662, 1975.
36. Bolen JL, Popp RL, French JW: Echocardiographic features of supravalvular aortic stenosis, *Circulation* 52:817, 1975.
37. Weisz D, Hartmann AF Jr, Weldon CS: Results of surgery for congenital supravalvular aortic stenosis, *Am J Cardiol* 37:73, 1976.
38. Keane JF, Fellows KE, LaFarge CG, et al: The surgical management of discrete and diffuse supravalvar aortic stenosis, *Circulation* 54:112, 1976.
39. Henry WL, Clark CE, Epstein SE: Asymmetric septal hypertrophy (ASH): the unifying link in the IHSS disease spectrum. Observations regarding its pathogenesis, pathophysiology, and course, *Circulation* 47:827, 1973.
40. Henry WL, Clark CE, Griffith JM, et al: Mechanism of left ventricular outflow obstruction in patients with obstructive asymmetric septal hypertrophy (idiopathic hypertrophic subaortic stenosis), *Am J Cardiol* 35:337, 1975.
41. Maron BJ, Gottdiener JS, Roberts WC, et al: Left ventricular outflow tract obstruction due to systolic anterior motion of the anterior mitral leaflet in patients with concentric left ventricular hypertrophy, *Circulation* 57:527, 1978.
42. Ferrans VJ, Morrow AG, Roberts WC: Myocardial ultrastructure in idiopathic hypertrophic subaortic stenosis: a study of operatively excised left ventricular outflow tract muscle in 14 patients, *Circulation* 45:769, 1972.
43. Maron BJ, Ferrans VJ, Henry WL, et al: Differences in distribution of myocardial abnormalities in patients with obstructive and nonobstructive asymmetric septal hypertrophy (ASH): light and electron microscopic findings, *Circulation* 50:436, 1974.
44. Maron BJ, Roberts WC: Quantitative analysis of cardiac muscle cell disorganization in the ventricular septum of patients with hypertrophic cardiomyopathy, *Circulation* 59:689, 1979.
45. Ross J Jr, Braunwald E, Gault JH, et al: The mechanism of the intraventricular pressure gradient in idiopathic hypertrophic subaortic stenosis, *Circulation* 34:558, 1966.
46. Harrison DC, Braunwald E, Glick G, et al: Effects of beta adrenergic blockade on the circulation, with particular reference to observations in patients with hypertrophic subaortic stenosis, *Circulation* 29:84, 1964.
47. Braunwald E, Ebert PA: Hemodynamic alterations in idiopathic hypertrophic subaortic stenosis induced by sympathomimetic drugs, *Am J Cardiol* 9:489, 1962.
48. Frank S, Braunwald E: Idiopathic hypertrophic subaortic stenosis: clinical analysis of 126 patients with emphasis on the natural history, *Circulation* 37:759, 1968.
49. Savage DD, Seides SF, Clark CE, et al: Electrocardiographic findings in patients with obstructive and nonobstructive hypertrophic cardiomyopathy, *Circulation* 58:402, 1978.
50. Henry WL, Clark CE, Epstein SE: Asymmetric septal hypertrophy: echocardiographic identification of the pathognomonic anatomic abnormality of IHSS, *Circulation* 47:225, 1973.
51. Shah PM, Gramiak R, Adelman AG, et al: Role of echocardiography in diagnostic and hemodynamic assessment of hypertrophic subaortic stenosis, *Circulation* 44:891, 1971.
52. Maron BJ, Henry WL, Roberts WC, et al: Comparison of echocardiographic and necropsy measurements of ventricular wall thicknesses in patients with and without disproportionate septal thickening, *Circulation* 55:341, 1977.
53. Martin RP, Rakowski H, French J, et al: Idiopathic hypertrophic subaortic stenosis viewed by wide-angle, phased-array echocardiography, *Circulation* 59:1206, 1979.
54. White CW, Zimmerman TJ: Prolonged left ventricular ejection time in the post-premature beat; a sensitive sign of idiopathic hypertrophic subaortic stenosis, *Circulation* 52:306, 1975.
55. Simon AL: Angiographic appearance of idiopathic hypertrophic subaortic stenosis, *Circulation* 46:614, 1972.
56. Adelman AG, McLoughlin MJ, Marquis Y, et al: Left ventricular cineangiographic observations in muscular subaortic stenosis, *Am J Cardiol* 24:689, 1969.
57. Redwood DR, Scherer JL, Epstein SE: Biventricular cineangiography in the evaluation of patients with asymmetric septal hypertrophy, *Circulation* 49:1116, 1974.
58. Stenson RE, Flamm MD Jr, Harrison DC, et al: Hypertrophic subaortic stenosis: clinical and hemodynamic effects of long-term propranolol therapy, *Am J Cardiol* 31:763, 1973.
59. Frank MJ, Abdulla AM, Canedo MI, et al: Long-term medical management of hypertrophic obstructive cardiomyopathy, *Am J Cardiol* 42:993, 1978.
60. Cohen LS, Braunwald E: Amelioration of angina pectoris in idiopathic hypertrophic subaortic stenosis with beta-adrenergic blockade, *Circulation* 35:847, 1967.
61. Cooley DA, Bloodwell RD, Hallman GL, et al: Surgical

treatment of muscular subaortic stenosis: results from septectomy in twenty-six patients, *Circulation* 35,36(suppl 1):124, 1967.
62. Morrow AG, Reitz BA, Epstein SE, et al: Operative treatment in hypertrophic subaortic stenosis: techniques, and the results of pre and postoperative assessments in 83 patients, *Circulation* 52:88, 1975.
63. Reis RL, Hannah H III, Carley JE, et al: Surgical treatment of idiopathic hypertrophic subaortic stenosis (IHSS): postoperative results in 30 patients following ventricular septal myotomy and myectomy (Morrow procedure), *Circulation* 56(suppl 2):128, 1977.
64. Maron BJ, Merrill WH, Freier PA, et al: Long-term clinical course and symptomatic status of patients after operation for hypertrophic subaortic stenosis, *Circulation* 57:1205, 1978.
65. Tajik AJ, Giuliani ER, Weidman WH, et al: Idiopathic hypertrophic subaortic stenosis: long-term surgical follow-up, *Am J Cardiol* 34:815, 1974.

CHAPTER 27

Aortico–Left Ventricular Tunnel

In this rare condition, a communication exists between the ascending aorta and left ventricle and causes a clinical picture of aortic insufficiency. It must be distinguished from ruptured sinus of Valsalva aneurysm and other aortic run-off lesions.

PATHOLOGIC ANATOMY[1]

A tunnel with appearance of a blood vessel arises above and to the left of the right coronary artery (Fig 27–1). Covered by a visceral pericardium, it may be 1.5 cm in diameter and resemble a saccular aneurysm. It is closely applied to the aorta and descends to the right of the pulmonary trunk to enter the infundibular septum. The aortico–left ventricular tunnel passes through the upper portion of the ventricular septum in the posterior wall, the right ventricular infundibulum, and empties into the left ventricular outflow tract. The tunnel bulges into the infundibular area, causing thickening of the endocardium and, occasionally, mild obstruction.

The left ventricle is enlarged, and the ascending aorta markedly dilated, because of the regurgitant flow into the left ventricle. The aortic valve may be normal or bicuspid. The coronary arteries are normal and do not arise from the tunnel.

Ventricular septal defect, pulmonary stenosis, and bicuspid pulmonary valve have been associated with aortico–left ventricular tunnel.

Pathophysiology

During ventricular systole there is forward flow through the tunnel into the aorta and during diastole flow back into the left ventricle. In addition, there is associated aortic valve regurgitation. The mechanism of aortic valve insufficiency is not fully understood. Several theories have been advanced: (1) relative insufficiency as a result of aortic dilatation, (2) intrinsic aortic valve disease such as bicuspid aortic valve, (3) lack of support of the right aortic cusp because of the close proximity of the tunnel, and (4) thickening of the aortic valve by turbulent flow. Lack of support of the right cusp may well be the main reason for aortic insufficiency.

THEORIES OF ORIGIN

An aortico–left ventricular tunnel may be either congenital or acquired. It may result from a dissecting hematoma of the ascending aorta that extends into the interventricular septum and ruptures into the left ventricle. However, the presence of aortic media in the wall of the tunnel, strongly suggests a congenital origin. The tunnel may represent an accessory coronary artery connecting with the left ventricle. The large regurgitating blood flow during diastole may result in aneurysmal dilatation, as in other coronary arterial fistulas.

Cases of aortico–atrial tunnels to either the left or right atrium have been reported. In these cases, however, coronary arteries arise from the tunnel, suggesting that the tunnels represent a coronary arterial fistula with marked dilatation of the main coronary artery rather than a true aortico–left ventricular tunnel.

The main anatomic distinction that must be made is with sinus of Valsalva aneurysm, which arises below the level of coronary arteries, whereas aortico–left ventricular tunnel arises above their origin.

Clinical Features

This anomaly has been reported primarily in boys. Cardiac disease is generally recognized by the presence of a "to-and-fro" murmur in infancy.[2,3] Congestive cardiac failure may develop in the neonatal period. Older patients may have exercise intolerance.

The physical examination reveals findings mimicking aortic insufficiency. The pulse pressure is wide. There are

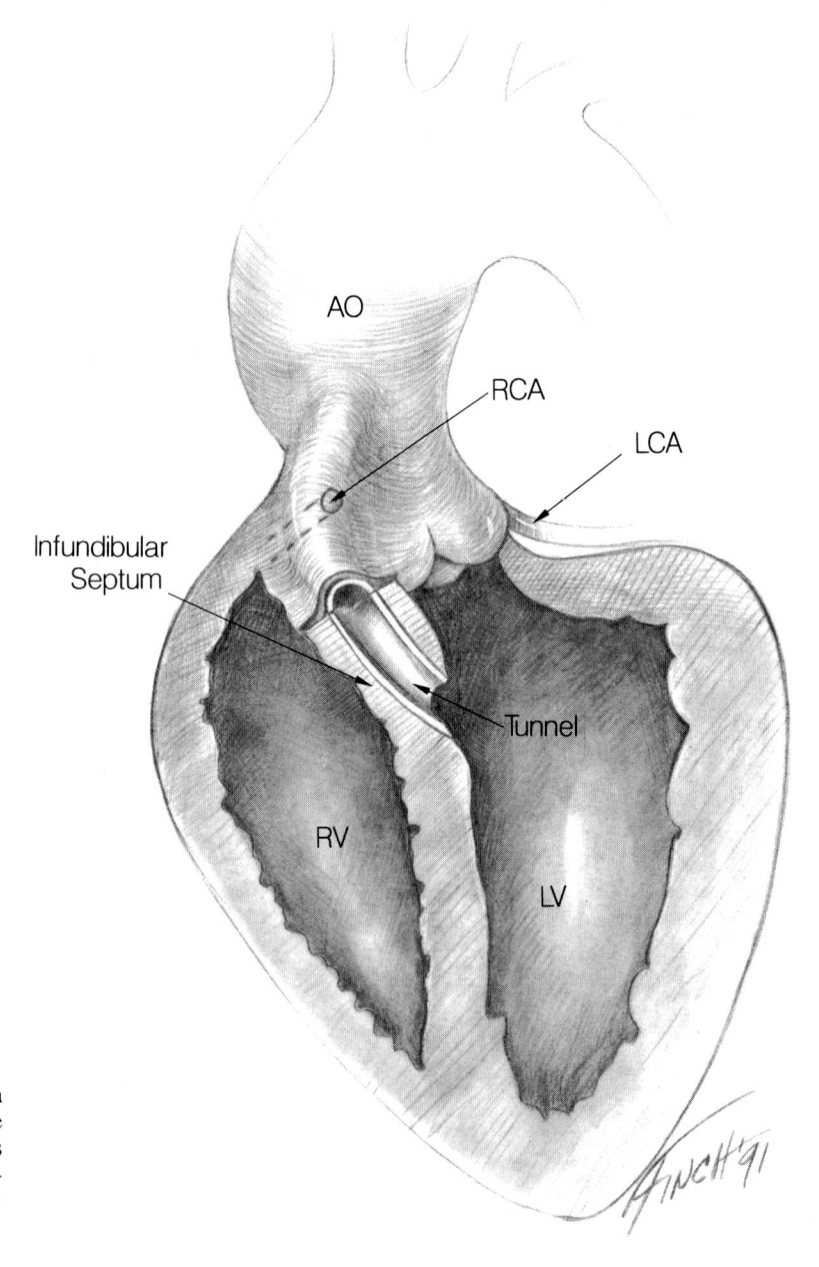

AORTICO-LEFT VENTRICULAR TUNNEL

FIG 27–1.
Aortico–left ventricular tunnel; diagram of aorta and opened ventricles in lateral projection. Large tunnel arises above coronary artery and passes through infundibular septum to enter the left ventricle tunnel covered by visceral pericardium. *AO* = aorta; *LV* = left ventricle; *RV* = right ventricle.

prominent murmurs associated with aortic regurgitation, an aortic ejection murmur related to the increased stroke volume across the aortic valve, and a prominent diastolic murmur of aortic insufficiency. The murmurs may be associated with thrills.

There is clinical evidence of cardiac enlargement and increased cardiac activity.

Electrocardiographic Features

The electrocardiogram may show slight left-axis deviation. There is left ventricular hypertrophy, often with ST-segment depression and inverted T waves in the left precordial leads.

Echocardiographic Features

The echocardiogram shows dilatation of the left atrium, left ventricle, and aortic root.[2] The valves, including the aortic, appear normal.

Radiographic Features

Because this condition is rare, it is not usually considered in the differential diagnosis of aortic runoff lesions,

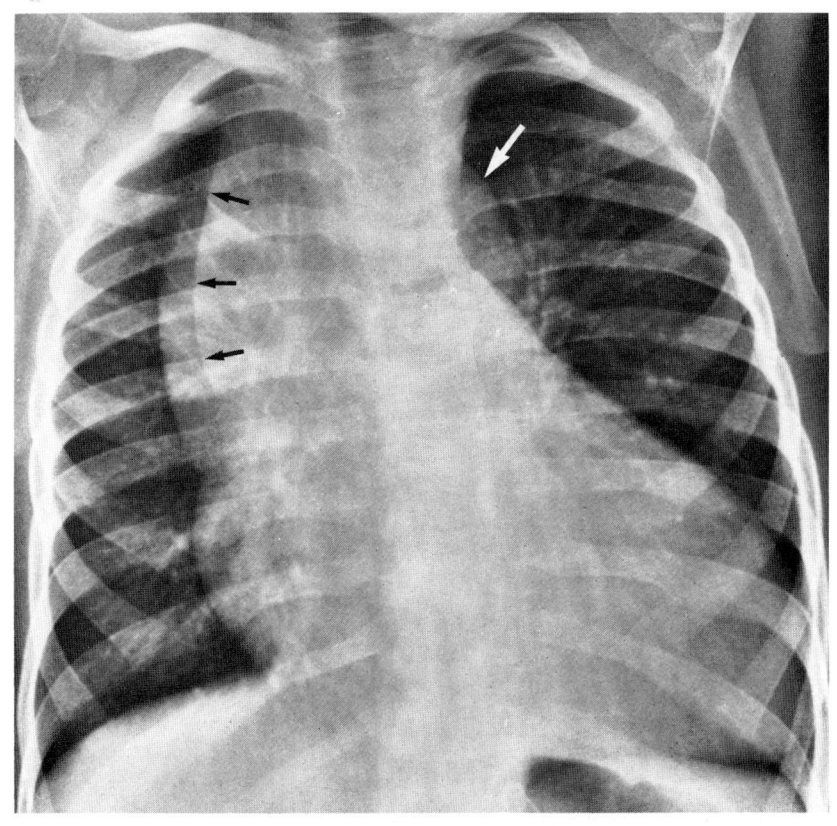

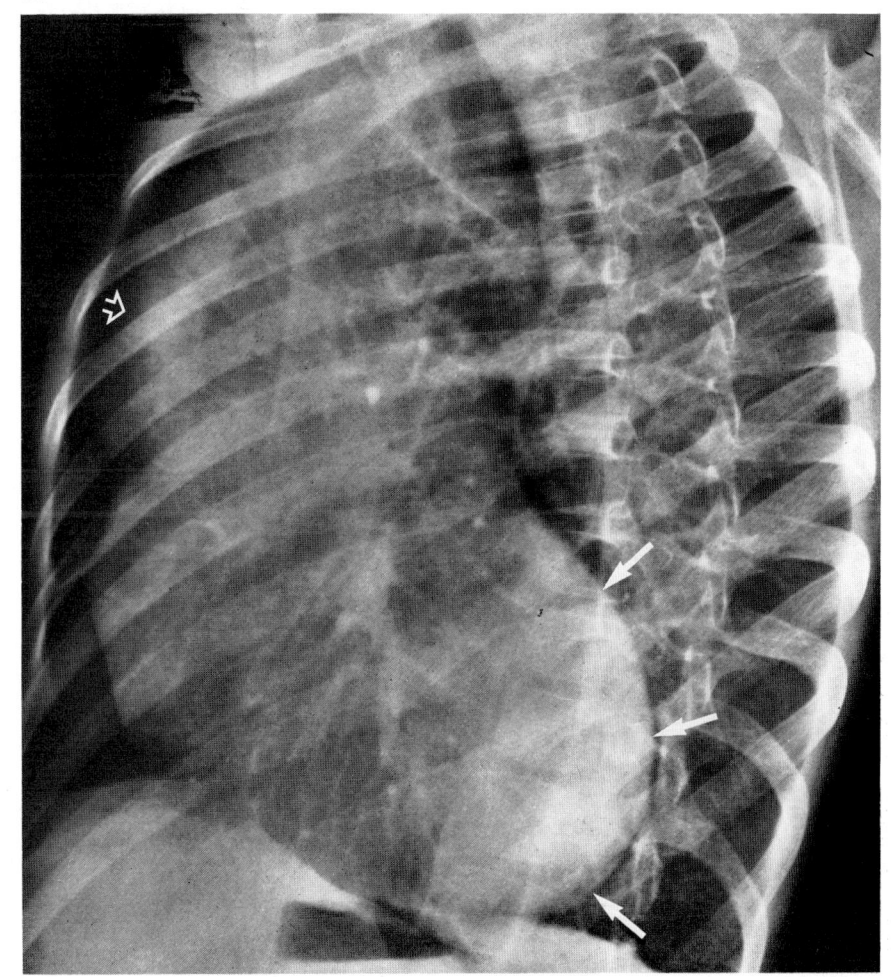

FIG 27–2.
Thoracic roentgenogram in aortico–left ventricular tunnel. **A,** posteroanterior projection; marked cardiomegaly because of left ventricular enlargement. Marked dilatation of the ascending aorta *(black arrows)* displacing the right superior vena cava, causing a double density. Normal pulmonary vasculature; prominent aortic knob *(white arrow)*. **B,** left anterior oblique projection; Enlarged left ventricle superimposed on the spine *(arrows)*. Marked prominence of the ascending aorta *(open arrow)*.
(Continued.)

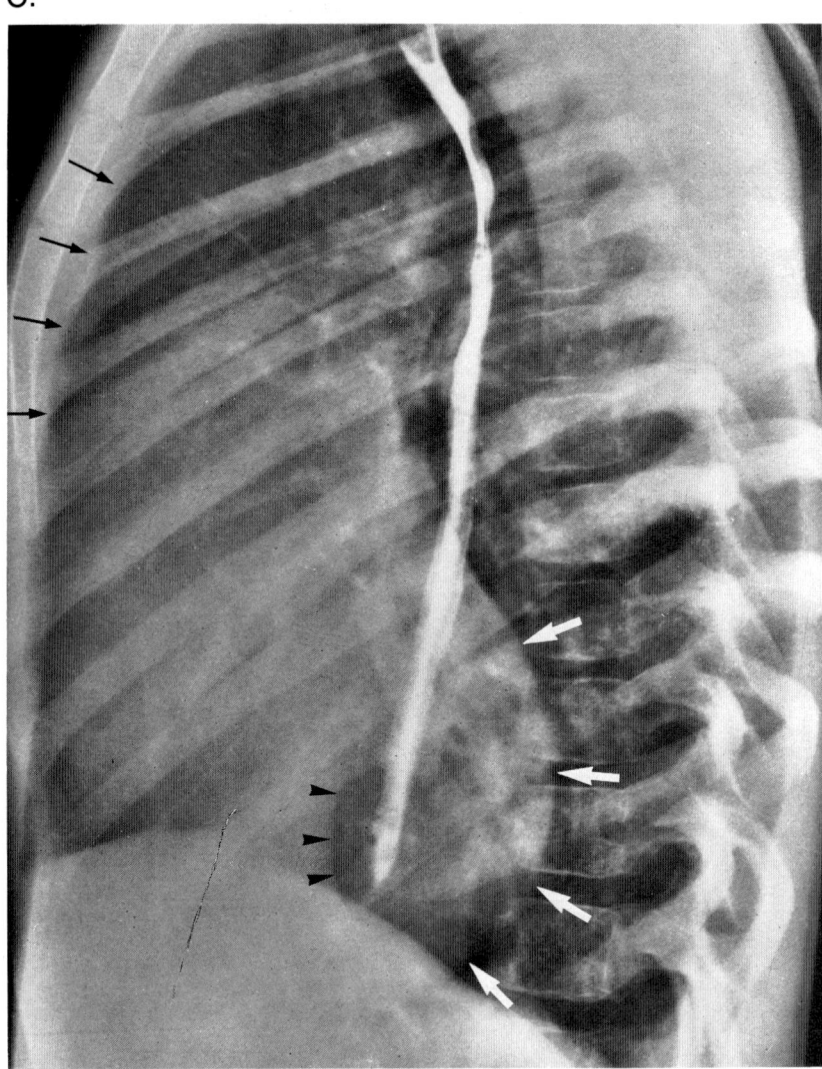

FIG 27-2 (cont.).
C, lateral projection; enlarged left ventricle extends behind the barium-filled esophagus and reflection of the inferior vena cava *(black arrows)*. Left atrium is not enlarged. Retrosternal space filled by the huge ascending aorta *(arrows)*.

although it should be considered in case of severe aortic insufficiency, which is rare in infancy and childhood. However, some radiographic findings suggest the correct diagnosis. Aortico–left ventricular tunnel leads to radiographic findings similar to those of severe aortic insufficiency.

1. The heart is markedly enlarged. REASON: An aortico–left ventricular tunnel is usually 1 to 1.5 cm in diameter and therefore allows a large flow to occur from the aorta into the left ventricle.

2. The left ventricle is markedly enlarged and observed best on posteroanterior and left anterior oblique projections (Fig 27–2).

3. Left atrial enlargement is absent. REASON: Provided left ventricular failure does not occur, left atrial pressure and volume are not increased.

4. The pulmonary vasculature is normal. REASON: Aortico–left ventricular tunnel is not associated with a shunt, so pulmonary blood flow is normal.

5. Severe dilatation of the ascending aorta results in a huge bulge along the right cardiac border (see Fig 27–2), particularly on the left anterior oblique projection. This finding is very suggestive of aortico–left ventricular tunnel, because severe aortic dilatation is not commonly seen.

6. In the right superior mediastinum, a double density may be observed because of displacement of the superior vena cava by the enlarged aorta. A bulge in the region of the main pulmonary artery is caused by the tunnel (see Fig 27–2,*A*).

7. Severe dilatation of the ascending aorta and the appearance of the tunnel mimicking a prominent pulmonary artery segment are the most helpful diagnostic findings. REASON: Because of the severe left ventricular enlarge-

ment, counterclockwise rotation of the heart occurs, placing the pulmonary artery more medially. Therefore, the pulmonary artery segment should not be prominent. Thus, a bulge in the region of the pulmonary artery should suggest a tunnel.

8. On the lateral projection (see Fig 27–2,C), the entire retrosternal space is filled by the huge ascending aorta.

9. The aortic knob tends to be prominent. REASON: Because of the large runoff, some dilatation of the aorta occurs, as in aortic valvar incompetence.

10. Chest roentgenographic findings are more suggestive if the left pulmonary artery can be seen through the prominent bulge caused by the tunnel (Fig 27–3).

11. Fluoroscopic observation shows markedly increased pulsation of the ascending aorta and left ventricle. REASON: Left ventricular stroke volume is increased by the severe aortic reflux.

CARDIAC CATHETERIZATION

The catheter course is normal. There is no evidence of a shunt. The right-sided cardiac pressures are normal. Aortic pressure tracings show a wide pulse pressure. Left ventricular end-diastolic pressure may be elevated if there is significant aortic regurgitation or left ventricular failure.

ANGIOGRAPHIC FEATURES

1. Left ventriculography demonstrates the enlarged and actively contracting left ventricle.

2. In the anteroposterior projection, the aortico–left ventricular tunnel is seen to the left of the aortic valve (Fig 27–4,A). On the lateral view, the tunnel is superimposed on the aorta (Fig 27–4,B). In both projections, the tunnel originates above the level of the coronary arteries. This feature distinguishes tunnel from a sinus of Valsalva aneurysm, which invariably arises below the level of the coronary arteries.

3. The aortic sinuses are not dilated, thereby excluding the diagnosis of Marfan syndrome, which also causes marked dilatation of the aortic sinuses.

4. The ascending aorta shows marked dilatation that does not involve the aortic sinuses.

5. Aortography demonstrates passage of contrast material from the aorta through the tunnel, with immediate opacification of the left ventricle.

6. The best view of the tunnel is obtained in a slight right anterior projection with selective injection into the tunnel.

7. On the left anterior oblique projection, the characteristic entry of the tunnel into the ventricular septum is demonstrated (see Fig 27–4).

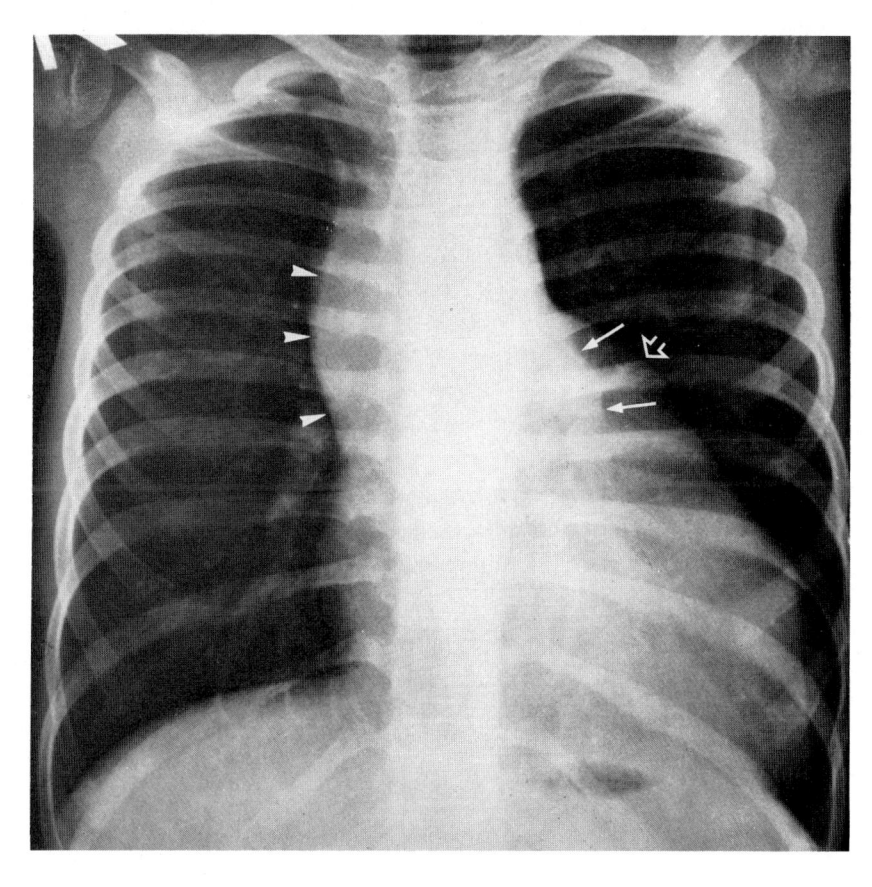

FIG 27–3.
Thoracic roentgenogram in aortico–left ventricular tunnel. Posteroanterior projection. Marked left ventricular enlargement, normal pulmonary vasculature, and dilatation of the ascending aorta *(white arrowheads)*. Large bulge in the region of the pulmonary artery segment is caused by the tunnel *(open arrow)*. The normal-sized left pulmonary artery *(black arrows)* can be seen through the prominent bulge, which does not exactly resemble a pulmonary artery segment. It could be confused with a distended left atrial appendage, but there are no other signs of left atrial enlargement. Normally, because the enlarged left ventricle causes counterclockwise rotation of the heart, the pulmonary artery segment should be concave. In this film, the prominent bulge suggests the diagnosis of aortico–left ventricular tunnel.

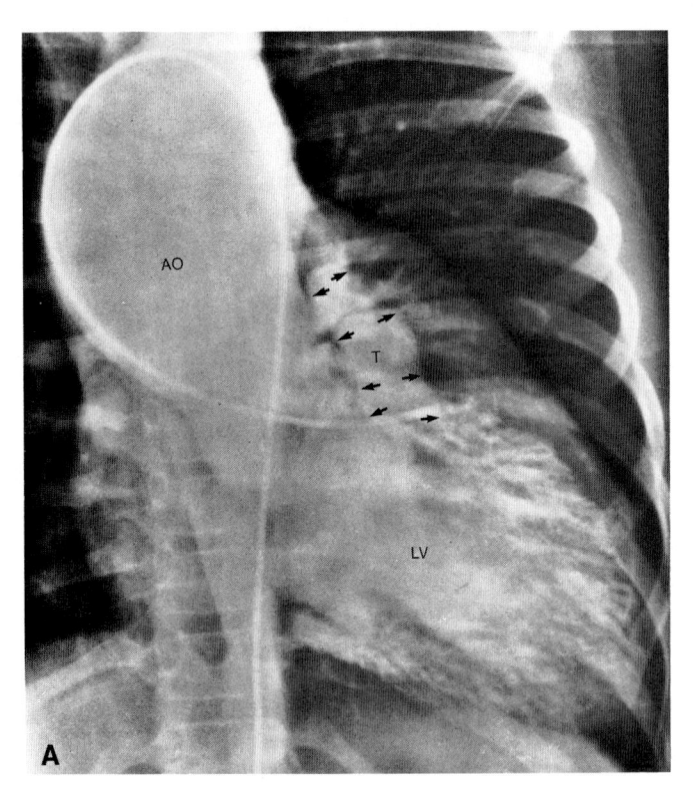

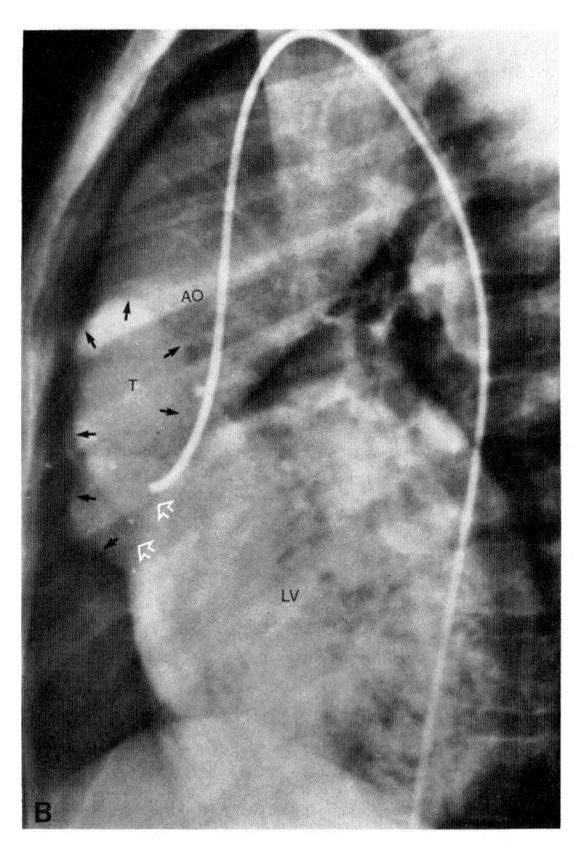

FIG 27-4.
Left ventriculogram in aortico-left ventricular tunnel. **A,** anteroposterior projection. Markedly enlarged left ventricle *(LV)*. The tunnel *(T) (arrows)* projects to the left of the aortic valve. The tunnel originates above the level of the sinus of Valsalva. Sinuses of Valsalva normal, excluding cystic medial necrosis. Relatively poor angiogram because of dilution of contrast medium by increased systolic and diastolic flow. **B,** lateral projection. Tunnel *(T)* outlined by arrows superimposed upon aorta. Enters the ventricular septum *(white arrows)*, which is characteristic for aortico-left ventricular tunnel. *AO* = aorta.

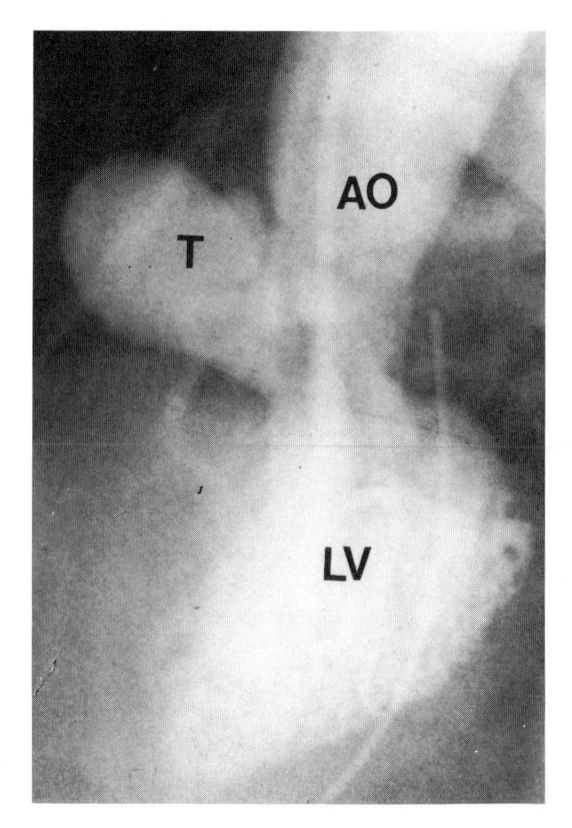

FIG 27-5.
Left ventriculogram with aortico-left ventricular tunnel forming a large aneurysm.

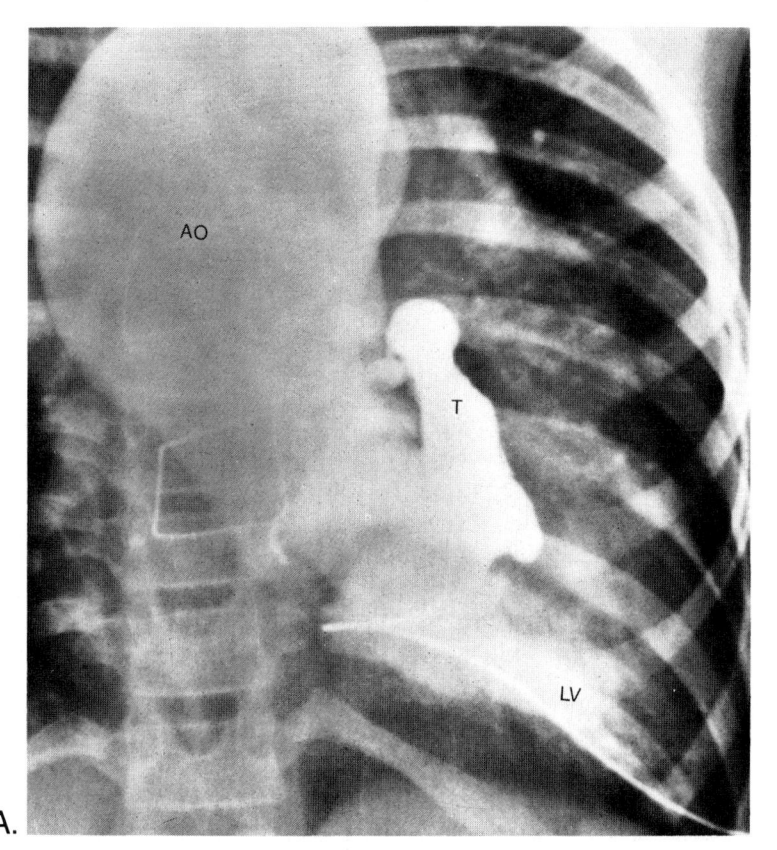

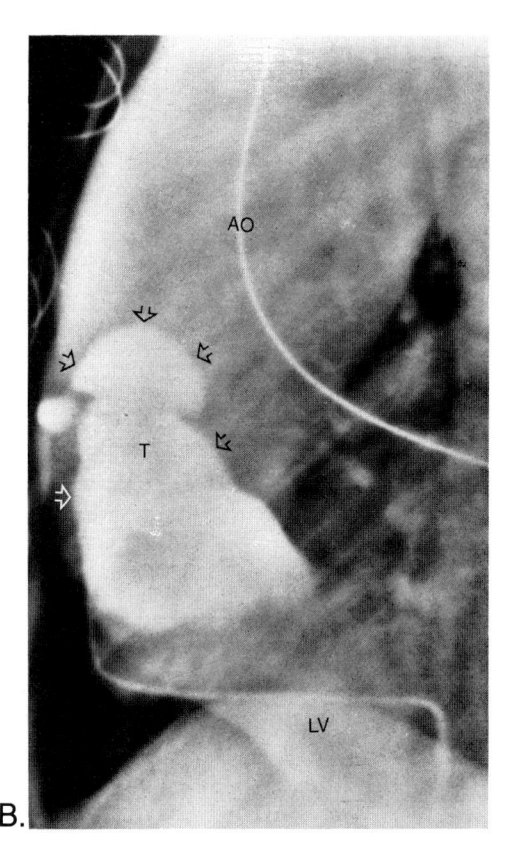

FIG 27-6.
Aortico–left ventricular tunnel, postoperative state seen in anteroposterior (**A**) and lateral (**B**) projections. Structure reminiscent of aortico–left ventricular tunnel apparent as a blind-ending pouch located anteriorly and lateral to aorta *(open arrows)*. Greatly dilated ascending aorta. The blind-ending tunnel is now densely opacified because flow has been obliterated by surgery. *AO* = aorta; *LV* = left ventricle.

8. Forward and backflow through the tunnel, as well as aortic reflux, can be observed on the left anterior oblique projection; the tunnel may form a large aneurysm (Fig 27–5).

OPERATION

With the identification of this anomaly, corrective operation should be undertaken.[3,4] Through an aortotomy, the tunnel orifice is sutured closed. C. Walton Lillehei repaired the first tunnel by suturing an Ivalon spindle into the tunnel, which resulted in closure, although some aortic reflux persisted. Postoperatively, a murmur of aortic regurgitation may still be heard. The murmur is considerably softer and probably related either to thickening of aortic valve cusps secondary to aortic root dilatation or to valvular changes secondary to turbulent flow across the aortic valve.[4] If only the aortic orifice is surgically closed, an aneurysm persists, with the likelihood of gradual enlargement with time. Consequently, the tunnel is incised, and the left ventricular orifice is also sutured closed.

This is one form of aortic regurgitation in infancy which carries a favorable operative risk, because valve replacement is not required.

POSTOPERATIVE FINDINGS

After closure of the tunnel, cardiac size gradually decreases. If only the aortic orifice of the tunnel is closed, the tunnel can still be seen after left ventriculography as a blind-ending conduit (Fig 27–6).

REFERENCES

1. Levy MJ, Lillehei CW, Anderson RC, et al: Aortico–left ventricular tunnel, *Circulation* 27:841, 1963.
2. Yu LC, Bharati S, Thilenius O, et al: Congenital aortico–left atrial tunnel, *Pediatr Cardiol* 1:153, 1980.
3. Mair DD, Fulton RE, McGoon DC: Successful surgical repair of aortico–left ventricular tunnel in an infant, *Mayo Clin Proc* 50:691, 1975.
4. Edwards JE: Aortico–left ventricular tunnel: the case for early treatment, *Chest* 70:5, 1976.

CHAPTER 28

Coarctation of the Aorta

Coarctation of the aorta (Latin cum—together—and arctare—to make tight) is a congenital anomaly of unknown etiology that occurs only at the junction of the distal aortic arch and the descending aorta. The term coarctation has also been applied to narrowings of other portions of the aorta and peripheral arteries, for example, abdominal coarctation or renal artery coarctation. Because the latter lesions are probably the result of arteritis or fibromuscular dysplasia, they should not be confused with classic coarctation, but they are included in this chapter because they represent abnormalities which may be confused with coarctation of the aorta.

INCIDENCE

Coarctation of the aorta accounts for 6% of congenital cardiac anomalies. The male/female ratio is 2.5:1 in patients with isolated coarctation,[1] but when coarctation is associated with other cardiac anomalies, there is no sex difference. In females with coarctation of the aorta, Turner's syndrome should be considered, because it occurs in 20% of these patients.[2]

ANATOMY

Coarctation of the aorta may be either a localized stenosis, located opposite the ductus arteriosus, or a hypoplastic stenotic segment, involving the entire aortic isthmus (Fig 28–1). Rarely, the descending aorta is hypoplastic from the area of the ductus to the level of the diaphragm. The location of the coarctation in relation to the ductus varies (Fig 28–1).

Localized Coarctation of the Aorta

In this form, a deformity of the aortic media projects into the aortic lumen, forming a diaphragm with an eccentric opening (Fig 28–2).[3] With age, secondary changes of intimal thickening develop, probably from eddies of blood through the narrowed area.[3] Externally, the coarctation site shows a localized depression around the greater curvature of the aorta, sparing the ventral portion of the lesser curvature side, and thus has been compared with the deformity that might be caused by pressing a butter knife along the greater curvature of the normal aorta (Fig 28–3). Involvement of the greater curvature of the aorta is always present but angiographically also involvement of the lesser curvature may be seen.

Diffuse Form of Coarctation of the Aorta (Tubular Hypoplasia)

In this form, a long, hypoplastic segment is present, usually from the left subclavian artery to the site of ductus arteriosus (Fig 28–4). Tubular hypoplasia is most common when the left subclavian artery arises from its normal position. REASON: The blood flow through the segment between the left subclavian artery and the coarctation consists only of the left subclavian flow; consequently, this segment is commonly of the same size as the left subclavian artery. A localized coarctation usually coexists at the site of the ductus, which is frequently patent. At times, the segment between the left carotid and left subclavian arteries is also hypoplastic. REASON: The left subclavian artery is perfused via a reversing ductus arteriosus and the innominate and left carotid arteries via ascending aorta. There is little flow in the segment between the left carotid and left subclavian arteries. Therefore, this segment does not grow and is hypoplastic.

The origin of the subclavian arteries in relation to the site of the coarctation of the aorta varies. The left subclavian artery usually arises proximal to the coarctation site. It is commonly dilated because of collateral flow (Fig 28–5,A). Rarely, it arises beyond the coarctation (Fig 28–5,E) or is involved in the coarctation site and its orifice narrowed (Fig 28–5,F). Rarely, the right subclavian

469

470 Outflow Obstructive Lesions

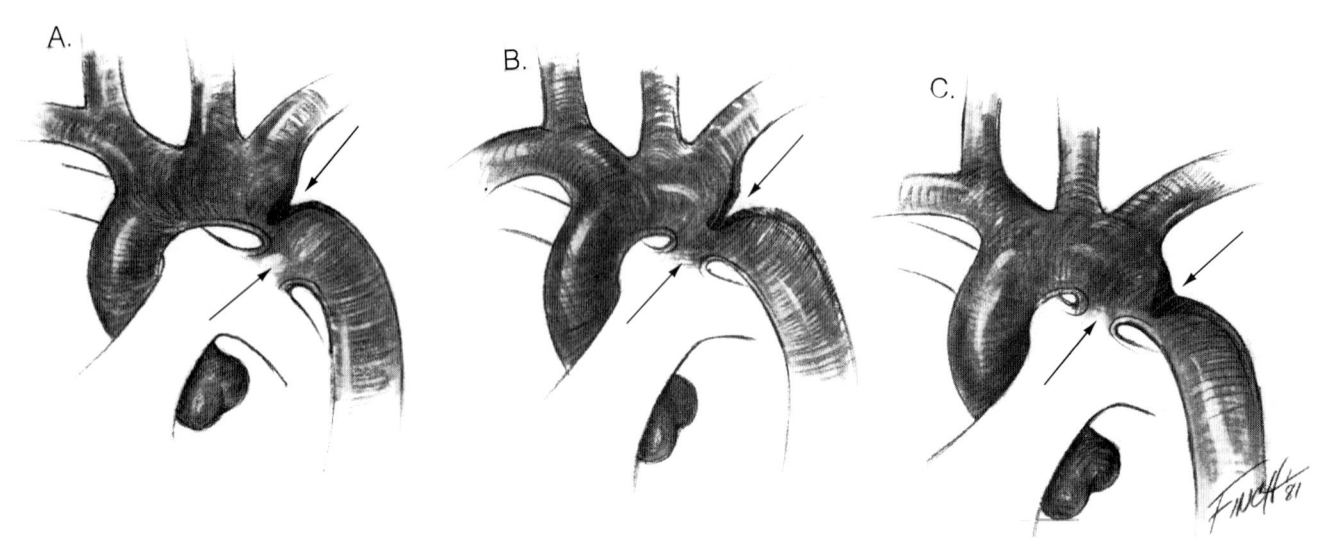

FIG 28–1.
Diagrams of relation of coarctation of aorta and ductus arteriosus. **A,** preductal; **B,** juxtaductal; and **C,** postductal.

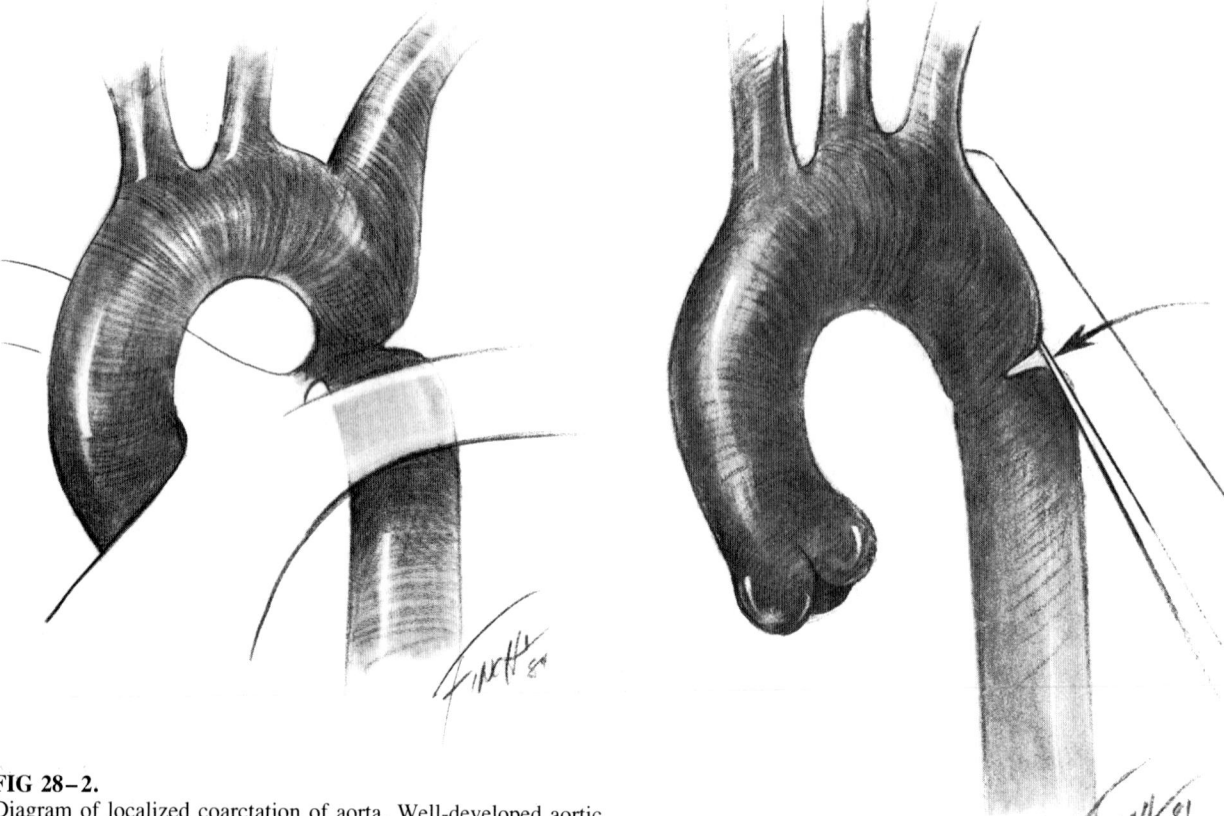

FIG 28–2.
Diagram of localized coarctation of aorta. Well-developed aortic arch; no tubular hypoplasia.

FIG 28–3.
Illustration of butter knife deformity of coarctation.

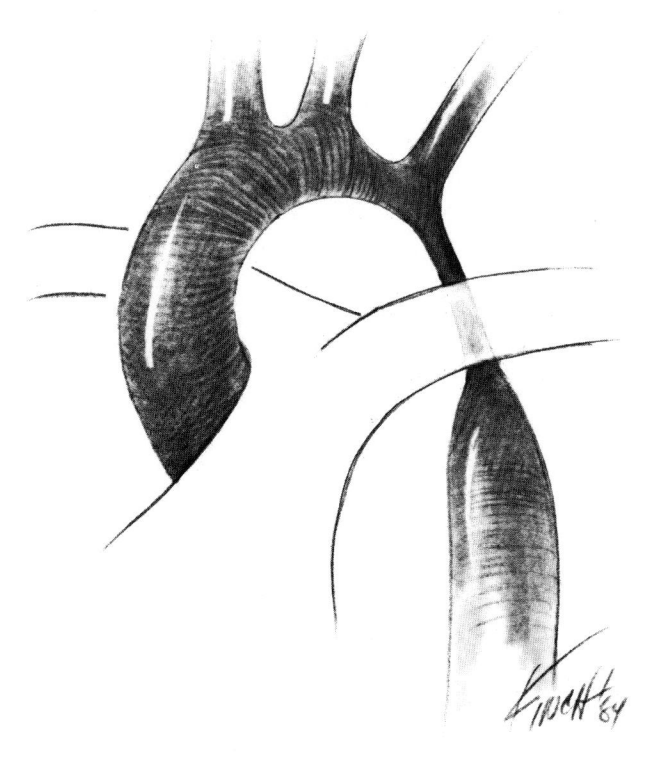

FIG 28-4.
Diagram of diffuse form of coarctation of aorta. Tubular hypoplasia of aortic isthmus; normal origin of left subclavian artery.

artery arises anomalously as the fourth branch from the descending aorta and is located beyond the coarctation site (Fig 28–5,*D*). Unilateral rib notching may coexist with the left subclavian artery arising from the same aortic level (see Fig 28–5,*E*). These variations of origin of subclavian arteries may give rise to unique blood pressure recordings and patterns of rib notching.

EMBRYOLOGY

The morphogenesis of coarctation of the aorta is unknown but probably differs for the two anatomic forms.

Localized coarctation of the aorta probably results from persistence of shelflike thickening of the media near the orifice of the left subclavian artery. As the aortic arches develop, the proximal migration of the left subclavian artery along the left aortic arch may result in a "spur" at the distal margin of this artery. On the other hand, the shelflike structure opposite the ductus arteriosus may be formed by division of ductal blood flow into proximal and distal streams early in the development.

The diffuse form of coarctation probably develops when blood flow through the aortic isthmus is markedly reduced during fetal life. In a normal fetus, only 10% of the cardiac output flows through the isthmus,[4] because the patent ductus arteriosus directs blood from the right ventricle into the descending aorta. In normal neonates, the diameter of the aortic isthmus is 25% smaller than either the ascending or the descending aorta. If coexisting cardiac anomalies further reduce flow across the isthmus, hypoplasia or atresia of the aortic isthmus may develop. Most patients with aortic isthmic narrowing (tubular hypoplasia of the aortic arch) have associated major intracardiac defects.[4, 5]

Because coarctation of the aorta is commonly juxtaductal or preductal, there is little change in fetal hemodynamics, and aortic obstruction is not evident before birth.

In either juxtaductal or preductal coarctation, the aorta immediately proximal to the ductus arteriosus may be narrowed and the flow through the isthmus less than normal. As the volume flowing through the isthmus decreases, a larger volume of blood flowing to the legs is derived from the right ventricle. There is a compensatory redistribution of blood flow across the foramen ovale, so more flow occurs into the right ventricle. This changed prenatal hemodynamic situation explains the common electrocardiographic findings of right ventricular hypertrophy at birth and the pathologic and radiologic evidence of right ventricular enlargement rather than of left ventricular hypertrophy.

In patients with localized juxtaductal coarctation, clinical evidence of obstruction develops only as the ductus closes (Fig 28–6). While the ductus remains patent, blood from the ascending aorta can readily pass to the descending aorta by traversing the aortic end of the open ductus arteriosus.[4] Constriction of the ductus arteriosus after birth abolishes the "bypass" through the aortic end of the duc-

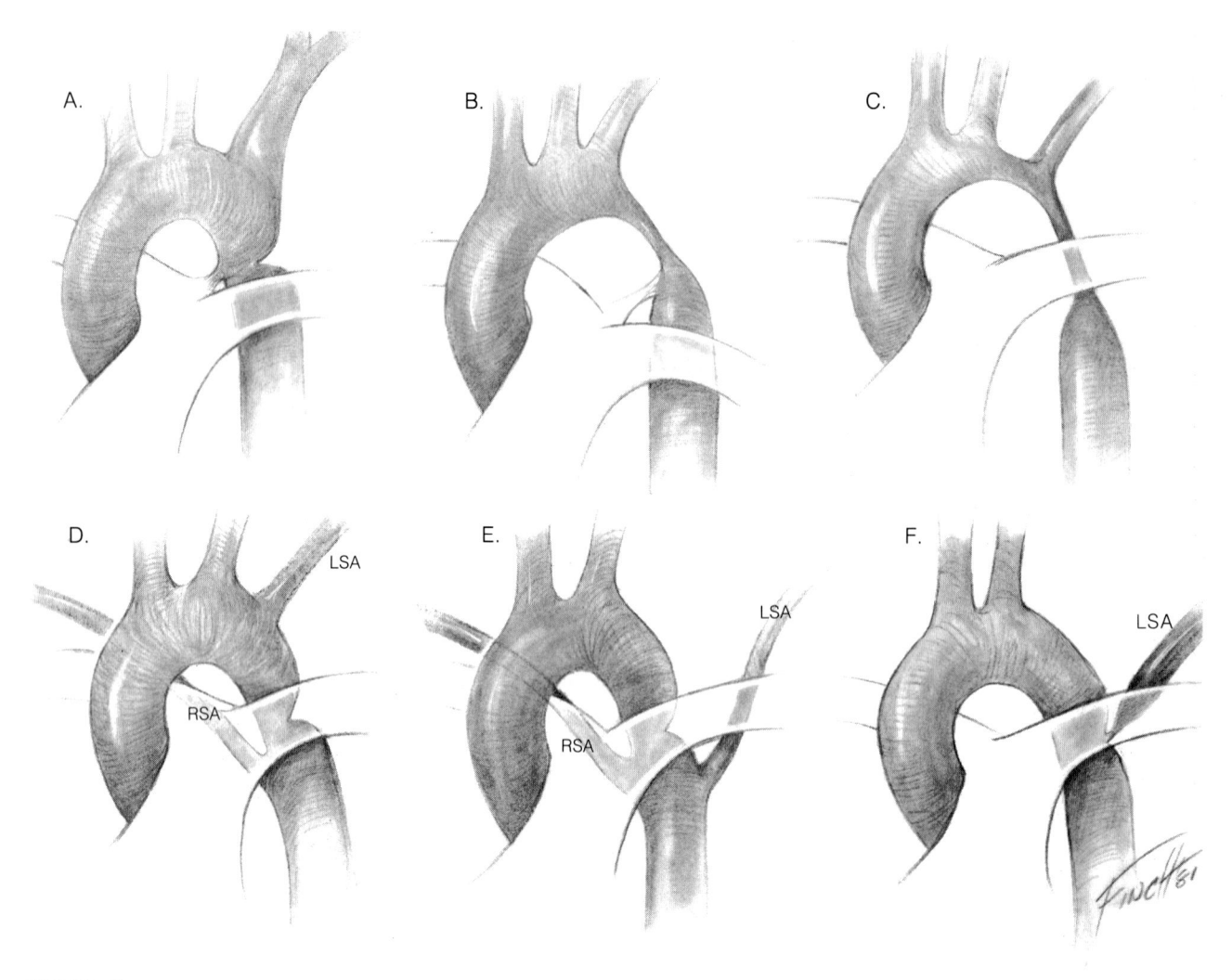

FIG 28–5.
Diagram of relation of coarctation of aorta to subclavian arteries. **A,** left subclavian arising proximal to coarctation; subcalvain artery is usually dilated because it carries collateral flow. **B,** left subclavian artery proximal to coarctation; diffuse hypoplasia distal to left carotid artery and distal to left subclavian artery. REASON: Prenatally, left subclavian artery was partially perfused through ductus arteriosus and ascending aorta. **D,** aberrant right subclavian artery *(RSA)* arising distal to coarctation. **E,** aberrant right subclavian artery *(RSA)* and left subclavian artery *(LSA)* arising distal to coarctation. **F,** left subclavian artery arising at coarctation site with stenosis of its origin. Some of these variations can be predicted by careful blood pressure measurements.

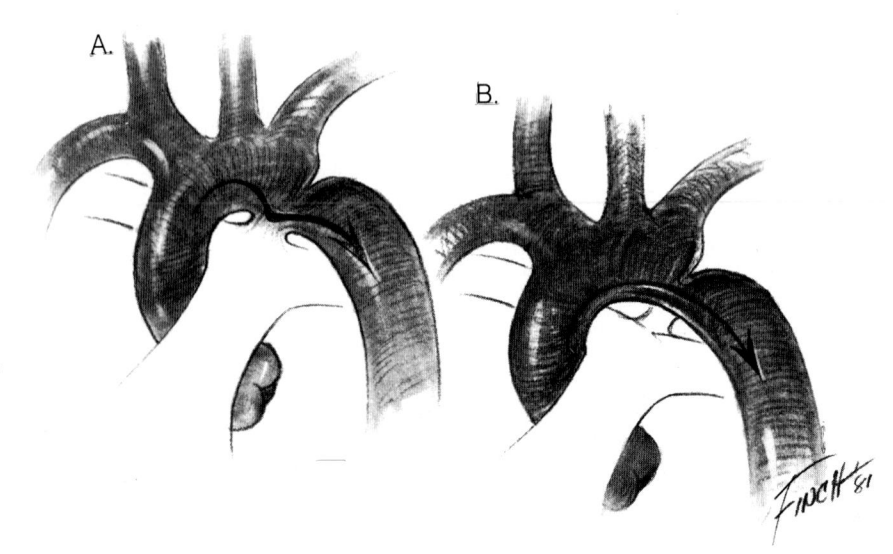

FIG 28–6.
Diagram of juxtaductal coarctation of aorta. **A,** prenatally. Because ductus arteriosus is patent, no gradient is present. Blood can flow from the ascending to descending aorta through the mouth of the ductus. **B,** postnatally. Ductus closed. Coarctation becomes evident clinically.

tus, and aortic obstruction develops. This has been shown in a few patients who had no signs of coarctation at the time of birth and who developed a pressure gradient as the ductus arteriosus obliterated.[4, 6]

PATHOPHYSIOLOGY

The hemodynamics are determined principally by the degree of obstruction, the relation of the coarctation to the site of the ductus arteriosus, the status of the ductus arteriosus, the presence of collateral circulation, and the type and severity of associated conditions.

In coarctation of the aorta, collateral vessels develop because of the pressure gradient across the area of the coarctation. Characteristically, at birth, the collateral circulation is absent or poorly developed, because the area below the coarctation has been supplied through the patent ductus arteriosus at systemic levels of pressure. Before birth, no pressure gradient existed between the ascending aorta and the descending aorta. Only in the extremely rare form of postductal coarctation is a pressure gradient present before birth so that collaterals may develop.

Almost immediately after birth, collateral flow can be demonstrated in all infants with coarctation of the aorta, but the collateral channels are small. They enlarge with age and in later childhood cause characteristic radiographic findings. The major collateral pathways involving primarily anterior arteries are demonstrated on the right of Figure 28–7, and those involving primarily posterior collaterals are demonstrated on the left of Figure 28–7. Obviously, both sets of arteries are present bilaterally but are not depicted simultaneously to avoid complicating the diagram. Below, the five major collateral pathways are described.

Spinal Artery

The spinal artery has segmental branches arising from the vertebral arteries and segmental connections with the intercostal and lumbar arteries. In coarctation of the aorta, blood from the high-pressure ascending aorta flows from the vertebral artery through segmental arteries into the anterior spinal artery. Blood flows toward the lower-pressure descending aorta and through the intercostal and lumbar arteries to the abdominal aorta. In most patients with coarctation of the aorta, the anterior spinal artery is markedly enlarged, and on rare occasions, this enlargement causes paraplegia.

Intercostal Collaterals

The intercostal collateral arteries play the primary role in supplying blood to the low-pressure descending aorta. The first two intercostal arteries are supplied by the costocervical trunk, although there may be bridging branches to the lower intercostal arteries. Consequently, the first two ribs are not notched. The other intercostal arteries originate from the abdominal aorta and communicate with the internal mammary artery. The internal mammary artery, arising from the high-pressure subclavian arteries, carries blood which then passes from the anterior through the posterior intercostal arteries into the lower-pressure descending aorta. These collateral channels gradually enlarge, become more tortuous, and cause erosions of the lower rib margin, which can be identified on thoracic roentgenograms. The shortest collateral pathways occur in the upper intercostal arteries. Their prominence gradually diminishes toward the lower ribs. Prominent notching of the lower ribs suggests an abdominal coarctation. Rib notching occurs bilaterally when both subclavian arteries arise proximal to the coarctation site. If one of the subclavian arteries arises at or below the coarctation, rib notching occurs only on the opposite side.

Epigastric Arteries

The internal mammary artery communicates not only with the anterior intercostal arteries but directly with the epigastric artery. Blood flows from the internal mammary artery then in a retrograde direction in the epigastric arteries to the low-pressure external iliac arteries.

Lateral Thoracic Artery

The lateral thoracic artery communicates with the intercostal arteries and carries blood from the high-pressure axillary artery to the low-pressure intercostals communicating with the thoracic aorta.

The Periscapular Network

A rich collateral network develops (demonstrated on the left inside of Fig 28–7) about the scapulae. The periscapular network is supplied from the subclavian arteries, primarily from the transverse scapular and transverse cervical arteries, and carries blood through connecting branches to the intercostal arteries to the descending aorta. If the periscapular network is unusually well developed, the scapulae may become notched, which may be apparent on thoracic roentgenograms.

In addition to these major collateral arteries, numerous smaller channels can be seen by aortography, but they are not discussed here because they contribute no major role in the collateral circulation.

Hypertension proximal to the coarctation of the aorta is common. There are two possible mechanisms:

1. Mechanical. Experimentally, when the diameter of the aorta is reduced by 50%, the pressure rises proximal to the narrowing.

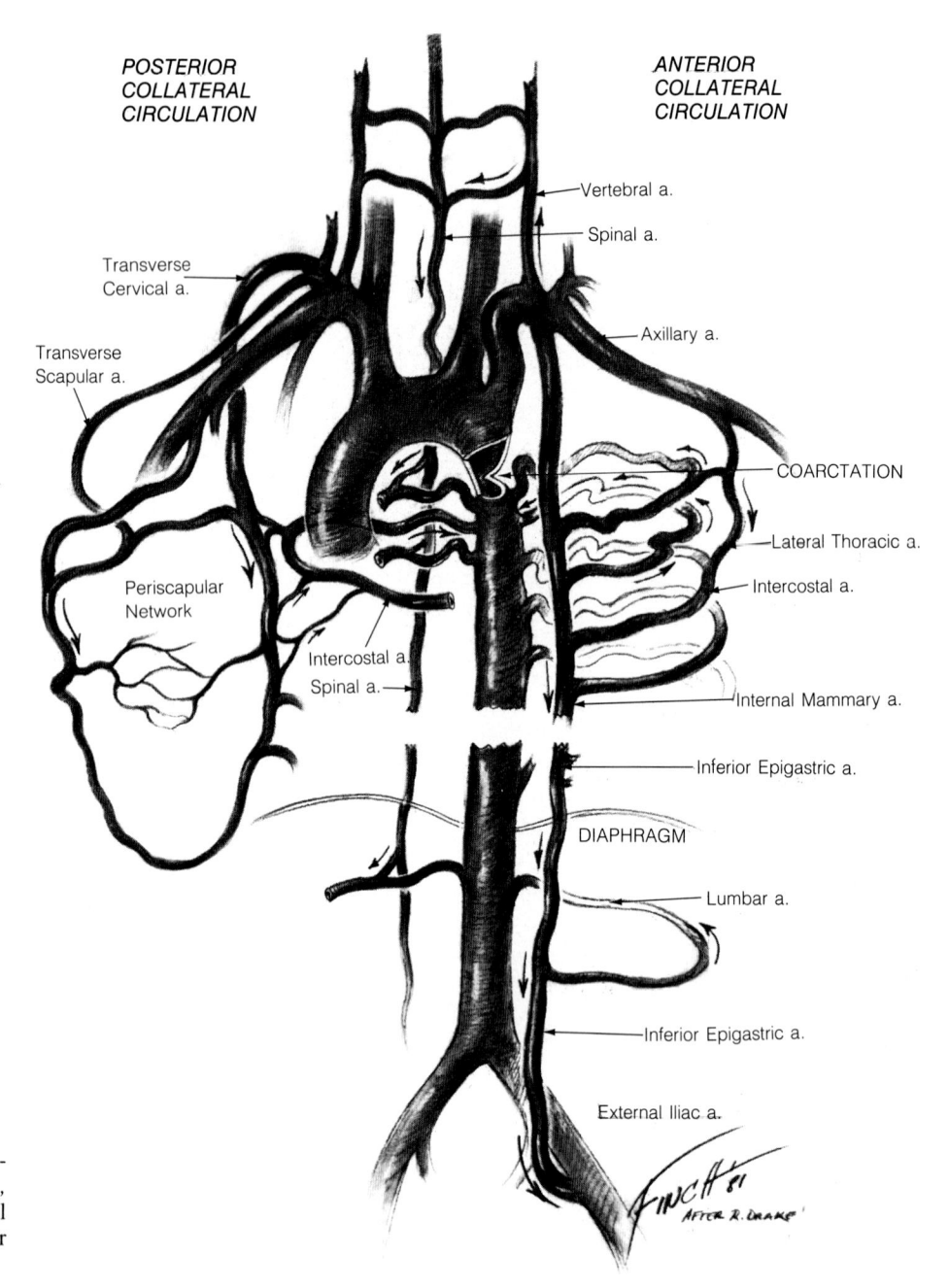

FIG 28–7.
Diagram of major collateral arteries in coarctation of aorta. *Left*, emphasizes posterior collateral system. *Right*, emphasizes anterior collateral system.

2. Renal. Hypertension in patients with coarctation of the aorta may arise on the basis of a Goldblatt kidney. Plasma renin levels are normal in patients with coarctation of the aorta.[16, 17] An abnormal elevation of plasma renin follows administration of furosemide as a hemodynamic stress.[18] As a compensatory mechanism to the renal hypoperfusion, the renin-angiotension-aldosterone mechanism is activated, increasing the intravascular fluid volume and cardiac index. With volume depletion by furosemide, there is an exaggerated renin response to maintain renal perfusion. Renin excretion is much more pronounced in patients with coarctation of the aorta than in normal individuals, suggesting a renin mechanism in addition to the mechanical theory to explain the patient's hypertension.

ASSOCIATED CONDITIONS

The incidence of associated malformation is related to the age of the patient at diagnosis. Patients with associated anomalies usually become symptomatic soon after birth, whereas patients with isolated coarctation become symptomatic in childhood.

The incidence of various anomalies in symptomatic

infants with coarctation is difficult to determine. The commonest coexisting problems include tubular hypoplasia in one half of cases, particularly if a ventricular septal defect is present, and a ventricular septal defect or patent ductus arteriosus, also in one half the cases.[5] Abnormalities of left ventricular outflow obstruction or left ventricular inflow obstruction from left ventricular or mitral hypoplasia are each present in about 20%. Bicuspid aortic valve is present in 50% of all cases of coarctation but is usually not stenotic hemodynamically.[3] Other than bicuspid aortic valve, associated valvar anomalies are uncommon. The one exception is Shone's syndrome,[7, 8] which includes supravalvar mitral ring, parachute mitral valve, and discrete subaortic stenosis.

Minor abnormalities of left ventricular papillary muscles[9] are present in most patients with coarctation of the aorta, but this is usually not clinically or hemodynamically significant.

Acquired cardiac abnormalities are common:

1. Endocardial fibroelastosis[10] is common in infants who die.
2. Mitral regurgitation, the result of papillary muscle dysfunction or abnormalities of chordae tendineae or mitral leaflets, is found in some severely ill neonates.[12, 13]
3. Intimal and medial thickening and atheroma of coronary arteries are common in older patients, presumably from systemic hypertension.[14]
4. Aortic aneurysm, developing either proximal or distal to the coarctation site, may arise from hypertension or bacterial endocarditis.[15] Also, the incidence of dissecting aneurysm is increased.
5. A jet lesion may develop in descending aorta below the coarctation and may be the site of subacute bacterial endocarditis.

Coarctation of the aorta may occur in patients with transposition of the aorta. For example, 1% of patients with transposition of the great vessels have coarctation of the aorta. These patients usually have a hypoplastic right ventricle.

Coarctation of the aorta occurs in 20% of patients with coexistent tricuspid atresia and transposition of the great vessels and in 25% of patients with Taussig-Bing heart.

CLINICAL FEATURES

The cardinal finding of coarctation of the aorta is differential blood pressure readings between the arms and the legs and stronger radial than femoral pulses. The leg recording should be at least 20 mm Hg lower than the arm to diagnose coarctation of the aorta. Blood pressure recordings should be made in both arms, because the readings may be different if either subclavian artery arises below the coarctation. No blood pressure difference is found between the arms and the legs when both subclavian arteries arise below the coarctation.

The blood pressure may be lower in the left arm than in the right arm when:

1. The left subclavian artery arises below the coarctation of the aorta.
2. The origin of left subclavian artery is involved in the coarctation.
3. Tubular hypoplasia occurs between the left carotid and left subclavian arteries.

The blood pressure may be lower in the right arm than in the left arm when:

1. The right subclavian artery arises anomalously from the descending aorta and beyond the coarctation.
2. Coarctation of the aorta and right arch coexist, with a mirror image of the patterns described above.

Two clinical pictures of coarctation are observed:

1. Symptomatic infants. As explained previously, coarctation of the aorta does not cause symptoms at birth. Congestive cardiac failure may develop in the neonatal period or early infancy, according to the rate of ductal closure, the severity of obstruction, and the presence of coexisting cardiac conditions. Cardiac failure develops either slowly or abruptly and may be precipitated by a respiratory infection. Neonates may be in cardiogenic shock, whereas infants initially show features of respiratory distress. The infant often appears cyanotic because of inadequate tissue perfusion. Blood pressure readings are low, and no difference is found between the arms and legs when the infant is in congestive cardiac failure. No mumurs are found. With treatment, the cardiac output improves, blood pressure rises, a pressure difference is found, and a soft systolic ejection murmur may be heard, often in the intrascapular area. A gallop is common, and the liver may be greatly enlarged.
2. Asymptomatic infants and children. If congestive cardiac failure is absent, most children are robust. Frequently the boys are athletic and rarely symptomatic. There may be complaints of headache but rarely of claudication or cold lower extremities. Angina is rare. Cardiac disease is recognized because of the discovery of either a murmur or elevated blood pressure.

Cardiac examination usually reveals a normal-sized heart. The aortic pulsations may be prominent in the suprasternal notch; and if a thrill is present in this location, an associated bicuspid valve should be suspected. A systolic ejection click also indicates a bicuspid aortic valve. A soft (grade 2–3/6) systolic ejection murmur may be heard over the back, particularly between the scapulae, at the cardiac apex, and in the aortic area. Because of the wide transmission of the murmur, it may be difficult to identify a bicuspid aortic valve. A short middiastolic murmur is present at the apex in one half of the patients. Its origin is unknown; perhaps it is related to minor abnormalities of the mitral valve apparatus.

ELECTROCARDIOGRAPHIC FEATURES

The QRS pattern varies with age. In symptomatic neonates and younger infants, the electrocardiogram (ECG) shows right ventricular hypertrophy and inverted T waves (left ventricular strain) in the left precordial leads. Reasons for the seemingly paradoxical right ventricular hypertrophy include hypoplasia of the left ventricle; postductal location of the coarctation, so that the right ventricle ejects against the coarctation prenatally; the effect of pulmonary hypertension on the right ventricle, and the volume load on the right ventricle before birth.

By 3 months of age, the ECG should show evidence of left ventricular hypertrophy. If isolated right ventricular hypertrophy persists, coexisting mitral stenosis should be suspected.

Most symptomatic older infants with isolated coarctation or those infants with large coexisting ventricular septal defect show biventricular hypertrophy.

In children with coarctation of the aorta, the ECG may be normal or show left ventricular hypertrophy. In 10%, a deeper than normal S wave may be present in lead V_6, but this does not indicate right ventricular hypertrophy. ST- and T-wave inversion in the left precordial leads indicates severe obstruction and, perhaps, left ventricular subendocardial ischemia.

The QRS axis and P waves are usually normal.

ECHOCARDIOGRAPHIC FEATURES

The details of the ascending, transverse, and descending aorta and the area of coarctation can be demonstrated by cross-sectional echocardiography performed from the suprasternal notch.[19, 20]

Echocardiography is also useful in identifying associated cardiac anomalies.[21] The most frequently identified anomaly is a bicuspid aortic valve, which shows eccentric diastolic closure. Occasionally, there is diastolic flutter of the mitral valve. Associated mitral valve anomalies and ventricular septal defect are the anomalies most commonly identified by echocardiography.

Echocardiographic studies are useful in demonstrating ventricular cavity size and function.[22] In neonates, as a residuum of the fetal hemodynamics, the right ventricle is dilated and hypertrophied, and the left ventricular cavity size and contractility are reduced (decreased stroke volume prenatally). With age, right ventricular size decreases, and the left ventricle enlarges, becomes hypertrophied, and shows improved contractility.

RADIOGRAPHIC FEATURES

The radiographic findings of coarctation of the aorta in neonates or young infants differ from the appearance in children or adults. REASON: In utero, because of the patent ductus arteriosus, no pressure gradient occurs across the coarctation; and consequently, there is no flow through collateral arteries (see Fig 28–6). Normally, 10% of the flow to the descending aorta crosses the aortic isthmus and so is ejected by the left ventricle. In coarctation of the aorta, the flow through the isthmus is less, and almost all blood flow to the descending aorta occurs through the ductus arteriosus and originates from the right ventricle. This results in volume overload and dilatation of the right ventricle.

As the ductus arteriosus closes after birth, a pressure gradient occurs in the aorta, and collateral arteries develop. The aortic obstruction causes left ventricular pressure overload. The size of the right ventricle gradually decreases.

The sudden pressure load on the left ventricle results in left ventricular decompensation, and severe congestive cardiac failure may develop. As collaterals enlarge and the infant survives, left ventricular size gradually decreases, but left ventricular hypertrophy invariably develops. In the older child and, particularly, in the adult with adequate collaterals, cardiac size is characteristically normal.

The radiographic findings for coarctation of the aorta can be divided into two categories: nonspecific and specific.

Nonspecific Features

These features, although not diagnostic of coarctation of the aorta, are found in a number of patients. The nonspecific features differ in infants and children.

Infants

The nonspecific radiographic features reflect the presence of congestive cardiac failure.

1. There is generalized cardiomegaly because both ventricles are enlarged (Fig 28–8).
2. The right ventricle is dilated. REASON: Residual dilatation of the right ventricle from the altered hemodynamics of the fetal circulation.

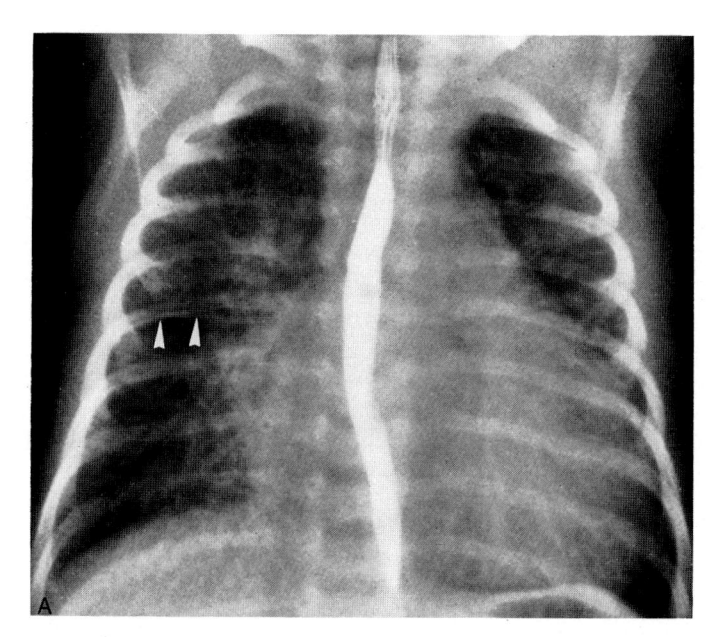

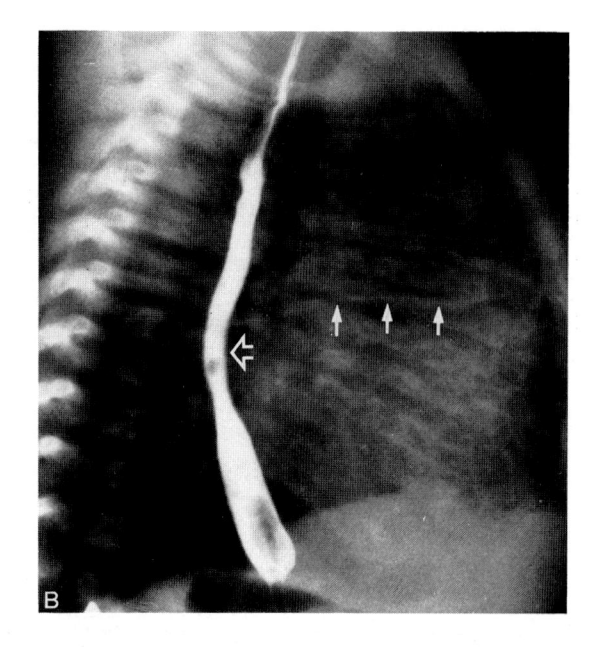

FIG 28–8.
Thoracic roentgenograms of an infant with coarctation of aorta and congestive cardiac failure. **A,** posteroanterior projection; marked cardiomegaly. Diffuse prominence of pulmonary vasculature which is indistinct. Prominent horizontal fissure *(arrows)* from small volume of pleural fluid or subpleural edema suggest cardiac failure rather than left-to-right shunt. **B,** lateral projection; increased cardiac size. Left atrial enlargement *(open arrow)*. Reticular pulmonary pattern at base suggests cardiac failure. No displacement of esophagus to allow specific diagnosis of coarctation of aorta.

3. The left ventricle is dilated. REASON: Immediately after birth, there are few collateral arteries, and the left ventricle usually fails.

4. The left atrium is enlarged. REASON: The failing left ventricle requires an increased filling pressure, which results in increased left atrial pressure.

5. The pulmonary vasculature is accentuated. REASON: The increased left atrial pressure is also transmitted to the pulmonary veins, which become engorged, resulting in "pulmonary congestion."

6. Pulmonary edema may occur, but pleural effusion is absent (see Fig 28–8). REASON: Left ventricular failure in infants does not cause pleural effusion, in contrast to adolescent and adult patients. The mechanism for the difference in response is unknown.

7. Specific radiologic findings for coarctation (discussed later) are usually subtle or absent in symptomatic infants. REASON: The aortic arch is usually overshadowed by thymic tissue, and poststenotic dilatation is usually absent immediately after birth, because there was virtually no flow through the area of coarctation prenatally. REASON: In utero, the pressure above and below the coarctation is equal because of the large patent ductus arteriosus. Only the very uncommon postductal coarctation causes a pressure differential in the fetal circulation.

Cardiomegaly, pulmonary congestion, and left atrial enlargement are observed in many other left-sided obstructive lesions and cardiomyopathies occurring in infants. These nonspecific roentgenographic findings are, therefore, "consistent" only with coarctation of the aorta but are more diagnostic when interpreted in light of the clinical findings. The radiographic differentiation between a left-sided obstructive lesion in congestive cardiac failure and a left-to-right shunt may be difficult.

The following radiographic findings are helpful to distinguish these two hemodynamic states, but the differentiation cannot always be made with certainty. In a left-sided obstructive lesion, the heart appears larger than the degree of the accentuation of the pulmonary vasculature seems to justify. In a left-to-right shunt, on the other hand, cardiac size is proportional to the degree of hypervascularity. In a left-to-right shunt, the pulmonary arteries appear distinct and well defined and cause numerous densities throughout both lung fields. REASON: In left-to-right shunt, the pulmonary arteries enlarge and become more tortuous, so that arteries are seen "on end." In contrast, in a left-sided obstructive lesion, the pulmonary vasculature tends to be more "fluffy," and a reticular pattern may sometimes be seen (see Fig 28–8). The distinction becomes impossible when a left-to-right shunt and coarctation of the aorta coexist.

Older Children and Adults

In older infants, children, and young adults, cardiac size is usually normal, but signs of left ventricular hyper-

478 Outflow Obstructive Lesions

FIG 28-9.
Thoracic roentgenogram, posteroanterior projection of coarctation of aorta in older patient. Characteristic cardiac contour with round left ventricular contour *(white arrows)*. Inconspicuous pulmonary artery. Normal cardiac size and pulmonary vasculature. Prominent ascending aorta *(black arrows)* suggests associated bicuspid aortic valve. Aortic arch and descending aorta inconspicuous, suggesting tubular hypoplasia and no poststenotic dilatation. Bilateral rib notching. No well-developed aortic knob. REASON: Density of dilated left subclavian artery *(small white arrows)* forms a straight density with distal aortic arch. This straight contour is common in coarctation. (see Fig. 28-16).

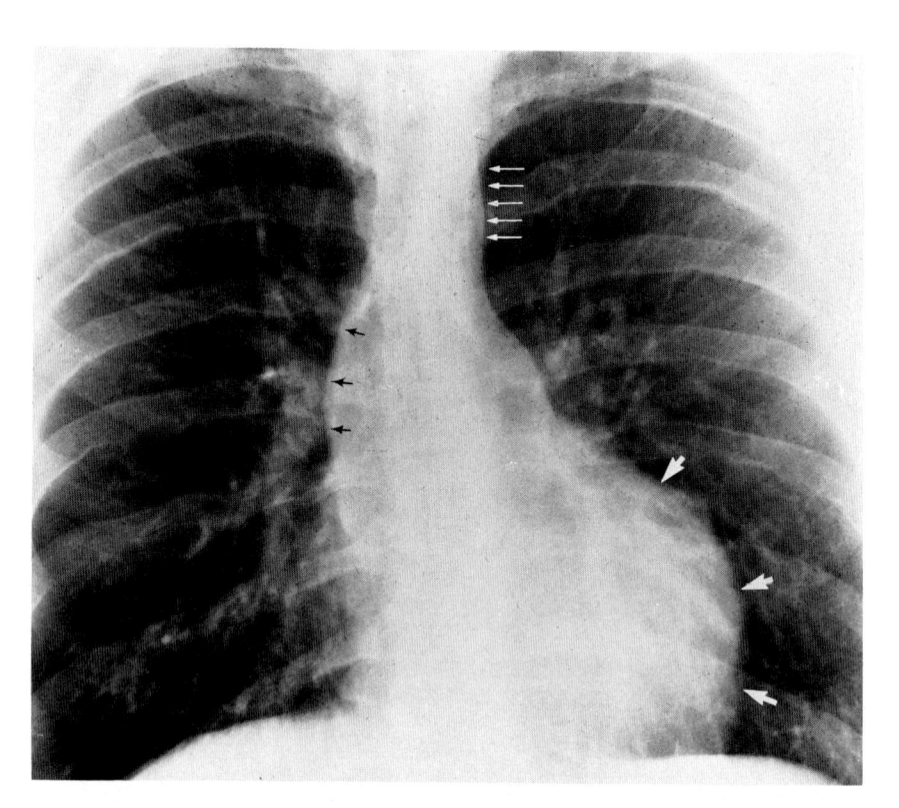

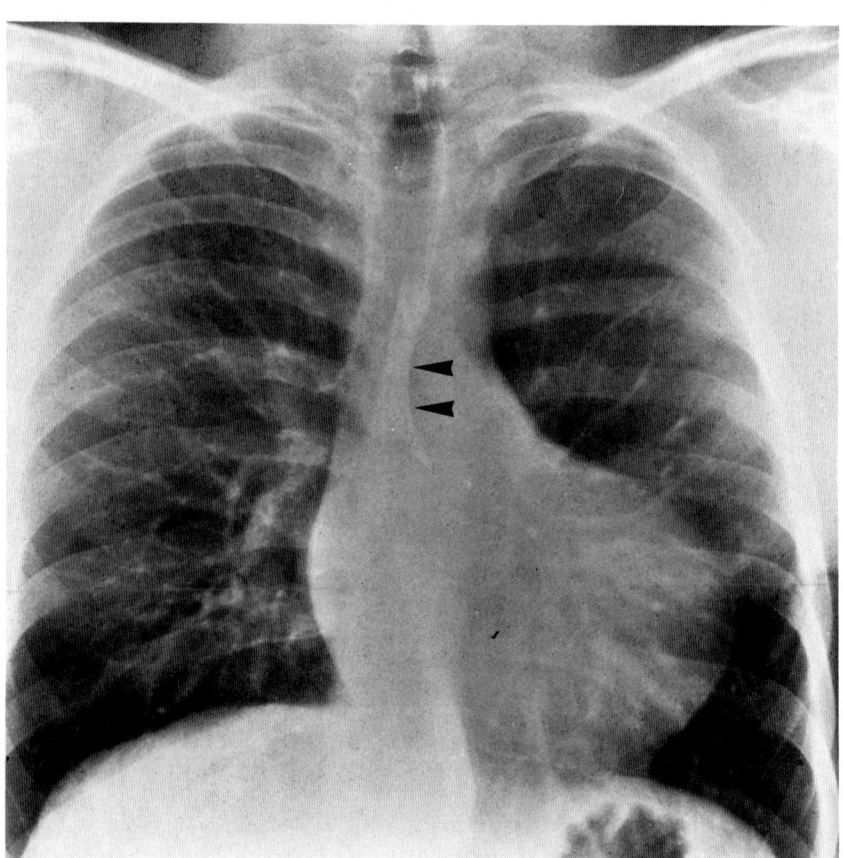

FIG 28-10.
Thoracic roentgenogram, posteroanterior projection of coarctation of aorta in young adult. Cardiac contour resembles that in tetralogy of Fallot, with concave pulmonary artery segment and elevated apex. Concave pulmonary artery due to counterclockwise rotation (left ventricular hypertrophy). Reason for elevated apex unknown. Inconspicuous aortic arch. Esophagus displaced to right *(arrows)* by poststenotic dilatation.

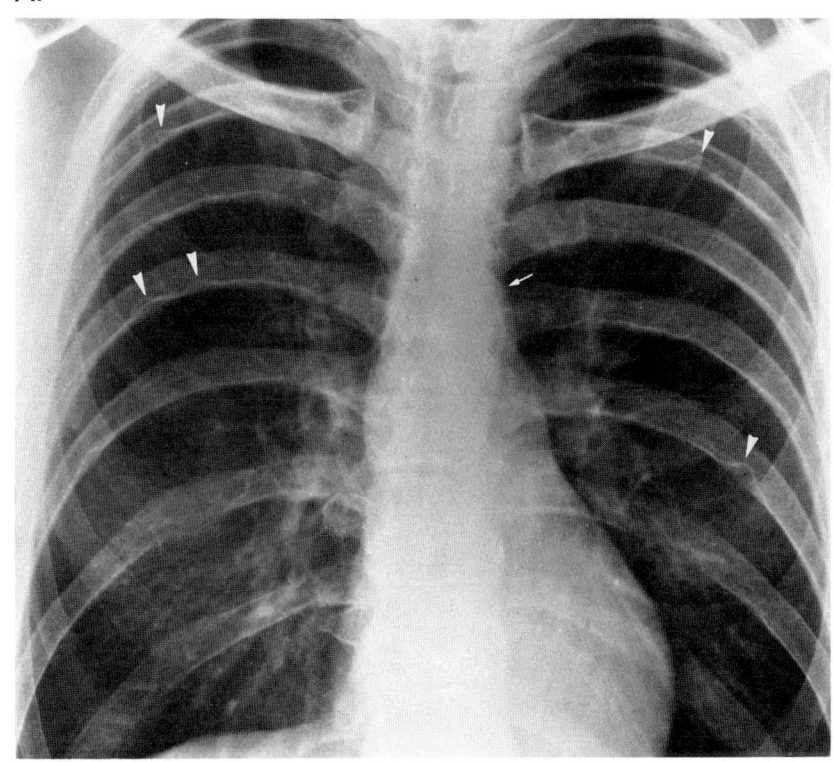

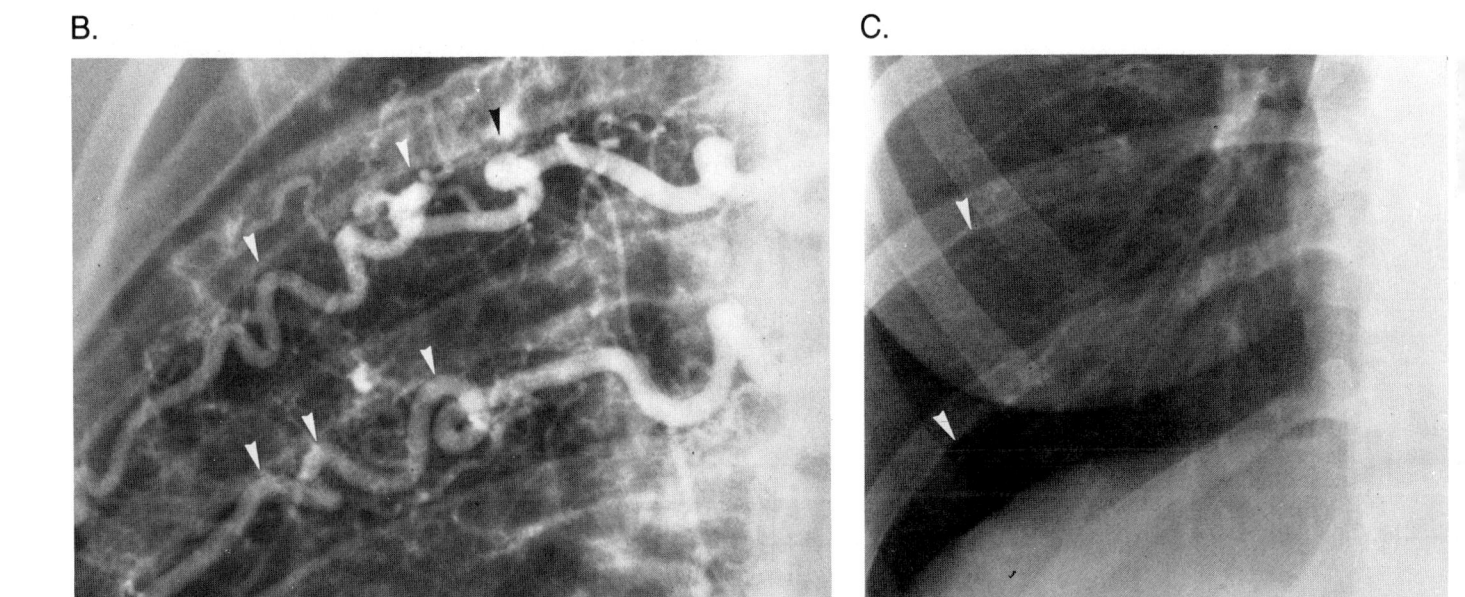

FIG 28–11.
Rib notching in coarctation of aorta. **A,** thoracic roentgenogram, posteroanterior projection. Notching of lower margin of ribs *(arrows);* also, "low arch sign" *(white arrow)*. The aortic arch is not visible because of tubular hypoplasia; what appears to be the aortic arch represents the poststenotic dilatation. **B,** selective aortogram, anteroposterior projection. Enlarged, tortuous intercostal arteries, eroding lower rib edges *(arrows)*. The true lower margin of ribs not seen because they are too thin. **C,** notching of only lower ribs in a patient with abdominal coarctation of aorta.

trophy develop. Because of the enlargement of collateral channels, the resistance on the left ventricle gradually decreases, resulting in left ventricular compensation and hypertrophy. The size of the right ventricle becomes normal.

1. The cardiac size is normal or insignificantly larger. REASON: The left ventricle is now compensated because of the gradual enlargement of collateral vessels, which decrease the resistance to left ventricular outflow.

2. The left ventricle has a rounded contour because of hypertrophy (Fig 28–9). REASON: The left ventricular systolic pressure remains increased.

3. Left atrial enlargement is not present. REASON: The left ventricle has compensated, and the left atrial pressure is normal.

4. The pulmonary vasculature is normal, because the left ventricle has compensated and there is no left-to-right shunt. Also, left ventricular end-diastolic, left atrial, and pulmonary venous pressure are normal.

5. The pulmonary artery segment is inconspicuous and the cardiac waist narrow. REASON: Left ventricular hypertrophy usually results in a counterclockwise rotation of the heart, causing the pulmonary artery segment to be rotated medially.

6. Sometimes the counterclockwise rotation of the heart is associated with an elevation of the apex (Fig 28–10), resulting in a configuration similar to that of tetralogy of Fallot. The reason for the elevation of the cardiac apex in some patients with coarctation is unknown.

Specific Features

There are specific radiologic findings that strongly suggest a diagnosis of coarctation of the aorta.

Rib Notching

Although rib notching may occur in any condition that causes enlargement and tortuosity of intercostal arteries, veins, or nerves, coarctation of the aorta is the most frequent cause. Therefore, rib notching is highly suggestive of coarctation, even if no poststenotic dilatation of the descending aorta can be observed. Rib notching is rare before the age of 10 years and is almost never observed before the age of 5 years. REASON: Notching is a manifestation of the collateral flow, which develops gradually with age and eventually causes pressure erosions of the ribs by tortuous intercostal arteries. Pathologically, the lower sulcus of the ribs appears irregular, whereas the lower margin of the rib is normal. Radiographically, however, the lower margin of the ribs appears notched, because the thinned normal rib margin is not seen, only the eroded thicker part of the rib.

1. Radiographically, rib notching is demonstrated along the lower margin of the ribs and is most prominent in the posterior aspect (Fig 28–11,A). REASON: The intercostal arteries lie in the costal sulcus. Because the intercostal arteries form the major collateral pathway, they become enlarged, elongated, and tortuous, causing pressure erosions of the cortical margin of the ribs, which can be demonstrated by angiography (Fig 28–11,B).

2. Notching is absent about the first and second ribs. REASON: The first two intercostal arteries arise from the costocervical trunk, not from the descending aorta below the area of coarctation. Therefore, the first two intercostal arteries are not collateral pathways.

3. Typically, notching is most visible in the upper ribs and becomes progressively less conspicuous in the

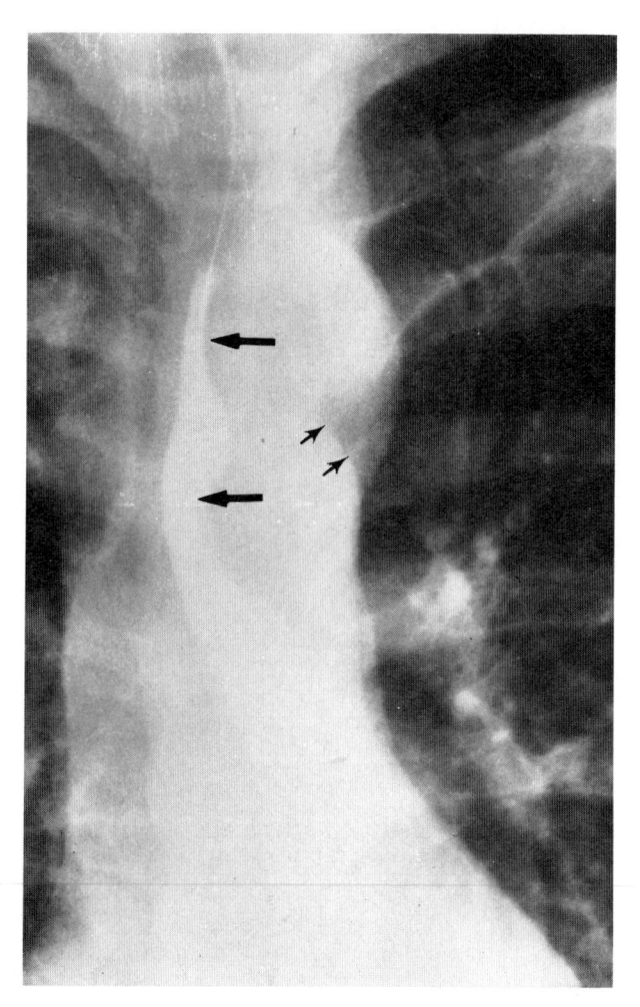

FIG 28–12.
Thoracic roentgenogram, posteroanterior projection in coarctation of aorta with well-developed aortic arch. Area of coarctation demonstrated by reversed figure-of-3 sign formed by aortic arch and poststenotic segment *(large black arrows)*. Double density formed by aortic arch and poststenotic segment *(small black arrows)*. Aortic knob normal.

lower ribs. REASON: The upper intercostal arteries represent the shortest collateral pathway and offer the least resistance and therefore have larger blood flow. Notching is best seen in the fourth through the seventh ribs. Prominent notching below the seventh rib suggests abdominal coarctation (Fig 28–11,C).

4. Rib notching is usually bilateral, although unilateral notching may be prominent when one of the subclavian arteries arises below the coarctation. Isolated notching of the right-sided ribs in the presence of a left aortic arch suggests either origin of the left subclavian artery below the coarctation or involvement of the left subclavian artery in the coarctation (see Fig 28–5). Absence of rib notching on the right side in the presence of a left aortic arch suggests an aberrant right subclavian artery arising below the level of the coarctation (see Fig 28–5). REASON: The subclavian artery arising below the coarctation is no longer under high pressure. The internal mammary artery, therefore, no longer feeds the intercostal arteries. If both subclavian arteries arise below the level of the coarctation (see Fig 28–5), rib notching is absent bilaterally. If a right aortic arch is present, the pattern of notching would be the opposite.

Mediastinum and Barium-Filled Esophagus

The most specific radiographic findings are obtained by observing the area of coarctation on thoracic roentgenograms. Scrutiny of the mediastinum and the barium-filled esophagus allows a diagnosis of coarctation of the aorta in most older infants, children, and adults. The radiographic

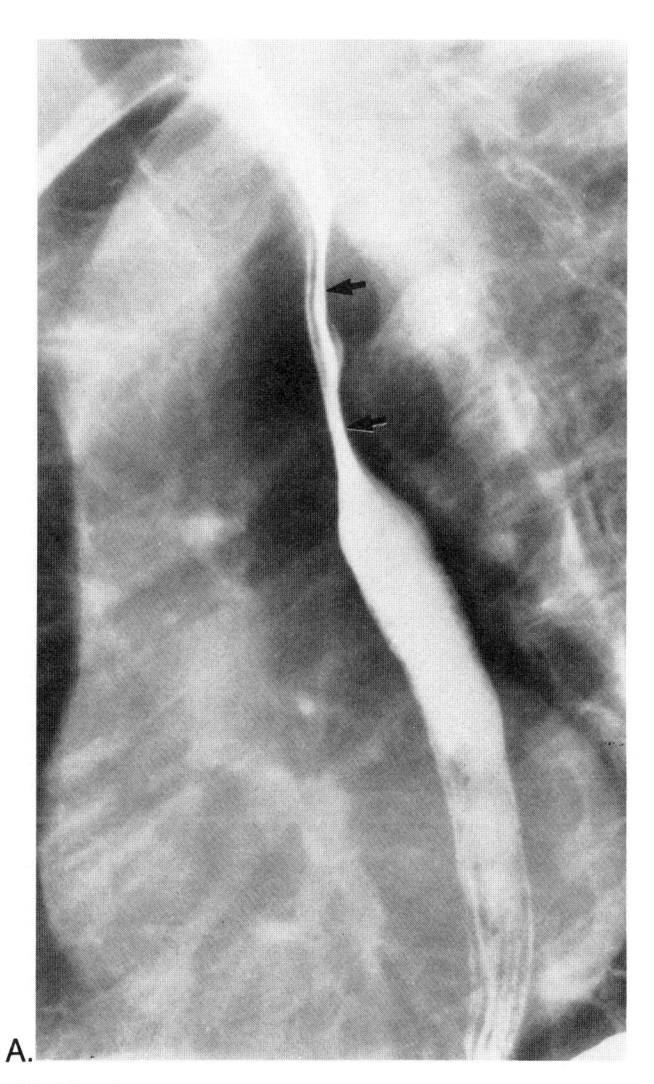

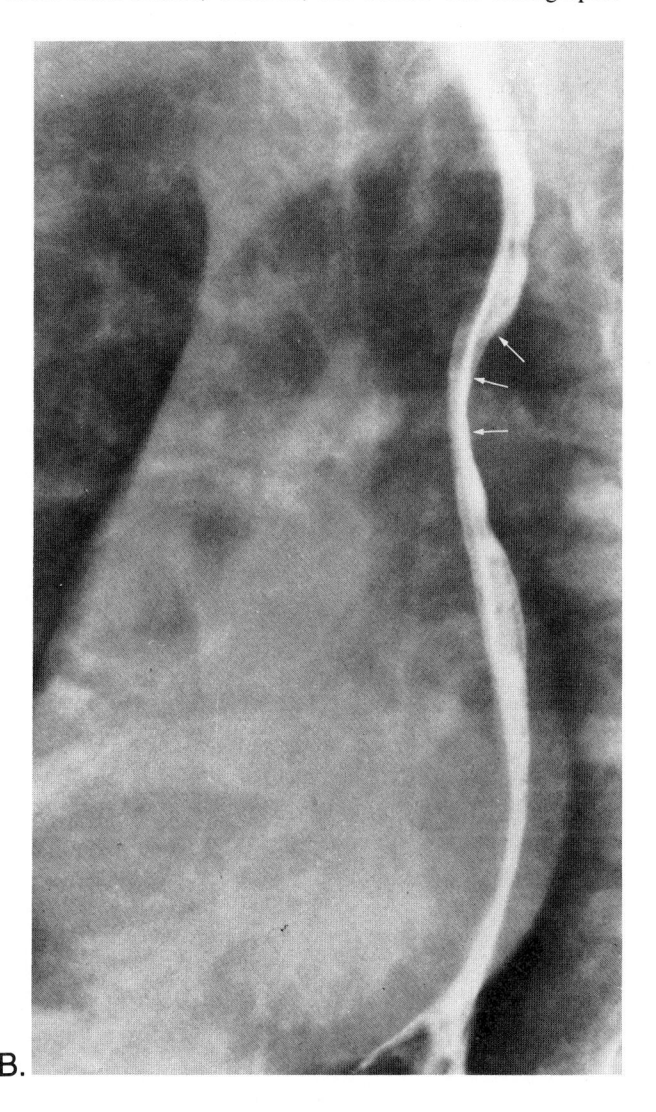

FIG 28–13.
Thoracic roentgenogram, left anterior oblique projection in coarctation of aorta. **A,** two indentations *(arrows)* of barium-filled esophagus create reverse figure-of-3 sign. Upper indentation is formed by aortic arch, lower indentation by poststenotic dilatation. **B,** poststenotic dilatation of aorta causes displacement of esophagus.

appearance varies, depending on the presence or absence of tubular hypoplasia, the location of the left subclavian artery, and the degree of poststenotic dilatation of the descending aorta.

Coarctation of Aorta With Normal Origin of the Left Subclavian Artery and Well-Developed Aortic Knob

This situation is uncommon and usually associated with tubular hypoplasia. This type has been presented as the classic textbook picture of coarctation (see Fig 28–2).

1. The distal aortic arch and poststenotic dilatation cause a notch along the left lateral margin of the aorta, yielding the figure-of-3 sign: displacement of the esophagus results in the reversed 3, epsilon, or E sign (Fig 28–12).

2. On lateral and left anterior oblique projections, the barium-filled esophagus is displaced anteriorly by the poststenotic segment above the level of the left mainstem bronchus (Fig 28–13,A).

3. With tubular hypoplasia, only the poststenotic segment is seen and may simulate the aortic arch (see Fig 28–11).

4. A characteristic notch, caused by the coarctation, can also be seen along the posterior wall of the aortic contour on the lateral projection (Fig 28–14). Therefore, both a posteroanterior and lateral projection should be obtained, although the best projection is the left anterior oblique.

Coarctation of the Aorta With Normal Origin of the Left Subclavian Artery and Tubular Hypoplasia

The hypoplasia involves the segment between left subclavian artery and the coarctation (see Fig 28–4).

1. The aortic arch is not seen. REASON: The arch is hypoplastic.

2. The poststenotic dilatation is demonstrated but may be misinterpreted as a normal but low-lying aortic arch (Figs 28–11,A and 28–15).

3. The barium-filled esophagus is displaced only by the poststenotic segment, creating only the lower portion of the 3 sign (see Fig 28–10).

Coarctation of the Aorta With Origin of the Subclavian Artery at the Level of Coarctation

Coarctation of the aorta with origin of the subclavian artery at the level of coarctation is a common occurrence (Fig 28–16).

1. The aortic arch is inconspicuous. REASON: The dilated origin of the left subclavian artery forms a straight upper left cardiac border, and the round density of the aortic arch is therefore not evident (Figs 28–9 and 28–17).

2. The poststenotic segment of the descending aorta beyond the coarctation of the aorta simulates a low-lying aortic arch.

3. The left subclavian artery tends to be enlarged and may reach aneurysmal proportions. REASON: The blood flow through the left subclavian artery is markedly in-

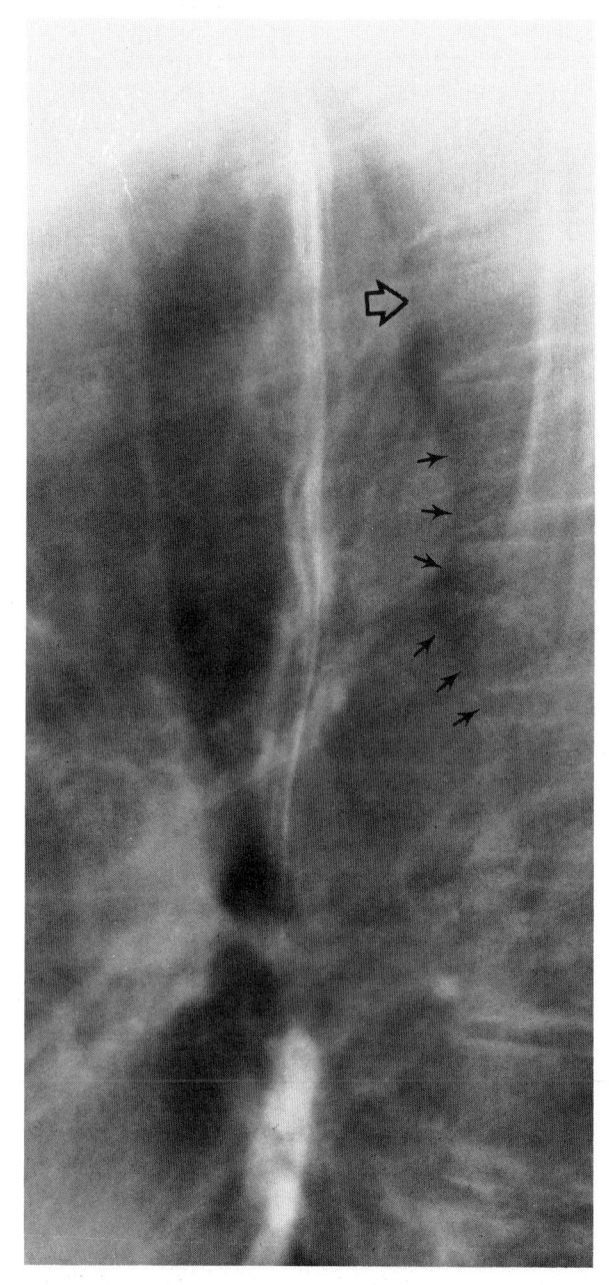

FIG 28–14.
Thoracic roentgenogram, lateral projection in coarctation of aorta. Figure-of-3 sign *(small arrows)* along the outer contour of aorta. Enlarged left subclavian artery *(open arrow)*. Barium-filled esophagus is not indented. Small black arrows outline the distal aortic arch and poststenotic segment of thoracic aorta.

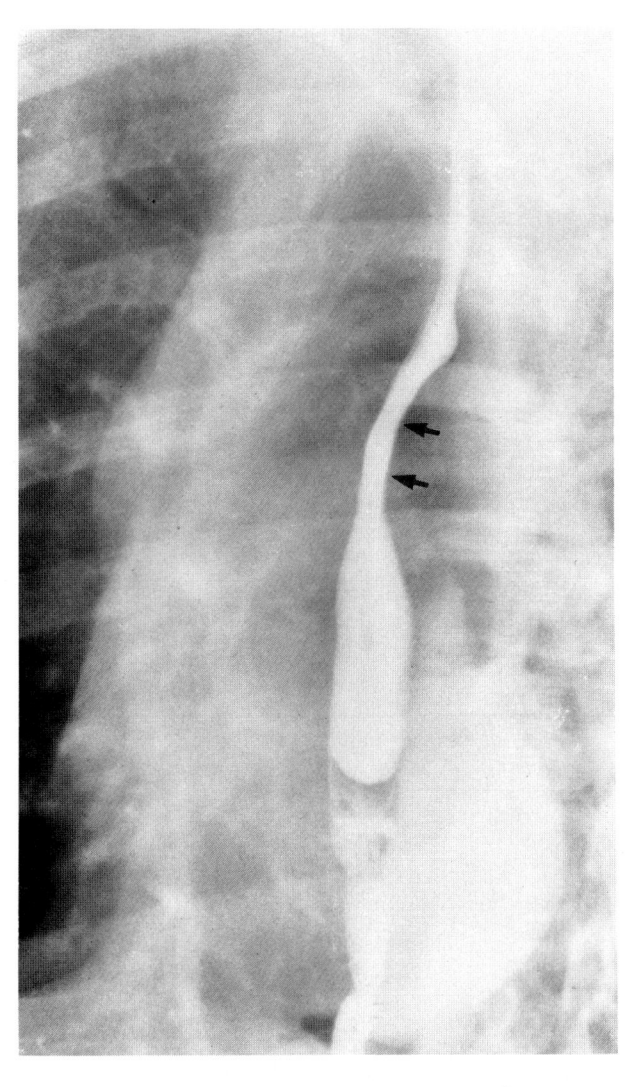

FIG 28–15.
Thoracic roentgenogram, left anterior oblique projection in coarctation of aorta. Marked anterior displacement of barium-filled esophagus *(arrows)* only by poststenotic dilatation. Because of tubular hypoplasia of aortic arch, esophagus not indented by aortic arch; may be misinterpreted as a low aortic arch.

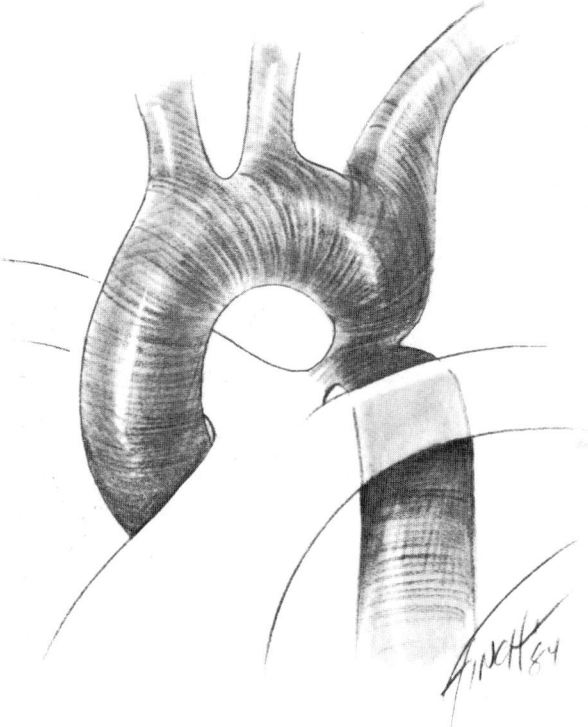

FIG 28–16.
Diagram of coarctation of aorta and origin of dilated left subclavian artery.

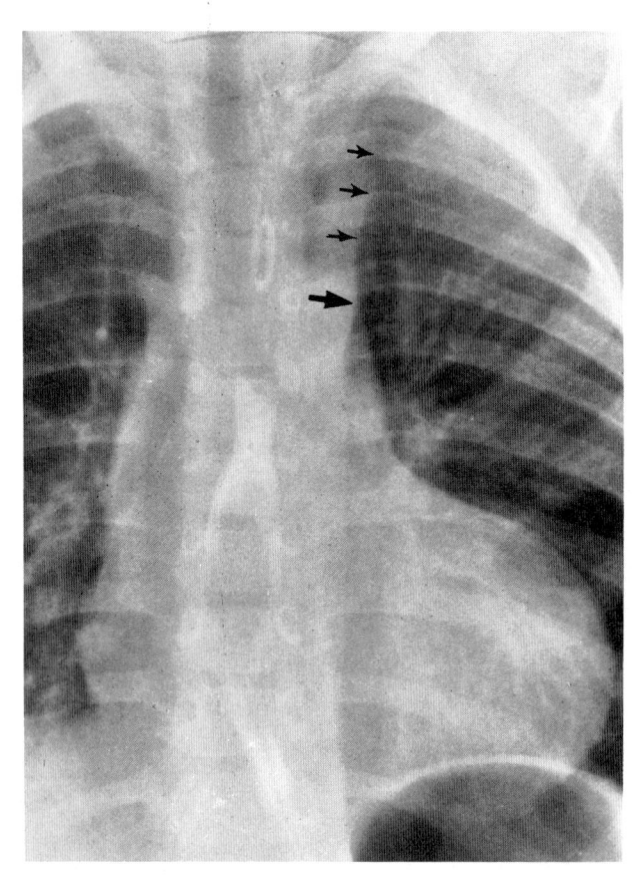

FIG 28–17.
Thoracic roentgenogram, posteroanterior projection in coarctation of aorta with low origin of prominent left subclavian artery. Straight left superior mediastinum *(small arrows)*. Poststenotic dilatation *(large arrow)* simulates low aortic arch.

creased because it represents a major collateral pathway. Sometimes, an aneurysm of the left subclavian artery is present (Fig 28–18).

Coarctation Without Tubular Hypoplasia and With No Poststenotic Dilatation

This type coarctation is rare. Usually, the entire descending aorta is hypoplastic (see Fig. 28–5,*C*).

1. Without rib notching, the diagnosis of coarctation cannot be made on a thoracic roentgenogram, because the esophagus is not displaced (Fig 28–19).
2. Angiography demonstrates the area of coarctation and, sometimes, diffuse hypoplasia of the entire thoracic aorta.

Coarctation of the Aorta Located Immediately Beyond the Left Subclavian Artery With Marked Poststenotic Dilatation

This type of coarctation is uncommon. In most patients, elongation of the ascending aorta occurs. REASON:

Unknown; possibly the increased aortic pressure is involved.

1. The poststenotic segment is visible. Because of its high position in the thorax, a prominent, normally located aortic arch is simulated (Fig 28–20).
2. The aortic arch itself is not seen because it is hypoplastic.

CARDIAC CATHETERIZATION

In neonates or infants with suspected coarctation of the aorta, we perform cardiac catheterization to locate the site and form of aortic obstruction, identify the origin of the brachiocephalic vessels in relation to the coarctation, and define the form and severity of any associated defects

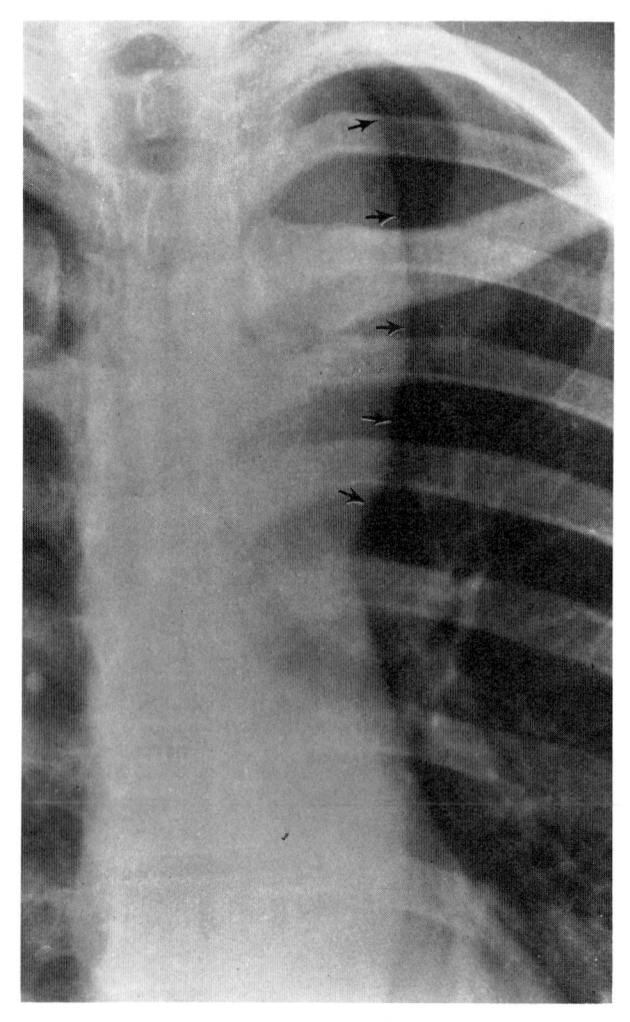

FIG 28–18.
Thoracic roentgenogram, posteroanterior projection in coarctation of aorta with low origin of left subclavian artery. Aneurysmal dilatation of left subclavian artery *(arrows)*, giving appearance of left superior mediastinal mass.

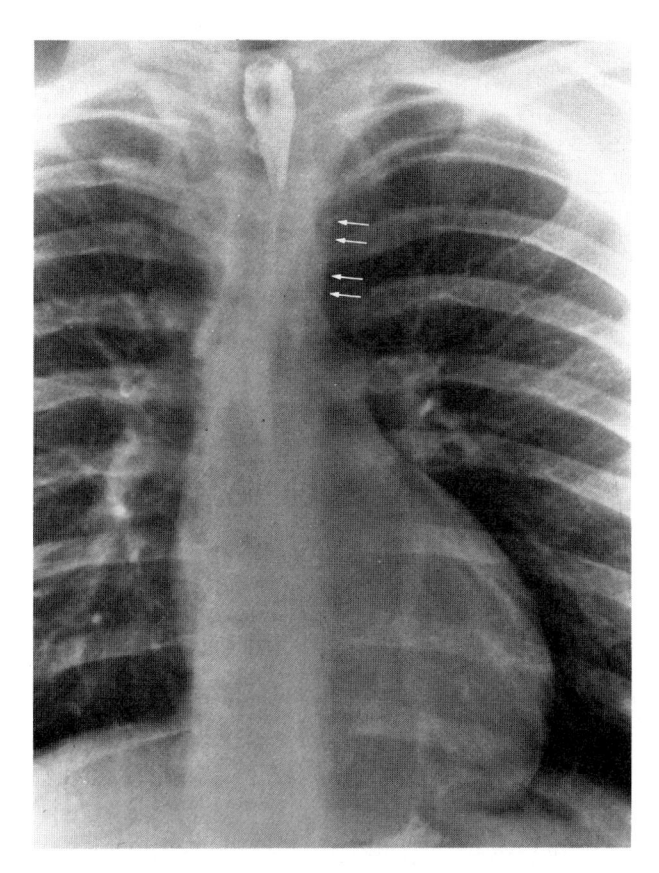

FIG 28-19.
Thoracic roentgenogram, posteroanterior projection in coarctation of aorta with tubular hypoplasia and without poststenotic dilatation. Inconspicuous aortic arch and descending aorta. Barium-filled esophagus not displaced. Diagnosis can be made only from the rib notching and straight left upper mediastinum *(arrow)* without aortic knob.

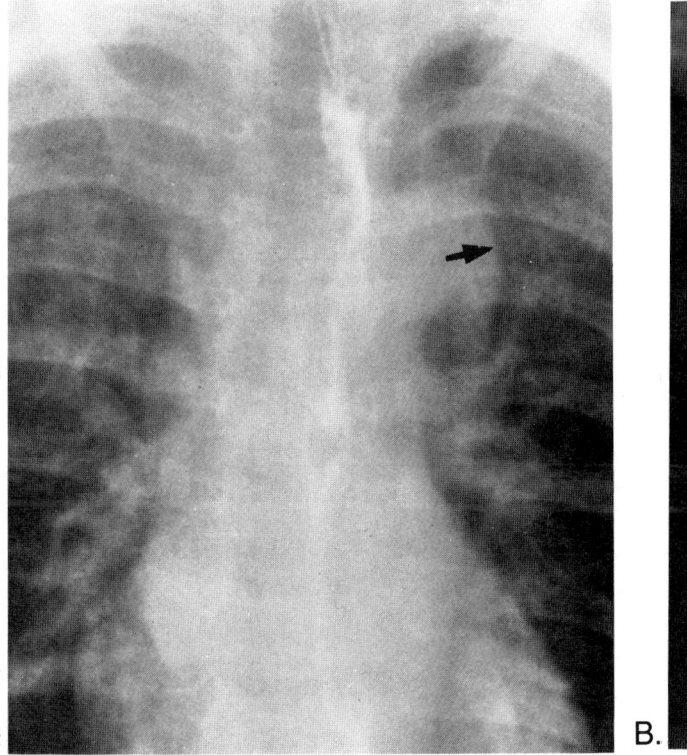

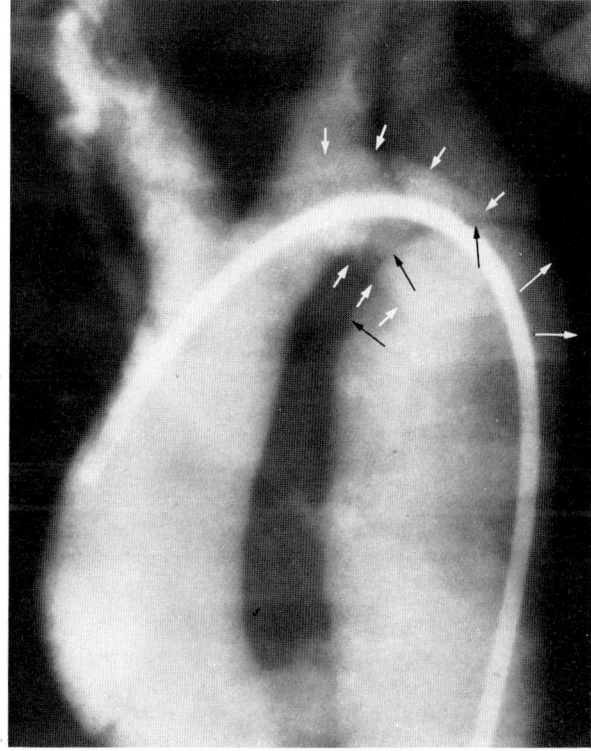

FIG 28-20.
Location of coarctation of aorta immediately beyond left subclavian artery. **A,** thoracic roentgenogram, posteroanterior projection; poststenotic dilatation *(black arrow)* simulates aortic arch. Aortic arch itself not seen because of tubular hypoplasia **B,** aortogram, anteroposterior projection; coarctation of aorta located immediately beyond origin of left subclavian artery. Tubular hypoplasia of distal arch *(white arrows)*. Marked poststenotic dilatation of ascending aorta from a bicuspid aorta valve.

that may require surgical treatment in addition to repair of the coarctation of the aorta. In children not in cardiac failure, we usually do not perform cardiac catheterization or even aortography, because coexisting cardiac conditions are less common in this population and most patients are improved by resecting the coarctation first. In addition, the site of coarctation can be determined accurately by a combination of radiologic findings, echocardiographic observation, or magnetic resonance imaging and blood pressure recordings. The poststenotic dilatation helps locate the distal site of the coarctation. If this is not identified on radiographs, we perform an aortogram.

Blood pressure recording in both arms also provides important information about the proximal site of the coarctation. If the blood pressure in the left arm equals that in the right arm, the coarctation is distal to the left subclavian artery. If the blood pressure reading is lower in the left arm, we perform an aortogram to demonstrate the reason, which may be:

1. Hypoplastic segment between the left common carotid and left subclavian arteries (see Fig 28–4).
2. Involvement of origin of the left subclavian artery in the coarctation.
3. Origin of the left subclavian artery beyond the coarctation.

In neonates and young infants, pulmonary hypertension is common and may be caused by coexisting ventricular septa defect, patent ductus arteriosus, or elevated pulmonary vascular resistance.

Pressures in the aorta are extremely variable. Values may be low both above and below the coarctation if congestive cardiac failure is present, or the pressure may be elevated proximal to the obstruction if cardiac output is normal.

Oximetry data may show a left-to-right shunt at the atrial level, probably from a stretched foramen ovale. If a ventricular septal defect coexists, a shunt is also found at the ventricular level. If the coarctation is severe and the ductus arteriosus is patent, a right-to-left shunt may be found into the descending aorta. The oxygen saturation in the descending aorta is then less than that in the ascending aorta.

From the catheterization data, it may be difficult to define precisely the relative roles of the various anomalies causing the congestive cardiac failure.

ANGIOGRAPHIC APPEARANCE

Various angiographic techniques can be used to demonstrate the area of the coarctation. In neonates and infants with small arteries, the introduction of arterial catheters is technically difficult, because the arteries are small. Consequently, it is better to study these patients by introducing catheters into the venous side and passing the catheter through the foramen ovale and patent or probe-patent ductus arteriosus into the descending aorta. The catheterization approach through a vein is almost invariably successful and yields adequate opacification of the aortic arch unless a large reversing patent ductus is present.

If a large reversing ductus arteriosus is present, the demonstration of the coarctation site may be inadequate. Under these circumstances, a balloon catheter can be passed from the pulmonary artery, through the ductus, into the descending aorta, so a balloon occlusion aortogram can be performed. With this technique, contrast medium is forced in retrograde fashion across the area of coarctation and patent ductus arteriosus (Fig 28–21).

The best views are a lateral view and shallow left anterior oblique with caudal angulation. Retrograde aortography of the right brachial artery or, preferably, the left brachial artery usually results in excellent delineation of the area of coarctation. However, in patients with adequate cardiac ouput, the ascending aorta and brachiocephalic vessels may be inadequately seen (Fig 28–22).

As long as a patent ductus is present, coarctation may be masked because of runoff into the pulmonary artery and the contribution of the mouth of the ductus to the cross-sectional (see Figs 28–6 and 28–21). The important finding is a notch along the greater curvature of the aorta (butter knife deformity; see Fig 28–3), which should establish the diagnosis of coarctation even without a pressure gradient. A notch on the greater curvature of the aorta is invariably present, but sometimes a ringlike constriction exists (see Fig 28–21).

In infants with decreased cardiac output, retrograde aortography may result in excellent imaging of the entire

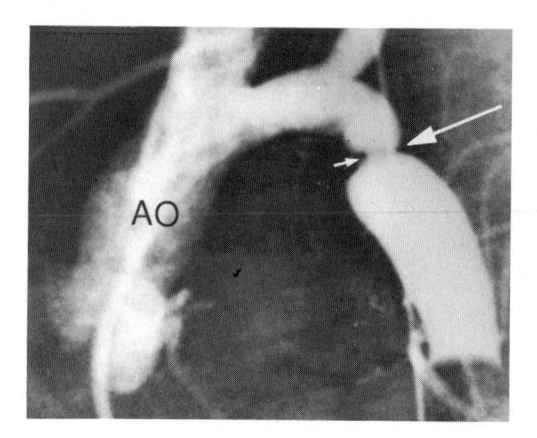

FIG 28–21.
Atypical coarctation. Neonate balloon occlusion aortogram. Lateral projection. Concentric ringlike ridge *(arrows)*. Indentation on greater curvature is always present. Collateral arteries absent despite severe aortic narrowing.

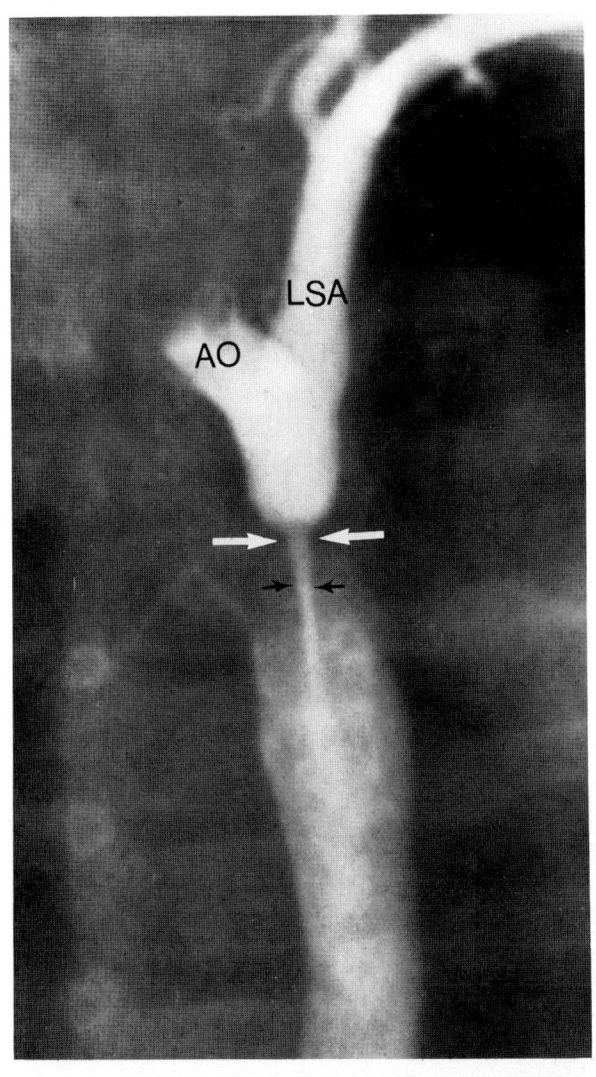

FIG 28–22.
Retrograde flush aortogram *(AO)*, anteroposterior projection in coarctation of aorta. Contrast material injected into left brachial artery opacifies left subclavian artery *(LSA)*, but there is incomplete opacification of aortic arch. Area of coarctation easily seen *(white arrows)*. Jet of contrast *(black arrows)* through coarctation site; poststenotic dilatation of descending aorta. This technique is adequate for demonstrating a coarctation without passing a catheter.

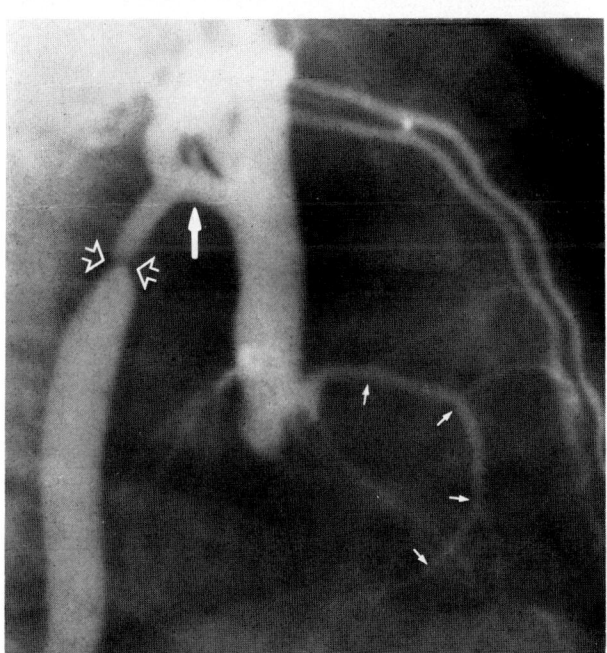

FIG 28–23.
Retrograde aortogram, lateral projection in coarctation of aorta. Opacification of aortic arch to level of aortic valve indicates decreased cardiac output. Tubular hypoplasia *(white arrow)* between left carotid and left subclavian arteries. Tubular hypoplasia of aortic isthmus and discrete coarctation with concentric narrowing *(open arrows)*. Sweeping course of right coronary artery indicates right ventricular enlargement *(small white arrows)* characteristic of infantile coarctation.

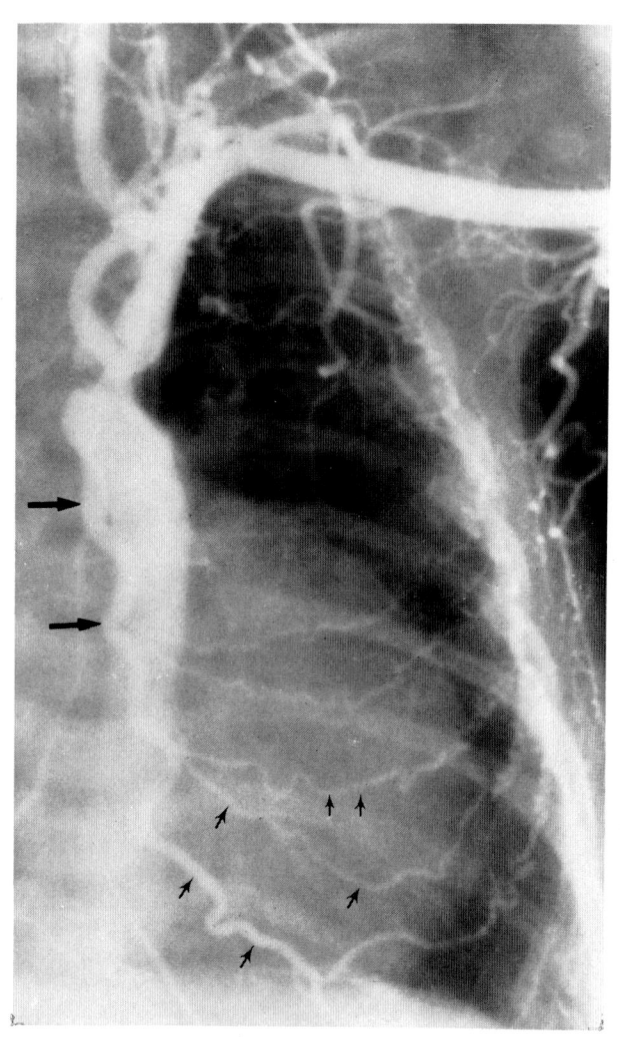

FIG 28–24.
Retrograde aortogram, anteroposterior projection in coarctation of aorta. Injection from left brachial artery. Discrete coarctation of aorta and well-developed collateral network. Major collateral blood flow occurs through enlarged internal mammary artery *(large arrows)*, anterior intercostal *(small arrows)*, and posterior intercostal arteries into descending aorta.

aortic arch and even filling of the coronary arteries (Fig 28–23). In infancy, collateral vessels are absent (see Fig 28–23), but they do develop during childhood (Fig 28–24).

There are several indications for angiography. In older children with clinical signs of coarctation but an atypical thoracic roentgenogram that does not show poststenotic dilatation, a chest film is mandatory, and the location of the aortic arch must be determined. If this is not evident, aortography can give important information about the descending aorta, which may (very rarely) be hypoplastic (Fig 28–25). Coarctation may occur with a right arch (Fig 28–26). An interesting and rare occurrence is coexistent coarctation and double aortic arch (Fig 28–27). When both arches are affected by the coarctation or if the uninvolved arch is hypoplastic, clinical signs of coarctation are evident.

MANAGEMENT

Management depends on the age of the patient and the presenting symptoms.

Symptomatic Neonate or Young Infant

In a symptomatic neonate or infant with congestive cardiac failure, the initial therapy is rapid digitalization and administration of a diuretic. Often, ventilatory assistance is given to neonates to reduce the respiratory effort. The neonate or infant must be observed carefully and catheterization performed on an emergency basis. If acidosis develops, prostaglandin E_1 should be administered in an attempt to open the ductus and increase perfusion of the

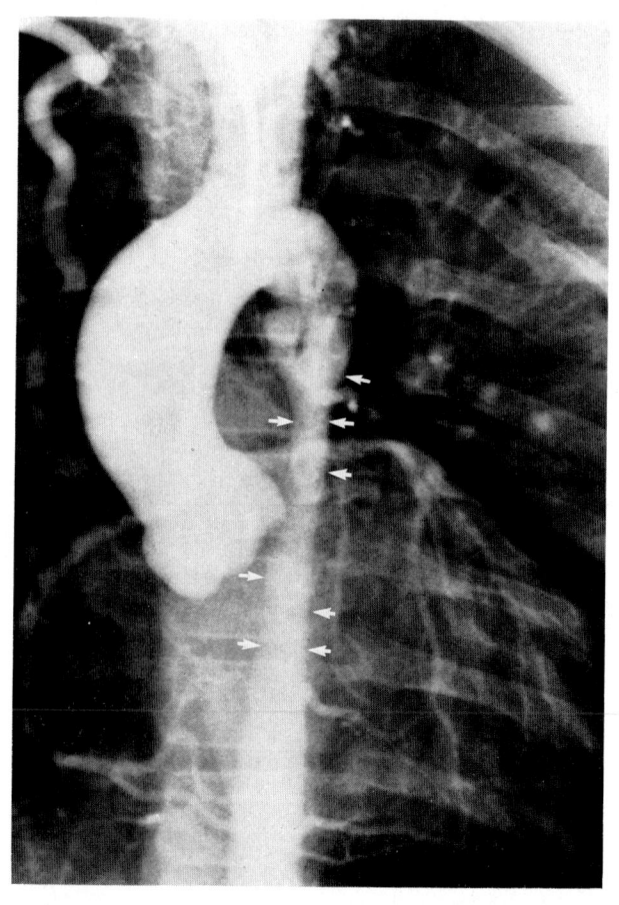

FIG 28–25.
Coarctation of aorta previously repaired without improvement. Note left rib resection and huge right mammary artery. Reason for surgical failure was diffuse hypoplasia of thoracic aorta *(arrows)*.

Coarctation of the Aorta 489

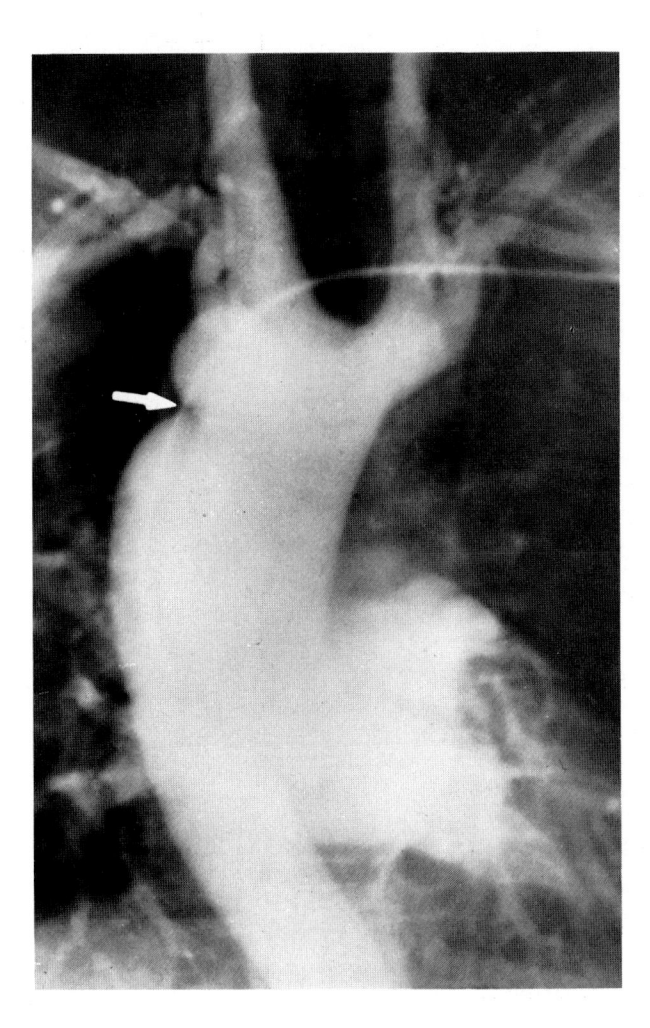

FIG 28–26.
Right ventriculogram, late phase, anteroposterior projection in coarctation of aorta and right aortic arch. Right aortic arch and coarctation of aorta *(arrow)*. Repair would require a right thoracotomy.

FIG 28–27.
Diagram of double aortic arch with coarctation. **A,** coarctation of both arches. Clinical sign of coarctation is present. **B,** coarctation of only one arch does not result in clinical signs of coarctation unless uninvolved arch is hypoplastic. Diagnosis is important because surgical division of uninvolved arch may result in clinical coarctation.

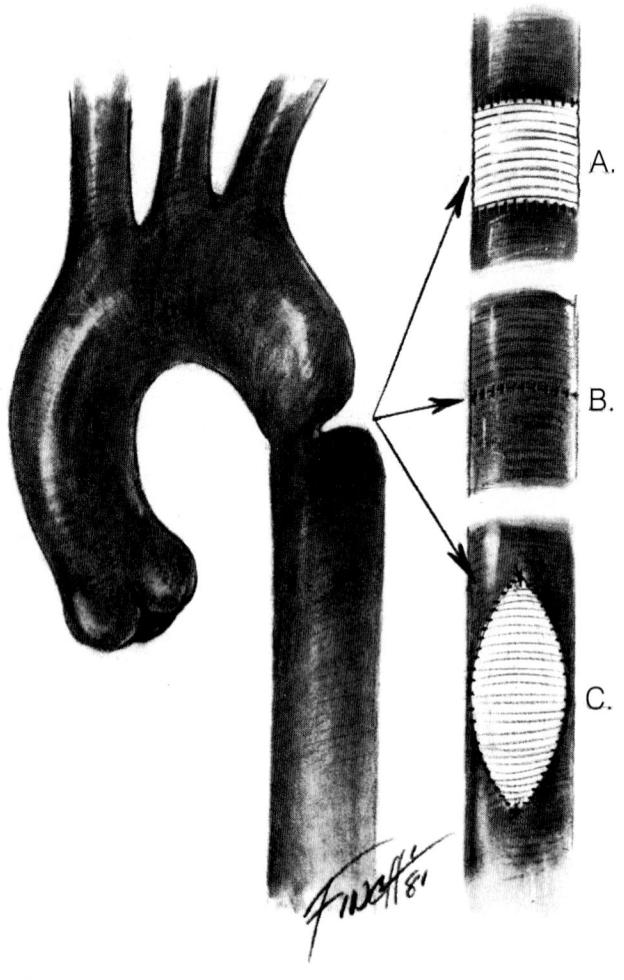

FIG 28–28.
Diagram of three types of operation for isolated coarctation of aorta. **A,** interposition of graft. **B,** end-to-end anastomosis. **C,** patch on-lay graft.

lower portion of the body. Most infants fail to respond fully to digitalization and require operation.

Four operative approaches have been used:

1. Resection of coarctation of the aorta and interposition of a tubular graft (Fig 28–28,*A*).

2. Resection of coarctation and end-to-end anastomosis (Fig 28–28,*B*); this was the initial form of treatment for coarctation of the aorta, but the anastomotic site may fail to grow.

3. Patch graft aortoplasty[23, 24] (Fig 28–28,*C*); this technique avoids circumferential anastomosis and preserves a portion of the aorta for growth. Little aortic mobilization is required, and it can be adapted to long areas of coarctation. Aneurysm of the patch may develop.

4. Subclavian flap technique (Fig 28–29). This has the advantages of not requiring a circumferential incision and of using living tissue to relieve the obstruction (an example of a postoperative aortogram is shown in Fig 28–32).

Recently, nonsurgical treatment by balloon dilatation of the coarctation has been attempted during cardiac catheterization. A balloon catheter is inflated to 10 to 15 atmospheres of pressure and the intima and media are ruptured at the level of the coarctation. The adventitia remains intact. At present, the clinical value of this nonsurgical technique is being evaluated (Fig 29–30). It is an attractive approach in recoarctation, where reoperation is technically difficult and carries a considerable risk.

The risk of operation in neonates is high, especially in those with coexisting conditions.[25–27] At the time of operation, banding of the pulmonary artery may be performed in infants with coexisting ventricular septal defect.

Asymptomatic Child

In older children, the usual approach is resection of the coarctation and end-to-end anastomosis. The operative risk is very low.

Operation is performed at age 2 years if marked hypertension is present or before school age in asymptomatic children.

COMPLICATIONS

There are a number of complications of coarctation of the aorta, including some serious postoperative problems. The full significance of the complications will be established only by longer clinical studies.

Postoperative Systemic Hypertension

In the immediate postoperative period, the blood pressure paradoxically increases. In the first 12 postoperative hours, the increase is related principally to sympathetic discharge,[28–30] because circulating catecholamine concentrations are markedly increased. Another explanation is overreaction of baroreceptors, which are suddenly submitted to elevated pressure in the descending aorta.

Postoperative hypertension may persist for several months.[31] Studies of exercise in postoperative patients have demonstrated an abnormal rise in blood pressure postoperatively,[32, 33] even in patients without residual coarctation.[34] The incidence of hypertension is greater in patients operated on when they are older.[35]

Mesenteric Arteritis

Mesenteric arteritis is an uncommon complication that characteristically develops on the third postoperative day.[36] The features are hypertension, abdominal pain and

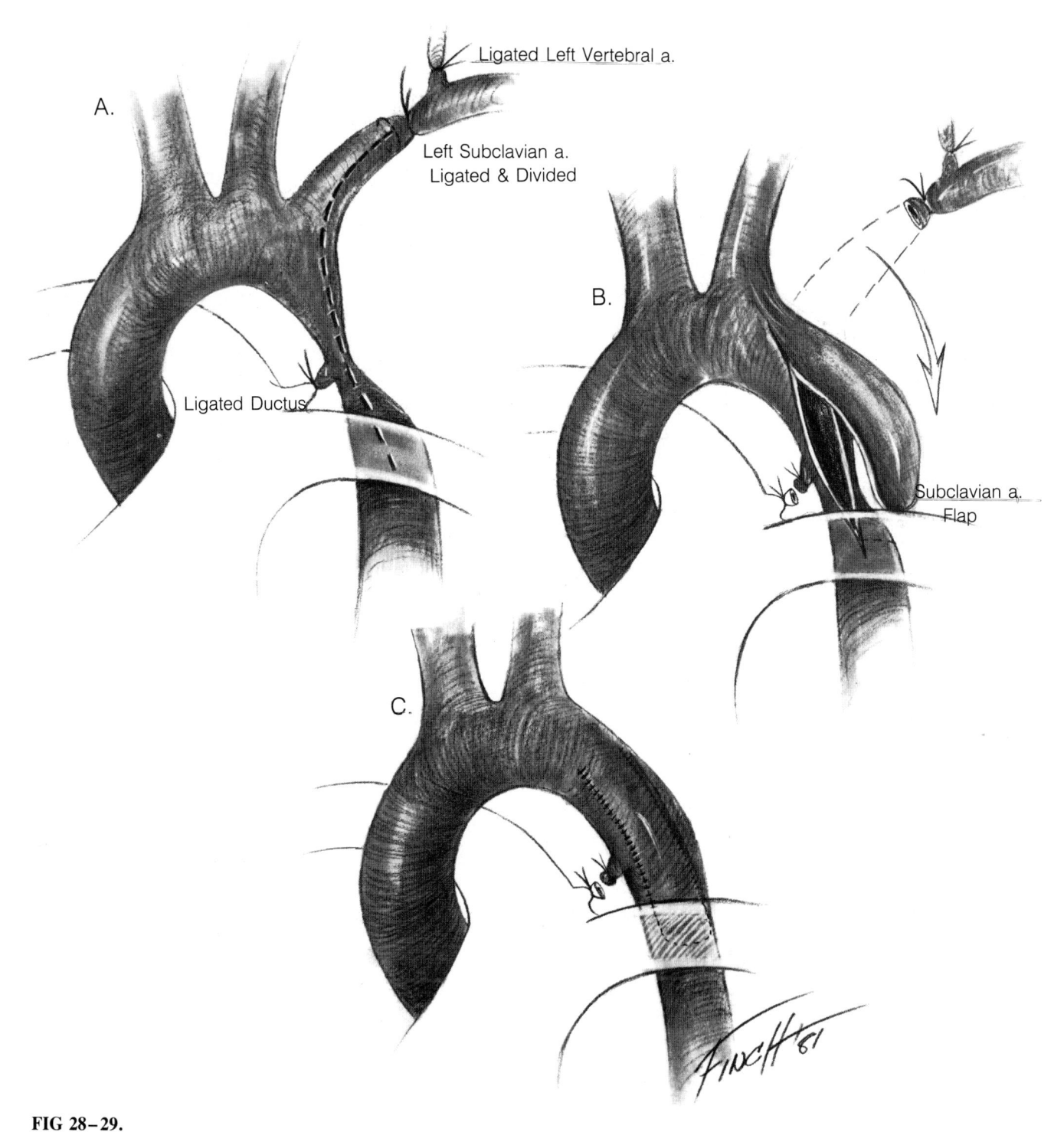

FIG 28–29.
Diagrams of repair of coarctation of aorta by subclavian flap technique. **A,** ductus and left subclavian artery ligated. Incision made along left subclavian artery across aortic isthmus into descending aorta. **B,** incised left subclavian artery opened and turned down as flap. **C,** flap of left subclavian artery sewn over opened isthmus and descending aorta.

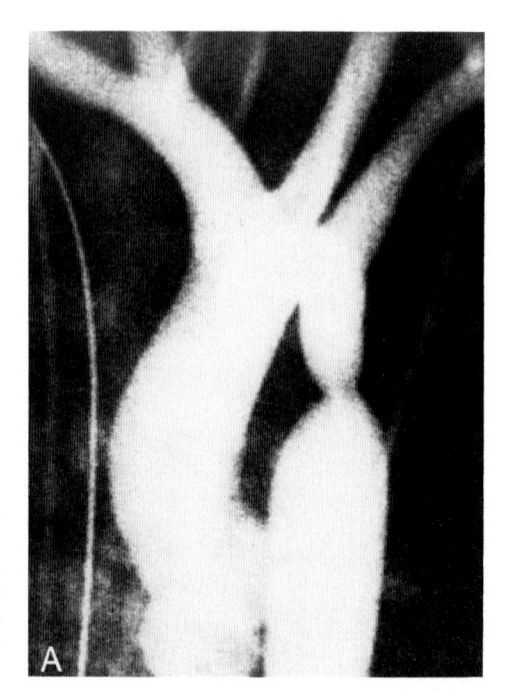

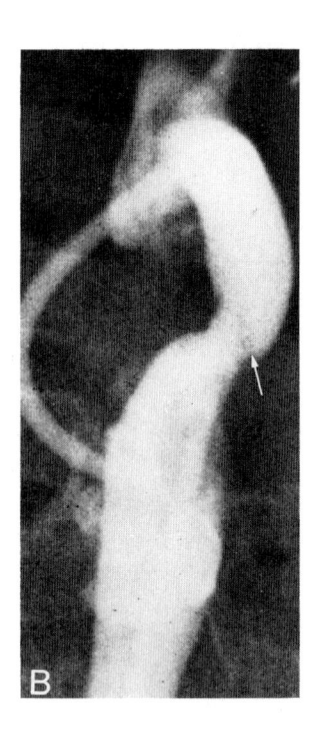

FIG 28–30.
A, severe coarctation of aorta (50 mm Hg gradient). Aortogram, anteroposterior projection. **B,** coarctation of aorta after balloon dilatation. Reduced narrowing; pressure gradient diminished to 5 mm Hg. Ruptured intima and media are seen as faint radiolucencies *(arrow)*.

tenderness, ileus, vomiting, abdominal bleeding, fever, and leukocytosis. Mesenteric arteritis can progress to intestinal necrosis and death.

Two theories have been proposed: (1) the effect of a sudden increase of blood pressure on the mesenteric arteries and (2) the effect of renin and angiotensin on the mesenteric arteries. Renin levels reach a maximum 2 to 5 days postoperatively and may constrict the mesenteric arteries.

Recoarctation of the Aorta

Recoarctation of the aorta has been attributed to failure of growth at the anastomotic site, fibrosis and scarring at the anastomotic site, and technically inadequate anastomosis. The exact incidence of this complication is unknown; the reported figures range from 6% to 48%. At our institution, it was 8.5% in all patients operated on,[37] but the complication is much more common in patients operated on in infancy.[38] If significant obstruction develops, reoperation may be required.

Spinal Cord Complications

This uncommon (0.5%) complication has been the subject of an excellent review.[39] Although spinal cord complications are more common in surgically treated patients, they may occur spontaneously. Aneurysms of the anterior spinal artery develop by collateral flow and may compress the spinal cord. In addition, because the blood flow to the spinal cord is segmental and the smallest numbers of segmental arteries occur in the thoracic area, this portion of the spinal cord is vulnerable during operation. Paralysis of the lower trunk and legs can develop after repair of coarctation; the extent and severity vary.

Vascular Complications

Premature myocardial infarction from coronary artery disease has been described,[40, 41] but these were usually patients who were older at the time of operation. Whether this will also be true of those operated on in infancy or childhood is unknown.

Cerebrovascular Complications

Cerebrovascular problems have also been reported, 42, 43 perhaps related to cerebrovascular disease. Other central nervous system vascular complications include ruptured berry aneurysm, a rare complication.

Aortic Dissection

Aneurysms may form by incomplete dissection or by true dissection.[3] It occurs secondary to hypertension and to cystic medial necrosis, which is more common in coarctation.

Bacterial Endocarditis

Bacterial endocarditis may occur on a coexisting bicuspid aortic valve or other cardiac anomaly at the jet lesion. It may also develop at the site of the coarctation repair.

POSTOPERATIVE RADIOGRAPHIC APPEARANCE

1. In infancy, cardiac enlargement, pulmonary congestion, and left atrial enlargement disappear.
2. Radiographic examinations several years later still show radiologic signs of coarctation from incomplete repair, lack of growth of the repair site, or recoarctation.
3. Coarctation may be hemodynamically and radiologically masked by the presence of a patent ductus (Fig 28–31,A). After ligation of the ductus, a pressure gradient may appear and the coarctation may be radiologically evident (Fig 28–31,B and C).
4. With the newer subclavian flap technique, recoarctation has been uncommon (see Fig 28–39), but the period of observation is too short to draw definite conclusions.

PSEUDOCOARCTATION (BUCKLING OR KINKING OF THE AORTA)

Pseudocoarctation is a distinct anatomic entity resulting from elongation of the aorta for unknown reasons. Be-

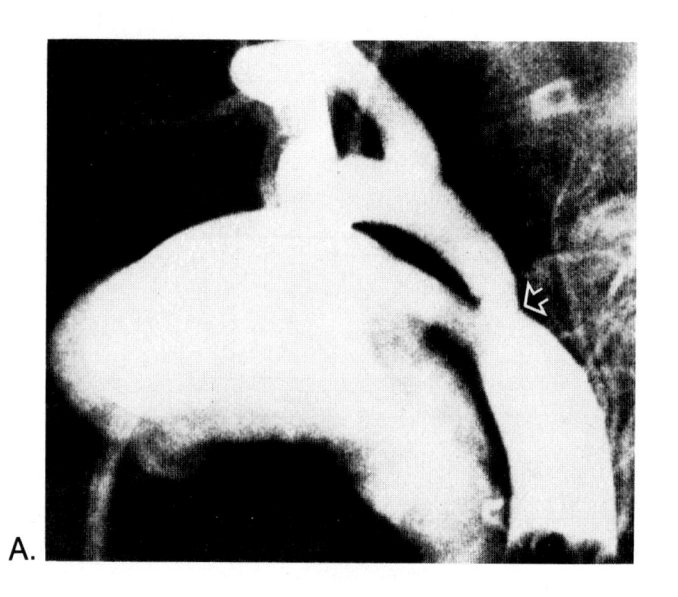

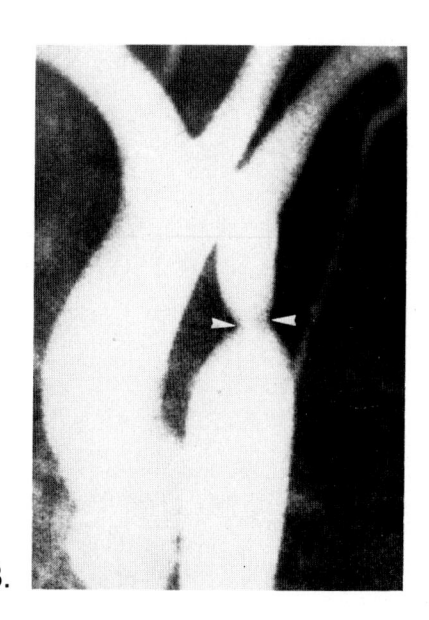

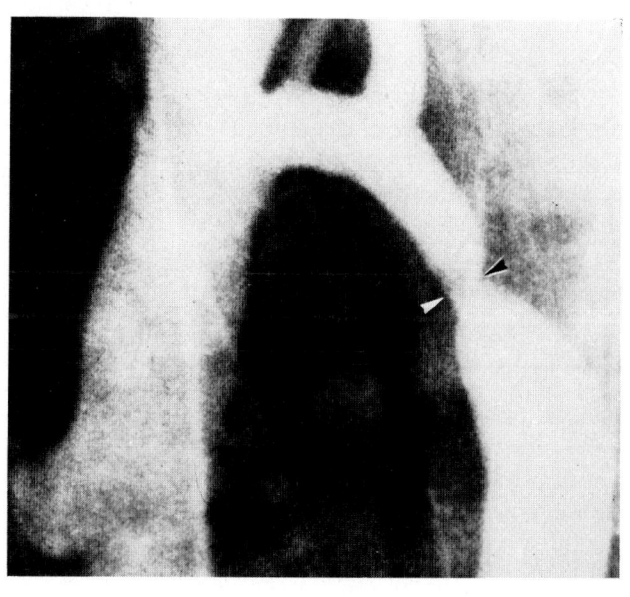

FIG 28–31.
A, balloon occlusion aortogram, lateral projection. Patent ductus *(white arrows);* coarctation and notch deformity along greater curvature of aorta in patient with no clinical signs of coarctation and mild tubal hypoplasia. Ductus was ligated; aortogram was done 1 year later. **B,** anteroposterior and, **C,** lateral protections. Coarctation became clinically and radiographically evident. Notch along greater curvature of aorta should have indicated coarctation.

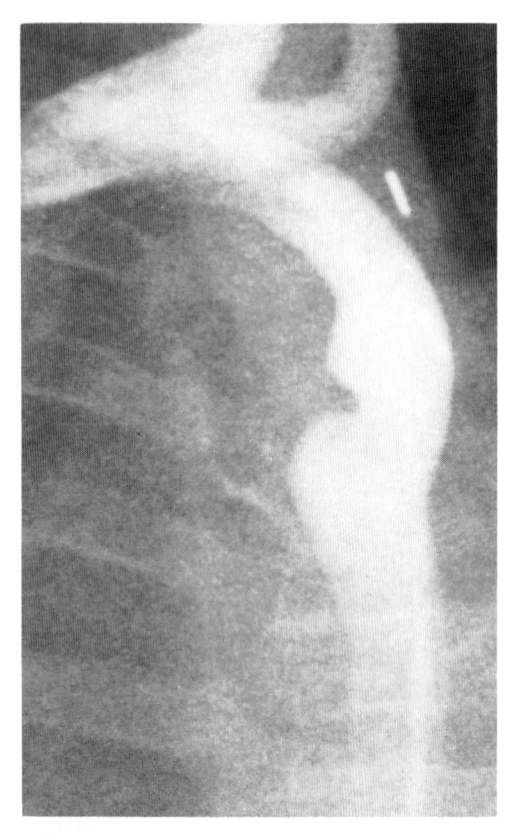

FIG 28–32.
Aortogram, anteroposterior projection of coarctation of aorta after repair by subclavian flap technique. Bulge on lesser curvature caused by entrance of previously large patent ductus arteriosus. Appearance should not be confused with incomplete repair, because greater curvature of aorta is normal. A characteristic finding for repair of coarctation by subclavian flap technique. Only innominate and left carotid arteries are opacified because left subclavian artery was used for repair.

FIG 28–33.
Diagram of pseudocoarctation of aorta. Elongation of aortic arch, with buckling proximal descending aorta. *LCA* = left carotid artery; *LPA* = left pulmonary artery; *LSA* = left subclavian artery; *PA* = pulmonary artery; *RCA* = right coronary artery; *RSA* = right subclavian artery.

cause the descending aorta is fixed by both the intercostal arteries and the ductus arteriosus, the aortic arch rises higher into the mediastinum and buckles at the level of the insertion of the ductus arteriosus (Figs 28–32 and 28–33). The angiographic appearance resembles that of coarctation of the aorta, so the term pseudocoarctation has been used. Kinking or buckling of the aorta are preferable and more descriptive terms. Although no pressure gradient exists, flow through the kinked area is turbulent, and an aneurysm of the proximal descending aorta may develop and require resection.

Pseudocoarctation of the aorta has been confused with true coarctation without a pressure gradient and with cervical aortic arch. Pseudocoarctation may be clinically differentiated from true coarctation of the aorta by the absence of systemic hypertension, collateral circulation, delayed femoral pulses, or a significant hemodynamic gradient across the kinked segment.[44–46]

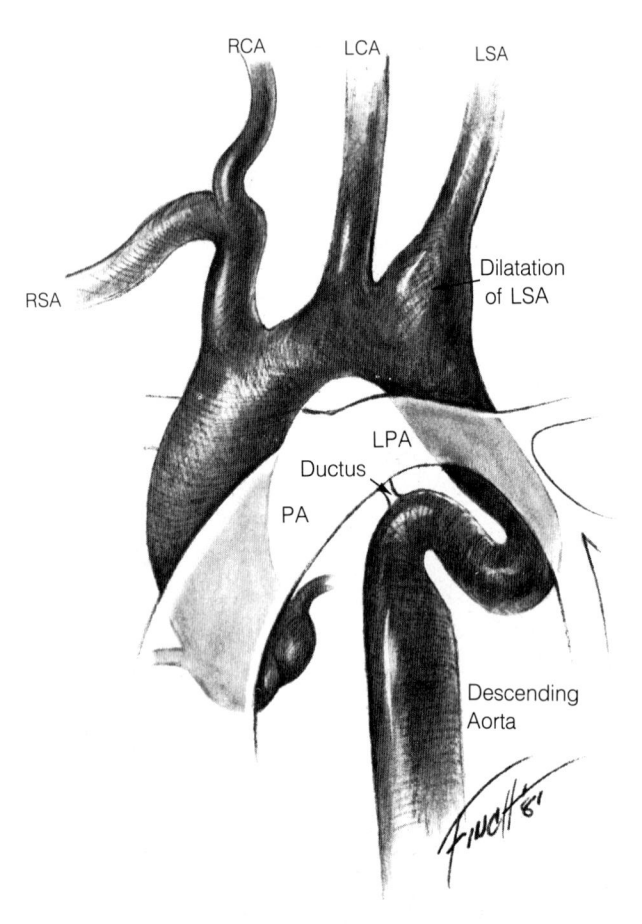

Radiographic Features

The thoracic roentgenographic findings of pseudocoarctation are identical to those of true coarctation and may be similar to cervical arch. The diagnosis can be established only by aortography.

Angiographic Appearance

Aortography is of particular importance to distinguish pseudocoarctation from true coarctation of the aorta or from cervical aortic arch. The angiographic findings are characteristic and show an elongated aorta that buckles at the insertion of the ductus ligament (Fig 28–34). The descending aorta below the ductus is dilated because of turbulent flow. In contrast to true coarctation, the characteristic butter knife deformity is absent. Pseudocoarctation can be differentiated from cervical arch, because the latter shows an increased number of arteries to the head, a ret-

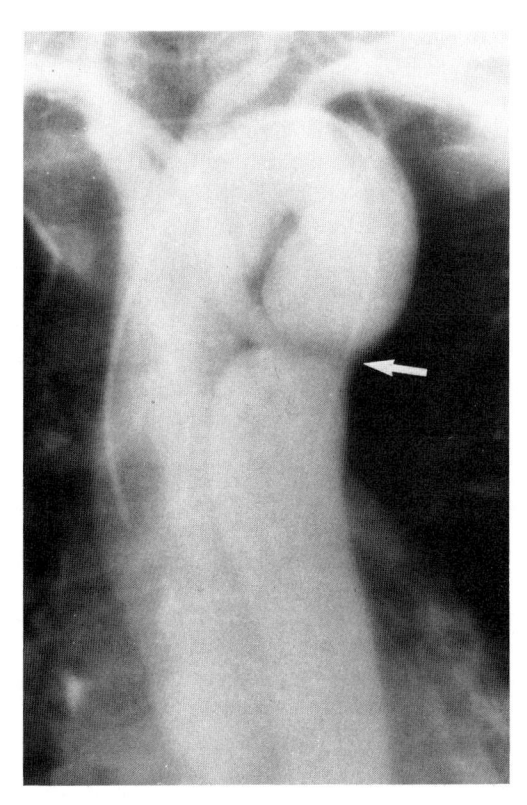

FIG 28-34.
Aortogram in pseudocoarctation of aorta. Elongation of aortic arch above ligamentum arteriosum; aberrant right subclavian artery. No pressure gradient.

roesophageal segment, and a descending aorta located on the side opposite the aortic arch. Pseudocoarctation also must not be confused with coarctation of the aorta without pressure gradient, which shows a butter knife deformity, no buckling, and no pressure gradient.

COARCTATION OF THE ABDOMINAL AORTA

This rare cause of left ventricular outflow tract obstruction produces its effects by causing systemic hypertension rather than by obstructing the abdominal aorta. Although called coarctation, it probably results from an arteritis.

Anatomy

There is either localized or diffuse narrowing of the abdominal aorta at or above the origin of the renal arteries.[47] Often the origins of the renal, superior mesenteric, or hepatic arteries are narrowed. Microscopic examination shows fibromuscular dysplasia, intimal proliferation, and nonspecific inflammation. Collateral circulation may develop between other visceral, thoracic, or abdominal wall arteries that arise proximal to the abdominal coarctation and the major visceral arteries originating from the coarcted site.

Bilateral renal arterial narrowing is usually present.
Bicuspid aortic valve is rare.

Hemodynamics

The degree of aortic narrowing is usually mild and causes little pressure gradient. The renal arterial narrowing reduces renal blood flow and causes systemic hypertension.

Clinical Features

Recognition of abdominal coarctation is important to prevent unnecessary thoracotomy. In contrast to coarctation of the thoracic aorta, abdominal coarctation occurs twice as commonly in females as in males.

Symptoms are usually mild in childhood. They may include headache, congestive cardiac failure (occasionally), and cerebrovascular accident.

The disease is usually recognized by the discovery of hypertension in a symptomatic or asymptomatic patient. A pressure difference may be found between the arms and legs, just as in classical coarctation.

There may be soft precordial ejection murmurs, but definite systolic murmurs are heard over the abdomen and lumbar areas. The aortic component of the second heart sound is accentuated (hypertension).

Electrocardiographic Features

The ECG is indistinguishable from that in thoracic coarctation of the aorta and shows left ventricular hypertrophy and, at times, a strain pattern.

Radiographic Features

Cardiac size and the pulmonary vasculature are normal. The cardiac contour may show left ventricular hypertrophy from chronic hypertension. There are no radiologic signs of classical coarctation.

Rib notching occurs, but, unlike in thoracic coarctation, it develops below the seventh rib (Fig 28–11C).
REASON: Collateral flow occurs primarily through the shortest pathways, which are the lower intercostal arteries in abdominal coarctation.

Angiographic Appearance

Angiographically, the narrowing differs from classic localized coarctation. Diffuse tapering of the abdominal

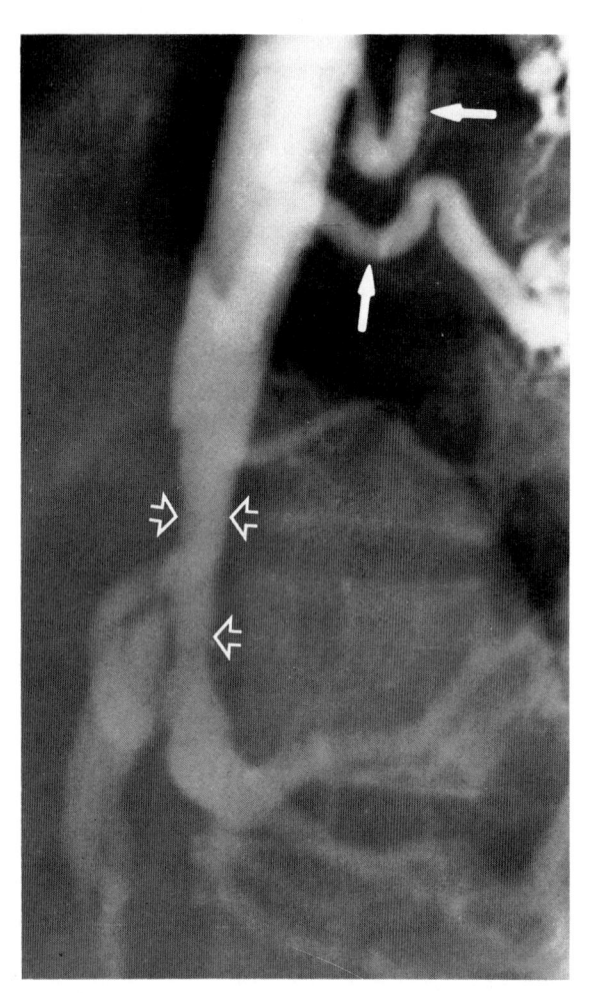

FIG 28–35.
Abdominal aortogram, lateral projection in coarctation of abdominal aorta. Markedly enlarged lower intercostal arteries *(arrows)*, diffuse narrowing of upper abdominal aorta *(open arrows),* and narrowing of celiac axis and superior mesenteric artery.

aorta involves the origins of the celiac axis and the superior mesenteric and renal arteries (Fig 28–35). Anteroposterior and lateral abdominal aortograms should be obtained.

Treatment

If the coarctation is localized, simple resection is carried out, but, unfortunately, such cases are rare. A variety of operations have been used—grafts, patch grafts, and bypass grafts. When the renal arteries are involved, bypass patch repair of renal arteries, autotransplantation, or nephrectomy have been performed.

Systemic hypertension may persist postoperatively, requiring evaluation of the renal arteries and the status of the renal parenchyma.

OTHER DISEASES OF THE AORTA

Other, more unusual, sites of narrowing have been described in the low thoracic aorta at the level of the diaphragm (hypoplasia of the thoracic aorta) and in the brachiocephalic arteries (Takayasu's disease or pulseless disease). The diffuse nature of the process and the association with aneurysms strongly suggest an acquired inflammatory process rather than a congenital disease. Therefore, these entities are not discussed in detail. Also, the diffuse nature of the narrowing and the histologic findings suggest arteritis rather than congenital disease, so this type of narrowing should not be classified as coarctation.

REFERENCES

1. Shinebourne EA, Tam ASY, Elseed TAM, et al: Coarctation of the aorta in infancy and childhood, *Br Heart J* 38:375, 1976.
2. Nora JJ, Torres FG, Sinha AK, et al: Characteristic cardiovascular anomalies of XO Turner's syndrome, XX and XY phenotype, and XO/XX Turner mosaic, *Am J Cardiol* 25:639, 1970.
3. Edwards JE, Carey LS, Neufeld HN, et al: *Congenital heart disease: correlation of pathologic anatomy and angiocardiography,* Philadelphia, 1965, Saunders, pp 677–698.
4. Rudolph AM, Heymann MA, Spitznas U: Hemodynamic considerations in the development of narrowing of the aorta, *Am J Cardiol* 30:514, 1972.
5. Becker AE, Becker MJ, Edwards JE: Anomalies associated with coarctation of aorta: particular reference to infancy, *Circulation* 41:1067, 1970.
6. Talner NS, Berman MA: Postnatal development of obstruction in coarctation of the aorta: role of the ductus arteriosus, *Pediatrics* 56:562, 1975.
7. Shone JD, Sellers RD, Anderson RC, et al: The developmental complex of "parachute mitral valve," supravalvular ring of left atrium, subaortic stenosis, and coarctation of aorta, *Am J Cardiol* 11:714, 1963.
8. Wood WC, Wood JC, Lower RR, et al: Associated coarctation of the aorta and mitral valve disease: nine cases with surgical correction of both lesions in three, *J Pediatr* 87:217, 1975.
9. Rosenquist GC: Congenital mitral valve disease associated with coarctation of the aorta: a spectrum that includes parachute deformity of the mitral valve, *Circulation* 49:985, 1974.
10. Moller JH, Lucas RV Jr, Adams P Jr, et al: Endocardial fibroelastosis: a clinical and anatomic study of 47 patients with emphasis on its relationship to mitral insufficiency, *Circulation* 30:759, 1964.
11. Arosemena E, Moller JH, Edwards JE: Scarring of the papillary muscles in left ventricular hypertrophy, *Am Heart J* 74:446, 1967.
12. Freed ME, Keane JF, VanPraagh R, et al: Coarctation of

the aorta with congenital mitral regurgitation, *Circulation* 49:1175, 1974.
13. Auger P, Wigle ED: Coarctation of the aorta associated with severe mitral insufficiency, *Am J Cardiol* 21:190, 1968.
14. Vlodaver Z, Neufeld HN: The coronary arteries in coarctation of the aorta, *Circulation* 37:449, 1968.
15. Edwards JE: Aneurysms of the thoracic aorta complicating coarctation, *Circulation* 48:195, 1973.
16. Strong WB, Botti RE, Silbert DR, et al: Peripheral and renal vein plasma renin activity in coarctation of the aorta, *Pediatrics* 45:254, 1970.
17. Amsterdam EA, Alberts WH, Christlieb AR, et al: Plasma renin activity in children with coarctation of the aorta, *Am J Cardiol* 23:396, 1969.
18. Alpert BS, Bain HH, Balfe JW, et al: Role of the renin-angiotension-aldosterone system in hypertensive children with coarctation of the aorta, *Am J Cardiol* 43:828, 1979.
19. Sahn DJ, Allen HD, McDonald G, et al: Realtime cross-sectional echocardiographic diagnosis of coarctation of the aorta: a prospective study of echocardiographic-angiographic correlations, *Circulation* 56:762, 1977.
20. Weyman AE, Caldwell RL, Hurwitz RA, et al: Cross-sectional echocardiographic detection of aortic obstruction: coarctation of the aorta, *Circulation* 57:498, 1978.
21. Scovil JA, Nanda NC, Gross CM, et al: Echocardiographic studies of abnormalities associated with coarctation of the aorta, *Circulation* 53:953, 1976.
22. Wing JP, Findlay WA, Sahn DJ, et al: Serial echocardiographic profiles in infants and children with coarctation of the aorta, *Am J Cardiol* 41:1270, 1978.
23. Fleming WH, Sarafian LB, Clark EB, et al: Critical aortic coarctation: patch aortoplasty in infants less than age 3 months, *Am J Cardiol* 44:687, 1979.
24. Reul GJ Jr, Kabbani SS, Sandiford FM, et al: Repair of coarctation of the thoracic aorta by patch graft aortoplasty, *J Thorac Cardiovasc Surg* 68:696, 1974.
25. Williams WG, Shindo G, Trusler GA, et al: Results of repair of coarctation of the aorta during infancy, *J Thorac Cardiovasc Surg* 79:603, 1980.
26. Connors JP, Hartmann AF Jr, Weldon CS: Considerations in the surgical management of infantile coarctation of aorta, *Am J Cardiol* 36:489, 1975.
27. Tawes RL Jr, Aberdeen E, Waterston DJ, et al: Coarctation of the aorta in infants and children: a review of 333 operative cases, including 179 infants, *Circulation* 49, 59(suppl I):173, 1969.
28. Benedict CR, Grahame-Smith DG, Fisher A: Changes in plasma catecholamines and dopamine beta-hydroxylase after corrective surgery for coarctation of the aorta, *Circulation* 57:598, 1978.
29. Rocchini AP, Rosenthal A, Barger AC, et al: Pathogenesis of paradoxical hypertension after coarctation resection, *Circulation*. 54:382, 1976.
30. Goodall M, Sealy WC: Increased sympathetic nerve activity following resection of coarctation of the thoracic aorta, *Circulation* 39:345, 1969.
31. March HW, Hultgren HN, Gerbode F: Immediate and remote effects of resection on the hypertension in coarctation of the aorta, *Br Heart J* 22:361, 1960.
32. Freed MD, Rocchini A, Rosenthal A, et al: Exercise-induced hypertension after surgical repair of coarctation of the aorta, *Am J Cardiol* 43:253, 1979.
33. James FW, Kaplan S: Systolic hypertension during submaximal exercise after correction of coarctation of aorta, *Circulation* 49, 50(suppl II):27, 1974.
34. Connor TM: Evaluation of persistent coarctation of aorta after surgery with blood pressure measurement and exercise testing, *Am J Cardiol* 43:74, 1979.
35. Pennington DG, Liberthson RR, Jacobs M, et al: Critical review of experience with surgical repair of coarctation of the aorta, *J Thorac Cardiovasc Surg* 77:217, 1979.
36. Ho ECK, Moss AJ: The syndrome of "mesenteric arteritis" following surgical repair of aortic coarctation: report of nine cases and review of the literature, *Pediatrics* 49:40, 1972.
37. Ibarra-Perez C, Castaneda AR, Varco RL, et al: Recoarctation of the aorta: nineteen year clinical experience, *Am J Cardiol* 23:778, 1969.
38. Hartmann AF Jr, Goldring D, Hernandez A, et al: Recurrent coarctation of the aorta after successful repair in infancy, *Am J Cardiol* 25:405, 1970.
39. Brewer LA III, Fosburg RG, Mulder GA, et al: Spinal cord complications following surgery for coarctation of the aorta: a study of 66 cases, *J Thorac Cardiovasc Surg* 64:368, 1972.
40. Cokkinos DV, Leachman RD, Cooley DA: Increased mortality rate from coronary artery disease following operation for coarctation of the aorta at a late age, *J Thorac Cardiovasc Surg* 77:315, 1979.
41. Maron BJ, Humphries JO, Rowe RD, et al: Prognosis of surgically corrected coarctation of the aorta: a 20-year postoperative appraisal, *circulation* 47:119, 1973.
42. Simon AB, Zloto AE: Coarctation of the aorta: longitudinal assessment of operated patients, *Circulation* 50:456, 1974.
43. Saalouke MG, Perry LW, Breckbill DL, et al: Cerebrovascular abnormalities in postoperative coarctation of aorta: four cases demonstrating left subclavian steal on aortography, *Am J Cardiol* 42:97, 1978.
44. Smyth PT, Edwards JE: Pseudocoarctation, kinking or buckling of the aorta, *Circulation* 46:1027, 1972.
45. Acevedo RE, Thilenius OG, Moulder PV, et al: Kinking of the aorta (pseudocoarctation) with coarctation, *Am J Cardiol* 21:442, 1968.
46. Gay WA Jr, Young WG Jr: Pseudocoarctation of the aorta—a reappraisal, *circulation* 37, 38(suppl VI):80, 1968.
47. Riemenschneider TA, Emmanouilides GC, Hirose F, et al: Coarctation of the abdominal aorta in children: report of three cases and review of the literature, *Pediatrics* 44:716, 1969.

CHAPTER 29

Pulmonary Stenosis

In patients with an intact ventricular septum, right-sided outflow obstruction can occur within the right ventricle, at the pulmonary valve, within the pulmonary arteries, and at the level of the pulmonary capillaries. By far the most common site is the pulmonary valve, the result from valvar stenosis. Less common forms of right ventricular obstruction are peripheral pulmonary arterial stenosis and infundibular pulmonary stenosis. The cardiac conditions associated with high pulmonary capillary resistance are discussed subsequently. Right ventricular outflow obstruction with an intact ventricular septum accounts for approximately 6% of congenital heart disease.

VALVAR PULMONARY STENOSIS[1, 2]

Pulmonary valvar stenosis can be caused by a dome-shaped, bicupsid, or dysplastic pulmonary valve. Regardless of its anatomic form, valvar pulmonary stenosis leads to certain anatomic and physiologic consequences. These can be seen from the formula:

$$PVA \cong \frac{CO}{\sqrt{K\ RVSP - PA}}$$

where PVA = pulmonary valve area,
CO = cardiac output,
K = constant,
$RSVP$ = right ventricular systolic pressure, and
PA = pulmonary arterial systolic pressure.

That is, as the size of the orifice of the stenotic pulmonary valve is reduced, the right ventricular systolic pressure increases to deliver the cardiac output.

Because of the increased right ventricular systolic pressure, right ventricular hypertrophy develops. The right ventricle becomes more trabeculated, and frequently the apical portion of the cavity is obliterated by hypertrophied muscle. Right ventricular subendocardial myocardial ischemia probably occurs, leading to right ventricular myocardial fibrosis, which is associated with right ventricular dilatation and, subsequently, with congestive cardiac failure.

The right atrial pressure may be elevated because of reduced right ventricular compliance from either right ventricular hypertrophy or fibrosis.

The elevated right atrial pressure may stretch the foramen ovale, permitting a right-to-left atrial shunt and cyanosis. Pulmonary stenosis with a right-to-left shunt at the atrial level and right ventricular hypertrophy has been known as "trilogy of Fallot." This is a cyanotic condition and is discussed subsequently.

Dome-Shaped Pulmonary Stenosis

In the normal pulmonary valve, there are three distinct cusps. Consequently, during systole, the pulmonary leaflets move freely, allowing unrestricted flow of blood without a pressure gradient (Fig 29–1). In pulmonary stenosis, movement of the valve cusps is limited, and flow through the valve is restricted, resulting in an outflow gradient.

In the most common anatomic form of pulmonary stenosis, three cusps are present but the commissures are fused, so that the valve has a small central orifice (Fig 29–2). The size of the orifice differs among cases, and its location often is slightly eccentric. During systole, the valve domes, and during diastole, three sinuses of Valsalva are formed, as in a normal valve (Fig 29–3). The stenotic pulmonary valve usually is thin, but sometimes it is thickened. Very rarely, it is calcified.

Clinical Features

Although a murmur is usually heard at birth or in the neonatal period, most patients are asymptomatic throughout childhood. If the right ventricle decompensates, congestive cardiac failure and cyanosis develop in infancy or, rarely, during childhood. Easy fatigability may be a symptom in patients with severe pulmonary stenosis.

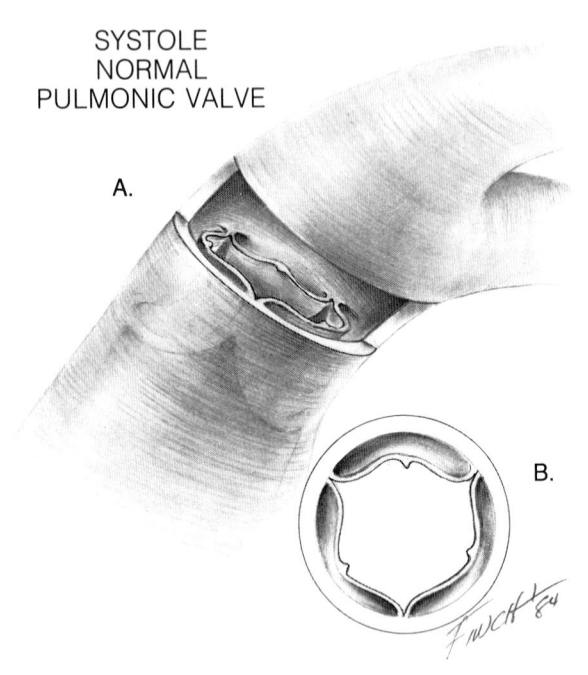

FIG 29-1.
Diagram of normal pulmonary valve during systole in lateral (**A**) and superior views (**B**). Blood flow is unrestricted from right ventricle because each of the three valve leaflets moves toward sinuses of Valsalva but does not touch wall of pulmonary artery.

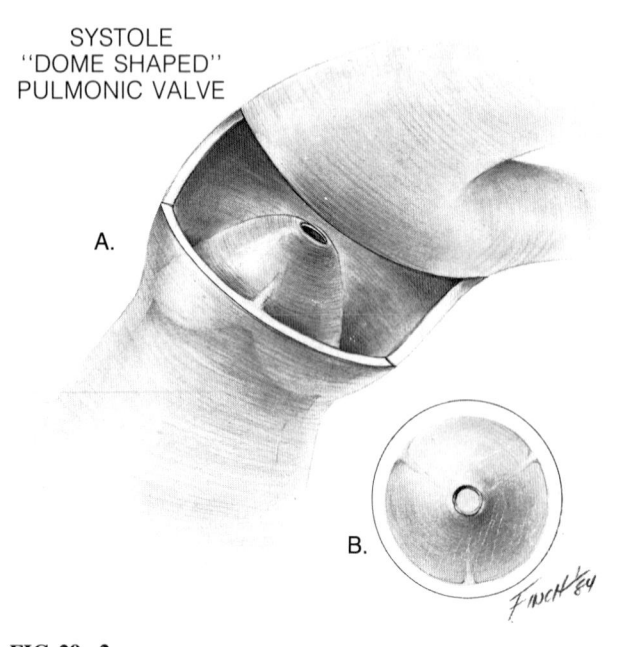

FIG 29-2.
Diagram of typical pulmonary valvar stenosis during systole in lateral (**A**) and superior (**B**) views. Small central orifice and doming of fused valve cusps.

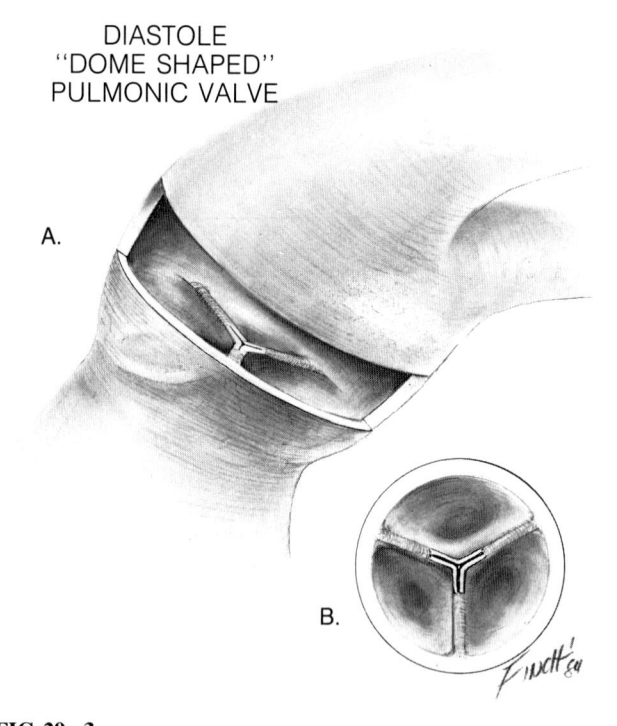

FIG 29-3.
Diagram of typical pulmonary valvar stenosis during diastole in lateral (**A**) and superior (**B**) views. Normal position of valve leaflets despite commissural fusion. Three normal-appearing sinuses of Valsalva are formed.

Physical Examination

Most patients show normal growth and development. There may be a right ventricular heave. Except in patients with mild stenosis, there is a thrill along the upper left sternal border and often in the suprasternal notch as well. There is a loud (grade 3–4/6) systolic ejection murmur beneath the left clavicle that radiates well to the left upper part of the back.[3, 4] The murmur usually begins with a pulmonary systolic ejection click, which occurs from the poststenotic dilatation of the pulmonary trunk. In severe stenosis, the pulmonary component of the second heart sound may be soft and delayed. In severe stenosis, a systolic murmur of coexisting tricuspid regurgitation may be heard.

Electrocardiographic Features

The electrocardiogram (ECG) roughly correlates with the severity of the stenosis. With increasing obstruction, a greater degree of right-axis deviation and right ventricular hypertrophy (manifested by a tall R wave in lead V_1) are found. The ECG is normal in mild stenosis, and although we have seen a normal tracing in a patient with a right ventricular systolic pressure of 100 mm Hg, most patients with moderate stenosis show an abnormal pattern. If the R wave in lead V_1 exceeds 30 mm, the stenosis is severe.

Right atrial enlargement is present in many patients

with severe stenosis because of decreased right ventricular compliance.

Abnormal T waves, in the form of deep inversion in the right precordial leads and inversion through the left precordial leads, indicate severe stenosis, and this pattern has been called "right ventricular strain." We believe this ECG change has serious import and should prompt cardiac catheterization and early operation.

Echocardiographic Features

The echocardiogram shows increased thickness of the right ventricular anterior wall, although this may be difficult to assess quantitatively because it is often impossible to distinguish the echoes from the chest wall from those of the right ventricular anterior wall. The right ventricular internal diameter may be increased with moderate or severe stenosis.

The normal pulmonary valve makes a small posterior movement, the *a* dip, with atrial systole.[5] The *a* dip is accentuated in patients with moderate or severe stenosis. This finding occurs in any patients with a low diastolic pulmonary arterial pressure and elevated right ventricular end-diastolic pressure. Thus, with atrial systole, the right ventricular end-diastolic pressure may exceed the pulmonary arterial pressure, causing this movement.

Radiographic Features

1. The cardiac silhouette is usually not enlarged (Fig 29–4,*A*). REASON: The hemodynamic consequence of valvar pulmonary stenosis is right ventricular hypertrophy, which does not increase overall cardiac size on posteroanterior roentgenograms.

2. The pulmonary vasculature is normal in most cases. REASON: Patients with pulmonary stenosis have a normal cardiac output, and consequently normal pulmonary flow, if no right-to-left shunt is present.

3. Patients with critical pulmonary stenosis have a tendency toward decreased pulmonary vasculature. REASON: Although cardiac output may be normal or low normal at rest, it is usually decreased during exercise because of the severe pulmonary obstruction.

4. Right ventricular hypertrophy may be evidenced on the lateral view, and the right atrium and left pulmonary artery may be prominent on left anterior oblique projection (Fig 29–4,*B*).

5. The heart is in a more vertical position, and the well-rounded left lower cardiac margin simulates left ventricular hypertrophy. REASON: Pulmonary stenosis causes hypertrophy and elongation of the right ventricle. Because that chamber rests on the diaphragm, it can elongate only in a cranial direction, resulting in a more vertical position of the heart. Because the heart is fixed by the superior and inferior venae cavae and the right ventricle is only hypertrophied and not grossly enlarged, counterclockwise rotation occurs (Fig 29–5). The counterclockwise rotation brings the more rounded posterior aspect of the left ventricle (obtuse margin) in profile along the left cardiac border of a posteroanterior projection, thus simulating left ventricular hypertrophy (Fig 29–6).

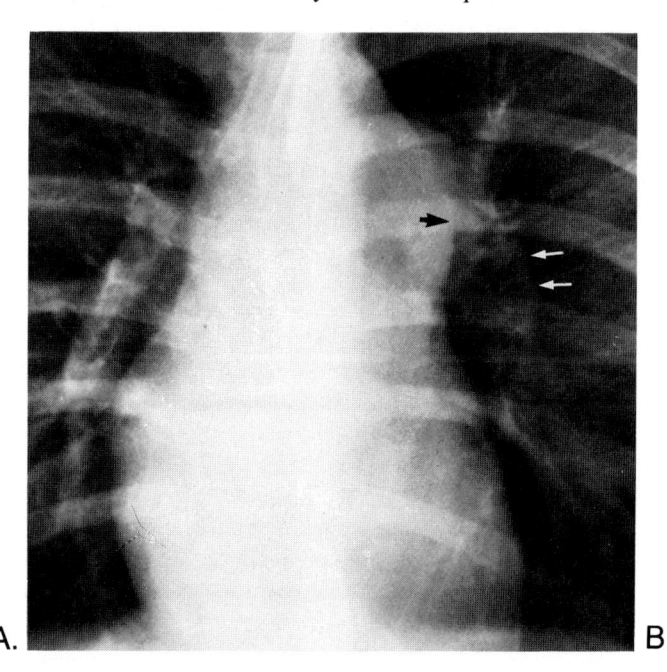

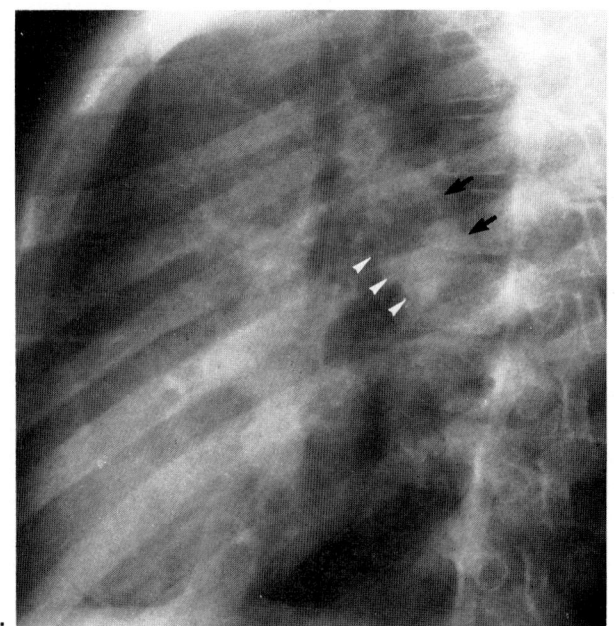

FIG 29–4.
Thoracic roentgenogram in valvar pulmonary stenosis. **A,** posteroanterior projection. Slight prominence of right atrium; marked prominence of main pulmonary artery segment *(black arrow)*. Poststenotic dilatation of left pulmonary artery *(white arrows)*. **B,** left anterior oblique projection. Poststenotic dilatation of left pulmonary artery *(arrows)* as it crosses over left mainstem bronchus.

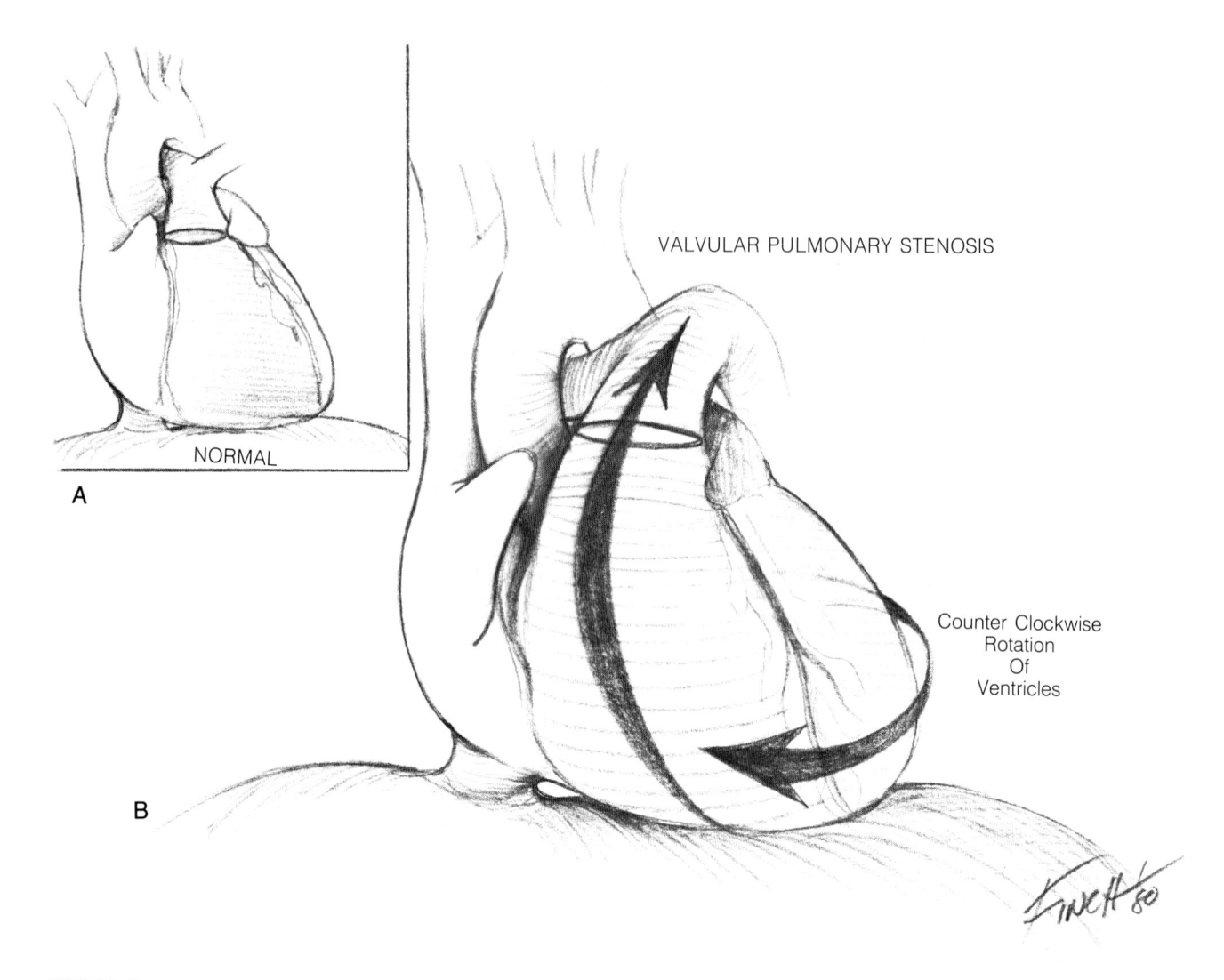

FIG 29–5.
A, diagram of normal heart on posteroanterior projection. Small portion of left ventricle forms lateral margin of heart. **B,** diagram of heart in anteroposterior projection of valvar pulmonary stenosis. Because right ventricle is elongated and hypertrophied, pulmonary valve is higher. Counterclockwise rotation of heart. Because of fixation of heart by superior and inferior venae cavae, counterclockwise rotation brings the more rounded posterior portion of left ventricle into profile, giving erroneous radiographic appearance of left ventricular hypertrophy.

6. Poststenotic dilatation of the pulmonary artery or of one of its major branches is virtually always present with valvar pulmonary stenosis except during infancy (Fig 29–7). REASON: In utero, only a small amount of blood flows through the stenotic pulmonary orifice because of the patent ductus arteriosus. Consequently, the force of the jet of blood through the stenotic valve is too small to cause poststenotic dilatation. Pulmonary arterial dilatation develops after the patent ductus closes, when the entire cardiac output passes through the stenotic pulmonary orifice and creates a forceful jet. In addition, during infancy, the main pulmonary artery segment is commonly overshadowed by thymic tissue.

7. In children and adults with pulmonary valvar stenosis, poststenotic dilatation of the main pulmonary artery and the left pulmonary artery are the most important diagnostic findings. In the normal adolescent, the pulmonary artery segment tends to be prominent, and the diagnosis can therefore be suggested only in the presence of a murmur.

8. Poststenotic dilatation almost invariably involves the main and left pulmonary artery. REASON: Because of the vertical position and counterclockwise rotation of the heart, the jet is most commonly directed from the main into the left pulmonary artery (Fig 29–8). Poststenotic dilatation of the left pulmonary artery can be seen on the posteroanterior or, better, the left anterior oblique projection (Fig 29–4,*B*).

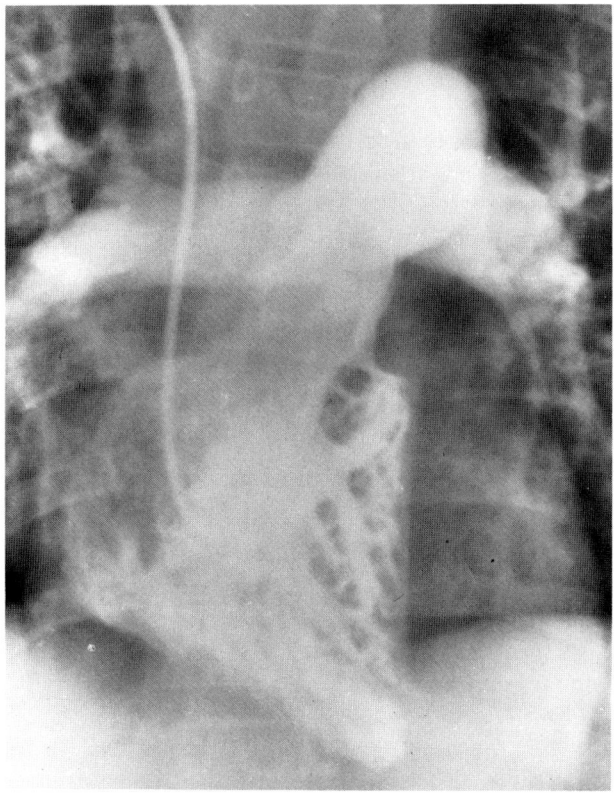

FIG 29–6.
Right ventriculogram, anteroposterior projection in valvar pulmonary stenosis. Counterclockwise rotation of heart results in right ventricle occupying medial position. Large portion of left ventricle forms left cardiac border and simulates left ventricular hypertrophy. Increased right ventricular trabeculations because of hypertrophy.

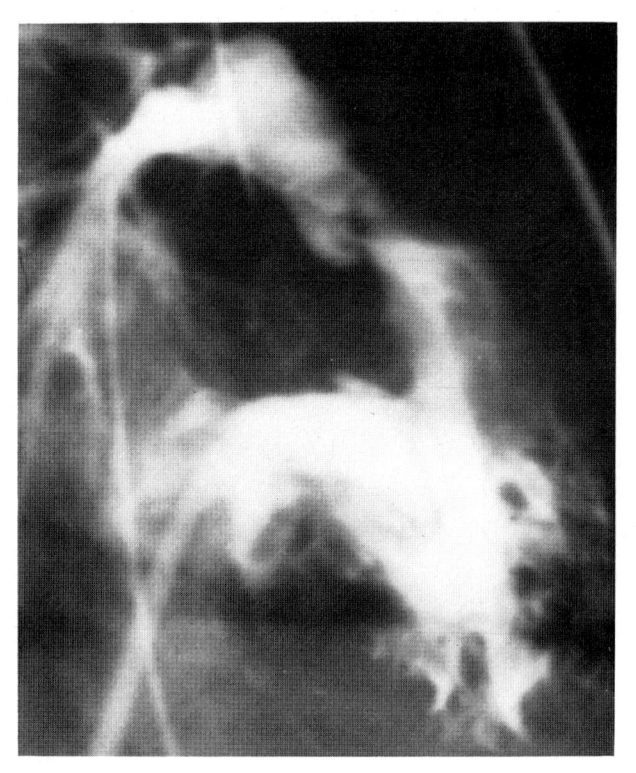

FIG 29–7.
Right ventriculogram, lateral projection in infant with critical valvar pulmonary stenosis. Marked thickening of pulmonary valve; minimal poststenotic dilatation of main pulmonary artery and ductus diverticulum.

9. There is no correlation between the degree of poststenotic dilatation and the pressure gradient across the pulmonary valve. On occasion, poststenotic dilatation of the main pulmonary artery is so great that it simulates a hilar mass. In the differential diagnosis, a lateral view is most helpful; masses are seen on the lateral projection as added abnormal densities, whereas the dilated main pulmonary artery does not cast an abnormal density.

10. The impact of the jet on the wall of the pulmonary artery causes a fibrotic reaction (jet lesion), which may later on calcify (Fig 29–9). A stenotic pulmonary valve may calcify later in life, but this is extremely rare.

11. Rarely, poststenotic dilatation of the main pulmonary artery is absent, and only the right or the left pulmonary artery shows dilatation (Fig 29–10,A). REASON: If the jet through the stenotic valve is centrally directed into the main pulmonary artery, it will extend unimpeded into the left pulmonary artery (Fig 29–10,B). Isolated poststenotic dilatation of the right pulmonary artery is rare because of the vertical orientation of the right ventricular outflow

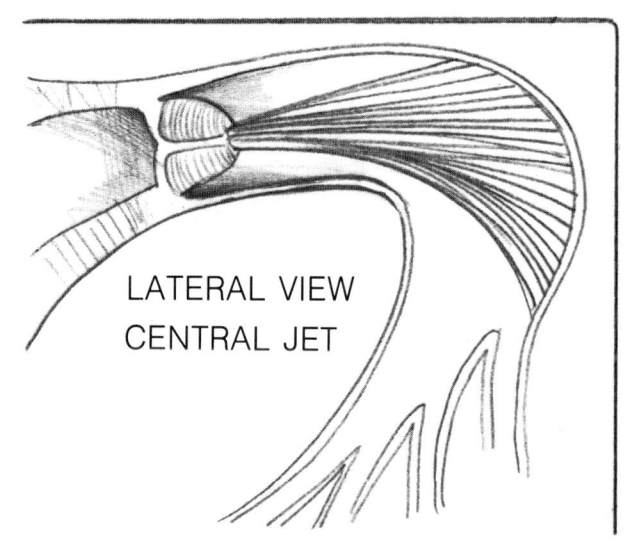

FIG 29–8.
Diagram of right ventriculogram in valvar pulmonary stenosis. Jet of contrast material is directed into left pulmonary artery because this artery is extension of main pulmonary artery. Right pulmonary artery branches at right angle from main pulmonary artery and is not dilated.

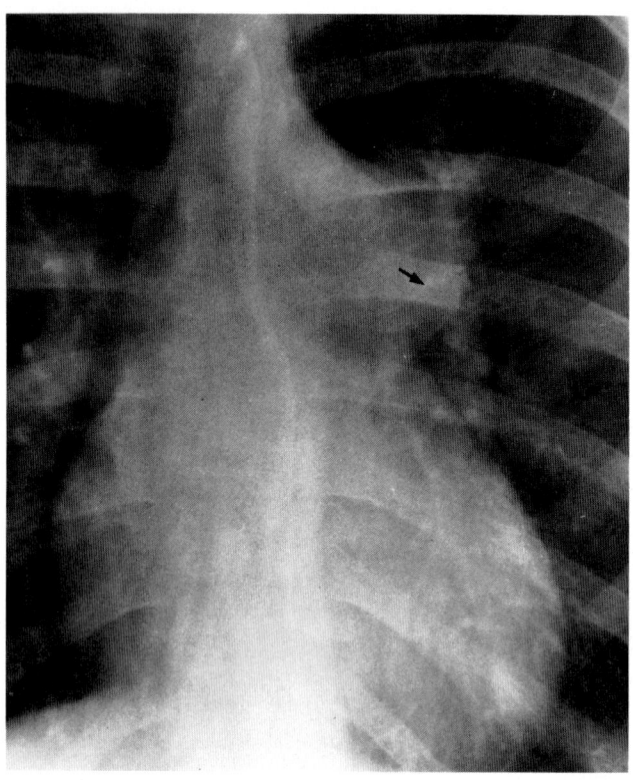

FIG 29-9.
Thoracic roentgenogram, posteroanterior projection in valvar pulmonary stenosis. Severe dilatation of main pulmonary arterial segment. Radiographic appearance is identical to that of hilar mass, but no mass was seen on other projections. Small fleck of calcium *(small arrow)* represents calcified jet lesion.

tract, in contradistinction to the rightward and more horizontal orientation in tetralogy of Fallot (see Chapter 30).

12. On fluoroscopy, the main pulmonary and the left pulmonary artery show increased pulsations. REASON: Impact of the forceful jet on the thin-walled main and left pulmonary arteries.

Cardiac Catheterization

The indications for cardiac catheterization are as follows:

1. Presence of cyanosis or congestive cardiac failure in an infant or child with a clinical pulmonary valvar stenosis.
2. As a routine procedure in an asymptomatic school-aged child with evidence of pulmonary valvar stenosis, in order to determine severity of the obstruction.
3. Balloon dilatation of pulmonary valve.

In most patients, the oximetry data are normal, but a right-to-left shunt, and sometimes also a small left-to-right shunt, may be found at the atrial level in patients with a stretched foramen ovale. The right ventricular systolic pressure is elevated, and there is a sharp pressure difference across the pulmonary valve, with a normal or low-normal pulmonary arterial pressure. The right ventricular systolic pressure characteristically shows a peaked contour, in contrast to the flat-topped pressure curve in patients with pulmonary stenosis and coexisting ventricular septal defect, as in tetralogy of Fallot.

The right ventricular end-diastolic pressure and the right atrial pressure are elevated in patients with marked right ventricular hypertrophy or with right ventricular decompensation. The cardiac output is normal at rest but may be less than normal with exercise.[7]

Angiographic Appearance:

1. Hypertrophy of the right ventricle is evidenced by increased trabeculations (Fig 29-6). There is a fair correlation between the degree of trabeculations and the severity of pulmonary stenosis, although the pressure gradient cannot be accurately predicted from the angiogram.

2. The right ventricle commonly assumes a more vertical and medial position. REASON: Pulmonary valvar stenosis causes a systolic overload of the right ventricle and secondary hypertrophy, primarily of the outflow portion. Hypertrophy of the right ventricle is also associated with elongation. Because the right ventricle cannot expand against the diaphragm, elongation results in a more vertical position of the heart, with a relatively high position of the pulmonary valve (see Figs 29-4,A, 29-5,B, and 29-6).

3. In addition to increased trabeculations, obstructive or nonobstructive muscle bundles may be present within the right ventricle. Muscle bundles should not be confused with trabeculations. Trabeculations are best seen along the periphery of the right ventricle, whereas muscle bundles lie in midstream and are perfectly round. Also, trabeculations tend to be more irregular (Fig 29-6).

4. Although the stenotic pulmonary valve may be as thin as a normal valve, commonly mild thickening occurs (Fig 29-11). Rarely, marked thickening may be present and mimic the angiographic appearance of a dysplastic pulmonary valve (Fig 29-12; see also Fig 29-24).

5. During systole, the stenotic pulmonary valve domes into the pulmonary artery. The angiographic appearance may vary. Ballooning of the valve starts in early systole, unlike the dysplastic valve, which may have a slightly domed appearance only at the end of systole.

6. If the contrast medium is expressed from the sinuses of Valsalva by the doming valve leaflet, a more square appearance is produced (see Fig 29-12, B and D).

7. A positive jet is seen during right ventriculography

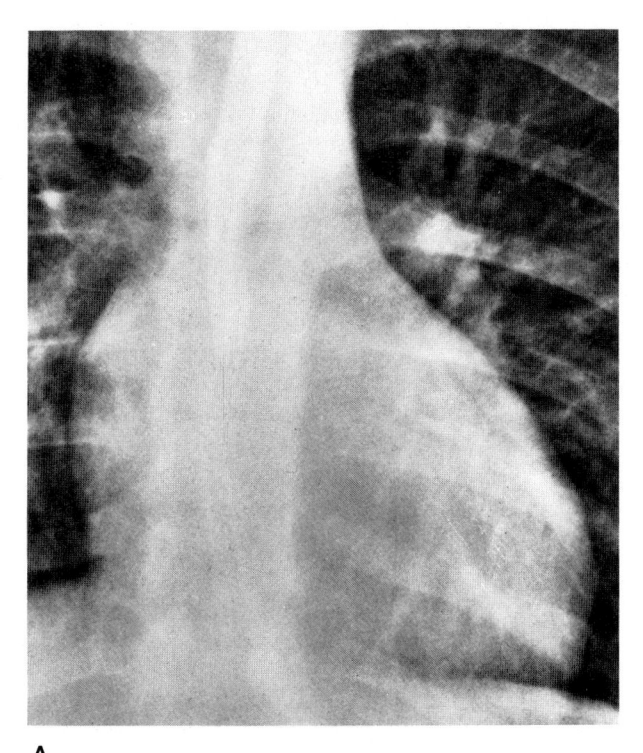

FIG 29–10.
A, posteroanterior roentgenogram of patient with valvar pulmonary stenosis in posteroanterior projection. The cardiac configuration is atypical, suggesting tetralogy of Fallot, because the pulmonary artery segment is concave. There is poststenotic dilatation of the left pulmonary artery. The atypical cardiac configuration is caused by an absent dilatation of the main pulmonary artery. **B,** explanatory diagram showing a central jet extending into the left pulmonary artery without impact on the main pulmonary artery. Main pulmonary artery is of normal size. **C,** diagram demonstrating poststenotic dilatation of the right and left pulmonary arteries without poststenotic dilatation of the main pulmonary artery (see also Fig 29–14). Isolated poststenotic dilatation of the right pulmonary artery is not observed in valvar pulmonary stenosis with intact septum. However, it is commonly seen in tetralogy of Fallot.

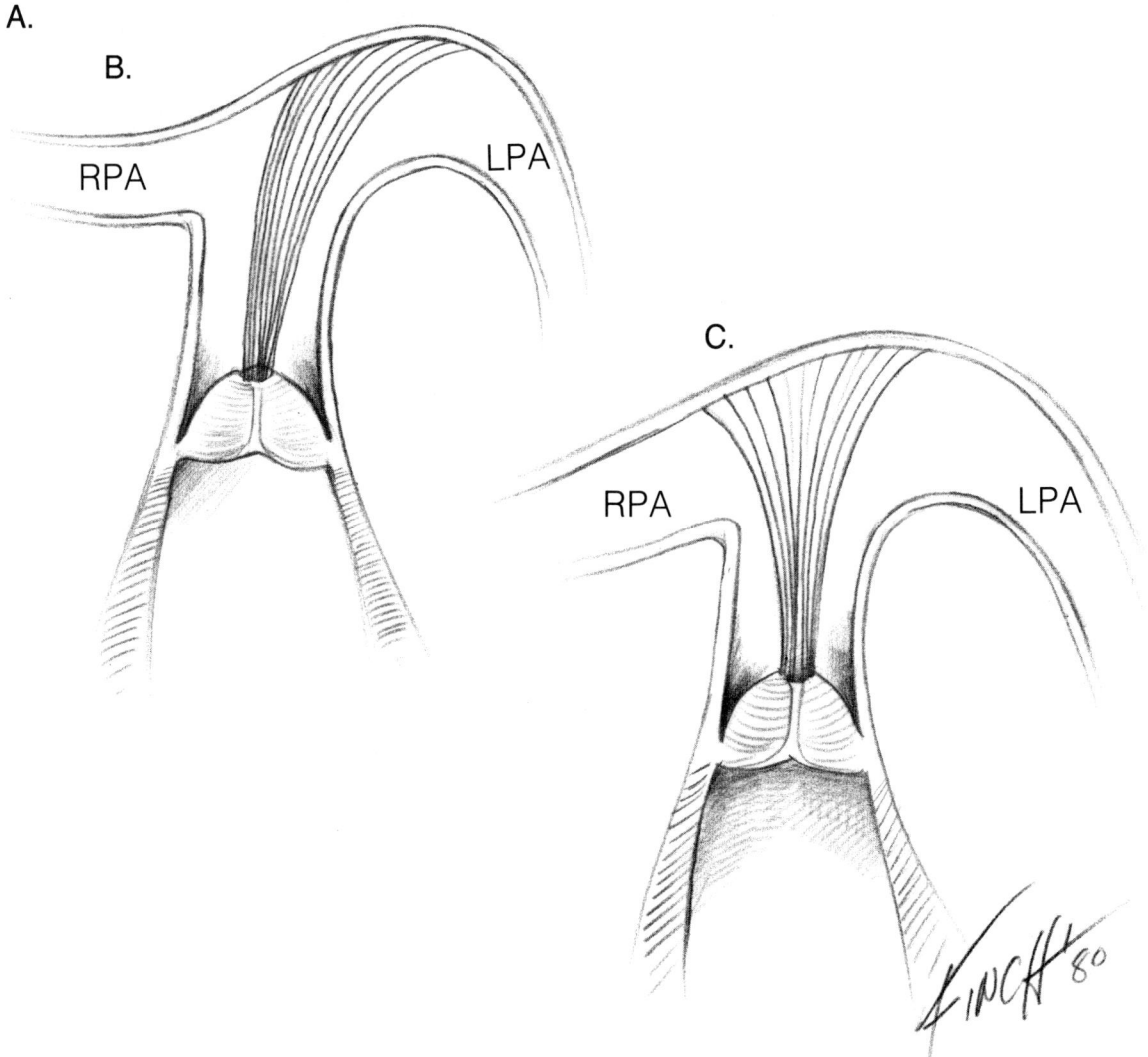

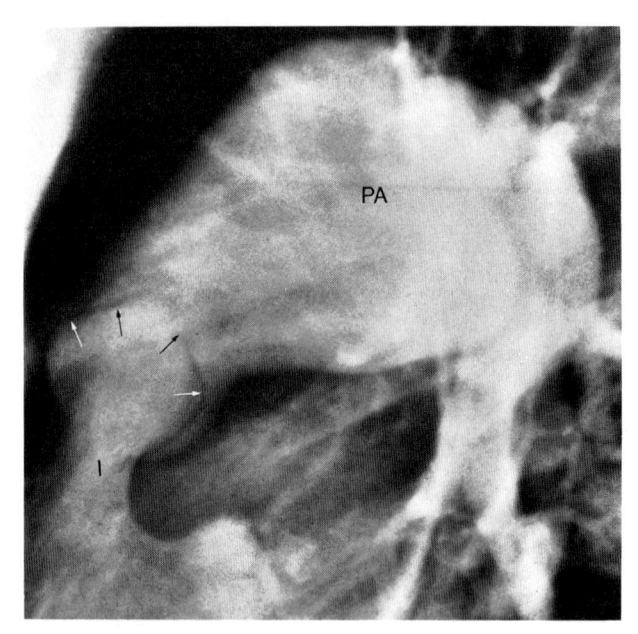

FIG 29-11.
Right ventriculogram, lateral projection in typical valvar pulmonary stenosis. Pulmonary valve *(arrows)* only minimally thickened. Enormous poststenotic dilatation of main pulmonary artery.

(Fig 29-13,*A*). After the contrast medium has cleared from the right ventricle, a negative jet may be seen (Fig 29-13,*B*).

8. Pulmonary valvar stenosis creates a forceful high-velocity jet, which results in poststenotic dilatation of the main and left pulmonary arteries (Figs 29-11 and 29-13). REASON: Maximum dilatation occurs at the site of impact of the jet on the wall of the pulmonary artery, which subsequently becomes dilated. Because the left pulmonary artery is a direct continuation of the main pulmonary artery, the jet is usually also directed into the left pulmonary artery, causing poststenotic dilatation of this artery as well (see Fig 29-8).

9. Rarely, poststenotic dilatation of the main pulmonary artery is absent, and only the left pulmonary artery is dilated. REASON: The stenotic pulmonary valve forms a jet, which lies in the center of the main pulmonary artery and extends directly into the left pulmonary artery. Therefore, the jet does not strike the pulmonary trunk (see Fig 29-10,*B*).

10. The jet may extend into the left and the right pulmonary arteries, resulting in poststenotic dilatation of both (rare) (Fig 29-14).

11. During diastole, the stenotic pulmonary valve leaflets invert normally, because they are usually thin and pliable (Fig 29-15).

12. During late systole, the hypertrophied infundibulum contracts forcefully and narrows considerably, simu-

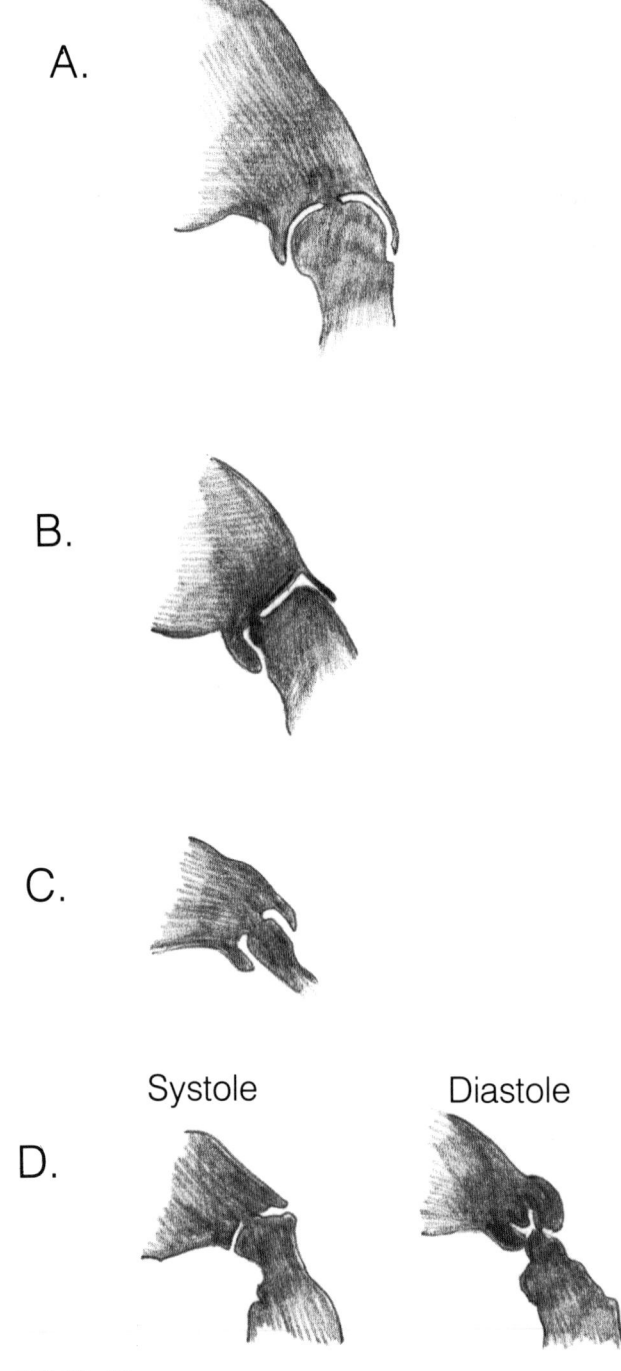

FIG 29-12.
Diagram of various appearances of stenotic pulmonary valve during systole. **A,** smooth, round, and domed appearance of pulmonary valve with either normal thickness or minimal thickening of the valve leaflets (most common). **B,** square appearance associated with obliteration of one of pulmonary sinuses of Valsalva. **C,** severely thickened pulmonary valve, resembling a dysplastic valve. Unlike dysplastic valve, however, size of the pulmonary anulus and supravalvar portion of pulmonary artery are normal, and poststenotic dilatation is present. **D,** atypical appearance association of obliteration of each of sinuses of Valsalva (rare).

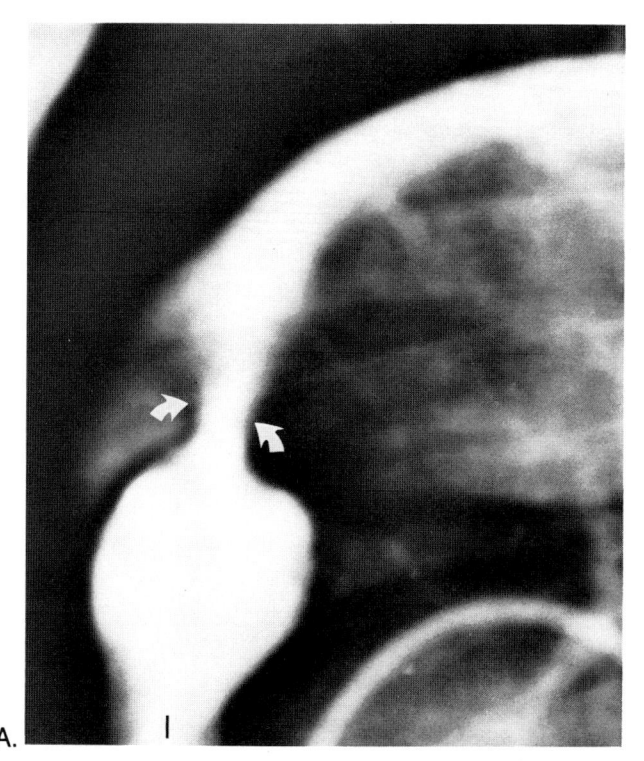

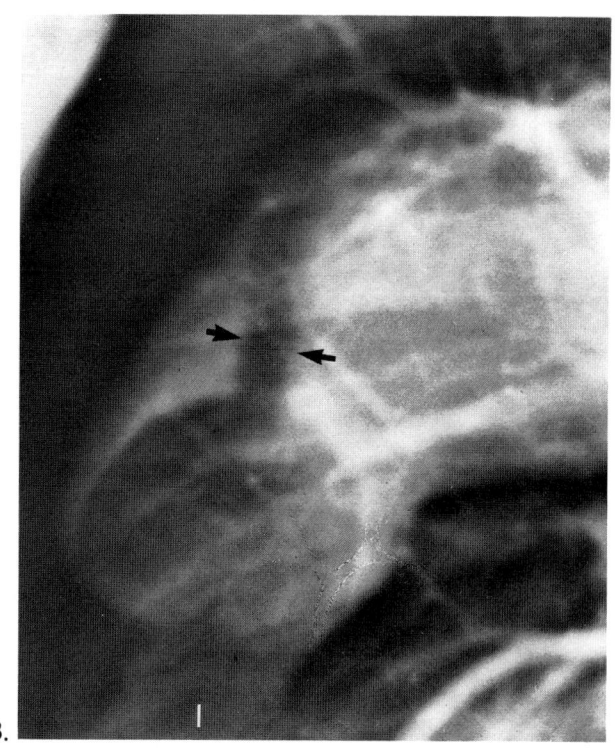

FIG 29–13.
Right ventriculogram, lateral projection of pulmonary valvar stenosis with domed-shaped valve. **A,** jet of contrast material ejected *(white arrows)* through stenotic pulmonary valve. Jet strikes roof of main pulmonary artery and extends into left pulmonary artery. **B,** late phase; negative jet *(black arrows)* caused by ejection of unopacified blood into still opacified pulmonary artery. Forceful contraction of infundibulum *(I)* simulating infundibular stenosis.

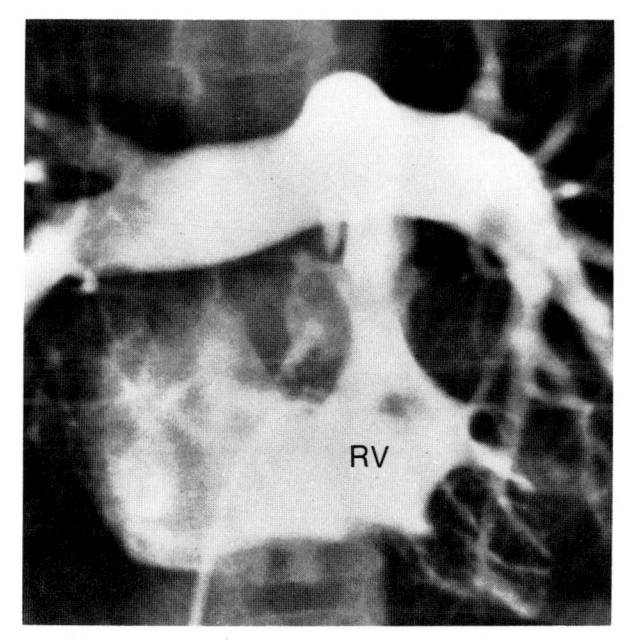

FIG 29–14.
Right ventriculogram *(RV)*, anteroposterior projection in valvar pulmonary stenosis. Centrally located jet causes poststenotic dilatation of both pulmonary arteries. Main pulmonary artery not dilated.

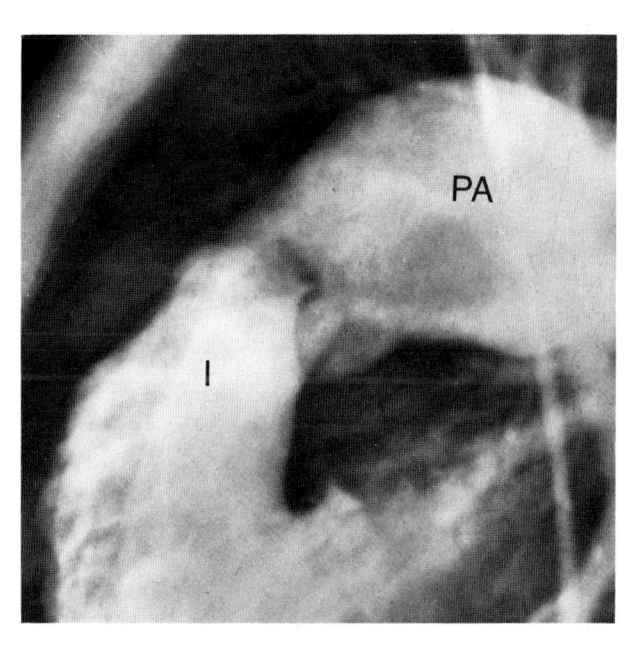

FIG 29–15.
Right ventriculogram, lateral projection during diastole in valvar pulmonary stenosis. Pulmonary valve cusps normally inverted. Infundibulum *(I)* widely patent. *PA* = pulmonary artery.

lating infundibular stenosis (Fig 29–14). However, the infundibulum relaxes completely during diastole (Fig 29–15), which distinguishes this secondary hypertrophy from true infundibular stenosis.

Operative Considerations

Pulmonary valvotomy is indicated as an emergency procedure in patients with congestive cardiac failure. Cyanosis is also an indication for urgent operation.

In asymptomatic patients, we recommend valvotomy when the gradient across the pulmonary valve exceeds 50 mm Hg or the pulmonary valve area is less than 0.5 cm^2/M^2.[1]

A commissurotomy is performed to increase the orifice size. This can be done using either cardiopulmonary bypass or the conditions of inflow stasis, in which inflow of blood into the heart is prevented by temporary occlusion of the superior and inferior venae cavae. A pulmonary arteriotomy can be done without significant blood loss, but the operation must be performed very rapidly because of the possibility of brain damage ($\leq$ 2 minutes).

Under direct vision, the fused commissures are carefully incised, converting the dome-shaped pulmonary valve into a bicuspid valve (Fig 29–16). Postoperatively, a gradient remains, but it is less than that present preoperatively. Pulmonary insufficiency is common but usually not a problem, because the pressure is low in the pulmonary artery, and the volume of regurgitating blood is not great.[8]

The operative risks, beyond infancy, are very low and the gradient is almost always reduced to low values.[9, 10]

Balloon dilation of dome-shaped pulmonary valvar stenosis has replaced surgery.

1. Angiography is carried out first and pressure measurements are recorded (Fig 29–17,*A*).
2. The pulmonary anulus is measured.
3. An angioplasty balloon catheter about 1.2 times the size of the pulmonary anulus or two balloon catheters are inserted and inflated in the stenotic pulmonary valve.
4. At low inflation pressures, a characteristic waist is seen at the level of the valve.
5. With higher pressures the valve ruptures, and the waist disappears at least on one side of the balloon.
6. Repeat right ventriculography and pulmonary angiography are carried out to assess the degree of pulmonary insufficiency, which is usually of a minor degree.
7. The split-valve leaflet may be seen as an open commissure during systole (Fig 29–17,*B*).

Right ventricular systolic pressure is reduced but generally less than with surgery. REASON: Unknown, but probably only one commissure may be split by the balloon compared with the surgical technique transforming the valve into a true bicuspid valve.

Balloon valvuloplasty is an established procedure in patients with a low gradient who would not be candidates for surgery. In recent years the indications for balloon an-

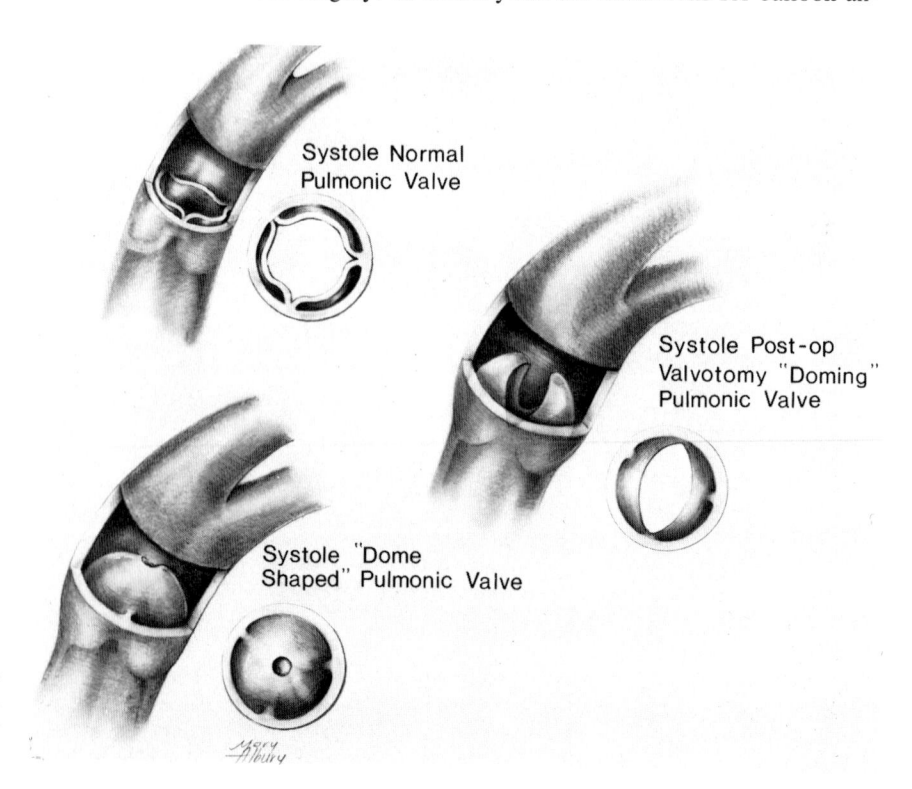

FIG 29–16.
Diagram comparing appearances of normal pulmonary valve, dome-shaped pulmonic valve, and bicuspid pulmonary valve after surgical incision of stenosis.

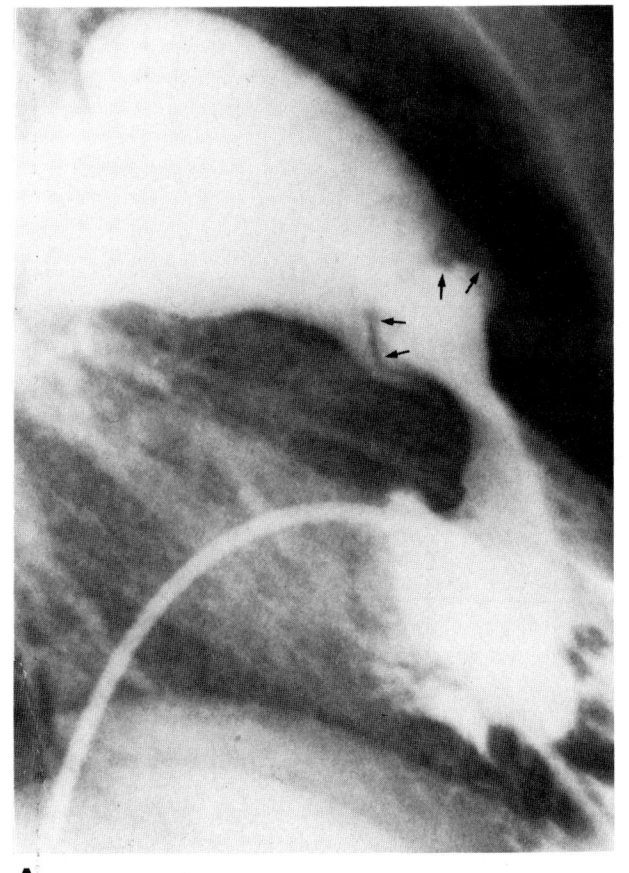

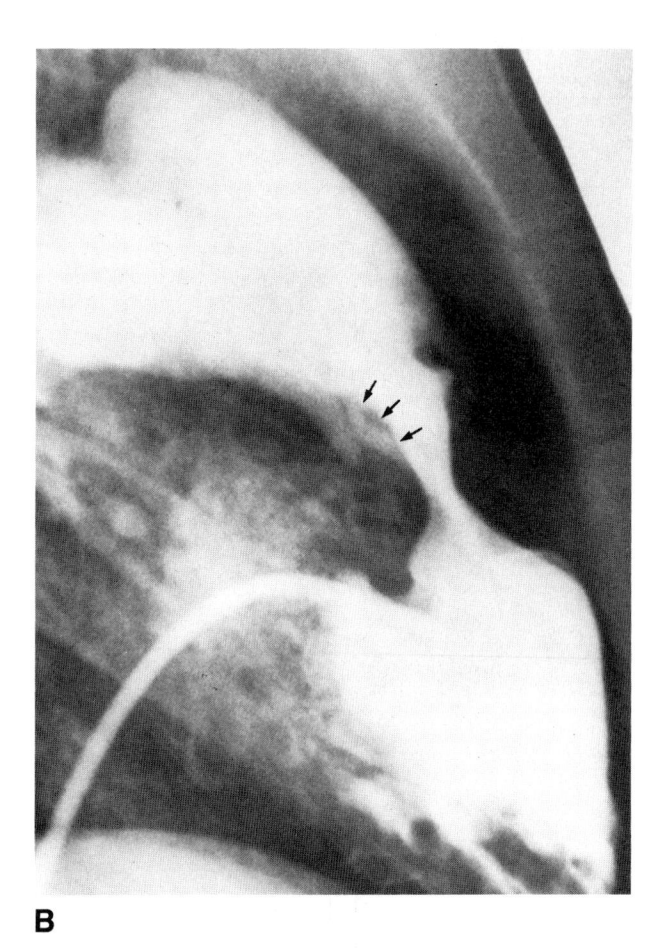

FIG 29-17.
A, lateral right ventriculogram in patient with 50 mm Hg gradient across the pulmonary valve and demonstration of a typical dome-shaped valvar pulmonary stenosis *(arrows)*. **B,** right ventriculogram after balloon valvuloplasty. During systole a commissure *(arrows)* is now demonstrated, created by balloon rupture of the dome-shaped valve. Pressure gradient dropped to 25 mm Hg.

gioplasty has been extended to patients with severe pulmonary stenosis.

Postoperative Appearance

1. In spite of relief of the pressure gradient by surgery, poststenotic dilatation does not regress.
2. The incised pulmonary valve shows persistent doming during systole, although the jet is no longer seen.
REASON: The surgeon has transformed the dome-shaped pulmonary valve into a bicuspid valve (Fig 29-16).

Dysplastic Pulmonary Valve

In 10% of cases of pulmonary valvar stenosis, the obstruction is caused by a dysplastic valve.

Pathology
In this form of stenosis, three valve leaflets are present and the commissures are not fused.[11] The obstruction results from the greatly thickened and redundant pulmonary valve leaflets. The bulky thickened valve lies in a small anulus, forming the obstruction (Fig 26-18). Histologic examination of the valve shows large, pale, stringy cells, resembling embryonic tissue (Fig 29-19).

Both the pulmonary anulus and the supravalvar portion of the main pulmonary artery are hypoplastic.

Hemodynamics
The dysplastic pulmonary valve has effects on the circulation similar to those of the dome-shaped pulmonary valve.

Clinical Features
As in domed-shaped pulmonary valvar stenosis, most patients are asymptomatic, although in an occasional patient cyanosis or congestive heart failure develop. In a few, there is a history of other family members with pulmonary stenosis.

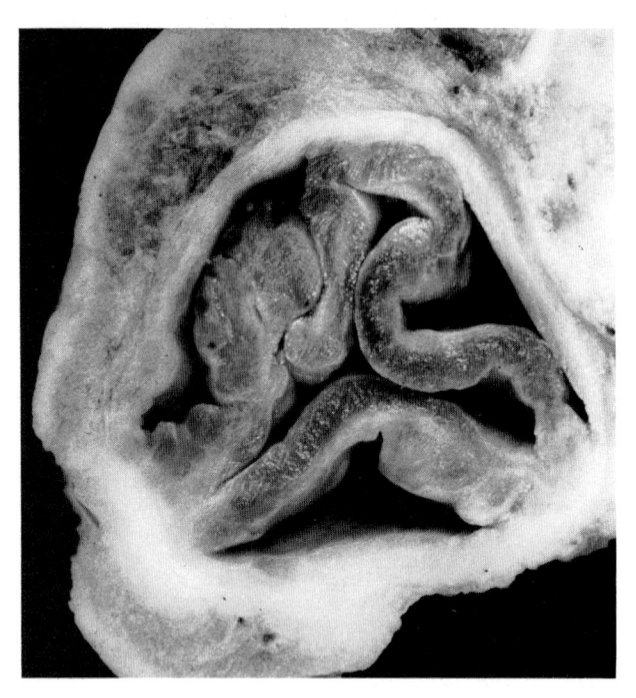

FIG 29–18.
Section through a dysplastic pulmonary valve viewed from pulmonary artery. Each pulmonary valve leaflet redundant and markedly thickened. Pulmonary anulus is hypoplastic. Sinuses of Valsalva narrowed.

Physical Examination

The physical findings resemble those of domed-shaped pulmonary valvar stenosis, with three differences:

1. A pulmonary systolic ejection click is rare, because poststenotic dilatation is not present.
2. Most patients are small, often less than the third percentile of height and weight (because of associated syndromes[12]).
3. There may be features of Noonan's syndrome or leopard syndrome.

Electrocardiographic Features

The ECG is in all respects similar to dome-shaped pulmonary valvar stenosis except the QRS axis is usually between -60 and -120 degrees. Probably, this is caused by an abnormality of the cardiac conduction system, and this finding helps to distinguish this form of stenosis from that caused by a domed-shaped valve, in which there is right-axis deviation, rarely more than $+180$ degrees.

Echocardiographic Features

The echocardiogram resembles that of typical pulmonary valvar stenosis, and the thickened dysplastic valve cannot be distinguished.

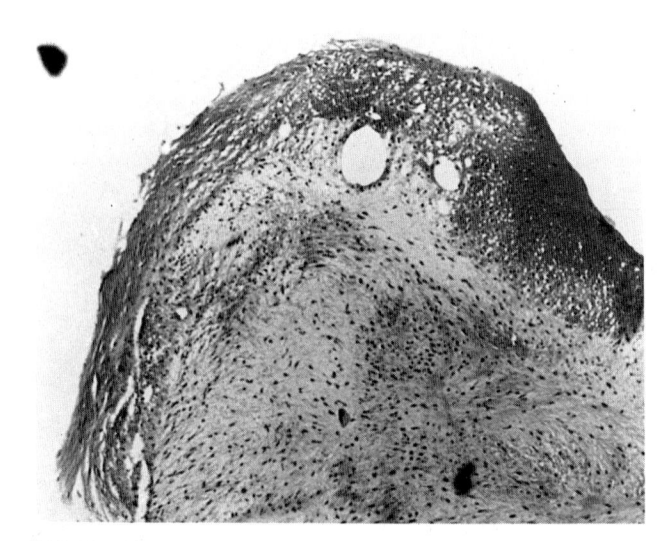

FIG 29–19.
Dysplastic pulmonary valvar tissue ($\times$ 100). Large pale cells with small central nuclei resemble embryonic tissue.

Radiographic Features

1. Right ventricular hypertrophy may be seen, as in domed-shaped valvar pulmonary stenosis.
2. Poststenotic dilatation of the pulmonary trunk is usually minimal or absent, although the right and left pulmonary arteries may show dilatation. REASON: Unlike the round jet created by a dome-shaped stenotic pulmonary

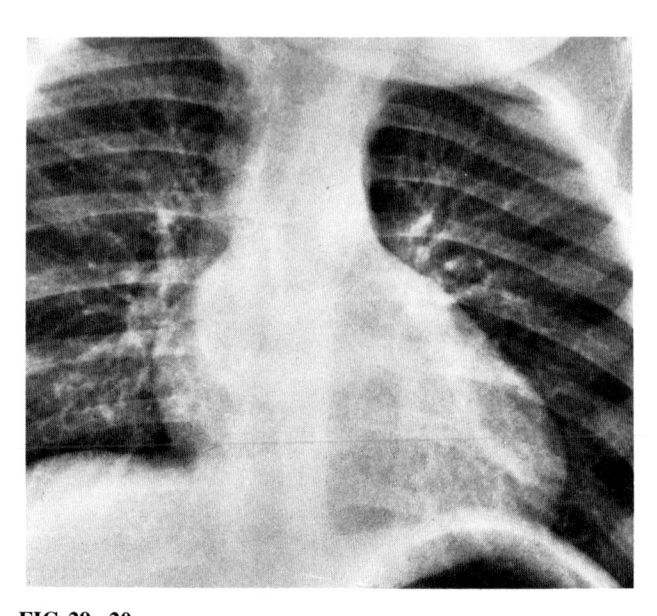

FIG 29–20.
Thoracic roentgenogram, posteroanterior projection of dysplastic pulmonary valve. Cardiac size and pulmonary vasculature normal. Pulmonary artery segment concave. Film resembles one from patient with tetralogy of Fallot. Poststenotic dilatation of main pulmonary artery is typically absent.

valve, the jet from the dysplastic valve has a Mercedes star cross section and usually does not impinge on the wall of the pulmonary trunk. The valve leaflets tend to guide the jet more centrally in the main pulmonary artery, as with the central jet in valvar pulmonary stenosis. The plain films of the dysplastic pulmonary valve may be normal or similar to those in tetralogy of Fallot (Fig 29–20).

Cardiac Catheterization

The indications and findings are similar to those in dome-shaped pulmonary stenosis.

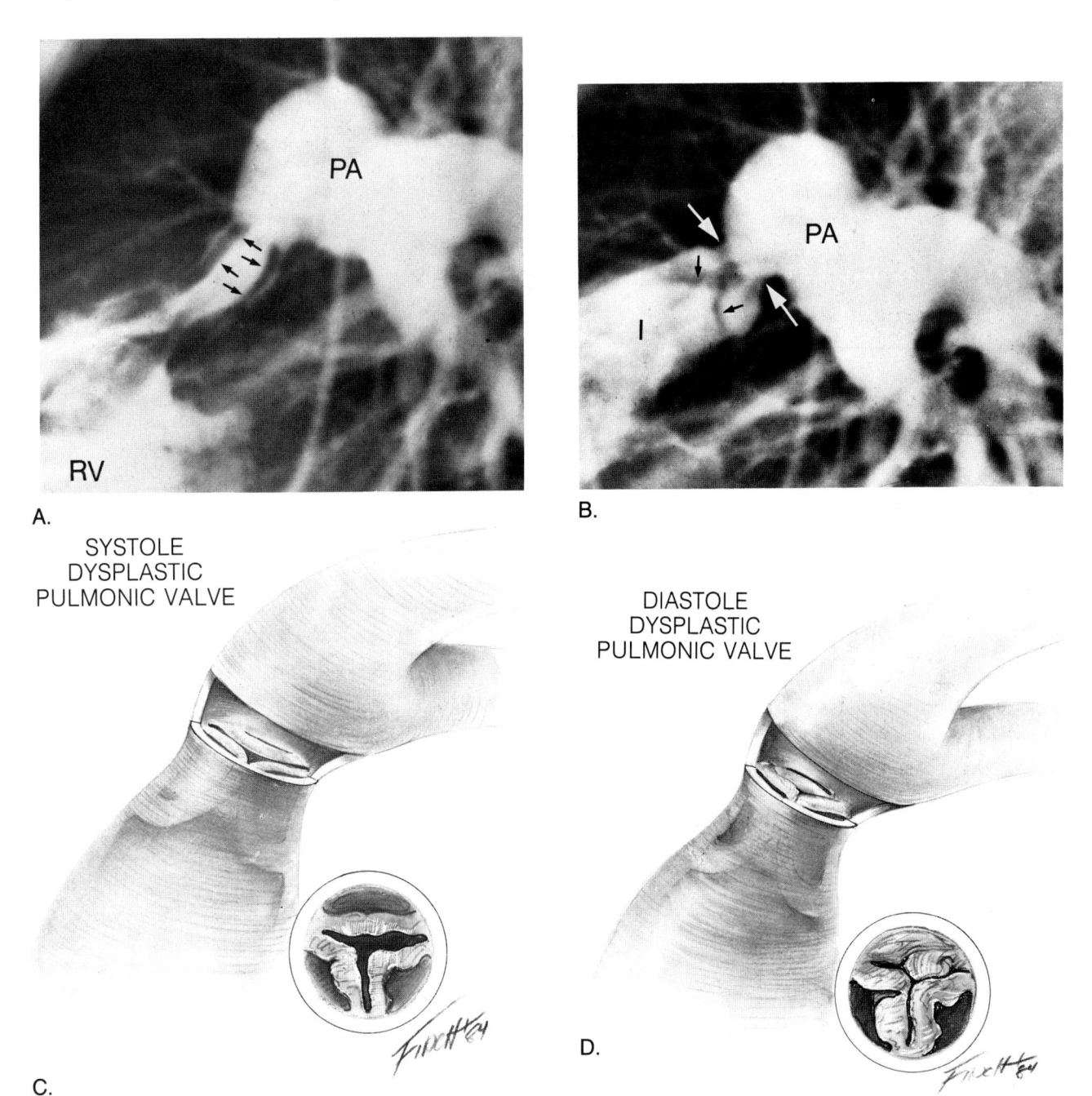

FIG 29–21.
Right ventriculogram, lateral projection of pulmonary stenosis with dysplastic valve. **A,** systolic view; markedly thickened leaflets *(arrows).* Small pulmonary anulus. **B,** diastolic view; thickened pulmonary valve leaflets *(small arrows).* Supravalvar narrowing *(white arrows).* Infundibulum *(I)* relaxed. Diagram of dysplastic pulmonary valve, systole **(C)** and diastole **(D).** *PA* = pulmonary artery; *RV* = right ventricle.

Angiographic Appearance

1. Right ventricular hypertrophy is evidenced by increased trabeculations.
2. The pulmonary anulus and proximal main pulmonary artery tend to be small, in contrast to domed-shaped valvular pulmonary stenosis (Fig 29–21,A). Previously dysplastic pulmonary valve was therefore termed "small pulmonary anulus syndrome."
3. The pulmonary valve is markedly thickened; this is the most consistent and characteristic angiographic finding of dysplastic pulmonary valve. Thickening becomes particularly obvious during diastole. REASON: Approximation of the valve leaflets results in a double thickness of valve tissue (Fig 29–21,B).
4. Irregular thickening may involve the free edge of the valve, giving a beaded appearance.
5. Longitudinal striations of the pulmonary valve leaflets may be seen (Fig 29–22), which is never seen in dome-shaped valvar stenosis. REASON: During systole, the thickened edges of the three valve leaflets are seen on end.
6. Rarely, longitudinal striations are not visible during systole, making differentiation from a severely thickened dome-shaped pulmonary valve difficult (Fig 29–23). Domed-shaped stenosis and dysplastic pulmonary valve may coexist.
7. The contrast medium may be completely displaced

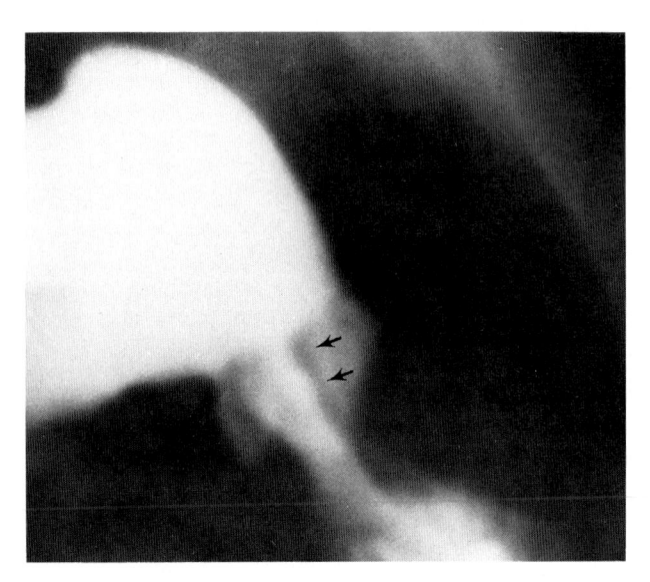

FIG 29–22.
Right ventriculogram, lateral projection; systolic view in dysplastic pulmonary valve. Longitudinal striations of thickened edges of pulmonary valve leaflet seen on end *(arrows)*. This is never seen in typical pulmonary valvar stenosis because the commissures are fused. Little contrast medium remains in sinuses of Valsalva because bulky valvar tissue obliterates this space. Marked contraction of right ventricular infundibulum.

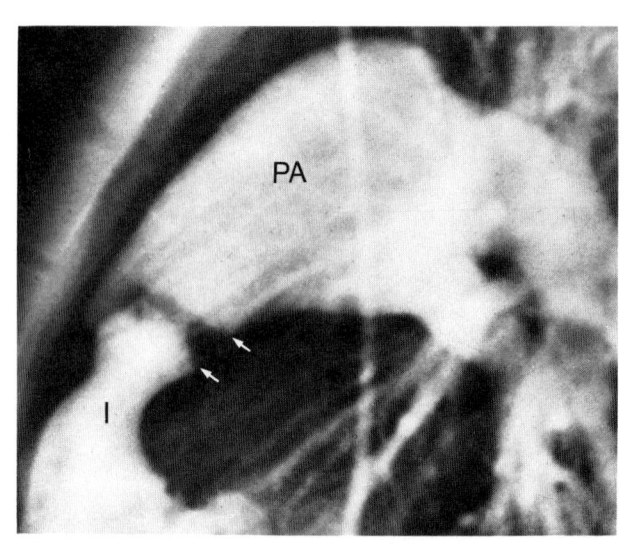

FIG 29–23.
Right ventriculogram, lateral projection; systolic view in valvar pulmonary stenosis and dysplastic valve. Markedly thickened, dome-shaped pulmonary valve *(arrows)*. Poststenotic dilatation of main pulmonary artery *(PA)* and of left pulmonary artery. Absence of supravalvar narrowing helps to distinguish this from dysplastic valve. However, this lesion should be surgically treated as dysplastic valve because commissurotomy alone may not relieve the pressure gradient. I = infundibulum.

from the sinuses of Valsalva during systole (Fig 29–24). REASON: The markedly thickened and redundant pulmonary valve leaflets are located in a small anulus and proximal main pulmonary artery. Therefore, the systolic configuration of the dysplastic valve is commonly square. The square appearance is rarely seen in dome-shaped pulmonary valvar stenosis (see Fig 29–12).

8. Apparent doming may be seen at the end of systole on the lateral view (Fig 29–24,A), but it is never as round and as smooth as in valvar pulmonary stenosis. The anteroposterior projection shows straightened valve leaflets (Fig 29–24,B).
9. A jet is rarely seen, although if present, it is not as well defined as in domed valvar pulmonary stenosis. REASON: The dysplastic pulmonary valve forms an irregular star-shaped orifice during systole, unlike the round orifice of a domed stenotic pulmonary valve (see Figs 29–2 and 29–16).
10. Poststenotic dilatation of the main pulmonary artery is absent, but poststenotic dilatation of the right and left pulmonary arteries may occur (Fig 29–24). REASON: The valve leaflets tend to guide the bloodstream through the center of the pulmonary valve, forming a central jet and preventing impact on the wall of the main pulmonary artery.
11. The main pulmonary artery is short and narrow.

In patients with dysplastic pulmonary valve, both the

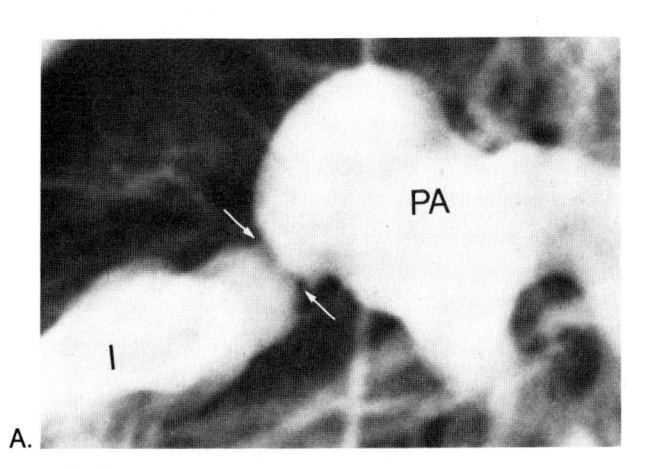

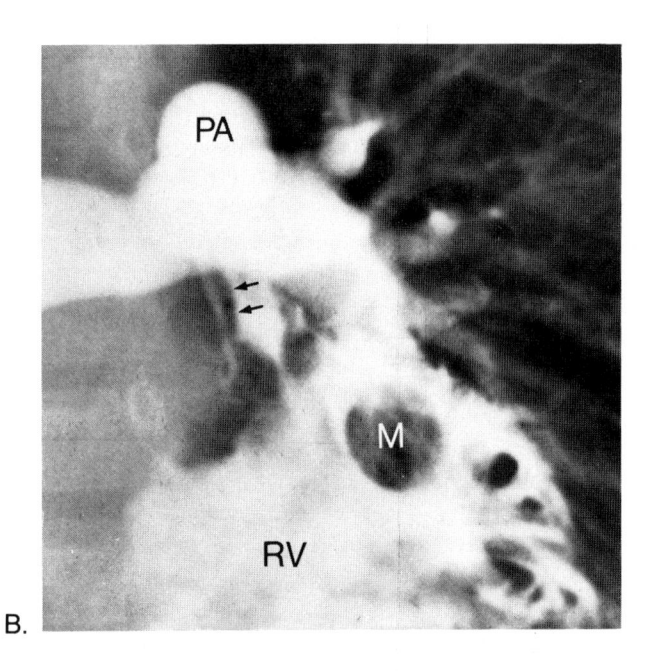

FIG 29–24.
Right ventriculogram *(RV)* of dysplastic pulmonary valve. **A,** lateral projection; typical appearance of dysplastic valve. Leaflets appear square because sinuses of Valsalva completely obliterated by redundant valvar tissue. Short main pulmonary artery *(PA)*; dilatation of right and left pulmonary arteries. Because of thickening of edges, valve appears to dome (pseudodoming), but this usually is not observed on anteroposterior projection. *I* = infundibulum. **B,** anteroposterior projection; normal-sized main pulmonary artery. Dilatation of right and left pulmonary arteries. Thickened valve leaflets straighten during systole *(black arrows)*. This finding distinguishes between valvar stenosis and dysplastic valve. Anomalous muscle bundle *(M)*.

pulmonary anulus and the proximal main pulmonary artery tend to be hypoplastic.

Operative Considerations

The indications for cardiac operation are the same as for domed-shaped pulmonary valvar stenosis, but the operation consists of excising one or more valve leaflets. If the anulus is small, a patch is sewn across it. Pulmonary insufficiency is common. The preoperative and postoperative angiographic appearance are identical. If a dysplastic pulmonary valve is diagnosed angiographically, the operation should not be performed by inflow stasis because of the longer time required to relieve the obstruction properly.

PERIPHERAL PULMONARY ARTERY STENOSIS

Peripheral pulmonary artery stenosis is an uncommon condition. A mild clinical form of this condition is present in about 5% of prematurely born infants, but it subsequently disappears.

Pathology

Peripheral pulmonary artery stenosis is almost always bilateral, and usually multiple stenotic areas are present. The anatomic lesion varies from a discrete, diaphragm-like, abrupt narrowing to a more diffuse fusiform stenotic type. Rarely, stenosis results from hypoplasia of the entire pulmonary arterial tree.

Four specific anatomic types have been described,[13] and each can be seen angiographically:

1. Stenosis of the pulmonary trunk.
2. Stenosis at the bifurcation extending into the left or right pulmonary artery or both.
3. Multiple peripheral stenoses.
4. Stenoses of both the pulmonary trunk and peripheral arteries.

Peripheral pulmonary artery stenosis may be associated with one of three recognized syndromes in which other cardiac anomalies are also common. Thus, it is the second most common cardiac condition in the rubella syndrome,[14, 15] patent ductus arteriosus being the most common. Peripheral pulmonary artery stenosis also is found in Noonan's syndrome, in which a dysplastic pulmonary valve is common. Peripheral pulmonary artery stenosis also may be associated with supravalvar aortic stenosis (Williams' syndrome) (see Chapter 26).

Peripheral pulmonary artery stenosis may coexist with other congenital cardiac malformations, such as tetralogy of Fallot, transposition of the great vessels, atrial septal defect, and ventricular septal defect.

In premature infants, a small (10 mm Hg) gradient may be found between the pulmonary trunk and branch pulmonary arteries. There are no anatomic changes other than marked discrepancy in caliber between the main pulmonary artery and the left and right main pulmonary arteries.[16]

Hemodynamics

Because of the obstruction, the systolic pressure increases in the right ventricle and in the pulmonary artery proximal to the stenosis. The pressure beyond the obstruction is normal or low. The diastolic pulmonary arterial pressure is identical proximal and distal to the stenosis, because there is free communication within the pulmonary arteries. As a result, a characteristic widened pulse pressure is found proximal to the obstruction.

Right ventricular hypertrophy develops in proportion to the degree of stenosis.

The other hemodynamic consequences, such as the development of cardiac failure or cyanosis, resemble those of valvar pulmonary stenosis, but the degree of obstruction usually is not as severe as in valvar pulmonary stenosis. Usually peripheral pulmonary artery stenosis is well tolerated, and there is no increase in gradient with age.[16, 17]

Clinical Features

Most patients are asymptomatic. The condition is detected either by a characteristic murmur or because the child has other stigmata such as those of rubella, Williams' syndrome, or Noonan's syndrome, or the mother gives a history of rubella in the first trimester of pregnancy. Occasionally the obstruction is severe enough to cause right-sided cardiac failure.

Physical Examination

The child may have the facies or other features of an associated syndrome. Usually there is neither a thrill nor a heave. The clue to the diagnosis is a high-pitched, grade 2 to 3/6 systolic ejection murmur heard well in the axillae, over the back, and at the base of the heart.[13] The murmur is rarely continuous, because there is no diastolic gradient across the stenosis. The second heart sound is normal.

Electrocardiographic Features

The ECG resembles that of valvar pulmonary stenosis.

Echocardiographic Features

The echocardiogram may show right ventricular hypertrophy, but the echo from the pulmonary valve appears normal. A specific diagnosis usually cannot be made.

Radiographic Features

In most cases, the diagnosis of peripheral pulmonary artery stenosis cannot be made from a thoracic roentgenogram. With the clinical information of a murmur heard over the lung fields and right ventricular hypertrophy on the ECG, careful scrutiny of a chest film may give a hint of the diagnosis by virtue of the following subtle findings:

1. Bizarre pulmonary vascular pattern. REASON: Multiple dilated poststenotic segments of the pulmonary arterial branches in both lung fields may be seen.
2. Regions of decreased pulmonary vasculature. REASON: Decreased pulmonary flow distal to areas of stenosis.
3. Decreased pulmonary vasculature in cases of diffuse pulmonary artery stenosis involving all branches of the pulmonary arteries.

Cardiac Catheterization

The oximetry data are normal. A systolic pressure gradient is present in the pulmonary arterial system, with a wide pulse pressure being found in the pulmonary artery proximal to the obstruction. The pulmonary arterial diastolic pressure is normal or low.

Angiographic Appearance

Areas of stenoses are usually well seen by selective pulmonary angiography. Determining the location of a pressure gradient at time of catheterization is most helpful,

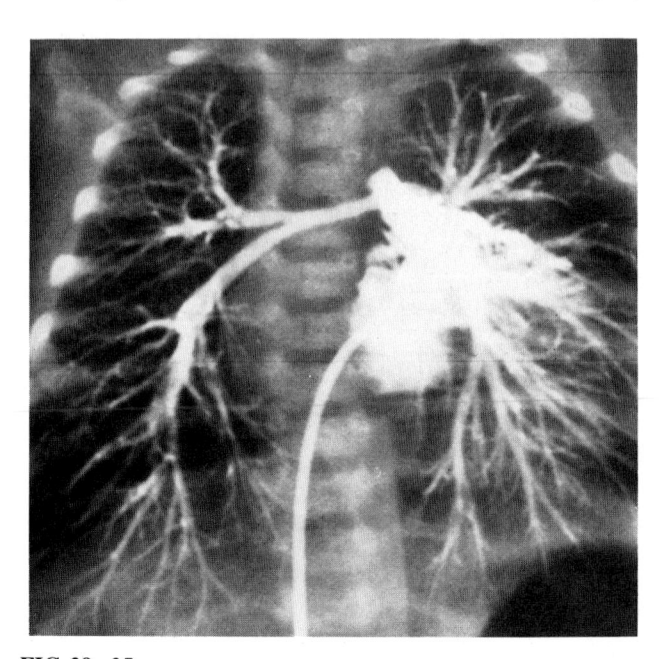

FIG 29-25.
Pulmonary arteriogram, anteroposterior projection of diffuse type of pulmonary artery stenosis. Hypoplasia of central pulmonary arterial tree.

because special views may be required to show the areas of narrowing.

1. The diffuse type of pulmonary artery stenosis, which may be the result of a diffuse arteritis, is characterized by diffuse narrowing of the main pulmonary artery and peripheral pulmonary arteries. Commonly, the main pulmonary artery is also small, giving the appearance of diffuse pulmonary hypoplasia (Fig 29–25).
2. Supravalvar pulmonary stenosis involving the main pulmonary artery is best seen in the lateral projection (Fig 29–26). This type occurs most commonly as part of the tetralogy of Fallot.
3. Single or multiple peripheral pulmonary artery stenoses of the tubular type are readily seen on the anteroposterior angiogram (Fig 29–27).
   Diaphragm-like stenosis may require oblique views to see the lesion clearly (Fig 29–28).
4. Stenosis involving the origin of the left pulmonary artery occurs most commonly in tetralogy of Fallot. Such stenoses are best demonstrated by a steep left anterior oblique projection with caudal beam angulation.
5. Rarely, a pressure gradient is recorded within a peripheral pulmonary artery during cardiac catheterization, yet no anatomic lesion can be demonstrated by careful angiography or even by postmortem examination. Such pressure gradients are probably caused by flow abnormalities without an anatomic lesion.
6. Peripheral pulmonary artery stenoses may be part of the rubella syndrome (Fig 29–29); the other angiographic findings of this syndrome are as follows:
   a. Patent ductus arteriosus.
   b. Shortened main pulmonary artery.
   c. A vertically positioned, thickened, insufficient, and sometimes dysplastic pulmonary valve.
7. The demonstration of peripheral pulmonary artery stenosis requires ascending aortography to exclude commonly associated supravalvar aortic stenosis (Williams' syndrome) (see Chapter 26).

Operative Considerations

Operation is indicated in patients with cyanosis or congestive cardiac failure, although operation is unfeasible in many patients because the stenoses are multiple and commonly in the periphery. If the stenosis is severe and operation is technically feasible, the normal arterial lumen can be restored by an end-to-end anastomosis or a patch angioplasty. Sometimes the hypertrophied intima is excised, in addition. Balloon arterial dilatation has been successful in treating peripheral pulmonary artery stenosis and lowering the gradient (Fig 29–30,A–C). However, in older children balloon dilatation commonly fails because of plastic recoil of the thick-walled pulmonary artery. Balloon dilatation, followed by placement of a stent, counteracts the plastic recoil (Fig 29–30,D–F).

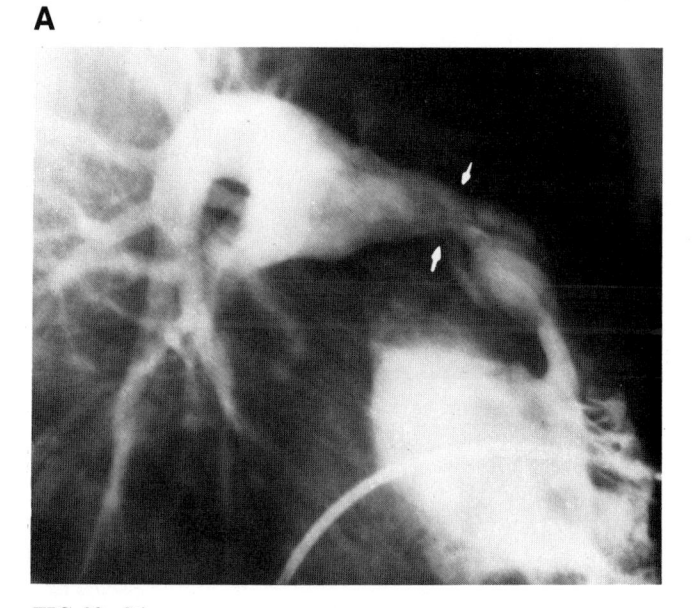

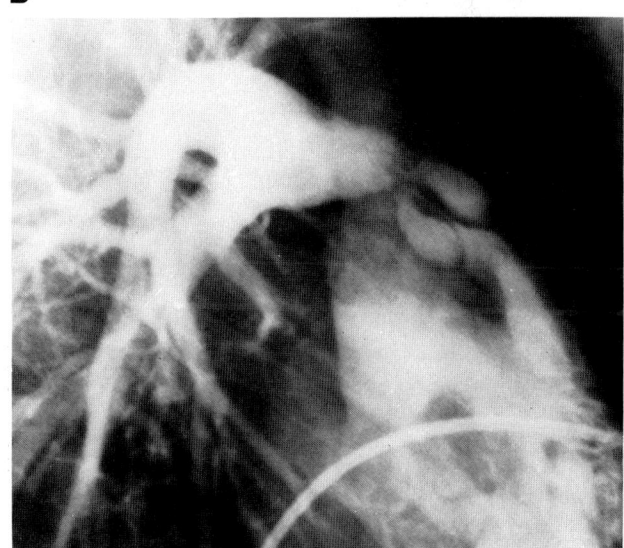

FIG 29–26.
Right ventriculogram, lateral projection of localized supravalvar pulmonary stenosis *(arrows)*. Tetralogy of Fallot and bicuspid pulmonary valve. Systolic **(A)** and diastolic **(B)** views. Note infundibular pulmonary stenosis and filling of the aorta through ventricular septal defect. Bicuspid pulmonary valve shows typical clamshell appearance.

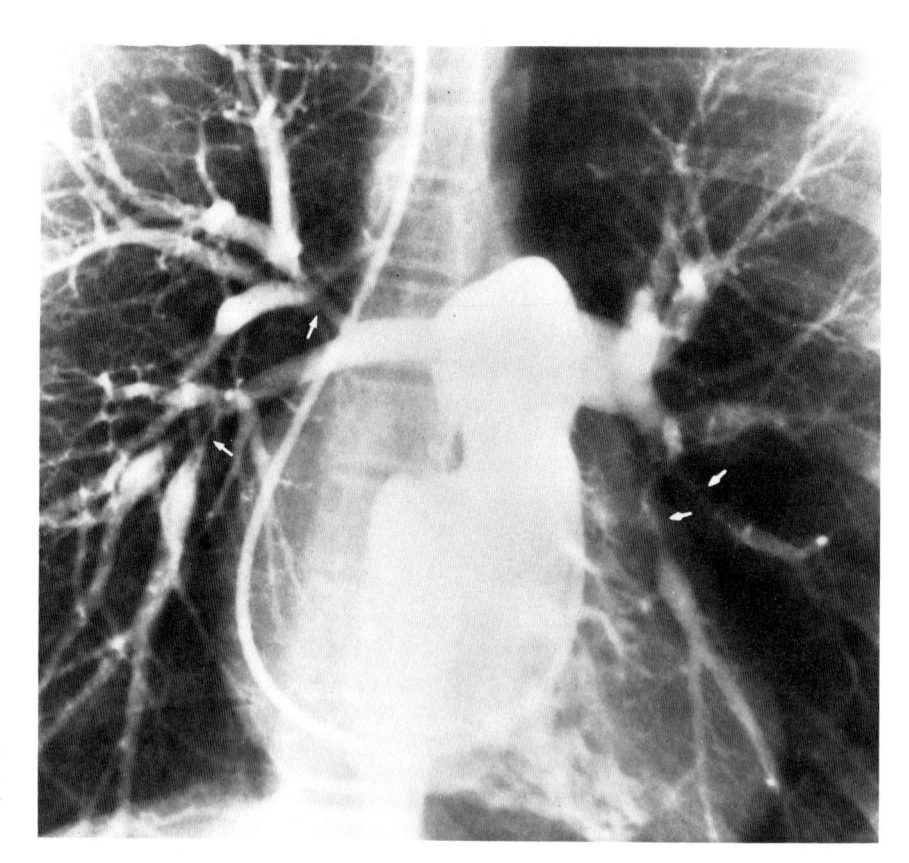

FIG 29–27.
Right ventriculogram, anteroposterior projection in peripheral pulmonary artery stenosis. Multiple bilateral pulmonary artery stenoses of tubular type *(arrows)*.

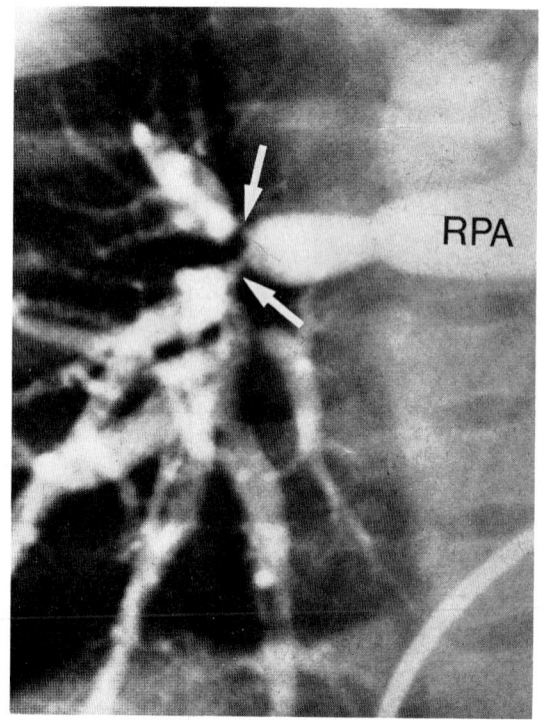

FIG 29–28.
Pulmonary arteriogram, slightly oblique projection in peripheral pulmonary artery stenosis. Diaphragm-like localized peripheral pulmonary artery stenosis *(arrows)*. Because of overlap of pulmonary arteries, this type can easily be overlooked unless oblique views are obtained.

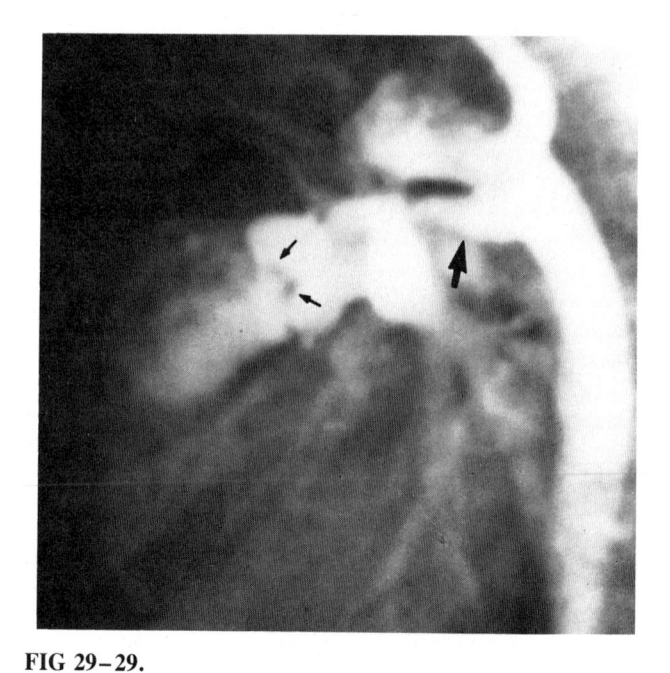

FIG 29–29.
Retrograde aortogram, lateral projection in rubella syndrome. Patent ductus arteriosus *(large arrow)*; short main pulmonary artery. Thickened vertical pulmonary valve *(small arrow)*, which allows regurgitation into right ventricle.

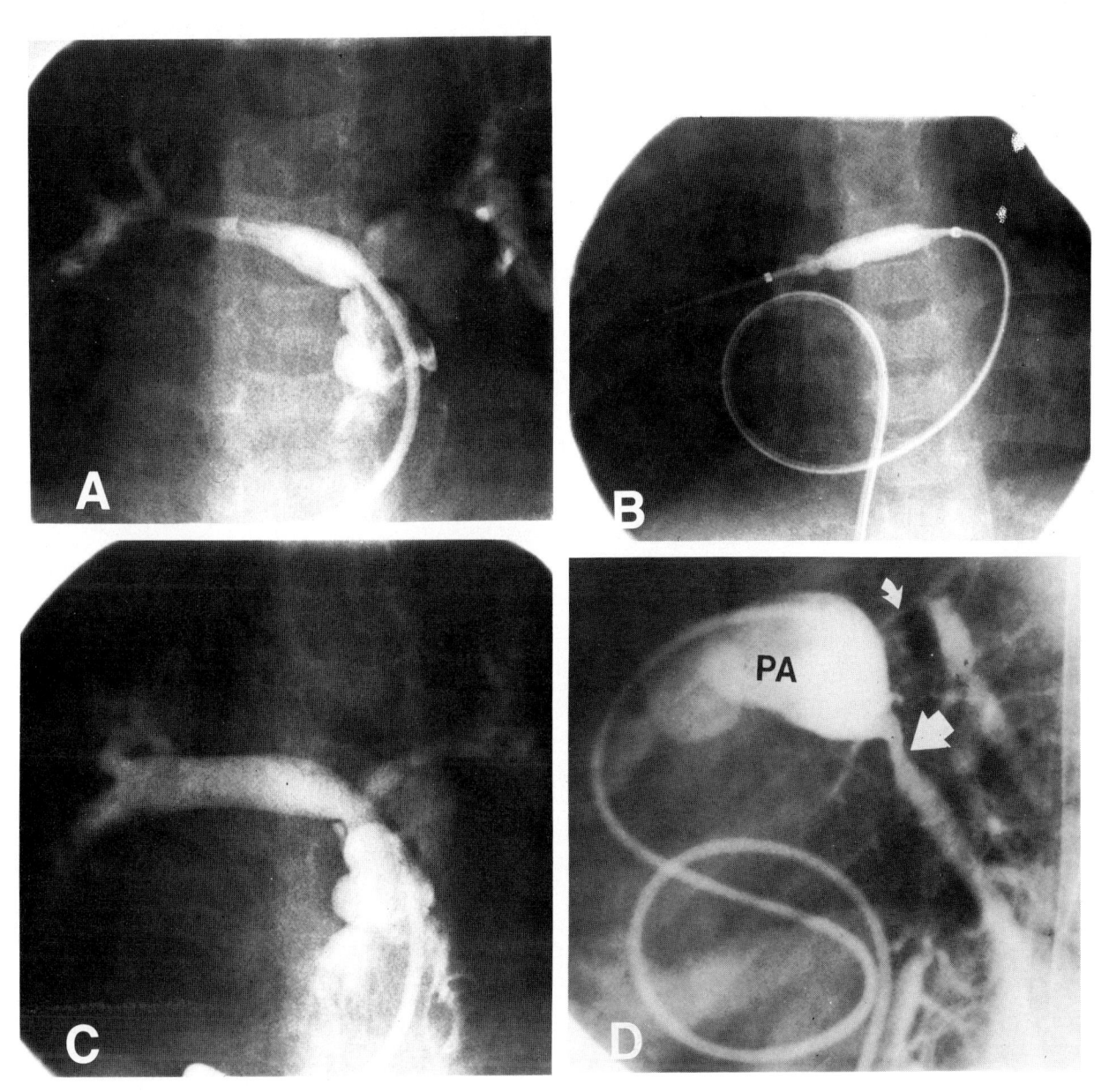

FIG 29–30.
Balloon dilatation technique for peripheral pulmonary artery stenosis seen in anteroposterior projection. **A,** pulmonary arteriogram before dilatation; stenosis of distal right main pulmonary artery. **B,** dilating catheter in place and slightly inflated demonstrating waist at stenotic site. **C,** after dilatation; increased caliber of right main pulmonary artery. However, in older children balloon dilatation commonly fails because of plastic recoil of the thick-walled pulmonary artery. Balloon dilatation, followed by placement of a stent, counteracts the plastic recoil. **D,** lateral pulmonary arteriogram with caudal beam angulation. Severe stenosis of the right *(solid arrow)* and left pulmonary artery *(small curved arrow)*. Before balloon dilatation had failed. **E,** anteroposterior view after placement of a Palmaz stent. **F,** repeat pulmonary arteriogram. Lateral projection. No residual stenosis after stent placement *(arrow)*.   *(Continued)*

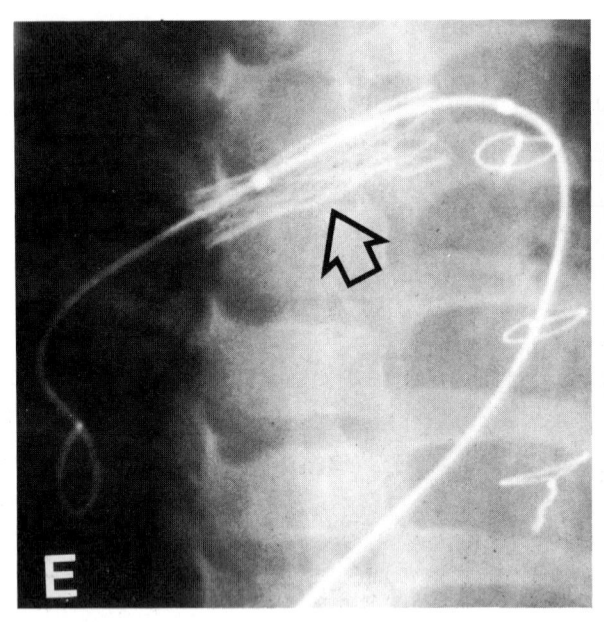

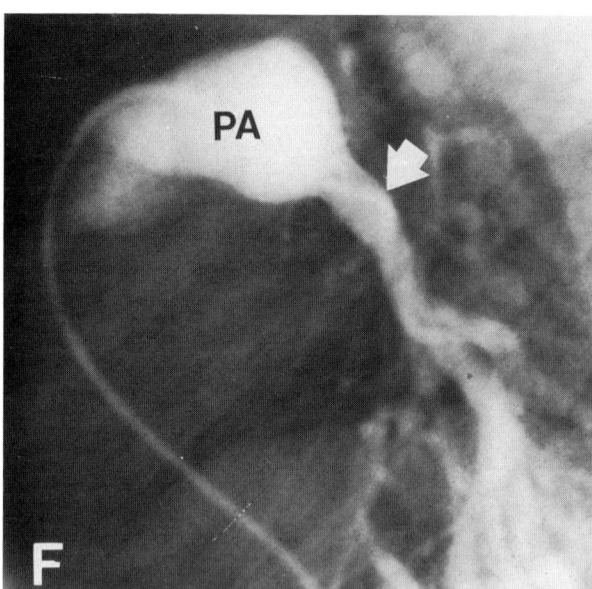

FIG 29-30 (cont.).

ISOLATED INFUNDIBULAR PULMONARY STENOSIS[18]

Usually, infundibular pulmonary stenosis coexists with ventricular septal defect (see Chapter 30). As an isolated lesion, it is an uncommon cause of right ventricular outflow obstruction.

Pathology

In stenosis of the os infundibuli, a localized narrowing of the infundibulum is present involving the junction of the right ventricle and the infundibulum (Fig 29-31).

Hemodynamics

The hemodynamic consequences of infundibular pulmonary stenosis resemble those of valvar pulmonary stenosis, but a pressure gradient is recorded below the level of the pulmonary valve.

Clinical Features

The history is indistinguishable from that in valvar pulmonary stenosis and depends on the severity of the obstruction. Cyanosis from a right-to-left shunt can develop in patients with moderate or severe stenosis and right-sided cardiac failure in patients with severe stenosis.

Physical Examination

Usually growth is normal. Although no clinical evidence of cardiac enlargement is found, on examination of the precordium, there may be a heave. The major auscul-

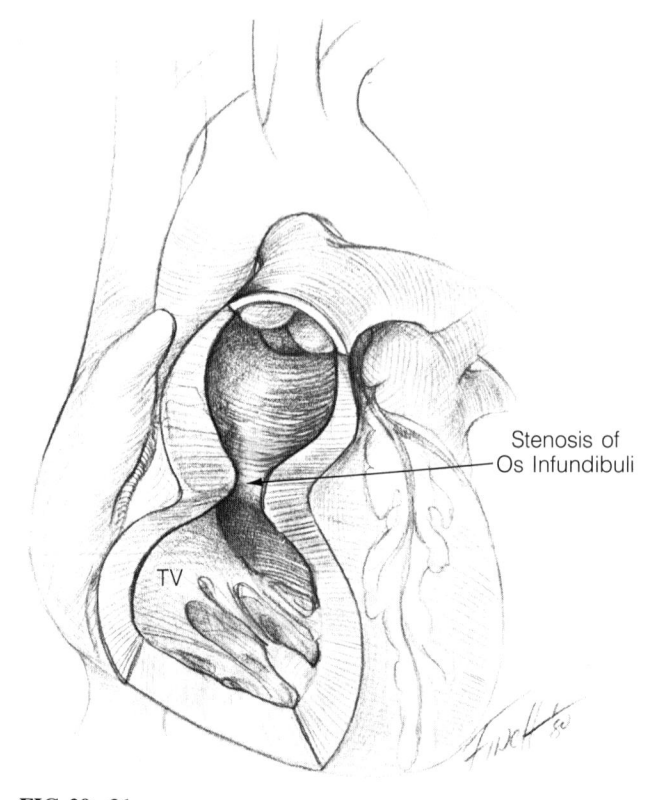

FIG 29-31.
Diagram of isolated infundibular pulmonary stenosis. Stenosis of os infundibulum. Right ventricle hypertrophied. Infundibular and pulmonary anulus normal size. *TV* = tricuspid valve.

tatory finding is a loud, usually grade 3 to 4/6 systolic ejection murmur, which is often associated with a thrill. This murmur may be located along the left sternal border rather than in the pulmonary area; but on the basis of the location of the murmur, infundibular stenosis cannot be distinguished from valvar stenosis. If the murmur is heard best along the left sternal border, it may be confused with that of a ventricular septal defect. The murmur may be widely transmitted.

Unlike the findings in valvar pulmonary stenosis, a pulmonary systolic ejection click is not heard because poststenotic dilatation is not present. Because of the stenosis, the pulmonary component of the second heart sound is delayed.

Electrocardiographic Features

The ECG is identical to that of valvar pulmonary stenosis.

Echocardiographic Features

The right ventricle may have an increased internal diameter and a thick wall. Unlike the findings in valvar pulmonary stenosis, echoes from the pulmonary valve are normal and do not show an accentuated *a* dip. The reason the *a* dip is absent is that the elevated right ventricular end-diastolic pressure is not transmitted beyond the obstruction and therefore does not reach the pulmonary valve.[19]

Fluttering of the pulmonary valve may be seen if there is a jet through the stenotic area that strikes the valve.

Radiographic Features

1. The cardiac configuration may be normal. REASON: Concentric hypertrophy does not enlarge the cardiac silhouette and may be difficult to see on thoracic roentgenograms.
2. Signs of right ventricular hypertrophy may be visible on a lateral or left anterior oblique projection.
3. The pulmonary vasculature is normal. REASON: The cardiac output is normal except in severe cases.
4. The pulmonary artery segment is normal or inconspicuous. REASON: Poststenotic dilatation of the pulmonary artery does not occur.
5. The roentgenographic findings may be identical to those of tetralogy of Fallot.

Cardiac Catheterization

The oximetry data are normal except in the occasional patient with a right-to-left shunt at the atrial level. A systolic gradient is found within the right ventricle at the level of the infundibulum. The systolic pressure beyond the obstruction is identical to the systolic pressure in the pulmonary artery.

In severe infundibular stenosis, the right ventricular end-diastolic and right atrial pressures are elevated.

Angiographic Appearance

1. Increased trabeculations of the right ventricle. REASON: Right ventricle hypertrophy secondary to infundibular obstruction.
2. Persistent narrowing of the infundibulum in the anteroposterior projection because of marked prominence of the parietal and septal bands of the crista (stenosis of the os infundibuli) (Fig 29–32).
3. Narrowing of the infundibulum on the lateral view. REASON: Narrowing caused by the crista supraventricularis posteriorly.

If the stenosis changes somewhat during systole and diastole, a muscular type of obstruction can be predicted. Stenosis of the os infundibuli should not be confused with an anomalous muscle bundle, which is outlined circumferentially by contrast medium and is more readily resectable. On rare occasion, an anomalous muscle bundle is in intimate contact with the wall of the ventricle, preventing circumferential delineation. Under those circumstances, the differentiation from isolated infundibular stenosis may be impossible.

Operative Considerations

Indications for operation include cyanosis, congestive cardiac failure, and a gradient of more than 50 mm Hg. Unlike valvar pulmonary stenosis, the degree of stenosis may increase with age because of increasing right ventricular hypertrophy.

The stenotic area can be excised through a right ventriculotomy. If the infundibulum is diffusely narrowed or the muscle cannot be sufficiently excised, an outflow patch is indicated to widen the infundibular area.

SUBINFUNDIBULAR PULMONARY STENOSIS

Stenotic lesions may occur in the body of the right ventricle below the infundibulum, causing stenosis, which may be severe. These stenotic lesions may occur either as an isolated lesion or in association with ventricular septal defect. The former are discussed here and include:

1. Anomalous muscle bundles.
2. Windsock deformity of the tricuspid valve.

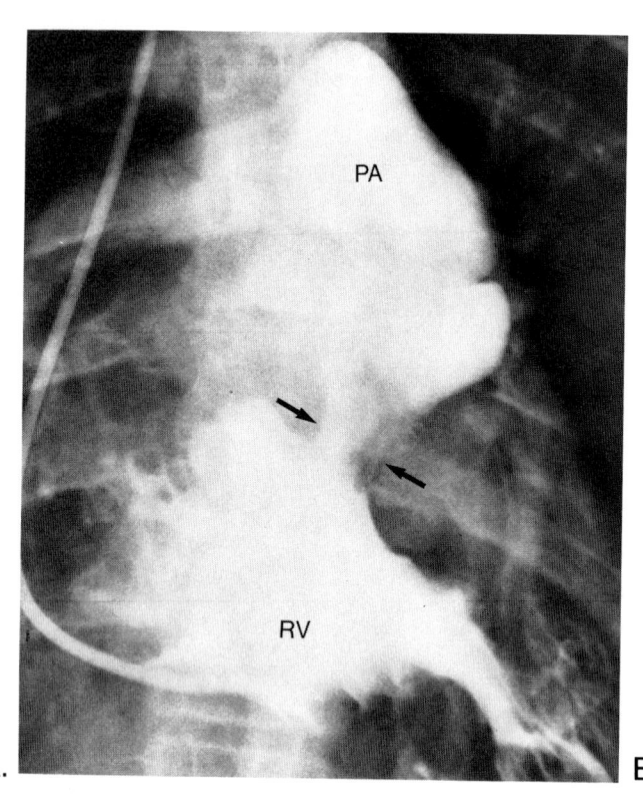

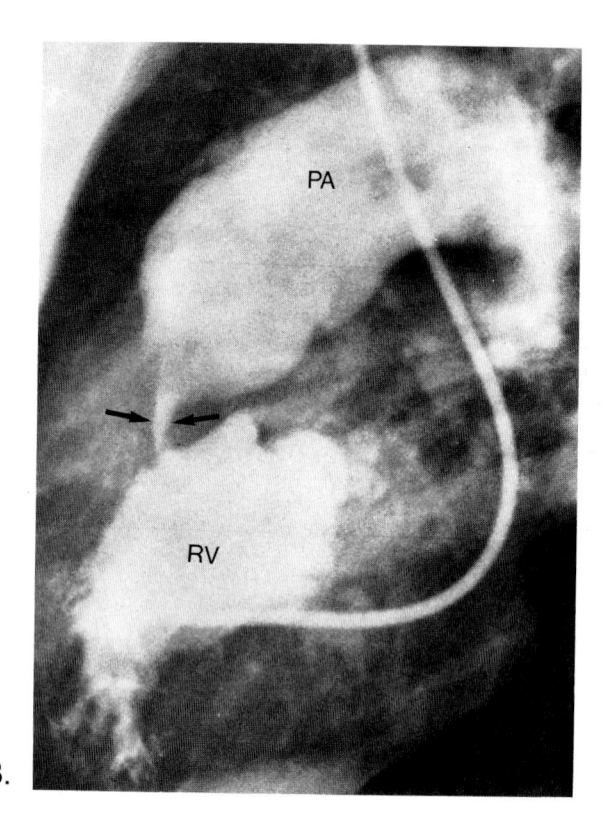

FIG 29–32.
Right ventriculogram *(RV)* in infundibular pulmonary stenosis in anteroposterior **(A)** and lateral **(B)** projections. Severe localized stenosis of os infundibulum *(arrows)*. Narrowing is concentric caused by a huge septal and parietal bands of the crista supraventricularis and did not change significantly between systole and diastole, in contrast to infundibular stenosis secondary to right ventricular hypertrophy. *PA* = pulmonary artery.

3. Accessory tricuspid valvar tissue.
4. Stenosis from thickened ventricular septum.

Anomalous Muscle Bundles in the Right Ventricle[20, 21]

This condition has also been called the "two-chambered right ventricle," because the right ventricular cavity is divided by muscle masses into a proximal high-pressure chamber and a distal low-pressure area.

Pathology

One or more muscle masses attach to the septal wall near the base of the anterior papillary muscle and pass in an anteroposterior direction to attach into the anterior wall of the right ventricle. Thus, these bundles cross the main stream of blood flow through the right ventricle and are located in the apical or inflow portion of the right ventricle (Fig 29–33). At the time of surgery, the attachment of the muscle bundle to the free right ventricular wall can be seen from the surface of the right ventricle as a "dimple." The hypertrophied moderator band originates lower, near the apex, and may not cause hemodynamic obstruction, which is also true of muscle bundles in other locations within the right ventricle.

Clinical Features

The history and physical examination resemble those of valvar and of infundibular pulmonary stenosis. The feature is a loud long ejection murmur, which is maximally heard along the midleft sternal border and is associated with a thrill. No click is present. The degree of splitting of the second sound and the intensity of P_2 may be normal in contrast to other forms of pulmonary stenosis.

Electrocardiographic Features

The ECG features are indistinguishable from those of infundibular stenosis.

Echocardiographic Features

No echocardiographic features have been reported to our knowledge; they may well be normal.

Radiographic Features

1. The thoracic roentgenogram may be entirely normal. REASON: Muscle bundles may be nonobstructive or cause only mild obstruction. Poststenotic dilatation of the main pulmonary artery is absent.

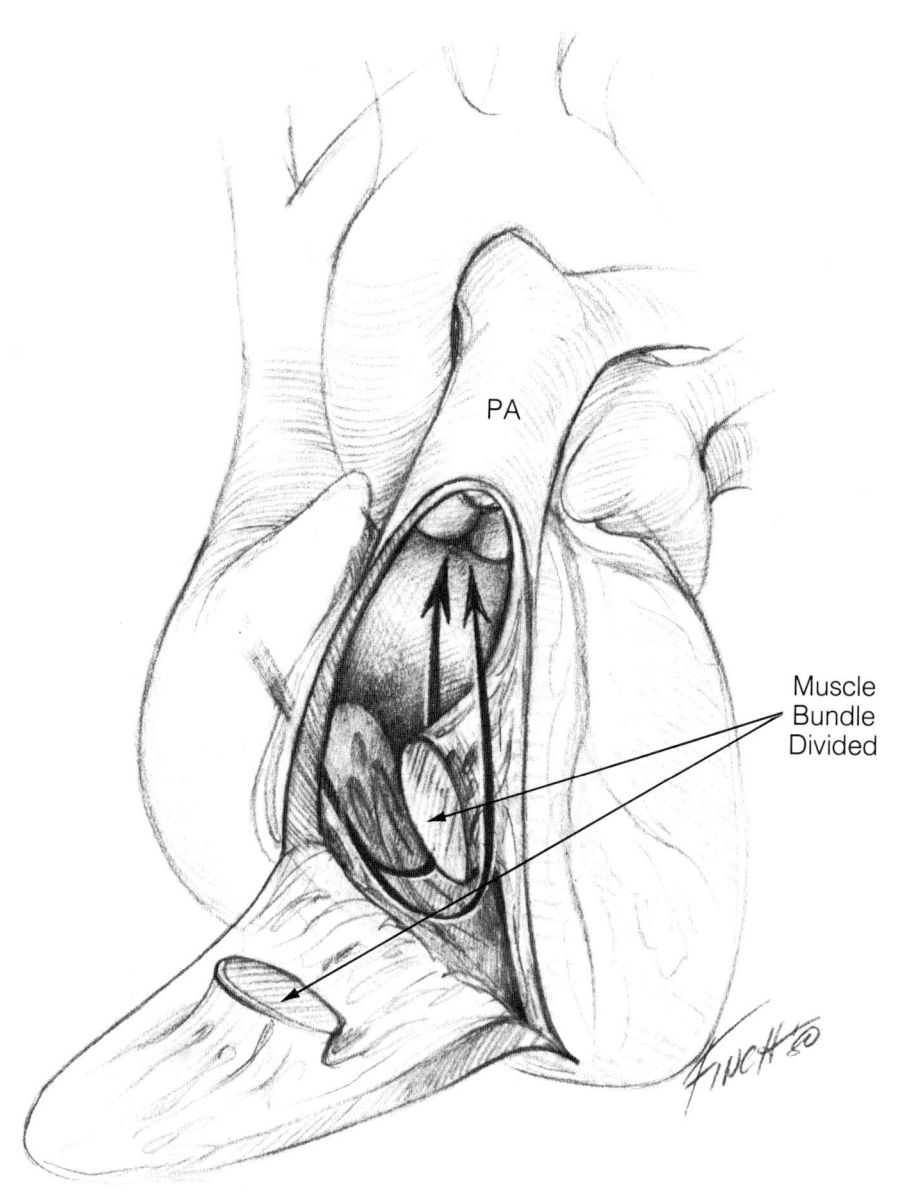

FIG 29-33.
Diagram of opened right ventricle showing a large anomalous muscle bundle that has been divided. Bundle extends from anterior wall to interventricular septum, dividing right ventricle into two chambers (two-chambered right ventricle). Blood flow around muscle bundle indicated by arrows. *PA* = pulmonary artery.

2. The pulmonary vasculature is normal. REASON: Pulmonary flow is normal provided there is no associated ventricular septal defect.

3. Muscle bundles may be part of other congenital defects. Associated ventricular septal defects are common above the muscle bundle, resulting in a left-to-right shunt.

Cardiac Catheterization

The oximetry data and catheter course are normal. The important data are obtained on withdrawal. A systolic pressure gradient is found low in the right ventricle, at times within a few centimeters of the tricuspid valve. This gradient may be missed if a continuous withdrawal pressure is not obtained through the right ventricle from the pulmonary artery to the right atrium.

Angiographic Appearance

Anomalous muscle bundles may be located in either the inflow portion or the outflow portion of the right ventricle. They should not be confused with increased right ventricular myocardial trabeculations, which are protruding muscle tissue seen along the edges of the right ventricle in patients with right ventricular hypertrophy (see Fig 29–6). Muscle bundles attach to the free wall of the right ventricle and extend across the right ventricular cavity to attach to the septal wall of the ventricle.

1. Anomalous muscle bundles form well-circumscribed round filling defects, which are outlined by contrast medium on an anteroposterior angiogram (Fig 29–34). REASON: Most muscle bundles course in an ante-

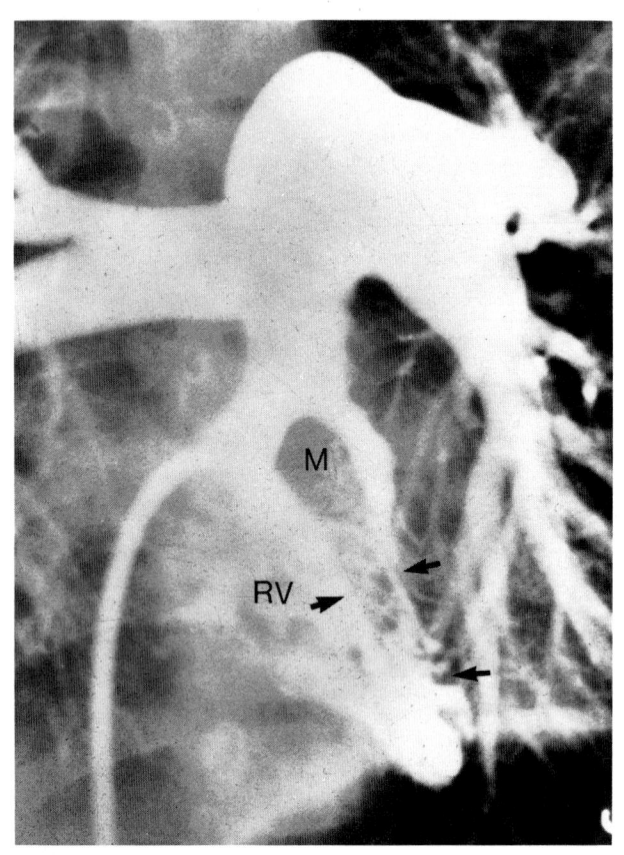

FIG 29–34.
Right ventriculogram *(RV)*, anteroposterior projection showing anomalous muscle bundle attached to free ventricular wall near apex. Typical muscle bundle *(M)* outlined by contrast medium. Note difference in appearance from increased trabeculations *(arrows)*.

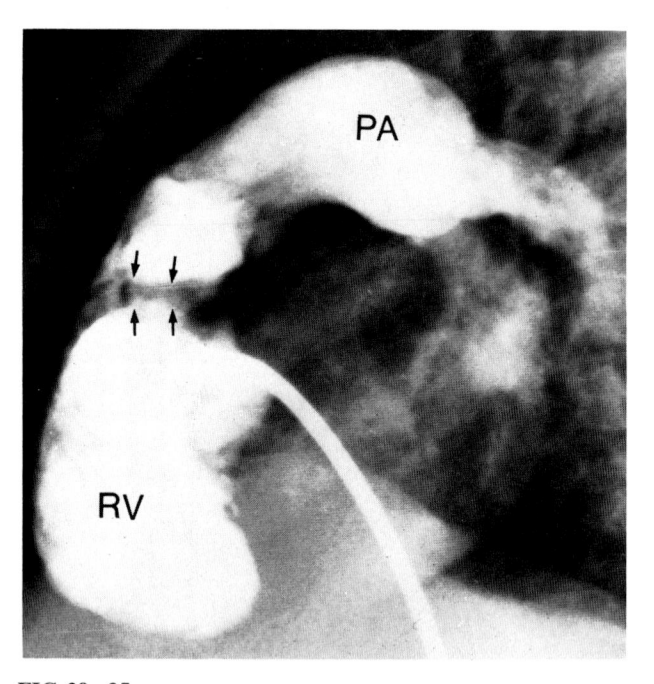

FIG 29–35.
Right ventriculogram *(RV)*, lateral projection showing anomalous muscle bundles. Radiolucent band *(arrows)* formed by muscle bundle, which extends from anterior right ventricular wall to interventricular septum. *PA* = pulmonary artery.

rior to posterior direction and lie more or less parallel to the x-ray beam, so they are seen on end. If the x-ray beam is angled toward the feet, muscle bundles are difficult to see on this projection. If muscle bundles are suspected on the basis of a pressure gradient, a right ventriculogram should be performed in a straight anteroposterior with no or caudal beam angulation.

2. On a lateral projection, muscle bundles form radiolucent bands which are less obvious (Fig 29–35).

3. Rarely, a muscle bundle is not circumferentially outlined by contrast medium if it touches the wall of the ventricle so that contrast medium cannot surround it.

4. Muscle bundles which extend obliquely from the apical area toward the septal wall (moderator bands) are not well seen on a lateral projection (Fig 29–36) and not well seen on an anteroposterior projection, because the direction of the muscle bundle is no longer parallel to the x-ray beam.

5. Muscle bundles may be either single or multiple (Fig 29–37).

6. When an anomalous muscle bundle coexists with a ventricular septal defect, it may partially occlude it and limit the volume of left-to-right shunt (Fig 29–38).

Two jets may be formed in the right ventricle, simulating two muscular septal defects (see Chapter 12), which could be erroneously interpreted as two separate ventricular septal defects.

Operative Considerations

The indications for operation are similar to those in infundibular stenosis but are perhaps more lenient, because anomalous muscle bundles tend to increase in severity with age and surgical excision results in cure.

Under cardiopulmonary bypass, a longitudinal ventriculotomy is performed. The muscle bundles may obscure the view of the tricuspid valve. The muscle bundles are divided from their attachment to the free wall of the right ventricle, and then their septal attachment is resected, taking care to avoid injury to the tricuspid valve. The attachment of the muscle bundle to the anterior ventricular wall can be seen by the surgeon without opening the ventricle, because it forms a dimple during systole.

The combination of a muscle bundle and a ventricular septal defect may present a confusing anatomical picture to the operating surgeon. Care must be taken to sew the patch over the true ventricular septal defect leading to the left ventricle.

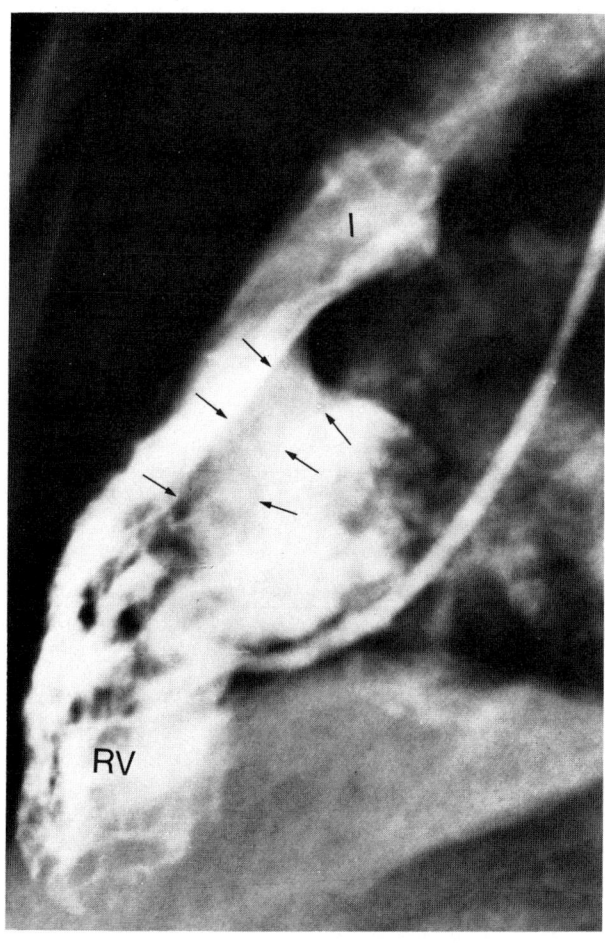

FIG 29–36.
Right ventriculogram *(RV)*, lateral projection showing anomalous muscle bundles. Anomalous muscle bundle extends obliquely from apical portion of right ventricle toward infundibulum and causes well-circumscribed radiolucent band *(arrows)*. Valvar pulmonary stenosis coexists. These oblique muscle bundles are usually referred to as hypertrophied moderator bands.

Rare Causes of Right Ventricular Outflow Obstruction

There are several rare causes of right ventricular outflow obstruction which can be identified correctly by angiography.[22-25]

Pouchlike Structures in the Right Ventricle

Pouchlike structures may originate from the right atrium or tricuspid valve. These saillike pouches prolapse during systole into the body of the right ventricle or, at times, into the infundibulum or to the level of the pulmonary valve, causing right-sided outflow obstruction.

There are three types of abnormalities:

1. Large saillike pouches originating from the right atrium Fig 29–39). This has been called a "spinnaker" or "windsock." In this rare type of obstruction, a pouch arises in the right atrium and passes through the tricuspid valve

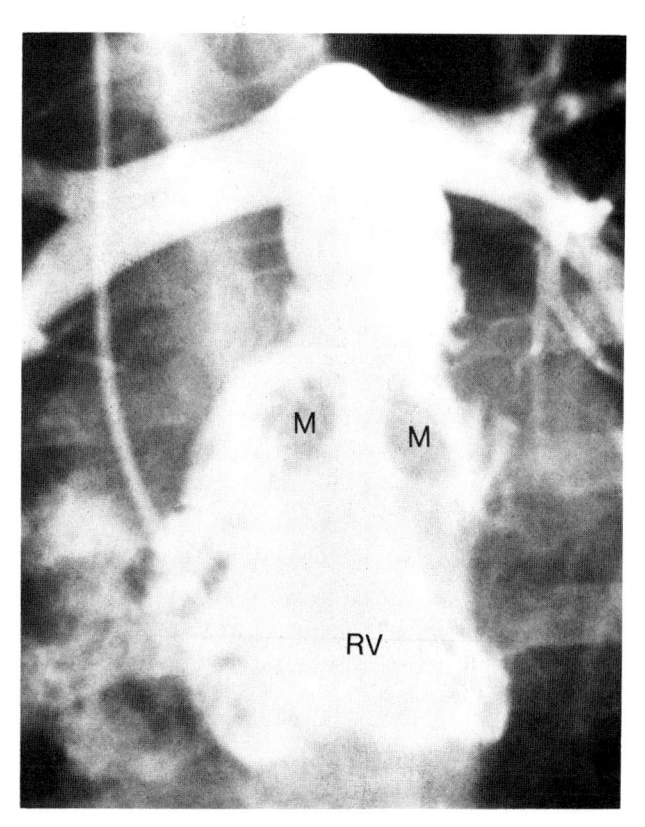

FIG 29–37.
Right ventriculogram *(RV)*, anteroposterior projection showing two anomalous muscle bundles *(M)*.

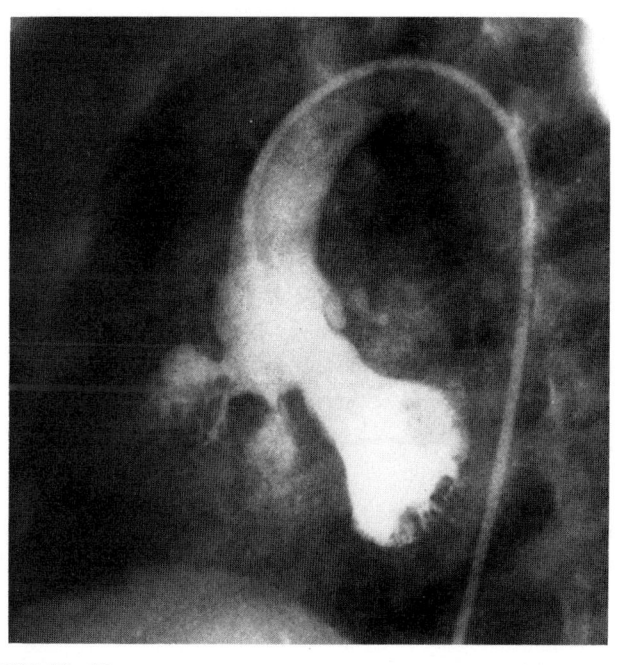

FIG 29–38.
Left ventriculogram, left anterior oblique projection showing anomalous muscle bundle and ventricular septal defect. Anomalous muscle bundles partially close ventricular septal defect, with jets of contrast material above and below muscle bundles.

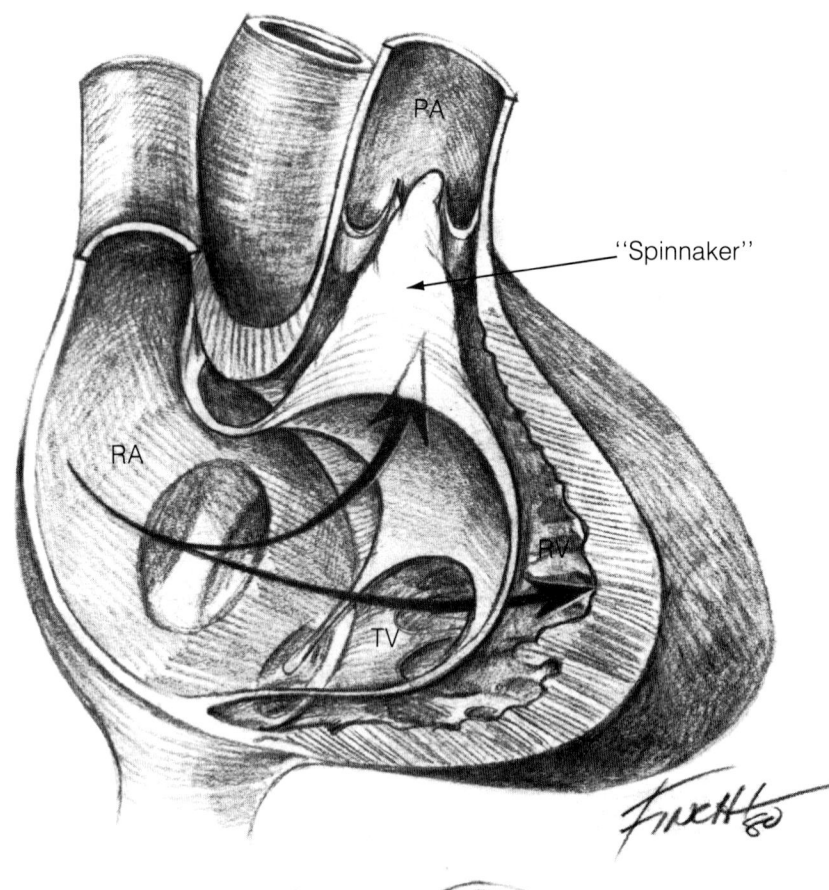

FIG 29–39.
Diagram of opened right atrium and ventricle. Spinnaker originates from right atrium and prolapses through tricuspid valve into right ventricle and through pulmonary valve. This saillike structure originates from right atrium and is believed to be a remnant of the sinus venosus valve. PA = pulmonary artery; RA = right atrium.

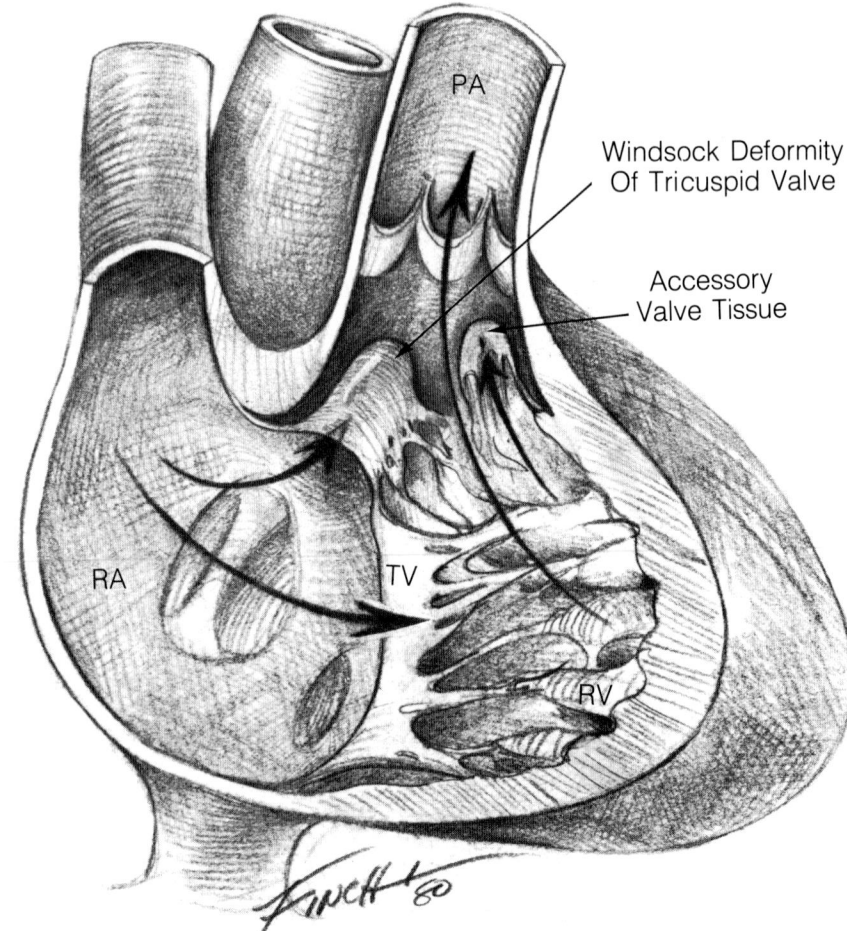

FIG 29–40.
Diagram of opened right atrium (RA) and ventricle (RV). Pouchlike extension (S) of tricuspid valve (TV) (windsock of tricuspid valve). Chordae tendineae attach edge of pouch to ventricular septum. Parachute-like structure of accessory tricuspid valve tissue (A) attaches directly to outflow of right ventricle, causing obstruction. PA = pulmonary artery.

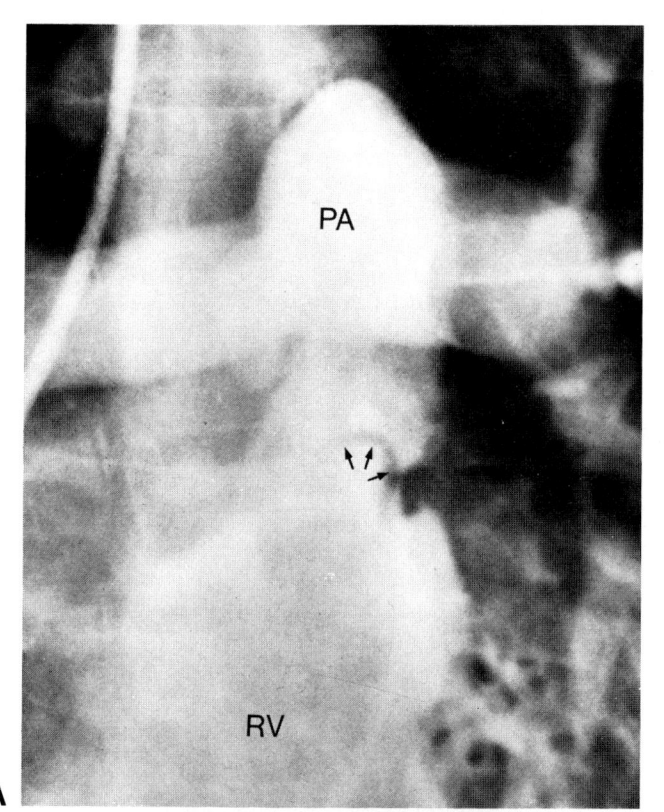

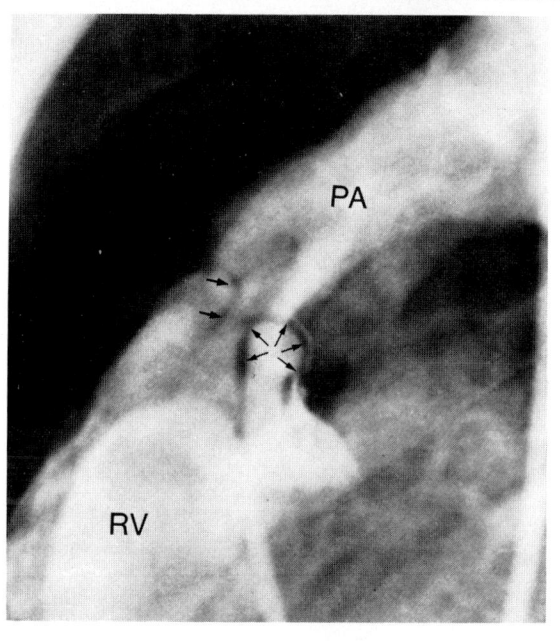

FIG 29–41.
Right ventriculogram *(RV)* showing pouches of tricuspid valve. **A,** anteroposterior projection; right ventricular outflow tract obstruction from saillike structures *(arrows)*. These are identified better on lateral projection. **B,** lateral projection; posterior pouch–like structure (windsock of the tricuspid valve). Anterior pouch *(small arrow)* attaches directly to outflow tract and represents acccessory tricuspid valve tissue. *PA* = pulmonary artery.

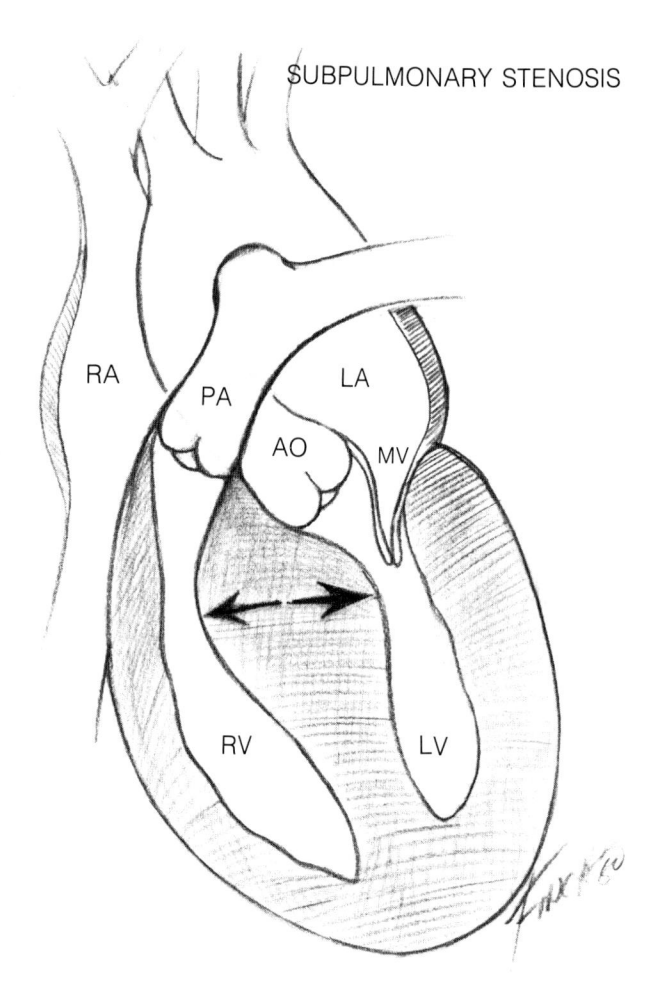

FIG 29–42.
Diagram of mechanism of right and left ventricular outflow obstruction caused by thickening of ventricular septum *(arrows)*. A symmetric septal hypertrophy (see Chapter 26) *AO* = aorta; *LA* = left atrium; *LV* = left ventricle; *MV* = mitral valve; *PA* = pulmonary artery; *RA* = right atrium; *RV* = right ventricle.

and prolapses during systole into the outflow tract or even through the pulmonary valve. This windsock or spinnaker attaches to the right atrium and is believed to represent a remnant of the right sinus venosus valve. Spinnakers may cause tricuspid insufficiency and, sometimes, hemodynamic right-sided obstruction.

2. Pouches arising from the tricuspid valve (Fig 29–40). Saillike structures and pouches may be formed by accessory tricuspid valve tissue. These parachute-like structures are attached by chordae tendineae to the right ventricle, the ventricular wall, the edge of the ventricular septal defect, or papillary muscle. They also prolapse during systole and may cause outflow obstruction. There are no distinctive clinical or laboratory features.

Angiograms performed within the right ventricle will show the accessory tricuspid valve leaflets by outlining both sides of the tissue by contrast material (Fig 29–41).

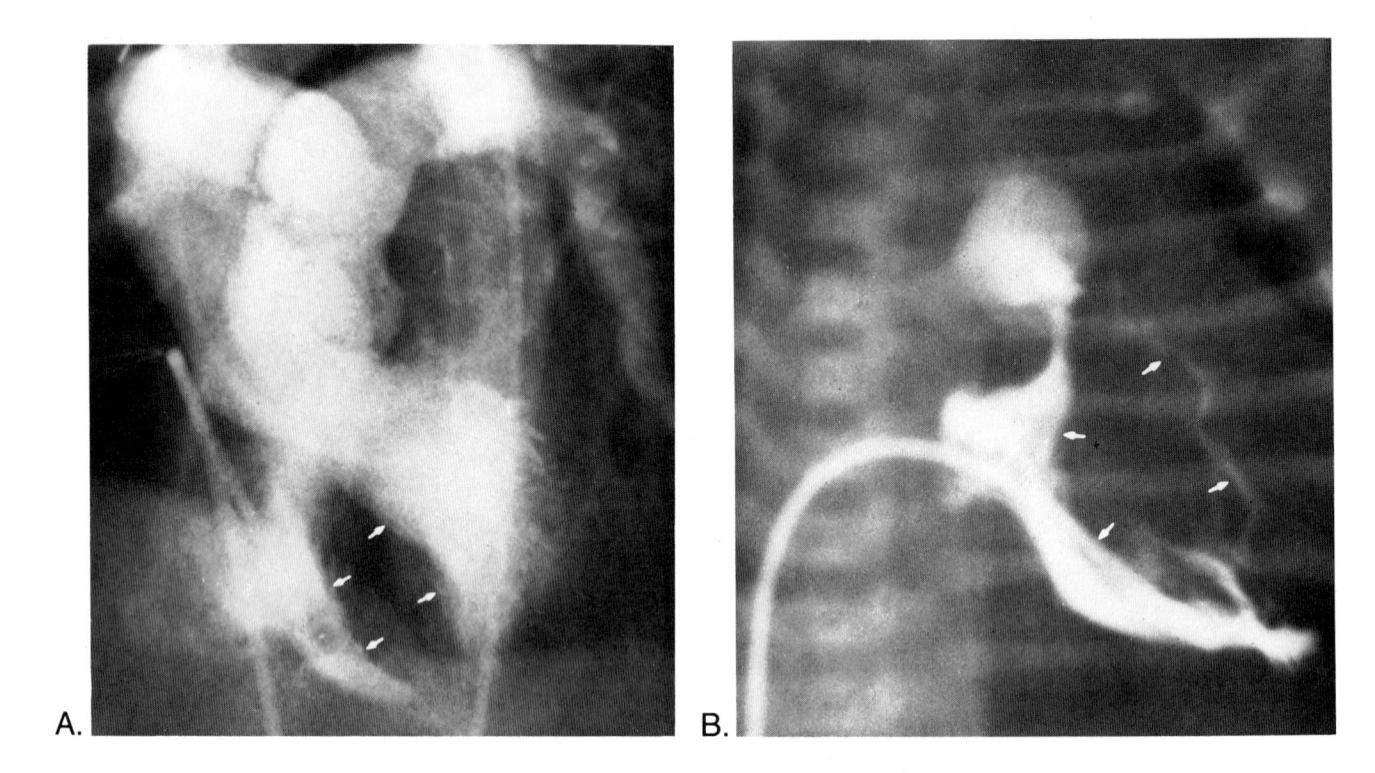

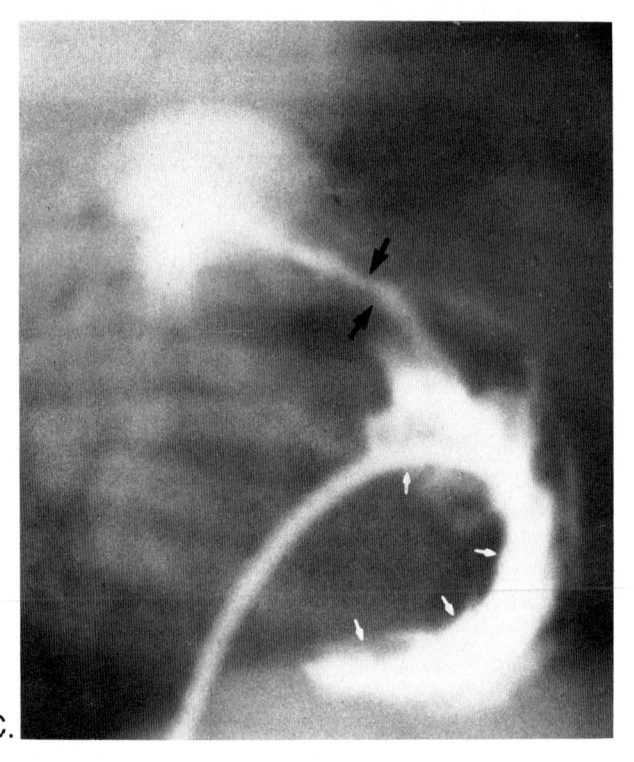

FIG 29-43.
Subpulmonary stenosis and hypertrophied interventricular septum. **A,** angiogram with simultaneous injection of right and left ventricles, left anterior oblique projection. Thickening of interventricular septum *(arrows)*. Significant right ventricular outflow gradient present. **B,** anteroposterior projection. Idiopathic hypertrophy of ventricular septum with encroachment on right ventricular cavity *(white arrows)*. **C,** lateral projection. Severe stenosis right ventricular outflow tract. Subvalvar jet *(black arrows)* formed. Subvalvar jet should not be confused with valvar pulmonary jet. (Pulmonary valve does not dome.)

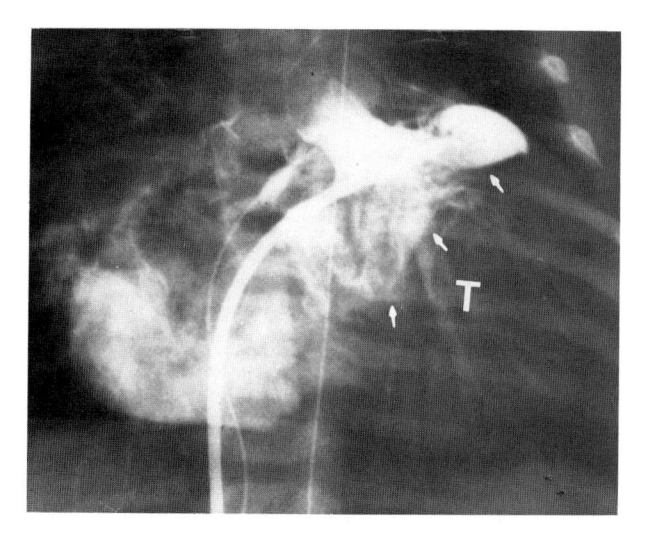

FIG 29–44.
Right ventriculogram, anteroposterior projection showing rhabdomyoma of interventricular septum. Marked encroachment on right ventricular cavity by large infiltrating tumor *(T) (arrows)*.

3. Accessory tricuspid valve tissue with attachment to the outflow tract of the right ventricle (see Fig 29–40).

Subpulmonary Stenosis Caused by Hypertrophied Interventricular Septum

Thickening of the ventricular septum may encroach on the left ventricular outflow tract, causing left-sided obstruction. Sometimes it also encroaches on the right ventricular outflow tract, causing right-sided outflow tract obstruction as well (Bernheim phenomenon) (Fig 29–42). Thickening of the ventricular septum may have many causes, such as asymmetric septal hypertrophy or glycogen storage disease. For unknown reasons, infants born of diabetic mothers have a thickened ventricular septum. A thickened septum is best seen by echocardiography or by simultaneous injection of the right and left ventricles (Fig 29–43). Rare causes of right outflow obstruction are cardiac tumors encroaching on the right ventricular outflow tract (Fig 29–44), prolapsing tumors arising in the right atrium, sinus of Valsalva aneurysm (Fig 29–46) (see

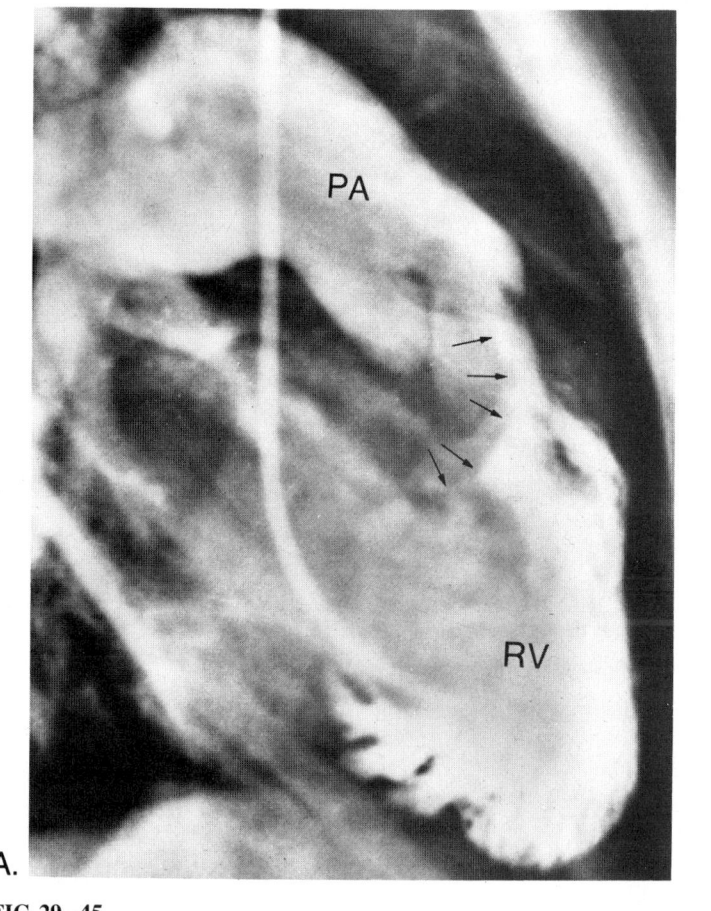

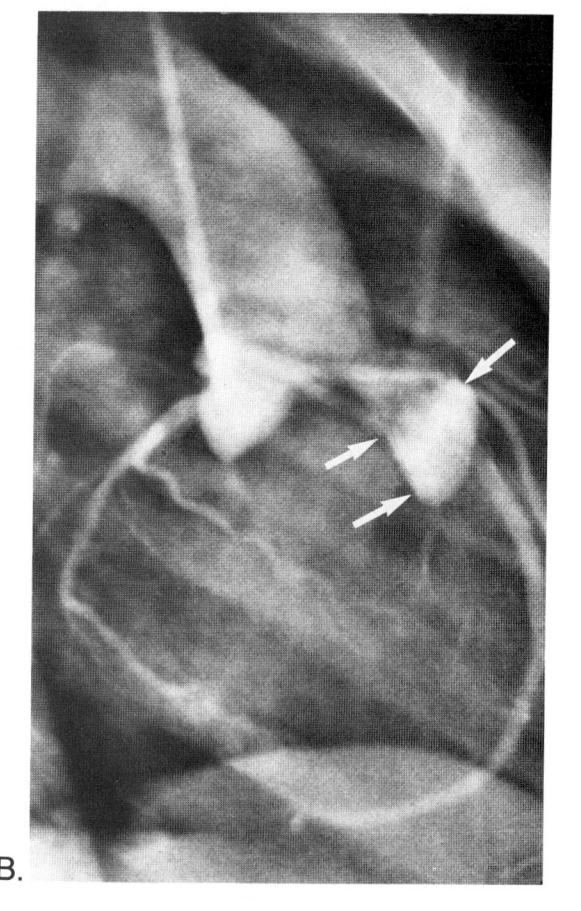

FIG 29–45.
Prolapse of aortic cusp through ventricular septal defect. **A,** right ventriculogram *(RV)*, lateral projection. Round filling defect *(arrows)* in right ventricular outflow tract causes significant obstruction. **B,** aortogram, lateral projection. Prolapse of aortic cusp *(arrow)* responsible for right-sided outflow tract obstruction. *PA* = pulmonary artery.

528 Outflow Obstructive Lesions

Chapter 24), aneurysm of the membranous septum (Fig 29–47) (see Chapter 12), and prolapsing aortic cusps (Fig 29–45) (see Chapter 26).

The typical angiographic features of subaortic stenosis causing left ventricular obstruction have been discussed in Chapter 26.

1. During right ventriculography, impingement on the right ventricle, as by a bulging septum, may be seen on the lateral projection.
2. Large filling defects are produced. REASON: The contrast medium is squeezed from the outflow tract because the septum impinges on the anterior wall of the right ventricle. Contrast is retained in trabeculations.

Prolapse of the Aortic Cusp

If a ventricular septal defect is located immediately beneath the aortic valve, one of the valve leaflets may lose its support and prolapse through the ventricular septal defect into the right ventricle. A negative filling defect can be demonstrated by right ventriculography (see Fig 29–45).

Sinus of Valsalva Aneurysm

An unruptured sinus of Valsalva aneurysm may extend into the right ventricular outflow tract and cause obstruction. An atypical round filling defect is demonstrated in the right ventricular outflow tract during right ventriculography (Fig 29–46). Aortography shows the aneurysm delineated by contrast medium. An aneurysm of the ventricular membranous septum (Fig 29–47) causes a similar but smaller filling defect.

Cardiac Tumors (See Chapter 73)

Rarely, a pedunculated right atrial myxoma prolapses through the tricuspid valve into the right ventricular out-

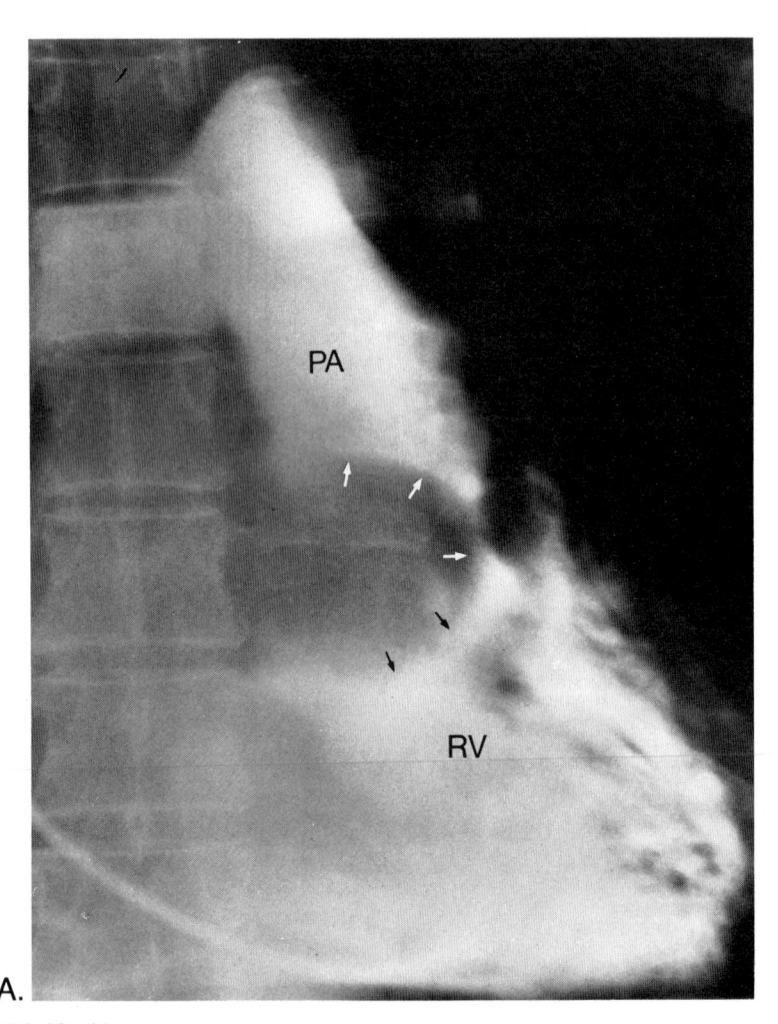

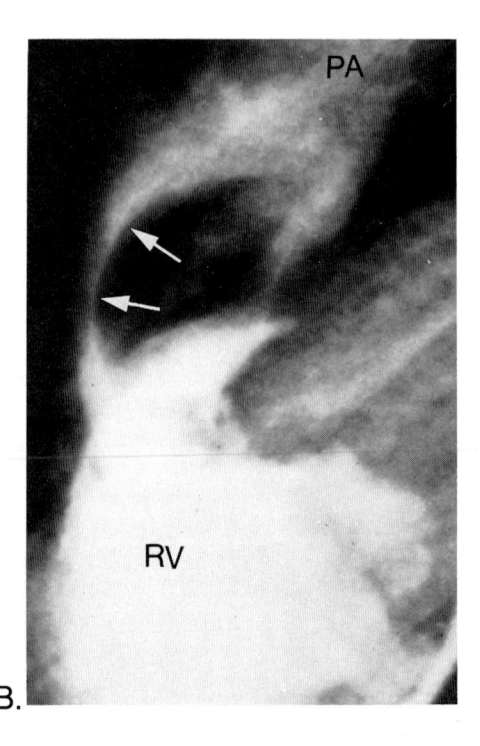

FIG 29–46.
Right ventriculogram *(RV)* showing sinus of Valsalva aneurysm. **A,** anteroposterior projection; atypical round filling defect *(arrows)* in high right ventricle, causing severe obstruction. **B,** lateral projection; encroachment on right ventricular outflow tract *(arrows)*. Aortography is required for differentiation from prolapsing aortic cusp. **C,** drawing of sinus of Valsalva aneurysm.   *(Continued.)*

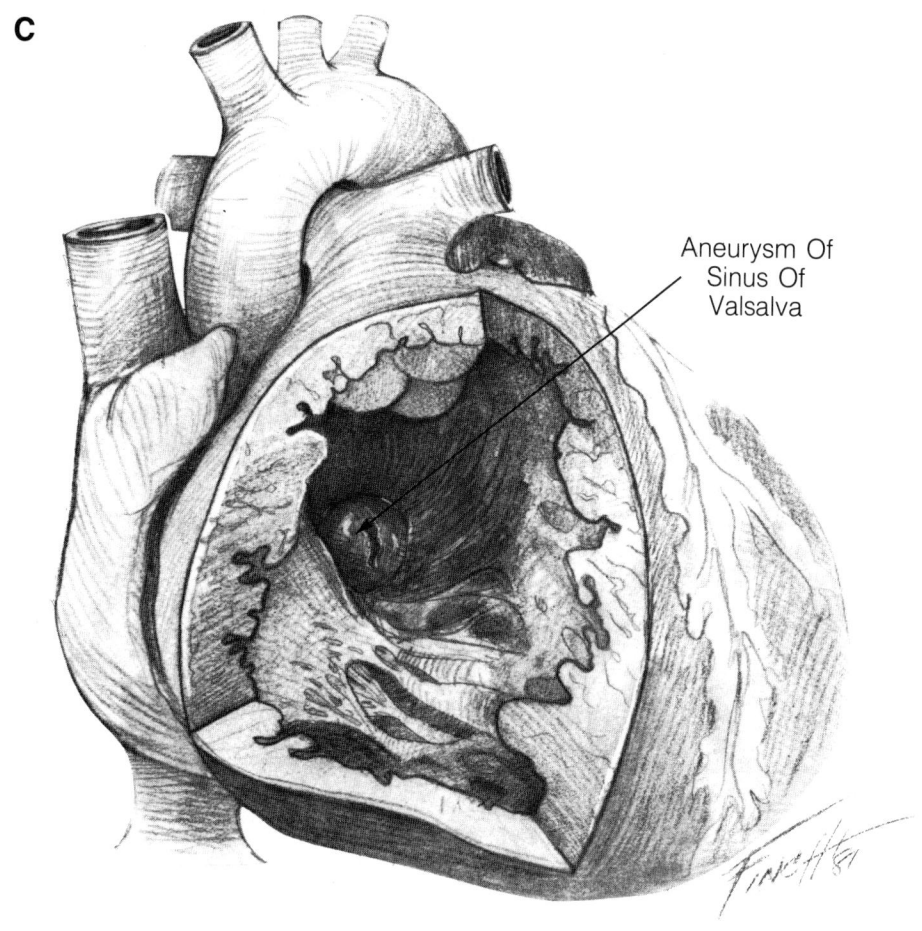

FIG 29-46 (cont.).

flow tract. Rhabdomyoma is a rare nonpedunculated tumor that infiltrates the myocardium. The right and left ventricular cavities may be encroached on by a large tumor mass.

Residual Stenosis After Removal of a Pulmonary Arterial Band

Pulmonary arterial bands may be placed too close to the pulmonary valve, which results in thickening of the pulmonary valve because of the impact of the valve leaflets on the constricted area of the pulmonary artery (Fig 29-48).

Properly placed bands may migrate toward the bifurcation of the main pulmonary artery and cause stenosis of the origin of the right, left, or both pulmonary arteries. Bands that migrate cause a characteristic angiographic diverticulum-like deformity of the main pulmonary artery. Stenosis of the right pulmonary artery is more common (Fig 29-49), because the origin of the right pulmonary artery from the pulmonary trunk is at a right angle. Stenosis of the left pulmonary artery occurs less commonly because of the direction of its origin from the main pulmonary artery.

IDIOPATHIC DILATATION OF THE PULMONARY ARTERY

Idiopathic dilatation of the pulmonary artery may represent a very mild form of pulmonary stenosis or be a primary abnormality of the pulmonary trunk. These patients are asymptomatic. Auscultatory findings are a pulmonary systolic ejection click and a short soft pulmonary systolic ejection murmur. The second heart sound is normal. A murmur of pulmonary insufficiency may be found.

Electrocardiographic Features

The ECG is normal.

Cardiac Catheterization

Cardiac catheterization data may be normal or show a small (10-15 mm Hg) gradient across the pulmonary valve.

Radiographic Features

Thoracic roentgenograms are indistinguishable from those in valvar pulmonary stenosis. In spite of the absence

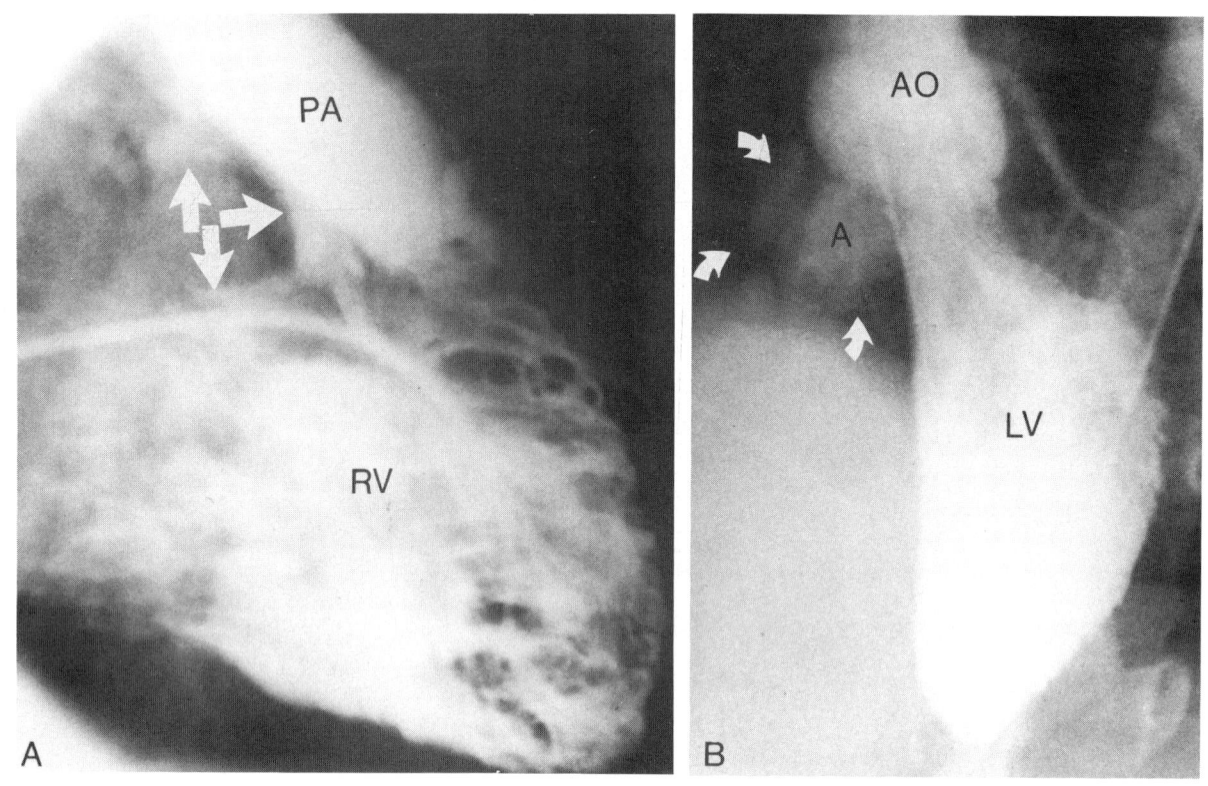

FIG 29–47.
A, right ventriculogram. Right anterior oblique projection. Large filling defect is present in the right ventricle *(arrows).* **B,** left ventriculogram. Left anterior oblique projection. A large aneurysm *(A) (arrows)* is demonstrated, accounting for the filling defect in the right ventricle.

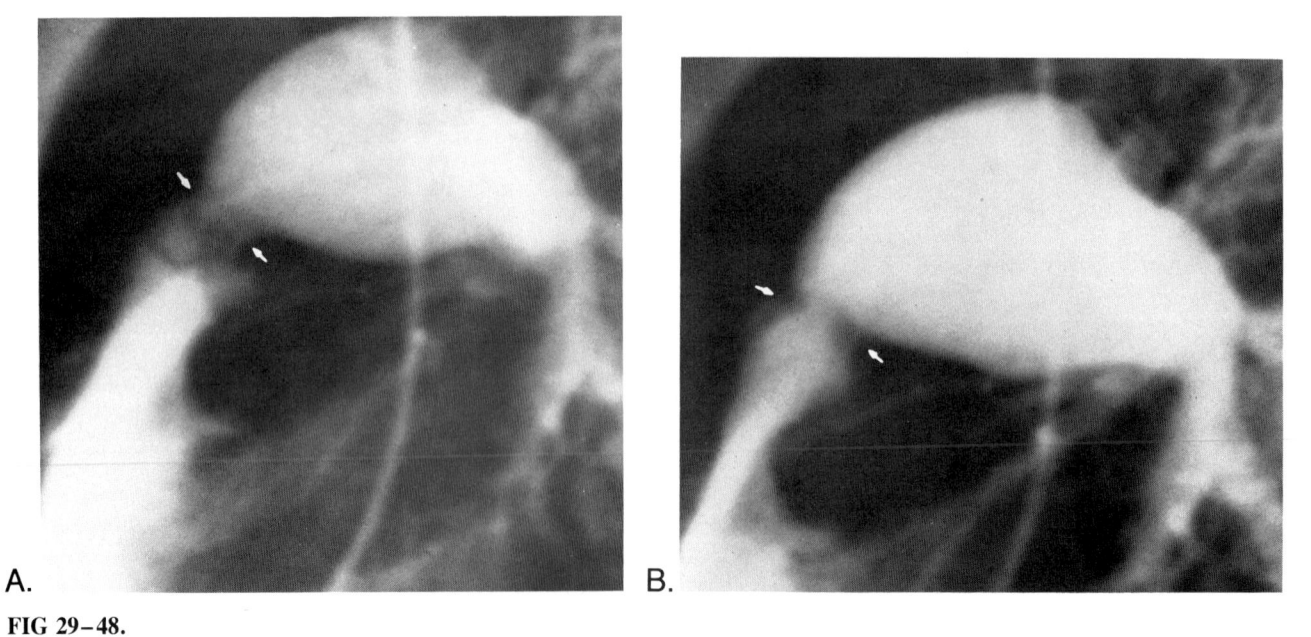

FIG 29–48.
Right ventriculogram, lateral projection showing pulmonary arterial band. **A,** diastolic view; pulmonary band *(arrows)* immediately above level of pulmonary valve. Thickening of pulmonary valvar leaflets caused by impact of valve leaflets against band. **B,** systolic view; pseudodoming of pulmonary valve because of impairment of motion of valve leaflets by constricting band *(arrows).*

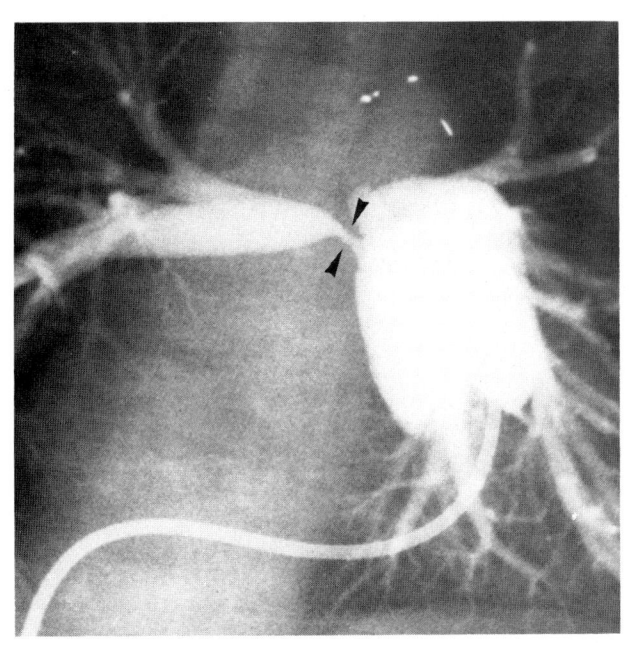

FIG 29-49.
Pulmonary arteriogram, cranially angulated anteroposterior projection showing pulmonary artery banding. Band located at bifurcation of pulmonary artery. Severe stenosis *(arrow)* of right pulmonary artery.

of a significant pressure gradient across the pulmonary valve, the pulmonary artery segment is markedly enlarged. Poststenotic dilatation of the left pulmonary artery may be absent. There is no correlation between the pressure gradient and the degree of poststenotic dilatation of the pulmonary artery.

Angiographic Appearance

1. The pulmonary valve is seen to dome as in valvar stenosis, supporting the concept that idiopathic pulmonary artery dilatation represents valvar pulmonary stenosis with no significant pressure gradient (Fig 29-50).

2. A well-defined jet is absent. REASON: Although the commissures of the valve are partially fused, the orifice is large, thus preventing the formation of a visible jet.

BICUSPID PULMONARY VALVE[26]

In a less common type of pulmonary stenosis, the pulmonary valve is bicuspid (Fig 29-51).[27] One of the commissures is fused or does not develop. Therefore, during systole, the pulmonary orifice is restricted, and the valve domes in a manner similar to a bicuspid aortic valve (see Chapter 26). Usually, the cusps are of equal size. As an isolated anomaly, bicuspid pulmonary valve is rare, but it is very common in tetralogy of Fallot, in which 90% of

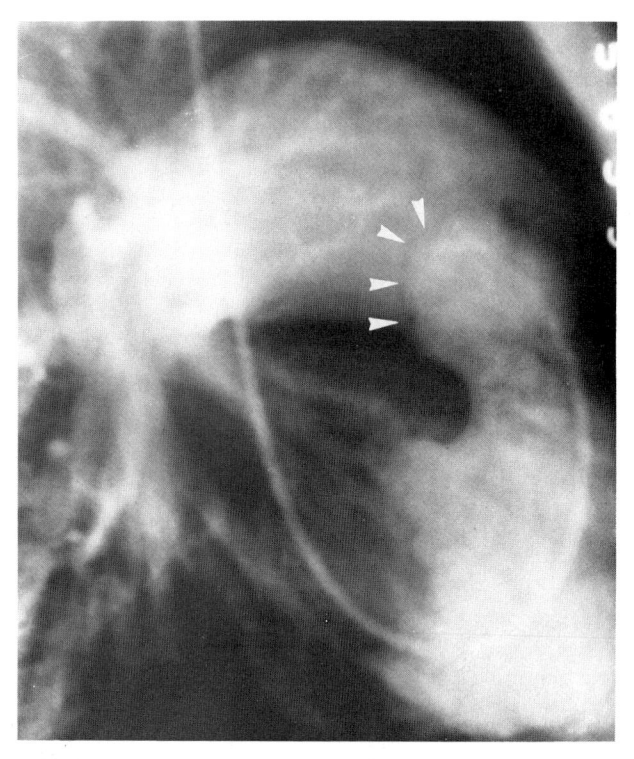

FIG 29-50.
Right ventriculogram, lateral projection showing idiopathic pulmonary dilatation. Doming of pulmonary valve *(arrows)*. Marked dilatation of main pulmonary artery but no dilatation of left pulmonary artery. No jet observed.

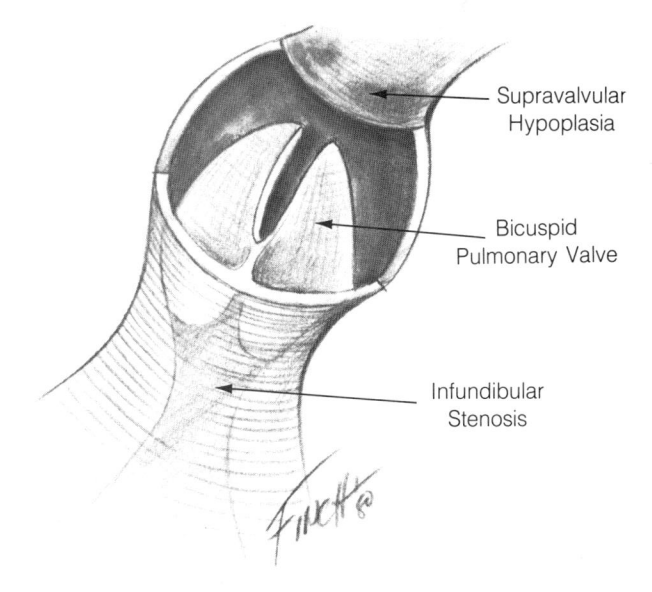

FIG 29-51.
Diagram of bicuspid pulmonary valve in tetralogy of Fallot and supravalvar narrowing of main pulmonary artery *(arrows)*.

532 Outflow Obstructive Lesions

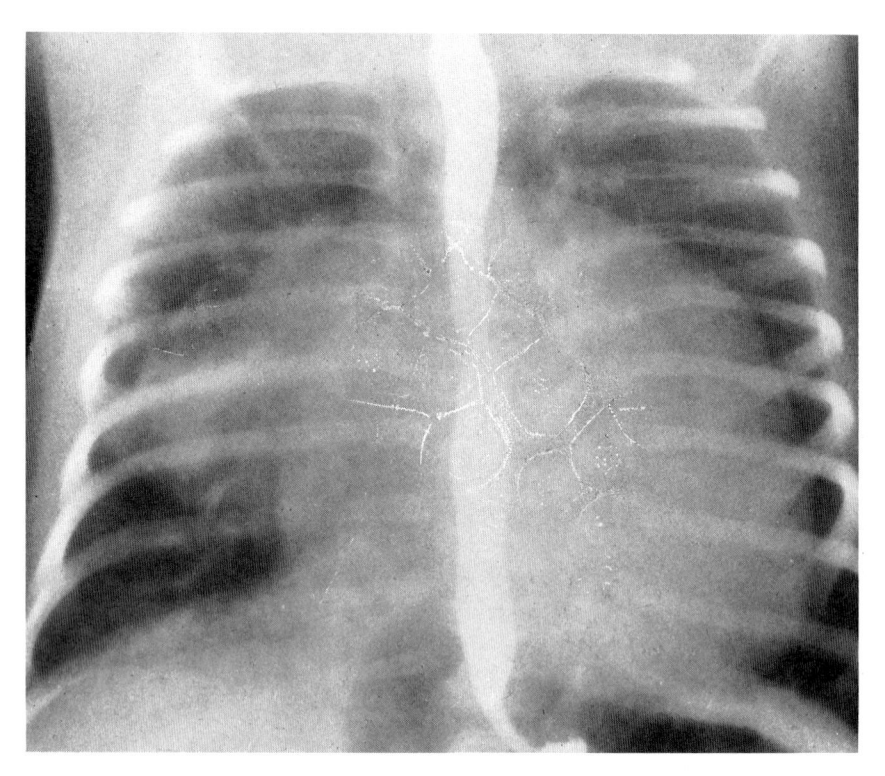

FIG 29–52.
Thoracic roentgenogram, posteroanterior projection in absence of pulmonary valve. Masslike structure in right hilum caused by massively dilated pulmonary artery.

patients have a bicuspid pulmonary valve. A bicuspid pulmonary valve may be a rare cause of isolated pulmonary insufficiency. The clinical and laboratory findings for this valvar anomaly are the same as a domed-shaped pulmonary valve. The angiographic features are as follows:

1. The bicuspid pulmonary valve is usually thickened.
2. During systole, doming can be seen.

3. A jet is seen, but it is usually less well defined.
REASON: The bicuspid pulmonary valve has a slitlike orifice similar to that of the bicuspid aortic valve.
4. Bicuspid valve in tetralogy of Fallot is usually associated with a small anulus and small supravalvar portion of the main pulmonary artery (see Fig 29–26).
5. The angiographic appearance of bicuspid pulmonary valve results in a characteristic "clamshell" deformity (see Fig 29–26).

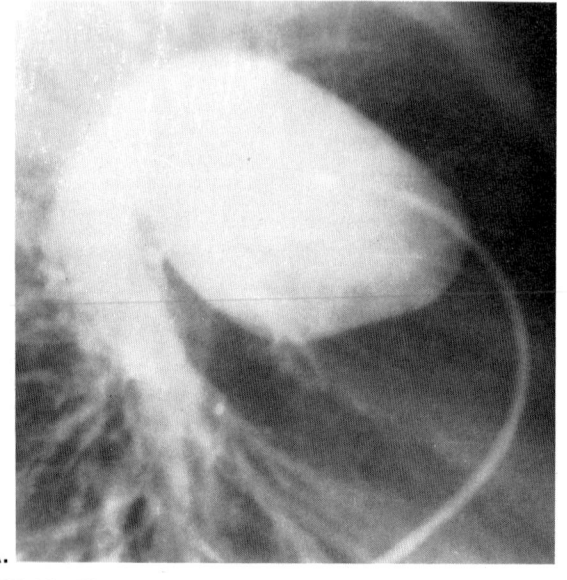

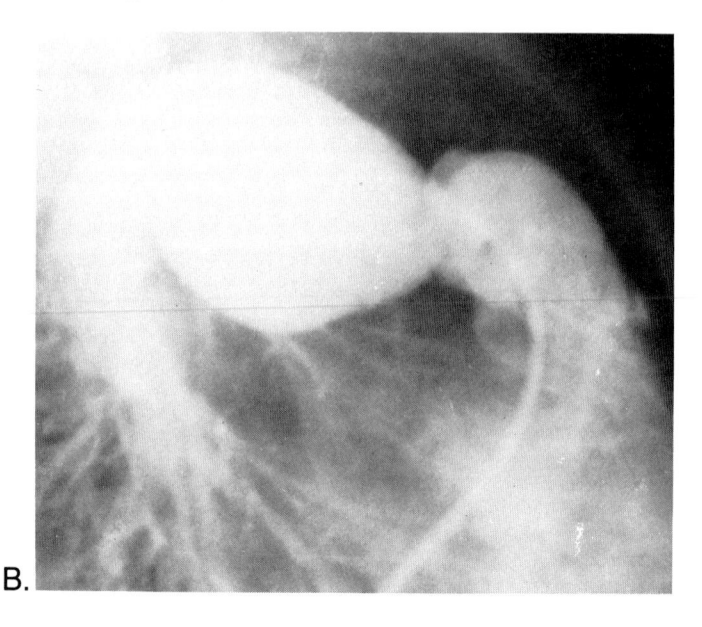

A.   B.

FIG 29–53.
Right ventriculogram, lateral projection; systolic view of absence of pulmonary valve. Enormous dilatation of main pulmonary artery; marked change in caliber observed between systole **(A)** and diastole **(B).** Pulmonary anulus but no valve leaflets are seen.

QUADRICUSPID PULMONARY VALVE

Quadricuspid semilunar valves are extremely rare. They may be either stenotic or incompetent.

ABSENCE OF THE PULMONARY VALVE

Absence of the pulmonary valve may occur as an isolated anomaly but more commonly is associated with tetralogy of Fallot (see Chapter 32). Pulmonary valve anomaly ranges from poorly developed, rudimentary pulmonary leaflets, to total absence of the valvar tissue. Consequently, the hemodynamic consequence of pulmonary stenosis and insufficiency are variable.

Clinical Features

When absence of the pulmonary valve is part of tetralogy of Fallot, a large left-to-right shunt usually occurs in infancy, and congestive cardiac failure may result. Later, mild cyanosis may develop because of a right-to-left shunt through the ventricular communication.

These patients have a loud systolic murmur from the ventricular septal defect and associated right ventricular outflow obstruction and also an early diastolic murmur of pulmonary insufficiency. The ECG may show right ventricular or biventricular hypertrophy, the latter in patients

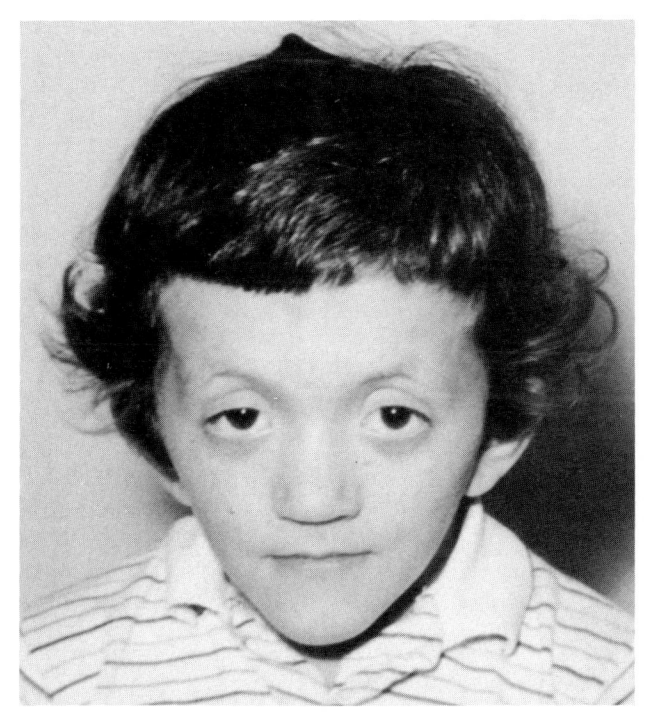

FIG 29–54.
Photograph of child showing characteristic features of Noonan's syndrome. Triangular face, hypertelorism, and ptosis.

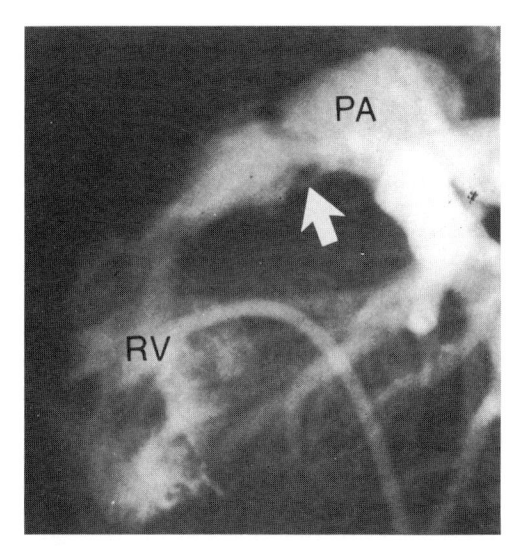

FIG 29–55.
Noonan's syndrome. Right ventriculogram. Lateral projection. Pulmonary valve *(arrow)* is redundant and does not dome. Poststenotic dilatation of pulmonary trunk is absent, indicating valvar dysplasia.

with a large left-to-right shunt. The condition can usually be diagnosed by echocardiography, which demonstrates the valvar anomaly and diastolic regurgitation.

Absence of the pulmonary valve is associated with aneurysmal dilatation of the pulmonary arteries, particularly the right pulmonary artery. The huge pulmonary arteries may cause bronchial compression, and the presenting clinical symptoms may be caused by recurrent pneumonia and atelectasis, particularly of the right lung.

Radiographic Features

The radiographic findings vary with the degree of pulmonary insufficiency.

1. The pulmonary trunk and right and left pulmonary arteries are enlarged and show increased pulsations on fluoroscopy. REASON: Increased stroke volume of the right ventricle, which is ejecting the cardiac output and the diastolic regurgitant volume.
2. Usually dilatation of the right pulmonary artery occurs (Fig 29–52).
3. The findings may be normal in patients with minimal pulmonary insufficiency
4. Aneurysmal dilatation of the left pulmonary artery may occur but is less common.

Angiographic Features

The angiographic findings vary with the degree to which pulmonary valvar tissue is absent.

534 Outflow Obstructive Lesions

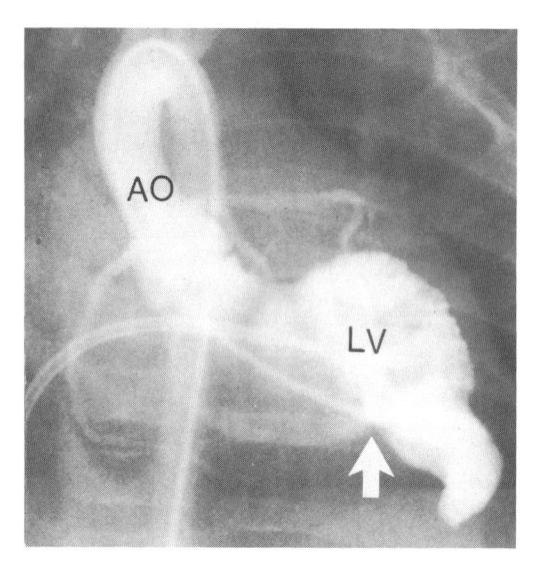

FIG 29–56.
Left ventriculogram. Same patient as in Figure 29–55. Note "ballerina slipper" deformity of left ventricle *(arrow)* because of hypertrophy of diaphragmatic portion of left ventricle.

1. The findings may be similar to that of valvar pulmonary stenosis, with doming of the pulmonary valve (partial absence of the valve of a minor degree.)
2. Remnants of the valve leaflets may be seen.
3. With complete absence of the valve, only the valve annulus (but no leaflets) can be identified. These patients tend to have severe pulmonary insufficiency (Fig 29–53).
4. In spite of absence of the pulmonary valve, the pulmonary annulus may be narrow, and both pulmonary stenosis and insufficiency may be present.
5. The aneurysmal dilatation of the pulmonary arteries is well seen, and markedly increased pulsations are demonstrated.
6. Pulmonary angiography demonstrates the degree of diastolic reflux (see Fig 29–53).

NOONAN'S SYNDROME

Noonan's syndrome (named after Jacqueline Noonan, a contemporary American cardiologist) is the name given to a constellation of features found in some patients with either pulmonary stenosis or left ventricular myopathy. The patients are usually small, being less than the tenth percentile for height and weight. The facies show rather

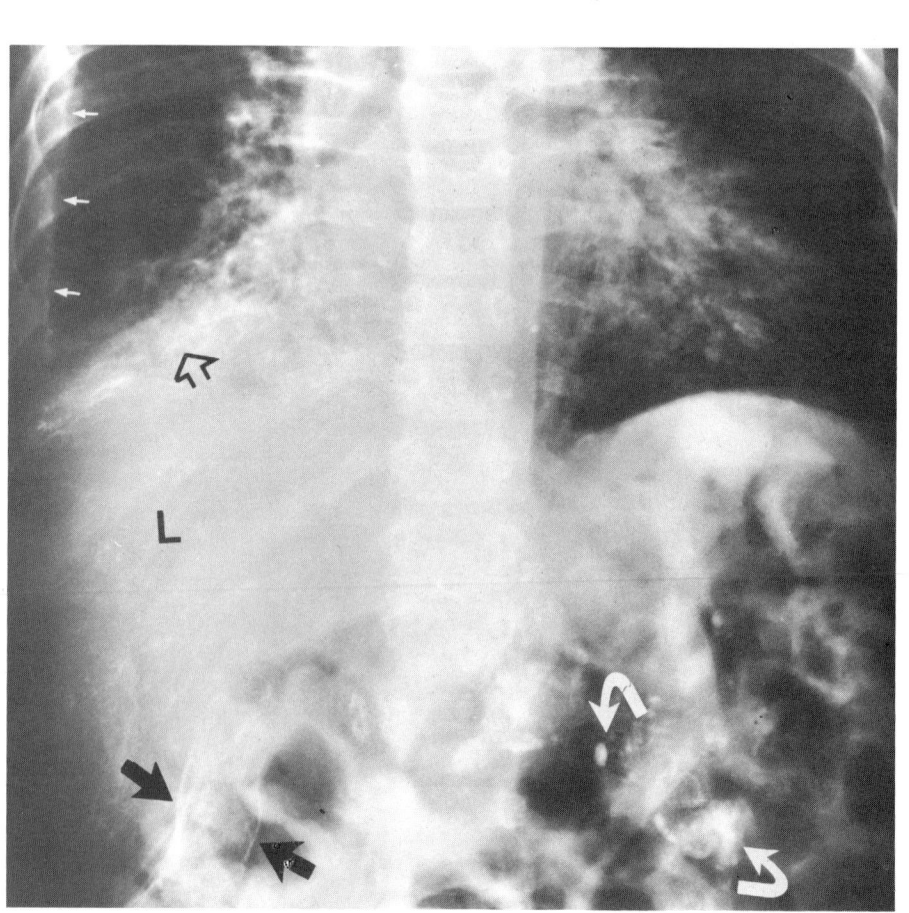

FIG 29–57.
Lymphangiogram in patient with Noonan's syndrome and extensive lymphatic abnormalities. Aplasia of para-aortic nodes with reflux of contrast medium into bowel *(curved arrows)*. Opacification of lymphatics of gallbladder *(solid black arrows)* and liver *(L)*. Demonstration of pulmonary lymphatics (pulmonary lymphangiectasia) *(open arrow)*. Right chylothorax *(small white arrows)*.

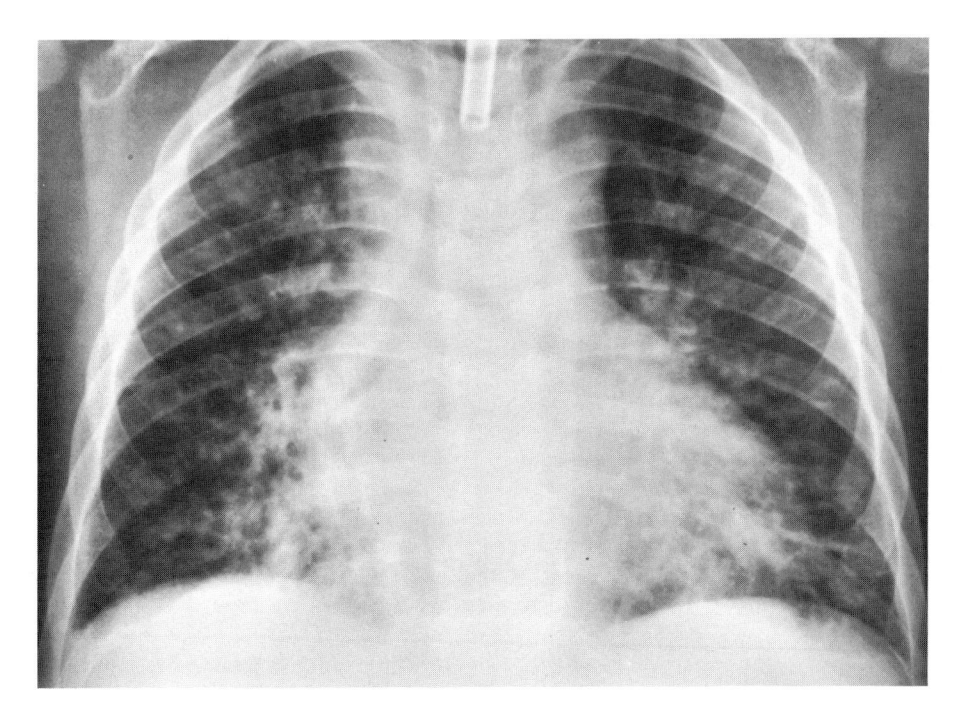

FIG 29-58.
Posteroanterior roentgenogram Noonan's syndrome and pulmonary lymphangiectasia. Thoracic roentgenogram. Posteroanterior projection. Extensive bilateral infiltrates are evident.

constant features: hypertelorism (92%), ptosis (21%), low-set ears (85%), low hairline (67%), abundant curly hair (26%), and short neck (90%) (Fig 29-54). One fourth of cases occur in families. Intelligence is normal.

Cardiovascular anomalies occur in three fourths of patients. Pulmonary stenosis caused by valvar dysplasia is the most common anomaly (Fig 29-55). Eccentric hypertrophy affecting the superior portion of the anterior wall, septum, and diaphragmatic portion of the left ventricle may be present. The angiogram gives an appearance described as "ballerina slipper" deformity (Fig 29-56).[28] The QRS axis is usually directed superiorly in patients with cardiac anomalies. Peripheral pulmonary artery stenosis may coexist with valvar pulmonary stenosis.

Dysplasia of the lymph channels is less frequent, and lymphangiography may demonstrate restricted lymph flow, aplasia or hypoplasia of the lymph channels, lymphangiectasia, ectasia and tortuosity of channels, chylous fistulas, and abnormal lymph nodes (Fig 29-57).[29, 30] Intestinal lymphangiectasia, which can be diagnosed by intestinal biopsy, is associated with malabsorption, protein-losing enteropathy with hypoproteinemia, and ascites. Pulmonary lymphangiectasia has been reported and associated with radiographic findings resembling pulmonary edema and pleural (chylous) effusion (Fig 29-58). Lymphedema may involve the extremities, particularly the lower, and the differential diagnosis is Milroy's disease. The result of the abnormality is lymphedema, which may be generalized and may manifest at birth, involving a particular organ, or may develop later.[30, 31] The pathogenesis is unknown.

REFERENCES

1. Lucas RV Jr, Moller JH: Pulmonary valvular stenosis. *Cardiovasc Clin* 2:156, 1971.
2. Levin OR, Blumenthal S: Pulmonic stenosis, *Circulation* 31-32(suppl III):33, 1965.
3. Vogelpoel L, Schrire V: Auscultatory and phonocardiographic assessment of pulmonary stenosis with intact ventricular septum, *Circulation* 22:55, 1960.
4. Leatham A, Weitzman D: Auscultatory and phonocardiographic signs of pulmonary stenosis *Br Heart J* 19:303, 1957.
5. Weyman AE, Dillon JC, Feigenbaum H, et al: Echocardiographic patterns of pulmonary valve motion in valvular pulmonary stenosis, *Am J Cardiol* 34:644, 1974.
6. Moller JH, Adams P Jr: The natural history of pulmonary valvular stenosis: serial cardiac catheterizations in 21 children, *Am J Cardiol* 16:654, 1965.
7. Stone FM, Bessinger FB Jr, Lucas RV Jr, et al: Pre and postoperative rest and exercise hemodynamics in children with pulmonary stenosis, *Circulation* 49:1102, 1974.
8. Talbert JL, Morrow AG, Collins NP, et al: The incidence and significance of pulmonic regurgitation after pulmonary valvulotomy, *Am Heart J* 65:590, 1963.
9. Lillehei CW, Simmons RL, Todd DB: Late hemodynamic response to correction of isolated pulmonary stenosis by open operation during pulmonary bypass, *Circulation* 32:258, 1965.
10. Tandon R, Nadas AS, Gross RE: Results of open-heart surgery in patients with pulmonic stenosis and intact ventricular septum: A report of 108 cases, *Circulation* 31:190, 1965.
11. Koretzky ED, Moller JH, Korns ME, et al: Congenital pul-

monary stenosis resulting from dysplasia of valve, *Circulation* 40:43, 1969.
12. Becu L, Somerville J, Gallo A: 'Isolated' pulmonary valve stenosis as part of more widespread cardiovascular disease, *Br Heart J* 38:472, 1976.
13. McCue CM, Robertson LW, Lester RG, et al: Pulmonary artery coarctations: a report of 20 cases with review of 319 cases from the literature, *J Pediatr* 67:222, 1965.
14. Rowe RD: Maternal rubella and pulmonary artery stenoses: report of eleven cases, *Pediatrics* 32:180, 1963.
15. Emmanouilides GC, Linde LM, Crittenden IH: Pulmonary artery stenosis associated with ductus arteriosus following maternal rubella, *Circulation* 29:514, 1964.
16. Danilowicz DA, Rudolph AM, Hoffman JIE, et al: Physiologic pressure differences between main and branch pulmonary arteries in infants, *Circulation* 45:410, 1972.
17. Hartmann AF Jr, Elliott LP, Goldring D: The course of peripheral pulmonary artery stenoses in children, *J Pediatr* 73:212, 1968.
18. Blount SG Jr, Vigoda PS, Swan H: Isolated infundibular stenosis, *Am Heart J* 57:684, 1959.
19. Weyman AE, Dillon JC, Feigenbaum H, et al: Cardiographic differentiation of infundibular from valvular pulmonary stenosis, *Am J Cardiol* 36:21, 1975.
20. Lucas RV Jr, Varco RL, Lillehei CW, et al: Anomalous muscle bundle of the right ventricle: hemodynamic consequences and surgical considerations, *Circulation* 25:443, 1962.
21. Rowland TW, Rosenthal A, Castaneda AR: Double-chamber right ventricle: experience with 17 cases, *Am Heart J* 89:445, 1975.
22. Cosio FG, Wang Y, Nicoloff DM: Membranous right ventricular outflow obstruction, *Am J Cardiol* 32:1000, 1973.
23. Pate JW, Ainger LE, Butterick OD: A new form of right ventricular outflow obstruction: case report, *Am Heart J* 68:249, 1964.
24. Pate JW, Richardson RL Jr, Giles HH: Accessory tricuspid leaflet producing right ventricular outflow obstruction, *N Engl J Med* 279:867, 1968.
25. Chesler E, Korns ME, Edwards JE: Anomalies of the tricuspid valve, including pouches, resembling aneurysms of the membranous ventricular septum, *Am J Cardiol* 21:661, 1968.
26. Ford AB, Hellerstein HK, Wood C, et al: Isolated congenital bicuspid pulmonary valve: clinical and pathologic study, *Am J Med* 20:474, 1956.
27. Miller RA, Lev M, Paul MH: Congenital absence of the pulmonary valve: the clinical syndrome of tetralogy of Fallot with pulmonary regurgitation, *Circulation* 26:266, 1962.
28. Baltaxe HA, Levin AR, Ehlers KH, et al: The appearance of the left ventricle in Noonan's syndrome, *Radiology* 109:155, 1973.
29. Hoeffel JC, Juncker P, Remy J: Lymphatic vessels dysplasia in Noonan's syndrome, *Am J Radiol* 134: 399, 1980.
30. White SW: Lymphedema in Noonan's syndrome, *Int J Dermatol* 23:656, 1984.
31. Witt DR, Hoyme HE, Zonana J, et al: Lymphedema in Noonan syndrome: Clues to pathogenesis and prenatal diagnosis and review of the literature, *Am J Med Genet* 27:841, 1987.

PART FOUR

Cyanosis and Decreased Pulmonary Arterial Vasculature

A variety of congenital cardiac malformations are associated with cyanosis and decreased pulmonary arterial vasculature. In common, each of the conditions has two components: obstruction to blood flow into the lungs and an intracardiac communication proximal to that obstruction. The obstruction is severe enough to limit pulmonary blood flow, so that a portion of systemic venous return is shunted into the aorta, causing the cyanosis. The obstruction to pulmonary blood flow may be located in either the outflow or the inflow portions of the right ventricle. In most cases the obstruction is located in the outflow tract of the right ventricle, at the level of the pulmonary valve or in the subvalvar area. Pulmonary arterial stenosis may coexist, but it is rarely the sole site of obstruction (such patients are discussed in Chapter 29). Obstruction may be partial (valvar stenosis or subvalvar stenosis) or complete (valvar atresia, e.g., pulmonary atresia). In the latter, the circulation depends on ductal patency. Many patients with conditions associated with pulmonary atresia develop severe hypoxemia in the neonatal period as the ductus arteriosus closes normally.

The pulmonary blood flow may be limited from obstruction to right ventricular inflow, with a shunt occurring proximally, that is, at the atrial level. Although less common, conditions such as Ebstein's malformation present such an example. In others, such as tricuspid atresia, obstruction to the right ventricular inflow is complete, and there is usually coexistent outflow obstruction to pulmonary blood flow (see Chapter 33).

Regardless of the site of obstruction, the volume of pulmonary blood flow is limited. Therefore, the pulmonary vasculature appears diminished on a thoracic roentgenogram.

The intracardiac communication allowing the right-to-left shunt may be located at the atrial or the ventricular level. The cardiac malformations classified here can be divided into two categories, depending on the location of the communication. The hemodynamics and clinical and laboratory features are similar among those with a ventricular level shunt and differ from those patients in whom the shunt is at the atrial level. The hemodynamic principles governing the blood flow through these communications are the same as discussed in Part 2 regarding cardiac conditions associated with a left-to-right shunt.

Conditions with an intraventricular communication are more common than those with an atrial communication and account for 10% of all instances of congenital cardiac malformations. Tetralogy of Fallot is the most frequent cause of cyanosis among the conditions with a ventricular communication and obstruction to pulmonary blood flow. A wide variety of other conditions have these general anatomic features with a ventricular communication and are called "tetrad variants" because they have a number of clinical and laboratory features in common. Cardiac size, whether determined clinically or radiographically, is normal, because the volume of blood within the heart is not increased. Cardiac failure does not occur in most instances, because the obstructed ventricle can readily decompress through the ventricular communication. Therefore, the pressure in the chamber proximal to the obstruction does not exceed systemic levels. The major auscultatory finding is a pulmonary systolic ejection murmur, related to turbulence of blood flow through the right ventricular outflow area. The loudness of this murmur is inversely related to the severity of the stenosis and therefore the volume of pulmonary blood flow. Therefore, the more severe the stenosis, the softer the murmur. This feature is very valuable to cardiologists in assessing the severity of the obstruction.

Other clinical, radiographic, and echocardiographic features allow distinction between the conditions grouped in this category, with cyanosis, decreased pulmonary vasculature, and normal cardiac size. Although the tetralogy of Fallot is the most common, other conditions that resemble it have sometimes been grouped as tetrad variants. Classification of cyanosis and decreased pulmonary vasculature is as follows:

I. Normal cardiac size
   A. Tetralogy of Fallot
   B. Tetrad variants
      1. Single ventricle with pulmonary stenosis (see Chapter 42)
         a. With transposition of great vessels
         b. Without transposition of great vessels
      2. Transposition of great vessels, ventricular septal defect, and pulmonary stenosis (see Chapter 38)
      3. L-Transposition of great vessels, ventricular septal defect, and pulmonary stenosis (see Chapter 39)
      4. Origin of both great vessels from right ventricle and pulmonary stenosis (see Chapter 41)
      5. Endocardial cushion defect and pulmonary stenosis (see Chapter 23)
      6. Cardiac malformations associated with asplenia syndrome (see Chapter 58)

In section 4, tetralogy of Fallot is discussed. Each of the other tetrad variants is discussed in other sections as indicated.

Among the malformations with a right-to-left shunt through an atrial communication, the clinical features are more variable because of the greater anatomic variety. In most instances, pulmonary blood flow is limited because of obstruction to blood flow into the right ventricle. This is in contrast to the group with a ventricular communication, where obstruction involves the right ventricular outflow. Often the inflow obstruction is from diminution of right ventricular cavity or tricuspid size.

Like any shunt at the atrial level, the relative ventricular compliances or the status of the atrioventricular valves determines the direction and magnitude of blood flow. If the atrial communication is narrow, systemic blood flow may be limited as well. In these instances, because of impedance of blood flow into the right ventricle, a right-to-left atrial shunt occurs.

In contrast to those conditions with a ventricular communication, the cardiac silhouette is often increased, principally because of right atrial enlargement. There may be signs of systemic venous congestion, with hepatomegaly and prominent jugular venous pulses. The murmurs are not as specific. Because many of the conditions grouped here have a small or hypoplastic right ventricle, the electrocardiogram may show a pattern of left ventricular hypertrophy or diminution of right ventricular forces. Because right atrial pressure is elevated, right atrial enlargement is present and electrocardiographically evidenced by tall peaked P waves.

The cardiac conditions grouped in this category are:

II. Cardiomegaly
   A. Tricuspid atresia (see Chapter 33)
   B. Pulmonary atresia with intact ventricular septum (see Chapter 34)
   C. Pulmonary stenosis with right-to-left atrial shunt (see Chapter 29)
   D. Hypoplasia of right ventricle (see Chapter 35)
   E. Ebstein's malformation (see Chapter 36)
   F. Transient tricuspid insufficiency (see Chapter 37)

Regardless of the level of right-to-left shunt, two clinical features reflect the volume of pulmonary blood flow. First, the degree of cyanosis is inversely related to the volume of pulmonary blood flow. Thus, the more severe the obstruction, the greater the cyanosis. Second, the loudness of the murmur also may reflect the severity of obstruction, particularly in those with a ventricular communication or those with tricuspid atresia. The murmur originates from the pulmonary stenosis in these conditions. Therefore, the more severe the stenosis, the less the volume of blood flow through the obstruction. The murmur then becomes softer.

In these conditions, symptoms develop principally from hypoxemia secondary to inadequate pulmonary blood flow. Symptoms of congestive cardiac failure are uncommon. If symptoms develop in the neonatal period, prostaglandin E_1 infusion may open the ductus arteriosus and improve pulmonary blood flow and hypoxemia. In older patients, a systemic pulmonary arterial shunt may be required to improve symptoms related to hypoxemia.

The conditions discussed in this section and sections 5 through 7 are associated with cyanosis. Cyanosis is the blue color imparted to the skin when more than 5 g/dL of reduced hemoglobin are present in capillary beds, which is one of the clinical manifestations of desaturation of systemic arterial blood. In response to the chronic hypoxemic state, the bone marrow is stimulated to produce erythrocytes, thereby increasing the oxygen-carrying capacity of blood. The hemoglobin and hematocrit values are elevated in these patients, the degree of elevation reflecting the extent of systemic arterial hypoxemia. At markedly elevated levels of hematocrit, there may be problems with hemostasis and intravascular thrombosis. Also as a result of chronic hypoxemia, growth is often slowed, but mental development appears normal, unless complicating neurologic problems occur.

Because of the right-to-left shunt, there is a potential for paradoxical embolus, brain abscess, or other cerebral complications. Fortunately these problems are becoming less frequent, because operative correction of most congenital cardiac malformations can be performed in infancy. Therefore, the period of risk is small, and the potential for adequate growth is maximized.

CHAPTER 30

Tetralogy of Fallot

The combination of ventricular septal defect, infundibular stenosis, overriding aorta, and right ventricular hypertrophy is commonly called tetralogy of Fallot. This combination was initially described by Nicholas Stensen (a Danish anatomist) in 1671 and was well known in the 1800s. In 1888, Fallot[1] (a 19th century French physician) made important observations in stating that patients with this combination of anomalies are cyanotic and furthermore that they constitute three fourths of the cyanotic patients beyond the second year of life. Tetralogy of Fallot accounts for 8% of all instances of congenital heart disease and is one of the two major forms causing cyanosis, the other being transposition of the great vessels.

PATHOLOGIC ANATOMY

Although tetralogy of Fallot classically has four components, Van Praagh et al.[2] considered it developmentally as a monology: Its various anomalies result from conal maldevelopment, resulting in hypoplasia of the right ventricular infundibulum. The enlarged aorta and hypoplasia of the right infundibulum and pulmonary artery can also be explained by an unequal division of the truncus by the conotruncal septum (see Fig 45–1). Others[3] have considered the key components to be ventricular septal defect and pulmonary stenosis. We, however, describe the traditional four components (Fig 30–1):

1. *Ventricular septal defect*. The ventricular septal defect is large except in a rare case in which it may be partially occluded by the septal leaflet of the tricuspid valve, accessory tricuspid valve tissue, or hypertrophied septal band.[1] The defect[4] involves both a part of the membranous septum and the muscular septum anterior to it (Fig 30–2). The defect lies beneath the crista supraventricularis and extends directly to the aortic root beneath the right and posterior aortic cusps. The conduction system passes along the inferior margin of the ventricular septal defect. Through the ventricular septal defect, the aortic, mitral, and tricuspid valves are in fibrous continuity. It is rare that muscular defects coexist.

2. *Overriding aorta* (also called "dextroposition of aorta"). Although aortic overriding, or straddling, was originally described as a component of tetralogy of Fallot, the extent is variable and presents no problem to the surgeon during operative repair. The aorta may arise almost exclusively from the left ventricle or nearly exclusively from the right ventricle (Fig 30–3). In the latter instance, the condition may be confused with double-outlet right ventricle, but mitral-aortic continuity is preserved in tetralogy of Fallot. There is a continuous spectrum from tetralogy of Fallot, with severe overriding of the aorta to double outlet right ventricle. If there is mitral-aortic discontinuity (Fig 30–3,D), the condition is classified as double-outlet right ventricle. Operative repair is identical to classic tetralogy of Fallot.

3. *Pulmonary stenosis*. An abnormality of the infundibular musculature is an important component of tetralogy of Fallot, which leads to infundibular stenosis in each patient. Van Praagh et al.[2] indicate that the hallmark of tetralogy of Fallot is an abnormally small subpulmonary infundibulum deviated anteriorly, superiorly, and in a leftward direction. Edwards[2] speaks of the vertical position of the crista supraventricularis, particularly the septal band. The crista supraventricularis is more prominent and more vertically oriented than normal. The septal band is hypertrophied, and the parietal band is displaced superiorly and is prominent anteriorly as it is directed leftward toward the septum. Above the crista supraventricularis and below the pulmonary valve lies the infundibular chamber. The form of stenosis varies (Fig 30–4). In some patients (10%), there is stenosis of the os infundibulum, with a localized narrowing at the inlet to the crista supraventricularis, whereas the infundibulum itself and pulmonary annulus are of normal caliber. In the other 90% of patients, the en-

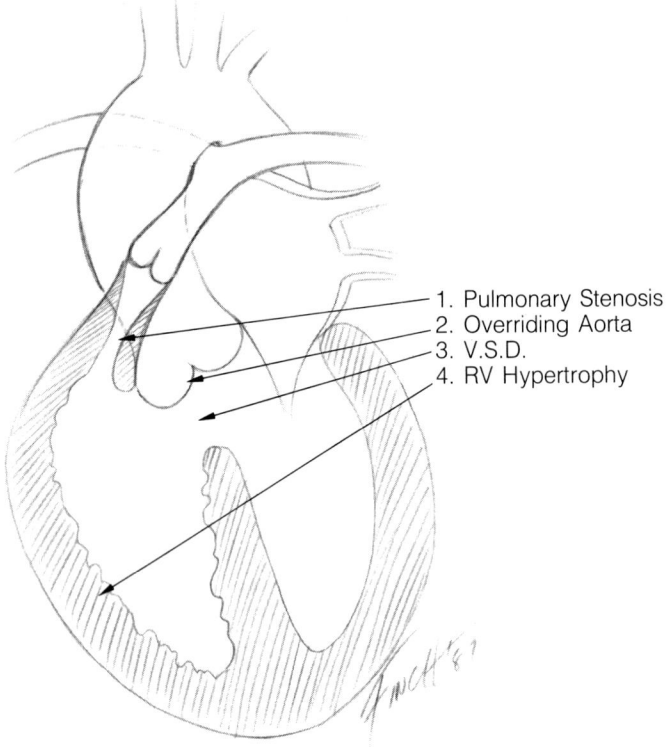

FIG 30–1.
Four components of tetralogy of Fallot. *1*, pulmonary stenosis; *2*, right ventricular *(RV)* hypertrophy; *3*, ventricular septal defect *(VSD)*; and *4*, overriding aorta.

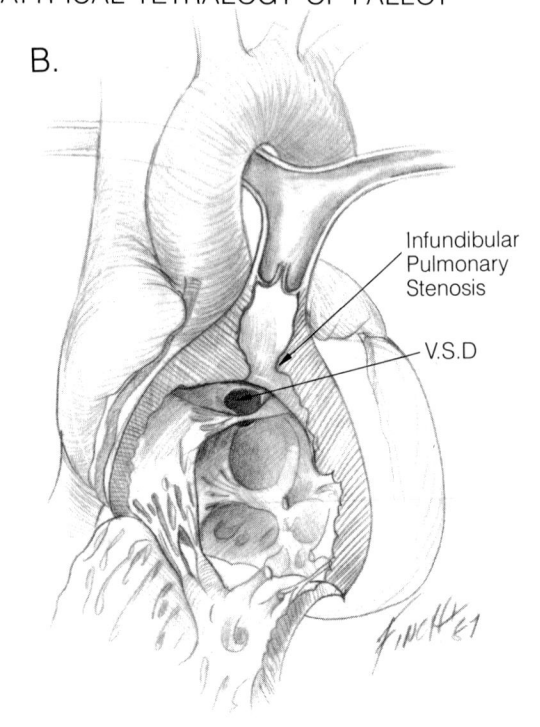

FIG 30–2.
Tetralogy of Fallot. **A,** typical form. Part of right ventricle has been removed. Large ventricular septal defect extending to aortic valve which can be seen through defect. Tricuspid valve, aortic valve, and mitral valve are in continuity. Right ventricular hypertrophy is evidenced by increased trabeculations. Stenosis of os infundibuli. **B,** atypical form. Infundibular stenosis with smaller ventricular septal defect *(VSD)* not related to aortic valve. This condition is better classified as "ventricular septal defect with pulmonary stenosis."

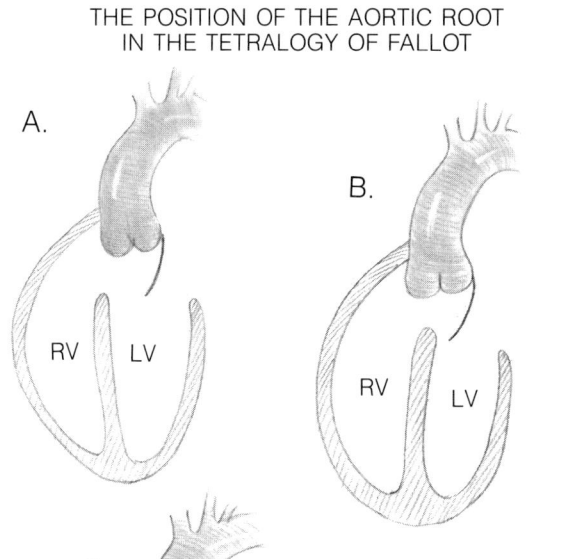

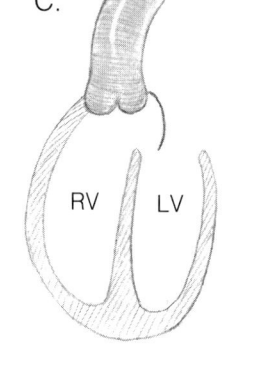

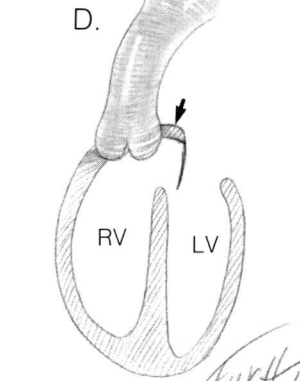

THE POSITION OF THE AORTIC ROOT
IN THE TETRALOGY OF FALLOT

FIG 30–3.
Tetralogy of Fallot with various degrees of overriding aorta. **A,** normal origin (no overriding) of aorta from left ventricle *(LV).* **B,** mild overriding of aorta (40%) and slightly more pronounced overriding of aorta **(C). D,** severe overriding of aorta with separation of anterior leaflet of mitral valve from aortic valve *(arrow)* by muscle. Because of this muscle, this form should be classified as double-outlet right ventricle. There is a continuous spectrum from severe overriding of aorta in tetralogy of Fallot to double-outlet right ventricle with pulmonary stenosis. *RV* = right ventricle.

tire infundibular area and pulmonary annulus are hypoplastic. Generally the infundibular stenosis progresses hemodynamically with time.

Pulmonary valvar anomalies are common (90%). The pulmonary valve is commonly bicuspid or unicommissural and stenotic. Hypoplasia of the pulmonary annulus usually coexists.

In at least three fourths of the patients, the major branches of the pulmonary arterial tree are hypoplastic or show stenotic areas involving the pulmonary trunk or its major branches, particularly the proximal left pulmonary artery (peripheral pulmonary artery stenosis).

The right ventricular outflow area and main pulmonary trunk are directed more toward the right side, which is in contrast to normal, where the right ventricular outflow tract is directed either vertically or slightly leftward.

Because of the low pulmonary arterial pressure, there is thinning of the medial coat of the pulmonary trunk and fragmentation of its elastic fibers. In the pulmonary trunk there may be a jet lesion, which is a potential site of bacterial endocarditis. Thrombi may be found in the pulmonary arterial tree.

4. *Right ventricular hypertrophy.* In response to the elevated right ventricular systolic pressure, the right ventricle shows concentric hypertrophy and prominent trabeculations.

Associated conditions include:

1. *Right aortic arch (25%).* Right aortic arch occurs in 25% of patients with tetralogy of Fallot. The incidence is greater among patients with severe degrees of pulmonary stenosis or with pulmonary atresia. The aortic arch passes to the right of the trachea and esophagus and above the right mainstem bronchus. The aorta descends on the right side but crosses the midline in the lower thorax and passes through the left hemidiaphragm (normal for situs solitus). Usually the right aortic arch shows mirror image branching (Fig 30–5). The aorta is large. Two theories have been advanced: (1) uneven division of the developmental truncus by the conotruncal septum into a large aortic and small pulmonary arterial component and (2) increased blood flow in utero. If pulmonary stenosis is severe, blood flow through the fetal ductus arteriosus is from left to right. Therefore, both the pulmonary and systemic blood flows pass through the ascending aorta. The more severe the degree of pulmonary stenosis, the larger the aorta.

Occasionally in tetralogy of Fallot the right aortic arch occurs with an aberrant left subclavian artery (Fig 30–6). Normally the aberrant left subclavian artery in a right aortic arch arises from an aortic diverticulum, but this is not the case in tetralogy of Fallot. This difference occurs because of patterns of fetal blood flow.[5] In a fetus without tetralogy of Fallot but with a right aortic arch and aberrant left subclavian artery, blood flows right to left through the ductus arteriosus, which connects to the proximal aberrant left subclavian artery. The large volume of blood that flows into the proximal left subclavian artery goes into the descending aorta. Therefore, the proximal left subclavian artery is enlarged, and its retroesophageal segment has been called an aortic diverticulum. In contrast, the fetal

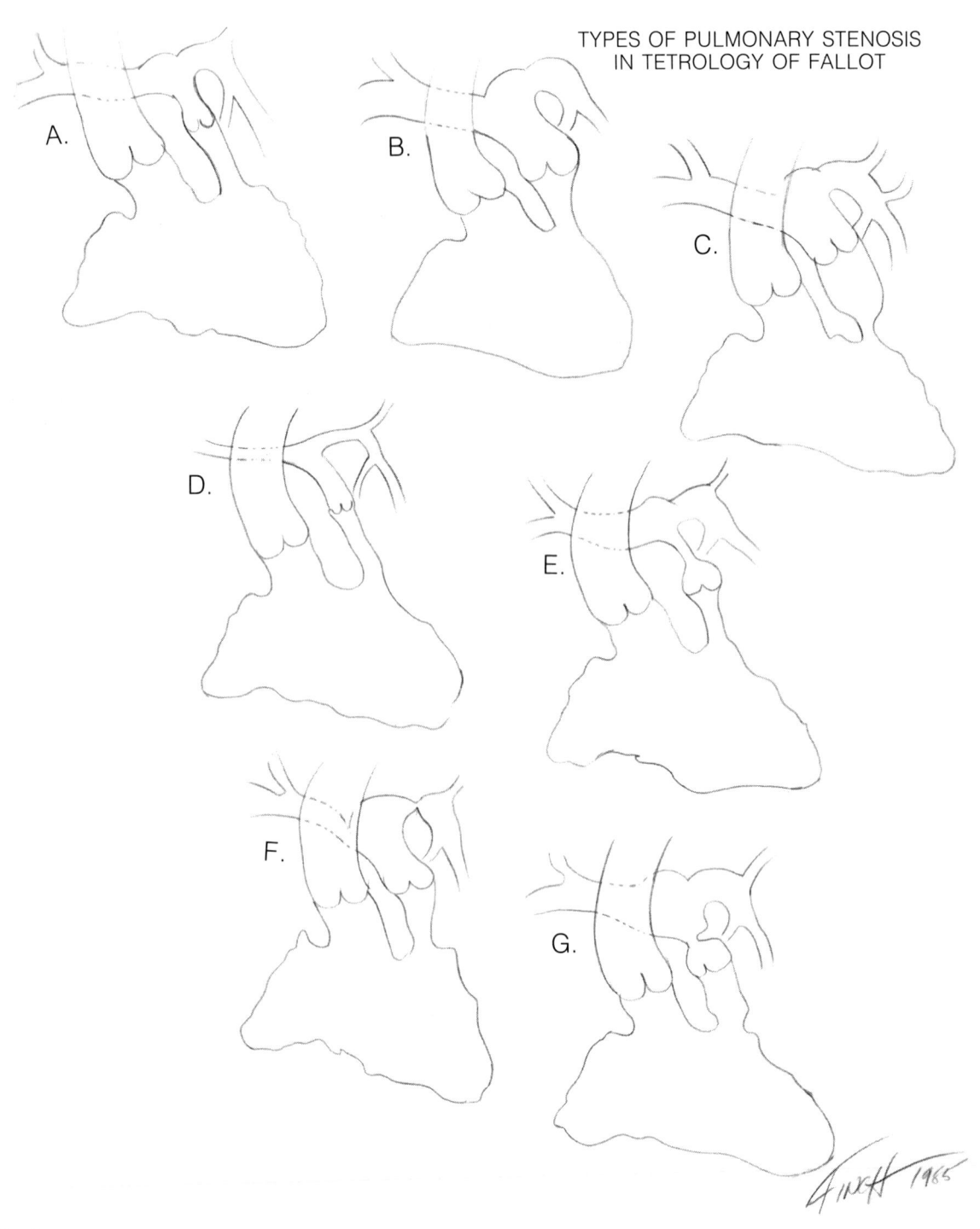

FIG 30-4.
Various types of infundibular pulmonary stenosis. **A,** typical tetralogy of Fallot. Diffuse tubular narrowing of the infundibulum, mild narrowing of pulmonary annulus and main pulmonary artery. Infundibulum, pulmonary annulus, and main pulmonary artery are commonly of same caliber. **B,** infundibular pulmonary stenosis with normal-size pulmonary annulus and main pulmonary artery. **C,** localized stenosis of inlet of infundibulum with normal-sized infundibular chamber, pulmonary annulus, and main pulmonary artery (stenosis of os infundibulum). **D,** severe tubular narrowing of infundibulum, severe hypoplasia of pulmonary annulus and main pulmonary artery, with hypoplasia of entire pulmonary arterial tree. **E,** tubular-type infundibular stenosis. Normal-sized pulmonary annulus. Tubular supravalar pulmonary hypoplasia. **F,** typical infundibular pulmonary stenosis. Normal-sized annulus. Normal main pulmonary artery. Peripheral right and left pulmonary artery stenoses. **G,** moderate infundibular pulmonary stenosis. Normal pulmonary annulus. Localized supravalvar pulmonary stenosis. On rare occasions infundibulum is normal and pulmonary stenosis is caused exclusively by stenotic pulmonary valve. Various combinations of these types of pulmonary stenosis may occur.

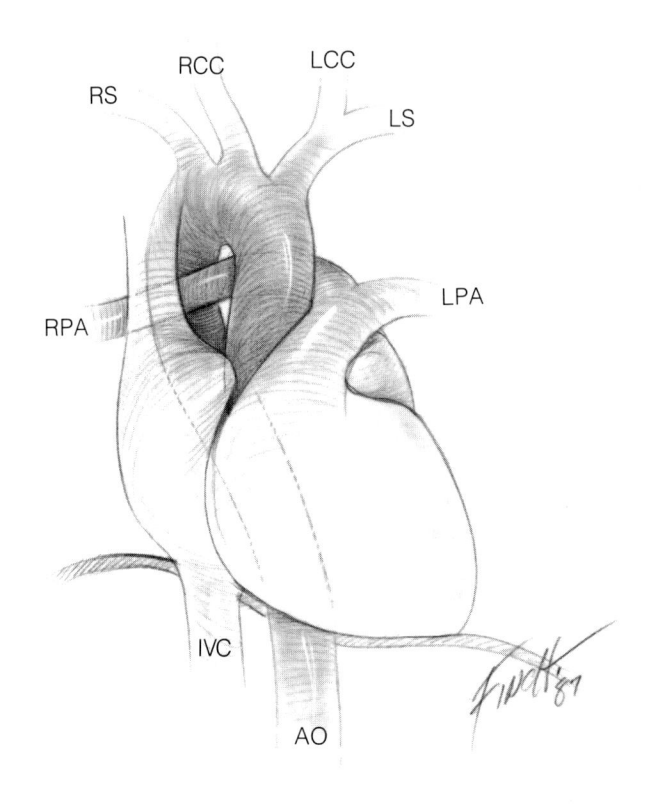

TETRALOGY OF FALLOT WITH RIGHT AORTIC ARCH

FIG 30–5.
Right aortic arch in tetralogy of Fallot. Mirror image branching of the brachiocephalic vessels. First branch from aorta is left innominate artery. Aortic arch lies to right of trachea and esophagus. Aorta descends on right side of spine but pierces diaphragm on left, indicating normal situs. Spatial relationship of inferior vena cava and descending aorta at level of diaphragm and in abdomen is normal (see Chapter 58). *RS* = right subclavian artery; *RCC* = right common carotid artery; *LCC* = left common carotid artery; *LS* = left subclavian artery; *LPA* = left pulmonary artery; *AO* = aorta; *IVC* = inferior vena cava; *RPA* = right pulmonary artery.

RIGHT AORTIC ARCH WITH ABERRANT LEFT SUBCLAVIAN ARTERY IN THE TETRALOGY OF FALLOT

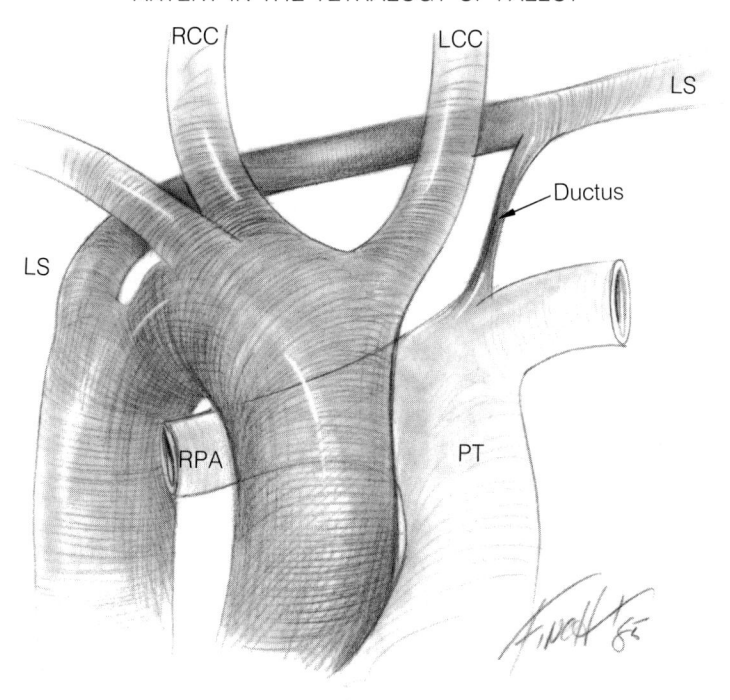

FIG 30–6.
Tetralogy of Fallot. Right aortic arch and aberrant left subclavian artery *(LS)*. Contrary to patients without pulmonary stenosis, aberrant subclavian artery does not arise from aortic diverticulum because ductal blood flow in utero is very small or even reversed. Ductus ligament to left pulmonary artery may be present, completing a vascular ring. *LCC* = left common carotid artery; *PT* = pulmonary trunk; *RCC* = right common carotid artery; *RPA* = right pulmonary artery.

circulation in tetralogy of Fallot is very different, particularly the pattern of flow through the ductus arteriosus. Flow occurs from the left subclavian artery through the ductus arteriosus into the pulmonary artery (i.e., from left to right). Therefore, the volume of flow through the proximal left subclavian artery is normal, and the retroesophageal segment is not dilated. No aortic diverticulum exists in patients with tetralogy of Fallot, right aortic arch, and aberrant left subclavian artery.

The ductus arteriosus may be either right sided, left sided, bilateral, or absent (Fig 30–7). In a right arch, the left-sided ductus arises from the left subclavian artery and extends to the left pulmonary artery. Infrequently, with a right aortic arch, isolation of the left subclavian artery occurs, which is associated with a subclavian steal (Fig 30–8). The subclavian artery does not originate from the aortic arch but is connected to the left pulmonary artery by a ligamentous ductus arteriosus. Isolation of the subclavian artery always occurs opposite the aortic arch. Its embryogenesis is discussed in Chapter 62. In tetralogy of Fallot, the ductus arteriosus rarely remains patent beyond the neonatal period. Persistent patency is much more common in patients with coexistent pulmonary atresia. If the ductus is located on the side opposite the aortic arch, it arises from the subclavian artery; the exception is the circumflex aortic arch (see Chapter 62). Other variations of ductal pattern include absence of the ductus and bilateral ductus, which may be either ligamentous or patent.

2. *Atrial septal defect.* Atrial septal defect occurs in about 10% of patients with tetralogy of Fallot. We have been impressed by the number of infants with this condition in whom a right-to-left atrial shunt was found at cardiac catheterization.

3. *Left superior vena cava (5%).* In these instances, the left superior vena cava connects to the coronary sinus and does not have hemodynamic significance.

4. *Coronary arterial anomalies (5%).* The right coronary artery may arise from the left anterior descending and cross anteriorly the right ventricular outflow tract (Fig 30–9,A), or the left anterior descending may arise from the right coronary artery and cross the outflow tract (Fig 30–9,B). Either of these coronary anomalies may severely restrict the ability to operate in the right ventricular outflow area because of their course. This may also be the

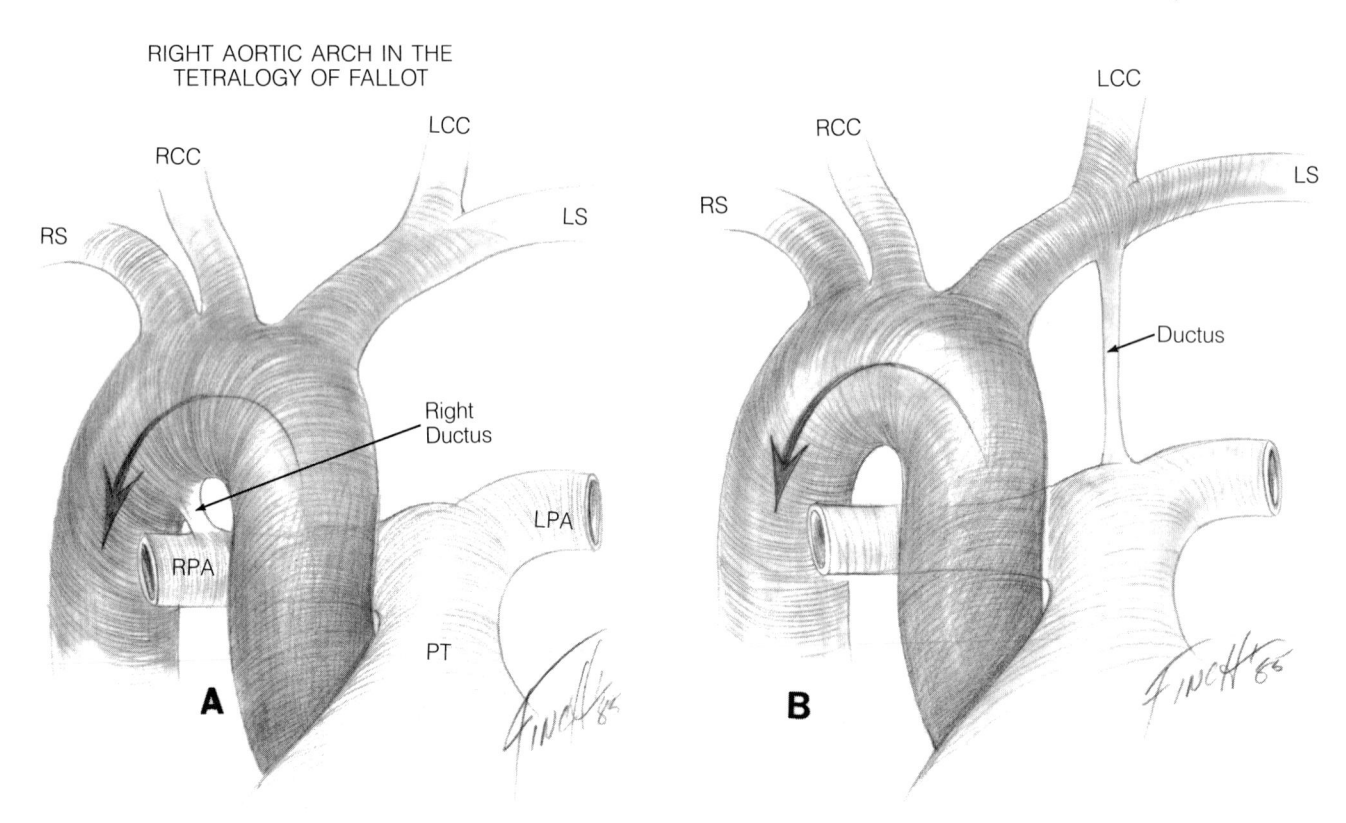

FIG 30–7.
Tetralogy of Fallot and right aortic arch. **A,** right-sided ductus. **B,** left-sided ductus, which typically arises from the left subclavian artery (opposite the aortic arch). Because the subclavian artery is anterior, this type of left-sided ductus arteriosus does not constitute a vascular ring. If the subclavian artery arises aberrantly and passes behind esophagus, a vascular ring is formed and completed by the ductus ligament (see Chapter 62). *LCC* = left common carotid artery; *LPA* = left pulmonary artery; *LS* = left subclavian artery; *RCC* = right common carotid artery; *RPA* = right pulmonary artery; *RS* = right subclavian artery; *PT* = pulmonary trunk.

TETRALOGY OF FALLOT—RIGHT ARCH AND ISOLATION OF LEFT SUBCLAVIAN ARTERY

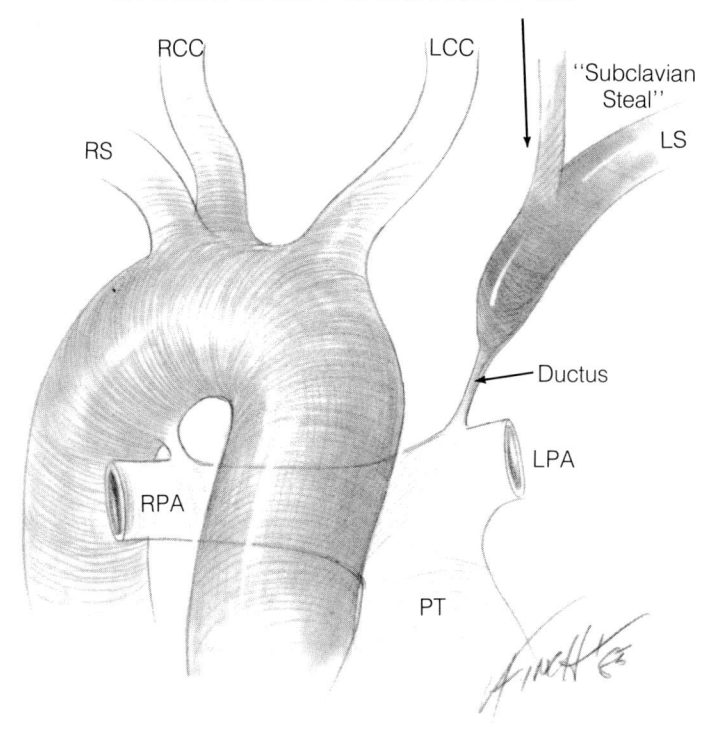

FIG 30–8.
Tetralogy of Fallot. Right aortic arch, isolation of left subclavian artery and bilateral ductus. Retroesophageal segment of left subclavian artery and left ductus arteriosus are atretic or absent. Blood flow occurs in retrograde fashion from vertebral artery into subclavian artery ("subclavian steal"). *LCC* = left common carotid artery; *LPA* = left pulmonary artery; *LS* = left subclavian artery; *RCC* = right common carotid artery; *RPA* = right pulmonary artery; *RS* = right subclavian artery.

case with single coronary arteries (Fig 30–10,A). However, not all single coronary arteries interfere with corrective surgery (Fig 30–10,B) (see Chapter 64).

5. *Enlarged bronchial arteries.* Enlarged bronchial arteries passing from the descending aorta into the lungs are common. Within the pulmonary parenchyma, the bronchial arteries ultimately join the pulmonary arterial tree. Bronchial arteries may be large and require ligation at operation. They are largest and most numerous in individuals with coexistent pulmonary atresia.

6. *Absence of a pulmonary artery (rare).* Generally if absence of a pulmonary artery occurs, it is found on the

IMPORTANT CORONARY VARIATIONS

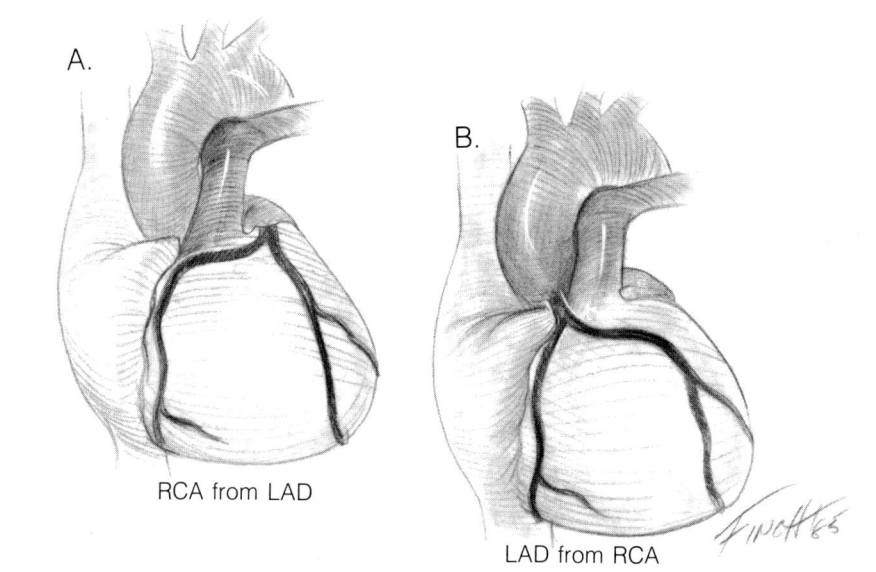

A. RCA from LAD

B. LAD from RCA

FIG 30–9.
Anomalous origin of coronary artery. **A,** right coronary artery *(RCA)* from left anterior descending artery *(LAD)*. Anomalous course of right coronary artery across right ventricular outflow tract makes a ventriculotomy impossible in most instances. **B,** anomalous origin of left anterior descending artery from right coronary artery. Anomalous course of left anterior descending artery across right ventricular outflow tract usually prevents operative incision of right ventricle.

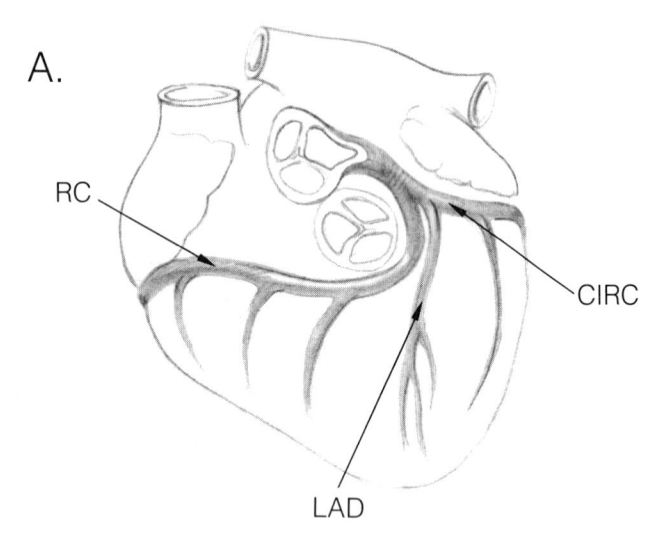

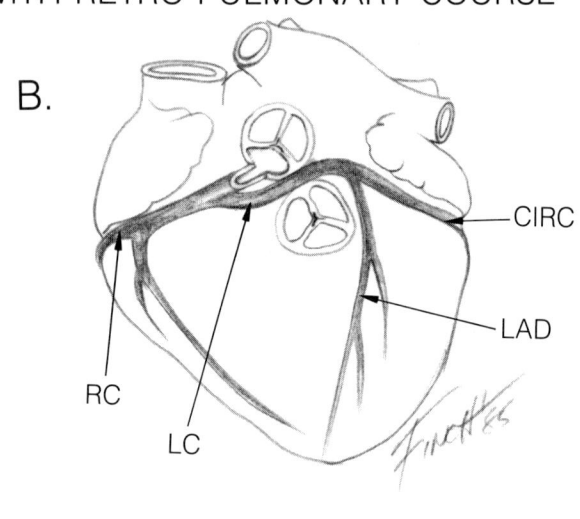

FIG 30–10.
Single coronary artery. **A,** arising above left aortic cusp. Anomalous anterior course of right coronary artery across right ventricular outflow tract. This condition is similar to the origin of the right coronary artery from the left anterior descending artery (see Fig 30–9,A). **B,** arising above right cusp. Retropulmonary course of left coronary artery. This anomaly does not prevent right ventriculotomy. More commonly, single coronary artery crosses in front of infundibulum, preventing a right ventriculotomy. Consequently, angiography and ultrasonography are important to determine course of aberrant branch in relation to pulmonary artery. Only certain coronary anomalies are of practical importance in operative management of tetralogy of Fallot. *CIRC* = circumflex coronary artery; *LC* = left coronary artery; *RC* = right coronary artery.

side opposite the aortic arch. In tetralogy of Fallot, however, absence of a pulmonary artery may occur either ipsilateral or contralateral to the aortic arch. When a pulmonary artery is absent and the involved lung is hypoplastic, the pulmonary trunk leads only to the single enlarged pulmonary artery, which supplies one lung. Although the involved lung is hypoplastic and lacks a proximal pulmonary artery, it contains a complete pulmonary arterial tree originating at the hilum. In the involved lung the pulmonary arterial system is supplied by bronchial and systemic collaterals. If the pleural space has been previously violated, pleural adhesions and systemic transpleural collaterals develop.

7. *Tricuspid insufficiency (rare).* The tricuspid valve can become thickened secondary to long-standing elevation of right ventricular systolic pressure. The tricuspid valve may also be involved by endocarditis. Either can lead to tricuspid regurgitation.

8. *Partial anomalous pulmonary venous connection (rare).*

9. *Double aortic arch (rare).*

10. *Ebstein's malformation of tricuspid valve (rare).*

11. *Mitral stenosis or other left ventricular inflow obstructive lesions (rare).* These may not be clinically evident because of the reduced pulmonary blood flow.

HEMODYNAMICS

In the presence of a large ventricular septal defect, the systolic pressures in the left and right ventricles are equal, and the systolic pressure is similar to the aortic systolic pressure. Because of the pulmonary stenosis, pulmonary arterial pressure is normal or low.

The direction and magnitude of shunt through the ventricular septal defect depend on the relationship between systemic vascular resistance and the resistance imposed by the pulmonary stenosis (Fig 30–11). If the pulmonary stenosis is mild, the shunt through the ventricular septal defect may be in a left-to-right direction resulting in a condition that has been called "acyanotic tetralogy," or "pink tetrad" (see Fig 30–11,A). When the degree of resistance to flow into the lungs and into the body are equal or nearly equal, bidirectional shunt may occur, yielding a balanced tetralogy of Fallot (see Fig 30–11,B). In patients with typical tetralogy of Fallot, the resistance imposed by the pulmonary stenosis exceeds systemic vascular resistance, and the shunt occurs in a right-to-left direction (see Fig 30–11;C).

The resistances caused by the pulmonary stenosis and the systemic vasculature vary in different physiologic states. The systemic vascular resistance varies consider-

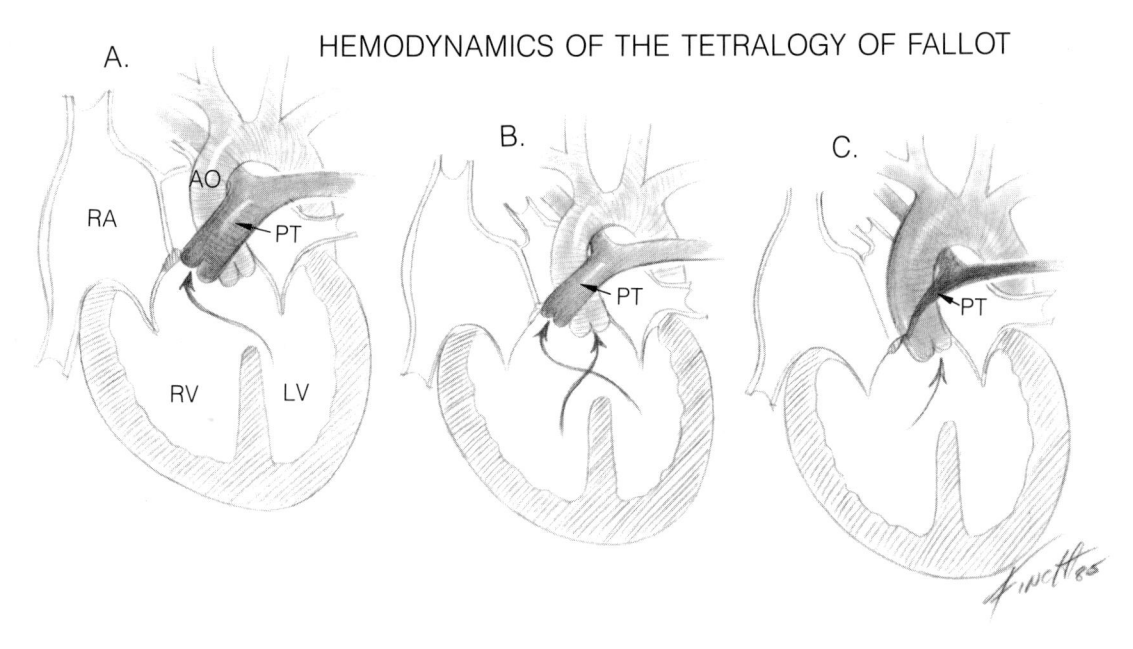

FIG 30-11.
Variations of tetralogy of Fallot. **A,** "Pink tetralogy of Fallot." Mild pulmonary stenosis and left-to-right shunt through ventricular septal defect. This condition is hemodynamically identical to ventricular septal defect. **B,** "Balanced tetrad." Degree of pulmonary stenosis limits pulmonary blood flow and may cause minimal right-to-left shunt. Radiographic findings may be within normal limits. **C,** typical tetralogy of Fallot. Severe pulmonary stenosis. Right-to-left shunt and cyanosis. Characteristic clinical, electrocardiographic, and radiographic findings are present. Hemodynamic conditions may change from **A** to **B** and **C** with age. Increasing degree of pulmonary stenosis because of lack of growth of infundibulum in proportion to increasing cardiac output with childhood growth. *AO* = aorta; *LV* = left ventricle; *PT* = pulmonary trunk; *RA* = right atrium; *RV* = right ventricle.

ably. For instance, during exercise it decreases. When a decrease in systemic vascular resistance occurs in a patient with tetralogy of Fallot, the right-to-left shunt increases and accentuates the cyanosis. Because the pulmonary stenosis results from hypertrophy and narrowing of the infundibulum, this obstruction is also not fixed and varies with the inotropic status of the infundibular myocardium. An increased contractile state, as from augmented β-adrenergic activity, narrows the infundibulum further and increases the right-to-left shunt. Variations in these two resistance factors account for some symptoms that occur in patients with tetralogy of Fallot.

Congestive cardiac failure is not a feature of uncomplicated tetralogy of Fallot. Although right ventricular systolic pressure is elevated, it has been functioning at this level from birth. Therefore, the hypertrophied state of the neonatal right ventricle persists throughout life. Because the ventricular septal defect is large, right ventricular systolic pressure cannot reach suprasystemic levels, regardless of the severity of the obstruction. Exceptions occur rarely with a small, pressure-limiting ventricular septal defect. Furthermore, left ventricular failure does not occur because this chamber is not submitted to volume overload. In fact, the volume load on cardiac chambers is normal, thereby accounting for the normal cardiac size found on a thoracic roentgenogram. Congestive cardiac failure can develop if another factor complicates the basic anatomy or physiology of tetralogy of Fallot, such as a large systemic pulmonary arterial shunt, myocarditis, or endocarditis.

CLINICAL FEATURES

Cyanosis is a major feature and usually appears by 6 months of age. The severity and age of onset of cyanosis vary with the degree of stenosis. Over a period of time, cyanosis usually progresses because of increasing severity of pulmonary stenosis. Clubbing appears after 6 months of age in cyanotic patients. The severity of cyanosis varies from day to day or with the time of day. Factors that lower systemic vascular resistance, such as hot weather, meals, or exercise, increase cyanosis.

Another symptom complex highly suggestive of tetralogy of Fallot is paroxysmal dyspnea or "tetrad spells." These episodes begin in infancy usually before 1 year of age, are initially brief, but become more prolonged and frequent by 1 year of age. Subsequently they disappear. These episodes are alarming, because the infant may become comatose, convulse or die because of severe hypoxemia. The spells occur more commonly in hot weather, in the morning, and with an infection. They are characterized by abrupt onset of hyperpnea, dyspnea, and then increasing degrees of cyanosis until the child becomes limp and unconscious.

The origin of these episodes is unknown, but during them, pulmonary blood flow is markedly reduced. One theory[6] purposes an acute increase in the degree of infundibular stenosis, perhaps caused by increased β-catecholamine activity. Another theory proposes that hyperventilation is the precipitating cause. According to the latter theory, any event that increases oxygen demands, such as feeding or defecation, can increase arterial Pco_2 and decrease pH and Po_2, because the degree of pulmonary stenosis is relatively fixed. The arterial changes in pH, Po_2, and Pco_2 stimulate the respiratory center of the brain, increasing ventilatory rate, further increasing oxygen demands and the right-to-left shunt. Depression of the respiratory center from sedation can break the spell.

Squatting is another characteristic feature of tetralogy of Fallot. Infants and small children tend to interrupt their activity to assume a squatting position to rest. In this position, arterial Po_2 rises. With squatting,[7] the volume of venous return from the lower extremities decreases, probably by reducing arterial flow to the legs. The systemic vascular resistance rises because of the gravitational effects on the circulation on assuming a squatting position. The resultant increase of systemic vascular resistance decreases the right-to-left shunt.[8]

As in most cyanotic conditions, growth is retarded, generally weight more than height. Brain abcess may occur, but in our experience only once in 500 patient years.

PHYSICAL EXAMINATION

Cyanosis, perhaps associated with clubbing, and small stature are noted. The degree of cyanosis varies from examination to examination, depending on the changing relationship between systemic vascular resistance and pulmonary stenosis. Findings of congestive cardiac failure are not present.

There may be a left precordial bulge because of right ventricular hypertrophy. The cardiac apex is normally located. A pulmonary systolic ejection murmur is present, its loudness being inversely related to the severity of the stenosis. During a severe tetrad spell or in patients with coexistent pulmonary atresia, no murmur is heard. This observation indicates that the origin of the murmur is from blood flow through the obstructed right ventricular outflow area and not through the ventricular septal defect. An accompanying thrill is uncommon.

Usually the second heart sound appears single. Because of the pulmonary stenosis and low pulmonary arterial pressure, the pulmonary component is inaudible. Therefore, the second heart sound is represented only by the aortic component. In about 10% of our patients (usually with severe stenosis), an apical systolic ejection click is present and related to the enlarged ascending aorta.

ELECTROCARDIOGRAPHIC FEATURES

The electrocardiographic pattern is remarkably similar among patients. There is right-axis deviation, usually between + 120 and + 150 degrees. Tall, peaked, pointed P waves are found in perhaps one third of older patients with tetralogy of Fallot. This P-wave pattern reflects atrial hypertrophy secondary to elevated right atrial pressure, because right ventricular compliance is reduced secondary to hypertrophy.

A pattern of right ventricular hypertrophy, usually with an rR' pattern in lead V_1, is found. The T waves are normal.

ECHOCARDIOGRAPHIC FEATURES

Echocardiography is an excellent method of diagnosis and permits satisfactory assessment of severity. Both M-mode and long-axis two-dimensional, apical, and subcostal views show an enlarged aorta overriding the ventricular septum. A ventricular septal defect is evident as dropout of echoes immediately below the aortic valve. The degree of aortic overriding can be assessed by studying the relationships between the aortic valve and ventricular septum. Aortic-mitral valve continuity is preserved. Suprasternal imaging allows determination of the position of the aortic arch. On cross-sectional views, right ventricular outflow obstruction at the infundibular, valvar, or supravalvar area can be assessed. Doppler techniques provide an estimate of the gradient across the right ventricular outflow tract. Doppler interrogation is also useful for assessment of the presence of systemic-pulmonary arterial shunts.

RADIOGRAPHIC FEATURES

Thoracic radiographic findings of tetralogy of Fallot vary depending on the degree of pulmonary stenosis. The more severe the pulmonary stenosis, the more characteristic the radiographic appearance. Pulmonary atresia with ventricular septal defect has the most characteristic cardiac silhouette.

We describe four radiographic appearances, which vary according to the severity of the stenosis, the volume of pulmonary blood flow, and associated malformations.

Ventricular Septal Defect, Pulmonary Stenosis, and Left-to-Right Shunt ("Pink Tetrad")

1. Depending on the degree of pulmonary stenosis, which may be mild, the pulmonary vasculature may be increased, and the radiographic findings are identical to those of a ventricular septal defect.

2. In spite of the left-to-right shunt, the pulmonary arterial segment is usually not prominent in contrast to a typical ventricular septal defect (in which pulmonary stenosis is not present). REASON: Because of the coexistent pulmonary stenosis, the volume of left-to-right shunt is limited. Furthermore, with infundibular pulmonary stenosis, the pulmonary annulus and main pulmonary artery tend to be small.

3. Cardiac size is normal or slightly enlarged. REASON: Pulmonary stenosis limits the left-to-right shunt. Left ventricular dilatation is absent or minimal.

Balanced and Slightly Cyanotic Tetralogy

The radiographic findings are normal (Fig 30–12). REASON: Because both ventricles are connected by a large ventricular septal defect, the systolic pressure in the ventricles are equal at a systemic level. Systolic pressures in the right ventricle do not exceed systemic levels. Thus, decompensation of the right ventricle does not occur. Because the volume of pulmonary blood flow is nearly normal, pulmonary vasculature and cardiac size are normal.

Tetralogy of Fallot With Right-to-Left Shunt

With increasing severity of pulmonary stenosis, a greater volume of blood is ejected from the right ventricle into the aorta. This direction of the ejection force (Fig 30–13) causes a clockwise rotation of the heart and elevation of the apex of the right ventricle. Together with the right ventricular enlargement, the clockwise rotation results in a typical wooden shoe (coeur en sabot[1])* appearance.

Clockwise rotation of the heart has the following consequences:

1. The cardiac apex is formed by the right ventricle instead of the left ventricle, as in the normal heart. This causes the round, upturned cardiac apex apparent on a thoracic roentgenogram.

2. The clockwise rotation displaces the pulmonary valve and right ventricular outflow tract toward the left.

3. The right pulmonary artery becomes the extension of the main pulmonary artery rather than the left pulmonary artery, as in a normal heart (see Fig 30–13,A). Therefore the ejection of blood through the pulmonary valve occurs principally into the right pulmonary artery (see Fig 30–13,B). This commonly causes the pulmonary vasculature to be more decreased in the left lung than in the right lung (Fig 30–14,B).

4. In spite of clockwise rotation of the heart, the left cardiac border is not round as in the clockwise rotation found in patients with atrial septal defect. REASON: The infundibulum is stenotic, and the main pulmonary artery is anatomically small. With dilatation of the infundibulum as in instances of stenosis of the os infundibulum, a small prominence in the region of the infundibulum may be visualized (Fig 30–14,A).

Anteroposterior Projection

1. The roentgenographic appearance of the pulmonary vasculature depends on the presence and extent of pulmonary stenosis and the degree of bronchial collateral arteries. Very large bronchial arteries, as can occur in some patients with coexistent pulmonary atresia, may result in increased pulmonary vasculature (see Chapter 31).

2. In many cases the pulmonary vasculature is either within normal limits or at the lower limits of normal (see Fig 30–12).

3. The apex of the heart tends to be elevated. REASON: Right ventricular hypertrophy causes clockwise rotation of the heart. The small infundibulum adds to this appearance (see Fig 30–14,B).

4. The pulmonary arterial segment tends to be concave. REASON: The pulmonary artery and infundibulum are

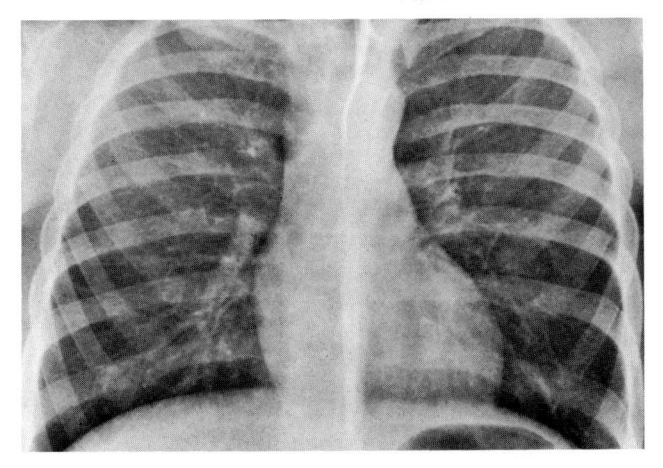

FIG 30–12.
Balanced tetralogy of Fallot. Thoracic roentgenogram. Posteroanterior projection. Normal cardiac size and pulmonary vasculature. Mild pulmonary stenosis and little right-to-left or left-to-right shunt.

*Sabot is a wooden shoe that was worn by peasants in Europe.

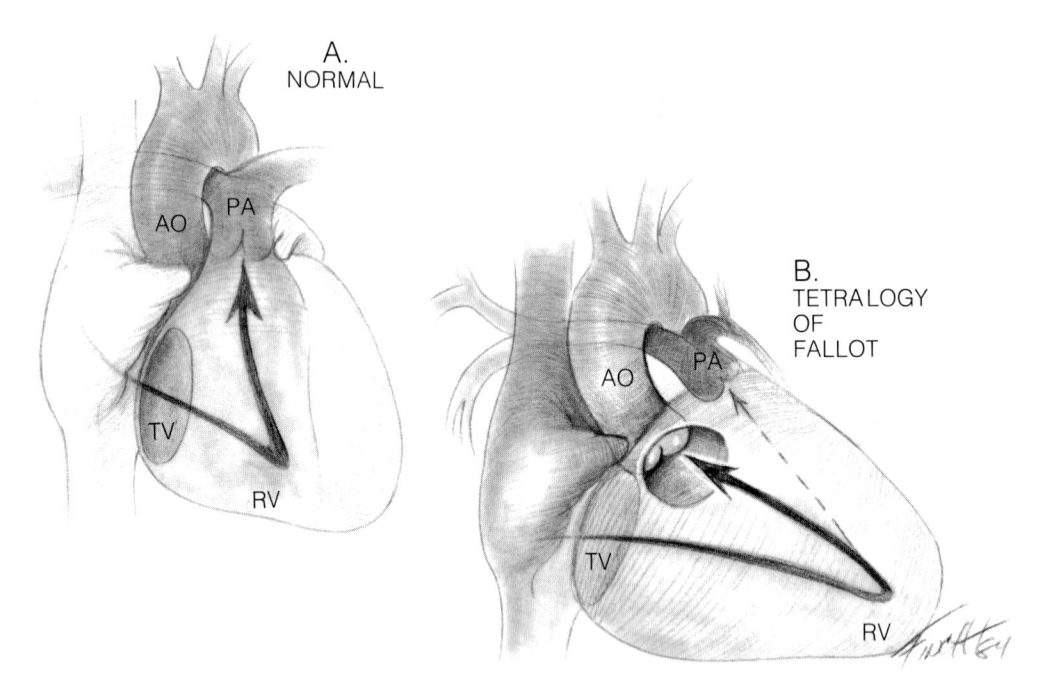

FIG 30–13.
Cross-section pattern of right ventricle. **A,** direction of blood flow *(arrow)* through right ventricle *(RV)* in normal heart. Ejection force is directed vertically into pulmonary artery, which has vertical position. Cardiac apex formed by left ventricle. **B,** tetralogy of Fallot and severe pulmonary stenosis. Small amount of blood is ejected into pulmonary artery *(PA) (dotted arrow)*. Most of blood ejected from right ventricle through ventricular septal defect into aorta *(AO)* (direction of ejection force indicated by solid arrow). Altered direction of blood flow induces clockwise rotation of heart, causing boot-shaped cardiac configuration. Cardiac apex is formed by right ventricle. Direction of main pulmonary artery is more horizontal. *TV* = tricuspid value.

anatomically small. The more severe the pulmonary stenosis, the more characteristic the cardiac silhouette.

5. The portion of the left cardiac border formed by the outflow portion of the right ventricle tends to be straight. REASON: The infundibulum is small (see Fig 30–14,B).

6. The cardiac apex is elevated. REASON: The ejection force of the right ventricle is directed into the ventricular septal defect. The more severe the pulmonary stenosis, the more elevated the cardiac apex (see Fig 30–14). This radiographic appearance varies depending on the projection whether lordotic or reversed lordotic (see Chapter 5).

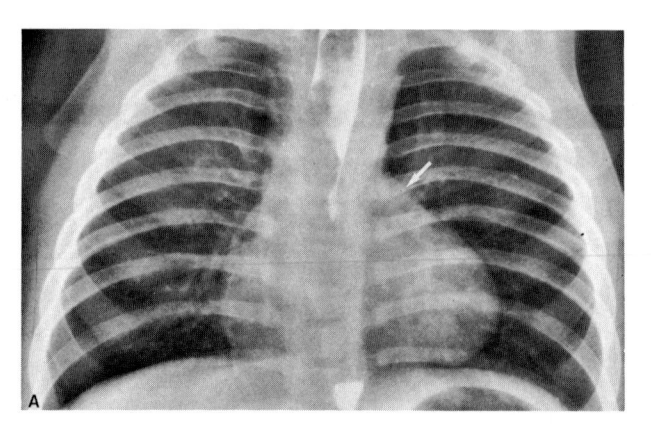

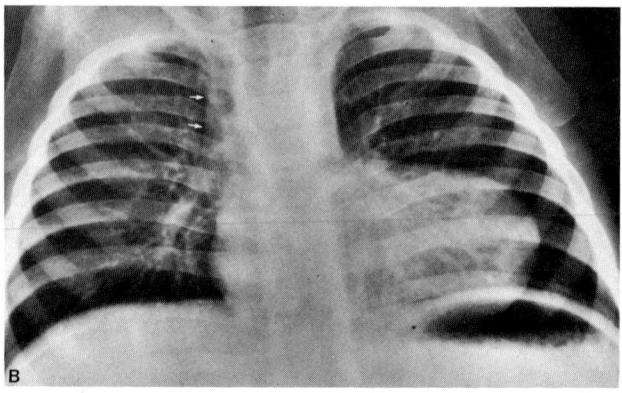

FIG 30–14.
Tetralogy of Fallot. Thoracic roentgenogram. Posteroanterior projection. **A,** Moderate severity. Pulmonary vasculature is at lower limits of normal. Heart is not enlarged. Slight elevation of cardiac apex. Left cardiac contour is unusually straight. Pulmonary arterial segment is not visualized (concave pulmonary artery segment). Small "bump" along upper cardiac border contour *(arrow)* suggests dilatation of infundibular chamber ("third ventricle"). **B,** diminished pulmonary vasculature, particularly in left lung. Heart is not enlarged. Clockwise rotation simulates cardiomegaly. Marked elevation of cardiac apex. Upper left cardiac border is unusually straight. Concave pulmonary arterial segment. Large ascending aorta displaces superior vena cava toward right *(arrows)*.

7. The aorta is enlarged, probably for two reasons. First, the volume of blood flow through the ascending aorta is increased because it consists of the cardiac output and bronchial arterial blood flow. Second, during development of the heart, the primitive truncus arteriosus is divided unequally into a larger aorta and a smaller pulmonary artery.

8. The superior vena cava may be prominent. REASON: The large ascending aorta displaces the adjacent right superior vena cava toward the right (see Fig 30–14,B).

9. The pulmonary vasculature is usually more decreased in the left lung compared with the right lung. REASON: Clockwise rotation of the heart, resulting in ejection of blood through the pulmonary valve directly into the right pulmonary artery (see Figs 30–13,B and 30–14,B), which may become dilated (poststenotic dilatation). In contrast, valvar in pulmonary stenosis with intact septum, post-stenotic dilatation of the left pulmonary is more common (see Chapter 29).

Left Anterior Oblique Projection

To obtain a satisfactory left anterior oblique view, one must obtain steep projections (Fig 30–15). REASON: The heart is rotated clockwise, particularly in patients with severe tetralogy of Fallot.

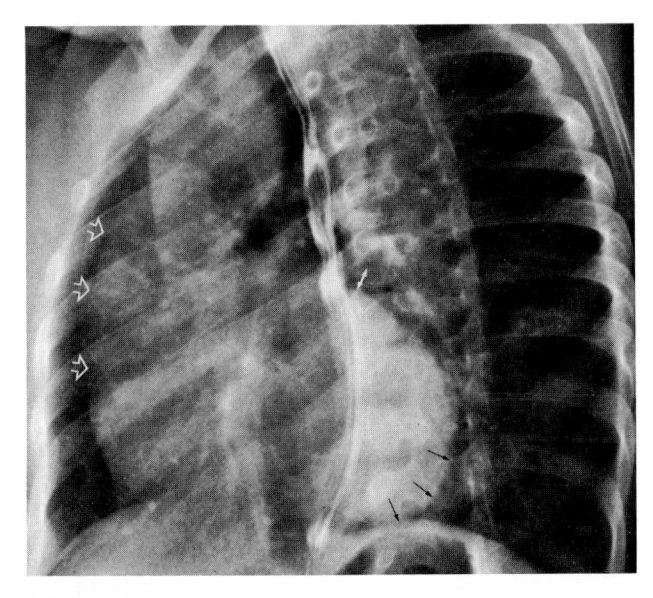

FIG 30–15.
Severe tetralogy of Fallot. Thoracic roentgenogram. Left anterior oblique projection. In spite of steep left anterior oblique projection, left ventricle overlies spine because of marked clockwise rotation. Clear space *(white arrows)* between left mainstem bronchus and heart because of small left atrium. Right atrial shadow blends with large ascending aorta *(open arrows)*. Classical radiographic findings of right-sided hypertrophy are lost. Cardiac apex is elevated *(black arrows)*.

1. There is a clear space between left mainstem bronchus and left atrium. REASON: The left atrium is not enlarged.

2. The typical radiographic findings for right-sided cardiac enlargement (bulging right cardiac border) are lost. REASON: Rotation of the heart and enlargement of the ascending aorta minimize the right atrial bulge.

Lateral Projection

1. The retrosternal space is obliterated by the hypertrophied right ventricle, and this may cause bulging of the sternum (Fig 30–16).

2. The left atrium is not enlarged. REASON: The flow through the lungs, left atrium, and left ventricle are decreased because of diminished volume of pulmonary blood flow.

3. The esophagus may be indented posteriorly by enlarged bronchial arteries, particularly in patients with severe tetralogy of Fallot or with coexistent pulmonary atresia.

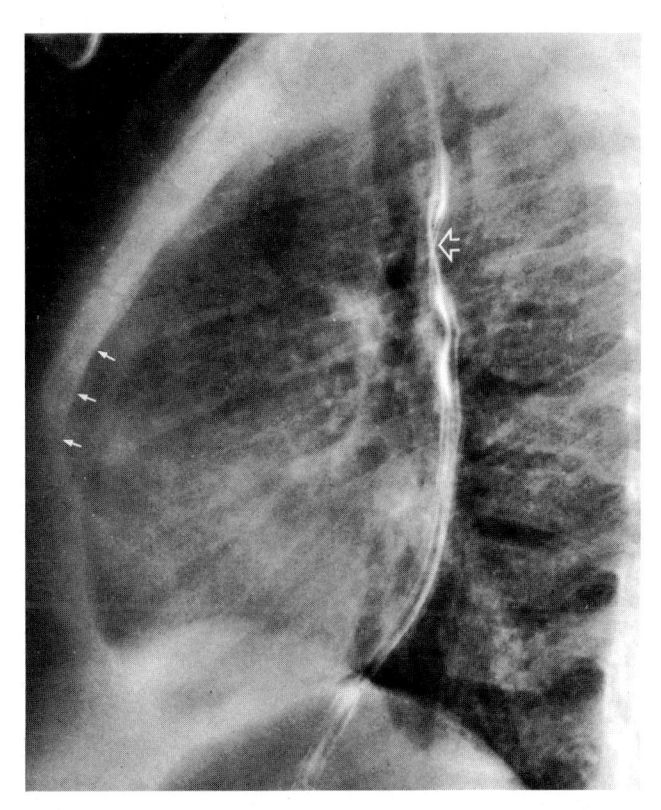

FIG 30–16.
Tetralogy of Fallot. Thoracic roentgenogram. Lateral projection. Increased contact of right side of heart with sternum. Anterior bowing of sternum *(solid arrows)* suggest right-sided hypertrophy. Esophagus is not displaced because left atrium is normal or small. Indentation of upper part of esophagus from behind *(open arrow)* suggests prominent bronchial artery.

Tetralogy of Fallot With Cardiomegaly

If tetralogy of Fallot is associated with cardiomegaly (Fig 30–17), an unusual coexistent condition should be considered:

1. The ventricular septal defect may be small. Therefore, right ventricular systolic pressure exceeds left ventricular systolic pressure, and right ventricular decompensation occurs. The ventricular septal defect may be anatomically small (rare), or it may be partially occluded by accessory tricuspid valve tissue, by an abnormally positioned large septal limb of the crista supraventricularis or an anomalous muscle bundle. Very rarely, a mitral valve abnormality may be the cause for cardiomegaly.
2. Insufficiency of a cardiac valve can cause cardiomegaly. This may result from absence of the pulmonary valve, from coexistent Ebstein's malformation, or from mitral regurgitation (if, for example, atrioventricular canal coexists with tetralogy of Fallot).

In each patient with tetralogy of Fallot, valuable diagnostic information can be obtained by reviewing the radiographic appearance of the bony thorax and identifying the location of the aortic arch.

The Bony Thorax

Careful scrutiny of the bony thorax is very valuable in patients with tetralogy of Fallot, particularly in the assessment of previous cardiac operations:

1. An abnormality or absence of an upper rib suggests previous resection and the presence of a systemic pulmonary shunt. This association is particularly strong if the resected rib is located on the side opposite the aortic arch, because a Blalock-Taussig procedure is usually performed contralateral to the arch (Fig 30–18,A). REASON: The subclavian artery arising from the innominate artery is less prone to kinking as it is turned down to be anastomosed to the pulmonary artery.
2. Unilateral rib notching suggests a previous Blalock-Taussig anastomosis. In this instance, collateral blood flow occurs to the distal subclavian artery in part from the descending aorta through the intercostal arteries. Rib notching can also indicate collateral blood flow through transpleural collateral arteries into a proximally obstructed pulmonary artery.
3. There is a higher incidence of the rib anomalies, hemivertebrae, scoliosis, faulty segmentation, premature fusion, and bowing of the sternum among patients with tetralogy of Fallot (Fig 30–19).

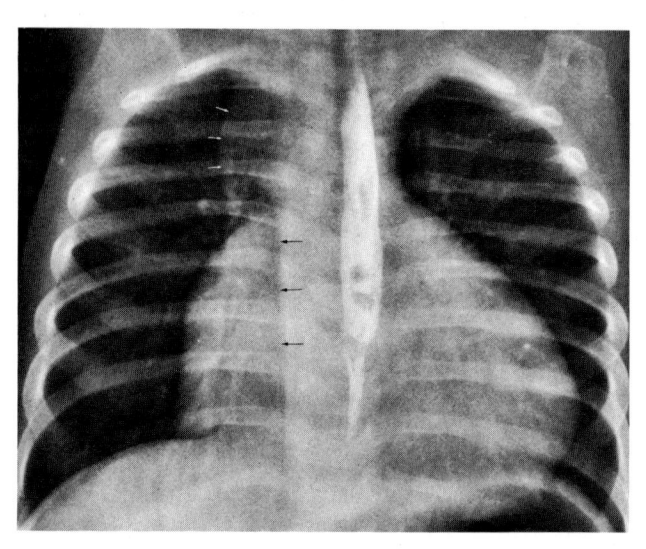

FIG 30–17.
Coexistent tetralogy of Fallot and atrioventricular canal. Thoracic roentgenogram. Posteroanterior projection. Marked cardiomegaly. Right aortic arch. Decreased pulmonary vasculature. Complicating factor must be considered to account for marked cardiomegaly. In this case, atrioventricular canal with pulmonary stenosis. NOTE: Displacement of trachea to left by right aortic arch. No indentation of esophagus by arch. Thoracic aorta descends on right (*black arrows*). Marked displacement of superior vena cava by right arch (*white arrows*).

Identification of the Aortic Arch

In the tetralogy of Fallot, the identification of the aortic arch is important because 25% of patients with cyanotic tetralogy of Fallot have a right aortic arch. The incidence of right arch increases with severity of pulmonary stenosis and is greatest among patients with coexistent pulmonary atresia. In right aortic arch:

1. The trachea and barium-filled esophagus are indented and slightly displaced to the left. The aorta descends on the right but pierces the diaphragm to the left of the spine (Figs 30–18,A and 30–20).
2. The right superior vena cava is displaced toward the right (see Fig 30–18,A and 30–20).
3. In most cases with right aortic arch, a retroesophageal vessel (aberrant left subclavian artery) is not present.
4. Among patients with a right aortic arch, no retroesophageal segment, and a right-sided descending aorta, 98% of cases are associated with a congenital cardiac anomaly. If the pulmonary vascular markings are decreased, tetralogy of Fallot is the most likely diagnosis. If the pulmonary vascular markings are increased, truncus arteriosus is the most likely diagnosis.

In patients with tetralogy of Fallot, a retroesophageal vessel (aberrant left subclavian artery) is rarely present.

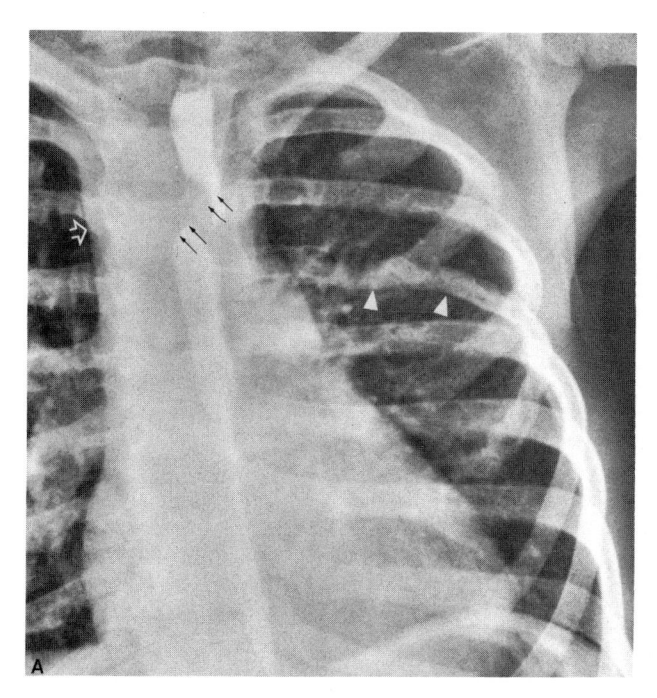

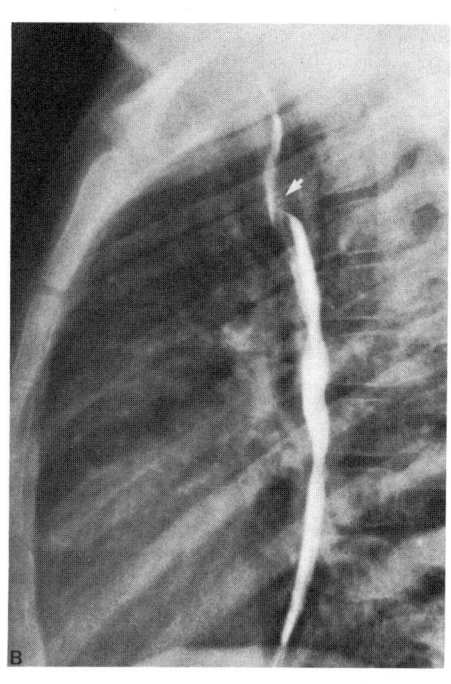

FIG 30–18.
Tetralogy of Fallot. Right aortic arch. Thoracic roentgenogram. **A,** posteroanterior projection. Previous rib resection *(white arrows)* indicates Blalock-Taussig anastomosis, which is characteristically performed opposite aortic arch. Barium-filled esophagus *(black arrows)* indented by aberrant left subclavian artery. In tetralogy of Fallot aberrant artery does not arise from an aortic diverticulum. Therefore, small indentation of barium-filled esophagus *(black arrows)* results. Superior vena cava displaced slightly by right aortic arch *(open arrow)*. **B,** lateral projection. Small indentation *(arrow)* of esophagus by aberrant left subclavian artery.

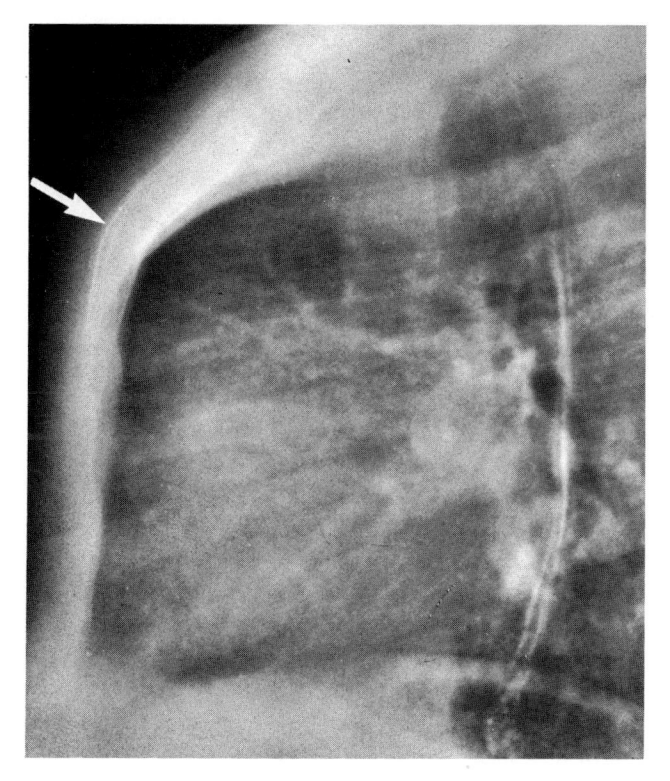

FIG 30–19.
Tetralogy of Fallot. Thoracic roentgenogram. Lateral projection. Premature fusion of manubrium, resulting in distinct bony bulge *(arrow)*.

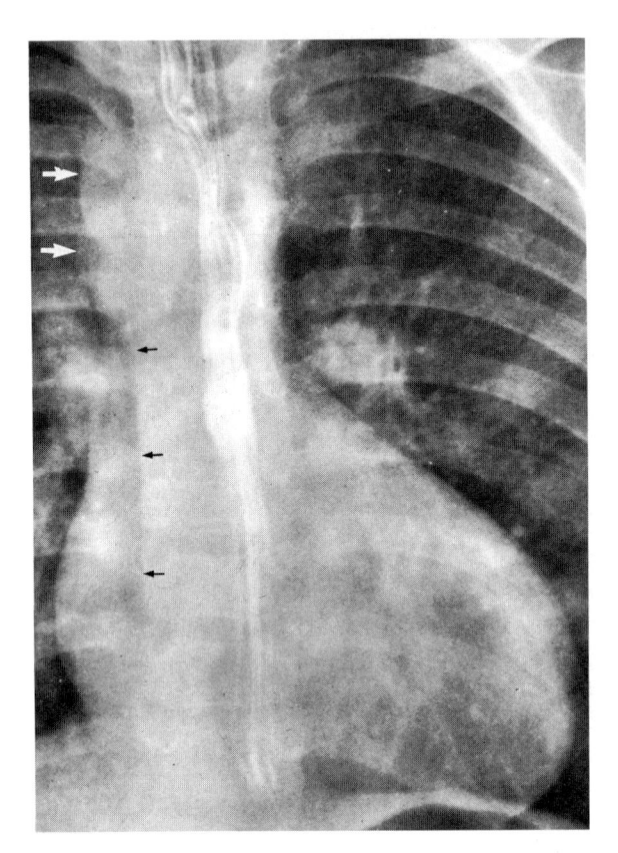

FIG 30-20.
Tetralogy of Fallot. Right aortic arch. Thoracic roentgenogram. Posteroanterior projection. Barium-filled esophagus and trachea are displaced by right aortic arch. No retroesophageal segment. Thoracic aorta descends on right *(black arrows)*. Superior vena cava is displaced toward right by right aortic arch *(white arrow).*

When present, the aberrant left subclavian artery does not arise from an aortic diverticulum as in patients without a congenital cardiac anomaly or in those with a coexistent left-to-right shunt (see Fig 30–18). Therefore, in patients with tetralogy of Fallot, the indentation on the esophagus from an aberrant left subclavian artery is small (see Fig 30–18,B). The appearance of a small esophageal indentation is virtually diagnostic of right arch, aberrant left subclavian artery, and tetralogy of Fallot. In an otherwise normal heart with right aortic arch and aberrant left subclavian artery, the retroesophageal portion of the aberrant subclavian artery is large (aortic diverticulum), because during fetal life this portion of the vessel carried a large volume of right-to-left blood flow through the ductus arteriosus. Conversely, during fetal life in tetralogy of Fallot, the flow through the ductus arteriosus is diminished or left to right because of the pulmonary stenosis. Therefore, the ductus arteriosus is either small or does not develop. Consequently, the retroesophageal segment of the left subclavian artery remains of normal size.

CARDIAC CATHETERIZATION

At many cardiac centers, most patients with tetralogy of Fallot undergo catheterization before a cardiac operation. The principal reason for cardiac catheterization is the angiographic demonstration of anatomic details, especially of the right ventricular outflow area, pulmonary arterial tree, and coexistent muscular ventricular septal defects of the coronary arterial anatomy.

During cardiac catheterization, care must be taken because the procedure may induce a tetrad spell. Thus, the operator must carefully observe the patient for restlessness and increase in cyanosis or respiratory rate and must monitor changes in arterial Po_2 and pH. Manipulation of the catheter in the right ventricular outflow area seems particularly capable of causing these spells.

The oxygen saturation of blood in the chambers of the right side of the heart is low in proportion to the degree of systemic oxygen desaturation. No evidence of a left-to-right shunt is found. A right-to-left shunt may be identified at the atrial level, with reduced left atrial and left ventricular oxygen saturations. Aortic oxygen saturation is reduced and may fall gradually or precipitously during the cardiac catheterization as changes in degree of pulmonary stenosis or systemic vascular resistance occur. Usually it is difficult to calculate the size of the right-to-left shunt because of the variability of aortic oxygen saturation during a cardiac catheterization.

Right atrial pressure, particularly the a wave is elevated. Right ventricular systolic pressure is elevated and at the same level as left ventricular and aortic systolic pressures. Pulmonary arterial pressure is reduced. Even with an end-hole catheter, it may be difficult to determine the site of stenosis on withdrawal pressure tracing from pulmonary artery through the right ventricle.

During the catheterization, balloon angiography may be performed to reveal sites of coexistent peripheral pulmonary arterial stenosis demonstrated angiographically. This technique may be particularly appropriate for stenotic areas that are difficult to approach operatively, as in the right pulmonary artery or in patients who have had a previous operation wherein the operative approach is rendered difficult because of adhesions.

ANGIOGRAPHIC FEATURES

In each patient with tetralogy of Fallot, right and left ventriculography and aortography are indicated, and often pulmonary angiography as well.

Right ventriculography is indicated:

1. To demonstrate the degree of infundibular pulmonary stenosis and coexistent obstructive right ventricular muscle bundles when they occur.
2. To demonstrate the size of the pulmonary annulus and main pulmonary artery.
3. To visualize the pulmonary arterial tree, which may be hypoplastic and may be unable to accept the entire cardiac output after closure of the ventricular septal defect.
4. To demonstrate associated branch pulmonary artery stenosis, which during cardiac operation may require extension of a patch beyond the level of pulmonary bifurcation.
5. To demonstrate the ventricular communications.

Left ventriculography is indicated to demonstrate an associated muscular ventricular communication. Depending on pulmonary and systemic resistance, the defect may not be demonstrated by right ventriculography. Although an associated muscular ventricular defect is rare, its demonstration is important because it may be overlooked at time of operation (see Fig 30–32).

Pulmonary angiography may be necessary, because stenotic lesions may be obscured by the opacified aorta. Special angiographic projections may be required to demonstrate these areas of stenosis. Rarely, pulmonary arteriography cannot be performed because the catheter in the pulmonary artery may induce a tetrad spell.

Aortography or selective coronary angiography should be performed. A catheter can be easily passed across the ventricular septal defect into the aorta to perform an aortogram, which demonstrates coronary anomalies (present in 5% of the cases)[9] that may make right ventriculotomy and complete repair difficult or impossible.

Finally, other injections may be required, depending on clinical and laboratory data of an individual case. For instance, a left ventriculogram should be performed to demonstrate atrioventricular valvular insufficiency as occurs in coexistent tetralogy of Fallot and atrioventricular canal (see Fig 30–17). It is also indicated to demonstrate a coexistent muscular defect.

ANGIOGRAPHIC POSITIONING

Because the infundibulum is foreshortened in both the anteroposterior and right anterior oblique projections, cranial beam angulation provides better visualization of this important area. With fixed biplane equipment, this angulation is accomplished by having the patient sit up. This projection also allows better demonstration of the main pulmonary artery and its bifurcation (see Chapter 7).

The standard lateral and a slightly rotated right anterior oblique projection also provide satisfactory demonstration of the anatomy of the right ventricular outflow tract. Because of the clockwise rotation of the heart, the ventricular septum lies in the direction of the x-ray beam and is therefore seen in profile on a lateral projection.

The branches of the pulmonary artery are best demonstrated by selective injection of the pulmonary artery to avoid superimposition of the aorta. A shallow right anterior oblique projection allows visualization of the origin of the right pulmonary artery. With cranial beam angulation, the left pulmonary artery may be seen without being obscured by other cardiac or vascular structures. The best view for the pulmonary bifurcation is a steep left anterior oblique projection with caudal beam angulation (see Fig 2–27).

ANGIOGRAPHIC APPEARANCE

Right ventriculography and aortography provide important information in tetralogy of Fallot.

Right Ventriculography

1. During a right ventriculogram, both the aorta and pulmonary artery opacify. If ventricular extrasystoles are induced during selective right ventriculography, the pulmonary artery opacifies but not the aorta (Fig 30–21). REASON: During a series of ventricular extrasystoles, the atrioventricular valves open for only a short period. Consequently, the ventricles receive a reduced volume of blood, and the stroke volume is reduced. As a result, ventricular systolic pressure may fall below the aortic diastolic pressure. Therefore, during extrasystoles, insufficient ventricular pressure is generated to open the aortic valve, and the aorta does not opacify. In contrast, the pulmonary valve opens because there is sufficient ventricular pressure to open the pulmonary valve against the low pulmonary arterial diastolic pressure. After a compensatory pause following the extrasystoles, the aortic valve opens with the next systole, and the aorta opacifies normally.
2. The infundibulum contracts forcefully during systole and relaxes during diastole. Even during diastole, the infundibulum remains narrower than normal, indicating infundibular stenosis (Fig 30–22).
3. The main pulmonary artery, infundibulum, and pulmonary annulus are smaller than normal and of similar caliber (see Fig 30–22). There is a variable degree of infundibular pulmonary stenosis from a localized stenosis of the os infundibulum to the diffuse fibrotic stenoses (Fig 30–23).
4. The crista supraventricularis is prominent and best

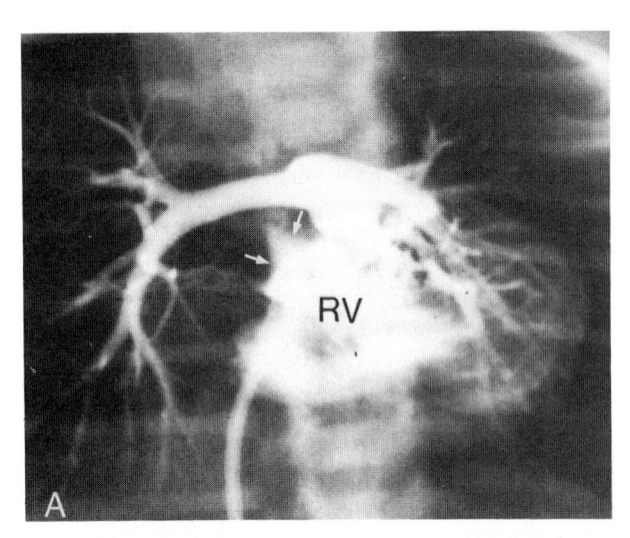

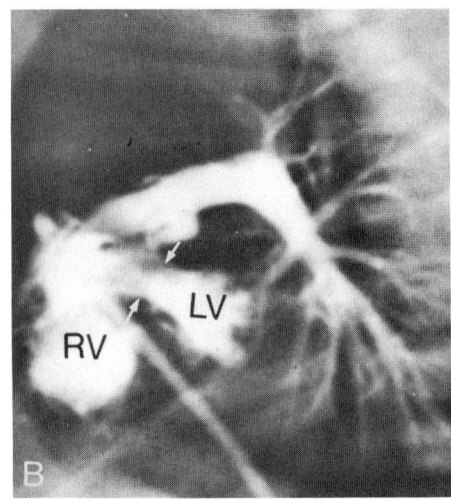

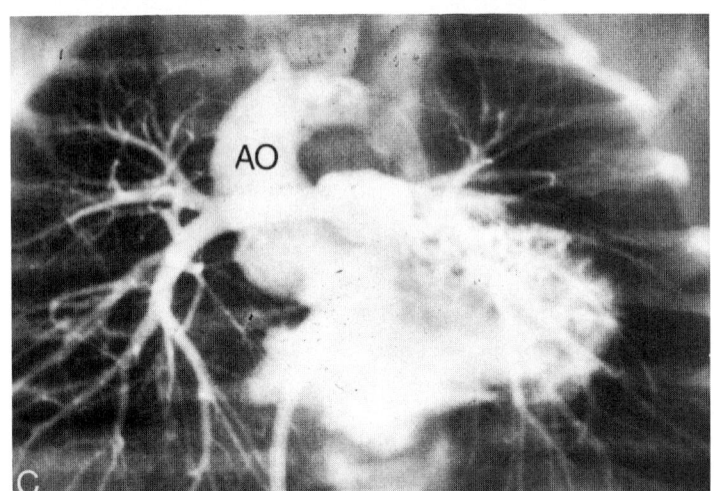

FIG 30–21.
Tetralogy of Fallot during a series of extrasystoles. Right ventriculogram *(RV)*. **A,** anteroposterior projection. Pulmonary arteries are well opacified, but aortic valve does not open. Aorta unopacified. Contrast medium immediately beneath closed aortic valve *(arrows)*. **B,** lateral projection. Large ventricular septal defect *(arrows)*. Contrast material fills left ventricle *(LV)* because of extrasystoles. Aorta unopacified. **C,** after compensatory pause. Dense opacification of aorta *(AO)*.

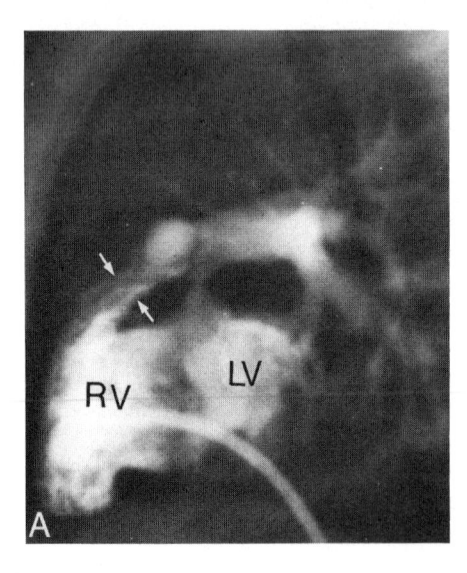

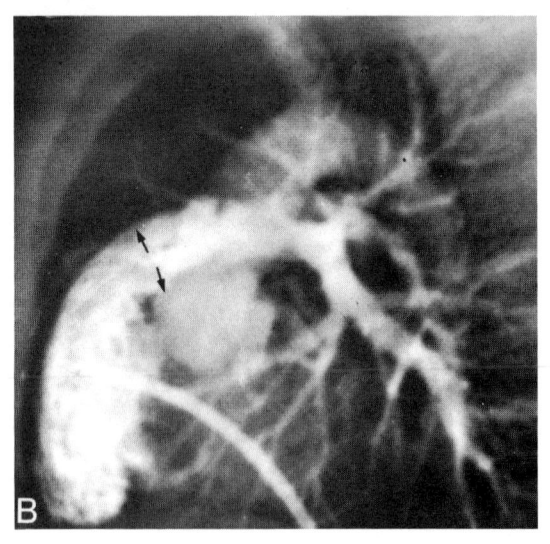

FIG 30–22.
Tetralogy of Fallot. Right ventriculogram *(RV)*. Lateral projection. **A,** during ventricular extrasystoles. Left ventricle *(LV)* fills densely through ventricular septal defect because of extrasystoles. Pulmonary artery is opacified. Infundibulum *(white arrows)* is contracted. Aorta is unopacified. **B,** after compensatory pause. Opacification of aorta. During diastole, infundibulum *(black arrows)* relaxes but is still stenotic. Aorta does not override (very uncommon). Extrasystoles also cause opacification of the left ventricle.

observed on a lateral projection, where it appears as a prominent posterior indentation (see Fig 30–23).

5. Right ventricle is hypertrophied and heavily trabeculated because of the hypertrophy (see Fig 30–23).

6. The pulmonary valve is thickened and stenotic in 90% of the cases. It is usually bicuspid and produces a fairly characteristic clamshell appearance on a lateral projection (see Fig 30–23).

7. Rarely, the pulmonary valve is normal.

8. With severe infundibular stenosis, the pulmonary annulus is also hypoplastic (see Fig 30–23).

9. Although the caliber of the main pulmonary artery is similar to that of the stenotic infundibulum and small pulmonary annulus, additional stenosis of the supravalvar portion of the main pulmonary artery may occur (see Fig 30–23).

10. Poststenotic dilatation of the main pulmonary artery or its major branches is rarely present.

11. Because the left pulmonary artery is located significantly more cephalad than the right (see Fig 30–23), this anatomic relationship facilitates demonstration of the pulmonary bifurcation on a lateral or steep left anterior oblique projection using caudad beam angulation.

12. Supravalvar pulmonary stenosis may be circumferential or may be caused by a stenotic fibrotic ridge (Fig 30–24). Rarely, a tubular type diffuse stenosis of the main pulmonary artery is present (Fig 30–25).

13. Stenoses of the right and left pulmonary arteries should be demonstrated to provide important information for operative repair. Because of anatomic variations, angiographic demonstration represents a challenge to the angiographer but is accomplished best by pulmonary arteriography (Fig 30–26) in anteroposterior projection and cranial beam angulation or left anterior oblique projection with caudal angulation (Fig 2–27).

14. The right pulmonary artery is usually larger than the left. REASON: Clockwise rotation orients the infundibulum toward the right pulmonary artery. Therefore, blood is ejected directly into the right pulmonary artery. The left pulmonary arterial tree tends to be smaller and may show delayed filling.

15. Diffuse severe pulmonary arterial stenoses or hypoplasia of the entire pulmonary arterial tree may be associated (Fig 30–28). In such patients, complete repair of the cardiac anomaly is contraindicated. A systemic pulmonary arterial shunt procedure is performed in the hope to stimulate pulmonary arterial growth. However, in spite of

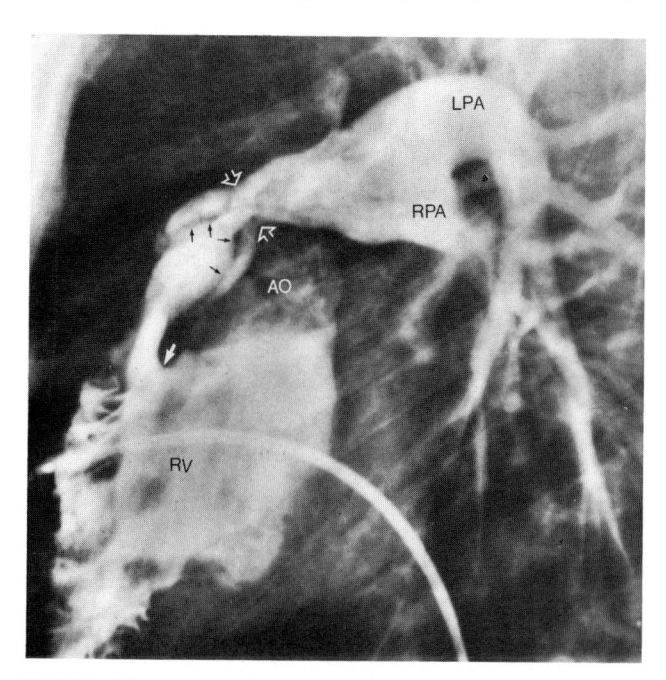

FIG 30–23.
Tetralogy of Fallot. Right ventriculogram during ventricular extrasystoles. Lateral projection. Increased trabeculations of right ventricle *(RV)* indicate right ventricular hypertrophy. Aorta *(AO)* is incompletely opacified because of ventricular extrasystoles. Crista supraventricularis *(white arrow)* narrows os infundibulum. Pulmonary valve is distinctly thickened *(small black arrows)* and has clamshell appearance typical of bicuspid pulmonary valve. Associated supravalvar pulmonary stenosis *(open arrows)*. Left pulmonary artery *(LPA)* shows poststenotic dilatation and is positioned considerably higher than right pulmonary artery *(RPA)*. Because of this anatomic relationship, origins of right and left pulmonary artery are well seen but could be better demonstrated by caudal beam angulation.

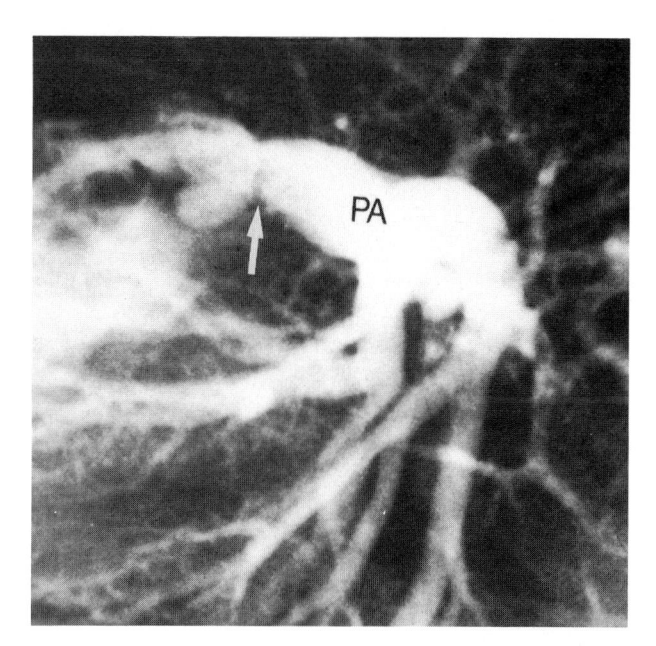

FIG 30–24.
Tetralogy of Fallot. Pulmonary arteriogram *(PA)*. Lateral projection. Well-defined fibrotic ridge *(arrow)* in supravalvar portion of pulmonary artery.

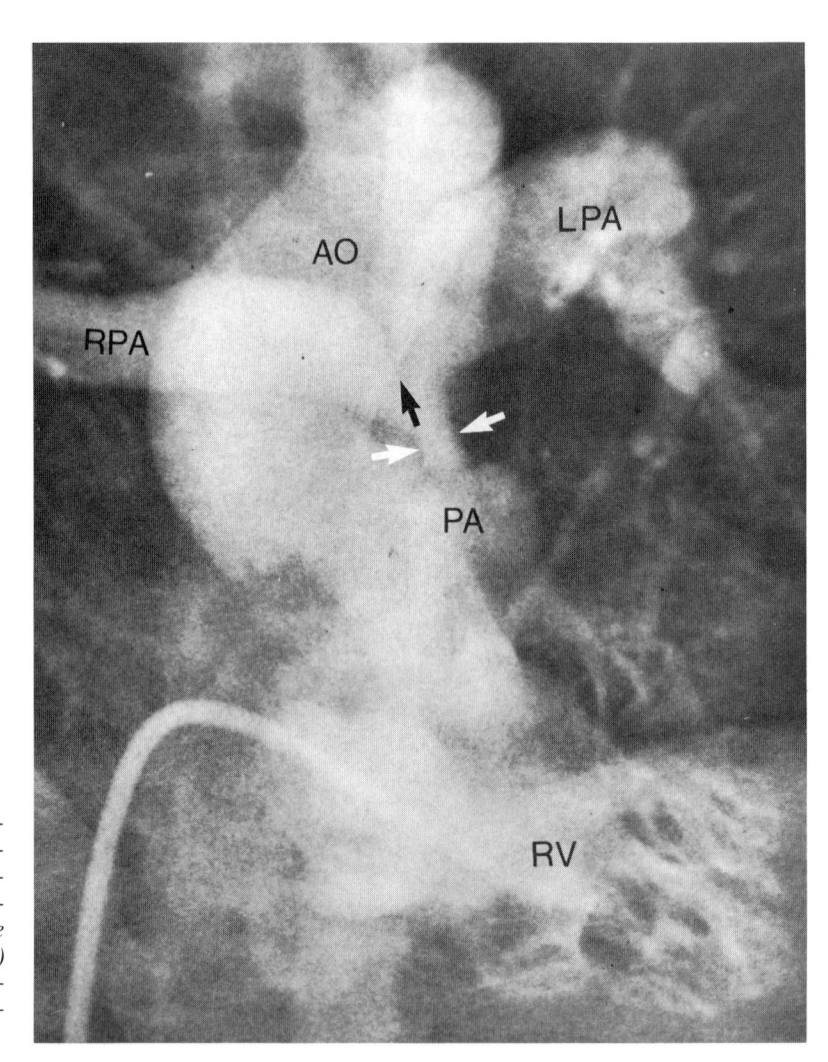

FIG 30–25.
Tetralogy of Fallot. Right ventriculogram. Anteroposterior projection. Heavily trabeculated hypertrophied right ventricle *(RV)*. Aorta *(AO)* and pulmonary arteries *(PA)* opacify simultaneously. Severe tubular supravalvar pulmonary stenosis *(white arrows)*. Large aorta. Left pulmonary artery *(LPA)* has abnormally high course and shows poststenotic dilatation. Right *(RPA)* and left pulmonary branch stenosis *(black arrow)*.

a systemic pulmonary arterial shunt, the pulmonary arteries may remain hypoplastic (see Fig 30–28).

16. Whether complete correction of tetralogy of Fallot is feasible depends largely on the cross-sectional area of the pulmonary artery. As measured on an anteroposterior projection of a right ventriculogram, the combined right and left pulmonary artery diameters should equal or be slightly larger than the diameter of the aorta at the level of the diaphragm. The operative correction is probably feasible (Fig 30–29).

17. In addition to infundibular and valvar pulmonary stenoses, anomalous right ventricular muscle bundles may be present and evident as large round radiolucencies in an anteroposterior projection of a right ventriculogram. Typically such muscle bundles are located below the level of the crista supraventricularis (Fig 30–30).

18. Characteristically the ventricular septal defect is large and extends to the level of the aortic valve. Therefore, it is located in a different position than the more common perimembranous septal defect (Fig 30–31). As a result, the aorta can override the septum to various degrees. Because of the subaortic location of the defect, care must be taken at time of operation to avoid damage to the aortic valve.

19. The degree to which the aorta straddles the ventricular septal defect varies from none (see Fig 30–23) to mild to severe. Most cases show some degree of overriding of the aorta. Patients with severe overriding tend to have a larger aorta.

20. Overriding of the aorta may be so severe that the distinction between tetralogy of Fallot with severe overriding of the aorta and double-outlet right ventricle may be difficult. In tetralogy of Fallot with severe overriding, the anterior leaflet of the mitral valve, however, remains in continuity with the aortic valve, whereas in double-outlet right ventricle, these two valves are separated by myocardial tissue (see Fig 30–3D).

21. The ventricular septal defect is large. Right and

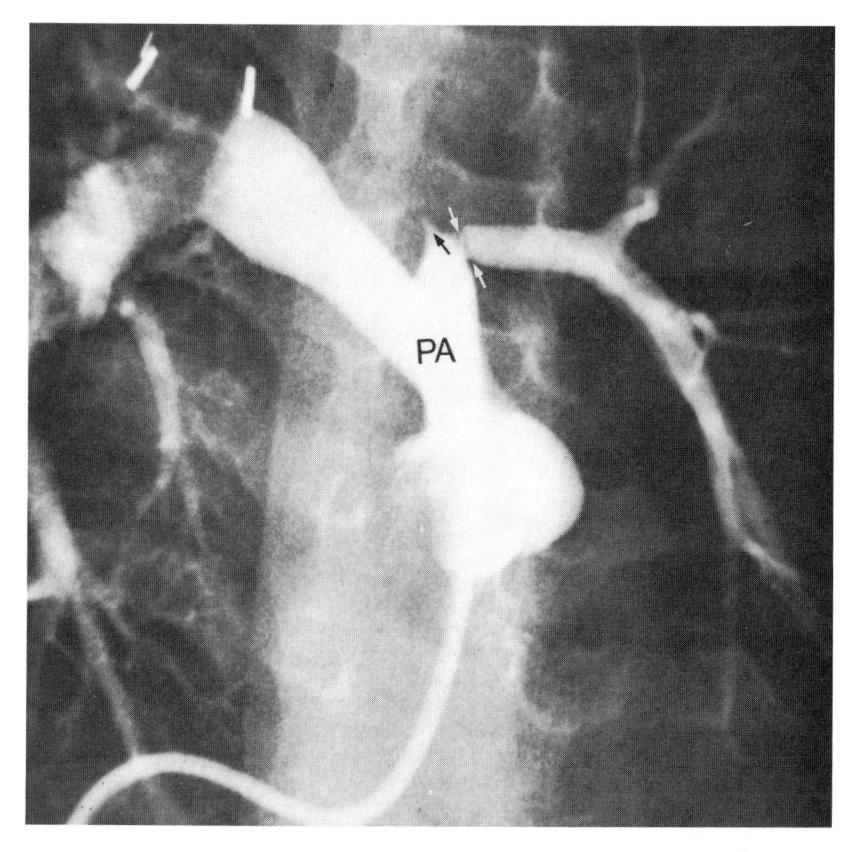

FIG 30–26.
Tetralogy of Fallot. Pulmonary arteriogram *(PA)*. Cranial beam angulation. Anteroposterior projection. Localized severe stenosis of left pulmonary artery *(white arrows)*. Small ductus diverticulum of left pulmonary artery *(black arrow)*. Main pulmonary artery shows mild tubular narrowing.

left ventricular systolic pressures are equal, and both ventricles eject blood into the aorta. Opacification of the left ventricle during right ventricular angiography is usually caused by extrasystoles and represents an angiographic artifact (see Fig 30–31). Without extrasystoles, significant opacification of the left ventricle does not occur (see Fig 30–31).

22. The association of muscular defects is rare. If the right ventricular pressure equals left ventricular pressure, such muscular defects can be seen on right ventriculography but they are best demonstrated by left ventriculography (Fig 30–32).

23. The association of a left-sided atrioventricular valve abnormality and the demonstration of ventricular communications with lower right ventricular pressure may require left ventriculography. The association of an atrioventricular canal can be expected from the electrocardiogram and echocardiography, but angiography should be carried out to demonstrate the degree of mitral incompetence (Fig 30–33).

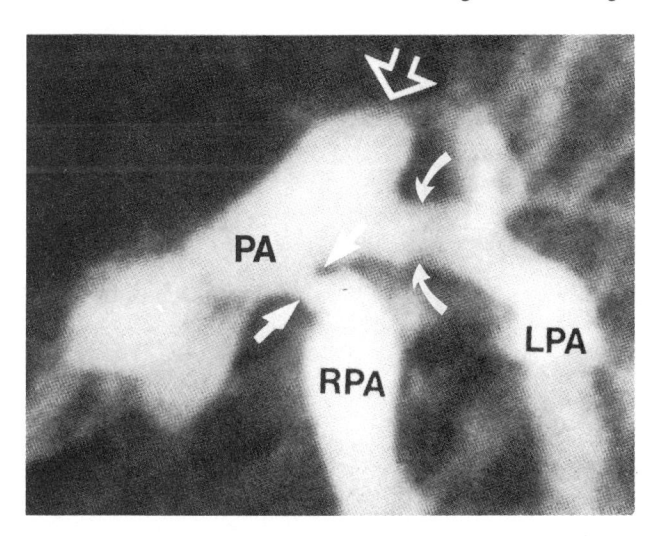

FIG 30–27.
Tetralogy of Fallot. Selective pulmonary arteriogram. Steep left interior oblique projection with caudal beam angulation. Pulmonary bifurcation is well demonstrated with severe stenosis of origin of right pulmonary artery *(straight arrows)*. Origin of left pulmonary artery is normal *(curved arrows)*. There is a prominent ductus diverticulum of pulmonary artery *(open arrow)*.

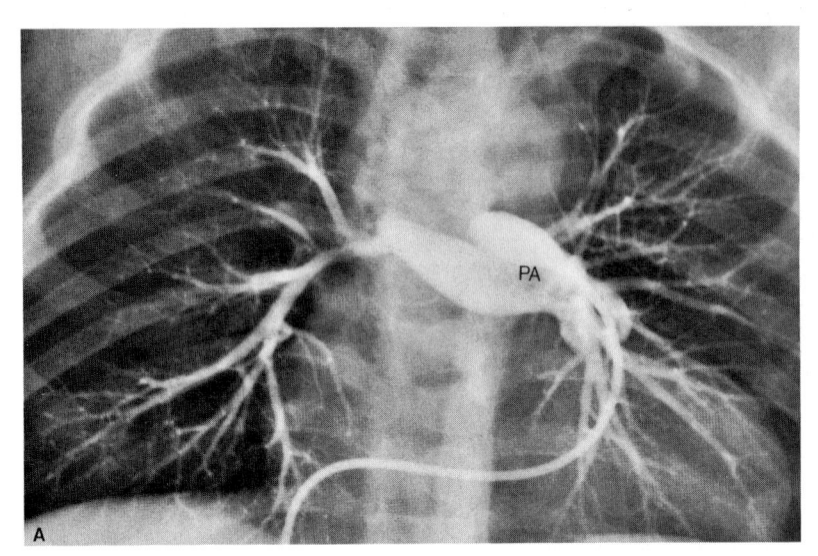

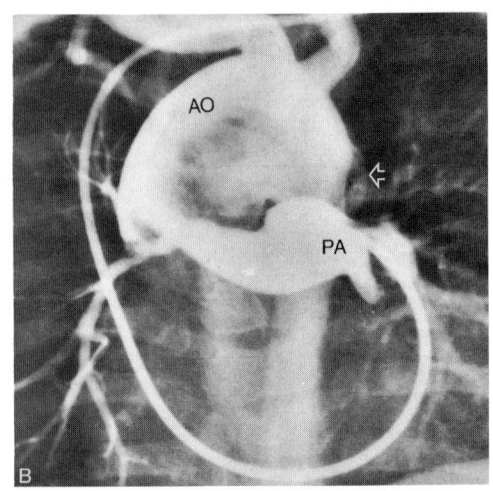

FIG 30–28.
Tetralogy of Fallot. Selective pulmonary arteriogram *(PA)*. Anteroposterior projection. **A,** severe diffuse right and left pulmonary artery stenosis (hypoplasia of pulmonary arterial tree). To stimulate growth, a left Blalock-Taussig and later on right Waterston anastomosis are performed. **B,** several years later. Opacification of aorta *(AO)* through a patent Waterston anastomosis, indicating high pulmonary arterial pressure. In spite of patent anastomosis, right pulmonary artery has not grown because of diffuse pulmonary hypoplasia. Left Blalock-Taussig anastomosis is patent *(open arrow),* Left pulmonary arterial tree has not grown.

ESTIMATION OF ADEQUATE PULMONARY ARTERIAL SIZE

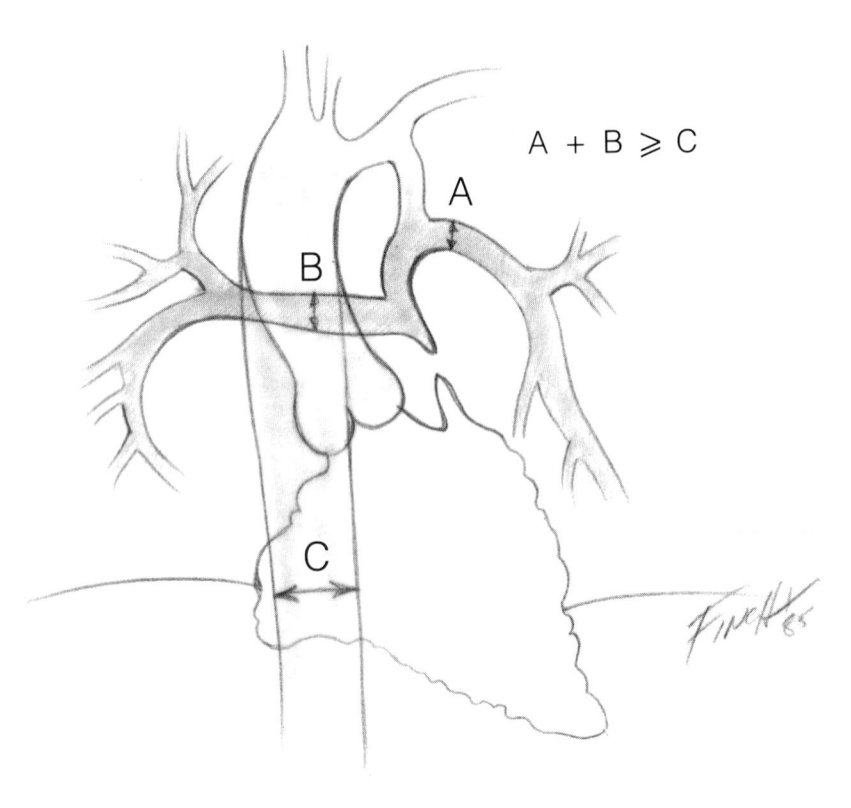

FIG 30–29.
Estimation of adequate pulmonary size for operative correction. Diameter of left pulmonary artery *(A)* plus diameter of right pulmonary artery *(B)* should equal or be larger than aortic diameter *(C)* at level of diaphragm.

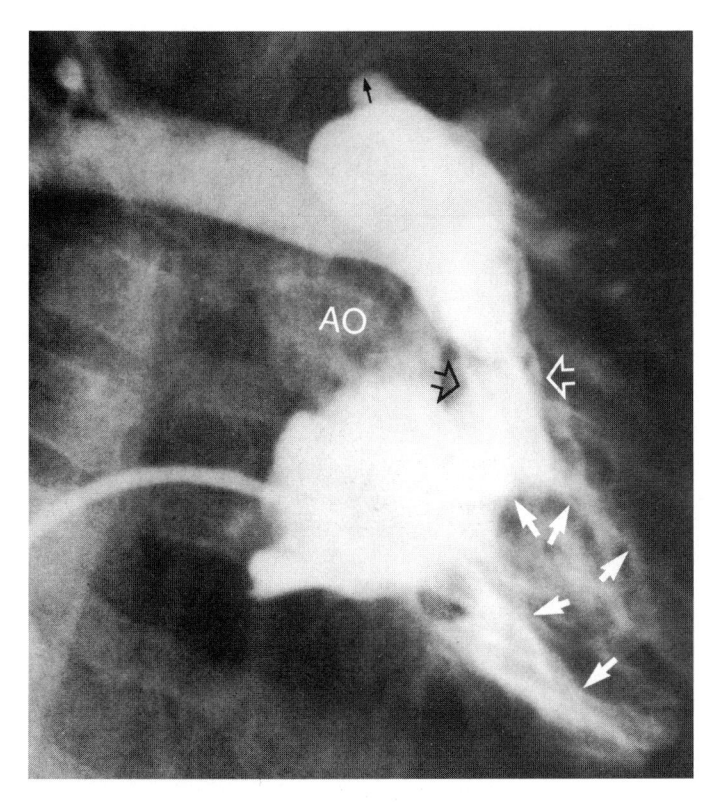

FIG 30-30.
Severe tetralogy of Fallot. Right ventriculogram. Right anterior oblique projection. Aorta *(AO)* opacifies faintly from ventricular extrasystoles. Large muscle bundle *(white arrows)* near apex of right ventricle. Nonobstructive. Hypertrophied septal band of crista supraventricularis *(open white arrow)* and parietal band *(open black arrow)*. Mild infundibular stenosis. Small ductus diverticulum *(small black arrow)* of main pulmonary artery (common finding because of jet).

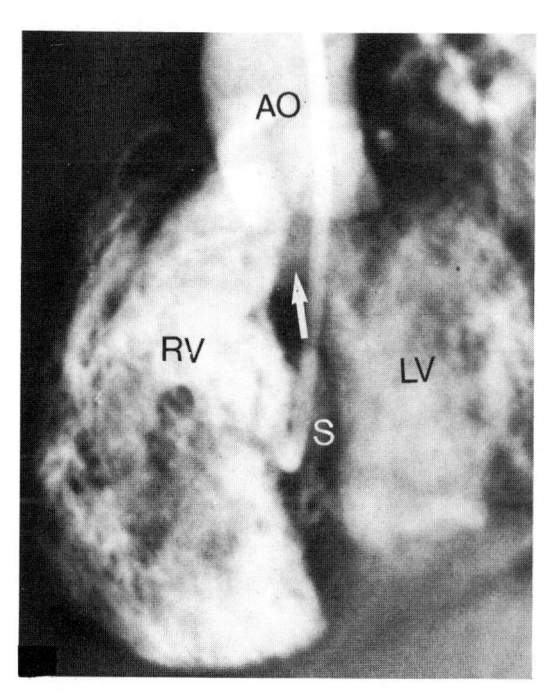

FIG 30-31.
Tetralogy of Fallot. Right ventriculograms *(RV)*. Steep left anterior oblique projection. Opacification of left ventricle *(LV)* through ventricular septal defect. Ventricular septal defect is located immediately beneath aortic valve and crest *(white arrow)* of septum *(S)*. Characteristic location of ventricular septal defect in tetralogy of Fallot. Mild overriding of aorta *(AO)*.

AORTOGRAPHY

Preoperative identification of the coronary arterial pattern is important because a branch of the coronary artery (either right or left) may pass across the anterior surface of the right ventricular outflow tract and prevent or complicate a right ventriculotomy. If this arterial branch is hidden in pericardial fat or the pericardial space has been obliterated because of a previous cardiac operation, the artery may be accidentally divided, resulting in myocardial infarction and death. Such an artery may also be mistaken for a large conal branch (conal branches are increased in size and number in tetralogy of Fallot) and intentionally ligated.

The most common coronary arterial anomalies are as follows:

1. Left anterior descending branch originating from the right coronary artery (see Fig 30-9,B). Under these circumstances, the left anterior descending coronary artery may pass either in front of or behind the pulmonary outflow tract. The anterior passage, which is much more common, prevents a right ventriculotomy to be extended across the outflow tract. Passage behind the pulmonary artery does not prevent right ventriculotomy.

2. Right coronary artery originating from the left coronary artery (see Fig 30-9,A). Under those circumstances, the left coronary artery arises normally above the

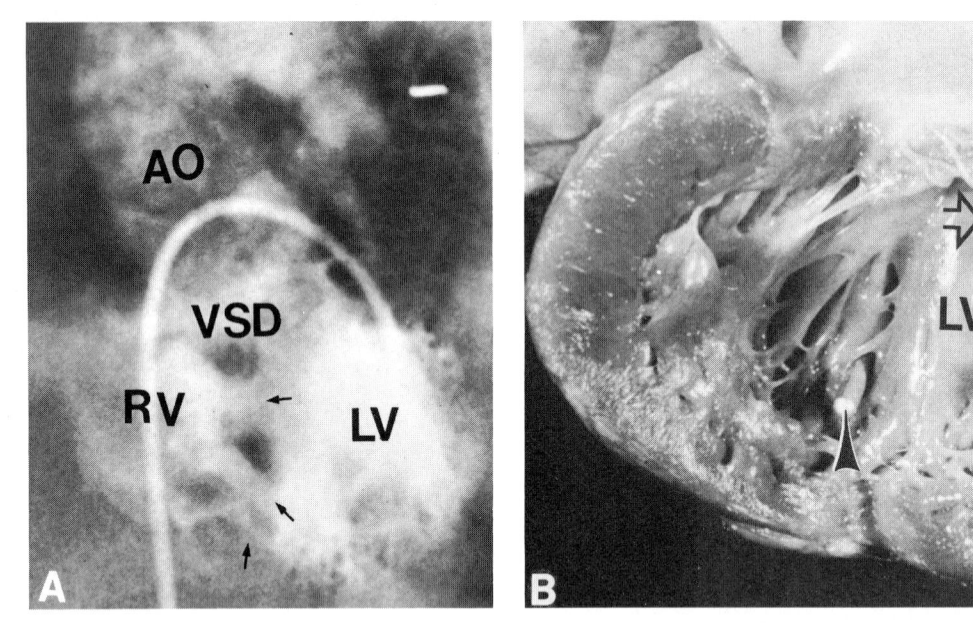

564 Cyanosis and Decreased Pulmonary Arterial Vasculature

FIG 30–32.
Tetralogy of Fallot. **A,** left ventriculogram *LV)*. Left anterior oblique projection with cranial beam angulation. Typical location of ventricular septal defect *(VSD)*. Three muscular ventricular septal defects *(arrows)*. *AO* = aorta; *RV* = right ventricle. **B,** postmortem specimen. Left atrium *(LA)* and left ventricle *(LV)* are opened. Ventricular septal defect *(arrow)*. Probes through muscular defects *(arrow head)*.

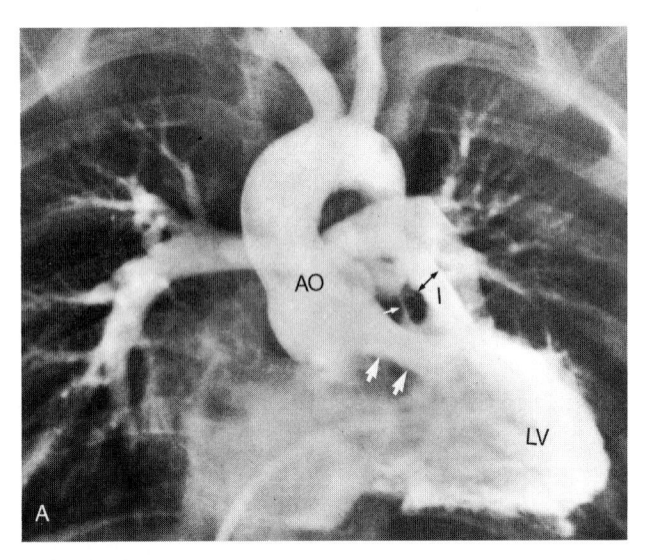

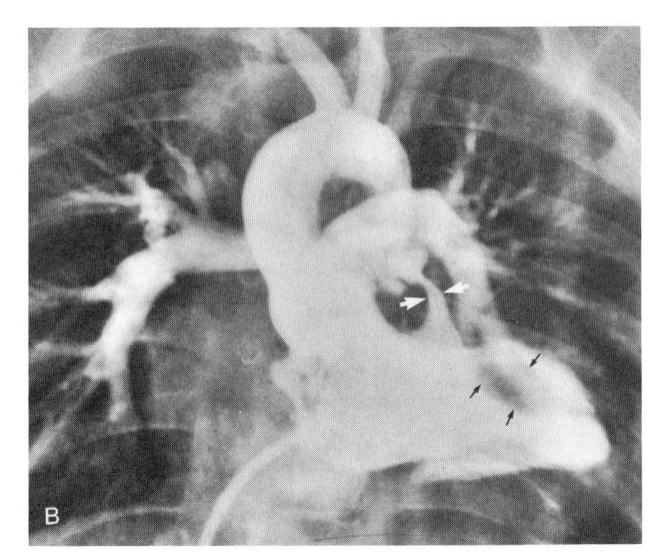

FIG 30–33.
Complete atrioventricular canal and pulmonary stenosis. Left ventriculogram *(LV)*. Anteroposterior projection. Left ventricle is injected to evaluate degree of atrioventricular valve insufficiency. **A,** diastole. Typical diastolic gooseneck deformity caused by superior portion of cleft anterior leaflet of mitral valve *(white arrows)*. Infundibulum *(I)* remains narrow and stenotic even during diastole *(black arrows)*. Aorta *(AO)* fills through ventricular septal defect. Hypertrophied muscle *(small white arrow)* splits the infundibulum. **B,** systole. No mitral incompetence. Forceful contraction of hypertrophied infundibulum *(white arrows)*. Large anterolateral papillary muscle in left ventricle forms filling defect *(black arrows)*.

left aortic cusp. The right coronary artery passes either in front of or behind the pulmonary artery and then in the right atrioventricular groove.

3. Single coronary artery. A single coronary artery may originate above either the right (see Fig 30–10,B) or left aortic cusp (see Fig 30–10,A). The right and left branches may pass in front or behind the pulmonary artery. Branches on the anterior surface of the ventricular outflow tract present a serious problem during cardiac operation.

Because of the incidence of coronary arterial anomalies,[9] their origin and course must be angiographically demonstrated as part of the preoperative evaluation of patients with tetralogy of Fallot. If aortography is not performed, the surgeon may mistake the aberrant artery for a large conal branch, and the artery may be unintentionally ligated (Fig 30–34). An abnormal course may make an operation impossible or require the insertion of a right ventricular conduit. In younger children, balloon occlusion aortography is sufficient, whereas in the adolescent and adult, selective coronary arteriography is preferable. Slight left anterior oblique and lateral projection are usually adequate to demonstrate coronary arterial anomalies, but additional angulated right and left anterior oblique projections may be required for localization of abnormal branches.

If an abnormal coronary artery pattern is recognized, the course of the aberrant branch either in front or behind the pulmonary outflow tract must be identified. This is a difficult angiographic task, and identification of an aberrant coronary artery may stump even the most experienced angiographer. Interpretation of the angiograms may be complicated by the severe clockwise rotation of the heart that may occur in tetralogy of Fallot. REASON: With marked clockwise rotation of the heart and a small hypoplastic infundibulum, the aberrant coronary artery may project far posteriorly on both the left anterior oblique and anteroposterior projections, mimicking a course behind the pulmonary artery (Fig 30–35).

Because the location of the aberrant coronary artery is of such importance, the placement of a second catheter with its tip in the right ventricular outflow tract is advisable. When a catheter tip is placed in the outflow tract at the level of the aberrant coronary arterial branch, an anteroposterior coronary arteriogram with caudad and cephalad angulation allows topographic localization by parallactic shift in relation to the catheter tip.

Usually it is evident from angiograms that the left anterior descending artery crosses anteriorly in front of the right ventricular outflow tract. This is particularly well seen in the right anterior oblique projection where the artery takes a distinct anterior and downward course (Fig 30–36). Other coronary anomalies such as coronary artery fistulas may occur, but these are less common than an anomalous origin (Fig 30–37).

MANAGEMENT

Propranolol, a β-adrenergic-blocking agent, has been used to treat acute episodes of hypoxia[10] and also has been used for long-term management,[11] but tachyphylaxis develops.

Treatment of tetralogy of Fallot is operative, either palliative or corrective, but valvar pulmonary artery stenosis and pulmonary branch stenosis can also be treated by balloon angioplasty (Fig 30–38).

Palliative Operations

A variety of palliative procedures are available, and their indications are as follows:

1. Infants less then 3 months of age who are symptomatic and require operation.
2. Patients with hypoplastic pulmonary arteries. The small caliber of the pulmonary arterial tree may be unable

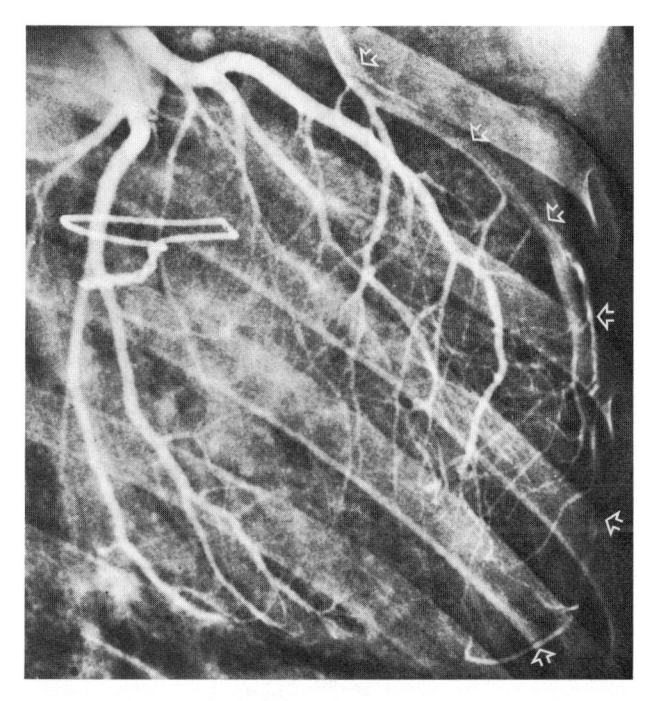

FIG 30–34.
Tetralogy of Fallot. Postoperative views. Coronary arteriogram. Right anterior oblique projection. Coronary angiogram not performed before operation. At operation, left anterior descending branch arising anomalously from right coronary artery was mistaken for a large conal branch and divided. Myocardial infarction occurred. Dense filling of circumflex circulation. Faint collateral filling of ligated left anterior descending *open arrows*).

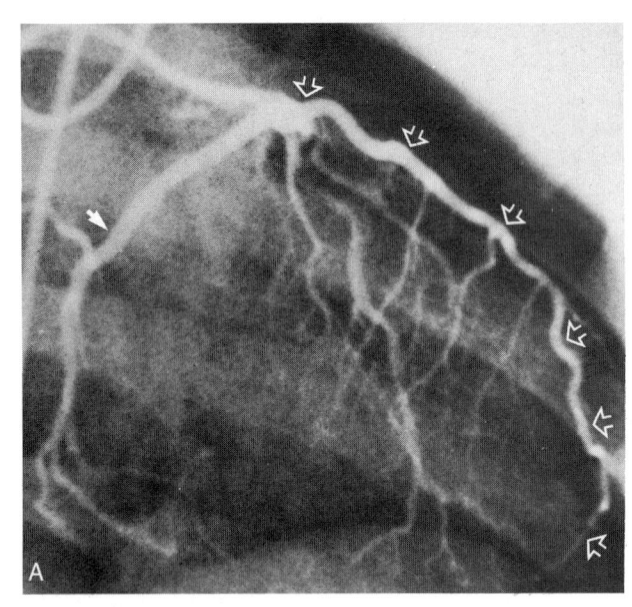

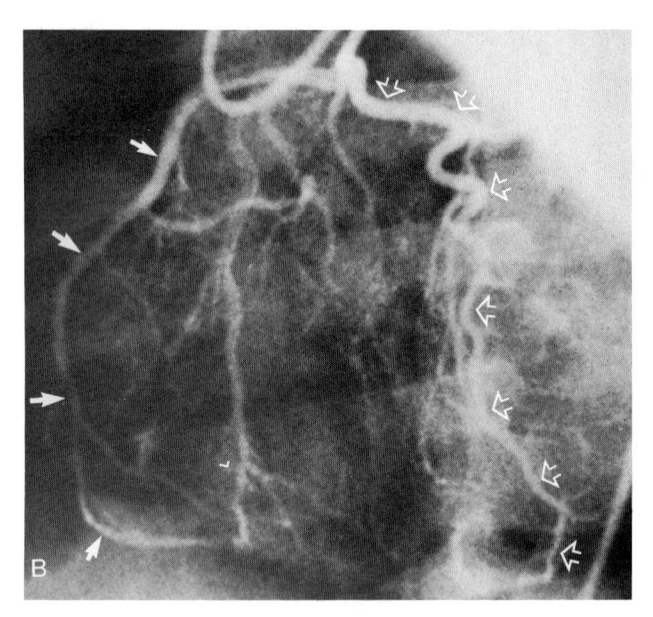

FIG 30–35.
Tetralogy of Fallot. Selective right coronary arteriogram. **A,** right anterior oblique projection. Right coronary artery *(solid white arrow)* gives rise to left anterior descending branch *(open white arrows)*. Location of artery either in front or behind infundibulum is impossible to determine. **B,** left anterior oblique projection. Right coronary artery *(solid white arrow)* projects anteriorly. Left anterior descending artery *(open white arrows)* appears to have a normal course. This was mistakenly interpreted as aberrant left coronary artery arising from right coronary artery crossing behind pulmonary artery. At operation, artery crossed in front of infundibulum. Definitive operation deferred.

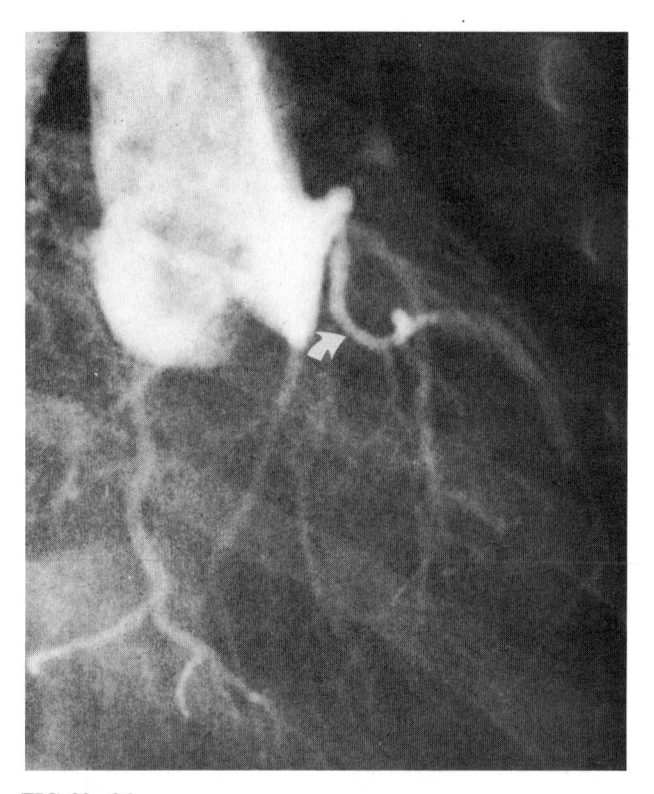

FIG 30–36.
Tetralogy of Fallot and anomalous origin of left anterior descending from right coronary artery. Aortogram. Right anterior oblique projection. Aberrant left anterior descending takes a distinct "low anterior dip" *(curved arrow)* while crossing right ventricular outflow tract.

to accept the entire cardiac output after complete correction.

3. An abnormal coronary arterial course in an infant.

4. Patients with hypoplastic pulmonary arteries and large bronchial arteries. The pulmonary arterial bed is increased in size by unifocalization (Fig 30–39).

Systemic pulmonary arterial shunts are an effective means to increase the pulmonary blood flow in patients with tetralogy of Fallot or other cyanotic malformations with reduced pulmonary blood flow. Such procedures increase the amount of fully oxygenated blood that the left ventricle delivers to the aorta. Consequently, the systemic arterial oxygen saturation increases, and the patient's condition generally improves. The procedure is most effective in patients with the lowest aortic saturation.

The increased pulmonary blood flow from the systemic pulmonary arterial shunt may stimulate growth of the pulmonary arterial tree, making subsequent corrective operation possible in patients with a hypoplastic pulmonary arterial tree. Unfortunately, this desired effect is not always achieved (see Fig 30–28).

Four complications can occur after creation of systemic-pulmonary shunts: (1) pulmonary edema and possible pulmonary hemorrhage caused by increased blood flow into a pulmonary vascular bed that previously carried a limited volume of pulmonary flow, (2) congestive cardiac failure if the shunt permits an excessive volume of pulmonary blood flow, (3) pulmonary vascular disease as a con-

FIG 30–37.
Tetralogy of Fallot. Right coronary arteriogram. Anteroposterior projection. Markedly enlarged right conal branch *(arrow)* caused by coronary artery fistula. Faint opacification of pulmonary artery *(PA)*.

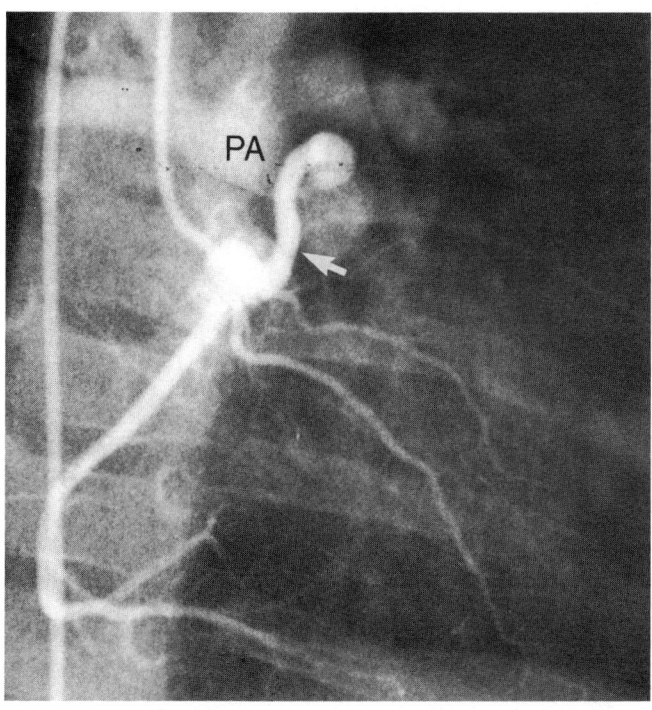

sequence of increased pulmonary blood flow and pulmonary arterial pressure, and (4) a significantly increased risk of bacterial endocarditis.

There are several types of systemic pulmonary arterial shunts, each with specific indications and limitations.

Blalock-Taussig Anastomosis

The Blalock-Taussig anastomosis (named after Alfred Blalock, a 20th century American surgeon, and Helen Taussig, a 20th century American pediatric cardiologist) was the first systemic pulmonary arterial shunt. The procedure involves the anastomosis of either the right or the left subclavian artery with the ipsilateral pulmonary artery (Fig 30–40). Preferably the subclavian artery located opposite the side of the aortic arch is used, because it arises from the innominate artery, which is longer than the ipsilateral subclavian artery, which arises directly from the same side as the aortic arch. If for some reason the subclavian artery arising from the aortic arch must be used, an arterioplasty may be necessary to prevent kinking of the subclavian as it is brought down to be anastomosed to the pulmonary artery (Fig 30–41). Another technique to circumvent the problem of kinking is the insertion of a synthetic Gortex or Dacron graft between subclavian and pulmonary arteries (Fig 30–42,A) or ascending aorta and main pulmonary artery (central shunt). The graft shown in Figure 30–42,B has the advantage that it may stimulate growth of the pulmonary artery.

The Blalock-Taussig anastomosis is a relatively straightforward procedure, particularly when it is performed in older children. It has an advantage over other shunts because the size and length of the subclavian artery offers resistance to flow. Thus, the development of congestive cardiac failure or pulmonary vascular disease are uncommon occurrences.[11] At the time of a corrective operation, the shunt can be taken down without technical difficulty, and it can be occluded by catheter techniques such as balloons or coils. Perhaps 10% of the shunts become occluded, usually immediately after the operation.

Potts Anastomosis

Potts (Willis Potts, a 20th century American surgeon) described another type of systemic pulmonary arterial shunt 1 year after Blalock first performed his historic operation in 1944. In the Potts anastomosis, a windowlike communication is created between the descending aorta and a branch pulmonary artery (Fig 30–43). In patients with a left aortic arch, the left pulmonary artery and, in those with a right aortic arch, the right pulmonary artery are anastomosed to the descending aorta.

The problem of kinking of the subclavian artery of the Blalock-Taussig shunt is avoided with the Potts anastomosis. The surgeon has to gauge the size of the shunt when it is created, and this is a major disadvantage of this operative technique. Because the Potts anastomosis has no length, the size of the communication becomes critical. It may be too little or, more commonly, too large, resulting in massive pulmonary blood flow, cardiac failure, and ultimately pulmonary hypertension.[12] Furthermore, it is more difficult to obliterate this anastomosis during correc-

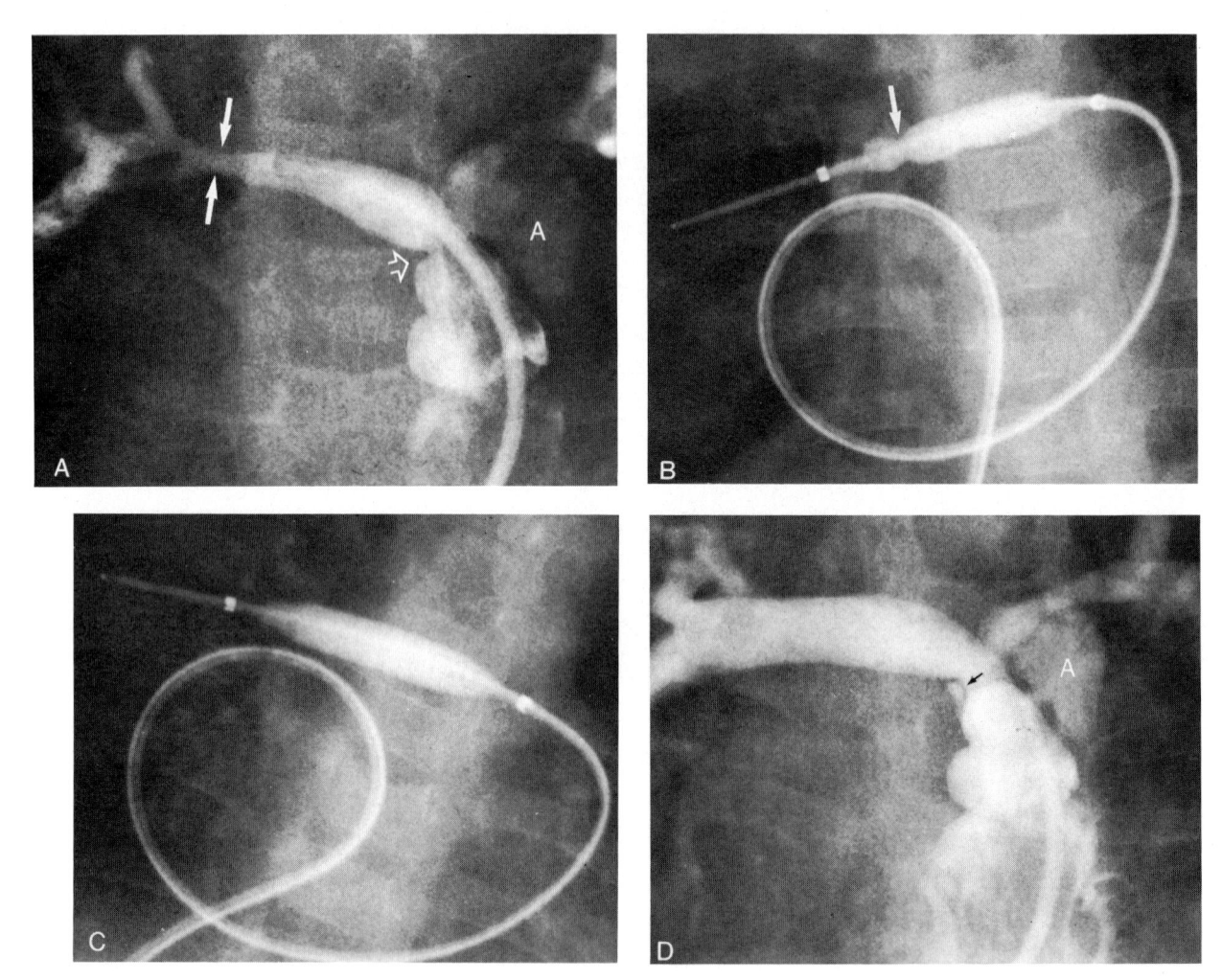

FIG 30–38.
Selective pulmonary arteriogram. Tetralogy of Fallot. Postoperative view. Suprasystemic pressure in right ventricle. **A,** pulmonary arteriogram. Anteroposterior projection. Marked stenosis of main pulmonary artery *(open arrow)*. Stenosis of right pulmonary artery *(solid arrows)*. Operative attempts to alleviate main pulmonary artery stenosis resulted in faintly opacified false aneurysm *(A)*. **B,** angioplasty balloon catheter passed into right pulmonary artery. Inflation produced distinct localized waist *(arrow)*. **C,** disappearance of waist in balloon, indicating successful dilatation. **D,** postdilatation pulmonary arteriogram. Marked enlargement of entire right pulmonary artery. Disappearance of localized stenosis. Dilatation of main pulmonary artery stenosis produced a small intimal flap *(arrow)*, which is commonly seen after balloon angioplasty. False aneurysm *(A)* remains unchanged.

tive operation. Because of these problems, this procedure is infrequently used.

Waterston-Cooley Shunt

The Waterston-Cooley shunt is named after Denis Waterston, a British surgeon, and Denton Cooley, an American surgeon of the 20th century. In this systemic pulmonary arterial shunt, the right pulmonary artery is anastomosed to the ascending aorta (Fig 30–44) and thus resembles the Potts procedure. As with the windowlike Potts anastomosis, the size of the communication is critical, and overperfusion of the lungs occurs when the anastomosis is too large.

The anastomosis is created by mobilizing the right pulmonary artery and drawing it anteriorly toward the aorta (Fig 30–45). Because of tension on the right pulmonary artery, it may become kinked or even interrupted. Generally, preferential blood flow occurs into the right pulmonary artery, and the left and main pulmonary arteries are not stimulated to grow. Congestive cardiac failure and pulmonary vascular disease are other complications.[13] Although previously used in infants, it has largely been replaced by the central shunt procedure.

Central Shunt

A central shunt is performed through a midline sternotomy, in contrast to other systemic pulmonary arterial shunts, which are performed through lateral thoracotomy.

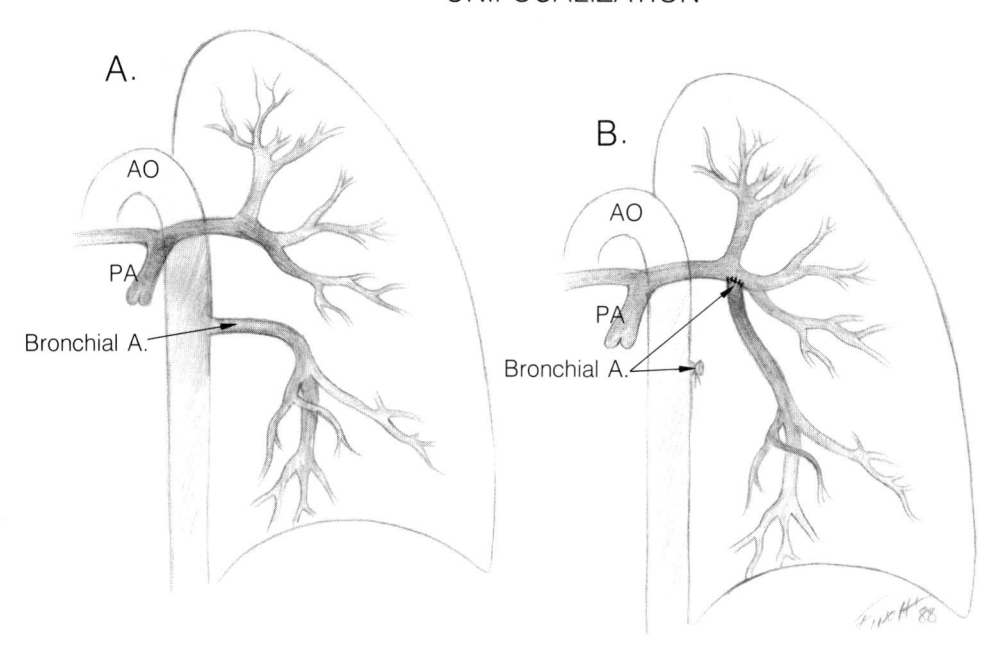

UNIFOCALIZATION

FIG 30-39.
Tetralogy of Fallot. Hypoplastic left pulmonary artery. **A,** diagram. Upper lobe is supplied by hypoplastic pulmonary artery and entire lower lobe by nonstenotic bronchial artery. **B,** unifocalization. Bronchial artery is ligated and anastomosed to pulmonary artery. This palliative operation enlarges pulmonary arterial bed for subsequent corrective operation. AO = aorta; PA = pulmonary artery.

In this technique, a connection is made between the main pulmonary artery and the ascending aorta. It has an advantage because blood flow into the main pulmonary artery is equally distributed to the right and left pulmonary arteries. Thus, the main pulmonary artery and both right and left pulmonary arteries may be stimulated to grow.

The shunt can be created in two ways. The anastomosis can be made by direct anastomosis in a windowlike fashion similar to the Potts and Waterston-Cooley anastomoses. When this fenestration is created, it is difficult to gauge the exact size of the communication.

Therefore, the procedure is usually performed by placing a short Gortex or Dacron tubular graft between the as-

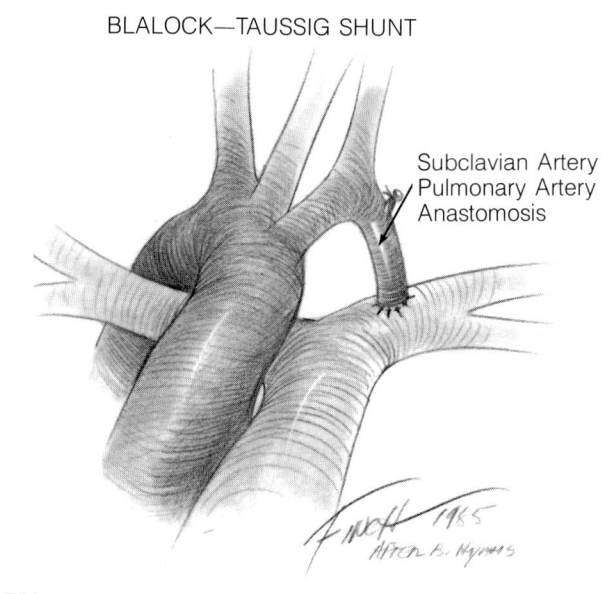

FIG 30-40.
Blalock-Taussig shunt. Opposite side of aortic arch. Right aortic arch. Vertebral artery has been ligated. Left subclavian artery is divided and anastomosed to left pulmonary artery.

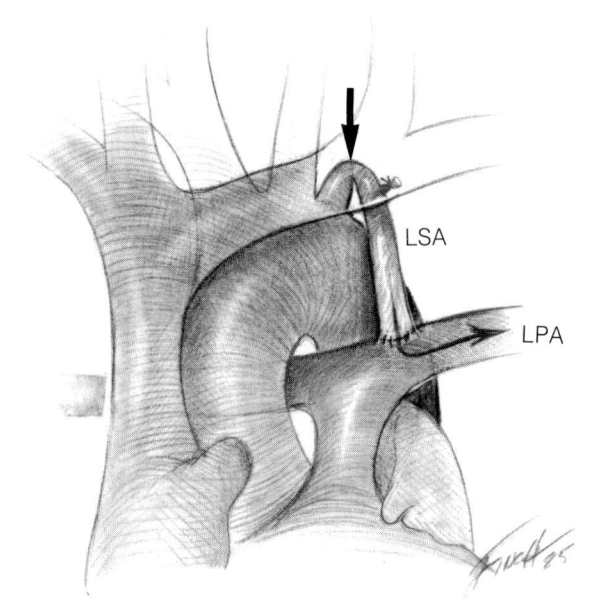

FIG 30-41.
Blalock-Taussig shunt. Same side as aortic arch. Left aortic arch. Left subclavian artery *(LSA)* is divided and anastomosed to left pulmonary artery *(LPA)*. Kinking of left subclavian artery may occur but can be prevented by arterioplasty.

570 *Cyanosis and Decreased Pulmonary Arterial Vasculature*

SYSTEMIC TO PULMONARY SHUNTS

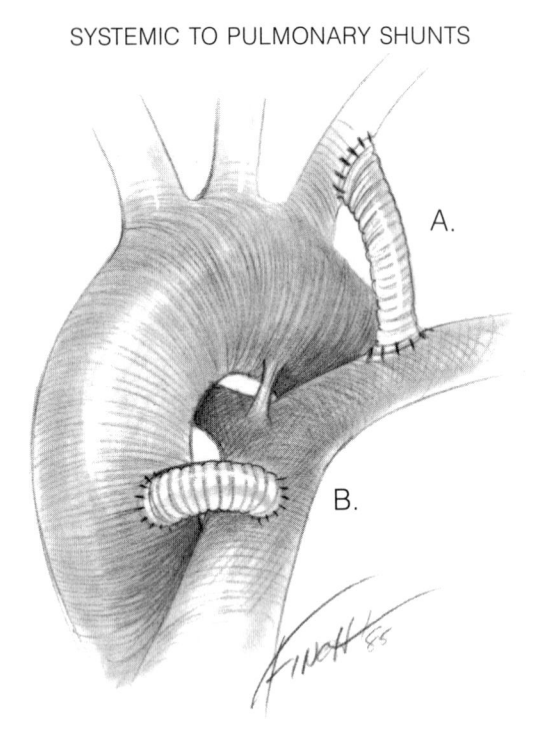

FIG 30-42.
A, graft is inserted between left subclavian and left pulmonary arteries. *B*, graft is inserted between ascending aorta and main pulmonary artery. This so-called central shunt may stimulate growth of main pulmonary artery.

cending aorta and pulmonary artery (see Fig 30-42,B). This technique has an advantage because the diameter of the graft can be carefully selected according to the size of the patient. Resistance to flow through the shunt can be increased by making the graft longer. The disadvantage of all synthetic grafts is lack of growth; therefore, as the child grows, the shunt becomes inadequate, because the size of the graft remains constant. In contrast, a Blalock-Taussig anastomosis usually becomes larger with time unless stenosis develops at the anastomotic site.

The central shunt has another disadvantage. The pericardial space must be entered to place the shunt. As a result, pericardial adhesions develop, which may complicate a subsequent corrective operation.

Corrective Operations

The first intracardiac correction of tetralogy of Fallot was performed by Dr. C. Walton Lillehei and colleagues in 1954 at the University of Minnesota. Lillehei exposed the heart through a transverse sternotomy. As initially described and subsequently modified, a longitudinal right ventriculotomy is carefully performed in the outflow area of the right ventricle. Care is taken to avoid damage to the left anterior descending coronary artery. Because the pulmonary annulus is often hypoplastic, the incision is extended across the annulus into the pulmonary artery. Through the ventriculotomy the ventricular septal defect is closed by a patch (Fig 30-46). Because the defect extends directly to the annulus of the aorta, care is taken to avoid damage to the aortic valve. The patch is carefully sutured to the lower margin of the defect to avoid damage to the atrioventricular bundle, which, if damaged, may result in complete heart block (Fig 30-47).

The stenotic right ventricular outflow tract is widened by excising part of the hypertrophied crista supraventricularis. The stenotic pulmonary valve is incised, and the outflow tract is further widened by insertion of either a pericardial or Dacron patch (Fig 30-48). Depending on the size of the main pulmonary artery and the right and left pulmonary arteries, the patch may have to be extended a variable distance into the main, right, or left pulmonary arteries (or combination thereof).

Operative repair of peripheral pulmonary artery

POTT'S SHUNT

Anastomosis Between Descending Aorta and Left Pulmonary Artery

FIG 30-43.
Potts' procedure. Communication between descending aorta and left pulmonary artery.

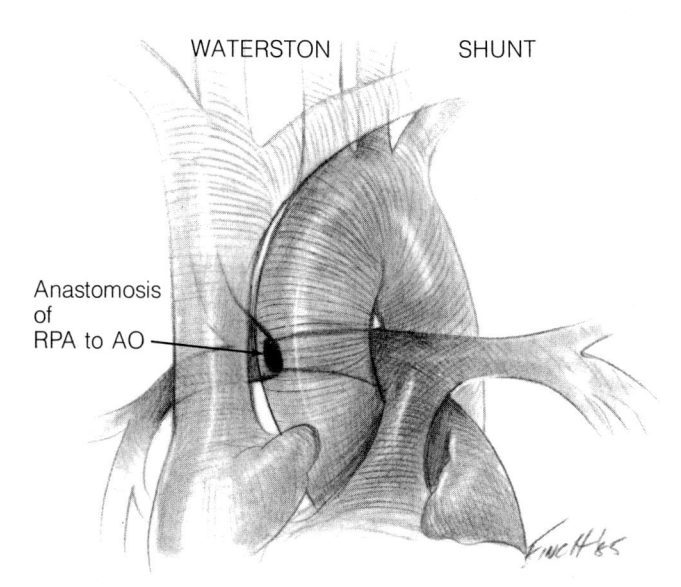

FIG 30–44.
Waterston-Cooley shunt. Communication between ascending aorta *(AO)* and right pulmonary artery *(RPA)*.

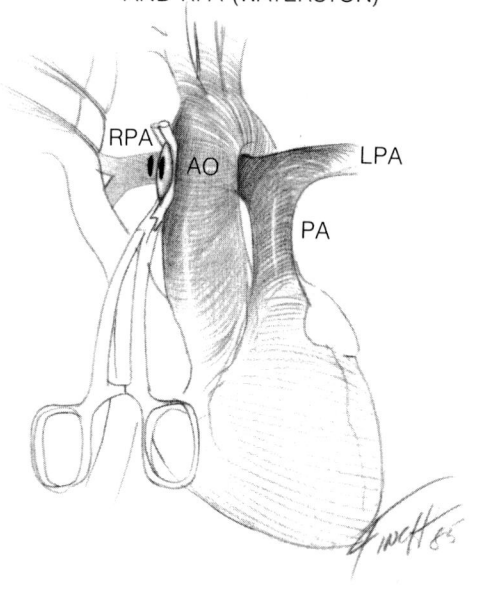

FIG 30–45.
Waterston-Cooley shunt. Right pulmonary artery *(RPA)* is mobilized and drawn toward ascending aorta *(AO)*. Openings are made in both arteries and anastomosed. *LPA* = left pulmonary artery; *PA* = pulmonary artery.

stenoses may be difficult to perform, particularly of the right pulmonary artery, because the right pulmonary artery is located behind the ascending aorta. Under those circumstances, the aorta may have to be divided to obtain access to the stenotic right pulmonary artery (Fig 30–49). Particularly in patients with a previous operation who have developed extensive adhesions, the operative approach to the peripheral pulmonary arterial stenosis becomes a very difficult task. Under those circumstances, balloon angioplasty is attempted before corrective operation.

In the relatively rare patient with a normal-sized pulmonary annulus and main pulmonary artery, the best results are obtained because patching across the annulus invariably results in pulmonary insufficiency and incomplete hemodynamic correction, particularly in patients with an extreme degree of infundibular pulmonary stenosis and hypoplastic main pulmonary artery. In some patients a conduit may be inserted. This is the most frequently used technique with pulmonary atresia and in patients with tetralogy of Fallot and a coronary arterial anomaly (Fig 30–50).

Although surgeons commonly speak of "complete correction" of the tetralogy of Fallot, operation almost never repairs the condition completely. A number of complications can occur from a corrective operation. An aneurysm, either true or false, is common in the infundibular area or pulmonary trunk or at the site of the right ventricular outflow tract patch. These aneurysms rarely enlarge with time or cause hemodynamic compromise.[14] Although the ventricular septal defect can be completely closed by a patch, a small residual shunt occurs more commonly than after repair of an isolated ventricular septal defect. The incidence of postoperative ventricular septal defect ranges from 10% to 20%[15,16]: Closure of the ventricular septal defect in tetralogy of Fallot is technically more difficult because the defect extends to and underlies the aortic valve leaflets (see Figs 30–46 and 30–67), which may be damaged during the repair. During repair, excessive tension on the sutures must be avoided and the sutures must be placed carefully to avoid damage to the bundles of His, which lies adjacent to the ventricular septal defect (see Fig 30–47). Usually the location of the residual ventricular septal defect is along the superior and posterior aspect of the defect.

Repair of the coexistent infundibular and valvar pulmonary stenoses rarely results in normal hemodynamics.[15,16] Particularly in patients with hypoplastic pulmonary annulus, severe infundibular stenosis, or pulmonary branch stenosis, operative repair results in pulmonary insufficiency.

Complete heart block, resulting from damage to the conduction system as it courses along the rim of the ventricular septal defect, is, fortunately, uncommon.[17] Inadvertent injury to coronary arterial branches is also rare, particularly with the improved angiographic visualization of coronary arterial branches preoperatively.

Right bundle block is found in nearly every postoperative patient and develops during the ventriculotomy. Sudden death may occur late.[18,19] The mechanism is un-

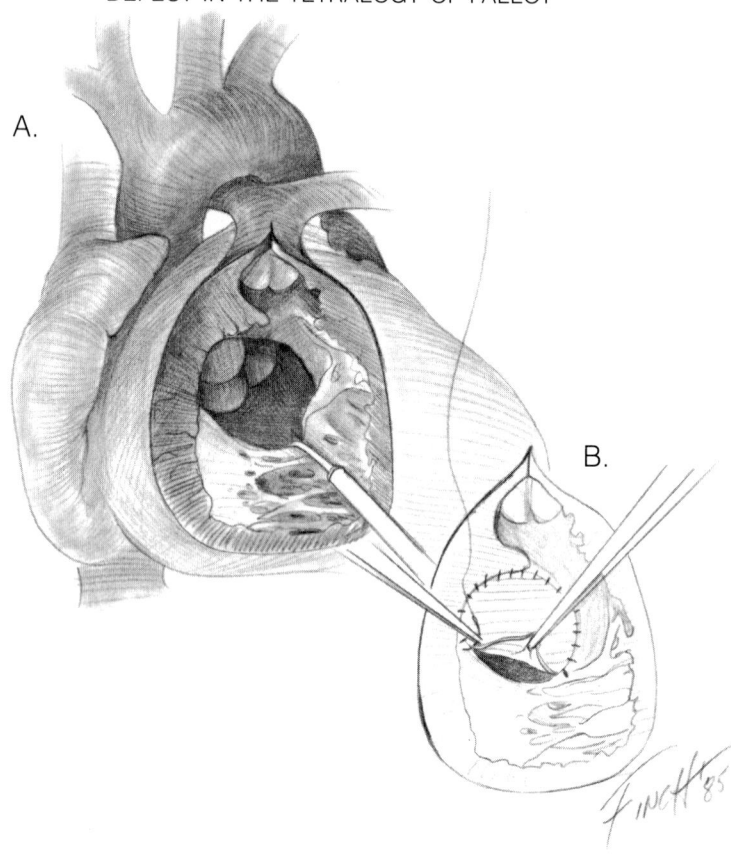

FIG 30–46.
Tetralogy of Fallot. **A,** location of ventricular septal defect. **B,** method of closure with patch.

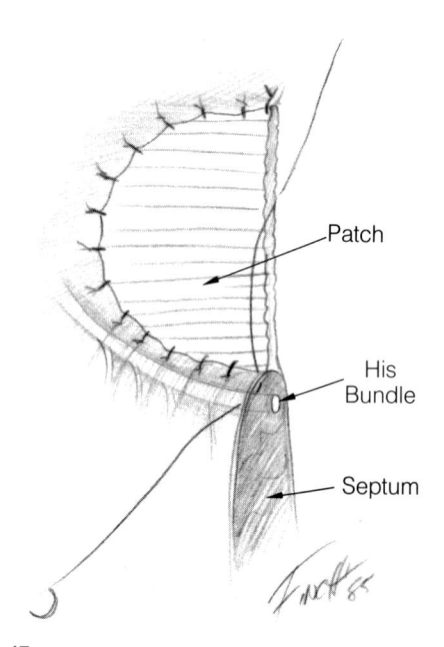

FIG 30–47.
Tetralogy of Fallot. Cross-section through ventricular septum and patch. Suture is inadvertently passed through conduction system along lower rim of defect *(arrow)*.

known, but it probably results from ventricular tachyarrhythmia.[20] Patients with ventricular ectopy should probably be treated with appropriate antiarrhythmic agents. Congestive heart failure[21] and depressed left ventricular function are rare postoperative problems.[22]

POSTOPERATIVE RADIOGRAPHIC FEATURES

Corrective Operation

1. Postoperatively the cardiac silhouette is larger than preoperatively, and it usually remains enlarged. REASON: Postoperative pulmonary insufficiency causes volume overload of the right ventricle. Incomplete relief of the outflow tract obstruction may result in right ventricular decompensation, particularly if there is a residual left-to-right shunt (Fig 30–51).

A second operation may be required to repair residual anomalies. Even with a second operation, residual anomalies may remain.[23–25]

2. The outflow tract patch may become calcified over a period of years (Fig 30–52), but this is without clinical

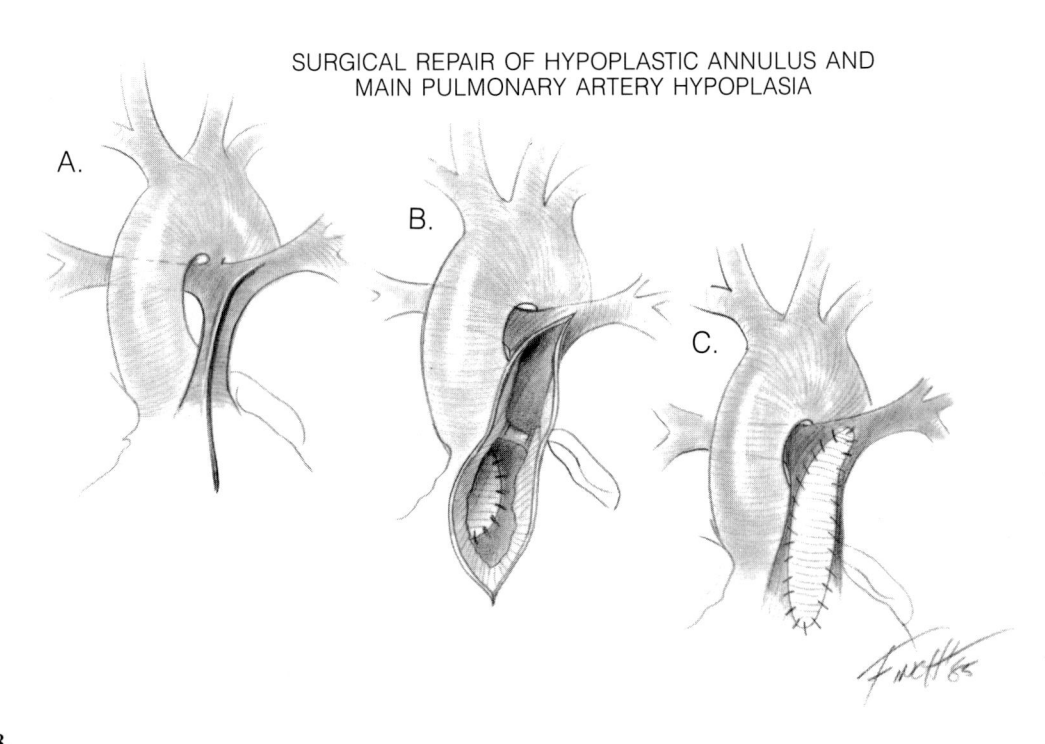

FIG 30-48.
Tetralogy of Fallot. Corrective operation. **A,** incision extends from right ventricular outflow tract through pulmonary annulus into main and left pulmonary arteries. **B,** ventricular septal defect is closed. Hypertrophied crista supraventricularis is excised. **C,** outflow tract, and main and left pulmonary arteries are further widened by insertion of patch.

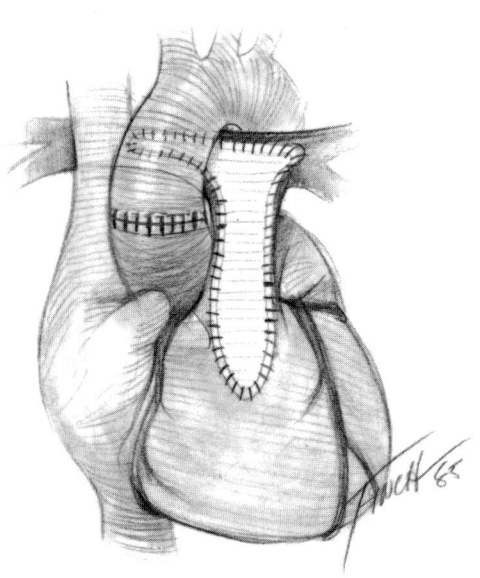

FIG 30-49.
Tetralogy of Fallot with hypoplastic main pulmonary artery and proximal right pulmonary artery stenosis. Operative repair. Ascending aorta is divided to repair peripheral right pulmonary artery stenosis.

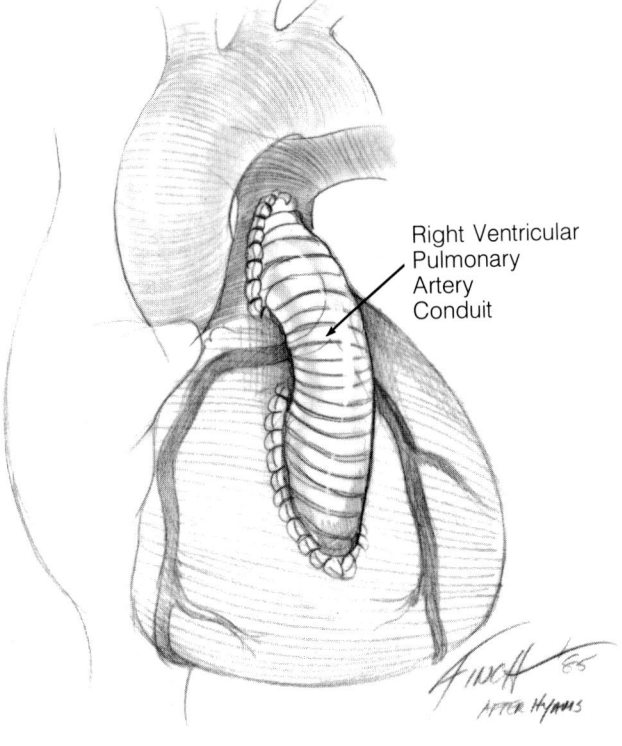

FIG 30-50.
Operative correction of tetralogy of Fallot and aberrant origin of right coronary artery crossing outflow tract. Bridging graft has been inserted. Same technique is used for correction of pulmonary atresia.

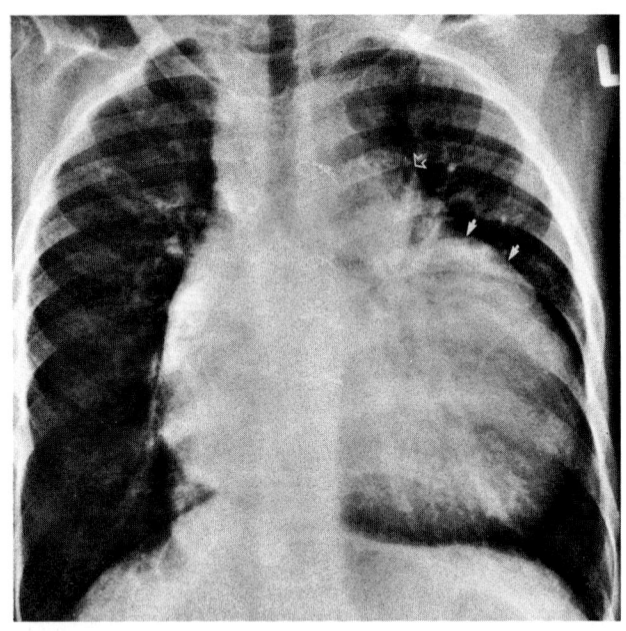

FIG 30–51.
Tetralogy of Fallot. Postoperative view. Thoracic roentgenogram. Posteroanterior projection. Typical radiographic appearance. Severe cardiomegaly. Prominent pulmonary arterial segment *(open arrow)* from patch repair of hypoplastic main pulmonary artery. Large bulge along left upper cardiac border *(white arrows)* is caused by outflow patch.

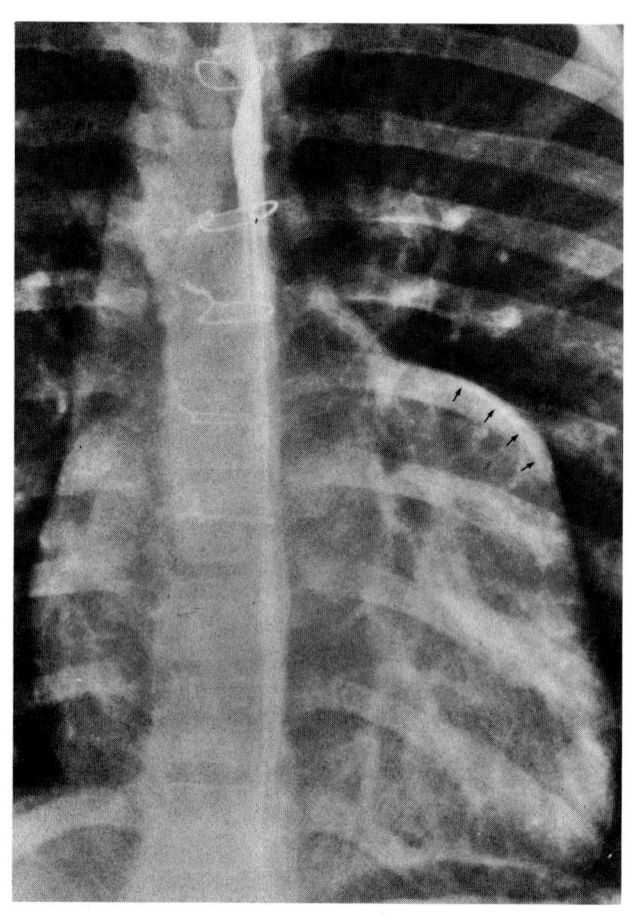

FIG 30–52.
Tetralogy of Fallot with right aortic arch. Postoperative view. Thoracic roentgenogram. Posteroanterior projection. Bulging right ventricular outflow patch has become calcified *(arrows)*.

significance. The patch closing the ventricular septal defect may also calcify.

3. A pericardial outflow patch may slowly progress into a right ventricular outflow tract aneurysm (Fig 30–53). A large aneurysm may be hemodynamically significant, because the aneurysm expands during systole and decreases the right ventricular output. These aneurysms have a broad base of origin from the right ventricle. If the bulge is very large, it may be difficult to differentiate between true and false aneurysm. Pericardial patches form aneurysms more commonly than do Dacron patches. Reoperation of the aneurysm may be required if it continues to grow.

4. A false aneurysm of the right ventricular outflow tract may develop from leakage of blood at the suture line. This type of aneurysm extends into the lung field. A false aneurysm is characterized by a small base at its origin from the right ventricle (Fig 30–54).

5. On a lateral projection, the right ventricular outflow tract may become adherent to the sternum (Fig 30–55). This adherence makes cardiac reoperation hazardous when the approach is through a midline sternotomy.

6. After repair of the outflow tract and pulmonary annulus, pulmonary insufficiency of a varying degree occurs. Pulmonary angiography shows the reflux into the right ventricle and increased systolic expansion of the pulmonary artery (increased stroke volume of the right ventricle).

7. The degree of pulmonary insufficiency is best evaluated by pulmonary arteriography. Care must be taken that all sideholes of the catheter are placed across the level of the pulmonary valve (Fig 30–56). Grading of the degree of pulmonary insufficiency is semiquantitative on a 1 to 4+ scale. Estimation is based on the amount of contrast medium regurgitating into the right ventricle at the beginning of the injection, the degree of diastolic distention of the right ventricle, and the degree of systolic distention of the pulmonary artery. REASON: Pulmonary insufficiency causes a wide pulmonary pulse pressure and increased stroke volume of the right ventricle.

Palliative Operation

Systemic pulmonary arterial shunts are usually performed to improve systemic oxygenation and promote growth of the pulmonary arteries so that complete correc-

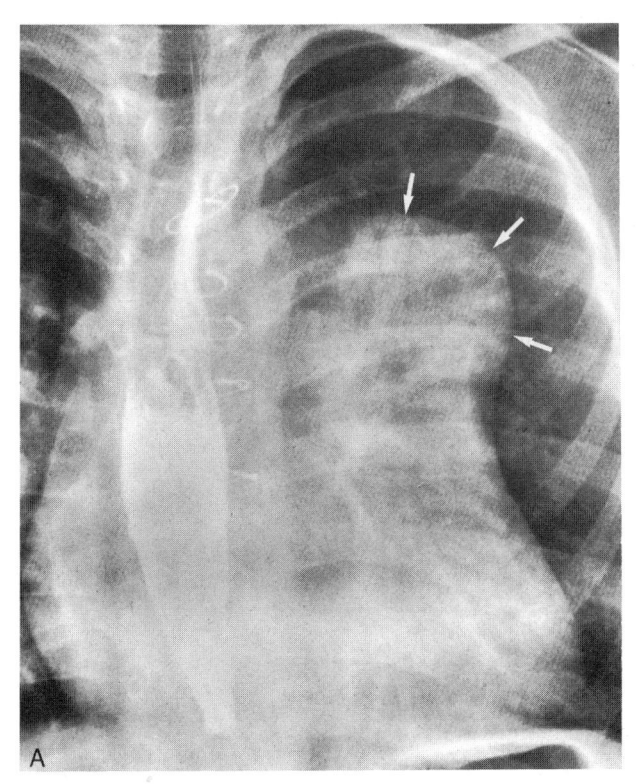

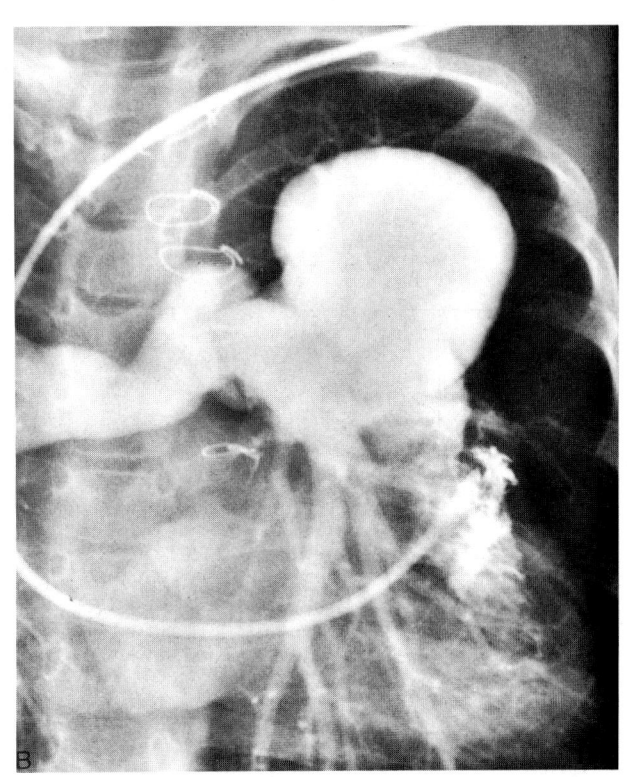

FIG 30–53.
Tetralogy of Fallot. Postoperative view. Right ventricular pericardial outflow patch. Same patient as in Figure 30–50. **A,** thoracic roentgenogram. Posteroanterior projection. Two years after operation, large aneurysm developed in region of repair *(white arrows)*. **B,** right ventriculogram. Anteroposterior projection. Three years after operation. Further growth of aneurysm. Aneurysm has broad communication with ventricle, suggesting a true rather than a false aneurysm.

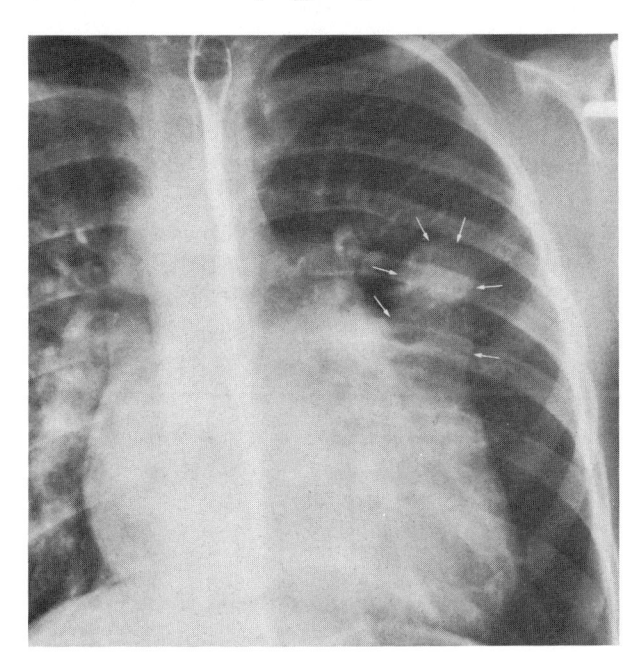

FIG 30–54.
Tetralogy of Fallot. Postoperative view. Thoracic roentgenogram. Posteroanterior projection. Right aortic arch. False aneurysm (pulsatile hematoma) *(arrows)* extends from suture line into lung field.

tion can be performed at a later date. Among the numerous complications of palliative procedures are kinking and occlusion of a branch pulmonary artery. If the shunt is too large, pulmonary congestion, cardiac failure, and pulmonary vascular disease may ensue.

1. A Blalock-Taussig shunt can be suspected on thoracic roentgenogram by finding evidence of a previous rib resection on the side opposite the aortic arch. REASON: The subclavian artery arising from the innominate artery provides more length for the anastomosis than the subclavian artery arising directly from the aortic arch, which is shorter and tends to kink during the operation. The latter may require an additional plastic procedure at the time of the original operation or subsequently. Another technique to avoid this complication is the insertion of a synthetic graft, which can be seen on a thoracic radiograph (Fig 30–57).

2. After a systemic pulmonary arterial shunt procedure, transient unilateral pulmonary edema may occur (Fig 30–58).

3. A large systemic pulmonary artery shunt may increase pulmonary vascular resistance, particularly

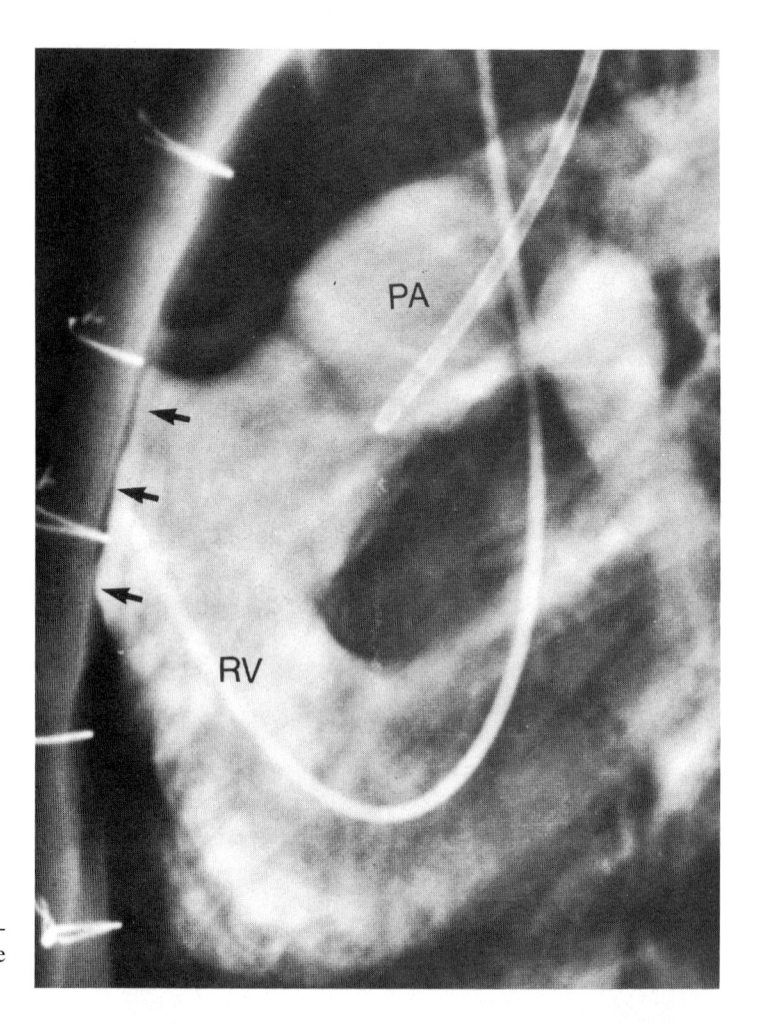

FIG 30-55.
Tetralogy of Fallot. Postoperative view. Right ventriculogram (RV). Lateral projection. Adherence of right ventricle to sternum (arrows). PA = pulmonary artery.

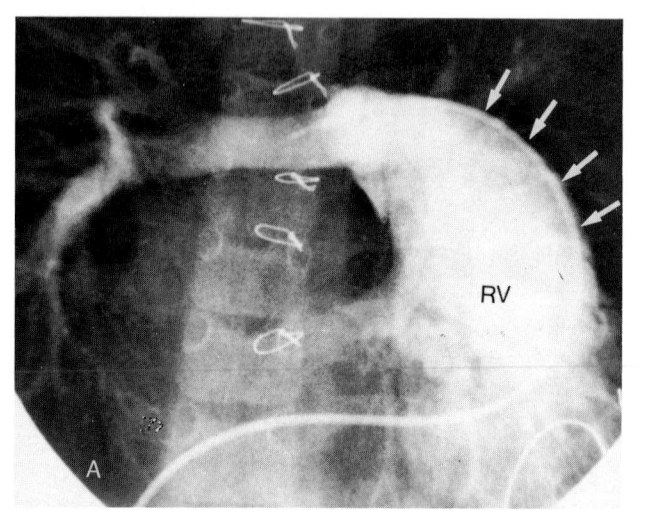

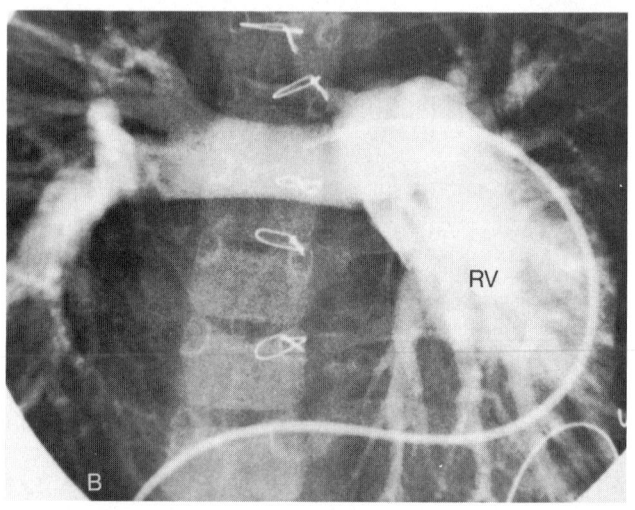

FIG 30-56.
Tetralogy of Fallot. Postoperative pulmonary annulus had been patched. Pulmonary arteriogram. **A,** Diastole. Ballooning of patched right ventricular outflow tract (RV) (arrows). Size of the right pulmonary artery is small, consistent with low diastolic pressure caused by pulmonary insufficiency. **B,** Systole. Outflow area remains large because outflow patch cannot contract. Marked systolic expansion of pulmonary arterial tree consistent with increased right ventricular stroke volume and wide pulse pressure. Angiographic appearance is consistent with 3+ pulmonary insufficiency.

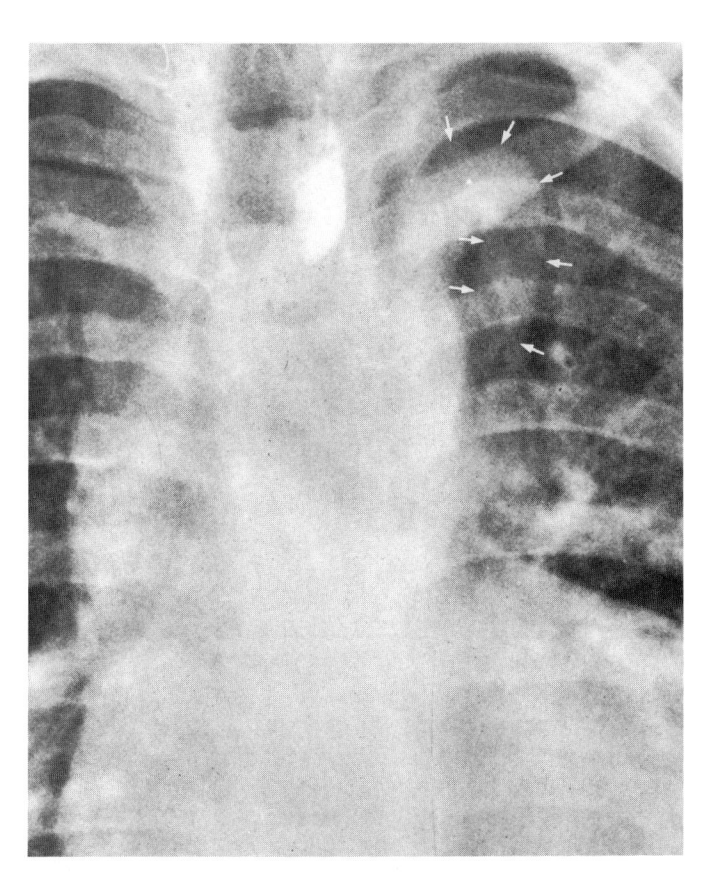

FIG 30–57.
Tetralogy of Fallot. Postoperative view. After placement of graft *(arrows)* from left subclavian artery to left pulmonary artery. Thoracic roentgenogram. Posteroanterior projection. Synthetic graft is clearly visualized *(arrows)*.

when the connection between the pulmonary artery and descending aorta has little length (Fig 30–59). In such shunts, such as a Waterston or a Potts, the size of the opening is very critical in determining the postoperative results and complications. On the other hand, the Blalock-Taussig anastomosis or a shunt using synthetic material offers resistance to blood flow because of the length. REASON: Resistance to flow is not only dependent on cross-sectional area of the conduit but also on its length. Therefore, pulmonary hypertension after creation of a Blalock-Taussig shunt and shunt using synthetic tubular grafts is infrequent.

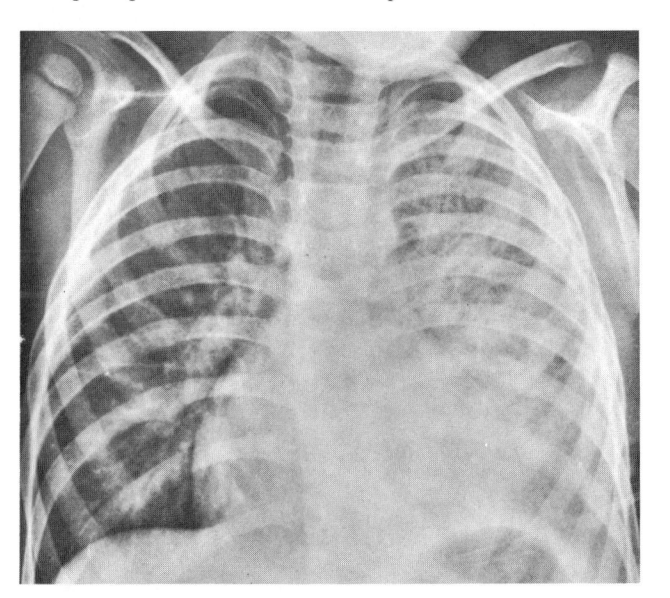

4. The Waterston-Cooley (ascending aorta to right pulmonary artery) shunt is also prone to development of pulmonary hypertension because it is a windowlike communication without length (Fig 30–60).

5. Stenosis or occlusion of a systemic pulmonary arterial shunt can be suspected radiographically by a change in the appearance of the pulmonary vasculature. In patients with a patent shunt, the pulmonary vasculature in the lung receiving the shunt tends to be increased. As the shunt becomes stenotic or closes, the pulmonary vasculature gradually decreases.

6. A much more serious complication, obstruction of a shunt and concomitant occlusion of the pulmonary artery, can be diagnosed on thoracic roentgenograms. A striking discrepancy of the pulmonary vasculature is apparent, and the occlusion of a pulmonary artery can be identified by isotopic perfusion studies. This

FIG 30–58.
Tetralogy of Fallot. One day after Potts' anastomosis. Thoracic roentgenogram. Posteroanterior projection. Extensive pulmonary edema of left lung. Edema was transient.

578 Cyanosis and Decreased Pulmonary Arterial Vasculature

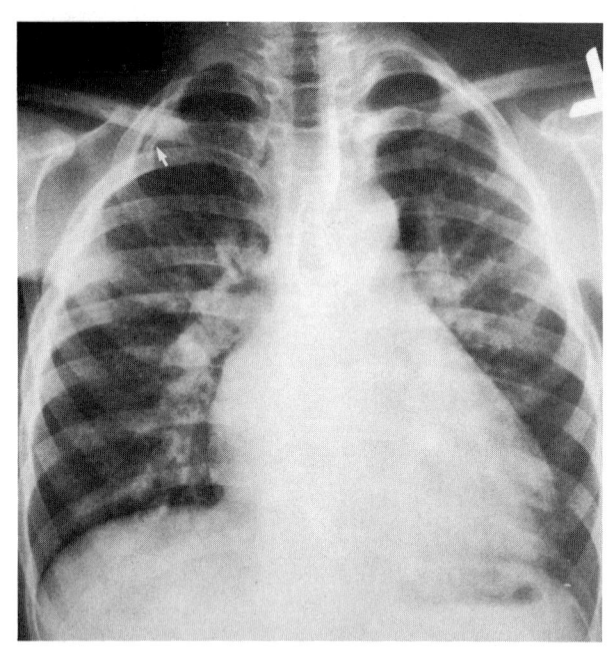

FIG 30–59.
Tetralogy of Fallot after Potts' anastomosis. Thoracic roentgenogram. Posteroanterior projection. Marked enlargement of central pulmonary arteries indicate pulmonary vascular disease. Previous right Blalock-Taussig anastomosis is evident by partial resection of third right rib *(arrow)*.

FIG 30–60.
Tetralogy of Fallot after Waterston-Cooley shunt. Right pulmonary arteriogram. Anteroposterior projection. Communication is evident as a negative filling defect *(arrows)* in opacified right pulmonary artery. Marked enlargement and tortuosity of pulmonary arteries indicate increased pulmonary blood flow and pulmonary hypertension.

complication is particularly common in patients with a Waterston-Cooley anastomoses because of kinking of the right pulmonary artery.

7. Even though a proximal pulmonary artery may become occluded, the distal pulmonary arterial tree almost invariably remains patent because of collateral bronchial arterial inflow. If the pleural space has previously been entered during an operation, the intercostal arteries may also supply the pulmonary arterial tree, through collateral arteries in pleural adhesions. Eventually the intercostal arteries enlarge and cause rib notching (Fig 30–61). The transpleural collaterals also result in pleural thickening. Occlusion of a pulmonary artery can be demonstrated by either a pulmonary arteriogram or a right ventriculogram (Fig 30–62).

8. Identification of patency of an occluded pulmonary artery to the level of the hilum is a difficult angiographic task. It is an important consideration for operative correction of the anomaly. Patency can be demonstrated angiographically by:
   a. Balloon occlusion descending aortography (Fig 30–63) and dense opacification of bronchial and intercostal arteries entering the pulmonary parenchyma.
   b. Pulmonary venous wedge angiography, with

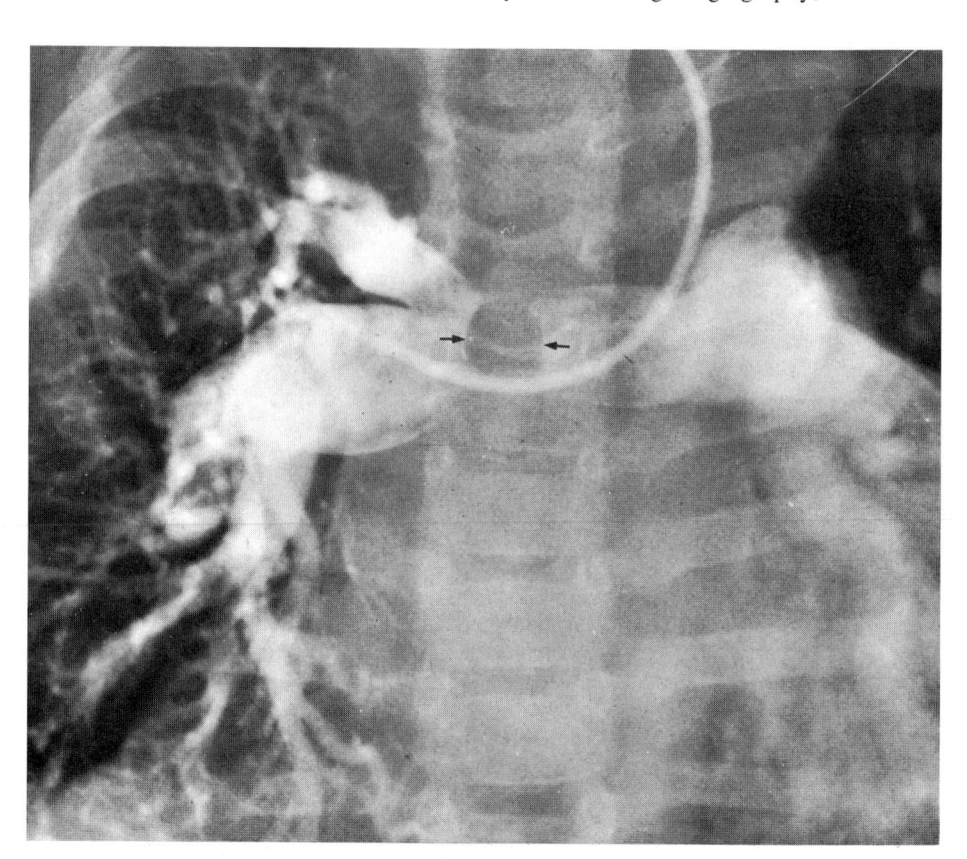

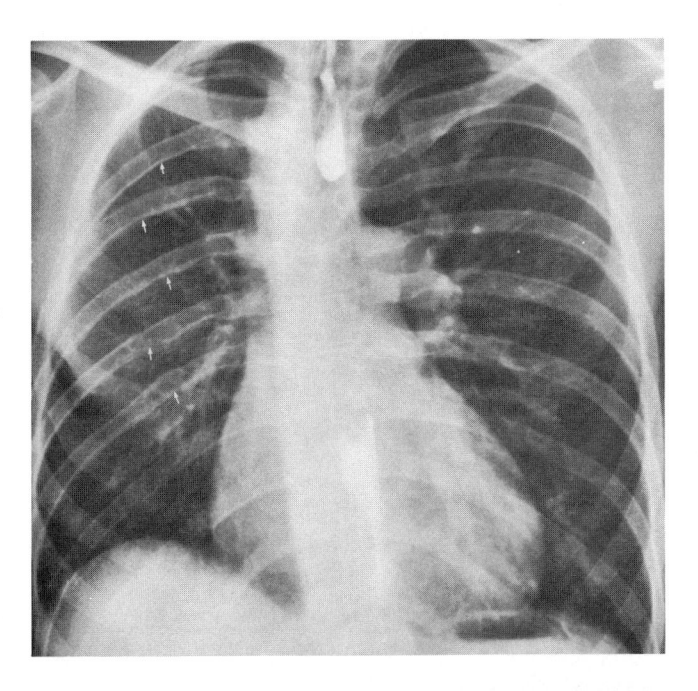

FIG 30–61.
Tetralogy of Fallot. Right aortic arch. Waterston anastomosis was performed 25 years ago. Thoracic roentgenogram. Posteroanterior projection. Normal cardiac size. Striking discrepancy between pulmonary vasculature of left lung, which is normal, and pulmonary vasculature of right lung, which is distinctly decreased. Extensive right rib notching *(arrows)* suggests collateral flow through enlarged intercostal arteries to patent right pulmonary artery.

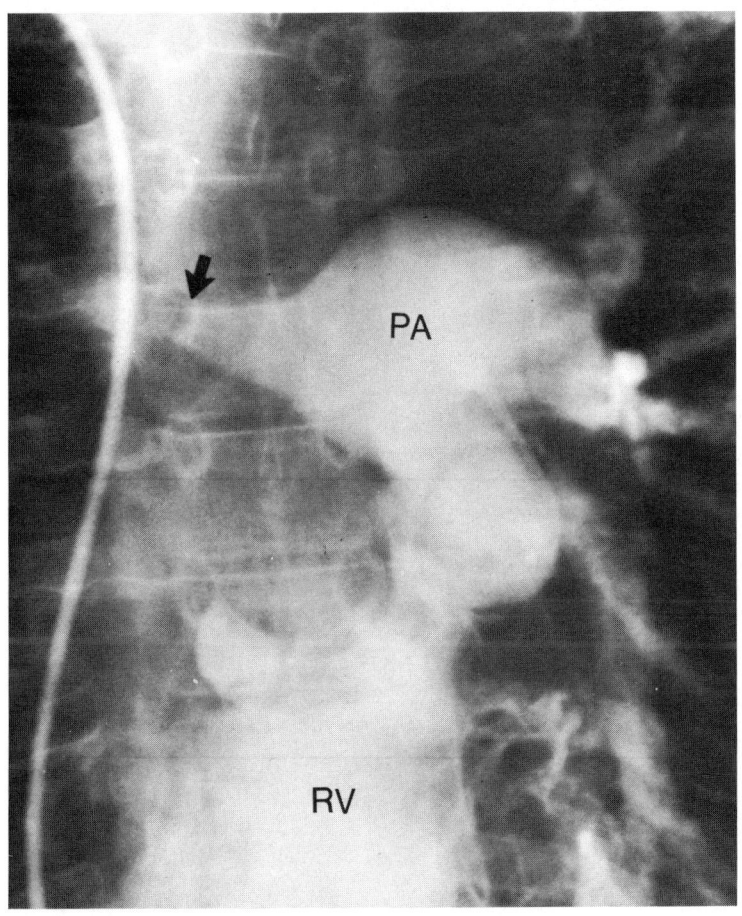

FIG 30–62.
Tetralogy of Fallot with Waterston-Cooley anastomosis. Right ventriculogram *(RV)*. Anteroposterior projection. Shunt and right pulmonary artery *(arrow)* are occluded. *PA* = pulmonary artery.

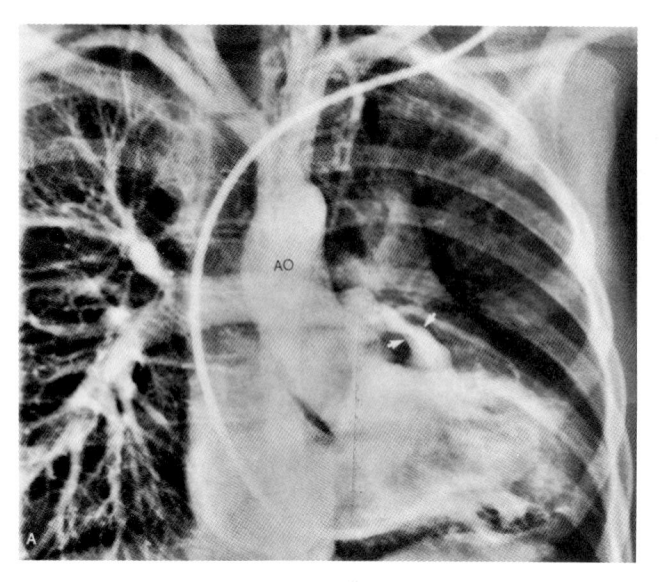

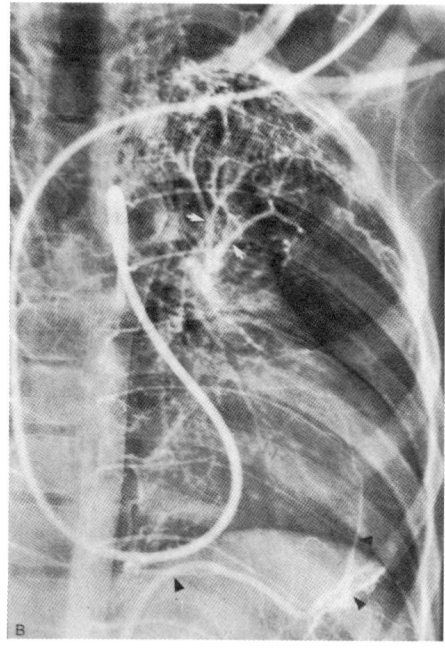

FIG 30-63.
Tetralogy of Fallot and absence of left pulmonary artery. **A,** right ventriculogram. Opacification of only right pulmonary artery. Marked infundibular pulmonary stenosis *(arrows).* Aorta *(AO)* is opacified through ventricular septal defect. Characteristically in tetralogy of Fallot, interruption of proximal pulmonary artery segment on same side as aortic arch (see Chapter 62). **B,** aortogram with balloon occlusion. Extensive transpleural collateral arteries with filling of central left pulmonary artery *(white arrows).* An arterial branch *(black arrow)* arises from abdominal aorta, traverses pleural space, and supplies pulmonary arterial branches. Transpleural collaterals develop only if the pleural space is obliterated by previous surgery.

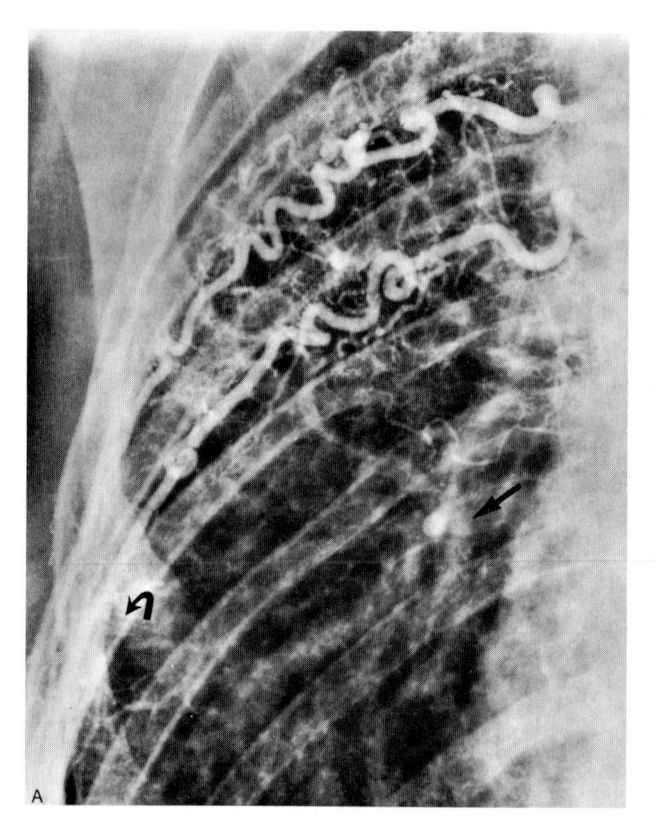

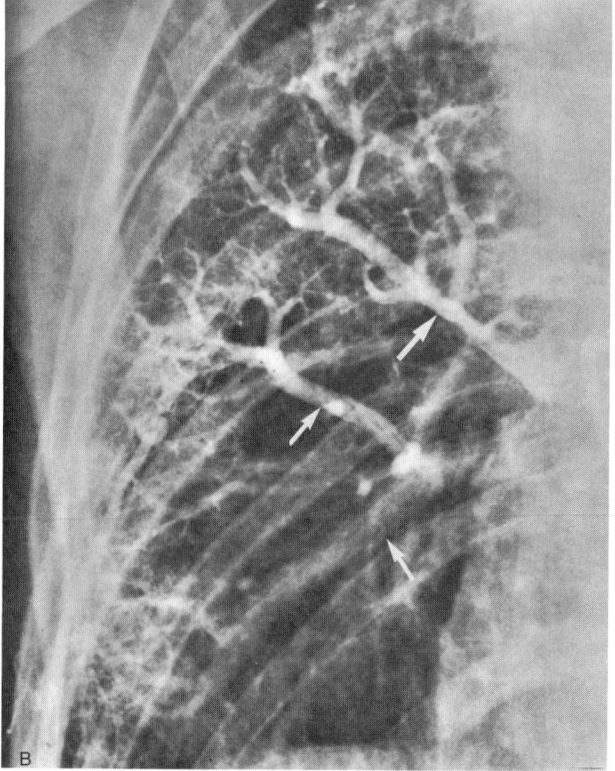

FIG 30-64.
Tetralogy of Fallot with occluded Waterston-Cooley shunt. **A,** selective injection into two intercostal arteries, which are enlarged and tortuous. Dense transpleural collateral network is clearly demonstrated *(curve arrow).* Early opacification of the right pulmonary artery *(black arrow).* **B,** later phase. Dense opacification of pulmonary artery branches proving patency facilitating operative correction.

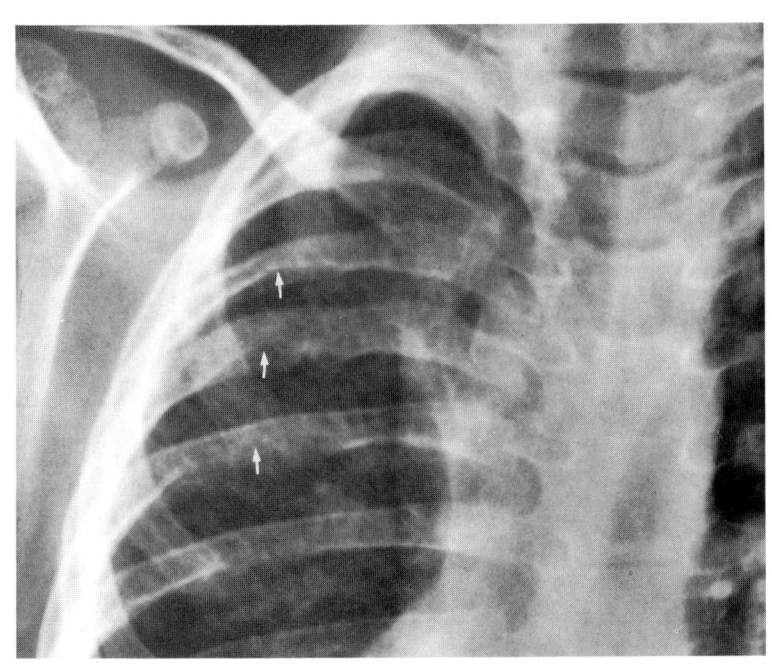

FIG 30-65.
Previous Blalock-Taussig anastomosis. Thoracic roentgenogram. Posteroanterior projection. Rib notching *(arrows)* caused by Blalock-Taussig anastomosis does not necessarily indicate pulmonary arterial occlusion.

  retrograde opacification of the pulmonary arterial tree.
  c. Simultaneous selective injection of several intercostal arteries (Fig 30–64) results in opacification of the pulmonary arterial tree through transpleural collaterals.
9. Rib notching after a Blalock-Taussig operation is a normal finding and does not necessarily indicate occlusion of the pulmonary artery (Fig 30–65).
  REASON: With division of a subclavian artery for the anastomosis, collateral blood flow to the ipsilateral upper extremity occurs primarily through intercostal arteries. These arteries enlarge, eroding the lower margin of the ribs and result in rib notching.
10. Nonopacification of the pulmonary artery does not necessarily indicate occlusion. REASON: A patent shunt may selectively supply one lung, resulting in nonopacification of the other lung. Therefore, occlusion of the shunt has to be proved by injection of the systemic circulation (Fig 30–66).
11. Occlusion of a pulmonary artery after a Blalock-Taussig anastomosis is much less common than after a Waterston or a Potts procedure.
12. The ventricular septal defect must be closed by an

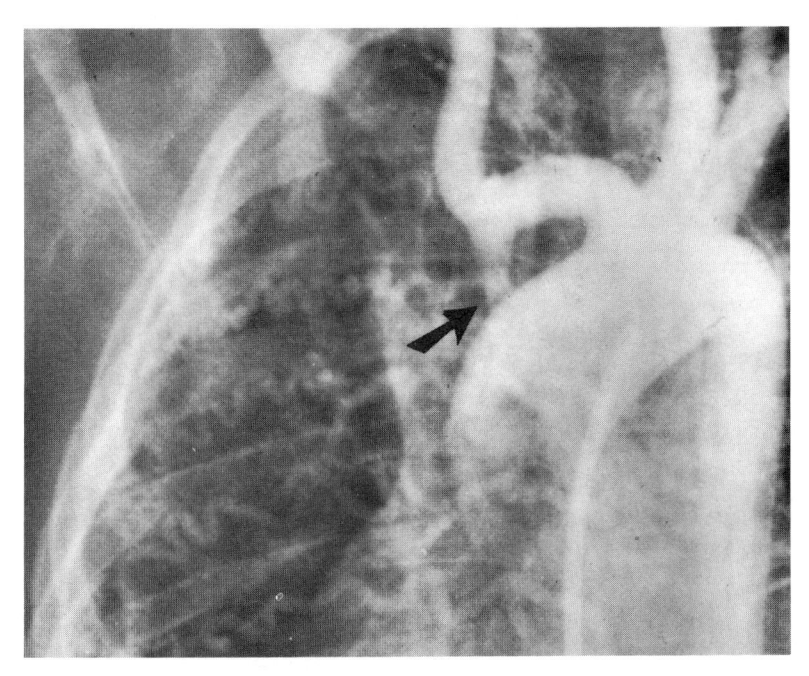

FIG 30-66.
Tetralogy of Fallot. Previous Blalock-Taussig anastomosis. Aortogram. Anteroposterior projection. Occluded shunt *(arrow)*. Typical kinking of innominate artery. Enlarged and tortuous intercostal arteries because of ligation of subclavian artery.

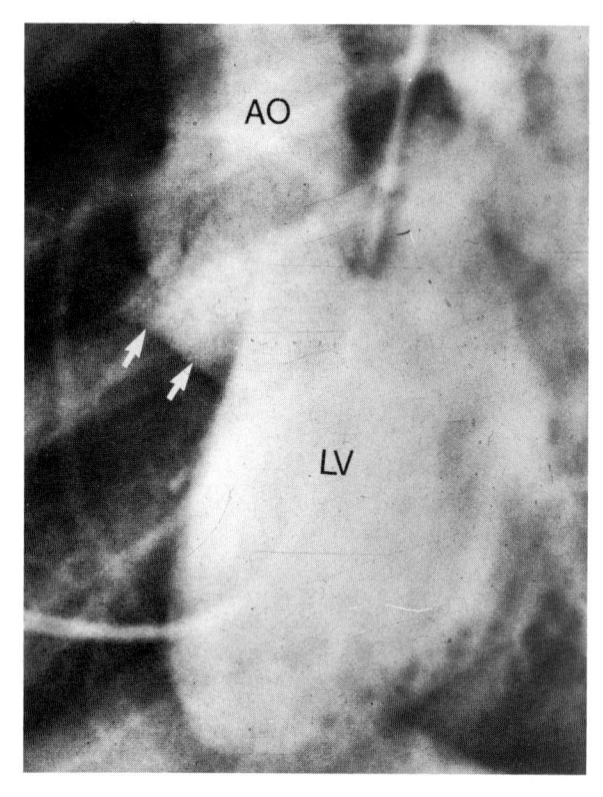

FIG 30–67.
Tetralogy of Fallot. Postoperative view. Closure of ventricular septal defect by patch. Left ventriculogram *(LV)*. Lateral projection. Patch is sewn obliquely across defect because of considerable overriding of aorta *(arrows)*. Complete closure of defect. Residual small shunt near aortic valve is more frequent than after closure of isolated ventricular septal defect. *AO* = aorta.

obliquely placed patch because of the overriding aorta. This patch can be well demonstrated by left ventriculography (Fig 30–67).

REFERENCES

1. Fallot A: Contribution a l'anatomie pathologique de la maladie bleue (cyanoses cardiaque), *Med Trop (Mars)* 25:138, 207, 341, 403, 1988.
2. Van Praagh R, Van Praagh S, Nebesar RA, et al: Tetralogy of Fallot: underdevelopment of the pulmonary infundibulum and its sequelae, *Am J Cardiol* 26:25, 1970.
3. Becker AE, Connor M, Anderson RH: Tetralogy of Fallot: a morphometric and geometric study, *Am J Cardiol* 35:402, 1975.
4. Rosenquist GC, Sweeney LJ, Stemple DR, et al: Ventricular septal defect in tetralogy of Fallot, *Am J Cardiol* 31:749, 1973.
5. Pisupatinath GV, Castaneda-Zuniga W, Amplatz K, et al: Aberrant left subclavian artery in tetralogy of Fallot, *Am J Cardiol* 45:811, 1980.
6. Guntheroth WG, Morgan BC, Mullins GL: Physiologic studies of paroxysmal hyperpnea in cyanotic congenital heart disease, *Circulation* 31:70, 1965.
7. Brotmacher L: Hemodynamic effects of squatting during repose, *Br Heart J* 19:559, 1957.
8. Guntheroth WG, Morgan BC, Mullins GL, et al: Venous return with knee chest position and squatting in tetralogy of Fallot, *Am Heart J* 75:313, 1968.
9. Fellows KE, Freed MD, Keane JF, et al: Results of routine preoperative coronary angiography in tetralogy of Fallot, *Circulation* 51:561, 1975.
10. Cumming GR, Carr W: Relief of dyspnoeic attacks in Fallot's tetralogy with propranolol, *Lancet* 1:519, 1966.
11. Ponie FE, Williams LC, Webb HM, et al: Propranolol palliation of tetralogy of Fallot: experience with long-term drug treatment in pediatric patients, *Pediatrics* 52:100, 1973.
12. Newfeld EA, Waldman JD, Paul MH, et al: Pulmonary vascular disease after systemic-pulmonary arterial shunt operations, *Am J Cardiol* 39:715, 1977.
13. Norberg WJ, Tadavarthy M, Knight L, et al: Late hemodynamic and angiographic findings after ascending aorta-pulmonary artery anastomosis, *J Thorac Cardiovasc Surg* 76:345, 1978.
14. Knight L, Joransen J, Marin-Garcia J, et al: Roentgenographic and angiocardiographic changes after total correction of the tetralogy of Fallot, *Am J Roentgenol, Radium Ther, Nucl Med* 123:691, 1975.
15. Joransen JA, Lucas RV Jr, Moller JH: Postoperative hemodynamics in tetralogy of Fallot: a study of 132 children, *Br Heart J* 41:33, 1979.
16. Ruzyllo W, Nihill MR, Mullins CE, et al: Hemodynamic evaluation of 221 patients after intracardiac repair of tetralogy of Fallot, *Am J Cardiol* 34:565, 1974.
17. Moss AJ, Klyman G, Emmanouilides GC: Late onset complete heart block. Newly recognized sequela of cardiac surgery, *Am J Cardiol* 30:884, 1972.
18. Gillette PC, Yeoman MA, Mullins CE, et al: Sudden death after repair of tetralogy of Fallot: electrocardiographic and electrophysiologic abnormalities, *Circulation* 56:566, 1977.
19. Marin-Garcia J, Moller JH: Sudden death after operative repair of tetralogy of Fallot, *Br Heart J* 39:1380, 1977.
20. Kobayashi J, Hirose H, Nakano S, et al: Ambulatory electrocardiographic study of the frequency and cause of ventricular arrhythmia after correction of tetralogy of Fallot, *Am J Cardiol* 54:1310, 1984.
21. Rocchini AP, Rosenthal A, Freed M, et al: Chronic congestive heart failure after repair of tetralogy of Fallot, *Circulation* 56:305, 1977.
22. Borow KM, Green LH, Castaneda AR, et al: Left ventricular function after repair of tetralogy of Fallot and its relationship to age at surgery, *Circulation* 61:1150, 1980.
23. Ebert PA: Second operations for pulmonary stenosis or insufficiency after repair of tetralogy of Fallot, *Am J Cardiol* 50:637, 1982.
24. Uretzky G, Puga FJ, Danielson GK, et al: Reoperation after correction of tetralogy of Fallot, *Circulation* 66(suppl I):I-202, 1982.
25. Castaneda AR, Sade RM, Lamberti J: Reoperation for residual defects after repair of tetralogy of Fallot, *Surgery* 76:1010, 1974.

CHAPTER 31

Tetralogy of Fallot With Pulmonary Atresia

VENTRICULAR SEPTAL DEFECT AND PULMONARY ATRESIA

In this form of tetralogy of Fallot, the connection between the right ventricle and distal pulmonary arterial tree is atretic. Pulmonary blood flow is derived from the aorta through either a patent ductus arteriosus, which may close in the neonatal period, systemic arteries, which connect with the pulmonary arterial tree, or bronchial collateral arteries. The condition is also known under "pseudotruncus arteriosus," because both ventricles eject solely into a single arterial vessel from which the pulmonary, systemic, and coronary arterial vasculature arise. The basic anatomic features are different, however.

PATHOLOGIC ANATOMY

The internal anatomy of the heart resembles tetralogy of Fallot, with the presence of a large ventricular septal defect, overriding aorta, and right ventricular hypertrophy. Right aortic arch is present in 50% of patients (greater than in patients with tetralogy of Fallot and pulmonary stenosis).

The site of pulmonary atresia varies (Fig 31–1). There may be infundibular atresia, or the infundibulum may be patent to the level of the pulmonary valve. In these instances, the main pulmonary artery may be patent to the level of the pulmonary valve. The main pulmonary artery may be atretic and manifest only as a fibrous strand that passes from the site of the pulmonary valve to a confluence of the left and right pulmonary arteries.

In other instances the fibrous strand representing the main pulmonary artery and the major pulmonary arterial branches to the left and right lungs may not even be confluent.

The vascular supply to the lungs may derive from a variety of systemic arteries called systemic pulmonary collateral arteries (Fig 31–2).

There are three basic types of systemic pulmonary collateral arteries:

1. The normal bronchial arterial branches, which are enlarged.
2. Arteries arising directly from the descending aorta, aortic arch, or abdominal aorta.
3. Arteries arising from other arterial branches of the aorta, such as subclavian, internal mammary, mediastinal, intercostal or coronary arteries (rare). These form an extrapulmonary anastomotic network.

These systemic collateral arteries anastomose with the pulmonary arterial tree in the region of the hilum, inside the lung, or at the periphery of the lung.[1-4] Sometimes anastomoses exist within the lung between pulmonary arteries of adjacent pulmonary segments or lobes.

There are four anatomic types of anatomoses:

1. Extrapulmonary, at the hilum and outside the lung.
2. Intrapulmonary to a branch of the pulmonary artery.
3. Intra-acinar in the periphery of the lung.
4. Direct aortic branches at the hilum, continuing as a single vessel with the same histologic characteristics and typical distribution of the pulmonary artery (Fig 31–3).

The origin of these arteries is uncertain. Segmental branch collateral arteries originate from intrasegmental branches of the embryonic dorsal aorta and are normally present during the third and fourth weeks of gestation. The site of the anastomoses is at the hilum. This type of anastomosis at the hilum is invariably stenotic at their junction,

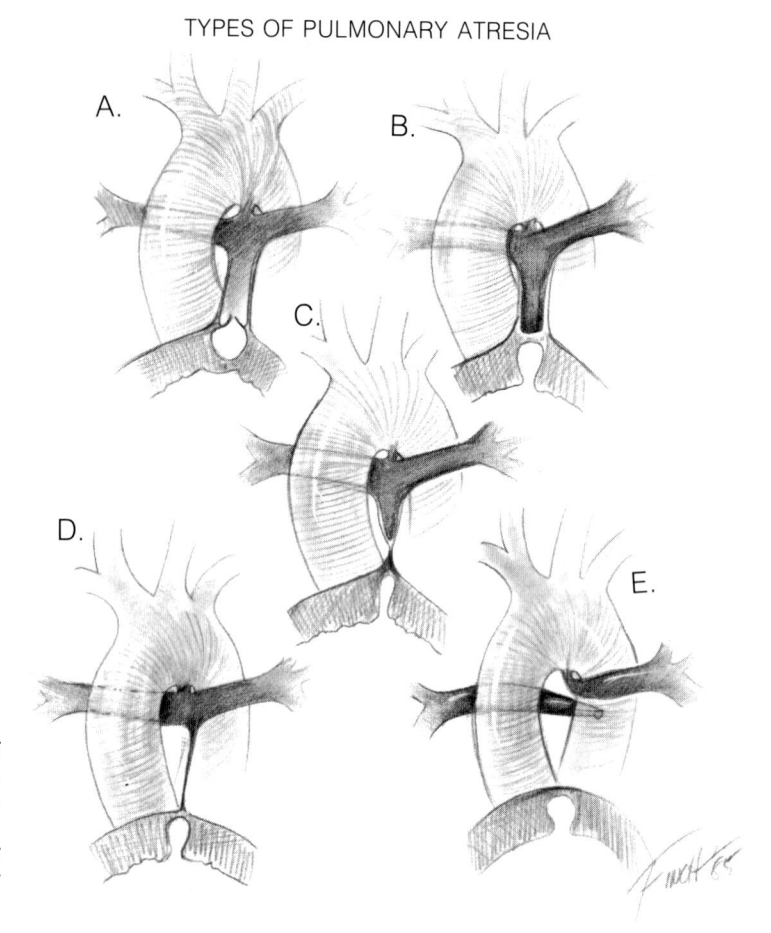

FIG 31–1.
Pulmonary atresia and ventricular septal defect. Types of atresia. **A,** infundibular atresia with patent pulmonary valve. **B,** Valvar atresia and patent stenotic infundibulum. **C,** atresia of pulmonary valve and proximal pulmonary artery. **D,** atresia of pulmonary valve and atresia of main pulmonary artery. **E,** valvar atresia and absence of main pulmonary artery.

with the pulmonary arterial tree perhaps representing involution of the intrasegmental artery. In contrast, direct aortic branches may provide the major blood supply to a lobe or a segment of a lobe. The developmental origin of such indirect aortic branches is less certain. All collaterals ultimately perfuse pulmonary alveoli.

Coronary arterial–right ventricular communications (sinusoids) occur much less frequently than in infants with severe pulmonary stenosis or pulmonary atresia with intact ventricular septum (see Chapter 34). Their presence, however, seems to negate the theory that such fistulas result from suprasystemic pressure in the right ventricle that reopens the sinusoids.

HEMODYNAMICS

Because of the pulmonary atresia, the entire right ventricular output is ejected into the aorta, where it mixes with the left ventricular output. The degree of cyanosis depends on the relative volume of blood being ejected from the right ventricle and the left ventricle, respectively. This volume depends on the relative amounts of venous return to the right and left atrium. The right ventricular output (i.e., systemic venous return) equals the cardiac output and is relatively constant among patients with tetralogy of Fallot and pulmonary atresia. In contrast, left ventricular output derived from the pulmonary venous return is extremely variable between patients with this condition because of the anatomic variations in the arterial vasculature supplying the pulmonary arterial tree. In most patients the systemic pulmonary arterial anastomoses are small, narrowed, and of limited number so that pulmonary blood flow is restricted. In addition, there may be stenotic areas at the junction of these systemic arteries with the pulmonary arterial tree. Each of these factors limits pulmonary blood flow, and cyanosis is usually intense.

In contrast, in a few patients the systemic pulmonary arterial anastomoses are large and unobstructed, and stenotic lesions are not present in the pulmonary arterial tree. In such patients, cyanosis is minimal. In fact, in an occasional patient the pulmonary blood flow is increased enough to cause cardiac failure from left ventricular volume overload.

In those with reduced pulmonary blood flow, pressure measured in the pulmonary arterial tree is either normal or

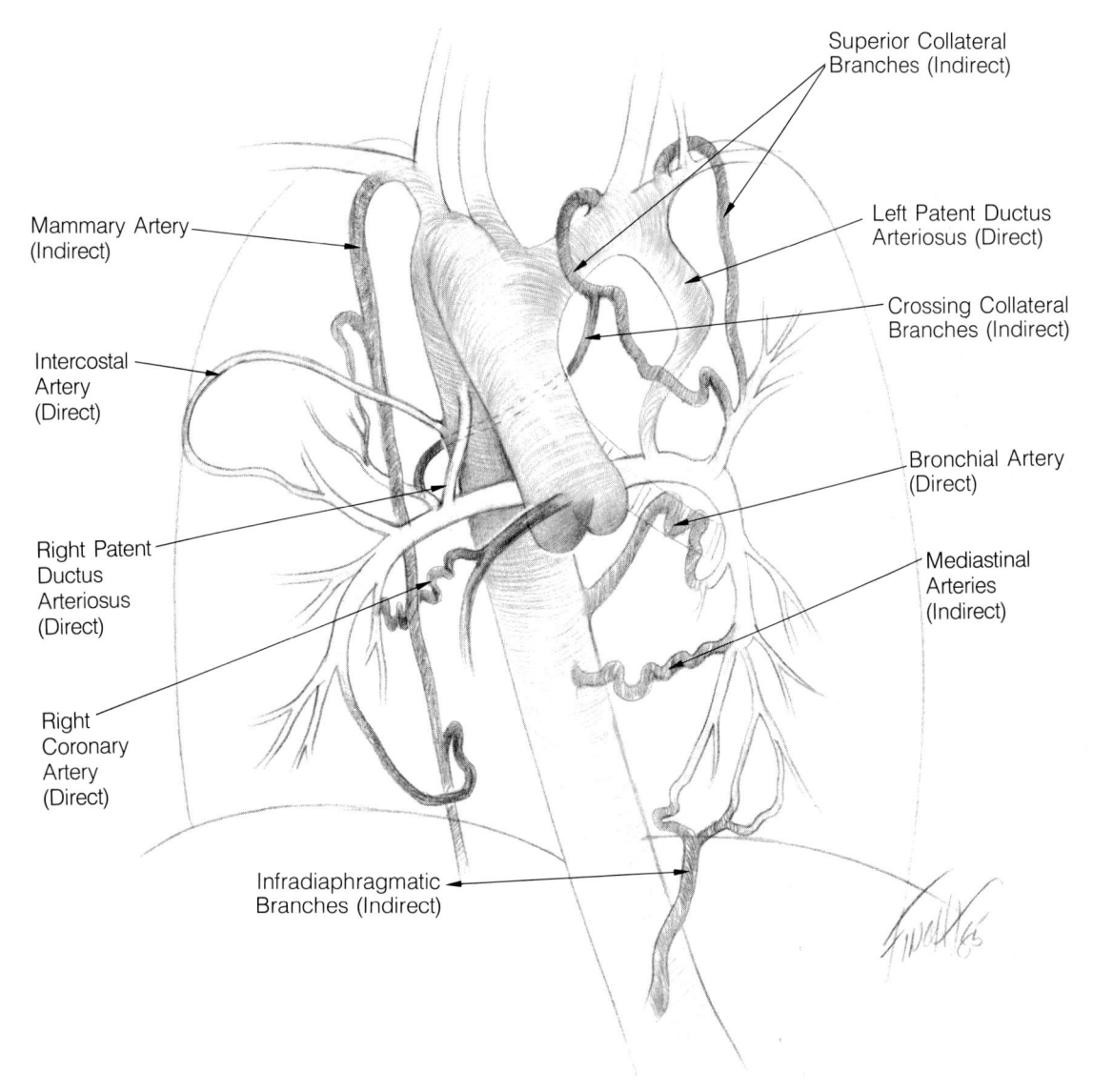

FIG 31–2.
Most common systemic collateral arteries in tetralogy of Fallot with pulmonary atresia.

low, whereas in those with increased pulmonary blood flow, pulmonary arterial pressure is elevated, may be at systemic levels, and may be associated with pulmonary vascular disease.

In neonates with tetralogy of Fallot and pulmonary atresia, the patent ductus arteriosus may be the major source of pulmonary blood flow. As the ductus closes in the neonatal period, intense cyanosis develops.

CLINICAL FEATURES

Cyanosis is the major clinical feature, and patients can be divided into three groups, depending on the severity of cyanosis: (1) intense cyanosis in the neonatal period or infancy; (2) persistent mild cyanosis throughout childhood associated with exercise intolerance; and (3) minimal cyanosis, perhaps associated with congestive cardiac failure. These three clinical types correlate with the caliber of communications between the aorta and pulmonary arterial tree.

4 TYPES OF SYSTEMIC-PULMONARY ANASTOMOSES

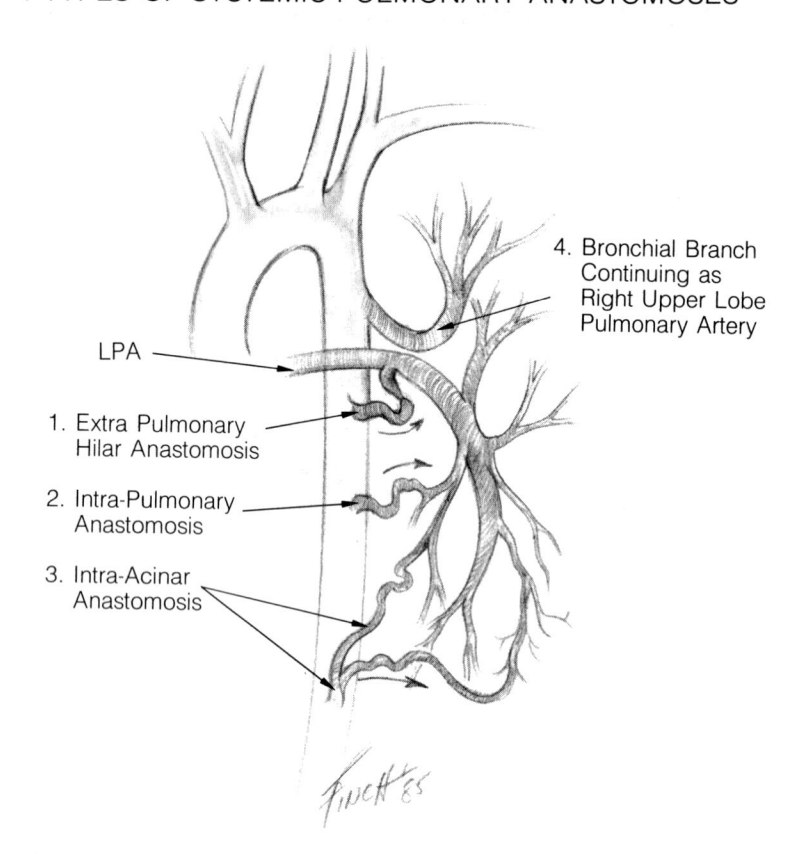

FIG 31-3.
Location of various systemic collateral arteries that ultimately reach the pulmonary capillary bed. *LPA* = left pulmonary artery.

In tetralogy of Fallot and pulmonary atresia, the second heart sound is single (representing aortic valve closure) and often loud even in the pulmonary area. An aortic systolic ejection click, reflecting the enlarged aorta, is heard at the cardiac apex.

The presence and loudness of the murmur correlate with the volume of pulmonary blood flow. The murmur is rarely more than grade 3/6. When present, the murmur is continuous because it reflects the blood flow through the systemic pulmonary arterial communication. In patients in whom the ductus arteriosus is the major connection, the murmur is heard best along the upper left sternal border and disappears if the ductus arteriosus closes. Continuous murmurs may be heard over other areas of the precordium or between the scapulae if major blood flow is through bronchial arterial communications. These murmurs often sound more shrill and closer to the ear than a patent ductus arteriosus.

ELECTROCARDIOGRAPHIC FEATURES

The electrocardiogram resembles that in a patient with tetralogy of Fallot. We have seen an occasional patient with a large volume of pulmonary blood flow who has shown a pattern of combined ventricular hypertrophy.

ECHOCARDIOGRAPHIC FEATURES

The echocardiogram shows the ventricular septal defect, overriding aorta, and right ventricular hypertrophy. The area of the pulmonary annulus is narrowed, and the pulmonary valve is not visualized. On Doppler interrogation of the pulmonary trunk, there is no antegrade flow from the right ventricle, and retrograde systolic and diastolic flows are seen, because pulmonary blood flow is derived through the ductus arteriosus.

Echocardiography is also helpful in outlining details of the location of the pulmonary arteries, the status of the pulmonary trunk and continuity between the left and right pulmonary arteries. Sinusoids with retrograde coronary blood flow can occasionally be demonstrated by color flow Doppler.

RADIOGRAPHIC FEATURES

Sometimes the diagnosis of tetralogy of Fallot with pulmonary atresia can be suggested from the thoracic roentgenogram. With increasing severity of infundibular pulmonary stenosis and increasing cyanosis, the radiographic appearance becomes more and more characteristic of tetralogy of Fallot, showing a boot-shaped cardiac contour, decreased pulmonary vasculature, and concave pulmonary arterial segment. In patients with pulmonary atresia and decreased pulmonary flow, the cardiac silhouette is characteristic.

In tetralogy of Fallot with pulmonary stenosis, there is a gradual decrease of pulmonary blood flow with an increasing degree of pulmonary stenosis. With pulmonary atresia, however, enlarged systemic arteries develop and supply blood to the pulmonary vascular bed. Consequently, the pulmonary vasculature may not be as decreased as might be expected. In fact, in 30% of patients, the large systemic arterial collaterals have no stenoses, resulting in normal to increased pulmonary vasculature.

1. Posteroanterior thoracic roentgenograms do not show significant cardiomegaly and are most commonly identical to tetralogy of Fallot. REASON: The right ventricle decompresses through the ventricular septal defect, and failure of the right ventricle does not occur. Exceptions rarely exist. Cases of pulmonary atresia and obstruction of the ventricular septal defect by either the septal limb of the crista supraventricularis or the tricuspid valve may cause cardiomegaly. Right ventricular enlargement then occurs because of the markedly elevated systolic pressure in the right ventricle or because of tricuspid insufficiency.

2. The cardiac silhouette is very characteristic for tetralogy of Fallot (Fig 31–4). REASON: The entire right ventricular output is delivered through the ventricular septal defect into the aorta. The ejection force of both the right and left ventricles is directed into the aorta, and elevation of the cardiac apex and clockwise rotation of the heart ensue (see Chapter 30).

3. The pulmonary arterial segment is concave. REASON: The main pulmonary artery is never enlarged because there is no flow as a result of pulmonary atresia. The main pulmonary artery is often atretic. Furthermore, all systemic pulmonary arterial anastomoses occur into the pulmonary arterial tree beyond the main pulmonary artery.

4. A right aortic arch is present in one half of the patients. This is a greater frequency than in tetralogy of Fallot (50% compared with 25%).

5. The appearance of the pulmonary vasculature varies according to the type of systemic pulmonary arterial collaterals and whether stenoses exist in the pulmonary arteries. If systemic arteries supply the lungs without anastomosis to the central pulmonary arterial tree, the typical comma-shaped shadows of the pulmonary arteries in both hilar areas are absent.

6. If systemic arterial collaterals have anastomotic connections with the pulmonary arteries in the region of the hilum, normal comma-shape shadows can usually be seen, although they tend to be small.

7. Usually the pulmonary vasculature appears either decreased or normal. In patients with fairly normal pulmonary blood flow, thoracic roentgenograms may be interpreted as normal. But commonly, however, an increased

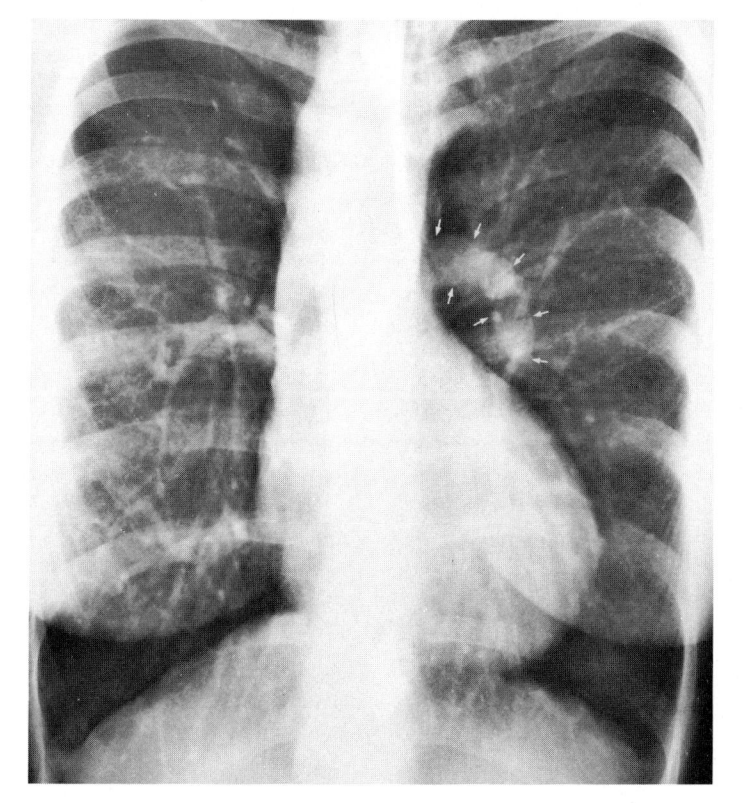

FIG 31–4.
Pulmonary atresia and ventricular septal defect. Thoracic roentgenogram. Posteroanterior projection. Right aortic arch. Decreased pulmonary vasculature. Normal cardiac size with upturned apex identical to tetralogy of Fallot. In the left lung is a characteristic hilar comma density *(arrows),* indicating the presence of a pulmonary artery. Bizarre pulmonary vasculature in right lung. No comma density is present to indicate bronchial collateral arteries.

number of vessels is seen on end in the lung fields (see Fig 31–4). REASON: Systemic collaterals and bronchial arteries have a more tortuous irregular course, and therefore more cross-sections are intersected by the x-ray beam. These form round densities in the lung fields. The irregular pattern of these tortuous vessels results in a bizarre appearance of the pulmonary vasculature.

8. Rarely with large systemic arterial collaterals without stenoses, the pulmonary blood flow is greatly increased. In these patients, particularly if a right aortic arch is present, the radiographic appearance is indistinguishable from persistent truncus arteriosus (Fig 31–5).

9. The barium-filled esophagus may be indented posteriorly (Fig 31–6). REASON: Bronchial arteries supplying the lungs are direct aortic collaterals, which may cross behind the esophagus and can cause indentations. These collateral arteries usually pass behind the esophagus, but very rarely they course between the trachea and the esophagus.

CARDIAC CATHETERIZATION

The purposes of cardiac catheterization are similar to tetralogy of Fallot without pulmonary atresia. In addition, pressure must be measured in systemic pulmonary arterial collaterals because it may be elevated. Furthermore, bronchial arteries can be occluded by catheterization techniques. The pressure and oximetry data obtained are similar to tetralogy of Fallot. Although the catheter tip can usually be advanced through the ventricular septal defect

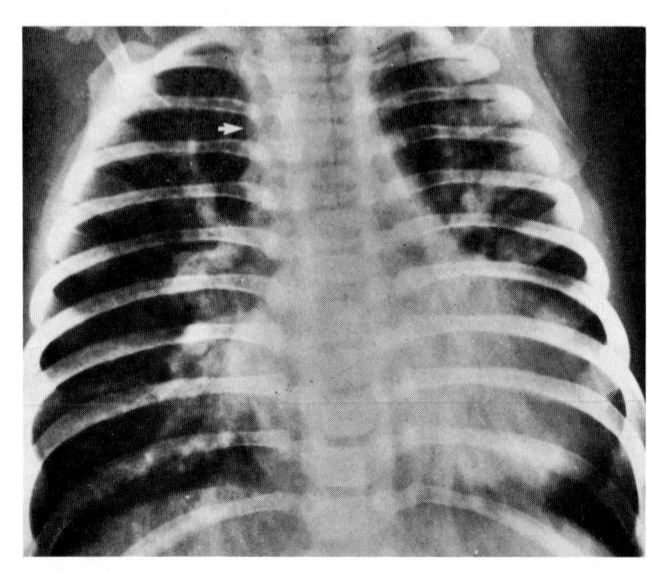

FIG 31–5.
Pulmonary atresia and ventricular septal defect. Thoracic roentgenogram. Posteroanterior projection. Increased pulmonary vasculature. Cardiomegaly. Because of increased vasculature and right aortic arch *(arrow)*, persistent truncus arteriosus is most likely radiographic diagnosis.

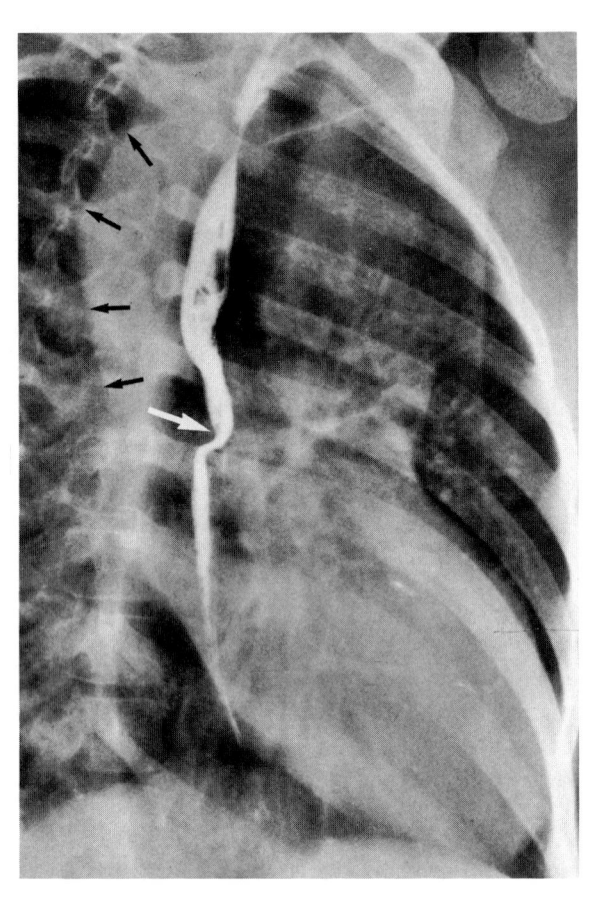

FIG 31–6.
Pulmonary atresia and ventricular septal defect. Thoracic roentgenogram. Right anterior oblique projection. Right aortic arch *(black arrows)*. Large bronchial artery *(white arrow)* indents esophagus posteriorly.

into the aorta, it cannot be advanced from the right ventricle into the pulmonary artery.

Various types of catheters can be used to selectively catheterize the collateral arteries supplying the lungs. The cobra, sidewinder, and the Amplatz left coronary configurations, as well as moveable core guidewires, are helpful to enter these arteries. It is preferable to approach these vessels with a catheter advanced from the femoral artery. Major arteries to the lungs should be catheterized and the catheter passed well into the lung field to identify the site and severity of stenotic lesions. In 70% of instances, distal pulmonary arterial pressure is either normal or low, whereas in the remainder, pressure is elevated, often to systemic levels. Pressure measurements in the bronchial and pulmonary arteries are essential to determine the presence of a pressure gradient. If stenoses are present, adequate blood flow would occur through an operatively inserted shunt. On the other hand, if there is associated pulmonary hypertension, a shunt procedure is contraindicated.

ANGIOGRAPHIC FEATURES

Careful angiography is necessary in each patient with pulmonary atresia and ventricular septal defect for the following reasons:

1. To demonstrate the size of both the right and left ventricles. REASON: After a corrective operation, each ventricle must be adequate to eject a normal cardiac output. If one ventricle is significantly hypoplastic, corrective operation is not feasible.

2. To demonstrate the type and location of infundibular or valvar pulmonary atresia (or both). Depending on the angiographic appearance, a pulmonary valvulotomy or a transannular patch can be performed to relieve the obstruction. On the other hand, if a long atretic segment is present, a right ventricular–pulmonary arterial conduit is required.

3. To demonstrate the degree of overriding of the aorta. With very severe overriding or double-outlet right ventricle, the operative risk increases.

4. To demonstrate the size of the proximal right and left pulmonary arteries. Placement of a systemic pulmonary arterial shunt may increase the size of diffusely hypoplastic pulmonary arteries. REASON: If hypoplastic, the pulmonary arterial tree may be inadequate to accept the entire cardiac output after closure of the ventricular septal defect (see Fig 30–29).

5. To measure the size of the proximal right and left pulmonary arteries and demonstrate continuity between right and left pulmonary arteries.

6. To demonstrate the commonly associated peripheral pulmonary artery stenosis, which may elevate right ventricular systolic pressure after complete repair.

7. To demonstrate both direct and indirect systemic collateral arteries into the lungs, their variations, and areas of stenosis. Because the degree of stenoses in the collateral arteries is difficult to assess angiographically, concomitant pressure measurements should be performed.

8. To demonstrate the coronary artery pattern. As in tetralogy of Fallot, the incidence of coronary anomalies with large and important arteries crossing the right ventricular outflow tract is about 5%. Such anomalies preclude correction by patch graft and require the insertion of a conduit (see Fig 30–49).

In patients with ventricular septal defect and pulmonary atresia, there are several unique features:

1. The appearance of the right and left ventricles are identical to tetralogy of Fallot. Either the right ventricular outflow tract, and the pulmonary valve, or the main pulmonary artery may be atretic.

2. The size of the aorta is larger than in tetralogy of Fallot. REASON: The entire systemic and pulmonary blood flows are carried through the ascending aorta throughout fetal life.

3. A remnant of the infundibulum is demonstrated (Fig 31–7,A and B), indicating that the malformation is developmentally a form of tetralogy of Fallot. At postmortem examination, in such instances, careful dissection reveals remnants of the right ventricular infundibulum or main pulmonary artery. This is not present in persistent true truncus arteriosus.

4. Rarely, the infundibulum, pulmonary valve, and main pulmonary artery are each atretic (Fig 31–7,C).

Demonstration of the Pulmonary Circulation

Angiography is important to determine the intrapulmonary distribution of arteries, the relationship of collateral arteries to the pulmonary arteries, and the presence of bronchopulmonary stenoses and to identify those collaterals allowing shunting that can be safely embolized or ligated during an operation. An ascending aortogram should be performed first. REASON: Great variability exists in the number and distribution of bronchial arteries. Because of the large volume of blood flow through the aorta, which represents the entire systemic and pulmonary blood flow, the injection must be very rapid, and a large amount of contrast medium must be used. Best results are obtained using balloon occlusion aortography.

Aortography serves as a roadmap for subsequent selective catheterization of individual collateral branches[5] to better document their relationship to the pulmonary artery and obtain pressure measurements. Only if a stenotic area is very severe can a pressure gradient and normal pulmonary arterial pressure beyond the area of stenosis be assumed. If only mild narrowing or no stenosis is observed, the pressure cannot be predicted angiographically.

Occasionally, even with satisfactory aortography, the pulmonary arterial branches cannot be opacified. Under those circumstances, angiography performed from the pulmonary venous wedge position is indicated (Fig 31–8).[6] In this technique, an end-hole or balloon catheter is passed through a patent foramen ovale into a pulmonary vein and wedged. Contrast material is injected at a rate of 2 to 4 mL/sec manually or with a power injector until the pulmonary artery fills to the level of the hilum. The amount of contrast medium can be minimized by layering it with saline solution. After the pulmonary veins are opacified, the saline solution pushes the contrast medium into the pulmonary arterial branches. Very rapid injections should be avoided, because they rupture pulmonary capillaries and cause extensive extravasation of contrast medium.

The systemic collateral arteries in the lungs must be

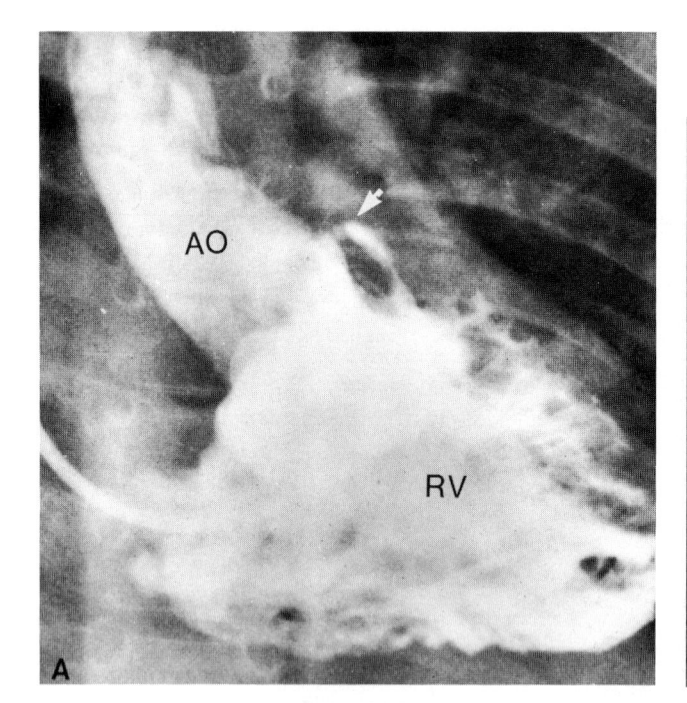

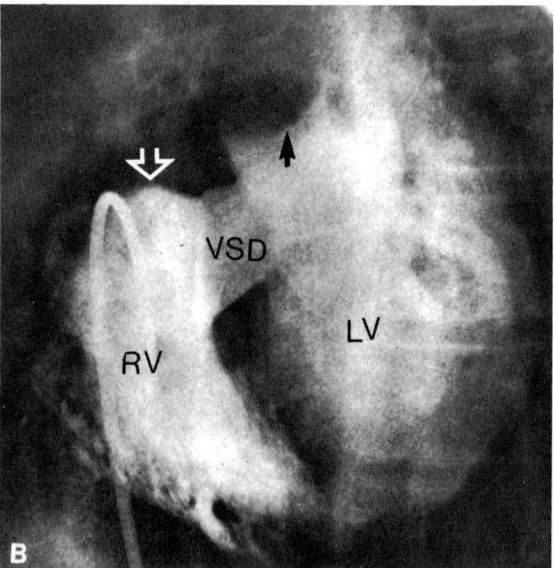

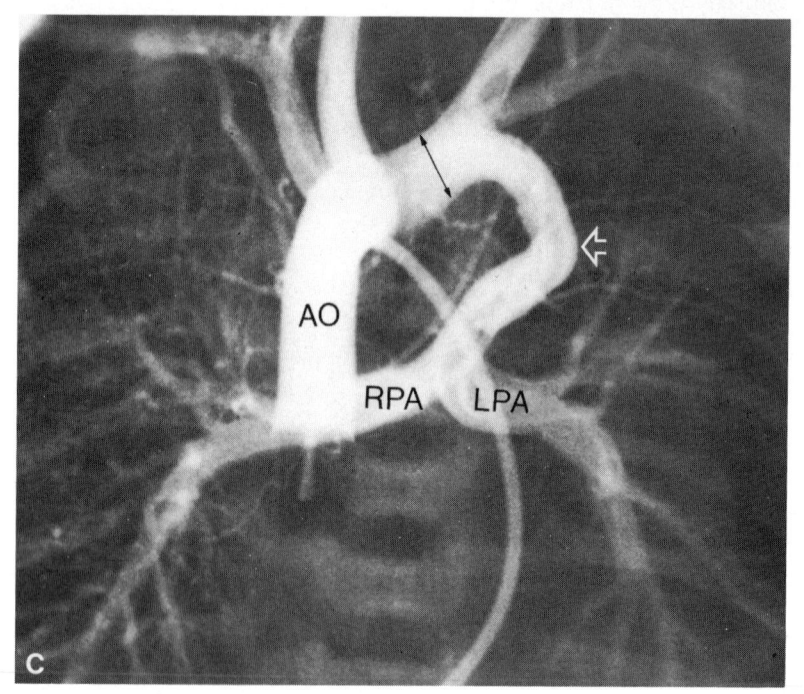

FIG 31–7.
Pulmonary atresia and ventricular septal defect. Typical findings: Right ventriculogram *(RV)*. **A,** right anterior oblique projection. Atretic infundibulum. Valvar pulmonary atresia *(arrow)*. Aorta *(AO)* opacifies through ventricular septal defect. **B,** right ventriculogram. Left anterior oblique projection. Atretic infundibulum *(open arrow)*. Left ventricle *(LV)* opacifies through ventricular septal defect *(VSD)*, outlining closed aortic valve *(black arrow)*. Aorta does not override (rare for this condition). **C,** balloon occlusion descending aortogram *(AO)*. Anteroposterior projection. Right aortic arch. From subclavian artery, large ductus arteriosus *(open arrow)* supplies right *(RPA)* and left pulmonary arteries *(LPA)*. Atretic main pulmonary artery. Ductus opposite side of aortic arch arises from subclavian artery (see Chapter 62). Markedly enlarged innominate artery *(black arrows)* because blood flow through this segment consists of left carotid arterial, left subclavian arterial, and total pulmonary blood flow through patent ductus arteriosus. Continuity between right and left pulmonary arteries.

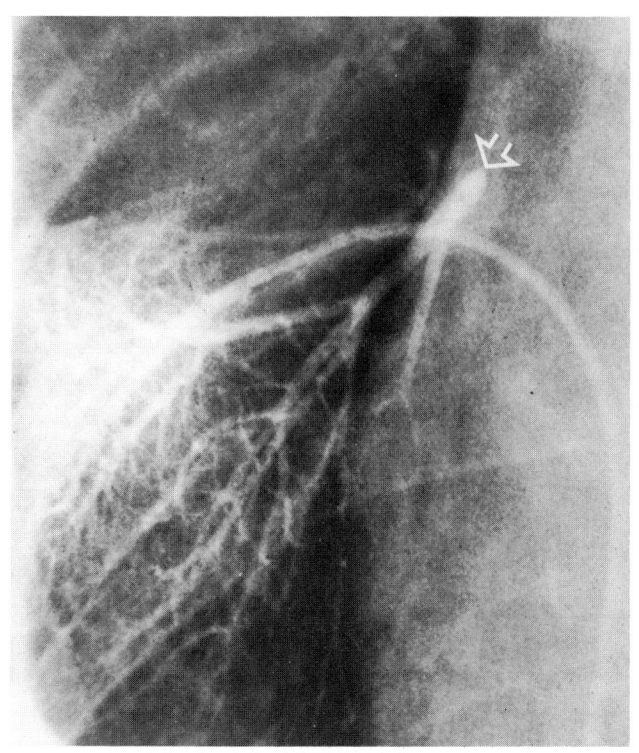

FIG 31–8.
Pulmonary atresia and ventricular septal defect. Right pulmonary venous wedge injection. Anteroposterior projection. Catheter is passed through atrial communication and wedged in right lower lobe pulmonary vein. Small and patent right pulmonary artery is opacified to level of right hilum *(arrow).*

differentiated from true pulmonary arteries. This distinction may be difficult. Generally the pulmonary arteries have a regular course and radiate from the hilum in a regular fashion. If a right or left pulmonary artery is present in the hilum, a characteristic commalike contour can be identified. Systemic collateral arteries pursue a more irregular and undulating course and enter the pulmonary parenchyma at various locations (see Figs 31–2 and 31–3).

There are several specific angiographic findings:

1. The major arterial supply to the pulmonary arteries may be through a patent ductus arteriosus. With a patent ductus arteriosus, demonstration of continuity between right and left pulmonary arteries is of paramount importance (Figs 31–9 and 31–10).

2. The ductus arteriosus may arise from either the ipsilateral side or the contralateral side of the aortic arch. When the ductus arises opposite the side of the aortic arch, it originates from a subclavian artery (see Chapter 62).

3. Rarely bilateral ductus are present (see Fig 31–9).

4. The identification of a ductal stenosis is important (see Fig 31–10) because it indicates that pulmonary arterial pressure is normal. In this situation, a systemic pulmonary arterial shunt can be inserted.

5. Rarely, a ductus arteriosus or a ductuslike collateral artery may be continuous with a single pulmonary artery, and stenosis is not present (Fig 31–11).

6. Rarely the ductus gives rise to the mammary artery (see Fig 31–10).

7. Typically direct or indirect systemic collateral ar-

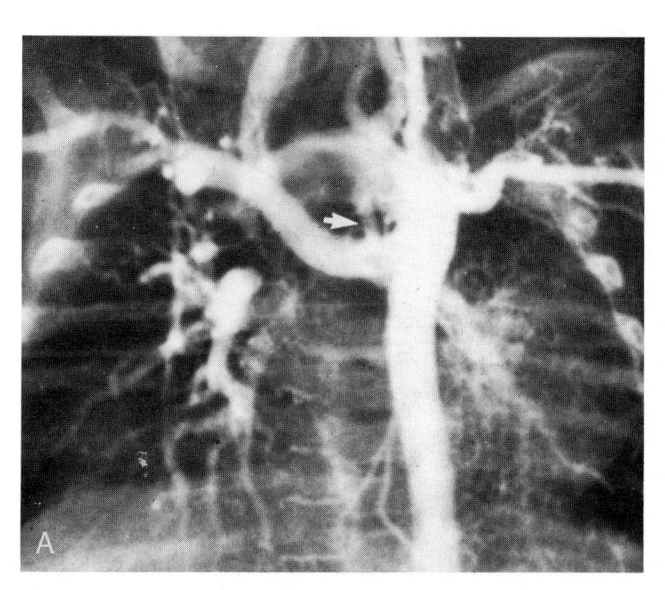

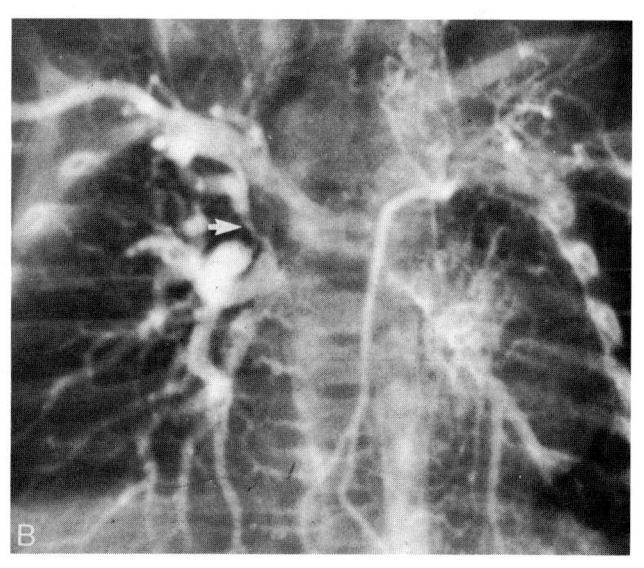

FIG 31–9.
Pulmonary atresia and ventricular septal defect. Retrograde aortogram. Anteroposterior projection. **A,** left aortic arch. Aberrant right subclavian artery. Bilateral ductus. Left-sided ductus arteriosus arises from aortic arch *(arrow)* and supplies left pulmonary artery. **B,** stenotic right ductus arteriosus *(arrow)* arises from subclavian artery and supplies right pulmonary artery. No continuity between right and left pulmonary arteries.

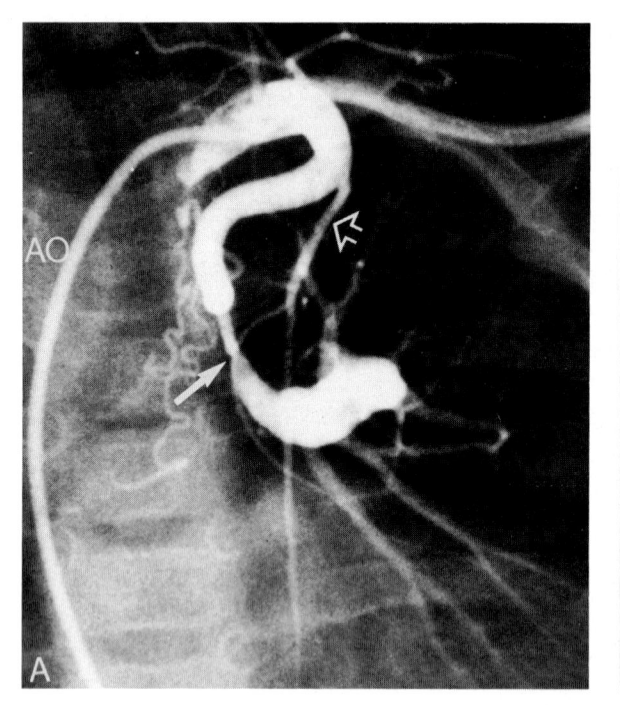

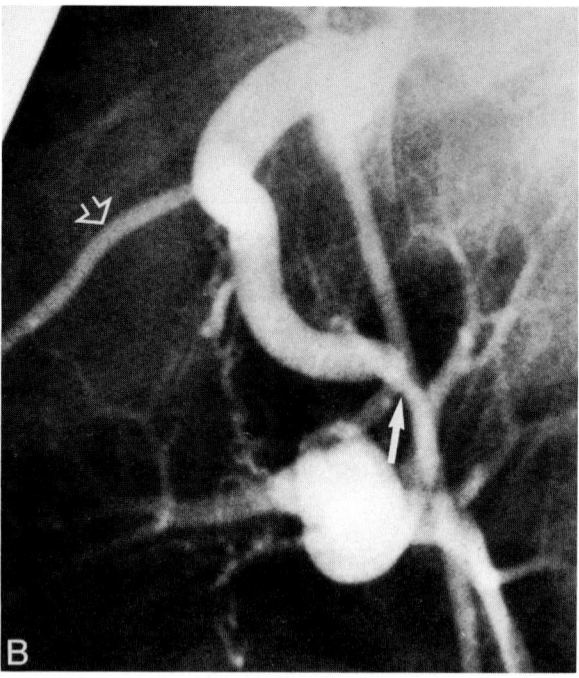

592 Cyanosis and Decreased Pulmonary Arterial Vasculature

FIG 31–10.
Pulmonary atresia and ventricular septal defect. Left subclavian arteriogram. **A,** anteroposterior and, **B,** lateral projections. Right aortic arch *(AO)*. Large patent ductus arteriosus arises from enlarged left subclavian artery. Stenosis of ductus at junction with pulmonary artery in hilum *(arrow)*. Because of stenosis, pulmonary arteries are protected from pulmonary hypertension. A systemic pulmonary arterial shunt could be placed advantageously. Mammary artery *(open arrow)* arises from ductus arteriosus.

FIG 31–11.
Pulmonary atresia and ventricular septal defect. Ascending aortogram. Anteroposterior projection. Right aortic arch. Ductuslike structure arises near origin of left innominate artery and continues as left pulmonary artery *(white arrow)*. No stenosis is present. Systemic pressure in left pulmonary artery. Developmental status of ductuslike structure can be determined only at operation or postmortem examination by identification of recurrent nerve encircling it. This artery is developmentally a true ductus arteriosus that arises at the origin of the left innominate from aortic arch. Right lung supplied by aortic collateral artery *(solid white arrow)* arising from descending aorta, which continues as right pulmonary artery. No stenosis. Right and left pulmonary arteries not in continuity.

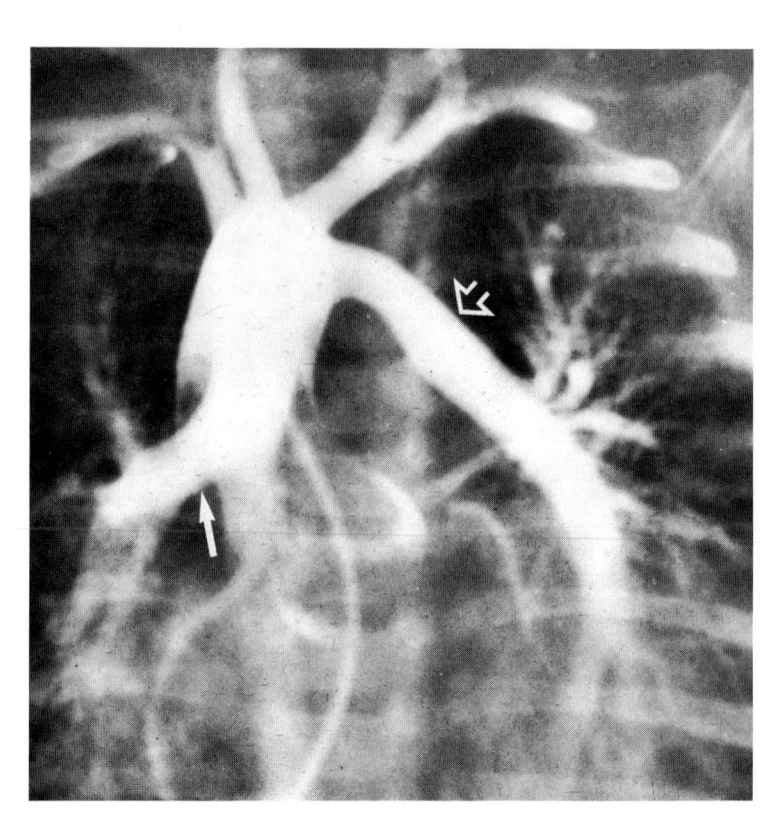

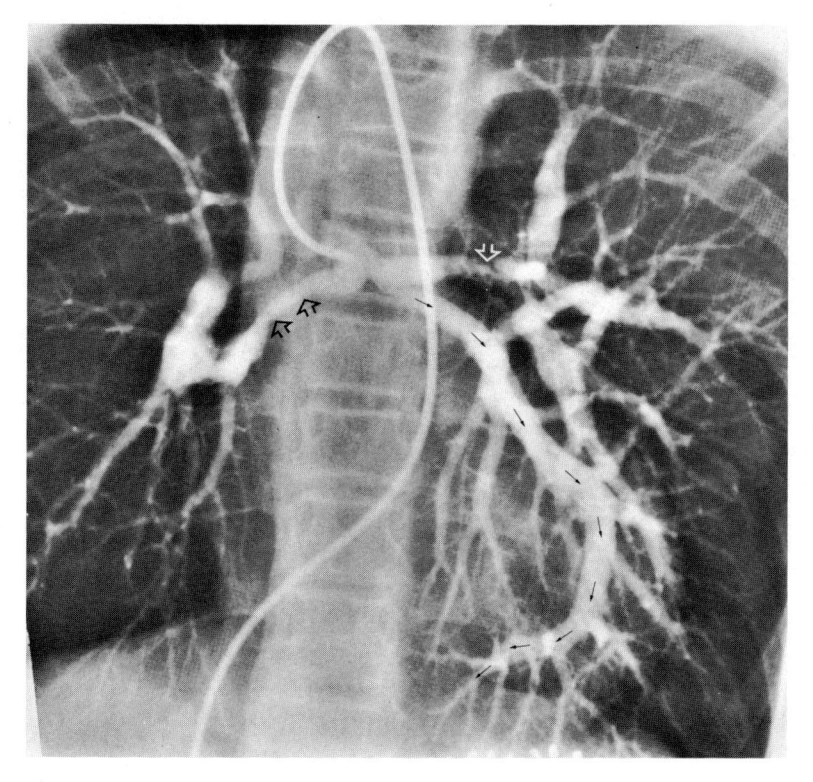

FIG 31–12.
Pulmonary atresia and ventricular septal defect. Right aortic arch. Selective injection of systemic collateral artery arising from descending aorta. Anteroposterior projection. Artery anastomoses with right and left pulmonary arteries near hilum. Numerous areas of stenoses *(arrows)*. One artery *(small black arrows)* with systemic pressure continues in unusual curved fashion with no significant stenosis. Latter is probably a bronchial artery with anastomotic connections with pulmonary artery at intra-acinar level. No opacification of main pulmonary artery.

teries show areas of stenosis at their junction with the pulmonary arterial tree (Fig 31–12). This situation is favorable for a systemic pulmonary arterial shunt or total correction.

8. Direct collateral arteries from the descending aorta are often termed "bronchial collaterals," although this term does not reflect their correct developmental origin. A more correct term is "direct systemic pulmonary arterial collaterals."

9. Rarely, either direct or indirect collateral arteries may supply a portion or an entire pulmonary lobe without connection to the pulmonary artery (Fig 31–13). Under those circumstances, ligation of the bronchial artery may result in pulmonary infarction (rare) (Fig 31–14).

10. Another rare cause of pulmonary infarction is inadvertent ligation of a distal bronchial and pulmonary artery that has no other source of bronchial inflow (Fig 31–15).

11. Indirect systemic pulmonary arterial collaterals may arise from various aortic branches, such as innominate, subclavian, intercostal, mammary, or other smaller arteries (Fig 31–16).

12. Direct collateral arteries may also arise from the abdominal aorta and pierce the diaphragm and communicate with pulmonary arterial branches (Fig 31–17). Similar to bronchial arteries, stenoses usually occur at the junction with pulmonary arterial branches.

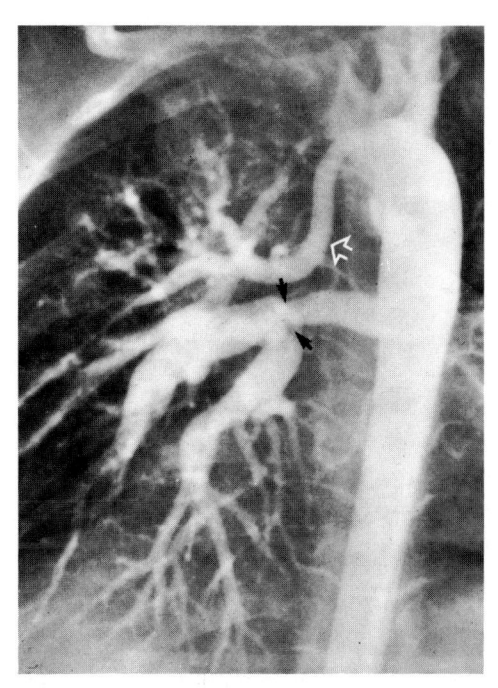

FIG 31–13.
Pulmonary atresia and ventricular septal defect. Aortogram. Anteroposterior projection. Direct systemic collateral artery *(open arrow)* supplies entire right upper lobe. No stenosis. Large bronchial artery connects with right pulmonary artery, and there is an area of stenosis *(black arrow)*. No connection exists between these two arteries. Ligation of upper artery *(open arrow)* could result in pulmonary infarction.

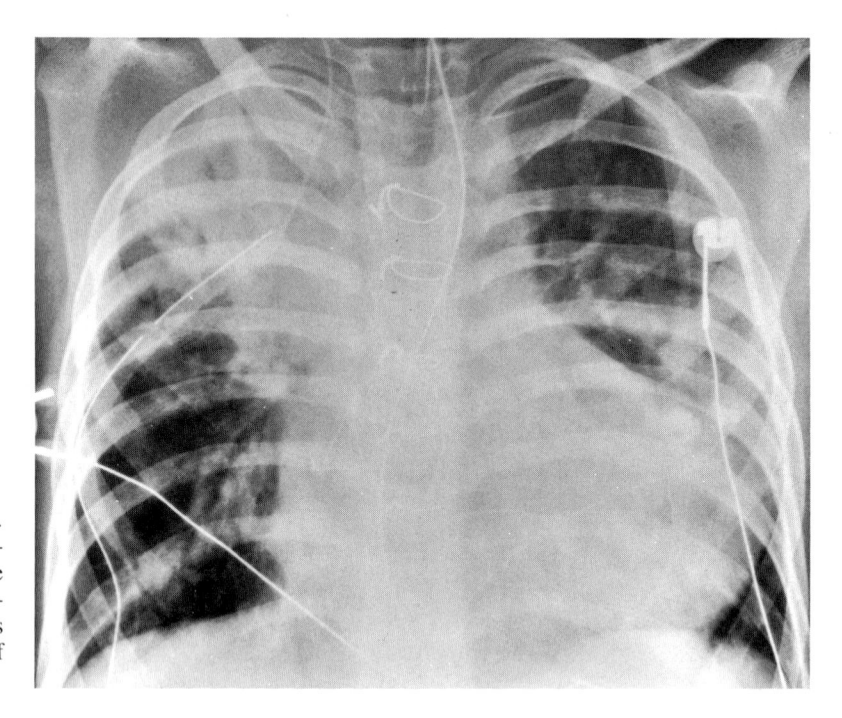

FIG 31–14.
Pulmonary atresia and ventricular septal defect. After corrective operation and ligation of bronchial artery, which was the only supply to the right upper lobe. Thoracic roentgenogram. Anteroposterior projection. Pulmonary infarction, as evidenced by opacification and consolidation of right upper lobe.

OPERATIVE CONSIDERATIONS

Both palliative and corrective operations have been used in patients with ventricular septal defect and pulmonary atresia. For operative correction of pulmonary atresia, the pulmonary artery must be of adequate size to receive the cardiac output. In infancy, a palliative operation is necessary to induce growth of the pulmonary arteries. We prefer a central shunt for this purpose because it stimulates growth of the main pulmonary artery.

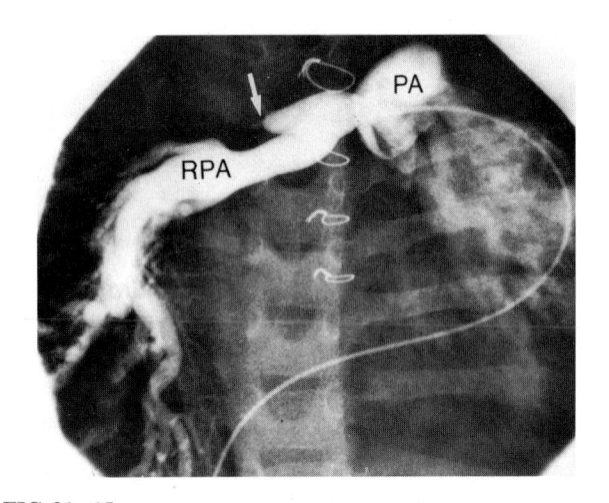

FIG 31–15.
Pulmonary atresia and ventricular septal defect. Postoperative pulmonary arteriogram (PA). Anterioposterior projection. Ligation of a bronchial artery in hilum, together with right pulmonary artery (RPA). Stump of ligated right upper lobe pulmonary artery is demonstrated (arrow).

In cases where the pulmonary arterial tree is inadequate to accept the total cardiac output, a systemic pulmonary arterial shunt is performed to enlarge the pulmonary arterial tree. The anastomosis must be performed beyond the site of narrowing or stenosis of a pulmonary artery.

Shunt procedures are carried out in identical fashion to tetralogy of Fallot. Waterston anastomoses or central shunts are preferred in infancy. The size of the pulmonary arteries can be determined angiographically. Although no exact means to determine the adequacy of the pulmonary arteries for corrective operation exists, generally if the diameters of the right and left pulmonary arteries in the hila are larger than the diameter of the descending aorta at the level of the diaphragm, their size is very likely adequate. Of course, this measurement represents only an approximation (see Fig 30–29).

During complete correction, operatively created and naturally occurring systemic pulmonary arterial shunts must be occluded because:

1. During cardiotomy, the return of blood from the lungs may be excessive.
2. As a result, the patient becomes underperfused, the surgical field flooded, and the left ventricle overdistended.

Ligation and repair of operatively created systemic pulmonary arterial shunt are comparatively simple. Bronchial collaterals, however, may not be readily accessible, and a thoracotomy may have to be performed in addition to the midline sternotomy. Bronchial arteries can be ligated in the hilum, but this may result in elimination of

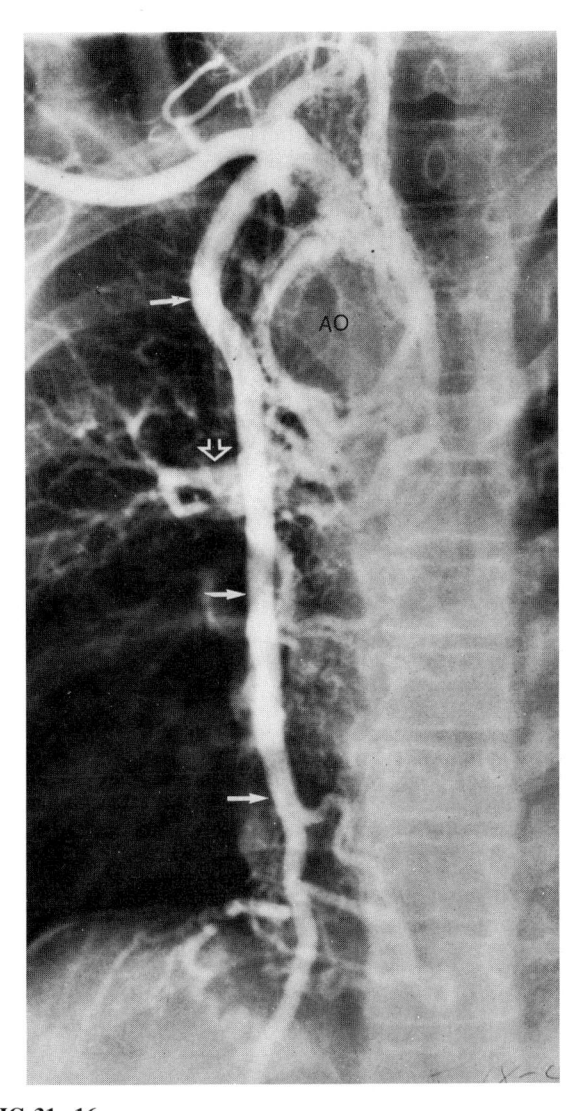

FIG 31–16.
Pulmonary atresia and ventricular septal defect. Right aortic arch *(AO)*. Right subclavian arteriogram. Anteroposterior projection. Aorta is encircled by numerous indirect collaterals arising from subclavian artery. Main collateral supply to lung occurs through markedly dilated *(solid white arrows)* internal mammary artery and its intercostal branches. Anastomoses *(open arrow)* with right pulmonary artery in hilum of lung are demonstrated.

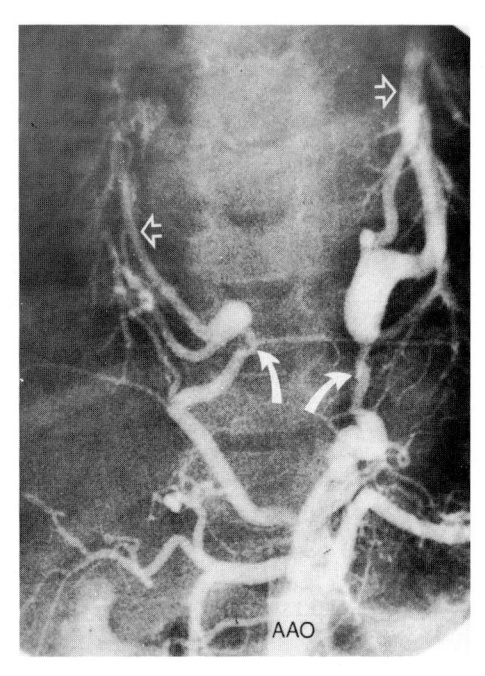

FIG 31–17.
Pulmonary atresia and ventricular septal defect. Abdominal aortogram *(AAO)*. Anteroposterior projection. Opacification of aorta. Systemic collateral arteries arise above level of the celiac axis and show severe stenoses *(curved arrows)*. Stenotic transdiaphragmatic connections to right and left lower lobe pulmonary arteries *(open arrows)*, which are well opacified. This anatomy is particularly suitable for catheter occlusion techniques.

blood flow to a pulmonary artery (see Fig 31–15). If bronchial arteries arise above the level of the left atrium, they can be exposed and ligated by an approach through a sternotomy and incising the posterior pericardium to reach their origin from the aorta.[7]

Catheter occlusion techniques are an alternative to ligation of systemic to pulmonary arterial shunts. Systemic pulmonary arterial shunts of adequate length, particularly when they communicate with a stenotic segment, can be obliterated by interventional catherization technics. The most suitable candidates for catheter occlusion are patients with an unusually long patent ductus arteriosus and stenoses at the junction with the pulmonary artery. Nonoperative closure of bronchial arteries is also feasible but technically more difficult in patients with short bronchial communications (Fig 31–18).

After occlusion of the arterial collaterals, an incision is made across the right ventricular outflow tract and extended across the atretic infundibulum and pulmonary valve into the pulmonary artery. A patch is then sewn over this area, expanding the circumference of the outflow tract. Because such patch grafts do not contain a valve, insufficiency is present. The decision whether the outflow tract is widened by a patch or a conduit[8] (see Fig 30–50) depends largely on the angiographic appearance of the right ventricular outflow tract and the main pulmonary artery. The leaflets of the porcine valve in the conduit commonly become thickened, insufficient, rigid, and sometimes calcified (Figs 31–19 and 31–20).

Conduits may have to be revised because:

1. The porcine valve malfunctions.
2. The patient outgrows the size of the conduit.
3. There is ingrowth of fibrous tissue, resulting in significant outflow obstruction.

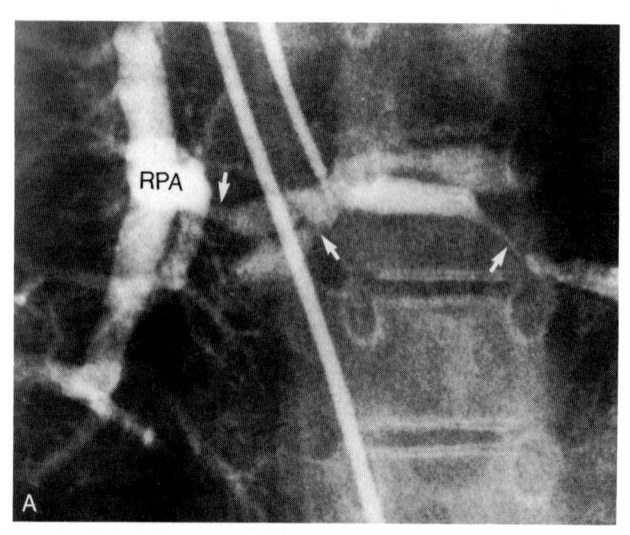

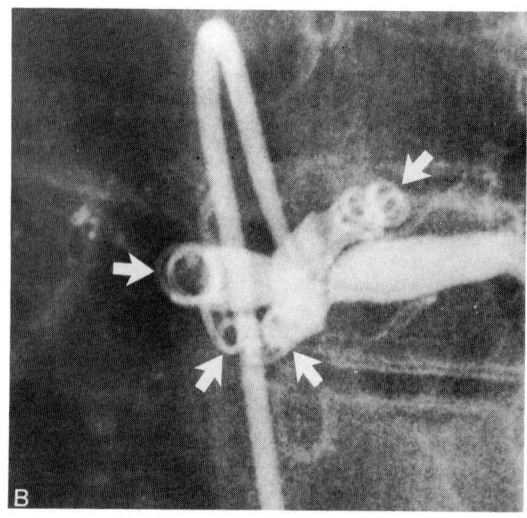

FIG 31-18.
Pulmonary atresia and ventricular septal defect. Right aortic arch. **A,** direct aortic systemic to pulmonary artery (?bronchialartery) communicating with right *(RPA)* and left pulmonary arteries. Numerous areas of stenoses *(white arrows)*. Bronchial arteries are short and therefore technically more difficult to occlude. **B,** second injection shows successful occlusion of communications by placement of steel coils *(arrows)*.

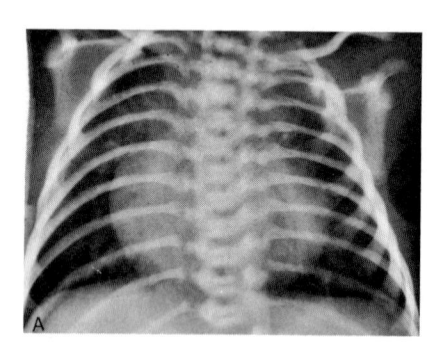

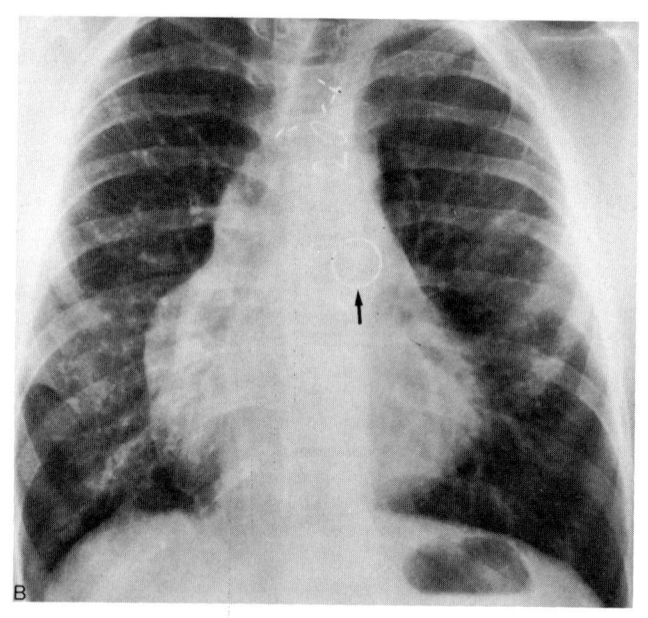

FIG 31-19.
Pulmonary atresia and ventricular septal defect. Thoracic roentenogram. Posteroanterior projection. **A,** marked cardiomegaly. Increased pulmonary vasculature. Atypical radiographic appearance. **B,** after Rastelli repair with valved conduit *(arrow)*. Several years later. Smaller cardiac size. Pulmonary vasculature lower limit of normal. Valved conduit demonstrated *(arrow)*.

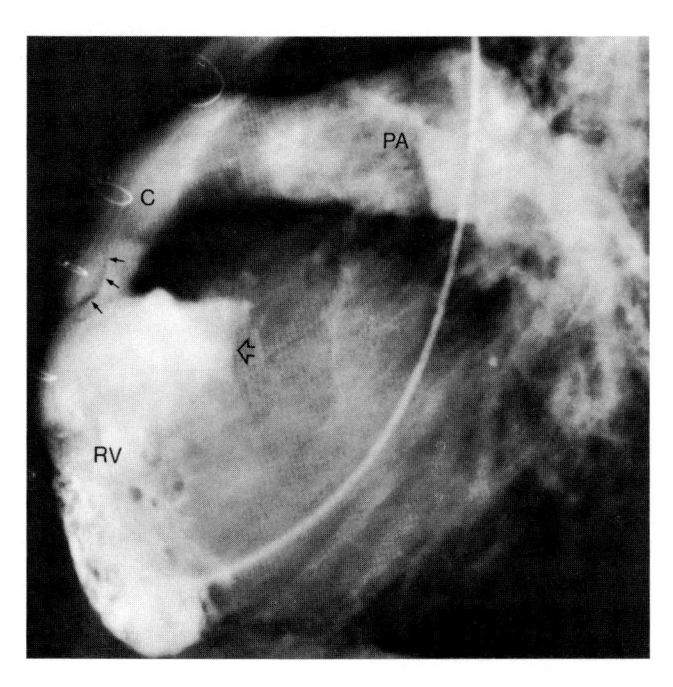

FIG 31–20.
Pulmonary atresia and ventricular septal defect after conduit repair. Right ventriculogram *(RV)*. Lateral projection. Leaflet of thickened porcine valve *(small black arrows)*. Patch of ventricular septal defect closure *(open arrow)*. Aorta is not opacified. C = conduit; PA = pulmonary artery.

Before a conduit can be placed in some patients, one or more preliminary procedures may be necessary to bring together the pulmonary arterial branches in each lung (see Fig 30–39). This concept of unifocalization was popularized by several surgeons. In the hilum of each lung, the major branches are anastomosed and connected to the aorta through a synthetic graft. This improves pulmonary blood flow and enhances growth of the pulmonary arterial tree. Subsequently the pulmonary arteries can be connected to the conduit during a reparative operation.

POSTOPERATIVE FINDINGS

1. After a corrective operation, the heart may become larger just as after correction of tetralogy of Fallot. On the other hand, in patients with increased pulmonary blood flow and cardiomegaly, cardiac size may decrease dramatically after repair.

2. Tissue valves in the conduit become thickened and rigid or even calcified. Insufficiency and stenosis follow (see Fig 31–20).

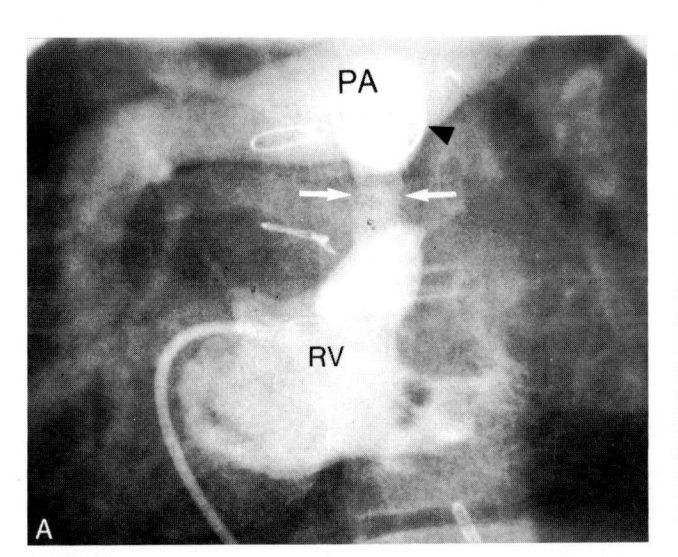

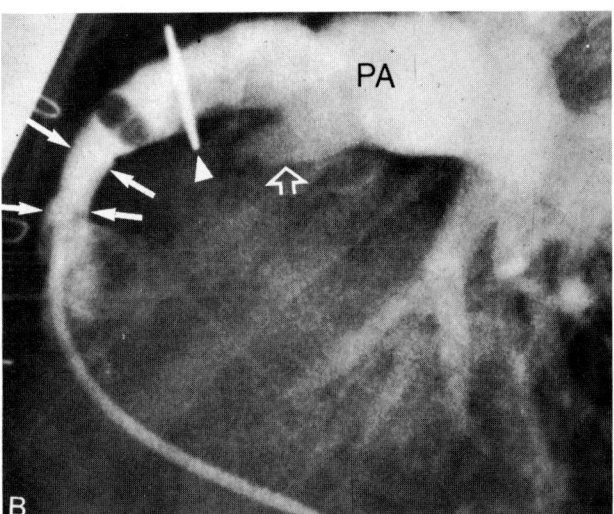

FIG 31–21.
Pulmonary atresia without ventricular septal defect. Repair by valved conduit. Right ventriculogram *(RV)*. **A,** anteroposterior and, **B,** lateral projections. Valve ring is well demonstrated *(arrowhead)*. Conduit *(white arrows)* is concentrically narrowed by ingrowth of fibrous tissue, causing right ventricular outflow obstruction. Atretic main pulmonary artery *(open arrow)* is opacified. PA = pulmonary artery.

3. Another common cause of conduit stenosis is ingrowth of fibrous tissue, usually starting at the anastomotic site with the right ventricle and progressing concentrically into the conduit (Fig 31–21).

REFERENCES

1. Rabinovitch M, Herrera-DeLeon V, Castaneda AR, et al: Growth and development of the pulmonary vascular bed in patients with tetralogy of Fallot with or without pulmonary atresia, *Circulation* 64:1234, 1981.
2. Thiene G, Frescura C, Bini RM, et al: Histology of pulmonary arterial supply in pulmonary atresia with ventricular septal defect, *Circulation* 60:1066, 1979.
3. McGoon MD, Fulton RE, Davis GD, et al: Systemic collateral and pulmonary artery stenosis in patients with congenital pulmonary valve atresia and ventricular septal defect, *Circulation* 56:473, 1977.
4. Liao PK, Edwards WD, Julsrud PR, et al: Pulmonary blood supply in patients with pulmonary atresia and ventricular septal defect, *J Am Coll Cardiol* 6:1343, 1985.
5. Chesler E, Beck W, Schrire V: Selective catheterization of pulmonary or bronchial arteries in the preoperative assessment of pseudotruncus arteriosus and truncus arteriosus type IV, *Am J Cardiol* 26:20, 1970.
6. Nihill MR, Mullins CE, McNamara DG: Visualization of the pulmonary arteries in pseudotruncus by pulmonary vein wedge angiography, *Circulation* 58:140, 1978.
7. McGoon DC, Baird DK, Davis GD: Surgical management of large bronchial collateral arteries with pulmonary stenosis or atresia, *Circulation* 52:109, 1975.
8. Alfieri O, Blackstone EH, Kirklin JW, et al: Surgical treatment of tetralogy of Fallot with pulmonary atresia, *J Thorac Cardiovasc Surg* 76:321, 1978.
9. Pacifico AD, Allen RH, Colvin EV: Direct reconstruction of pulmonary artery arborization anomaly and intracardiac repair of pulmonary atresia with ventricular septal defect, *Am J Cardiol* 55:1647, 1985.
10. Millikan JS, Puga FJ, Danielson GR, et al: Staged surgical repair of pulmonary arteries, ventricular septal defect, and hypoplastic pulmonary arteries, *J Thorac Cardiovasc Surg* 91:818, 1986.

CHAPTER 32

Tetralogy of Fallot With Absent Pulmonary Valve

In the condition tetralogy of Fallot with absent pulmonary valve, the anatomic details resemble tetralogy of Fallot. The clinical features, however, are different, because cyanosis is mild, pulmonary symptoms are prominent, and congestive cardiac failure may occur. The thoracic roentgenogram has a characteristic appearance and is usually diagnostic.

PATHOLOGIC ANATOMY

The basic cardiac anatomy is that of tetralogy of Fallot, but the infundibular stenosis is mild. The pulmonary stenosis is usually mild and caused by a hypoplastic and stenotic pulmonary annulus. There is a spectrum of the severity of the abnormality ranging from nearly complete to partial absence of the pulmonary valve. Accordingly the degree of pulmonary insufficiency varies. In the most severe form, at the location of the pulmonary valve, a rudimentary ridge of nodular fibrous tissue is present. This tissue does not show structural features of a normal pulmonary valve and has a histologic appearance of large, pale, grainy, myxoma-appearing cells. In contrast to tetralogy of Fallot, the right ventricle is dilated from the pulmonary regurgitation.

The pulmonary trunk and major pulmonary arteries, particularly the right, are dilated, often to aneurysmal proportions. The left pulmonary artery may be of normal size because of the orientation of the pulmonary trunk toward the right pulmonary artery. The dilated pulmonary arteries may compress adjacent bronchi. When they are compressed by a dilated pulmonary artery, atelectasis or emphysema of the associated lobe or lobes, particularly of the right middle lobe, occurs. Bronchiomalacia may coexist.[1]

The ductus arteriosus, either ligamentous or patent, is frequently absent. Lack of continuity of left pulmonary artery with pulmonary trunk also occurs.

HEMODYNAMICS

Because the obstruction to right ventricular outflow is usually mild, the shunt through the ventricular septal defect is usually left to right or predominantly so. Therefore, the aortic oxygen saturation is only minimally decreased. As the pulmonary vascular resistance decreases after, birth, the volume of pulmonary blood flow becomes excessive and causes left ventricular failure, unless counterbalanced by pulmonary stenosis.[2] The other major hemodynamic abnormality is related to the associated pulmonary regurgitation through the rudimentary pulmonary valve. This increases right ventricular stroke volume, resulting in increased pulsation of the pulmonary arterial tree. The regurgitant volume augments the diastolic right ventricular volume, leading to right ventricular dilatation.

CLINICAL FEATURES

In the neonatal period, cyanosis and a precordial murmur are found. The cyanosis improves as pulmonary vascular resistance falls. Cyanosis is not severe and is unassociated with hypoxemic symptoms or complications. Cyanosis reappears within weeks or by 3 months as pulmonary complications develop.[3, 4] Then the cyanosis is associated with tachypnea, wheezing, grunting, stridor, and retractions. New respiratory symptoms rarely occur after 3 months of age and may clear completely by 18 months of age in patients who have not required an operation. Patients with minimal pulmonary regurgitation have few respiratory symptoms.

Respiratory distress and features of congestive cardiac failure are common on physical examination. There is usually a precordial bulge and heave related to right ventricular enlargement.

The cardiac findings are those of pulmonary stenosis and insufficiency. The loudness of these murmurs are related to the amount of left-to-right shunt and the volume of regurgitant flow. There is a long pulmonary systolic ejection murmur, which is well heard throughout the thorax, probably because of transmission throughout the pulmonary arterial tree. The second heart sound is loud and single, representing only the aortic valve closure sound, because there are no valve cusps to cause a pulmonary closure sound. The second heart sound is followed by an early diastolic murmur of pulmonary insufficiency, heard best in the second and third left intercostal spaces.[5] The length and loudness of the murmurs are directly related to the degree of pulmonary insufficiency, and they may be quite prominent. A pulmonary systolic ejection click may be heard, reflecting the dilated pulmonary trunk.

Auscultation over the lung fields may reveal localized findings of pulmonary consolidation, emphysema, or pneumonia. REASON: The huge pulmonary artery compresses major bronchi, usually the right mainstem bronchus.

ELECTROCARDIOGRAPHIC FEATURES

The electrocardiogram resembles tetralogy of Fallot with right-axis deviation, right atrial enlargement, and right ventricular hypertrophy. In those patients with a large volume of pulmonary blood flow, left ventricular hypertrophy may be associated.

ECHOCARDIOGRAPHIC FEATURES

In addition to the usual findings of tetralogy of Fallot, the pulmonary trunk and proximal branches are markedly dilated, and Doppler studies show marked pulmonary regurgitation. Echoes from the pulmonary valve are often not recorded, but failure to find this structure is not diagnostic in itself, because rudimentary leaflets may be present. The right ventricle is dilated. Paradoxical septal motion may be present.

RADIOGRAPHIC FEATURES

The findings of a patient with congenital absence of the pulmonary valve are usually characteristic. Diagnosis can be made on the basis of radiographic findings in most cases. Because the extent of pulmonary valvar anomaly varies from partial to complete absence, the hemodynamic and radiographic findings are not uniform. The presence of coexistent conditions can also modify the radiographic appearance. For instance, severe stenosis of the pulmonary annulus or right ventricular infundibulum reduces the degree of pulmonary insufficiency. In such cases the radiographic findings are subtle, and radiographic differentiation from classical tetralogy of Fallot may be impossible. In most patients, however, the pulmonary insufficiency is massive, causing characteristic radiographic features:

1. Typically the heart is markedly enlarged in contrast to the normal-sized cardiac silhouette in uncomplicated tetralogy of Fallot (Fig 32–1). REASON: The right ventricular volume is markedly increased because of pulmonary regurgitation, and left ventricular volume may be increased because of augmented pulmonary blood flow. Because of the

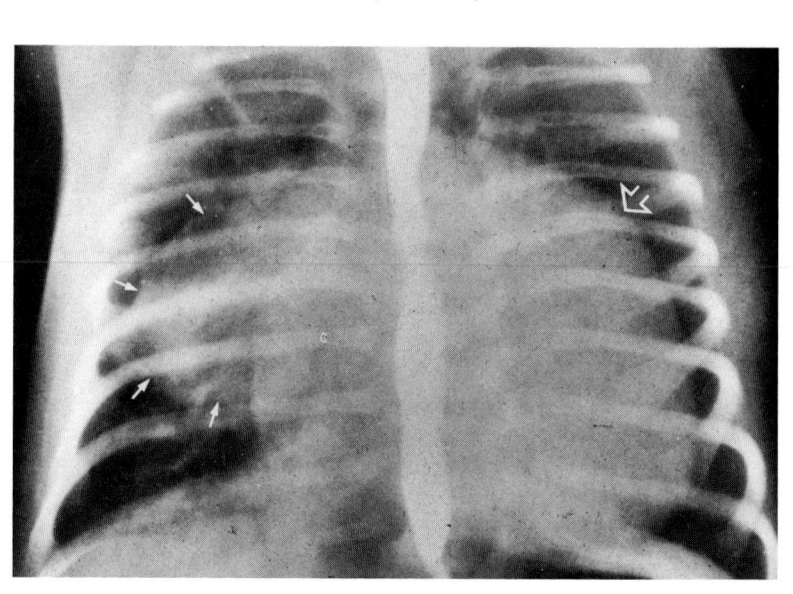

FIG 32–1.
Tetralogy of Fallot and absent pulmonary valve. Thoracic roentgenogram. Posteroanterior projection. Aneurysmal right pulmonary artery forms huge mass in right midlung field *(white arrows)*. Fluoroscopically this mass pulsates vigorously. Severe cardiomegaly. Bulging right ventricular outflow tract *(open arrow)*. Characteristic configuration of tetralogy of Fallot is lost.

different hemodynamics, the characteristic configuration of tetralogy is lost (see Fig 32–1).

2. The main pulmonary artery and right ventricular infundibulum are markedly enlarged (see Fig 32–1). REASON: The increased right ventricular stroke volume during systole and the large regurgitant volume during diastole enlarge both the right ventricle and the main pulmonary artery.

3. The proximal right pulmonary artery shows characteristic aneurysmal dilatation (see Fig 32–1). REASON: The markedly increased stroke volume and severe regurgitant flow enlarge one or both pulmonary arteries (increased blood flow tends to enlarge arteries). If the infundibulum is directed toward the right pulmonary artery, as is common in tetralogy of Fallot with clockwise rotation of the heart, aneurysmal dilatation occurs primarily in the right pulmonary artery (most common) (see Fig 32–1). If the infundibulum is oriented more vertically, the main and both proximal pulmonary arteries show aneurysmal dilatation. If the infundibulum is oriented toward the left, the left pulmonary artery shows aneurysmal dilatation, which is least common (Fig 32–2).

4. Massive dilatation of the proximal right and left pulmonary arteries may not be evident on a thoracic roentgenogram (see Fig 32–2), because this portion of these arteries lies within the mediastinum not outlined by air. They are not visible without contrast injection.

5. The peripheral pulmonary arterial vasculature is normal in spite of aneurysmal dilatation of the central pulmonary arteries.

6. The aneurysmal dilatation of the proximal portion of a pulmonary artery may compress the corresponding bronchus and cause pulmonary symptoms (Fig 32–3). The lungs show areas of emphysema, atelectasis, or generalized pneumonia.

7. Because the aneurysmal dilatation of pulmonary arteries may radiographically simulate a mass, fluoroscopy is helpful to establish the mass as a vascular structure. Because of the increased pulse pressure caused by pulmonary insufficiency, active pulsations of the mass can be observed fluoroscopically.

8. The degree of pulmonary insufficiency is governed not only by the anatomic status of the pulmonary valve but by the degree of infundibular pulmonary stenosis. Severe stenosis prevents significant reflux. Under those circumstances the pulmonary artery is minimally dilated, cardiac size remains normal, and the findings are normal or identical to tetralogy of Fallot (Fig 32–4).

9. If dilatation involves primarily the main pulmonary artery and if the pulmonary artery is located medially it may not be seen on a posteroanterior thoracic roentgenogram (Fig 32–5).

CARDIAC CATHETERIZATION

Cardiac catheterization is performed to confirm diagnosis and exclude coexisting conditions. It is usually possible to pass the catheter across the ventricular septal defect into the aorta. When the catheter is in the major pulmonary arteries, its tip shows a wide to-and-fro motion with each cardiac cycle because of the large regurgitant flow.

Pressure data reveal equal left and right ventricular systolic pressures identical to tetralogy of Fallot. Across the pulmonary annulus a pressure difference is found that

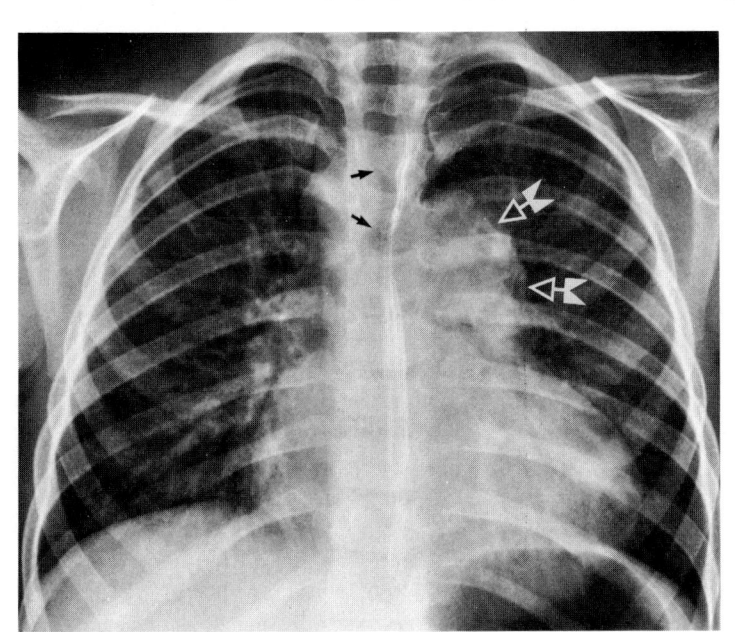

FIG 32–2.
Tetralogy of Fallot and absent pulmonary valve. Thoracic roentgenogram. Posteroanterior projection. Right aortic arch displaces trachea to left *(black arrows)*. Cardiac configuration atypical for tetralogy of Fallot. Heart larger than in tetralogy of Fallot. REASON: Absence of pulmonary valve results in volume overload of right ventricle. Aneurysmal dilatation of left pulmonary artery *(open arrows)* without dilatation of right pulmonary artery. This is the least common finding in this condition.

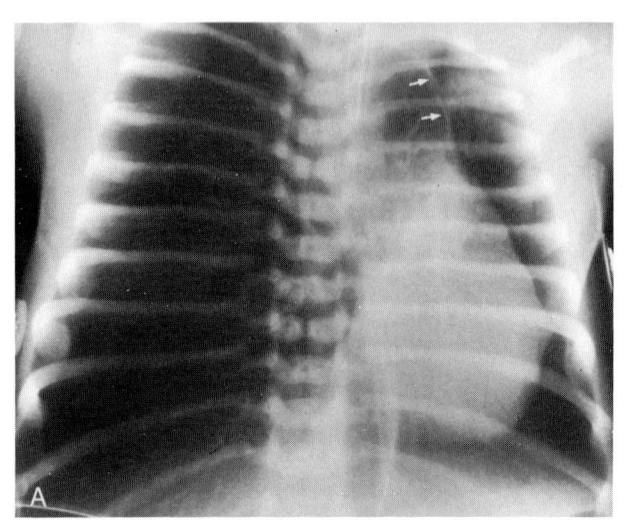

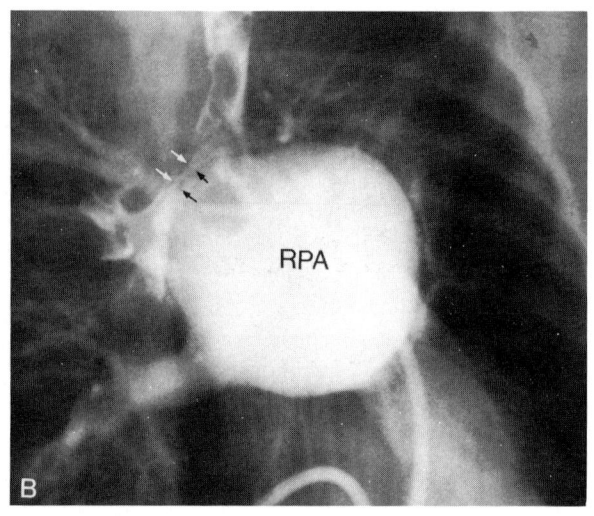

FIG 32–3.
Tetralogy of Fallot and absence of the pulmonary valve. **A,** thoracic roentgenogram. Posteroanterior projection. Mediastinal shift and depression of right diaphragm, indicating obstructive emphysema of right lung. Herniation of right lung to the left *(arrows)*. **B,** pulmonary arteriogram and simultaneous bronchogram. Anteroposterior projection. Marked mediastinal shift and compression of the right bronchus by huge right pulmonary artery *(RPA) (arrows)*.

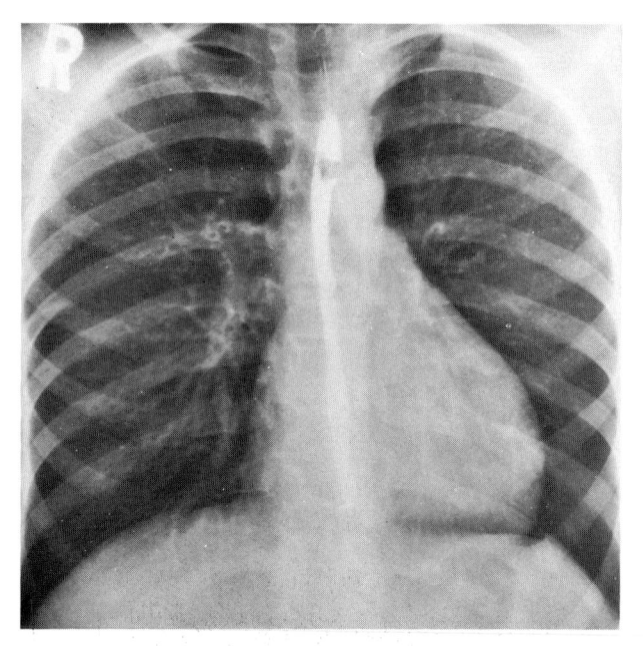

FIG 32–4.
Tetralogy of Fallot and partial absence of pulmonary valve. Thoracic roentgenogram. Posteroanterior projection. Normal cardiac size and configuration. Normal pulmonary vasculature. Diagnosis of absent pulmonary valve cannot be made. REASON: In spite of absence of pulmonary valve, severe stenoses at pulmonary annulus and infundibulum prevented significant pulmonary regurgitation. Dilatation of pulmonary arterial tree involved only intramediastinal portion of right and left pulmonary arteries and consequently was not visualized. Pulmonary vasculature in left lung is slightly less than right lung as occasionally seen in tetralogy of Fallot.

is caused by the large volume of flow across the narrowed pulmonary annulus. The pulmonary arterial pulse pressure is widened, the systolic pressure being elevated because of the large stroke volume, and the diastolic pressure lowered by the pulmonary regurgitation. The pulmonary arterial diastolic pressure may equal right ventricular end-diastolic pressure.

Oximetry data reveal a predominant left-to-right shunt, but there may be a small right-to-left shunt desaturation of aortic blood.

ANGIOGRAPHIC APPEARANCE

Selective right ventriculography and pulmonary angiography are essential to establish a precise diagnosis. Right ventriculography demonstrates the infundibular area, narrowed pulmonary annulus, and the ventricular septal defect, whereas pulmonary angiography demonstrates the status of the pulmonary valve and degree of pulmonary regurgitation.

1. The right ventricular anatomy is identical to tetralogy of Fallot except that the infundibulum is usually dilated. REASON: Increased stroke volume of the right ventricle and the diastolic regurgitant volume cause dilatation of the entire right ventricle.

2. The massively dilated right pulmonary artery opacifies densely (Fig 32–6).

3. If only the intramediastinal portions of the right and left pulmonary arteries are dilated, as when the in-

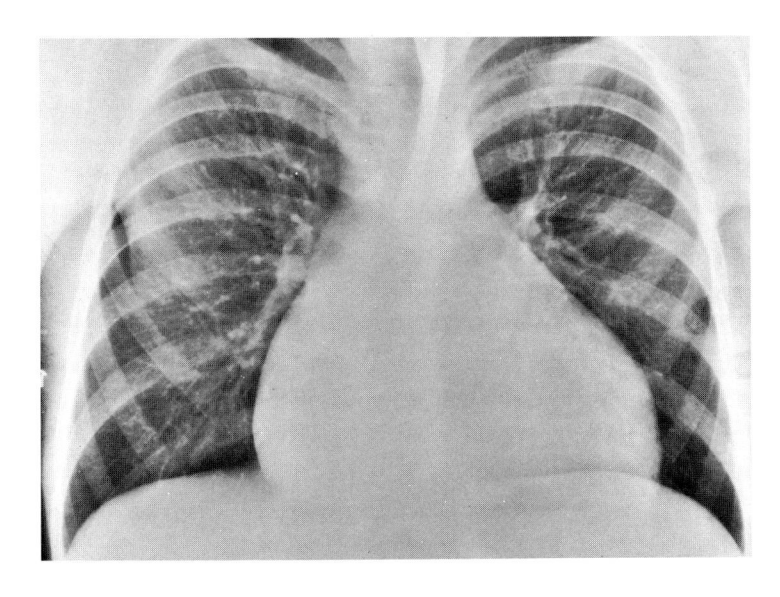

FIG 32-5.
Tetralogy of Fallot with absence of pulmonary valve. Posteroanterior projection. Moderately enlarged heart. Pulmonary vasculature is slightly decreased. Cardiomegaly is caused by pulmonary insufficiency. Dilated main and right pulmonary arteries are located centrally and therefore not seen (see Fig 32-6).

fundibulum is directed vertically, angiography is the only method to demonstrate the size of the central pulmonary arteries (Fig 32-7).

4. In a lateral projection, either right ventriculography or pulmonary angiography demonstrates the anatomy of the infundibulum and pulmonary valve. At this site narrowing is found that is related to the stenotic pulmonary annulus. A varying amount of valve tissue is demonstrated and the degree of pulmonary regurgitation can be estimated.

5. If the pulmonary valve is completely absent, rudimentary tiny valve leaflets or only a pulmonary annulus can be demonstrated (Fig 32-8).

6. When the infundibulum is directed toward the left pulmonary artery, dilatation involves only the left pulmonary artery (least common) (Fig 32-9). Because of clockwise rotation of the heart in patients with tetralogy of Fal-

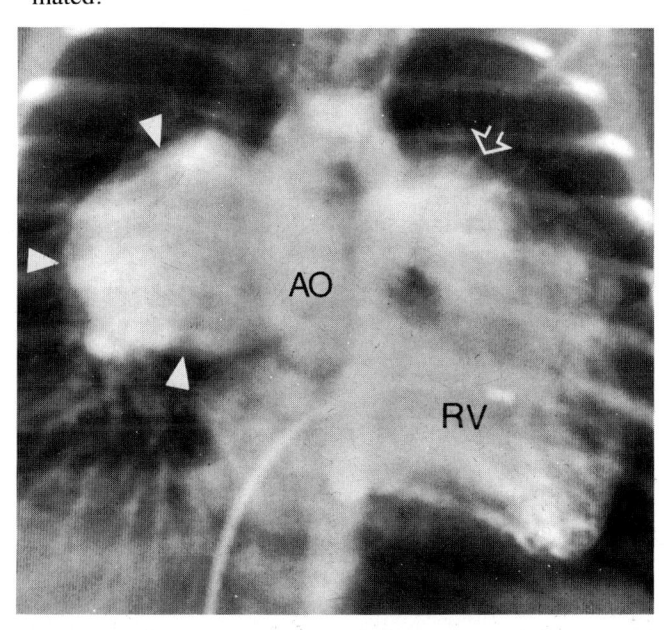

FIG 32-6.
Tetralogy of Fallot and absence of pulmonary valve. Right ventriculogram. Anteroposterior projection. Classic appearance with aneurysmal right pulmonary artery *(arrowhead)* (most common form). Dilated right ventricle *(RV)* and infundibulum *(open arrow)*. Aorta *(AO)* opacifies through ventricular septal defect.

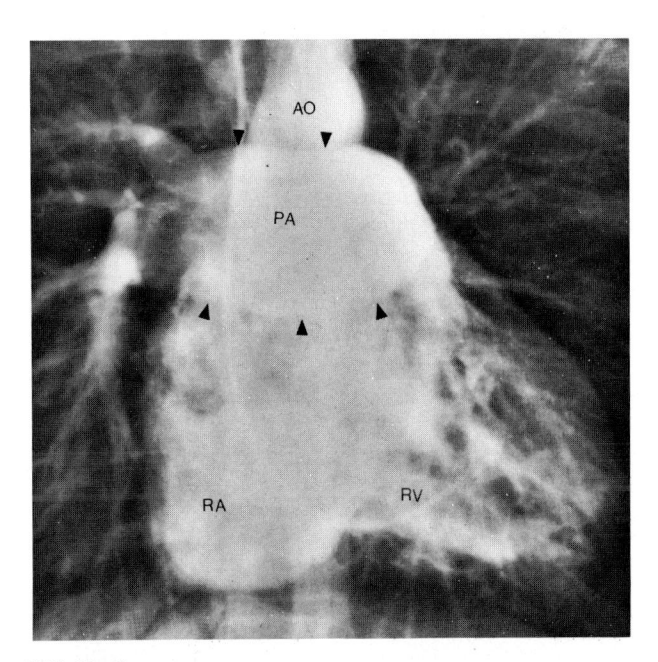

FIG 32-7.
Tetralogy of Fallot and absence of pulmonary valve. Right ventriculogram *(RV)*. Anteroposterior projection. Dilatation of only intramediastinal portions of right and left pulmonary arteries *(arrowheads)*, which were not visible on thoracic roentgenograms (see Fig 33-5). Aorta is opacified through ventricular septal defect. Tricuspid reflux outlines right atrium *(RA)*. AO = aorta; PA = pulmonary artery.

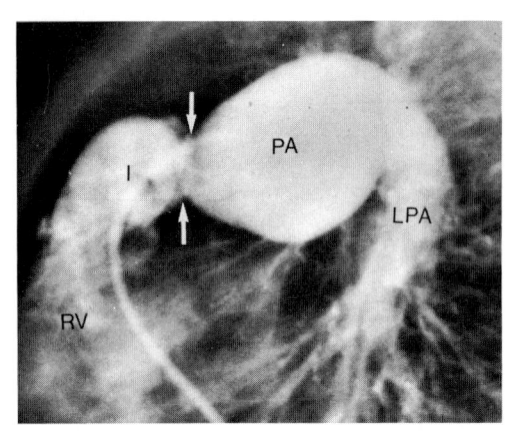

604 Cyanosis and Decreased Pulmonary Arterial Vasculature

FIG 32–8.
Complete absence of pulmonary valve. Pulmonary arteriogram. Lateral projection. Marked dilatation of main pulmonary artery. Left pulmonary artery normal size *(LPA)*. Free reflux outlines infundibulum *(I)* and right ventricle *(RV)*. Pulmonary valve leaflets not visualized. Stenotic pulmonary valve annulus *(arrows)* demark right ventricular infundibulum from pulmonary artery *(PA)*.

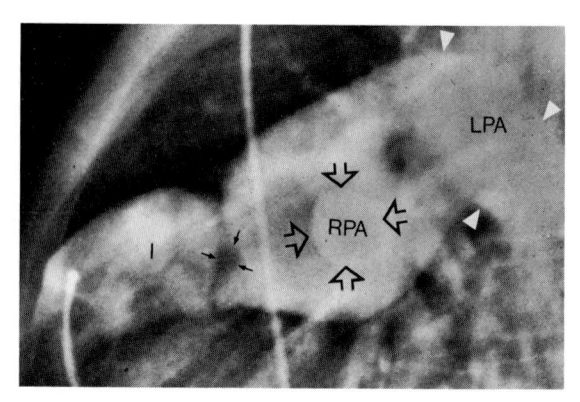

FIG 32–9.
Tetralogy of Fallot and partial absence of pulmonary valve. Right ventriculogram. Lateral projection. Rudimentary nodular valve consisting of myxomatous tissue is visualized *(black arrows)*. Dilatation of main pulmonary artery and left pulmonary artery *(LPA) (white arrowheads)*. Right pulmonary artery *(RPA)* is normal size. *I* = infundibulum.

lot, dilatation of the right pulmonary artery is much more common.

7. There is a continuous spectrum from complete absence of the pulmonary valve to valvular stenosis with pulmonary insufficiency. A partially stenotic valve ring may be present (Fig 32–10). Such a ringlike structure limits the degree of pulmonary insufficiency. Rarely, partial absence is an isolated finding without the tetralogy of Fallot.

8. If the fibrous valve plate is more developed, it becomes stenotic and produces a jet (Fig 32–11). Under such circumstances, the degree of pulmonary insufficiency is minor.

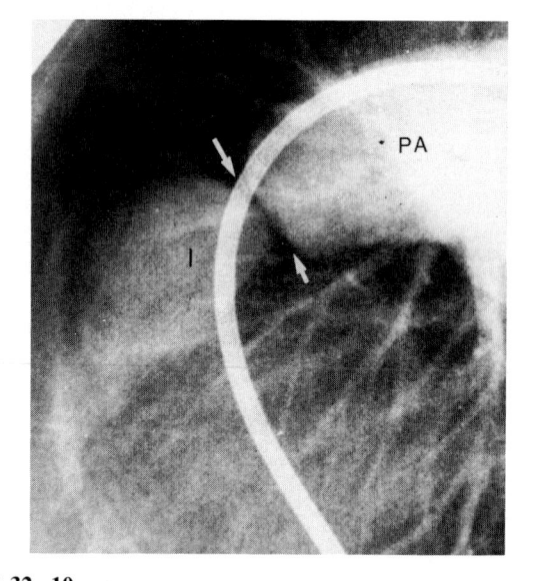

MANAGEMENT

The management of a symptomatic infant with this condition should be aggressive and prompt, aimed at treatment of cardiac failure and respiratory symptoms.[6] After this initial medical care, an operation to relieve tracheal and bronchial compression should follow to prevent progressive bronchiomalacia and pulmonary complications.

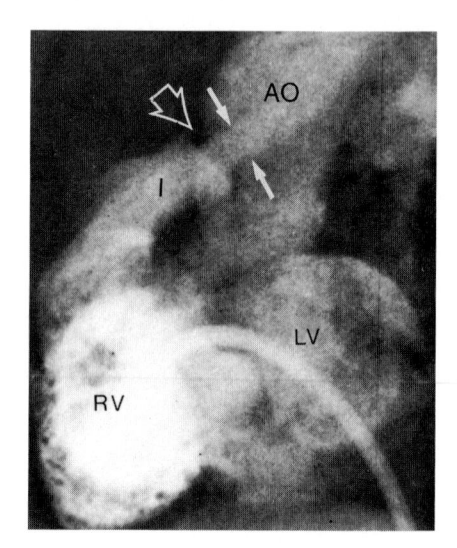

FIG 32–10.
Partial absence of pulmonary valve without tetralogy of Fallot. Right ventriculogram. Lateral projection. A fibrous ring *(arrows)* limits degree of pulmonary insufficiency. *PA* = pulmonary artery; *I* = infundibulum.

FIG 32–11.
Tetralogy of Fallot and partial absence of pulmonary valve. Right ventriculogram. Lateral projection. Thick dysplastic stenotic valve *(open arrow)* produces distinct jet *(arrows)*, indicating pulmonary stenosis. Aorta *(AO)* is opacified through ventricular septal defect. *RV* = right ventricle; *LV* = left ventricle.

Previously, operation was often delayed so the infant required prolonged ventilatory support, with its resulting problems and complications, including poor nutrition and debilitation.

One of the reasons for this procrastination with operation was the lack of consensus for the preferable operation and the variety of operations[6,7] proposed; namely, plication of the aneurysm, suspension of the dilated pulmonary artery to the retrosternal fascia, placement of a graft from the main to the right pulmonary artery passing anteriorly to the aorta, Glenn procedure, repair of the ventricular septal defect without replacement of the pulmonary valve, and repair of the ventricular septal defect with replacement of the pulmonary valve. Each operation has advantages and drawbacks, and as yet a single large series with satisfactory results has not been described.

Currently we favor closure of the ventricular septal defect without operative repair of the pulmonary valve. This reduces the left-to-right shunt and the volume of blood flow through the pulmonary arteries. This operation converts the condition into pulmonary insufficiency and intact ventricular septum, a malformation that has a good prognosis. We do not replace the pulmonary valve because of the eventual necessity of replacing this valve as the child grows and the difficulty we have experienced in finding a satisfactory replacement pulmonary valve, whether tissue or prosthetic. Furthermore, because isolated pulmonary insufficiency is so well tolerated in individuals without pulmonary hypertension, we do not believe the added problems for "complete repair" are warranted. Neither do we believe placement of a conduit or plication of the pulmonary arterial aneurysms directly addresses the major hemodynamic problems.

CONDITIONS SIMULATING TETRALOGY OF FALLOT

A number of other conditions have a ventricular communication and severe pulmonary stenosis in which a right-to-left shunt is present. These conditions, sometimes called "tetrad variants," must be considered in the differential diagnosis of tetralogy of Fallot[8] and identified, because the operative approach varies considerably. Usually the clinical and laboratory findings obtained before cardiac catheterization and angiography are sufficiently different to either suspect or be fairly confident that such a variant is present. Echocardiography is particularly helpful in this regard. Armed with this information, the cardiologist can thoughtfully plan the appropriate angiograms to clearly delineate the abnormality.

The basic anatomic conditions in which a ventricular septal communication and pulmonary stenosis coexist have each been described in other chapters and include:

1. Ventricular septal defect and anomalous right ventricular muscle bundles.
2. Ventricular septal defect not typical of tetralogy of Fallot and pulmonary stenosis.
3. Ventricular septal defect and peripheral pulmonary arterial stenosis.
4. Double-outlet right ventricle and pulmonary stenosis.[9]
5. Tetralogy of Fallot and endocardial cushion defect.[10]
6. Single ventricle and pulmonary stenosis.[11,12]
   a. Normally related great vessels.
   b. Transposition of great vessels.
7. Complete transposition of great vessels, ventricular septal defect, and pulmonary stenosis.[13-18]
8. Corrected transposition of great vessels, ventricular septal defect, and pulmonary stenosis.[19,20]
9. Complex congenital heart disease associated with asplenia.

Although the basic conditions have been described elsewhere, there are certain features in common. Cyanosis is the major clinical feature, and its severity correlates directly with the severity of the stenosis. A history of physical findings of congestive cardiac failure is rare, because regardless of the severity of the stenosis, the obstructed ventricle always has an exit through the ventricular communication. Exceptions occur, such tetralogy of Fallot with a small ventricular septal defect and tetralogy of Fallot with endocardial cushion defect; congestive cardiac failure may develop in these two conditions. In each of the tetrad variants, a systolic ejection murmur is present and related to blood flow through the pulmonary stenosis. The loudness of the murmur is inversely related to the degree of pulmonary stenosis. The second heart sound is usually single.

Cardiac size is usually normal, although its contour may be abnormal and diagnostic, as in single ventricle or corrected transposition of great vessels. The pulmonary vasculature is diminished. Like tetralogy of Fallot, right aortic arch is common among these conditions.

Operations are available for these patients and, depending on the anatomic details, may involve a corrective procedure or palliation by either a Fontan procedure or a systemic pulmonary arterial shunt.

REFERENCES

1. Bove EL, Shaher RM, Alley R, et al: Tetralogy of Fallot with absent pulmonary valve and aneurysm of the pulmonary artery: report of two cases presenting as obstructive lung disease, *J Pediatr* 81:339, 1972.
2. Lakier JB, Stanger P, Heymann MA, et al: Tetralogy of Fallot with absent pulmonary valve: natural history and hemodynamic considerations, *Circulation* 50:167, 1974.
3. Fischer DR, Neches WH, Beerman LB, et al: Tetralogy of

Fallot with absent pulmonic valve: analysis of 17 patients, *Am J Cardiol* 53:1433, 1984.
4. Miller RA, Lev M, Paul MH: Congenital absence of the pulmonary valve: the clinical syndrome of tetralogy of Fallot with pulmonary regurgitation, *Circulation* 26:266, 1962.
5. Fontana ME, Wooley CF: The murmur of pulmonic regurgitation in tetralogy of Fallot with absent pulmonic valve, *Circulation* 57:986, 1978.
6. Pinsky WW, Nihill MR, Mullins CE, et al: The absent pulmonary valve syndrome: considerations of management, *Circulation* 57:159, 1978.
7. Stafford EG, Mair DD, McGoon DC, et al: Tetralogy of Fallot with absent pulmonary valve: surgical considerations and results, *Circulation* 47,48(suppl 3):24, 1973.
8. Rao BNS, Edwards JE: CPC: conditions simulating the tetralogy of Fallot, *Circulation* 49:173, 1974.
9. Zamora R, Moller JH, Edwards JE: Double-outlet right ventricle: anatomic types and associated anomalies, *Chest* 68:672, 1975.
10. Tandon R, Moller JH, Edwards JE: Tetralogy of Fallot associated with persistent common atrioventricular canal (endocardial cushion defect), *Br Heart J* 36:197, 1974.
11. Marin-Garcia J, Tandon R, Moller JH, et al: Common (single) ventricle with normally related great vessels, *Circulation* 49:565, 1974.
12. Marin-Garcia J, Tandon R, Moller JH, et al: Single ventricle with transposition, *Circulation* 49:994, 1974.
13. Shaher RM, Puddu GC, Khoury G, et al: Complete transposition of the great vessels with anatomic obstruction of the outflow tract of the left ventricle: surgical implications of anatomic findings, *Am J Cardiol* 19:658, 1967.
14. Layman TE, Edwards JE: Anomalies of the cardiac valves associated with complete transposition of the great vessels, *Am J Cardiol* 19:247, 1967.
15. Reimenschneider TA, Goldberg SJ, Ruttenberg HD, et al: Subpulmonic obstruction in complete d-transposition produced by redundant tricuspid tissue, *Circulation* 39:603, 1969.
16. Vidine BA, Subramanian S, Wagner HR: Aneurysm of the membranous ventricular septum in transposition of the great arteries, *Circulation* 53:157, 1976.
17. Mathew R, Rosenthal A, Fellows K: The significance of right aortic arch in d-transposition of the great arteries, *Am Heart J* 87:314, 1974.
18. Rastelli GC, Wallace RB, Ongley PA: Complete repair of transposition of the great arteries with surgical technique, *Circulation* 39:83, 1969.
19. Levy MJ, Lillehei W, Elliott LP, et al: Accessory valvular tissue causing subpulmonary stenosis in corrected transposition of the great vessels, *Circulation* 27:494, 1963.
20. Krongrad E, Ellis K, Steeg CN, et al: Subpulmonary obstruction in congenitally corrected transposition of the great arteries due to ventricular membranous septal aneurysms, *Circulation* 54:679, 1976.

CHAPTER 33

Tricuspid Atresia With Normally Related Great Vessels

Although tricuspid atresia accounts for about 1.5% of instances of congenital cardiac malformations, it is an important cause of death and cyanosis in the neonatal period. The diagnosis can be made by clinical and laboratory findings, and ultimately for many patients, operative palliation is an option. Tricuspid atresia is at one end of a spectrum that ranges from tricuspid atresia to severe tricuspid stenosis and mild tricuspid stenosis.

PATHOLOGIC ANATOMY

In tricuspid atresia the tricuspid valve is absent and so is the sinus or inflow portion of the right ventricle. Typically the right ventricle consists of only the conus portion and usually appears as an outpouching of the left ventricle. Rarely a portion of the inflow portion of the right ventricle is present. No communication exists between the right atrium and right ventricle.[1] The site of the tricuspid valve is evident as a dimple on the floor of the right atrium, and tricuspid valvar tissue is not evident. The atretic area is usually muscular and rarely membranous. Hemodynamic atresia of the tricuspid valve may rarely be acquired by vegetations on the tricuspid valvar leaflets or an obstructing right atrial or right ventricular tumor.

Tricuspid atresia has been classified according to associated cardiac anomalies[2]:

Type I: Normally related great vessels (70%)
    a. Intact ventricular septum and pulmonary atresia (Fig 33–1,A)
    b. Small ventricular septal defect (VSD) and pulmonary stenosis (Fig 33–1,B)
    c. Large VSD without pulmonary stenosis (Fig 33–1,C)

Type II: Transposition of great vessels (25%)
    a. Intact ventricular septum and pulmonary atresia
    b. Small VSD and pulmonary stenosis
    c. Large VSD without pulmonary stenosis

Type III: Corrected transposition of great vessels (5%)

The pathologic features of tricuspid atresia with transposition of the great vessels (types II and III) are discussed in Chapter 43. Among those with normally related great vessels, the anterior leaflet of the mitral valve is in continuity with the aortic valve, and the pulmonary artery arises anteriorly from the hypoplastic conus portion of the right ventricle. The size of the right ventricle varies, depending on the degree of obstruction to the right ventricular outflow, which may occur at the VSD, at the infundibulum, or pulmonary valvar level (see Fig 33–1).[3] Obstruction to pulmonary blood flow is common (75% of all cases) and may be related to one of three mechanisms: a small VSD, small and hypoplastic right ventricle, and infundibular or valvar pulmonary stenosis.

In the patients with coexistent pulmonary atresia (Types Ia and IIa), pulmonary blood flow depends on patency of the ductus arteriosus. The right ventricle varies from a slitlike, endothelial-lined chamber in individuals with an intact ventricular septum to an adequate-size chamber (see Fig 33–1,A). In patients without pulmonary stenosis and nonobstructing VSD, the right ventricular cavity may show less hypoplasia and may even approach normal size (see Fig 33–1,C).

The size of the right ventricle varies directly with the degree of obstruction. Also the radiographic appearance of the pulmonary vasculature ranges from being markedly decreased to increased. The pulmonary artery is hypoplastic in patients with a small VSD and pulmonary stenosis but

TYPES OF TRICUSPID ATRESIA

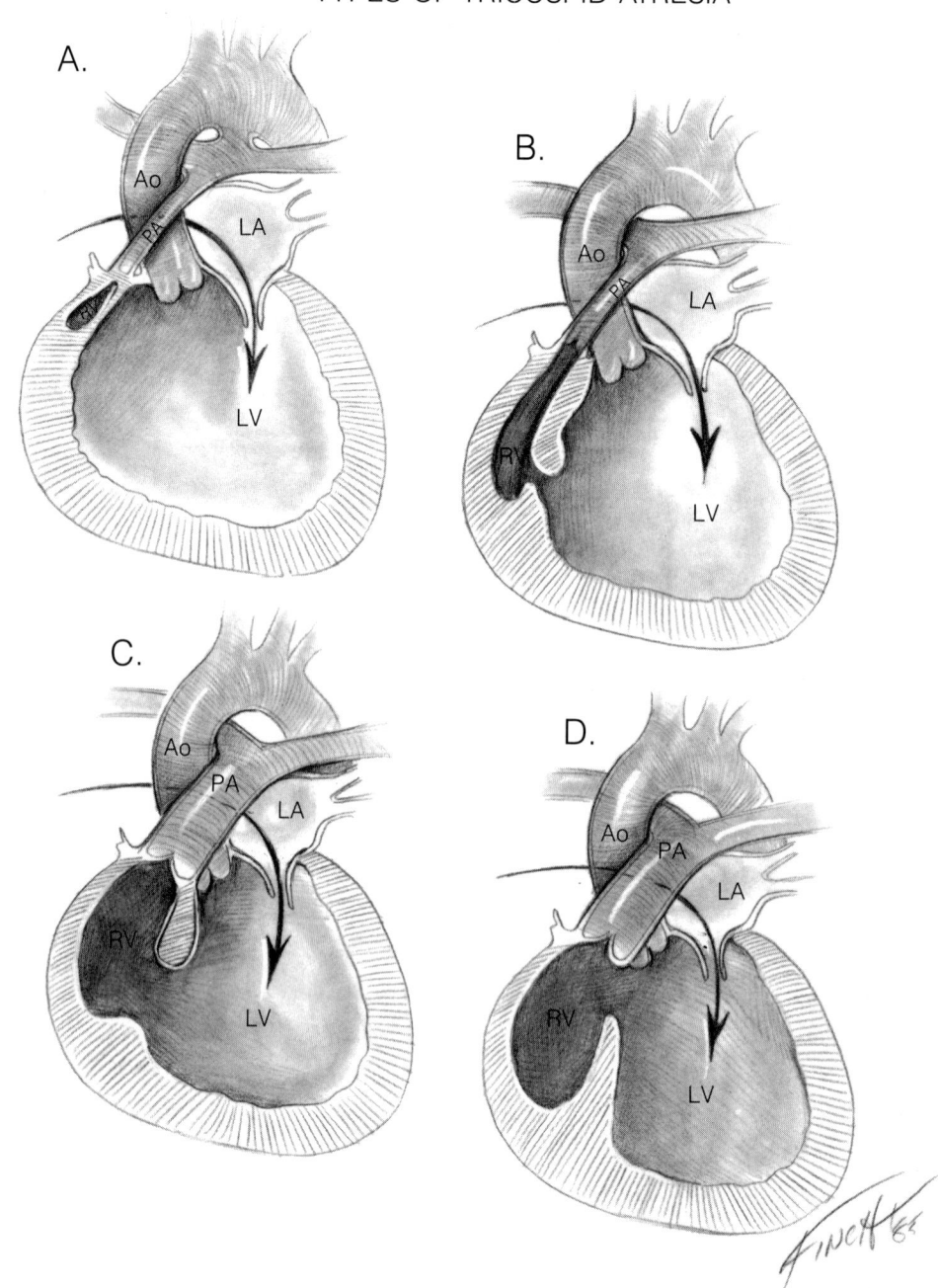

FIG 33–1.
Tricuspid atresia. Central circulation. **A,** coexistent pulmonary atresia. Intact ventricular septum. Right ventricle, tiny blind pouch. Patent ductus arteriosus perfuses pulmonary arteries. **B,** small pressure limiting ventricular septal defect. Small pulmonary arteries. Associated infundibular or valvar pulmonary stenosis. **C,** large ventricular septal defect. No pulmonary stenosis. Large pulmonary arteries, increased pulmonary blood flow. **D,** large ventricular septal defect immediately below aortic valve (overriding), as in tetralogy of Fallot. Ao = aorta; LA = left atrium; LV = left ventricle; RV = right ventricle; PA = pulmonary artery.

enlarged in patients without obstruction. The status of the ventricular septum varies. In less than 5% of instances, the ventricular septum is intact (see Fig 33–1,A). In the remaining, a VSD is present, the location and size of which varies. The defect is usually located in the membranous portion of the ventricular septum. Because it is usually small, it causes obstruction to pulmonary blood flow either alone or in combination with associated infundibular or valvar pulmonary stenosis. Rarely, the VSD is located immediately beneath the aortic valve, similar to the location of the ventricular defect in tetralogy of Fallot (see Fig 33–1,D).

An atrial communication is present and provides the only exit from the right atrium. In two thirds of patients the communication is present in the form of a patent foramen ovale, which because of its small size may obstruct egress of blood from the right atrium. Indeed, in some instances the foramen ovale may herniate to the left. In most of the remaining cases, an ostium secundum type of atrial septal defect is found or, less commonly, an ostium primum defect. Rarely, the atrial septum is intact, and the right-to-left atrial shunt occurs with blood flowing in a retrograde direction through the coronary sinus, which communicates with the left atrium through a fenestration (see Chapter 20).

Additional anatomic changes reflect the altered hemodynamics. The right atrium is enlarged and its wall thickened. Usually the left atrium and left ventricle are enlarged, because they receive the entire systemic and pulmonary blood flows.

Right aortic arch with mirror-image branching occurs in 5% of cases. Double aortic arch is rarely found.

HEMODYNAMICS

The systemic venous return enters the right atrium through the superior and inferior venae cavae and the coronary sinus. This entire blood volume passes from right atrium to left atrium through the atrial communication (see Fig 33–1), which may be restricted, in which case right atrial pressure is elevated.

Right-to-left shunting in tricuspid atresia occurs during atrial systole. Virtually all the blood shunted right to left is transported during atrial contraction. Right atrial systole also contributes significantly to left ventricular filling and produces regurgitant venous flow into the inferior vena cava and hepatic veins.[4] As a result, the supradiaphragmatic portion of the inferior vena cava tends to be larger than normal.

The systemic venous return mixes with the pulmonary venous return in the left atrium, and the combined volume passes into the left ventricle. The left ventricle is dilated in proportion to the volume of pulmonary blood flow.

Mixing of the two venous returns is usually uniform, so that the oxygen saturation of blood samples from the aorta and the pulmonary artery are similar. Thus, tricuspid atresia is an admixture lesion, and like admixture lesions, the degree of cyanosis depends on the volume of systemic venous return (cardiac output), oxygen saturation of systemic venous return, the volume of pulmonary venous return, and the oxygen saturation of pulmonary venous return. Therefore, in a patient at rest and without pulmonary parenchymal disease, the degree of cyanosis is inversely related to the volume of pulmonary blood flow. When the pulmonary blood flow is diminished because of pulmonary stenosis or atresia, cyanosis is readily identifiable. The age of onset and severity of cyanosis reflect the degree of obstruction to pulmonary blood flow. For instance, patients with coexistent pulmonary atresia become intensely cyanotic in the neonatal period as the ductus arteriosus closes.

Among those without stenosis, the volume of pulmonary blood flow is governed by the pulmonary vascular resistance. Thus, immediately after birth, pulmonary vascular resistance is elevated and pulmonary blood flow is limited. As a result, cyanosis is intense. When the pulmonary vascular resistance falls, pulmonary blood flow increases, and cyanosis lessens.

Clinical, radiographic, and other findings vary with the size of the VSD (commonly stenotic), the presence or absence of pulmonary stenosis, and transposition of the great vessels. Cases of tricuspid atresia have generally been divided into two categories according to the status of the pulmonary vasculature as either decreased (75% of patients) or increased (25% of patients). According to the classification previously present, patients with pulmonary atresia or stenosis show decreased pulmonary vasculature, and those without obstruction to pulmonary blood flow show increased pulmonary vasculature. This division occurs regardless of whether the great vessels are transposed or not. Most patients, however, with normally related great vessels have decreased pulmonary blood flow, and most patients with transposition of great vessels increased pulmonary blood flow. Because of the important differences in clinical and radiographic findings and in the management between these two categories, we present them separately. Tricuspid atresia with normally related great vessels is discussed in this chapter, and those with coexistent transposition of the great vessels are discussed in Chapter 43.

CLINICAL FEATURES

Most patients with tricuspid atresia and decreased pulmonary blood flow are identified by 1 week of age because of the presence of either cyanosis or a murmur.[5, 6] The age of onset and severity of cyanosis correlate with the severity of the pulmonary stenosis. With age, cyanosis progresses, as the obstruction to pulmonary outflow increases and the volume of pulmonary blood flow decreases. In those with coexistent pulmonary atresia, cyanosis becomes intense as the ductus arteriosus closes in the neonatal period. In these neonates, hypoxemia may be severe and associated with acidosis. Thus, neonates showing severe cyanosis may require an early operation, whereas those with mild cyanosis may be relatively asymptomatic for several months to years.

Dyspnea, hyperpnea, and clubbing develop in association with the hypoxemia. Squatting and hypoxic spells occur but with much less frequency than in patients with tetralogy of Fallot.

On physical examination, the features are often not diagnostic of tricuspid atresia but merely reflect the severity of the pulmonary stenosis and volume of pulmonary blood flow. There are cyanosis, clubbing, and hyperventilation. The neck veins may be distended and show prominent a waves, but this is difficult to observe in neonates and infants because of their short chubby necks. In patients with tricuspid atresia and decreased pulmonary blood flow, the liver is not enlarged, except in an occasional patient with a small foramen ovale.

The first heart sound is single and may be prominent. The second heart sound is also single. Usually a midsystolic murmur is present in the third and fourth left intercostal spaces. The murmur is created by blood flow through the obstructed pathway between the left ventricle and the pulmonary artery. With age the murmur becomes softer, indicating increasing severity of pulmonary stenosis or closing of the ventricular septal defect. A thrill is uncommon.

Occasionally no murmur is heard. Absence of a murmur is ominous, because it indicates a markedly reduced pulmonary blood flow. Rarely a continuous murmur of the associated patent ductus arteriosus is present in patients with coexistent pulmonary atresia.

ELECTROCARDIOGRAPHIC FEATURES

The electrocardiogram (ECG) in most patients is diagnostic, showing a characteristic pattern of left-axis deviation, right atrial enlargement, and left ventricular hypertrophy (or absence of right ventricular forces).

About 85% of patients with tricuspid atresia and decreased pulmonary blood flow have left-axis deviation between 0 and -90 degrees.[7,8] In the remaining patients the axis may be normal but never directed to the right. Left-axis deviation is related to an abnormality of the conduction system in which the left bundle branches originate close to the nodal-bundle junction and the right bundle is markedly elongated.[9] With the left-axis deviation, characteristically a Q wave is found in leads I and aVL. This has been a major distinguishing feature from pulmonary atresia, wherein a Q wave is found in leads III and aVF.

Right atrial enlargement, manifested by tall peaked P waves, is present in 75 percent of patients, but its presence does not correlate with the status of the atrial septum. The P-R interval is short in one half of the patients.

In the precordial leads, the major QRS forces are directed posteriorly and leftward, yielding a predominant S wave in lead V_1 and a tall R wave in lead V_6. This pattern reflects the combination of hypoplasia of the right ventricle and the enlargement of the left ventricle, because the latter chamber receives the entire systemic and pulmonary venous returns. The T waves are inverted in the left precordial leads in one half of the patients. They may change in amplitude during the patient's course, but we have been unable to correlate the changes with alterations in the patient's status or hemodynamics.

ECHOCARDIOGRAPHIC FEATURES

On cross-sectional echocardiography, the diagnosis can be made with reasonable certainty and the coexistent conditions assessed. Four features are characteristic: (1) absence of echoes from the tricuspid valve (in normal individuals, even in infants, the tricuspid valve can be readily identified echocardiographically); (2) a large posteriorly located atrioventricular valve (mitral valve) that shows wide excursion: (3) mitral-semilunar valve continuity; and (4) a small, anteriorly located right ventricular chamber.[10]

The left atrium and left ventricle are enlarged. A patent foramen ovale is visualized best from the subcostal location and is usually associated with an aneurysm-like stricture of redundant atrial septum that billows into the left atrium. Doppler shows right-to-left atrial shunting. In older patients, evidence of decreased left ventricular contractility may be present. The origin of this is unknown but may relate to myocardial alterations from the combination of increased left ventricular volume and myocardial hypoxemia.

The location and size of the ventricular septal defect can be observed. Pulmonary stenosis and hypoplasia of the pulmonary trunk may be found. The flow into the pulmonary artery either through a ductus arteriosus or in an antegrade direction can be assessed by Doppler. The relationship of the great vessels to the ventricular chambers can be identified whether transposed or normally related.

RADIOGRAPHIC FEATURES

In most patients, the radiographic features are characteristic enough to suggest the correct diagnosis. Enough variability of the cardiac contour exists, however, that in some patients the diagnosis can be suspected only when the radiographic appearance is considered in the light of the clinical information of cyanosis and left-axis deviation on the ECG.

1. The most characteristic feature of the cardiac contour is a rounded left cardiac border that has a much larger diameter (Fig 33–2,A and C) than the diameter of the apex in tetralogy of Fallot (Fig. 33–2,B) or other conditions with right ventricular hypertrophy.

2. The large rounded contour of the left ventricle is also seen on a left anterior oblique projection (Fig 33–2,D). REASON: The left ventricle is dilated because it receives the entire systemic and pulmonary venous return.

3. On a left anterior oblique projection the space between the left atrium and left mainstem bronchus is oblit-

DIFFERENTIAL DIAGNOSIS BETWEEN TRICUSPID ATRESIA AND TETRALOGY OF FALLOT

A. TRICUSPID ATRESIA
AP

B. TETRALOGY OF FALLOT
AP

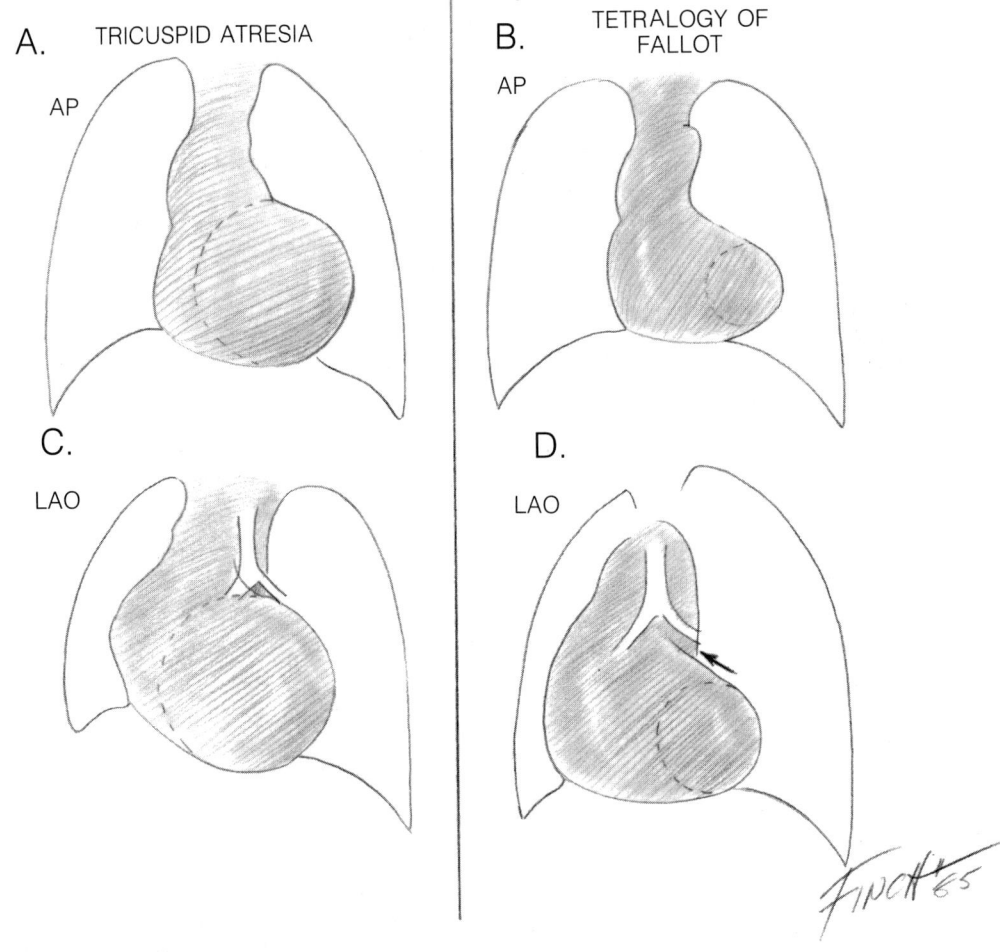

C. LAO

D. LAO

FIG 33–2.
Diagrams of cardiac contours. **A,** typical tricuspid atresia. Posteroanterior projection. Rounded contour formed by left ventricle can be fitted into circle with large diameter. **B,** tetralogy of Fallot. Posteroanterior projection. Cardiac apex can be fitted into circle with much smaller radius than with tricuspid atresia. **C,** tricuspid atresia. Left anterior oblique *(LAO)* projection. Enlarged left atrium and left ventricle from circle with large diameter. Left atrium in contact with left stem bronchus. **D,** tetralogy of Fallot. Left anterior oblique projection. Cardiac apex fitted into circle with much smaller diameter. Clear space *(arrow)* between left atrium and left mainstem bronchus (see Fig 30–15).

erated. REASON: The size of the left atrium is either normal or enlarged. This is another distinguishing feature from tetralogy of Fallot, which typically has a clear space between left heart border and left main bronchus (see Figs 33–2,D and 30–15).

4. On the left anterior oblique projection, the right atrial border has an increased diameter. REASON: The right atrium is enlarged because of the obligatory right-to-left atrial shunt and frequently elevated right atrial pressure. Obstruction at the level of the atrial communication may increase right atrial pressure further.

5. The right superior mediastinum tends to be prominent (Fig 33–3). REASON: Counterclockwise rotation of the heart occurring from left ventricular enlargement displaces the aorta and superior vena cava toward the right.

6. The pulmonary arterial segment is not prominent (see Fig 33–3). REASON: The pulmonary artery is small anatomically and displaced medially by counterclockwise rotation of the heart.

7. On a left anterior oblique projection the large left ventricular contour is well seen. The right atrial border is prominent (Fig 33–4).

8. In infants, the cardiac apex may appear elevated. REASON: In this age group, films are taken in a lordotic projection.

9. The presence of a right aortic arch does not exclude tricuspid atresia (Fig 33–5). Although the incidence (25%) of right arch is higher in tetralogy of Fallot, it is also present in tricuspid atresia (5%).

10. Usually, the cardiac size is normal or only slightly enlarged (Figs 33–3, 33–5, and 33–6). REASON: More than 75% of patients have either pulmonary stenosis or a narrowed ventricular septal defect, which limits pulmonary blood flow.

11. The size of the left atrium is either normal or only slightly enlarged (see Fig 33–6). REASON: Although the volume of blood that flows through the left atrium consists of the entire systemic and pulmonary venous returns, this

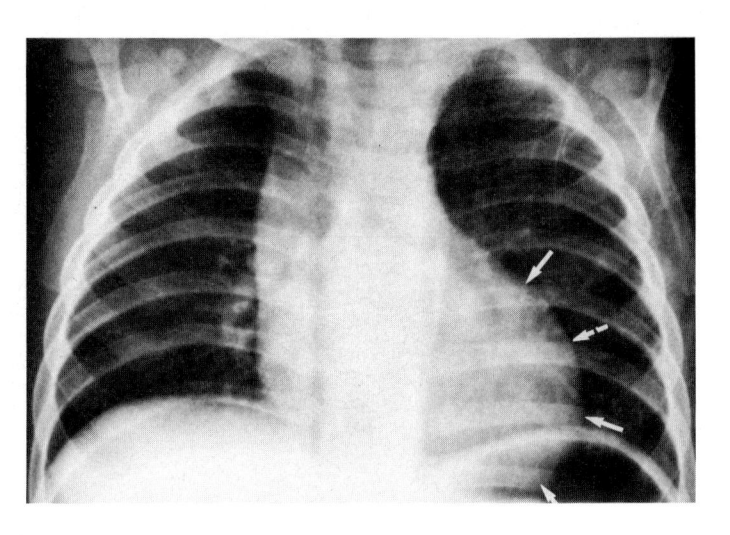

FIG 33–3.
Tricuspid atresia with pulmonary stenosis. Thoracic roentgenogram. Posteroanterior projection. Decreased pulmonary vasculature. Cardiac size is only minimally enlarged. Characteristic rounded left ventricular contour *(arrows)*. Concave pulmonary arterial segment. Contrary to tetralogy of Fallot, aortic knob not prominent. Prominent right superior mediastinum because of counterclockwise rotation.

volume is usually not greatly increased because the pulmonary blood flow is limited by obstruction.

12. The pulmonary vasculature varies from decreased to normal. Three fourths of patients have at least slight reduction of pulmonary arterial vasculature (see Figs 33–3, 33–5, and 33–6).

13. Patients without obstruction to pulmonary blood flow whether the great vessels are transposed or normally related have a significantly enlarged cardiac silhouette, increased pulmonary arterial vasculature, and left atrial enlargement (Fig 33–7).

14. When the pulmonary arterial vasculature is increased in a cyanotic patient with left-axis deviation (see Fig 33–7), the differential diagnosis includes tricuspid atresia with a large ventricular septal defect, without pulmonary stenosis, and tricuspid atresia with transposition of great vessels and single ventricle.

15. There is a higher incidence of juxtaposition of the atrial appendages, particularly with tricuspid atresia and transposition. Rarely, a notch may be seen between the displaced atrial appendage and the left ventricular contour (Fig 33–8).

CARDIAC CATHETERIZATION

Cardiac catheterization in neonates and infants is undertaken to establish the diagnosis and distinguish tricus-

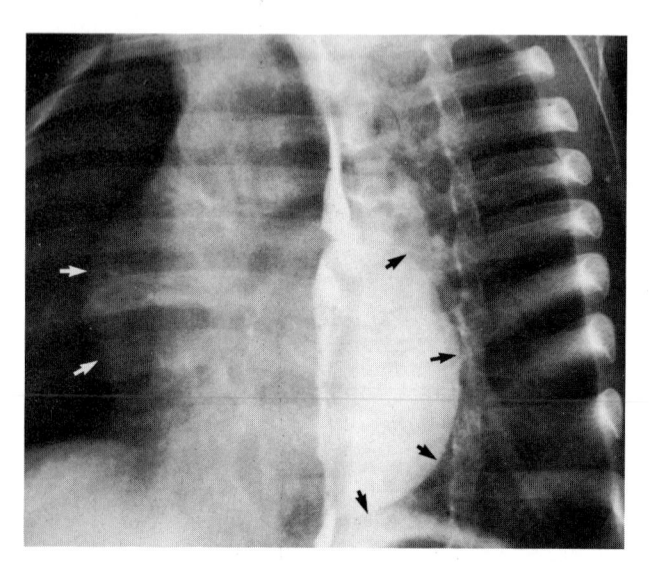

FIG 33–4.
Tricuspid atresia. Thoracic roentgenogram. Left anterior oblique projection. Space beneath left mainstem bronchus is obliterated by left atrium. Left atrium and left ventricle form rounded contour *(arrows)*. Prominent right atrial segment *(white arrows)* from right atrial enlargement.

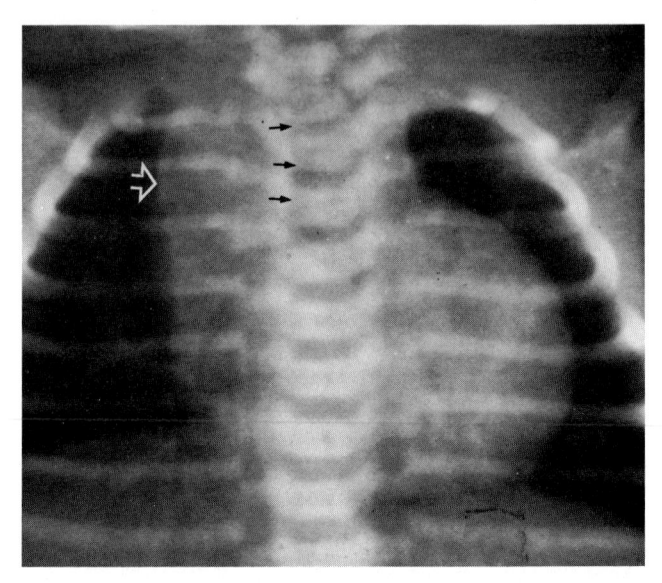

FIG 33–5.
Tricuspid atresia and right aortic arch. **A,** thoracic roentgenogram. Posteroanterior projection. Right arch displaces trachea *(black arrows)* toward left and causes mass density along right superior mediastinum *(open arrow)*. Circular left ventricular contour.

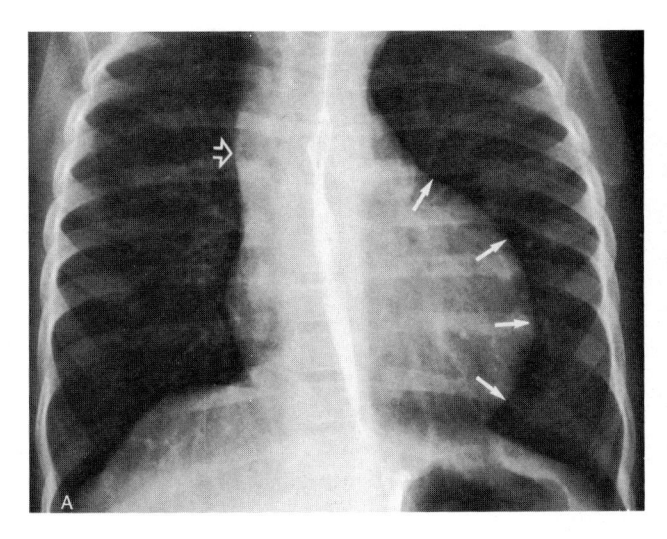

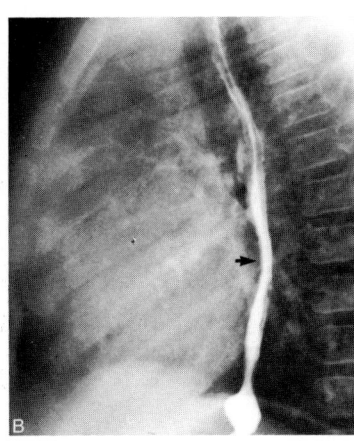

FIG 33-6.
Tricuspid atresia and obstructing ventricular septal defect. Thoracic roentgenogram. **A,** posteroanterior projection. Slight cardiomegaly. Decreased pulmonary vasculature. Unusually round left cardiac contour *(small white arrows),* characteristic of tricuspid atresia. Right superior mediastinum *(open arrow)* is prominent because of counterclockwise rotation of heart. Aortic knob is inconspicuous, in distinction to tetralogy of Fallot. **B,** lateral projection. Minimal left atrial enlargement *(arrow).*

pid atresia from similar conditions associated with right ventricular hypoplasia. During cardiac catheterization of neonates, balloon atrial septostomy is also performed.

The preferable catheter approach is through the femoral vein, because by this route the catheter can easily be advanced into the left atrium and left ventricle. With a balloon-tipped catheter, the tip may be advanced from the left ventricle across the ventricular septal defect into the pulmonary artery or into the aorta.

In neonates, right atrial pressure, particularly the a wave, is elevated and exceeds left atrial pressure.[5] This

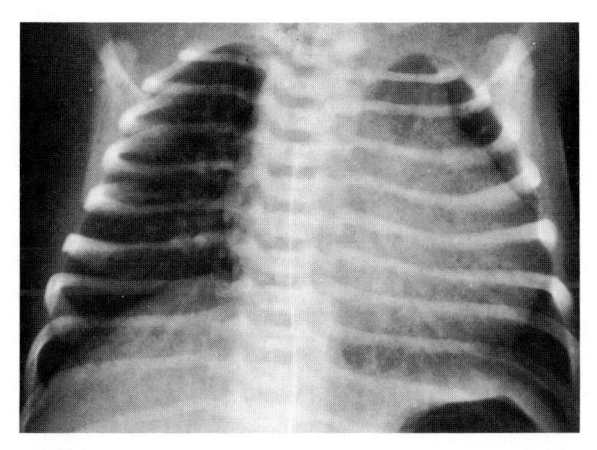

FIG 33-7.
Tricuspid atresia without obstruction to pulmonary blood flow. Thoracic roentgenogram. Posteroanterior projection. Pulmonary vasculature markedly increased. Severe cardiomegaly. Nonspecific cardiac contour. Diagnosis suggested only by history of cyanosis and left axis deviation. Statistically the most likely radiographic diagnosis is tricuspid atresia with transposition of great vessels.

pressure difference indicates obstruction at the foramen ovale. In neonates and infants, left atrial and left ventricular pressures are normal.

In patients with reduced pulmonary blood flow, pulmonary arterial pressure is usually normal, because there is obstruction between the left ventricle and the pulmonary artery from either a small size of the ventricular septal defect or pulmonary stenosis.

Oximetry data show a lower than normal oxygen saturation in the right atrium because the saturation of blood returning from the body is reduced. There is evidence of a right-to-left atrial shunt, with the left atrial oxygen saturation being significantly lower than the pulmonary venous oxygen saturation. Because uniform mixing occurs, oxygen saturation in the left ventricle, aorta, and pulmonary artery is virtually identical.

During cardiac catheterization in a neonate, balloon atrial septostomy is performed to create or enlarge the atrial communication,[11] allowing an unobstructed atrial right-to-left shunt.

In patients with tricuspid atresia, cardiac catheterization may be repeated before operative procedures, particularly the Fontan procedure. At subsequent catheterizations, particular attention is directed to pressure measurements, which may alter the effectiveness of a Fontan operation. Left ventricular dysfunction may develop[12, 13] and elevate left ventricular end-diastolic and left atrial pressures. Pulmonary arterial pressure should always be measured if the patient is considered for a Fontan procedure. In such a patient, the volume of pulmonary blood flow must be determined, to calculate the pulmonary vascular resistance. Elevation of either left ventricular end-diastolic pressure or

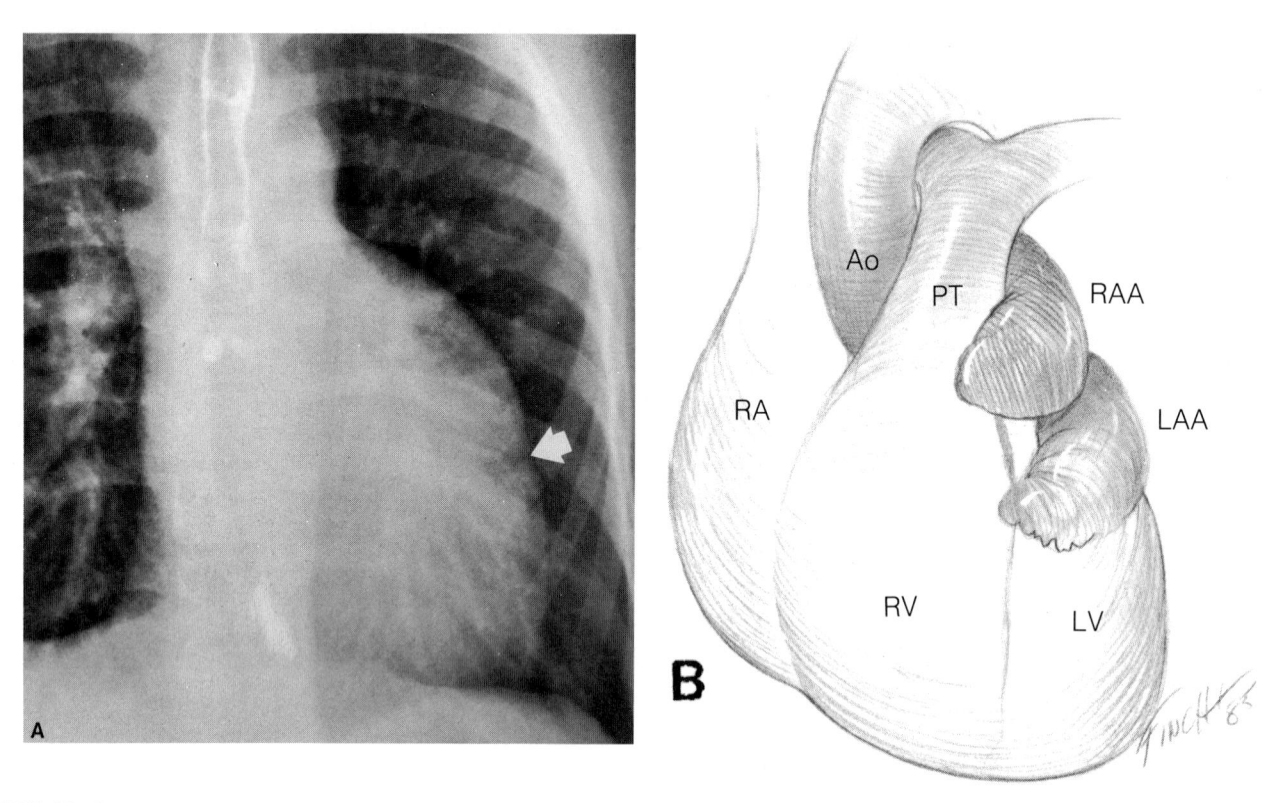

FIG 33–8.
Tricuspid atresia and juxtaposition of atrial appendages. Thoracic roentgenogram. Posteroanterior projection. **A,** subtle notch *(arrow)* below left atrial appendage. Identical radiographic finding is seen in common ventricle with ventricular inversion (see Chapter 39). **B,** juxtaposition of atrial appendages. Ao = aorta; PT = pulmonary trunk; RAA = right atrial appendage; LAA = left atrial appendage; LV = left ventricle; RV = right ventricle; RA = right atrium.

pulmonary vascular resistance increases the risk of a Fontan procedure.

Angiography is an important aspect of cardiac catheterization.

ANGIOGRAPHIC FEATURES

Selective right atrial injection or venous angiography demonstrates the right-to-left atrial shunt at the atrial level. Although anteroposterior and lateral positions are adequate to demonstrate the atrial level shunt, the location and size of the atrial communication can be observed only on an angled left anterior oblique projection.

During cardiac catheterization, attempts must be made to pass the catheter from the right atrium into the right ventricle because angiography may be misleading about patency of the tricuspid valve. For instance, with associated pulmonary atresia and intact ventricular septum (see Fig 33–1,A), there is little flow into the right ventricle. Thus, after right atrial injection in such patients, the right ventricle may not opacify and the diagnosis of tricuspid atresia may erroneously be made. But if a catheter can be advanced into the right ventricle from the right atrium, patency of the tricuspid valve is established. We have incorrectly diagnosed tricuspid atresia in a neonate with severe tricuspid stenosis and in another patient with a tumor occluding the tricuspid valve.

1. Right atrial injection demonstrates an enlarged right atrium. The left atrium is immediately opacified (Fig 33–9,A).
2. In patients without a narrowed atrial communication, the increased right atrial pressure may cause the fossa ovalis to herniate into the left atrium (Fig 33–9,B), allowing the obligatory right-to-left shunt. A rare mode of egress of blood from the right atrium is through a fenestrated coronary sinus (see Chapter 20).
3. The supradiaphragmatic portion of the inferior vena cava is commonly enlarged (see Fig 33–9). REASON: Increased right atrial pressure and forceful atrial systole.
4. After selective right atrial injection, opaque material refluxes into the hepatic veins and sometimes into a dilated coronary sinus. REASON: Increased right atrial pressure and atrial systole.

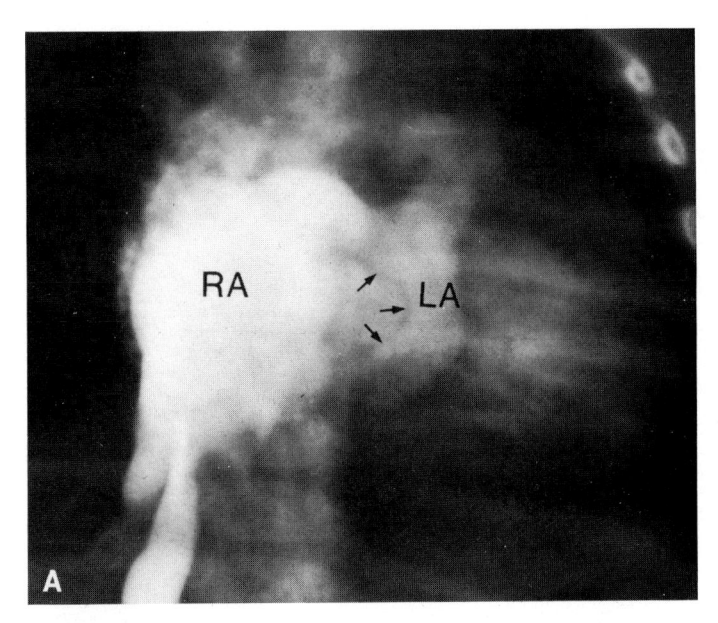

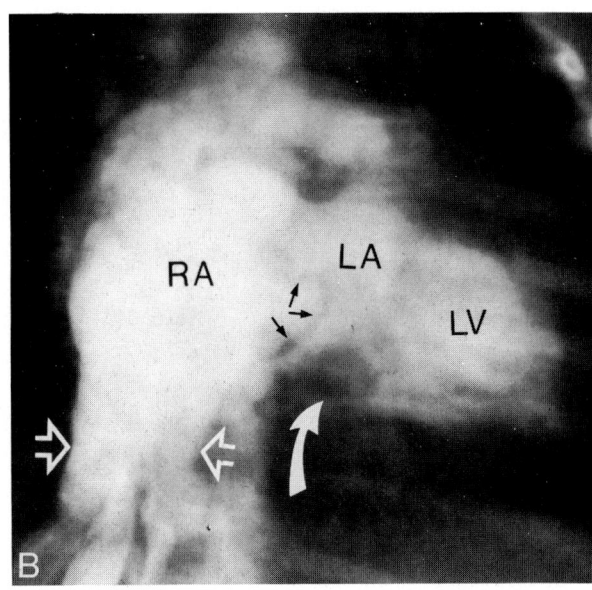

FIG 33–9.
A, Tricuspid atresia and herniation of fossa ovalis. Right atrial *(RA)* angiogram. Anteroposterior projections. Immediate opacification of enlarged left atrium *(LA)*. Enlarged right atrium. Herniation of fossa ovalis *(black arrows)* because small atrial communication is present. **B,** reflux of contrast medium into inferior vena cava. Enlarged supradiaphragmatic portion of inferior vena cava *(open arrow)*. At the normal location of right ventricle a radiolucency ("right ventricular window") is present, a characteristic feature of tricuspid atresia *(white arrow)*. LV = left ventricle.

5. Juxtaposition of the atrial appendages is well seen after right atrial injection (Fig 33–10).

6. Right arch occurs in about 5% of the cases, much less frequently than with tetralogy (see Fig 33–10).

7. From the left ventricle, both great vessels fill simultaneously, the pulmonary artery through a ventricular septal defect present in most patients and the aorta directly from the left ventricle (Fig 33–11).

8. Left ventriculography is indicated to demonstrate the size of the ventricular septal defect, the size of the hypoplastic right ventricle, and the presence or absence of pulmonary stenosis.

9. Typically the left ventricle is slightly enlarged, and the right ventricle is severely hypoplastic and consists of only the conus portion (infundibulum) (see Fig 33–11).

10. The ventricular septal defect may be the major site of obstruction to pulmonary blood flow (Fig 33–12), or pulmonary stenosis may be present at either the infundibular or valvar level (see Fig 33–12).

11. Rarely, the ventricular septal defect is large and nonobstructive, and the sinus portion of the right ventricle is more fully developed (see Fig 33–12). If there is no infundibular or valvar stenosis, pulmonary blood flow may be normal or increased. Cyanosis is less pronounced in such patients. Consequently, the size of the right ventricle varies considerably, but typically the sinus portion is absent.

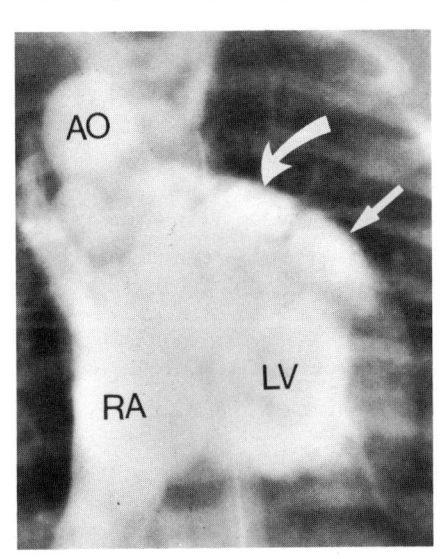

FIG 33–10.
Right atriogram. Juxtaposition of atrial appendages. Right atriogram. Anteroposterior projection. Right and left atrial appendage *(straight arrow)*. Note right aortic arch. *Ao* = aorta; *RA* = right atrium; *LV* = left ventricle.

MANAGEMENT

The prognosis for patients with tricuspid atresia and decreased pulmonary blood flow is one of the poorest of all forms of congenital heart disease. One half of these pa-

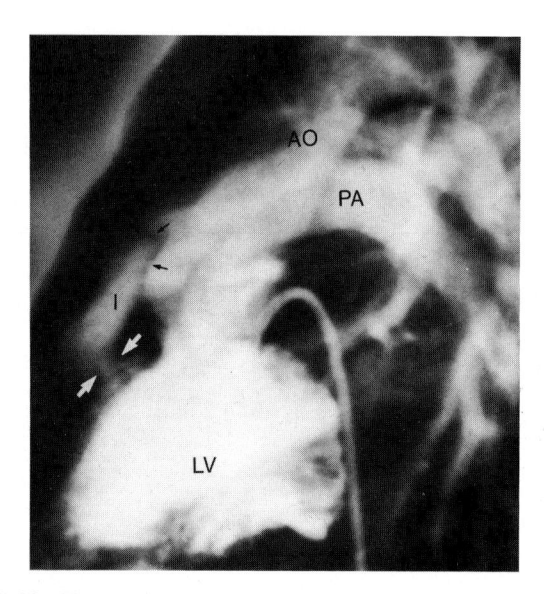

FIG 33–11.
Tricuspid atresia with obstruction to pulmonary blood flow. Left ventriculogram *(LV)*. Lateral projection. Small obstructing ventricular septal defect *(white arrows)*. Right ventricle consists only of outflow portion. Absent inflow portion. Diffusely narrowed infundibulum *(I)*. Slightly thickened bicuspid pulmonary valve *(black arrows)*. Obstructions are present at level of ventricular septal defect, infundibulum, and pulmonary valve. *AO* = aorta; *PA* = pulmonary artery (see Fig 33–8,B).

FIG 33–12.
Tricuspid atresia and large ventricular septal defect *(arrows)*. Left ventriculogram. Left anterior oblique projection. Well developed sinus portion of right ventricle. Example of wide variability of right ventricular hypoplasia. *PA* = pulmonary artery; *RV* = right ventricle; *LV* = left ventricle.

tients die by 6 months of age and two thirds by 1 year. There are occasional reports of survival to the fifth decade. Thus, most patients require an operation in infancy. Operative procedures for the treatment of tricuspid atresia are designed to remove obstruction to intracardiac blood flow and to increase pulmonary blood flow. The long-term goal of these initial palliative procedures is to allow survival of the patient without the development of pulmonary vascular disease or distortion of the pulmonary arterial tree so that a physiologic operation (Fontan procedure) can be performed when the child is older.

The initial palliative step is usually taken during the first cardiac catheterization, when a balloon atrial septostomy is performed. We perform this step routinely, whereas others limit its use to infants with a gradient between the right and left atria. In older infants or children in whom the foramen ovale is restricted, an atrial communication may be operatively created with the Blalock-Hanlon operation. This may be performed in conjunction with a systemic pulmonary arterial shunt. A blade atrial septostomy is an option for older infants and children and can be performed by cardiac catheterization.

In patients with tricuspid atresia and decreased pulmonary blood flow, a systemic pulmonary arterial shunt procedure is indicated if there are hypoxic spells or in cases of progressive hypoxemia.

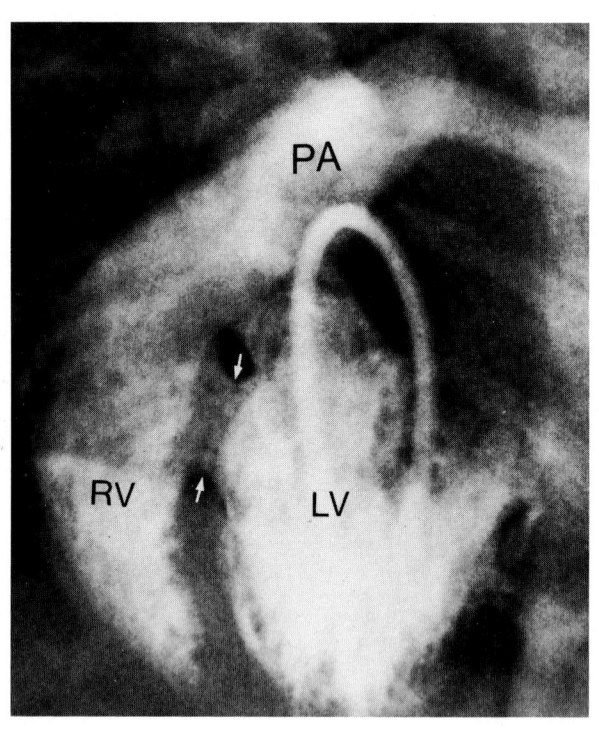

A variety of palliative procedures have been used to improve pulmonary arterial blood flow in patients with tricuspid atresia[14, 15]:

1. Blalock-Taussig shunt (subclavian to pulmonary artery).
2. Central (or Gortex) shunt.
3. Potts' procedure (descending aorta to left pulmonary artery).
4. Waterston procedure (ascending aorta to right pulmonary artery).
5. Glenn procedure (superior vena cava to pulmonary artery).

Development of pulmonary vascular disease and distortion of the pulmonary arterial tree should be avoided. Thus, care should be exercised in selecting the appropriate procedure. At our institution we avoid the use of the Potts and the Waterston procedures for several reasons. In both procedures, it is difficult to create a proper-sized communication between the aorta and pulmonary arterial tree. The shunts tend to be too large and may further increase with growth of the child. Because of their large size, the volume of pulmonary blood flow is often excessive, leading to congestive cardiac failure and left ventricular dysfunction. Pulmonary arterial pressure is usually elevated, and pulmonary vascular disease may develop. Furthermore, with growth, there may be changes in the relationship between the aorta and the respective branch pulmonary artery involved in the shunt, so that distortion of the proximal pulmonary artery occurs. Pulmonary hypertension and pulmonary artery distortion complicate or eliminate the possibility of a subsequent Fontan procedure.

The Glenn procedure (named after William Glenn, a contemporary American surgeon) is an end-to-end anastomosis of the superior vena cava to the right pulmonary artery (Fig 33–13,A), with ligation of the azygos vein to prevent collateral blood flow. This classic operation and its modifications have been available as a palliative procedure for a couple of decades. In one modification (bilateral Glenn or modified Glenn) the superior vena cava is anastomosed end to side to the right pulmonary artery (Fig 33–13,B). This establishes blood flow to both lungs and maintains continuity of the major pulmonary arteries.

Thus, the pulmonary arterial bed has the potential to develop normally for eventual Fontan procedure. It has the advantage of being an obligatory shunt where the left ventricle does not have to pump the volume of shunted blood as with other systemic pulmonary arterial shunts. Three conditions must be met to be a suitable candidate for a Glenn procedure: (1) the lungs should be free of pulmonary parenchymal disease that could affect oxygenation and also elevate pulmonary vascular resistance, (2) there should be a single superior vena cava (in the presence of bilateral superior venae cavae, venous collaterals develop between the right and left superior venae cavae, which will eventually carry blood away from the lung), and (3) the pulmonary vascular resistance should be normal. If pulmonary resistance is elevated, superior vena caval pressure increases, leading to superior vena caval syndrome. Thus, the Glenn procedure is contraindicated in neonates and indeed has to be carefully considered in infants less than 6 months of age because of the normally elevated pulmonary vascular resistance. Long-term complications of the Glenn

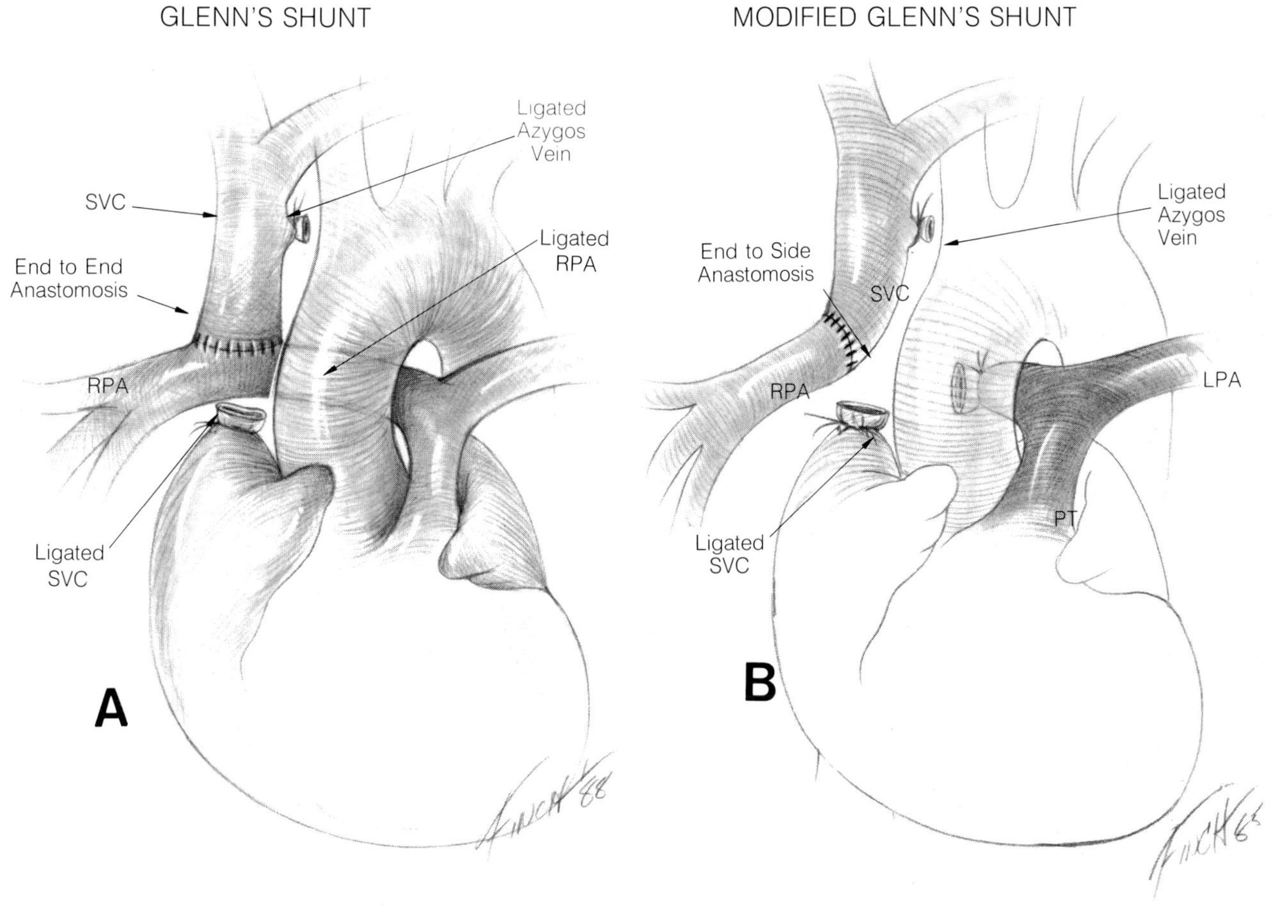

FIG 33–13.
Glenn procedure. **A,** end-to-end anastomosis between superior vena cava *(SVC)* and right pulmonary artery *CRPA)*. Proximal right pulmonary artery and azygos vein have been ligated (classic Glenn). **B,** modified or bilateral Glenn with end-to-side anastomosis between superior vena cava and right pulmonary artery. *LPA* = left pulmonary artery; *PT* = pulmonary trunk.

procedure include progressively decreased perfusion of the right lung because of development of collaterals to other systemic veins, underperfusion of right upper lobe because of inflow from bronchial collaterals, and development of stenoses or occlusions of the shunt.

Another late complication of the classic Glenn procedure is the development of arteriovenous fistulas within the right lung (ultimately about 20% of patients), which decrease arterial oxygen saturation. With time cyanosis increases and the clinical condition deteriorates. Although the cause for the development of these intrapulmonary shunts is unknown, gravitational effects, nonpulsating blood flow, and hypoxemia have been suggested. Gravitational forces probably play a role because the intrapulmonary shunts develop in the right lower lobe and not in the right upper or right middle lobes. The fistulas can be readily detected by selective pulmonary angiography, ultrasonic techniques, or isotopic techniques. The modified Glenn procedure is frequently performed for tricuspid atresia or other cyanotic conditions as the first stage before the Fontan operation. It tends to have fewer complications than the classic Glenn.

The Blalock-Taussig and the central shunts are generally the preferred palliative procedures. With either technique the size of the shunt can be carefully controlled by either the normal diameter of the subclavian artery or selection of the appropriate caliber of the graft. As a result, pulmonary arterial pressure is rarely elevated, and development of pulmonary vascular disease is uncommon. Furthermore, the size of the shunt is usually adequate to improve systemic oxygen saturation and the patient's condition.

In neonates and young infants we perform a central shunt and reserve the Blalock-Taussig shunt for older infants and children, because it is technically more difficult to perform an arterial anastomosis in small infants.

Tricuspid atresia can be corrected physiologically by the Fontan operation (named after Frances Fontan, a contemporary French surgeon.)[16, 17] In this procedure the right atrium is connected to the main pulmonary artery or right pulmonary artery either by direct anastomosis of the right atrial appendage or, less commonly, with a graft containing a tissue valve that tends to be functional for only a short period (Fig 33–14). The atrial communication is closed, which forces the systemic venous return into the pulmonary artery. In a variation the tube graft is embedded in the right ventricle in hopes that the right ventricle will generate some propulsive force to blood flow into the lungs. Another variation is the retroaortic anastomosis of the main pulmonary artery to the right atrium (Fig 33–15). This operation is feasible only if the pulmonary artery is of fair size. In all Fontan procedures, the atrial septal defect is closed operatively, so that the entire systemic venous return passes into the pulmonary arterial tree. Four conditions must be present for a satisfactory result from this operation: (1) normal pulmonary vascular resistance with a mean pulmonary arterial pressure less than 20 mm Hg, (2) adequate-sized pulmonary arterial tree without stenotic areas (e.g., after a shunt procedure), (3) normal left ventricular function with an end-diastolic pressure less than 10 mm Hg, and (4) normal sinus rhythm.

Postoperatively there may be evidence of increased right atrial pressure, superior vena caval syndrome, hepatomegaly, protein-losing enteropathy, ascites, and right pleural effusion. It may take several months for these features to disappear.

The long-term results of the Fontan procedure are unknown. Although the patients are no longer cyanotic, we

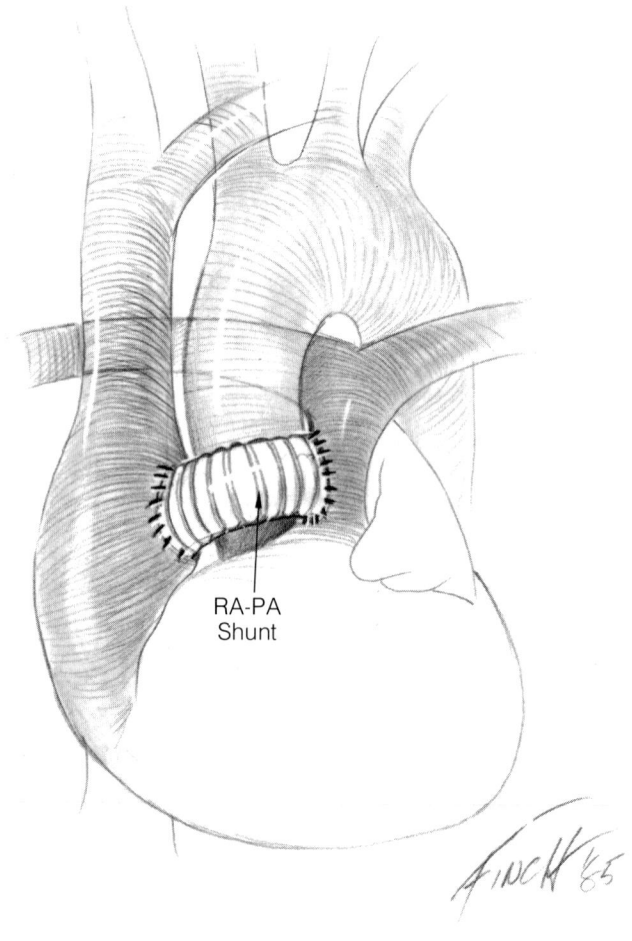

FIG 33–14.
Fontan procedure with right atrial–pulmonary arterial connection. RA = right atrium; PA = pulmonary artery. AO = aorta; IVC = inferior vena cava; LA = left atrium; LPA = left pulmonary artery; LV = left ventricle; RA = right atrium; RPA = right pulmonary artery; RV = right ventricle; SVC = superior vena cava.

VARIATION OF THE FONTAN PROCEDURE

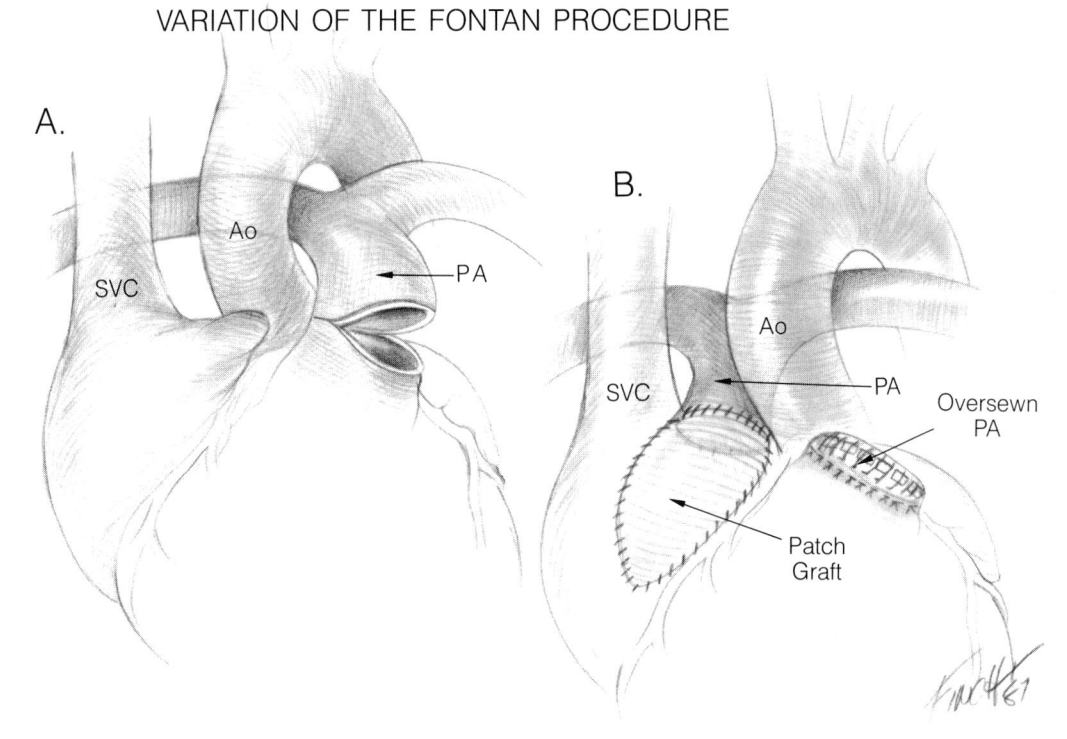

FIG 33–15.
Fontan modification for large main pulmonary arteries. **A,** main pulmonary artery divided. **B,** anastomosis behind aorta to right atrium. Anastomosis is enlarged by patch graft. Right ventricular portion of pulmonary artery is oversewn. *Ao* = aorta; *SVC* = superior vena cava; *PA* = pulmonary artery.

have found that the patients may be unable to increase cardiac output with exercise. Generally the Fontan procedure is performed in school-aged children, although about 20% of the procedures are performed in children less than 4 years of age but rarely less than 1 year of age.

POSTOPERATIVE ROENTGENOGRAPHIC FEATURES

1. Systemic to pulmonary arterial shunts (Potts, Blalock-Taussig, or central shunts) give identical radiographic findings to those for the palliation of tetralogy of Fallot (Fig 33–16) (see Chapter 30).

2. After systemic to a pulmonary arterial shunt, pulmonary vasculature and cardiac size may increase.

3. After Fontan procedure and its modifications, there is usually no change of the radiographic findings.

4. The Fontan conduit is usually not recognized on a thoracic roentgenogram.

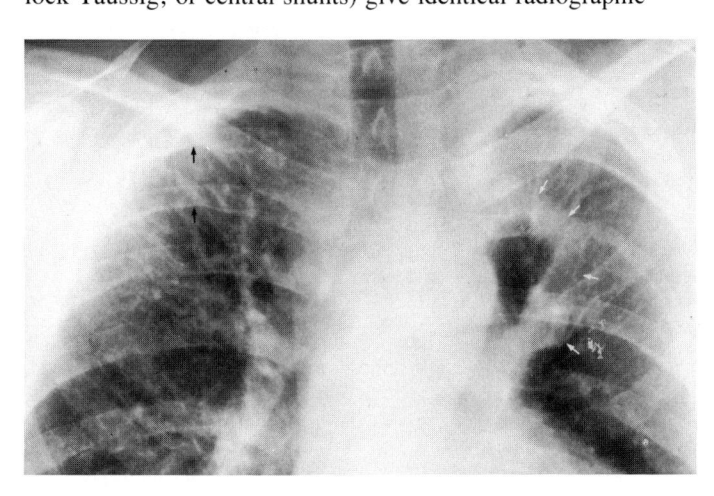

FIG 33–16.
Tricuspid atresia. Systemic to pulmonary artery shunt. Thoracic roentgenogram. Posteroanterior projection. Rib resection on left. Synthetic graft *(white arrows)*. Previous right Blalock-Taussig anastomosis resulted in rib notching *(small black arrows)*. Pleural thickening and stringy parenchymal pattern in right upper lobe suggest thrombosis of anastomosis and systemic transpleural collaterals to right pulmonary artery. Findings are identical to shunt procedures performed for tetralogy of Fallot.

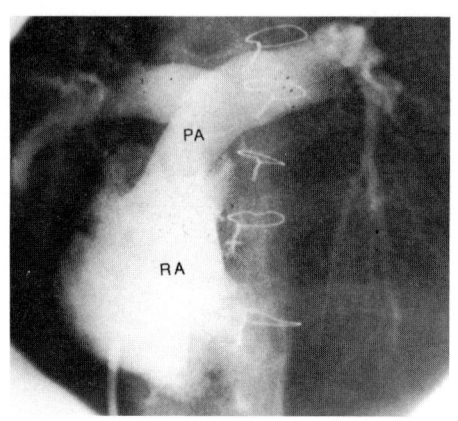

FIG 33-17.
Modified Fontan procedure. Right atriogram. Anteroposterior projection. Pulmonary artery *(PA)* with native valve anastomosed to right atrium *(RA)*. Normal opacification of pulmonary artery. No reflux into coronary sinus, suggesting near-normal right atrial pressure.

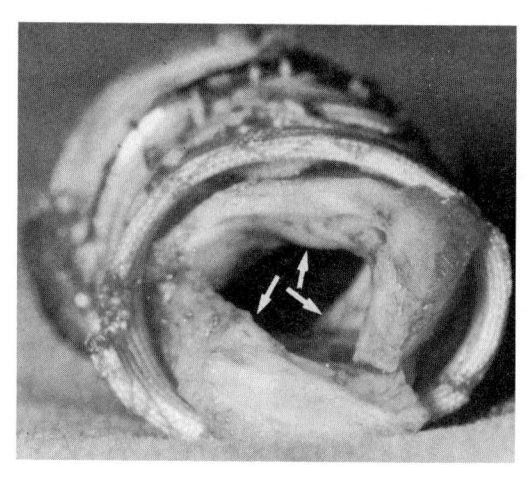

FIG 33-19.
Operatively placed Fontan conduit. Severe stenosis of conduit at right ventricular anastomosis. Close-up view. Stenosis is caused by ingrowth of fibrous tissue *(arrows)*.

POSTOPERATIVE ANGIOGRAPHIC APPEARANCE

1. With a well-functioning Fontan anastomosis there is satisfactory opacification of the pulmonary arteries after a right angiogram (Fig 33-17). If the right atrial pressure is low, there is no reflux into the coronary sinus. Such excellent results are achieved if the native and nonstenotic pulmonary valve can be used.

2. With a direct anastomosis of the right atrial appendage to the pulmonary artery, flow of contrast material tends to be more sluggish because of pulmonary insufficiency (Fig 33-18).

3. Angiography is indicated after a Fontan procedure if the patient's condition deteriorates. When a conduit containing a porcine valve is used, the porcine leaflets may become thickened, calcified, immobile, and stenotic. Furthermore, ingrowth of fibrous tissue into the conduit may cause stenosis (Fig 33-19).

4. Competence of the tissue valve can be evaluated by passing the catheter through the conduit and performing a pulmonary arteriogram (Fig 33-20).

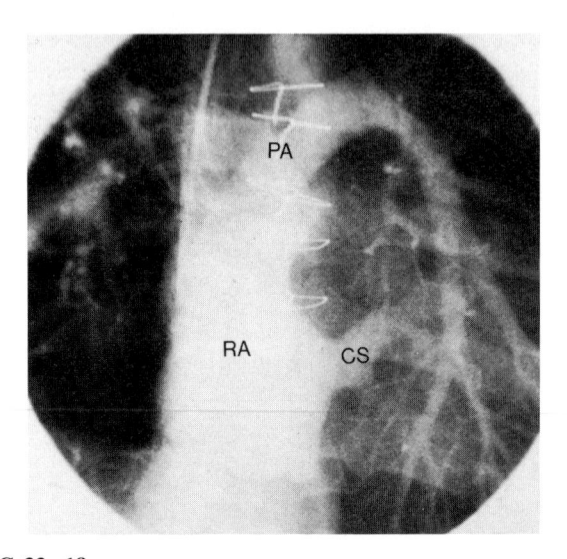

FIG 33-18.
Tricuspid atresia. Modified Fontan anastomosis. Direct anastomosis between right atrial *(RA)* appendage and pulmonary artery *(PA)*. Right atriogram. Anteroposterior projection. Sluggish antegrade flow into pulmonary artery. Coronary sinus *(CS)* is opacified by reflux of contrast medium, suggesting elevated right atrial pressure.

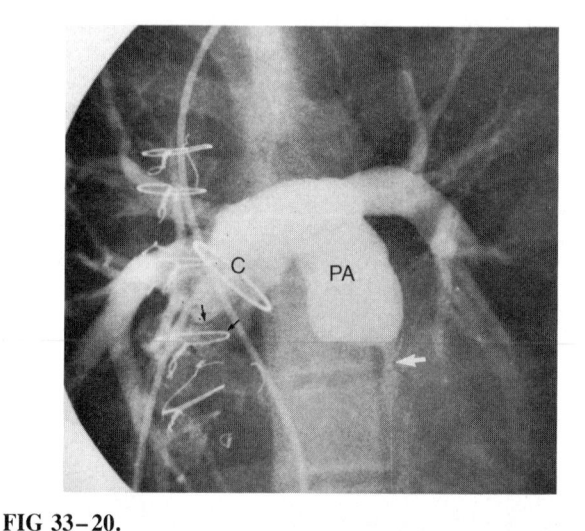

FIG 33-20.
Tricuspid atresia. Valved conduit. Catheter is passed through conduit *(C)*. Pulmonary arteriogram *(PA)*. Anteroposterior projection. Slightly thickened porcine valve *(black arrows)*. Pulmonary valve is oversewn with minor leak *(white arrow)*. Competent valve conduit.

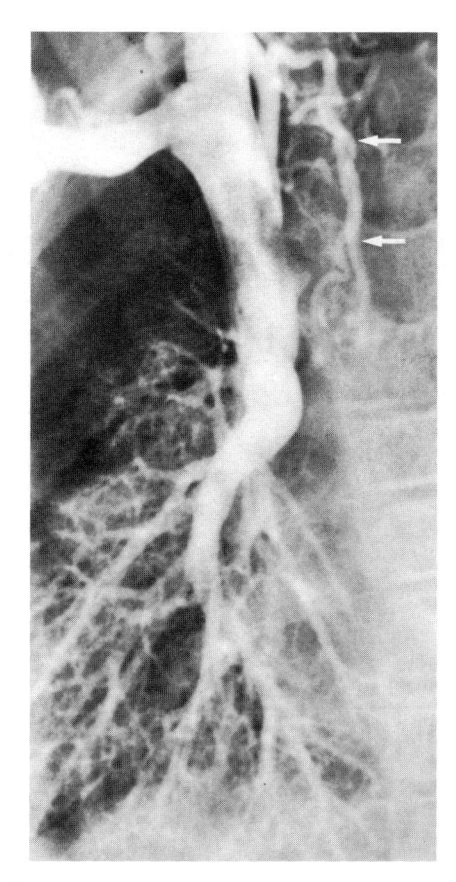

FIG 33-21.
Tricuspid atresia. Recent classic Glenn anastomosis. Injection of contrast media into right superior vena cava. Anteroposterior projection. Antegrade flow of contrast medium and opacification of entire right pulmonary arterial tree. Systemic collateral arteries are absent.

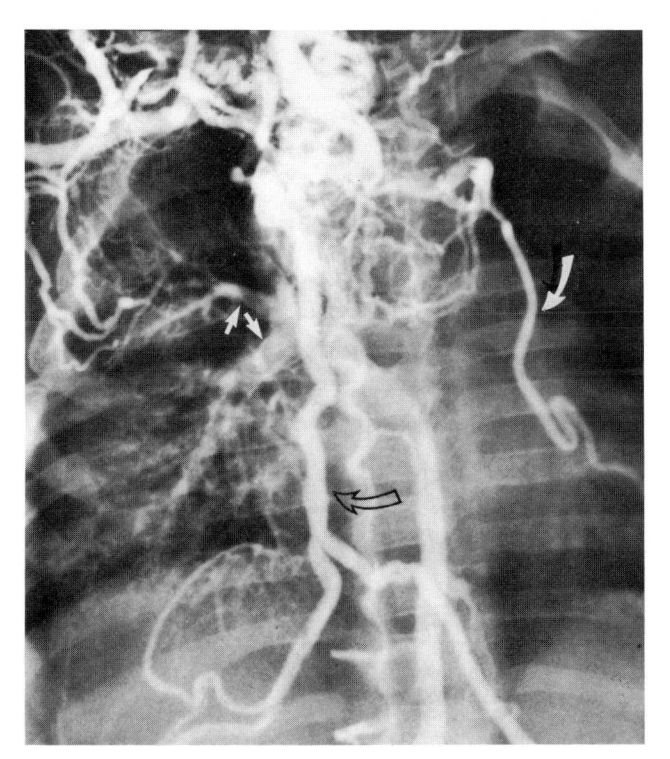

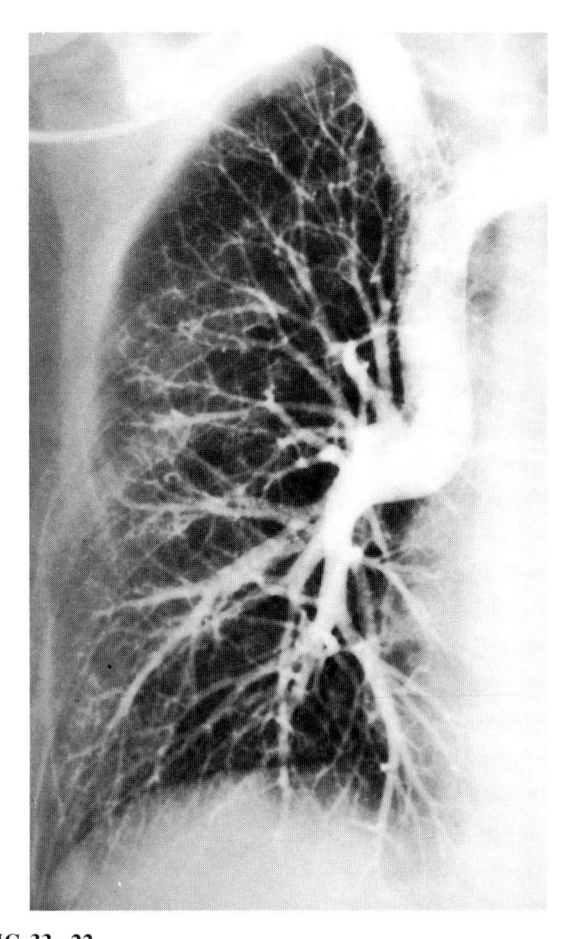

FIG 33-22.
Tricuspid atresia. Glenn anastomosis 2 years later. Same patient as Figure 33-21. Injection of contrast media into right antecubital. vein. Anteroposterior projection. Early systemic venous collaterals *(arrows)*. Nonfilling of right upper lobe pulmonary artery because of bronchial arterial collateral inflow. Retrograde blood flow through right upper pulmonary artery could be observed cineangiographically by dilution of contrast medium. Blood sample drawn at this site may show a high oxygen content.

FIG 33-23.
Tricuspid atresia. Glenn anastomosis was done many years previously. Same patient as Figure 33-21. Injection of contrast media into right brachial vein. Anteroposterior projection. Extensive systemic collateral arteries. Little antegrade flow into right pulmonary artery *(white arrows)*. Systemic venous collateral blood flow occurs primarily through mammary vein *(curved arrow)*, azygos vein and paravertebral plexus. Flow is through opposite side *(curved white arrow)* via periaortic venous network into pericardial vein.

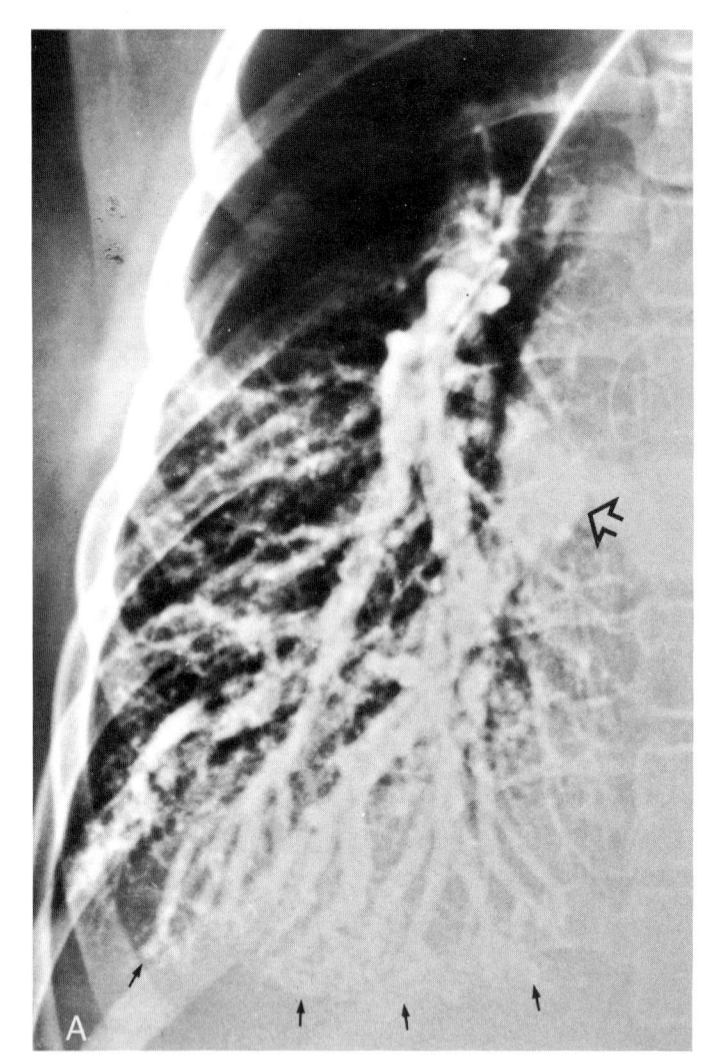

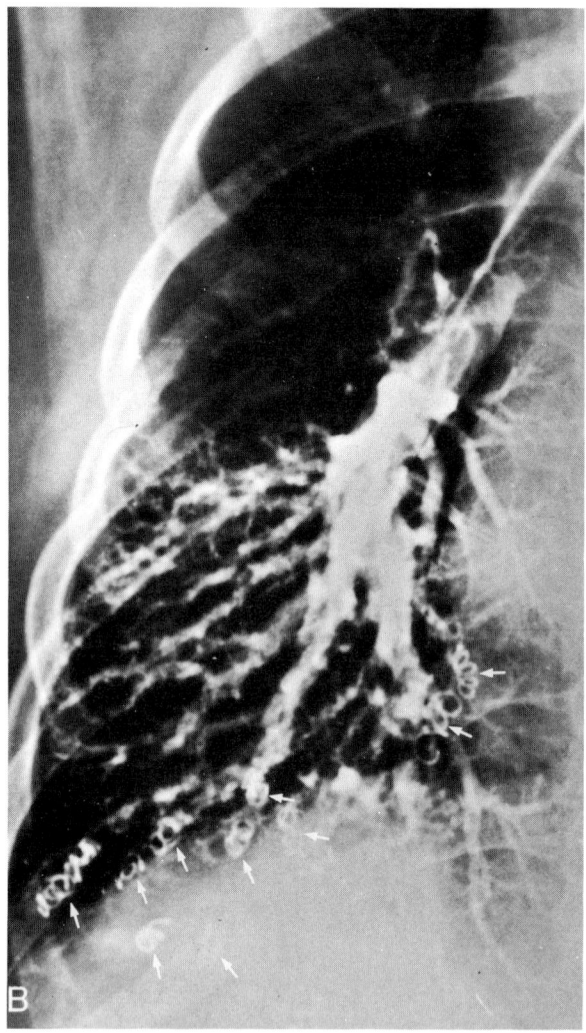

FIG 33–24.
Tricuspid atresia. Late Glenn anastomosis. Anteroposterior projection. **A,** injection of contrast medium into right pulmonary artery. Prompt filling of right lower pulmonary vein *(open arrow)* through multiple pulmonary arteriovenous fistulae *(black arrows).* Nonopacification of right upper lobe because of bronchial inflow. **B,** after embolization of arteriovenous fistulas with stainless steel coils *(arrows).* Pulmonary veins no longer opacify early. Patient's cyanosis was improved. (Courtesy of Dr. Antoinette Gomez, University of California–Los Angeles.)

5. Valve stenosis or insufficiency is the rule rather than the exception.

6. The appearance of a Glenn anastomosis depends largely on its duration. Shortly after operation, the entire right pulmonary arterial tree opacifies after injection of contrast material into the superior vena cava (Fig 33–21).

7. A few years after placement of a Glenn anastomosis, systemic arterial collaterals develop. The arterial branches to the right upper lobe no longer opacify (Fig 33–22). REASON: Bronchial collateral arteries into the right upper lobe supply the pulmonary artery in retrograde direction. The retrograde flow can be seen cineangiographically by a negative jet in the injected anastomosed pulmonary artery after selective injection of the right upper lobe pulmonary artery demonstrating retrograde flow or by a systemic arterial injection that opacifies the right upper lobe bronchial arteries.

8. After the Glenn procedure, with further development of venous collateral vessels and systemic to pulmonary arterial shunts, blood flow into the right pulmonary artery gradually decreases. Eventually there is very little antegrade flow into the right pulmonary artery (Fig 33–23).

9. A rare long-term complication of the Glenn procedure is the development of pulmonary arteriovenous fistulas. These can be treated nonsurgically by embolization

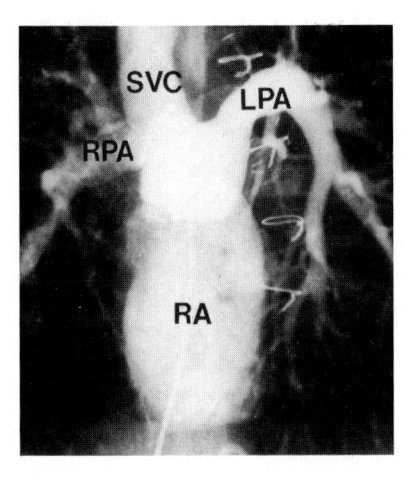

FIG 33–25.
Tricuspid atresia. Postoperative modified Glenn and Fontan procedures. Pulmonary arteriogram. Anteroposterior projection. Right atrial and superior vena caval inflow are visualized. *SVC* = superior vena cava; *LPA* = left pulmonary artery; *RA* = right atrium; *RPA* = right pulmonary artery.

with stainless coils or detachable balloons. Embolization improves the clinical status and peripheral oxygen saturation (Fig 33–24).

10. In patients who had a staged operation (modified Glenn, followed by Fontan) pulmonary arteriography demonstrates both anastomoses (Fig 33–25).

REFERENCES

1. Scalia D, Russo P, Anderson RH, et al: The surgical anatomy of hearts with no direct communication between the right atrium and the ventricular mass—so-called tricuspid atresia, *J Thorac Cardiovasc Surg* 87:743, 1984.
2. Edwards JE, Burchell HB: Congenital tricuspid atresia: a classification, *Med Clin North Am* 33:1177, 1949.
3. Guller B, Titus JL: Morphological studies in tricuspid atresia, *Circulation* 38:977, 1968.
4. Levin AR, Spach MS, Canent RV, et al: Dynamics of interatrial shunting in children with obstruction of the tricuspid and pulmonic valves, *Circulation* 41:503, 1970.
5. Dick M, Fyler DC, Nadas AS: Tricuspid atresia: clinical course in 101 patients, *Am J Cardiol* 36:327, 1975.
6. Patel R, Fox K, Taylor JFN, et al: Tricuspid atresia: clinical course in 62 cases (1967–1974), *Br Heart J* 40:1408, 1978.
7. Guller B, Titus JL, DuShane JW: Electrocardiographic diagnosis of malformations associated with tricuspid atresia: correlation with morphologic features, *Am Heart J* 78:180, 1969.
8. Davachi F, Lucas RV Jr, Moller JH: The electrocardiogram and vectorcardiogram in tricuspid atresia: correlation with pathologic anatomy, *Am J Cardiol* 25:18, 1970.
9. Guller B, DuShane JW, Titus JL: The atrioventricular conduction system in two cases of tricuspid atresia, *Circulation* 40:217, 1969.
10. Seward JB, Tajik AJ, Hagler DJ, et al: Echocardiographic spectrum of tricuspid atresia, *Mayo Clin Proc* 53:100, 1978.
11. Rashkind W, Waldhausen J, Miller W, et al: Palliative treatment in tricuspid atresia: combined balloon atrioseptostomy and surgical alteration of pulmonary blood flow, *J Thorac Cardiovasc Surg* 57:812, 1969.
12. Nishioka K, Kamiya T, Ueda T, et al: Left ventricular volume characteristics in children with tricuspid atresia before and after surgery, *Am J Cardiol* 47:1105, 1981.
13. LaCorte MA, Dick M, Scheer G, et al: Left ventricular function in tricuspid atresia: angiographic analysis in 28 patients, *Circulation* 52:996, 1975.
14. Rao PS: Natural history of the ventricular septal defect in tricuspid atresia and its surgical implications, *Br Heart J* 39:276, 1977.
15. Kyger ER III, Reul GJ Jr, Sandiford FM, et al: Surgical palliation of tricuspid atresia, *Circulation* 52:685, 1975.
16. Shemin RJ, Merrill WH, Pfeifer JS, et al: Evaluation of right atrial—pulmonary artery conduits for tricuspid atresia: experimental study, *J Thorac Cardiovasc Surg* 77:684, 1979.
17. Gale AW, Danielson GK, McGoon DC, et al: Fontan procedure for tricuspid atresia, *Circulation* 62:91, 1980.

CHAPTER 34

Pulmonary Atresia With Intact Ventricular Septum

Pulmonary atresia with intact ventricular septum is an uncommon (1%–3%) type of congenital cardiac malformation but an important cause of neonatal cyanosis. Its importance lies in the fact that patients with this condition can be successfully corrected or palliated. It must be distinguished from tricuspid atresia, which it resembles hemodynamically and clinically. The condition of coexistent severe pulmonary stenosis, hypoplastic right ventricle, and atrial right-to-left shunt represents a variant of pulmonary atresia and is not discussed as a separate condition.

Pulmonary atresia may be acquired after a systemic to pulmonary arterial shunt because of the lack of antegrade blood flow through the pulmonary valve or because the elevated pulmonary artery pressure from the shunt exceeds that in the right ventricle, so the pulmonary valve cannot open. A similar phenomenon occurs in patients with tetralogy of Fallot and a systemic to pulmonary arterial shunt. In these situations the infundibulum becomes narrowed and eventually atretic. Functional pulmonary atresia, diagnosed at the time of right ventriculography, is another variant, found in neonates with elevated pulmonary vascular resistance, in whom the right ventricle is incapable of developing sufficient systemic pressure to open the pulmonary valve.

FETAL CIRCULATION

In spite of the complete obstruction, pulmonary atresia is well tolerated during fetal life. The right ventricle is bypassed and does not contribute to systemic circulation as in a normal fetus. The left ventricle provides the entire cardiac output as in instances of tricuspid atresia.

The aorta and its isthmus are enlarged because they receive the entire cardiac output in contrast to the normal fetal circulation. The lungs are supplied from left-to-right flow through the patent ductus arteriosus and through bronchial arteries. Because of this reverse flow through the patent ductus arteriosus, the ductus arteriosus arises higher from the aortic arch and has a more vertical direction than the ductus arteriosus in a normal fetus (Fig 34–1). The volume of blood flow to lung is determined by the size of the patent ductus arteriosus and affects the size of the pulmonary arterial tree. The smaller the caliber of the ductus, the more hypoplastic the pulmonary arterial tree. The size and status of the ductus arteriosus are also very important for postnatal survival. The ductus arteriosus tends to be narrow in most patients and constricts in response to the postnatal increase of arterial Po_2. Immediately after birth, blood flow across the atrial communication becomes reduced because of the elimination of placental blood flow. The atrial communication is usually adequate for a few weeks or months, allowing an obligatory right-to-left shunt. Admixture of systemic and pulmonary venous returns occurs in the left atrium and further in the left ventricle.

When pulmonary blood flow is not limited, left atrial pressure may rise and impede the blood flow from the right atrium. Therefore, right atrial pressure rises and maintains the right-to-left shunt.

PATHOLOGIC ANATOMY

In pulmonary atresia with intact ventricular septum, the pulmonary leaflets are completely fused, and the pulmonary valve is present as a diaphragm with two or three raphaes. The diaphragm is thick and fibrotic. Atresia is localized to the valve in 80% of cases, whereas in the other 20% infundibular atresia coexists.[1, 2] The pulmonary annulus is usually hypoplastic.

Prominent muscle bundles in the right ventricle may

DUCTUS IN PULMONARY ATRESIA

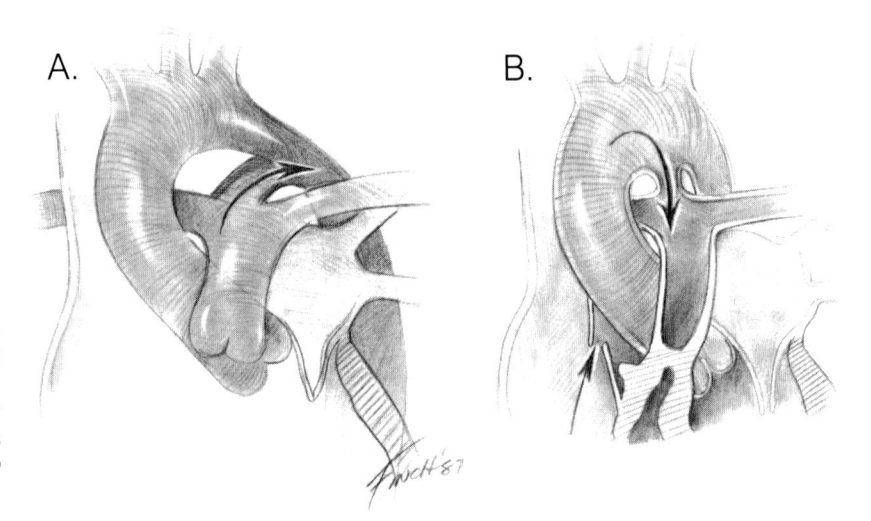

FIG 34–1.
Fetal circulation. **A,** normal. Patent ductus passes in horizontal direction to descending aorta. Direction of blood flow is right to left. Isthmus is normally narrowed. **B,** pulmonary atresia. Ductus arises more vertically from aortic arch. Direction of blood flow is left to right.

extend to the pulmonary valve, particularly the right and left cusps.[3] This muscular tissue has to be considered during pulmonary valvotomy, because an incision through either the right or left pulmonary sinus leads into underlying muscle and creates a narrowed tract. Although such muscle bundles are also present in a normal right ventricle, they are not as prominent as in pulmonary atresia because the infundibulum is narrowed from the marked right ventricular hypertrophy. The muscle bundles related to the pulmonary valve are termed the right posterior muscle bundle and the left posterior muscle bundle. An anterior muscle bundle usually cannot be identified.

The major anatomic variations of pulmonary atresia are related to the size of the right ventricle and its associated features.[1–6] The volume of blood flow into and out of the right ventricle determine its size. Traditionally patients with pulmonary atresia have been classified as having either a hypoplastic or an enlarged right ventricle.[6] The size of the right ventricle among these patients is really a spectrum from diminutive to greatly enlarged, with the right ventricle being of normal size in some. The two categories are, however, helpful clinically, hemodynamically and angiographically, because most patients have or resemble more closely one of these two types. In describing the anatomic characteristics of the right ventricle, the inlet, trabecular, and outlet portions must be discussed. The details of the tricuspid valve are also an important consideration.

Hypoplastic Right Ventricle

In two thirds of the cases, the right ventricle is smaller than normal, and the hypoplasia involves each of the three portions of the right ventricle: the inlet, trabeculated, and outflow areas (Fig 34–2).[1, 2] A correlation exists between the degree of tricuspid obstruction, right ventricular cavity size, and the level of right ventricular systolic pressure. In a hypoplastic right ventricle, each component of the tricuspid valve is abnormal and diminutive. The tricuspid annulus is hypoplastic, the leaflets are thickened, chordae tendineae are shortened, and the papillary muscle hypoplastic (see Fig 34–2). Tricuspid stenosis may result, but not regurgitation. The trabeculated portion is often obstructed by hypertrophied myocardium. Infundibular stenosis or atresia usually coexists. The pulmonary trunk, although patent to the level of the pulmonary valve, may be hypoplastic (10%).[1, 2] Hypoplasia of major pulmonary arterial branches may coexist.

A unique feature among patients with a hypoplastic right ventricle are right ventricular–coronary arterial communications (Fig 34–3), which provide egress of blood from the blindly ending right ventricle. These communications reflect the elevated right ventricular systolic pressure.[2, 6, 7] They represent enlarged myocardial sinusoids that communicate with branches of either the right, left, or both coronary arteries. Blood flows from the right ventricle into the coronary arteries during systole.[8] During diastole, blood flows from the aorta into the coronary arteries. If right ventricular systolic pressure is decreased by an operation, coronary right ventricular fistulas may be present.

Connections may occur between the coronary arteries and the right ventricle, but no connection may exist between the coronary arteries and aorta (see Fig 34–3,B).[7] Under this circumstance, if right ventricular systolic pressure is reduced by an operation, myocardial infarction may occur. The myocardium in the distribution of the involved coronary artery may be ischemic and show necrosis.[9]

Enlarged Right Ventricle

Among patients with pulmonary atresia, intact ventricular septum, and dilated right ventricle, tricuspid regurgitation is present, communications of sinusoids to coronary

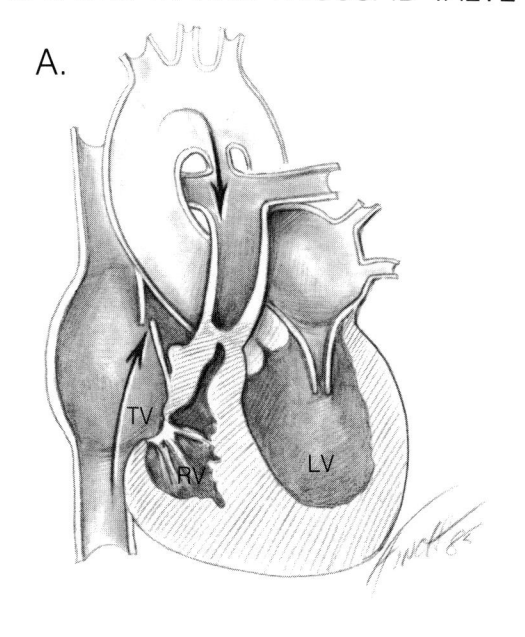

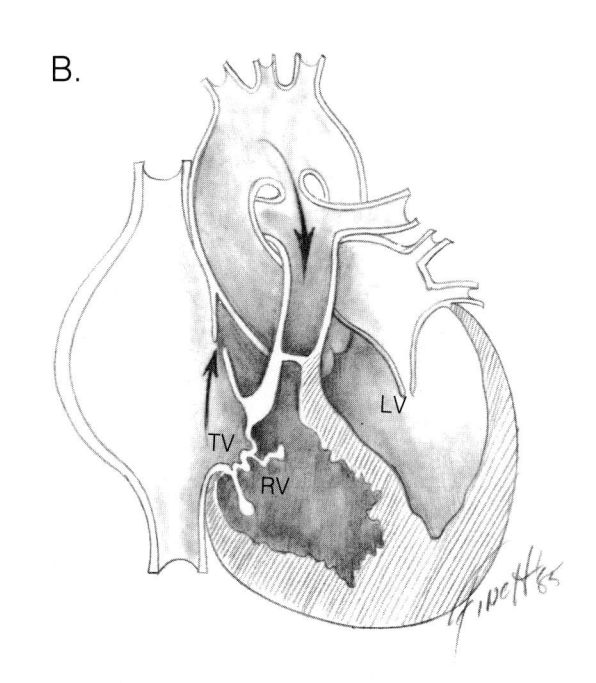

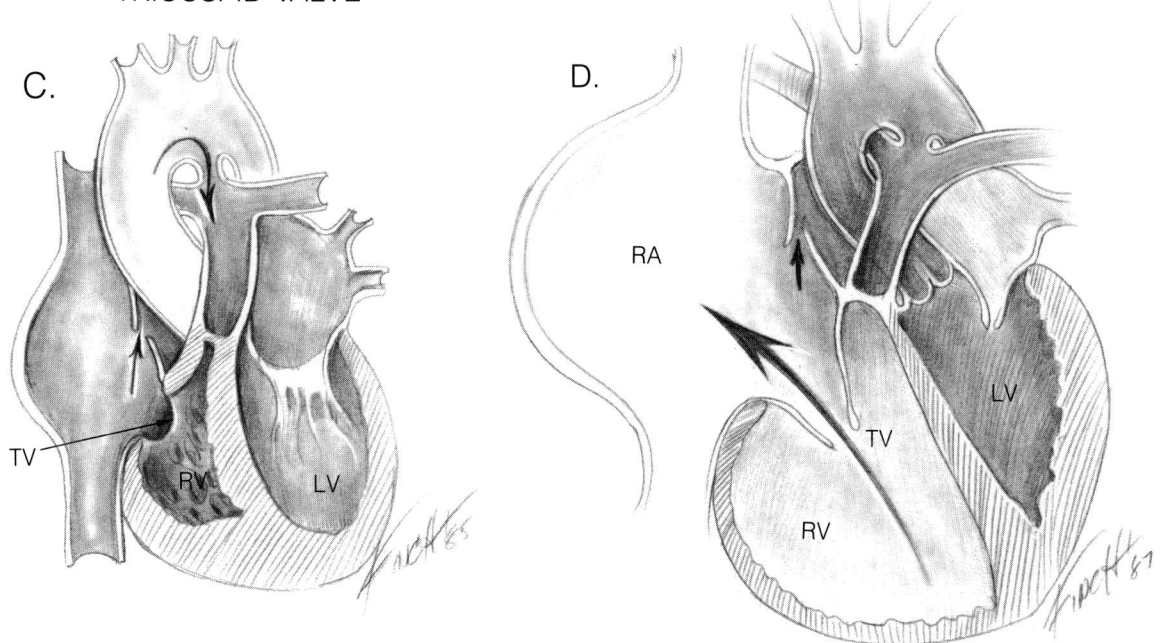

FIG 34–2.
Pulmonary atresia and intact ventricular septum. Central circulation. **A,** hypoplasia of right ventricle *(RV)* and tricuspid valve *(TV)*. **B,** normal-sized right ventricle. Dysplastic pulmonary valve. Tricuspid regurgitation. **C,** congenitally unguarded tricuspid valve. **D,** incompetent tricuspid valve. *LV* = left ventricle. *RA* = right atrium.

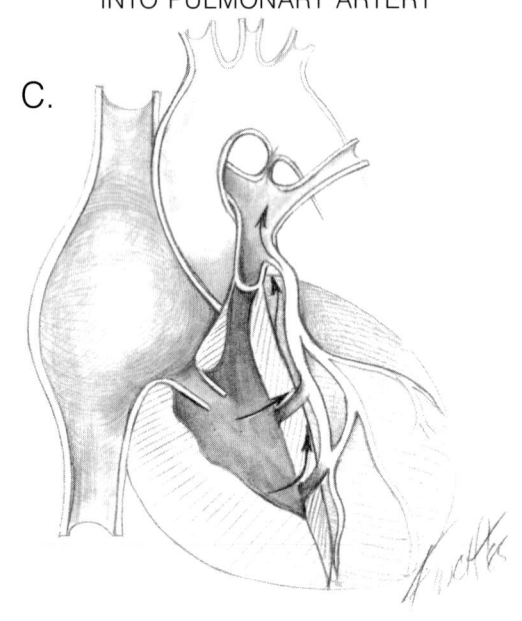

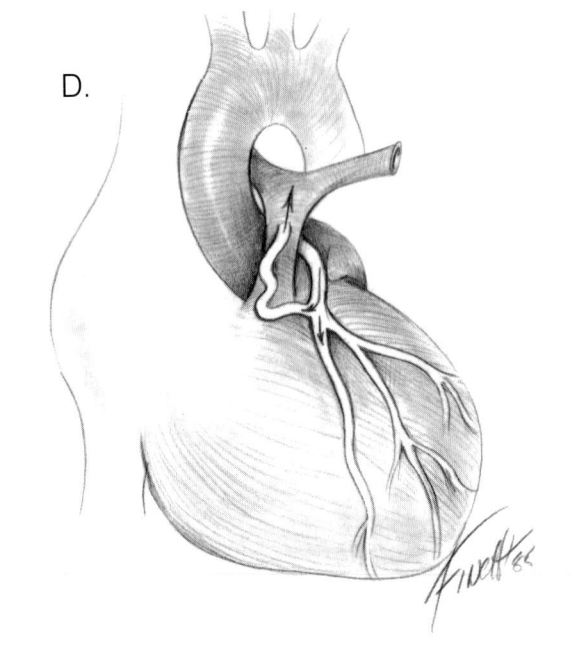

FIG 34–3.
Pulmonary atresia. Coronary arterial circulation. **A,** hypoplastic right ventricle *(RV)*. Myocardial sinusoids communicate with left coronary arterial circulation. Retrograde flow into ascending aorta during systole. **B,** hypoplastic right ventricle. Discontinuity of proximal left coronary artery. **C,** hypoplastic right ventricle. Aberrant left coronary artery is communicating with pulmonary artery. **D,** hypoplastic right ventricle. Fistula between left coronary artery and pulmonary artery is providing blood flow into lungs even after closure of ductus arteriosus. *TV* = tricuspid valve.

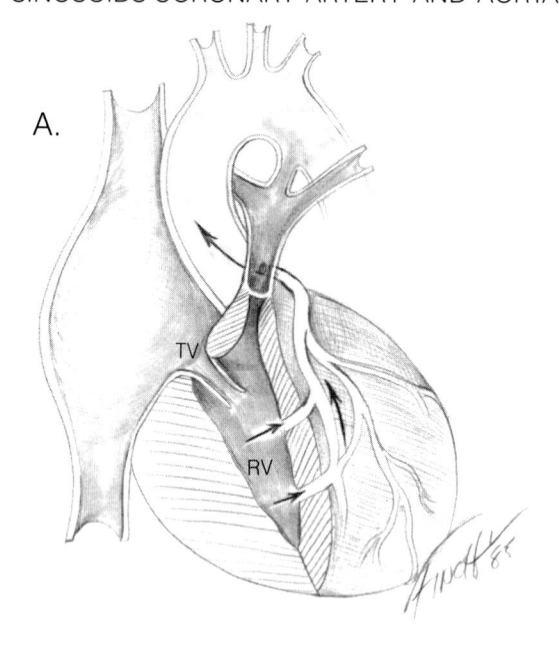

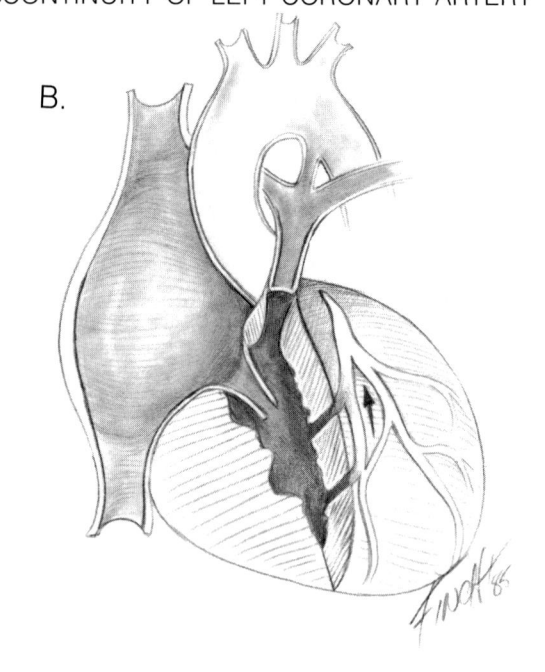

arteries are absent, and right ventricular systolic pressure is below aortic systolic pressure (see Fig 34–2,D). Both the right atrium and right ventricle are greatly enlarged proportionally to the degree of tricuspid regurgitation. The tricuspid valve may show features of Ebstein's malformation or dysplastic features of leaflets and chordae tendinae (or both) (see Fig 34–2,B).[6, 10] Rarely, tricuspid valvar tissue and papillary muscles are absent, although a tricuspid valve orifice exists. This condition is called "congenitally unguarded tricuspid orifice," with coexistent pulmonary atresia (see Fig 34–2,C),[11] and it is associated with major tricuspid regurgitation. In all patients with a dilated right ventricle, the right ventricular wall is normal or thinned, and infundibular atresia is not present.

Between the extremes of hypoplasia and dilatation of the right ventricle, there are a few patients with a right ventricle of normal size, architecture, and valve apparatus.

OTHER ANATOMIC FEATURES

The size of the tricuspid annulus correlates with right ventricular size, but no correlation exists between size of the pulmonary artery and the right ventricle. The size of the right ventricle is related to flow through the tricuspid valve, whereas the size of the pulmonary annulus is related to flow through the patent ductus arteriosus. The size of the major pulmonary arteries may reflect the caliber of the ductus arteriosus in utero.

The size of the left atrium and left ventricle depend on the degree of pulmonary flow. In patients with a small patent ductus arteriosus, the chambers of the left side of the heart are normal sized.

In all patients with pulmonary atresia, the right atrium is enlarged and its wall thickened, particularly among those patients with an enlarged right ventricle.[1, 2, 6] There is an atrial communication, usually a patent foramen ovale, which may be restrictive. If restrictive, the valve of the foramen ovale may herniate into the left atrium, or, rarely, retrograde blood flow may be present through a fenestrated coronary sinus into the left atrium (see Chapter 20).

A rare association of pulmonary atresia is aberrant left coronary artery arising from the pulmonary artery (see Fig 34–3,C). Under these circumstances, blood flow to the lungs is established from the right coronary artery through intracoronary anastomoses to the aberrant left coronary artery and pulmonary artery. In spite of closure of the patent ductus arteriosus, pulmonary blood flow may be adequate, with survival as long as 21 years.[12] The same hemodynamics are present if there is a coronary artery fistula with the pulmonary artery (see Fig 34–3,D).

Among the variants are pulmonary stenosis and hypoplastic right ventricle, in which the pulmonary valve has a small central opening.[13, 14] The rare case of pulmonary valve atresia and a tiny ventricular septal defect clinically and radiographically resembles pulmonary atresia with an intact ventricular septum.

HEMODYNAMICS

The basic circulatory pattern resembles coexistent tricuspid and pulmonary atresia. The systemic venous return passes predominately from right to left through the atrial communication. In the left atrium it mixes with the pulmonary venous return (which is usually small) and passes through the left ventricle to the aorta (see Fig 34–2). The pulmonary blood flow is tenuous and depends on patency of the ductus arteriosus. As the ductus arteriosus closes during the neonatal period, pulmonary blood flow becomes markedly reduced. With reduction of pulmonary blood flow, systemic hypoxemia and its complications occur and the neonate may die.

In patients with a hypoplastic right ventricle, right ventricular systolic pressure exceeds aortic systolic pressure. The volume of blood that enters the right ventricle equals the small volume of blood that leaves the ventricle through the coronary arteries during systole. During diastole, blood can flow from the aorta back into the right ventricle.

In contrast, when the tricuspid valve is incompetent, the right ventricle does not generate an elevated systolic pressure. The volume of blood entering the right ventricle is large, because it equals the regurgitant volume. As a result, both the right atrium and right ventricle are dilated and markedly pulsatile (see Fig 34–2,D).

CLINICAL FEATURES[6, 15]

At birth, the infant appears normal. As the ductus arteriosus closes, generally during the first day of life, progressive cyanosis, tachypnea, and hyperpnea develop and progress, often rapidly. With hypoxemia, acidosis develops, and the infant becomes ashen and has gasping respirations. We have observed an occasional patient in whom the ductus arteriosus remained patent. Minimal cyanosis and few symptoms were present.

Tricuspid regurgitation (or the hypoplastic right ventricle and small foramen ovale) elevates right atrial pressure. Signs such as hepatomegaly and peripheral edema result from the elevated pressure.

In those patients with a hypoplastic right ventricle, cardiac activity is normal. Usually no murmur is heard, but there may be a soft murmur, either systolic or continuous, from blood flow through the patent ductus arteriosus. With tricuspid regurgitation, cardiac activity is increased, and there is a prominent systolic murmur, perhaps associated with a thrill along the lower left sternal border, and a middiastolic murmur in the same area. The second heart sound is single, but this is the expected finding in a neonate during the first 2 days of life.

The auscultatory findings are not diagnostic but should raise the possibility of pulmonary atresia either because the continuous murmur suggests ductal dependency or because a murmur of tricuspid regurgitation is present. These clinical findings suggest the differential diagnosis of pulmonary atresia, tricuspid regurgitation, Ebstein's malformation of the tricuspid valve, transient tricuspid regurgitation of the newborn, or intrinsic anomalies of the tricuspid valve, perhaps associated with right ventricular abnormalities.

ELECTROCARDIOGRAPHIC FEATURES[15, 16]

The QRS axis is usually normal, or directed slightly to the right, in contrast to the left axis deviation found in tricuspid atresia. Another feature distinguishing these two conditions is the presence of a qR pattern in lead aVF in the former and a qR pattern in lead I of the latter.

The P waves are often tall, peaked, and pointed, indicating right atrial enlargement. In patients surviving operation, this may remain the only electrocardiographic finding.

The precordial leads show a variable QRS pattern. Among those with a hypoplastic right ventricle, the precordial leads show an rS pattern in lead V_1 and a predominant R wave in lead V_6 (a pattern resembling tricuspid atresia). In those with a dilated right ventricle, the precordial leads may be normal or show right ventricular hypertrophy.

The T waves are normal.

ECHOCARDIOGRAPHIC FEATURES

The two-dimensional echocardiogram is quite useful in reaching a diagnosis of pulmonary atresia, in identifying other major anatomic features, and distinguishing anatomic from functional pulmonary atresia.[17] On the subcostal and short-axis views, the right ventricular outflow area and pulmonary artery are visualized, and the pulmonary valve is seen as a precordial platelike membrane, which may be mobile but does not open. This is in contrast to the aortic valve, often seen en face in the same view that shows normal movement of the leaflets. The caliber of the pulmonary trunk and proximal pulmonary arteries can be measured and the area beneath the pulmonary valve evaluated for coexistent infundibular atresia. On a subcostal or apical view, the right ventricular cavity size can be assessed.[18] The subcostal view shows the details of the atrial septum, including diameter of the atrial communication.

Echo Doppler is an excellent means of detecting and assessing the severity of coexistent tricuspid regurgitation, determining right-to-left atrial shunting, showing pulmonary arterial filling from the ductus and occasionally demonstrating intramyocardial sinusoids and retrograde coronary flow.

RADIOGRAPHIC FEATURES

The radiographic appearance of pulmonary atresia with intact ventricular septum is not uniform and is determined largely by the competency of the tricuspid valve. In patients without tricuspid regurgitation, in which the only egress of blood from the right ventricle is through myocardial sinusoids, the right ventricle is diminutive and the right atrium not greatly enlarged. Cardiac size is normal in such patients.

Because tricuspid regurgitation allows free flow of blood into and out of the right ventricle, the right ventricle and right atrium are significantly enlarged. The enlarged right atrium contributes to the overall cardiac size on a thoracic roentgenogram. A large degree of tricuspid regurgitation causes severe right atrial and right ventricular enlargement and massive cardiomegaly.

Pulmonary atresia with intact ventricular septum can present one of the largest cardiac silhouettes found among neonates. Cardiomegaly is present in many patients, because the right atrium is usually enlarged as a result of elevated right atrial pressure from a narrow foramen ovale or tricuspid regurgitation.

1. Cardiac size may be normal (Fig 34–4), making differentiation from the more commonly occurring tetralogy of Fallot difficult. With a competent tricuspid valve, the right ventricle is diminutive and the right atrium not significantly enlarged unless there is obstruction at the level of the fossa ovalis (rare).

2. The left cardiac border tends to be rounded (see Fig 34–4), identical to tricuspid atresia because it has the same hemodynamics. REASON: The left ventricle carries the entire pulmonary and systemic blood flows, resulting in various degrees of left ventricular enlargement, depending on the volume of pulmonary blood flow. Because of left ventricular enlargement, counterclockwise rotation of the heart occurs, displacing the right ventricle medially. The rounded left cardiac contour in pulmonary atresia with intact septum is not as marked as in patients with tricuspid atresia in whom pulmonary blood flow is greater and the left ventricle larger.

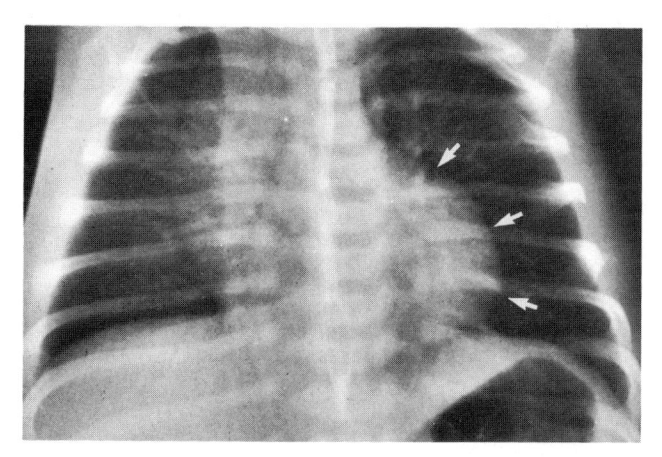

FIG 34-4.
Pulmonary atresia and intact ventricular septum. Neonate. Thoracic roentgenogram. Anteroposterior projection. Normal cardiac size. Pulmonary vasculature is at the lower limits of normal because ductus arteriosus is still patent. Round left cardiac border *(arrows)* is similar to tricuspid atresia. Concave pulmonary arterial segment. Prominence of right cardiac border because of thymus. Radiologic differentiation from more common tetralogy of Fallot cannot be made with certainty, although round cardiac contour is more consistent with pulmonary atresia or tricuspid atresia.

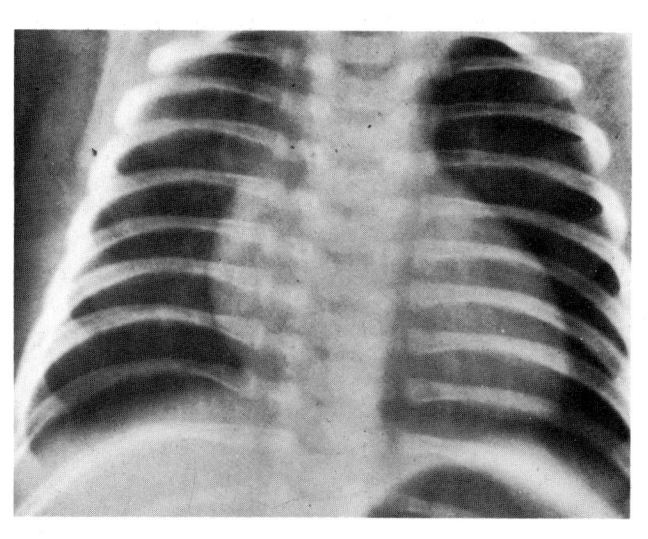

FIG 34-5.
Pulmonary atresia and mild tricuspid regurgitation. Thoracic roentgenogram. Posteroanterior projection. Mild enlargement of cardiac silhouette. Left cardiac border has rounded left ventricular configuration. Pulmonary arterial segment is not prominent. Decreased pulmonary vasculature. Prominent right atrial border.

3. The pulmonary vasculature is decreased but may appear within normal limits for a neonate. REASON: Adequate blood flow through the patent ductus arteriosus may be present, and the radiographic appearance of the pulmonary vasculature in a neonate is normally sparse. In spite of the patent ductus arteriosus, however, the pulmonary vasculature is not increased because of the elevated fetal pulmonary vascular resistance and the normal tendency for closure of the ductus arteriosus.

4. The pulmonary arterial segment is concave. REASON: With this condition the main pulmonary artery is always small and located more centrally because of counterclockwise rotation of the heart.

5. In one half of neonates with pulmonary atresia, cardiac size is nearly normal. After birth, however, there is progressive and rapid cardiac enlargement. REASON: Associated tricuspid regurgitation causes increasing distention of the right atrium and dilatation of the right ventricle.

6. There may be mild cardiomegaly (Fig 34-5). REASON: Most patients with pulmonary atresia have some degree of tricuspid regurgitation resulting in right atrial enlargement.

7. The right atrial border tends to be prominent. REASON: Tricuspid insufficiency increases right ventricular and right atrial size.

8. There may be moderate or severe cardiomegaly (Fig 34-6). REASON: With increasing degrees of incompetence of the tricuspid valve, there is a continuum of right atrial and right ventricular enlargement. The presence of moderate or marked cardiomegaly on a thoracic roentgenogram suggests the association of either severe tricuspid valvar dysplasia or Ebstein's malformation of the tricuspid valve.

9. There may be massive cardiomegaly (Fig 34-7). REASON: The combination of severe tricuspid regurgitation and a failing right ventricle leads to the largest cardiac silhouettes seen in neonates. This cardiac silhouette is indistinguishable from Ebstein's malformation of the tricuspid

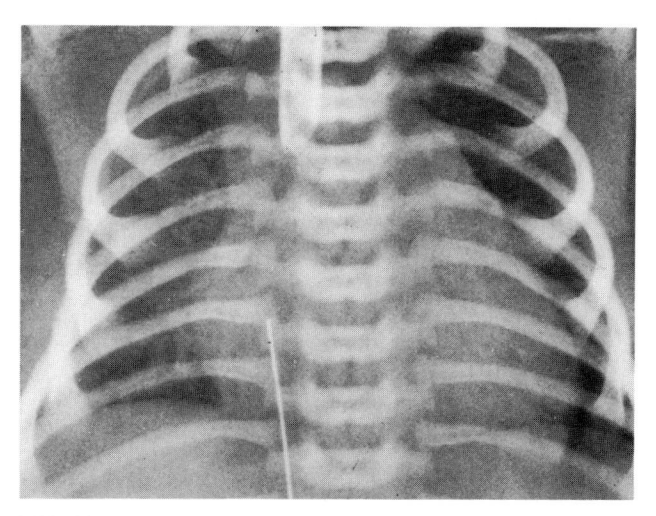

FIG 34-6.
Pulmonary atresia, intact ventricular septum, and severe tricuspid regurgitation. Thoracic roentgenogram. Posteroanterior projection. Severe cardiomegaly. Pulmonary vasculature is extremely sparse. Cardiac configuration is not characteristic of pulmonary atresia.

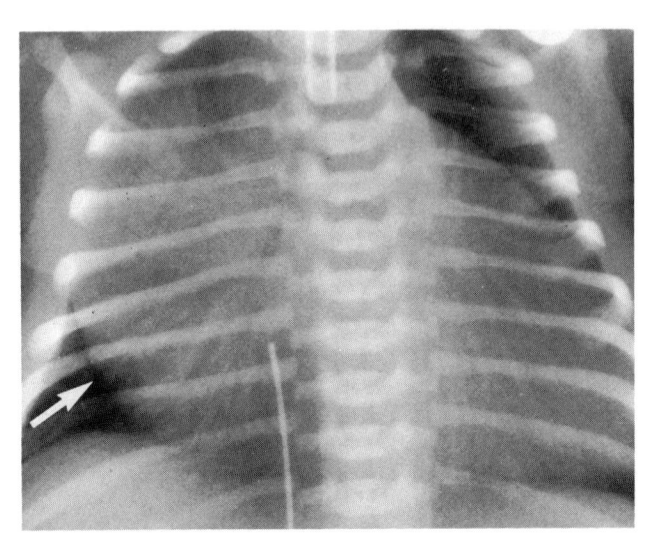

FIG 34–7.
Pulmonary atresia, intact ventricular septum, and associated Ebstein's malformation of the tricuspid valve. Severe tricuspid regurgitation. Thoracic roentgenogram. Posteroanterior projection. Heart is massively enlarged, occupying almost entire thoracic cavity. Right cardiac border is formed by a huge dilated right atrium *(arrow).*

valve or isolated tricuspid insufficiency of the newborn (see Chapters 36 and 76). Sometimes pericardial effusion (very rare in neonates) or a mediastinal tumor may also produce a massively enlarged cardiac silhouette.

10. The aortic arch is virtually always on the left side. When a right arch is present, pulmonary atresia with ventricular septal defect is much more likely.

11. The left atrium is of normal size or only slightly enlarged. REASON: Although left atrial blood flow consists of the entire systemic and pulmonary venous returns, in most patients pulmonary blood flow is so small that the left atrium is only minimally enlarged. Left atrial enlargement is therefore less common than in tricuspid atresia, which tends to have much larger pulmonary blood flow.

12. With increasing degrees of cardiomegaly, the barium-filled esophagus may be significantly displaced by the enlarged right side of the heart, giving the appearance of left atrial enlargement (pseudo left atrial enlargement). Differentiation between true and false left atrial enlargement may be impossible radiographically.

13. In older patients with pulmonary atresia, if the pleural space has been entered during a thoracotomy, collateral arteries may develop through the adhesions. Unilateral rib notching may develop (rare).

CARDIAC CATHETERIZATION

Cardiac catheterization is performed to distinguish among the various conditions and to determine the size of the right ventricle, and to assess the character of the tricuspid valve.

The catheter can easily be advanced from the inferior vena cava through the right atrium into the left atrium and left ventricle in a fashion similar to tricuspid atresia. It may be impossible to advance the catheter tip into a hypoplastic right ventricle. If the right ventricle is dilated, the catheter can enter the right ventricle. With excessive tricuspid regurgitation, the catheter may show an exaggerated to-and-fro movement into and out of the right ventricle. Although it may be possible to manipulate an arterial catheter from the aorta through the ductus arteriosus into the pulmonary artery, this is inadvisable, because it may obstruct a narrowed ductus and thereby increase the hypoxemia.

The oxygen saturations in the right side of the heart are quite low. Evidence of right-to-left shunt is present at the atrial level. Systemic arterial desaturation is present, the severity being inversely related to the volume of pulmonary blood flow.

Right atrial pressures, particularly the a wave, are elevated. In patients with a hypoplastic right ventricle, right ventricular systolic pressure may reach 120 to 130 mm Hg, whereas in those with tricuspid regurgitation, it is only slightly or moderately elevated. Right ventricular end-diastolic pressure may be elevated to 15 mm Hg.

After pulmonary valvotomy, right ventricular size may become normal, although right-to-left shunting may remain because of persistently decreased compliance of the right ventricle. The shunt may be eliminated by closing the foramen ovale operatively, but the right ventricle must be adequate to handle the systemic cardiac output. Adequacy of the right ventricle can be determined during a postoperative cardiac catheterization by occluding the foramen ovale with a balloon and measuring the cardiac output and the pressures in the right atrium and ventricle.[16] Although right ventricular volume can also be measured by biplane angiography, such techniques are less accurate for the right ventricle than for the left ventricle because of the more complex shape of the former. Furthermore, in the calculation of right ventricular volume, it is difficult to compensate for the heavy trabeculations.

ANGIOGRAPHIC FEATURES

Angiography plays an important role in the preoperative assessment of patients with pulmonary atresia with intact ventricular septum. Right ventricular and aortic injections should be made and usually a right atrial injection provides additional information. The angiographic findings largely determine the type of operative procedure.

Right Atriography

The right atrium can be opacified by either venous angiography or selective injection through a catheter.

1. The right atrium is invariably enlarged. REASON: Because of the obligatory right-to-left shunt at the atrial level, right atrial pressures are elevated or equal left atrial pressures provided the atrial communication is of adequate size.

2. In most patients, a pressure gradient does not exist across the atrial communication, and the right atrium is therefore only slightly enlarged (Fig 34–8).

3. In patients with tricuspid regurgitation, the right atrium may be huge (see Fig 34–18). This occurs particularly if Ebstein's malformation of the tricuspid valve coexists (see Fig 34–19).

4. Immediate opacification of the left atrium and left ventricle occurs in diastole (see Fig 34–8).

5. The left atrium and the left ventricle are slightly enlarged, and the left ventricle shows mild left ventricular hypertrophy. Left ventricular size depends largely on the amount of pulmonary blood flow.

6. The right ventricle may not opacify. REASON: In patients without tricuspid regurgitation, the only exit of blood from the right ventricle is through myocardial sinusoids. The inflow of blood into the right ventricle may be minute; consequently, little opaque material enters this chamber during angiography. Nonopacification of the right ventricle on right atriography therefore does not always indicate tricuspid atresia.

7. If there is sufficient inflow of blood into the right ventricle as in instances with tricuspid regurgitation, the right ventricle, including its inflow portion, opacifies (see Fig 34–18). This is an important differential diagnostic point, because most patients with tricuspid atresia lack an inflow portion of the right ventricle, although exceptions exist (see Chapter 33).

8. When the right ventricle is opacified, the characteristic clear space between the right atrium and the left ventricle commonly seen in tricuspid atresia (right ventricular window) is obliterated by the contrast material (see Fig 34–8).

9. The size of the foramen ovale can be determined by right atrial injection in a left anterior oblique projection with cranial beam angulation (Fig 34–9,A). It can also be gauged by drawing a balloon-tipped catheter across the plane of the atrial septum and measuring balloon diameter.

10. The size of the hypoplastic tricuspid annulus and status of the tricuspid valve are evaluated in right anterior oblique projection (Fig 34–9,B).

11. Obstruction at the level of the foramen ovale may result in herniation of the atrial septum toward the left atrium, forming an aneurysm of the fossa ovalis (Fig 34–10).

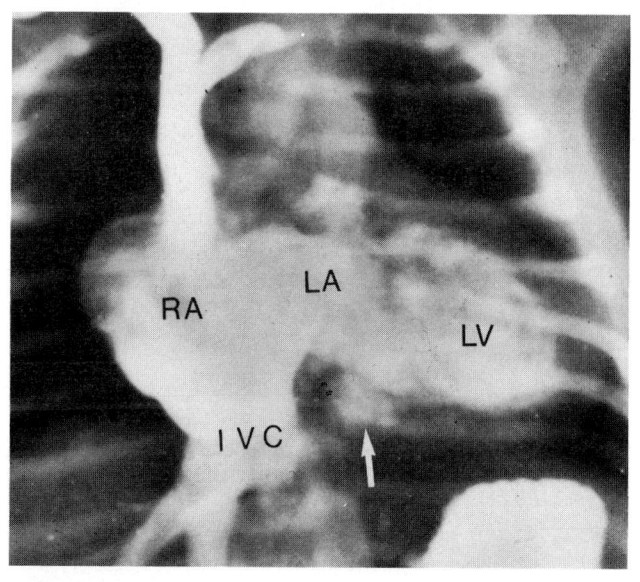

Right Ventriculography

Right ventriculography is the most important angiographic evaluation. Consequently, vigorous attempts should be made to pass the catheter into the right ventricle. In patients with associated tricuspid stenosis or hypoplasia of the tricuspid annulus, this may not be possible.

Once the catheter has entered the right ventricle, a small amount of opaque material should be injected manually to estimate the size of the right ventricle. Then standard right ventriculography can be performed using a proper amount of contrast medium and delivery rate. In patients with a diminutive right ventricle, a small amount of contrast medium should be injected comparatively slowly, whereas patients with significant tricuspid regurgitation require a large amount of contrast medium to be delivered rapidly. In patients with a competent tricuspid valve, a diminutive right ventricle, and coronary sinusoids, adequate opacification can be obtained by manual injection, although a power injection is preferred.

Right ventriculography is important, because it allows visualization of the following:

1. Right ventricular size.[19] Both anteroposterior and lateral projections are necessary to assess right ventricular

FIG 34–8.
Pulmonary atresia and intact ventricular septum. Venous angiogram. Anteroposterior projection. Enlarged right atrium *(RA)* and inferior vena cava *(IVC)*. Opacification of left atrium *(LA)* and slightly enlarged left ventricle *(LV)*. Small right ventricle *(arrow)* is also opacified. In contrast to tricuspid atresia, sinus portion of right ventricle *(arrow)*, although small is developed.

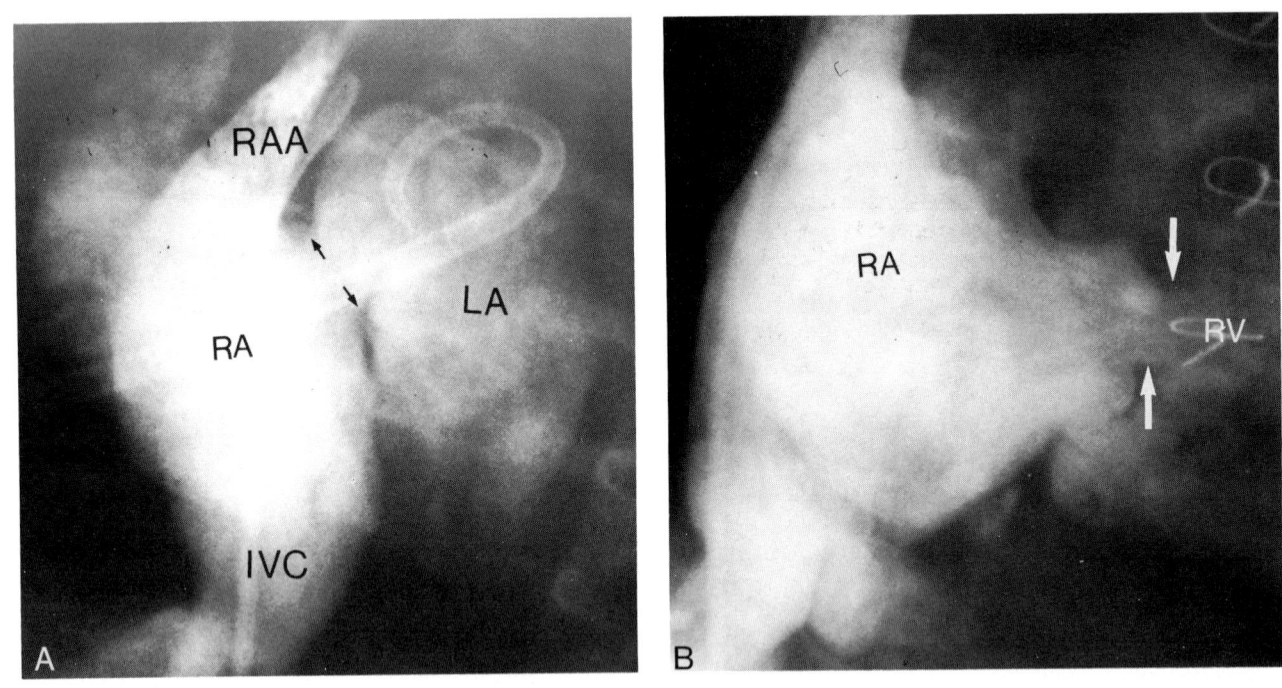

FIG 34–9.
Pulmonary atresia and intact ventricular septum. **A,** right atriogram *(RA).* Left anterior oblique projection with cranial beam angulation. Adequate-sized atrial communication *(arrows).* **B,** right atriogram, right anterior oblique projection. After operation. Atrial communication is closed. Tricuspid valve is stenotic *(arrows).* LA = left atrium; *IVC* = inferior vena cava; *RAA* = right atrial appendage; *RV* = right ventricle.

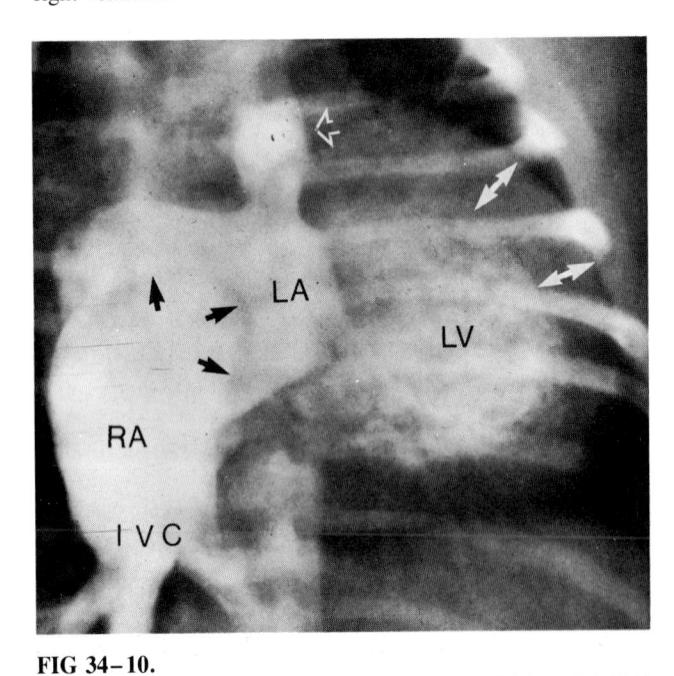

FIG 34–10.
Pulmonary atresia and intact ventricular septum. Right atrial *(RA)* angiogram. Anteroposterior projection. Herniation of the fossa ovalis *(black arrows)* is forming aneurysm of fossa ovalis. Enlarged inferior vena cava *(IVC).* Right ventricle is not opacified. Opacification of a structure *(open arrow)* in region of right ventricular outflow tract is an atypical left atrial appendage. Enlarged and thick-walled left ventricular *(LV)* cavity *(white arrows).* LA = left atrium.

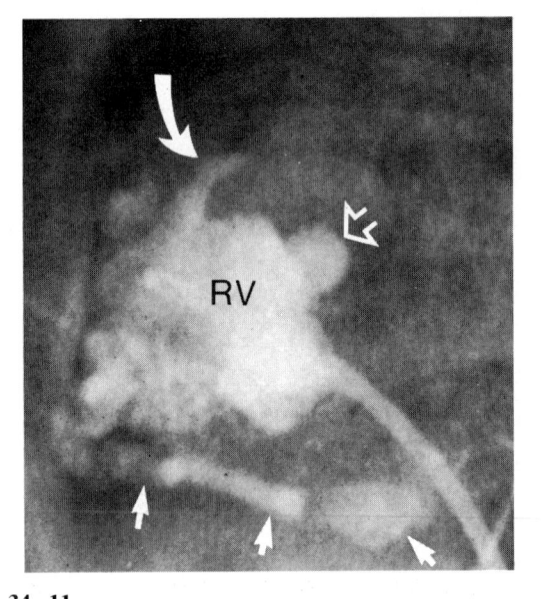

FIG 34–11.
Pulmonary atresia and competent tricuspid valve. Right ventriculogram *(RV).* Lateral projection. Hypoplastic atretic infundibulum *(curved arrow).* Filling of coronary artery through sinusoids *(white solid arrows).* Aneurysm of membranous septum *(open arrow)* is bulging into left ventricle during systole, indicating that right ventricular systolic pressure exceeds left ventricular systolic pressure. Normally, aneurysms of membranous septum bulge into right ventricle, because left ventricular pressure exceeds right ventricular pressure (see Chapter 14).

size. If right ventricular volume measurements are contemplated, biplane views are mandatory. Right ventricular size and function are important for operative management.

2. Functional assessment (together with pressure measurements) of the tricuspid valve.

3. Ventricular contractility, which may be decreased.

4. The infundibulum and atretic pulmonary valve.[20] A markedly narrowed or atretic infundibulum may alter the operative approach, because valvulotomy and incision of the annulus may not relieve the obstruction.

The size of the right ventricular cavity varies, depending on the volume of blood flow through the tricuspid valve.[21] The size and competency of the tricuspid valve, therefore, largely determine right ventricular size.

1. The right ventricle may be diminutive. REASON: In such patients, the tricuspid valve is competent, and the only egress of blood from the right ventricle occurs through myocardial sinusoids (Fig 34–11).

2. In a patient with a diminutive right ventricle, the tricuspid annulus is hypoplastic. REASON: A small right ventricle can accept only a small tricuspid annulus.

3. With a small right ventricular cavity, the infundibulum is usually diminutive (see Fig 34–11) or it may be completely obliterated by myocardium (infundibular atresia).

4. Myocardial sinusoids provide the only egress of blood from the right ventricle and usually occur from the right ventricle to the coronary arteries (Fig 34–12,A). Contrast medium leaves the right ventricle during systole

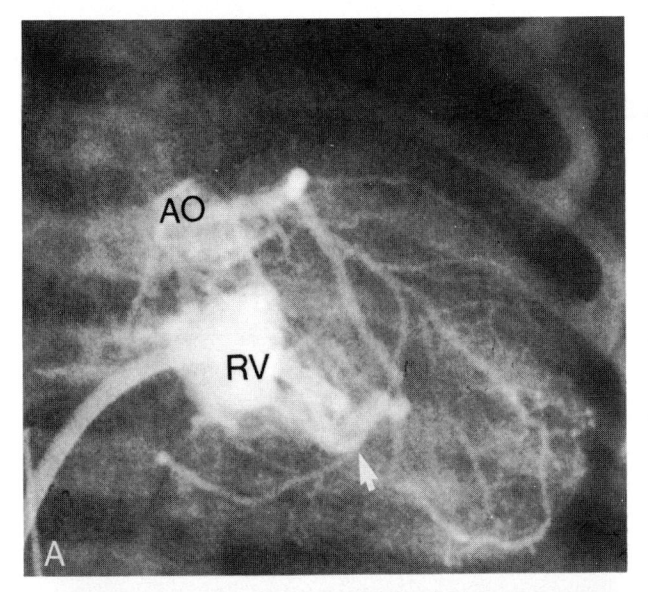

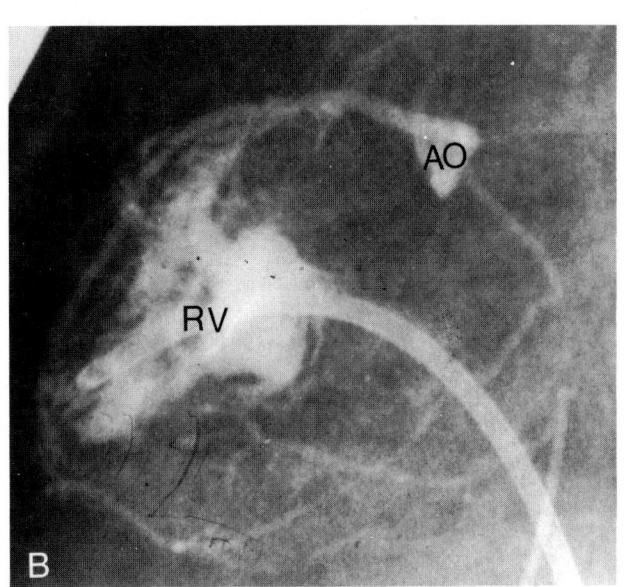

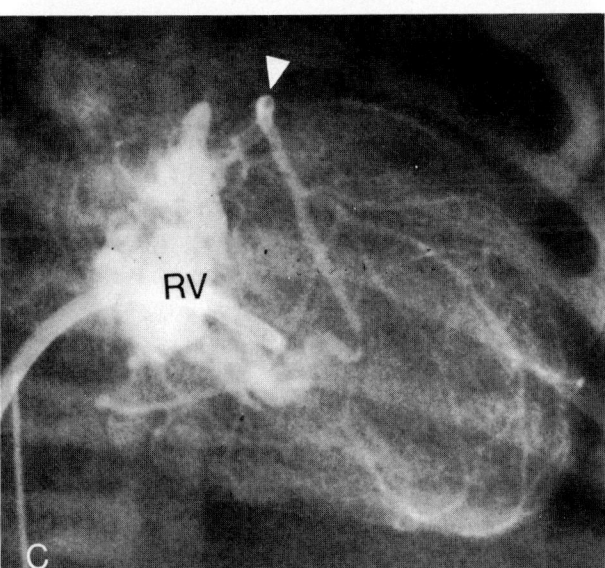

FIG 34–12.
Pulmonary atresia and intact ventricular septum. Diminutive right ventricle. Egress of blood only through well-developed sinusoids. Right ventriculograms *(RV)*. **A,** anteroposterior projection. Systole. Sinusoids *(arrows)* are well opacified. Coronary blood flow occurs into aorta *(AO)*. **B,** lateral projection. Systole. Large left anterior descending and circumflex coronary artery branches carry blood to aorta. **C,** anteroposterior projection. Diastole. Unopacified blood *(arrowhead)* from aorta enters left anterior descending and circumflex coronary arterial branches. Retrograde blood flow during diastole from aorta into right ventricle.

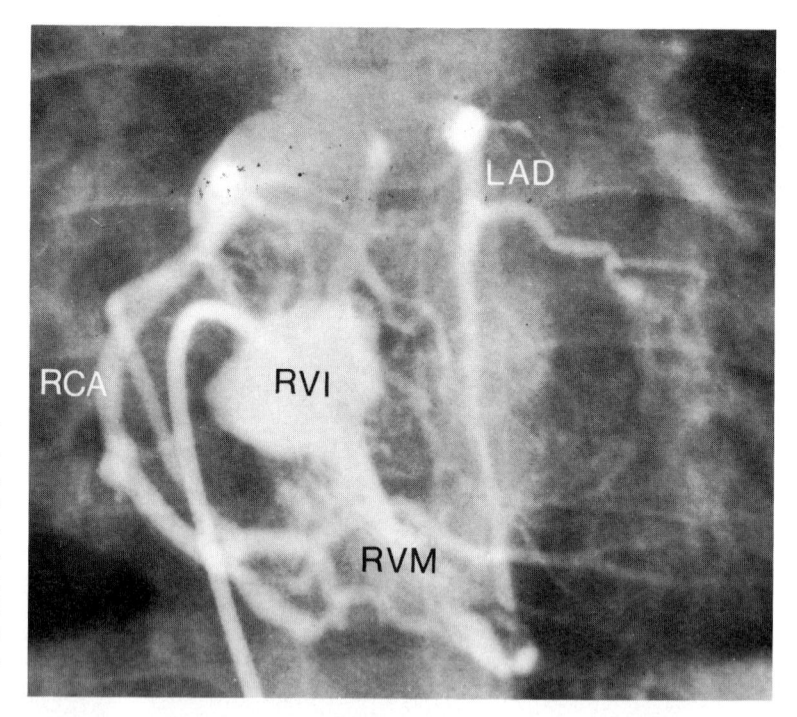

FIG 34–13.
Pulmonary atresia, intact ventricular septum, and infundibular atresia. Hypoplasia of right ventricle. Right ventriculogram. Anteroposterior projection. Egress of blood through unusually well-developed sinusoids, including right coronary arterial tree. Because of counterclockwise rotation of heart, right ventricular cavity occupies medial position. Smooth right ventricular inflow portion *(RVI)* and trabeculated muscular portion *(RVM)*. Atretic infundibulum. *LAD* = left anterior descending; *RCA* = right coronary artery.

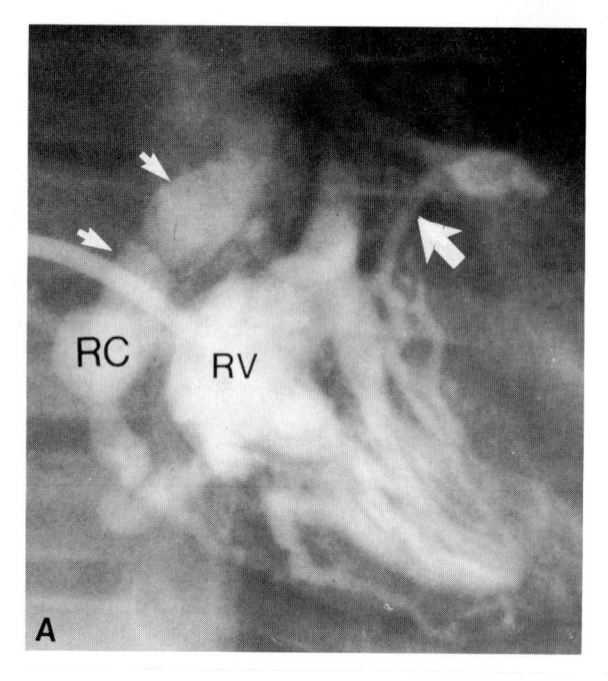

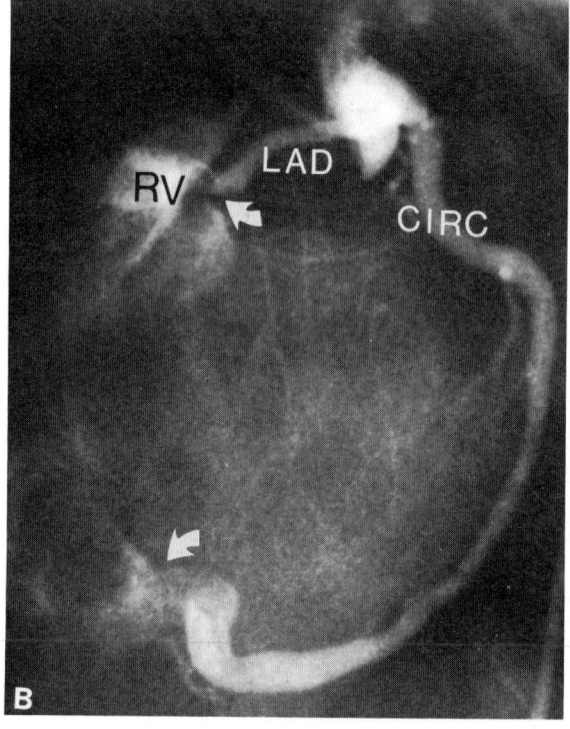

FIG 34–14.
Pulmonary atresia and hypoplastic right ventricle. **A,** right ventriculogram. Anteroposterior projection. Hypoplastic right ventricle with characteristic division between sinus *(RV)* and muscular portion. Right *(small arrows)* and left *(large arrow)* coronary arteries are filled through sinusoids. Right coronary artery *(RC)* shows aneurysmal dilatation. **B,** selective left coronary arteriogram. Left anterior oblique projection. The left descending artery *(LAD)* and circumflex branch *(CIRC)* have fistulous communications *(arrows)* with right ventricle *(RV)*. There is complete interruption of left anterior descending branch *(upper arrow)*.

since right ventricular systolic pressure exceeds that in the aorta. Retrograde flow of blood then occurs into the aorta (see Fig 34–12,B).

5. During ventricular diastole (see Fig 34–12,C), blood flows back from the aorta into the coronary arteries and sometimes into the right ventricle. REASON: Aortic diastolic pressure exceeds right ventricular diastolic pressure.

6. Although sinusoids occur more commonly to the left coronary arterial system, they may also be present in the right coronary artery (Fig 34–13) or the entire coronary arterial tree.

7. Blood flow through the coronary arteries may be very large, resulting in aneurysmal dilatation of the coronary tree (Fig 34–14,A). After operation and decrease of right ventricular systolic pressure, an aortic runoff (coronary artery fistula) into the right ventricle may be present (see Fig 34–29).

8. There may be complete interruption of a coronary artery (Fig 34–14,B). Demonstration of the coronary arteries by selective injection is therefore important before operation.

9. Patients with prominent myocardial sinusoids may have marked left ventricular enlargement and hypertrophy. REASON: The left ventricle carries systemic and pulmonary blood flow, and the left ventricle is perfused with desaturated blood from the right ventricle.

10. Because of marked right ventricular hypertrophy, the three portions of the ventricle are usually well delineated (see Figs 34–14 and 34–15). These include the sinus portion, which is usually smooth; the trabecular portion, which is highly trabeculated with very little capacity; and infundibular or outflow portion.

11. There is a continuous spectrum from critical pulmonary stenosis with adequate-sized right ventricle to critical pulmonary stenosis with right ventricular hypoplasia (Fig 34–15) to pulmonary atresia with severe right ventricular hypoplasia.

12. When the trabecular portion of the right ventricle is unusually well developed, estimation of right ventricular

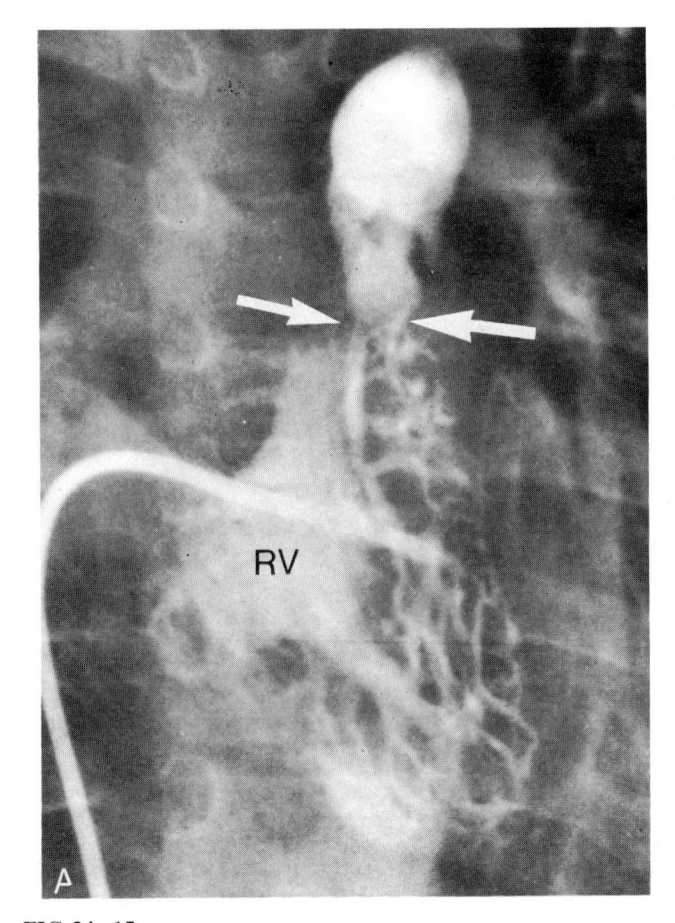

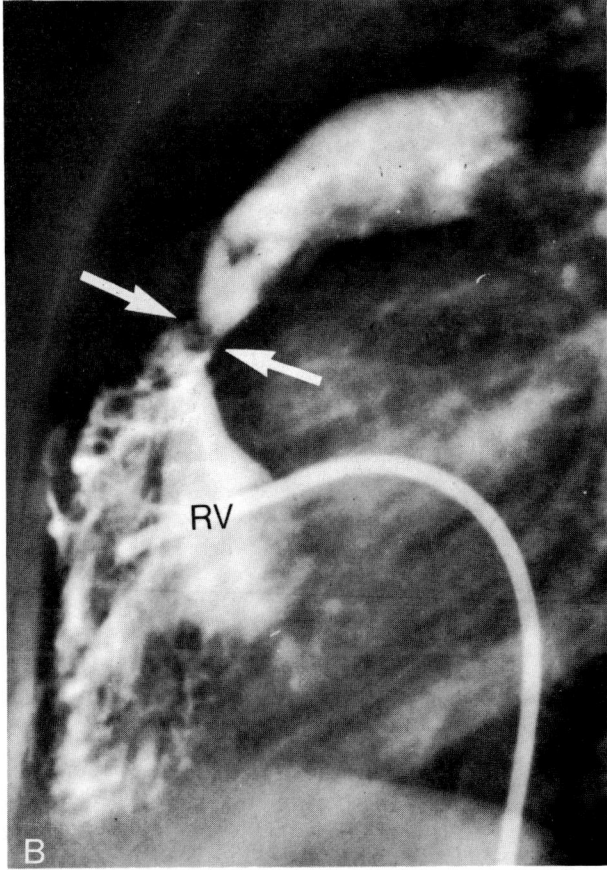

FIG 34–15.
Critical valvar pulmonary stenosis and right-to-left shunt at atrial level. Right ventriculogram. **A,** anteroposterior and **B,** lateral projections. Most of right ventricle consists of an unusually well-developed muscular portion. Very small inflow portion *(RV)*. Almost complete infundibular obstruction *(arrows)*. Because right ventricular cavity is obliterated by muscle, it is judged as hypoplastic. Left pulmonary artery is not opacified because of patent Blalock-Taussig shunt.

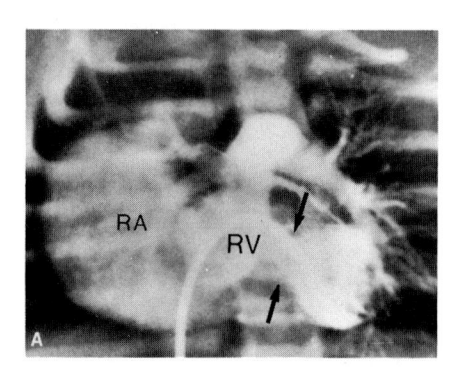

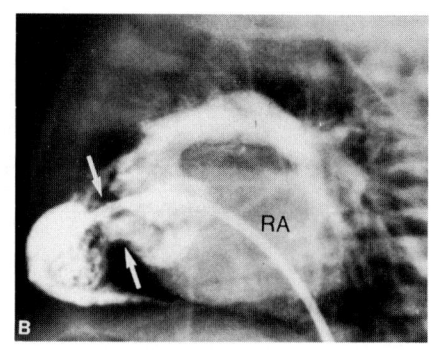

FIG 34–16.
Critical valvar pulmonary stenosis and right-to-left shunt at atrial level. Right ventriculogram *(RV)*. **A,** anteroposterior and, **B,** lateral projections. Severe tricuspid regurgitation but no evidence of Ebstein's malformation. Large muscle mass in right ventricle causes hourglass deformity *(arrows)*. RA = right atrium.

size may be difficult (see Fig 34–15). The capacity of the right ventricle may be overestimated.

13. In patients with pulmonary atresia or critical pulmonary stenosis and an intact septum, large muscle masses may give a characteristic hourglass deformity to the right ventricle (Fig 34–16).

14. The right ventricle and right atrium are greatly enlarged in patients with massive tricuspid regurgitation as a result of either coexistent dysplasia (Figs 34–17 and 34–18), Ebstein's malformation of the tricuspid valve (Fig 34–19) or other tricuspid valve abnormalities.

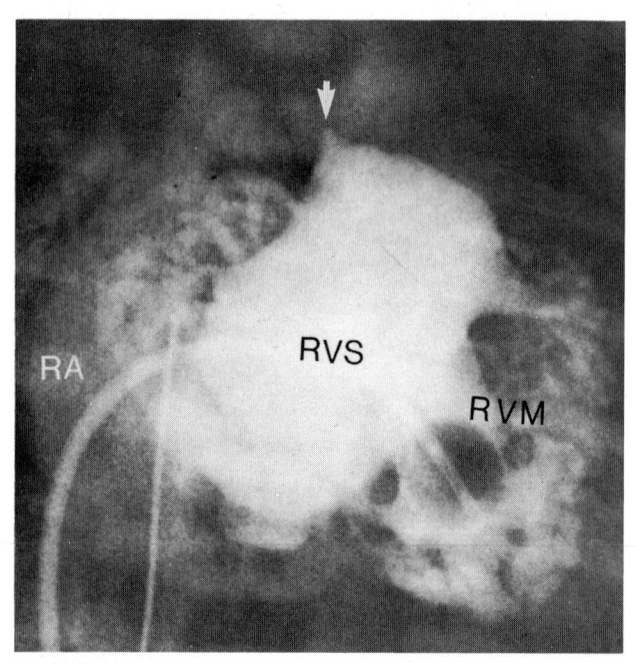

15. The infundibulum may be atretic, severely stenotic, or widely patent (see Fig 34–19).

16. Neonates with massive tricuspid regurgitation and a normal pulmonary valve may generate insufficient right ventricular systolic pressure to open the pulmonary valve. This angiographic appearance simulates pulmonary atresia. In this circumstance, the normally elevated pulmonary arterial pressure because of pulmonary resistance of the neonate, hold the valve closed. Therefore, in a neonate with a low right ventricular systolic pressure from massive tricuspid reflux, nonopacification of the pulmonary artery after right ventriculography has been termed "functional pulmonary atresia." In such patients, pulmonary arteriography or aortography may demonstrate reflux through the pulmonary valve (Fig 34–20), thereby excluding anatomic pulmonary atresia.[22]

17. With an increasing degree of tricuspid regurgitation, the right ventricle enlarges. Right ventricular size depends on blood flow into that chamber.

18. Differentiation between a dysplastic tricuspid valve and Ebstein's anomaly of the tricuspid valve may be difficult. Sometimes only small remnants of downward displaced valvar leaflets are demonstrated. There is a spectrum of malformations from severe dysplasia of the tricuspid valve to Ebstein's malformation and unguarded orifice of the tricuspid valve (complete absence of valve tissue) (Fig 34–21).

19. Occasionally an aneurysm of the membranous ventricular septum may coexist. It bulges into the left ventricular outflow tract, if right ventricular systolic pressure is markedly elevated (see Fig 34–11). If the tricuspid valve is competent, the right ventricle develops suprasystemic pressure, which causes the aneurysm of the membranous septum to bulge from right to left. Normally such an aneurysm would bulge into the right ventricle (see Chapter 14).

FIG 34–17.
Pulmonary atresia, intact ventricular septum, and tricuspid regurgitation. Anteroposterior projection. Enlarged right ventricle. Smooth sinus portion *(RVS)* is well delineated from heavily trabeculated right ventricular muscular portion *(RVM)*. Huge muscle bundles. Valvar pulmonary atresia *(white arrow)*. RA = right atrium.

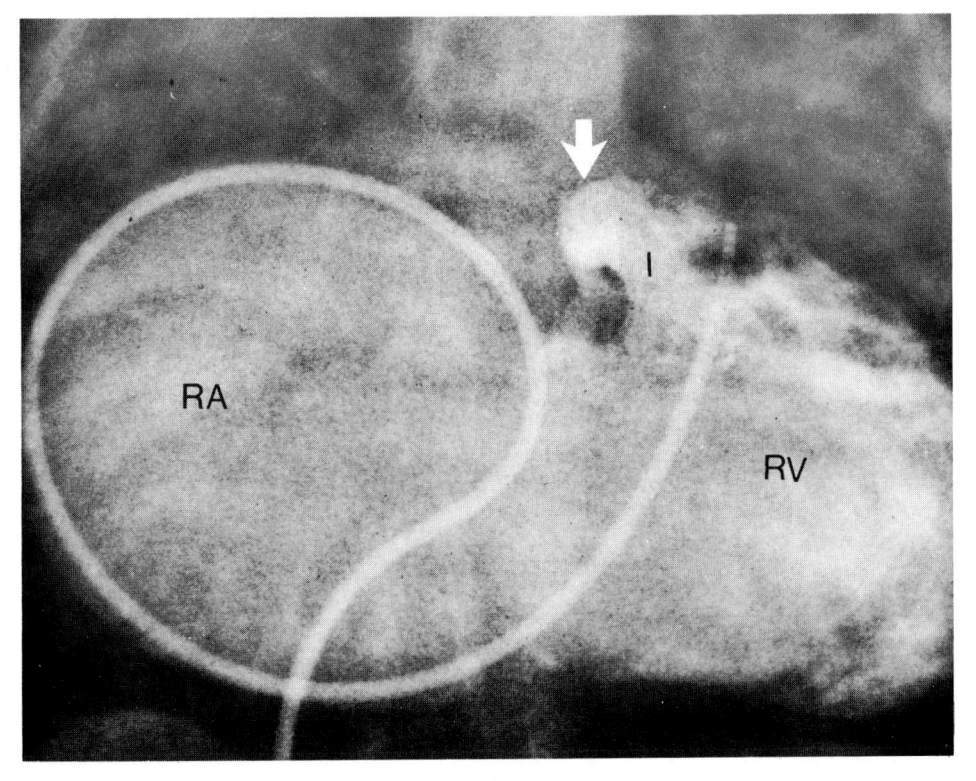

FIG 34–18.
Pulmonary atresia, intact ventricular septum, and tricuspid regurgitation. Right ventriculogram (RV). Anteroposterior projection. Massive right ventricular enlargement. Catheter is coiled in giant right atrium (RA). Mechanism for tricuspid regurgitation uncertain. No evidence of Ebstein's malformation. I = infundibulum. Arrow indicates atretic pulmonary valve.

Aortography

Aortography is required to demonstrate the status of the ductus arteriosus, the pulmonary arterial tree, and the coronary arteries. Best results are obtained with balloon occlusion aortography, in which a balloon is momentarily inflated in the descending aorta beyond the patent ductus arteriosus while an injection is made proximally.

Demonstration of the coronary arteries is important. REASONS: First, there may be no connection of a coronary artery with the aorta (see Figs 34–3,B and 34–14,B). Under this circumstance, operative correction and consequent decrease of right ventricular systolic pressure may result in nonperfusion of a coronary artery and massive myocardial

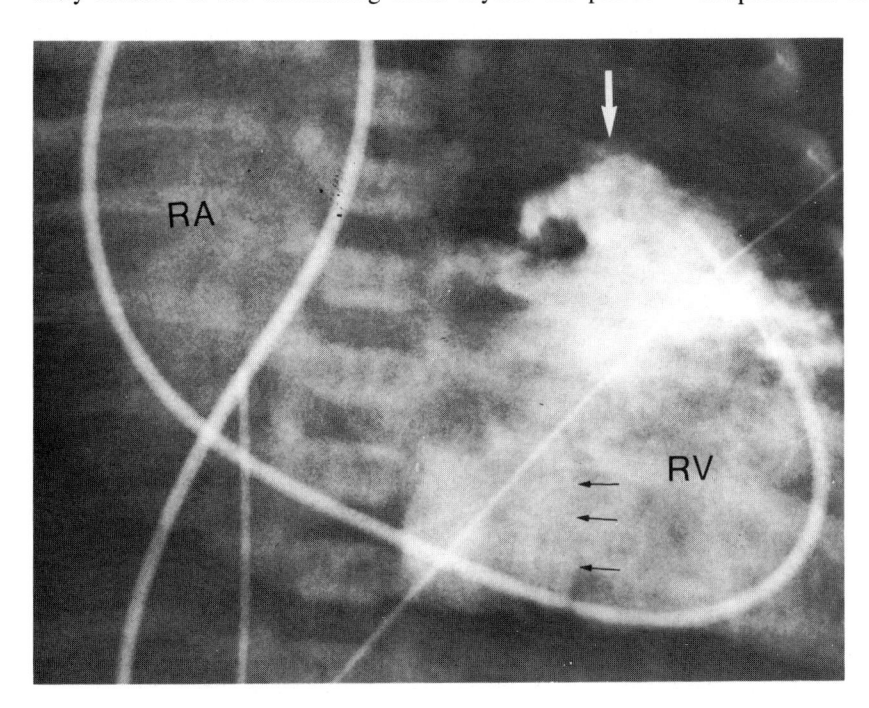

FIG 34–19.
Pulmonary atresia (arrow), intact ventricular septum, large infundibulum, and tricuspid regurgitation from Ebstein's malformation. Right ventriculogram (RV). Anteroposterior projection. Downwardly displaced tricuspid valve leaflet (black arrows). Catheter is coiled in giant atrium (RA), which is opacified because of tricuspid regurgitation.

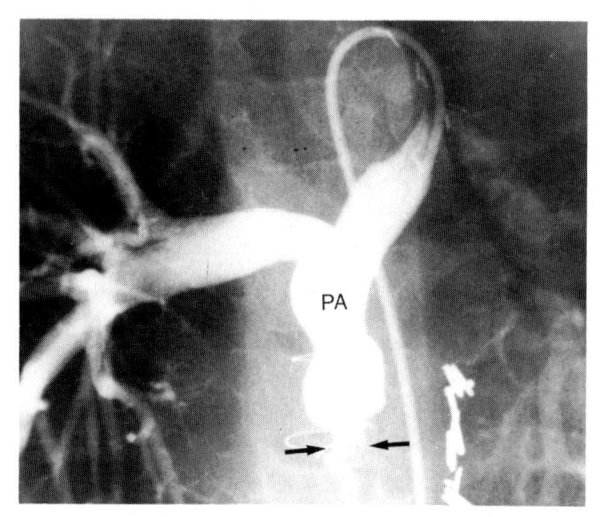

FIG 34-20.
Functional pulmonary atresia and Blalock-Taussig anastomosis. Catheter passed through anastomosis into main pulmonary artery *(PA)*. Small amount of reflux *(arrows)* through pulmonary valve. Right ventriculography in neonatal period failed to opacify pulmonary artery. Erroneous diagnosis of anatomic pulmonary atresia was made.

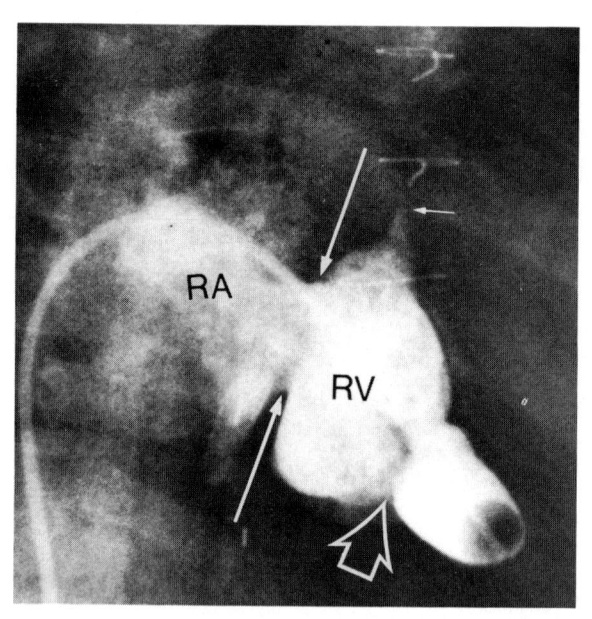

FIG 34-21.
Pulmonary infundibular atresia *(small white arrow)* and unguarded tricuspid valve. Right ventriculogram *(RV)*. Right anterior oblique projection. Tricuspid annulus *(long arrows)* visualized. Opacification of right atrium *(RA)* because of regurgitation. At postmortem examination, a tiny remnant of valve tissue was found near the apex *(open arrow)*. This condition was diagnosed pathologically as pulmonary atresia with unguarded tricuspid valve and severe form of Ebstein's malformation.

infarction. Second, the sinusoidal connection of the coronary artery with the ventricle may be huge, allowing a large diastolic flow from the aorta into the right ventricle. Under this circumstance, ligation or patch closure of the anomalous connection is indicated to prevent a large coronary fistula after operation. Third, only a segment of a coronary artery may communicate with the right ventricle, resulting in interruption of the artery (see Fig 34-14,B).

1. The patent ductus arteriosus varies in size, is more tortuous, and arises higher on the aortic arch than normal (Figs 34-1,B and 34-22). The ductus appears more like a branch arising from the aortic arch than a continuation of the left pulmonary artery (see Fig 34-22). During fetal life the ductus arteriosus carries blood from the aorta into the pulmonary arteries, in contrast to the normal ductus arteriosus, which carries blood from the pulmonary artery primarily into the descending aorta. This difference of blood flow in patients with pulmonary atresia very likely accounts for the different shape and orientation of the ductus arteriosus (see Fig 34-1).

2. The main pulmonary artery and pulmonary annulus are hypoplastic. The degree varies among patients. REASON: Lack of blood flow through this segment of the pulmonary artery.

3. Opacification of the pulmonary arterial tree shows varying degrees of hypoplasia.

4. If reflux of contrast medium occurs through the pulmonary valve, differentiation of functional atresia (no forward flow on right ventriculography) from anatomic atresia (complete obliteration of the pulmonary valve) (see Fig 34-20) can be made. Two angiographic features may allow distinction of some cases. The course of the ductus arteriosus may be normal, and the aortic isthmus is smaller than either the ascending or the descending aorta. Both of these features indicate a normal fetal pathway of blood, making anatomic pulmonary atresia unlikely.

5. Atresia of the main pulmonary artery may be encountered in patients with pulmonary atresia associated with asplenia (Fig 34-23).

6. Simultaneous aortography and right ventriculography may demonstrate the distance between the opacified right ventricle and atretic pulmonary valve, allowing the diagnosis of associated infundibular atresia.[23] This may be important for operative management, because incision of the pulmonary valve, annulus, and infundibulum may not relieve the infundibular obstruction.

OPERATIVE CONSIDERATIONS

Because the pulmonary circulation depends on patency of the ductus arteriosus, prostaglandin E_1 should be administered in the neonatal period. This promptly improves oxygenation and makes cardiac catheterization and operation safer. Acidosis associated with hypoxemia

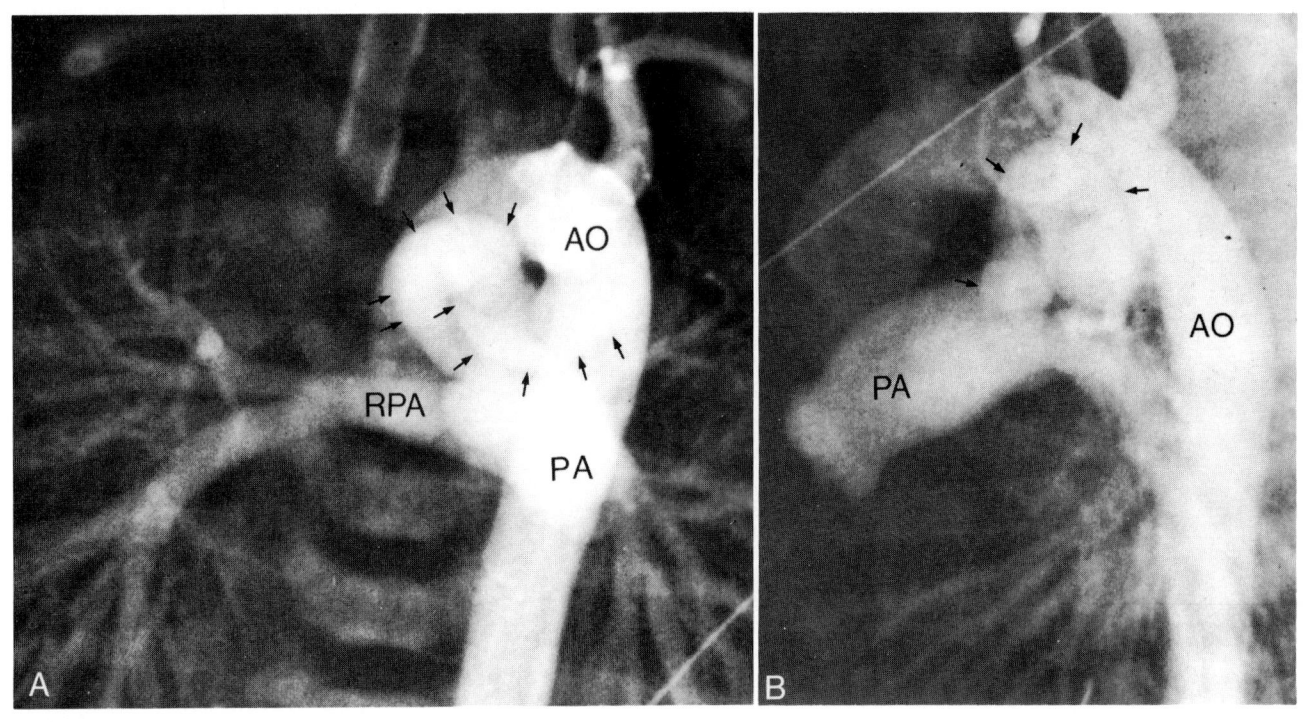

FIG 34-22.
Pulmonary atresia and intact ventricular septum. Aortogram *(AO)*. **A,** anteroposterior and, **B,** lateral projections. Long tortuous patent ductus arteriosus *(arrows)*. Ductus arises higher from aortic arch than normal. Main pulmonary artery *(PA)* is well developed. *RPA* = right pulmonary artery.

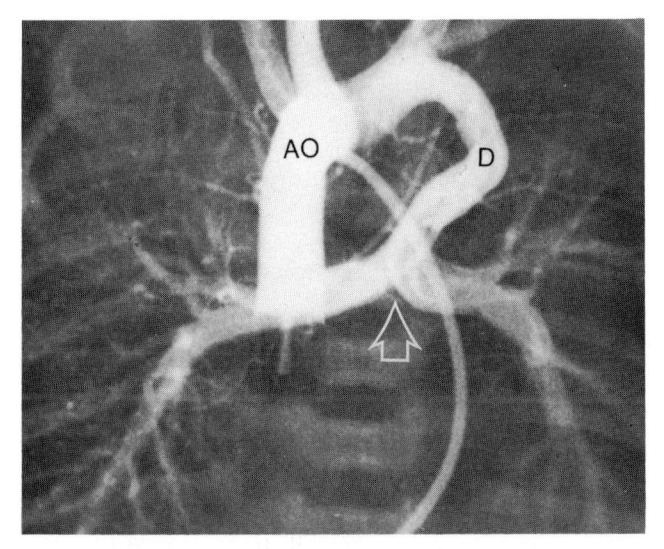

FIG 34-23.
Pulmonary atresia in asplenia syndrome. Aortogram *(AO)*. Balloon occlusion technique. Anteroposterior projection. Catheter from common ventricle through ascending aorta into descending aorta. Right aortic arch and large patent ductus *(D)* arises from left subclavian artery. Both pulmonary arteries opacify. Atresia of main pulmonary artery *(open arrow)*. Symmetric nature of the right and left pulmonary arteries suggests "bilateral right-sidedness" (see Chapter 58), as in asplenia.

should be treated with bicarbonate and glucose. Prostaglandin allows stabilization of the child in preparation for these procedures.

After cardiac catheterization, operation is indicated. A variety of operative procedures have been used in infants with pulmonary atresia, the selection of the procedure depending on the size of the right ventricle, degree of tricuspid regurgitation, and the experience and preference of the surgical team.[1, 2, 20, 24, 25] With this knowledge, certain decisions must be made during cardiac catheterization. Among those patients with a very hypoplastic right ventricle, a balloon atrioseptostomy is generally performed to create an adequate atrial communication.

In infants with a very hypoplastic right ventricle, a systemic pulmonary arterial shunt is performed. The advantages and disadvantages of each of these shunt procedures was discussed previously (see Chapter 30). Shunt procedures allow adequate pulmonary circulation and permit the child to grow. Some centers subsequently perform a pulmonary valvotomy in hope that a hypoplastic right ventricle may increase in size, but a limiting factor for success may be the hypoplastic tricuspid annulus.

When the size of the right ventricle is normal or near normal, pulmonary valvotomy is indicated if there is neither infundibular atresia or stenosis. Valvotomy should be performed even if tricuspid regurgitation coexists. If there

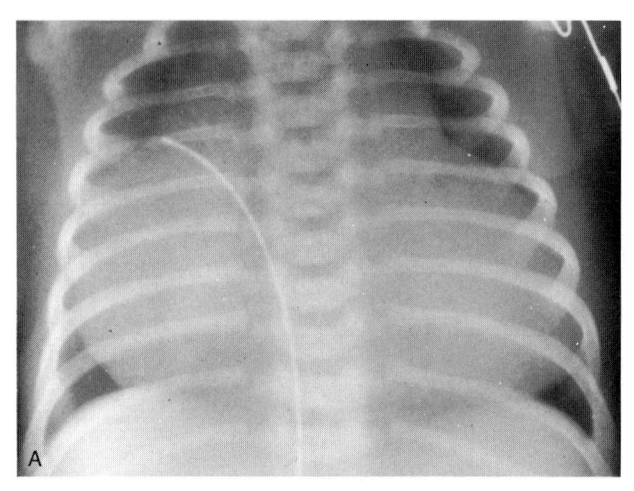

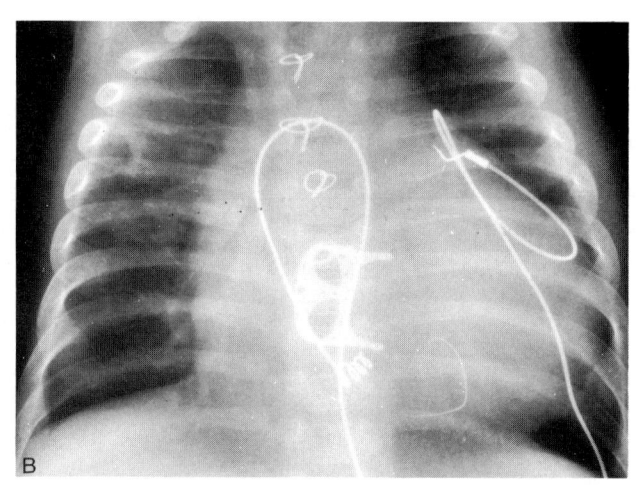

FIG 34–24.
Pulmonary atresia, intact ventricular septum, and tricuspid insufficiency. Thoracic roentgenogram. Posteroanterior projection. **A,** massive cardiomegaly. Cardiac silhouette fills entire thoracic cavity. **B,** after pulmonary valvotomy and insertion of prosthetic tricuspid valve. Striking decrease of cardiac size and improvement of pulmonary vasculature.

is infundibular obstruction or a narrowed pulmonary annulus, a patch across the right ventricular outflow tract and pulmonary annulus is used.

The careful selection of an appropriate operation and the use of prostaglandins, preoperatively, intraoperatively, and postoperatively have significantly decreased the operative mortality and improved clinical and hemodynamic results.[26]

Patients with a markedly hypoplastic right ventricle may ultimately be candidates for a Fontan procedure. Those patients with near normal–sized right ventricle may show an increase in the size of the right ventricle after valvotomy. Those with a dilated right ventricle and marked tricuspid regurgitation have a poor prognosis.

POSTOPERATIVE RADIOGRAPHIC FEATURES

After a pulmonary valvulotomy or an aorticopulmonary shunt, pulmonary blood flow increases and cardiac size decreases. REASON: Improved oxygenation decreases myocardial hypoxia.

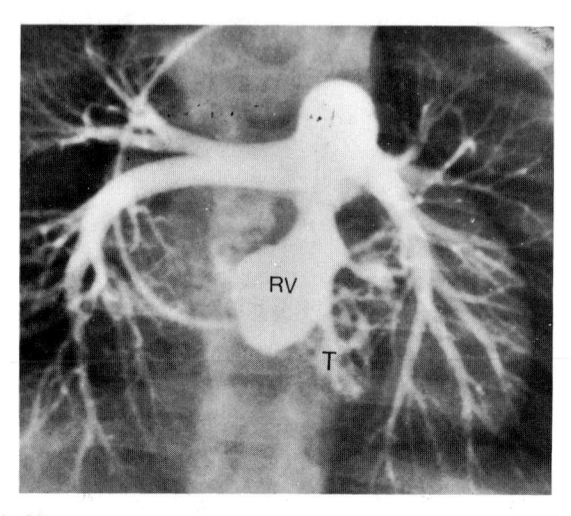

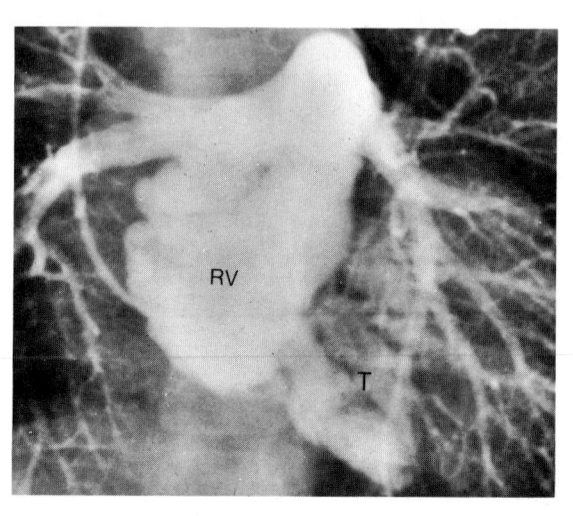

FIG 34–25.
Postoperative pulmonary atresia and intact ventricular septum. Right ventriculogram *(RV)*. Anteroposterior projection. **A,** immediately after pulmonary valvotomy. Very small right ventricle. Trabeculated portion is sharply *(T)* separated from smooth sinus portion. Adequate antegrade pulmonary blood flow. Right-to-left atrial shunt persisted because of small hypertrophied and noncompliant right ventricle. **B,** 3 years later. Considerable growth of right ventricular cavity. Characteristic internal architecture retained. Balloon occlusion of atrial communication during cardiac catheterization proved adequacy of right ventricular chamber. Subsequent atrial defect was closed by an operation.

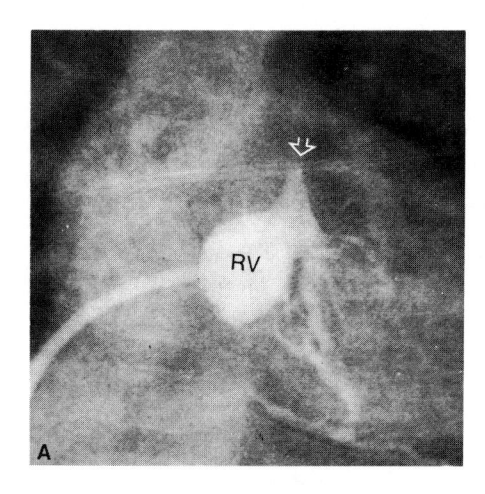

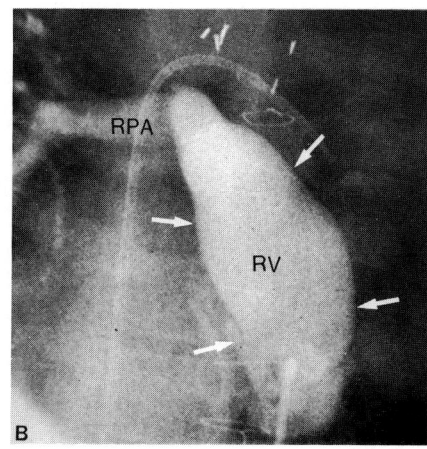

FIG 34–26.
Pulmonary valvar and infundibular atresia *(arrow)*. Diminutive right ventricle. Right ventriculogram *(RV)*. Anteroposterior projection. **A,** because of inadequacy of right ventricle, left-sided systemic-pulmonary artery shunt was performed *(arrow)*. **B,** after operation with insertion of large patch. There is marked enlargement of right ventricular cavity, but right ventricle has not grown *(arrows)*. RPA = right pulmonary artery.

1. The most striking change in cardiac size occurs in patients with massive tricuspid regurgitation who have tricuspid valve replacement (Fig 34–24).

2. After operative relief of the outflow obstruction, the right ventricle may grow[27] but retains its characteristic angiographic architecture, with a sharp delineation between trabecular and sinus portions (Fig 34–25). The right ventricle usually also retains it hemodynamic characteristic of decreased compliance.

3. Patients with a markedly hypoplastic right ventricle treated with either pulmonary valvulotomy or an aorticopulmonary shunt show little or no ventricular growth. Right ventricular capacity can be increased by enlarging the cavity by an outflow patch (Fig 34–26).

4. In patients with infundibular atresia and atresia of the main pulmonary artery, a conduit may be inserted (Fig 34–27). Such conduits must ultimately be replaced, because the infants may outgrow its size or the conduit may become narrowed by tissue ingrowth.

5. Sinusoids usually do not function after operative decompression of the right ventricle. Large sinusoids of the lacunar type may persist as coronary arterial fistula.

The termination of the coronary arteries in the myocardium may take at least two different patterns (Fig 34–28): Capillaries may form lakes, also called "coronary sinusoids" (see Fig 34–28,A), which finally communicate with the left ventricle, or a dense capillary network (see Fig 34–28,B), which has small communications with the left ventricular cavity. These small communications tend to close after operative correction of pulmonary atresia. These communications can be seen normally at time of postmortem examination in the left ventricle and are nonfunctional. Sometimes, however, a puff of contrast medium can be seen to enter the left ventricular cavity during coronary arteriography in normal patients. If the intracavitary pressure in either the right or the left ventricle increases, as in pulmonary or aortic atresia, retrograde flow may occur through these normally present communications into the coronary arteries and aorta. During diastole, blood flow occurs from the coronary arteries into the right ventricle. Sometimes these communications are huge and form coronary artery–right ventricular fistulas after surgery (Fig 34–29).

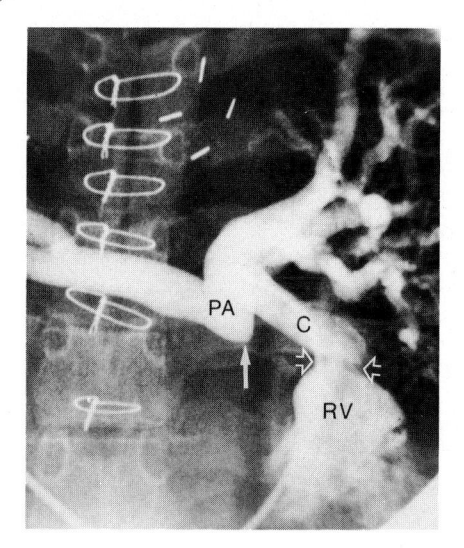

FIG 34–27.
Pulmonary atresia with atresia of main pulmonary artery *(arrow)*. Postoperative view. Right ventriculogram *(RV)*. Right anterior oblique projection. Conduit *(C)* is inserted from right ventricular outflow tract to pulmonary artery *(PA)*. Mouth of conduit is somewhat narrowed by ingrowth of fibrous tissue *(open arrows)*.

FIG 34-28.
A, cross-section through myocardium demonstrating "sinusoids," which are formed by capillaries communicating with either right or left ventricle. With normal left or right ventricular systolic pressure, sinusoids are not functioning. **B,** variation of sinusoids forming a capillary network communicating with ventricular cavity. With elevated right or left ventricular systolic pressure, coronary sinusoids remain patent, and a bidirectional blood flow occurs *(arrows)*. *RV* = right ventricle.

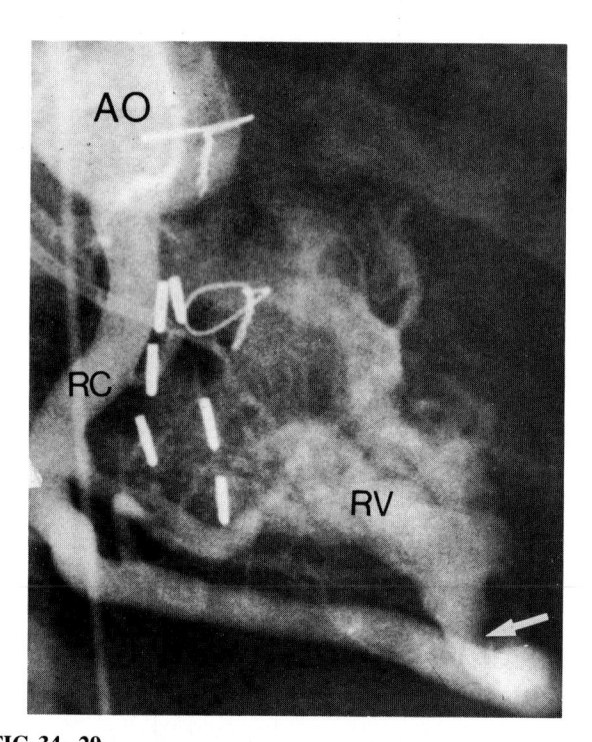

FIG 34-29.
Pulmonary atresia. Postoperative. Aortogram *(AO)*. Right anterior oblique projection. Huge right coronary artery *(RC)* fills right ventricle *(RV)* through large sinusoidal connection *(arrow)*, representing large coronary artery–right ventricular fistula. Operative ligation of right ventricular sinusoidal connections is therefore advisable.

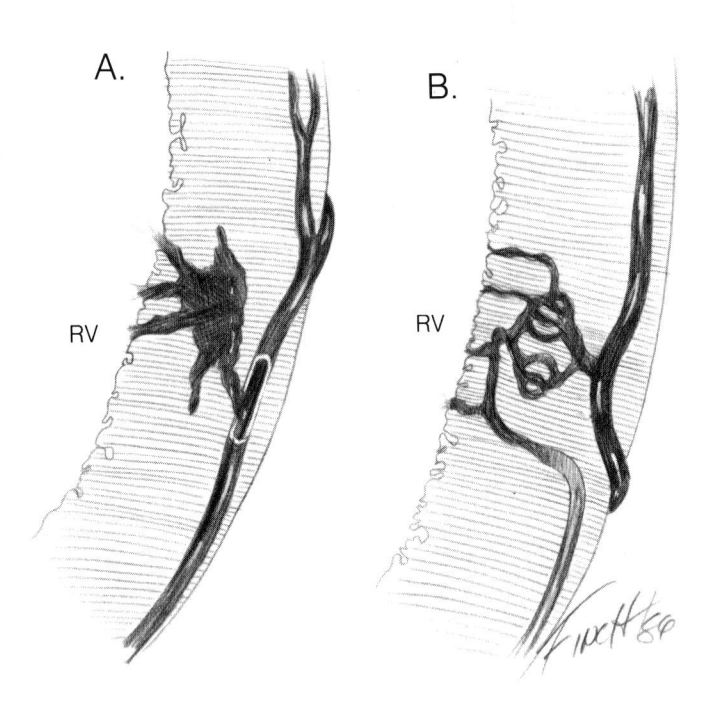

REFERENCES

1. McArthur JD, Munsi SC, Sukumar IP et al: Pulmonary valve atresia with intact ventricular septum: report of a case with long survival and pulmonary blood supply from an anomalous coronary artery, *Circulation* 44:740, 1971.
2. Freedom RM, Wilson G, Trusler GA, et al: Pulmonary atresia and intact ventricular septum, *Scand J Thorac Cardiovasc Surg* 17:1, 1983.
3. Cobanoglu A, Metzdorff MT, Pinson CW, et al: Valvotomy for pulmonary atresia with intact ventricular septum: a disciplined approach to achieve a functioning right ventricle, *J Thorac Cardiovasc Surg* 89:482, 1985.
4. Elliott LP, Adams P Jr, Edwards JE: Pulmonary atresia with intact ventricular septum, *Br Heart J* 25:489, 1963.
5. Kanjuh VI, Stevenson JE, Amplatz K, et al: Congenitally unguarded tricuspid orifice with coexistent pulmonary atresia, *Circulation* 30:911, 1964.
6. Patel RG, Freedom RM, Moes CAF, et al: Right ventricular volume determinations in 18 patients with pulmonary atresia and intact ventricular septum: Analysis of factors influencing right ventricular growth, *Circulation* 61:428, 1980.
7. Davignon AL, Greenwold WE, DuShane JW, et al: Congenital pulmonary atresia with intact ventricular septum: clinicopathologic correlation of two anatomic types, *Am Heart J* 62:591, 1961.
8. Sissman NJ, Abrams HL: Bidirectional shunting in a coronary artery–right ventricular fistula associated with pulmonary atresia and an intact ventricular septum, *Circulation* 32:582, 1965.
9. Freedom RM, White RI Jr, Ho CS et al: Evaluation of patients with pulmonary atresia and intact ventricular septum by double catheter technique, *Am J Cardiol* 33:892, 1974.
10. Bharati S, McAllister HA Jr, Chiemmongkoltip P, et al:

Congenital pulmonary atresia with tricuspid insufficiency: morphologic study, *Am J Cardiol* 40:70, 1977.
11. Zuberbuhler JR, Anderson RH: Morphological variations in pulmonary atresia with intact ventricular septum, *Br Heart J* 41:281, 1979.
12. Lauer RM, Fink HP, Petry EL, et al: Angiographic demonstration of intramyocardial sinusoids in pulmonary-valve atresia with intact ventricular septum and hypoplastic right ventricle, *N Engl J Med* 271:68, 1964.
13. Freedom RM, Culham G, Moes F, et al: Differentiation of functional and structural pulmonary atresia: role of aortography, *Am J Cardiol* 41:914, 1978.
14. Arom KV, Edwards JE: Relationship between right ventricular muscle bundles and pulmonary valve: significance in pulmonary atresia with intact ventricular septum, *Circulation* 54(suppl 3):III–79, 1976.
15. Graham TP Jr, Bender HW, Atwood GF, et al: Increase in right ventricular volume following valvulotomy for pulmonary atresia or stenosis with intact ventricular septum, *Circulation* 49–50(suppl II):II–69, 1974.
16. O'Connor WN, Cottrill CM, Johnson GL, et al: Pulmonary atresia with intact ventricular septum and ventriculocoronary communications: surgical significance, *Circulation* 65:805, 1982.
17. de Leval M, Bull C, Stark J, et al: Pulmonary atresia and intact ventricular septum: surgical management based on a revised classification, *Circulation* 66:272, 1982.
18. Haworth SG, Silove ED: Pulmonary arterial structure in pulmonary atresia after prostaglandin E_2 administration, *Br Heart J* 45:311, 1981.
19. Blackman MS, Schneider B, Sondheimer HM: Absent proximal left main coronary artery in association with pulmonary atresia, *Br Heart J* 46:449, 1981.
20. Lewis AB, Wells W, Lindesmith GG: Evaluation and surgical treatment of pulmonary atresia and intact ventricular septum in infancy, *Circulation* 67:1318, 1983.
21. Kutsche LM, Van Mierop LHS: Pulmonary atresia with and without ventricular septal defect: a differential etiology and pathogenesis for the atresia in the two types? *Am J Cardiol* 51:932, 1983.
22. Bass JL, Fuhrman BP, Lock JE: Balloon occlusion of atrial septal defect to assess right ventricular capability in hypoplastic right heart syndrome, *Circulation* 68:1081, 1983.
23. Freedom RM: The morphologic variations of pulmonary atresia with intact ventricular septum: guidelines for surgical intervention, *Pediatr Cardiol* 4:183, 1983.
24. Bull C, De Leval MR, Mercanti C, et al: Pulmonary atresia and intact ventricular septum: a revised classification, *Circulation* 66:266, 1982.
25. De Leval M, Bull C, Hopkins R, et al: Decision making in the definitive repair of the heart with a small right ventricle, *Circulation* 72 (suppl II):II–52, 1985.
26. Milliken JC, Laks H, Hellenbrand W, et al: Early and late results in the treatment of patients with pulmonary atresia and intact ventricular septum, *Circulation* 72(suppl II):II–61, 1985.
27. Fyfe DA, Edwards WD, Driscoll DJ: Myocardial ischemia in patients with pulmonary atresia and intact ventricular septum, *J Am Coll Cardiol* 8:402, 1986.

CHAPTER 35

Isolated Hypoplasia of Right Ventricle

Hypoplasia of the right ventricle is found commonly among patients with either tricuspid or pulmonary atresia. It coexists less commonly with pulmonary stenosis, complete transposition of the great vessels, ventricular septal defect, or tetralogy of Fallot. As an isolated condition, hypoplasia of the right ventricle is rare but must be considered in the differential diagnosis of cyanosis and decreased pulmonary vascularity. It shows a familial tendency.[1-4] It appears most frequently in the neonatal period and is rare in infants or older individuals.

PATHOLOGIC ANATOMY

The tricuspid annulus and tricuspid valve, although normally formed, are hypoplastic. The size of the right ventricular cavity is reduced.[1-4] There is a right-to-left shunt at the atrial level and cyanosis.[5]

Left-sided cardiac chambers are normal in form but may be slightly enlarged because of a right-to-left shunt at the atrial level. There are several anatomic variations[4]:

Type I: Medium-sized right ventricle, tricuspid stenosis, normal pulmonary valve (Fig 35–1).
Type II: Small right ventricle, rudimentary tricuspid valve, atresia of the pulmonary orifice (see Chapter 34).
Type III: Medium-sized right ventricle, tricuspid stenosis, ventricular septal defect.
Type IV: Isolated hypoplasia of the right ventricle, anatomically normal tricuspid and pulmonary valves.

The condition should not be confused with Holmes' heart (see Chapter 42), which also shows ventricular hypoplasia, but both atrioventricular valves empty into the left ventricle. In primary hypoplasia of the right ventricle, the right atrioventricular (tricuspid) valve connects with the hypoplastic right ventricle.

HEMODYNAMICS

Because of the hypoplasia of the right ventricle, the volume of blood that enters the right ventricle is reduced; consequently, the volume of pulmonary blood flow is limited. Elevation of right atrial pressure and a right-to-left shunt through the foramen ovale occur, causing cyanosis. The hemodynamic derangement is greatest among those patients with the smallest right ventricles. Although right atrial pressure is elevated, right ventricular systolic pressure is normal.

CLINICAL FEATURES

Patients with severe hypoplasia of the right ventricle appear in the neonatal period with intense cyanosis and other features that resemble pulmonary atresia. In these neonates there are no murmurs and only a single second sound.[1-4] Hepatomegaly may be present.

Occasionally adults are recognized as having a hypoplastic right ventricle, which may be described as tricuspid stenosis. In such patients, cyanosis may be minimal or inapparent, and the major clinical features are signs of systemic venous obstruction, with prominent neck veins and hepatomegaly.

ELECTROCARDIOGRAPHIC FEATURES

The electrocardiogram (ECG) is not characteristic. On an electrocardiogram, a small R wave and deep S wave in

PRIMARY HYPOPLASIA OF THE RIGHT VENTRICLE

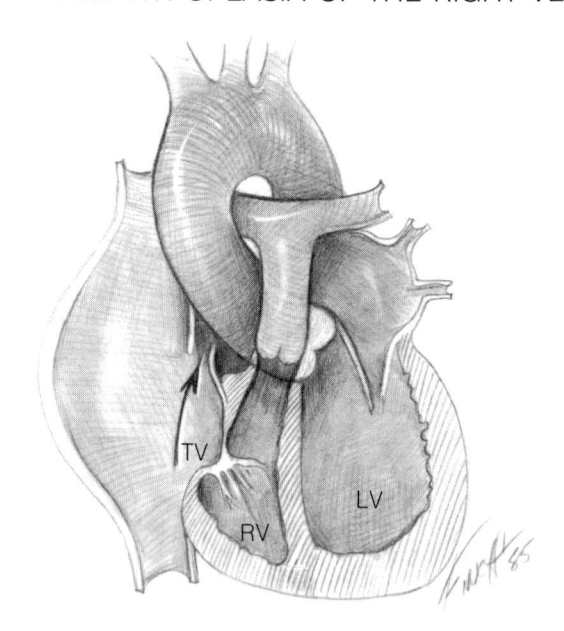

FIG 35–1.
Hypoplasia of right ventricle. Anatomic features. Size of right ventricular cavity *(RV)* is markedly reduced, and tricuspid annulus is hypoplastic. Hypoplastic right ventricle cannot accept a normal-sized tricuspid annulus. Tricuspid valve *(TV)* anatomically is either normal or stenotic. LV = left ventricle.

lead I and tall R wave and small or absent S wave in lead V_6 may be observed. The findings are identical to left ventricular hypertrophy. The P waves are tall and peaked, indicating right atrial enlargement.

ECHOCARDIOGRAPHIC FEATURES

Echocardiography is most helpful in distinguishing this condition from pulmonary atresia, tricuspid atresia, or Ebstein's malformation. In the latter two conditions, clinical features (and particularly electrocardiography) are fairly typical. On subcostal and apical cross-sectional views, the appearance is very typical, with an enlarged left ventricle adjacent to a hypoplastic right ventricle. The size of the atrial communication can be assessed. The reduced diameter of the tricuspid annulus is seen. Doppler interrogation of the tricuspid and pulmonary valves helps to determine their status and demonstrate antegrade flow without a gradient.

RADIOGRAPHIC FEATURES

In many older patients, the thoracic roentgenogram is normal. In these instances, the hypoplasia of the right ventricle and tricuspid valve are minimal, and the right-to-left shunt at the atrial level is small and does not significantly enlarge the left ventricle. The pulmonary vasculature is normal.

With more severe right ventricular hypoplasia, cardiomegaly and decreased pulmonary vasculature are found. The cardiac silhouette has a left ventricular contour and a prominent right atrial border (Fig 35–2).[1–3] REASON: The heart is rotated in a counterclockwise direction, and the left ventricle is anatomically enlarged because of the right-to-left shunt at the atrial level. The left ventricular blood volume therefore consists of the total pulmonary venous return and part of the systemic venous return shunted at

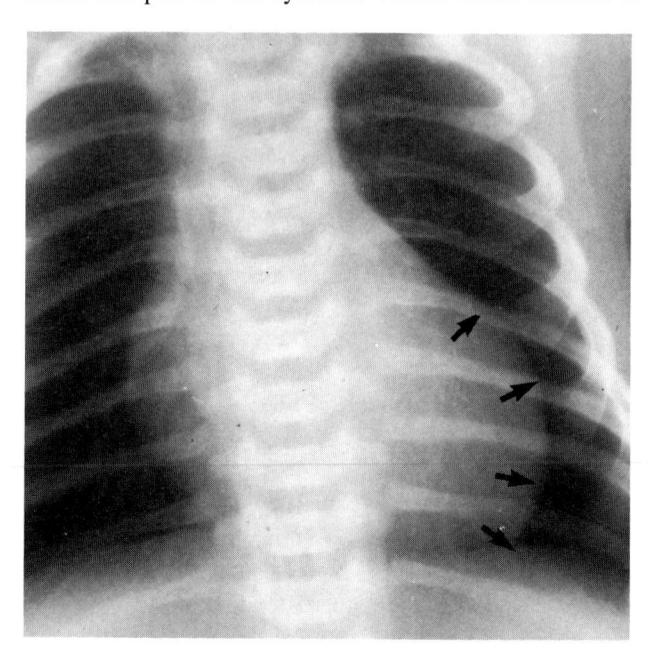

FIG 35–2.
Hypoplasia of right ventricle. Thoracic roentgenogram. Posteroanterior projection. Minimally enlarged heart. Left ventricular configuration *(arrows)* is identical to tricuspid atresia. Decreased pulmonary vasculature. Inconspicuous main pulmonary artery because of its more central position secondary to counterclockwise rotation.

the atrial level. In very severe cases the roentgenographic appearance is identical to pulmonary atresia with intact septum or tricuspid atresia, which show the same anatomy. Differentiation is impossible.

CARDIAC CATHETERIZATION

When the catheter is advanced from the inferior vena cava into the heart, it tends to pass from the right atrium into the left atrium and left ventricle, as in pulmonary or tricuspid atresia. It may be difficult to pass the catheter into the hypoplastic right ventricle.

Right atrial pressure may be elevated, whereas right ventricular and pulmonary arterial pressures are normal. A right-to-left shunt is present at the atrial level. Few conditions are associated with a right-to-left atrial shunt and normal right ventricular systolic pressures. These conditions are total anomalous pulmonary venous connection, Ebstein's malformation, and pulmonary atresia with tricuspid regurgitation. Usually the clinical and laboratory findings of these cardiac malformations are characteristic enough that distinction is evident when the hemodynamics are measured.

Attempts should be made to enter the right ventricle during cardiac catheterization, because a dense right-to-left shunt at the atrial level may obscure the right ventricle during atrial angiography and lead to a false diagnosis of either tricuspid or pulmonary atresia.

ANGIOGRAPHIC FEATURES

Hypoplasia of the right ventricle may be difficult to recognize angiographically. It is important to clearly define the tricuspid and pulmonary valves.

1. Injection in the right atrium or a systemic demonstrates a right-to-left shunt at the atrial level.
2. The hypoplastic right ventricle is demonstrated best by right ventriculography (Fig 35–3). It is small, narrow, and oriented vertically. Because of its small size, the distance of the right ventricular cavity from the diaphragm is increased.
3. Hypoplasia of the tricuspid annulus is best seen on right anterior oblique or lateral projection during diastole (Fig 35–4).
4. The degree of tricuspid hypoplasia can be accurately assessed on a lateral right ventriculogram (Fig 35–4) by measuring the diameter of the tricuspid annulus.
5. Ventricular hypoplasia may be associated with pulmonary stenosis. The stenotic pulmonary valve can be recognized on a lateral right ventriculogram (Fig 35–5).[5]

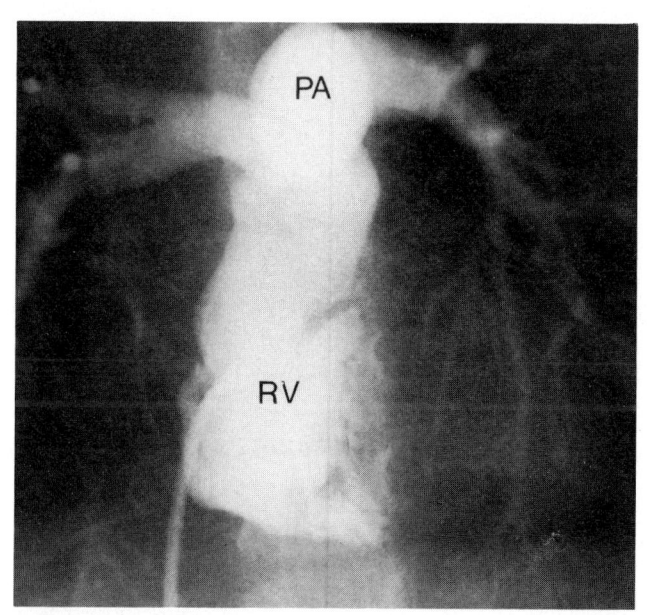

FIG 35–3.
Hypoplasia of right ventricle. Right ventriculogram (RV). Anteroposterior projection. Small right ventricular cavity. Hypoplasia involves primarily trabeculated portion of right ventricle and apical recess. Right ventricle has vertical orientation and is displaced medially by counterclockwise rotation. Normal pulmonary artery (PA) occupying medial midline position. On thoracic roentgenogram, pulmonary arterial segment is inconspicuous.

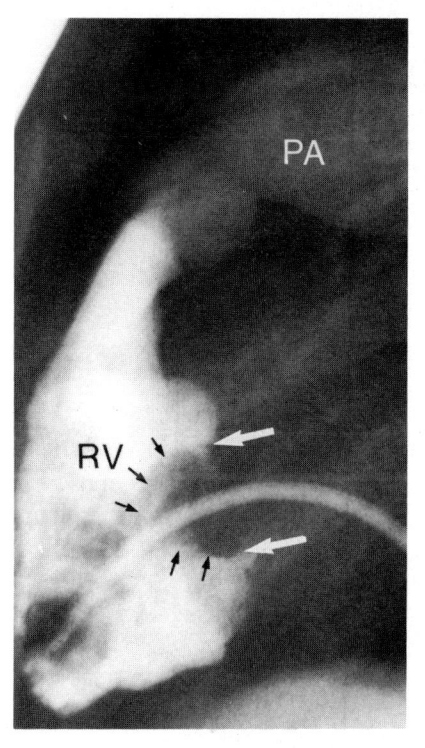

FIG 35–4.
Hypoplasia of right ventricle. Same patient as in Figure 35–3. Right ventriculogram (RV). Lateral projection. Right ventricle does not appear as hypoplastic as on anteroposterior projection. Distinct hypoplasia of tricuspid annulus (arrows). PA = pulmonary artery.

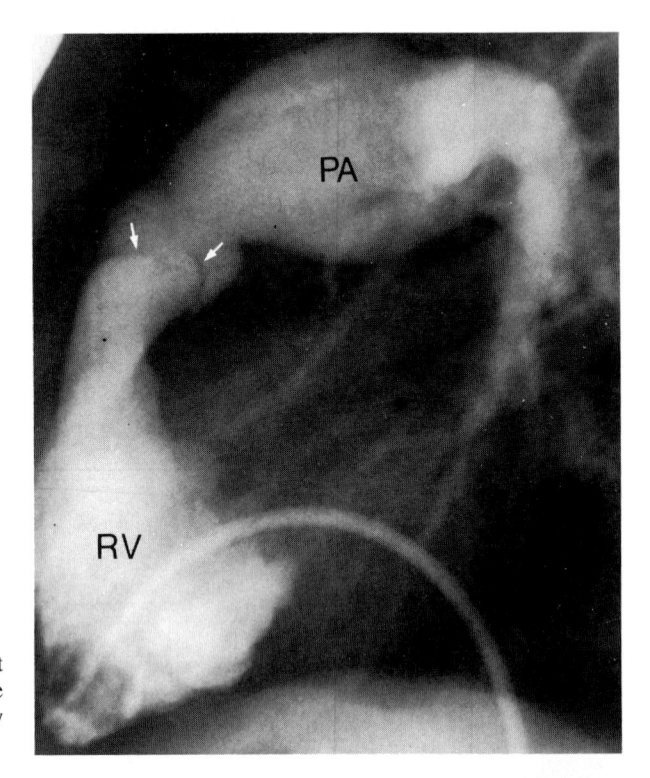

FIG 35–5.
Hypoplasia of right ventricle with valvar pulmonary stenosis. Right ventriculogram *(RV)*. Lateral projection. Doming of pulmonary valve *(arrows)*. Moderate poststenotic dilatation of main pulmonary artery *(PA)*.

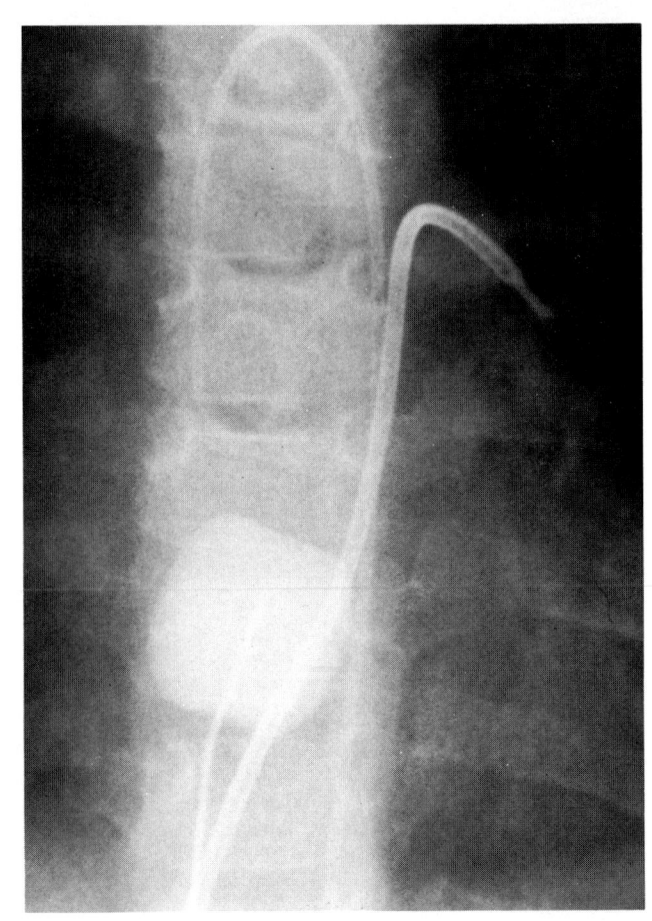

FIG 35–6.
Hypoplasia of right ventricle. Roentgenogram during cardiac catheterization. Anteroposterior projection. Balloon catheter is passed into left atrium. Balloon has been inflated and pulled snugly against the atrial septum, occluding atrial communication. Therefore, right-to-left atrial shunt is eliminated, and right ventricle must carry entire cardiac output. During balloon occlusion, patient is closely monitored by blood pressure measurement and systemic arterial oxygen saturation.

6. Adequacy of the right ventricle to carry the entire cardiac output is very difficult to judge by angiography and volume measurements. The best physiologic test to prove adequate size of the right ventricular chamber is occlusion of the foramen ovale with a balloon catheter during cardiac catheterization (Fig 35–6). Peripheral arterial and right atrial pressures and oxygen saturation are monitored. If right atrial pressure rises and the arteriovenous oxygen difference widens, the right ventricle cannot sustain adequate cardiac output. If the right ventricle can accept the entire systemic venous return, the foramen ovale can be closed operatively or by a device, eliminating cyanosis and other complications of the right-to-left atrial shunt.

7. Hypoplasia of the right ventricle may be severe. The large right-to-left shunt causes left ventricular enlargement (Fig 35–7) and generalized cardiomegaly. REASON: The increased blood flow through the left side of the heart resembles the hemodynamics of tricuspid atresia or pulmonary atresia with intact septum.

8. Hypoplasia of the tricuspid annulus and functional tricuspid stenosis may be associated with other congenital abnormalities such as ventricular septal defect, transposition of the great vessels, and tetralogy of Fallot (Fig 35–8).

OPERATIVE CONSIDERATIONS

In the neonatal period, the usual treatment is creation of a systemic to pulmonary arterial shunt. When the child is older, and if the pulmonary vascular resistance is low, the atrial communication can be closed and a Fontan operation can be performed. In patients with an adequate-sized

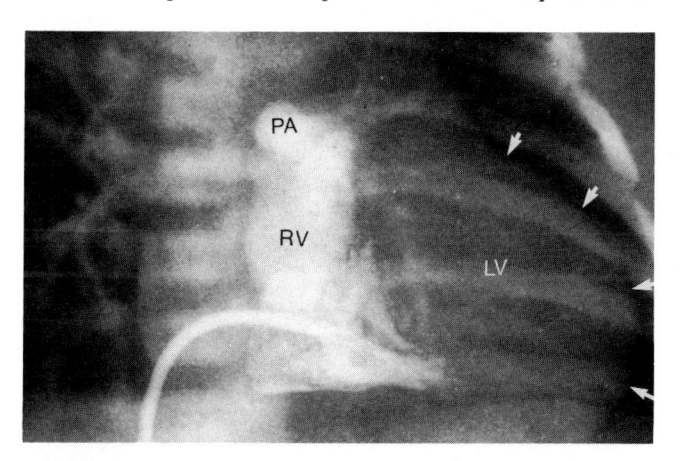

FIG 35–7.
Severe hypoplasia of right ventricle. Right ventriculogram *(RV)*. Anteroposterior projection. Very small right ventricular cavity. Trabeculated portion of right ventricle is virtually absent. Massive enlargement of left ventricle *(arrows)* because of large right-to-left atrial shunt. At time of cardiac catheterization, right ventricle proved to be inadequate to carry entire cardiac output. LV = left ventricle; PA = pulmonary artery.

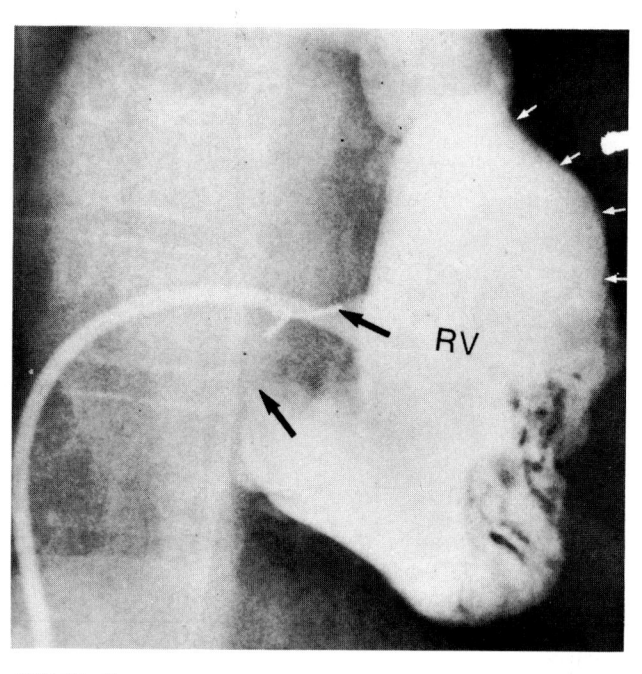

FIG 35–8.
Tetralogy of Fallot. Postoperative right ventriculogram (RV). Anteroposterior projection. Ventricular septal defect has been closed and right ventricular outflow tract enlarged by pericardial patch *(white arrows)*. Hypoplastic tricuspid annulus *(black arrows)*.

right ventricle as determined by balloon occlusion of the atrial communication, the operative approach is closure of the atrial septal defect.

POSTOPERATIVE FEATURES

After operative closure of foramen ovale, there is no significant change in cardiac size or the appearance of the pulmonary vasculature.

REFERENCES

1. Raghib G, Amplatz K, Moller JH, et al: CPC: hypoplasia of right ventricle and of tricuspid valve, *Am Heart J* 70:806, 1965.
2. Davachi F, McLean RH, Moller JH, et al: Hypoplasia of the right ventricle and tricuspid valve in siblings, *J Pediatr* 71:869, 1967.
3. Becker AE, Becker MJ, Moller JH, et al: Hypoplasia of right ventricle and tricuspid valve in three siblings, *Chest* 60:273, 1971.
4. Medd WE, Neufeld HN, Weidman WH, et al: Isolated hypoplasia of the right ventricle and tricuspid valve in siblings, *Br Heart J* 23:25, 1961.
5. Sackner MA, Robinson MJ, Jamison WL, et al: Isolated right ventricular hypoplasia with atrial septal defect or patent foramen ovale, *Circulation* 24:1388, 1961.

CHAPTER 36

Ebstein's Malformation

In 1866, Ebstein (Wilhelm Ebstein, a 19th Century German physician) described a downward displacement of the tricuspid valve, which is a rare congenital cardiac anomaly. It presents a wide anatomic and clinical spectrum. Individuals with this condition may be asymptomatic into the sixth or seventh decade of life, but it has also been associated with fetal cardiac failure. Ebstein's malformation usually occurs as an isolated lesion, but it can coexist with pulmonary atresia or stenosis and, rarely, tetralogy of Fallot or endocardial cushion defect.

PATHOLOGIC ANATOMY

The major pathologic feature relates to the septal and posterior leaflets of the tricuspid valve. These are adherent to the right ventricular wall, so that the free portion of the valve leaflets originates at a variable distance below the atrioventricular annulus and within the right ventricle.[1–3] This feature is called "downward displacement" of the tricuspid valve (Fig 36–1). The maximum point of displacement is at the commissure between these two leaflets. These leaflets are often dysplastic,[4] and although variable in size, they are frequently enlarged. The anterior leaflet, although normally attached, is usually abnormal, being large and saillike. It is abnormally attached between the anterolateral papillary muscle and an abnormal chordal attachment to the crista supraventricularis (Fig 36–2).

The commissures may all be fused, and the orifice through the valve may be narrowed or at times imperforate,[5] in which instance the tricuspid valve is atretic. Fusion of the commissures may also result in tricuspid stenosis.

The degree to which the valve is displaced varies greatly and may be so extreme that the displaced valve attaches in the right ventricle at the level of the crista supraventricularis and its associated septal and parietal bands (Fig 36–3).

Because of the displacement of the tricuspid valve, the right side of the heart becomes tripartite: the right atrium, the atrialized right ventricle (portion between the tricuspid annulus and the displaced tricuspid valve), and the right ventricle (Fig 36–4).[1] The effective size of the right atrium is enlarged, whereas the right ventricular chamber is reduced. Usually the right atrium, atrialized portion of the right ventricle, and the right atrioventricular annulus are enlarged. The enlargement results from insufficiency of the tricuspid valve and may be extreme. Enlargement of the right atrium and atrialized right ventricle progresses with age. The musculature of the atrialized right ventricle progressively thins, becoming a huge, smooth thin-walled chamber (Figs 36–5 and 36–6).[6] If the tricuspid valve is stenotic, the size of the right ventricle is reduced.

An atrial communication, either patent foramen ovale or atrial septal defect, is usually present through which a right-to-left shunt occurs. Associated intracardiac malformations are rare. Ebstein's malformation has been associated with pulmonary stenosis, pulmonary atresia, and ventricular septal defect. Ebstein's malformation may be associated with mitral valvar abnormalities, particularly mitral prolapse. One case of Ebstein's malformation with a right aortic arch has been described. Additional anomalies (in order of frequency) are ventricular septal defect, pulmonary atresia, ventricular septal defect coexisting with pulmonary stenosis, isolated pulmonary stenosis, patent ductus arteriosus, coarctation of the aorta, sinus venosus atrial septal defect, atrioventricular canal, and cor triatriatum.

Ebstein's malformation must be differentiated from dysplasia of the tricuspid valve, which also causes tricuspid regurgitation. Dysplasia of the tricuspid valve consists of (1) focal or diffuse thickening of the valve leaflets, (2) deficient development of chordae tendineae and papillary muscles and tethering of the free margin of the tricuspid valve, (3) improper separation of valvar components from the ventricular wall, and (4) focal agenesis of valvar tissue. Various combinations of these four anatomic features

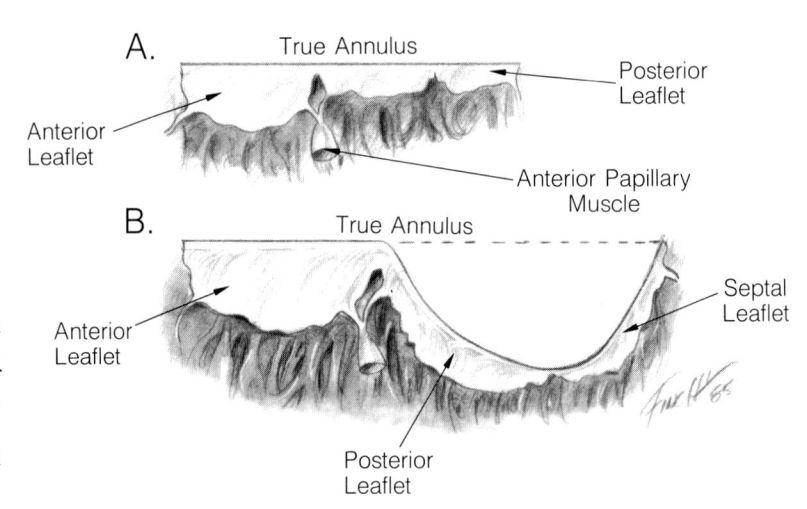

FIG 36–1.
Tricuspid valve attachment. **A,** normal. Attachment of all tricuspid valve leaflets to annulus. **B,** Ebstein's malformation. Downward displacement of posterior and septal leaflets that do not attach to annulus. Portion of anterior leaflet attaches normally. Depending on severity of malformation, downward displacement may involve only a single leaflet.

are possible and can lead to tricuspid regurgitation. In contrast to Ebstein's malformation, the valve attaches normally to the true annulus.

HEMODYNAMICS

The hemodynamic consequences of Ebstein's malformation vary considerably.[7] Generally, the more extreme the degree of displacement of the tricuspid valve, the more significant the hemodynamic changes. The other major anatomic variable relates to the status of the tricuspid valve, whether it is stenotic or regurgitant. If the displacement is mild and the valve function normal, the hemodynamics are essentially normal.

In Ebstein's malformation, the volume of the right ventricle distal to the tricuspid valve is reduced in contrast

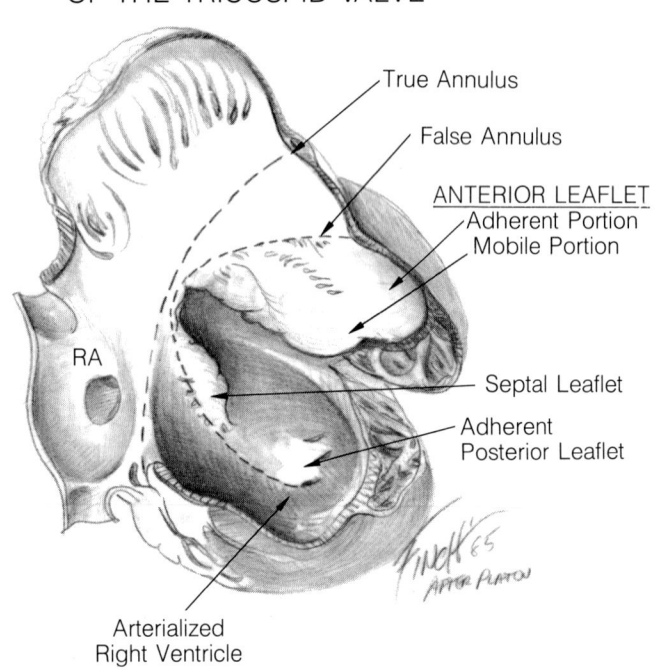

FIG 36–2.
Severe Ebstein's malformation. Opened right ventricle. Dysplastic septal leaflet. Posterior leaflet is hypoplastic and adherent to right ventricular wall. Anterior leaflet is saillike, is markedly enlarged, and may cause outflow tract obstruction. *RA* = right atrium.

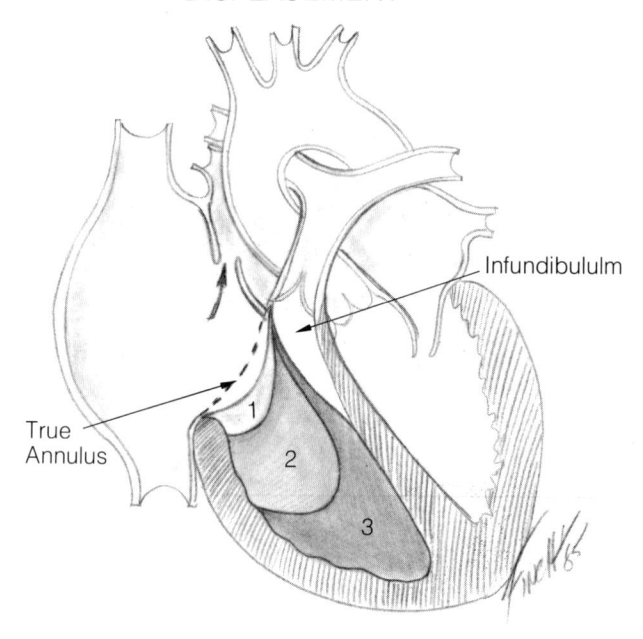

FIG 36–3.
Ebstein's malformation. Variations in downward displacement of tricuspid valve. *Grade 1*, minimal downward displacement. *Grade 2*, moderate downward displacement. *Grade 3*, severe downward displacement. Right ventricle proper, consists only of right ventricular infundibulum. Right-to-left shunt through foramen ovale.

EBSTEIN'S ANOMALY WITH TRICUSPID STENOSIS

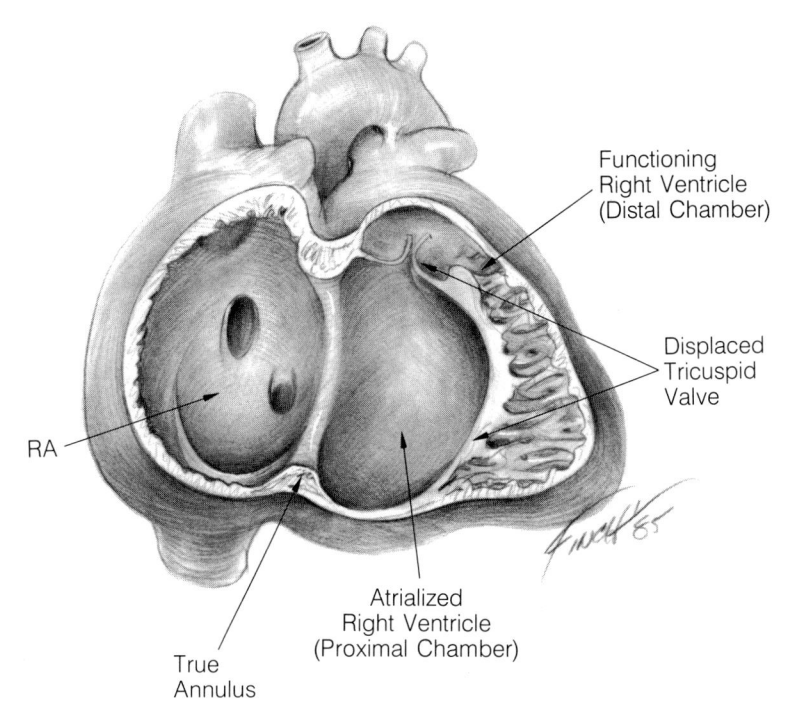

FIG 36–4.
Severe Ebstein's malformation. Anterior walls of right ventricle and atrium *(RA)* have been removed. Severe downward displacement of tricuspid valve has created tripartite right side of heart. Right atrium proper atrialized portion of right ventricle, which is dilated, and right ventricle proper, which consists only of infundibulum and a small portion of trabeculated right ventricle.

to primary tricuspid insufficiency, where the true right ventricle is enlarged. The saillike anterior leaflet may obstruct the right ventricular outflow tract, resulting in tricuspid stenosis (see Fig 36–2).

Because of the right-to-left atrial shunt, which is related to elevated right atrial pressure, cyanosis is a feature. The elevation may occur from tricuspid stenosis, elevated pulmonary vascular resistance, tricuspid insufficiency, or decreased right ventricular compliance. Cyanosis may be intense in the neonatal period. At this age pulmonary vascular resistance is elevated and the right ventricle hypertrophied and therefore less compliant. The reduced compliance accentuates the right-to-left shunt and the degree of tricuspid insufficiency. Tricuspid regurgitation may be extreme and lead to congestive cardiac failure and marked cardiomegaly. Postnatally as pulmonary vascular resistance falls, the right ventricle becomes more compliant. Therefore, pulmonary blood flow increases, and the degree of tricuspid insufficiency decreases. The cardiac failure improves, cardiomegaly decreases, and cyanosis lessens.

Patients with Ebstein's malformation may develop episodes of paroxysmal supraventricular tachycardia, related to a dilated right atrium, or coexistent Wolff-Parkinson-White syndrome. Tachycardia shortens the diastolic filling period, impeding right ventricular filling, increasing right atrial pressure, and increasing tricuspid insufficiency if it

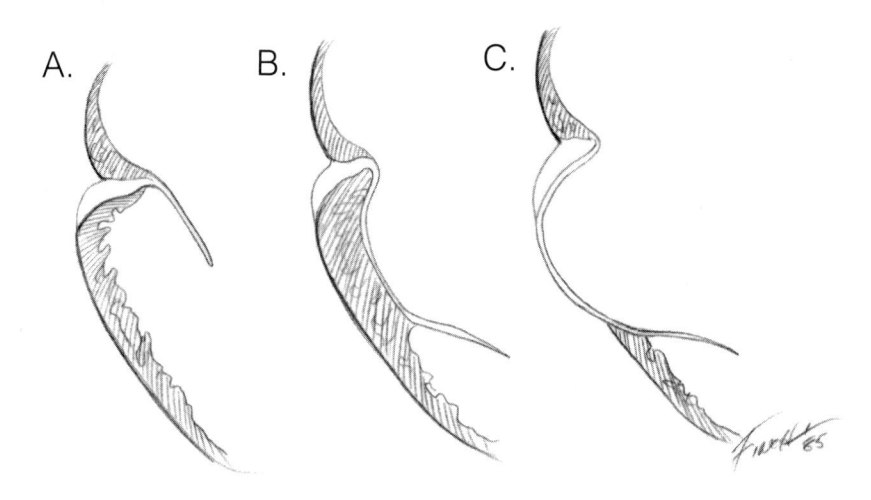

FIG 36–5.
Progressive thinning and enlargement of atrialized right ventricle. **A,** normal. Right ventricle remains of normal size throughout life. **B,** Ebstein's malformation of tricuspid valve. Valve leaflet adherent to normal right ventricular musculature. **C,** many years later. Marked thinning of musculature and progressive dilatation.

EBSTEIN'S ANOMALY

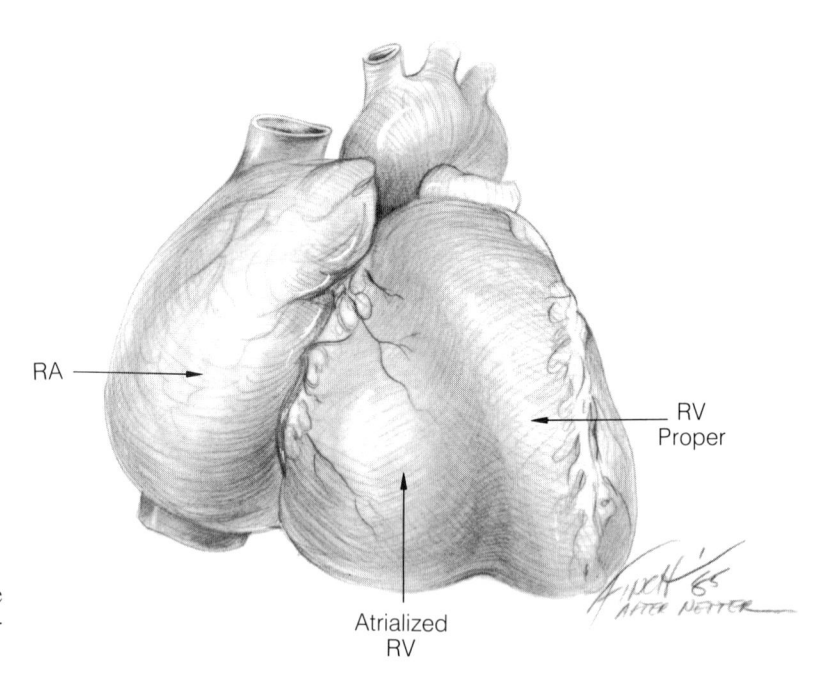

FIG 36–6.
Ebstein's malformation. Comparatively early stage of dilatation. Enlarged right atrium (RA). Dilatation of atrialized portion of right ventricle (RV).

coexists. Cyanosis and symptoms increase during episodes of supraventricular tachycardia.

With time, symptoms, including cyanosis, become worse. The tricuspid insufficiency tends to increase because of progressive right ventricular dilatation and perhaps because of hypoxic effects on the myocardium.

CLINICAL FEATURES[7–10]

Symptoms often occur in the neonatal period, with cyanosis, congestive cardiac failure, and a murmur. As pulmonary vascular resistance falls, the cyanosis and cardiac failure improve and may disappear entirely. Other neonates or infants with Ebstein's malformation are asymptomatic and initially recognized at an old age as having a congenital cardiac malformation because of a murmur, cyanosis, or both. Later during childhood or early adulthood, cyanosis reappears and may be associated with easy fatigability. Subsequently in such patients, cardiac failure appears, which is an ominous sign. Symptoms may also be produced or precipitated at any age by episodes of paroxysmal tachycardia, which may lead to cardiac failure, intensified cyanosis, and syncope or palpitation.

In the neonate, cyanosis may be intense, but in older patients, there may be only a malar flush or red-cheeked appearance, reflecting mild cyanosis. Clubbing may coexist. In those patients with more severe forms, the heart is enlarged and there is a precordial bulge. The auscultatory findings may be normal in patients with mild disease or in whom the condition is stable.

Often the cardiac sounds give a characteristic triple or quadruple rhythm, with prominent third and fourth heart sounds, often combined with split first and second heart sounds from complete right bundle branch block. The pulmonic component may be soft or absent in patients with markedly decreased pulmonary blood flow. Occasionally a midsystolic click is present as well.

A panoply of murmurs may also be present. A systolic murmur probably representing tricuspid insufficiency or right ventricular outflow tract obstruction is found in most patients. Located along the left sternal border, the loudness varies from grade 1 to 5/6 among patients. The murmur may be harsh, may be rough, and may occupy most of the systole. A middiastolic murmur is present, similar to that of an atrial septal defect, and probably results from increased antegrade flow across the tricuspid valve. A soft, variable extracardiac scratchy sound is often heard, the origin of which is uncertain.

ELECTROCARDIOGRAPHIC FEATURES

The electrocardiogram (ECG) is always abnormal and usually very diagnostic.[7–10] The QRS complex shows one of two patterns: right bundle branch block or Wolff-Parkinson-White syndrome (type B). The height of R wave in lead V_1 does not exceed 11 mm. Because of the abnormality of intraventricular conduction, the QRS axis is usually abnormal and may be directed either to the right or to the left.

P waves are often tall and broad, and some of the tallest P waves are found in this condition. The P-R interval is prolonged.

Paroxysmal supraventricular tachycardia, atrial flutter, or other dysrhythmias may be found.

ECHOCARDIOGRAPHIC FEATURES

Two-dimensional echocardiography is diagnostic in most cases.[11–13] On an apical view, the three portions of the right side of the heart can be visualized (i.e., right atrium, atrialized right ventricle and right ventricle). The attachment of the anterior and septal leaflets, as well as the normal tricuspid annulus, can be seen. Thus, the degree of downward displacement can be estimated. Because of the dilated right ventricle, the left ventricle may be rotated posteriorly. On a long-axis view, the thickened anterior leaflet of the tricuspid valve and its chordae tendineae can be identified. On a short-axis view, the exaggerated movement of the anterior leaflet is visualized. Dilatation of the right ventricle and paradoxical septal motion can be seen. The degree of tricuspid regurgitation can be assessed by Doppler techniques.

RADIOGRAPHIC FEATURES

The roentgenographic findings of Ebstein's malformation vary from normal to a characteristic cardiac contour, which allows roentgenographic diagnosis with high accuracy.[8, 10] This variation reflects the wide range of the functional and anatomic abnormality of the tricuspid valve. In addition, varying degrees of tricuspid regurgitation or tricuspid stenosis may be present, which affect right atrial size.

Only patients with a marked hemodynamic abnormality have a characteristic cardiac contour, which may be present even in the neonatal period (Fig 36–7). Tricuspid regurgitation results in progressive enlargement of the right atrium and eventually enlargement and thinning of the right ventricular outflow tract. This combination of chamber enlargement causes the characteristic boxlike cardiac contour. Typically the clinical findings and roentgenographic appearance improve after birth and gradually progress during adulthood. REASON: At birth the elevated pulmonary vascular resistance affects the right ventricle, and the degree of cyanosis is particularly severe because of the exaggerated tricuspid regurgitation and the decreased right ventricular compliance.

The specific radiographic findings include the following:

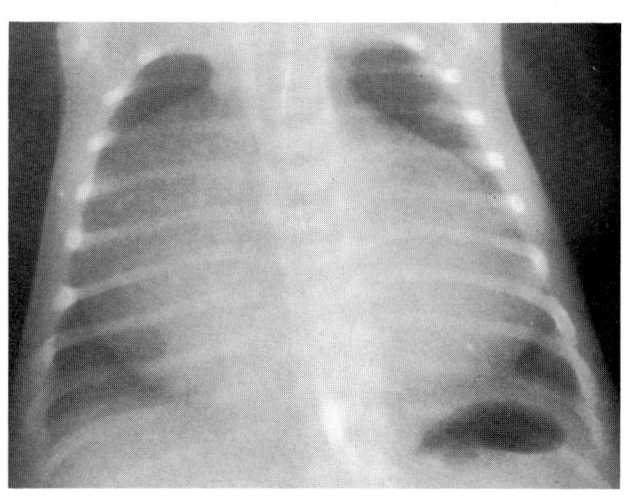

FIG 36–7.
Ebstein's malformation. Severe. Thoracic roentgenogram. Posteroanterior projection. Deeply cyanotic neonate. Massive cardiomegaly. Decreased pulmonary vasculature. Findings indistinguishable from pulmonary atresia with intact ventricular septum.

1. The cardiac contour may be entirely normal. In these patients, the anatomic abnormality of the tricuspid valve is mild and does not result in significant tricuspid regurgitation or stenosis.

2. In patients with significant tricuspid insufficiency, the right atrium and atrialized portion of the right ventricle enlarge, causing proportional cardiomegaly (see Fig 36–7). Active pulsations are seen on fluoroscopy.

3. With severe displacement of the tricuspid valve and major tricuspid regurgitation, the cardiac silhouette is huge because of massive right atrial enlargement. In neonates, Ebstein's malformation is associated with the largest cardiac silhouettes among this age group. Although a similar cardiac contour may be found in neonates with pulmonary atresia and intact ventricular septum (see Fig 36–7), the enormous size of the right atrium is more consistent with Ebstein's malformation.

4. In the early stages of Ebstein's malformation when less marked tricuspid regurgitation is present, the right atrium may not be prominent on the posteroanterior roentgenogram because of the clockwise rotation of the heart. In fact, the posteroanterior roentgenogram may easily be mistaken for prominence of the left side of the heart (Fig 36–8).

5. Oblique and lateral projections are valuable in demonstrating the enlargement of the right side of the heart.

6. The pulmonary vasculature varies from normal in mild cases to decreased in severe cases (see Figs 36–7 and 36–8). The presence of decreased pulmonary vasculature helps to distinguish Ebstein's malformation from other more common causes of generalized cardiomegaly, such

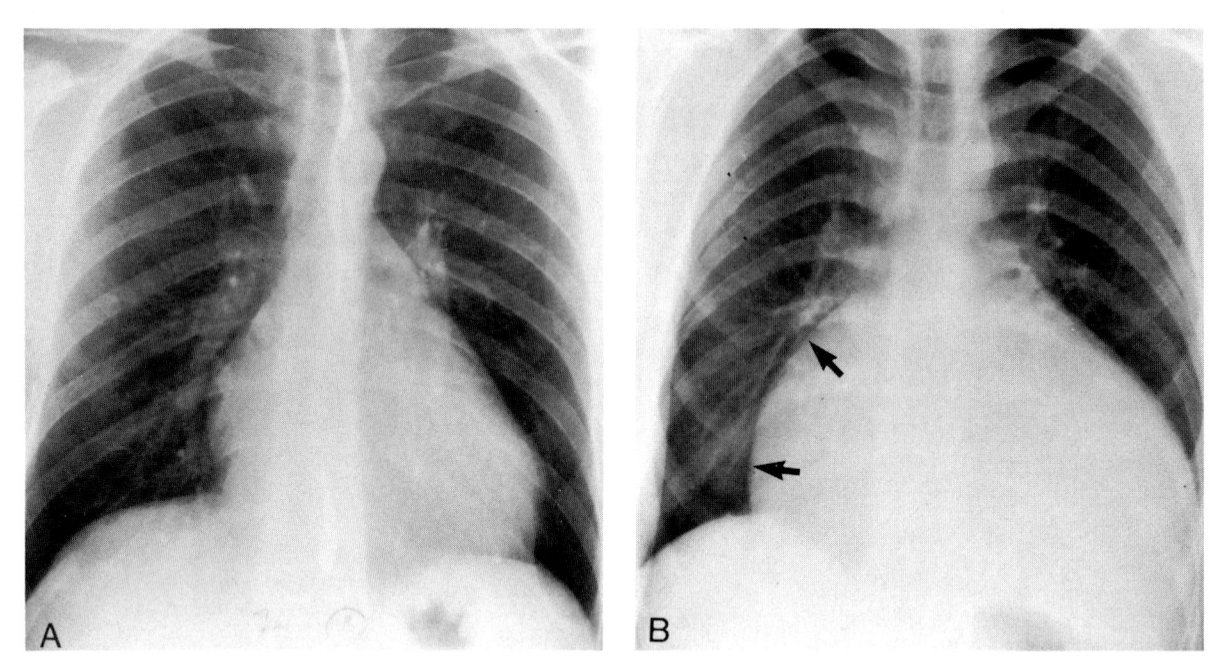

FIG 36–8.
Ebstein's malformation. Mild. Thoracic roentgenograms. Posteroanterior projection. **A,** slightly enlarged heart. Contour is radiographically suggestive of a left-sided cardiac lesion because of clockwise rotation secondary to right-sided enlargement. Normal pulmonary vasculature. Correct roentgenogram diagnosis cannot be suggested without oblique projections. **B,** same patient later in life. Progressive cardiomegaly. Decreased pulmonary vasculature and right atrial enlargement *(arrows)* suggest correct diagnosis in spite of left ventricular contour.

as cardiomyopathy, mitral valvar disease, and congestive cardiac failure.

7. In more advanced cases, dilation of the right ventricular outflow tract is particularly well seen on a right anterior oblique projection.

8. With more severe right atrial enlargement, the right atrium may form the border in each of the four standard projections, even the lateral view, making the recognition of individual cardiac chambers impossible (Fig 36–9).

9. Enlargement of the right atrium, atrialized portion of the right ventricle, and, finally, dilation of the right ventricular outflow tract progresses (see Fig 36–8,B) during life.

10. Left atrial enlargement is absent. REASON: Unlike tricuspid atresia where the entire systemic venous return passes through the left atrium, the volume of the right-to-left shunt in Ebstein's malformation is usually not large enough to significantly enlarge the left atrium. This is an important differential diagnostic sign to exclude mitral valvular disease, which may result in a similar cardiac contour because of distention of the left atrial appendage.

11. The right atrium may become so large that on a lateral projection it extends behind the barium-filled esophagus, simulating a displaced and enlarged left ventricle (see Fig 36–9).

12. The superior mediastinum is narrow, and the ascending aorta is not prominent. The superior vena cava rather than the ascending aorta forms the upper right cardiac border. REASON: As with other cardiac conditions with dilated right-sided cardiac chambers, the heart is rotated clockwise (see Chapter 19). This rotation displaces the ascending aorta medially and within the cardiac silhouette.

13. Later in life, progressive dilation of the right ventricular outflow tract results in a very characteristic squared off, boxlike, or pumpkinlike appearance of the cardiac silhouette (Fig 36–10).

CARDIAC CATHETERIZATION

It has been considered dangerous to catheterize patients with Ebstein's malformation because of deaths associated with this procedure. Arrhythmias may be induced during cardiac catheterization in perhaps 25% of patients with Ebstein's malformation, and some of them have been associated with death. With improved techniques, better monitoring equipment, and defibrillators, the risk has decreased significantly, and catheterization is carried out in a fashion identical to patients with other cardiac malformations.

One diagnostic feature of catheterization is the localization of the tricuspid valve. The catheter is slowly withdrawn from the apex of the right ventricle, and transition is recorded between right ventricular and right atrial pressures. Normally this point of transition is located over the spine, but in Ebstein's malformation it is displaced to the left (Fig 36–11). The use of an electrode catheter has enhanced the diagnostic reliability of this technique. With this catheter a simultaneous pressure tracing and intracardiac electrogram are recorded as the catheter is withdrawn from the pulmonary artery through the right ventricle into the right atrium. In the right ventricle, a typical right ventricular pressure curve and ECG are recorded. In the atrialized right ventricle, an atrial pressure contour is found, whereas a ventricular ECG is recorded, and finally in the right atrium, an atrial electrical recording is found.

The catheter may form a large loop in the right atrium, and it may pass readily into the right ventricle. Oximetry data show a right-to-left atrial level shunt, and a left-to-right shunt may be found as well.

Beyond the neonatal period, right ventricular systolic pressure is usually normal. Right atrial pressure is often elevated with a large v wave with predominant tricuspid regurgitation or large a wave with predominant tricuspid stenosis.

ANGIOGRAPHIC FEATURES

Angiography is helpful in delineating the size of the cardiac chambers, the malformation of the tricuspid valve,

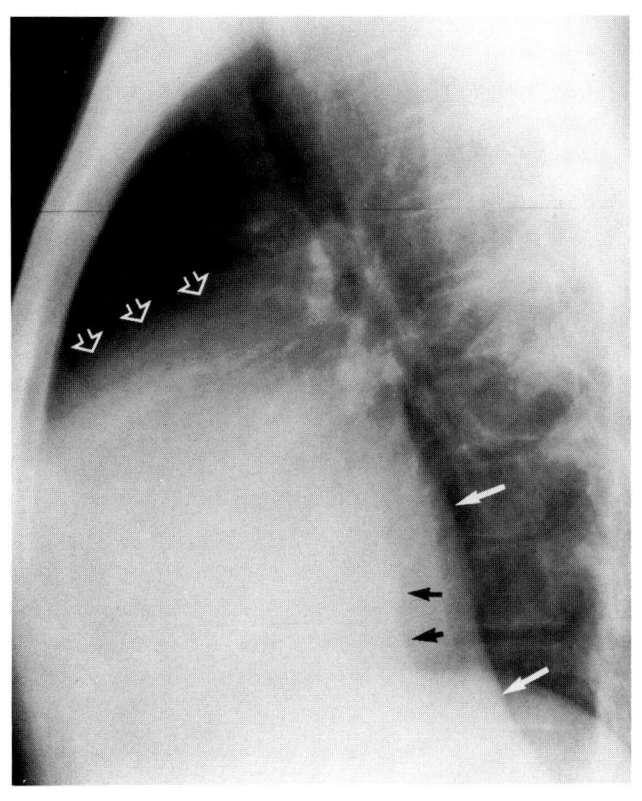

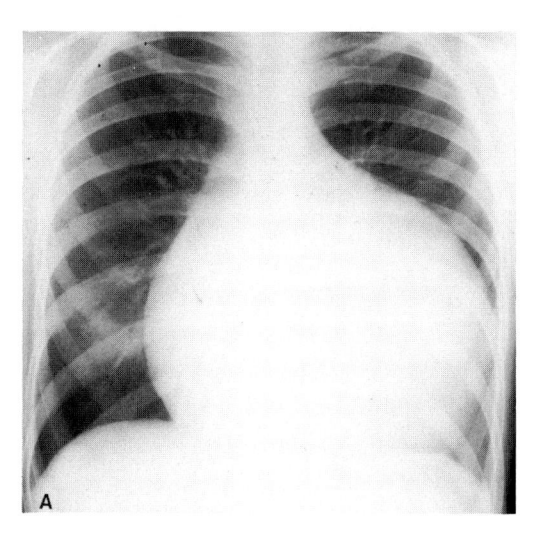

FIG 36–9.
Ebstein's malformation. Severe tricuspid regurgitation. Thoracic roentgenogram. Lateral projection. Right atrium forms cardiac border anteriorly *(open arrows)* and posteriorly *(white arrows),* preventing individual chamber recognition. Cardiac silhouette extends beyond caval reflection *(black arrows),* simulating left ventricular enlargement.

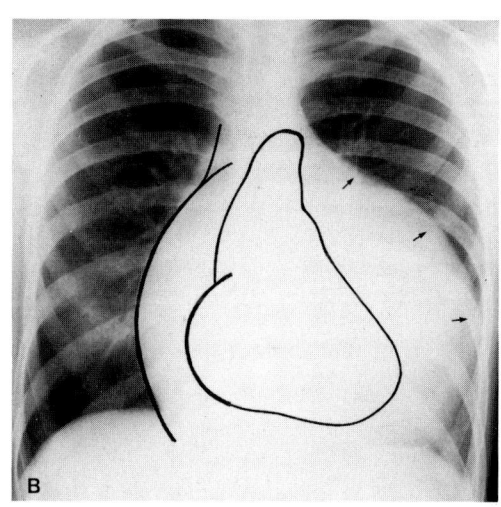

FIG 36–10.
Ebstein's malformation. Late stage. **A,** thoracic roentgenogram. Anteroposterior projection. Huge cardiac silhouette. Sparse pulmonary vasculature. Right atrial border increased. Cardiac contour has assumed characteristic squared-off appearance from dilation of right ventricular outflow tract. Superior vena cava forms right superior mediastinal border. Findings are characteristic of late-stage Ebstein's malformation. **B,** diagram demonstrating the difference between the cardiac silhouette in a normal individual and in Ebstein's malformation.

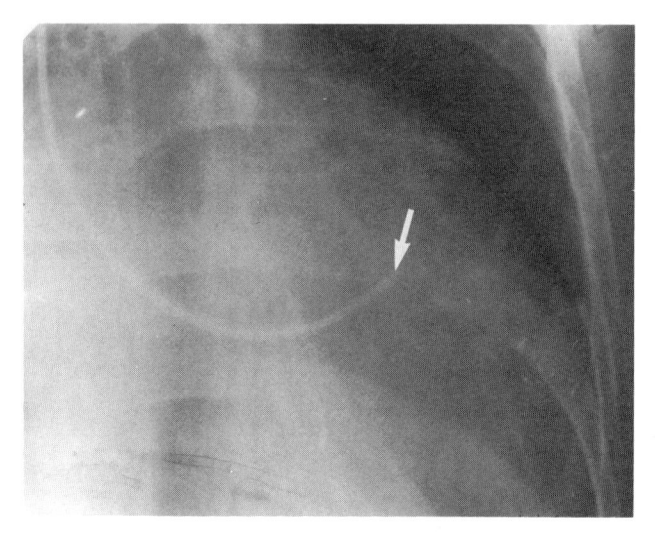

FIG 36–11.
Roentgenogram during cardiac catheterization. Catheter tip at position where pressure change occurred between right ventricle and right atrium. Normally the tricuspid valve is located over the thoracic spine. In this patient, pressure change occurs far to left *(arrow)* of spine, confirming diagnosis of Ebstein's malformation with marked downward displacement of valve apparatus.

and the degree of tricuspid regurgitation. Left ventricular angiography should be performed to exclude associated mitral valve prolapse.

Right-sided angiography must be performed through a large-bore catheter to allow the rapid delivery of a large amount of contrast medium. REASON: The right-sided cardiac chambers may be huge because of tricuspid regurgitation, which markedly dilutes the contrast material.

The diagnosis can usually be established angiographically by identifying the tripartite appearance of the right side of the heart. The components are as follows:

1. An enlarged, smooth-walled right atrium.
2. A thin and smooth-walled atrialized portion of the right ventricle.
3. A trabecular outflow portion of the right ventricle, which may be small or large, depending on the stage of the disease.

During catheterization the catheter has a tendency to become stuck at the level of the downward displaced tricuspid valve. If this occurs, a small injection of contrast medium suffices to establish a diagnosis, because in Ebstein's malformation, the portion of the right ventricle at the level of the valve is smoothwalled and has other anatomic characteristic of an atrium. The demonstration of this smooth-walled portion is characteristic of Ebstein's malformation.

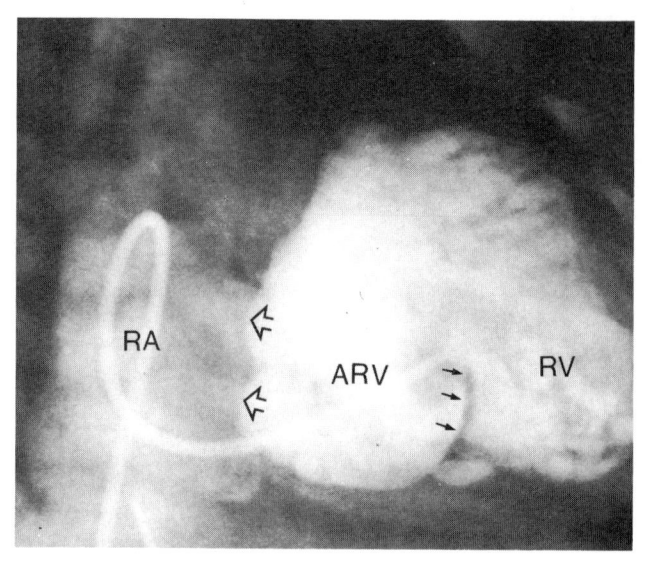

FIG 36–12.
Ebstein's malformation. Right ventriculogram. Slight right anterior oblique projection. Diastole. Catheter tip in smooth atrialized portion of right ventricle *(ARV)*. Moderately severe downward displacement of tricuspid valve. Valve is slightly thickened and distinctly visualized *(arrows)*. Trabeculated portion of right ventricle *(RV)* (right ventricle proper) is dilated. Tricuspid annulus *(open arrows)* is distinctly visualized. Almost no tricuspid reflux, very likely because of a well-formed large anterior leaflet. RA = right atrium.

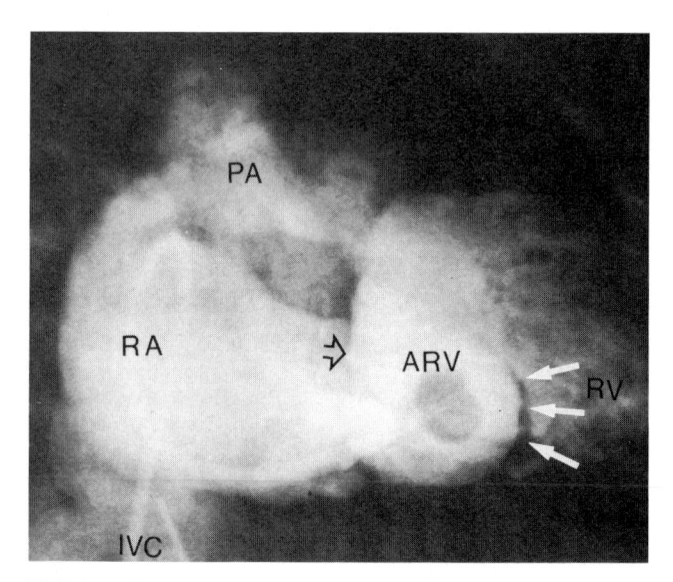

FIG 36–13.
Ebstein's malformation. Moderately severe. Injection of contrast medium into smooth atrialized portion of right ventricle *(ARV)*. Systole. Regurgitation into enlarged right atrium and inferior vena cava *(IVC)*. Right atrium *(RA)* shows systolic expansion. True tricuspid annulus with attachment of anterior leaflet of tricuspid valve *(open arrow)*. Displaced thickened valve leaflet is distinctly demonstrated *(white arrows)*. PA = pulmonary artery.

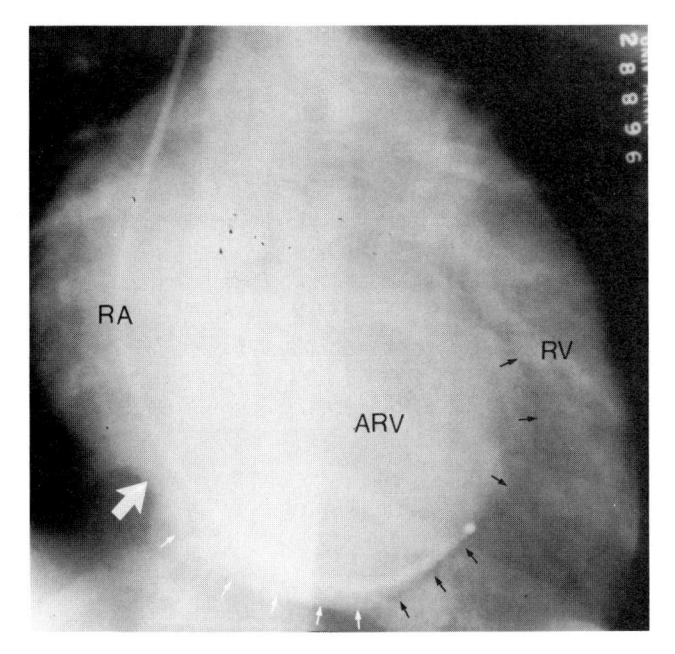

FIG 36–14.
Ebstein's malformation. Angiogram is performed in low-pressure area. Catheter is resting on displaced valve leaflet. Huge dilated atrialized portion of right ventricle *(ARV) (small white arrows)*. Tricuspid valve leaflets are not well identified *(black arrows)*. Transition between bulging atrialized ventricle and right atrium *(RA)* is distinctly seen as a notch *(large white arrow)*. Massive tricuspid reflux. The two bulges can be seen from exterior of heart during cardiac operation (see Fig 36–6). *RV* = right ventricle distal to tricuspid valve.

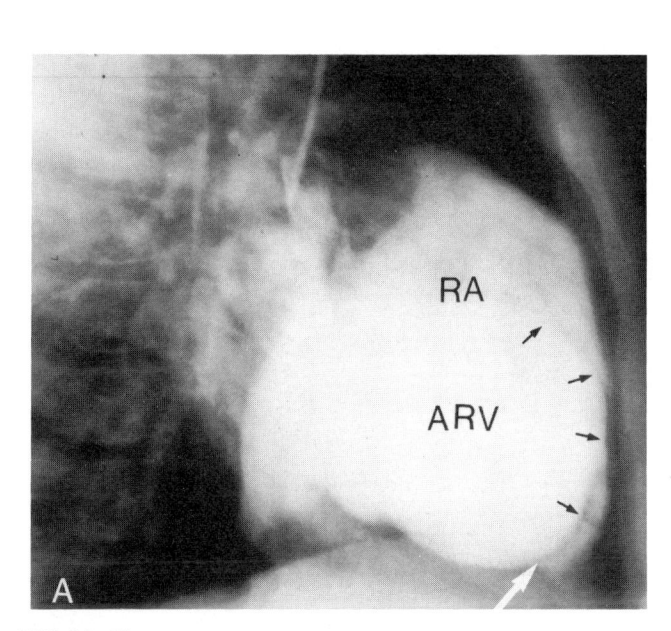

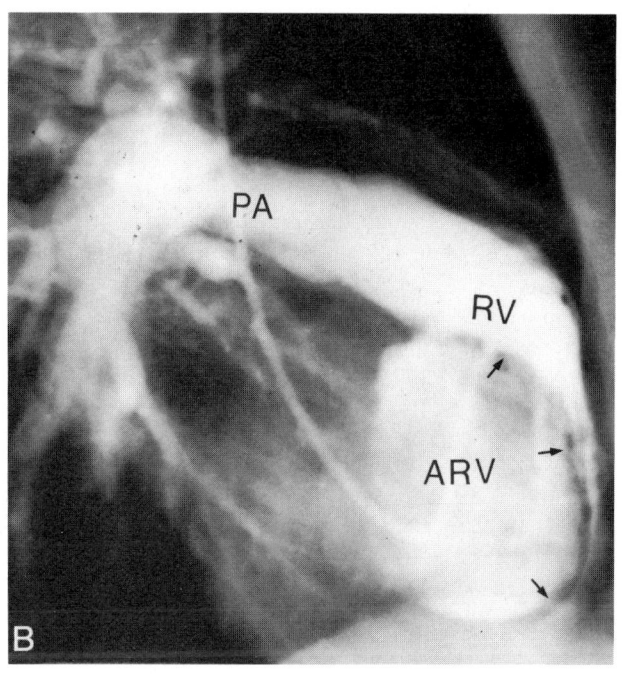

FIG 36–15.
Ebstein's malformation of tricuspid valve. Lateral projection. Injection of atrialized portion of right ventricle. **A,** systole. Atrialized portion *(ARV)* and right atrium *(RA)* superimposed on opacified right ventricle. Consequently, round double density is formed *(black arrows)*. Displaced tricuspid valve leaflet is difficult to see *(white arrow)*. **B,** diastole. After completion of injection of contrast material. Atrialized portion now filled with blood is clearly separated from right ventricle proper, which is still filled with dense contrast medium. Right ventricle consisting only of the infundibulum, indicating severe (grade 3) valve displacement. Displaced valve *(arrows)* is better visualized. *PA* = pulmonary artery.

Specific angiographic features are as follows:

1. The atrialized portion of the right ventricle varies in size, and the leaflets of the downwardly displaced tricuspid valve are usually distinctly visible (Fig 36–12). The degree of downward displacement is variable, and the size of the valve leaflets is inconstant. Sometimes only rudimentary valvar tissue is present.

2. The valve tissue may be paper thin. Most patients with Ebstein's malformation have some degree of tricuspid regurgitation (Fig 36–13).

3. Even if the displaced valve leaflets are not well seen, the diagnosis can be established by the demonstration of the smooth atrialized portion of the right ventricle, which may be huge (Fig 36–14). The dilated atrialized right ventricle forms a distinct bulge, which can also be seen from the outside of the heart (see Fig 36–6).

4. Demarcation between the smooth atrialized portion of the right ventricle and the right ventricle proper and the downwardly displaced tricuspid valve leaflets can also be seen on a lateral projection. In a lateral projection, however, the smooth atrialized portion of the right ventricle and right atrium are superimposed on the right ventricle proper, causing a double density (Fig 36–15,A).

5. When blood enters the atrialized portion of the right ventricle, it dilutes the contrast medium and the atrialized portion (Fig 36–15,B). The displaced valve and right ventricle proper can be distinctly seen.

6. A left ventriculogram, performed to exclude the rare association of a ventricular septal defect or mitral valve prolapse, demonstrates the displaced and squeezed left ventricle by the huge right side of the heart (Fig 36–16).

TREATMENT

In symptomatic neonates, supportive measures are necessary during the first few days of life until pulmonary vascular resistance has fallen sufficiently that right ventricular compliance and tricuspid regurgitation improve and cyanosis lessens. Digitalization, administration of diuretics, treatment of acidosis, and use of mechanical ventilation may be required. Tachyarrhythmias may require treatment.

Most patients are asymptomatic for a long period of time and require neither medical or operative treatment. Systemic pulmonary arterial shunts should not be used because they elevate pulmonary arterial pressure, and even a small elevation may be sufficient to keep the pulmonary valve closed and accentuate tricuspid insufficiency. A Glenn procedure (superior vena cava to pulmonary artery communication) has been used in older children who are symptomatic from cyanosis. The complications of a Glenn procedure have been discussed previously (See Chapters 30 and 33) and are significant.

Direct operative procedures have been applied on the tricuspid valve.[14] These have involved plication of the right atrial free wall and closure of the atrial septal defect. The tricuspid valve may be replaced by a mechanical or tissue valve. A tricuspid annuloplasty and realignment of the tricuspid leaflets may be performed. Construction of a monocusp valve using the anterior leaflet has been carried out. Selection of proper patients for operation is difficult, and the criteria are not well defined. The type of procedure depends largely on the findings at time of operative exploration.

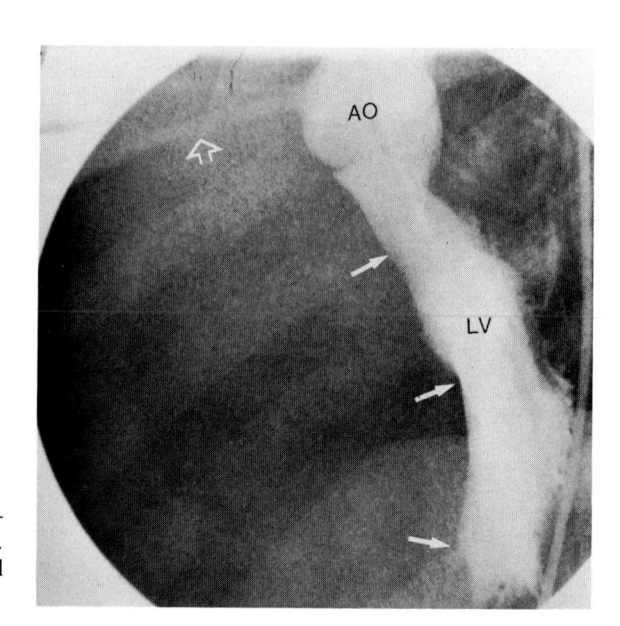

FIG 36–16.
Ebstein's malformation. Left ventriculogram. Left anterior oblique projection. Left ventricle (LV) is compressed by huge right side of heart. Ventricular septum, normally convex, is concave (arrows). No mitral valve prolapse and no ventricular septal defect. AO = aorta.

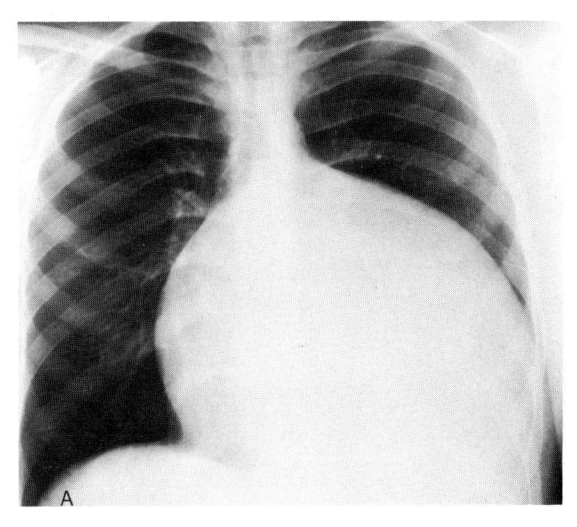

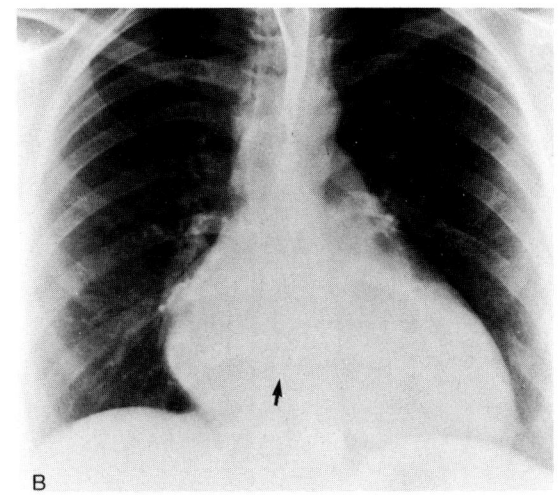

FIG 36-17.
Ebstein's malformation of tricuspid valve. **A,** preoperative. Characteristic features of late-stage Ebstein's disease. **B,** after operative replacement of tricuspid tissue valve *(arrow)*. Dramatic reduction in cardiac size.

POSTOPERATIVE RADIOGRAPHIC FEATURES

After the operative replacement of the tricuspid valve there may be a dramatic decrease of the cardiomegaly (Fig 36-17). Plication and other plastic procedures are hemodynamically less rewarding.

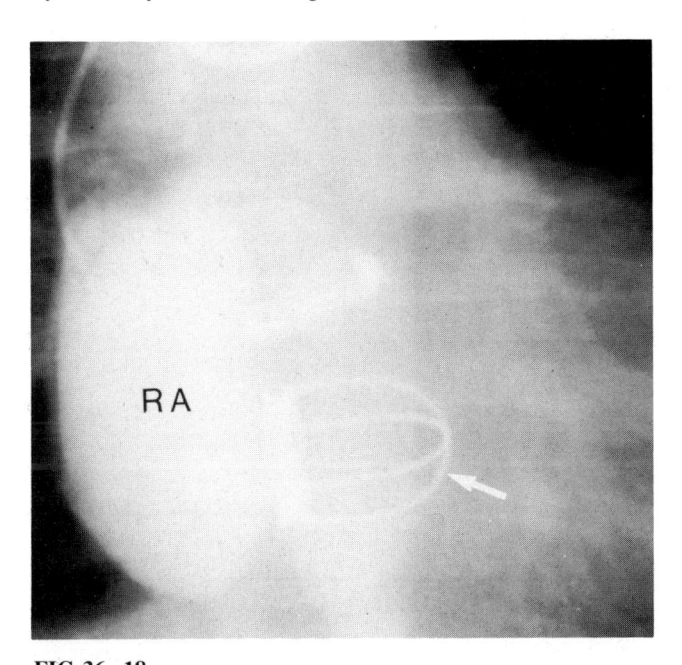

Angiography demonstrates the reduction of right atrial size to normal, particularly if valve replacement is combined with atrial plication (Fig 36-18).

REFERENCES

1. Anderson KR, Lie JT: Pathologic anatomy of Ebstein's anomaly of the heart revisited, *Am J Cardiol* 41:739, 1978.
2. Anderson KR, Zuberbuhler JR, Anderson RH, et al: Morphologic spectrum of Ebstein's anomaly of the heart: a review, *Mayo Clin Proc* 54:174, 1979.
3. Zuberbuhler JR, Allwork SP, Anderson RH: The spectrum of Ebstein's anomaly of the tricuspid valve, *J Thorac Cardiovasc Surg* 77:202, 1979.
4. Becker AE, Becker MJ, Edwards JE: Pathologic spectrum of dysplasia of the tricuspid valve, *Arch Pathol* 91:167, 1971.
5. Lev M, Liberthson RR, Joseph RH, et al: The pathologic anatomy of Ebstein's disease, *Arch Pathol* 90:334, 1970.
6. Anderson KR, Lie JT: The right ventricular myocardium in Ebstein's anomaly: a morphometric histopathologic study, *Mayo Clin Proc* 54:181, 1979.
7. Giuliani ER, Fuster V, Brandenburg RO, et al: Ebstein's anomaly: the clinical features and natural history of Ebstein's anomaly of the tricuspid valve, *Mayo Clin Proc* 54:163, 1979.
8. Takayasu S, Obunai Y, Konno S: Clinical classification of Ebstein's anomaly, *Am Heart J* 95:154, 1978.
9. Schiebler GL, Adams P Jr, Anderson RC, et al: Clinical study of twenty-three cases of Ebstein's anomaly of the tricuspid valve, *Circulation* 19:165, 1959.
10. Bialostozky D, Horwitz S, Espino-Vela J: Ebstein's malformation of the tricuspid valve: a review of 65 cases, *Am J Cardiol* 29:826, 1972.

FIG 36-18.
Ebstein's malformation. Right atriogram *(RA)*. Anteroposterior projection. Right atrium is plicated. Tricuspid valve is replaced by Starr-Edwards valve *(arrow)*, and right atrium is plicated. Valve sewn above orifice of coronary sinus, which was incorporated into the ventricle. No adverse sequelae occurred.

11. Matsumoto M, Matsuo H, Nagata S, et al: Visualization of Ebstein's anomaly of the tricuspid valve by two-dimensional and standard echocardiography, *Circulation* 53:69, 1976.
12. Gussenhoven WJ, Spitaels SEC, Bom N, et al: Echocardiographic criteria for Ebstein's anomaly of the tricuspid valve, *Br Heart J* 43:31, 1980.
13. Ports TA, Silverman NH, Schiller NB: Two-dimensional echocardiographic assessment of Ebstein's anomaly, *Circulation* 58:336, 1978.
14. Danielson GK, Maloney JD, Devloo RAE: Surgical repair of Ebstein's anomaly, *Mayo Clin Proc* 54:185, 1979.

CHAPTER 37

Primary Tricuspid Insufficiency

Tricuspid insufficiency may result from a variety of cardiac conditions and should not be considered as a primary diagnosis until specific causes have been excluded.

In this chapter we discuss only those instances in which a primary anomaly of the tricuspid valve is present. A brief classification[1] of tricuspid insufficiency follows. Many of the listed conditions are described elsewhere in these volumes.

I. Tricuspid insufficiency as a component of another cardiac anomaly.
   A. Endocardial cushion defect (see Chapter 23).
   B. Ebstein's malformation of the tricuspid valve (see Chapter 36).
   C. Endocarditis.
II. Tricuspid insufficiency secondary to a right ventricular abnormality.
   A. Conditions increasing right ventricular systolic pressure.
      1. Pulmonary stenosis or atresia (see Chapter 34).
      2. Pulmonary hypertension.
   B. Conditions increasing right ventricular volume.
      1. Cardiomyopathy.
      2. Premature closure of foramen ovale (see Chapter 76).
      3. Endocardial fibroelastosis (see Chapter 56).
III. Primary tricuspid insufficiency.

Tricuspid insufficiency as an isolated or primary entity is uncommon and generally produces major symptoms in the neonatal period.

PATHOLOGIC ANATOMY

Primary tricuspid insufficiency usually results from either of two abnormalities. First, called "tricuspid valve dysplasia," a wide variation of tricuspid valvar anomalies are found, ranging from merely nodularity of valve cusps to irregular thickening of cusps, short or absent chordae tendineae, and small papillary muscles.[2] The valve may be even more rudimentary and evident only as a nodular ring at the tricuspid annulus. The valve originates from the tricuspid annulus or slightly below it.

The second is *transient tricuspid insufficiency* of the *neonate*.[3,4] Tricuspid insufficiency, often quite severe, is present in the neonatal period and subsequently disappears during the first year of life. Necrosis of the anterior papillary muscle of the tricuspid valve may be found. Most neonates with transient tricuspid insufficiency have a history of transient perinatal distress and neonatal asphyxia.[5] At birth such neonates often have hypoxemia, hypoglycemia, and elevated serum creatinine phosphokinase fraction 2 levels (supporting evidence of myocardial infarction).[6] Hypoxemia and depletion of cardiac glycogen stores have been postulated as potential causes for papillary muscle damage and dysfunction.

In both forms, the right atrium and right ventricle are dilated. The foramen ovale is open. The left ventricle may be enlarged as well, and its contractility decreased, both features suggesting additional damage to the left ventricular myocardium.

HEMODYNAMICS (FIG 37–1)

In older individuals without other cardiac anomalies, tricuspid insufficiency is well tolerated. Right ventricular systolic pressure is low (25 mm Hg), and therefore there is not a large propelling force for the regurgitant flow. In neonates or individuals with a coexistent condition that raises right ventricular systolic pressure, congestive cardiac failure can occur,[7–9] because the elevated right ventricular systolic pressure augments the degree of tricuspid regurgitation. In neonates, pulmonary vascular resistance elevates right ventricular systolic pressure. Subsequently, as pul-

TRANSIENT TRICUSPID INSUFFICIENCY OF THE NEWBORN

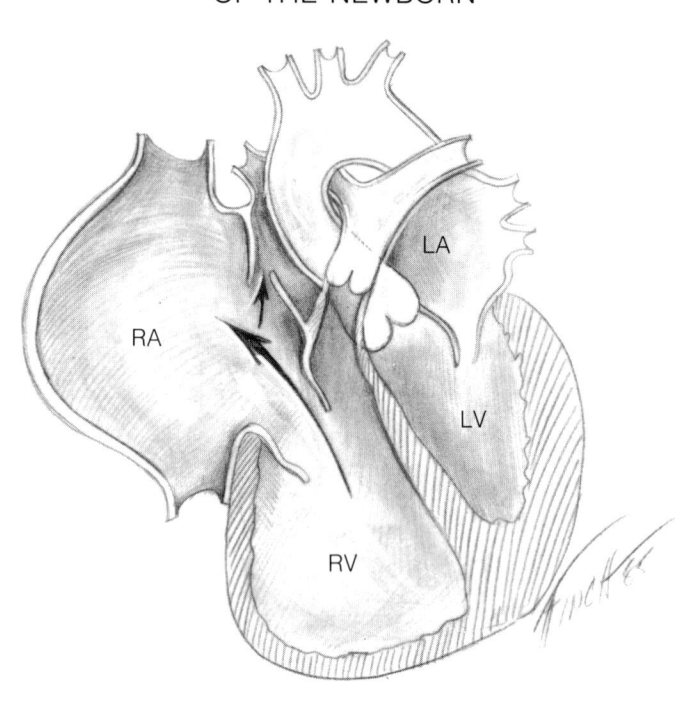

FIG 37–1.
Transient tricuspid insufficiency. Central circulation. Regurgitation from enlarged right ventricle *(RV)* to huge right atrium *(RA) (large arrow)*. Right-to-left shunt at atrial level *(smaller arrow)*. *LA* = left atrium; *LV* = left ventricle.

monary vascular resistance declines, tricuspid regurgitation decreases and may disappear. In addition, improved oxygenation and reduced tension of the papillary muscle improve the status of papillary muscle. A right-to-left shunt occurs through the foramen ovale, causing cyanosis. With the reduction of the tricuspid insufficiency, right atrial pressure falls, the right atrium becomes smaller, and the foramen ovale, which was held open, closes, eliminating the potential for a shunt.

CLINICAL FEATURES

Symptoms are often present during the first day of life. Cyanosis is the initial symptom. It may be associated with findings of congestive cardiac failure. Tachypnea and tachycardia are present. A systolic murmur, which may be loud, is present along the lower left sternal border and radiates to the right precordium. Classically the murmur is high pitched and pansystolic. Hepatomegaly is common.

ELECTROCARDIOGRAPHIC FEATURES

There may be right-axis deviation and right ventricular hypertrophy, but they are difficult to distinguish from the normal pattern of a neonate. In each of our personally observed symptomatic patients, the P waves were tall and peaked (right atrial enlargement). Changes in the ST segments and T waves may be present, reflecting myocardial ischemia.

ECHOCARDIOGRAPHIC FEATURES

Little echocardiographic data are available, but such an examination would help to exclude other conditions with tricuspid abnormalities. Distinction between coexistant pulmonary atresia with tricuspid insufficiency and severe isolated tricuspid insufficiency may be difficult. With significant tricuspid insufficiency the right ventricle may develop insufficient pressure to open the pulmonary valve, and consequently on an echocardiogram, the pulmonary valve appears closed. A Doppler study can show the tricuspid regurgitation and can be used to estimate right ventricular systolic pressure. The foramen ovale may be evident as drop out of atrial septal echoes. Left ventricular contractility may be reduced.

RADIOGRAPHIC FEATURES

Although the radiographic features are typical, they are not diagnostic. The appearance is identical to Ebstein's malformation, pulmonary atresia with intact septum or critical pulmonary stenosis.

1. The heart is greatly enlarged (Fig 37–2). REASON:
    a. Tricuspid regurgitation is usually severe and results

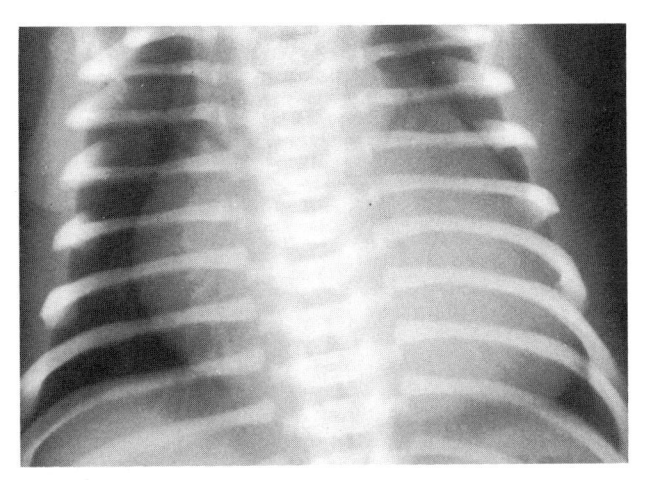

FIG 37–2.
Transient tricuspid insufficiency. Thoracic roentgenogram. Posteroanterior projection. Massively enlarged heart. Decreased pulmonary vasculature. Appearance is identical to Ebstein's malformation or pulmonary atresia with intact ventricular septum.

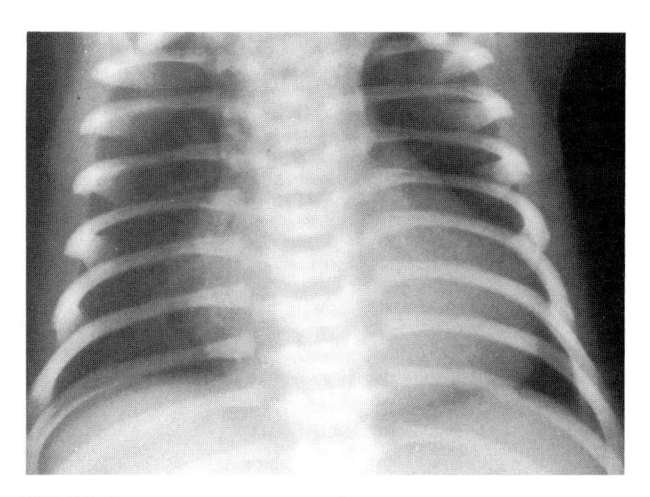

FIG 37–3.
Transient tricuspid insufficiency. Same patient as Figure 37–2. After improvement of tricuspid regurgitation. Thoracic roentgenogram. Posteroanterior projection. Marked decrease in cardiac size and improvement of pulmonary vasculature.

in major right ventricular and right atrial enlargement.
  b. Associated left ventricular enlargement, as a consequence of myocardial ischemia, coexists.
2. The pulmonary vasculature is decreased (see Fig 37–2). REASON: A right-to-left shunt occurs at the atrial level as in neonates with Ebstein's anomaly or with pulmonary atresia with intact ventricular septum.
3. Fluoroscopically the heart is very active. REASON: Increased stroke volume of the right ventricle and systolic expansion of the right atrium.
4. After improvement and the disappearance of tricuspid regurgitation, cardiac size decreases and the pulmonary vasculature becomes normal (Fig 37–3).

CARDIAC CATHETERIZATION

Cardiac catheterization is performed to define the anomaly and exclude coexistent conditions. The catheter tip can be easily advanced into the right ventricle, excluding tricuspid atresia. The catheter rocks freely back and forth across the tricuspid valve because of the tricuspid regurgitation.

Right ventricular systolic pressure is less than systemic and is commonly near normal. If right ventricular systolic pressure is elevated, coexistent pulmonary stenosis must be considered. Right atrial pressures are elevated.

Oxygen saturation in the left atrium and left ventricle are reduced, reflecting the right-to-left atrial shunt at the atrial level.

ANGIOGRAPHIC FEATURES

A large volume of contrast material should be injected rapidly into the right ventricle to avoid dilutional effects of the tricuspid regurgitation. Usually anteroposterior and lateral projections are sufficient for the diagnosis.

1. Right ventriculography (Fig 37–4) shows massive regurgitation through the tricuspid valve during each sys-

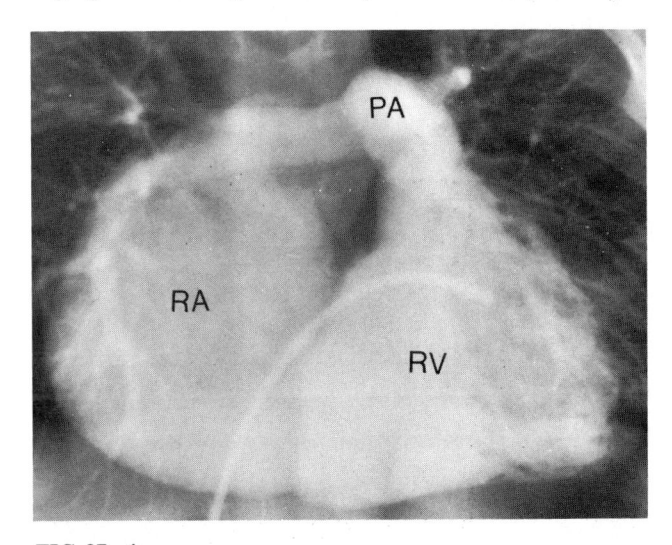

FIG 37–4.
Transient tricuspid insufficiency. Right ventriculogram (RV). Anteroposterior projection. Dense opacification of right atrium from tricuspid regurgitation. Markedly enlarged right atrium (RA) and right ventricle. Tricuspid annulus and valve are in normal location. There is no atrialized portion of right ventricle; therefore, diagnosis of Ebstein's malformation is unlikely. PA = pulmonary artery.

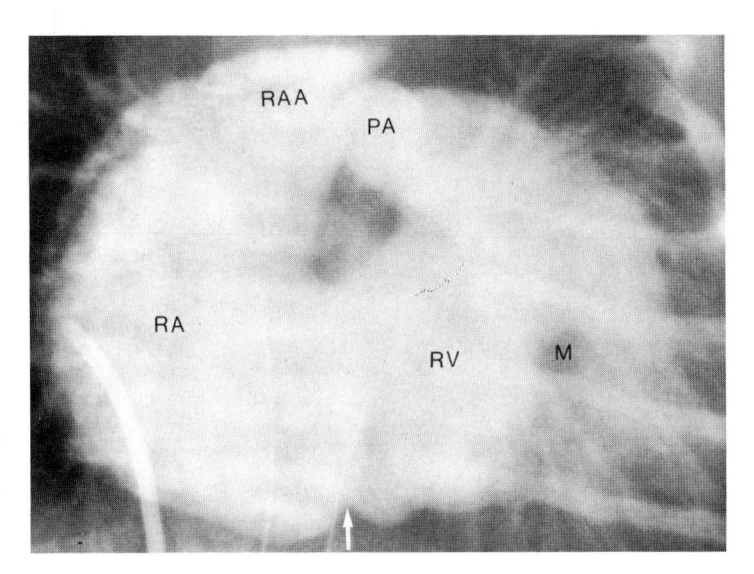

FIG 37–5.
Transient tricuspid insufficiency. Right atriogram (RA). Anteroposterior projection. Massively enlarged right atrium and appendage (RAA). Tricuspid annulus is well demonstrated (arrow). No evidence for Ebstein's malformation. Incidental nonobstructing muscle bundle (M). PA = pulmonary artery; RV = right ventricle.

tole. The right atrium expands during systole, and contrast material may reflux into the venae cavae.

2. The right ventricle is greatly enlarged and pulsatile. The pulmonary valve opens during systole, contrary to instances with coexistent pulmonary atresia.

3. Right atriogram may show a greatly enlarged, pulsatile right atrium (Fig 37–5). The tricuspid annulus is of normal size and the valve normally located (in contrast to Ebstein's malformation).

4. Contrast material passes from right-to-left atrium through a foramen ovale, opacifying the left atrium and left ventricle, thereby demonstrating the right-to-left shunt.

5. On improvement of the tricuspid insufficiency, right ventriculography demonstrates less tricuspid regurgitation and marked decrease in right ventricular and right atrial size (Fig 37–6).

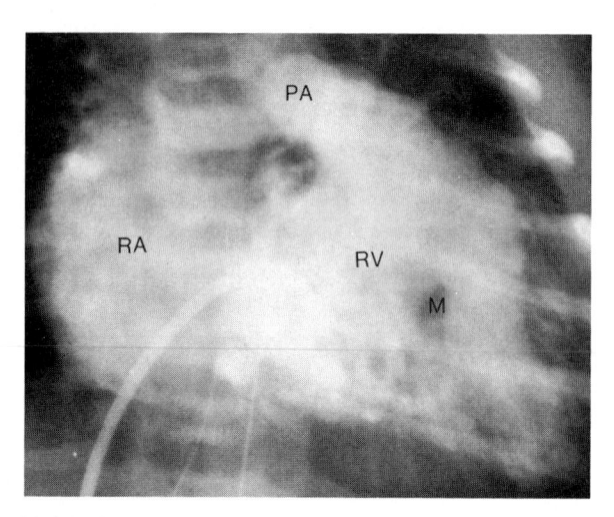

MANAGEMENT

Neonates with transient tricuspid insufficiency and some neonates with tricuspid dysplasia improve as the pulmonary vascular resistance declines to a normal level. In neonates, treatment is directed at improving hypoxemia, acidosis, and hypoglycemia, lowering pulmonary vasculature resistance, and improving myocardial contractility. Digitalis or other inotropic support should be given. In most neonates, the murmur disappears and cardiac size returns to normal during infancy. In symptomatic neonates or infants with tricuspid dysplasia who fail to improve, management is difficult. The mortality in such infants is considerable. Replacement of the tricuspid valve may be attempted in severely ill infants, but this is difficult and associated with a high mortality.

FIG 37–6.
Transient tricuspid insufficiency. Same patient as Figure 37–5 after improvement. Anteroposterior projection. Marked reduction in right ventricular size. Minor tricuspid regurgitation is still present. PA = pulmonary artery; RV = right ventricle; M = muscle bundle; RA = right atriogram.

REFERENCES

1. Shrivastava S, Moller JH: Severe isolated tricuspid regurgitation in the neonate. Unpublished observations, 1985.
2. Becker AE, Becker MJ, Edwards JE: Pathologic spectrum of dysplasia of the tricuspid valve: features in common with Ebstein's malformation, Arch Pathol 91:167, 1971.
3. Boucek RJ Jr, Graham TP Jr, Morgan JP, et al: Spontaneous resolution of massive congenital tricuspid insufficiency, Circulation 54:795, 1976.
4. Freymann R, Kallfelz HC: Transient tricuspid incompetence in a newborn, Eur J Cardiol 2:467, 1975.
5. Bucciarelli RL, Nelson RM, Egan EA II, et al: Transient tricuspid insufficiency of the newborn: a form of myocardial dysfunction in stressed newborns, Pediatrics 59:330, 1977.

6. Nelson RM, Bucciarelli RL, Eitzman DV, et al: Serum creatine phosphokinase MB fraction in newborns with transient tricuspid insufficiency, *N Engl J Med* 298:146, 1978.
7. Barr PA, Celermajer JM, Bowdler JD, et al: Severe congenital tricuspid incompetence in the neonate, *Circulation* 49:962, 1974.
8. Sanayl SK, Bhargava SK, Saxena HMK, et al: Congenital insufficiency of the tricuspid valve: a rare cause of massive cardiomegaly and congestive cardiac failure in neonate, *Indian Heart J* 20:214, 1968.
9. Reisman M, Hipona FA, Bloor CM, et al: Congenital tricuspid insufficiency: a cause of massive cardiomegaly and heart failure in the neonate, *J Pediatr* 66:869, 1965.

PART FIVE

Cyanosis and Increased Pulmonary Arterial Vasculature

The cardiac conditions resulting in cyanosis and increased pulmonary arterial vasculature have been called "admixture lesions," indicating the potential for mixture of systemic and pulmonary venous returns. In common, therefore, each of these conditions have bidirectional shunts, a right-to-left shunt, as indicated by cyanosis, and a left-to-right shunt, as indicated by the usually present increased pulmonary blood flow on a thoracic roentgenogram. The admixture may be virtually complete, resulting in equal aortic and pulmonary arterial oxygen saturations or incomplete admixture as occurs in the most common anomaly in this group of admixture lesions, transposition of the great vessels. Although patients with transposition show evidence of a portion of the systemic venous blood entering the left atrium or ventricle and a portion of pulmonary venous return entering the right atrium or ventricle, the volume of blood going in either direction is limited. Therefore, the aortic and pulmonary arterial oxygen saturations are dissimilar. In fact, early treatment of this condition is designed to improve the admixture.

Complete mixture occurs in the less common lesions of the group, and in these, aortic and pulmonary arterial oxygen saturations are equal or nearly so. In these lesions the entire systemic and pulmonary venous returns empty into a common chamber before being distributed into the systemic and pulmonary arterial circuits, respectively. Complete admixture may occur at any level of the heart: at the level of veins—total anomalous pulmonary venous connection, at the level of the atrium—single atrium, at the level of the ventricle—single ventricle, or at the level of the great vessels—truncus arteriosus. In these instances the shunts are obligatory because of the anatomic connections.

Among patients with admixture lesions other than transposition of the great vessels, there is an inverse relationship between the volume of pulmonary blood flow and the degree of cyanosis. Therefore, the greater the volume of pulmonary blood flow, the less the degree of cyanosis and vice versa. Thus, observation about the degree of cyanosis provides information about the factors, such as pulmonary vascular resistance, influencing pulmonary blood flow.

The hemodynamics of admixture lesions result from an anatomic lesion that allows mixture of the two major venous returns. In cardiac conditions with an atretic cardiac valve, whether atrioventricular or semilunar valve, admixture occurs. Tricuspid atresia and mitral atresia have uniform mixing at the atrial level, and pulmonary atresia and aortic atresia could also be considered admixture lesions, because the aorta and pulmonary artery also have uniform mixing of blood at the atrial level. We have not grouped them as admixture lesions, however, because their basic hemodynamic, clinical, and laboratory findings are individually different, and none closely resembles the other admixture conditions. Besides, their pattern of pulmonary vasculature is different, being decreased in pulmonary atresia and in tricuspid atresia, and showing mixed pulmonary arterial and venous vasculature in mitral atresia and in aortic atresia. Other conditions such as single ventricle with pulmonary stenosis or truncus arteriosus with stenosis of the pulmonary arteries may have decreased pulmonary blood flow, but the principle of uniform mixing and inverse relationship between cyanosis and magnitude of pulmonary blood flow still exists.

The hemodynamic factors that govern the shunts at the atrial, ventricular, or great vessel level are similar to those governing the conditions associated with a left-to-right shunt at these levels. Relative ventricular compliance governs shunts at the atrial level and relative vascular resistances for shunts at the ventricular or great vessel level. Similarly many of the clinical and laboratory features resemble those of comparable left-to-right shunts.

In conditions with atrial admixture, such as total anomalous pulmonary venous connection or single atrium, the major features reflect increased blood flow through the structures of the right side of the heart, namely, pulmonary systolic ejection murmur, tricuspid mid-diastolic murmur, wide splitting of the second heart sound, and an electrocardiographic pattern of incomplete right bundle branch block. Fixed splitting of the second heart sound and the absence of left atrial enlargement reflect the communication in the atrial septum. Pulmonary hypertension is uncommon in cases of atrial admixture.

In anomalies with admixture at either the ventricular or great vessel level, the magnitude of pulmonary blood flow is generally determined by the relationship between pulmonary and systemic vascular resistances. These patients usually have evidence of pulmonary hypertension and features reflecting increased blood flow through the left-sided cardiac chambers—left atrial enlargement, apical middiastolic murmur, and left ventricular hypertrophy on the electrocardiogram. The development of congestive cardiac failure, which commonly occurs in these patients, appears at 2 to 3 months of age, when the pulmonary vascular resistance has declined to such a point to allow left ventricular dilatation and cardiac failure.

Patients with admixture lesions have potential complications, such as brain abscess and paradoxical embolism. Because of the increased pulmonary blood flow, they have increased respiratory tract infections and episodes of pneumonia. Congestive cardiac failure is common. The combination of hypoxemia and cardiac failure lead to slow growth.

In this section, we discuss transposition of the great vessels and its variants first, before turning our attention to the less common, and more anatomically variable forms of admixture lesions.

In the interpretation of angiograms of patients with an admixture lesion, particularly if there are abnormalities of the relative position of the great vessels, it is helpful to use a logical method to analyze the structures of the heart, identifying each segment of the heart and its relation to the next portion of the heart (segmental approach).

Angiographically the heart can be submitted to segmental analysis allowing identification of cardiac structures and relationships.

1. Analysis starts on the venous side of the circulation with the identification of the right (venous) atrium. Almost invariably the right atrium is an extension of the inferior vena cava; although rarely, the inferior vena cava enters the left atrium directly, most commonly seen in syndrome.

2. The right atrium connects to a ventricle that can be either an anatomic right ventricle or an anatomic left ventricle. The former is called "concordant atrioventricular connection" and the latter "discordant atrioventricular connection."

3. The atrioventricular valves correspond to the respective ventricles. Thus, the right ventricle has a tricuspid valve, and a left ventricle has a mitral valve. Whether the atrioventricular connection is concordant or disconcordant, the ventricle connected to the right atrium is a venous ventricle and receives desaturated blood.

4. From the ventricles the great arteries arise, and the connection may be concordant or disconcordant at this site also. If the right ventricle gives rise to the pulmonary artery, the ventriculoarterial connection is normal (i.e., concordant). If the right ventricle gives rise to the aorta, the ventriculoarterial connection is discordant (i.e., the great vessels are transposed).

This segmental approach to cardiac structures is useful in the analysis of complex forms of transposition. Both the physiology and the anatomy should be considered in the diagnostic analysis of angiograms. A uniform terminology has not been agreed on to describe transposition of the great vessels, so we will use three terminologies: One using traditional terms, such as complete or corrected transposition; a second describing position of the great vessels and relative position of the ventricles, such as D-transposition or L-transposition of great vessels with ventricular inversion; and a third describing connections, such as atrioventricular concordance and ventricular arterial discordance.

ANGIOGRAPHIC ANALYSIS

In the analysis of angiographic films of patients with malposition of the great vessels, two steps are important:

1. Disregard purely anatomic terms that may lead to a misinterpretation. Replace the term "right" ventricle with "venous" ventricle. The venous ventricle receives systemic venous blood and may anatomically be either

a right or a left ventricle. Therefore, it is important to determine if the venous or arterial ventricle has been injected. Information about the blood oxygen determination measured from the ventricle just before angiography and the anatomic angiographic appearance of the ventricle are helpful as well. In doubtful cases, the right atrial injection or venous angiography will identify the right atrium and atrioventricular connection. Angiographic identification of the anatomic right atrium is usually unnecessary, because the inferior vena cava connects to the anatomic right atrium.

Once we have determined which ventricle has been injected, we determine the great artery that arises from the ventricle. If the aorta arises from the venous ventricle, the diagnosis is a form of transposition of the great vessels. If the pulmonary artery arises from the venous ventricle, the basic hemodynamic pattern is that of a normal heart. If a transposition is present and the hemodynamics are correct, L-loop transposition (discordant atrioventricular connection with transposition or corrected transposition of the great vessels) should be considered.

2. Identify the anatomic characteristics of the ventricles.
   a. Angiographic features of a morphologic right ventricle include the following:
      (1) Coarse trabeculations.
      (2) Although the tricuspid valve has three papillary muscles, these are usually not seen on angiograms.
      (3) The tricuspid valve annulus, which is readily identified during diastole as a round or oval filling defect (blood entering the opacified ventricle), is separated from the pulmonary artery by the infundibulum.
      (4) Rarely, the semilunar valve is in continuity with the right atrioventricular valve because of deficient development of the conus.
   b. The angiographic identification of a morphologic left ventricle include the following:
      (1) Left ventricular free wall shows fine trabeculations, whereas the left ventricular outflow tract and septal surface show virtually no trabeculations.
      (2) During systole two papillary muscles of the mitral valve are usually seen as filling defects.
      (3) The mitral valve is in fibrous continuity with the semilunar valve, because there is no infundibulum in a left ventricle.
      (4) Rarely, the semilunar valve is not in continuity with the atrioventricular valve because of persistence of the left conus. Because in this case the right ventricle also has an infundibulum, this condition is usually referred to as "double coni." The conus can also be deficient bilaterally.
      (5) A triangular shape.

Using this physiologic and anatomic approach to the angiogram should allow precise definition of the cardiac malformation. Malformations with transposition can be described using various terminologies currently employed by various authors. Because of the variable backgrounds of the readers we use all three terminologies in the following chapters.

CHAPTER 38

Complete Transposition of the Great Vessels

Complete transposition of the great vessels accounts for 8% of all instances of congenital cardiac malformations. It occurs twice as often in males as females. Without treatment, 90% of infants die by 1 year of age.

In this common congenital cardiac malformation causing cyanosis, the aorta arises from the right ventricle and the pulmonary artery from the left ventricle. The term transposition (trans + ponere) means placed across, and when it is applied to the great vessels, it indicates that they are misplaced across the ventricular septum.

The term transposition has been defined and described in various ways. Transposition as applied to the great vessels has been used to indicate that the aorta is the anterior blood vessel and the pulmonary artery the posterior blood vessel (the opposite of normal). This definition of transposition is inaccurate, because in some patients with a circulatory pattern of complete transposition of the great vessels, the aorta lies posterior to the pulmonary artery but arises from the right ventricle.

The term "D-transposition" of the great vessels has also been applied to complete transposition of the great vessels. D-Transposition was defined to indicate that the aorta is positioned anteriorly and to the right of the pulmonary artery. Although in most patients with complete transposition of the great vessels, the term accurately defines the interrelationships between the aorta and pulmonary artery (Fig 38–1,A), this is not invariable. In this condition, the aorta may be anteriorly (Fig 38–1,B) and leftward (Fig 38–1,C), side by side (Fig 38–1,D) or posterior (Fig 38–1,E) to the pulmonary artery (posterior transposition). Furthermore, the D- in the term D- transposition should not be confused with the D used to describe ventricular looping.

Transposition has also been defined using a segmental anatomic approach, in which the relationship between various segments of the heart is described. In complete transposition of the great vessels, there is concordant atrioventricular connection, but there is ventriculoarterial discordance, indicating that there is an incorrect connection between the great arteries and the respective ventricles. This definition is the most satisfactory because it describes the interrelationship between anatomic structures and is not based merely on external relationships.

PATHOLOGIC ANATOMY

Complete transposition of the great vessels has been considered to result from abnormal conal development and abnormal conoventricular positioning.[1] Initially, conal tissue lies beneath both semilunar valves in the embryo. Normally the subpulmonary portions of the conus develops while the subaortic portion involutes. As a result, the pulmonary artery normally arises from an infundibulum, which is positioned anteriorly and to the left, whereas the aorta arising from the left ventricle does not have an infundibulum. Transposition of great vessels has been considered to result from absorption of the left-sided subpulmonary portion of the conus and development of the right-sided subaortic portion of the conus.

The interrelationships between the atria and ventricles are normal. The aorta arises from the infundibulum of the right ventricle and the pulmonary artery from the left ventricle (Fig 38–2). Fibrous continuity may exist between the mitral valve and the transposed pulmonary valve (Fig 38–3), but often there is a narrow muscular separation (left-sided conus) separating the mitral and pulmonary valves.

In 60% of patients, the ventricular septum is intact, and in the other 40%, a ventricular septal defect is present.

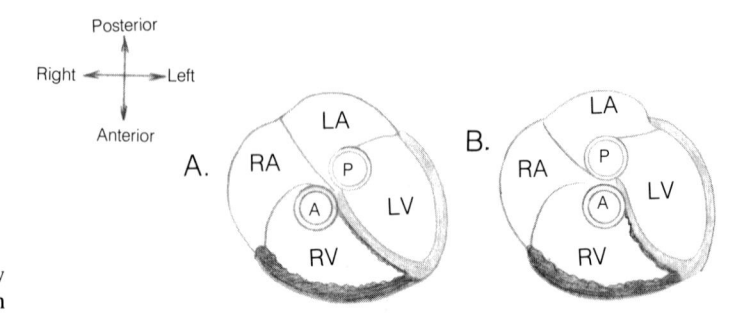

676 *Cyanosis and Increased Pulmonary Arterial Vasculature*

FIG 38–1.
Transposition of great vessels. View from above. Diagram showing relation of aorta *(A)* and pulmonary artery *(P)*. **A,** aorta is anterior and to the right of pulmonary artery. **B,** aorta is directly anterior of pulmonary artery. **C,** aorta is anterior and to the left of pulmonary artery. **D,** aorta is to the right and lateral to pulmonary artery. **E,** aorta is to the right and posterior of pulmonary artery. *LA* = left atrium; *LV* = left ventricle; *RA* = right atrium; *RV* = right ventricle.

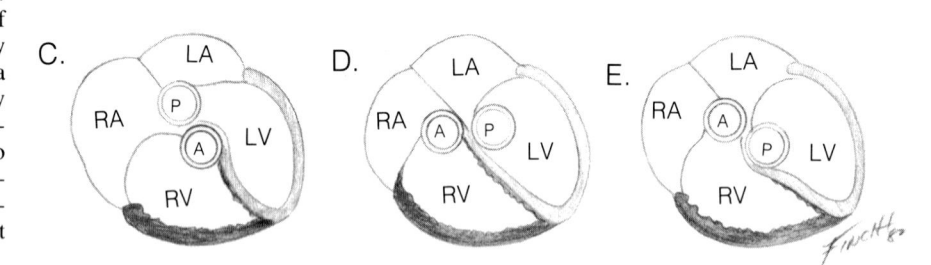

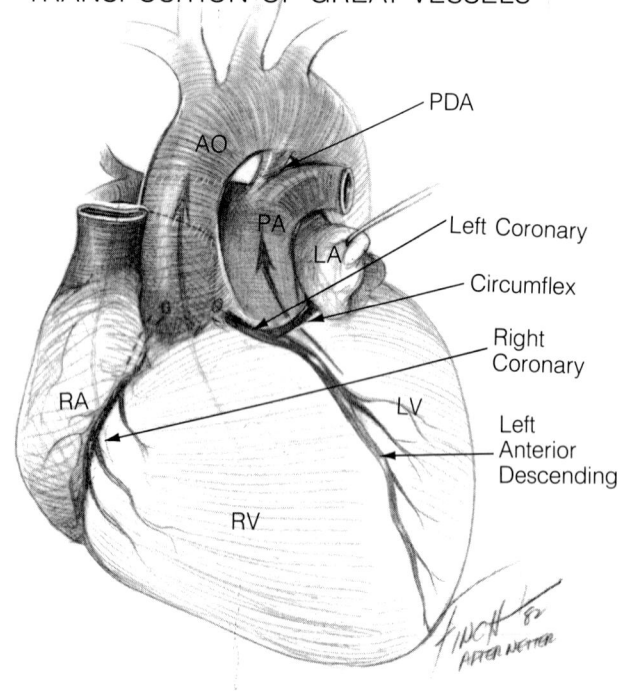

FIG 38–2.
Transposition of great vessels. Diagram showing anatomic relationships. Aorta *(AO)* arises from right ventricle *(RV)*. Pulmonary artery *(PA)* arises from left ventricle *(LV)*. Coronary arteries arise posteriorly from aorta. *LA* = left atrium; *PDA* = patent ductus arteriosus; *RA* = right atrium.

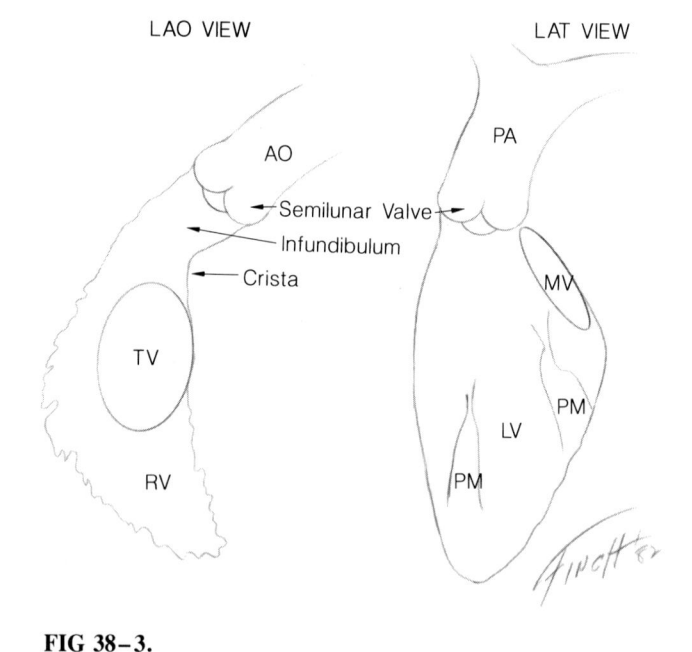

FIG 38–3.
Transposition of great vessels. Diagram showing outline of right ventricle *(RV)* in left anterior oblique view and left ventricle *(LV)* in lateral view as they would appear angiographically. Tricuspid valve *(TV)* is separated from semilunar valve. Mitral valve *(MV)* is continuous with semilunar valve. *PM* = papillary muscle.

An atrial septal defect and patent ductus arteriosus are uncommon after the neonatal period.

Subpulmonary stenosis is common and may be either fixed or dynamic. Fixed pulmonary stenosis is present in one third of patients with a coexistent ventricular septal defect. Stenosis may result from valvar stenosis, subpulmonary membrane, accessory mitral valve tissue, tethering of the anterior leaflet of the mitral valve by abnormal chordae tendineae to the ventricular septum, or, rarely, herniation of septal leaflet of the tricuspid valve through the ventricular septal defect.

Dynamic subpulmonary stenosis may develop during the first year of life, primarily in infants with an intact ventricular septum (Fig 38–4,A). In such patients left ventricular systolic pressure is considerably lower than right ventricular systolic pressure. Therefore, after birth as the left ventricle thins, the interventricular septum bulges into the left ventricle, causing subpulmonary narrowing. Other causes of left-sided obstruction are demonstrated in Figure 38–4.

The origins of both coronary arteries is different from the normal heart. Normally the anterior cusp gives rise to the right coronary artery. In transposition, however, the anterior cusp does not give rise to a coronary artery and is therefore the noncoronary cusp (Fig 38–5). The posterior origin of the coronary arteries allows the surgeon to switch the great vessels and transplant the coronary arteries (see later discussion of arterial switch operation). In most cases the left coronary artery gives rise to the circumflex and anterior descending branch, but in contrast to normal, it passes anteriorly to the pulmonary artery. Less frequently the circumflex branch arises from the right, or there may be a single coronary artery as in the normal heart.

HEMODYNAMICS

Because of the transposition of the great vessels, two largely independent circulations, the pulmonary and systemic, exist. These circulations are in parallel rather than in series as in a normal individual. Thus, systemic venous return entering the right atrium from the vena cavae flows predominately to the aorta, whereas pulmonary venous blood is returned principally to the pulmonary artery and lungs. Survival depends on bidirectional shunting between the two sides of the heart. The bidirectional shunting may occur at either the atrial or the ventricular level, depending on the coexistent anomalies. If more than one communication is present, the shunt at the atrial level is usually from left to right.

Because of these features, the major hemodynamic abnormalities are deficient oxygen delivery to tissues and abnormal left and right ventricular workloads related to increased systolic pressures and to increased diastolic volumes.

In patients with an intact ventricular septum, blood flows through the ductus arteriosus from the aorta to the pulmonary artery in early neonatal life. Thus, the volume of blood returning to the left atrium is increased, and fully saturated blood flows from the left atrium to the right atrium. When the ductus arteriosus closes (on the first or second day of life), a bidirectional shunt exists at the atrial level, being from right to left during ventricular diastole, and left to right during ventricular systole.[2] Factors that control this exchange are not understood, but over a period of time, the volume passing from left to right and from right to left are equal, but there are phasic differences.

In patients with transposition of the great vessels and large ventricular septal defect, the level of arterial oxygen saturation depends in large part on the volume of pulmonary blood flow, with a large flow being associated with a higher systemic oxygen saturation.[3] If pulmonary stenosis or pulmonary vascular disease develop, reducing pulmonary blood flow, cyanosis intensifies.

Factors influencing the volume of pulmonary blood flow are unknown but have generally been considered related to ventricular compliance (e.g., in atrial septal defect) in patients with intact ventricular septum or relative resistances to ventricular outflow (e.g., in ventricular septal defect) if there is a large ventricular communication.

Left ventricular failure may occur in patients with a large volume of pulmonary blood flow, as in patients with an isolated ventricular septal defect.

Bronchopulmonary arterial collaterals develop in patients with transposition of the great vessels. Bronchial arterial blood thus enters the pulmonary arterial bed at a site proximal to the pulmonary capillaries. This may serve as an additional site of right-to-left shunt.

Natural History

Four events occur with time among patients with transposition of the great vessels.

1. Development of pulmonary vascular obstructive disease. Patients with complete transposition of the great vessels develop pulmonary vascular obstructive disease in greater frequency and at an accelerated rate compared with other types of congenital cardiac malformations with a similar level of pulmonary blood flow and pulmonary arterial pressure.[4-6] Vascular disease develops most frequently in patients with coexistent ventricular septal defect but also among those with intact ventricular septum[7] or with associated pulmonary stenosis. Microthrombi have been identified in pulmonary arterioles and are considered a contributing factor. Prolonged hypoxemia and poly-

LEFT SIDED OBSTRUCTIONS
IN COMPLETE TRANSPOSITION OF THE GREAT VESSELS

FIG 38–4.
Transposition of great vessels. Anatomic causes of left ventricular outflow obstruction as they would appear on left ventriculogram, lateral projection. **A,** dynamic subpulmonary stenosis between ventricular septum and anterior leaflet of mitral valve, which moves anteriorly during systole. **B,** normal systolic posterior motion of mitral valve peripheral pulmonary artery stenosis. **C,** valvar pulmonary stenosis. **D,** discrete membranous subpulmonary stenosis. **E,** dysplastic pulmonary valve. **F,** aneurysm of membranous septum. **G,** accessory mitral valve tissue. **H,** Supravalvar stenosis. **I,** pulmonary artery branch stenosis.

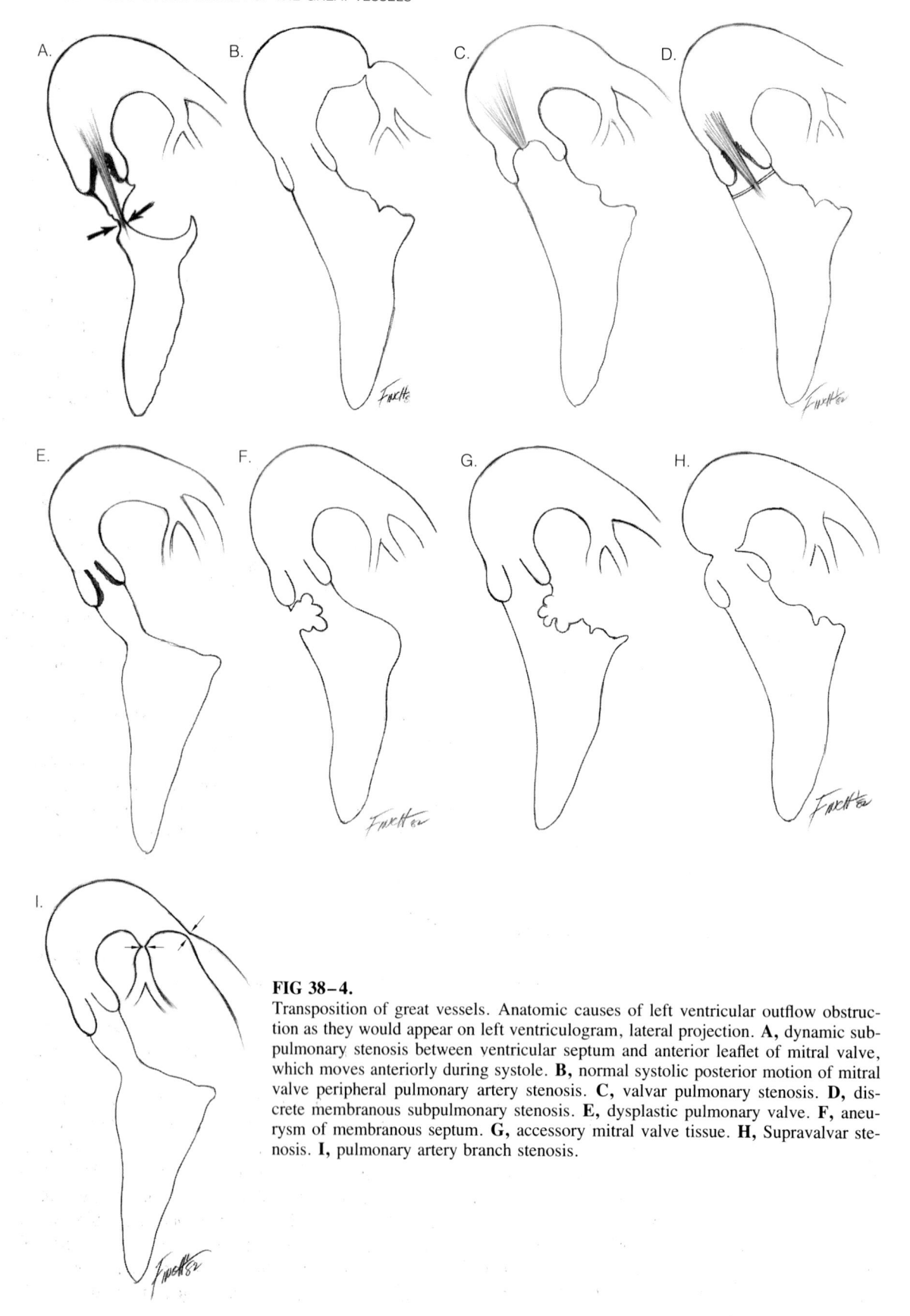

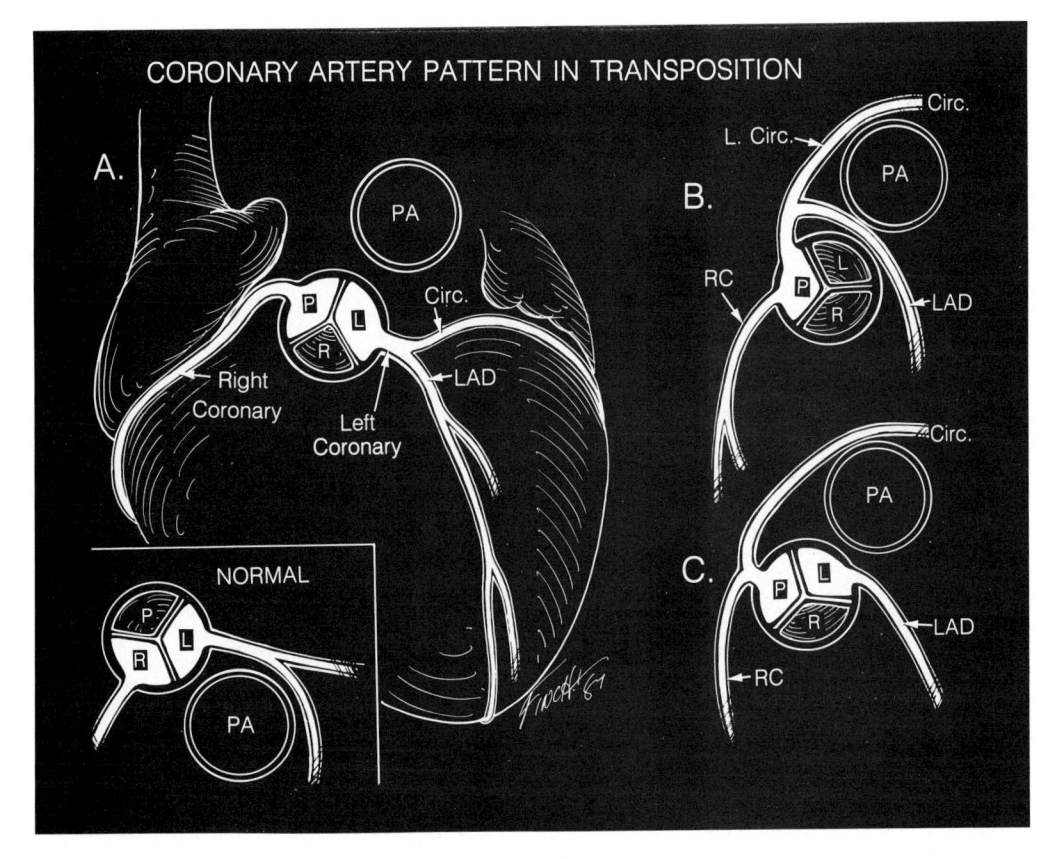

FIG 38–5.
Transposition of great vessels. Coronary arterial pattern. **A,** most common pattern. Right coronary artery arises above posterior *(P)* cusp and left coronary artery arises above left *(L)* cusp. Right *(R)* cusp is noncoronary. **B,** variant. Both coronary arteries arise above posterior cusp. **C,** variant. Right coronary *(RC)* artery and circumflex artery *(CIRC)* arise from common trunk above posterior cusp. Left anterior descending *(LAD)* coronary artery arises above left cusp. *Insert,* coronary artery pattern in normal. Posterior cusp in noncoronary. *PA* = pulmonary artery.

cythemia are other potential factors in patients with intact ventricular septum.

In patients with a ventricular septal defect, pulmonary vascular changes may be noted by 6 months of age. Hypoxemia of the pulmonary vascular bed may be a factor in the development of these changes. Particularly because of the bronchial-pulmonary arterial anastomosis, desaturated blood perfuses pulmonary arterioles.[8] In addition, the pulmonary arterioles contain thinner media and show less hypertrophy in response to elevated pressure than other conditions with similar level of pulmonary arterial pressure. The other disturbing feature is that pulmonary vascular disease may progress after successful correction of the anomaly with an atrial switch procedure.[9]

Assessment of pulmonary vascular resistance by cardiac catheterization remains difficult because of the inaccuracies in the application of the Fick principle to this circulatory pattern.

2. Development of subpulmonary stenosis. In patients with intact ventricular septum, subpulmonary stenosis may develop during the first year of life. Because left ventricular systolic pressure is low, with time the interventricular septum bows into the left ventricle, causing subpulmonary stenosis.[10] In addition, the mitral valve moves anteriorly towards the septum during systole. The reason is unknown. The severity of subpulmonary stenosis tends to be exaggerated before corrective operation.

3. Deterioration of ventricular function. Angiographic and echocardiographic measurements of right ventricular dimensions show an increased right ventricular end-diastolic volume, low ejection fraction, and prolonged right ventricular ejection time,[11] suggesting depressed right ventricular myocardial function. This has been taken to indicate that the right ventricle is poorly adapted to serve as a systemic pump. The etiology of these changes remains unknown and is in contrast to the apparently normal right ventricular function in patients with tetralogy of Fallot.

4. Spontaneous closure of ventricular septal defect. The ventricular septal defect may undergo spontaneous closure or diminution in size.[12] This event occurs more commonly than among patients with isolated ventricular septal defect. This may be related to the fact that most infants with transposition of the great vessels undergo cardiac catheterization, whereas only selected patients with a large ventricular septal defect receive cardiac catheterization.

CLINICAL FEATURES

Cyanosis is the major clinical finding on both history and physical examination. It becomes clinically evident by 48 hours of age in patients with an intact ventricular septum, because at this age the ductus arteriosus has closed, eliminating a major route of shunting. In neonates, the cyanosis is often intense and complicated by acidosis. In infants with a large ventricular septal defect or a large patent ductus arteriosus, cyanosis is less intense, but the major symptoms and findings are those of congestive cardiac failure from left ventricular volume overload.

On physical examination, the neonate is often heavy, may be chubby, and has tachypnea (because of hypoxemia). Subsequently, growth may be slowed until corrective operation is performed.

In the neonatal period, auscultation usually shows no murmur or, at best, a soft, nonspecific systolic murmur along the left sternal border. The heart sounds may seem normal for a neonate, but the second heart sound is usually single and loud because the aortic valve is anteriorly placed and therefore close to the anterior thoracic wall. If the ductus arteriosus is patent, a continuous murmur may be heard.

Among infants with associated ventricular septal defect, a grade 3 to 4/6 pansystolic murmur may be present. Usually these patients are less cyanotic but have findings of congestive cardiac failure. An apical middiastolic murmur may be present as well.

In patients with subpulmonary stenosis, a grade 2 to 3/6 systolic ejection murmur is heard along the left sternal border, and this is transmitted to the right side of the back. This murmur may appear in patients who develop subpulmonary stenosis.

ELECTROCARDIOGRAPHIC FEATURES

Most patients show right-axis deviation and right ventricular hypertrophy. In patients with ventricular septal defect and increased pulmonary blood flow, left ventricular hypertrophy may coexist. In the neonate, the electrocardiogram is identical with that of a normal neonate. In the normal infant, the axis shifts toward the normal, and the R wave in lead V_1 decreases in amplitude; in transposition of the great vessels, however, these changes persist and represent right ventricular hypertrophy.

ECHOCARDIOGRAPHIC FEATURES

Cross-sectional echocardiography allows easy identification of transposition, because the great vessels can be followed to their major branching, especially when subcostal imaging is employed.[13-15] Thus, it is usually easy to follow the great vessel arising from the left ventricle to its major bifurcation into left and right pulmonary arteries.

Cross-sectional echocardiography is also useful in determining the size of the atrial communication both before and after septostomy, the presence of larger ventricular septal defects, and some forms of subpulmonary obstruction.[16, 17] In dynamic subpulmonary stenosis there is abnormal septal motion and anterior systolic motion of the anterior leaflet of the mitral valve. Doppler analysis shows retrograde diastolic flow in the pulmonary artery if the ductus is patent. This offers confirmation that the posterior great artery is the pulmonary artery. Flows across the foramen ovale can also be assessed, especially with subcostal imaging.

RADIOGRAPHIC FEATURES

Transposition of the great vessels is the most common cyanotic lesion associated with increased pulmonary blood flow and presents a fairly characteristic radiographic appearance. Therefore, because of its high frequency, a correct diagnosis can usually be made from a posteroanterior thoracic radiograph if the pulmonary vasculature is increased. In patients with complete transposition and decreased pulmonary flow as a result of pulmonary stenosis, the radiographic appearance may be identical to severe tetralogy of Fallot.

Complete Transposition of Great Vessels With Increased Pulmonary Blood Flow

1. The pulmonary vasculature is increased (Fig 38–6). REASON: The systemic and pulmonary circuits com-

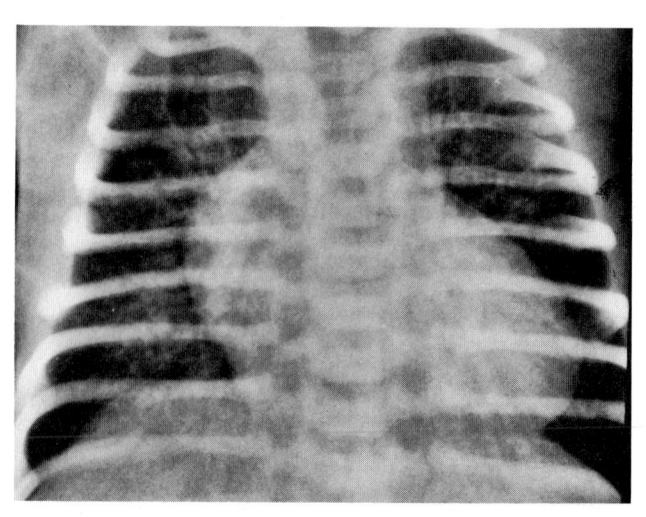

FIG 38–6.
Complete transposition of great vessels without pulmonary stenosis. Thoracic roentgenogram. Posteroanterior projection. Marked cardiomegaly. Increased pulmonary vasculature. Pulmonary arterial segment is not evident. Narrow mediastinum from small amount of thymic tissue and abnormal position of great vessels. Prominent right atrial border. Cardiac configuration with a narrow mediastinum has been called "egg on its side" or "apple on a string."

municate through a foramen ovale, ventricular septal defect, or patent ductus arteriosus. Because the pulmonary vascular resistance is less than the systemic vascular resistance, there is an increased blood flow through the lungs, which distend the pulmonary vasculature.

2. At birth, the pulmonary vasculature appears normal (Fig 38–7). REASON: The elevated neonatal pulmonary vascular resistance precludes an increased pulmonary blood flow.

3. As the pulmonary vascular resistance decreases, the pulmonary vasculature increases (Fig 38–8) and cardiac size increases. There is little relationship between the degree of increased pulmonary vasculature and the volume of bidirectional shunting.

4. Cardiac size is increased. REASON: The volume of blood in the pulmonary circulation is increased, and the left ventricle dilates. The right ventricle is hypertrophied because it is subjected to systemic level of pressure.

5. The right lower cardiac border is prominent because of right atrial enlargement (see Fig 38–6). REASON: The right ventricle is hypertrophied and its compliance reduced. Consequently, right atrial pressure increases.

6. The pulmonary arterial segment is usually concave. REASON: The pulmonary artery, although enlarged, is located centrally and behind the aorta. Consequently, it does not form the left cardiac border as in a normal patient. This is particularly striking, because in most patients with increased pulmonary blood flow, the pulmonary artery forms a prominent bulge along the upper left cardiac border.

7. The increased pulmonary vasculature, absence of the pulmonary arterial segment, and absence of the thymus

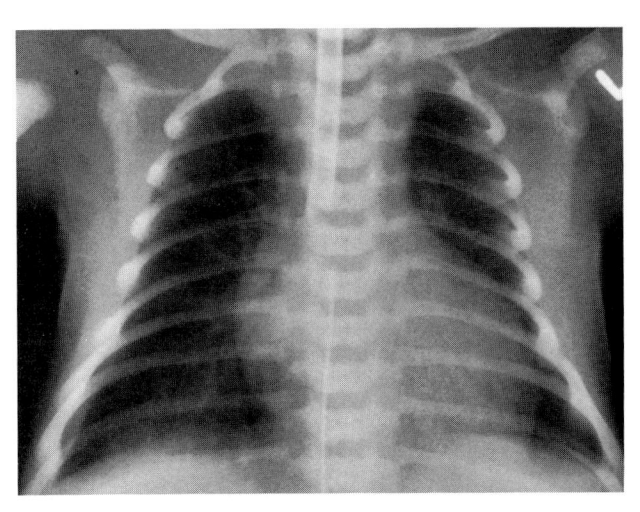

FIG 38–8.
Complete transposition of great vessels. Infant. Same patient as Figure 38–7. Thoracic roentgenogram. Posteroanterior projection. Increased pulmonary vasculature secondary to decreasing pulmonary vascular resistance. Increase in cardiac size.

are the key radiographic features of complete transposition of the great vessels (Fig 38–9,A). Because transposition of the great vessels is a severe cardiac malformation, it may result in stress related shrinkage of the thymus.

8. Depending on the volume of pulmonary blood flow, left atrial enlargement is present (Fig 38–9,B). REASON: Because of increased pulmonary blood flow, the left atrium is distended as a result of the increased volume of blood it receives.

9. Rarely, the thymus is prominent, and this finding precludes the correct radiographic diagnosis (Fig 38–10).

10. In an infant the appearance of the pulmonary vasculature is identical to a left-to-right shunt. In older patients, however, the peripheral pulmonary arteries may appear fluffy and indistinct (see Figs 38–9 and 5–11). This pattern is sometimes called "admixture vasculature" and can also be observed in other cyanotic cardiac anomalies and is not specific for complete transposition of great vessels. REASON: Not definitely known but probably caused by extensive bronchopulmonary arterial communications, which have been demonstrated both pathologically and angiographically. Hypoxemia generally causes an overgrowth of the capillary bed and also reflex vasospasm of the pulmonary arteries. Also overgrowth of bronchial arteries occurs, resulting in bronchopulmonary arterial shunting.

Because of the orientation of the left ventricle, the blood flow is directed primarily into the right pulmonary artery. Blood flow through the right lung, therefore, is commonly increased compared with the left lung, which can be proved by perfusion scans.

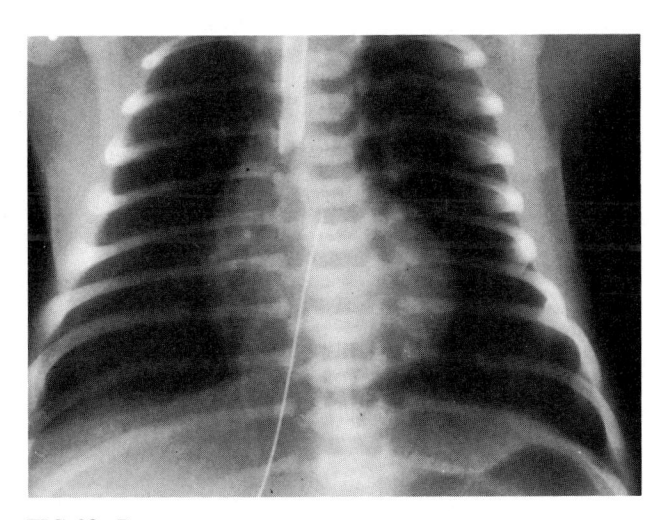

FIG 38–7.
Complete transposition of great vessels. Neonate. Thoracic roentgenogram. Posteroanterior projection. Normal pulmonary vasculature. Normal cardiac size.

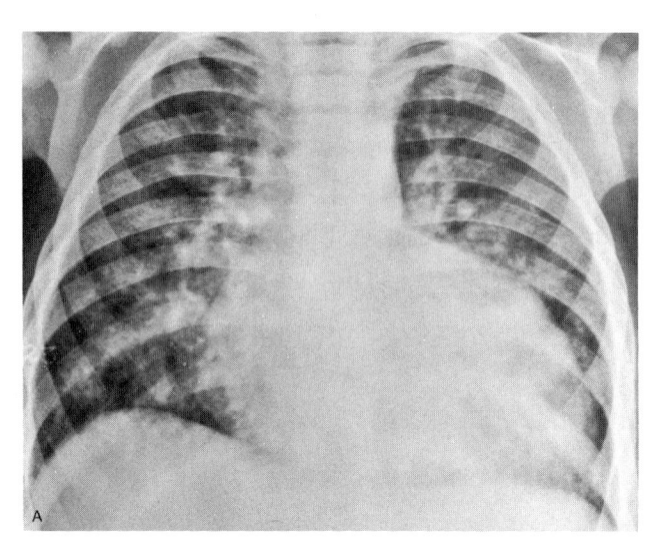

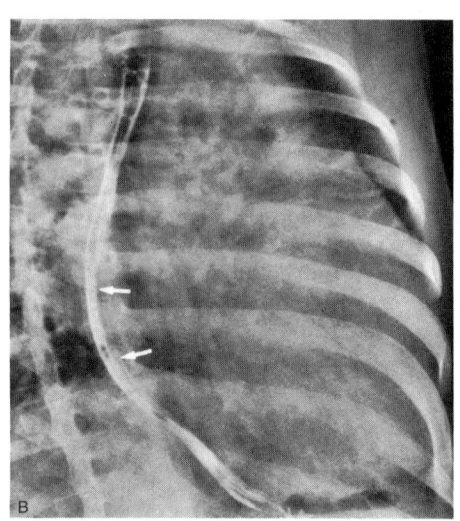

FIG 38–9.
Complete transposition of great vessels. Thoracic roentgenogram. **A,** posteroanterior projection. Marked increased pulmonary vasculature and cardiomegaly. In spite of increased pulmonary flow, pulmonary arterial segment is concave because main pulmonary artery is located medially. (Increased pulmonary vasculature without a prominent pulmonary arterial segment always suggests an abnormally placed pulmonary artery.) The pulmonary vasculature has a fluffy appearance consistent with an admixture lesion. **B,** right anterior oblique projection. Left atrial enlargement *(arrows)*.

Transposition of the Great Vessels With Obstruction of Pulmonary Flow

In 10% of patients with complete transposition of great vessels, pulmonary stenosis, particularly subpulmonary obstruction, and ventricular septal defect are present. Normal or decreased pulmonary blood flow results. The radiographic appearance is therefore different from complete transposition of the great vessels with increased pulmonary flow.

1. The pulmonary vasculature is normal or decreased (Fig 38–11).
2. Cardiac size is usually normal. Cardiac configuration may be entirely normal (see Fig 38–11). A patient may have a severe cyanotic congenital malformation but a normal thoracic roentgenogram.
3. The cardiac apex may be elevated and the aortic arch right sided, simulating the roentgenographic findings of tetralogy of Fallot (Fig 38–12).

In tetralogy of Fallot, however, the degree of cyanosis correlates with the amount of pulmonary flow. In contrast, in complete transposition, normal or prominent pulmonary vasculature can be found in severely cyanotic patients, particularly if pulmonary stenosis is present.

CARDIAC CATHETERIZATION

The initial cardiac catheterization is usually performed in the neonatal period. At this age the patients are frequently very hypoxemic and perhaps acidotic. This cardiac catheterization procedure is often performed quickly, without an effort to obtain detailed hemodynamic information. The purposes of the initial study are to:

1. Establish the diagnosis (by angiography).
2. Identify major coexistent conditions.
3. Perform a balloon atrial septostomy.

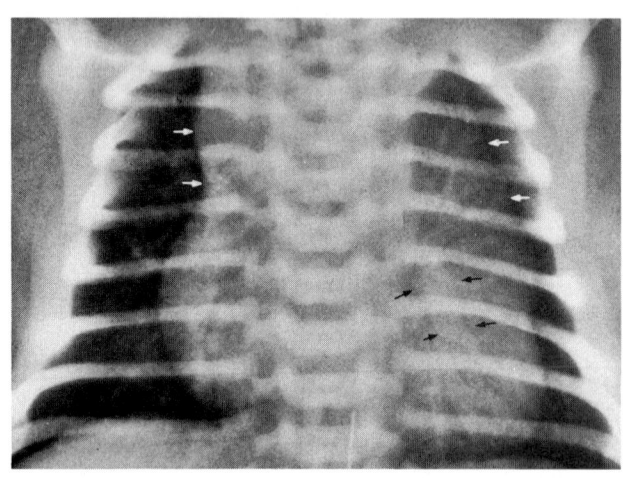

FIG 38–10.
Complete transposition of great vessels. Thoracic roentgenogram. Posteroanterior projection. Cardiomegaly and increased pulmonary vasculature. Large left pulmonary arteries *(small black arrows)* are seen through cardiac silhouette. Thymus *(small white arrows)* is enlarged. Therefore, characteristic radiographic appearance of complete transposition of great vessels is no longer present. Correct diagnosis cannot be suggested from this roentgenogram.

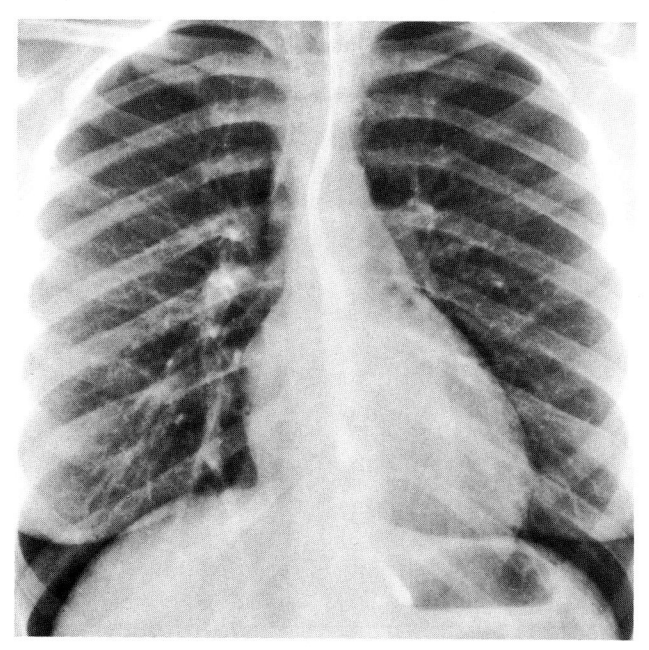

FIG 38–11.
Complete transposition of great vessels and pulmonary stenosis. Deeply cyanotic patient. Thoracic roentgenogram. Posteroanterior projection. Normal cardiac size and pulmonary vasculature. No radiographic evidence of a congenital cardiac malformation.

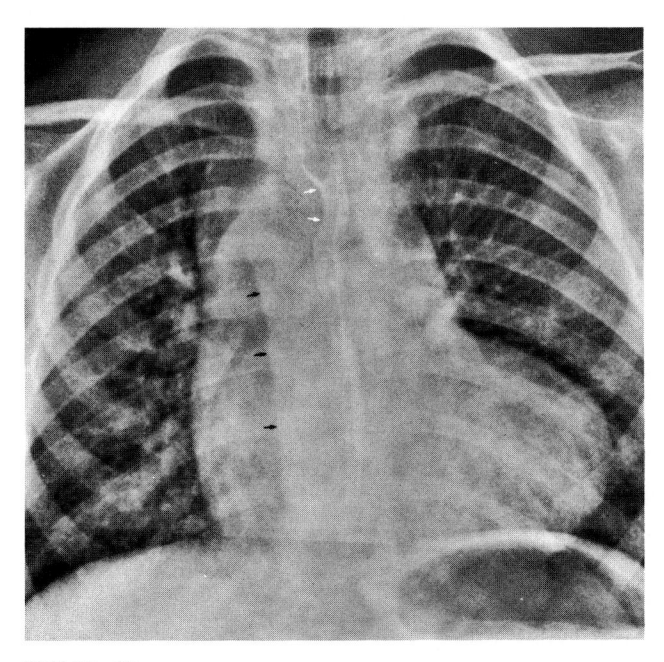

FIG 38–12.
Complete transposition of great vessels and pulmonary stenosis. Thoracic roentgenogram. Posteroanterior projection. Boot-shaped cardiac configuration. Indentation of right side of esophagus *(white arrows)* from right aortic arch and visualization of right descending aorta *(black arrows)*. Roentgen findings mimic tetralogy of Fallot. However, this patient had extremely severe degree of cyanosis, which is more consistent with transposition and pulmonary stenosis than tetralogy because of the adequate pulmonary vasculature.

The bidirectional shunting in neonates with transposition of the great vessels is improved by performing a balloon atrioseptostomy (Rashkind procedure). The tip of a balloon-tipped catheter is advanced into the left atrium and the balloon inflated. The inflated balloon is then withdrawn forcefully across the atrial septum in an effort to enlarge the atrial communication (Fig 38–13).[18] This procedure, which can be performed at low risk, often provides sufficient interatrial mixing, so that the infant can grow and live to 1 year of age or longer before severe hypoxemia recurs.

At a subsequent cardiac catheterization in preparation for operation, more detailed hemodynamic information is obtained.

The catheter course in complete transposition of the great vessels is diagnostic (see Chapter 6). The catheter tip can be advanced from the right ventricle into the aorta. Before the development of balloon-tipped catheters, it was difficult to catheterize the pulmonary artery because of the 180-degree turn that the catheter had to take in the left ventricle to enter the pulmonary artery. If a ventricular septal defect coexists, the catheter may be passed through it into the pulmonary artery.

Oximetry data are useful in identifying the site and amount of bidirectional shunt. In neonates with an intact ventricular septum and closed ductus arteriosus, there may

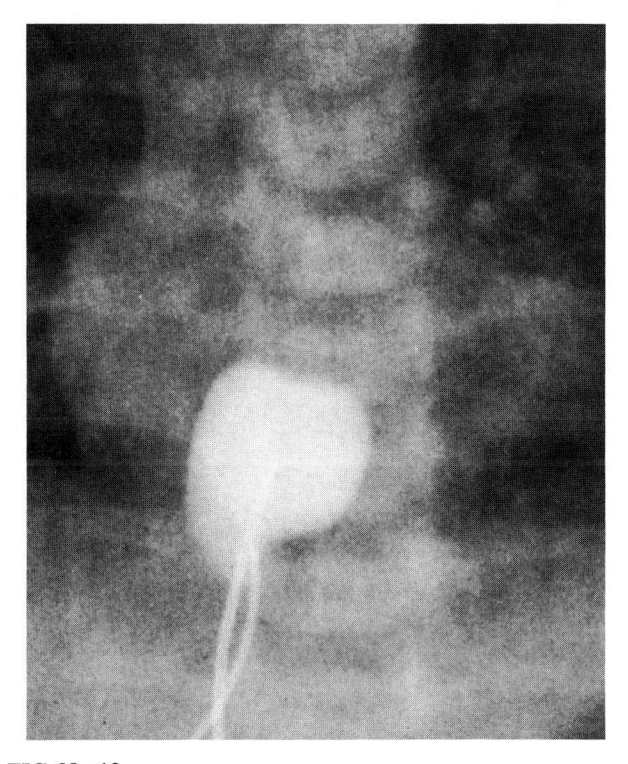

FIG 38–13.
Transposition of great vessels during balloon septostomy. Large inflated balloon has been withdrawn across atrial septum, causing a tear and enlargement of atrial communication.

not be an appreciable increase in oxygen saturation in the right atrium and only a small decrease in oxygen saturations in the left side of the heart between the pulmonary veins and left ventricle. The oxygen saturation is lower in the aorta than in the pulmonary artery. Even on inhalation of 100% oxygen, the aortic saturation usually does not rise significantly. This useful diagnostic test is often employed before catheterization. Failure to increase arterial oxygen saturation on inhalation of high concentration of oxygen is highly suggestive of transposition of the great vessels and tends to exclude pulmonary parenchymal disease as the cause of the cyanosis.

In patients with a large ventricular septal defect or patent ductus arteriosus, there is a significant increase in oxygen saturation in the right side of the heart and significant decrease on the left side of the heart, reflecting the large volume of the bidirectional shunt.

The oxygen data have often been used to calculate pulmonary and systemic blood flows by the Fick principle, but the calculations are often inaccurate because of the narrowed systemic and pulmonary arteriovenous oxygen differences. Small errors in the oxygen values can cause large differences in calculating blood flows. Therefore, calculation of vascular resistance yields inaccurate results as well. Bronchopulmonary communications also contribute to blood flow through pulmonary capillaries and are not accounted for by the oxygen saturations used in calculation of blood flows.

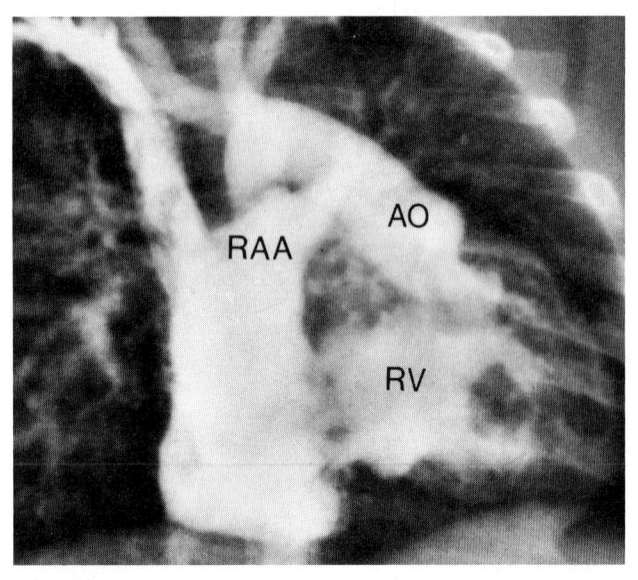

FIG 38–14.
Complete transposition of great vessels. Venous angiogram. Anteroposterior projection. Superior vena cava connects to anatomic right atrium, which can be identified by its broad-based atrial appendage *(RAA)*. Right atrium connects to a heavily trabeculated anatomic right ventricle *(RV)*, which gives rise to aorta *(AO)*. Aorta ascends on left. This sequence of flow of contrast media is characteristic for complete transposition of great vessels.

Atrial pressures may be unequal before balloon atrial septostomy. Right atrial pressure is greater than left atrial pressure, but after successful septostomy, the pressures should be equal. Right ventricular systolic pressure is elevated to systemic levels. Subaortic stenosis is rare. Left ventricular systolic pressure varies considerably among patients. In neonates with an intact ventricular septum, it may be elevated to systemic levels because of the normally elevated pulmonary vascular resistance or patent ductus arteriosus of a neonate. Within days, the left ventricular systolic pressure falls to 25 to 30 mm Hg. In such patients in the first year of life, left ventricular systolic pressure may increase because of the development of subpulmonary stenosis or, less frequently, the development of pulmonary vascular disease. In patients with a large ventricular septal defect, left ventricular systolic pressure is elevated often to the level of right ventricular systolic pressure.

When the systolic pressure is elevated in the left ventricle, pulmonary arterial pressure must be measured to distinguish between elevated pulmonary resistance and subpulmonary stenosis.

ANGIOGRAPHIC FEATURES

Although the diagnosis of complete transposition of the great vessels can be made by venous angiography (Fig 38–14), by clinical means and echocardiography, only selective angiography can firmly establish the diagnosis and demonstrate associated anomalies. An exact assessment of the anatomy and physiology are mandatory before a palliative or corrective operative procedure.

Right Ventriculography

Right ventriculography is indicated for the following reasons:

1. Demonstration of the size and function of the right ventricle. Transposition of the great vessels may be associated with significant hypoplasia of the right ventricle (Fig 38–15). Such a case does not lend itself to corrective operative procedures.

2. Many patients with complete transposition of the great vessels and intact ventricular septum have abnormal right ventricular function, which is manifested by a decreased ejection fraction and increased end-systolic volume.

3. Dilatation of the right ventricle may result in tricuspid regurgitation (Fig 38–16).

4. A coexistent ventricular septal defect can usually be demonstrated by right ventriculography. REASON: Most commonly right ventricular pressure exceeds left ventricular pressure.

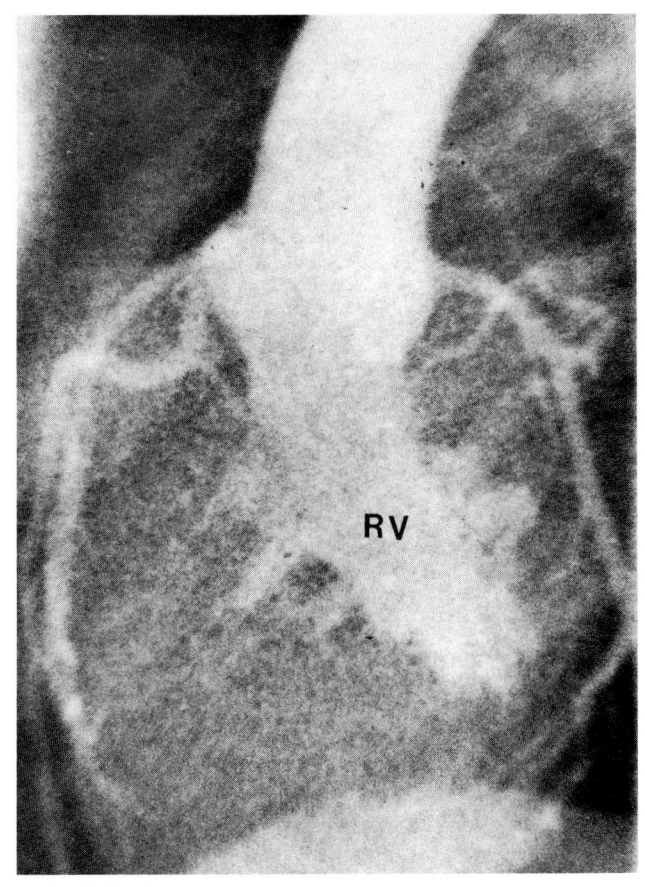

FIG 38–15.
Complete transposition of great vessels and hypoplastic right ventricle *(RV)*. Right ventriculogram.

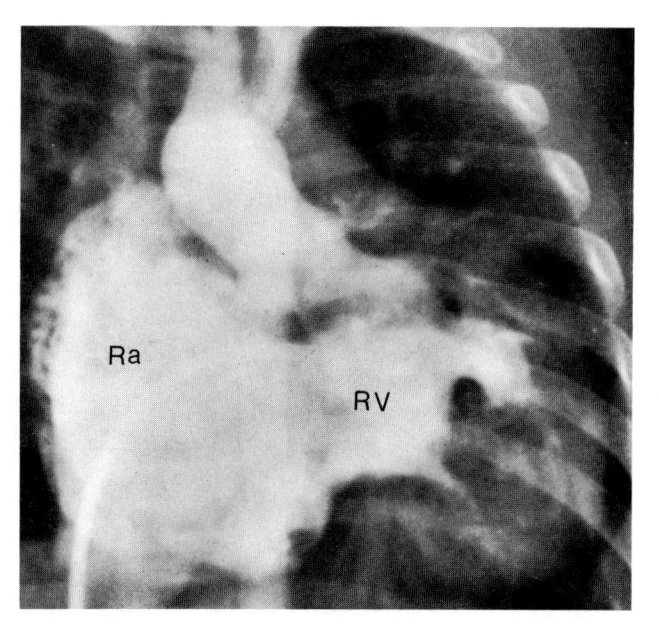

FIG 38–16.
Complete transposition of great vessels. Right ventriculogram. Anteroposterior view. Marked tricuspid insufficiency. Tip of catheter in right ventricle *(RV)*. Right atrium *(Ra)* densely opacifies. This degree of regurgitation is uncommon. When tricuspid insufficiency is present in transposition of great vessels, it is usually of a minor degree.

5. Demonstration of the right ventricular outflow tract for visualization of coexistent subaortic stenosis, which may require a Damus-Kaye-Stansel operation for repair.

In complete transposition of the great vessels, the angiographic findings of the right ventricle are as follows:

1. The right ventricle shows increased trabeculations. REASON: Because the aorta connects to the right ventricle, the systemic pressure induces right ventricular hypertrophy, which is evidenced by increased trabeculations (Fig 38–17).

2. The right ventricle is enlarged. REASON: Unknown. Contrary to compensated pulmonary stenosis, which produces concentric right ventricular hypertrophy and a reduced right ventricular cavity, in complete transposition right ventricular enlargement develops in addition to hypertrophy. Perhaps the combination of a systemic level of pressure and the perfusion of the right ventricular myocardium by desaturated blood results in right ventricular enlargement.

3. The aorta arises from the infundibulum. The aortic valve is separated from the tricuspid valve by the infundibulum. Therefore, these two valves are not in continuity.

4. Because the aorta arises from the infundibulum, the aortic valve lies in a higher and more anterior plane than the pulmonary valve (exceptions exist).

5. The outflow tracts of the right and left ventricle no longer cross as in the normal heart. In complete transposition of the great vessels, the outflow tracts have a more parallel and anteroposterior relationship (Figs 38–18 and 38–22,B).

6. The aortic valve plane is tilted anteriorly (see Fig 38–17).

7. The right (anterior) coronary cusp does not give rise to the right coronary artery as in the normal heart.

8. The pulmonary artery usually lies directly behind or slightly to the right of the aorta. Consequently, the pulmonary artery is commonly superimposed on the aorta. Because the aorta lies in front of the pulmonary artery, a slight degree of rotation of the thorax or the heart (see Fig 38–18) projects the aorta to either the right or left of the pulmonary artery.

9. The relative position of the great vessels is variable (see Fig 38–1). Usually the pulmonary artery lies directly behind the aorta, but it may also be to the left and right of the aorta.

10. Tricuspid insufficiency (about 1% of the cases)

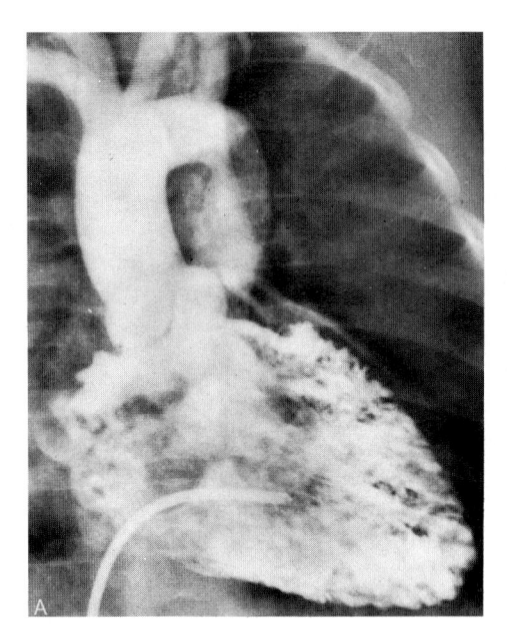

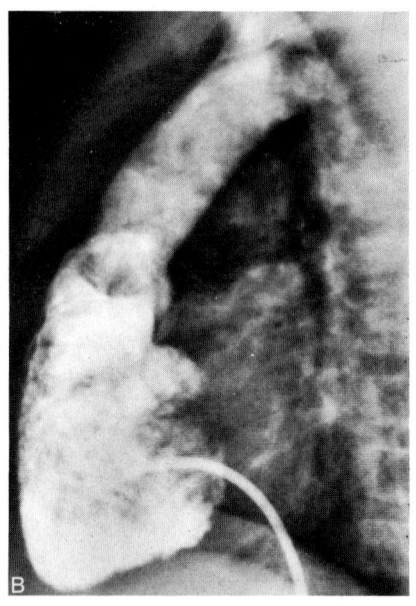

FIG 38–17.
Complete transposition of great vessels. Right ventriculogram. **A,** anteroposterior and, **B,** lateral projections. Enlarged and heavily trabeculated right ventricle. Aorta arises from right ventricular infundibulum separated from tricuspid valve. Aortic valve plane is high and tilted. Ascending aorta lies anteriorly and immediately behind sternum. Right coronary artery does not arise from anterior aortic cusp.

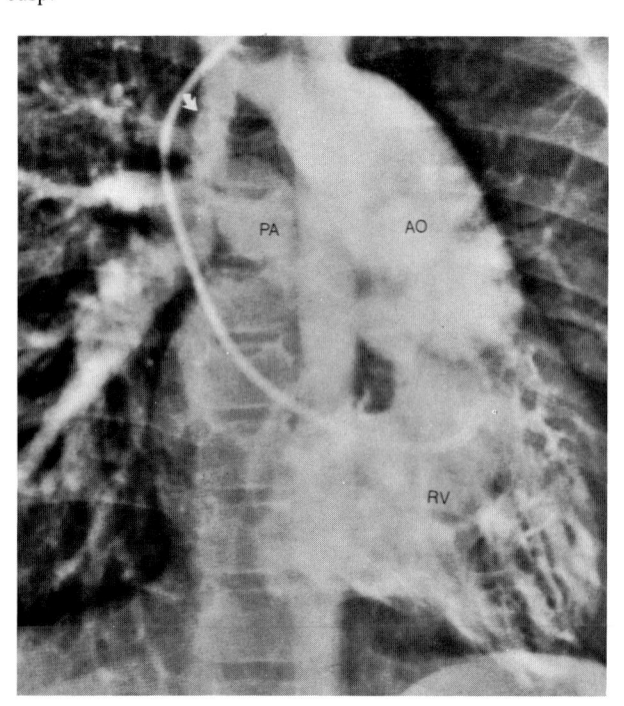

FIG 38–18.
Complete transposition of great vessels and pulmonary atresia. Right ventriculogram. Anteroposterior projection. Blalock-Taussig operation had been performed *(curved arrow)*. Heavily trabeculated right ventricle *(RV)* with infundibulum (concordant atrioventricular connection). Infundibulum gives rise to aorta (discordant ventriculoarterial connection, D-transposition). Because of clockwise rotation of heart, anteriorly placed aorta *(AO)* projects to left of pulmonary artery *(PA)*, as in corrected transposition of great vessels.

may be present. It is usually mild and probably occurs secondary to right ventricular dilatation. Rarely, tricuspid reflux is severe (see Fig 38–16).

11. Rarely, the right ventricle has a poorly developed infundibulum (Fig 38–19). In such patients the aortic valve lies in the same plane or is lower than the pulmonary valve. The relative position of the great vessels is variable and not as important diagnostically as the fact that the aorta arises from the heavily trabeculated (anatomic) right ventricle. (This anatomic relationship is called "concordant atrioventricular connection" with discordant ventriculoarterial connection.)

12. Typically the right ventricle shows decreased contractility (Fig 38–20). REASON: Myocardial hypoxia and systemic level of pressure.

13. Rarely, the right ventricular contractility is normal (Fig 38–21).

Left Ventriculography

Left ventriculography is performed to:

1. Demonstrate the size of the left ventricle.
2. Demonstrate left ventricular obstructions.
3. Exclude mitral insufficiency.
4. Demonstrate the relationship of anterior mitral and aortic valve leaflets.

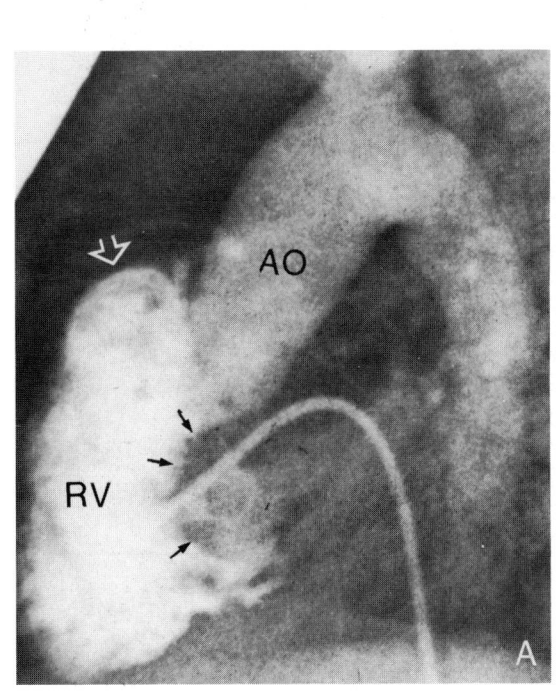

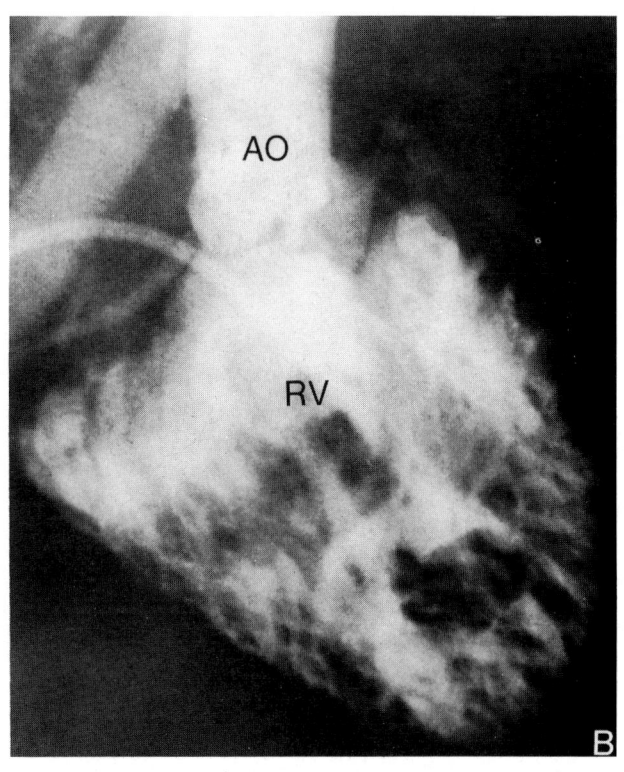

FIG 38–19.
Complete transposition of great vessels. Right ventriculogram (RV). **A,** lateral projection. Hypoplasia of infundibulum. Aortic valve is lower and appears in close proximity to tricuspid valve *(black arrows)*. Aorta *(AO)* does not arise from infundibular region *(open arrow)*. Nevertheless, it is transposed (placed across ventricular septum). **B,** right anterior oblique projection. Aorta lies very close to catheter, which has been passed through tricuspid valve. Poorly developed infundibulum.

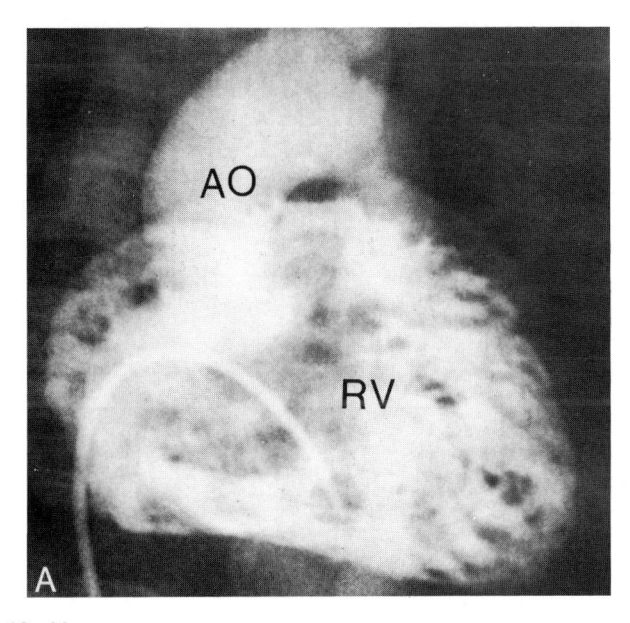

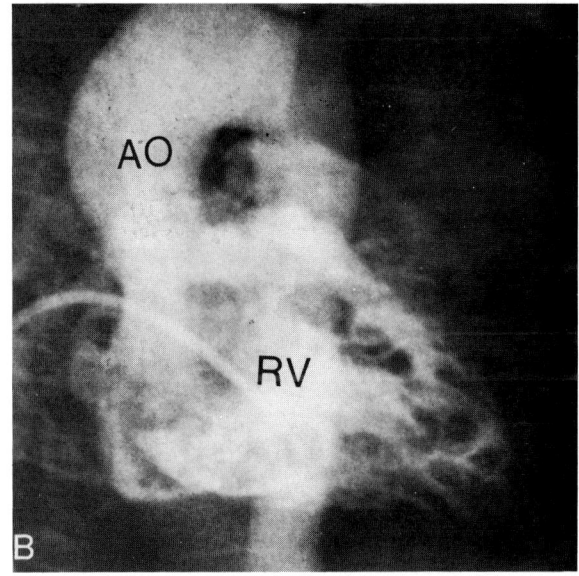

FIG 38–20.
Complete transposition of great vessels. Right ventriculogram. **A,** diastole. **B,** systole. Right ventricle *(RV)* shows decreased contractility, which is almost always in this condition. AO = aorta.

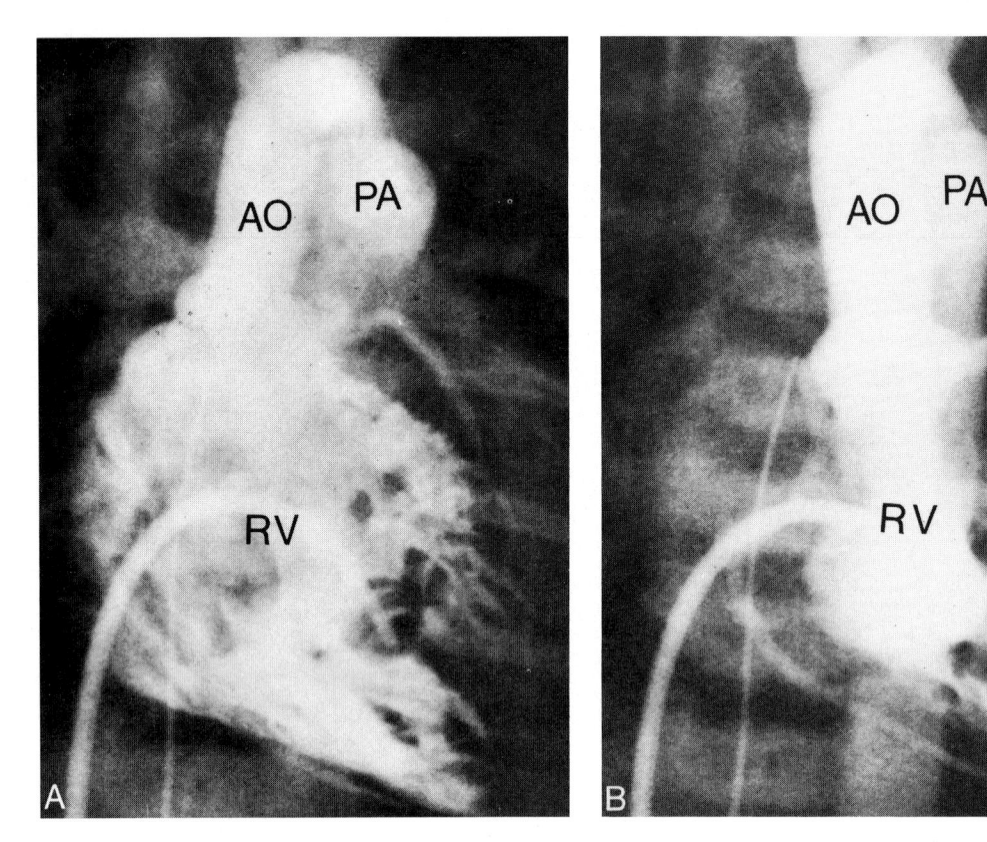

FIG 38–21.
Complete transposition of great vessels. Patent ductus arteriosus. Right ventriculogram. Anteroposterior projection. **A,** diastole. **B,** systole. Excellent contractility of right ventricle *(RV)*. Pulmonary artery *(PA)* opacifies through patent ductus arteriosus. *AO* = aorta.

Demonstration of Ventricular Septal Defects

Before operative correction, the location, size, and number of ventricular septal defects must be demonstrated. As with isolated ventricular septal defect, an angled left anterior oblique view is preferred for demonstration. The angiographic demonstration of ventricular septal defects in patients with complete transposition of the great vessels is simplified because the outflow tracts of the two ventricles lie parallel to one another and no longer cross as in the normal heart (Fig 38–22). Consequently, the configuration of the septum is less complex than in patients with normally related great vessels.

1. Ventricular septal defects can be visualized by either right or left ventriculography. REASON: Right ventriculography demonstrates the ventricular septal defect during systole because of the elevated right ventricular systolic pressure (Fig 38–23). Left ventriculography can also demonstrate the ventricular septal defect. During diastole, blood shunts from left to right through the defect because of the greater compliance of the right ventricle.

2. Most ventricular septal defects are located in the area of the membranous septum and near the septal leaflet of the tricuspid valve. The membranous septum is no longer related to the aorta as in the normal heart. REASON: The aorta arises from the right ventricular infundibulum and is remote from the membranous septum. The tricuspid valve may become partially adherent and occlude the defect and form a pouch (see Figs 38–23,A and 38–4,F). These deformities of the septal leaflet of the tricuspid valve are similar to aneurysm of the membranous septum present in patients with isolated ventricular septal defect. Because the right ventricular systolic pressure exceeds left ventricular systolic pressure in many patients with complete transposition of the great vessels, the septal leaflet of the tricuspid valve may herniate through the ventricular septal defect into the left ventricle, causing subvalvar pulmonary obstruction (see Fig 38–23,B). The herniating septal leaflet of the tricuspid leaflet may partially or completely occlude the ventricular septal defect. Systolic herniation of the aneurysm of the membranous septum causes a distinct filling defect in the left ventricular outflow tract (see Fig 38–23,C).

3. Multiple ventricular septal defects may be present.

4. Muscular septal defects are uncommon (Fig 38–24).

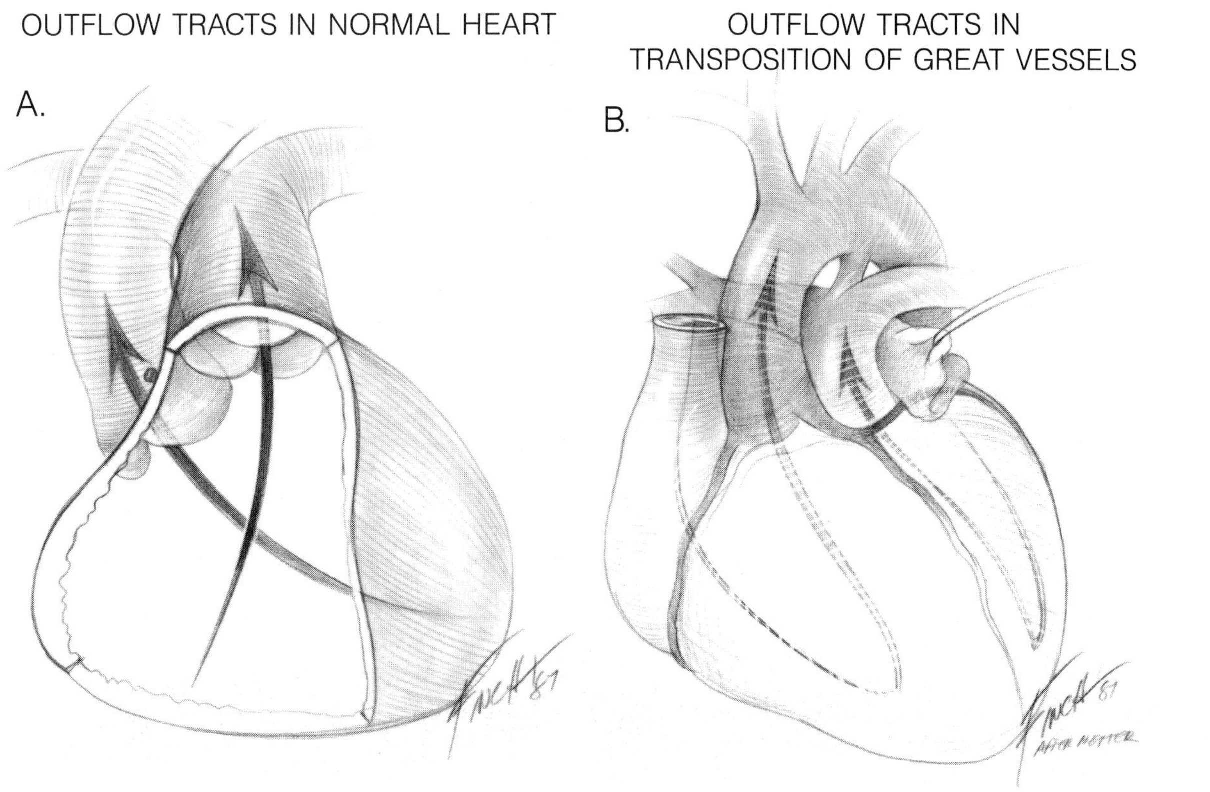

OUTFLOW TRACTS IN NORMAL HEART

A.

OUTFLOW TRACTS IN TRANSPOSITION OF GREAT VESSELS

B.

FIG 38–22.
Diagram demonstrating orientation of great vessels. **A,** normal. Outflow tracts cross and consequently septum has a complex spiral shape. **B,** complete transposition of great vessels. Outflow tracts are parallel, and ventricular septum is straighter.

Demonstration of Left Ventricular Outflow Obstruction

Left ventricular outflow tract obstruction must be demonstrated by pressure measurements and angiography to properly plan operative correction. Some forms of left ventricular outflow obstruction such as valvar pulmonary stenosis and discrete subpulmonary membrane may lend themselves to direct operative approach, but other types of obstruction cannot be removed. Consequently, the operative procedure is different among such patients.

There are eight types of left ventricular outflow tract obstruction (see Fig 38–4):

1. Valvar pulmonary stenosis.
2. Discrete subpulmonary membrane.
3. Accessory mitral valvar tissue.
4. Herniation of the septal leaflet of tricuspid valve through the ventricular septal defect.
5. Dynamic obstruction (similar to muscular subaortic stenosis).
6. Localized muscular subpulmonary stenosis similar to the stenosis of the os infundibulum (double coni).
7. Supravalvar pulmonary stenosis.
8. Peripheral pulmonary arterial stenosis.

Left ventriculography may show a number of appearances, depending on the specific type of obstructive lesion:

1. Valvar pulmonary stenosis is readily identified by left ventriculography. The pulmonary valve domes as in isolated pulmonary stenosis (Fig 38–25).

2. A discrete subpulmonary membrane forms a linear radiolucency immediately beneath the pulmonary valve. The membrane can be best visualized on anteroposterior and angulated left anterior oblique projections (Fig 38–26).

3. Accessory mitral valvar tissue, such as a pouch, may be identified as a filling defect attached to the anterior leaflet of the mitral valve prolapsing into the left ventricular outflow tract (Fig 38–27).

4. Herniation of the tricuspid valve through a ventricular septal defect forms an anterior narrowing of the subpulmonary area (Fig 38–28). This is in contrast to accessory mitral valvar tissue observed posteriorly in the left ventricular outflow tract.

5. The most common cause of left ventricular outflow tract obstruction is dynamic narrowing caused by anterior motion of the mitral valve. This gives an appearance similar to idiopathic hypertrophic subaortic stenosis. During

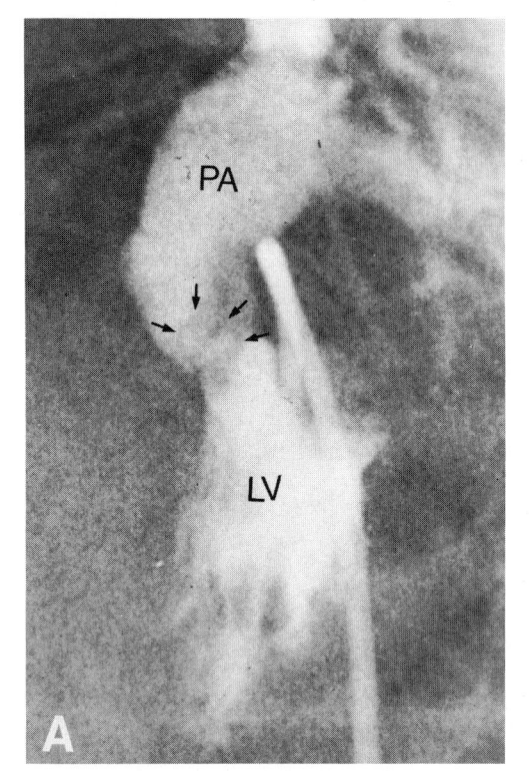

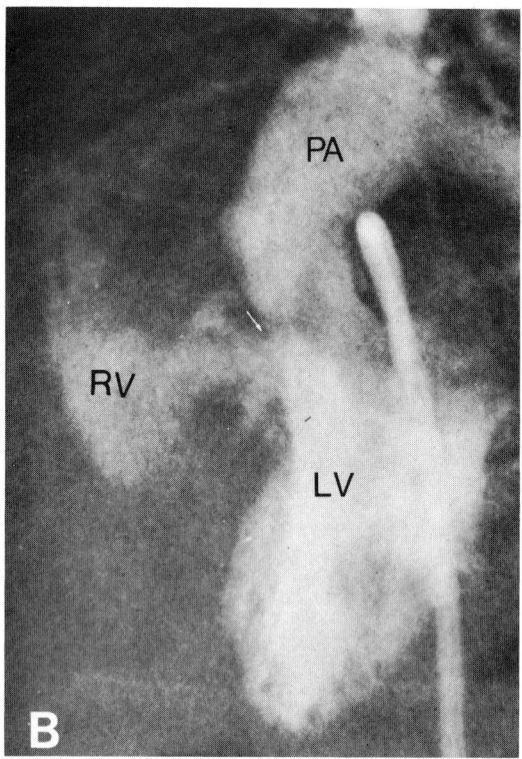

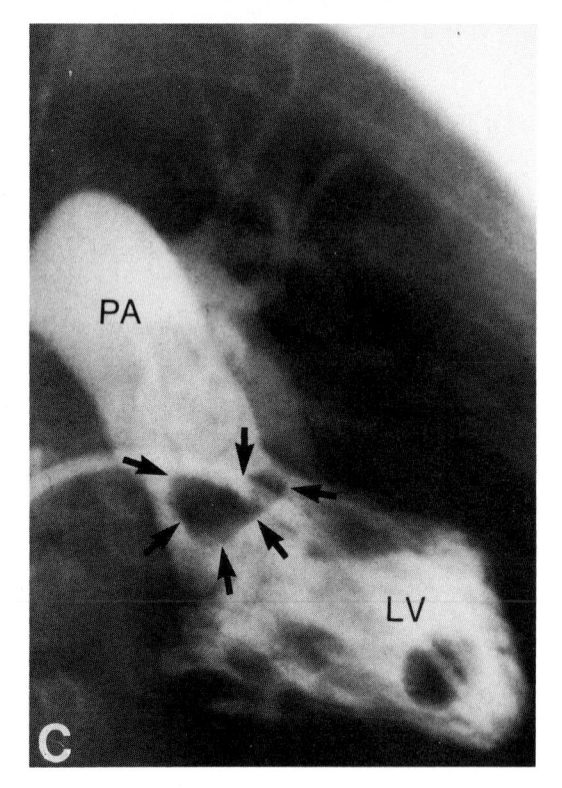

FIG 38–23.
Complete transposition of great vessels with ventricular septal defect. Left ventriculogram (LV). Left anterior oblique projection. **A,** systole. Septal leaflet of tricuspid valve is seen to herniate through defect, causing a well-defined obstructing radiolucency in left ventricular outflow tract (arrows). **B,** diastole. Left-to-right shunt through membranous defect (arrow), which is in close proximity to septal leaflet of tricuspid valve. **C,** left ventriculogram. Anteroposterior projection. Systole. Aneurysm of membranous septum forms well-defined obstructing defect (arrows). PA = pulmonary artery; RV = right ventriculogram.

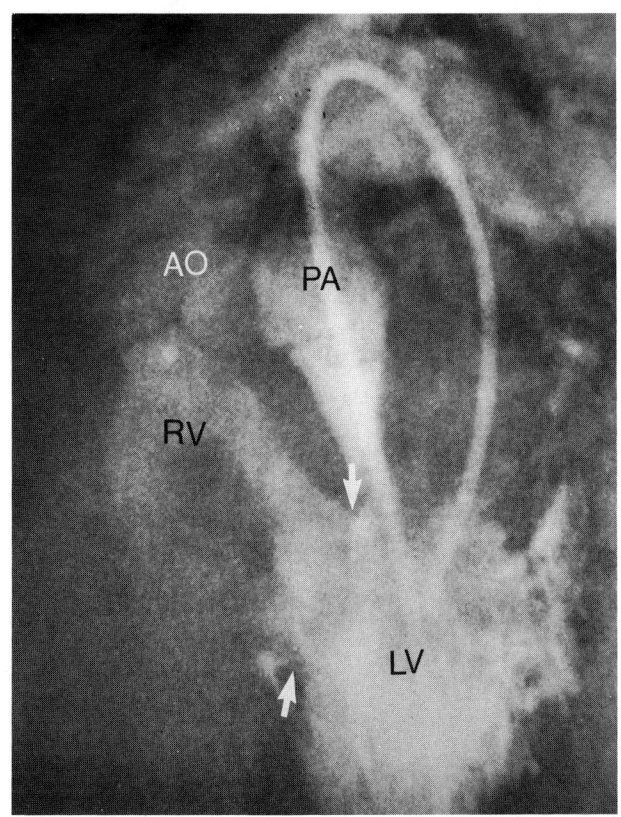

FIG 38–24.
Transposition of great vessels. Left ventriculogram *(LV)*. Left anterior oblique projection. Large single muscular septal defect *(arrows)*. AO = aorta; PA = pulmonary artery; RV = right ventricle.

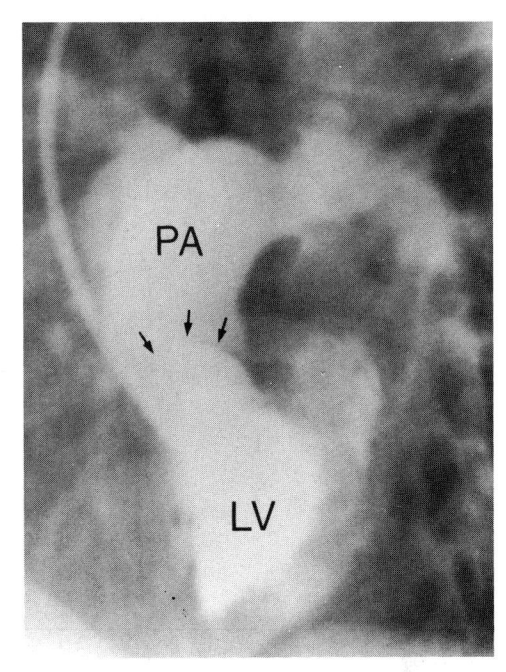

FIG 38–25.
Complete transposition of great vessels. Left ventriculogram *(LV)*. Left anterior oblique projection. Valvar pulmonary stenosis, as indicated by doming pulmonary valve *(arrows)*. PA = pulmonary artery.

diastole the left ventricular outflow tract appears normal (Fig 38–29,A). But during systole the mitral valvar apparatus moves anteriorly (Fig 38–29,B). The anterior leaflet of the mitral valve and the bulging ventricular septum narrow the outflow tract resulting in a pressure gradient, which may be severe. This type of obstruction is not correctable by operation.

6. The impact of the mitral valve striking the ventricular septum causes thickening of the mitral valve and development of a fibrous ridge along the ventricular septum. The fibrous ridge causes a characteristic filling defect. This can be seen on the anteroposterior projection of a left ventriculogram during systole when the mitral valve makes impact with the septum. This should not be confused with a subpulmonary membrane, which forms a narrow radiolucent line persisting during systole and diastole. Excision of a broad ridge is unadvisable, because this operation does not relieve the dynamic obstruction.

7. Systolic anterior motion of the mitral valve and fibrous thickening of the septum develop with time. Both the fibrous ridge and thickened mitral valve may increase the degree of subpulmonary outflow obstruction (see Fig 38–29).

8. Localized muscular subpulmonary stenosis may be caused by incomplete absorption of the left ventricular conus during embryologic development. A fixed area of narrowing is present immediately beneath the pulmonary valve. The pulmonary valve is not in fibrous continuity with the mitral valve (Fig 38–30). Valvar pulmonary stenosis commonly coexists. The pulmonary valve is usually thickened by the subvalvar jet (see Fig 38–30). The angiographic appearance of this type of subvalvar stenosis is very similar to the stenosis of os infundibulum observed in tetralogy of Fallot.

Demonstration of Coronary Arterial Pattern

The coronary arterial pattern is important in distinguishing between complete and partial transposition of the great vessels (i.e., double-outlet right ventricle). In complete transposition of the great vessels, the right coronary artery does not originate from the right (anterior) cusp, as in a normal heart. Therefore, in complete transposition of the great vessels, the anterior cusp is the noncoronary cusp. In patients with forms of partial transposition, the coronary arterial pattern is usually normal (see Fig 38–5).

In 60% of patients the left coronary artery divides into a left anterior descending and a circumflex branch (Fig

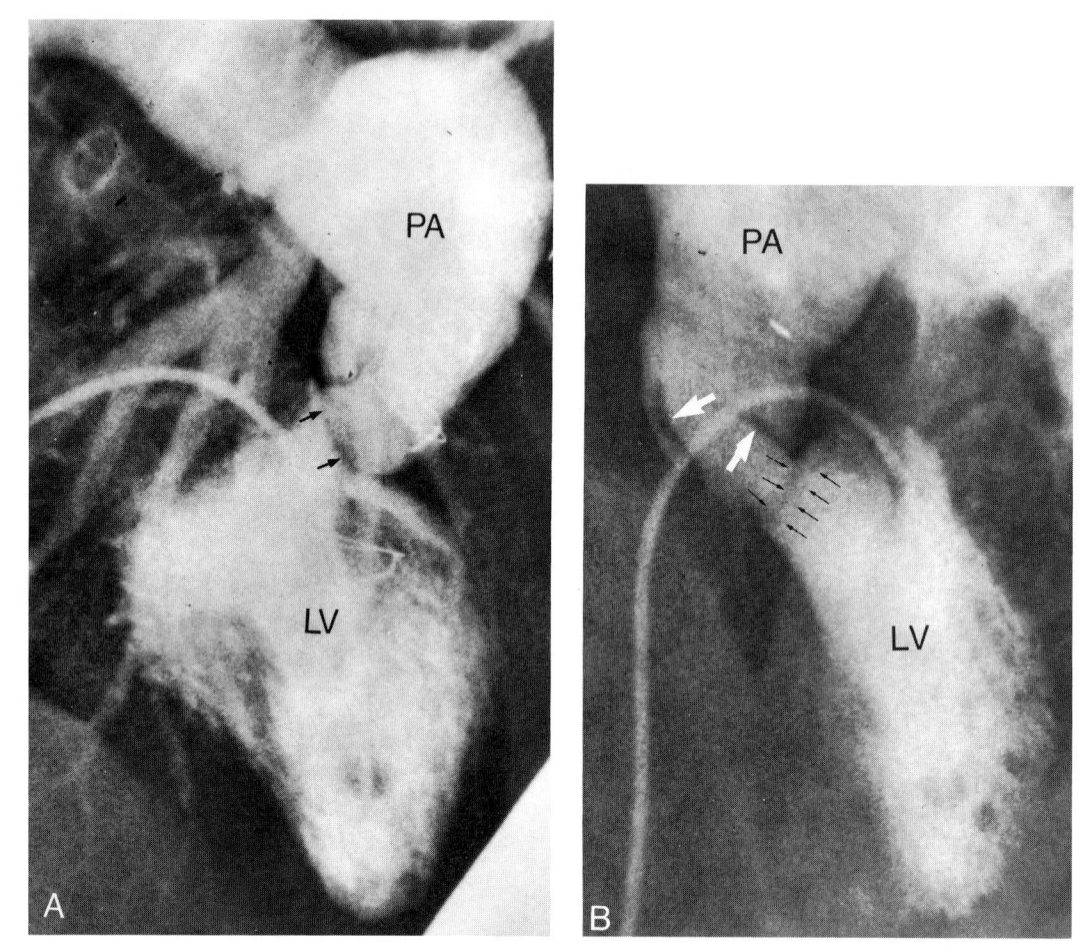

FIG 38–26.
Complete transposition of great vessels. Left ventriculogram *(LV)*. **A,** right anterior oblique and, **B,** left anterior oblique projections. Fine radiolucent line *(arrows)* beneath pulmonary valve is typical for discrete membranous subpulmonary stenosis. Pulmonary valve is thickened because of subvalvar jet formed by diaphragm *(white arrows)*. *PA* = pulmonary artery.

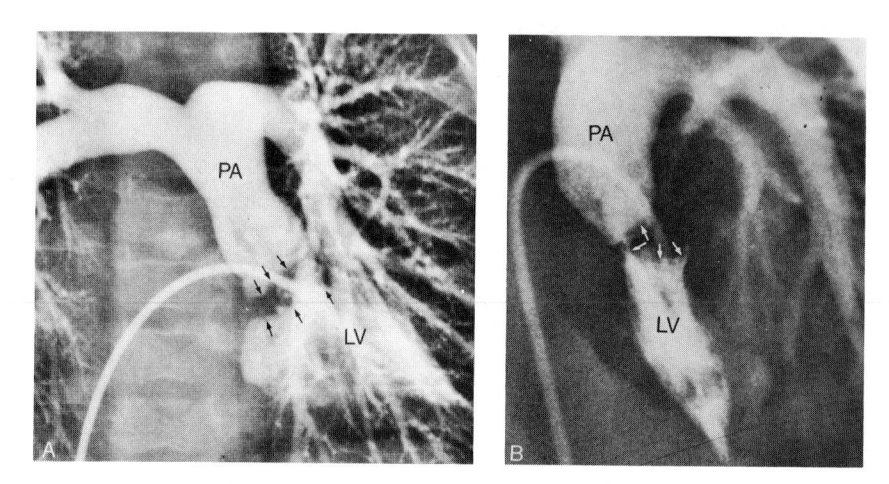

FIG 38–27.
Complete transposition of great vessels. Left ventriculogram *(LV)*. **A,** anteroposterior projection. Smooth-walled left ventricle *(LV)*. Catheter is passed through foramen ovale and mitral valve into the left ventricle. Pulmonary artery *(PA)* is opacified. Immediately beneath pulmonary valve is lobulated radiolucency *(arrows)*, caused by accessory mitral valvar tissue. Similar filling defect occurs with systolic anterior motion of mitral valve and with prolapse of tricuspid valve through a ventricular septal defect. **B,** left anterior oblique projection. Accessory valve tissue of mitral valve forms a large pouch *(arrows)*.

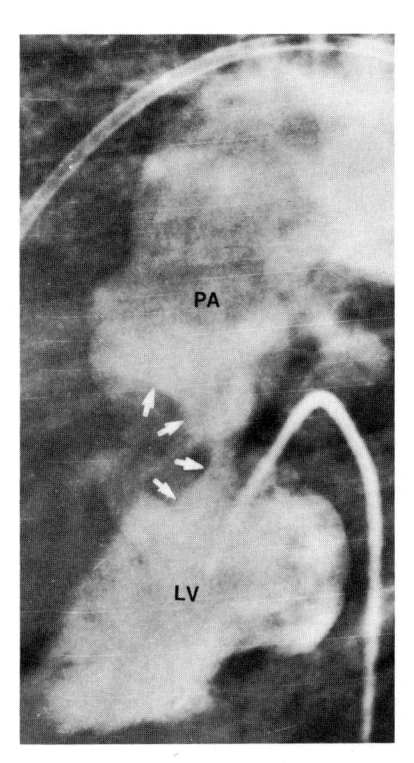

FIG 38-28.
Complete transposition of great vessels. Left ventriculogram (LV). Left anterior oblique projection. Herniation of septal leaflet of tricuspid valve through ventricular septal defect, causing subpulmonary stenosis (arrows). Stenosis is located anteriorly along septum. This should not be confused with accessory mitral valve tissue, which lies posteriorly. LV = left ventricle; PA = pulmonary artery.

38-5), as in the normal heart, but the left anterior descending branch crosses in front of the pulmonary artery. The circumflex branch may lie either in front of or behind the pulmonary artery (see Fig 38-5). In the other 40% of patients, the circumflex artery arises from the right coronary artery, whereas the left anterior descending artery is a single artery that arises above the left cusp (Fig 38-31). Rarely, there is a single coronary artery that gives rise to the right, anterior descending, and circumflex branches.

Demonstration of the exact coronary anatomy is very important if an arterial switch operation is being contemplated. The best view for visualizing the origins of the coronary arteries is the anteroposterior projection with caudal angulation. Balloon occlusion of the ascending aorta with injection proximal to the balloon will provide excellent visualization (see Fig 38-33). REASON: The aortic valve plane is tilted posteriorly, thereby projecting the right (noncoronary) cusp above the other two cusps from which the coronary arteries arise. In addition, a lateral or steep left anterior oblique projection with cranial angulation is helpful, but sometimes the posterior origins of the coronary arteries are superimposed.

Aortography in a lateral projection is diagnostic of complete transposition of the great vessels. Normally in this view, the right coronary ostium is seen in profile arising above the right (anterior) aortic cusp. Because in complete transposition of the great vessels the right coronary artery does not arise from the right (anterior) cusp, its origin is not visualized in this projection (see Fig 38-31).

1. On the lateral view of an aortogram, the right coronary artery arises from the posterior cusp (the noncoronary cusp in the normal heart).
2. The most common pattern is identical to the normal heart. The circumflex and left anterior descending branches arise from the left circumflex coronary artery (Fig 38-32).
3. Rare patterns include single coronary artery, both coronary arteries arising above the same cusp, or the circumflex branch arising from the right coronary artery (Fig 38-33). With a single coronary artery arising from the posterior cusp, it is important to determine whether the left coronary artery crosses in front or behind the aorta as it passes to the left. Its position in front may make arterial switch technically impossible.
4. If the circumflex branch arises from the right coronary artery, the anteroposterior projection is characteristic because both arteries divide and outline the atrioventricular grooves (see Fig 38-33).
5. Origin of the right coronary artery above the anterior cusp is exceedingly rare in complete transposition (Fig 38-34) but usual in partial transposition. This finding is therefore helpful in distinguishing these two conditions.

MANAGEMENT

Neonates with complete transposition of the great vessels are treated with prostaglandin E_1.[19] This maintains patency of the ductus arteriosus, improves bidirectional shunting, and results in a considerably higher arterial Po_2 and better condition of the neonate. Beyond 1 week of age, prostaglandin E_1 is no longer as effective in opening the ductus arteriosus. During the initial cardiac catheterization to aid in the diagnosis, balloon atrial septostomy is performed to improve oxygenation. Prostaglandin E_1 is discontinued after the catheterization. If the neonate redevelops symptoms, particularly intense hypoxemia, a Blalock-Hanlon procedure (Fig 38-35) may be performed.[20] During this operative procedure an atrial septal defect is created without the use of cardiopulmonary bypass.

Either the balloon atrial septostomy or Blalock-Hanlon procedure[21] provides sufficient palliation so that the infant can grow. Often by the time the infant is 1 year old, the hypoxemia has increased so that a corrective procedure is

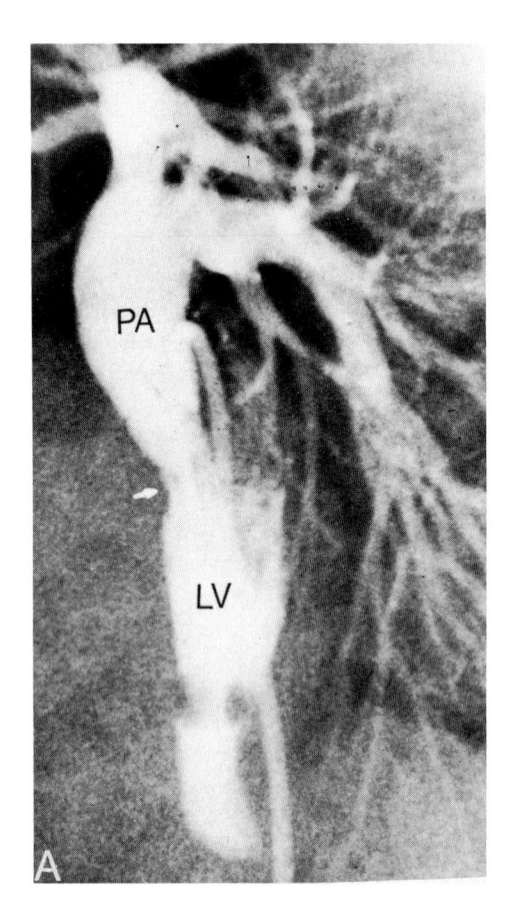

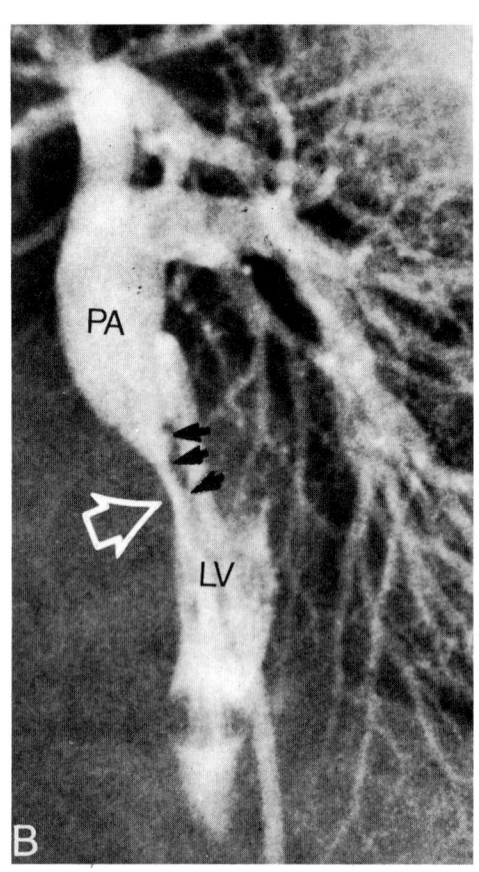

FIG 38-29.
Complete transposition of great vessels. Left ventriculogram *(LV)*. Left anterior oblique projection. **A,** diastole. Left ventricular outflow tract is slightly narrowed as a result of bulging ventricular septum because of high right ventricular systolic pressure. Fibrous ridge *(arrow)* is present on interventricular septum because of impact of mitral valve. **B,** systole. Marked anterior motion of mitral valve *(black arrows)*. Anterior leaflet of mitral valve *(black arrows)* makes contact with septum *("kissing mitral valve")*. Marked systolic inward bulge of ventricular septum *(open white arrow)* and anterior motion of mitral valve cause severe dynamic subpulmonary stenosis. Pulmonary artery *(PA)* is well opacified.

necessary. Atrial switch operations are the most widely used corrective procedures. In such procedures a baffle is created in the atria, so that blood from the superior and inferior venae cavae is directed through the mitral valve, and pulmonary venous blood is directed through the tricuspid valve. Thus, a series circulation is created. Three different procedures are currently used:

1. Mustard procedure,[22] in which a patch of pericardium or Dacron is used to create the baffle (Fig 38-36).
2. Schumacher procedure,[23] in which a pedicle graft of right atrial free wall is used.
3. Senning procedure,[24] in which atrial septum and right atrial free wall are used to create the baffle.

All atrial switch operations have the disadvantage that the right ventricle is subjected to systemic pressure. Life expectancy data of these operations are not available as yet. If a ventricular septal defect coexists, it can be closed during the atrial switch operation. Subpulmonary stenosis is difficult to relieve, because the subpulmonary region is a difficult anatomic area to approach during an operation. Furthermore, the types of subpulmonary stenosis vary considerably, and some of them such as systolic anterior motion of the mitral valve are not correctable.

Another variety of corrective operations, the arterial switch procedure, is widely used. In such a procedure, the circulation is corrected by changing the blood flow at the level of the great vessels.[25, 26] The most direct approach was initially described by Jatene in which the proximal portions of the aorta and pulmonary artery are divided above the sinuses of Valsalva and then reattached to the origin of the other vessel (Fig 38-37). It is necessary to move the coronary arteries so that they are attached to the new "aortic" root and perfused at a systemic level of pressure. This is done by excising a button of aortic tissue about the orifice of each coronary artery and then inserting this tissue into the opposite great vessel (old pulmonary ar-

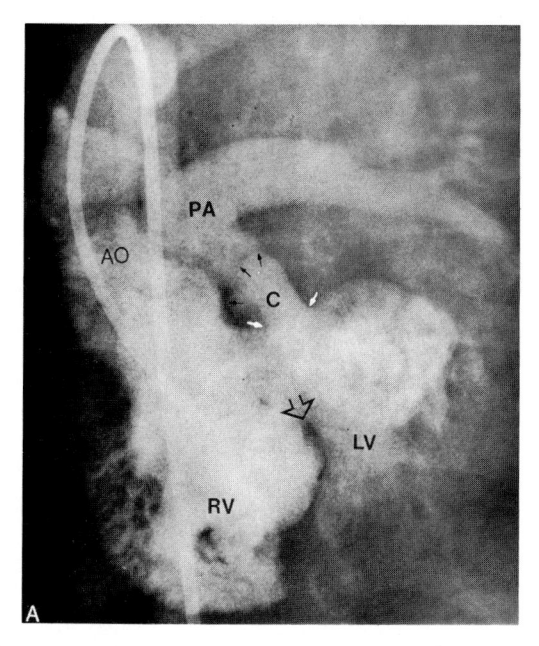

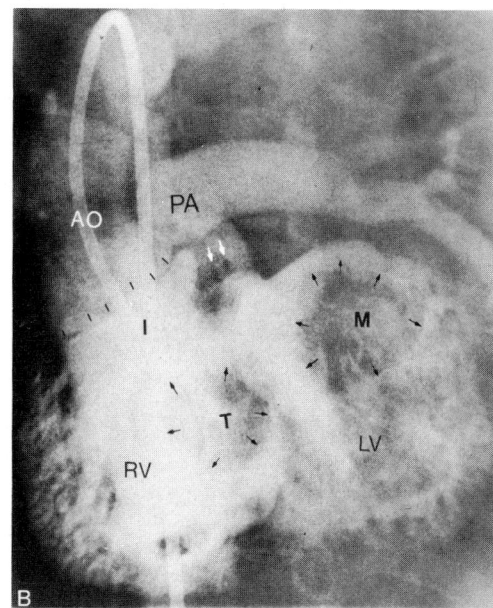

FIG 38-30.
Complete transposition of great vessels. Right ventriculogram. Left anterior oblique projection. Catheter is passed through aortic valve *(AO)* into right ventricle *(RV)*. **A,** systole. Injection into right ventricle. Left ventricle *(LV)* is opacified through ventricular septal defect. Pulmonary artery *(PA)* opacifies from left ventricle. Pulmonary artery arises from left ventricular conus *(C)*, which is stenotic *(white arrows)*. Pulmonary valve domes *(small black arrows)*. Edges of pulmonary valve are distinctly thickened. Edge of ventricular septum is clearly visualized *(open black arrow)*. **B,** diastole. Mitral *(M)* and tricuspid *(T)* annuli *(small black arrows)*, shown by blood entering ventricles. Aortic valve *(black accent lines)* is separated from tricuspid valve by right ventricular conus (infundibulum [I]). Pulmonary valve *(white arrows)* is separated from mitral valve by left ventricular conus. Therefore, double coni are present.

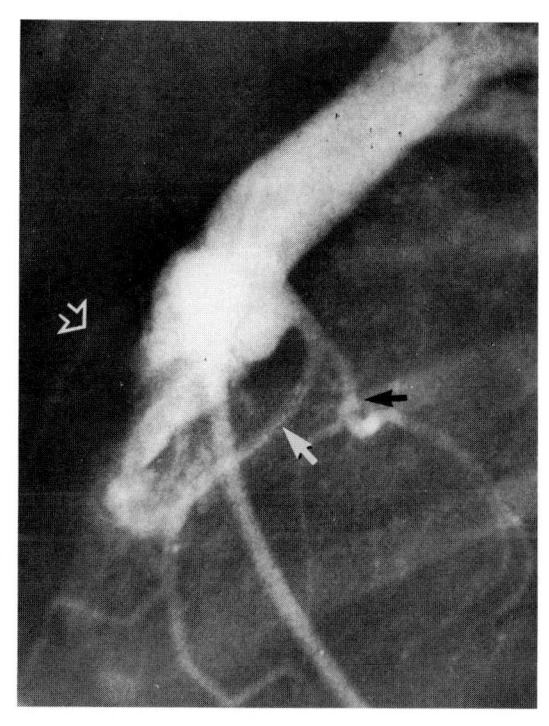

FIG 38-31.
Complete transposition of great vessels. Aortogram. Lateral projection. Anterior cusp does not give rise to coronary artery. Circumflex *(black arrow)* arising from right coronary *(white arrow)* occurs in about 40% of cases. Posterior origin of right coronary artery is typical for complete transposition of great vessels. Left anterior branch is projected anteriorly *(open arrow)*.

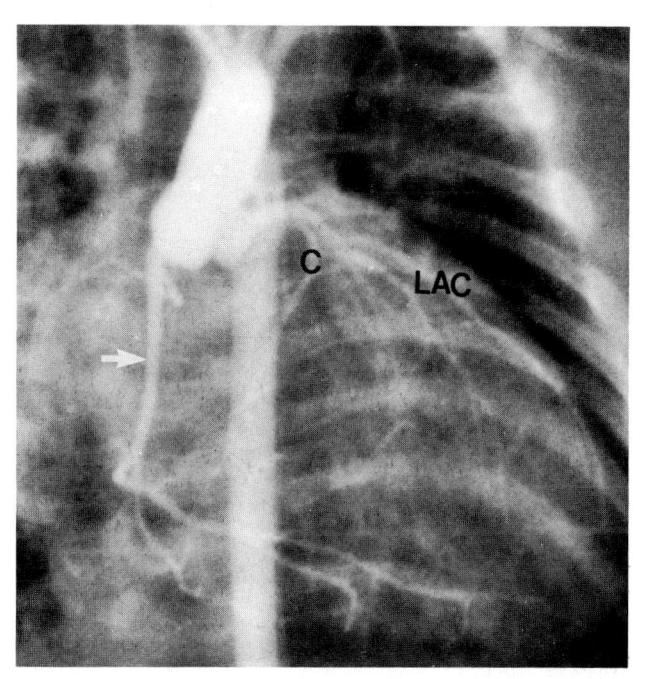

FIG 38-32.
Transposition of great vessels. Aortogram. Anteroposterior projection. Normal coronary distribution with common origin of circumflex branch *(C)* and left anterior descending branch *(LAC)* from left main coronary. Normal location of right coronary *(white arrow)* in atrioventricular groove.

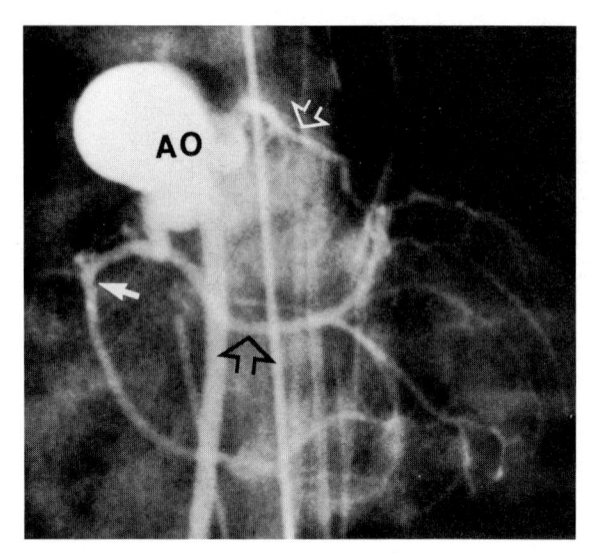

FIG 38–33.
Transposition of great vessels. Aortogram *(AO)*. Anteroposterior projection with caudal beam angulation (looking up). Circumflex branch *(black arrow)* arising from right *(white arrow)*. Both arteries outline atrioventricular grooves. Left anterior descending *(open arrow)* is an isolated branch and projects much higher.

terial root, new aortic root). This procedure must be performed in neonates, because in infants and older children the left ventricular wall is thin because of the low level of pressure and is incapable of developing a systemic level of pressure.[27] This fact prompted Yacoub[26] to develop a two-stage procedure. In the first stage, the pulmonary artery is banded during the neonatal period. This maintains a high systolic pressure in the left ventricle, so its wall retains its thickness and degree of hypertrophy. Subsequently, when the infant is older, the band is removed, and an arterial switch procedure is performed. The long-term effects of these procedures need to be evaluated.

If the patient has a large coexistent ventricular septal defect whether with or without pulmonary stenosis, an operative approach to change the circulation at the great vessel level is possible. In these procedures the coronary arteries do not need to be moved, but a conduit is required.[28] If subpulmonary stenosis is not present, the pulmonary trunk is divided and its proximal end sewn into the side of the ascending aorta (Fig 38–38). Thus, left ventricular (oxygenated) blood enters the aorta and supplies the coronary arteries. A right ventriculotomy is then performed, through which the ventricular septal defect is closed. A conduit is then sewn into the right ventriculotomy to connect the right ventricle to the distal segment of the pulmonary trunk. The circulation is thereby corrected.

When a ventricular septal defect coexists with pulmonary stenosis, a right ventriculotomy is performed, and a patch is placed in such a way that blood is directed

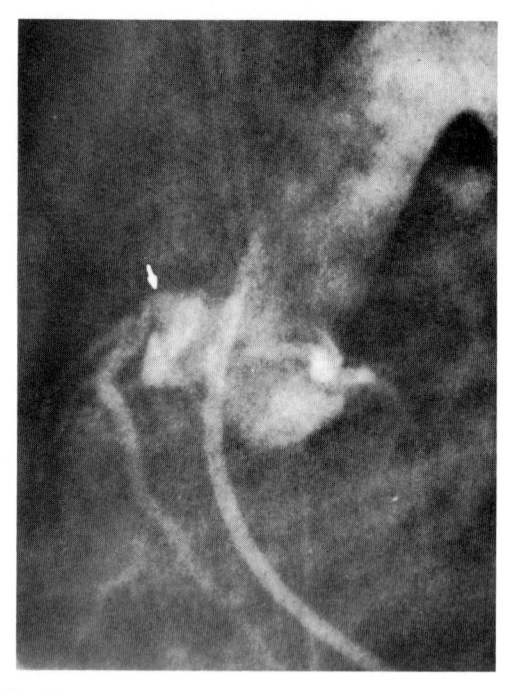

FIG 38–34.
Complete transposition of great vessels. Aortogram. Lateral projection. Right coronary *(white arrow)* arising above right cusp, which is exceedingly rare in complete transposition.

through the ventricular septal defect into the aorta.[29] From the proximal part of the right ventricle, a conduit is inserted and the distal end connected to the pulmonary artery (Fig 38–39). Occasionally the problem of subpulmonary stenosis can be approached using a left ventricular-pulmonary artery conduit (Fig 38–40) and an atrial switch operation.[30] In patients with subaortic obstruction, a Damus-Kaye-Stansel repair is performed. Left ventricular blood flows into the aorta by anastomosing the pulmonary artery end to side to the aorta. The pulmonary arteries are perfused from the right ventricle via valved conduit (Fig 38–41).

The long-term postoperative status of atrial switch operations has been studied to considerable extent. There are four major long-term complications:

1. Obstruction to venous return.[31–34] Either systemic or pulmonary venous return can be obstructed by improper placement of the baffle or by scarring and contraction. Superior vena caval obstruction is by far the most common and generally occurs at the site where the superior aspect of the baffle crosses beneath the rim of the atrial septal defect. Pulmonary venous obstruction, particularly of the left pulmonary veins can occur, because the baffle is sutured close to them. This can be recognized radiographically or by radioisotopic technique in finding a significant discrepancy of pulmonary blood flow between the two lungs.

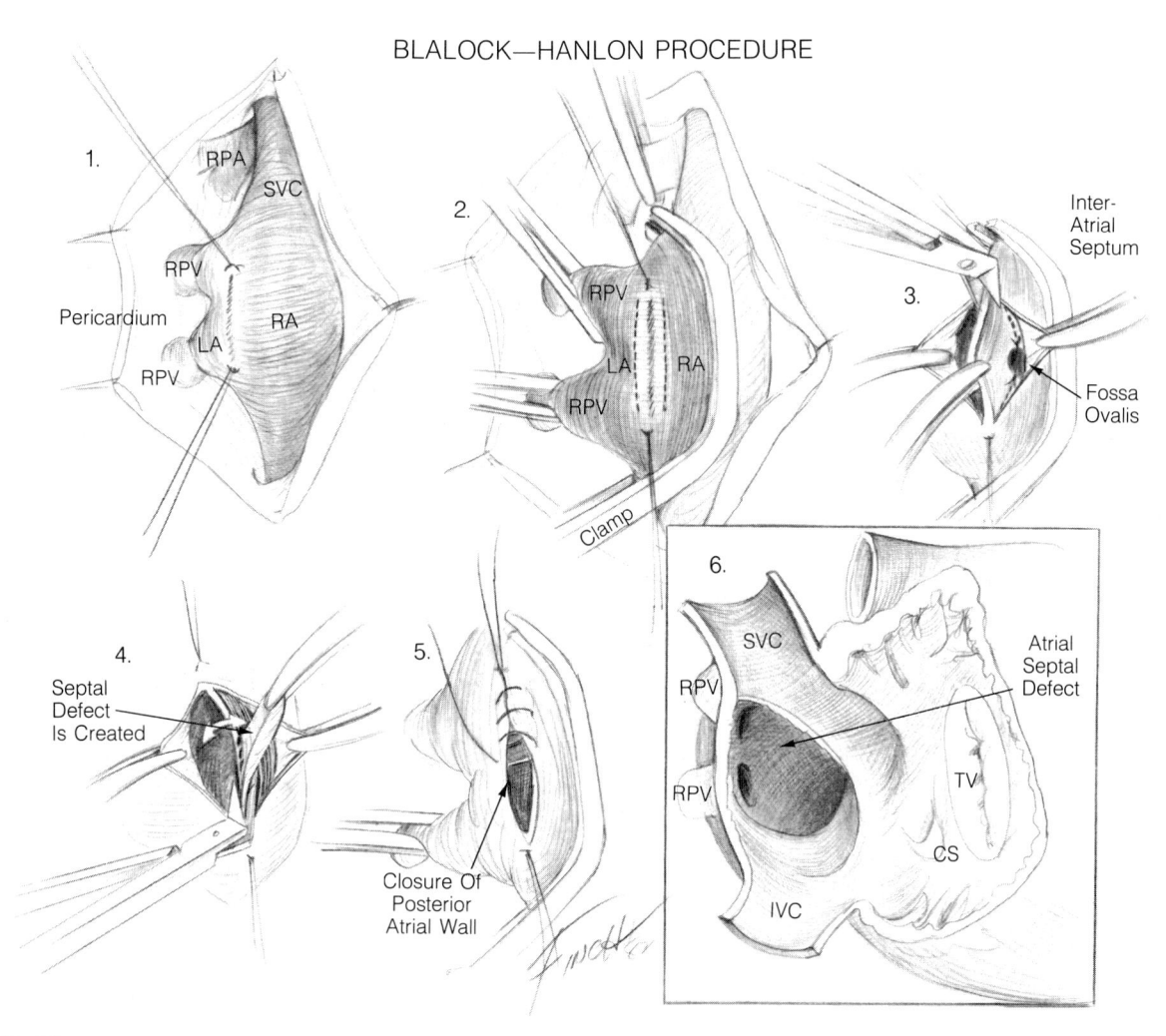

BLALOCK—HANLON PROCEDURE

FIG 38–35.
Blalock-Hanlon procedure. **1,** through right thoracotomy, posterior wall of right atrium *(RA)*, left atrium *(LA)*, superior vena cava *(SVC)* and right pulmonary veins *(RPV)* are exposed. **2,** clamp is placed across back wall of atria, including atrial septum. Incisions *(dashed lines)* are made on either side of atrial septum. **3,** atrial septum is partially withdrawn from atria. **4,** portion of atrial septum is excised. **5,** posterior atrial wall is closed. **6,** lateral view illustrates operatively created posteriorly positioned atrial septal defect. **CS** = coronary sinus; *IVC* = inferior vena cava; *TV* = tricuspid valve; *RPA* = right pulmonary artery.

2. Arrhythmias.[35–37] Sick sinus syndrome, junctional rhythm, and supraventricular tachycardia are each common after any of the types of atrial switch operations. The sinoatrial node or its artery can be injured as the superior limb of the baffle is sutured, or the atrial conduction pathways can be disrupted as the atrial septum is incised. These rhythm disturbances may account for the occurrence of sudden death reported after atrial switch operations.

3. Decreased right ventricular function.[11, 38] Echocardiographic, angiographic, and exercise data suggest depressed right ventricular function. This has been assumed to reflect inability of the right ventricle to develop systemic levels of pressure. Despite these measurements, most children carry on a normal active life. Perhaps with time, more patients will develop symptoms.

4. Progression of pulmonary vascular disease. One reason for performing a corrective operation is to arrest the progression of pulmonary vascular disease. Reports have indicated that it may progress even though the operation is successful.[9] This finding is perhaps not unexpected, because many patients have pulmonary vascular obstructive disease, and progression has been described in cases of isolated ventricular septal defect after a successful operation.

POSTOPERATIVE RADIOGRAPHIC FEATURES

1. After successful balloon atrial septostomy or a Blalock-Hanlon operation, there may be a striking decrease in cardiac size.

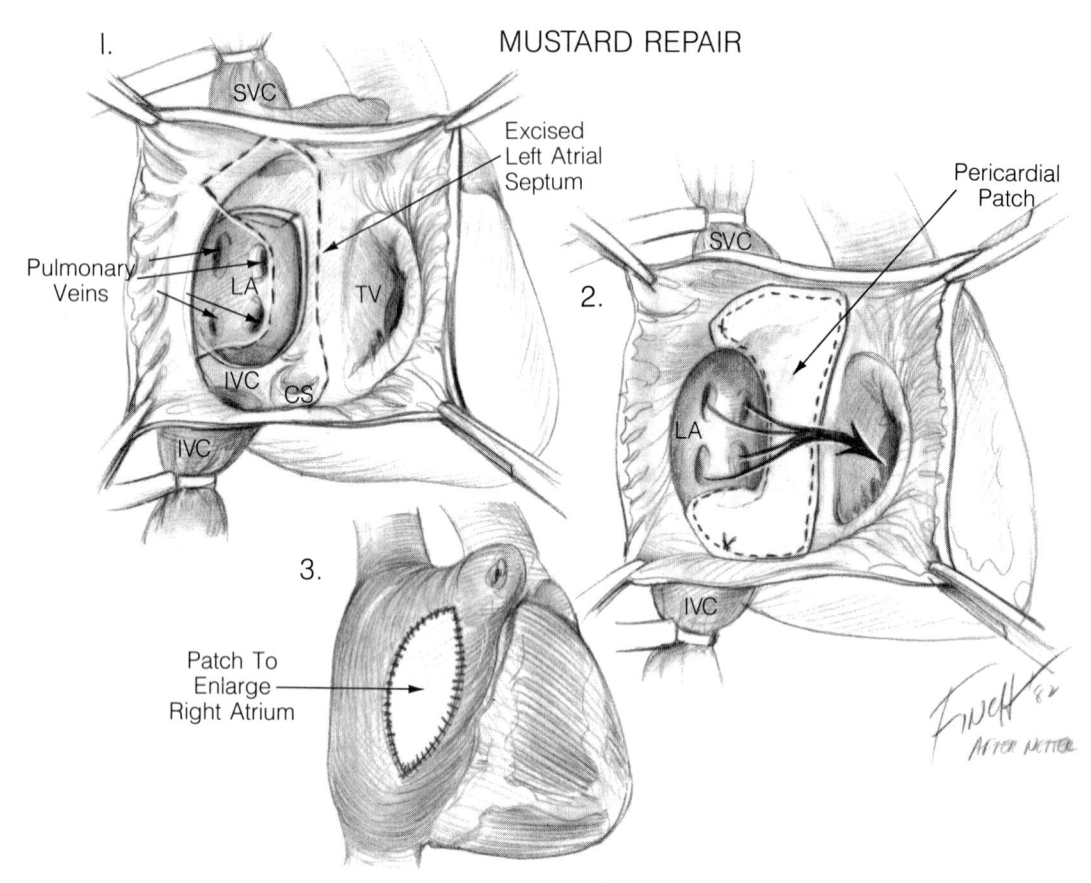

698   *Cyanosis and Increased Pulmonary Arterial Vasculature*

FIG 38–36.
1–3, Mustard procedure. Through right atriotomy, atrial septum is excised. Pericardial patch is sewn along dotted line, forming baffle. Pulmonary venous blood flows over baffle into tricuspid valve *(TV)*. Vena caval blood flows behind baffle through mitral valve. *LA* = left atrium; *SVC* = superior vena cava.

2. After operative correction or palliation there may be marked regrowth of thymic tissue (Fig 38–42). "Rebound" thymic growth may also occur after correction of other congenital cardiac anomalies, but it never appears as pronounced as in infants with complete transposition of the great vessels.

3. If radiographic evidence of a right thoracotomy (absent or deformed rib) is present in a cyanotic patient, either a Blalock-Hanlon operation (Fig 38–43) or a Blalock-Taussig operation (commonly performed for tetralogy of Fallot) is suggested.

4. The appearance of a mass at the right cardiophrenic angle after an atrial switch operation strongly suggests obstruction of the inferior limb of the interatrial baffle (see Fig 38–43).

5. Prominence of the superior vena cava and enlargement of the azygos vein suggest obstruction of the superior aspect of the baffle.

6. The appearance of a venous obstructive pattern, particularly in the left lung, suggests compromise of the left pulmonary veins.

7. Conduits may become densely calcified and clearly visible on chest x-ray films (Fig 38–44).

POSTOPERATIVE ANGIOGRAPHIC APPEARANCE

Postoperative cardiac catheterization and angiography have been used to evaluate operative results.

1. In patients with an atrial switch operation, injection of either the superior or inferior vena cava outlines the baffle. The contrast material then passes into the anatomic left ventricle and pulmonary artery, indicating hemodynamic correction (Fig 38–45).

2. The late phase of the angiograms demonstrates the pulmonary veins, which is followed by opacification of the remaining atrium. Visualization of the anatomic right ventricle and aorta then occurs (see Fig 38–45).

3. After insertion of the baffle, particularly its superior limb, a shunt may occur, indicated by leakage of con-

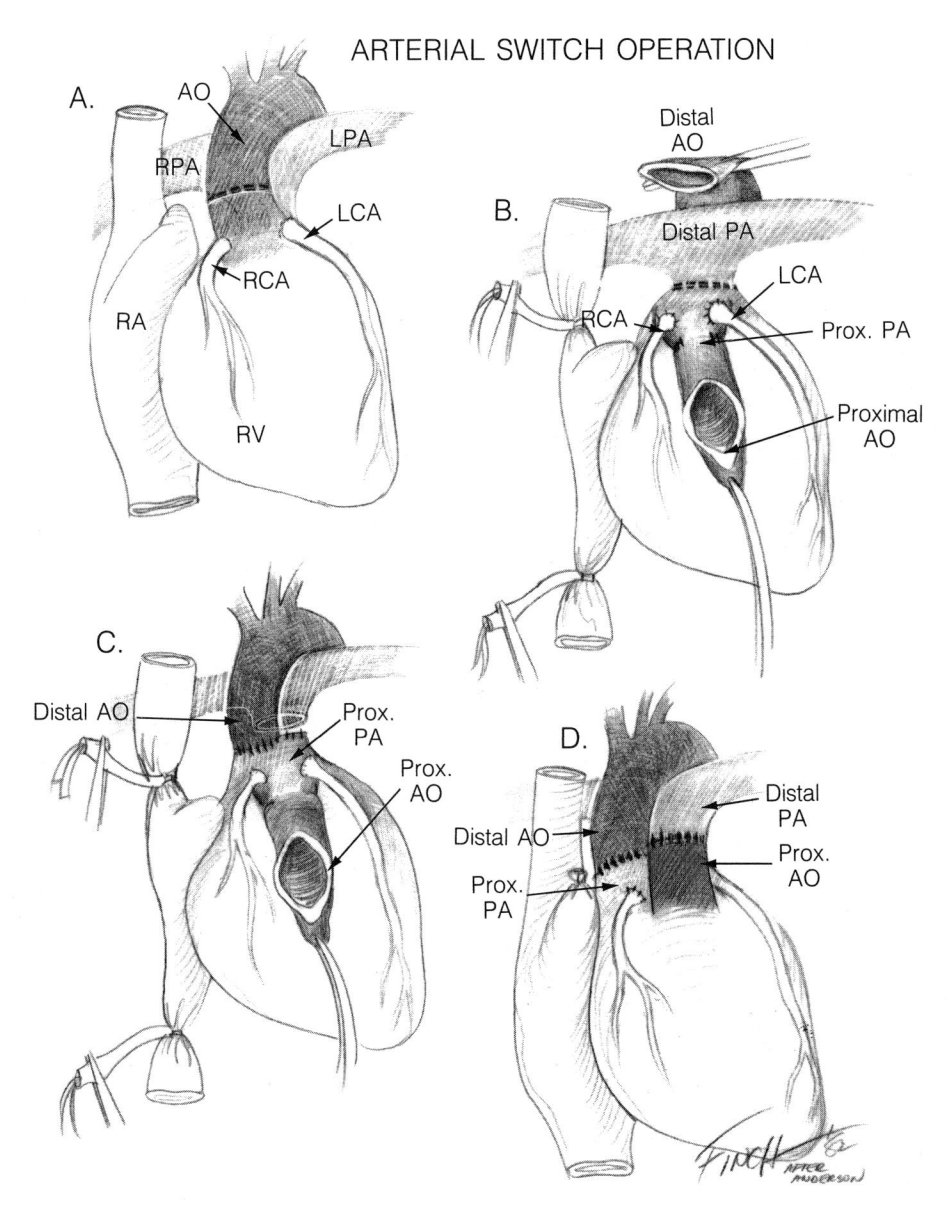

FIG 38–37.
Arterial switch operation. **A,** circumferencial incision is made around aortic root *(AO)* above orifices of coronary arteries *(LCA* and *RCA)* **B,** proximal aorta retracted anteriorly. Coronary arteries are removed from posterior aortic wall and attached to anterior wall of pulmonary artery *(PA)*. **C,** distal orifice of ascending aorta is anastomosed to proximal pulmonary artery. **D,** proximal aorta is anastomosed to distal pulmonary artery. *RA* = right atrium; *RPA* = right pulmonary artery; *RV* = right ventricle.

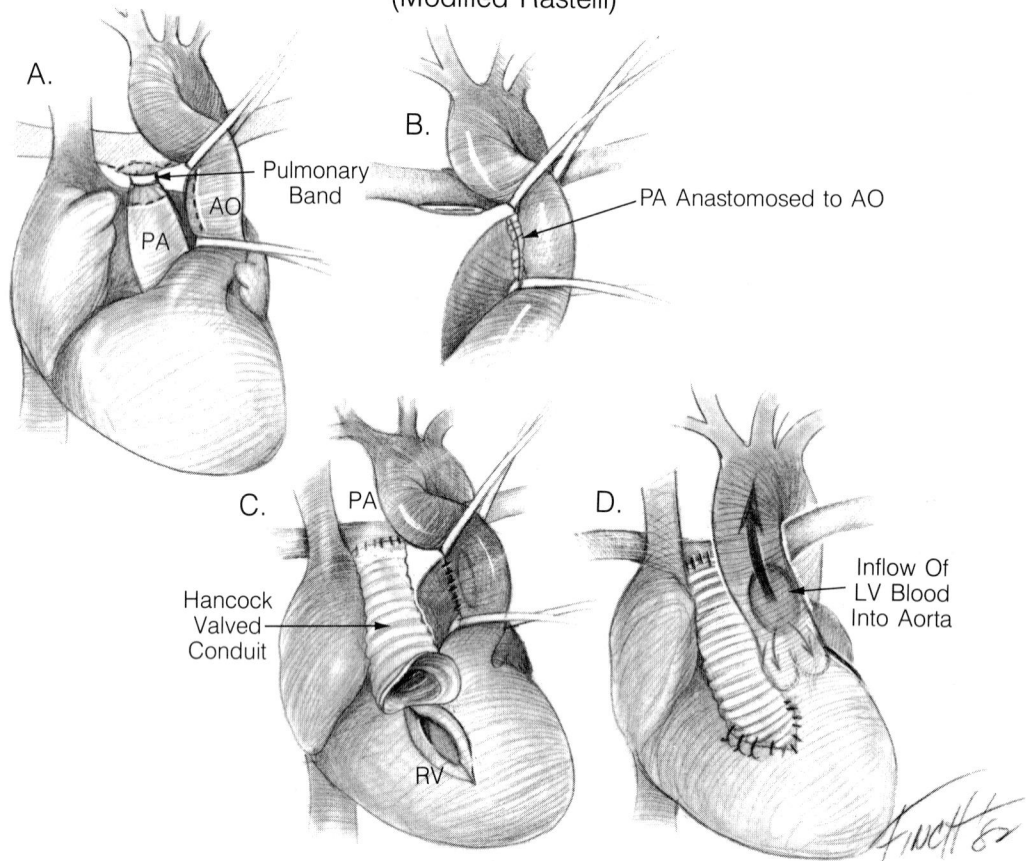

700 Cyanosis and Increased Pulmonary Arterial Vasculature

FIG 38-38.
Arterial switch procedure (modified Rastelli). **A,** Aorta *(AO)* and pulmonary artery *(PA)* are identified, and incision is made in ascending aorta. **B,** pulmonary artery is divided, and distal end of proximal pulmonary artery is anastomosed to posterior aspect of ascending aorta. **C,** right ventricle *(RV)* is opened and conduit anastomosed between *RV* and *PA*. **D,** completed operation. Blood from pulmonary artery flows into aorta, perfusing coronary arteries. Aortic pressure maintains closure of aortic valve. *LV* = left ventricle.

RASTELLI REPAIR OF TRANSPOSITION WITH VSD AND SUBPULMONARY STENOSIS

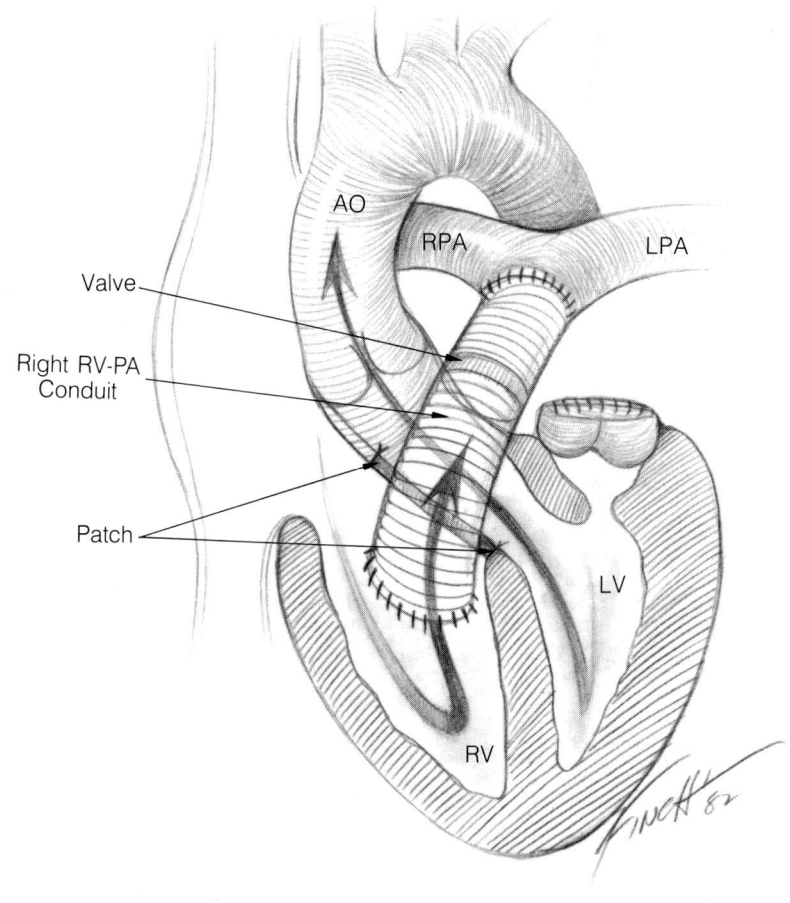

FIG 38–39.
Rastelli procedure for transposition of great vessels, ventricular septal defect, and pulmonary stenosis. Ventricular septal defect *(VSD)* is closed so left ventricular *(LV)* blood is delivered to aorta *(AO)*. Blood from right atrium and right ventricle *(RV)* passes through valved conduit into right pulmonary artery *(RPA)* and left pulmonary artery *(LPA)*. Distal end of proximal pulmonary artery is oversewn.

REPAIR OF TRANSPOSITION WITH SUBPULMONARY STENOSIS

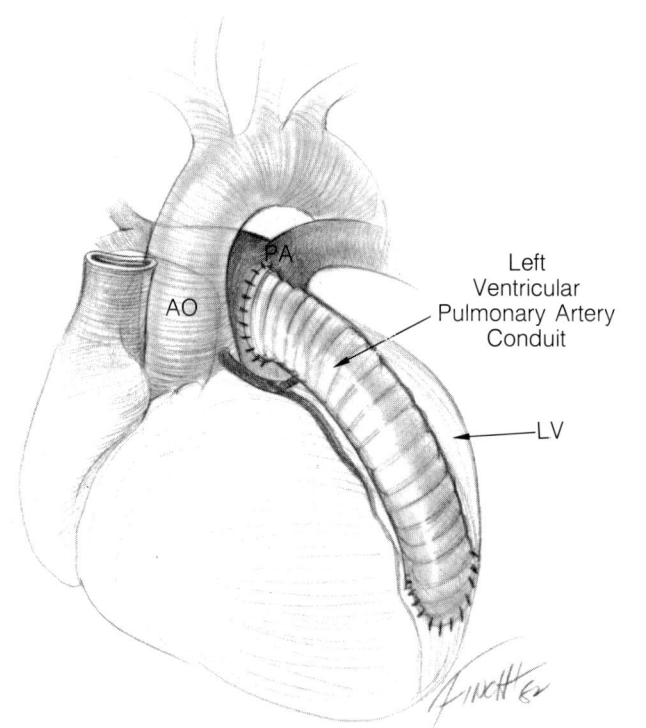

FIG 38–40.
Left ventricular *(LV)*–pulmonary artery *(PA)* conduit for complete transposition of great vessels. *AO* = aorta.

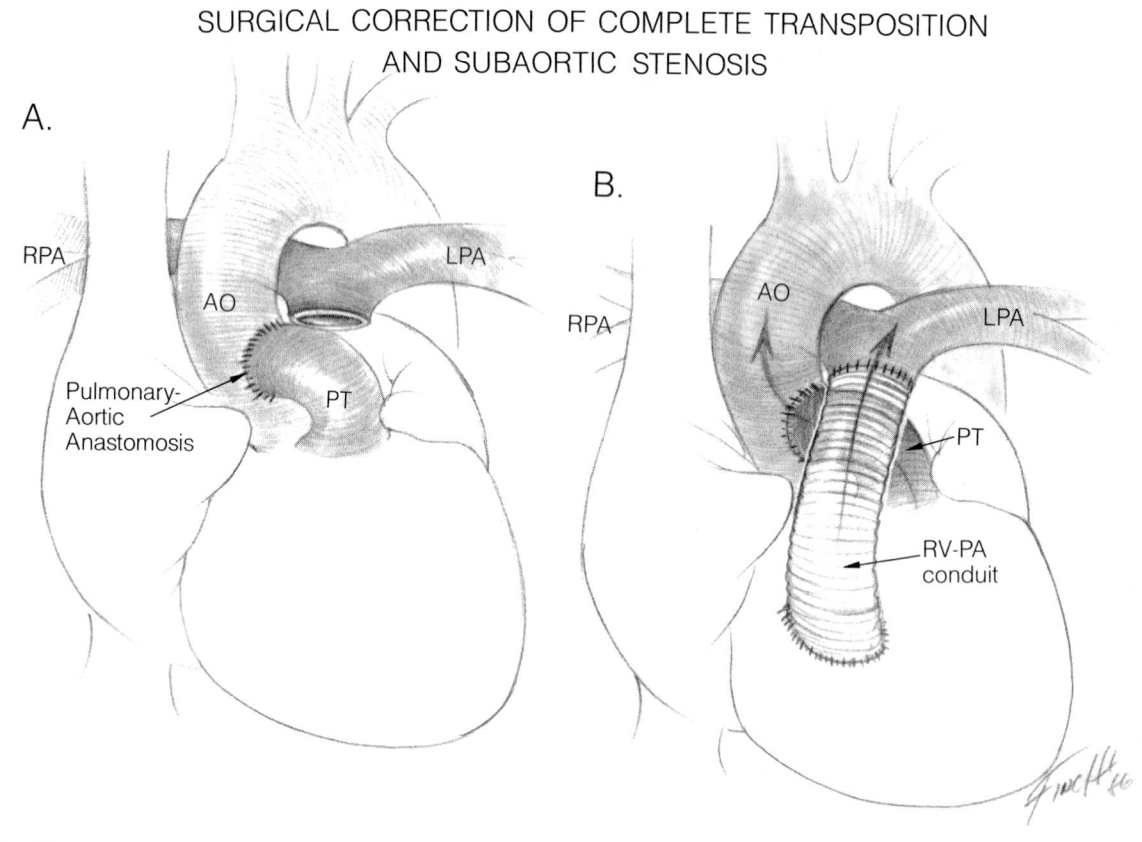

FIG 38–41.
Damus-Kaye-Stansel repair for transposition of great vessels and subaortic obstruction. Pulmonary trunk *(PT)* is divided and sewn to side of ascending aorta *(AO)*. Conduit is placed between right ventricle *(RV)* and pulmonary artery *(PA)*. LPA = left pulmonary artery; RPA = right pulmonary artery.

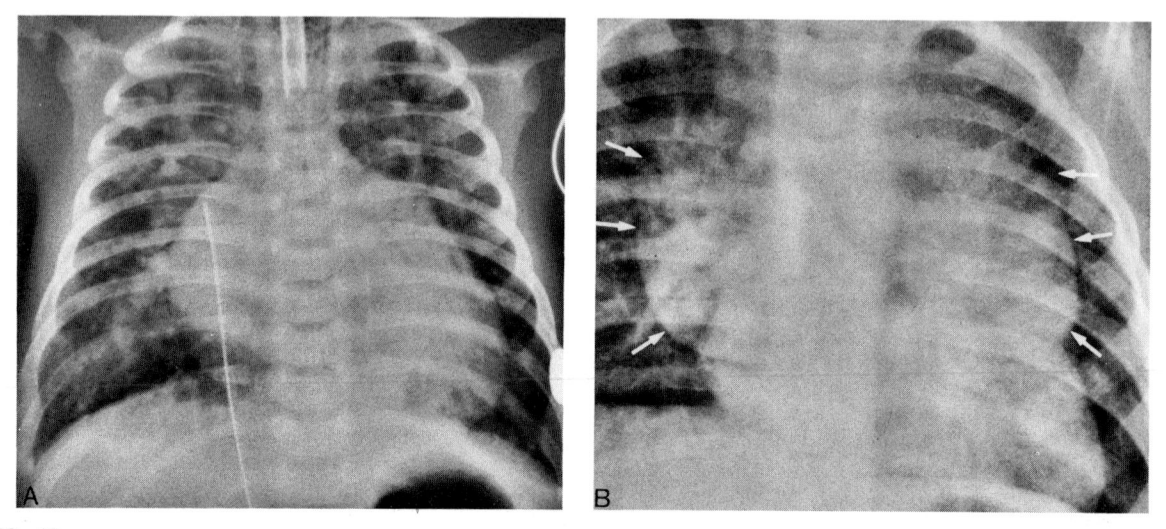

FIG 38–42.
Complete transposition of great vessels in infant. **A,** before and, **B,** after Rashkind procedure. Exuberant regrowth of thymus *(white arrows)*. "Rebound thymus."

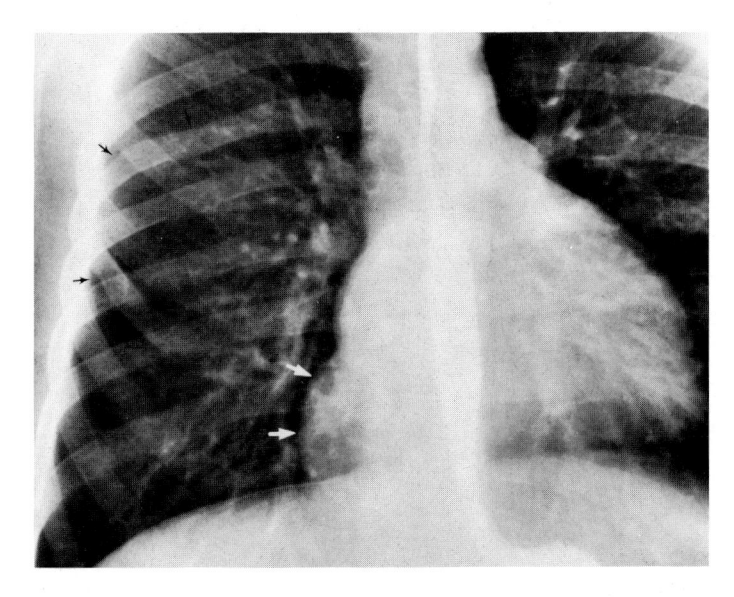

FIG 38-43.
Complete transposition of great vessels. Thoracic roentgenogram. Posteroanterior projection. Rib irregularities *(black arrows)* suggest previous right thoracotomy. Wire sutures in sternum suggest corrective operation. After atrial switch operation (Mustard procedure), mass appeared at the right cardiophrenic angle *(white arrows),* which was caused by obstruction of inferior limb of baffle (dilatation of inferior vena cava).

trast medium from the baffle into the atrium receiving pulmonary venous blood (Fig 38-46). Usually the shunts are small and of no hemodynamic significance.

4. The most common problem with the baffle is narrowing with obstruction. Minor degrees of narrowing without hemodynamic significance are commonly visualized. More severe narrowing or complete obstruction of the baffle (Fig 38-47) may occur and cause the superior vena cava syndrome.

5. Rarely the baffle is completely occluded (Fig 38-48).

6. Another complication is occlusion on the left pulmonary veins by the baffle. Under these circumstances, after left ventriculography, the left pulmonary artery does not opacify because of the large inflow of blood from bronchial arteries. Oxygen saturation in the left pulmonary artery is higher than in the right. Nonopacification of a pulmonary artery does not necessarily indicate anatomic

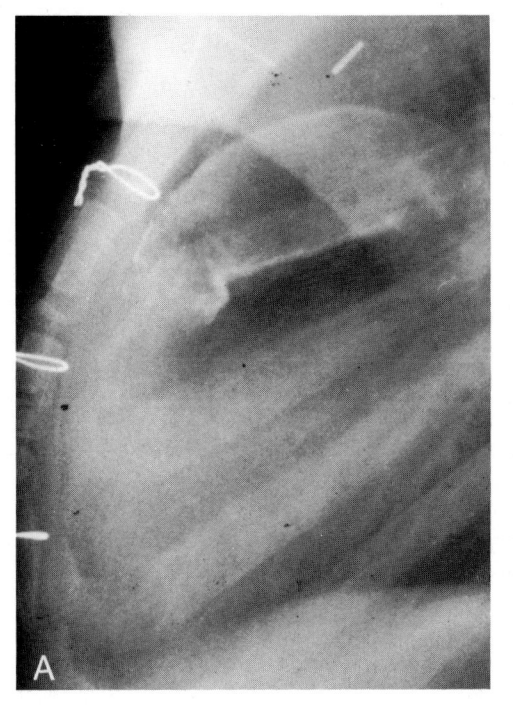

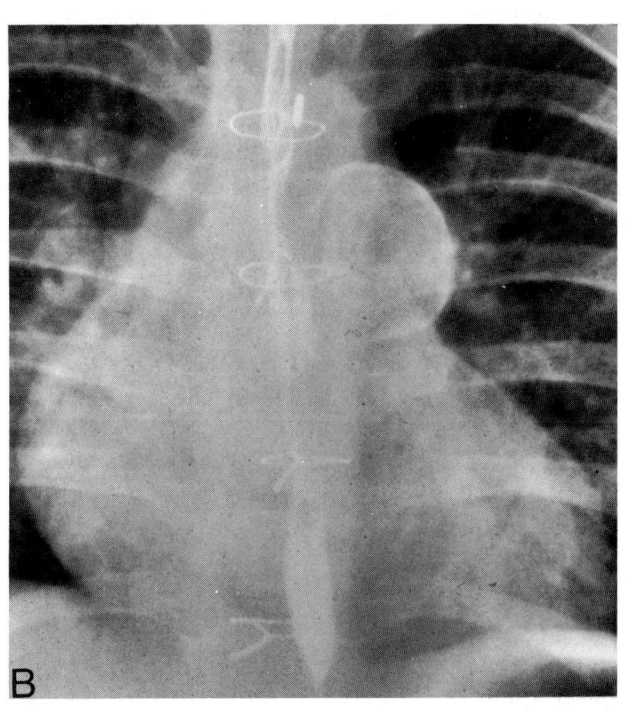

FIG 38-44.
Repair of transposition of great vessels with interrupted aortic arch. Thoracic roentgenogram. **A,** anteroposterior and, **B,** lateral projections. Conduit has become densely opacified and is clearly visible.

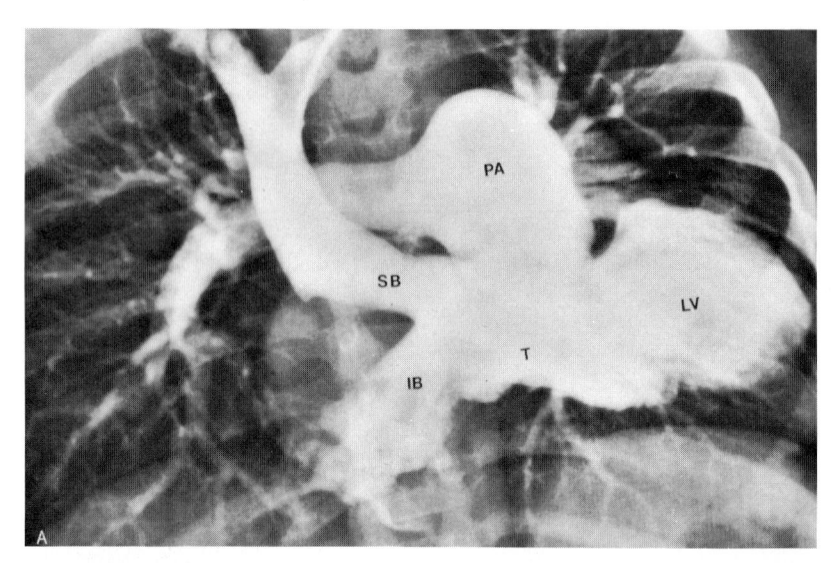

FIG 38–45.
Complete transposition of the great vessels after a Mustard procedure. Injection into superior vena cava. Anteroposterior projection. **A,** superior limb of baffle *(SB)* of normal size. Reflux of contrast material occurs into inferior limb of baffle *(IB)*. Both baffles provide a conduit for systemic blood through mitral valve into left ventricle *(LV)* and pulmonary artery *(PA)*. (T = tricuspid valve.) **B,** late phase. Opacification of pulmonary veins *(PV)* and remaining atrium *(A)*. Opacification of anatomic right ventricle *(RV)* and aorta *(AO)* occurs. Therefore, malformation has been physiologically but not anatomically corrected.

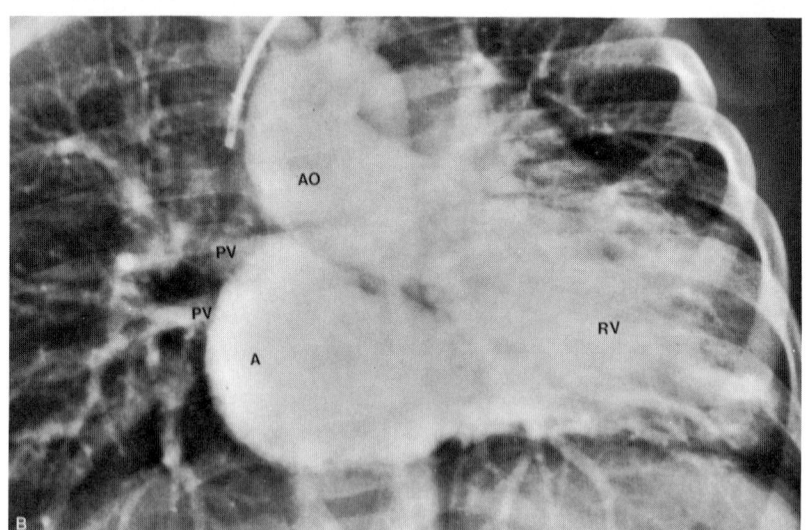

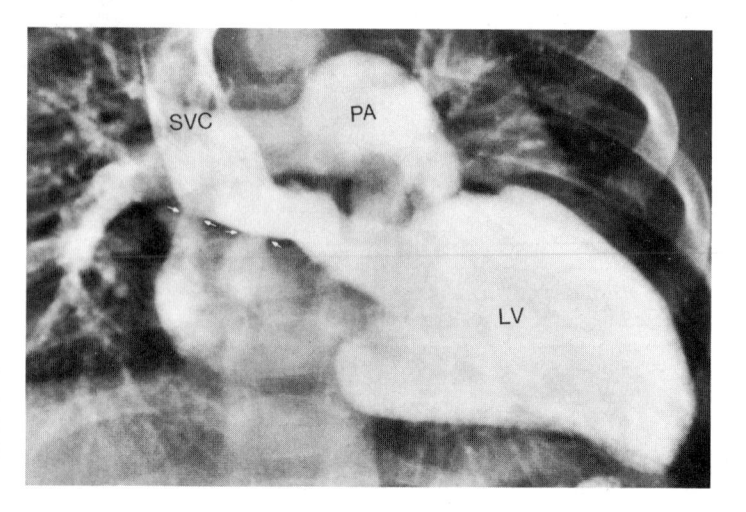

FIG 38–46.
Complete transposition of great vessels after Mustard procedure. Injection into superior vena cava *(SVC)*. Anteroposterior projection. Contrast material passes through superior limb of baffle *(small arrows)* into other atrium, indicating a shunt. LV = left ventricle; PA = pulmonary artery.

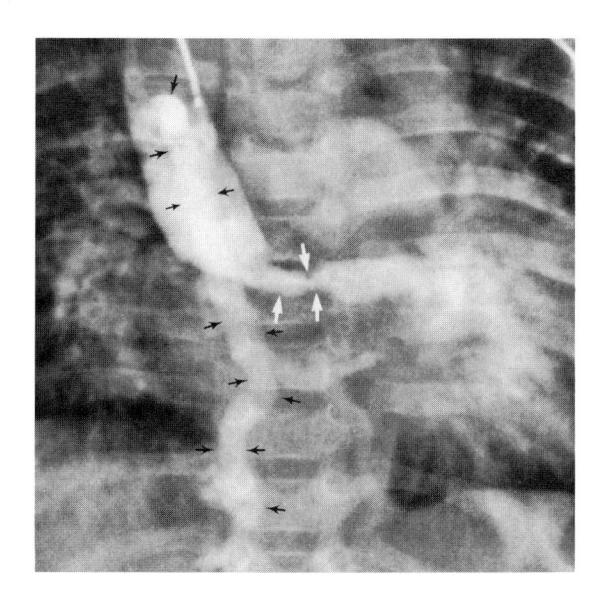

FIG 38–47.
Complete transposition of great vessels after Mustard procedure. Injection into superior vena cava. Anteroposterior projection. Severe narrowing of superior limb of baffle *(white arrows)*. Drainage of contrast medium through markedly enlarged azygos vein *(black arrows)*. This patient had symptoms of superior vena caval obstruction.

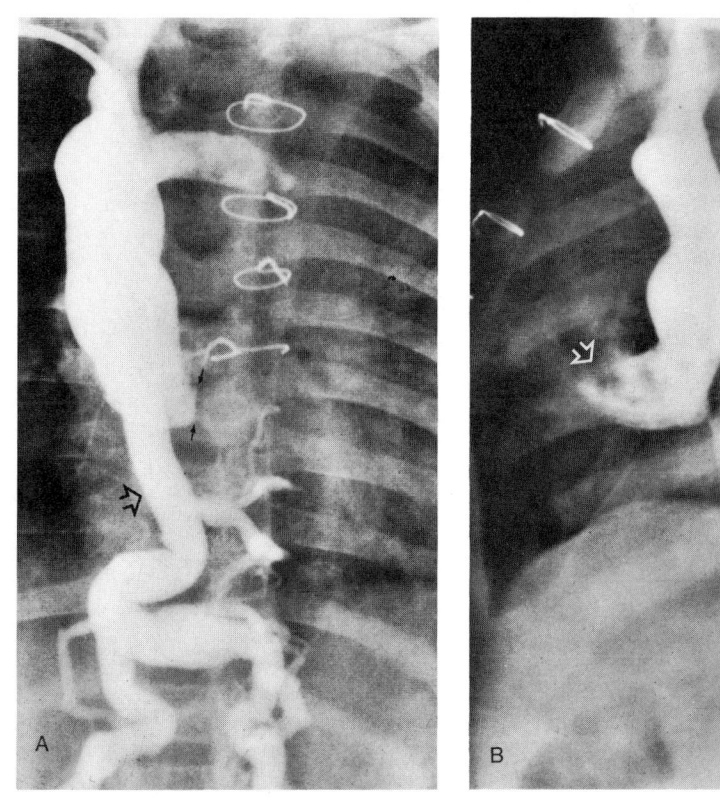

FIG 38–48.
Superior vena cavogram after Mustard procedure. **A,** anteroposterior projection. Complete occlusion of superior limb of baffle *(open white arrow)*. Collateral retrograde flow through huge azygos vein *(open black arrow)*. **B,** lateral projection showing azygos vein to better advantage.

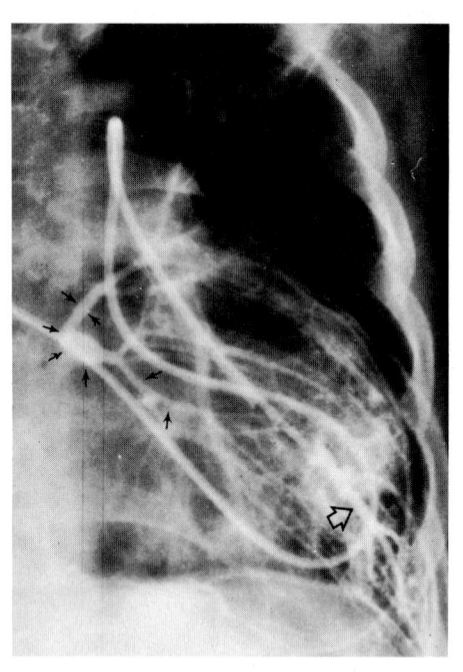

FIG 38-49.
Complete transposition of great vessels after Mustard procedure. Right pulmonary arteriogram. Anteroposterior projection. Previous thoracic roentgenograms had shown progressively decreasing pulmonary vasculature in left lung. Catheter is passed through superior limb of baffle into left ventricle and pulmonary artery. Left lower lobe pulmonary artery is occluded with balloon. Contrast material is injected. Opacification of pulmonary artery *(open arrow)* distal to balloon. Opacification of very small pulmonary veins follows *(black arrows)*. Left pulmonary vein is not patent because it became obstructed by insertion of baffle.

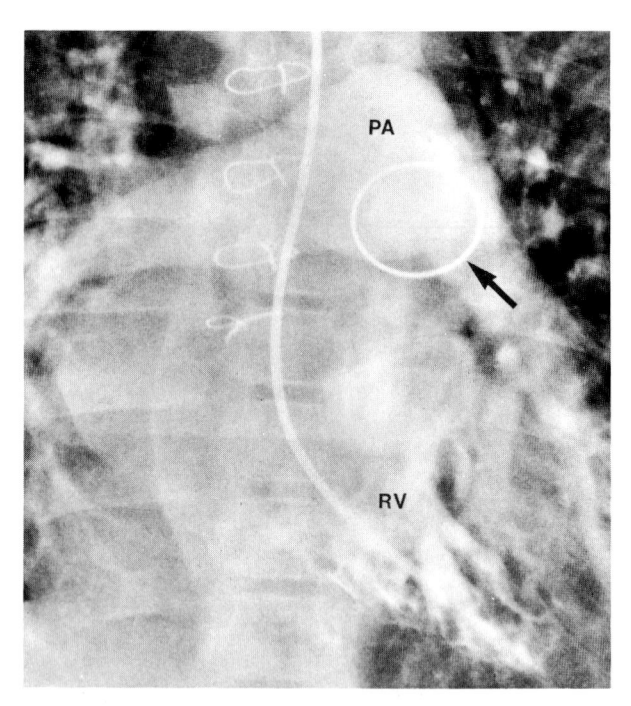

FIG 38-50.
Complete transposition of great vessels after Rastelli procedure. Right ventriculogram. Anteroposterior projection. Right ventricle *(RV)* and pulmonary artery *(PA)* are opacified. Valve in conduit is recognized by metal ring *(arrow)*.

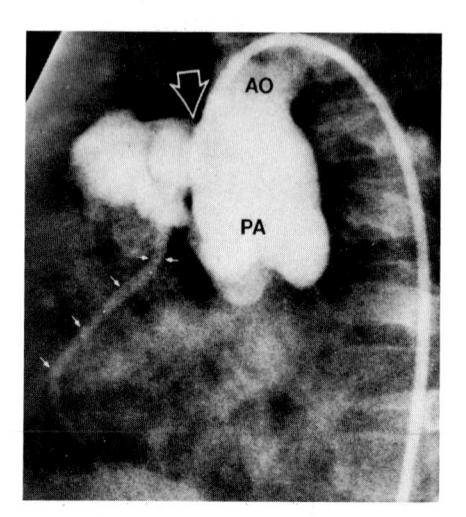

obstruction of the artery. The nonopacification may occur from blood flowing from the left pulmonary artery into the right pulmonary artery. In this instance, occlusion of pulmonary veins results in bronchial arterial inflow into the pulmonary arterial system. This can be proved by balloon occlusion angiography of a peripheral pulmonary artery (Fig 38-49).

7. After a conduit operation, blood flows from the right ventricle to the pulmonary artery through a composite graft. This is readily demonstrated by right ventriculography (Fig 38-50).

8. The angiographic appearance after a classic arterial switch operation is fairly normal. However, angiography with a modified arterial switch operation may be confusing. Through an aortic approach the catheter passes through the aortic arch and into the ascending aorta, which has been anastomosed to the proximal pulmonary artery (Fig 38-51). Aortography outlines both the pulmonary and aortic valves. The aortic root can be identified by opacification of the coronary arteries.

9. As with other thoracic operative procedures, the patient may develop a chylothorax. Obstruction of the tho-

FIG 38-51.
Complete transposition of great vessels after modified arterial switch operation. Aortogram. Lateral projection. Catheter is passed from descending aorta through aortic arch *(AO)* into proximal pulmonary artery *(PA)*, which has been anastomosed to aorta. From opacified pulmonary artery, contrast medium passes into aortic root, which has been anastomosed to pulmonary artery *(white open arrow)*, forming an aortic pulmonic window. From aortic root, coronary arteries opacify *(small white arrows)*.

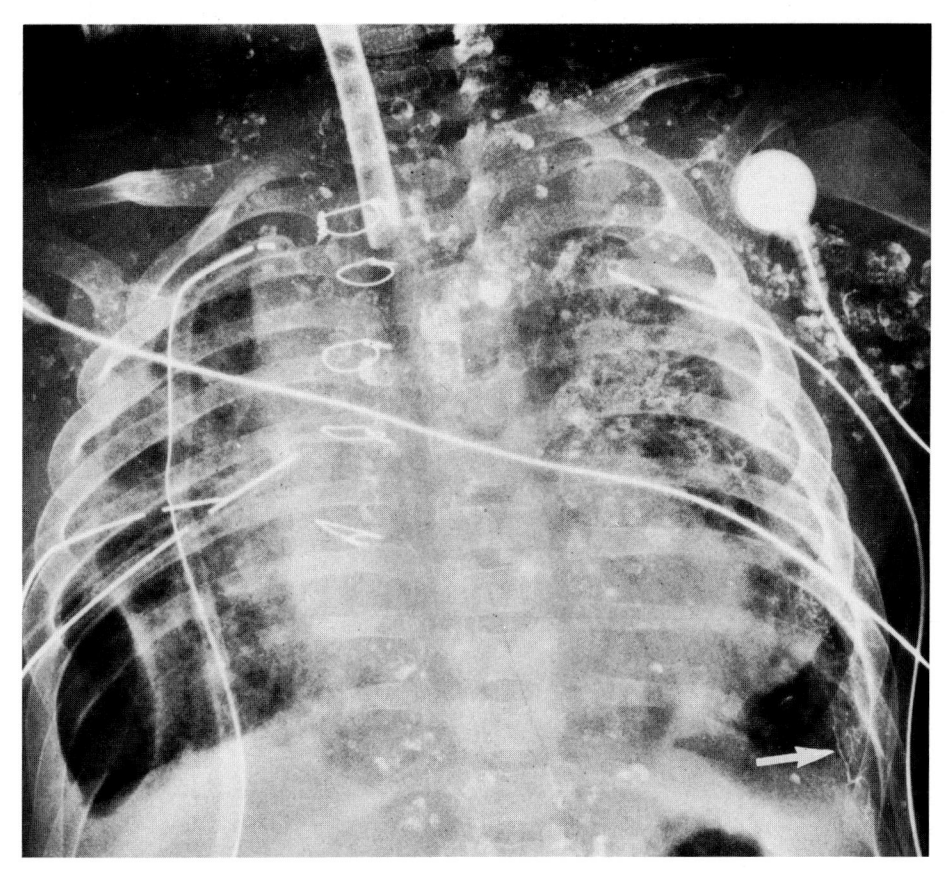

FIG 38–52.
Transposition of great vessels after Mustard procedure. Bilateral chylothorax. Thoracic roentgenogram. Posteroanterior projection. Lymphangiogram. Numerous mediastinal and pulmonary nodes are opacified. Pleural lymphatics *(arrow)* are visible, indicating drainage into pleural space because of thoracic duct obstruction.

racic duct can be proved by lymphangiography (Fig 38–52).

REFERENCES

1. Goor DA, Edwards JE: The spectrum of transposition of the great arteries: with specific reference to developmental anatomy of the conus, *Circulation* 48:406, 1973.
2. Plauth WH Jr, Nadas AS, Bernhard WF, et al: Changing hemodynamics in patients with transposition of the great arteries, *Circulation* 42:131, 1970.
3. Mair DD, Ritter DG: Factors influencing intercirculatory mixing in patients with complete transposition of the great arteries, *Am J Cardiol* 30:653, 1972.
4. Yamaki S, Tezuka F: Quantitative analysis of pulmonary vascular disease in complete transposition of the great arteries, *Circulation* 54:805, 1976.
5. Edwards WD, Edwards JE: Hypertensive pulmonary vascular disease in d-transposition of the great arteries, *Am J Cardiol* 41:921, 1978.
6. Newfeld EA, Paul MH, Muster AJ, et al: Pulmonary vascular disease in complete transposition of the great arteries: a study of 200 patients, *Am J Cardiol* 34:75, 1974.
7. Lakier JB, Stanger P, Heymann MA, et al: Early onset of pulmonary vascular obstruction in patients with aortopulmonary transposition and intact ventricular septum, *Circulation* 51:875, 1975.
8. Aziz KU, Paul MH, Rowe RD: Bronchopulmonary circulation in d-transposition of the great arteries: possible role in genesis of accelerated pulmonary vascular disease, *Am J Cardiol* 39:432, 1977.
9. Berman W Jr, Whitman V, Pierce WS, et al: The development of pulmonary vascular obstructive disease after successful Mustard operation in early infancy, *Circulation* 58:181, 1978.
10. Aziz KU, Paul MH, Idriss FS, et al: Clinical manifestations of dynamic left ventricular outflow tract stenosis with D-transposition of the great arteries with intact ventricular septum, *Am J Cardiol* 44:290, 1979.
11. Graham TP Jr, Atwood GF, Boucek RJ Jr, et al: Right heart volume characteristics in transposition of the great arteries, *Circulation* 51:881, 1975.
12. Plauth WH Jr, Nadas AS, Bernhard WF, et al: Transposition of the great arteries: clinical and physiological observations on 74 patients treated by palliative surgery, *Circulation* 37:316, 1968.
13. Aziz KU, Paul MH, Muster AJ: Echocardiographic assess-

ment of left ventricular outflow tract in d-transposition of the great arteries, *Am J Cardiol* 41:543, 1978.
14. Dillon JC, Feigenbaum H, Konecke LL, et al: Echocardiographic manifestations of d-transposition of the great arteries, *Am J Cardiol* 32:74, 1973.
15. Bierman FZ, Williams RG: Prospective diagnosis of d-transposition of the great arteries in neonates by subxiphoid, two-dimensional echocardiography, *Circulation* 60:1496, 1979.
16. Nanda NC, Gramiak R, Manning JA, et al: Echocardiographic features of subpulmonic obstruction in dextrotransposition of the great vessels, *Circulation* 51:515, 1975.
17. Marino B, DeSimone G, Pasquini L, et al: Complete transposition of the great arteries: Visualization of left and right outflow tract obstruction by oblique subcostal two-dimensional echocardiography, *Am J Cardiol* 55:1140, 1985.
18. Rashkind WJ: Balloon atrioseptostomy, *Adv Cardiol* 11:2, 1974.
19. Freed MD, Heymann MA, Lewis AB, et al: Prostaglandin E$_1$ in infants with ductus arteriosus–dependent congenital heart disease. *Circulation* 64:899, 1981.
20. Blalock A, Hanlon CR: The surgical treatment of complete transposition of the aorta and the pulmonary artery, *Surg Gynecol Obstet* 90:1, 1950.
21. Clark EB, Sweeney LJ, Rosenquist GC: Atrial defect size after Blalock-Hanlon atrioseptectomy, *Am J Cardiol* 40:405, 1977.
22. Mustard WT: Successful two-stage correction of transposition of the great vessels, *Surgery* 55:469, 1964.
23. Waldhausen JA, Pierce WS, Berman W Jr, et al: Modified Shumacker repair of transposition of the great arteries, *Circulation* 60:(suppl I):110, 1979.
24. Senning A: Correction of transposition of the great arteries, *Ann Surg* 182:287, 1975.
25. Mamiya RT, Moreno-Cabral RJ, Nakamura FT, et al: Retransposition of the great vessels for transposition with ventricular septal defect and pulmonary hypertension, *J Thorac Cardiovasc Surg* 73:340, 1977.
26. Yacoub MH: The case for anatomic correction of transposition of the great arteries, *J Thorac Cardiovasc Surg* 78:3, 1979.
27. Smith A, Wilkinson JL, Arnold R, et al: Growth and development of ventricular walls in complete transposition of the great arteries with intact septum (simple transposition), *Am J Cardiol* 49:362, 1982.
28. Danielson GK, Tabry IF, Mair DD, et al: Great-vessel switch operation without coronary relocation for transposition of great arteries, *Mayo Clin Proc* 53:675, 1978.
29. Rastelli GC: A new approach to "anatomic" repair of transposition of the great arteries, *Mayo Clin Proc* 44:1, 1969.
30. Crupi G, Anderson RH, Ho SY, et al: Complete transposition of the great arteries with intact ventricular septum and left ventricular outflow tract obstruction: surgical management and anatomic considerations, *J Thorac Cardiovasc Surg* 78:730, 1979.
31. Berman MA, Barash PS, Hellenbrand WE, et al: Late development of severe pulmonary venous obstruction following the Mustard operation, *Circulation* 56(suppl II):91, 1977.
32. Stark J, Silove ED, Taylor JFN, et al: Obstruction to systemic venous return following the Mustard operation for transposition of the great arteries, *J Thorac Cardiovasc Surg* 68:742, 1974.
33. Takahashi M, Lindesmith GG, Lewis AB, et al: Long-term results of the Mustard procedure, *Circulation* 56(suppl 3):85, 1977.
34. Rodriguez-Fernandez HL, Kelly DT, Collado A, et al: Hemodynamic data and angiographic findings after Mustard repair for complete transposition of the great arteries, *Circulation* 46:799, 1972.
35. Schiller MS, Levin AR, Haft JI, et al: Electrophysiologic studies in sick sinus syndrome following surgery for d-transposition of the great arteries, *J Pediatr* 91:891, 1977.
36. Saalouke MG, Rios J, Perry LW, et al: Electrophysiologic studies after Mustard's operation for d-transposition of the great vessels, *Am J Cardiol* 41:1104, 1978.
37. Bharati S, Molthan ME, Veasy LG, et al: Conduction system in two cases of sudden death two years after the Mustard procedure, *J Thorac Cardiovasc Surg* 77:101, 1979.
38. Hagler DJ, Ritter DG, Mair DD, et al: Clinical, angiographic, and hemodynamic assessment of late results after Mustard operation, *Circulation* 57:1214, 1978.

CHAPTER 39

Congenital Corrected Transposition of Great Vessels: L-Transposition of Great Vessels

The term corrected transposition of the great vessels names two important features that characterize this condition: (1) correct circulatory pattern, because systemic venous return is delivered to the pulmonary artery and pulmonary venous return to the aorta; and (2) transposition of the great vessels, indicating that the aorta arises from an anatomic right ventricle and the pulmonary artery arises from an anatomic left ventricle. The heart is functionally normal, but associated cardiac anomalies are almost always present that cause cardiovascular signs and symptoms. Other names for the condition are "l-transposition of the great vessels"[1] and "atrioventricular discordance with ventricular-arterial discordance."[2]

PATHOLOGIC ANATOMY

Ventricular inversion is a key anatomic feature of corrected transposition of the great vessels. This term indicates a change in lateral relationships. Thus, the anatomic right ventricle lies to the left of the anatomic left ventricle (Fig 39–1). The right atrium communicates with the left ventricle through a mitral valve (the atrioventricular valves have the features of the related ventricles). This ventricle is smooth walled, it lacks an infundibulum, and fibrous continuity exists between the atrioventricular and semilunar (the inverted mitral and the pulmonary) valves. This ventricle carries systemic venous blood from the right atrium to the pulmonary artery. The main pulmonary artery arises from this ventricle in a posterior and midline position.

The pulmonary veins join the posterior wall of the normally positioned left atrium. The left atrium is connected to the inverted right ventricle through the tricuspid valve. The right ventricle is trabeculated and possesses an infundibulum that separates the atrioventricular and semilunar (the inverted tricuspid and the aortic) valves. The ascending aorta originates from the infundibulum and is located anteriorly and to the left of the pulmonary trunk. The aortic valve is located at a higher plane than the pulmonary valve.

In corrected transposition of great vessels, not only are the ventricles inverted, but the atrioventricular valves and coronary arteries are also. The anatomic left (venous) ventricle lies to the right in the cardiac mass and is supplied by a coronary arterial system, which arises above the right aortic cusp (Fig 39–2). It resembles a left coronary arterial system because it has two branches, the anterior descending, which descends along the anterior surface of the heart in the interventricular groove, and an inverted circumflex branch, which crosses the outflow area of the venous ventricle to lie in the right atrioventricular groove. The latter, because of its course, is often called the "right coronary artery," but developmentally it represents the circumflex artery. Both arteries supply the anatomic left ventricle. The course of the right coronary artery across the outflow area of the venous ventricle presents a major difficulty to operative correction of interventricular anomalies requiring a ventriculotomy.

The anatomic right (systemic) ventricle is also supplied by an artery passing in an atrioventricular groove. It arises above the left aortic cusp. It is commonly referred to as the "circumflex artery," but developmentally it represents the inverted right coronary artery.

The anterior aortic cusp, as in all instances of transposition of great vessels, is the noncoronary cusp.

710 Cyanosis and Increased Pulmonary Arterial Vasculature

ANATOMIC FEATURES OF CORRECTED TRANSPOSITION
(L-Transposition)

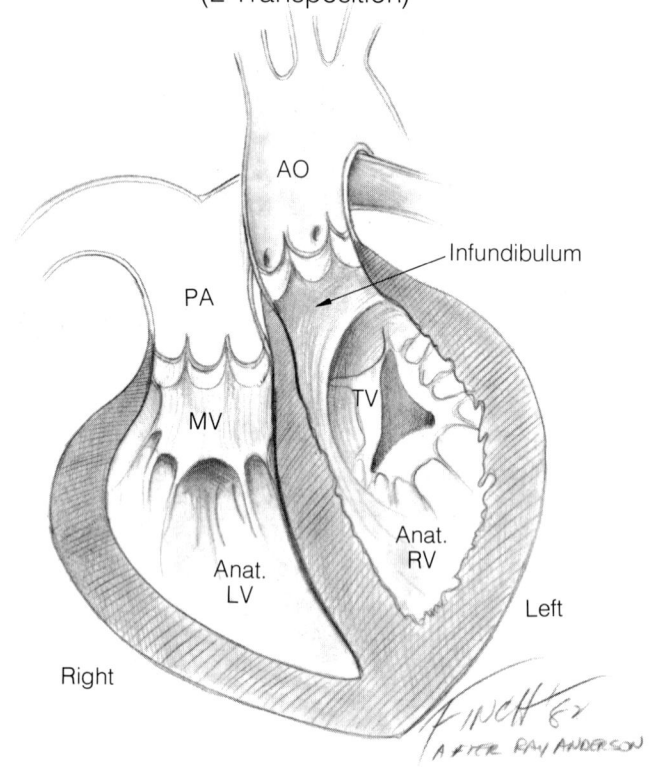

FIG 39–1.
Congenital corrected transposition of great vessels. *AO* = aorta; *Anat. LV* = anatomic left ventricle; *MV* = mitral valve; *PA* = pulmonary artery; *Anat. RV* = anatomic right ventricle; *TV* = tricuspid valve. Pulmonary valve in fibrous continuity with mitral valve. Aortic valve separated from tricuspid valve by infundibulum.

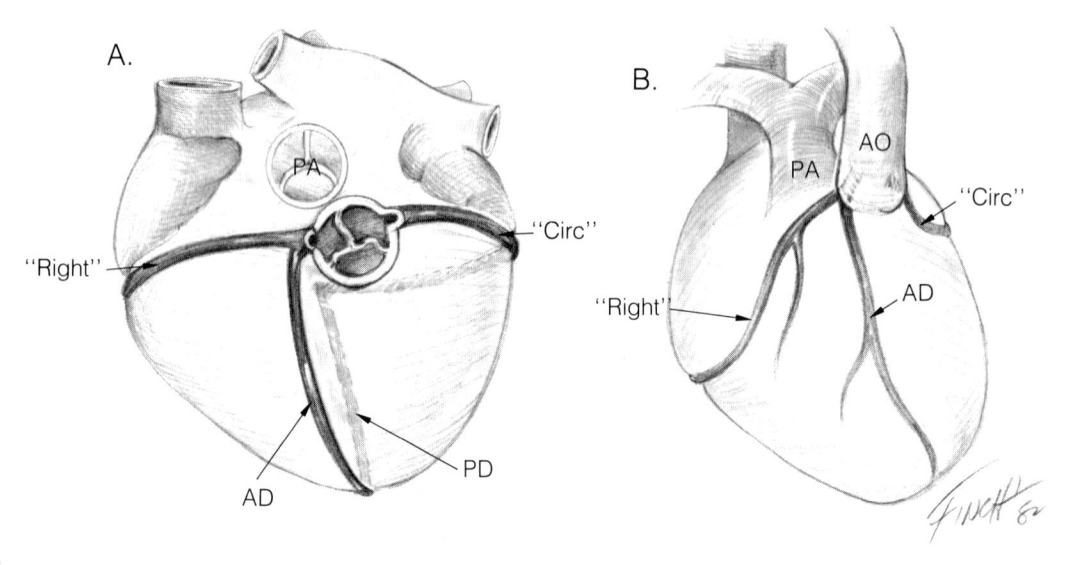

FIG 39–2.
Congenital corrected transposition of great vessels. Coronary arterial system. Superior (**A**) and frontal (**B**) views. Venous (anatomic left) ventricle supplied by anterior descending *(AD)* and circumflex "right" coronary arteries. Arterial (anatomic right) ventricle supplied by right "circumflex" *(CRC)* artery. "Right" coronary artery crosses outflow area of venous ventricle, complicating cardiac operation. Anterior cusp, which normally gives rise to right coronary artery, is noncoronary cusp. *AO* = aorta; *PA* = pulmonary artery; *PD* = posterior descending.

The coronary arteries and atrioventricular valves remain with the proper inverted ventricles.

COEXISTENT CARDIAC MALFORMATIONS

Congenitally corrected transposition of the great vessels is common in patients with malposition of the heart,[3, 4] particularly those with either dextroversion or levoversion (see Chapter 58).

Ventricular septal defect is the most common coexistent malformation.[3, 4] The defect may be located in various positions in the ventricular septum and is usually large. Pulmonary stenosis either isolated or with ventricular septal defect is common, and the stenosis results from valvar stenosis or subpulmonary stenosis from redundant subvalvar tissue.[5–8] Pulmonary atresia may be present. Congenital abnormalities found in the normal heart may be found in corrected transposition, but they occur in the opposite ventricle (ventricular equivalents).

In nearly every patient, some degree of Ebstein's malformation of the tricuspid valve is present.[3, 9, 10] This may lead to significant left atrioventricular valvar regurgitation ("mitral" insufficiency) in about one third of patients.

The size of the ventricles varies (Fig 39–3), depending on the location of the atrioventricular valves, especially the left, in relation to the ventricular septum. A spectrum exists ranging from two equal-sized ventricles to single ventricle with L-malposition of the great vessels and a hypoplastic subpulmonary chamber.

Inverted Malformations[11]

In hearts with noninverted ventricles, some cardiac anomalies occur typically in either the anatomic right or the anatomic left ventricle. These anomalies can also occur in the inverted ventricles of the heart of corrected transposition of great vessels. Such cardiac anomalies are usually referred to as inverted malformations, because they occur in the same anatomic structures but are located on the opposite side of the heart and therefore lead to a different set of clinical findings. Specific inverted malformations are described as follows:

1. Downward displacement of the tricuspid valve, similar to Ebstein's malformation. Because the tricuspid valve is located in the systemic ventricle, insufficiency of this valve gives a clinical picture of mitral insufficiency and leads to left atrial enlargement.

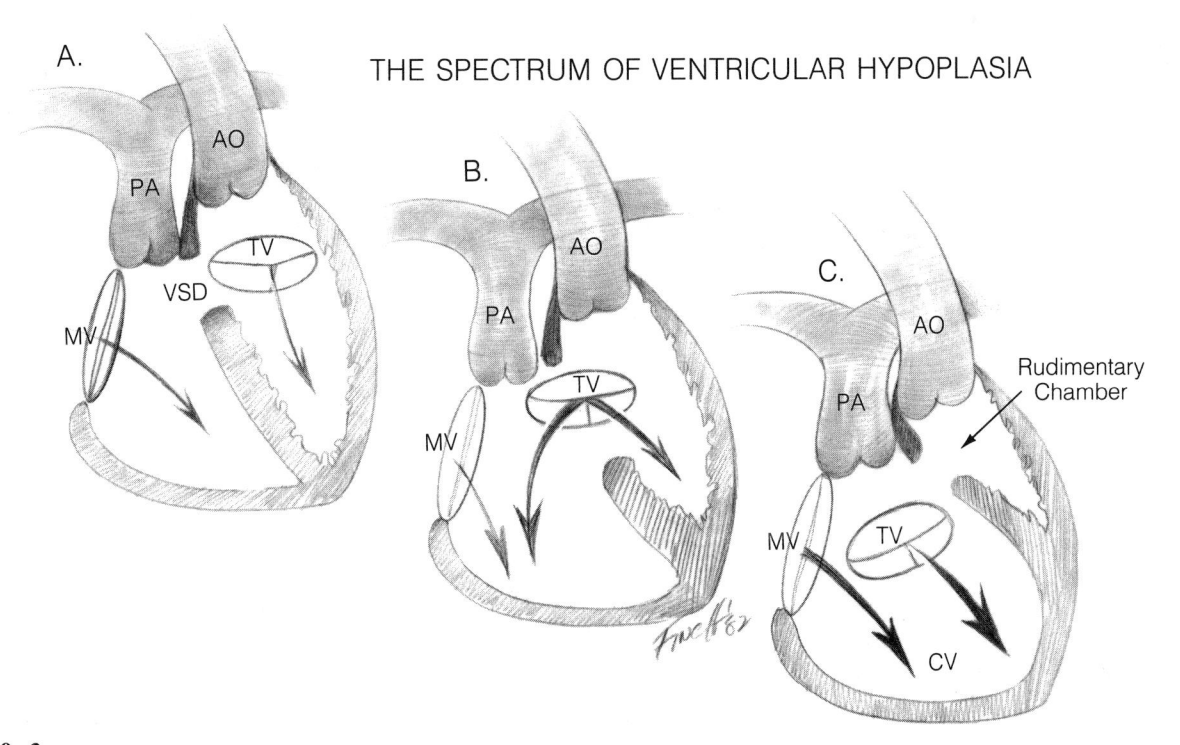

FIG 39–3.
Spectrum of ventricular hypoplasia when great vessels in position of L-transposition. **A,** congenitally corrected transposition of great vessels and ventricular septal defect *(VSD)*. Equal-sized ventricles. **B,** congenitally corrected transposition of great vessels and straddling left (tricuspid) atrioventricular valve. Hypoplasia of inverted right ventricle. **C,** single ventricle *(CV)* with L-malposition of great vessels. Both atrioventricular valves empty into single ventricle. Hypoplastic subaortic chamber. *AO* = aorta; *MV* = mitral valve; *PA* = pulmonary artery; *TV* = tricuspid valve.

2. Anomalous right ventricular muscle bundles. In corrected transposition, anomalous right ventricular muscle bundles are located in the anatomic right ventricle and therefore cause subaortic stenosis.

3. Accessory mitral tissue. This tissue is located in the inverted left ventricular outflow tract. It can cause obstruction, yielding a clinical picture of subpulmonary stenosis.

4. Accessory tricuspid valve tissue. This can form a windsock deformity, causing obstruction to outflow in the inverted right (arterial) ventricle.

5. Prolapse of the mitral valve. Prolapse of the mitral (right) atrioventricular valve presents a clinical picture of tricuspid insufficiency.

6. Prolapse of the tricuspid valve. Prolapse of the tricuspid (left) atrioventricular valve in the right (arterial) ventricle gives a clinical picture of mitral insufficiency.

7. Double-outlet right ventricle. Double-outlet inverted right (systemic) ventricle is the inverted malformation of double-outlet (Fig 39–4) right ventricle.[12] It presents a similar clinical picture. Both the aorta and pulmonary artery arise from the systemic ventricle.

8. Parachute mitral valve. This deformity of the right (mitral) valve gives a clinical picture of tricuspid stenosis.

DEVELOPMENTAL ASPECTS

Congenitally corrected transposition of the great vessels is believed to result from an abnormal pattern of looping of the embryonic bulboventricular loop. The primitive bulboventricular loop rotates to the left in contrast to normal, where it rotates to the right (Fig 39–5). Thus, the primitive right ventricle is displaced to the left and the primitive left ventricle to the right.[13] This process has been called "L-ventricular looping," and the position of the resultant ventricles has been called "L-ventricular loop." The atrioventricular valves, bundles of His, and coronary arteries are also inverted in this process.

The primitive truncus arteriosus is then divided in such a fashion so that aorta and pulmonary artery arise from the inverted right and inverted left ventricles, respectively.

HEMODYNAMICS

The basic circulatory pattern is that of a normal heart. Because most patients have coexistent cardiac anomalies, the normal pattern is altered by these anomalies. Therefore, the hemodynamics within an individual patient depend on the type of associated malformations.

CLINICAL FEATURES

The clinical features of patients with corrected transposition of the great vessels depend on the type and severity of associated cardiac anomalies.[3, 14] A few patients with either no or minimal associated anomalies live normal

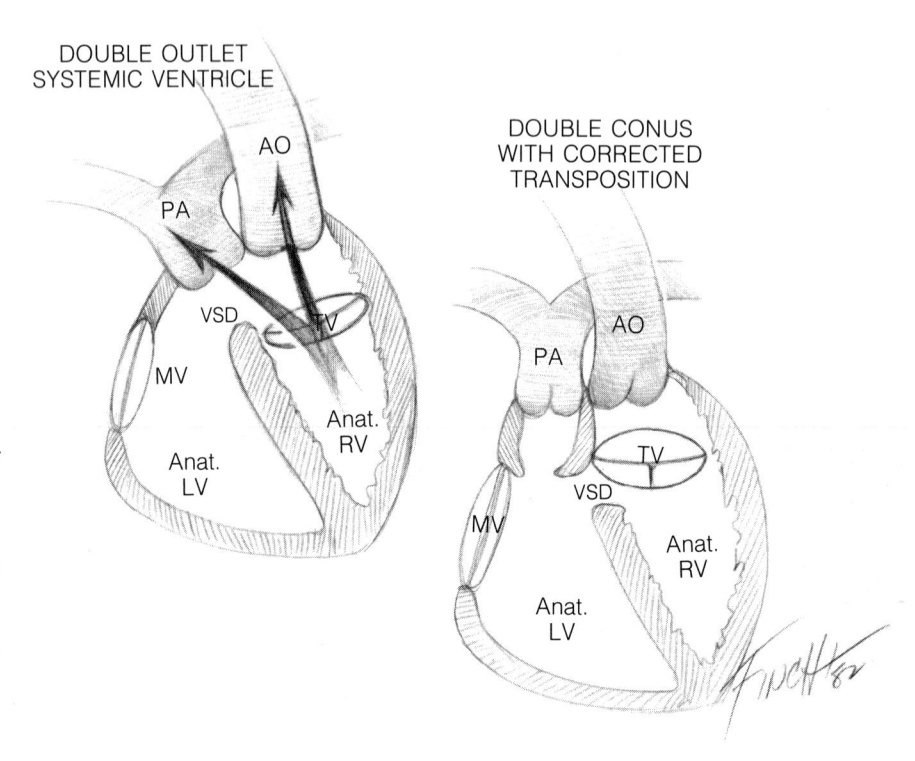

FIG 39–4.
Variants of corrected transposition of great vessels. **Left,** double-outlet systemic ventricle. Both great vessels originate from inverted anatomic right ventricle (Anat. RV) and are separated from atrioventricular valves by muscle tissue. **Right,** double conus. Both great vessels originate above conus tissue. AO = aorta; MV = mitral valve; PA = pulmonary artery; TV = tricuspid valve; Anat. LV = anatomic left ventricle.

DEVELOPMENTAL ASPECTS OF L-TRANSPOSITION

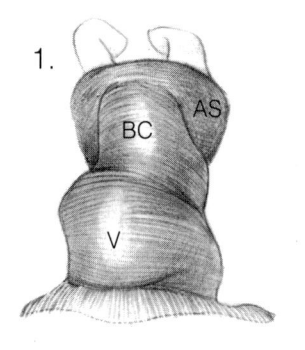

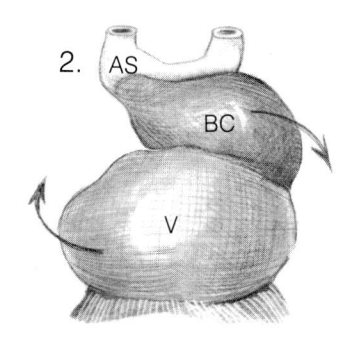

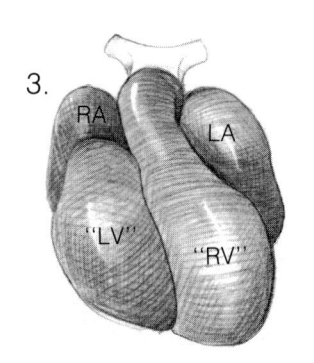

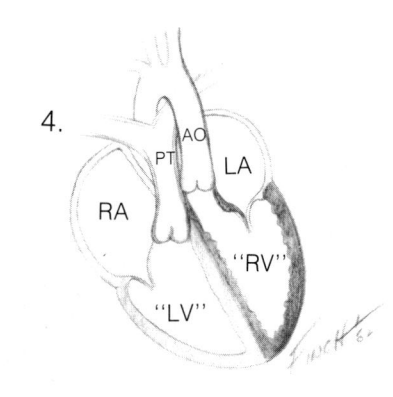

FIG 39-5.
1-4, development of congenitally corrected transposition of great vessels. Primitive bulboventricular loop rotates to left. Bulbus cordis *(BC)*, which becomes anatomic right ventricle *("RV")* deviates to left, whereas ventricularis *(V)*, which becomes anatomic left ventricle *("LV")*, shifts toward right, leading to ventricular inversion (**3** and **4**). *AO* = aorta; *AS* = aortic sac; *LA* = left atrium; *PT* = pulmonary trunk; *RA* = right atrium.

lives, but most patients develop symptoms during infancy. The symptoms are related to either congestive cardiac failure from a left-to-right shunt through a ventricular septal defect or from severe left atrioventricular valvar insufficiency or cyanosis from a combination of ventricular septal defect and pulmonary stenosis resembling tetralogy of Fallot.

Auscultatory findings are those of the associated cardiac condition. The unique auscultatory feature of corrected transposition of the great vessels is the presence of a very loud second heart sound located in the second left intercostal space. This sound represents the closure of the anteriorly and leftward placed aortic valve.

ELECTROCARDIOGRAPHIC FEATURES

The electrocardiogram usually is very suggestive of the diagnosis. Because of the inversion of the bundles of His,[14] the initial depolarization of the ventricular septum is in the opposite direction of normal. This leads to a characteristic pattern with a q wave present in lead V_1 and no q wave in lead V_6.[15-17] Large q waves are found in leads III and aVF. The remainder of the QRS complex varies but usually shows a pattern of ventricular hypertrophy. Tall R waves in the left precordial leads, resembling left ventricular hypertrophy, are found in those patients with Ebstein's malformation of the tricuspid valve, leading to left atrioventricular valve insufficiency. Tall R waves in the right precordial leads of right ventricular hypertrophy are found when the hemodynamics resemble tetralogy of Fallot. In 10% of patients, complete heart block is present, which may be present at birth or develop suddenly.

Cross-sectional echocardiography confirms the diagnosis by demonstrating side-by-side ventricle, three leaflets in the left-sided atrioventricular valve, lack of continuity between the left atrioventricular valve and the anterior and leftward greater artery, and continuity between the right atrioventricular valve and the posterormedial great artery. The ventricular septum is oriented obliquely to the sagittal plane. The ventricle receiving systemic venous blood is smooth, whereas the other ventricle is trabeculated. Often papillary attachment of the left atrioventricular valve is to the interventricular septum. Associated cardiac malformations include Ebstein's malformation of the left atrioventricular valve, ventricular septal defect, and pulmonary stenosis.

RADIOGRAPHIC FEATURES

Careful analysis of the cardiac silhouette may suggest the diagnosis of corrected transposition of the great vessels, but none of the radiographic findings is diagnostic or always present. In many patients the diagnosis cannot be made radiographically.

1. Cardiac size, cardiac contour, and pulmonary vasculature may be normal (Fig 39–6). This occurs in patients with minimal hemodynamic abnormalities or ventricular septal defect and pulmonary stenosis ("balanced tetralogy").

2. In most patients, cardiomegaly is present, and the pulmonary vasculature is abnormal, because corrected transposition usually coexists with other major cardiac anomalies. The pulmonary vasculature may be either increased or diminished, depending on the type of associated condition.

3. The pulmonary arterial segment is absent. REASON: The main pulmonary artery is located centrally and does not contribute to the cardiac border. The left cardiac border therefore has two components—the aorta and the ventricle—rather than three (aortic knob, pulmonary arterial segment, and ventricle) of the normal heart (Fig 39–7). Differences between normal and corrected transposition are summarized in Figure 39–7.

4. The aortic segment may be prominent along the upper left cardiac border. REASON: The aortic valve lies to the left of the pulmonary artery, and the ascending aorta commonly forms a convex arc (Fig 39–8).

5. The aorta may also ascend more medially, in which case the ascending aorta does not form a prominent bulge (Figs 39–6 and 39–9).

6. A prominent bulge along the lower left cardiac border may be formed by the inverted right ventricle. Commonly the cardiac silhouette is different from normal (Fig 39–9).

7. In patients with marked enlargement of pulmonary arteries from increased pulmonary blood flow, the right hilum is prominent and elevated. From this hilum, enlarged branches descend into the right lower lung field, giving a horsetail or waterfall appearance (Fig 39–10).

8. A markedly enlarged main pulmonary artery may also cause localized displacement of the trachea and esophagus posteriorly (Fig 39–11).

9. An abnormal cardiac position, such as mesocardia, and particularly dextroversion, strongly suggests the presence of corrected transposition of the great vessels because these cardiac malpositions have a high incidence of corrected transposition of the great vessels (Figs 39–12 and 39–13).

10. The left (anatomic tricuspid) atrioventricular valve commonly shows features of Ebstein's malformation, which is associated with valvar insufficiency. If it is significant, cardiomegaly, left atrial enlargement, and increased pulmonary venous markings are present (Fig 39–14).

CARDIAC CATHETERIZATION

The diagnosis rests on cardiac catheterization and angiography. The catheter course is diagnostically helpful. It may be difficult to advance a venous catheter from the ventricle into the pulmonary artery because of the sharp angle that the catheter must take. Once in the pulmonary artery, the catheter course is typical (Fig 39–15). In the anteroposterior projection, the catheter course lies in the midline, and on lateral view it lies posteriorly. An arterial catheter advanced into the ascending aorta passes along the upper left cardiac border and is located anteriorly on the lateral projection.

The oximetry and pressure data are similar to those

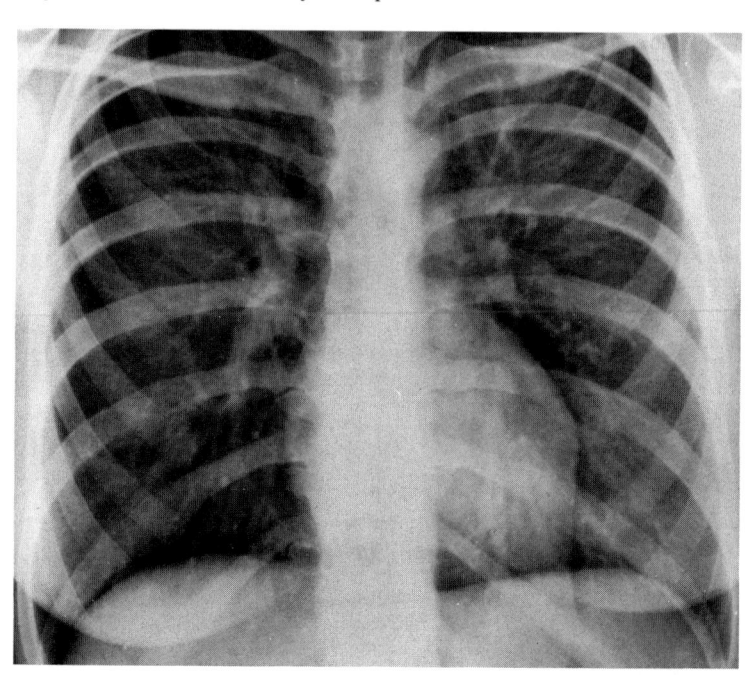

FIG 39–6.
Congenital corrected transposition of great vessels with ventricular septal defect and pulmonary stenosis. Thoracic roentgenogram. Posteroanterior projection. Normal cardiac contour and vasculature.

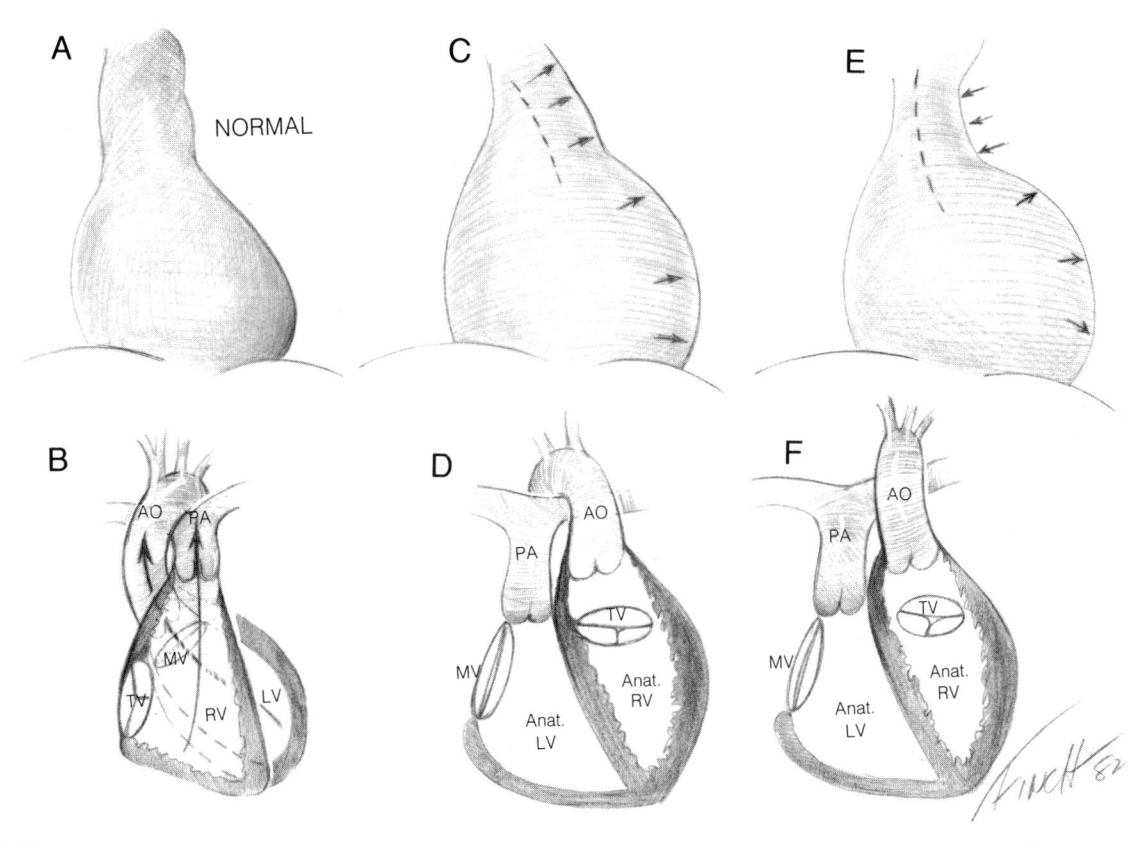

FIG 39-7.
Cardiac contours and intracardiac relationships. **A,** normal heart. Left cardiac contour consists of three segments: aortic arch, main pulmonary artery, and left ventricle. **B,** right ventricle *(RV)* lies anterior. Tricuspid valve *(TV)* is separated from pulmonary valve by infundibulum. Left ventricle *(LV)* lies posteriorly. Mitral valve *(MV)* and aortic valve are in fibrous continuity. Spiral interventricular septum separates ventricles, and outflow tracts cross. Pulmonary valve is located anteriorly, superiorly, and to left of aortic valve. **C,** congenital corrected transposition of great vessels. Left cardiac border consists of two segments: ascending aorta and inverted right ventricle. Aorta ascends toward left forming prominent bulge. **D,** venous ventricle has anatomic features of a left ventricle. Right (mitral) atrioventricular valve *(MV)* is in fibrous continuity with pulmonary valve. Arterial ventricle has anatomic features of right ventricle. Left (tricuspid) atrioventricular valve *(TV)* is separated from aortic valve by infundibulum. Ventricular septum is perpendicular to anterior chest wall, and outflow tracts do not cross. Aortic valve and ascending aorta are located anteriorly, superiorly, and to left of pulmonary valve and pulmonary artery. **E,** in congenital corrected transposition of great vessels, aorta may ascend more medially. As a result upper left cardiac contour is either less convex or concave. Inverted right ventricle may cause prominent ventricular segment simulating left ventricular hypertrophy. **F,** same anatomic relationships as **D,** but aorta located more centrally placed.

described elsewhere for the associated cardiac conditions, such as ventricular septal defect, pulmonary stenosis, or atrioventricular valve insufficiency. The pulmonary arterial wedge or left atrial pressure should be measured because of the frequency of left atrioventricular valvar insufficiency.

ANGIOGRAPHIC FEATURES

Because of the anatomic complexity of this condition and the associated cardiac anomalies, ventriculography should be performed in both ventricles. To prevent misdiagnosis, the angiograms should be analyzed in three steps:

1. Hemodynamic assessment. The venous and the arterial ventricles should be identified using oximetry data, angiographic identification of the venous or arterial atrium, and catheter course. This information provides information about the circulatory pattern, which should be normal in this condition.

2. Anatomic analysis. The anatomic right and left ventricles and the relative position of the great vessels should be identified.

3. Associated anomalies. The presence of associated anomalies is then assessed.

In corrected transposition of the great vessels, although the great vessels are anatomically transposed, the inversion of the ventricles physiologically corrects the circulation and results in a normal hemodynamic pattern. Thus, opacification of the venous ventricle on an angiogram is followed by opacification of the pulmonary artery,

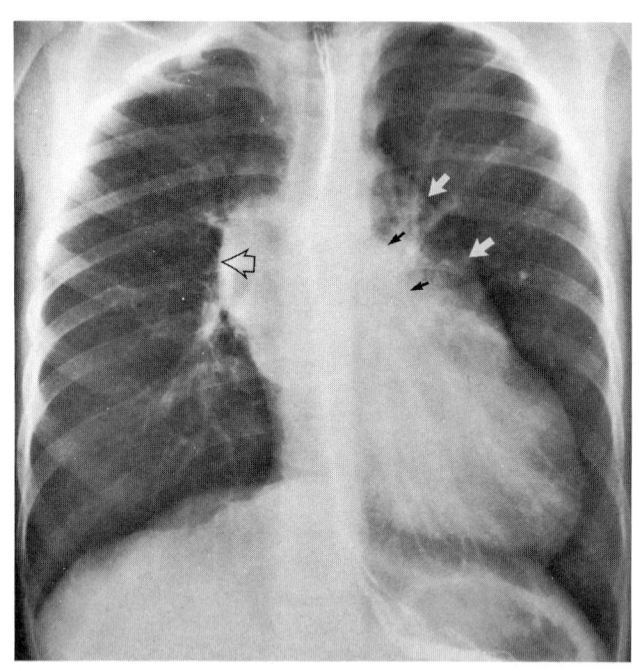

FIG 39–8.
Congenital corrected transposition of great vessels. Thoracic roentgenogram. Posteroanterior projection. Left cardiac border has two segments, formed by inverted ascending aorta *(arrows)* above and systemic ventricle below. Medial position of left pulmonary artery *(small arrows)*. Density right hilum *(open arrow)* is caused by inverted, large main pulmonary artery.

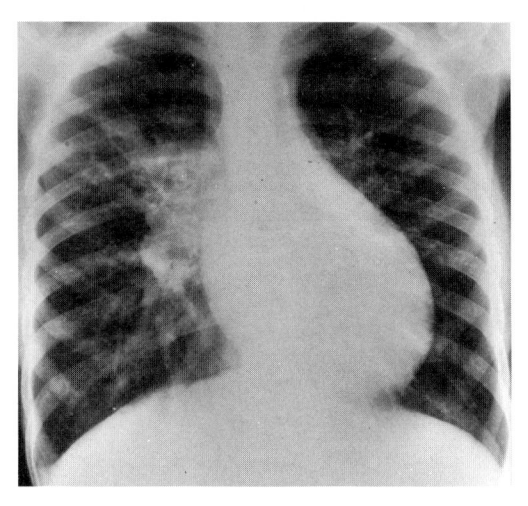

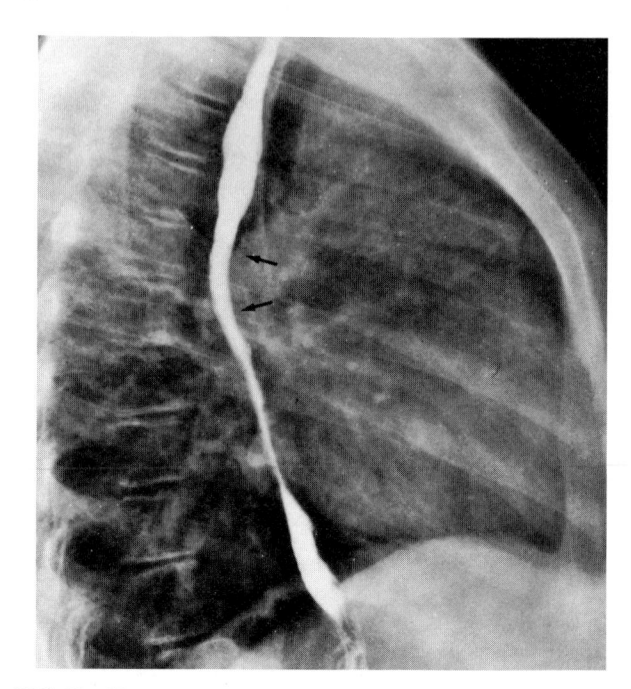

FIG 39–10.
Congenital corrected transposition of great vessels with large ventricular septal defect. Thoracic roentgenogram. Posteroanterior projection. Right pulmonary artery is enlarged, elevated, and displaced toward the right, giving a waterfall or horsetail appearance. Absent pulmonary arterial segment despite increased pulmonary arterial vasculature. REASON: Pulmonary artery in central position.

except in patients with coexistent pulmonary atresia. On the late phase of a venous angiogram, the left atrium, arterial ventricle, and aorta are sequentially opacified. The sequence of opacification reflects a normal pattern of hemodynamics. Ventriculography commonly results in some degree of atrioventricular valvar regurgitation, a feature that is helpful because it allows identification of the corresponding atrium supplying the injected ventricle.

In corrected transposition of the great vessels, the right atrium connects to a ventricle with the anatomic fea-

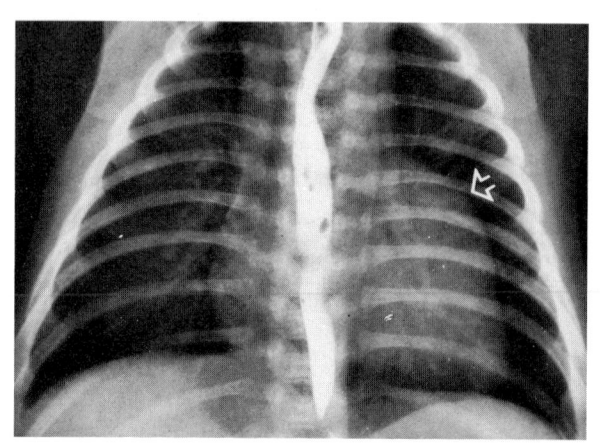

FIG 39–9.
Congenital corrected transposition of great vessels. Thoracic roentgenogram. Posteroanterior projection. Prominent bulge of left cardiac border *(arrow)* is caused by systemic (inverted right) ventricle. Pulmonary arterial segment is absent. Ascending aorta does not form upper left cardiac border, because it ascends more medially in this patient.

FIG 39–11.
Congenital corrected transposition of great vessels and large ventricular septal defect. Thoracic roentgenogram. Lateral projection. Enlarged posteriorly located pulmonary artery causes localized displacement of barium-filled esophagus *(arrows)*.

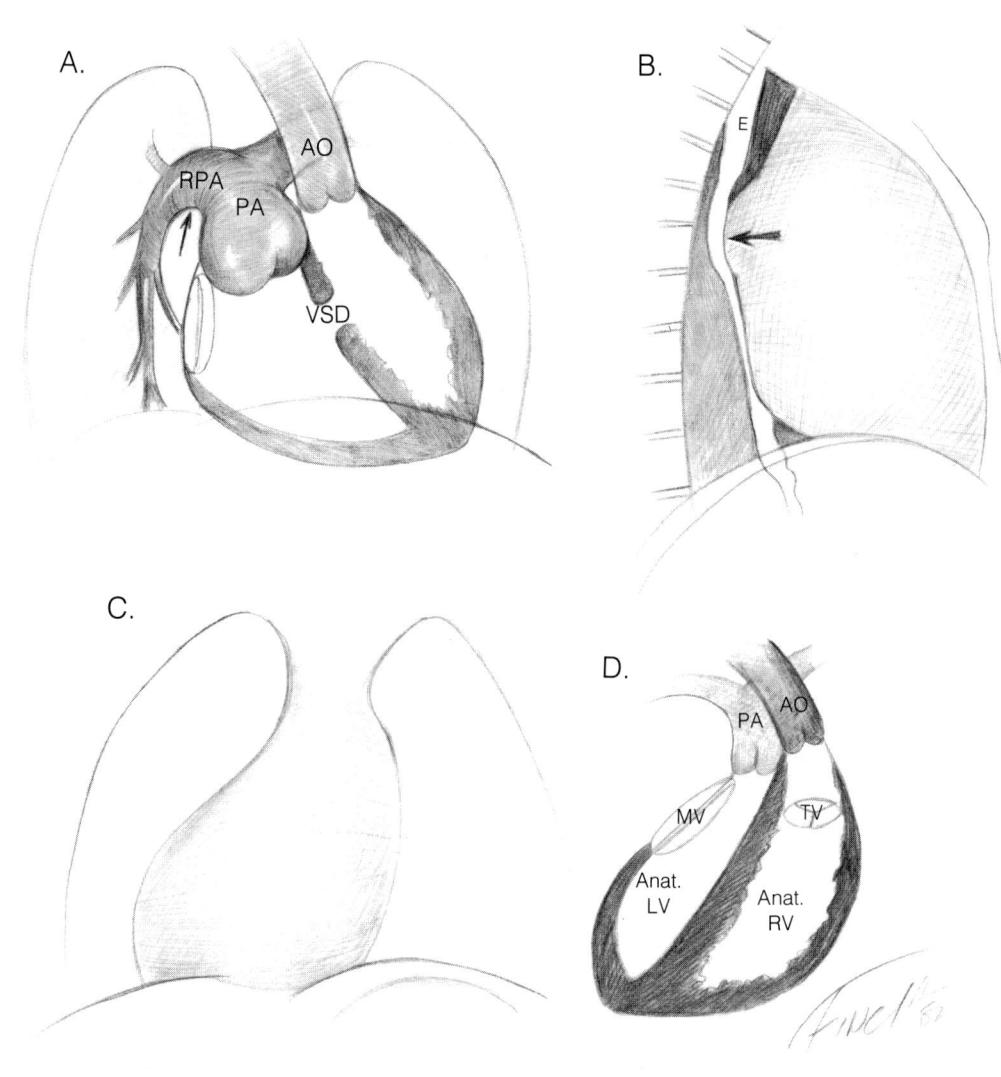

FIG 39–12.
Congenital corrected transposition of great vessels with ventricular septal defect. **A,** Waterfall appearance. **B,** localized displacement of esophagus posteriorly. **C,** with dextroversion. **D,** internal anatomy of corrected transposition and dextroversion. *Anat. LV* = anatomic left ventricle; *Anat. RV* = anatomic right ventricle; *AO* = aorta; *MV* = mitral valve; *PA* = pulmonary artery; *RPA* = right pulmonary artery; *TV* = tricuspid valve; *VSD* = ventricular septal defect; *E* = esophagus.

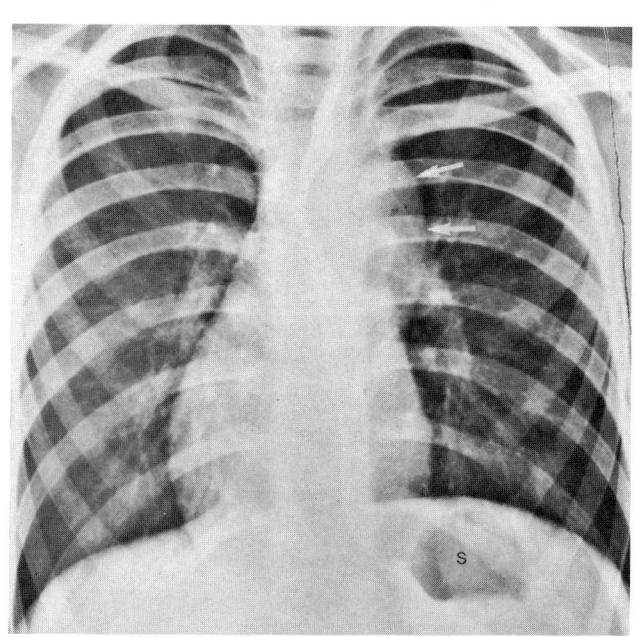

FIG 39–13.
Dextroversion of situs solitus with associated congenital corrected transpositon of great vessels. Thoracic roentgenogram. Posteroanterior projection. Left aortic arch and stomach *(S)* lie on left, indicating situs solitus. Cardiac apex is in right hemithorax. Pulmonary arterial segment is absent. Prominence of ascending aorta *(arrows)* is consistent with congenital corrected transposition of great vessels.

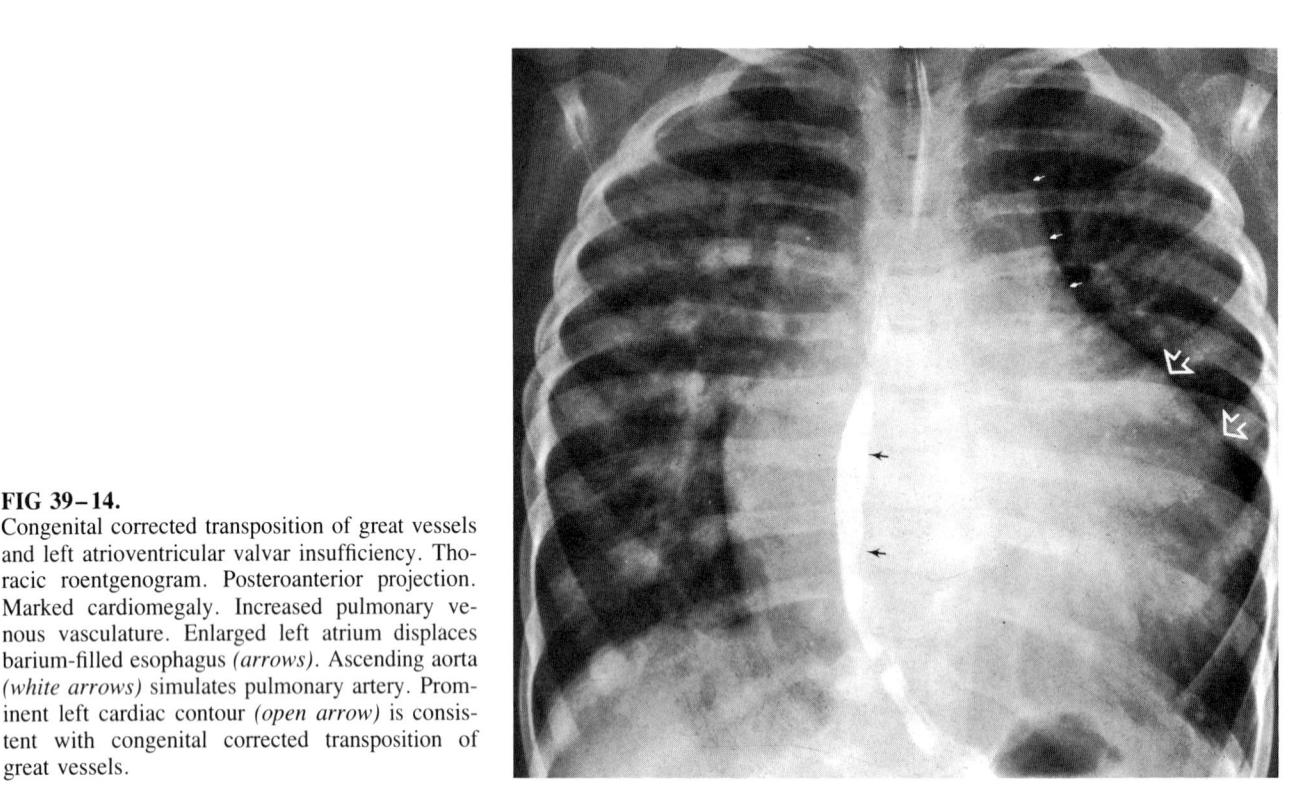

FIG 39–14.
Congenital corrected transposition of great vessels and left atrioventricular valvar insufficiency. Thoracic roentgenogram. Posteroanterior projection. Marked cardiomegaly. Increased pulmonary venous vasculature. Enlarged left atrium displaces barium-filled esophagus *(arrows)*. Ascending aorta *(white arrows)* simulates pulmonary artery. Prominent left cardiac contour *(open arrow)* is consistent with congenital corrected transposition of great vessels.

tures of a left ventricle, and the left atrium connects to a ventricle with anatomic features of a right ventricle. The atrioventricular connection is therefore *discordant*. Discordant atrioventricular connections almost invariably exist with a discordant ventriculoarterial connection (i.e., transposition of the great vessels); the latter feature corrects the circulation, yielding a hemodynamically corrected transposition of the great vessels. Discordant atrioventricular connection (inversion of the ventricles, L-loop) with arterioventricular concordance (i.e., without transposition) is ex-

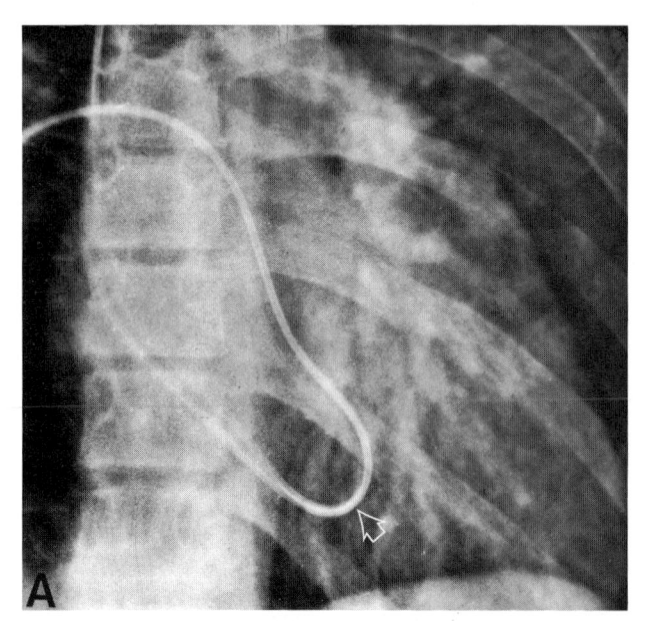

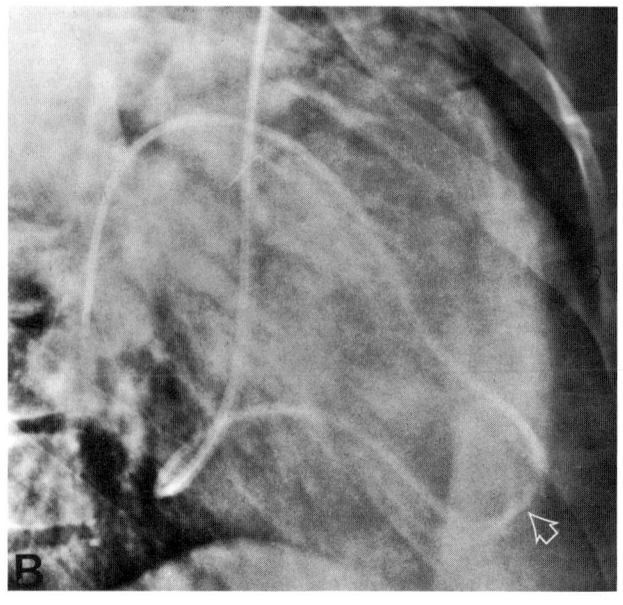

FIG 39–15.
Congenital corrected transposition of great vessels. Catheter course into pulmonary artery. **A,** anteroposterior projection. Catheter has a medial course. Narrow loop *(open arrow)* outlines apex of inverted ventricles. **B,** Lateral projection. Catheter has posterior course. Taillike ventricle is outlined by catheter *(open arrow)*.

tremely rare and results in cyanosis. This malformation has been called "clinical transposition," or "isolated inversion of the ventricles" (see Chapter 40). After the hemodynamics have been clarified by catheterization data and the anatomic details of the ventricles identified angiographically, the position of the great vessels should be analyzed. The relationship of the great vessels to the ventricles must be identified. The relative position of the great vessels to each other on the anteroposterior projection, although usually quite characteristic of L-loop transposition, is less important because the relative position of the great arteries is not as constant as the atrioventricular discordance (see Chapter 59). The ventricles can be identified and distinguished angiographically.

Venous (Inverted Left Ventricle) Ventriculography

1. The catheter course is normal from the superior vena cava through the right atrium into the venous ventricle (see Fig 39–15).
2. The long axis of the ventricle is more horizontal than normal. This gives the ventricle a taillike (or wedge-shaped) appearance (Fig 39–16). REASON: The outflow tract of the venous ventricle is more medial than in a normal heart.

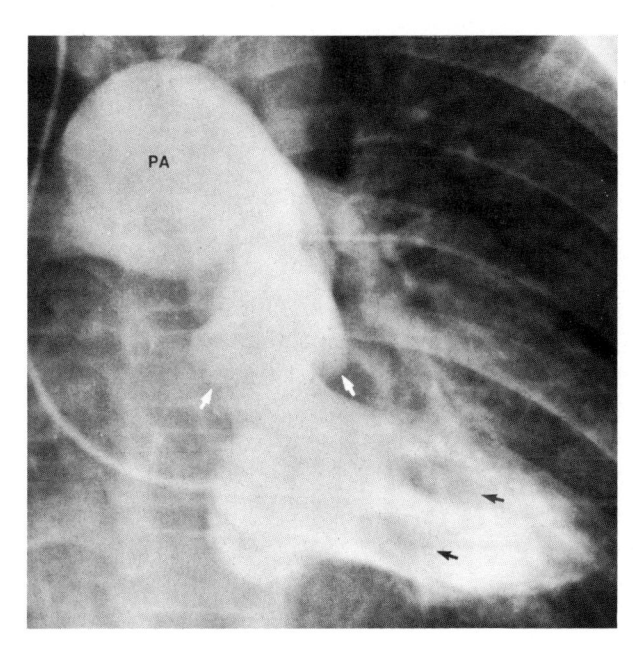

FIG 39–16.
Congenital corrected transposition of great vessels. Angiogram from venous ventricle. Anteroposterior projection. Normal catheter course from superior vena cava through right atrium to venous ventricle. Smooth-walled, triangular, tail-shaped ventricular cavity. Two papillary muscles *(black arrows)* indicate presence of a mitral valve. Pulmonary valve annulus *(white arrows)* is located in low position in continuity with right (mitral) atrioventricular valve. Pulmonary artery *(PA)* lies medially and is enlarged.

3. The wall of the ventricle is smooth. REASON: This ventricle is anatomically a left ventricle because it normally has fewer trabeculations than an anatomic right ventricle.
4. Two papillary muscles (Fig 39–16) can usually be identified during systole. This finding indicates that the atrioventricular valve is an anatomic mitral valve. REASON: Inversion of the ventricle is associated with inversion of the atrioventricular valves. The right atrioventricular valve is therefore a mitral valve.
5. Although visualization of two papillary muscles indicates the presence of a mitral valve, failure to identify them does not exclude the presence of a mitral valve. The much smaller papillary muscles of the tricuspid valve are not identifiable angiographically in the more trabeculated anatomic right ventricle.
6. The outflow tract of the venous ventricle is more medially placed than in a normal heart.
7. The pulmonary valve is located medially and lower than normal (see Fig 39–16). It is in continuity with the right atrioventricular valve (mitral valve). REASON: Because the venous ventricle is an anatomic left ventricle, it lacks an infundibulum.
8. The pulmonary artery (see Fig 39–16) is usually large even in patients without pulmonary stenosis or a left-to-right shunt. REASON: Unknown. The pulmonary artery is located medially in the mediastinum. Because it does not form a border of the heart, it cannot be seen on a thoracic roentgenogram, and therefore the pulmonary arterial segment is absent.
9. The size of the pulmonary artery may be aneurysmal (Fig 39–17). REASON: Unknown.
10. Because of the medial position of the pulmonary trunk, the left pulmonary artery is also more medially placed than normal.
11. On a lateral view the venous ventricle projects anteriorly but usually not as much as in a normal heart (Fig 39–18).
12. The pulmonary artery arises relatively posteriorly (see Fig 39–18). The pulmonary valve is located in a low position and in continuity with the atrioventricular valve.
13. The infundibulum, which is normally located anteriorly, is not observed. There is, however, a characteristic anterior recess of the ventricle that is regularly entered during venous catheterization.
14. Angiographic appearance of left and right pulmonary arteries is normal.
15. Rarely in this condition the pulmonary artery may arise from the infundibulum, resulting in "double coni" (Fig 39–19), similar to particular instances of complete transposition of the great vessels.
16. Mesocardia or dextroversion of the heart is commonly associated with corrected transposition of the great

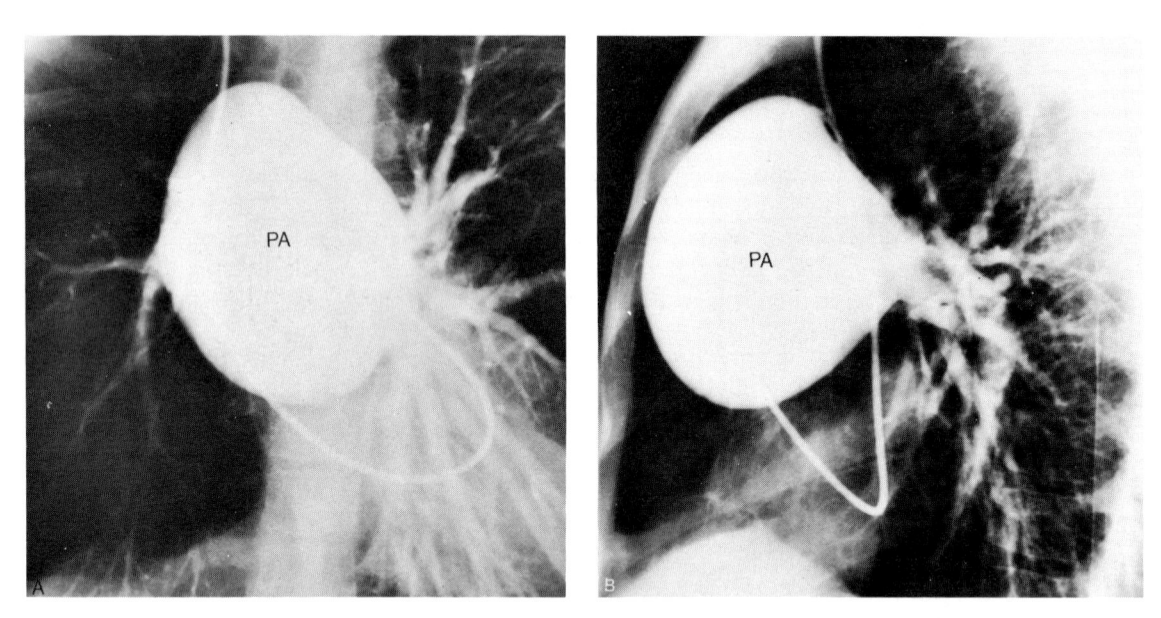

FIG 39–17.
Corrected transposition of great vessels. Pulmonary arteriogram. **A,** anteroposterior and, **B,** lateral projections. Aneurysmal dilatation of medially placed pulmonary artery *(PA)*.

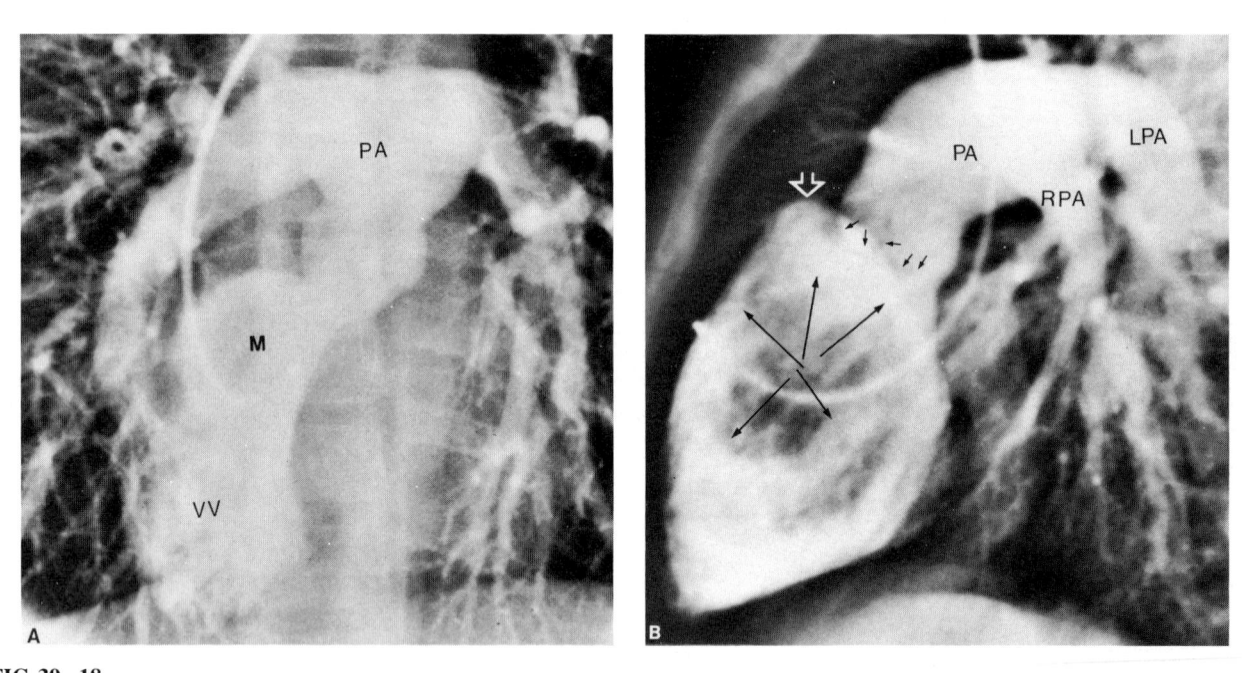

FIG 39–18.
Congenital corrected transposition of great vessels without associated cardiac anomalies (very rare). Angiogram from venous ventricle. **A,** anteroposterior projection. Venous ventricle *(VV)* has anatomic characteristics of left ventricle. Pulmonary valve in continuity with right AV valve (mitral valve [*M*]). **B,** lateral view. Ventricular cavity is smooth walled. Unopacified blood outlines orifice of right (mitral) atrioventricular valve *(long black arrows)*. Pulmonary valve *(small black arrows)* is located posteriorly, in low position, in continuity with right atrioventricular valve. No infundibulum. Shoulderlike recess *(open white arrow)* is located anteriorly. Normal division of right *(RPA)* and left *(LPA)* pulmonary arteries. *PA* = pulmonary artery.

vessels, particularly in patients with coexistent ventricular septal defect and pulmonary stenosis (see Fig 39–19).

17. On the late phase of a venous ventriculogram or pulmonary arteriogram, the left atrium, the systemic ventricle, and aorta opacify, indicating normal hemodynamics characteristic for corrected transposition (see Fig 39–25).

18. Ventricular septal defect, pulmonary stenosis, or both are commonly associated with corrected transposition of the great vessels (see Figs 39–19 and 39–26).

Arterial (Anatomic Right Ventricle) Ventriculography

1. The arterial ventricle lies superiorly to the venous ventricle and forms the left cardiac border. The ventricular septum lies in a plane perpendicular to the anterior chest wall. On anteroposterior angiograms, the septum is clearly outlined separating the ventricles (see Figs 39–25 and 39–26).

2. The left atrioventricular valve, which is anatomically a tricuspid valve, is not in continuity with the aortic valve. REASON: The arterial ventricle is an anatomic right ventricle. Therefore, an infundibulum separates the atrioventricular valve from the semilunar valve. The anatomic right ventricle has a tricuspid valve.

3. Papillary muscles cannot be identified in this ventricle. REASON: This ventricle has a tricuspid valve. Papillary muscles of a tricuspid valve usually cannot be visualized angiographically.

4. The surface of this ventricle shows diffuse trabeculations characteristic of an anatomic right ventricle (Fig 39–20, see also Figs 2–19 and 2–21).

5. The aortic valve is located higher and to the left of the lower and medially positioned pulmonary valve (see Fig 34–20). REASON: The aorta arises from the infundibulum of the anatomic right ventricle, and there is inversion (L-loop transposition), with the aortic valve lying to the left of the pulmonary valve.

6. The position of the ascending aorta is variable. It may ascend along the upper left cardiac border (more common) or may ascend more medially.

7. On a lateral projection, the arterial ventricle lies above the venous ventricle, being separated by a relatively horizontal septum (Fig 39–21).

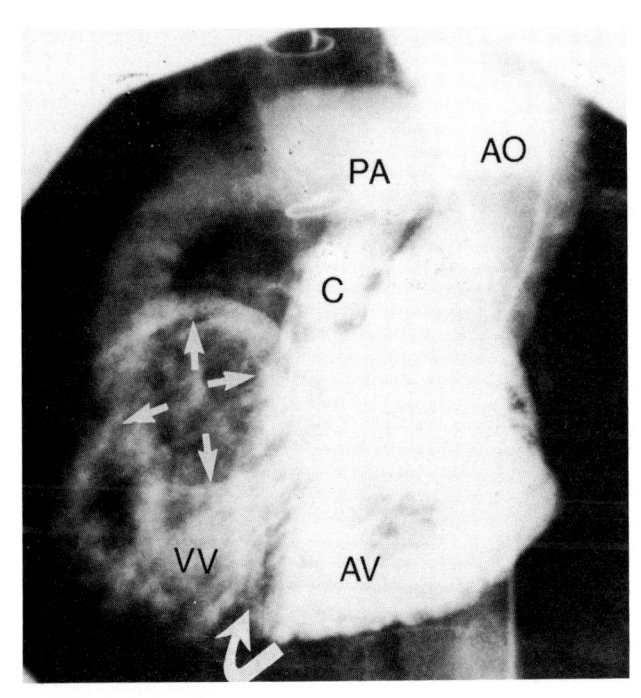

FIG 39–19.
Corrected transposition of great vessels, double conus, and dextroversion of heart. Arterial ventricle *(AV)* injected via transaortic catheter. Anteroposterior projection. Venous ventricle *(VV)* is opacified via ventricular septal defect. Ventricular septum *(curved arrow)*. Both great vessels are opacified. Pulmonary artery *(PA)* is separated from right AV valve *(arrows)* by a conus. *AO* = aorta; *C* = conus.

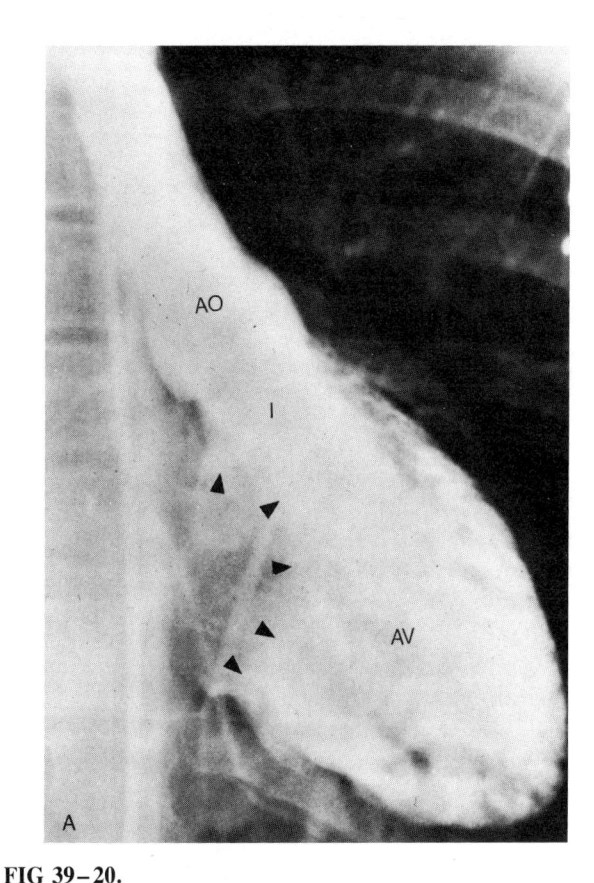

FIG 39–20.
Congenital corrected transposition of great vessels. Angiogram from arterial ventricle *(AV)*. Anteroposterior projection. Systemic (anatomic right ventricle) located superiorly and to left of venous ventricle (anatomic left ventricle). Ventricular septum in horizontal position. Aortic valve separated from left atrioventricular valve *(arrowheads)* by infundibulum *(I)* and located superiorly and to left of pulmonary valve. *AO* = aorta.

FIG 39–21.
Congenital corrected transposition of great vessels. Angiogram from arterial ventricle. Lateral view. Trabeculated wall of anatomic right ventricle. Ventricle positioned superiorly. Aorta *(AO)* arises from infundibulum *(I)*. Aortic valve is not in continuity with left (tricuspid) atrioventricular valve *(arrowheads)*. Aorta lies anteriorly, typical of most instances of transposition of great vessels.

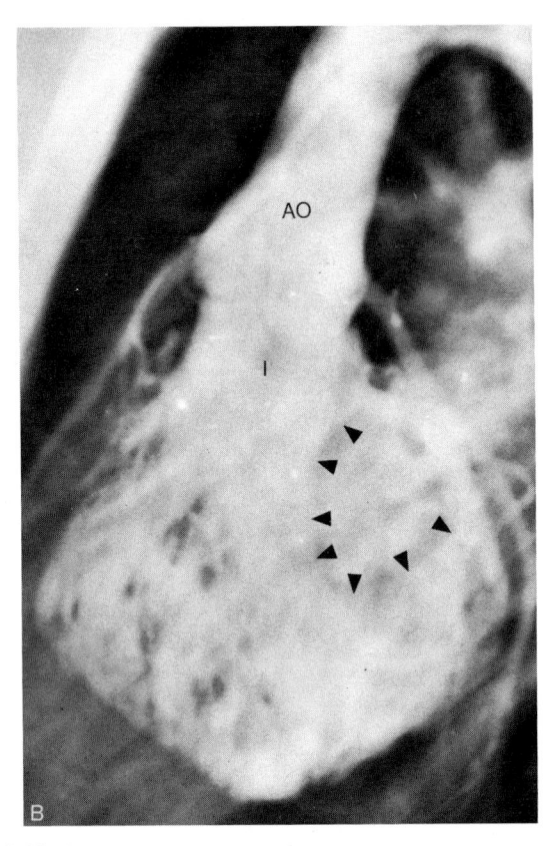

8. On lateral view the aortic valve lies anterior and above the level of the pulmonary valve (see Fig 39–21). REASON: Because the aorta is transposed and arises from the anatomic right ventricle, it is located anteriorly.

9. Insufficiency of the left atrioventricular valve (tricuspid valve) because of displaced leaflets (left-sided Ebstein's) is commonly present (Fig 39–22). Injection of contrast material into the arterial ventricle allows semiquantitative assessment of the degree of left atrioventricular valvar regurgitation. Rarely, displaced valve leaflets (Ebstein's malformation) are clearly seen (see Fig 39–22).

10. The size of the arterial ventricle is variable in corrected transposition of the great vessels. The systemic ventricle may be hypoplastic (Fig 39–23). Performing a ventriculogram is important to demonstrate the size of the systemic ventricle. Hypoplasia may occur from a left-to-right shunt at the atrial level if no ventricular septal defect is present or, more commonly, with an associated ventricular septal defect.

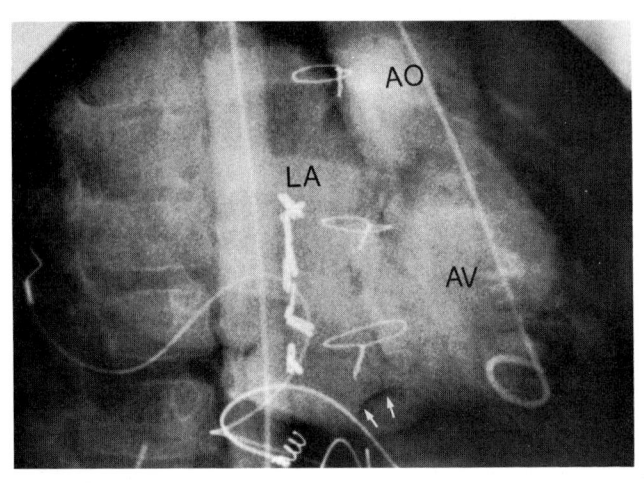

FIG 39–22.
Congenital corrected transposition of great vessels and insufficiency of left atrioventricular valve because of Ebsteinlike anomaly. Angiogram from arterial ventricle *(AV)*. Transaortic catheter. Right anterior oblique projection. Marked regurgitation and dense opacification of left atrium *(LA)*. Displaced valve leaflet is clearly seen *(arrows)*. *AO* = aorta.

11. In corrected transposition of the great vessels with a ventricular communication, the size of the systemic ventricle varies from normal to mild hypoplasia (double-inlet systemic ventricle) to marked hypoplasia (common ventricle).

12. Before operation, angiographic assessment of the size of the systemic ventricle is important because closure

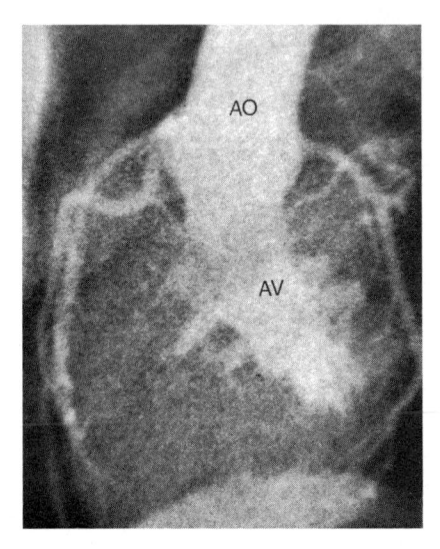

FIG 39–23.
Congenital corrected transposition of great vessels and hypoplasia of arterial (right) ventricle. Angiogram from arterial ventricle *(AV)*. Lateral projection. Typical coronary arterial pattern. Common origin of anterior descending and "right" coronary arteries. Circumflex artery arises posteriorly as a single branch. *AO* = aorta.

of the ventricular septal defect may be fatal if the ventricle is too small (see Fig 39–23).[18]

13. Hypoplasia of the systemic ventricle may be suspected on a thoracic roentgenogram by a more localized and bulge high along the upper left cardiac border (Fig. 39–24).

14. The left (tricuspid) atrioventricular valve may straddle the ventricular septal defect (Fig 39–25). This anomaly is termed "double-inlet venous ventricle," or "double-inlet inverted left ventricle." (A straddling tricuspid valve and ventricular septal defect in the normal heart are also called "double-inlet left ventricle" (see Chapter 44).

15. There are many valvar abnormalities—Ebstein's malformation of the left atrioventricular valve being the most common (see Fig 39–22).

16. In the venous ventricle, a membrane, as in subaortic stenosis, may be seen lying beneath the pulmonary valve (Fig 39–26). The malformation is inverted.

17. Mitral valve prolapse also occurs in the venous ventricle because the mitral valve is also inverted (Fig 39–26).

18. Aneurysms of the membranous septum bulge into the venous ventricle and project in the subpulmonary area, where they may cause outflow tract obstruction (Fig

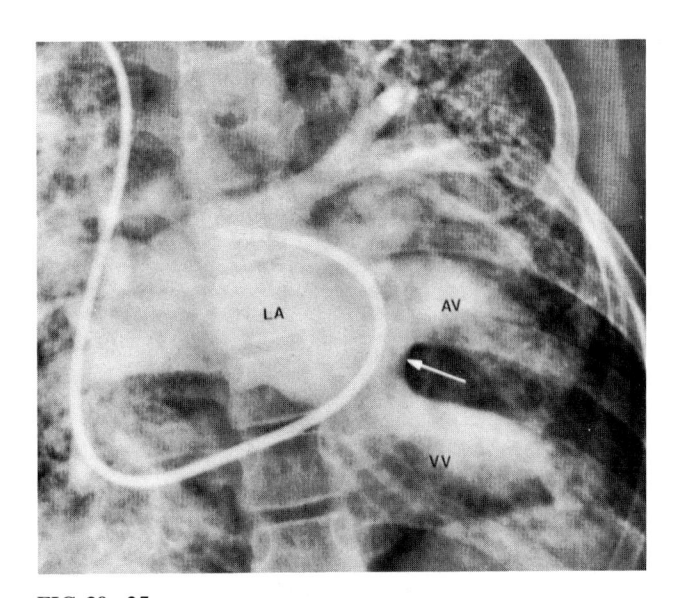

FIG 39–25.
Congenital corrected transposition of great vessels, ventricular septal defect, and straddling left (tricuspid) atrioventricular valve. Angiogram from venous ventricle. Late phase. Anteroposterior projection. Double-inlet inverted left ventricle. From left atrium *(LA)*, simultaneous opacification of arterial ventricle *(AV)* and venous ventricle *(VV)* occurs. Ventricles are separated by horizontally positioned septum. Ventricular septal defect *(arrow)*.

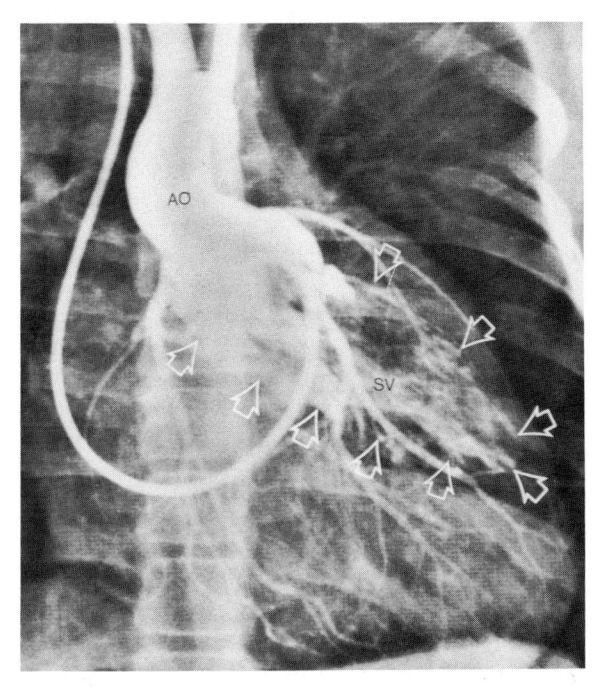

FIG 39–24.
Congenital corrected transposition of great vessels and hypoplastic systemic ventricle. Angiogram from systemic ventricle *(SV)*. Anteroposterior projection. Catheter course from venous ventricle through ventricular septal defect. Hypoplastic ventricle is indicated by open white arrows. *AO* = aorta.

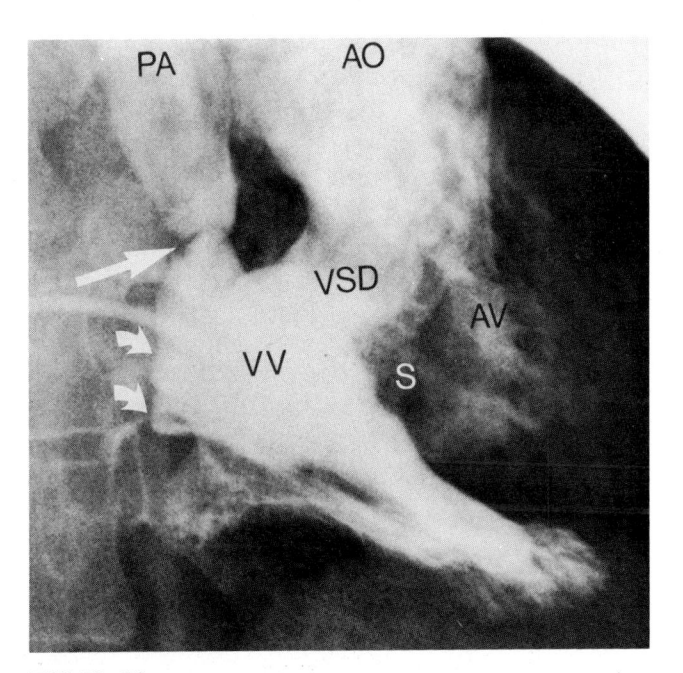

FIG 39–26.
Corrected transposition of great vessels. Angiogram from venous ventricle *(VV)*. Discrete subpulmonary membrane *(large white arrow)*. Mild prolapse of mitral valve *(curved arrows)*. Arterial ventricle *(AV)* fills via ventricular septal defect *(VSD)*. Septum *(S)* is seen on end. Both great vessels are opacified. *AO* = aorta; *PA* = pulmonary artery.

39–27). REASON: The venous ventricle does not have an infundibulum. In the normal heart a ventricular aneurysm projects below the crista supraventricularis at the level of the septal leaflet of the tricuspid valve.

Coronary Arterial Angiography

Identification of the coronary arterial pattern is helpful in making the diagnosis of corrected transposition of great vessels.

1. The "right" (developmentally left) coronary artery lies in the right atrioventricular groove (Fig 39–28). This artery gives rise to the anterior descending coronary artery, which passes in the interventricular groove and extends to the cardiac apex. In anteroposterior projection it bisects obliquely the cardiac silhouette.

2. The "right" (developmentally left) coronary artery arises above the right posterior aortic cusp. The origin of the coronary artery is not seen in profile on anteroposterior projection.

3. The "left" (developmentally right) coronary artery arises above the left posterior aortic cusp and extends toward the left in the atrioventricular groove, giving off branches to the systemic (right) ventricle. Its most important branch is the posterior descending coronary artery, which extends toward the cardiac apex.

4. On lateral projection, the anterior (noncoronary) cusp does not give rise to a coronary artery (Fig 39–29), as is characteristic for all transpositions of the great vessels.

OPERATIVE CONSIDERATIONS

Corrective operations are complicated by (1) the abnormal course of the right coronary artery crossing the venous ventricular outflow tract, (2) the abnormal course of the bundles of His, (3) the more complicated forms of coexistent cardiac conditions, and (4) the frequency of cardiac malposition. Formerly the development of complete heart block after intracardiac operation was very high, but with cardiac mapping during operation and improved knowledge of anatomic details of the conduction tissue, this is much less of a problem.[19] When the ventricular septal defect is closed, the patch is placed on the systemic (right) ventricular aspect of the defect to avoid the conduction system.[20] Ventricular septal defects are generally closed through either the right atrium or the left ventricular apex. Replacement of the left atrioventricular valve is performed in patients with symptoms caused by significant re-

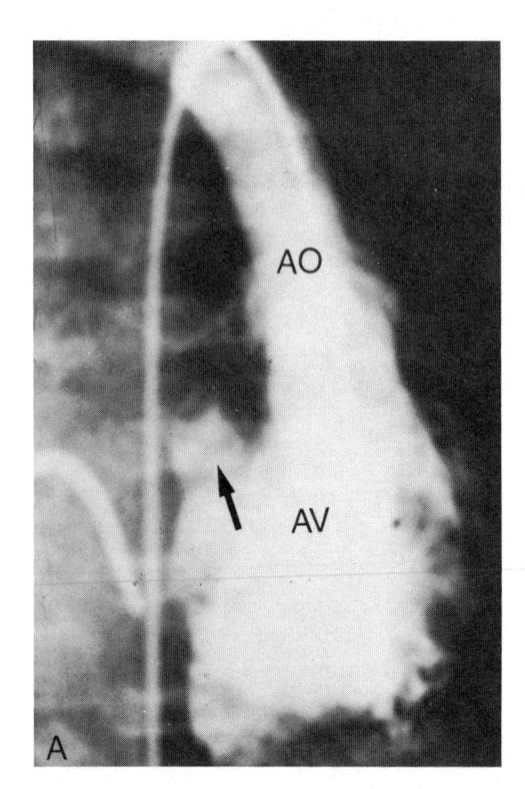

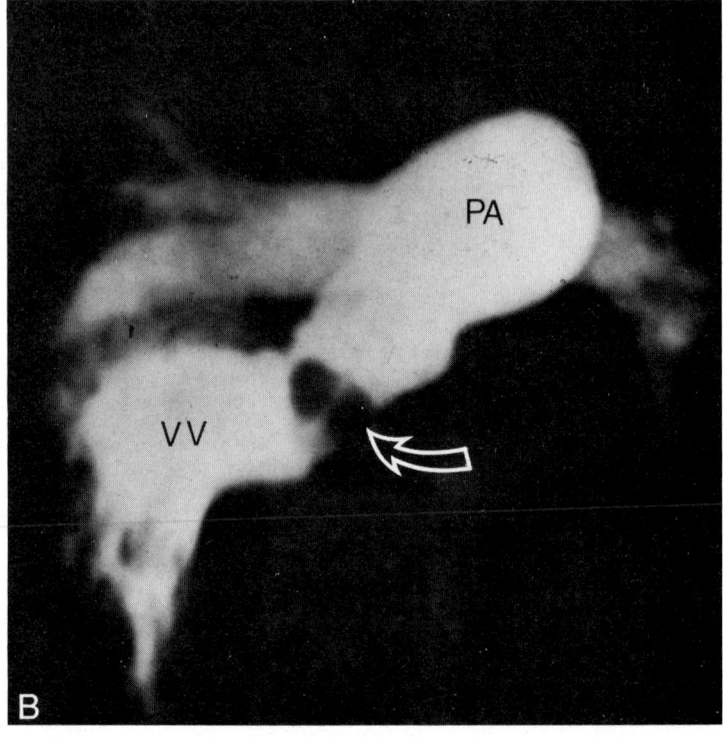

FIG 39–27.
Corrected transposition of great vessels. Ventriculograms. Anteroposterior projections. **A,** arterial ventricle *(AV)* via transaortic catheterization. Aneurysm of ventricular septum *(arrow).* **B,** venous ventricle *(VV).* Large subpulmonary filling defect *(arrow)* is caused by aneurysm of septum. *AO* = aorta; *PA* = pulmonary artery.

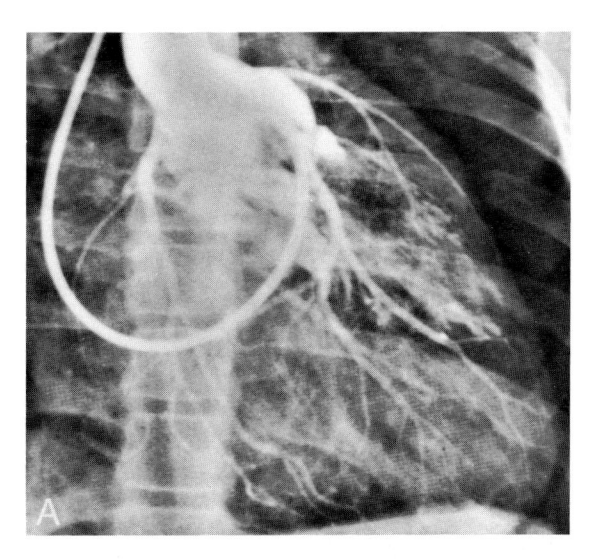

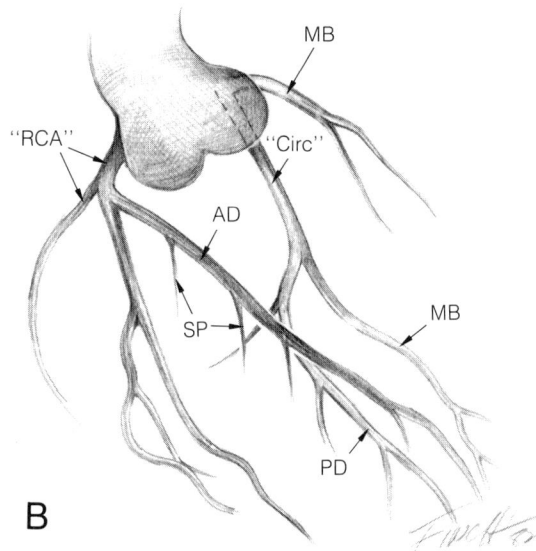

FIG 39-28.
Congenital corrected transposition of great vessels. Coronary arterial pattern. **A,** aortogram. Anteroposterior projection and, **B,** diagram to identify coronary arterial branches. *"RCA"* = right coronary artery; *AD* = anterior descending; *MB* = muscular branches; *PD* = posterior descending; *"CRC"* = circumflex; *SP* = septal branch.

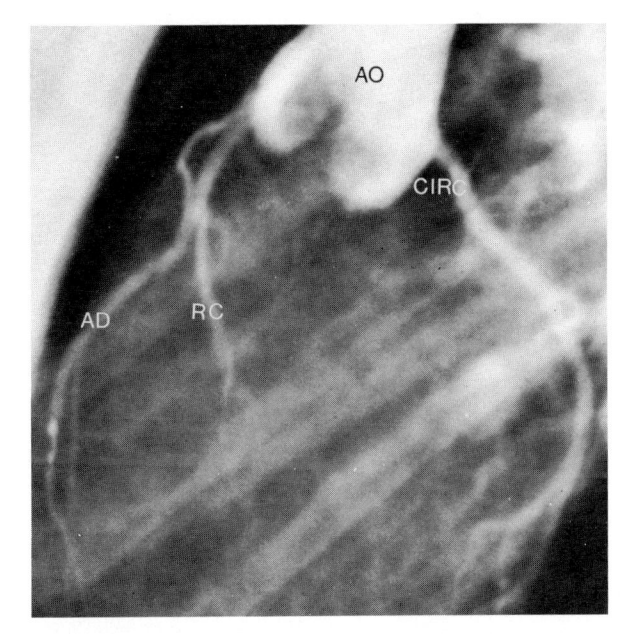

FIG 39-29.
Congenital corrected transposition of great vessels. Aortogram. Lateral projection. Posterior origin of circumflex *(arrow)*, which does not give rise of anterior descending artery. Anterior aortic cusp is noncoronary. Origin of right coronary artery is not seen in profile. Anterior descending *(AD)* arises from right coronary *(RC)* artery. Origin of circumflex *(CIRC)* is seen in profile posteriorly. *AO* = aorta.

gurgitation. Obstruction to pulmonary outflow can be repaired using a conduit.

Palliative procedures, similar to those used in patients with congenital cardiac malformations with normally related ventricles, are used in many infants with this condition.

REFERENCES

1. Van Praagh R: Terminology of congenital heart disease: glossary and commentary, *Circulation* 56:139, 1977.
2. Shinebourne EA, Macartney FJ, Anderson RH: Sequential chamber localization: the logical approach to diagnosis in congenital heart disease, *Br Heart J* 38:327, 1976.
3. Schiebler GL, Edwards JE, Burchell HB, et al: Congenital corrected transposition of the great vessels: a study of 33 cases, *Pediatrics* 27(part II):851, 1961.
4. Allwork SP, Bentall HH, Becker AE, et al: Congenitally corrected transposition of the great arteries: morphologic study of 32 cases, *Am J Cardiol* 38:910, 1976.
5. Summerall CP, Clowes GHA, Boone JA: Aneurysm of ventricular septum with outflow obstruction of the venous ventricle in corrected transposition of great vessels, *Am Heart J* 72:525, 1966.
6. Levy MJ, Lillehei CW, Elliott LP, et al: Accessory valvular tissue causing subpulmonary stenosis in corrected transposition of great vessels, *Circulation* 27:494, 1963.
7. Anderson RH, Becker AE, Gerlis LM: The pulmonary outflow tract in classically corrected transposition, *J Thorac Cardiovasc Surg* 69:747, 1975.
8. Krongrad E, Ellis K, Steeg CN, et al: Subpulmonary ob-

struction in congenitally corrected transposition of the great arteries due to ventricular membranous septal aneurysms, *Circulation* 54:679, 1976.
9. Anderson KR, Danielson GK, McGoon DC, et al: Ebstein's anomaly of the left-sided tricuspid valve: pathological anatomy of the valvular malformation, *Circulation* 58(part 2):87, 1978.
10. Dekker A, Mehrizi A, Vengsarkar AS: Corrected transposition of the great vessels with Ebstein malformation of the left atrioventricular valve: an embryologic analysis and two case reports, *Circulation* 31:119, 1965.
11. Todd DB, Anderson RC, Edwards JE: Inverted malformations in corrected transposition of the great vessels, *Circulation* 32:298, 1965.
12. Ruttenberg HD, Anderson RC, Elliott LP, et al: Origin of both great vessels from the arterial ventricle: a complex with ventricular inversion, *Br Heart J* 26:631, 1964.
13. de la Cruz MV, Miller BL: Double inlet left ventricle, *Circulation* 37:249, 1968.
14. Anderson RH, Becker AE, Arnold R, et al: The conducting tissues in congenitally corrected transposition, *Circulation* 50:911, 1974.
15. Anderson RC, Lillehei CW, Lester RG: Corrected transposition of the great vessels of the heart: a review of 17 cases, *Pediatrics* 20:626, 1957.
16. Ruttenberg HD, Elliott LP, Anderson RC, et al: Congenital corrected transposition of the great vessels: correlation of electrocardiograms and vectorcardiograms with associated cardiac malformations and hemodynamic states, *Am J Cardiol* 17:339, 1966.
17. Victorica BE, Miller BL, Gessner IH: Electrocardiogram and vectorcardiogram in ventricular inversion (corrected transposition), *Am Heart J* 86:733, 1973.
18. Erath HG Jr, Graham TP Jr, Hammon JW Jr, et al: Hypoplasia of the systemic ventricle in congenitally corrected transposition of the great arteries: preoperative documentation and possible implications of operation, *J Thorac Cardiovasc Surg* 79:770, 1980.
19. Hallman GL, Gill SS, Bloodwell RD, et al: Surgical treatment of cardiac defects associated with corrected transposition of the great vessels, *Circulation* 35(suppl I):133, 1967.
20. de Leval MR, Bastos P, Stark J, et al: Surgical technique to reduce the risks of heart block following closure of ventricular septal defect in atrioventricular discordance, *J Thorac Cardiovasc Surg* 78:515, 1979.

CHAPTER 40

Clinical Transposition: Ventricular Inversion With Nontransposition or Isolated Ventricular Inversion

In conditions with ventricular inversion (discordant atrioventricular connection), the ventricle receiving systemic venous blood has anatomic features of a left ventricle, whereas the ventricle receiving pulmonary venous blood has anatomic features of a right ventricle. Ventricular inversion is almost invariably associated with transposition of the great vessels (discordant ventriculo-arterial connection). Thus, the pulmonary artery arises from the venous (anatomic left) ventricle and the aorta from the systemic (anatomic right) ventricle, resulting in congenitally corrected transposition of the great vessels that has a normal circulatory pattern (Fig 40–1,A).

Rarely, inversion of the ventricles (discordant atrioventricular connection) is not associated with transposition of the great vessels.[1] Therefore, concordant ventriculoarterial relationships are present. When this combination occurs, the venous (anatomic left) ventricle gives rise to the aorta, and the other ventricle (anatomic right) gives rise to a pulmonary artery. Thus, the great vessels are not transposed, and concordant ventriculoarterial connection exists. As a result, systemic venous blood enters through the right atrioventricular valve (mitral valve) into the venous ventricle (anatomic left ventricle) and passes into the aorta. Pulmonary venous blood passes through the left atrioventricular valve (tricuspid) into the right ventricle and then to the pulmonary artery. Therefore, the circulation is hemodynamically identical to complete transposition of the great vessels and causes deep cyanosis (Fig 40–1,B). The great vessels, because they connect to appropriate ventricles, are normally related. Therefore, the pulmonary artery lies anterior to the aorta. As a consequence, this rare condition has been called by several names: clinical transposition, ventricular inversion with nontransposition, and isolated ventricular inversion.

This anomaly should not be confused with the even rarer condition, complete transposition of the great vessels (concordant atrioventricular and discordant ventricular arterioventricular connection, D-loop transposition) in which the aorta is located posteriorly to the pulmonary artery, also called "posterior transposition" (see Chapter 38). These two conditions are identical hemodynamically, but in clinical transposition the venous ventricle is an inverted anatomic left ventricle, whereas in complete transposition the venous ventricle is an anatomic right ventricle. As in other forms of transposition, a ventricular septal defect, pulmonary stenosis, or both may coexist. Clinical transposition of the great vessels should not be confused with congenital corrected transposition of the great vessels. There are no unique clinical features to identify clinical transposition of the great vessels. The history and physical examination resemble complete transposition of the great vessels.

RADIOGRAPHIC FEATURES

The appearance of the thoracic roentgenogram is identical to congenital corrected transposition of the great vessels (L-loop transposition). There is a prominent bulge of the left cardiac border, and the pulmonary arterial segment

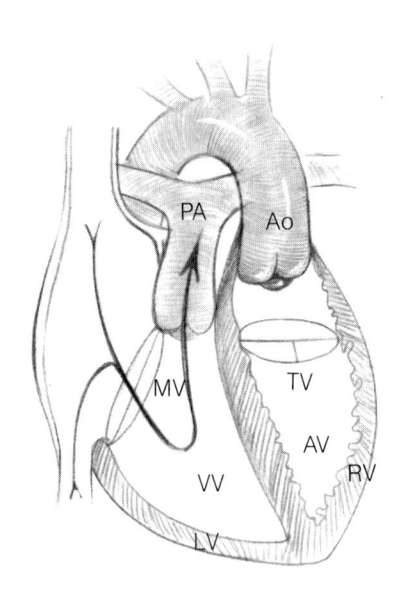

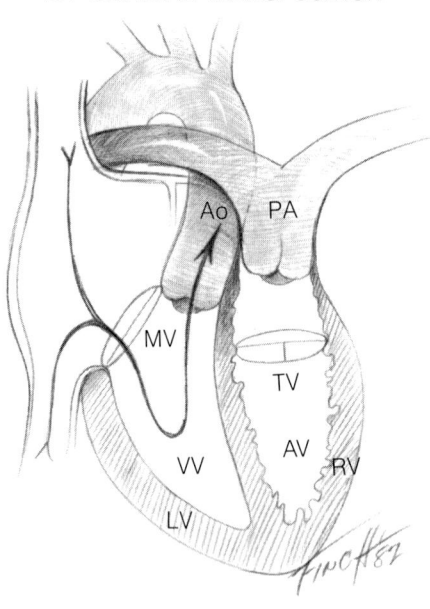

728 *Cyanosis and Increased Pulmonary Arterial Vasculature*

FIG 40–1.
A, congenital corrected transposition of great vessels with ventricular inversion (discordant atrioventricular and ventriculoarterial connections). Hemodynamically normal heart. **B,** clinical transposition of great vessels. Ventricular inversion (discordant atrioventricular connection) and concordant ventriculoarterial connection. Aorta *(Ao)* arises from venous (anatomic left) ventricle. Therefore, aorta is not transposed (concordant ventriculoarterial connection). Pulmonary artery *(PA)* arises from pulmonary (anatomic right) ventricle *(AV)*. Connection of aorta to venous ventricle *(VV)* results in hemodynamics of complete transposition of great vessels. *MV* = mitral valve; *TV* = tricuspid valve; *LV* = left ventricle; *RV* = right ventricle.

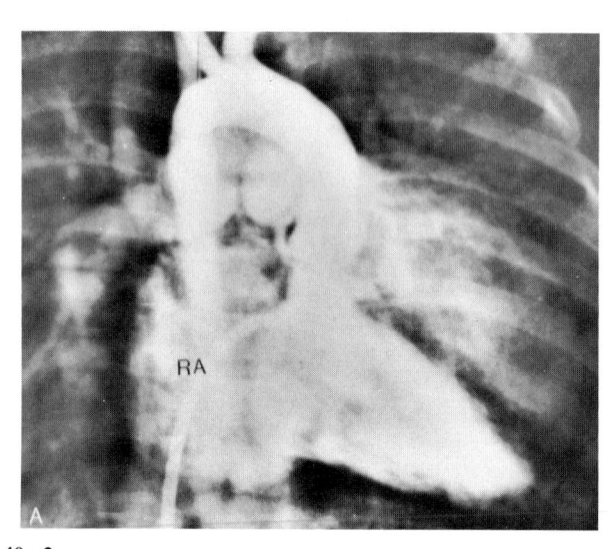

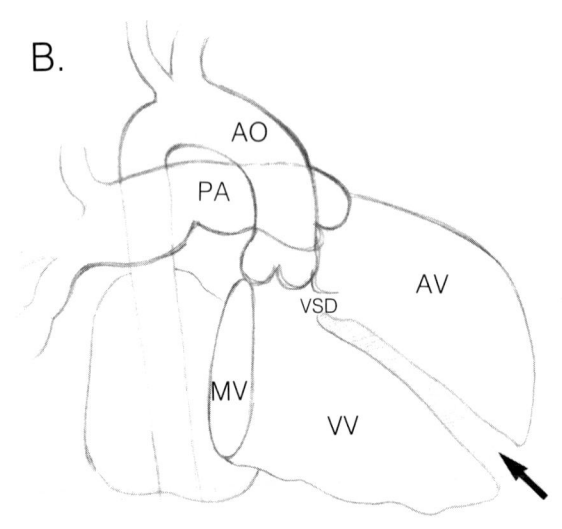

FIG 40–2.
Clinical transposition of great vessels. **A,** ventriculogram. Anteroposterior projection. **B,** accompanying diagram. Catheter is passed through right atrioventricular valve into smooth-walled (anatomic left) ventricle. Slight reflux of contrast medium into right atrium *(RA)*, indicating that this ventricle *(VV)* receives the systemic venous blood. Aorta *(AO)* arises from this inverted ventricle. Aortic valve is positioned low because it does not arise from an infundibulum. Faint opacification of arterial ventricle *(AV)* through ventricular septal defect *(VSD)*. Ventricular septum is seen on end *(arrow)*, as in corrected transposition of great vessels. Right aortic arch. *MV* = mitral valve; *PA* = pulmonary artery.

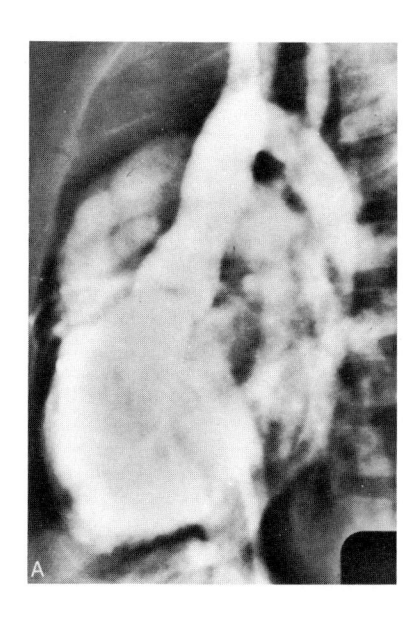

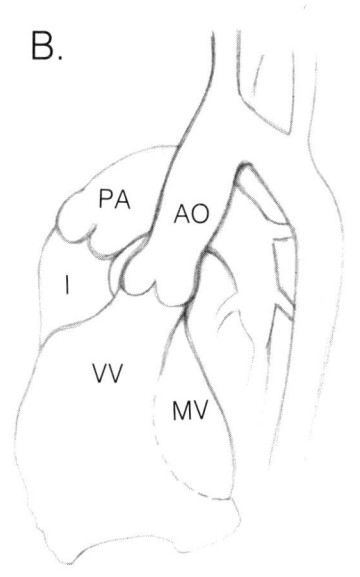

FIG 40–3.
Clinical transposition of great vessels. **A,** venous ventriculogram. Lateral projection and, **B,** diagram. Normally placed (nontransposed) aorta *(AO)*. Pulmonary artery *(PA)* fills faintly through ventricular septal defect. Aortic valve is positioned lower than pulmonary valve because aorta *(AO)* arises from anatomic left ventricle *(VV)*. *I* = infundibulum; *MV* = mitral value.

is absent. The pulmonary vasculature varies, depending on the associated cardiac conditions.

ANGIOGRAPHIC FEATURES

1. Injection of the venous ventricle demonstrates features of a left ventricle. It is smooth and triangular in shape. The aorta arises from this chamber (Fig 40–2) and passes to the left of the pulmonary artery.

2. On the lateral projection, the aorta is located posteriorly (Fig 40–3). There is continuity between the aortic and atrioventricular valve. The plane of the aortic valve lies lower than the pulmonary valve, because the anatomic left ventricle has no infundibulum.

3. Injection of the ventricle beneath the pulmonary artery outlines a chamber with features of a right ventricle. It has an infundibulum from which the pulmonary artery arises. This ventricle lies to the left of the ventricle supplying the aorta and forms the upper left cardiac border, as typically seen in a patient with ventricular inversion (Fig 40–4). The ventricular septum lies in a plane perpendicular to the anterior thoracic wall.

4. On a lateral projection, the pulmonary artery lies

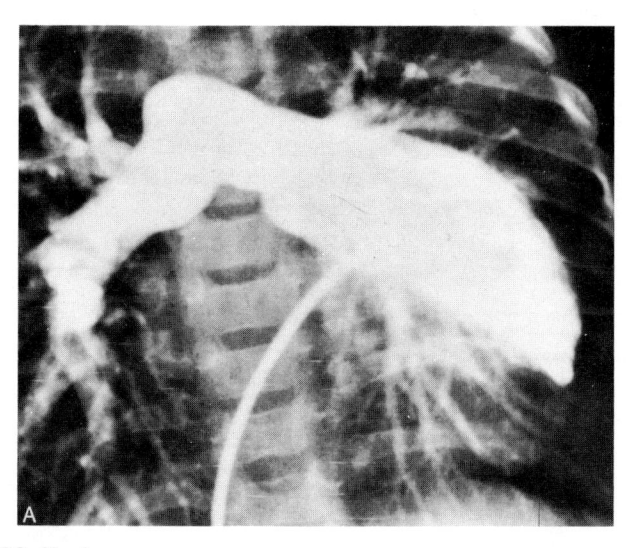

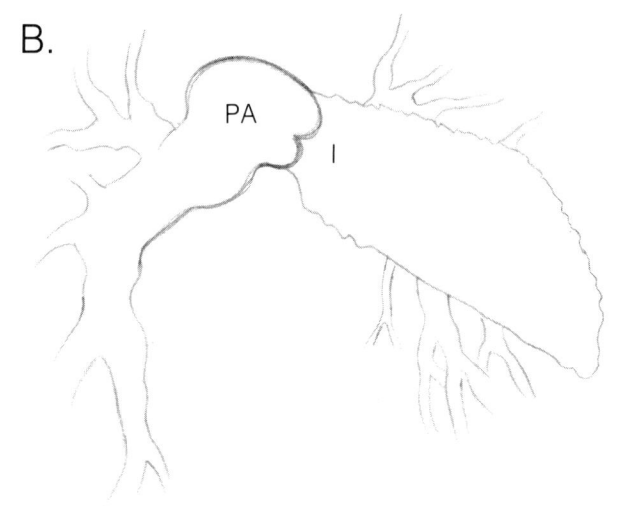

FIG 40–4.
Clinical transposition of great vessels. **A,** ventriculogram of inverted right ventricle. Anteroposterior projection and **B,** accompanying diagram. Position of ventricle characteristic of right ventricle in ventricular inversion. Pulmonary artery *(PA)* is densely opacified. *I* = infundibulum.

anteriorly, and its valve plane is higher than the aortic valve (see Fig 40–3).

5. On late films after injection into the pulmonary ventricle, the ventricle and pulmonary artery reopacify, consistant with the hemodynamics of complete transposition of the great vessels.

SUMMARY

Clinical transposition of the great vessels is a rare cardiac anomaly that results from ventricular inversion without associated transposition of the great vessels, and causes in cyanosis. It should not be confused with congenital corrected posterior transposition of the great vessels or with a crisscross heart.

REFERENCE

1. Quero-Jimenez M, Raposo-Sonnenfeld I: Isolated ventricular inversion with situs solitus, *Br Heart J* 37:293, 1975.

CHAPTER 41

Double-Outlet Ventricle

The term double-outlet ventricle refers to conditions in which one great vessel and more than 50% of the other arise from one ventricle. In virtually all instances a ventricular septal defect exists, and usually both great vessels arise from a morphologic right ventricle.

This chapter presents several forms of double-outlet ventricle and conditions that may be confused with it. The following are discussed herein:

1. Double-outlet right ventricle.
2. Double-outlet right ventricle with pulmonary stenosis.
3. Double-outlet and double-inlet right ventricle.
4. Transposition of the aorta and biventricular origin of the pulmonary trunk.
5. Double-outlet inverted right ventricle.
6. Double-outlet left ventricle.

DOUBLE-OUTLET RIGHT VENTRICLE

Double-outlet right ventricle, also called "origin of both great vessels from the right ventricle," is an uncommon congenital cardiac anomaly in which a positional anomaly of the great vessels and ventricular septum are present. Both the pulmonary artery and aorta originate from the right ventricle. A ventricular septal defect is usually present. Depending on anatomic details, the clinical and hemodynamics may resemble a large ventricular septal defect, tetralogy of Fallot, or complete transposition of the great vessels.

Pathologic Anatomy

Certain basic anatomic features are present in each patient with double-outlet right ventricle[1,2] (1) the pulmonary trunk and aorta show a normal external appearance; (2) at least 50% of the aortic root originates from the right ventricle, and the aortic valve lies to the right of the pulmonary valve; (3) the plane of the aortic valve is higher and more anterior than normal and is at the same level as the pulmonary valve; and (4) the aortic and mitral valves are separated by muscular tissue. Thus, fibrous continuity between the aortic and mitral valves is absent. A ventricular septal defect is present except in rare circumstances. A muscle band passes from the anterior to posterior walls of the right ventricle and separates the subaortic and subpulmonary outflow tracts (trunco-conal septum).

Double-outlet right ventricle has been classified(1-4) according to the location of the ventricular septal defect (Fig 41-1).

Type I: Ventricular septal defect below the crista supraventricularis
  A. Subaortic ventricular septal defect. The defect lies below the septal limb of the crista supraventricularis and to the right of the muscular band separating the subpulmonary and subaortic outflow tracts (trunco-conal septum).
  B. Remote noncommitted ventricular septal defect. The ventricular septal defect is located below the crista supraventricularis and is not related closely to either the subpulmonary or subaortic areas.

Type II: Ventricular septal defect above the crista supraventricularis
  A. Subpulmonary ventricular septal defect. The defect is located above the crista supraventricularis and immediately below the pulmonary valve.[5] This is considered the Taussig-Bing anomaly.[1]
  B. Subpulmonary and subaortic ventricular septal defect, also called "double committed" ventricular septal defect. The defect is centered below the muscle mass separating the outflow tracts.

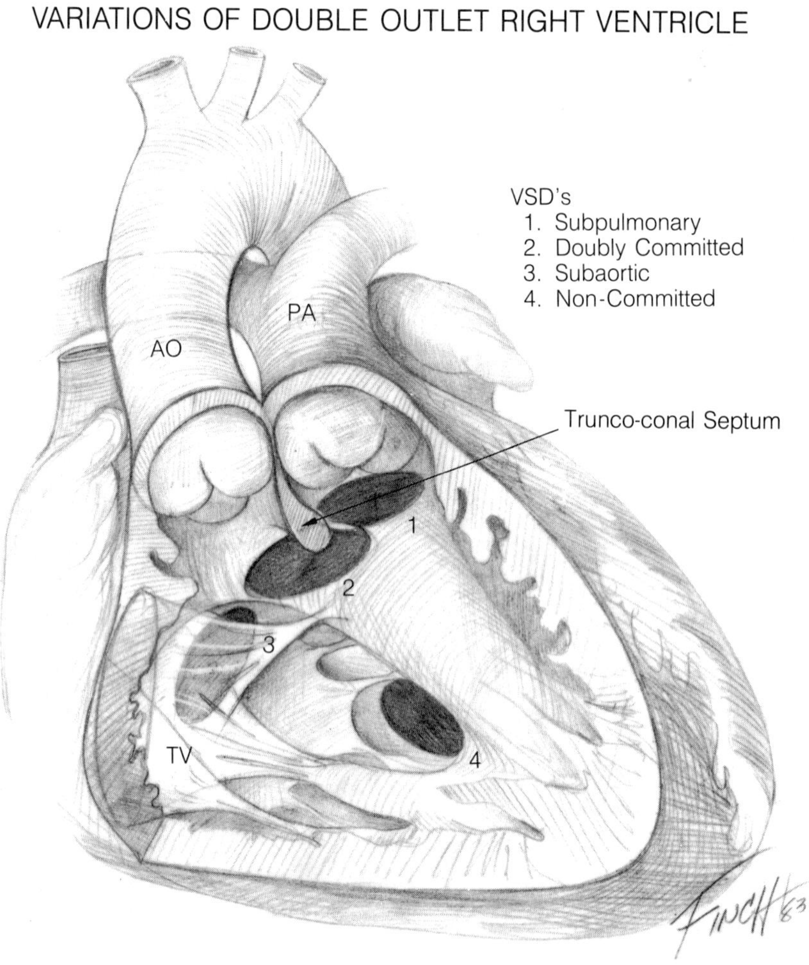

VARIATIONS OF DOUBLE OUTLET RIGHT VENTRICLE

VSD's
1. Subpulmonary
2. Doubly Committed
3. Subaortic
4. Non-Committed

FIG 41–1.
Double-outlet right ventricle. Diagram of opened right ventricle showing most common locations of ventricular septal defect. Outflow tracts separated by conal-truncal septum. Pulmonary and aortic valves are at same level. *AO* = aorta; *PA* = pulmonary artery; *TV* = tricuspid valve.

Usually the ventricular septal defect is large and the only exit of blood from the left ventricle. The ventricular septal defect may become smaller with age, thus obstructing left ventricular outflow. Rarely the ventricular septum is intact.[6, 7] The latter form is associated with an atrial level shunt and either a hypoplastic left ventricle or mitral insufficiency (Fig 41–2).

Associated Conditions

Pulmonary stenosis, either valvar or subvalvar, occurs in 50% of cases. It is much more common with a subaortic ventricular septal defect than with a subpulmonary ventricular septal defect.[1–4]

Coarctation of the aorta, interruption of the aortic arch, and aortic stenosis are also common, being present principally among patients with subpulmonary ventricular septal defect.[3, 4] Subaortic stenosis may be present because of hypertrophy of the subaortic conus. Abnormalities of the mitral valve apparatus are common, including parachute mitral valve, supravalvar stenosing ring, and features of the Shone syndrome.[3] Mitral valve anomalies (or aortic obstruction) rarely occur in the presence of a co-existent subaortic ventricular septal defect and pulmonary stenosis.

Atrial septal defect is present in one fourth of the patients. In about 10% of cases, double-outlet right ventricle is associated with L-malposition of the great vessels and ventricular inversion, so that the aorta lies to the left of the pulmonary artery (Fig 41–3,D).[8] In L-transposition, the right ventricle underlies the aorta and thus supplies the systemic circulation, and at least 50% of the pulmonary artery also originates from this ventricle. Most of these cases are associated with pulmonary stenosis. In this circumstance the ventricular septal defect may be either infracristal or supracristal, thus being subpulmonary or subaortic, respectively. This relationship of the anatomic position of the ventricular septal defect to the great vessels is hemodynamically the opposite from double outlet with noninversion (Fig 41–3).

Rarely, double-outlet right ventricle coexists with double-inlet right ventricle. In these patients, the ventricu-

DOUBLE OUTLET RV WITH INTACT SEPTUM

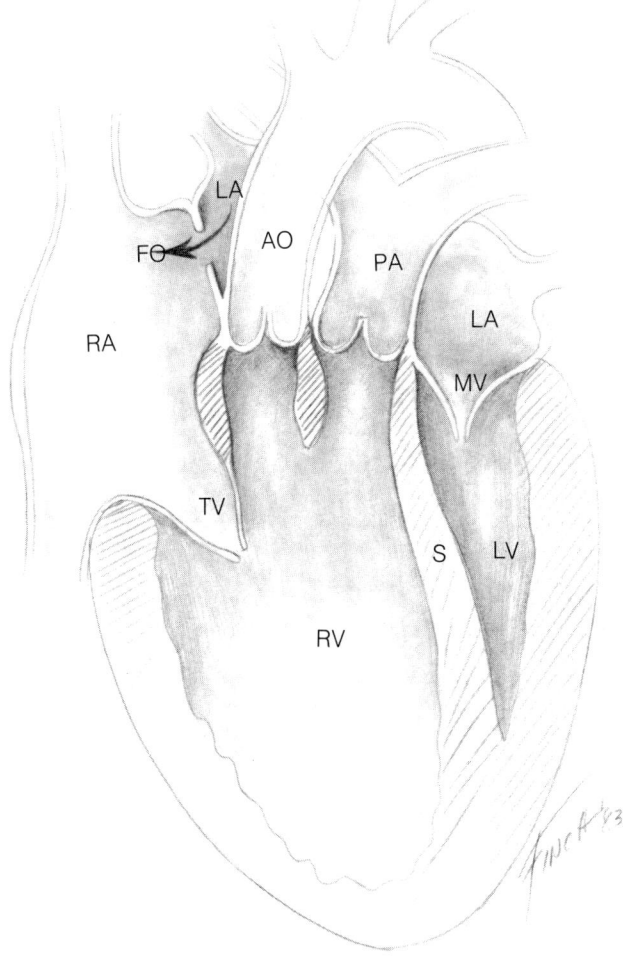

FIG 41–2.
Double-outlet right ventricle with intact ventricular septum. Hypoplastic left ventricle *(LV)*. Left-to-right shunt through foramen ovale *(FO)*. *AO* = aorta; *LA* = left atrium; *MV* = mitral valve; *RA* = right atrium; *RV* = right ventricle; *S* = interventricular septum; *TV* = tricuspid valve; *PA* = pulmonary artery.

lar septal defect lies posteriorly, and the mitral valve straddles the ventricular septum. As a result, left atrial blood enters both ventricles (see Chapter 44).

Embryogenesis

Early in the embryo, the truncus overlies the primitive right ventricle, with the portion that ultimately becomes the aorta lying to the right and the portion that becomes the pulmonary artery lying to the left. The portion of the ventricular conus lying under the aortic valve normally rotates posteriorly and to the left, whereas the conus below the aortic valve reabsorbs and the junction between the conus and ventricle shifts to the left. These events lead to the aorta arising from the left ventricle and establishes aortic-mitral continuity.

Double-outlet right ventricle probably results from failure of this process to take place, and absorption to some degree of each conus takes place. The presence of a large subpulmonary conus is associated with a subaortic ventricular septal defect and vice versa.

Hemodynamics

Three basic hemodynamic patterns are found among patients with double-outlet right ventricle, which may be modified by the presence of coexistent conditions such as aortic obstruction, or mitral valve anomalies:

1. Double-outlet right ventricle with subaortic ventricular septal defect. In this hemodynamic pattern the ventricular septal defect is located below the subaortic conus. In the usual form of double-outlet right ventricle, the defect is infracristal (see Fig 41–3,A). In associated L-malposition, a supracristal defect yields similar hemodynamics (see Fig 41–3,C).

The hemodynamic pattern resembles a large ventricular septal defect and pulmonary hypertension. Fully saturated left ventricular blood passes through the ventricular septal defect and furnishes most of the blood flowing into the aorta and also contributes a major portion of the pulmonary blood flow. The systemic venous return enters the right ventricle and passes principally to the pulmonary artery. Therefore, little or no clinical cyanosis is present. Aortic oxygen saturation exceeds pulmonary arterial oxygen saturation, reflecting the pattern of streaming in the right ventricle.

Occasionally the ventricular septal defect becomes smaller, restricting flow from the left ventricle. In these circumstances, left ventricular systolic pressure rises and may exceed 200 mm Hg.

2. Double-outlet right ventricle with subpulmonary ventricular septal defect. In the usual patient with this form of double outlet, the defect is located above the crista supraventricularis (see Fig 41–3,B), but in those with L-malposition, an infracristal defect yields similar hemodynamics (see Fig 41–3,D). The hemodynamic pattern resembles that of complete transposition of the great vessels and ventricular septal defect. Left ventricular blood flows through the ventricular septal defect predominantly into the pulmonary artery. Only a small portion reaches the aorta. The systemic venous return passes principally to the aorta. Thus, the patient is intensely cyanotic, and pulmonary arterial oxygen saturation is greater than aortic saturation, reflecting the pattern of streaming in the right ventricle. Pulmonary hypertension is present. Coarctation or interruption of the aortic arch are common.

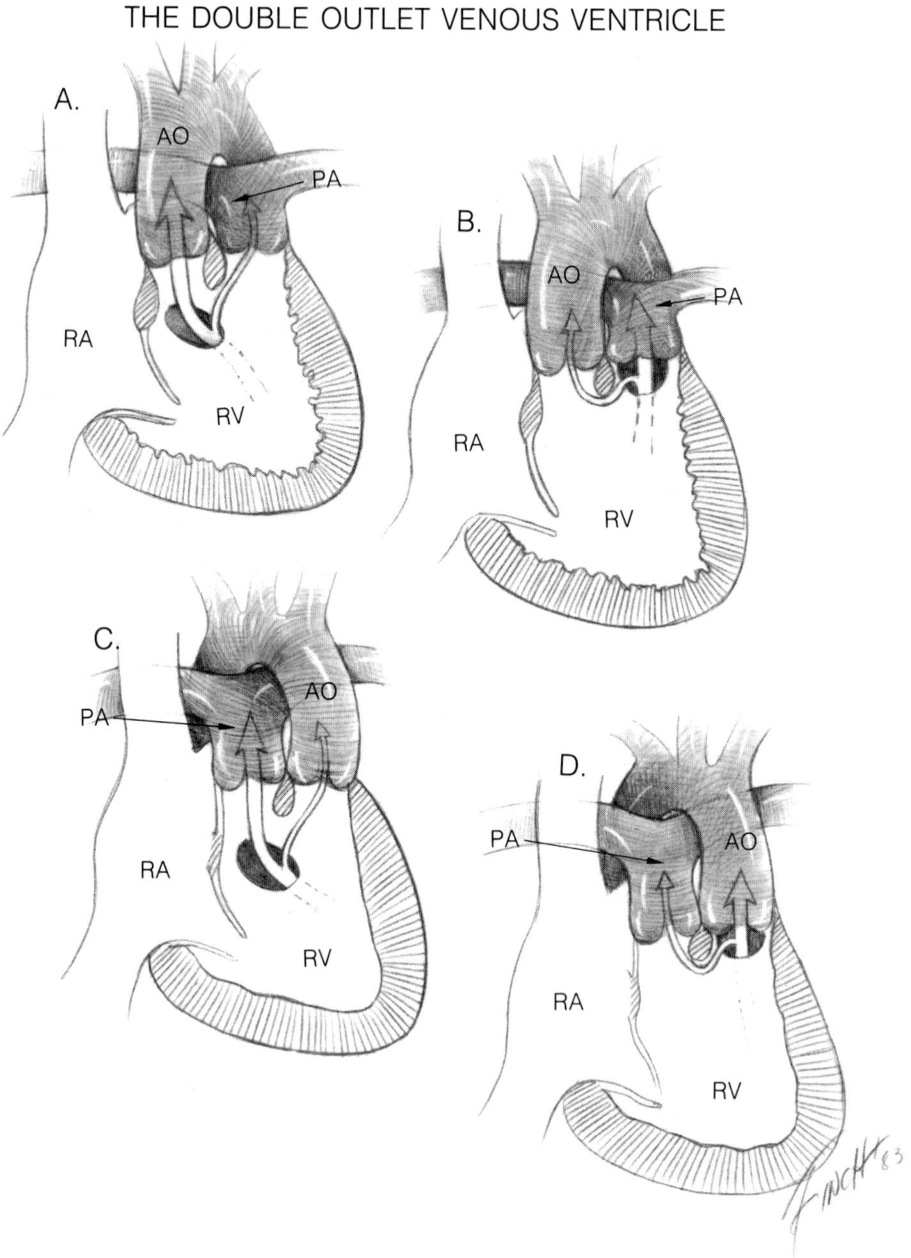

THE DOUBLE OUTLET VENOUS VENTRICLE

FIG 41–3.
Types of double-outlet right ventricle showing relationships between location of ventricular septal defect and position of great vessels. **A** and **B**, normally related great vessels. **C** and **D**, L-malposition of great vessels. **A** and **C**, infracristal ventricular septal defect. **B** and **D**, supracristal ventricular septal defect. Hemodynamics of L-transposition (**C** and **D**) are opposite of normally related great vessels (**A** and **B**). AO = aorta; PA = pulmonary artery; RA = right atrium; RV = right ventricle.

3. Double-outlet right ventricle with pulmonary stenosis. In virtually all patients with coexistent pulmonary stenosis, the ventricular septal defect is subaortic, and the hemodynamics resemble tetralogy of Fallot. The ventricular systolic pressures are equal, whereas pulmonary arterial pressure is low. Because of the pulmonary stenosis, pulmonary blood flow is limited. The oxygen saturation of aortic blood is low and may be lower than pulmonary arterial oxygen saturation.

Several factors may modify these basic hemodynamic patterns:

1. In patients with doubly committed or remote ventricular septal defect, the oxygen saturations in the great vessels may be more nearly equal, which may help identify the location of the ventricular septal defect.
2. Coexistent conditions influence the hemodynamics. The presence of either coarctation of the aorta or interruption of the aortic arch increases resistance to aortic flow and therefore increases the volume of pulmonary blood flow. Mitral valve anomalies increase pulmonary venous pressure and total pulmonary vascular resistance, which reduces pulmonary blood flow and may cause pulmonary edema.

3. As in any patient with pulmonary hypertension secondary to a large volume of pulmonary blood flow, pulmonary vascular disease may develop. The development may be hastened by coexistent mitral valve disease.

4. Subaortic stenosis from an hypertrophied subaortic conus can increase in severity, augmenting the volume of pulmonary blood flow.

Clinical Features

The clinical picture of double-outlet right ventricle varies and depends on three factors: the location of the ventricular septal defect relative to the great vessels, the presence or absence of pulmonary stenosis, and the presence of coexistent cardiac anomalies.[9]

Three clinical pictures that parallel the basic hemodynamic patterns are described:

1. Subaortic ventricular septal defect. The clinical features resemble a large ventricular septal defect and pulmonary hypertension. Cyanosis is not present. As the pulmonary vascular resistance falls, with symptoms manifesting during infancy with congestive cardiac failure. There is clinical evidence of cardiomegaly. A loud pansystolic murmur and accentuated pulmonary component of the second heart sound are heard. The murmur is associated with a thrill. Usually an apical middiastolic murmur secondary to increased pulmonary venous return across the mitral valve is heard.

2. Subpulmonary ventricular septal defect. The clinical picture resembles complete transposition of the great vessels, with symptoms manifesting early in life with cyanosis and congestive cardiac failure. Growth is significantly delayed. Respiratory tract infections are common.

The heart is greatly enlarged and commonly causes a precordial bulge. There is a loud pansystolic murmur along the left sternal border and an accentuated pulmonary component of the second heart sound. An apical middiastolic murmur from increased flow across the mitral valve is usually present.

Among these patients coarctation of the aorta and interruption of the aortic arch are common. This produces profound cardiac failure. Often infants present with a shocklike picture during the first couple of weeks of life. In such patients, the pulses and blood pressure are diminished in the legs. Subaortic stenosis and mitral stenosis also coexist among these patients and are evident on auscultation by an aortic systolic ejection murmur and an apical late diastolic murmur, respectively.

3. Subaortic ventricular septal defect and pulmonary stenosis. The clinical features resemble tetralogy of Fallot. Patients have cyanosis but not congestive cardiac failure, because the pulmonary stenosis limits the volume of pulmonary blood flow. In addition to cyanosis, there is delayed growth and exercise intolerance. The age of onset and severity of cyanosis depend directly on the degree of pulmonary stenosis.

4. Cardiac size is usually normal. There is a loud pulmonary systolic ejection murmur along the middle to upper left sternal border, which is associated with a thrill. The second heart sound is single. Diastole is clear.

Electrocardiographic Features

The QRS axis is usually directed toward the right. Although Neufeld et al.[1] described a high frequency of left-axis deviation among patients with this condition, this is the exception rather than the rule. Right ventricular hypertrophy is present. It may be associated with left ventricular hypertrophy when there is greatly increased pulmonary blood flow. A pattern of left ventricular hypertrophy and strain is found in patients whose ventricular septal defect becomes smaller and who have markedly elevated left ventricular systolic pressure.

Echocardiographic Features

The echocardiographic imaging in double-outlet ventricle reflects the anatomic detail.[10,11] The preferred view is subcostal. A systematic approach is necessary. After identification of vena caval flow into the right atrium and then into the ventricles, ventricular anatomy should be assessed for degree of trabeculation and position of great arteries because of the potential for ventricular inversion. In double-outlet right ventricle, both great arteries arise anteriorly, the great artery with a more posterior position having at least 50% commitment to the right ventricle. There is aortic-mitral valve discontinuity. Malalignment ventricular septal defect is usually present. Coexistent pulmonary stenosis can be assessed by imaging and confirmed by Doppler analysis.

Radiographic Features

The diagnosis of double-outlet right ventricle cannot be made correctly by analysis of the thoracic roentgenogram. A cardiac silhouette, however, which resembles ventricular septal defect in a patient with cyanosis, strongly suggests double-outlet right ventricle. REASON: Complete transposition of the great vessels with increased pulmonary vasculature does not have a prominent pulmonary arterial segment, and other cyanotic lesions with increased pulmonary blood flow (admixture lesions) usually have other diagnostic radiographic features.

1. The heart is enlarged, and the pulmonary vasculature is increased (Fig 41–4). REASON: The hemodynamics

FIG 41–4.
Double-outlet right ventricle. Thoracic roentgenogram. Posteroanterior projection. Features are identical to ventricular septal defect. Increased pulmonary vasculature. Enlarged pulmonary artery segment *(white arrow)*. Inconspicuous aorta. Displacement of esophagus *(arrows)* because of enlarged left atrium. With history of cyanosis, the possibility of double-outlet right ventricle can be suggested.

in double-outlet right ventricle without pulmonary stenosis resemble ventricular septal defect, with increased pulmonary blood flow and increased flow through the left-sided cardiac chambers.

2. Depending on the location of the ventricular septal defect, there may be no clinical diagnosis. The radiographic and clinical diagnosis with subaortic communication is therefore commonly ventricular septal defect.

3. The left atrium is enlarged (see Fig 41–4). REASON: Pulmonary flow is increased, and the left atrium is distended as in ventricular septal defect.

4. The pulmonary arterial segment is prominent. REASON: The pulmonary artery is dilated by the increased pulmonary blood flow, and in double-outlet right ventricle the left-to-right relationship of aorta and pulmonary artery is normal in most patients. The pulmonary artery is therefore normally positioned along the upper left cardiac border in distinction to complete transposition of the great vessels.

5. The aorta is inconspicuous. Although the cardiac output is normal, the aorta is partially overshadowed by the enlarged main pulmonary arterial segment, as in ventricular septal defect.

6. Rarely, the main pulmonary arterial segment is not prominent as in complete transposition of the great vessels. REASON: The side-by-side relationship between the aorta and pulmonary artery is inconsistent. Occasionally the pulmonary artery lies either behind or to the right of the aorta. Therefore, the pulmonary arterial segment may not appear enlarged despite anatomic dilatation of the pulmonary artery from the increased pulmonary blood flow and pressure. In these circumstances, the cardiac silhouette is identical to that of complete transposition of the great vessels.

7. In patients with coexistent pulmonary stenosis, the cardiac contour is similar to tetralogy of Fallot, because the pulmonary artery is not enlarged, and cardiac size is normal (Fig 41–5).

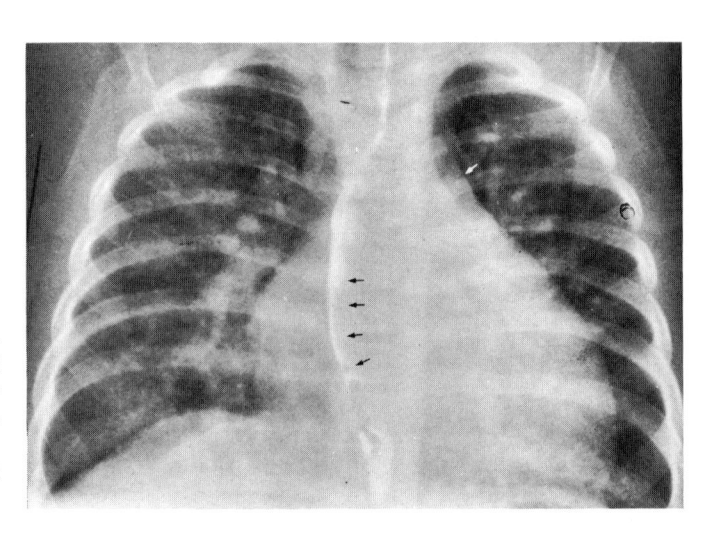

8. The appearance of double outlet with L-malposition is identical to corrected transposition of the great vessels (Fig 41–6).

Cardiac Catheterization

Cardiac catheterization and angiography are performed to:

1. Establish the diagnosis.
2. Locate the position of the ventricular septal defect.
3. Measure intracardiac pressures and calculate blood flows and vascular resistances.
4. Identify associated cardiac conditions.

From the right ventricle it is possible to advance the catheter into each great vessel. When a catheter is advanced in a retrograde direction across the aortic valve, it usually can be advanced into the left ventricle through a subaortic or doubly committed ventricular septal defect but not through a subpulmonary ventricular septal defect.

There is oximetry evidence of a bidirectional ventricular shunt, with blood in the aorta being desaturated to a variable extent, and an increase in oxygen saturation in the right ventricle from the left-to-right shunt. Usually the pulmonary arterial and aortic oxygen saturations are different. In subpulmonary ventricular septal defect, pulmonary arterial saturation is considerably higher than aortic saturation, the latter often being less than 80%. Among patients with subaortic ventricular septal defect, usually the aortic saturation is higher than pulmonary arterial saturation; it may be as high as 95%. There is considerable variation among those patients with subaortic ventricular septal defect, particularly when pulmonary vascular disease is present. An atrial left-to-right shunt may be found in patients with coexistent atrial septal defect.

Systemic pressure is found in the right ventricle. Pul-

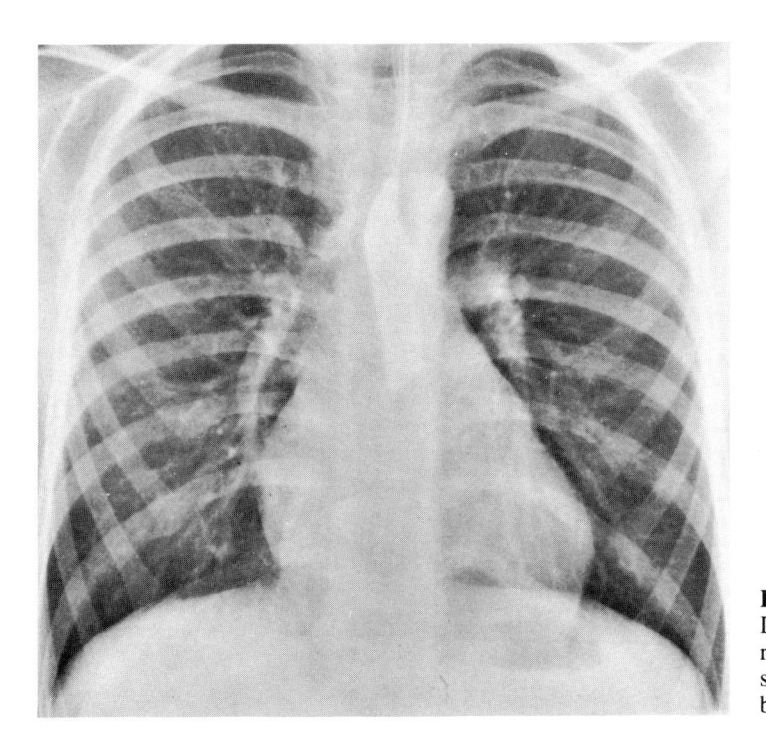

FIG 41–5.
Double-outlet right ventricle with pulmonary stenosis. Thoracic roentgenogram. Posteroanterior projection. Cardiac silhouette is indistinguishable from normal heart or from balanced tetralogy of Fallot.

monary hypertension is present except in patients with coexistent pulmonary stenosis. The pulmonary capillary pressure must be measured because of the increased incidence of mitral obstructive lesions in this condition. Left ventricular systolic pressure equals that in the right ventricle except in patients with a small ventricular septal defect, in which case, left ventricular systolic pressure is elevated.

Angiographic Features

Exact angiographic diagnosis of double-outlet right ventricle is important to the surgeon because the operative repair varies depending on the location of the ventricular septal defect in respect to the great vessels and complicating coexistent conditions. Right and left ventriculography are required to demonstrate the location of the ventricular septal defect and the anatomic details of the outflow tracts.

Location of Ventricular Septal Defect

The location of the ventricular septal defect can be determined by the following:

1. Visualization of the defect and its relationship to the great arteries in two angiographic projections.
2. The degree of opacification of the great vessels after right and left ventriculography reflects their oxygen concentrations. When the ventricular septal defect is located beneath the aortic valve, the aortic blood is nearly fully saturated, and therefore the aorta opacifies densely after a left ventriculogram, whereas the pulmonary artery

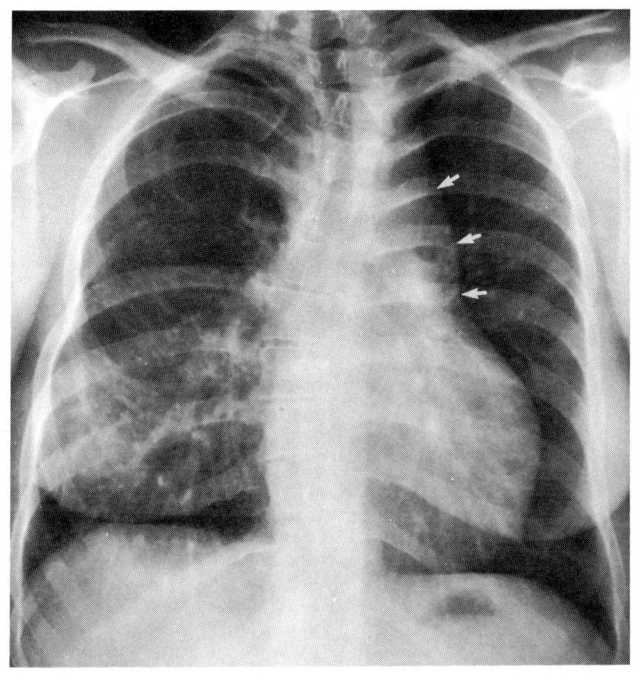

FIG 41–6.
Double-outlet right ventricle and L-malposition (corrected transposition) of great vessels and pulmonary stenosis. Thoracic roentgenogram. Posteroanterior projection. Decreased pulmonary vasculature. Prominent bulge *(arrows)* along left cardiac border (ascending aorta) is consistent with corrected transposition. Roentgen findings are identical to corrected transposition of great vessels with pulmonary stenosis.

is minimally opacified. On the other hand, when the ventricular septal defect lies beneath the pulmonary valve, a left v entriculogram densely opacifies the pulmonary trunk and faintly opacifies the aorta. Such a patient is significantly cyanotic. In a doubly committed ventricular septal defect, both great vessels are opacified equally (Fig 41–7). The late phase of a pulmonary arteriogram reflects the hemodynamics more reliably, because ventriculograms are often associated with extrasystoles or streaming effects, depending on the site of injection.

3. Right ventriculography also reflects the hemodynamics. The location of the ventricular septal defect is evidenced by a localized dilution of the contrast material.

4. Catheter course. The location of the defect can be identified as just discussed.

Right Ventriculography

1. The right ventricle is heavily trabeculated and enlarged. REASON: The right ventricle ejects not only the systemic venous return but also a portion of the pulmonary venous return. Therefore, right ventricular volume load is increased. Right ventricular hypertrophy occurs because the systolic pressure is elevated in the right ventricle, as with any large ventricular communication (see Fig 41–7).

2. Both great vessels opacify after right ventriculography. The degree of opacification depends on the location of the ventricular septal defect in relation to the great arteries.

3. The aortic and pulmonary valves are located approximately at the same level. REASON: In double-outlet right ventricle, the pulmonary artery and the aorta arise from separate coni, and therefore the aortic valve is higher than normal. In the normal heart the aorta does not arise from a conus, and the aortic valve is located lower than the pulmonary valve.

4. The main pulmonary artery is usually enlarged. REASON: Hemodynamically double-outlet right ventricle is usually associated with a left-to-right shunt and pulmonary hypertension. The exception is double-outlet right ventricle with coexistent pulmonary stenosis.

5. The outflow tracts to the aorta and the pulmonary artery are separated by a prominent muscular spur (truncoconal septum) (see Fig 41–7). The spur is seen well on an anteroposterior projection of a right ventriculogram.

6. The muscular conus leading to the aorta may be hypertrophied, causing subaortic stenosis (Fig 41–8).

7. The subaortic area must be visualized before a corrective operation to exclude stenosis at this site. The subaortic conus is best visualized if injected selectively (Fig 41–9).

8. The relationship between aorta and pulmonary artery are almost always normal in the anteroposterior projection.

9. On the lateral projection, both semilunar valves are located at the same body level because each artery arises

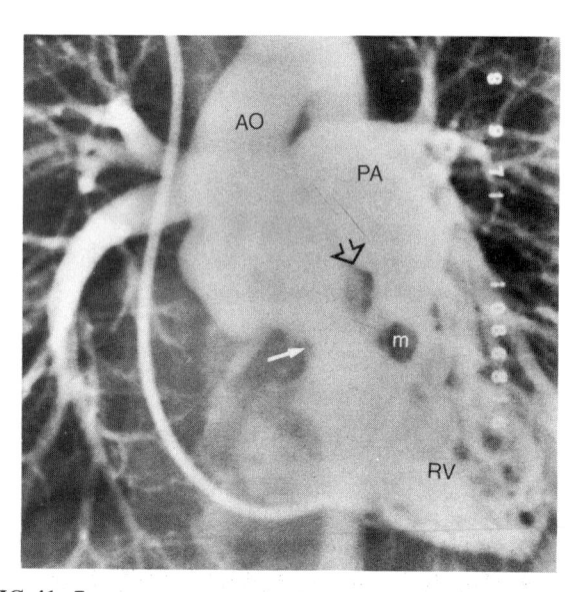

FIG 41–7.
Double-outlet right ventricle. Doubly committed ventricular septal defect. Right ventriculogram (RV). Both great vessels are opacified to same degree. Anteroposterior projection. Coni are located below both pulmonary artery (PA) and aorta (AO). Marked right ventricular hypertrophy. Entrance (white arrow) to subaortic conus is hypertrophied, causing subaortic stenosis. Coni are separated by a characteristic muscular spur (open arrow) (trunco-conal septum). Muscle bundle (m) causes subpulmonary stenosis.

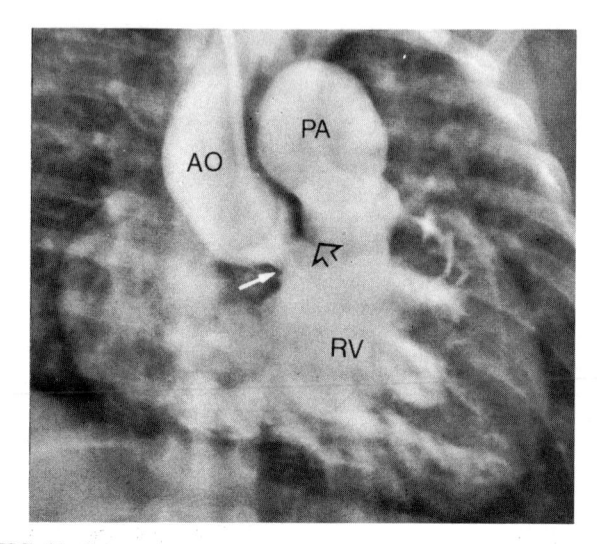

FIG 41–8.
Double-outlet right ventricle and muscular subaortic stenosis. Right ventriculogram. Anteroposterior projection. Hypertrophied right ventricle (RV). Both great vessels opacified with same intensity. Truncal-conal septum (open arrow). Marked subaortic stenosis (solid arrow). Bicuspid aortic valve. AO = aorta; PA = pulmonary artery.

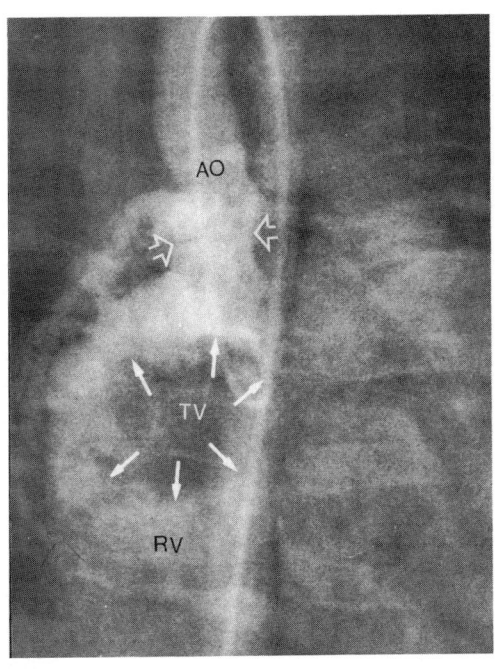

FIG 41-9.
Double-outlet right ventricle. Right ventriculogram *(RV)*. Selective injection of subaortic conus, which is normal. Diastole. Aortic valve *(open arrows)* is separated from open tricuspid valve *(TV) (arrows)*. *AO* = aorta.

FIG 41-10.
Double-outlet right ventricle and subpulmonary ventricular septal defect (Taussig-Bing heart). Right ventriculogram *(RV)*. Lateral projection. Aorta *(AO)* is densely opacified, reflecting low aortic desaturation and cyanosis. Pulmonary artery *(PA)* is less densely opacified, indicating higher oxygen concentration. Aorta arises from right ventricle and is superimposed on pulmonary artery, which projects slightly anteriorly to aorta *(open arrow)*. Aortic valve plane *(white arrow)* is tilted anteriorly. Left ventricle *(LV)* and pulmonary artery are faintly opacified through ventricular septal defect. Dense opacification of aorta and faint opacification of pulmonary artery on a right ventriculogram strongly suggest double-outlet right ventricle with subpulmonary ventricular septal defect (Taussig-Bing heart). Ventricular septal defect is not visualized on this nonangulated projection.

from a separate conus. In this projection the aorta and pulmonary artery are superimposed, although either vessel may project slightly more anteriorly (Fig 41-10). In the normal heart the aorta projects posteriorly to the pulmonary artery.

10. The plane of the aortic valve is tilted anteriorly (see Fig 41-10). REASON: The aorta arises from the anterior right ventricle.

11. The semilunar valves are separated from the anterior leaflet of the mitral valve by muscular tissue (Fig 41-11). Fibrous continuity between the mitral valve and one of the semilunar valves is not present, as is the case in the normal heart or in complete transposition of the great vessels.

12. In the presence of a subaortic ventricular septal defect, right ventriculography densely opacifies the pulmonary trunk and faintly opacifies the aorta (Fig 41-12) (aortic saturation is higher than pulmonary artery saturation).

13. In the presence of a subpulmonary ventricular septal defect (Taussig-Bing heart), the right ventriculogram densely opacifies the aorta and faintly opacifies the pulmonary artery (see Fig 41-10). REASON: The pulmonary artery receives largely unopacified left ventricular blood (pulmonary artery saturation is higher than the aortic saturation, as in complete transposition). Because of streaming and induced arrhythmias with ventriculography,

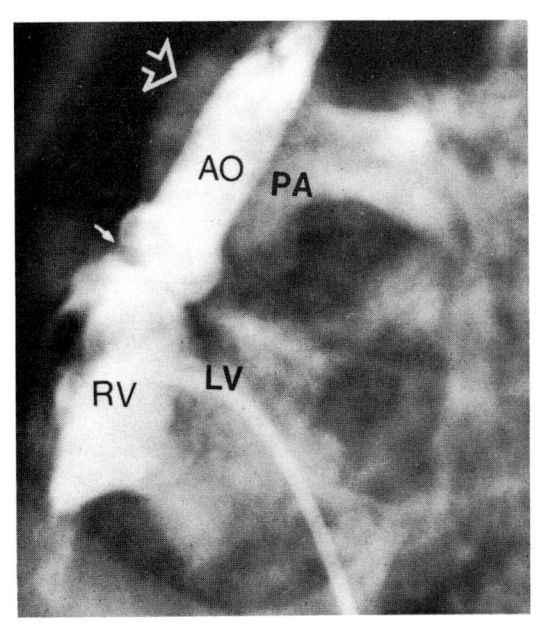

late-phase angiograms more reliably show the hemodynamics.

Left Ventriculography

1. Differentiation of double-outlet right ventricle from either ventricular septal defect or complete transposition of the great vessels hinges on the demonstration of muscular separation of the aortic or pulmonary valve from the mitral valve. This separation can be demonstrated best on an angulated left ventriculogram (Fig 41-13).

2. Depending on the location of the ventricular septal defect, one great vessel is more densely opacified. The degree of opacification of the great vessels is the opposite of the contrast density seen on right ventriculography. In the presence of a subpulmonary defect (Taussig-Bing heart), the pulmonary artery densely opacifies. In the presence of a subaortic defect, the aorta is more densely opacified.

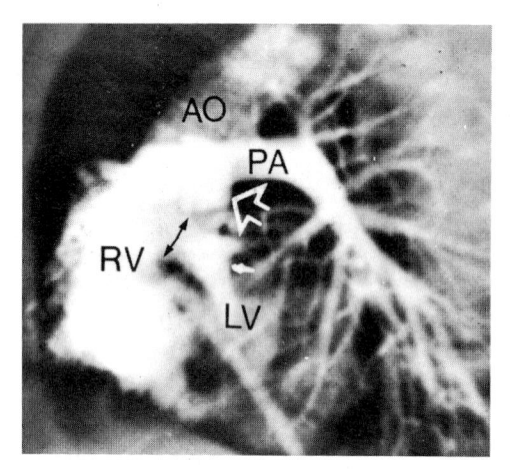

FIG 41–11.
Double-outlet right ventricle with pulmonary stenosis and subaortic ventricular septal defect. Right ventriculogram *(RV)*. Normal size pulmonary artery *(PA)* superimposed on aorta *(AO)*, which is less densely opacified, indicating a higher oxygen concentration. Subaortic ventricular septal defect *(black arrows)*. Anterior leaflet of mitral valve is separated *(white arrow)* from aortic valve, indicating double-outlet right ventricle rather than tetralogy of Fallot with severe overriding of aorta. A continuous spectrum exists from severe overriding to aorta to double-outlet right ventricle. *LV* = left ventricle.

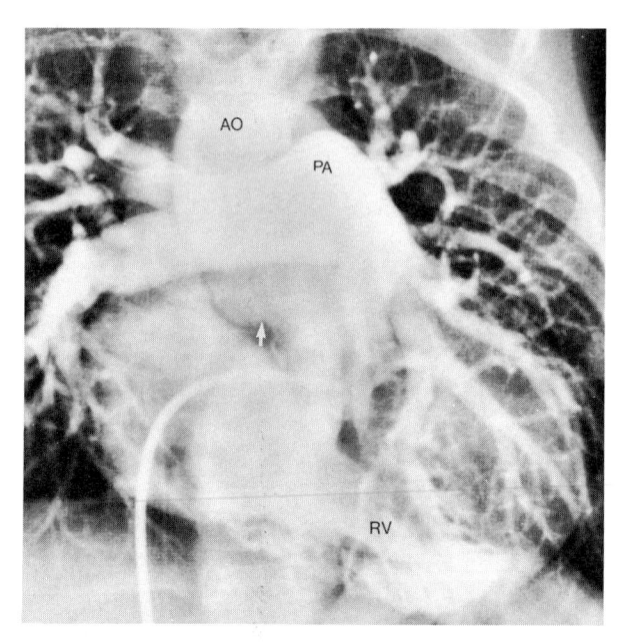

FIG 41–12.
Double-outlet right ventricle. Right ventriculogram *(RV)*. Pulmonary artery *(PA)* is denser than aorta *(AO)*, consistent with subaortic location of ventricular septal defect. Subaortic stenosis *(arrow)*.

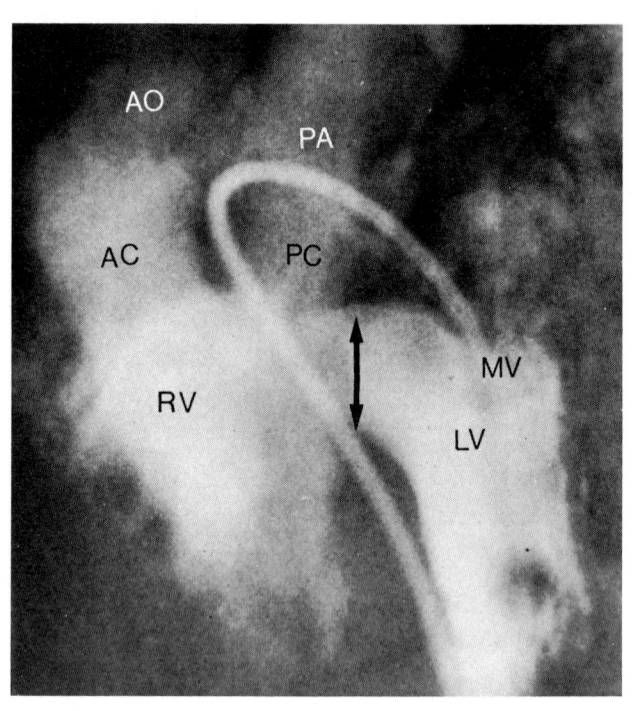

FIG 41–13.
Double-outlet right ventricle. Subpulmonary ventricular septal defect (Taussig-Bing heart). Left ventriculogram *(LV)*. Both great vessels are opacified through large ventricular septal defect *(black arrow)*. Aortic conus *(AC)* and pulmonary conus *(PC)* are demonstrated. Catheter passed through mitral valve *(MV)* is not in continuity with either semilunar valve. *AO* = aorta; *PA* = pulmonary artery; *RV* = right ventricle.

Doubly committed ventricular septal defect results in fairly equal opacification of both great vessels (Fig 41–14).

3. Double-outlet right ventricle should not be confused with complete transposition of the great vessels and bilateral coni in which case fibrous continuity between the mitral and pulmonary valves does not exist but the pulmonary artery arises exclusively from the left ventricle (Fig 41–15).

4. Double-outlet right ventricle should also not be confused with transposition of the aorta and biventricular origin of the pulmonary trunk (Fig 41–16). In this condition, mitral-pulmonary continuity exists and the pulmonary artery overrides the ventricular septal defect but does not arise from a conus, as in Taussig-Bing heart (Fig 41–17).

Aortography

Aortography is indicated to exclude coexistent patent ductus arteriosus, which often cannot be detected clinically. REASON: Because of pulmonary hypertension, the murmur of a patent ductus arteriosus is not heard.

Aortography should also be performed to exclude coarctation of the aorta, which is commonly present in dou-

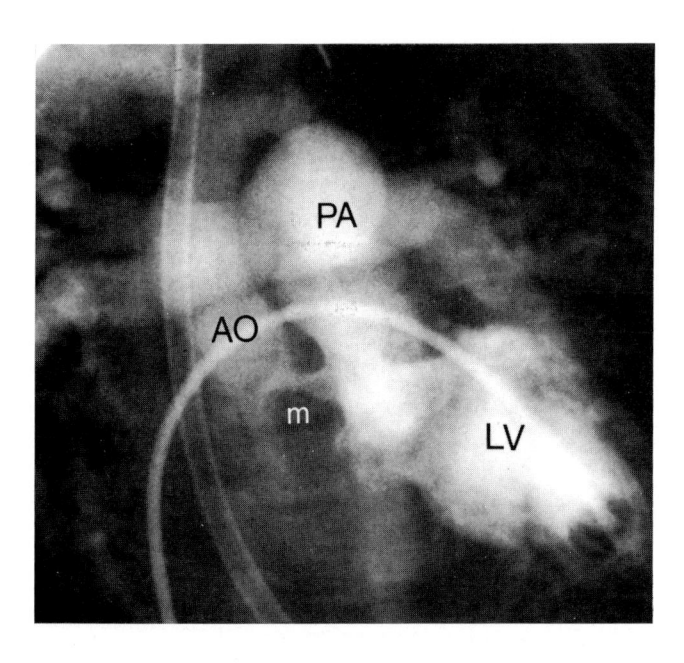

FIG 41–14.
Double-outlet right ventricle. Doubly committed ventricular septal defect. Left ventriculogram *(LV)*. Anteroposterior projection. Both great vessels opacify with same density (pulmonary artery slighty denser because it is much larger). Large muscle bundle *(m)* causes subaortic stenosis. *AO* = aorta; *PA* = pulmonary artery.

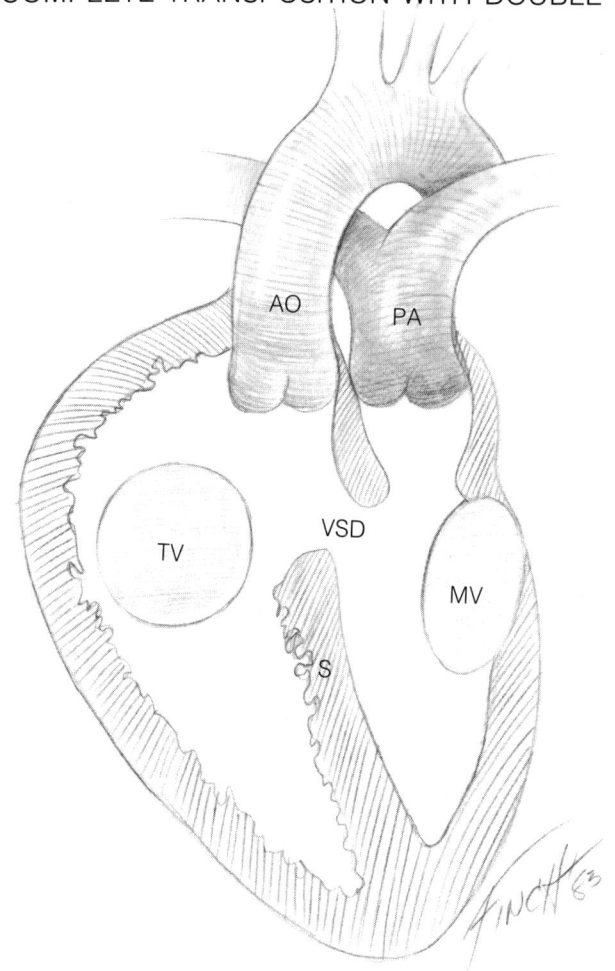

COMPLETE TRANSPOSITION WITH DOUBLE CONI

FIG 41–15.
Complete transposition with double coni. Aorta *(AO)* arises from conus of right ventricle and pulmonary artery *(PA)* from left ventricular conus. No fibrous continuity between pulmonary artery and mitral valve *(MV)*. Pulmonary valve is lower than aorta. *S* = interventricular septum; *TV* = tricuspid valve; *VSD* = ventricular septal defect.

BIVENTRICULAR ORIGIN OF PA

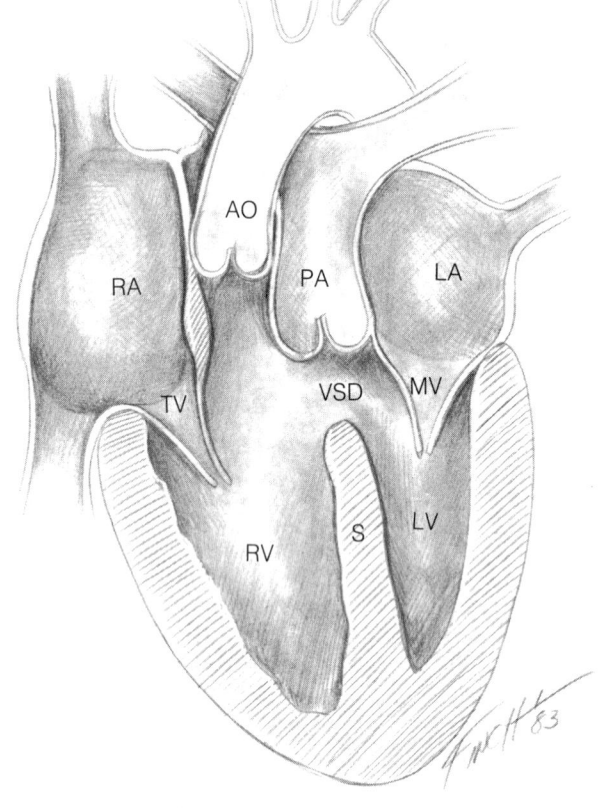

FIG 41–16.
Transposition of aorta with biventricular origin of pulmonary artery, which overrides ventricular septum. Fibrous continuity between mitral and pulmonary valve is present as in complete transposition. *AO* = aorta; *LA* = left atrium; *LV* = left ventricle; *MV* = mitral valve; *PA* = pulmonary artery; *RA* = right atrium; *RV* = right ventricle; *S* = interventricular septum; *TV* = tricuspid valve; *VSD* = ventricular septal defect.

DOUBLE OUTLET RV TAUSSIG—BING TYPE

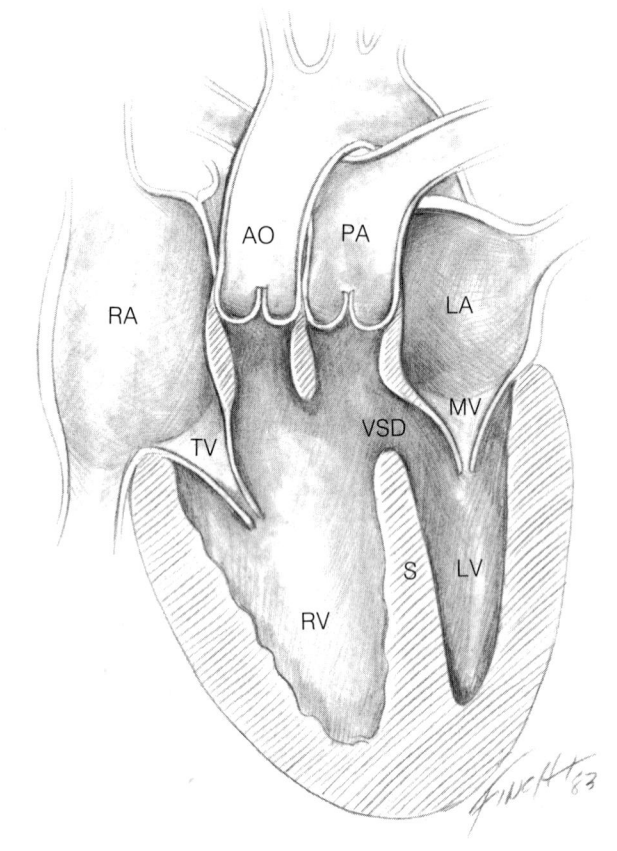

FIG 41–17.
Double-outlet right ventricle (Taussig-Bing heart). Both great vessels arise from separate coni, which are separated by conal septum. No mitral pulmonary artery continuity. Aortic and pulmonary valves are at same level. Typically ventricular septal defect is supracristal and subpulmonary. *AO* = aorta; *LA* = left atrium; *LV* = left ventricle; *MV* = mitral valve; *PA* = pulmonary artery; *RA* = right atrium; *RV* = right ventricle; *S* = interventricular septum; *TV* = tricuspid valve; *VSD* = ventricular septal defect.

ble-outlet right ventricle, particularly with a subpulmonary ventricular septal defect.

1. On the anteroposterior projection, the aortic valve lies in a plane higher than in the normal heart and at the level of the pulmonary valve (Figs 41–18 and 41–19). REASON: In double-outlet right ventricle, the aorta arises from a separate conus.
2. The plane of the aortic valve is more horizontal and lies slightly more toward the right than normal (see Fig 41–19). REASON: The aorta arises from the right ventricle in a position medial to the pulmonary artery. The aorta arises from a separate conus and does not curve posteriorly toward the left ventricle.
3. On the lateral projection, the aorta lies more anteriorly than normal, and the valve plane is tilted anteriorly (see Fig 41–19).
4. As in complete transposition of the great vessels, a right aortic arch is extremely rare except in the presence of associated pulmonary stenosis.

The angiographic demonstration of the coronary arterial pattern may be helpful in distinguishing between double-outlet right ventricle and complete transposition of the great vessels. The angiographic differentiation between the two may be difficult, particularly when there is biventricular origin of the pulmonary trunk. In complete transposition of the great vessels, the anterior aortic cusp is noncoronary, and both coronary arteries arise posteriorly, whereas in double-outlet right ventricle, the coronary arterial pattern is normal, with the right coronary artery arising from the anteriorly placed right cusp, the left coronary artery arising from the left cusp, and the posterior cusp is the

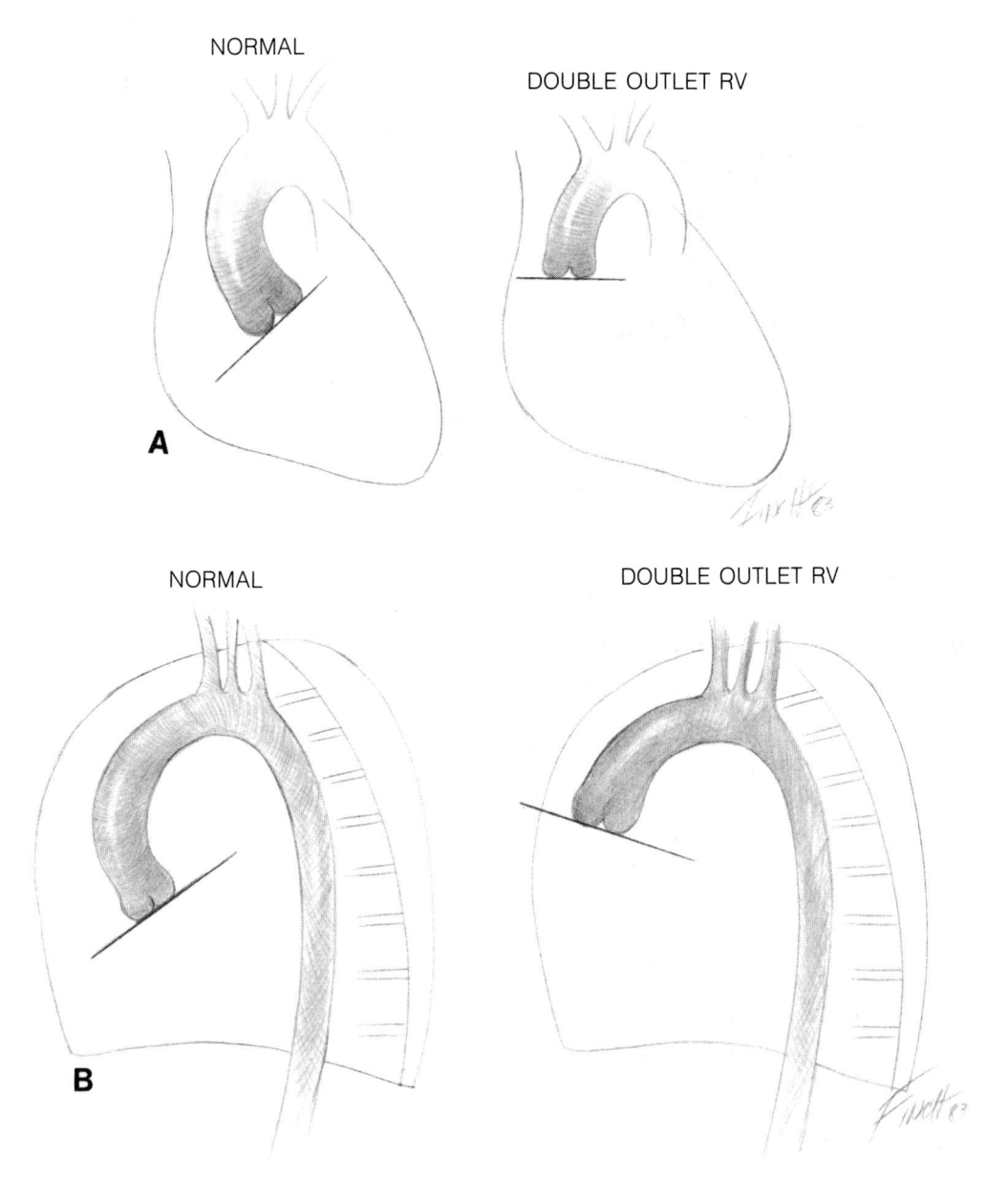

FIG 41–18.
Double-outlet right ventricle. Aortogram *(AO)*. **A,** anteroposterior and, **B,** lateral projections. Normal tilt of aortic valve plane is lost, and aorta is located more toward right and anteriorly.

noncoronary cusp. Rare exceptions exist. Variations such as single coronary artery or both coronary arteries arising above the same aortic cusp may be present as in a normal heart.

Unfortunately, the coronary arterial pattern is not uniform in double-outlet right ventricle; rarely, the coronary arterial pattern is identical to complete transposition of the great vessels (See Chapter 64).

OPERATIVE CONSIDERATIONS

Depending on the anatomy, various surgical options are viable:

1. Diverting the blood from the left ventricle into the pulmonary artery, to be followed by an atrial switch operation (Fig 41–20).

2. Diverting the blood from the left ventricle to the aorta by wide excision of the conal septum and insertion of a scimitar-shaped large patch (Fig 41–21).

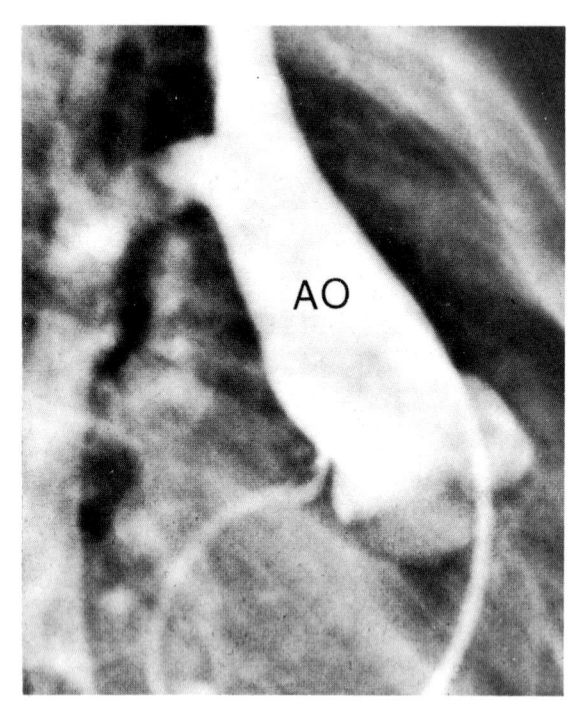

FIG 41–19.
Double-outlet right ventricle. Aortogram *(AO)*. Lateral projection. Anterior location and tilt of aortic valve plane.

3. Diverting the flow from the left ventricle into the pulmonary artery and performing an inflow switching operation (see Fig 41–20). (Both of the latter two options have the disadvantage that the conal septal spur is not removed. The potential complication is the development of subaortic or subpulmonary stenosis.)

4. Removing the truncoconal septum and diverting left ventricular blood flow via patch into the aorta (Fig 41–22).

5. Closing the tricuspid valve by patch, closing the pulmonary valve and performing a Fontan procedure (Fig 41–23). This operation is usually carried out in two stages. The first stage is a modified Glenn anastomosis of the superior vena cava to the right pulmonary artery (see Chapter 33).

The type of operation depends on the location of the defect and the presence of associated malformations. Among patients with subaortic ventricular septal defect, a tunnel is created along the posterior wall of the right ventricle between the ventricular septal defect and the subaortic conus (see Fig 41–22).[12–14] If the ventricular septal defect is restrictive, the defect can be enlarged anteriorly. If the tunnel seems to narrow the subpulmonary area, a right ventricular outflow tract patch can be placed or a conduit inserted (see Fig 41–22).

The timing of this operation varies. Some centers prefer to place a pulmonary artery band in infancy and perform corrective surgery when the child is older, whereas other centers correct the abnormality in infancy.

In patients with a subaortic ventricular septal defect and pulmonary stenosis, the repair of the defect is basically the same. The right ventricular outflow tract is repaired as in patients with tetralogy of Fallot. In some infants a palliative shunt is placed to delay a corrective procedure until the patient is older.

In patients with a subpulmonary ventricular septal defect, an interventricular patch is sewn, excluding the pulmonary artery from the right ventricle and directing left ventricular blood into the pulmonary artery. This creates a circulation-like complete transposition of the great vessels. Then an atrial baffle is inserted as in complete transposition of the great vessels (see Fig 41–20).

Depending on anatomy, it is also possible to excise the conal septum, which does not contain conduction system, and sew a patch from ventricular septal defect to the aorta similar to correction of tetralogy of Fallot (see Fig 41–21).

In double-outlet right ventricle with subaortic stenosis, an arterial switch operation such as the Damus-Kaye-Stensel procedure can be performed (see Fig 38–41).

POSTOPERATIVE RADIOGRAPHIC FEATURES

After correction of double-outlet right ventricle, cardiac size and pulmonary vasculature decrease just as after repair of any condition with increased pulmonary blood flow.

If a conduit has been inserted, it can be recognized by the radiopaque valve ring. Conduits in place for several years commonly show calcification. Another late complication is narrowing of the conduit by ingrowth of tissue, which results in stenosis. Replacement of the stenotic conduit is often needed. Finally, the porcine valve of the conduit may become rigid and calcified, resulting in either stenosis or insufficiency.

DOUBLE-OUTLET RIGHT VENTRICLE WITH PULMONARY STENOSIS

Among patients with tetralogy of Fallot there is a continuous spectrum of the position of the aorta in relation to the ventricular septum. This ranges from no overriding to maximal overriding of the aorta, a form that closely approaches double outlet with pulmonary stenosis. In this form the aorta arises from the right ventricle but not from a conus, and aortic-mitral continuity does not exist (see Fig 41–12). This form of double-outlet right ventricle

SURGICAL CORRECTION OF TAUSSIG-BING ANOMALY

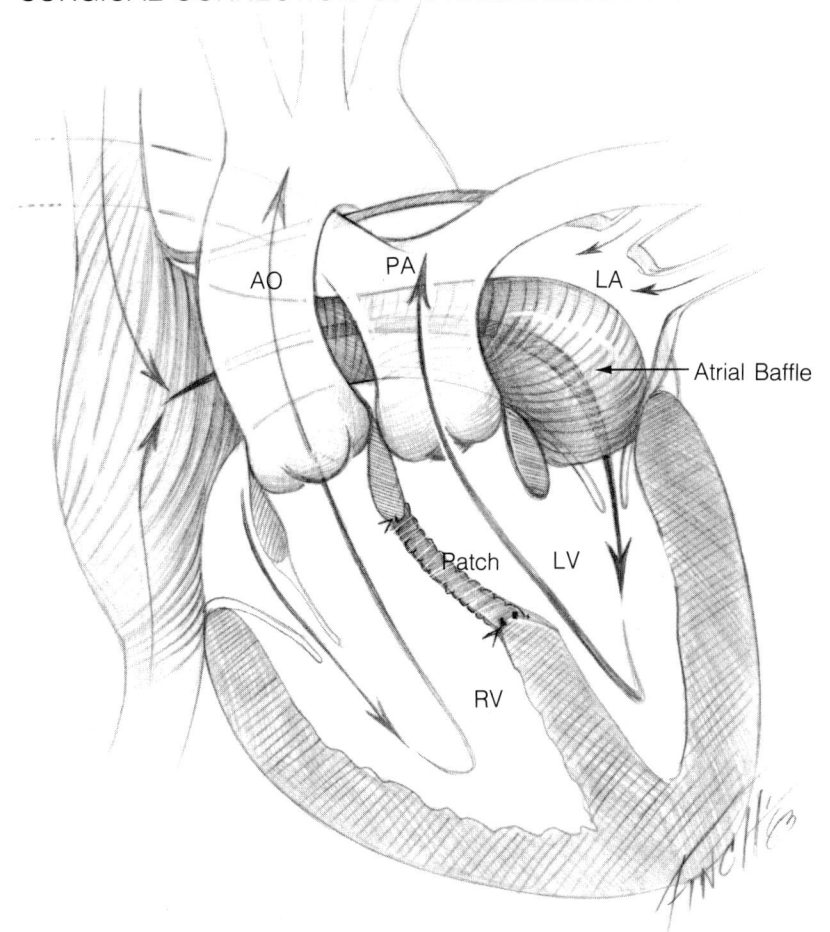

FIG 41–20.
Operative correction of double-outlet right ventricle with subpulmonary ventricular septal defect. Patch is placed so that left ventricular blood passes exclusively to pulmonary artery. Atrial baffle procedure is performed to switch venous inflows. AO = aorta; PA = pulmonary artery; LA = left atrium; LV = left ventricle; RV = right ventricle.

with pulmonary stenosis hemodynamically resembles tetralogy of Fallot and has identical radiographic findings. This form has to be distinguished angiographically from the usual type of double-outlet right ventricle in which the aorta arises from a separate infundibulum. The aorta does not arise from a conus, the aortic valve is located lower than the pulmonary valve, and a band of myocardial tissue does not separate the aortic and pulmonary outflow areas. The aortic valve is, however, separated from the mitral valve by muscular tissue. Operative correction is identical to the repair of tetralogy of Fallot.

COEXISTENT DOUBLE-OUTLET AND DOUBLE-INLET RIGHT VENTRICLE

Double-outlet right ventricle may rarely be associated with double-inlet right ventricle. Under those circumstances, the ventricular septal defect is located posteriorly, and the mitral valve straddles or overrides the ventricular septum. Left atrial blood enters not only the left ventricle but also the right ventricle (Fig 41–24).

TRANSPOSITION OF THE AORTA AND BIVENTRICULAR ORIGIN OF PULMONARY TRUNK

Transposition of the aorta and biventricular origin of the pulmonary trunk, a rare anomaly, is an intermediate anatomic form between complete transposition of the great vessels and double-outlet right ventricle with subpulmonary ventricular septal defect.[15, 16] In this condition, the aorta arises anteriorly from the right ventricle, and the pulmonary trunk straddles a ventricular septal defect (see Fig 41–16). Continuity exists between the pulmonary and mitral valves. Therefore, the aortic valve lies more cephalad than the pulmonary valve. The great vessels may be side by side, or the aorta slightly more anteriorly. Obstructive lesions may be present in the aortic outflow tract.

The hemodynamic and clinical features resemble double-outlet right ventricle with subpulmonary ventricular septal defect. It can be distinguished angiographically by identifying the valvar continuity on the left side of the heart, the low position of the pulmonary valve, and the overriding of the pulmonary trunk.

INTRAVENTRICULAR REPAIR OF TAUSSIG-BING ANOMALY WITH SIDE-BY-SIDE AORTA AND PULMONARY ARTERY

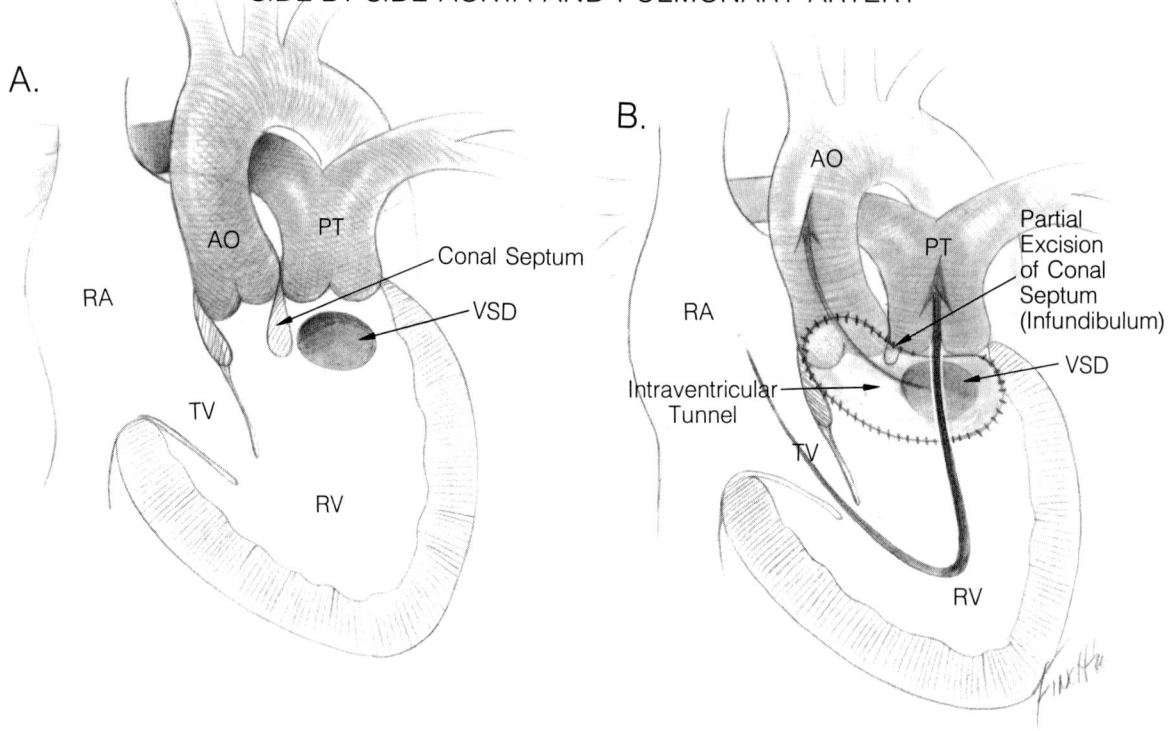

FIG 41–21.
Operative correction of double-outlet right ventricle by intraventricular patch. Truncoconal septum is partially excised, and patch is sewn from ventricular septal defect to aorta, directing fully saturated blood into aorta. Venous blood passes over patch into pulmonary artery. *AO* = aorta; *PT* = pulmonary trunk; *VSD* = ventricular septal defect; *RV* = right ventricle; *TV* = tricuspid valve; *RA* = right atrium.

SURGICAL CORRECTION OF DOUBLE OUTLET RIGHT VENTRICLE WITH SUB AORTIC V.S.D. AND SUB PULMONARY STENOSIS

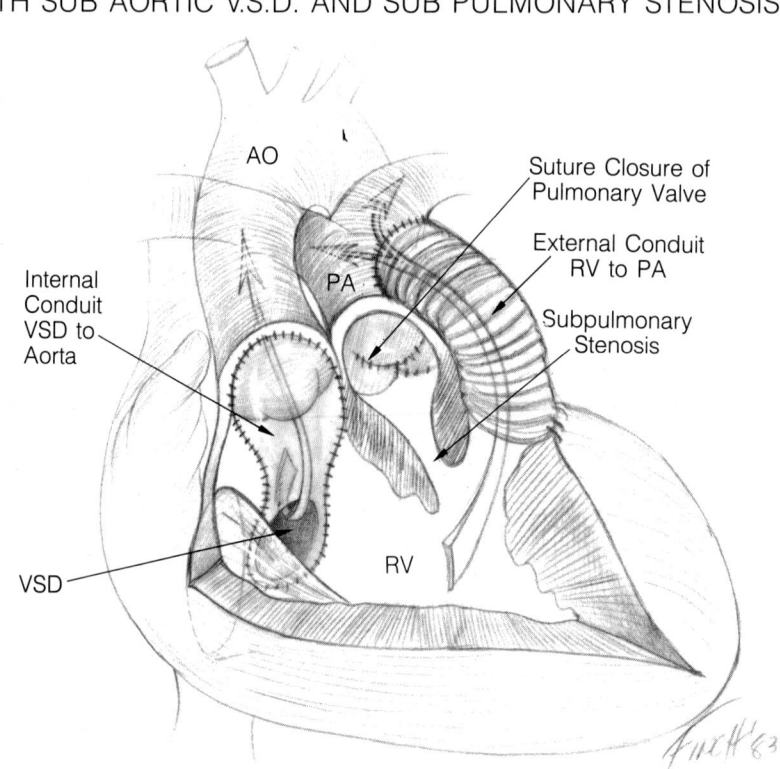

FIG 41–22.
Operative correction of double-outlet right ventricle with subaortic ventricular septal defect and subpulmonary stenosis. Intraventricular patch is sewn into right ventricle. Blood passing through ventricular septal defect *(VSD)* into aorta *(AO)*. Pulmonary valve is closed, and an external conduit is placed between right ventricle *(RV)* and pulmonary artery *(PA)*.

SURGICAL CORRECTION OF DOUBLE OUTLET RIGHT VENTRICLE

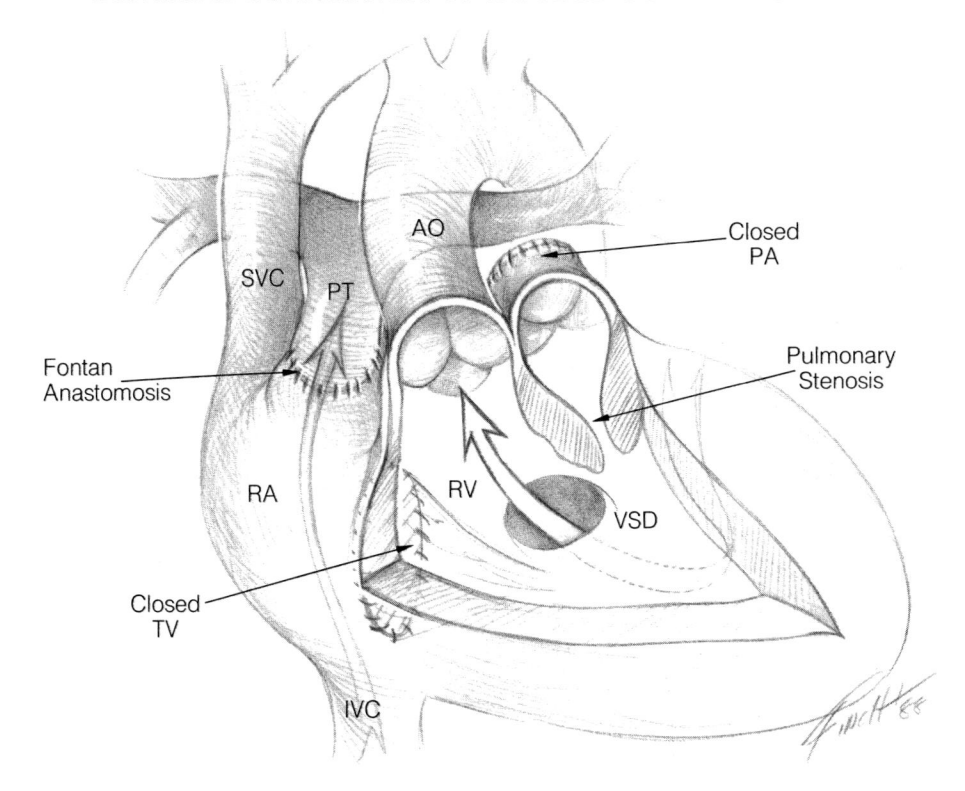

FIG 41–23.
Operative correction of double-outlet right ventricle, noncommitted ventricular septal defect, and subpulmonary stenosis. The tricuspid valve has been closed by patch. Pulmonary artery is closed and anastomosed to right atrium (Fontan procedure). Left ventricular blood passes to ventricular defect into aorta (arrow). PT = pulmonary trunk; AO = aorta; RV = right ventricle; IVC = inferior vena cava; SVC = superior vena cava; VSD = ventricular septal defect; RA = right atrium; TV = tricuspid valve; PA = pulmonary artery.

DOUBLE INLET RV
DOUBLE OUTLET RV

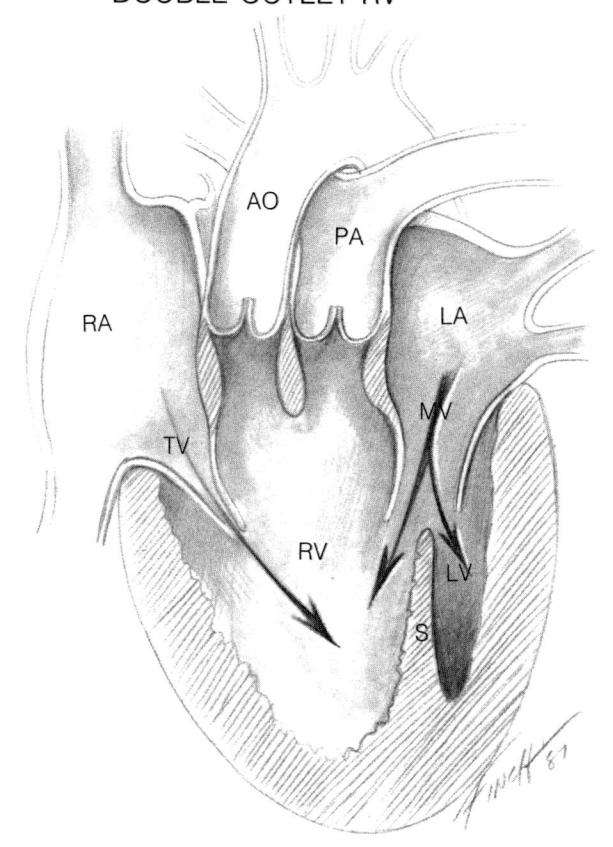

FIG 41–24.
Double inlet-double outlet right ventricle. Mitral valve straddles or overrides a posterior ventricular septal defect. Left ventricle tends to be smaller than normal. Both great vessels arise from right ventricle. AO = aorta; PA = pulmonary artery; LA = left atrium; MV = mitral valve; LV = left ventricle; S = interventricular septum; RV = right ventricle; TV = tricuspid valve; RA = right atrium.

DOUBLE-OUTLET SYSTEMIC VENTRICLE

Double-outlet systemic ventricle (discordant atrioventricular connection with double outlet, double-outlet right ventricle with corrected transposition, or origin of both great vessels from the inverted arterial ventricle) is also considered in Chapter 39.

Pathologic Anatomy

This anomaly is a variant of corrected transposition of the great vessels, because the ventricles are inverted. Both the aorta and pulmonary artery arise from the systemic ventricle, which in this condition has the morphologic details of a right ventricle. The pulmonary valve is not in continuity with the right (mitral) atrioventricular valve. There is always a ventricular septal defect through which the venous (anatomic left) ventricle empties. The location of the defect varies in relation to the crista supraventricularis, which is located in the systemic ventricle. The hemodynamics vary accordingly. The cardiac anomalies commonly present in corrected transposition of the great vessels may also coexist. The thoracic roentgenographic findings are identical to congenital corrected transposition of the great vessels (L-loop transposition).

Angiographic Features

1. Selected injection of the venous ventricle allows identification of the right atrioventricular (mitral) valve. The pulmonary valve is not in continuity with this atrioventricular valve.

2. The pulmonary valve lies in a higher than normal plane and at the same level as the aortic valve (see Fig 39–19).

3. Injection of the systemic ventricle shows simultaneous opacification of the aorta and the pulmonary artery.

4. The aorta lies to the left of the pulmonary artery, and on a lateral projection, they are superimposed.

5. The venous ventricle is smooth walled, whereas the systemic ventricle is heavily trabeculated. The plane of the ventricular septum lies perpendicular to the anterior thoracic wall.

DOUBLE-OUTLET LEFT VENTRICLE

Double-outlet left ventricle is a rare condition in which both great vessels arise either completely or almost exclusively from a morphologic left ventricle (Fig 41–25). This condition should not be confused with double-outlet inverted right ventricle, which is a variant of congenital corrected transposition of the great vessels, in which the morphologic right ventricle is inverted and located along the left side of the heart.

Although double-outlet left ventricle has been reported with atrioventricular discordance, in most patients atrioventricular concordance is present.[17–19] A ventricular septal defect has been reported in all but one case (Fig 41–26).[20] The defect is usually located below the aortic valve and has characteristics of the ventricular septal defect of tetralogy of Fallot. The defect may also be subpulmonary, committed to both great vessels, or remote.

The position of the great vessels is variable. The aorta is usually located to the right of the pulmonary artery and may be either anterior or posterior to it.[17] Both great vessels may override the ventricular septal defect and contribute to the upper margin of the defect. This occurs if the conal septum is deficient between the aorta and pulmonary artery.

Conal anatomy is variable, usually the subaortic conus is absent, and there is a stenotic subpulmonary conus. Pulmonary stenosis, either valvar or subvalvar, is present in most patients.

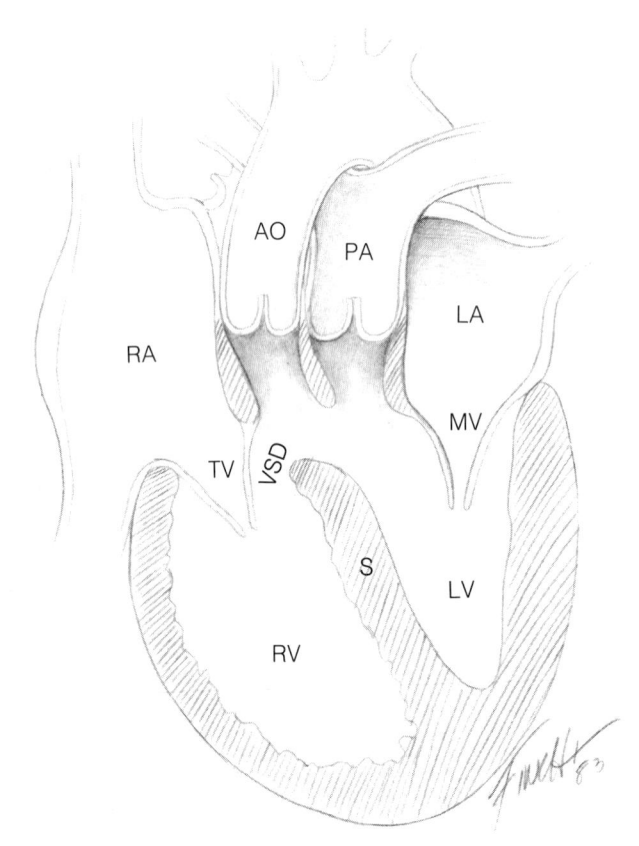

FIG 41–25.
Double-outlet left ventricle. Both aorta and pulmonary artery arise to left of ventricular septum and above ventricular septal defect. *AO* = aorta; *PA* = pulmonary artery; *LA* = left atrium; *MV* = mitral valve; *LV* = left ventricle; *S* = interventricular septum; *RV* = right ventricle; *VSD* = ventricular septal defect; *TV* = tricuspid valve; *RA* = right atrium.

DOUBLE OUTLET LV WITH INTACT SEPTUM

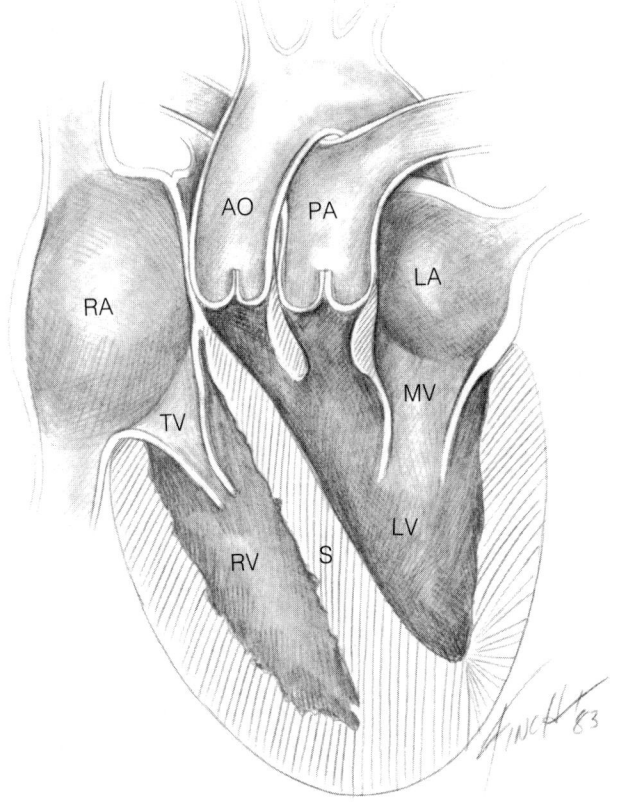

FIG 41–26.
Double-outlet left ventricle with intact ventricular septum. Right ventricle not connected to a great vessel. Blood exits right ventricle through either tricuspid regurgitation or myocardial sinusoids. *AO* = aorta; *PA* = pulmonary artery; *LA* = left atrium; *MV* = mitral valve; *LV* = left ventricle; *S* = interventricular septum; *RV* = right ventricle; *TV* = tricuspid valve; *RA* = right atrium.

Anomalies of the tricuspid valve occur commonly and include tricuspid stenosis, atresia, straddling, and Ebstein's malformation.[17] Double-outlet left ventricle also may occur in patients with either situs inversus or situs ambiguous.

Hemodynamics

The hemodynamic patterns resemble those of double-outlet right ventricle and depend on the relationship of the ventricular septal defect to the great vessels and the presence of pulmonary stenosis. Because most patients have pulmonary stenosis, the resultant hemodynamics resemble tetralogy of Fallot. In the occasional patient without pulmonary stenosis, the hemodynamics resemble isolated ventricular septal defect, and congestive cardiac failure may develop.

Clinical Features

The clinical features resemble those of double-outlet right ventricle and vary in a similar way according to the presence of pulmonary stenosis and the location of the ventricular septal defect in relation to the aorta. Most patients in the neonatal period or in infancy have a murmur, cyanosis (if pulmonary stenosis coexists), or cardiac failure (if pulmonary stenosis is not present). The murmur is loud, and often the second heart sound appears single.

Electrocardiographic Features

Very few electrocardiograms have been described. Usually the QRS axis is normal. Biventricular hypertrophy may be found as in double-outlet right ventricle.

Echocardiographic Features

Although we are aware of no reports of echocardiographic findings in double-outlet left ventricle, the imaging analysis follows the anatomy.

Radiographic Features

There are no characteristic features that allow the diagnosis of double-outlet left ventricle from analysis of thoracic roentgenograms. Usually cardiac size is normal, and pulmonary vasculature is either normal or decreased. REASON: Most patients with double-outlet left ventricle have associated pulmonary stenosis, and, consequently, the hemodynamic features resemble tetralogy of Fallot.

Cardiac Catheterization

The pressures in the right and left ventricles are equal. A gradient may be found across the pulmonary valve. A right-to-left shunt is present at the ventricular level, and a left-to-right shunt is also present if pulmonary stenosis is not present.

Angiographic Features

Right and left ventriculography, particularly in the left anterior oblique position, are required to establish the diagnosis of double-outlet left ventricle.[19] Attempts must be made to outline both the conal septum on end and the edge of the ventricular septal defect.

1. In a shallow left anterior oblique projection, both great arteries opacify densely from the left ventricle and before the right ventricle is filled through a ventricular septal defect (Fig 41–27).
2. There is almost invariably a stenotic subpulmonary conus. The ventricular septal defect is located immediately below the aorta, as in cases of tetralogy of Fallot.

DOUBLE OUTLET LV

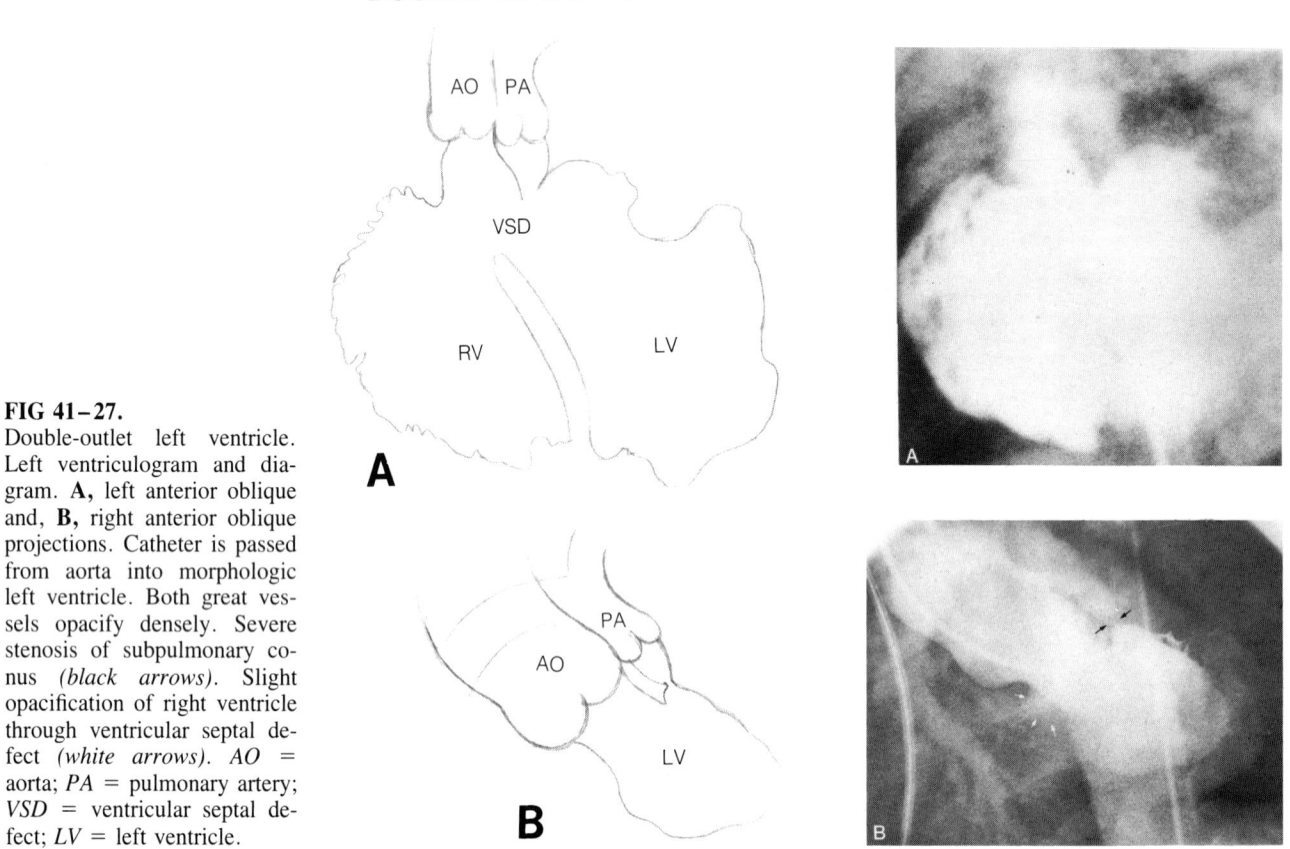

FIG 41-27.
Double-outlet left ventricle. Left ventriculogram and diagram. **A,** left anterior oblique and, **B,** right anterior oblique projections. Catheter is passed from aorta into morphologic left ventricle. Both great vessels opacify densely. Severe stenosis of subpulmonary conus *(black arrows)*. Slight opacification of right ventricle through ventricular septal defect *(white arrows)*. *AO* = aorta; *PA* = pulmonary artery; *VSD* = ventricular septal defect; *LV* = left ventricle.

3. In the left anterior oblique projection, the ventricular septum is located to the right of the origin of both the aorta and pulmonary artery. This indicates that both great arteries arise from the left ventricle (see Fig 41-27).

Operative Considerations

Operative treatment depends on the number, size, and location of ventricular septal defects and the interrelationship between the aorta and pulmonary artery.[17, 21] Usually at operation, the ventricular septal defect can be closed so left ventricular blood passes into the aorta. In these cases a conduit is then placed between the right ventricle and the pulmonary artery to circumvent the pulmonary stenosis.

In patients without pulmonary stenosis, the ventricular septal defect may be closed in such a fashion so that the right ventricle is connected to the pulmonary artery and left ventricle to the aorta.

If there is a subaortic ventricular septal defect and pulmonary stenosis can be relieved internally, the defect may be closed, leaving the pulmonary artery arising from the left ventricle and the aorta connected to the right ventricle, thus converting the circulation to that of complete transposition of the great vessels. Then an atrial baffle procedure is performed to correct the circulation.

SUMMARY

1. Double-outlet right ventricle is also called origin of both great vessels from the right ventricle. Both great arteries arise from the morphologic right ventricle, and the mitral valve and the aortic and pulmonary valve are not in continuity (see Fig 41-1).
   a. Double-outlet right ventricle is almost invariably associated with a ventricular septal defect (see Fig 41-1).
   b. The location of the ventricular septal defect varies. It may be related to the aorta, to both great vessels, to the pulmonary artery, or to neither great vessel (see Fig 41-3).
   c. Taussig-Bing complex is a specific type of double-outlet right ventricle with two coni and a supracristal ventricular septal defect located beneath the pulmonary valve (see Fig 41-18).
   d. Double-outlet right ventricle with intact ventricular septum rarely occurs. Blood leaves the left ventricle through either mitral regurgitation or myocardial sinusoids. The left ventricle is hypoplastic in these cases.
2. Transposition of the aorta and biventricular origin of the pulmonary artery (see Fig 41-17). In this form of

transposition, the pulmonary artery is located immediately above a ventricular septal defect and overrides the interventricular septum to a varying degree. This type of transposition differs from the Taussig-Bing heart in that the pulmonary artery does not arise from a conus and the pulmonary and mitral valves are in continuity. Cases in which the pulmonary artery overrides the ventricular septum by more than 50% are sometimes classified as double-outlet right ventricle.
3. Double-outlet left ventricle is a very rare condition that is almost always associated with a ventricular septal defect and usually subpulmonary stenosis. Both great vessels arise from a morphologic left ventricle, and the ventricular septal defect is commonly located beneath the aorta in a position resembling tetralogy of Fallot (see Fig 41–25).
   a. Double-outlet left ventricle with intact ventricular septum has been reported once and was associated with tricuspid regurgitation (see Fig 41–26).
4. Each of these types of double-outlet right or left ventricle may occur with situs inversus.
5. Double-outlet inverted right ventricle may occur. Although equivalents of the various types of double-outlet ventricle could occur theoretically with discordant atrioventricular connection (ventricular inversion with transposition, corrected transposition, L-loop transposition), only double-outlet inverted right ventricle has been reported. In this situation, both great vessels arise from an inverted morphologic right ventricle, which is the systemic ventricle. Neither great vessel is in continuity with the right (mitral) atrioventricular valve (see Fig 41–3).

REFERENCES

1. Neufeld HN, DuShane JW, Wood EH, et al: Origin of both great vessels from the right ventricle: I, without pulmonary stenosis, *Circulation* 23:399, 1961.
2. Neufeld HN, Lucas RV Jr, Lester RG, et al: Origin of both great vessels from the right ventricle without pulmonary stenosis, *Br Heart J* 24:393, 1962.
3. Zamora R, Moller JH, Edwards JE: Double-outlet right ventricle: anatomic types and associated anomalies, *Chest* 68:672, 1975.
4. Sridaromont S, Ritter DG, Feldt RH, et al: Double-outlet right ventricle: anatomic and angiocardiographic correlations, *Mayo Clin Proc* 53:555, 1978.
5. Hightower BM, Barcia A, Bargeron LM Jr, et al: Double-outlet right ventricle with transposed great arteries and subpulmonary ventricular septal defect: the Taussig-Bing malformation, *Circulation* 39 and 40(suppl I):207, 1969.
6. Ainger LE: Double-outlet right ventricle: intact ventricular septum, mitral stenosis, and blind left ventricle, *Am Heart J* 70:521, 1965.
7. Davachi F, Moller JH, Edwards JE: Origin of both great vessels from right ventricle with intact ventricular septum, *Am Heart J* 75:790, 1968.
8. Lincoln C, Anderson RH, Shinebourne EA, et al: Double outlet right ventricle with l-malposition of the aorta, *Br Heart J* 37:453, 1975.
9. Sondheimer HM, Freedom RM, Olley PM: Double outlet right ventricle: clinical spectrum and prognosis, *Am J Cardiol* 39:709, 1977.
10. Hagler DJ, Tajik AJ, Seward JB, et al: Double-outlet right ventricle; wide-angle two-dimensional echocardiographic observations, *Circulation* 63:419, 1981.
11. DiSessa TG, Hagan AD, Pope C, et al: Two dimensional echocardiographic characteristics of double outlet right ventricle, *Am J Cardiol* 44:1146, 1979.
12. Stewart RW, Kirklin JW, Pacifico AD, et al: Repair of double-outlet right ventricle: an analysis of 62 cases, *J Thorac Cardiovasc Surg* 78:502, 1979.
13. Gomes MMR, Weidman WH, McGoon DC, et al: Double-outlet right ventricle without pulmonic stenosis: surgical considerations and results of operation, *Circulation* 43 and 44(suppl I):31, 1971.
14. Kirklin JK, Castaneda AR: Surgical correction of double-outlet right ventricle with noncommitted ventricular septal defect, *J Thorac Cardiovasc Surg* 73:399, 1977.
15. Elliott LP, Adams P Jr, Levy MJ, et al: Right ventricular aorta and biventricular pulmonary trunk, an uncommon form of transposition, *Am J Cardiol* 66:478, 1963.
16. Beuren A: Differential diagnosis of the Taussig-Bing heart from complete transposition of the great vessels with a posteriorly overriding pulmonary artery, *Circulation* 21:1071, 1960.
17. Bharati S, Lev M, Stewart R, et al: The morphological spectrum of double outlet left ventricle and its surgical significance, *Circulation* 58:558, 1978.
18. Coto EO, Jimenez MQ, Castaneda AR, et al: Double outlet from chamber of left ventricular morphology, *Br Heart J* 42:15, 1979.
19. Brandt PWT, Calder AL, Barratt-Boyes BG, et al: Double outlet left ventricle: morphology, cineangiocardiographic diagnosis and surgical treatment, *Am J Cardiol* 38:897, 1976.
20. Paul MH, Muster AJ, Sinha SN, et al: Double-outlet left ventricle with an intact ventricular septum: clinical and autopsy diagnosis and developmental implications, *Circulation* 41:129, 1970.
21. Pacifico AD, Kirklin JW, Bargeron LM Jr, et al: Surgical treatment of double-outlet left ventricle: report of four cases, *Circulation* 48(suppl III):19, 1973.

CHAPTER 42

Single Ventricle

Single ventricle has long been of interest to anatomists and pathologists and with the past 20 years has held considerable interest to cardiologists and surgeons as well, because operative treatment has become available. Although an uncommon condition, it has sparked extensive discussions in the past decade. These discussions have related to nomenclature and to basic anatomic definitions, such as what a ventricle is.[1-3] The interested reader is referred to other sources for information about these controversial issues. A number of terms have been used to describe the condition or its variants, such as single ventricle, common ventricle, rudimentary ventricle, cor triloculare biatriatum, single ventricle with rudimentary outflow chamber, double-inlet ventricle. These names reflect an anatomic focus on the ventricular structure. In contrast, clinicians and surgeons are interested in the coexistent conditions present in almost all cases. The associated anomalies result in a variety of clinical and laboratory features and require various operative approaches. Thus, although the ventricular anatomy provides a unifying theme for this chapter, the clinical and radiographic features are diverse.

We choose to distinguish single ventricle from univentricular heart, a term used to describe hearts in which one ventricular chamber receives the entire venous return to the heart. This category includes tricuspid atresia and mitral atresia. We prefer to consider them separately because of the unique clinical and laboratory findings. Thus, in this chapter, some of the hearts classified by others as univentricular heart are discussed.

PATHOLOGIC ANATOMY

The hearts discussed in this chapter have double-inlet atrioventricular connection. This connection may be through either two separate or a common atrioventricular valve (Fig 42–1). The separate valves are usually patent, but rarely one may be represented as an imperforate membrane. Because in single ventricle the anatomic features of the two atrioventricular valves do not allow distinction between mitral or tricuspid valve, they are referred to as left and right atrioventricular valves, respectively. With a definition of single ventricle possessing a common or two distinct atrioventricular valves, mitral atresia and tricuspid atresia are excluded. These latter two conditions do possess many morphologic similarities to single ventricle but are discussed elsewhere (see Chapters 33 and 51), because they each have distinctive and well-described hemodynamic and clinical features. Likewise, there are similarities between single ventricle and straddling atrioventricular valves, which are also discussed in a separate chapter (see Chapter 44). Single ventricle, straddling atrioventricular valve, and atretic atrioventricular valve are often considered as points on a continuum.

Single ventricle has been subdivided on the basis of ventricular morphology, origin of the great vessels, and associated malformations.[4, 5] Three morphologic forms of single ventricle are well recognized (Fig 42–2):

1. Left ventricular type, usually with a rudimentary chamber right ventricle. This, the most frequent type (75%), was classed as type A by Van Praagh, or called "double-inlet left ventricle." The single ventricle has morphologic features of a left ventricle. A small rudimentary chamber is present as well, and separated from the single ventricle by a trabecular septum. These two chambers communicate through a bulboventricular foramen. The small chamber is believed to represent a rudimentary right ventricle, but it lacks the sinus portion and is principally the right ventricular infundibulum. The rudimentary chamber lies anteriorly and may be located to either the right or left. In 90% of left ventricular–type single ventricle, transposition of the great vessels coexists, and outflow obstruction is frequent.

2. Right ventricular type, usually with a rudimentary chamber of left ventricular type (20%). This is Van

A-V CONNECTION MODE IN UNIVENTRICULAR HEART

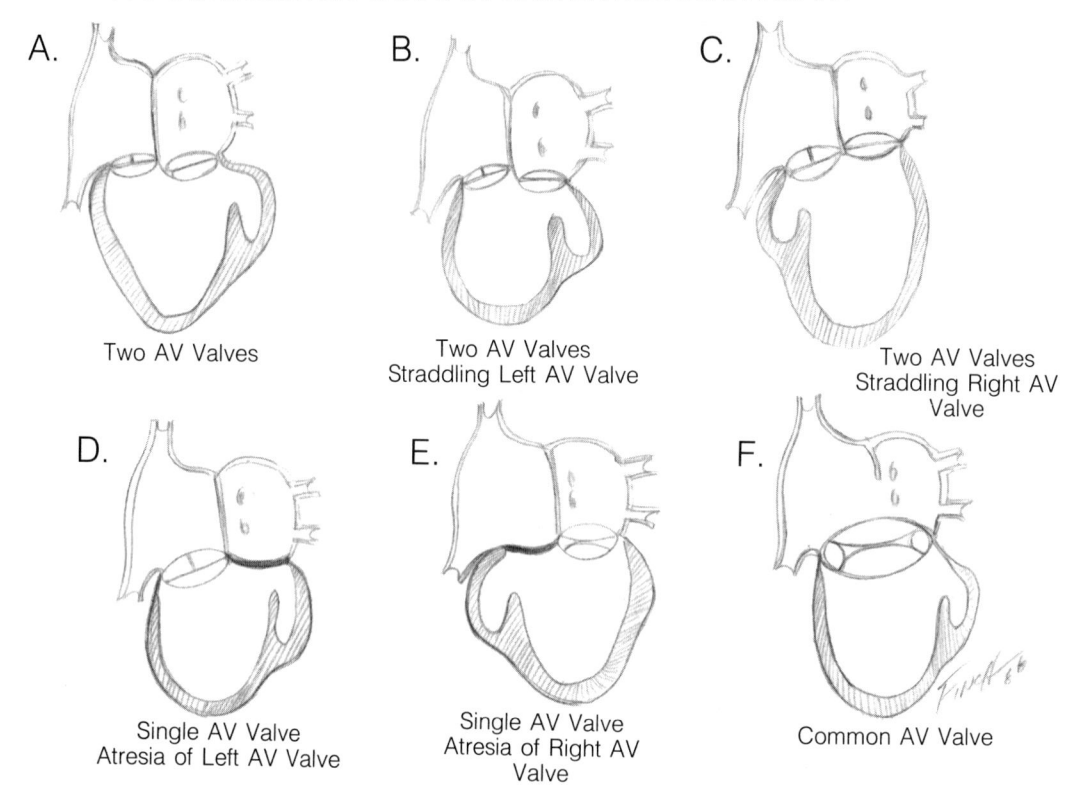

A. Two AV Valves

B. Two AV Valves Straddling Left AV Valve

C. Two AV Valves Straddling Right AV Valve

D. Single AV Valve Atresia of Left AV Valve

E. Single AV Valve Atresia of Right AV Valve

F. Common AV Valve

FIG 42–1.
Type of atrioventricular connection in univentricular heart. **A,** two atrioventricular *(AV)* valves connecting to single ventricle. **B,** two atrioventricular valves with straddling of left atrioventricular valve. **C,** two atrioventricular valves with straddling right atrioventricular valve. **D,** single atrioventricular valve and atresia of left atrioventricular valve. **E,** Single atrioventricular valve and atresia of right atrioventricular valve. **F,** common atrioventricular valve.

Praagh's type B, or double-inlet right ventricle.[6,7] The morphologic features of the single ventricle resemble those of a right ventricle in having coarse trabeculations. A rudimentary chamber (left ventricle) is located posteriorly. The size of this chamber varies from being hypoplastic to only a tiny slit. Straddling of the atrioventricular valves is common. Double outlet from the single ventricle is usually present, with each great vessel arising from an infundibulum.

3. Indeterminate type (5%). In this form, there are morphologic features of neither a left nor a right ventricle, and a rudimentary chamber is not present. The relationship of the great vessels is extremely variable, but usually the aorta is anterior.

In each type of single ventricle, the great vessel connections are variable.

1. Concordant, with the pulmonary artery arising from the rudimentary chamber and the aorta from the single ventricle (Fig 42–3).
2. Discordant with the aorta arising from the rudimentary chamber, and the pulmonary artery from the single ventricle (transposition) (Fig 42–4).
3. Double outlet from either the single ventricle or the rudimentary chamber.
4. Single outlet such as occurs in coexistent truncus arteriosus, aortic atresia, or pulmonary atresia.

Transposition of the great vessels is present in 85% of patients. The aorta may be located either anteriorly and to the right (D-transposition) or anteriorly and to the left (L-transposition).

Outflow obstruction to either great vessel is frequently present, and its severity varies widely. For instance, pulmonary stenosis may be mild, or there may be pulmonary atresia. Furthermore, stenotic lesions tend to progress. Obstruction to pulmonary blood flow may be related to narrowing of the bulboventricular foramen (in concordant great vessels), to valvar pulmonary stenosis, perhaps with a hypoplastic pulmonary annulus, or subpulmonary stenosis. Coarctation and interruption of the aortic arch occur more commonly when the aorta arises from the rudimen-

TYPES OF SINGLE VENTRICLES

INFUNDIBULAR INVERSION

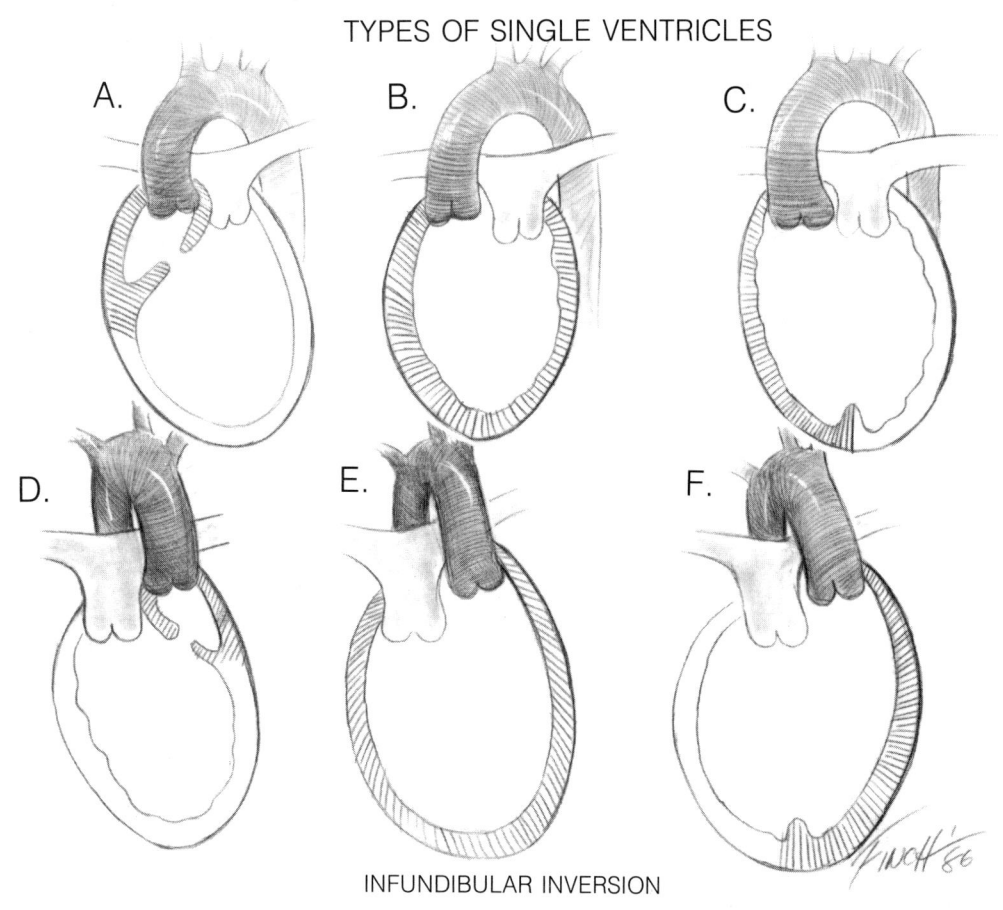

FIG 42–2.
Types of single ventricle: right ventricular musculature shaded. D-malposition (**A, B,** and **C**) and L-malposition (**D, E,** and **F**). **A** and **D,** single ventricle of left ventricular type. Subaortic area represents rudimentary right ventricle. **B** and **E,** single ventricle of right ventricular type. **C** and **F,** single ventricle of intermediate type. Morphologic features of neither right nor left ventricles.

tary chamber (transposition) and the bulboventricular foramen is narrowed, which in itself causes obstruction to systemic blood flow.

Anomalies of atrioventricular valves are common and include atresia, straddling, stenotic, or regurgitant valves.

The atria may show features of situs solitus, situs inversus, or atrial isomerism, either right or left. Particularly in types of isomerism, anomalies of systemic or pulmonary venous connection are found.

HEMODYNAMICS

The entire systemic and entire pulmonary venous returns flow into the single ventricle. Blood is ejected from the single ventricle into the aorta and pulmonary artery, depending on the relative resistances to flow. The resistance to flow is governed by the status of the pulmonary and systemic arteriolar beds and anatomic lesions in the respective outflow areas or great arteries. As in other admixture lesions, arterial oxygen desaturation is present. Four factors influence aortic oxygen saturation: (1) volume of systemic blood flow, (2) mixed venous oxygen saturation, (3) pulmonary venous oxygen saturation, and (4) volume of pulmonary blood flow. The first three factors are relatively constant, so that the major determinant of aortic oxygen saturation is the volume of pulmonary blood flow.

An inverse relationship exists between the volume of pulmonary blood flow and the degree of cyanosis. This principle is illustrated in patients with single ventricle without anatomic outflow obstructive lesions. In the neonatal period, pulmonary vascular resistance is elevated; thus, pulmonary blood flow is limited. With the normal maturation of the pulmonary arterioles, pulmonary vascular resistance declines, pulmonary blood flow increases, and cyanosis lessens. Conditions such as coexistent coarctation of the aorta or stenosis of the bulboventricular foramen limit systemic blood flow and increase the pulmonary blood flow. Similarly, pulmonary or subpulmonary stenosis reduces pulmonary blood flow.

HOLMES HEART

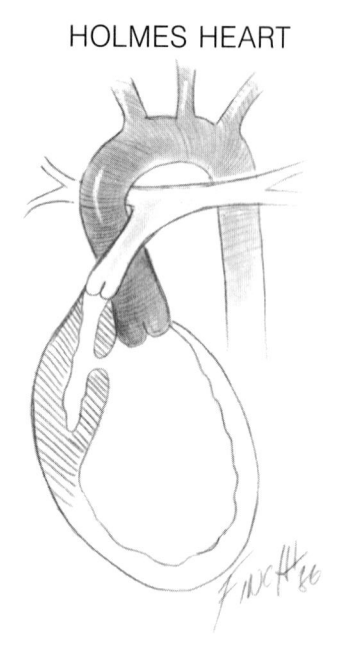

FIG 42-3.
Single ventricle with normally related great vessels (Holmes' heart). Pulmonary artery fills from rudimentary chamber.

Congestive cardiac failure can occur among patients with single ventricle. The usual reason is volume overload of the ventricle, which is caused by excessive pulmonary blood flow, but it may also develop from atrioventricular valvular insufficiency. On occasion, cardiac failure develops in patients who have undergone pulmonary arterial banding and develop stenosis of the bulboventricular foramen.[9, 10] In this situation, a pressure gradient is found across each outflow area, and the pressure in the single ventricle becomes suprasystemic.

CLINICAL FEATURES

The clinical features of patients with single ventricle can generally be divided into two categories, which depend on the volume of pulmonary blood flow.

Patients without obstruction to pulmonary blood flow resemble those with a large left-to-right shunt at the ventricular level. Symptoms of congestive cardiac failure appear early in infancy (as pulmonary vascular resistance declines). Dyspnea, frequent respiratory tract infections, slow growth, and easy fatiguability during feeding are present. Cyanosis is prominent in the neonatal period but lessens as the pulmonary vascular resistance falls.

On physical examination, the infant is small for age and minimally cyanotic. Features of congestive cardiac failure, tachypnea, tachycardia, and hepatomegaly are present. Frequently there is a precordial bulge. The first heart sound is normal, and the second heart sound is usually single and loud, because of the anterior position of the transposed aorta. There is often a thrill, associated with a grade 2 to 4/6 long systolic murmur. A middiastolic murmur is present at the cardiac apex, reflecting the large volume of blood flow across the mitral valve.

Some of these patients have severe cardiac failure in the neonatal period because of a coexistent coarctation or interruption of the aorta. The pulmonary blood flow is more increased in these patients than in those without aortic obstruction. A blood pressure differential is found between arms and legs.

The signs and symptoms are more variable among those individuals with pulmonary outflow obstruction but tend to increase in severity, because the stenosis usually progresses with age. If stenosis is severe or there is pulmonary atresia, intense cyanosis develops in the neonatal pe-

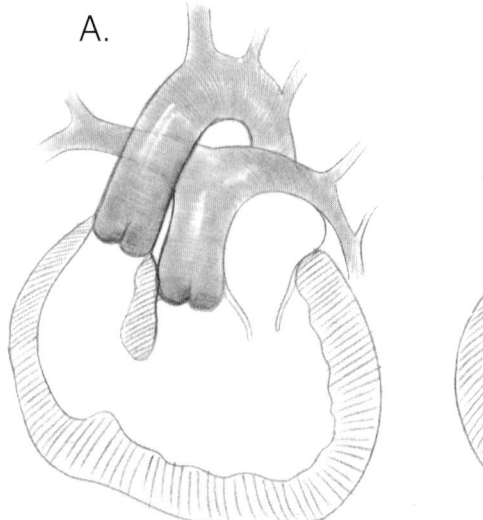

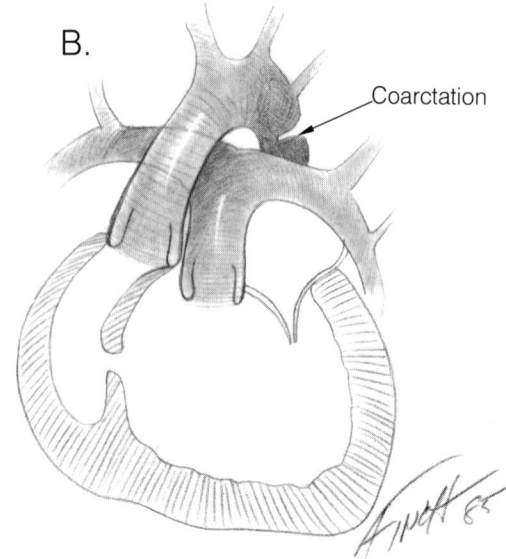

FIG 42-4.
Single ventricle and transposition of great vessels. Aorta arises from rudimentary chamber. **A**, large bulboventricular foramen. **B**, narrowed bulboventricular foramen. Coarctation of aorta associated.

riod as the ductus arteriosus closes. In the latter patients there may be either no murmur or a continuous murmur of a patent ductus arteriosus. In individuals with less severe stenosis, an ejection systolic murmur, which may be prominent, is present over the back in those with coexistent transposition of the great vessels because the pulmonary artery is located posteriorly. Neither congestive cardiac failure nor cardiomegaly is found in these patients.

ELECTROCARDIOGRAPHIC FEATURES

The electrocardiographic QRS patterns described in single ventricle are variable.[11] The picture is confusing because the electrocardiograms have been described in relation to the position of the great vessels and not the ventricular anatomy. The location of the conduction tissue varies according to the ventricular anatomy.[12, 13] In most patients the initial QRS forces are directed abnormally and not rightward and anteriorly; therefore, q waves are not found in the left precordial leads.

The precordial leads show a pattern of right ventricular hypertrophy, left ventricular hypertrophy, tall isodiphasic RS, or an rS across the precordial leads. The QRS axis may be directed leftward, or superiorly (in cases with a common atrioventricular valve), or rightward.

Patterns of atrial enlargement may be present, reflecting associated cardiac conditions. Left atrial enlargement may be present in patients with left atrioventricular valve insufficiency or long-standing increased pulmonary blood flow. Right atrial enlargement may be found in patients with right atrioventricular valvar insufficiency or pulmonary stenosis.

ECHOCARDIOGRAPHIC FEATURES[14-17]

Echocardiographic studies provide important information in the study of patients with single ventricle, particularly regarding the relationship of atrioventricular valves and the ventricular chamber. A septum is not found in the ventricular chamber, and no septum separates the atrioventricular valves. The outflow chamber can be demonstrated and the position of great vessels located. With Doppler techniques, turbulence across outflow areas can be identified and gradients estimated. Doppler techniques are valuable in identifying atrioventricular valvar insufficiency.

Similar to Doppler, contrast echocardiography is very helpful. After injection into a systemic vein, the microbubbles pass through an atrioventricular valve and fill the entire ventricular cavity.

RADIOGRAPHIC FEATURES

The correct diagnosis of single ventricle cannot be suggested from thoracic roentgenograms. REASON: The internal architecture of the ventricle can be identified only by the injection of contrast medium.

The roentgenographic findings of single ventricle with D-transposition are identical to those of complete transposition of the great vessels.[18] In these instances there is cardiomegaly with a narrow superior mediastinum (see Chapter 38). The appearance of common ventricle with L-transposition is identical to congenital corrected transposition of the great vessels. In these patients the upper left cardiac border may show a distinct bulge because of the origin of the aorta from the left aspect of the heart (see Chapter 39). Rarely, along the left cardiac border a small notch may be seen that marks the demarcation between the rudimentary (outflow) chamber and the common ventricle (Fig 42–5).

Patients without pulmonary stenosis have pulmonary hypertension, increased pulmonary vascular markings, and markedly enlarged pulmonary arteries (Fig 42–6).

In patients with pulmonary stenosis, depending on the degree of the obstruction, the pulmonary vasculature may be either normal or decreased (Fig 42–7). If pulmonary

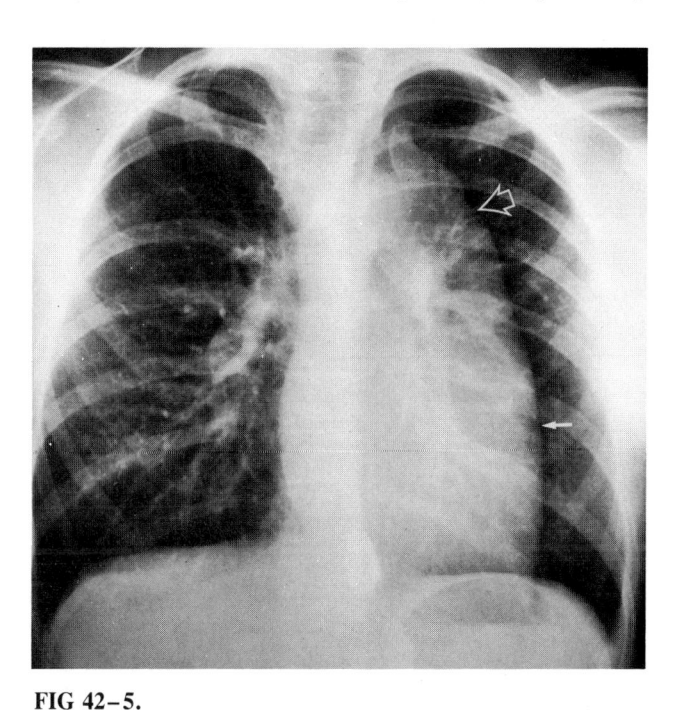

FIG 42–5.
Single ventricle with L-transposition and pulmonary stenosis. Thoracic roentgenogram. Posteroanterior projection. Characteristic large bulge along left cardiac border is formed by inverted (L-transposed) aorta *(open arrow)* identical to corrected transposition of great vessels. Small notch *(arrow)* along ventricular contour represents demarcation between rudimentary chamber and common ventricular chamber. In most patients this finding is so subtle that correct diagnosis cannot be suggested.

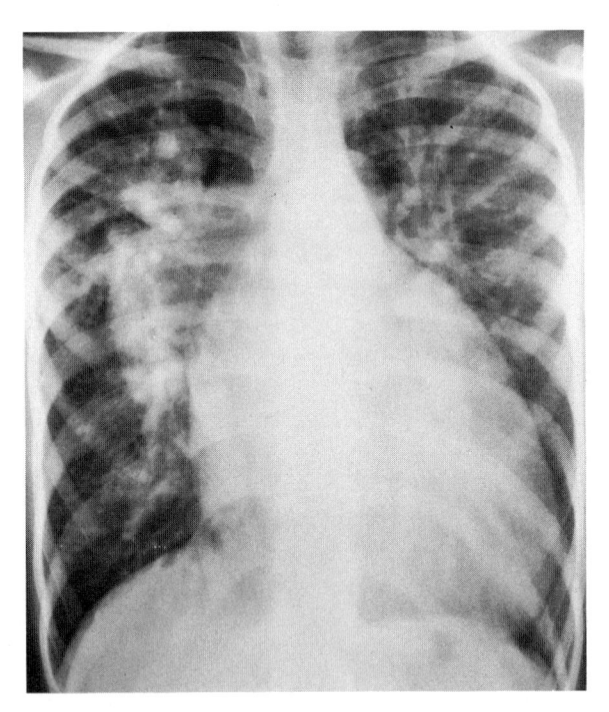

FIG 42-6.
Single ventricle, D-transposition of great vessels without pulmonary stenosis. Thoracic roentgenogram. Posteroanterior projection. Markedly enlarged heart. Pulmonary vasculature is greatly increased. REASON: Systemic pressure of single ventricle is transmitted to pulmonary circulation. Coexistence of huge hilar pulmonary arteries and lacking main pulmonary artery segment suggests an abnormal position of the pulmonary artery, as in transposition of the great vessels. Roentgenographic findings are indistinguishable from D-transposition of great vessels with well-developed ventricles.

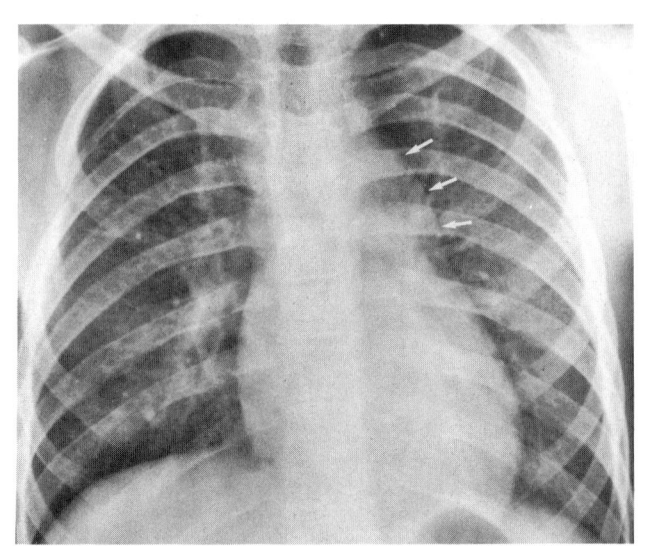

FIG 42-7.
Single ventricle, pulmonary stenosis, and L-transposition of great vessels. Thoracic roentgenogram. Posteroanterior projection. Heart is not enlarged. Normal pulmonary vasculature. L-transposition of aorta *(arrows)* mimics the pulmonary arterial segment so perfectly that radiographic diagnosis of this radiograph might be valvar pulmonary stenosis. The correct diagnosis cannot be suggested.

atresia coexists, the pulmonary vasculature is markedly decreased. The combination of single ventricle and pulmonary atresia is commonly found in the asplenic syndrome.

In patients with normally related great vessels (Holmes' heart) and pulmonary stenosis, the pulmonary vasculature is decreased. Without pulmonary stenosis the pulmonary vasculature is increased. The heart is not significantly enlarged, and its configuration is indistinguishable from tetralogy of Fallot or transposition of the great vessels with pulmonary stenosis (Fig 42-8).

CARDIAC CATHETERIZATION

Cardiac catheterization is used to diagnose the single ventricle, identify and measure severity of outflow obstruction, and calculate vascular resistances. With the use of balloon-tipped catheters, it is usually possible to catheterize both great vessels. During the procedure the catheter course should be carefully observed, because this can provide information about abnormal systemic venous connection. In addition, the course of the catheter into the great vessels can provide information if they are transposed. In patients with the aorta located anteriorly and leftward (L-transposition of great vessels), the catheter course along the upper left cardiac border is characteristic. In those patients with coexistent transposition of the great vessels on a lateral projection, the catheter course into the aorta is anterior.

Pressures should be measured during withdrawal of

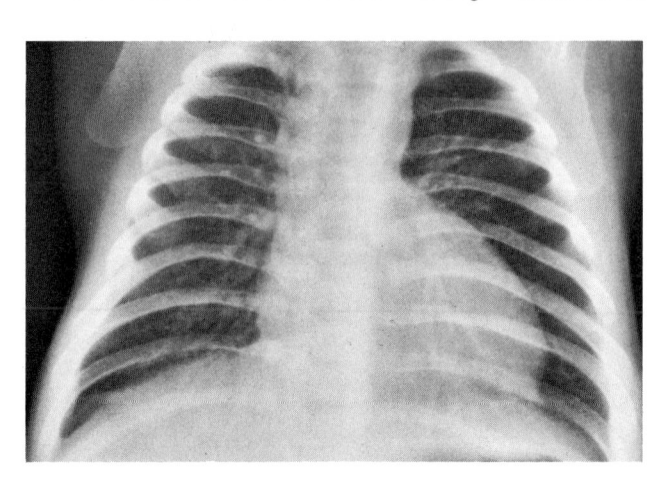

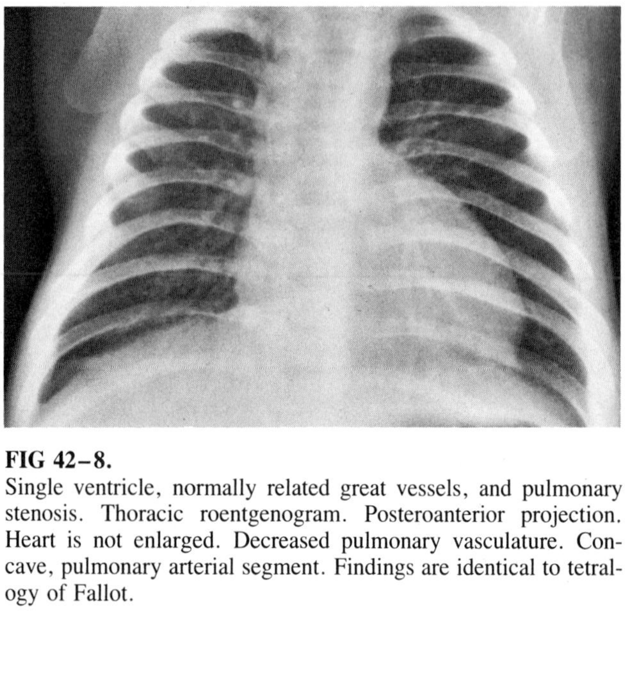

FIG 42-8.
Single ventricle, normally related great vessels, and pulmonary stenosis. Thoracic roentgenogram. Posteroanterior projection. Heart is not enlarged. Decreased pulmonary vasculature. Concave, pulmonary arterial segment. Findings are identical to tetralogy of Fallot.

the catheter from each great vessel to identify outflow obstructive lesions. Without an obstruction, systolic pressures are identical in the single ventricle and both great vessels, but with an obstruction, a gradient is found across the respective outflow area. Pressures measured in the great arteries, combined with oxygen data, can be used to calculate vascular resistances. Careful measurement of the end-diastolic pressure in the single ventricle is important if the patient is being considered for a modified Fontan procedure.

Oximetry data show a bidirectional shunt at the ventricular level but rarely at the atrial level, an important finding helping to distinguish single ventricle from some other conditions with a univentricular heart, such as tricuspid or mitral atresia.

In patients without pulmonary outflow obstruction, there is a large increase of oxygen saturation between the right atrium and the single ventricle, and aortic oxygen saturation is high. If obstruction to pulmonary blood flow is present, the increase is less and aortic oxygen saturation lower. Although mixing of the systemic and pulmonary venous returns should be uniform, it is often incomplete, and the saturation in the great vessels differ. When the rudimentary chamber is located laterally, aortic oxygen saturation exceeds that in the pulmonary artery,[8] and the opposite is found when the rudimentary chamber is medially located.

ANGIOGRAPHIC FEATURES

Angiography in patients with a single ventricle should delineate the following:

1. Ventricular anatomy.
2. Outflow chamber and great vessels.
3. Mechanisms of aortic or pulmonary outflow obstruction.
4. Status of atrioventricular junction and valves.
5. Nature of systemic and pulmonary venous connections.

Angiography is important for identification of the type of single ventricle. A single ventricle can exist without a rudimentary chamber (most common in asplenia) and could be divided by an operation into two ventricular chambers. Anteroposterior and lateral angiographic projections are usually adequate to identify the ventricular anatomy. The injection of contrast material into a single ventricle should be performed through a large catheter, with a large amount of contrast medium being delivered rapidly. The volume of the single ventricle is considerably greater than the normal ventricles because the entire systemic and pulmonary venous returns pass through this chamber. In addition, increased pulmonary blood flow may be present, further diluting the contrast medium. Aortography is often indicated in patients with single ventricle to identify the coronary arterial pattern, which can provide important information before an operation to divide the single ventricle or to insert a conduit.[19]

In transposition of the great vessels, the anterior aortic cusp is the noncoronary cusp and the coronary arteries arise from the posterior and left cusps, respectively. In a single ventricle, without inversion of the infundibulum (D-transposition), the left coronary artery divides into the anterior descending and circumflex branches, which have essentially a normal distribution. In a single ventricle with L-transposition, the coronary arterial pattern may be either normal or identical to that of congenital corrected transposition of the great vessels, with the anterior descending coronary artery arising from the "right coronary artery."

Pressure measurements and demonstration of the size of the bulboventricular foramen are important, because this communication between the single ventricle and the rudimentary chamber may be restrictive (Fig 42–9).

About 20% of patients with single ventricle do not have a rudimentary chamber. In these patients a remnant of a ventricular septum may be present in normal location at the floor of the common ventricle, or no septal remnant is found at all. Both of these types of common ventricle

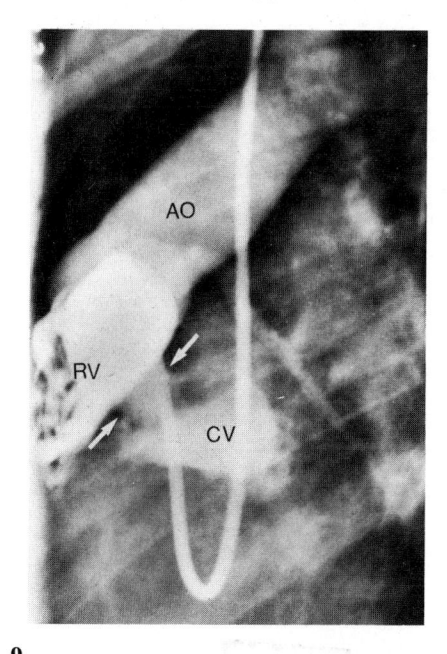

FIG 42–9.
Single ventricle with D-transposition. Selective angiogram. Lateral projection. Small trabeculated rudimentary chamber *(RV)*. Reflux through ventricular communication (bulboventricular foramen) *(arrows)* into single ventricle *(CV)*, which is incompletely filled. Stenotic communication. Great vessels are transposed. *AO* = aorta.

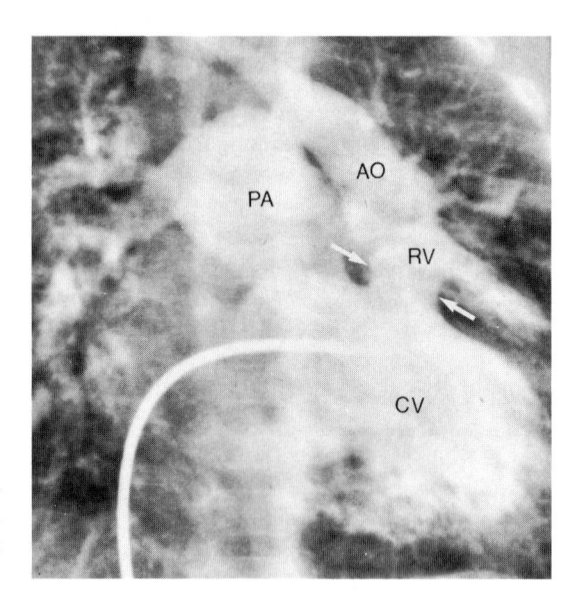

760 Cyanosis and Increased Pulmonary Arterial Vasculature

FIG 42–10.
Single ventricle *(CV)*, with L-transposition. Ventriculogram. Anteroposterior projection. Pulmonary artery *(PA)* is located medially to aorta *(AO)*. Hypoplastic right ventricle *(RV)* fills through an adequate-sized communication *(arrows)*, being approximately the size of the aorta.

are often present in patients with the asplenia and are potentially correctable by operation.

The angiographic features can be described according to the location of great vessels:

1. Transposition of great vessels with D-transposition. In a single ventricle with D-transposition, the small hypoplastic chamber is well visualized on a lateral projection (see Fig 42–9). The rudimentary chamber is located anteriorly, giving rise to the aorta. It has a trabeculated internal architecture like a right ventricle (see Fig 42–9). As with complete transposition (see Chapter 38), the side-by-side relationship on the anteroposterior projection is variable.

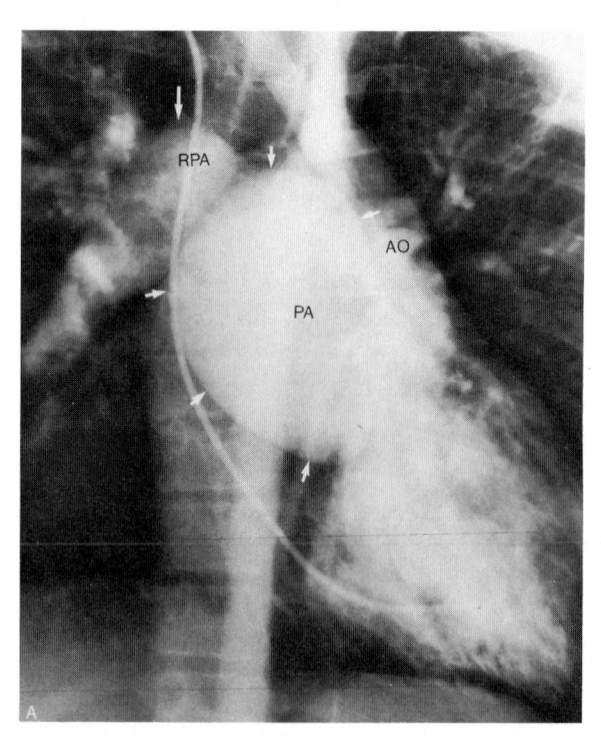

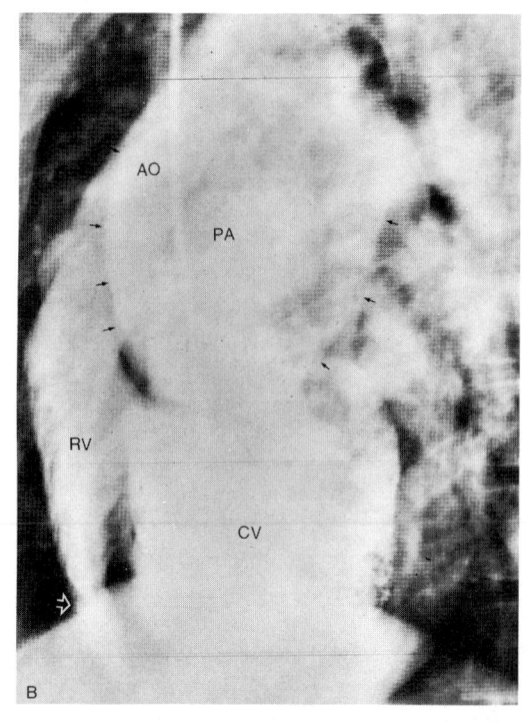

FIG 42–11.
Single ventricle *(CV)* and L-transposition. Ventriculogram. **A,** anteroposterior and, **B,** lateral projections. Medially placed huge pulmonary artery *(PA)* *(arrows)*. Aorta *(AO)* lies to left of pulmonary artery as in L-transposition. Right pulmonary artery *(RPA)* has unusually high *(white arrow)* waterfall appearance. Right ventricle *(RV)* is hypoplastic but has an inflow portion *(open arrow)*. Communication between hypoplastic right ventricle and common ventricle is fairly large *(white arrows)*.

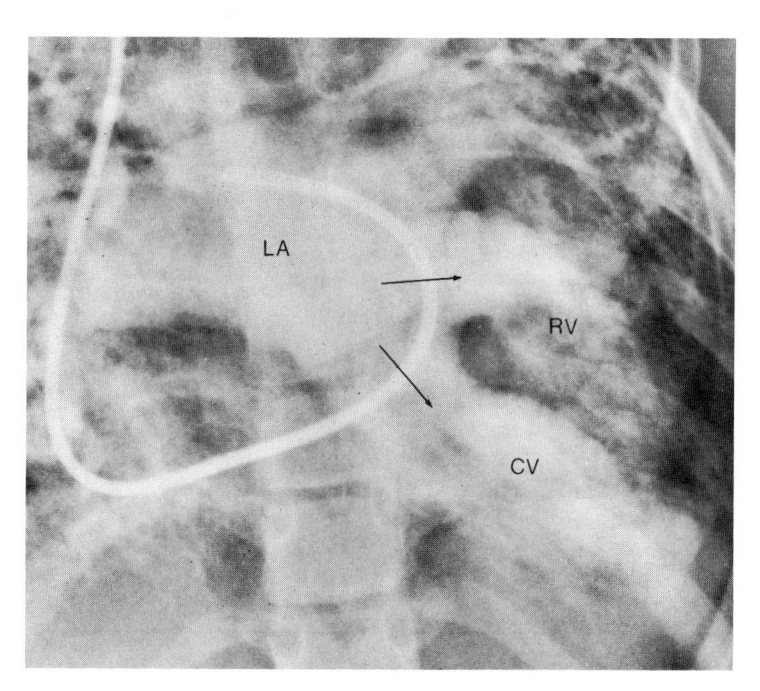

FIG 42–12.
Single ventricle. Pulmonary arteriogram. Late phase. Anteroposterior projection. Opaque returning from lungs fills left atrium *(LA)* and enters *(arrows)* rudimentary chamber *(RV)* and single ventricle *(CV)*, indicating straddling or overriding left atrioventricular valve with hypoplasia of systemic (right) ventricle.

2. Transposition of great vessels with L-transposition. Whereas the infundibular chamber is *almost* always small in patients with a noninverted infundibulum (D-transposition), its size varies considerably among individuals with L-transposition. There is a continuous spectrum from L-transposition with ventricular septal defect, through L-transposition with straddling left atrioventricular valve, to single ventricle with L-transposition. Determination of the size of the subaortic chamber (anatomic right ventricle) is of practical importance, because an adequate-sized subaortic ventricular chamber allows operative correction.

   a. On an anteroposterior projection after injection of contrast medium into the single ventricle, both great vessels and the communication between the single ventricle and outflow chambers are well visualized (Fig 42–10).
   b. Characteristically, the medially located pulmonary artery is enlarged and may occasionally be aneurysmal (Fig 42–11). REASON: Unknown.
   c. The aneurysmal pulmonary artery may not be seen on a thoracic roentgenogram. REASON: In L-transposition the main pulmonary artery occupies a medial position, and its borders are not outlined by air.
   d. A levophase of a pulmonary angiogram is very helpful in defining the size of the subaortic chamber. When the systemic ventricle is of adequate size and receives the left atrioventricular valve, pulmonary venous blood drains exclusively into that ventricle. On the other hand, with a true single ventricle, contrast medium drains into the common ventricular chamber, and the subaortic chamber (Fig 42–12).
   e. The location of the left atrioventricular valve in relation to the ventricular chamber or chambers can be better demonstrated by selective injection into the left atrium (Fig 42–13).
   f. Because the aorta is located anteriorly, slight rotation of either the heart or the thorax to the right

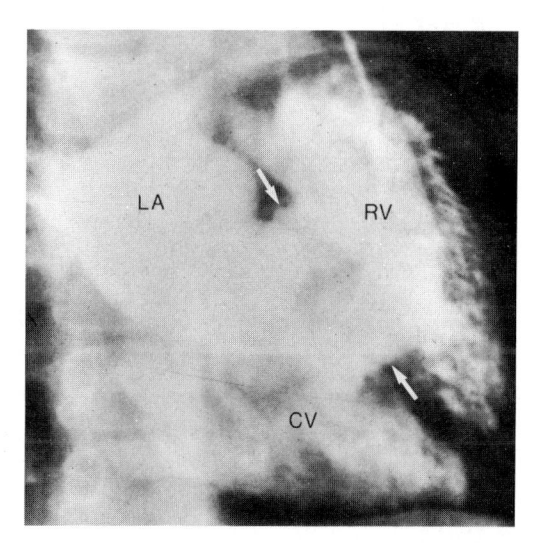

FIG 42–13.
Single ventricle. Left atriogram. Anteroposterior projection. Catheter is passed from aorta through huge bulboventricular foramen *(arrows)*, single ventricle *(CV)*, into left atrium *(LA)*. Right ventricle *(RV)* is of fair size, but left atrioventricular valve is related to common ventricle, which also receives right atrioventricular valve.

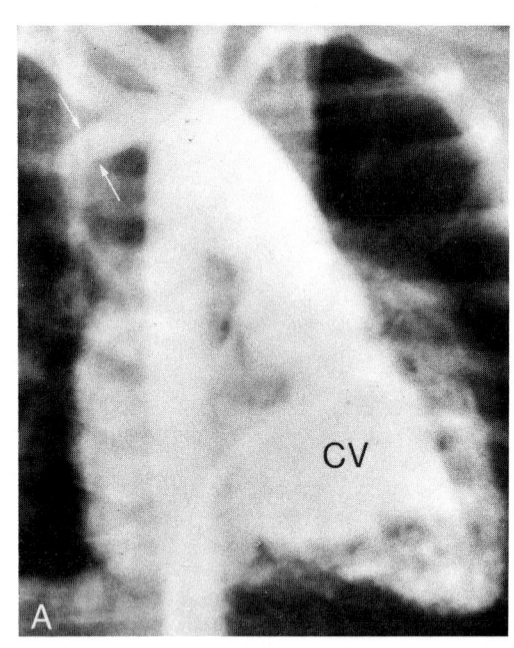

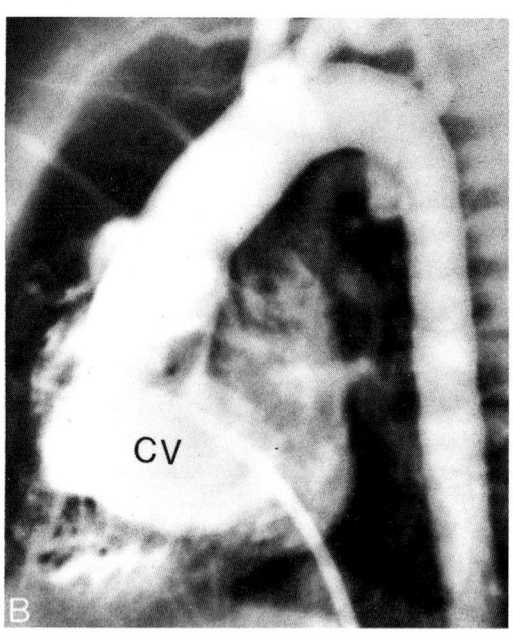

FIG 42–14.
Single ventricle without rudimentary chamber transposition of great vessels and pulmonary atresia. Ventriculogram *(CV)*. **A,** anteroposterior projection. Trabeculated outflow chamber related to transposed aorta. Left-sided position of aorta occurs from rotation of heart and should not be confused with L-transposition. Severely stenotic left-sided ductus arteriosus *(arrows)* arises from left subclavian artery. **B,** lateral projection. Single ventricle without rudimentary chamber. Transposed aorta. Pulmonary arteries are not opacified because ductus arteriosus is severely stenotic.

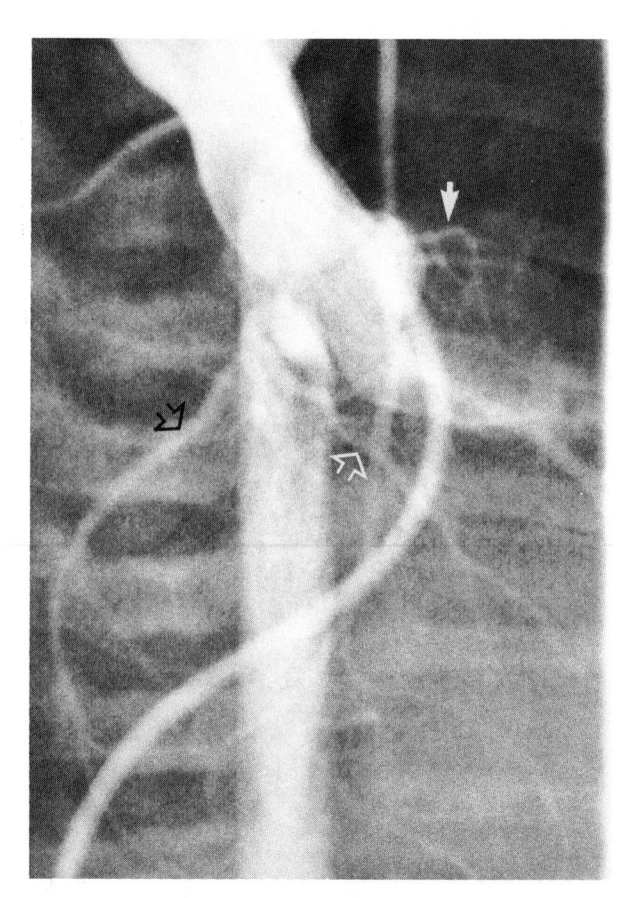

FIG 42–15.
Single ventricle. Aortogram. Anteroposterior projection. Coronary arterial pattern is identical to congenital corrected transposition of great vessels. Left anterior descending artery *(open white arrow)* arises from "right" (inverted circumflex) *(open black arrow)*. Circumflex artery *(white arrow)* arising from left cusp as single vessel. This coronary arterial pattern distinguishes between L-transposition and D-transposition.

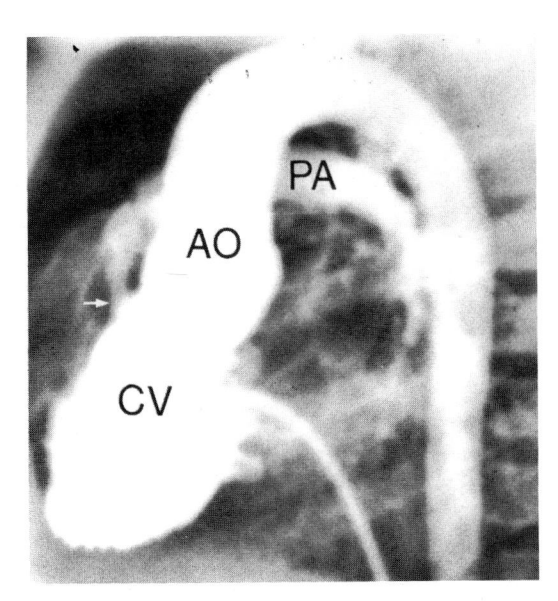

FIG 42–16.
Single ventricle, normally related great vessels, and pulmonary stenosis. Ventriculogram. Lateral projection. Both atrioventricular valves empty into single ventricle *(CV)*. Anterior rudimentary chamber consists only of outflow portion, which connects to single ventricle by severely stenotic ventricular *(arrow)* communication. *AO* = aorta; *PA* = pulmonary artery.

may project the ascending aorta to the left, producing a false picture of L-position (Fig 42–14). The coronary arterial pattern is helpful in distinguishing between L and D-transposition (Fig 42–15) by identifying the origin of the anterior descending artery from either the right or left coronary artery, respectively.
3. Normally related great vessels (Holmes' heart). In this anatomic form, the great vessels are normally related, with the aorta arising posteriorly from the single ventricle and the pulmonary artery arising anteriorly from the outflow chamber. Pulmonary stenosis coexists in most cases, and the major differential consideration is tetralogy of Fallot.[20] Both atrioventricular valves enter a morphologic left ventricle, and the rudimentary right outflow chamber is severely hypoplastic.
   a. The outflow chamber is invariably hypoplastic, and the single ventricle is slightly enlarged. In most instances, the sinus portion (inflow portion) of the right ventricle is absent, and the outflow chamber consists only of the infundibulum (Fig 42–16).
   b. Pulmonary stenosis may be caused by a small communication between the single ventricle and outflow chamber (see Fig 42–16), infundibular or valvar pulmonary stenosis, or a combination thereof. Infundibular pulmonary stenosis is the most common obstructive mechanism (Fig 42–17).
   c. A well-developed sinus portion of the right ventricle is rare (Fig 42–18). Single ventricle (normally great vessels) without pulmonary stenosis is exceedingly rare, resulting in increased pulmonary flow and pulmonary hypertension; it requires operative palliation by pulmonary arterial banding (see Fig 42–18).

OPERATIVE CONSIDERATIONS[21, 22]

In infants with congestive cardiac failure, aggressive treatment with digitalis and diuretics is indicated. Al-

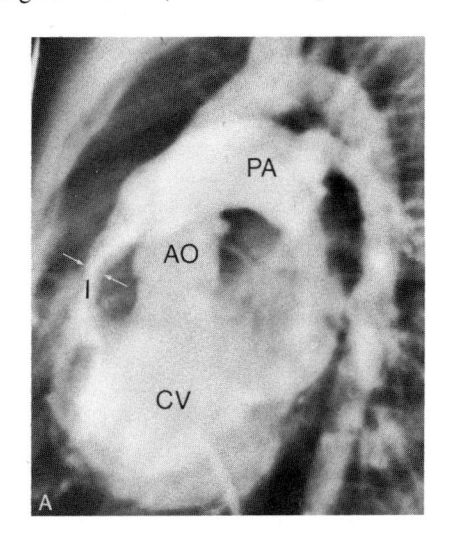

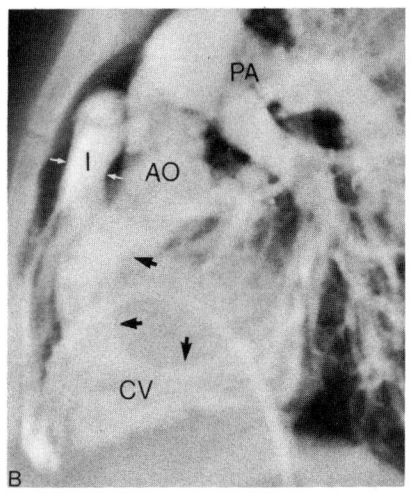

FIG 42–17.
Single ventricle and normally related great vessels. Ventriculogram. Anteroposterior projection. **A,** systole. Diminutive outflow chamber filled through ventricular communication. Severe systolic narrowing of infundibulum *(I) (arrows)*. **B,** diastole. Catheter passed through right atrioventricular valve *(black arrows)*, which enters common ventricle *(CV)*. Narrowed infundibulum *(I)* of hypoplastic rudimentary right chamber *(arrows)* is well demonstrated. *AO* = aorta; *PA* = pulmonary artery.

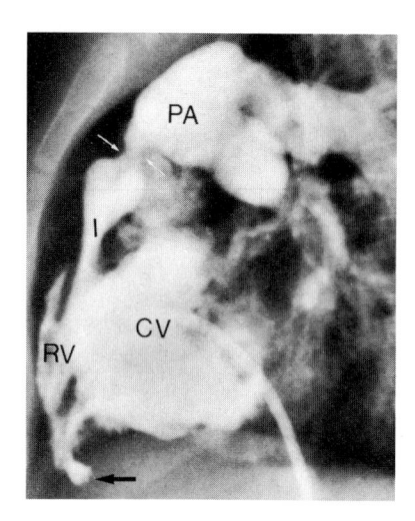

FIG 42–18.
Single ventricle and normally related great vessels without pulmonary stenosis and with pulmonary hypertension. Ventriculogram (CV). Lateral projection. Patient was paliated by band around main pulmonary artery (PA). Outflow chamber (I) has severely hypoplastic. Inflow portion of hypoplastic right ventricle (RV) is developed (black arrow).

though a few patients with mild pulmonary stenosis respond, cardiac failure is chronic in most. Palliation with a pulmonary artery band is required for most infants with congestive cardiac failure secondary to excessive pulmonary blood flow. Although this procedure can successfully relieve cardiac failure and protect the pulmonary vasculature from development of vascular disease, it has a serious

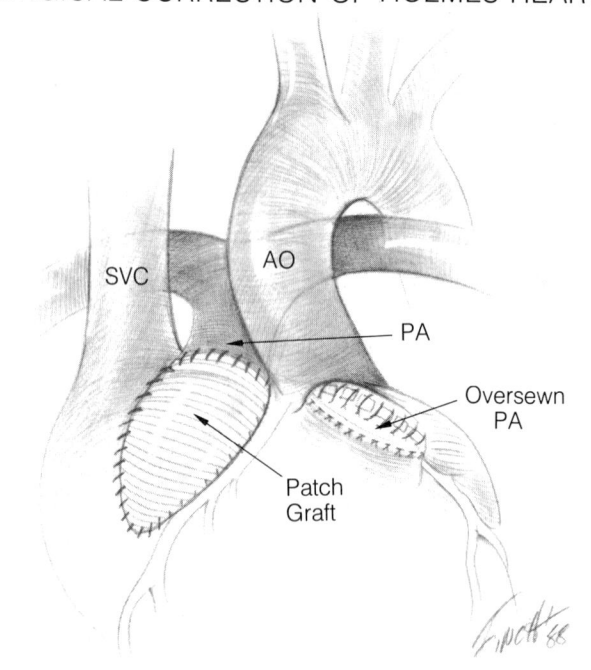

SURGICAL CORRECTION OF HOLMES HEART

FIG 42–20.
Single ventricle and normally related great vessels, repaired by modified Fontan procedure. Atrial septal defect and tricuspid valve closed by patches. An anastomosis is made between right atrium and pulmonary artery, or other modifications of Fontan procedure are performed. *AO* = aorta; *PA* = pulmonary artery; *SVC* = superior vena cava.

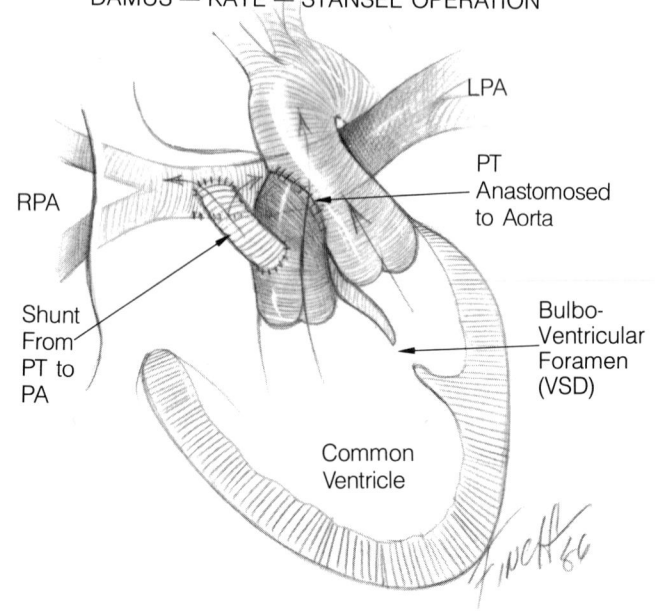

SURGICAL PALLIATION OF COMMON VENTRICLE WITH STENOTIC BULBO-VENTRICULAR FORAMEN
DAMUS — KAYE — STANSEL OPERATION

FIG 42–19.
Operative palliation of single ventricle with stenotic bulboventricular foramen (VSD). Proximal part of pulmonary trunk (PT) is divided and sewn end to side of aorta. Small central shunt is performed from pulmonary trunk to confluence between right pulmonary artery (RPA) and left pulmonary artery (LPA), preventing development of pulmonary hypertension.

FIG 42–21.
Operative repair of single ventricle. Left atrioventricular valve is sewn shut. Atrial patch is sewn to exclude vena caval return from entering ventricle. Right atrium *(RA)* is anastomosed to pulmonary artery *(PA)* as in a Fontan procedure. *Ao* = aorta; *LA* = left atrium.

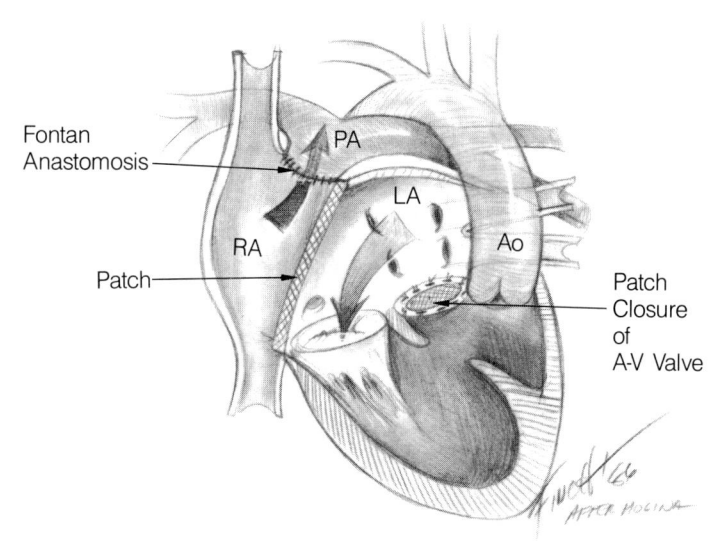

complication, namely the development of subaortic obstruction. With banding of the pulmonary artery, severe hypertrophy of the ventricle occurs, which can narrow the outflow chamber leading to the aorta. Fibrous proliferation may be found at this site as well.[9, 10] Thus, obstruction exists to both outlets from the ventricle. Surgically the stenotic bulboventricular foramen can be enlarged, a conduit from the ventricle to the aorta can be inserted, or a modified Damus-Kaye-Stansel (Fig 42–19) or the Fontan procedure can be performed.[21,23]

Among those patients with decreased pulmonary blood flow, a systemic-to-pulmonary arterial shunt is performed. The specific type depends principally on the patient's age and the preference of the surgeon.

These palliative procedures are designed to improve the patient's condition, so they can grow to an age when the systemic and pulmonary circulatory systems can be separated. Two operative approaches have been used, primarily in children beyond 5 years of age.

One of these is the Fontan procedure,[24] namely, creat-

SURGICAL REPAIR OF SINGLE VENTRICLE

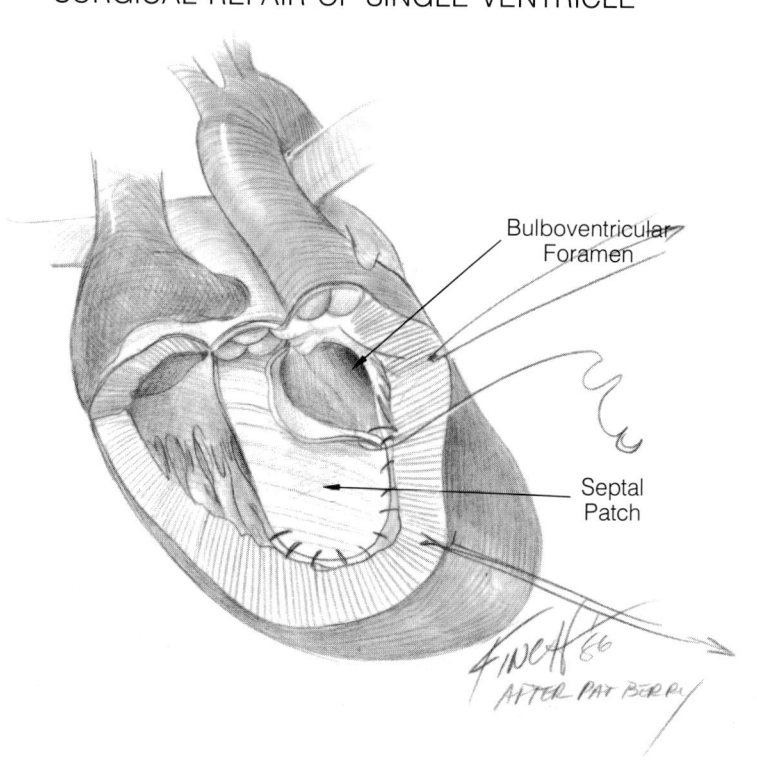

FIG 42–22.
Operative repair of single ventricle by septation technique. A septal patch is placed between atrioventricular valves and continued toward cardiac apex, dividing single ventricle into two equal-sized chambers. Septum allows blood from left atrium to flow through bulboventricular foramen into aorta.

ing a communication between the right atrium and pulmonary artery and oversewing the right atrioventricular valve (Fig 42–20), or partitioning the right atrium in the presence of atrioventricular valve insufficiency (Fig 42–21). To be a candidate for this procedure, the patient must have a pulmonary vascular resistance of less than 5 units/M,^{2} pulmonary artery pressure less than 20 mm Hg, normal ventricular function, and no obstructive lesions in the pulmonary arterial tree. The operative mortality is 10%, and intermediate term follow-up is satisfactory.

The other approach is septation of the ventricle,[25] which has an operative mortality as high as 50%. In this operation, the single ventricle is divided by a patch into two equal ventricular chambers (Fig 42–22). The presence of outflow obstruction increases the risk. Knowledge of the location of the cardiac conduction system and intracardiac mapping techniques can reduce the incidence of postoperative block.

REFERENCES

1. Anderson RH, Becker AE, Macartney FJ, et al: Is "tricuspid atresia" a univentricular heart? *Pediatr Cardiol* 1:51, 1979.
2. Bharati S, Lev M: The concept of tricuspid atresia complex as distinct from that of the single ventricle complex, *Pediatr Cardiol* 1:57, 1979.
3. Van Praagh R, David I, Van Praagh S: What is a ventricle? The single-ventricle trap, *Pediatr Cardiol* 2:79, 1982.
4. Van Praagh R, Van Praagh S, Vlad P, et al: Diagnosis of the anatomic types of single or common ventricle, *Am J Cardiol* 15:345, 1965.
5. Van Praagh R, Ongley PA, Swan HJC: Anatomic types of single or common ventricle in man: morphologic and geometric aspects of 60 necropsied cases, *Am J Cardiol* 13:367, 1964.
6. Keeton BR, Macartney FJ, Hunter S, et al: Univentricular heart of right ventricular type with double or common inlet, *Circulation* 59:403, 1979.
7. Shinebourne EA, Lau K-C, Calcaterra G, et al: Univentricular heart of right ventricular type: clinical, angiographic and electrocardiographic features, *Am J Cardiol* 46:439, 1980.
8. Rahimtoola SH, Ongley PA, Swan HJC: The hemodynamics of common (or single) ventricle, *Circulation* 34:14, 1966.
9. Freedom RM, Sondheimer H, Dische R, et al: Development of "subaortic stenosis" after pulmonary arterial banding for common ventricle, *Am J Cardiol* 39:78, 1977.
10. Somerville J, Becu L, Ross D: Common ventricle with acquired subaortic obstruction, *Am J Cardiol* 34:206, 1974.
11. Davachi F, Moller JH: The electrocardiogram and vectorcardiogram in single ventricle: anatomic correlations, *Am J Cardiol* 23:19, 1969.
12. Wilkinson JL, Anderson RH, Arnold R, et al: The conducting tissues in primitive ventricular hearts without an outlet chamber, *Circulation* 53:930, 1976.
13. Anderson RH, Arnold R, Thapar MK, et al: Cardiac specialized tissue in hearts with an apparently single ventricular chamber (double inlet left ventricle), *Am J Cardiol* 33:95, 1974.
14. Smallhorn JF, Tommasini G, Macartney FJ: Two-dimensional echocardiographic assessment of common atrioventricular valves in univentricular hearts, *Br Heart J* 46:30, 1981.
15. Bisset GS III, Hirschfeld SS: The univentricular heart: Combined 2-dimensional-pulsed Doppler (duplex) echocardiographic evaluation, *Am J Cardiol* 51:1149, 1983.
16. Seward JB, Tajik AJ, Hagler DJ, et al: Contrast echocardiography in single or common ventricle, *Circulation* 55:513, 1977.
17. Seward JB, Tajik AJ, Hagler DJ, et al: Echocardiogram in common (single) ventricle: angiographic-anatomic correlation, *Am J Cardiol* 39:217, 1977.
18. Elliott LP, Gedgaudas E: The roentgenologic findings in common ventricle with transposition of the great vessels, *Radiology* 82:850, 1964.
19. Keeton BR, Lie JT, McGoon DC, et al: Anatomy of coronary arteries in univentricular hearts and its surgical implications, *Am J Cardiol* 43:569, 1979.
20. Saalouke MG, Perry LW, Okoroma EO, et al: Primitive ventricle with normally related great vessels and stenotic subpulmonary outlet chamber: angiographic differentiation from tetralogy of Fallot, *Br Heart J* 40:49, 1978.
21. Chen S, Pennington G, Nouri S, et al: Management of infants with univentricular heart, *Am Heart J* 107:1252, 1984.
22. Moodie DS, Ritter DG, Tajik AH, et al: Long-term follow-up after palliative operation for univentricular heart, *Am J Cardiol* 53:1648, 1984.
23. Penkoske PA, Freedom RM, Williams WG, et al: Surgical palliation of subaortic stenosis in the univentricular heart, *J Thorac Cardiovasc Surg* 87:767, 1984.
24. Yacoub MH, Radley-Smith R: Use of a valved conduit from right atrium to pulmonary artery for "correction" of single ventricle, *Circulation* 54(suppl 3):63, 1976.
25. Edie RN, Ellis K, Gersony WM, et al: Surgical repair of single ventricle, *J Thorac Cardiovasc Surg* 66:350, 1973.

CHAPTER 43

Tricuspid Atresia With Transposition of Great Vessels

About 25% of patients with tricuspid atresia have coexistent transposition of the great vessels. In most of these the pulmonary vasculature is increased. Thus, this lesion must be considered in the differential diagnosis of the admixture lesions. Generally the finding of left-axis deviation in a patient with cyanosis and increased pulmonary vasculature strongly suggests tricuspid atresia with transposition of the great vessels. Tricuspid atresia may be associated with truncus arteriosus and with double outlet from either the rudimentary chamber or the left ventricle. These rare combinations are also associated with increased pulmonary blood flow and may be discovered during the study of a patient with suspected tricuspid atresia and transposition of the great vessels.

PATHOLOGIC ANATOMY

The usual features of tricuspid atresia (see Chapter 33) are present, but other anatomic features differ when the great vessels are transposed. In contrast to most instances of tricuspid atresia with normally related great vessels, the pulmonary artery, left atrium, and left ventricle are greatly enlarged because of the increased pulmonary blood flow. Histologic examination of the lungs may show pulmonary vascular disease. The transposed great vessels may be in the relationship of either complete transposition or corrected transposition of the great vessels.

Complete Transposition of Great Vessels

Among those with coexistent complete transposition of the great vessels, the aorta arises from an anteriorly located chamber, which is usually rudimentary. The pulmonary artery arises posteriorly from the left ventricle, and the pulmonary valve is in continuity with the anterior leaflet of the mitral valve (Fig 43–1).[1] Thus, the aortic valve is located more cephalad than the pulmonary valve. With time, obstruction may be present or may develop between the left ventricle and the aorta, limiting systemic blood flow and enhancing pulmonary blood flow. As in tricuspid atresia without transposition of the great vessels, this obstruction may be present at the level of the ventricular septal defect, rudimentary right ventricle (subaortic stenosis), or aortic valve. Various combinations of these obstructions are found, but they are much less common than the subpulmonary obstruction found among patients with tricuspid atresia and normally related great vessels.

Among patients with coexistent tricuspid atresia and complete transposition of the great vessels, coarctation of the aorta, hypoplasia of the aortic arch, and patent ductus arteriosus occur in 5% to 10% of cases.[2,3] Pulmonary outflow obstruction is present in a few of these patients. The pulmonary valve may be atretic, the pulmonary valve or pulmonary annulus may be stenotic, or there may be subpulmonary stenosis because of a conus below the pulmonary valve. Under the latter circumstances, the mitral valve is no longer in continuity with the pulmonary valve. Rarely, transposition of the great vessels may be associated with a double conus.

Corrected Transposition of Great Vessels

Tricuspid atresia may also coexist with forms of L-transposition. The term "corrected transposition with tricuspid atresia" is inadequate to define anatomy or physiology, because three anatomically and physiologically different conditions might carry this designation.[4–6] Because of this confusing terminology, it is preferable to speak of

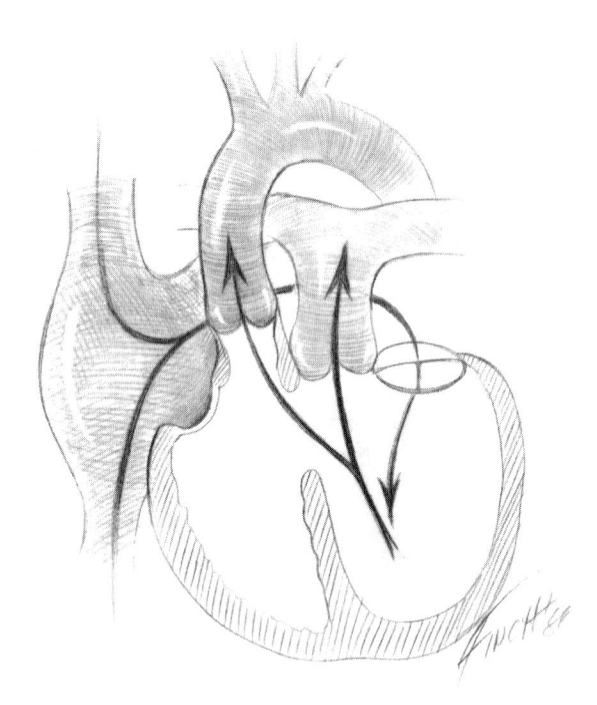

FIG 43-1.
Tricuspid atresia with complete transposition of great vessels. Central circulation. Obligatory right-to-left shunt at the atrial level. Both great vessels fill via atrial septal defect. Aorta arises from a conus and is not in continuity with atretic tricuspid valve. Pulmonary valve is in continuity with mitral valve as in complete transposition. Rarely, two coni, pulmonary stenosis, or atresia may be present.

right or left atrioventricular valve atresia or to use a sequential approach:

1. Classical L-transposition of the great vessels (corrected transposition of the great vessels or discordant atrioventricular and ventriculoarterial connection) bulboventricular inversion with left atrioventricular valve (tricuspid) atresia (Fig 43-2).
2. Tricuspid atresia with isolated bulbar inversion (Fig 43-3).
3. Corrected transposition (L-transposition of the great vessels or discordant atrioventricular valve and ventriculoarterial connection) with right atrioventricular valve (mitral) atresia (Fig 43-4).

Each of three conditions has a single characteristic anatomic finding: The great vessels are transposed, and the aorta lies anteriorly and to the left of the pulmonary artery. This results in the characteristic configuration of the great vessels found in corrected transposition of the great vessels.

Each of the three conditions may be associated with pulmonary stenosis or pulmonary atresia, increasing the number of anatomic variations. Each of these well-defined anatomic entities is discussed.

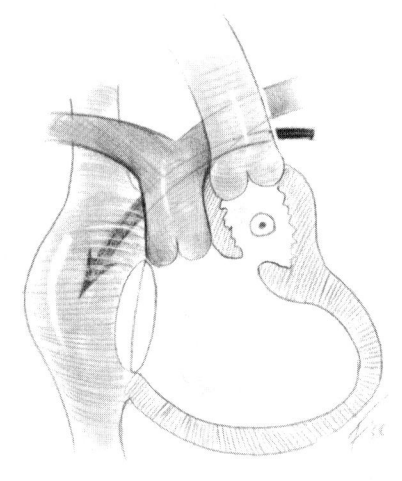

FIG 43-2.
L-Transposition of great vessels with tricuspid atresia. Anatomic tricuspid valve (hemodynamic mitral valve) is atretic. Obligatory left-to-right shunt is at atrial level. Because of atretic left atrioventricular valve, systemic anatomic right ventricle is hypoplastic.

Corrected Transposition With Left Atrioventricular (Tricuspid) Valve Atresia (See Fig 43-2)

The ventricles and great vessels are inverted and the great vessels are transposed. Therefore, the ventricle connected to the pulmonary artery anatomically resembles a left ventricle and lacks a conus. The ventricle connected to the aorta (the systemic ventricle) anatomically resembles a right ventricle. The left atrioventricular valve (tricuspid valve) is separated from the aorta by a conus (infundibulum).

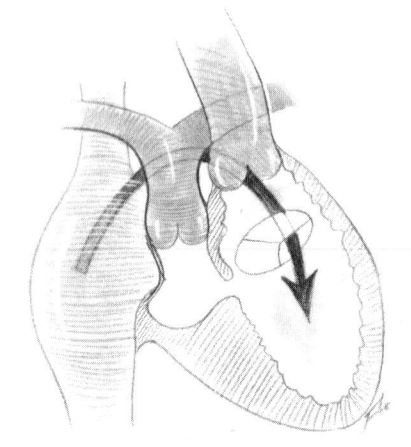

FIG 43-3.
Tricuspid atresia with isolated bulbar inversion. Right atrioventricular valve (tricuspid valve) is atretic. Obligatory right-to-left shunt is at atrial level. Aorta is located anterior and to left of pulmonary artery.

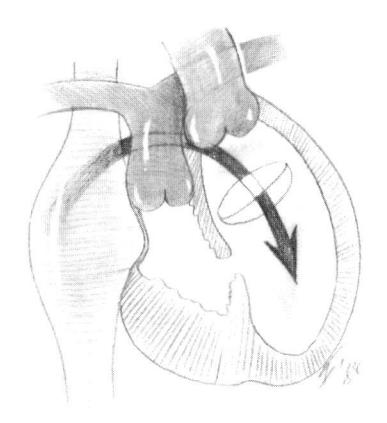

FIG 43-4.
Corrected transposition with right atrioventricular valve atresia (anatomic mitral atresia). Atrioventricular discordance and ventriculoarterial discordance. Obligatory right-to-left shunt at atrial level.

In this condition the left atrioventricular valve (tricuspid valve) is atretic, therefore the term "tricuspid atresia with L-transposition of the great vessels" (see Fig 43-2). Hemodynamically, however, this condition differs from tricuspid atresia, because a left-to-right shunt occurs at the atrial level, and the circulation is identical to mitral atresia.

Because ventricular inversion involves both the inflow and outflow tracts, this anatomic situation has also been termed as "bulboventricular inversion."

Isolated Bulbar Inversion (See Fig 43-3)

In this form of tricuspid atresia, only the bulbar portion (outflow tract) of the ventricles is inverted, whereas the sinus portion (inflow tract) and related atrioventricular valves are not inverted. Thus, atrioventricular concordance exists. The right atrioventricular valve (tricuspid valve) is atretic. The left (mitral) atrioventricular valve joins the left ventricle. A conus separates the left atrioventricular valve (mitral valve) from the aorta, and usually a conus is found in the pulmonary ventricle (double coni) as well. The aorta arises anteriorly and to the left. Therefore, the term "tricuspid atresia with corrected transposition" (L-transposition) might apply. Hemodynamically, this condition is identical to tricuspid atresia without transposition of the great vessels.

Corrected Transposition of the Great Vessels With Right Atrioventricular Valve Atresia (See Fig 43-4)

In this condition, inversion of the ventricles and the atrioventricular valves coexists, with inversion and transposition of the great vessels identical to classical corrected transposition (L-transposition of the great vessels). Atresia of the right atrioventricular valve results in a right-to-left atrial shunt. Because the right atrioventricular valve is anatomically a mitral valve, this condition physiologically mimics tricuspid atresia but anatomically is mitral atresia.

Juxtaposition of the Atrial Appendages

Among the patients with tricuspid atresia and coexistent transposition of the great vessels, juxtaposition of the atrial appendages is common (10%-40%) (Fig 43-5). It occurs slightly more often in females and with various other congenital cardiac malformations.[6] Juxtaposition of the atrial appendage without major cardiac anomalies is extremely rare.

In juxtaposition of the atrial appendages, both atrial appendages lie on one side of the great arteries in contrast to normal, where an atrial appendage lies on each side of the great vessels.

Juxtaposition of the atrial appendages occurs six times more commonly to the left of the great vessels than to the right. When they both lie to the left of the great vessels, the left atrial appendage is in a normal position, and the right atrial appendage passes behind the great vessels and lies above the left atrial appendage along the left cardiac border.

JUXTAPOSITION OF ATRIAL APPENDAGES

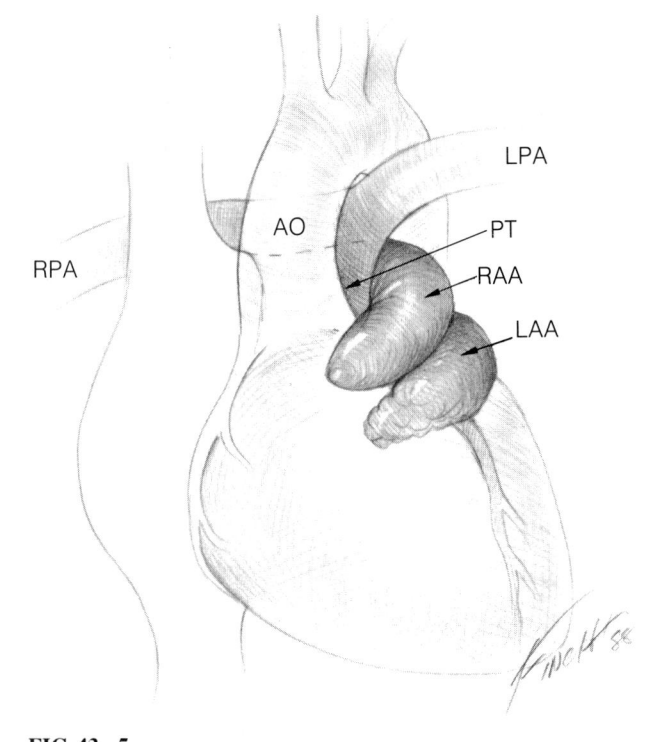

FIG 43-5.
Juxtaposition of atrial appendages. *RPA* = right pulmonary artery; *AO* = aorta; *LPA* = left pulmonary artery; *PT* = pulmonary trunk; *RAA* = right atrial appendage; *LAA* = left atrial appendage.

The malformation is important for two reasons:

1. During cardiac catheterization, confusion may exist if desaturated blood is sampled from a low-pressure area while the catheter tip lies along the left cardiac border, in an area expected to be left atrium.

2. The juxtaposed atrial appendages form a prominent bulge along the upper left cardiac contour, closely simulating the configuration of tricuspid atresia.

HEMODYNAMICS

The intracardiac hemodynamics and the volume of systemic and pulmonary blood flows are influenced by relative resistance to flow into aorta and pulmonary artery, respectively. In tricuspid atresia with transposition of the great vessels, pulmonary blood flow is determined principally by the pulmonary vascular resistance. Because the pulmonary resistance is elevated in the neonate, pulmonary blood flow is limited. By 3 months of age when pulmonary vascular resistance has declined to a lower level, the volume of pulmonary blood flow is greatly increased. Congestive cardiac failure is often present in patients with tricuspid atresia and transposition of the great vessels because of the excessive volume load placed on the left ventricle. Left ventricular dysfunction develops in older children with this condition, perhaps from the combined effects of left ventricular dilatation and myocardial perfusion with desaturated blood. The presence of subaortic stenosis or lesions such as coarctation of the aorta accentuates the pulmonary blood flow and hastens the onset of cardiac failure.

CLINICAL FEATURES

Signs and symptoms of hypoxemia are minimal, and the patient may not appear cyanotic, because the degree of cyanosis is inversely related to the volume of pulmonary blood flow, which in this instance is excessive.

Congestive cardiac failure is present and develops between 2 to 3 months of age.[2, 7] Respiratory difficulties, slow feeding, frequent respiratory tract infections, and slow growth are features of cardiac failure.

The combination of minimal or absence of cyanosis, the presence of congestive cardiac failure, and the auscultatory findings lead to the common misdiagnosis of ventricular septal defect.

There may be a pulse or blood pressure difference between the arms and legs if coarctation of the aorta coexists. Clinical evidence of cardiomegaly with a laterally displaced cardiac apex, precordial bulge, or both is present.

There is a prominent long systolic murmur along the mid-left sternal border. An apical middiastolic murmur is present, reflecting the increased pulmonary blood flow resulting from the large volume of blood flow across the mitral valve. The first heart sound is loud, and the second heart sound is single and loud, because the aorta and the aortic valve lie anteriorly.

ELECTROCARDIOGRAPHIC FEATURES

Although most patients with tricuspid atresia and transposition of the great vessels show left-axis deviation, 30% have an axis in the normal range.[8] Left atrial enlargement, often combined with right atrial enlargement, is found in older patients. The precordial leads show a pattern of left ventricular hypertrophy. The QRS pattern in lead V_6 often shows a large q wave and tall R wave. The R wave in lead V_1 tends to be taller than that found in lead V_1 of patients with tricuspid atresia with decreased pulmonary blood flow.

ECHOCARDIOGRAPHIC FEATURES

The findings resemble those of patients with tricuspid atresia and decreased pulmonary blood flow, except that the left atrial, left ventricular, and pulmonary artery dimensions are larger, and the great vessels are transposed.

Juxtaposed atrial appendages can be observed, if present. Doppler analysis reflects the flow dynamics across the atrial septum and pulmonary outflow area.

RADIOGRAPHIC FEATURES

In most patients, thoracic roentgenograms are not specific enough to allow a correct diagnosis. The combination of cyanosis, left-axis deviation, and increased pulmonary vasculature, however, strongly suggests tricuspid atresia with transposition of the great vessels. Exceptions exist, because tricuspid atresia with normally related great vessels can occur without obstruction to pulmonary flow and, therefore, show increased pulmonary vasculature (see Chapter 33). Likewise, tricuspid atresia with transposition of the great vessels rarely has decreased pulmonary blood flow from associated pulmonary stenosis.

1. In patients with tricuspid atresia and transposition of the great vessels with subpulmonary or valvar pulmonary stenosis, the radiographic findings are identical to tricuspid atresia and normally related great vessels. Decreased pulmonary vasculature is found (rare).

2. Usually the pulmonary vasculature is increased (Fig 43–6). REASON: The pulmonary artery arises unobstructed from the left ventricle.

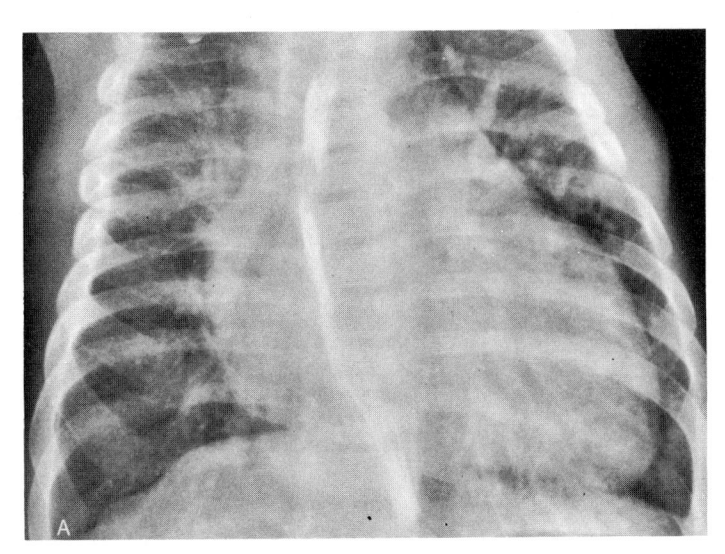

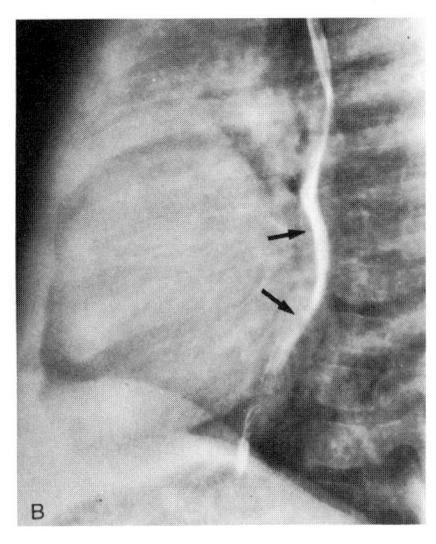

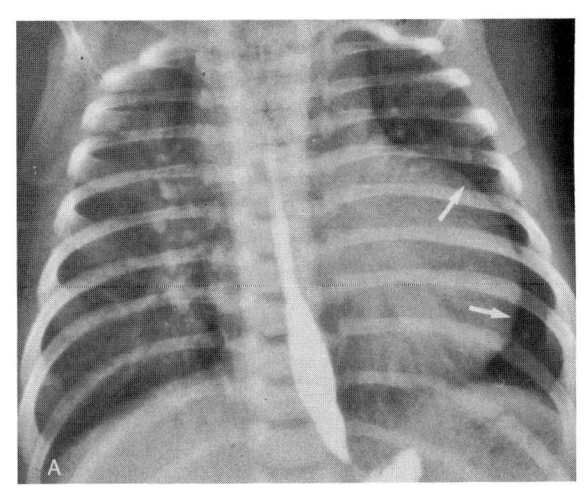

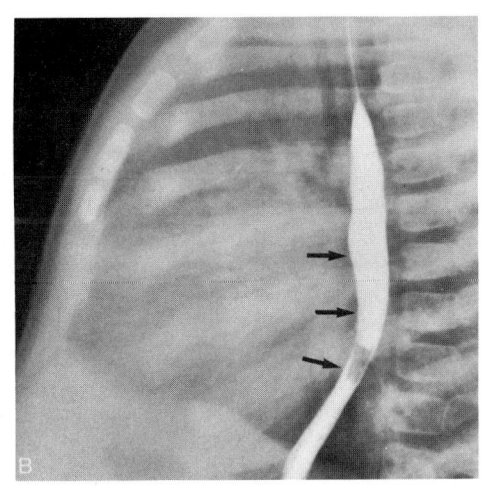

FIG 43-6.
Tricuspid atresia and D-transposition of great vessels. Thoracic roentgenogram. **A,** posteroanterior and, **B,** lateral projections. Markedly enlarged heart. Increased pulmonary vasculature. Left atrial enlargement. Findings are nonspecific and consistent with other admixture lesions except for total anomalous venous return. With the clinical information of left-axis deviation on electrocardiogram and cyanosis, tricuspid atresia with transposition of great vessels can be suggested.

3. The left atrium is enlarged (Figs 43–6 and 43–7). REASON: Blood flow through the lung and left atrium is increased because of the large volume of pulmonary blood flow (see Fig 43–7), and the left atrium receives also total systemic venous return.

4. The radiographic finding of left atrial enlargement resembles other admixture lesions except total anomalous pulmonary venous connection.

5. The cardiac configuration may be highly suggestive of tricuspid atresia because of the rounded, spherical left cardiac border (see Fig 43–7).

6. In spite of increased pulmonary blood flow, the pulmonary artery is not prominent. REASON: The main pulmonary artery, although enlarged, lies within the mediastinum and does not form a portion of the cardiac border.

7. The cardiac configuration is particularly suggestive of coexistent corrected transposition (L-transposition of the great vessels) in patients with juxtaposition of the atrial appendages (Fig 43–8).

8. In patients with tricuspid atresia and corrected transposition of the great vessels, the ascending aorta usually forms a prominent bulge along the left upper cardiac border (see Fig 43–8).

FIG 43-7.
Tricuspid atresia and D-transposition of great vessels. Thoracic roentgenogram. **A,** posteroanterior and, **B,** lateral projections. Increased pulmonary vasculature. Enlarged left atrium *(arrow)*. Left cardiac border is spherical *(arrows)* because of enlarged left ventricle. Pulmonary arterial segment is concave because enlarged pulmonary artery is in medial position.

FIG 43–8.
Tricuspid atresia and D-transposition of great vessels. Thoracic roentgenogram. **A,** posteroanterior projection. Increased pulmonary vasculature. Concave pulmonary arterial segment suggests transposition of great vessels. Prominent bulge along left upper cardiac border with a notch *(arrow)* suggests either corrected transposition of great vessels or juxtaposition of atrial appendages. **B,** venous angiography. Anteroposterior projection. Dense right-to-left shunt at atrial level. Juxtaposition of arterial appendages forms prominent bulge and notch seen in **A.** Right aortic arch. *RAA* = right atrial appendage; *LAA* = left atrial appendage.

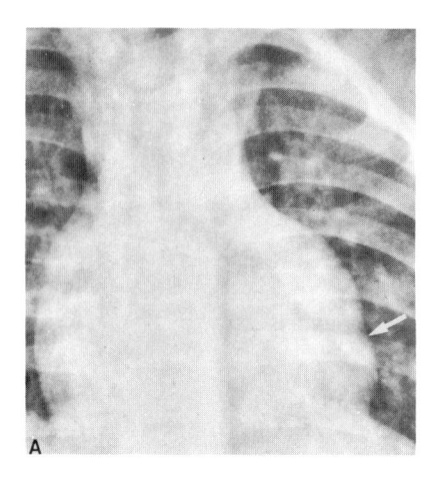

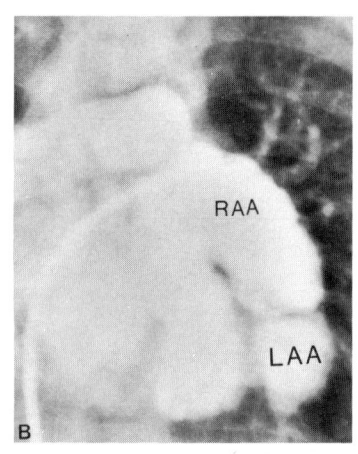

CARDIAC CATHETERIZATION

The basic cardiac catheterization and angiographic features are similar to those discussed in Chapter 33. There are, however, notable exceptions:

1. The oxygen saturation in the aorta and pulmonary artery are higher than in tricuspid atresia with reduced pulmonary blood flow. The large volume of fully saturated pulmonary blood mixes with the volume of systemic venous return. Therefore, the resultant oxygen saturation is high.
2. The pulmonary arterial pressure is elevated, and the pulmonary arterial systolic pressure usually equals aortic systolic pressure, because there is free transmission of ventricular pressure into the pulmonary arterial bed (pulmonary stenosis is absent).
3. Left ventricular end-diastolic pressure is elevated because of the large volume of pulmonary venous return. This elevation does not necessarily indicate myocardial dysfunction.

ANGIOGRAPHIC FEATURES

Cardiac catheterization and angiography are essential to determine the anatomic details, including degree of pulmonary stenosis, position of the great vessels, and size of the ventricular communication. These features are important in the selection and timing of cardiac operation:

1. A right atrial injection shows an immediate dense right-to-left shunt at the atrial level (Fig 43–9). The size of the atrial communication varies and can be visualized on a left anterior oblique projection.
2. The supradiaphragmatic portion of the inferior vena cava tends to be enlarged as in tricuspid atresia and normally related great vessels (see Fig 43–9).
3. If juxtaposition of the atrial appendages is present, confusing densities may be formed along the left cardiac border. On a lateral projection the left atrial appendage occupies a fairly normal, usually slightly lower position, and the right atrial appendage projects posteriorly (Fig 43–10).

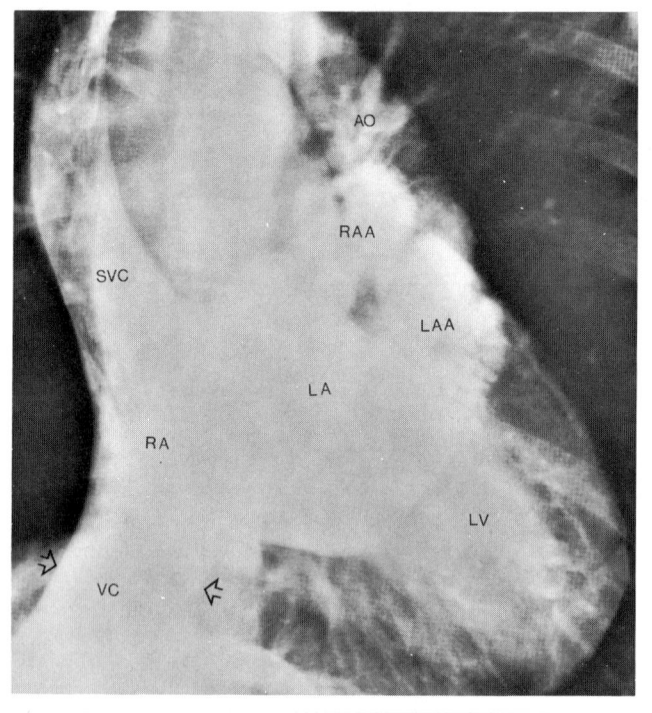

FIG 43–9.
Right atrioventricular valvar atresia and juxtaposition of the atrial appendages. Injection into superior vena cava. Anteroposterior projection. Markedly enlarged inferior vena cava *(open arrows).* Right atrial appendage *(RAA)* projects above left atrial appendage *(LAA)* along left cardiac border. Thick-walled left ventricle *(LV)* gives rise to aorta *(AO),* forming left cardiac border. Therefore, diagnosis is corrected transposition of great vessels with right atrioventricular valvar atresia ("mitral atresia"). Hemodynamically identical to tricuspid atresia without transposition of great vessels. *LA* = left atrium; *RA* = right atrium; *VC* = vena cava; *SVC* = superior vena cava.

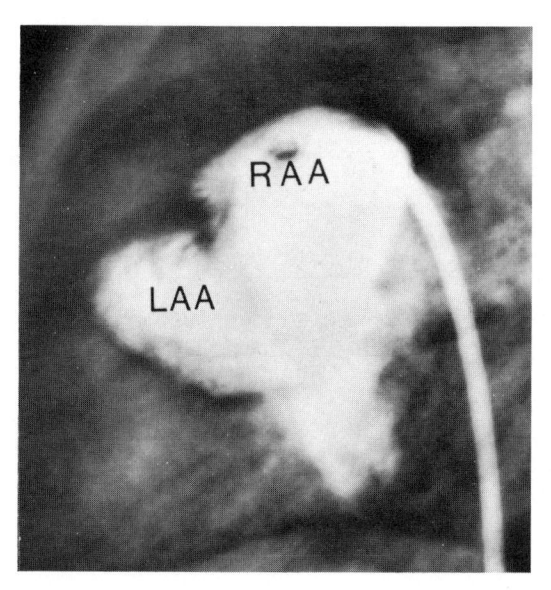

FIG 43–10.
Tricuspid atresia and transposition of great vessels. Right atriogram. Lateral projection. Right atrial appendage *(RAA)* is located posteriorly behind expected course of great vessels. Left atrial appendage *(LAA)* is slightly lower but in otherwise normal position.

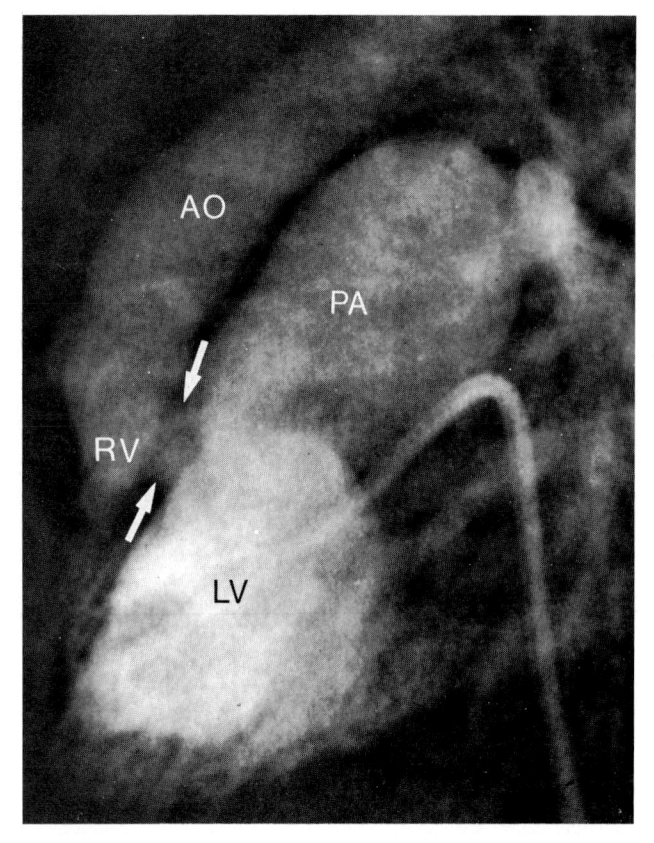

FIG 43–11.
Tricuspid atresia and transposition of great vessels. Left ventriculogram. Lateral projection. Enlarged posteriorly placed left ventricle *(LV)* gives rise to large pulmonary artery *(PA)*. Pulmonary valve is in continuity with mitral valve. Hypoplastic anterior subaortic chamber fills via ventricular communication *(arrows)*. Aorta *(AO)* is transposed and arises from hypoplastic chamber. RV = right ventricle.

4. Angiographic interpretation may be particularly difficult if the juxtaposed appendages project toward the right or if one of them occupies an atypically low position simulating a ventricular chamber or ventricular diverticulum (see Fig 43–8). Under those circumstances, the asynchronous contraction of the atrial appendage is most helpful in the exclusion of a ventricular struction.
5. As previously described (see Chapter 33), a medially located nonopacified ventricular area corresponds to the absent inflow portion of the venous ventricle ("right ventricular window").
6. Ventriculography from the posterior ventricle demonstrates an enlarged smooth-walled anatomic left ventricle but no infundibulum. The pulmonary artery arises posteriorly from this ventricle and is usually enlarged and in continuity with the mitral valve (Fig 43–11).
7. As with other types of transposition of the great vessels, double coni may exist (see Chapter 38).
8. The anteriorly located and usually hypoplastic chamber is the outflow area of the right ventricle and gives rise to the transposed aorta (Fig 43–12).
9. Careful pressure measurements and angiographic demonstration of the ventricular septal defect are of paramount importance, because the ventricular communication may be restrictive and influence the operative procedure.
10. The ventricular communication is best seen by left ventriculography. If it is nonobstructive, it is also demonstrable by injection into the subaortic hypoplastic chamber because pressures in the ventricles are equal (Fig 43–13).
11. The degree of hypoplasia of the subaortic chamber varies. With large ventricular communication, the right ventricle may be well developed as in tricuspid atresia with normally related great vessels.
12. With marked hypoplasia of the subaortic chamber, the hypoplastic ventricle may be visible on the anteroposterior projection. REASON: Marked counterclockwise rotation of the heart.
13. A rare form of tricuspid atresia with transposition is isolated bulbar inversion (see Figs 43–3 and 43–14). The tricuspid valve is atretic and overlies the hypoplastic anatomic right ventricle. The mitral valve connects normally to an anatomic left ventricle. Inversion and transposition of the outflow portions of both ventricles are present. Consequently, the aorta

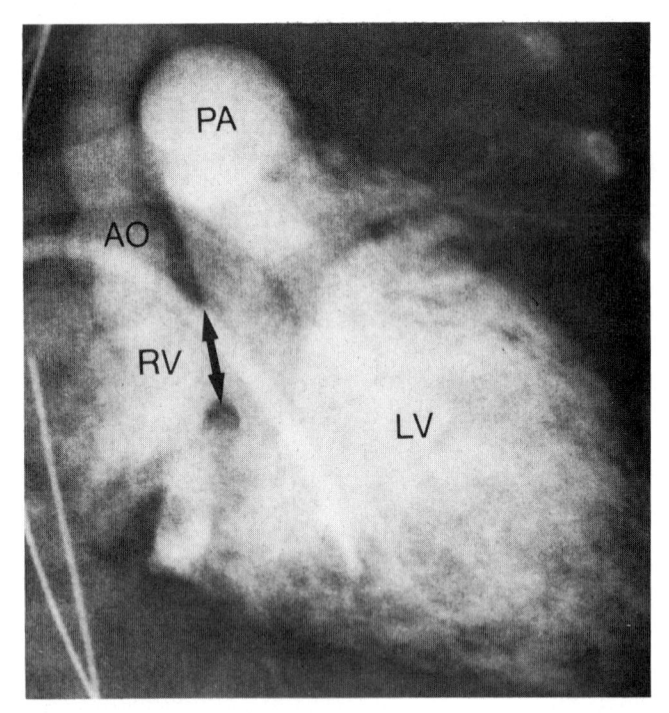

FIG 43–12.
Tricuspid atresia with transposition of great vessels. Left ventriculogram. Anteroposterior projection. Huge left ventricle *(LV)* gives rise to large pulmonary artery *(PA)*. Hypoplastic subaortic chamber fills via large ventricular communication *(arrows)*. Aorta *(AO)* is transposed and arises from hypoplastic chamber. *RV* = right ventricle.

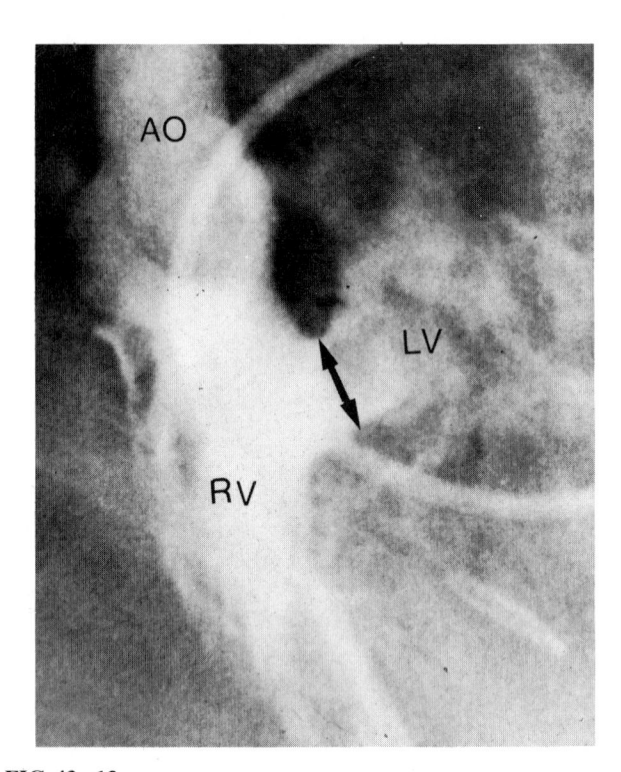

FIG 43–13.
Tricuspid atresia with D-transposition of great vessels. Right ventriculogram. Left anterior oblique projection with cranial angulation. Inflow portion of right ventricle *(RV)* is fairly well developed and only minimally hypoplastic. Ventricular communication *(arrows)*. *AO* = aorta; *LV* = left ventricle.

arises from an infundibulum lying along the left cardiac border, and the aortic valve is not in continuity with the mitral valve. The pulmonary valve, on the other hand, is positioned lower than the aortic valve in spite of the fact that it arises from an anatomic right ventricle. This chamber, however, does not have an infundibulum. Exceptions exist because each ventricle may have an infundibulum (double coni).

14. The aorta is located anteriorly and the pulmonary artery posteriorly. On an anteroposterior projection, the relative lateral positions of the great vessels can be determined. The aorta may be positioned either to the right (D-transposition) or to the left (L-transposition) of the pulmonary artery. Both types of transposition of the great vessels may occur with a conus below each great vessel (double coni).
15. Differentiation between the three types of tricuspid atresia with corrected transposition (L-transposition) can usually be made:
    a. Corrected transposition with right atrioventricular valve atresia (anatomically mitral atresia). The large posterior ventricle is an anatomic right ventricle, which can usually be recognized angiographically. A right-to-left shunt is present at the atrial level.
    b. Corrected transposition with tricuspid atresia (left atrioventricular valve). A large obligatory left-to-right shunt occurs at the atrial level, resembling hemodynamically mitral atresia. This direction of atrial shunt is opposite of the expected right-to-left shunt of tricuspid atresia.
    c. Isolated bulbar inversion. The angiographic findings are identical to corrected transposition with right atrioventricular valve atresia, but the large ventricle has the anatomic characteristics of a left ventricle.

MANAGEMENT

The principles of management include treatment of the congestive cardiac failure by digitalis and other measures, reduction of pulmonary blood flow by pulmonary arterial banding, and relief of obstruction to systemic blood flow that may be present in the form of coarctation of the aorta. Among the patients with complete transposition of the great vessels, pulmonary arterial banding is usually needed around 2 to 3 months of age to reduce the pulmonary blood flow.[7,9] It has an additional advantage in some patients of protecting against the development of pulmonary vascular disease, but this protective effect is not always achieved.

Ultimately some patients may be candidates for Fontan procedure if pulmonary arterial pressure is normal and the pulmonary arterial tree has not been distorted by previous palliative procedures.

POSTOPERATIVE RADIOGRAPHIC FEATURES

The principles of treatment of tricuspid atresia with transposition of the great vessels are similar to tricuspid atresia with normally related great vessels, and the postoperative appearance is similar. Because most patients with tricuspid atresia and transposition of the great vessels have increased pulmonary vasculature, the most common palliative operative procedure is pulmonary artery banding. Palliative treatment of the rarer cases of tricuspid atresia with transposition and pulmonary stenosis is by an aorticopulmonary shunt. The postoperative radiographic appearance in these patients is identical to other cyanotic lesion with decreased flow (see Chapters 30 and 33).

REFERENCES

1. Tandon R, Edwards JE: Tricuspid atresia, *J Thorac Cardiovasc Surg* 67:530, 1974.
2. Marcano BA, Riemenschneider TA, Rutterberg HD, et al: Tricuspid atresia with increased pulmonary blood flow, *Circulation* 40:399, 1969.
3. Kessler A, Adams P Jr: Association of transposition of the great vessels and rudimentary right ventricle with and without tricuspid atresia, *Pediatrics* 19:851, 1957.
4. Restivo A, Ho SY, Anderson RH, et al: Absent left atrioventricular connection with right atrium connected to morphologically left ventricular chamber, rudimentary right ventricular chamber, and ventriculoarterial discordance: problem of mitral versus tricuspid atresia, *Br Heart J* 48:240, 1982.
5. Tandon R, Marin-Garcia J, Moller JH, et al: Tricuspid atresia with L-transposition, *Am Heart J* 88:417, 1974.
6. Scalia D, Russo P, Anderson RH, et al: The surgical anatomy of hearts with no direct communication between the right atrium and the ventricular mass—so-called tricuspid atresia, *J Thorac Cardiovasc Surg* 87:743, 1984.
7. Dick M, Fyler DC, Nadas AS: Tricuspid atresia: clinical course in 101 patients, *Am J Cardiol* 35:327, 1975.
8. Davachi F, Lucas RV Jr, Moller JH: The electrocardiogram and vectorcardiogram in tricuspid atresia: correlation with pathologic anatomy, *Am J Cardiol* 25:18, 1970.
9. Williams WG, Rubis L, Fowler RS, et al: Tricuspid atresia: results of treatment in 160 children, *Am J Cardiol* 38:235, 1976.

CHAPTER 44

Double-Inlet Ventricle

Double-inlet ventricle is a rare condition in which one of the atrioventricular valves overrides a ventricular septal defect. Therefore, one ventricle receives blood from both atria. Double-inlet ventricle is commonly associated with hypoplasia of the ventricle underlying the involved valve because of the reduced blood flow into that chamber. Double-inlet left ventricle occurs more commonly than double-inlet right ventricle.

Two terms have been used in double-inlet ventricle to describe the relationship of the involved atrioventricular valve to the ventricular septum. Overriding atrioventricular valve describes the condition in which the valve orifice faces both ventricles, but the papillary muscle and chordae tendineae insert into the appropriate ventricle. Straddling atrioventricular valve describes the situation where a valve may or may not override a ventricular septal defect but has a papillary muscle or chordal attachment to the opposite ventricle. Straddling atrioventricular valves have also been described in patients with ventricular inversion (corrected transposition of the great vessels).

DOUBLE-INLET LEFT VENTRICLE

In double-inlet left ventricle, the left ventricle receives the entire volume of flow from the left atrium and a portion of the systemic venous return from the right atrium.

Pathologic Anatomy

The atrial septum is usually intact. A ventricular septal defect, generally of the atrioventricular canal type, is present.[1] This defect extends under the septal leaflet of the tricuspid valve and to the level of the atrioventricular annulus.

Double-inlet left ventricle results from tricuspid valvar malalignment and presents a spectrum of anomalies, with three anatomic types[1,2]:

1. The tricuspid valve orifice may be displaced so it overrides the ventricular septal defect, but the chordal attachments are normal and attach into the right ventricle (central straddling) (Fig 44–1).

2. The tricuspid valve orifice is displaced, and some chordae tendineae pass through the ventricular septal defect and are attached in the left ventricle (Fig 44–2).

3. The tricuspid valve orifice may be normally positioned in relation to the ventricular septal defect, but chordae tendineae pass through the ventricular septal defect to attach in the left ventricle (peripheral straddling).

In double-inlet left ventricle, the atrial septum is abnormally oriented and forms an angle of nearly 90 degrees with the ventricular septum, thereby allowing the right atrium to communicate with both ventricles. Normally the angle formed between the atrial and the ventricular septae is less than 90%. Mitral valvar abnormalities such as incompetence, stenosis, cleft, hypoplasia, and atresia may coexist.

This anomaly probably results from failure or incomplete medial migration of the primitive common atrioventricular canal to override the developing ventricular septum. Therefore, the atrioventricular canal joins the ventricles unequally.

Hemodynamics

This condition is characterized by a bidirectional shunt. The right-to-left shunt occurs from the right atrium into the left ventricle through the straddling valve. A left-to-right shunt, which is usually large, occurs through the coexistent ventricular septal defect. Pulmonary hypertension and congestive cardiac failure are common because of the large ventricular septal defect.

Clinical Features

In patients without a major associated cardiac condition, the history and physical examination are indistin-

DOUBLE INLET LV WITH OVERRIDING TV

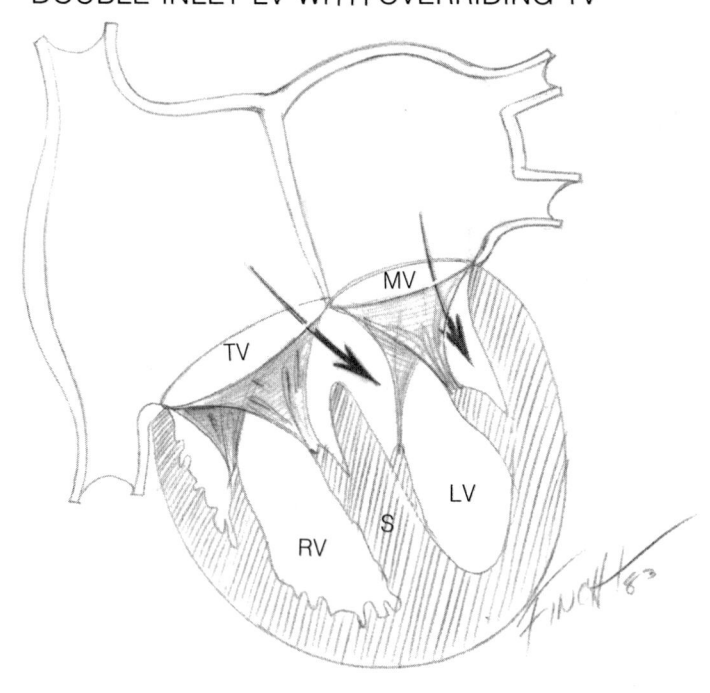

FIG 44–1.
Double-inlet left ventricle *(LV)* with overriding tricuspid valve *(TV)*. Defect in ventricular septum *(S)*. Tricuspid valve partially faces left ventricle, but chordal attachments are normal. *MV* = mitral valve; *RV* = right ventricle.

guishable from those of a large ventricular septal defect. The features of congestive cardiac failure develop in early infancy. Despite the presence of a right-to-left shunt from the right atrium to the left ventricle, cyanosis is not a feature of the history or physical examination, because the left-to-right shunt is usually large. There is a loud harsh pansystolic murmur along the left sternal border associated with a thrill. The pulmonic component of the second heart sound is accentuated because of pulmonary hypertension. An apical middiastolic murmur representing the increased blood flow across the mitral valve, secondary to the shunt, is heard.

DOUBLE INLET LV WITH STRADDLING TV

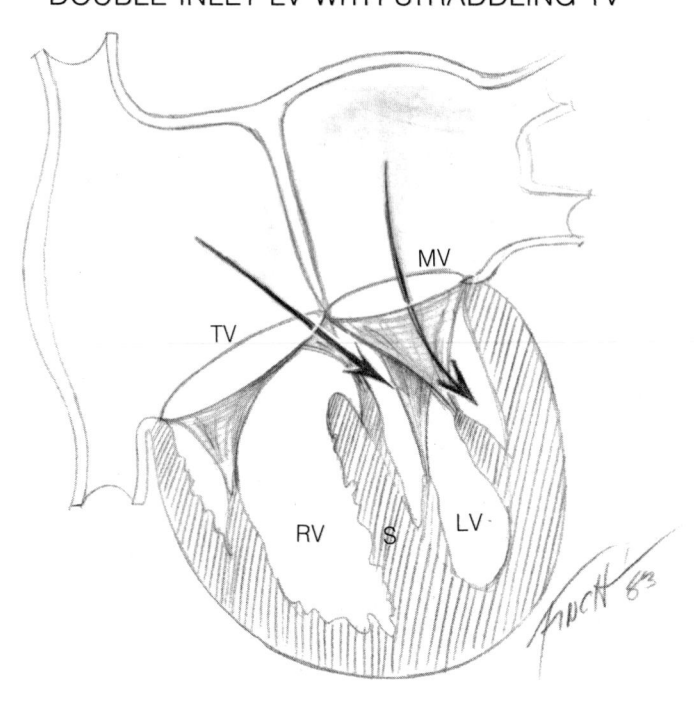

FIG 44–2.
Double-inlet left ventricle *(LV)* with straddling tricuspid valve *(TV)*. Chordal attachments of TV to left side of interventricular septum *(S)*. *MV* = mitral valve; *RV* = right ventricle.

If the straddling tricuspid valve is associated with right ventricular outflow tract obstruction, the clinical findings resemble tetralogy of Fallot.

Electrocardiographic Features

The electrocardiogram reflects the hypoplasia of the right ventricle. Although the QRS axis is usually normal, the precordial leads show an rS pattern in the right and an Rs pattern in the left precordial leads.

Echocardiographic Features

Echocardiographic tracings are extremely important in the diagnosis of straddling tricuspid valve, and care must be taken to distinguish it from endocardial cushion defect. The following features are noted on echocardiography[3, 4]:

1. Echoes can be recorded from two atrioventricular valves without noting an intervening ventricular septum.
2. The septal leaflet of the tricuspid valve opens posteriorly with reference to the plane of the interventricular septum.
3. The anterior leaflet of the tricuspid valve may cross the plane of the interventricular septum during diastole.
4. The size of the right ventricle (or more rarely, the left ventricle) is reduced.
5. A large posterior defect can be identified in the ventricular septum.

Doppler color flow measurements can assess direction of blood flow into the ventricle. The left atrioventricular valve is often stenotic. The status of both the atrial septum and pulmonary outflow must be evaluated.

Radiographic Features

There are no roentgenographic findings that permit the distinction of double-inlet left ventricle from isolated ventricular septal defect.

Cardiac Catheterization

The passage of the catheter directly from the right atrium into the left ventricle in a low position is consistent with the diagnosis, but such a catheter course is identical to the catheter passage in patients with an endocardial cushion defect.

Unless there are coexistent cardiac anomalies, the hemodynamics resemble a large ventricular septal defect, with a large left-to-right shunt at the ventricular level and pulmonary hypertension. The one distinguishing feature is a right-to-left shunt, which causes minimal systemic arterial desaturation. Arterial saturations may range from 85% to 93%, depending on the degree of straddling and the volume of pulmonary blood flow.

Angiographic Features

The angiographic diagnosis of straddling tricuspid valve (double-inlet left ventricle) is difficult, but nevertheless a diagnosis can be firmly established using both right and left ventriculography. In addition, right atrial injection of contrast medium is important, because after injection of this chamber, both ventricles opacify simultaneously. REASON: Normally right atrial blood flows only into the right ventricle, but in this condition a portion is diverted by the straddling tricuspid valve into the left ventricle.

Angiograms should be obtained in a shallow left anterior oblique projection with beam angulation. REASON: Straddling tricuspid valve is associated with a ventricular septal defect in the posterior aspect of the septum (atrioventricular canal type). This portion of the septum is best demonstrated by this projection (see Chapter 12).

Right Ventriculography

1. During systole, the ventricular septal defect is demonstrated immediately beneath the straddling tricuspid valve.
2. The annulus of the straddling tricuspid valve is incompletely visualized. REASON: The part of the tricuspid annulus that overrides the left ventricle is not outlined by contrast medium.
3. During diastole, unopacified blood entering the tricuspid valve outlines only the right ventricular portion of the valve. The normal round radiolucency outlining the entire tricuspid annulus is not present.
4. If the left ventricle is also opacified on a right ventriculogram, the entire overriding tricuspid annulus and also the mitral annulus can be identified as two complete radiolucent circles.

Left Ventriculography

1. During systole, because of the left-to-right shunt through the ventricular septal defect, the inflow portion of the right ventricle is visualized.
2. The right ventricle is well opacified. REASON: Most patients have a large left-to-right shunt through the ventricular septal defect.
3. In the tricuspid area, immediately above the ventricular septal defect, an irregularly bulging pouch resembling an aneurysm of the membranous septum is outlined. REASON: The straddling leaflet of the tricuspid valve lies immediately above the ventricular septal defect and may

balloon during systole. The lower margin of the valve leaflet is outlined by contrast medium below (Fig 44–3).

4. During diastole the tricuspid annulus is identified as a circular filling defect that clearly overrides the ventricular septum. This appearance differs from aneurysm of the membranous septum, in which the entire tricuspid annulus is situated above the right ventricle. Diastolic frames obtained after left ventriculography demonstrate overriding of the tricuspid annulus as well (see Fig 44–3). This is the most important finding in diagnosing straddling tricuspid valve. Occasionally a steeper left anterior oblique projection is required to visualize the straddling tricuspid valvar annulus.

5. An overriding valve cannot be differentiated from a straddling valve.

Operative Considerations

Operative repair of double-inlet left ventricle is difficult (Fig 44–4). Every effort should be made to preserve the tricuspid valve, but in cases with severe incompetence, it must be replaced.[5] Repair of the ventricular septal defect by patch should be carried out in such a fashion that the entire tricuspid valve empties into the right ventricle. By doing so, the capacity of the right ventricle is enlarged. Left ventricular outflow tract obstruction, mitral incompetence, or tricuspid stenosis are complications of the opera-

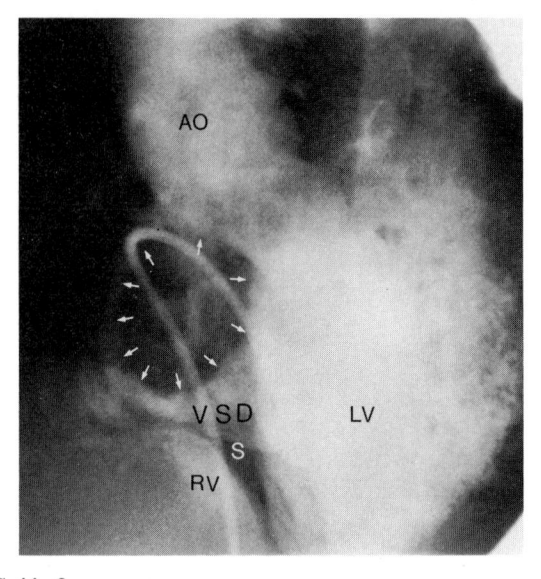

FIG 44–3.
Double-inlet left ventricle. Left ventriculogram. Shallow left anterior oblique projection. Diastolic frame. Enlarged left ventricle *(LV)*. REASON: It receives total pulmonary flow and part of systemic flow. Hypoplastic right ventricle *(RV)*. Ventricular septal defect *(VSD)* lies immediately beneath tricuspid valve. Tricuspid annulus *(arrows)* is outlined by blood entering ventricles. Tricuspid valve straddles or overrides septum *(S)*. *AO* = aorta.

FIG 44–4.
Operative correction of double-inlet left ventricle *(LV)* with straddling tricuspid valve *(TV)*. Patch sewn obliquely to include papillary muscles of TV into right ventricle *(RV)*. *MV* = mitral valve. *S* = septum.

tive repair. The risk of developing heart block is greater than in repair of uncomplicated ventricular septal defect. In patients with severe hypoplasia of the right ventricle, a Fontan procedure may be performed combined with operative closure of the tricuspid valve.[6]

Because of the increased risk of an operation, operative treatment is usually delayed until the patient is about 5 years of age.

DOUBLE-INLET RIGHT VENTRICLE

Double-inlet right ventricle with straddling mitral valve occurs less frequently than double-inlet left ventricle with straddling tricuspid valve.

Pathologic Anatomy

As in double-inlet left ventricle, an abnormality of the common atrioventricular valve occurs in relation to the plane of the ventricular septum. During development the atrioventricular canal migrates too far to the right so that a portion of the mitral valve overlies the right ventricle.

A ventricular septal defect is an integral part of this malformation. It is located posteriorly and immediately below the mitral valve. Double-inlet right ventricle presents a spectrum of malformations, with three anatomic types:

1. The orifice of the mitral valve overrides the ventricular septal defect, but the chordal attachments are normal (Fig 44–5).
2. The orifice of the mitral valve overrides the ventricular septal defect, and a part of the mitral valve apparatus, papillary muscles, and chordae tendineae attach either to the edge of the ventricular septum or in the right ventricle (Fig 44–6).
3. The entire mitral valve overlies the right ventricle (total commitment of mitral valve). The entire left atrial volume enters the right ventricle. The ventricular septum may be intact (Fig 44–7), or there may be a ventricular septal defect (Fig 44–8) remote from the mitral annulus. In this form the left ventricle is diminutive.

In the first two types, flow from the left atrium occurs simultaneously into both ventricles. The right ventricle receives blood from two sources, therefore the term double-inlet right ventricle.

The size of the left ventricle varies considerably be-

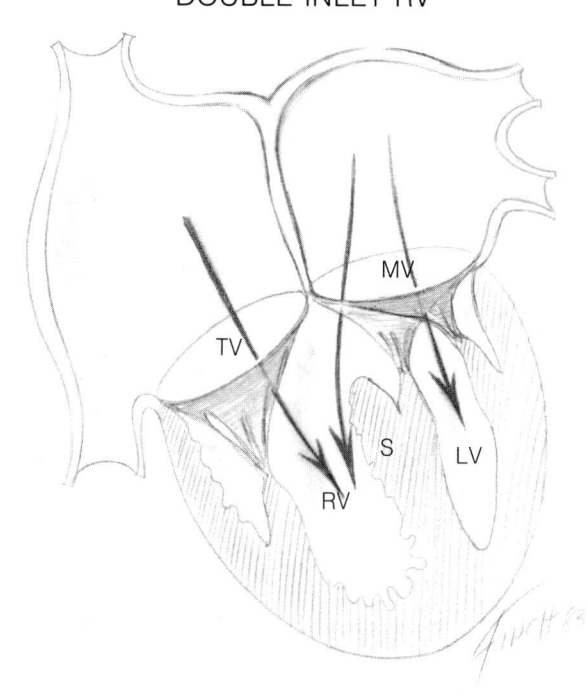

FIG 44–5.
Double-inlet right ventricle *(RV)* with overriding mitral valve *(MV)*. Mitral valve partially faces RV but chordal attachments are to left ventricle *(LV)* exclusively. S = septum; TV = tricuspid valve.

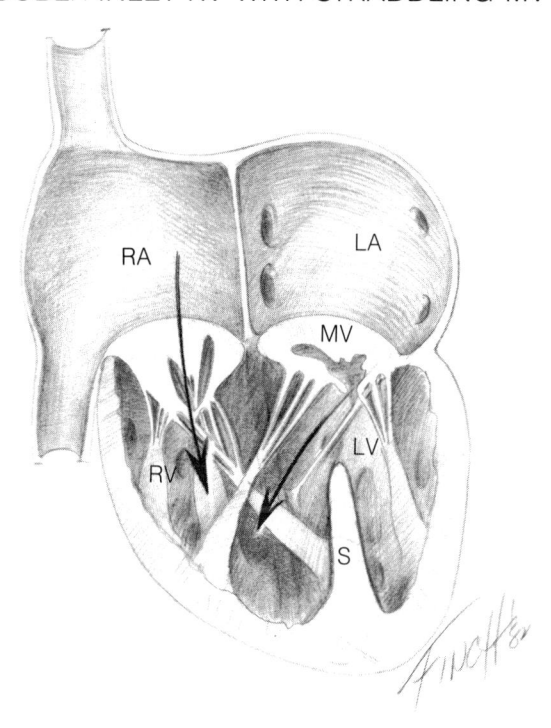

FIG 44–6.
Double-inlet right ventricle *(RV)* with straddling mitral valve *(MV)*. Ventricular septum *(S)* displaced to left, reducing size of left ventricle *(LV)* and enlarging right ventricle *(RV)*. Blood through both tricuspid *(TV)* and mitral valve *(MV)* enters right ventricle.

DOUBLE INLET RV WITH INTACT SEPTUM

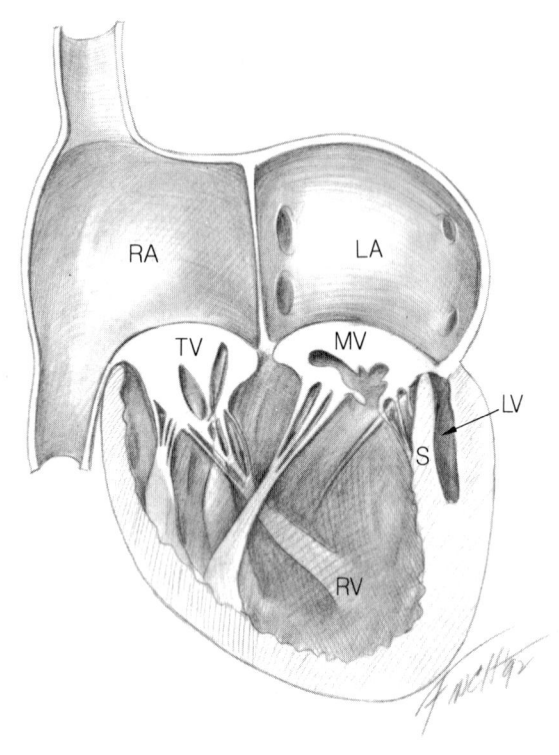

FIG 44–7.
Double-inlet right ventricle *(RV)* with intact ventricular septum *(S)*. Both mitral *(MV)* and tricuspid *(TV)* valves face RV. Hypoplastic left ventricle *(LV)*.

DOUBLE INLET RV WITH TOTAL COMMITMENT OF MV AND VSD

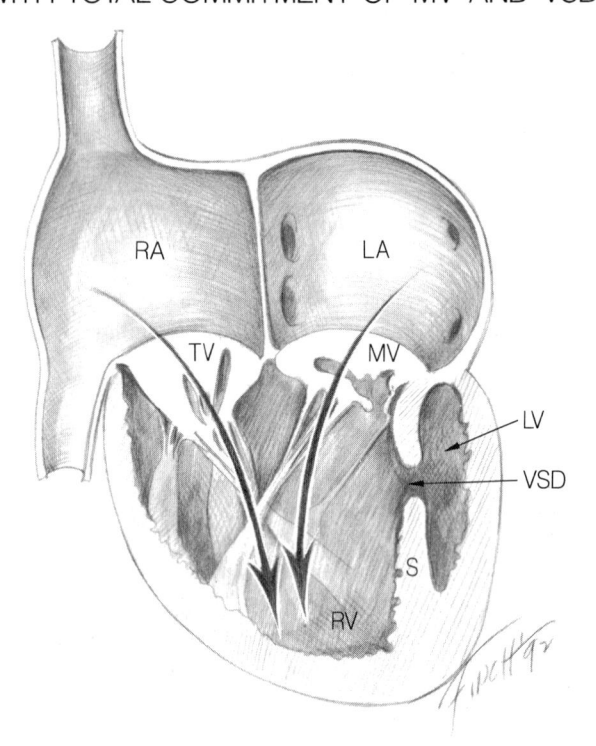

FIG 44–8.
Double-inlet right ventricle *(RV)* with total commitment of mitral valve *(MV)*. Through ventricular septal defect *(VSD)* hypoplastic left ventricle *(LV)* receives blood. S = interventricular septum; TV = tricuspid valve.

cause it depends on the volume of inflow but, it is usually hypoplastic. In the presence of major overriding of the mitral valve, the left ventricle is severely hypoplastic, the heart resembling single ventricle of a right ventricular type.

Because of the left ventricular hypoplasia and the location of ventricular septal defect, either double-outlet right ventricle with subpulmonary ventricular septal defect or complete transposition of the great vessels is commonly associated (Fig 44–9).[7,8] Double-inlet right ventricle occurs frequently in crisscross heart. Among patients with straddling mitral valve and double-outlet right ventricle, subpulmonary stenosis is frequent, and the straddling mitral valve may cause subpulmonary obstruction.[3] The condition has also been described with complete atrioventricular canal, in which case subaortic obstruction is found.[8]

Hemodynamics

It is difficult to describe a hemodynamic picture of double-inlet right ventricle, because the condition usually coexists with other major congenital cardiac anomalies that dominate the hemodynamic findings. Double-inlet right ventricle causes an obligatory left-to-right shunt at the ventricular level and, depending on the type of associated malformation, can lead to either subaortic or subpulmonary stenosis.

Clinical Features

Because of the few cases with this condition, there are no clear-cut clinical or electrocardiographic findings of double-inlet right ventricle.

Echocardiographic Features

There is limited echocardiographic experience with this condition. The left ventricle is hypoplastic, and the mitral valve overrides the plane of the ventricular septum and the coexistent ventricular septal defect.

The following features may be noted:

1. Echoes can be recorded from two atrioventricular valves without intervening ventricular septum.
2. The septal leaflet of the tricuspid valve opens anteriorly to the plane of the ventricular septum.

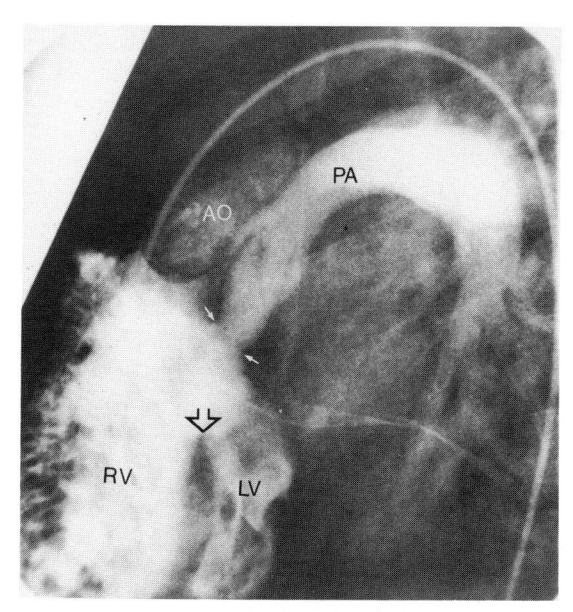

FIG 44-9.
Double-inlet right ventricle. Subpulmonary conus. Right ventriculogram. Steep left anterior oblique projection. Enlarged right ventricle *(RV)* and small left ventricle *(LV)*. Large ventricular communication *(white arrows)*. Edge of ventricular septum *(open arrow)*. Mitral valve empties partially into right ventricle. Aorta *(AO)* anterior to pulmonary artery *(PA)*.

3. The size of the left ventricle is reduced.
4. A large ventricular septal defect can be identified.

Radiographic Features

The correct diagnosis cannot be suspected from clinical findings or an analysis of thoracic roentgenograms. Marked cardiomegaly and increased pulmonary vasculature are present. Left atrial enlargement is expected because of the left-to-right shunt from the left atrium to the right ventricle.

Angiographic Features

Injection into both the right ventricle and the left atrium are necessary to establish the diagnosis of double-inlet right ventricle. The condition may be misdiagnosed as mitral atresia because of severe hypoplasia of the left ventricle. If the mitral valve is of normal size, contrast medium enters both ventricles simultaneously. In the presence of associated hypoplasia of the mitral valve, a left-to-right shunt can be demonstrated at the atrial level as well.

1. Injection of the left atrium demonstrates opacification of the right ventricle and simultaneous opacification of the right atrium because of a left-to-right shunt at the atrial level. The opening into the left ventricle is often obstructed, caused by a hypoplastic mitral valve.

2. The posteriorly placed left ventricle, which is usually smaller than the enlarged anteriorly placed right ventricle, may be better seen on the late films of a pulmonary arteriogram.

3. In patients with total commitment of mitral valve to the right ventricle, direct opacification of the left ventricle does not occur.

4. Right ventriculography demonstrates the enlarged right and the hypoplastic left ventricles. In cases of double-inlet right ventricle with intact ventricular septum, the diminutive left ventricle does not opacify.

5. Both great vessels usually arise from the enlarged right ventricle (see Fig 44-9). REASON: Because the left ventricle is diminutive, the right ventricle usually gives rise to both great arteries. Double-inlet right ventricle is therefore commonly associated with double-outlet right ventricle.

6. The great arteries are usually in a transposed position and have separate coni (see Fig 44-9).

7. Selective injection of the left ventricle with cranial angulation should show the orifice of the mitral valve overriding the plane of the ventricular septum.

The diagnosis of double-inlet right ventricle must be considered as a possible coexistent condition in patients with various forms of transposition of the great vessels, with left ventricular hypoplasia, or with endocardial cushion defect. Careful echocardiographic and angiographic studies should diagnose this rare coexistent condition.

Operative Considerations

This condition is potentially correctable. If there is straddling of the mitral valve and the left ventricle is near normal size, a patch can be sewn to the right side of the ventricular septum, so that the mitral apparatus is retained in relation to the left ventricle (Fig 44-10). In total commitment or near total commitment of the mitral valve, the essentially single ventricle can be divided by a patch, the patch being placed between the papillary muscle of the tricuspid and the mitral valve.

SUMMARY

Double-inlet right ventricle and double-inlet left ventricle are variations of an endocardial cushion defect in which a ventricular communication is present in the ventricular septum and lies beneath the tricuspid valve (double-inlet left ventricle) or the mitral valve (double-inlet right ventricle). The anomaly develops by an abnormal migration of the embryonic common atrioventricular valve toward either the right (double-inlet right ventricle) or the left (double-inlet left ventricle).

SURGICAL CORRECTION OF DOUBLE INLET RV WITH STRADDLING MITRAL VALVE

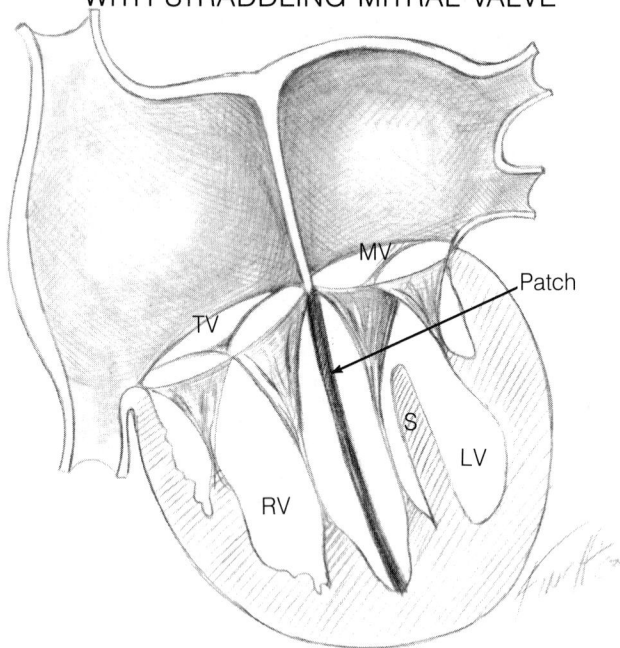

FIG 44–10.
Surgical correction of double inlet right ventricle *(RV)* with straddling mitral valve *(MV)*. Ventricular septal patch sewn to include straddling papillary muscle attachment of MV into left ventricle *(LV)*. S = interventricular septum; TV = tricuspid valve.

Double inlet occurs commonly in patients with corrected transposition of the great vessels (see Chapter 39).

Hemodynamically double-inlet left ventricle results in a right-to-left shunt and double-inlet right ventricle in a left-to-right shunt. Because of the dual inflow, one ventricle is enlarged, and the other ventricle is hypoplastic because it receives less blood. Therefore, double-inlet left ventricle occurs with hypoplasia of the right ventricle, and double-inlet right ventricle occurs with hypoplasia of the left ventricle. The diagnosis is suggested angiographically by diastolic filling of both ventricles after selective angiography into the atrium.

Several terms are redefined:

1. Overriding atrioventricular valve. An atrioventricular valve overrides a ventricular septal defect when its orifice faces both ventricles, but the papillary muscle and chordae tendineae of this valve insert into the appropriate ventricle (see Figs 44–1 and 44–5).

2. Straddling atrioventricular valve. An atrioventricular valve may or may not override a ventricular septal defect but has papillary muscle or chordal attachment to the opposite ventricle (see Figs 44–2 and 44–6).

3. Double-inlet right ventricle. A ventricular septal defect is located in posterior atrioventricular canal position and immediately adjacent to both the tricuspid and the mitral annuli. The mitral valve straddles the ventricular septal defect, and left atrial blood enters both the morphologic right and left ventricles. The mitral valve may either straddle (see Fig 44–6) or override (see Figs 44–5 and 44–9).

4. Double-inlet left ventricle. A ventricular septal defect is located in posterior (atrioventricular canal) position, which the tricuspid valve straddles. Right atrial blood enters both ventricles. Both types of double inlet are variations of an endocardial cushion defect.

5. Total commitment of both atrioventricular valves to one ventricle (see Fig 44–8). This is a rare type of double-inlet right ventricle or double-inlet left ventricle. A ventricular septal defect is distant from the atrioventricular valvar annuli. Therefore, the atrioventricular valves do not straddle the defect and are totally committed to one of the ventricles (see Fig 44–8). There may be a ventricular septal defect (see Fig 44–8), or the ventricular septum may be intact (see Fig 44–7).

6. Double-inlet ventricle may coexist with double-outlet ventricle (see Fig 44–9).

7. Double-inlet ventricle may coexist with ventricular inversion.

REFERENCES

1. Bharati S, McAllister HA Jr, Lev M: Straddling and displaced atrioventricular orifices and valves, *Circulation* 60:673, 1979.
2. Aziz KU, Paul MH, Muster AJ, et al: Positional abnormalities of atrioventricular valves in transposition of the great arteries including double outlet right ventricle, atrioventricular valve straddling and malattachment, *Am J Cardiol* 44:1135, 1979.
3. Seward JB, Tajik AK, Ritter DG: Echocardiographic features

of straddling tricuspid valve, *Mayo Clin Proc* 50:427, 1975.
4. LaCorte MA, Fellows KE, Williams RG: Overriding tricuspid valve: echocardiographic and angiocardiographic features, *Am J Cardiol* 37:911, 1976.
5. Pacifico AD, Soto B, Bargeron LM Jr: Surgical treatment of straddling tricuspid valve, *Circulation* 60:655, 1979.
6. Tabry IF, McGoon DC, Danielson GK, et al: Surgical management of straddling atrioventricular valve, *J Thorac Cardiovasc Surg* 77:191, 1979.
7. Kitamura N, Takao A, Ando M, et al: Taussig-Bing heart with mitral valve straddling: case reports and postmortem study, *Circulation* 49:761, 1974.
8. Freedom RM, Bini R, Dische R, et al: The straddling mitral valve: morphological observations and clinical implications, *Eur J Cardiol* 8:27, 1978.

CHAPTER 45

Truncus Arteriosus

Truncus arteriosus, although accounting for only 1% to 4% of instances of congenital cardiac anomalies, is important because it causes severe symptoms in infancy and can be operatively corrected. Crupi et al.[1] have defined truncus as a single arterial trunk that leaves the heart by way of a single arterial valve and gives rise to the coronary, systemic, and one or both pulmonary arteries.

Three other trunco-conal lesions may be confused with truncus arteriosus, in part because of terminology. Tetralogy of Fallot and pulmonary atresia have been called "pseudotruncus arteriosus" (see Chapter 31), but it has different embryogenesis. Origin of a pulmonary artery from the ascending aorta has been termed hemitruncus and likewise has a different embryologic origin (see Chapter 18). Aorticopulmonary septal defect (window) (see Chapter 17) represents partial separation of the primitive truncus rather than total absence of conotruncal septum. Each of these may cause confusion in angiographic diagnosis, particularly when a ventricular septal defect coexists. Yet in each of these three conditions, two semilunar valves are present, although one may be atretic.

PATHOLOGICAL ANATOMY

This malformation results from faulty development of the primitive truncus arteriosus, which lies between the conal region and the aortic sac.

In the fifth week of gestation, endocardial ridges form in the bulbus cordis and primitive truncus arteriosus (Fig 45–1,A). These ridges fuse (Figs 45–1,A and 45–2), forming the aorticopulmonary septum, which divides the truncus arteriosus into pulmonary and aortic channels. For unknown reasons, the aortic pulmonary septum forms in a spiral fashion (Fig 45–1,B), causing the great arteries to normally twist around each other. The bulbus cordis becomes the right ventricular outflow tract.

Various abnormalities in the development of the truncoconal septum (aorticopulmonary septum) may occur, resulting in various cardiac anomalies. The division of the truncus by the truncal ridges may be uneven and result in either a large aorta and hypoplastic pulmonary artery channel (see Figs 45–1,B and 45–2) (tetrology of Fallot) or a hypoplastic aorta and large pulmonary artery, as in aortic atresia (see Chapter 50).

There may be incomplete development and lack of fusion of the aorticopulmonary septum, resulting in a fenestration, as in aorticopulmonary window (Figs 45–1,B and 45–3) (see Chapter 17).

The aorticopulmonary septum may not develop in a spiral fashion, which results in complete transposition of the great vessels (Figs 45–1,B and 45–4) (see Chapter 38).

The aorticopulmonary septum may be largely absent and fail to fuse, which results in persistent truncus arteriosus (Figs 45–1,B and 45–5), or the septum may be malpositioned, resulting in aortic origin of the pulmonary artery (hemitruncus) (Figs 45–1,B and 45–6).

In truncus arteriosus, a single arterial vessel arises from the heart and receives blood from both ventricles, because a ventricular septal defect coexists. This vessel supplies the aorta, pulmonary arteries, and coronary arteries (see Fig 45–11).

Truncus arteriosus has been classified according to the pattern of origin of the pulmonary arteries[2]:

Type I: Origin of pulmonary arteries from a short pulmonary trunk (see Fig 45–2).

Type II: Origin of pulmonary arteries from the truncus itself, with their origins being separate but close together (see Fig 45–3).

Type III: Origin of pulmonary arteries from truncus, with separate and widely spaced origins (rare) (see Fig 45–4).

Type IV: Origin of pulmonary arteries from descending aorta (see Fig 45–5).

Most cases of truncus arteriosus are probably an inter-

A. PARTITION OF THE TRUNCUS ARTERIOSUS

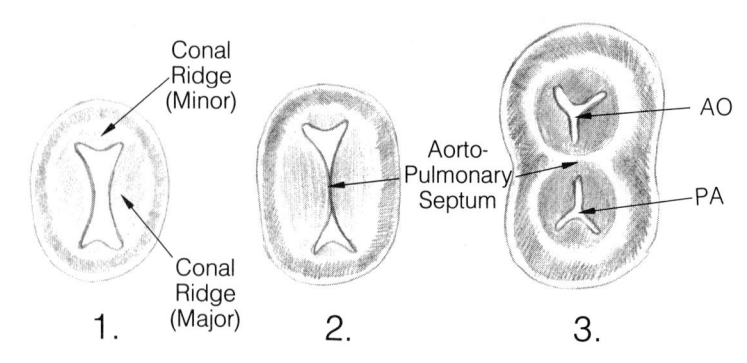

B. THE TRUNCO—CONAL SEPTUM

1. Normal
2. Unequal Division
3. Defect — A-P Window
4. No Spiraling — Transposition
5. Absence — Truncus Arteriosus
6. Malposition — Aortic Origin of Pulmonary Artery (Hemitruncus)

Tetralogy of Fallot or Aortic Atresia

FIG 45–1.
Development processes dividing truncus arteriosus and variants. **A,** normal development. *1,* endocardial ridges develop in bulbus cordis (two major and two minor endocardial ridges). *2,* fusion of major ridges. *3,* formation of aorticopulmonary-septum dividing truncus into separate pulmonary and aortic channels. **B,** development of congenital variations. *1,* normally truncoconal-septum develops in a spiral fashion, dividing primitive truncus into two equal-sized channels, namely, the pulmonary artery and the aorta. Normal cardiac anatomy results *(below)* and ventricles and great vessel wrap around each other. *2,* unequal division of truncus arteriosus. Large aortic channel and small pulmonary channel result in tetralogy of Fallot. Spiral development of septum is preserved. Great vessels and ventricles twist around each other normally. *3,* normal development of truncoconal-septum but incomplete fusion of truncal ridges. Defect in septum as in aorticopulmonary *(A-P)* window *(below)*. *4,* absent twist of truncoconal-septum divides truncus and outflow tracts into two parallel channels. Complete transposition of great vessels results *(below)*. Ventricles and great vessels are behind one another. Great vessels no longer twisted around each other. *5,* absence of truncoconal-septum. Truncus arteriosus and ventricular septal defect immediately beneath truncal valve. *6,* malposition of septum causes one of pulmonary arteries to arise from aortic channel. Result is aortic origin of pulmonary artery (hemitruncus).

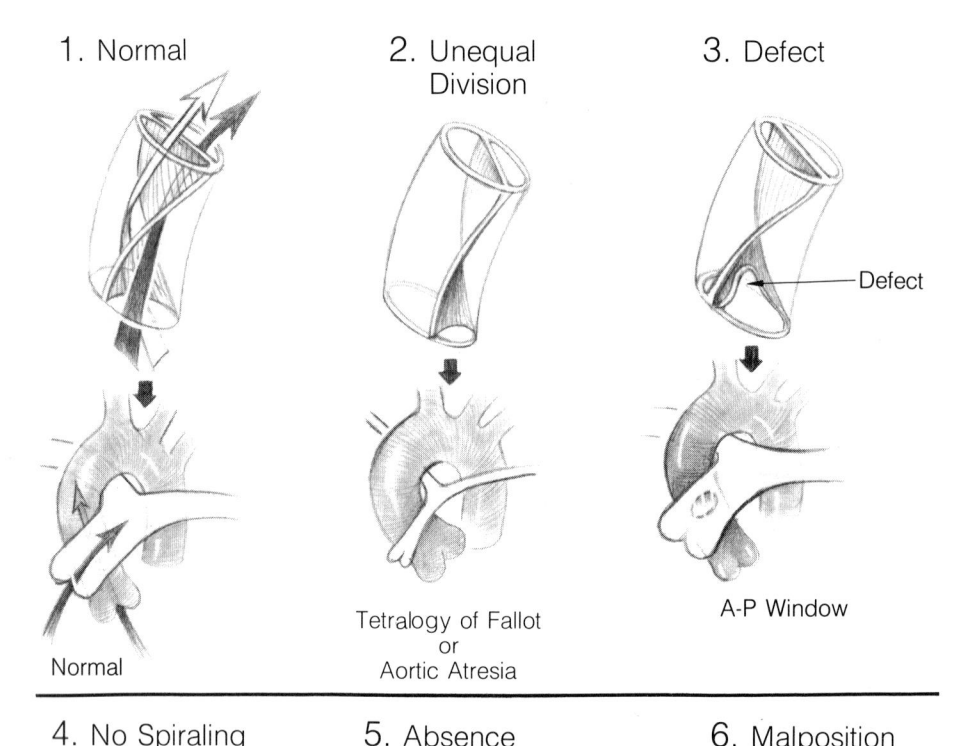

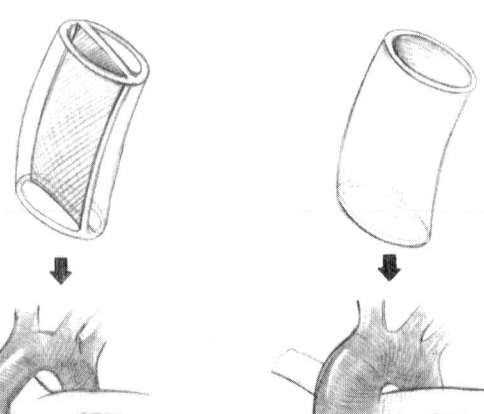

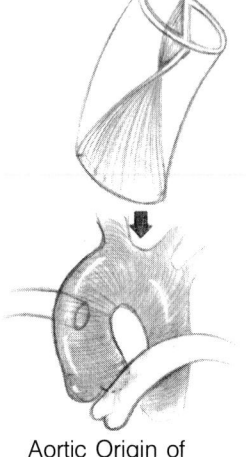

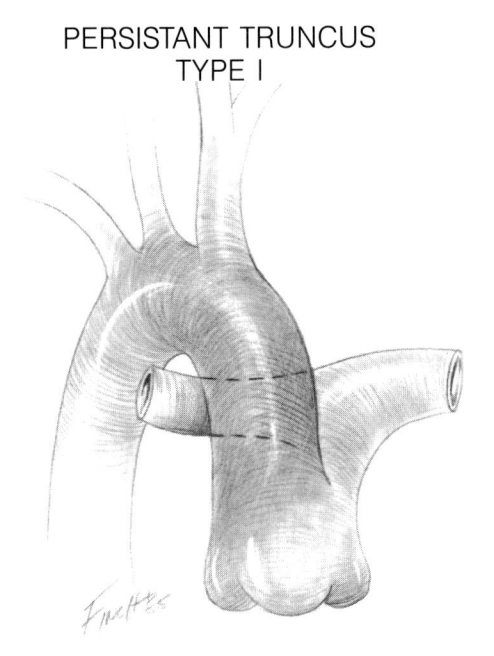

FIG 45–2.
Persistent truncus arteriosus type I. Pulmonary arteries arise from truncus through short common vessel.

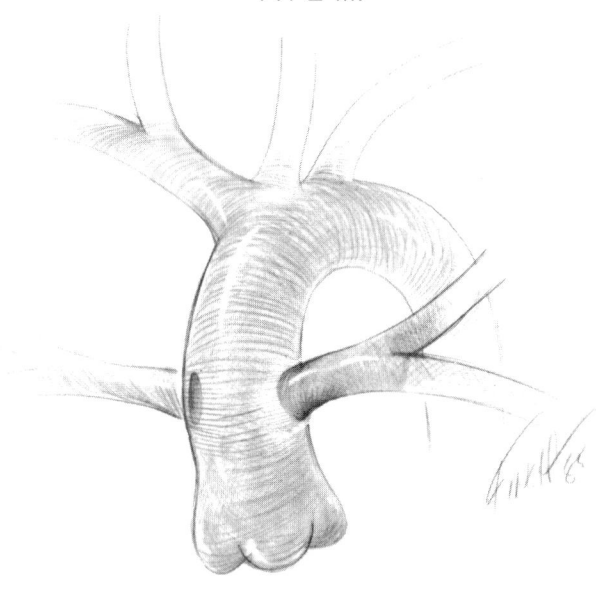

FIG 45–4.
Persistent truncus arteriosus type III. Pulmonary arteries arise from separate orifices from posterior wall of truncus.

mediate form between types I and II. Probably all cases classified as truncus arteriosus type IV represent developmentally tetralogy of Fallot with pulmonary atresia.[2, 3] Careful examination of such cases reveals an infundibulum that ends blindly and a fibrous strand passing from the infundibulum to the pulmonary arteries. This strand represents the atretic main pulmonary artery. In truncus arteriosus, an infundibulum is not present, and this feature serves to distinguish truncus type IV from tetralogy of Fallot with pulmonary atresia (see Chapter 31).

Unilateral absence of a pulmonary artery (hemitruncus), may coexist on either the same side (see Fig 45–6)

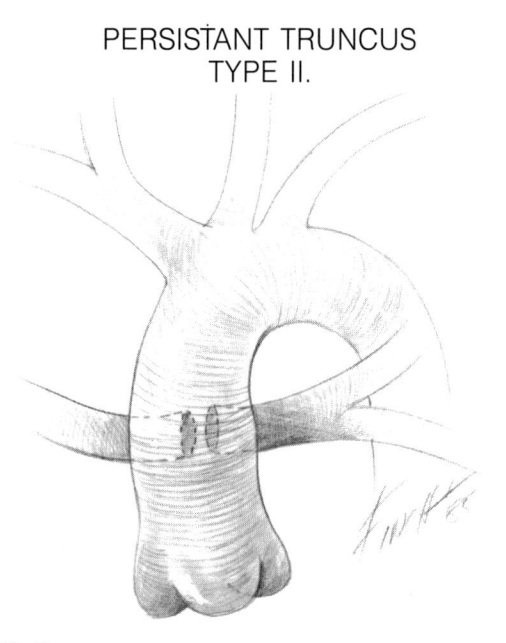

FIG 45–3.
Persistent truncus arteriosus type II. Pulmonary arteries arise adjacent to one another from the truncus.

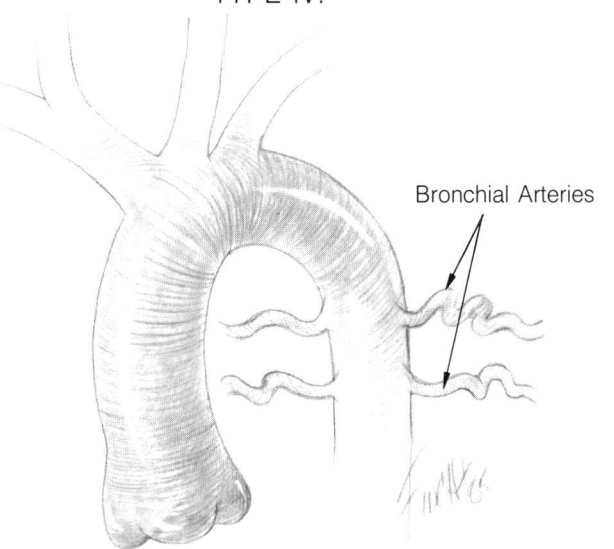

FIG 45–5.
Persistent truncus arteriosus type IV. Bronchial arteries from descending aorta supply pulmonary arterial tree.

LEFT HEMITRUNCUS

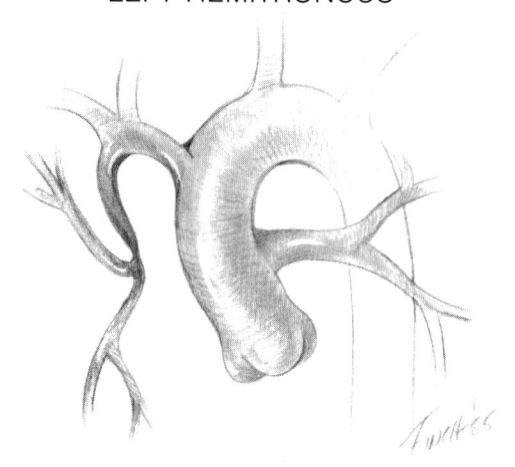

FIG 45-6.
Persistent truncus arteriosus with proximal interruption of right pulmonary artery. Left pulmonary artery arises from truncus arteriosus. Right pulmonary artery arises from right patent ductus arteriosus.

or opposite the side from the aortic arch (Fig 45-7). Under those circumstances, the contralateral pulmonary artery may be supplied by a patent ductus (see Fig 45-6). Sometimes origin of a pulmonary artery from the ascending aorta may coexist with a patent contralateral pulmonary artery (Fig 45-8) (see Chapter 18). Rarely truncus arteriosus has an interrupted aortic arch (Fig 45-9). The origin of a pulmonary artery may be narrowed.

RIGHT HEMITRUNCUS

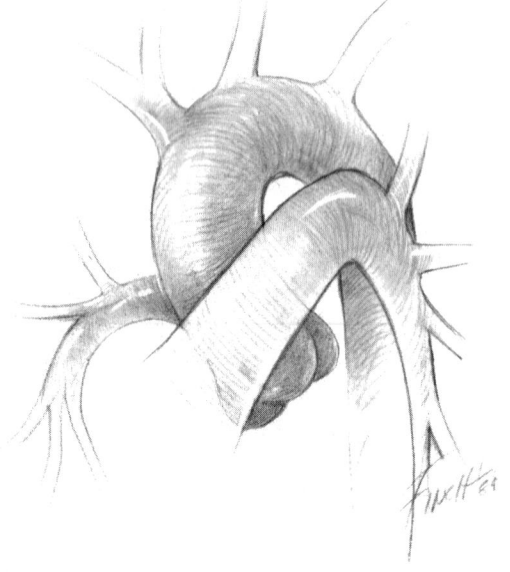

FIG 45-7.
Persistent truncus arteriosus with proximal interruption of left pulmonary artery. Right pulmonary artery arises from truncus arteriosus.

HEMITRUNCUS ORIGIN OF RPA FROM AORTA

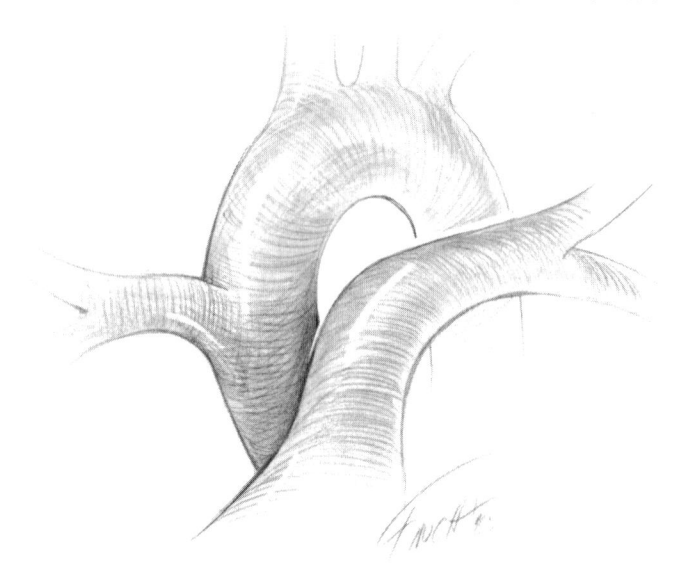

FIG 45-8.
Origin of right pulmonary artery from ascending aorta. Left pulmonary artery originates normally from pulmonary trunk.

A ventricular septal defect is an integral part of the malformation. It is almost always large and is located immediately below the truncal valve but does not involve the membranous septum. The truncus arteriosus usually straddles the ventricular septal defect, but in one third of the

TRUNCUS WITH INTERRUPTION OF AORTIC ARCH

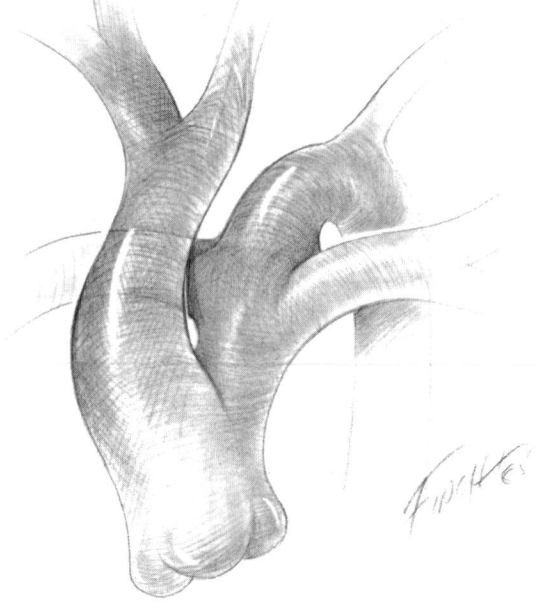

FIG 45-9.
Truncus arteriosus with interruption of aortic arch. Interruption between left carotid and left subclavian arteries. Descending aorta is supplied by large reversing patent ductus arteriosus.

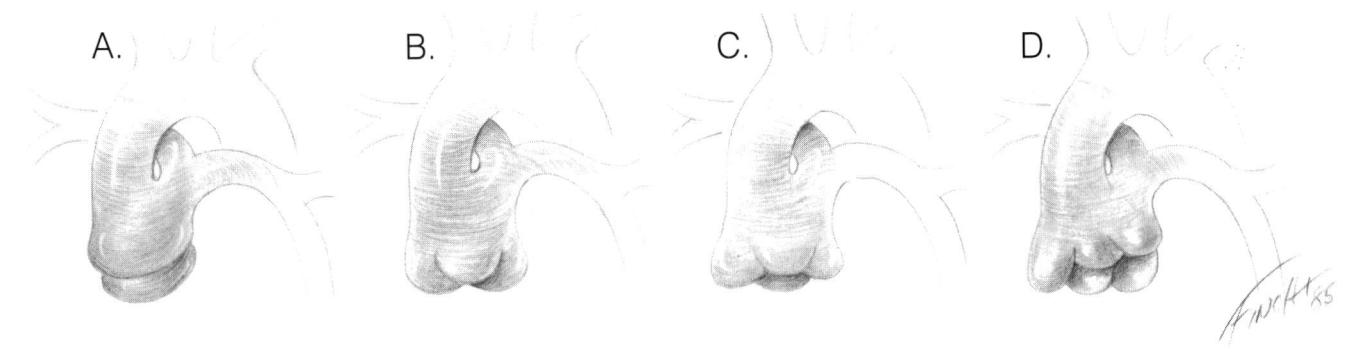

VARIATIONS OF TRUNCAL VALVE

FIG 45–10.
Persistent truncus arteriosus. Variations of truncal valve. **A**, bicuspid; **B**, tricuspid; **C**, tetracuspid; and **D**, pentacuspid.

cases, it originates almost exclusively from one ventricle the right ventricle more often than the left.

The number of cusps of the truncal valve varies from two to six, with approximately two thirds having three cusps and another fourth having four cusps (Fig 45–10).[4,5] The truncal valve may be either stenotic or insufficient. If present, truncal stenosis is usually noted in neonates and results from thickened, nodular, poorly differentiated valve cusps.[6,7] Insufficiency, present in about one fourth of patients, results from a variety of anatomic causes: inequality of cusps, lack of support of valve cusps because of the ventricular defect, fusion of cusps, or thickening of cusps.[8] Histologically the nodular truncal valve shows abundant mucoid material and appears similar to a dysplastic pulmonary valve.

The mitral valve is usually in continuity with the truncal valve, but the tricuspid valve is usually separate. The atrioventricular valves are usually normal.

The status of the ductus arteriosus varies. In one half of the patients, the ductus arteriosus is absent. In the other half it is patent in many, and ligamentous in the others.

About one third of patients have a right aortic arch, almost always with mirror image branching, but with a few instances of aberrant left subclavian artery. Truncus arteriosus may coexist with interruption of the aortic arch, in which the pulmonary artery and descending aorta are in continuity through a patent ductus arteriosus (see Fig 45–9).

The origin of the coronary arteries is extremely variable, and the pattern does not seem to correlate with the number of semilunar valve leaflets.[9,10] Usually, however, the left coronary artery arises from the left side of the truncus and the right coronary artery from the right side of the truncus arteriosus. Variations include single coronary artery, origin of a coronary artery above the sinotubular ridge, and origin of both coronary arteries above a single cusp.

Truncus arteriosus may coexist with either mitral or tricuspid atresia or with discordant ventricles. Coexistent atrial septal defect and left superior vena cava may each be present in 10% of patients.

Right ventricular hypertrophy is present because the right ventricle develops a systemic level of pressure. The left atrium and left ventricle are usually dilated because of the increased volume of blood flow or truncal regurgitation.

Myocardial ischemia may develop in the presence of normal coronary arteries, perhaps because of such factors as the large myocardial mass, desaturated coronary arterial blood, and low diastolic perfusion pressure secondary to truncal insufficiency and diastolic runoff into pulmonary arteries.

HEMODYNAMICS

The major hemodynamic consequences are pulmonary hypertension, ventricular volume overload from increased pulmonary blood flow or truncal insufficiency, and systemic arterial desaturation.

Both ventricles eject exclusively into the truncus arteriosus. Some streaming of the blood flow occurs, so the aorta may receive a greater portion of blood from the left ventricle, whereas the pulmonary arteries receive a greater portion from the right ventricle (Fig 45–11). Thus, aortic oxygen saturation may be higher than pulmonary arterial saturation. The distribution of blood flow from the truncus arteriosus is determined by the relative pulmonary and systemic vascular resistances, because pulmonary and aortic pressures are almost always equal. In patients with stenosis of the origin of the pulmonary arteries from the truncus arteriosus, pulmonary arterial pressure may be normal. In such patients the pulmonary stenosis is the principal determinant of pulmonary blood flow. At birth and in the neo-

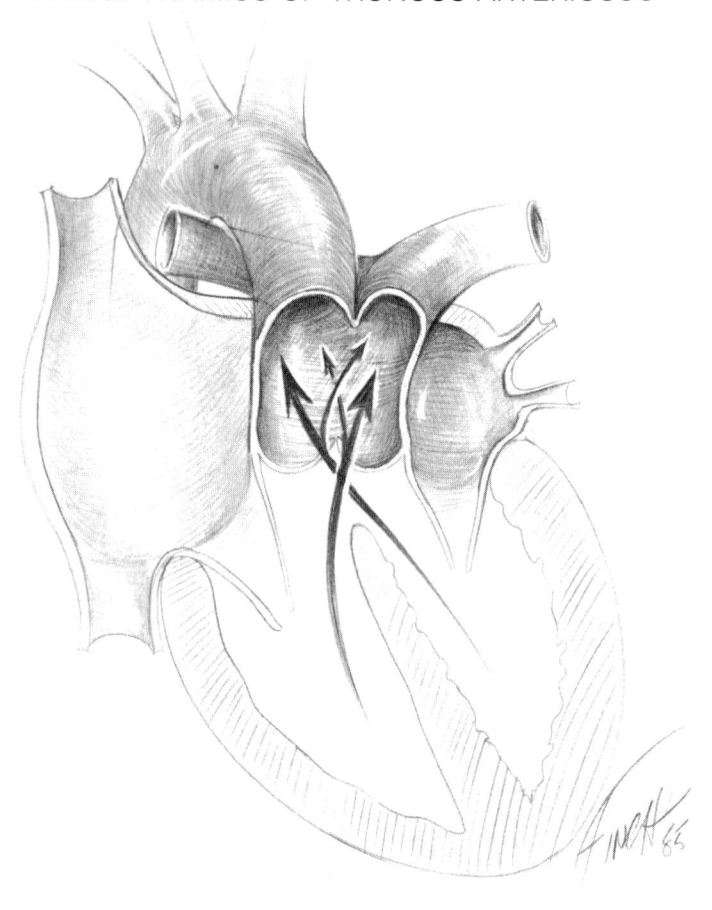

HEMODYNAMICS OF TRUNCUS ARTERIOSUS

FIG 45–11.
Persistent truncus arteriosus. Central circulation. Left ventricle ejects predominately into aorta. Right ventricle ejects predominately into pulmonary artery. Therefore, aortic saturation is usually higher than pulmonary arterial saturation.

natal period, because the pulmonary vascular resistance is elevated, pulmonary blood flow is limited. With the postnatal decline of pulmonary vascular resistance, the volume of pulmonary blood flow increases. This increased blood flow enlarges the left atrium and left ventricle. Because of left ventricular dilatation, congestive cardiac failure develops. Pulmonary vascular disease[11] occurs in these patients often at a rate faster than in individuals with an isolated ventricular septal defect.[12] As the pulmonary vascular disease progresses, the pulmonary blood flow becomes limited.

The degree of systemic arterial desaturation is in part determined by streaming and in part by the volume of the pulmonary blood flow, as in other admixture lesions. Cyanosis is inversely related to the volume of pulmonary blood flow.

Anomalies of the truncal valve may have a profound effect on the underlying hemodynamics of truncus arteriosus. Truncal insufficiency can augment the volume overload of the left ventricle, and truncal stenosis causes a gradient to outflow from both ventricles.

Because of diastolic blood flow from the truncus arteriosus into the pulmonary arteries, ventricles, or both because of truncal insufficiency, a wide aortic pulse pressure is found.

CLINICAL FEATURES

The presence of a cardiac malformation is suspected in almost all patients during infancy, usually in the neonatal period.[5] The age of onset depends on the status of the pulmonary vasculature and the status of the truncal valve. Neonates with truncal stenosis or severe truncal insufficiency have symptoms during the first few days of life.

In neonates, a cardiac anomaly may be recognized by the finding of a murmur or the presence of cyanosis. As pulmonary vascular resistance declines, cyanosis improves and eventually may disappear, but the findings of cardiac failure develop because of left ventricular volume overload. Tachypnea, tachycardia, slow growth, fatigue on feeding, and excessive perspiration are noted. Symptoms of failure develop in the neonatal period in patients with either truncal stenosis or severe truncal insufficiency. As pulmonary vascular disease develops in older patients, cyanosis increases and cardiac failure improves, unless truncal insufficiency coexists.

In many infants cyanosis is minimal or absent, and therefore the diagnosis of truncus arteriosus is not readily apparent. Aortic stenosis or ventricular septal defect often may be diagnosed because of the similar auscultatory findings. There is a long loud systolic murmur along the left sternal border, which radiates widely. An apical middiastolic murmur is heard because of increased flow across the mitral valve. These two features resemble those in ventricular septal defect. An apical systolic ejection click from the enlarged truncus is heard and may suggest a diagnosis of aortic stenosis.

The second heart sound is single, the pulse pressure is wide, and the arterial pulses are accentuated. These features help to distinguish truncus arteriosus from most conditions with which it might be confused. If the truncal valve is insufficient, an early high-pitched diastolic murmur is heard, and the pulse pressure is even wider.

If cyanosis is evident or intense, either pulmonary vascular disease or, rarely, stenosis of the origin of the pulmonary artery is present.

ELECTROCARDIOGRAPHIC FEATURES

The electrocardiogram is not diagnostic and merely reflects the hemodynamics. The QRS axis is normal or directed to the right. The precordial leads show a pattern of either right or combined ventricular hypertrophy. The pattern of left ventricular hypertrophy correlates with increased pulmonary blood flow. The T waves may be inverted in the left precordial leads in individuals with either truncal stenosis or severe truncal insufficiency.

ECHOCARDIOGRAPHIC FEATURES

The echocardiogram is usually diagnostic[13-15] and allows distinction of truncus arteriosus from other cardiac conditions that have similar anatomic or hemodynamic features.

A long-axis parasternal projection shows a large arterial vessel leaving the heart and overriding a ventricular septal defect. A similar appearance is found with tetralogy of Fallot, but the left atrium and left ventricle are enlarged in patients with truncus arteriosus. The subcostal and parasternal short-axis projections allow truncus arteriosus to be distinguished from tetralogy of Fallot. The pulmonary arteries arise from the posterior aspect of the truncus arteriosus, whereas on this view the right ventricular outflow tract and pulmonary trunk course 120 degrees around the ascending aorta in tetralogy of Fallot. The presence and degree of truncal insufficiency can be assessed by Doppler echocardiography.

RADIOGRAPHIC FEATURES

The radiographic features of truncus arteriosus are not uniform. REASON: The hemodynamics of truncus arteriosus vary considerably. The volume of pulmonary blood flow, may be limited by elevated pulmonary vascular resistance or stenosis of the pulmonary arteries.

Although the roentgenographic hallmark of truncus arteriosus should be absence of the main pulmonary arterial segment, it is difficult to recognize radiographically because the left pulmonary artery may cast an identical shadow and simulate the main pulmonary arterial segment. Furthermore, in infancy, thymic tissue may overshadow this portion of the cardiac contour. In some patients the truncus arteriosus consists predominantly of a large pulmonary component simulating a pulmonary arterial segment (see Fig 45-19).

The roentgenographic diagnosis of truncus arteriosus can be made with great certainty in a cyanotic patient who shows increased pulmonary blood flow and a right aortic arch. REASON: Almost one third of patients with truncus arteriosus have a right aortic arch. Right aortic arch in complete transposition of the great vessels without pulmonary stenosis or other cyanotic conditions with increased pulmonary blood flow is very rare.

1. The cardiac silhouette is invariably enlarged (Fig 45-12). REASON: Except for the very rare cases of pulmonary stenosis, the pulmonary blood flow is greatly increased, and predominately the left ventricle is dilated.

2. The degree of cardiomegaly varies with the volume of pulmonary blood flow and reflects the degree of pulmonary vascular resistance. In patients with low pulmonary vascular resistance and greatly increased pulmonary blood flow, severe cardiomegaly is present (see Fig 45-12).

3. Pulmonary vascular disease develops in patients with truncus arteriosus, and pulmonary vascular resistance increases with time. Decrease in pulmonary blood flow results, cardiac size decreases, and left atrial enlargement disappears. In patients with elevated pulmonary vascular resistance, the cardiac size tends to be smaller (Fig 45-13).

4. With increasing pulmonary vascular resistance, the peripheral pulmonary arterial branches become sparse, giving the radiographic appearance of "pruning" (see Fig 45-13).

5. With low pulmonary vascular resistance, the left atrium and both ventricles are enlarged. REASON: Increased pulmonary blood flow enlarges the left ventricle and elevates right ventricular systolic pressure, increasing right ventricular size.

6. The distribution of pulmonary blood flow may be unequal between the lungs, with the left lung having rela-

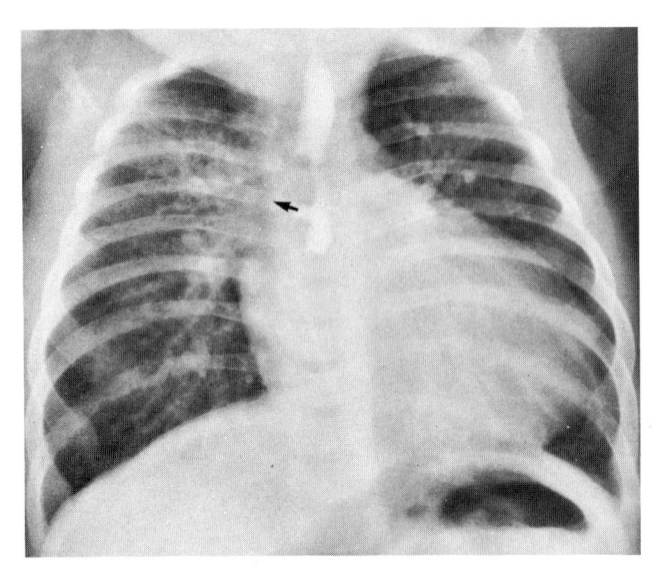

FIG 45–12.
Truncus arteriosus. Low pulmonary resistance. Thoracic roentgenogram. Posteroanterior projection. Marked cardiomegaly. Elevated cardiac apex. Increased pulmonary vascularity. Both hilar shadows, particularly the right, are unusually high in position *(arrow)*. Unequal pulmonary blood flow between right and left lungs.

FIG 45–13.
Truncus arteriosus. Increased pulmonary vascular resistance. Thoracic roentgenogram. Posteroanterior projection. Enlarged heart but smaller than in figure 45–12. Discrepancy between central and peripheral pulmonary arteries suggests increased pulmonary vascular resistance. Distinct disparity between pulmonary vasculature in right lung and left lung, a common finding in truncus arteriosus. Inconspicuous superior vena cava and ascending aorta because of clockwise rotation of heart. Pulmonary arterial segment has slightly different shape but is distinctly seen. A fairly large aortic arch and discrepancy between right and left pulmonary vasculature are consistent with truncus arteriosus.

tively less flow. Thus, a discrepancy in the lung fields is noted (see Figs 45–12 and 45–13). REASON: Unknown, possibly a streaming phenomenon similar to patent ductus arteriosus (see Chapter 16). Rarely, this discrepancy in blood flow is caused by unilateral truncal stenosis.

7. Sometimes there is a discrepancy not only in the size of the hila but also in their position, the right hilum being higher than the left (see Fig 45–12).

8. The aorta is anatomically enlarged because truncus arteriosus is an aortic runoff lesion, but the ascending aorta is usually not prominent radiographically (see Figs 45–12 and 45–13). REASON: Because of right ventricular enlargement, clockwise rotation of the heart occurs, placing the truncus more midline. However, the aortic arch itself is usually prominent. REASON: Truncus arteriosus is an aortic runoff lesion with wide pulse pressure and diastolic aortic back flow, which tends to enlarge the aorta.

9. The diagnosis of truncus arteriosus becomes almost certain in a patient with cyanosis, increased pulmonary flow, and a right aortic arch (Fig 45–14). REASON: In all cyanotic conditions with increased pulmonary flow, a right aortic arch is very rare. On the other hand, one third of patients with truncus arteriosus have a right aortic arch.

10. The right arch almost invariably has a right-sided descending aorta and no retroesophageal segment. Rarely, there is an aberrant left subclavian artery passing in a retroesophageal position. Interruption of the aortic arch may also coexist and have a retroesophageal segment.

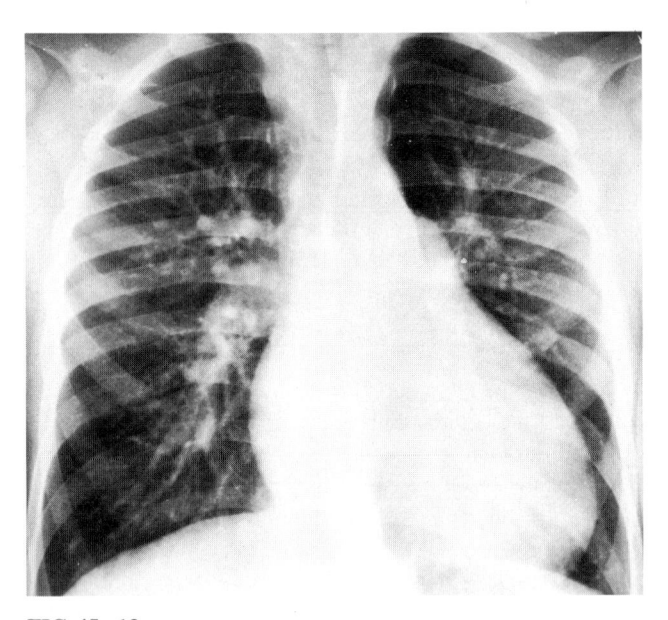

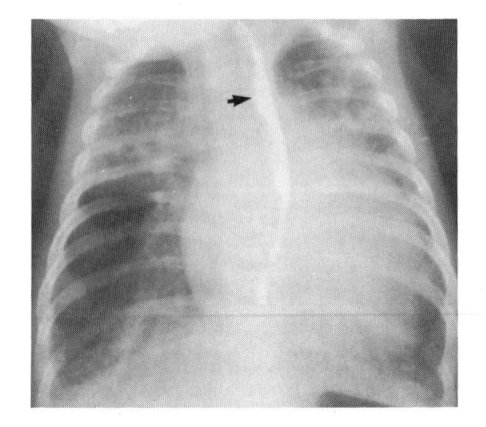

FIG 45–14.
Truncus arteriosus. Thoracic roentgenogram. Anteroposterior projection. Combination of cyanosis, increased pulmonary blood flow, and right aortic arch suggests truncus arteriosus. Right aortic arch can be suspected by lack of a density to the left of barium-filled esophagus *(black arrow)*. Trachea is not well seen. Marked cardiomegaly. Markedly increased pulmonary vasculature. High right hilar density.

11. The appearance of the pulmonary arterial segment is variable and complicates the radiographic diagnosis of truncus arteriosus. REASON: The anatomic details of the pulmonary arteries arising from the truncus vary. Also, the left pulmonary artery may simulate a normal-appearing pulmonary arterial segment.

12. On the posteroanterior projection, the pulmonary arterial segment may be simulated so perfectly that the radiographic appearance is identical to that of a large left-to-right shunt and normally related great vessels (see Fig 45–13).

13. On close scrutiny, the pulmonary arterial segment usually appears bizarre. The pulmonary arterial segment may have an unusual contour. It may be formed by either an abnormally positioned short main (type I) or the left pulmonary artery rather than the main pulmonary artery (Fig 45–15).

14. In a right anterior oblique projection the pulmonary arterial segment is absent anteriorly (Fig 45–16). REASON: Even in truncus type I, which may have a short main pulmonary artery, the infundibulum and supravalvar portion of the main pulmonary artery are absent. This absence also results in an unusual tetradlike configuration on the left anterior oblique projection (Fig 45–17).

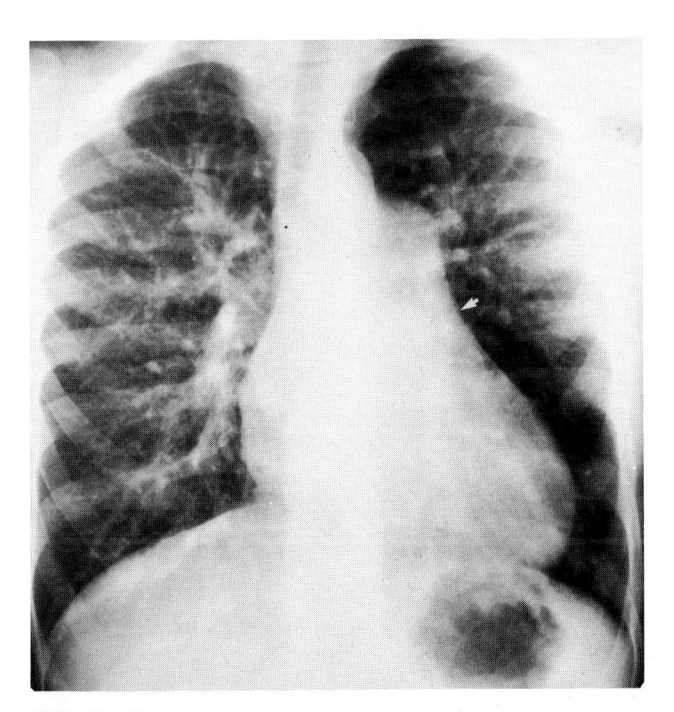

FIG 45–16.
Truncus arteriosus. Thoracic roentgenogram. Right anterior oblique projection. Distinct shelflike concavity in region of pulmonary arterial segment *(arrow)*. REASON: Pulmonary artery is abnormal in configuration and location.

15. Rarely, the left pulmonary arterial density (comma shadow) (truncus type II) is completely separated from the aortic density, which results in a distinctly concave pulmonary arterial segment (Fig 45–18). Under those circumstances, the cardiac configuration closely mimics that of tetralogy of Fallot (rare).

16. Occassionally, right ventricular enlargement causes upturning of the apex as in tetralogy of Fallot (see Figs 45–12 and 45–18).

17. Truncus arteriosus type IV is in most cases tetral-

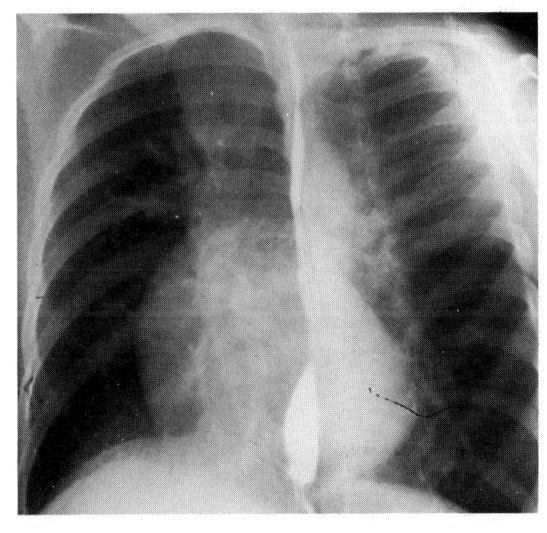

FIG 45–15.
Truncus arteriosus. Increased pulmonary vascular resistance. Thoracic roentgenogram. Posteroanterior projection. Only slightly increased cardiac size. Less pulmonary blood flow to left lung than right lung. Pulmonary arterial segment is prominent but unusual in configuration. Concavity in region of right ventricular outflow tract *(arrow)* because infundibulum is absent. Pulmonary arterial segment is formed by left pulmonary artery.

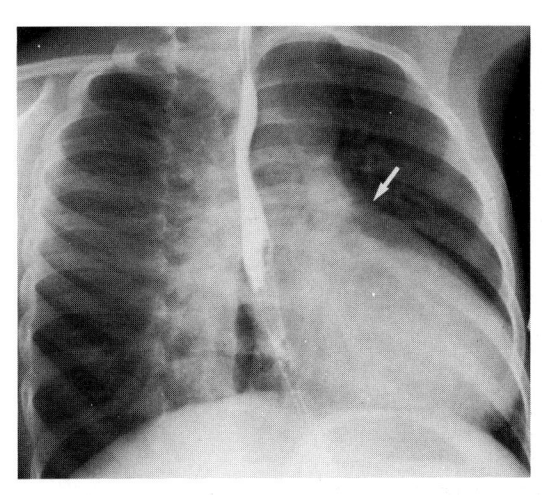

FIG 45–17.
Truncus arteriosus. Thoracic roentgenogram. Left anterior oblique projection. Clockwise rotation of heart causes left ventricle to overlie spine even in this steep left anterior oblique projection. Right-sided cardiac enlargement. Slight elevation of cardiac apex closely simulating configuration of tetralogy of Fallot.

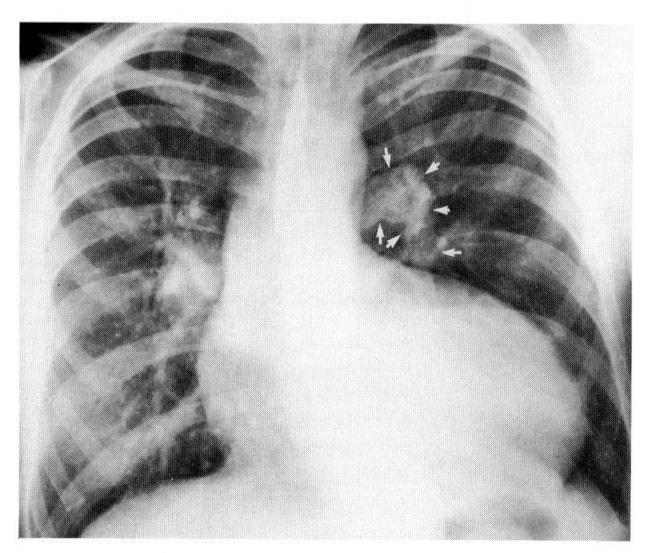

FIG 45–18.
Truncus arteriosus type II. Thoracic roentgenogram. Posteroanterior projection. Absence of pulmonary arterial segment results in concavity simulating configuration of tetralogy of Fallot. Hilar comma densities are at unequal position. Elevation of left hilum *(arrows)*. Low position of right hilum. Decreased peripheral pulmonary vasculature, particularly in left lung, suggests elevated pulmonary vascular resistance.

ogy of Fallot with pulmonary atresia. The radiographic findings of the very rare, persistent truncus arteriosus type IV are indistinguishable from tetralogy of Fallot (see Chapter 31).

CARDIAC CATHETERIZATION

Although the diagnosis can usually be made accurately by echocardiography, cardiac catheterization is necessary to determine the hemodynamics. The catheter can readily be passed from the venous side of the circulation through the ventricular septal defect into the truncus arteriosus. The catheter tip should be advanced into both pulmonary arteries from the truncus arteriosus. Pressure and oxygen saturations should be measured in each pulmonary artery to identify stenosis of the origin of a pulmonary artery or differences in oxygen saturation. A balloon-tipped catheter may be needed to catheterize both arteries, or specially shaped catheters may have to be introduced in retrograde fashion.

In virtually all patients, the systolic pressure is the same in both ventricles, the truncus, and both pulmonary arteries. A wide pulse pressure is found in the pulmonary artery and truncus if pulmonary resistance is low or truncal insufficiency is present. As pulmonary vascular disease develops, diastolic pressure rises. A systolic gradient is found between the ventricles and truncus arteriosus in individuals with truncal stenosis.

Oximetry data show an increased oxygen saturation in the right ventricle compared with the right atrium. Evidence of a left-to-right atrial shunt may be present through a foramen ovale or atrial septal defect, particularly in patients less than 1 year of age. Oxygen saturation of blood in the left ventricle is less than that of the left atrium because of the right-to-left shunt. Usually a difference is found between the oxygen saturation of the aorta and pulmonary artery with the aorta being higher.

Careful pressure measurements should be made in the great vessels. Oxygen saturations in pulmonary artery, aorta, mixed venous, and a site reflecting pulmonary venous blood allow calculation of vascular resistances in the systemic and pulmonary circulations.

ANGIOGRAPHIC FEATURES

Ventriculography is performed to define the ventricular septal defect, evaluate atrioventricular valvular competency, and establish the common origin of the aorta and pulmonary trunk. The rare combination of aorticopulmonary window and ventricular septal defect may be difficult to distinguish angiographically from persistent truncus arteriosus.

Aortography is required to demonstrate the anatomy of the truncus and the truncal valve. The knowledge of truncal anatomy aids the surgeon in making operative decisions. In addition, knowledge of the anatomy of the coronary arteries is important when a corrective operation is considered.

A catheter can be advanced into the truncus in either retrograde direction or antegrade direction through the ventricular septal defect, because the ventricular septal defect lies immediately beneath the truncal valve, which generally overrides the ventricular septum. For satisfactory angiography, large-bore catheters must be used to allow the rapid delivery of a large amount of contrast medium. The volume of blood flow through the truncus arteriosus is large; that is, the entire systemic and pulmonary blood flows pass through the truncus arteriosus. Blood flow and therefore dilution of contrast medium occurs in both systole and diastole. Coexistent truncal insufficiency further increases blood flow through the truncus. Thus, contrast medium may be diluted in this large volume of blood, yielding an inadequately opacified angiogram.

Either left or right ventriculography is adequate to define the location of the ventricular septal defect. REASON: The pressures in the ventricles are equal, and both ventricles eject blood into the truncus arteriosus. Because of clockwise rotation of the heart, a slight right anterior oblique and a very steep left anterior lateral projection with cranial angulation are excellent to demonstrate anatomic details.

Right Ventriculogram

1. Both the aortic and pulmonary arterial trees fill simultaneously after right ventriculography. Because of streaming, a greater portion of the contrast medium enters the pulmonary artery (see the discussion of hemodynamics). The truncal valve usually occupies a low position and overrides the ventricular septal defect to a variable degree. The defect is immediately beneath the truncal valve.

2. An infundibulum cannot be identified in the right ventricle because it is anatomically absent.

3. On a lateral projection, ventricular septum is seen on end because of clockwise rotation of the heart from right ventricular enlargement (Fig 45–19).

4. The truncal valve is commonly thickened.

5. The degree of overriding of the truncal valve varies. Commonly there is some degree of overriding.

6. The division of the truncus into a pulmonary and aortic portion is variable. The truncus may consist mostly of an enlarged pulmonary portion. This variation has been termed "truncus pulmonicus" (see Fig 45–19).

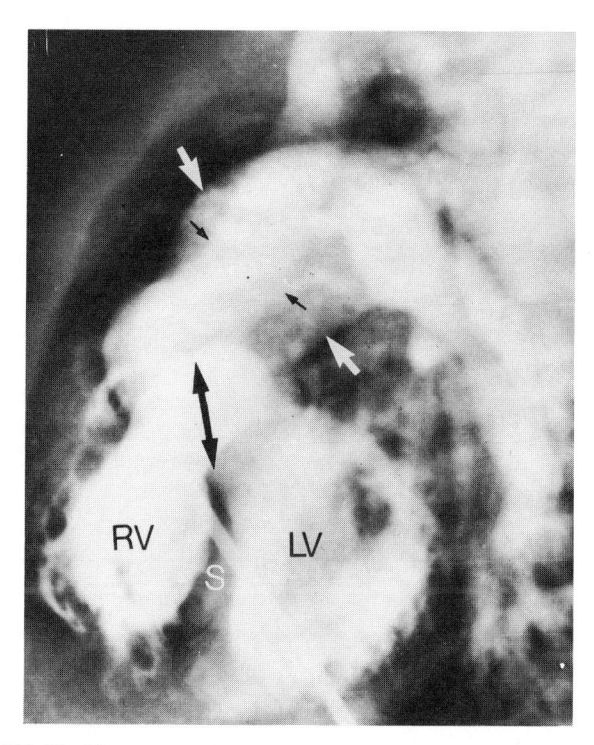

Left Ventriculogram

Unless abnormalities of the left artrioventricular valve are suspected, left ventriculography does not add additional information.

Aortography

A very rapid injection of contrast material into the truncus arteriosus allows the demonstration of the truncal valve and its function. Because the coronary arterial anatomy is extremely variable, it also should be demonstrated.

1. The pulmonary arteries may arise as a single trunk (truncus type I), which has a varying degree of length. If the pulmonary trunk is fairly long, it can be distinctly seen as a separate structure from the truncus arteriosus, particularly if it is injected selectively (Fig 45–20).

2. In truncus arteriosus, type I, the pulmonary artery arises from either the lateral or posterior aspect of the truncus arteriosus (see Fig 45–19).

3. The pulmonary trunk may be fairly long. There may be a completely separate valve leaflet for this trunk, but the valve is contiguous with the remaining truncal valve leaflets (see Fig 45–20).

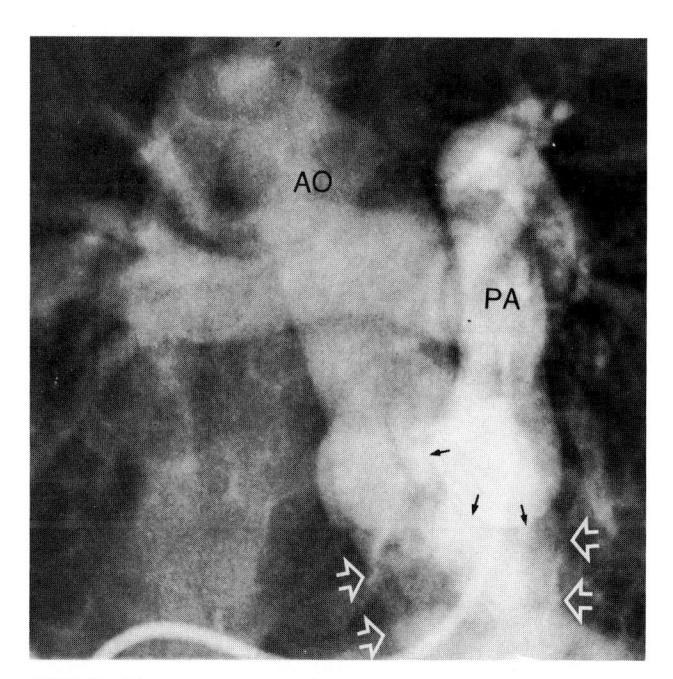

FIG 45–19.
Truncus arteriosus. Right ventriculogram *(RV)*. Lateral projection. Fifty percent overriding of truncal valve. Ventricular septum *(S)* is well visualized. Large ventricular septal defect immediately beneath truncal valve *(long double arrow)*. No right ventricular outflow tract. Truncus consists of large pulmonary *(white arrows)* and normal-sized aortic division *(small black arrows)* "truncus pulmonicus". *LV* = left ventricle.

FIG 45–20.
Truncus arteriosus, type I. Pulmonary arterial injection. Anteroposterior projection. Right aortic arch. Long separate origin of pulmonary artery *(PA)*. Common valve leaflet *(black arrows)* is present for pulmonary artery. This valve leaflet is continuous with remaining truncal valve leaflets and at same level. Four truncal valve leaflets are present. Considable truncal insufficiency *(open arrows)*. *AO* = aorta.

4. If the pulmonary artery arises separately along the left border of the truncus arteriosus and has its own valve leaflet, differentiation from aorticopulmonary window may be difficult. In aorticopulmonary window, however, the pulmonary valve is completely separated and higher than the aortic valve, and an infundibulum is present in the right ventricle. In truncus arteriosus, the infundibulum is absent.

5. Although more than three truncal valve leaflets may be present, the valve is most commonly tricuspid (65%) and competent (75%) (Fig 45–21).

6. Rarely, truncus arteriosus coexists with interruption of the aortic arch (Fig 45–22).

7. Stenosis of the origin of the pulmonary arteries may involve one or both pulmonary arteries (Fig 45–23). It is consequently important to obtain pressures in both pulmonary arteries.

8. The truncal valve may not only be insufficient but also stenotic (Fig 45–24).

9. A right arch is commonly found (one third of the cases).

10. Proximal interruption of a pulmonary artery may occur (hemitruncus). Interruption may be on either the same or opposite side of the aortic arch (Fig 45–25). The interrupted pulmonary artery stays patent and

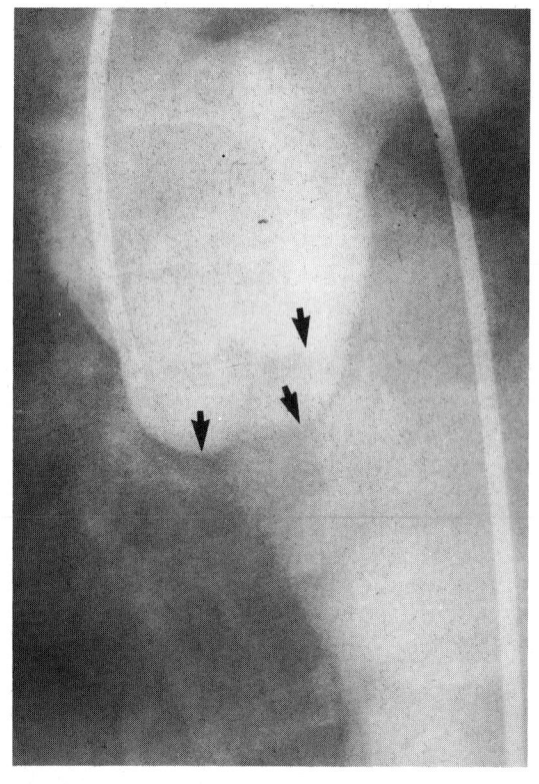

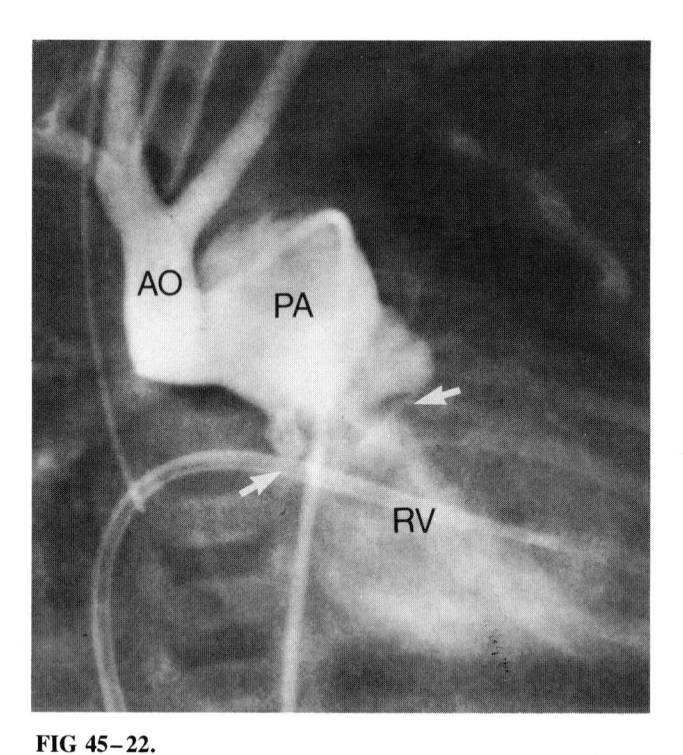

FIG 45–22.
Truncus arteriosus and interruption of aortic arch. Injection in truncus arteriosus. Anteroposterior projection. Catheter passed through reversing patent ductus arteriosus from descending aorta. Pulmonary division of truncus is unusually large ("truncus pulmonicus"). Absent distal aortic arch. Thickened insufficient truncal valve *(white arrows)*. *AO* = ascending aorta; *PA* = pulmonary artery; *RV* = right ventricle.

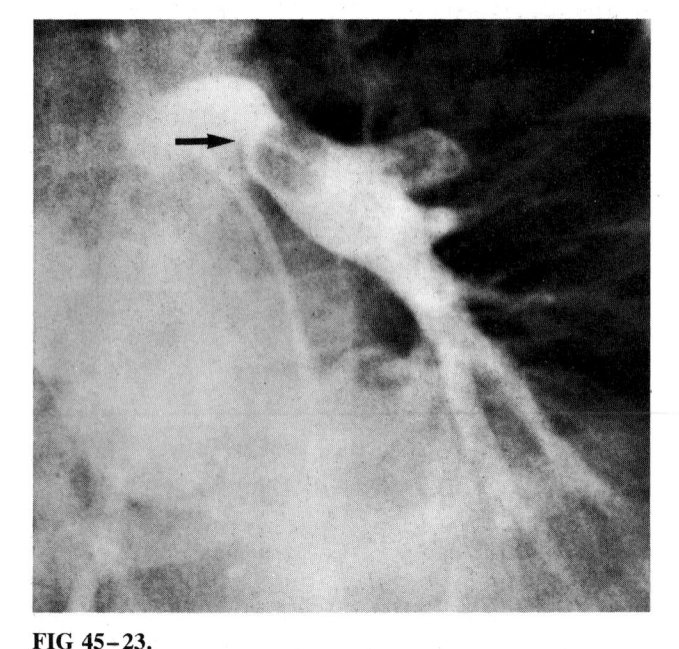

FIG 45–21.
Truncus arteriosus. Aortogram. Anteroposterior projection. Three competent valve leaflets *(arrows)*.

FIG 45–23.
Truncus arteriosus, type II. Selective left pulmonary arteriogram. Anteroposterior projection. Left pulmonary arterial pressure is normal because of localized stenosis of origin of left pulmonary artery *(arrow)*.

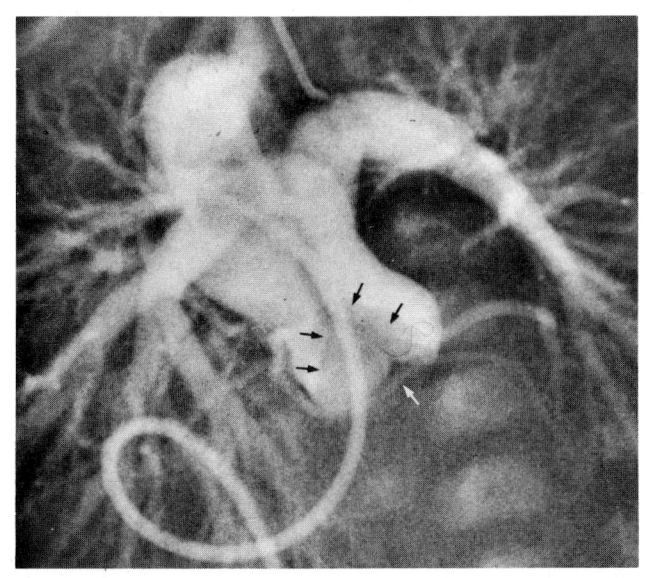

FIG 45–24.
Truncus arteriosus, type I. Truncal injection. Anteroposterior projection. Doming of common truncal valve *(arrows)*, indicating truncal stenosis. Right aortic arch and right descending aorta. Origin of left circumflex artery is from right coronary artery *(white arrows)*.

fills late through collateral arteries or a patent ductus arteriosus.

11. Because of the large volume of blood flow through the truncus arteriosus and superimposition of contrast medium of various structures, the coronary arteries may not fill adequately. Selective coronary arteriography may be required for better demonstration (Fig 45–26).

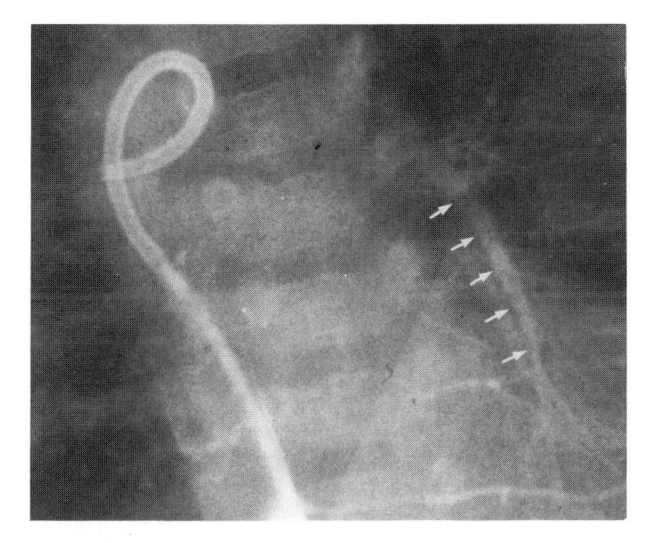

FIG 45–25.
Truncus arteriosus with interruption of proximal left pulmonary artery and right aortic arch. Aortogram. Late phase. Anteroposterior projection. Small patent left pulmonary artery opacifies via collateral arteries *(arrows)*.

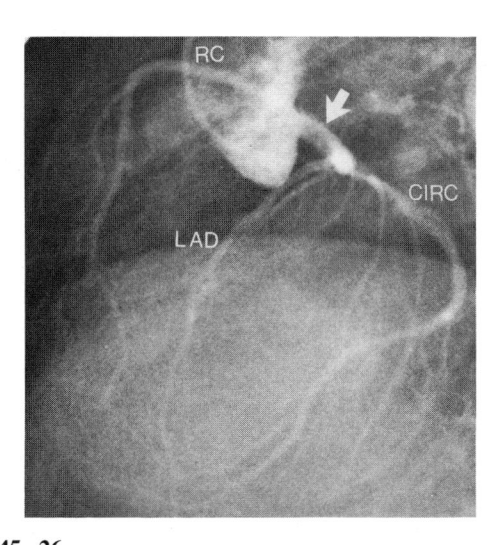

FIG 45–26.
Truncus arteriosus, type I. Selective left coronary arteriogram. Left anterior oblique projection. Single coronary artery *(arrow)*, giving rise to left circumflex *(CIRC)* and right coronary arteries *(RC)*. Origin of coronary arteries is more posterior than normal, common in persistent truncus arteriosus. *LAD* = left anterior descending branch.

Truncus Arteriosus Type IV

Truncus arteriosus type IV is a disputed entity but probably exists. In most suspected cases, an infundibulum can be demonstrated angiographically or microscopically at the time of postmortem examination, disproving that it

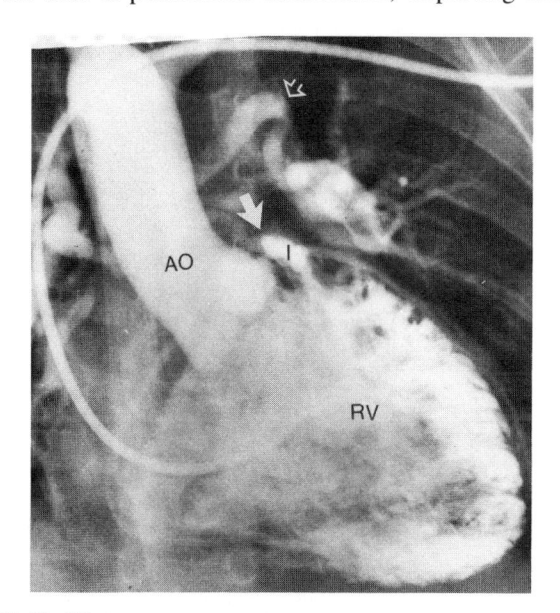

FIG 45–27.
Ventricular septal defect and pulmonary atresia. Right ventriculogram. Anteroposterior projection. Differentiation between truncus arteriosus and tetralogy of Fallot with pulmonary atresia made by demonstration of infundibulum *(I) (arrow)*. Circulation to pulmonary arteries via bronchial arteries *(open arrow)*. *AO* = aorta; *RV* = right ventricle.

represents persistent truncus arteriosus. Although the hemodynamics of truncus arteriosus type IV and tetralogy of Fallot with pulmonary atresia are identical, many times angiography can determine the developmental etiology by visualization of an infundibulum (Fig 45–27). If an infundibulum is not demonstrated angiographically, tetralogy of Fallot with pulmonary atresia (pseudotruncus) cannot be excluded, because infundibular atresia may be present. However, an atretic infundibulum and main pulmonary artery may be found at postmortem examination, disproving the diagnosis of persistent truncus arteriosus type IV.

OPERATIVE CONSIDERATIONS

The infant in congestive cardiac failure should be treated vigorously with digitalis and diuretics. When the patient has improved, an operation should be considered. In the past, pulmonary arterial banding was widely used to provide palliation.[16, 17] This procedure was associated with a number of problems: a high operative mortality, distortion of pulmonary arteries, ineffectiveness associated with development of pulmonary vascular disease, and the need for a subsequent corrective operation, which was associated with a higher mortality than if a banding had not been performed.

Thus, at most centers the approach is a corrective procedure using a conduit. In this procedure, an elliptical incision is made in the outflow area of the right ventricle, through which the ventricular septal defect is patched. The pulmonary arteries are removed from the truncus and the resultant defect in the truncus is closed. Then a woven Dacron conduit is interposed between the right ventriculotomy and the pulmonary arteries. Usually the conduit contains a biologic valve (Fig 45–28). Whereas previously this procedure was delayed until the child was of school age, it is currently performed in infants when they become symptomatic.[18–20] This early operation prevents the development of pulmonary vascular disease, which increases the risk of operation in older children. This was a sufficient factor, so that one center (Mayo Clinic) did not perform this procedure if pulmonary vascular resistance exceeds 8 units.[2] In infants the conduit will need replacement, because the conduit becomes inadequate as the child grows or the conduit becomes obstructed by ingrowth of fibrous tissue. The operative mortality is about 10%.

If there is a major truncal insufficiency, the truncal valve needs to be replaced with a prosthetic valve.[21]

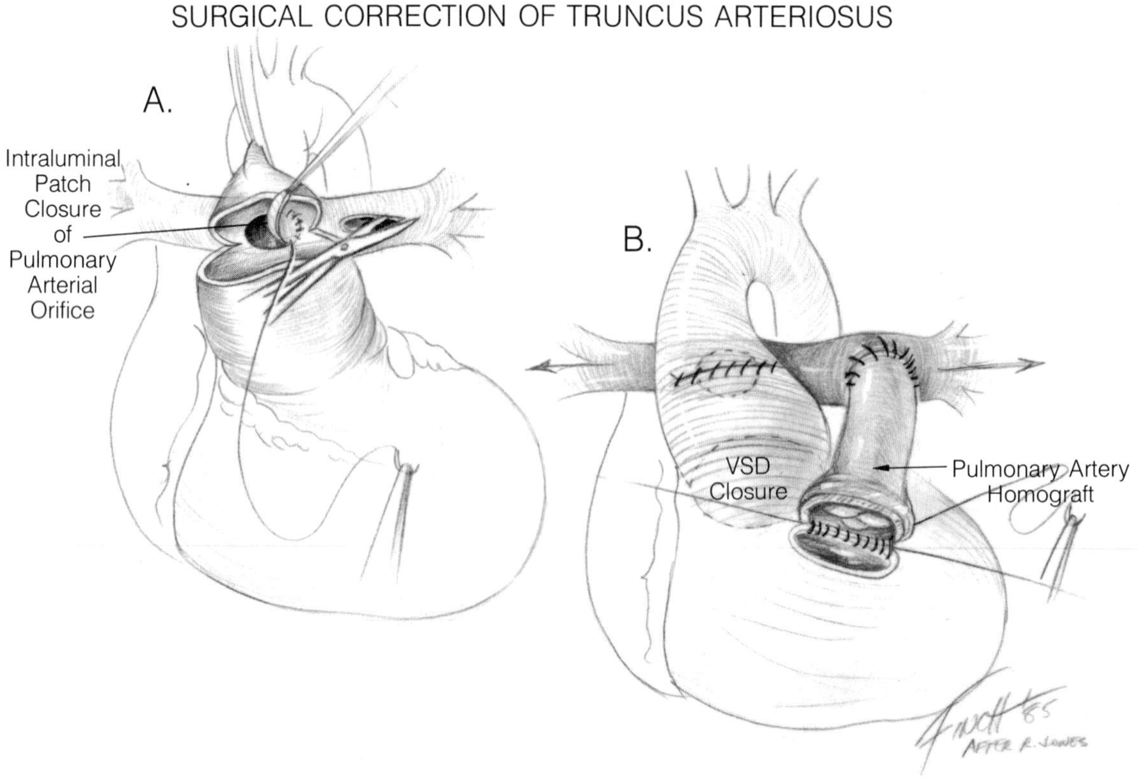

FIG 45–28.
Persistent truncus arteriosus. Operative correction. **A,** truncus arteriosus is opened. Communication to pulmonary arteries is closed. **B,** valved conduit is placed between right ventricle and pulmonary arteries. *VSD* = ventricular septal defect.

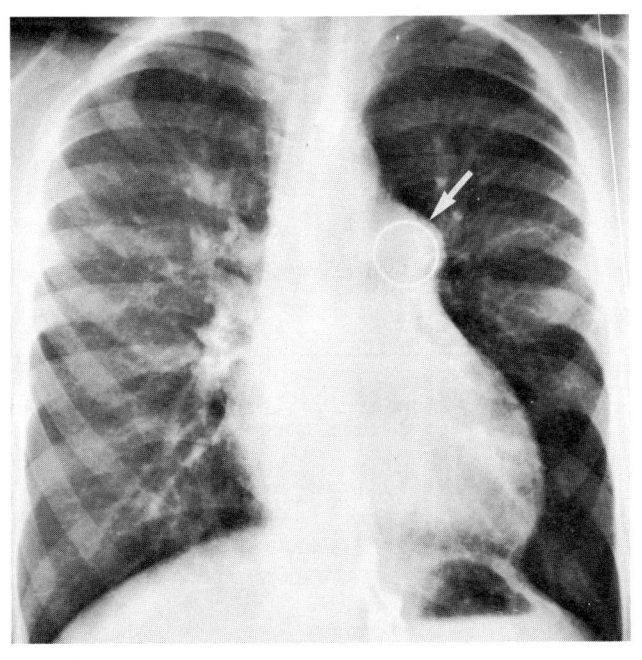

FIG 45–29.
Truncus arteriosus after corrective operation. Thoracic roentgenogram. Posteroanterior projection. Pulmonary vasculature and cardiac size have returned to normal. Discrepancy between pulmonary vasculature in right and left lung remains. Ring of prosthetic valve in pulmonary artery conduit is demonstrated *(arrow)*.

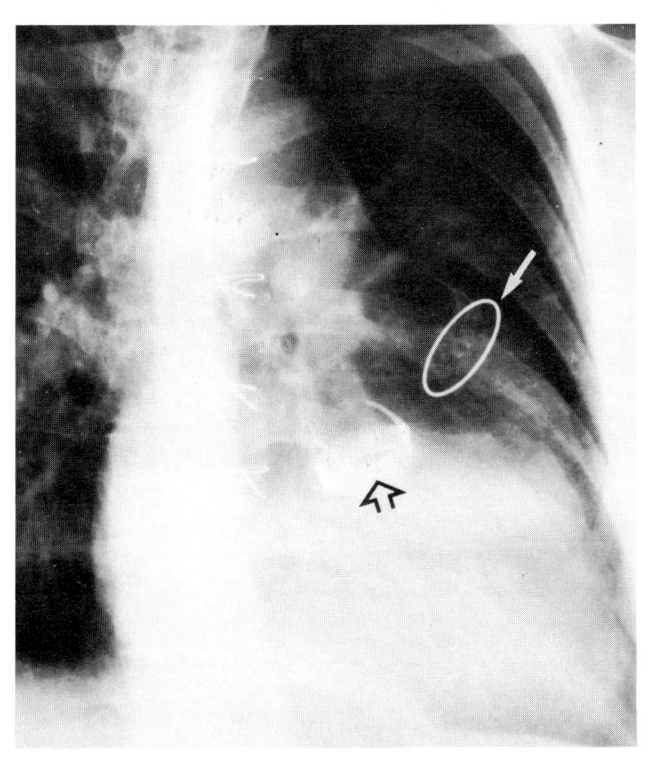

FIG 45–31.
Truncus arteriosus type II after banding of both pulmonary arteries. Right pulmonary arteriogram. Anteroposterior projection. Marked constriction of right pulmonary artery *(arrows)* by band.

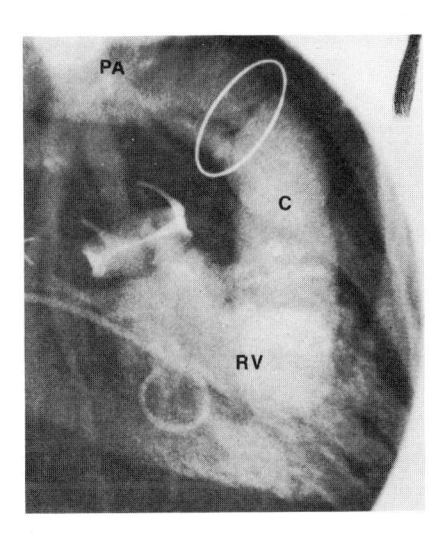

FIG 45–32.
Truncus arteriosus and truncal insufficiency after corrective operation. Right ventriculogram. Right anterior oblique projection. Normal-sized right ventricle *(RV)*. Normal flow through valved conduit *(C)* into pulmonary artery *(PA)*. Aortic valve is replaced by prosthetic valve.

FIG 45–30.
Truncus arteriosus and truncal valve insufficiency after corrective operation. Thoracic roentgenogram. Posteroanterior projection. Prosthetic valve *(black arrow)* and tissue valve *(white arrow)*. This appearance is virtually diagnostic for repair of truncus arteriosus with truncal insufficiency.

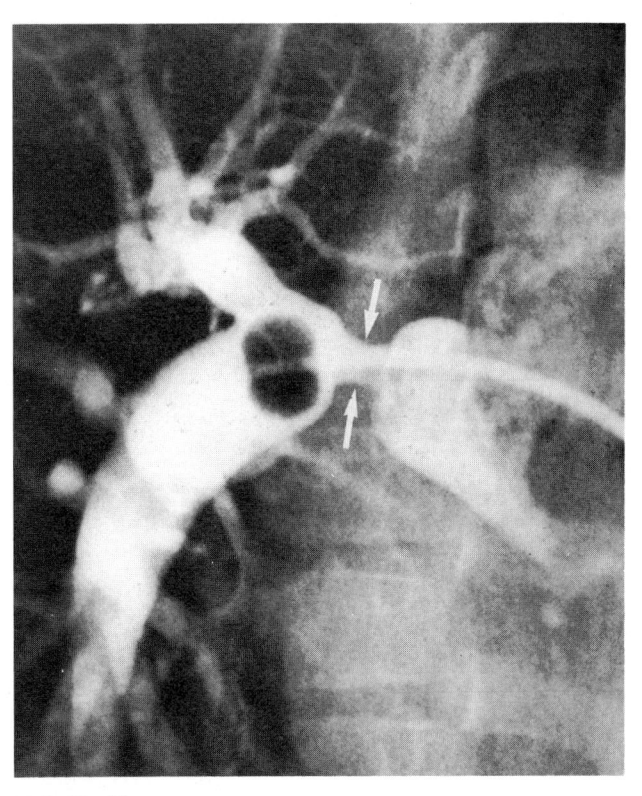

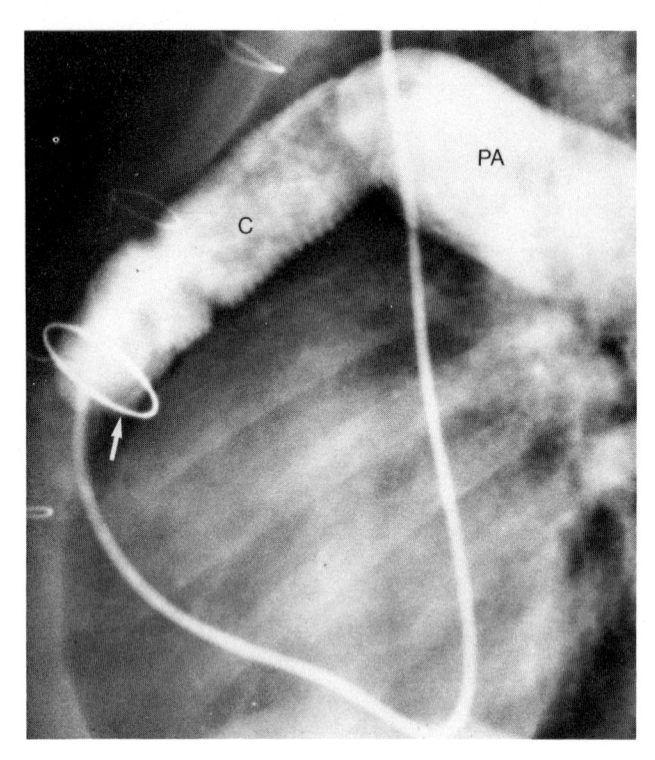

FIG 45–33.
Truncus arteriosus after operation. Conduit *(C)* is injected selectively to evaluate competency of tissue valve. Lateral projection. Catheter is passed through right ventricle into graft. Graft is well outlined. No insufficiency of valve *(arrow)*. PA = pulmonary artery.

POSTOPERATIVE RADIOGRAPHIC FEATURES

1. After complete repair of truncus arteriosus, cardiac size and pulmonary vasculature may rapidly regress to normal (Fig 45–29).
2. In patients requiring valve replacement of the truncal valve, the roentgenographic findings are virtually diagnostic in showing two valves, the second being in the conduit (Fig 45–30).
3. With elevated pulmonary vascular resistance, pulmonary banding is performed before corrective surgery (Fig 45–31).
4. Conduits may become densely calcified with time.
5. Right ventriculography shows the anatomy of the conduit after operation (Fig 45–32) and is particularly useful in evaluating competence of the conduit valve (Fig 45–32).
6. Conduits may become narrowed by ingrowth of fibrous tissue, and tissue valve may become stiff, stenotic, and insufficient (Fig 45–33).
7. Competency of the prosthetic truncal valve can be evaluated by aortography.

REFERENCES

1. Crupi G, Macartney FJ, Anderson RH: Persistent truncus arteriosus: a study of 66 autopsy cases with special reference to definition and morphogenesis, *Am J Cardiol* 40:569, 1977.
2. Collett RW, Edwards JE: Persistent truncus arteriosus: a classification according to anatomic types, *Surg Clin North Am* August:1245, 1949.
3. Edwards JE: Persistent truncus arteriosus: a comment, *Am Heart J* 92:1, 1976.
4. Becker AE, Becker MJ, Edwards JE: Pathology of the semilunar valve in persistent truncus arteriosus, *J Thorac Cardiovasc Surg* 62:16, 1971.
5. Calder L, Van Praagh R, Van Praagh S, et al: Truncus arteriosus communis: clinical, angiocardiographic, and pathologic findings in 100 patients, *Am Heart J* 92:23, 1976.
6. Gerlis LM, Wilson N, Dickinson DF, et al: Valvar stenosis in truncus arteriosus, *Br Heart J* 52:440, 1984.
7. Patel RG, Freedom RM, Bloom KR, et al: Truncal or aortic valve stenosis in functionally single arterial trunk: a clinical, hemodynamic and pathologic study of six cases, *Am J Cardiol* 42:800, 1978.
8. Rosenquist GC, Bharati S, McAllister HA et al: Truncus arteriosus communis: truncal valve anomalies associated with small conal or truncal septal defects, *Am J Cardiol* 37:410, 1976.
9. Shrivastava S, Edwards JE: Coronary arterial origin in persistent truncus arteriosus, *Circulation* 55:551, 1977.
10. Anderson KR, McGoon DC, Lie JT: Surgical significance of the coronary arterial anatomy in truncus arteriosus communis, *Am J Cardiol* 41:76, 1978.
11. Juaneda E, Haworth SG: Pulmonary vascular disease in children with truncus arteriosus, *Am J Cardiol* 54:1314, 1984.
12. Marcelletti C, McGoon DC, Mair DD: The natural history of truncus arteriosus, *Circulation* 54:108, 1976.
13. Rice MJ, Seward JB, Hagler DJ, et al: Definitive diagnosis of truncus arteriosus by two-dimensional echocardiography, *Mayo Clin Proc* 57:476, 1982.
14. Houston AB, Gregory NL, Murtagh E, et al: Two-dimensional echocardiography in infants with persistent truncus arteriosus, *Br Heart J* 46:492, 1981.
15. Hagler DJ, Tajik AJ, Seward JB, et al: Wide-angle two-dimensional echocardiographic profiles of conotruncal abnormalities, *Mayo Clin Proc* 55:73, 1980.
16. Oldham HN Jr, Kakos GS, Jarmakani MM, et al: Pulmonary artery banding in infants with complex congenital heart defects, *Ann Thorac Surg* 13:342, 1972.
17. Singh AK, DeLeval MR, Pincott JR, et al: Pulmonary artery banding for truncus arteriosus in the first year of life, *Circulation* 54(suppl 3):III-17, 1975.

18. Spicer RL, Behrendt D, Crowley DC, et al: Repair of truncus arteriosus in neonates with the use of a valveless conduit, *Circulation* 70(suppl I):I-26, 1984.
19. Stark J, Gandhi D, deLeval M, et al: Surgical treatment of persistent truncus arteriosus in the first year of life, *Br Heart J* 40:1280, 1978.
20. Musumeci F, Piccoli GP, Dickinson DF, et al: Surgical experience with persistent truncus arteriosus in symptomatic infants under 1 year of age: report of 13 consecutive cases, *Br Heart J* 46:179, 1981.
21. DeLeval MR, McGoon DC, Wallace RB, et al: Management of truncal valvular regurgitation, *Ann Surg* 180:427, 1974.

CHAPTER 46

Total Anomalous Pulmonary Venous Connection

In total anomalous pulmonary venous connection (TAPVC), the pulmonary veins do not connect to the left atrium but instead connect to a systemic venous structure. Thus, the pulmonary venous blood returns to the right side of the heart. An atrial septal defect is present and provides the only source of blood to the left side of the heart. Because pulmonary and systemic venous returns mix thoroughly in the right atrium, TAPVC is considered an admixture lesion. It is associated with two clinical and laboratory pictures, depending on the status of the pulmonary venous connection: those with pulmonary venous obstruction and those without.

EMBRYOLOGY

The embryology of the heart, particularly concerning the incorporation of the pulmonary veins into the left atrium, is reviewed. The lung buds develop as outpouchings of the foregut, and thus their early venous connection is derived from the splanchnic plexus and does not connect directly to the heart (Fig 46–1,A). The early venous connections are to the anterior cardinal veins or the umbilical-vitelline system. Later in the embryo a projection, the common pulmonary vein, develops from the left atrium and ultimately makes contact with the primitive pulmonary venous system (Fig 46–1,B and C). Normally the pulmonary veins are incorporated into the posterior wall of the left atrium, and the connections to the systemic venous system disappear. In contrast, in TAPVC the common pulmonary vein either does not form or does not make contact with the pulmonary venous system. Thus, connections of the pulmonary venous system persist to the systemic venous system. These connections are to remnants of the right anterior cardinal vein, left anterior cardinal vein, the umbilical-vitelline system, or their major tributaries.[1] No direct connection exists between the pulmonary veins and the left atrium.

PATHOLOGIC ANATOMY

Although the pulmonary veins do not connect to the left atrium, generally they converge in the mediastinum directly behind the left atrium. The individual pulmonary veins join together and form confluence located immediately posterior to the left atrium. From this confluence a channel connects to a major venous tributary either above or below the diaphragm. Occasionally the venous connection may be to more than one site or directly to the right atrium.

Total anomalous pulmonary venous connection has been divided into anatomic subtypes based on the site of anomalous connection[1–3]:

1. Supracardiac connection
   a. Right superior vena cava (Fig 46–2,A) (less common)
   b. Azygous vein or hemiazygous vein (Fig 46–2,B) (rare)
   c. Left superior vena cava or left innominate vein (Fig 46–2,C) (common)
   d. Right innominate vein (very rare)
2. Cardiac connection
   a. Coronary sinus (Fig 46–2,D) (more common)
   b. Right atrium (Fig 46–2,E) (less common)
3. Infracardiac (infradiaphragmatic) connection
   a. Portal venous system (Fig 46–2,F) (more common)
   b. Ductus venosus (Fig 46–2,G) (less common)
   c. Inferior vena cava (Fig 46–2,H) (rare)

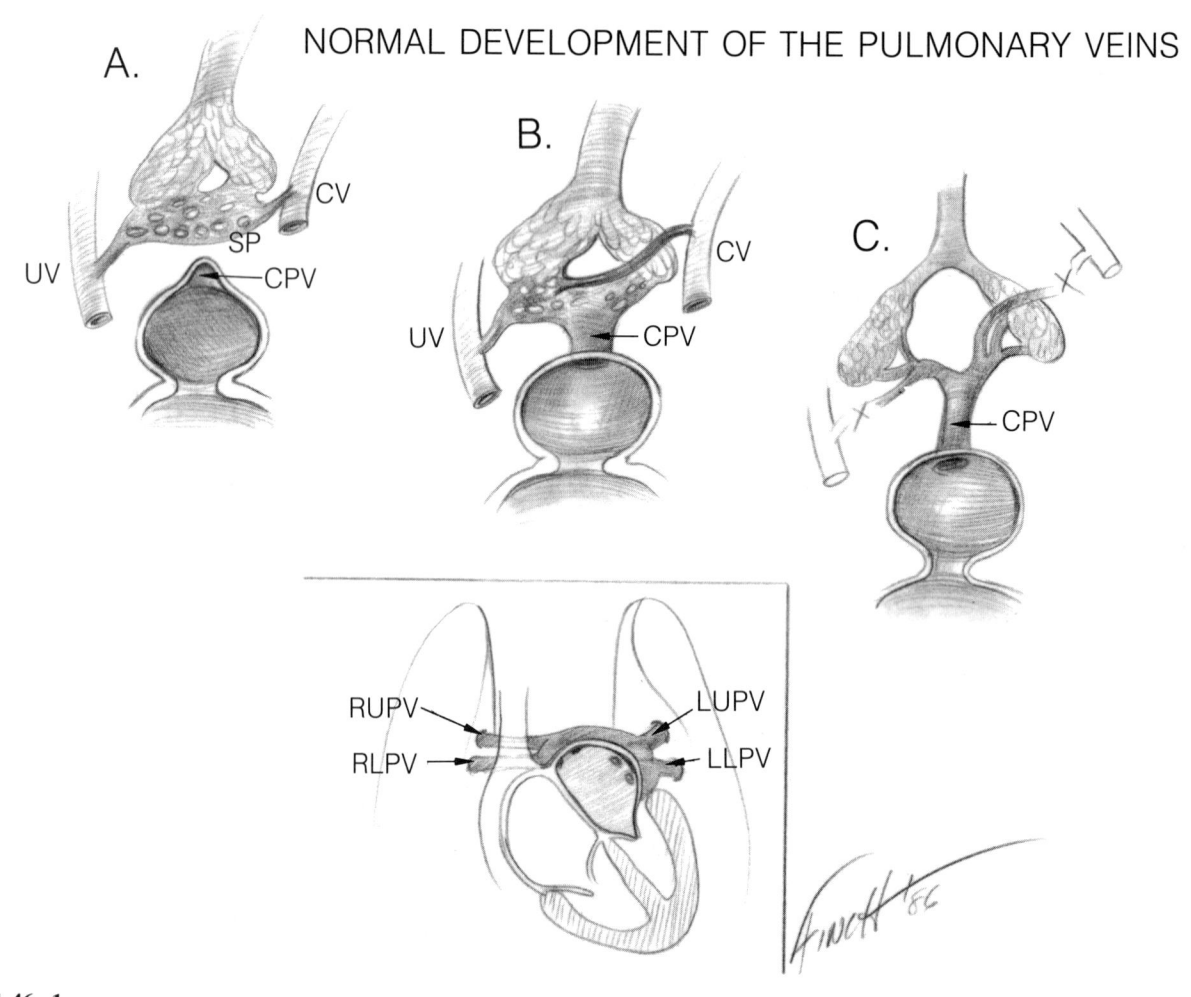

FIG 46–1.
Total anomalous pulmonary venous connection. **A–C,** embryologic development. *UV* = umbilical vein; *CV* = cardinal vein; *SP* = splanchnic plexus; *CPV* = common pulmonary vein; *RUPV* = right upper pulmonary vein; *LUPV* = left upper pulmonary vein; *RLPV* = right lower pulmonary vein; *LLPV* = left lower pulmonary vein.

    d. Hepatic vein (very rare)
    e. Left gastric vein (very rare)
4. Mixed type
    a. Pulmonary veins from various lobes may connect to different sites

In approximately three fourths of the cases, the connecting vein is widely patent and does not obstruct pulmonary venous return. In these cases the right atrium, right ventricle, and pulmonary artery are dilated because there is increased pulmonary blood flow. The left ventricle is smaller than normal, because the ventricular septum is displaced toward the left ventricle because of right ventricular dilatation. In each case of TAPVC, left atrial volume is reduced. During normal development, the confluence of pulmonary veins is incorporated into the posterior wall of the left atrium and adds to the volume of that chamber.

In the remaining one fourth of the cases, the vein connecting the pulmonary venous confluence to the systemic venous system is narrowed and obstructed from either an intrinsic stenotic area or extrinsic compression. One site of extrinsic compression occurs when the connecting left vertical vein passes between the left mainstem bronchus and left pulmonary artery. This situation is called "hemodynamic vise." The vein becomes compressed as pulmonary arterial pressure increases (Fig 46–3).[4, 5] The vein may also pass in front of the pulmonary artery (persistent left superior vena cava), which usually does not cause venous obstruction. Another form of compression occurs in infradiaphragmatic connection, where the venous channel passes through the esophageal hiatus through the diaphragm.[2, 6] The esophageal hiatus is narrowed by diaphragmatic contraction or by swallowing when the esophagus is distended. Other causes of pulmonary venous obstruction include a narrowed foramen ovale and the increased resistance to flow through a long narrow venous

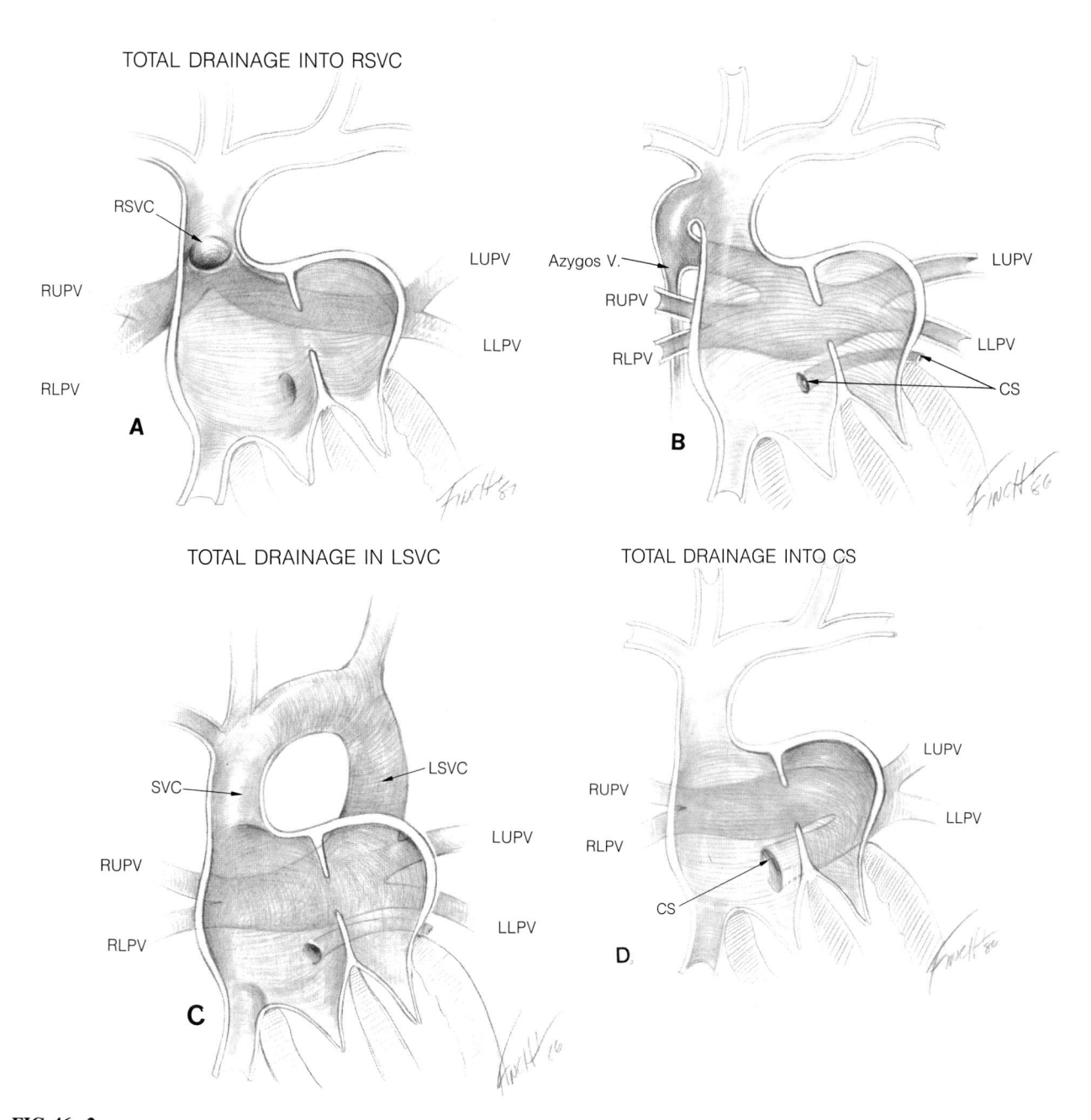

FIG 46–2.
Total anomalous pulmonary venous connection. Anatomic types with various sites of connection. **A,** right superior vena cava *(RSVC).* **B,** azygos vein. **C,** left superior vena cava *(LSVC).* **D,** coronary sinus *(CS). LA* = left atrium; *LH* = left hepatic vein; *LLPV* = left lower pulmonary vein; *LUPV* = left upper pulmonary vein; *RH* = right hepatic vein; *LH* = left hepatic vein; *RLPV* = right lower pulmonary vein; *RUPV* = right upper pulmonary *vein.*

(Continued.)

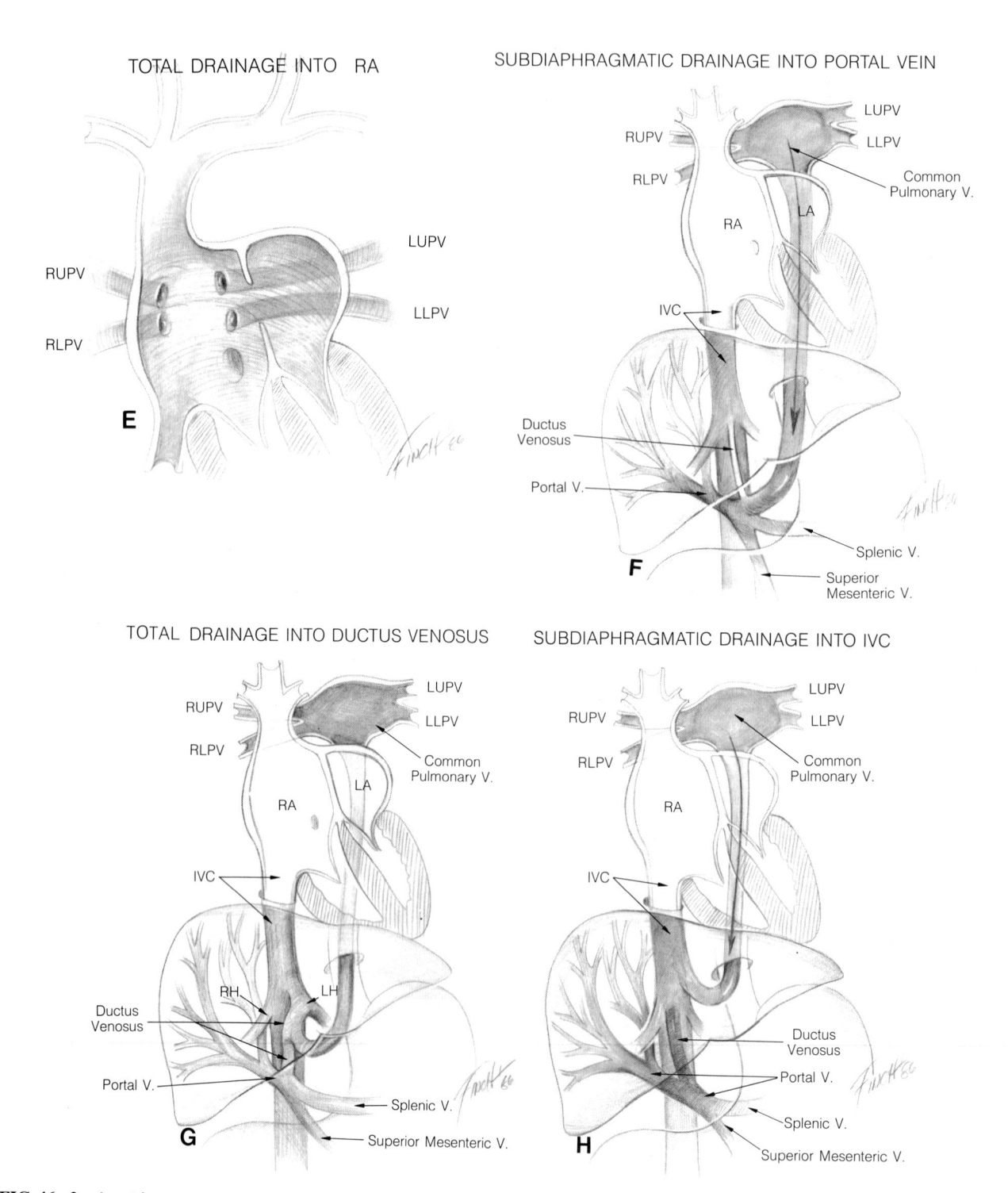

FIG 46-2 (cont.).
E, right atrium *(RA).* **F,** portal venous system. **G,** ductus venosus. **H,** inferior vena cava *(IVC).*

HEMODYNAMIC VISE

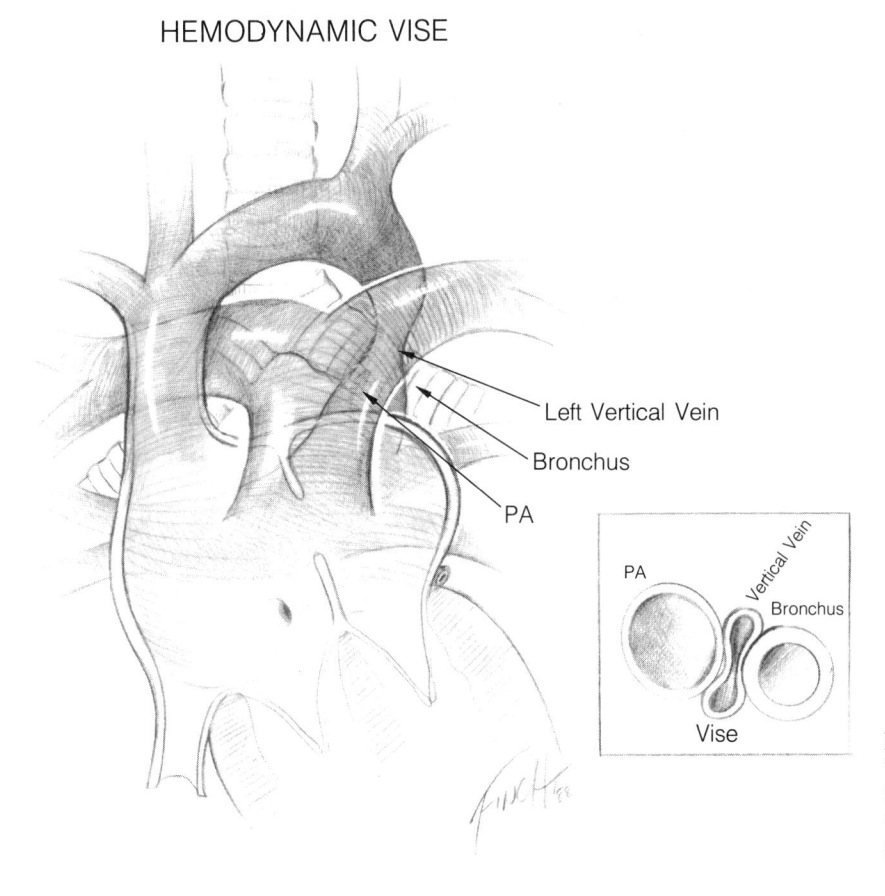

FIG 46–3.
"Hemodynamic vise." Diagram demonstrating compression of connecting left vertical vein between left mainstem bronchus and pulmonary artery *(PA)*.

channel as occurs in the infradiaphragmatic form. Pulmonary venous obstruction is invariably present in total anomalous connection to the portal vein because of the high resistance of the hepatic parenchymal circulation. Total connection into the ductus venosus may not be obstructive during the first few days of life. REASON: The ductus venosus extends from the portal vein to the left hepatic vein and bypasses the hepatic parenchyma. As the ductus venosus closes postnatally, venous obstruction develops. Connection to the hepatic vein or inferior vena cava is usually nonobstructive because the venous return does not pass through the hepatic parenchyma or closing ductus venosus.

When pulmonary venous obstruction is present, the right ventricle is hypertrophied, but the right side of the heart is not dilated, because the pulmonary blood flow is limited. In these patients, histologic examination of the lungs shows edema, dilated lymphatics, and medial hypertrophy of arterioles.[7]

An atrial communication is an integral component of total anomalous pulmonary venous connection and is usually through a foramen ovale or secundum atrial septal defect. Rarely, an ostium primum defect is present.

Total anomalous pulmonary venous connection can coexist with other cardiac malformations, particularly those associated with splenic anomalies.[2, 3, 6] In asplenia, TAPVC occurs in three fourths of patients. It is usually not evident clinically, because the hemodynamics in most instances are influenced by other major coexistent cardiac anomalies, particularly pulmonary stenosis or atresia, which limit pulmonary blood flow.

In polysplenia, partial anomalous pulmonary venous connection occurs more commonly than total anomalous connection. In the latter the total connection is directly to the right atrium. Indeed, polysplenia is virtually the only circumstance in which this form of TAPVC occurs (Fig 46–2,E).

HEMODYNAMICS

The right atrium receives the entire systemic and pulmonary venous blood flows. These volumes mix almost uniformly in the right atrium, although some streaming may occur. The mixed venous blood flows both across the tricuspid valve into the right ventricle and through the atrial communication into the left atrium (Fig 46–4). Atrial pressures are equal. Therefore, the volume of blood flow into the left and right ventricles depends largely on the respective ventricular compliances, which, in turn, are

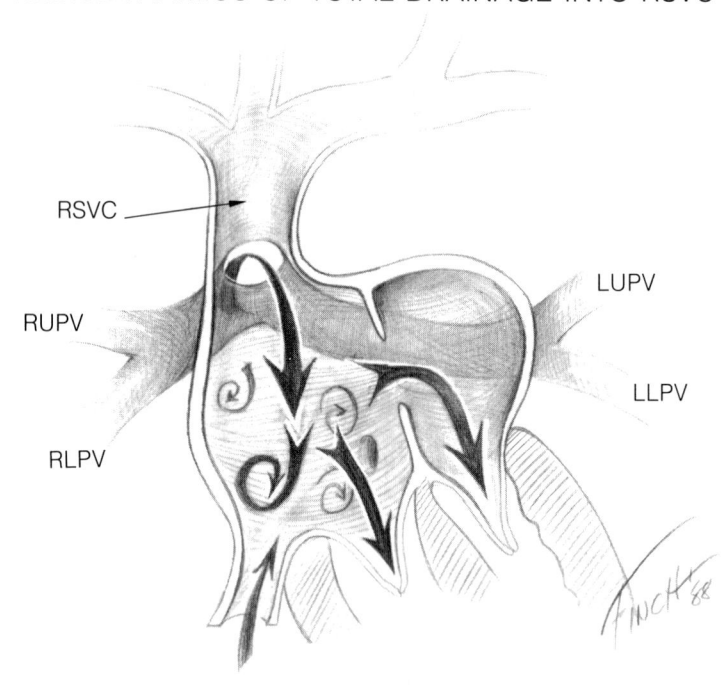

FIG 46-4.
Total anomalous pulmonary venous connection to superior vena cava. Central circulation. Mixed blood flows into right ventricle and through an atrial communication into left atrium and systemic circulation *(arrows)*. RSVC = right superior vena cava; RUPV = right upper pulmonary vein; LLPV = left lower pulmonary vein; RLPV = right lower pulmonary vein; LUPV = left upper pulmonary vein.

influenced principally by the thickness of the right and left ventricular walls.

Before birth, aortic and pulmonary arterial pressures and right and left ventricular wall thicknesses are equal. Therefore, ventricular compliances are relatively equal. The volume of pulmonary and systemic blood flow should also be relatively equal. After birth, the pulmonary vascular resistance normally declines, and the right ventricle becomes thinner. This causes the right ventricle to become more compliant and the pulmonary blood flow to increase significantly. In many cases of TAPVC the hemodynamics resemble those of an atrial septal defect, because in both conditions blood flow depends on relative ventricular compliances. Because in atrial septal defect and in many cases of TAPVC pulmonary arterial pressure is normal or near normal, the ratio of pulmonary to systemic blood flow may exceed 3:1.

In patients with obstruction to pulmonary venous return, pulmonary arterial pressure is elevated. In some patients the elevation is slight and related merely to the large volume of pulmonary venous blood flow through the connecting venous channel or occasionally narrowing of the foramen ovale. Because of the elevation of pulmonary arterial pressure, the right ventricle is more hypertrophied and less compliant. The pulmonary blood flow is therefore limited.

In patients with an anatomic cause of pulmonary venous obstruction, pulmonary arterial pressure is maintained at systemic levels. Therefore, resistance to pulmonary blood flow remains elevated, and right ventricular hypertrophy is maintained. As a result, right ventricular compliance is reduced, and the volume of pulmonary blood flow is limited.

Total anomalous pulmonary venous connection is an admixture lesion. Therefore, the degree of cyanosis is inversely related to the volume of pulmonary blood flow. In a neonate or an infant with significant pulmonary venous obstruction, the degree of cyanosis is marked, whereas in those with a large volume of pulmonary blood flow, cyanosis is minimal.

Some infants with TAPVC without pulmonary venous obstruction develop congestive cardiac failure, which is unusual for conditions causing a volume load on the right ventricle. Most patients, however, are asymptomatic. In the pulmonary arterioles, medial hypertrophy and eventually intimal proliferation develop slowly, causing pulmonary vascular disease.[7]

CLINICAL FEATURES

There are two distinct clinical pictures of patients with total anomalous pulmonary venous connection, depending on whether pulmonary venous obstruction is absent or present.

Without Pulmonary Venous Obstruction

Patients without pulmonary venous connection show a combination of mild cyanosis and congestive cardiac failure, usually developing in early infancy. Growth is slow, and respiratory tract infections are frequent. There is a precordial bulge and clinical evidence of cardiomegaly. The auscultatory findings resemble those of an atrial septal defect. There is a soft pulmonary systolic ejection murmur, a middiastolic murmur, and wide fixed splitting of the second heart sound. The pulmonary component may be slightly increased.

With Pulmonary Venous Obstruction

These patients show marked cyanosis in the neonatal period, and most die by 1 month of age unless an operation is performed.[6] The principle findings are respiratory: tachypnea and dyspnea. Symptoms progress, and the neonate may develop acidosis and disseminated intravascular coagulation from the extreme hypoxemia.

There may be either no murmur or a soft nonspecific murmur. The pulmonary component of the second heart sound is accentuated. Rales may be heard over the lung fields. The clinical picture is that of neonatal respiratory disease rather than cardiac disease.

ELECTROCARDIOGRAPHIC FEATURES

The major hemodynamic effects are on the right side of the heart. In the neonatal period, the electrocardiogram is indistinguishable from normal. Subsequently in those patients without pulmonary venous obstruction, a pattern of right ventricular enlargement is found. There is an rSR′ pattern with terminal delay found in lead V_1.

In those patients with obstruction, right-axis deviation and right ventricular hypertrophy with a tall R wave in lead V_1 are present.

ECHOCARDIOGRAPHIC FEATURES[8-13]

The echocardiographic findings are very helpful in establishing a diagnosis of TAPVC. Pulmonary veins entering the left atrium are not identified. Although this finding is highly reliable, it may be related to inexperience of the echocardiographic technician. If only one pulmonary vein is identified entering the left atrium, the diagnosis of TAPVC can be excluded. Doppler interrogation of the left atrium is also useful in identifying pulmonary veins in individuals with normally connecting veins. Left atrial volume is small, and a defect is found in the atrial septum through which right-to-left flow can be detected. The left ventricle may appear reduced in size. The right ventricle is principally hypertrophied in those with obstruction and dilated in those without. Paradoxical septal motion is found in the latter. Commonly the pulmonary venous confluence is identified as an echo-free space behind the left atrium. The connecting venous channel is often identified. Doppler interrogation of the connecting venous channel is very helpful in identifying the direction of blood flow in this vessel and thereby distinguishing it from other vascular structures.

RADIOGRAPHIC FEATURES

The radiographic appearance of TAPVC is not uniform and varies with the degree of obstruction to the pulmonary venous system. If no obstruction occurs, the pulmonary arterial vasculature and cardiac size are greatly increased. In contrast, with obstruction to pulmonary venous return the pulmonary vasculature may be normal and the heart size minimally enlarged, or the cardiac size is normal and the lung fields show significant pulmonary venous congestion.

Because most patients with TAPVC have normal pulmonary vascular resistance and pulmonary arterial pressure, markedly increased pulmonary blood flow and cardiomegaly are commonly observed. This group of patients are described first and then those with pulmonary venous obstruction.

Normal Pulmonary Arterial Pressure and Nonobstructed Venous Connection

The radiographic features of those without obstruction are described in two sections. The first presents the general features in each patient and the second presents features specific to an individual type of connection.

General Features

1. The heart is greatly enlarged. REASON: Pulmonary blood flow is markedly increased. Both systemic and the increased pulmonary venous return pass through the right side of the heart, resulting in marked right atrial and right ventricular dilatation.

2. In spite of right atrial dilatation, the right atrium is not uniformly prominent (Fig 46–5). REASON: Enlargement of the right atrium and right ventricle against the sternum results in clockwise rotation as in atrial septal defect (see Chapter 19).

3. The ascending aorta does not form the upper right cardiac border, and the superior mediastinum is narrow unless obscured by venous structures. REASON: Clockwise rotation of the heart.

4. The left cardiac border commonly has a rounded appearance (Fig 46–5) because of marked dilatation of the right ventricular outflow tract and clockwise rotation of the heart. The main pulmonary arterial segment may not be distinctly visible because of the dilated outflow tract.

5. The radiographic appearance is indistinguishable

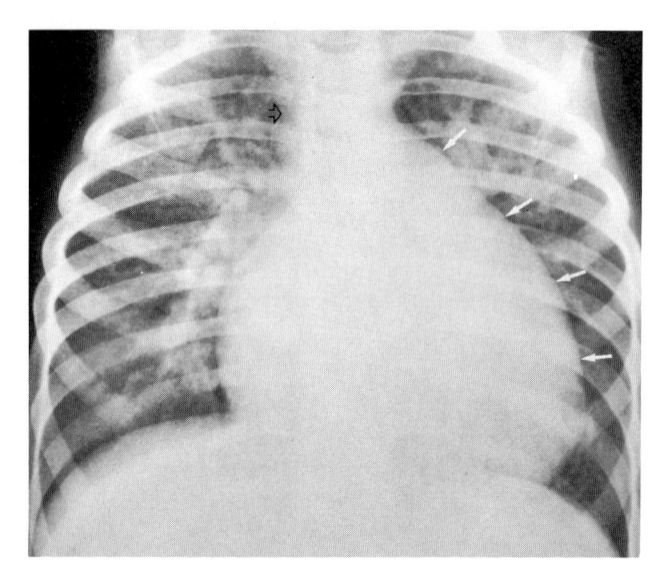

FIG 46–5.
Total anomalous pulmonary venous connection to coronary sinus. Thoracic roentgenogram. Posteroanterior projection. Markedly enlarged heart. Pulmonary vasculature is greatly increased. Typical rounded left cardiac border *(arrows)* is caused by marked dilatation of right ventricle. Right ventricle forms left cardiac border as in secundum atrial septal defect. Pulmonary arterial segment is overshadowed by markedly dilated right ventricular outflow tract. In spite of severe enlargement of right atrium, right atrial border is only slightly prominent because of clockwise rotation of heart. Ascending aorta is not visualized. Superior vena cava forms right mediastinal border *(open black arrow).*

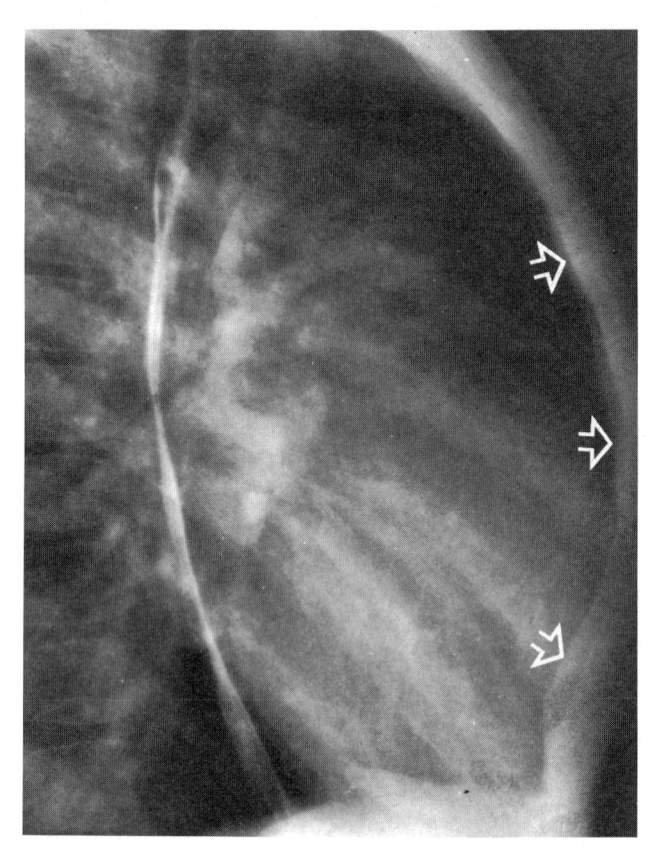

FIG 46–6.
Total anomalous pulmonary venous connection. Thoracic roentgenogram. Lateral projection. Barium-filled esophagus is not displaced. Left atrium is not enlarged in this condition. Anterior bowing of sternum *(open arrows)* is caused by right-sided enlargement as in atrial septal defect.

from an ostium secundum or primum atrial septal defect with a large left-to-right shunt. Differentiation from atrial septal defect can be made only if an enlarged connecting vein is visible.

6. Barium swallow is helpful because left atrial enlargement is never present (Fig 46–6). REASON: The entire systemic and pulmonary venous return occurs through the right side of the heart. As long as the pulmonary resistance is low and the right ventricle is compliant, most of the venous return enters the right ventricle, and a volume of blood equal to the cardiac output is shunted through the foramen ovale to the left side of the heart, which tends to be anatomically small.

7. The presence of left atrial enlargement excludes total anomalous pulmonary venous connection.

Specific Types

Specific types of TAPVC can be diagnosed from radiographic features by visualization of the anomalous connecting vein.

1. Total anomalous pulmonary venous connection to coronary sinus. The enlarged coronary sinus may be seen on a lateral thoracic roentgenogram with barium swallow (Fig 46–7) by an indentation of the esophagus at a site lower than the left atrium. In most cases, however, the coronary sinus may not be sufficiently enlarged to indent the esophagus.

2. Total anomalous venous connection to the superior vena cava or azygos vein. The superior vena cava is dilated and markedly prominent along the upper right cardiac border on the posteroanterior roentgenogram (Fig 46–8).

3. Total anomalous pulmonary venous connection to the azygos vein may result in a mass density in the region of the azygos vein immediately above the right mainstem bronchus (Fig 46–9). In most cases differentiation from total connection to superior vena cava cannot be made.

4. Total anomalous pulmonary venous connection to a persistent left superior vena cava results in enlargement of the left superior vena cava or left vertical vein and right superior vena cava, resulting in the typical figure-of-8 appearance or "snowman heart" (Fig 46–10).

5. The appearance on the posteroanterior roentgenogram may closely mimic a superior mediastinal mass, particularly lymphoma. To aid in the differential diagnosis, a

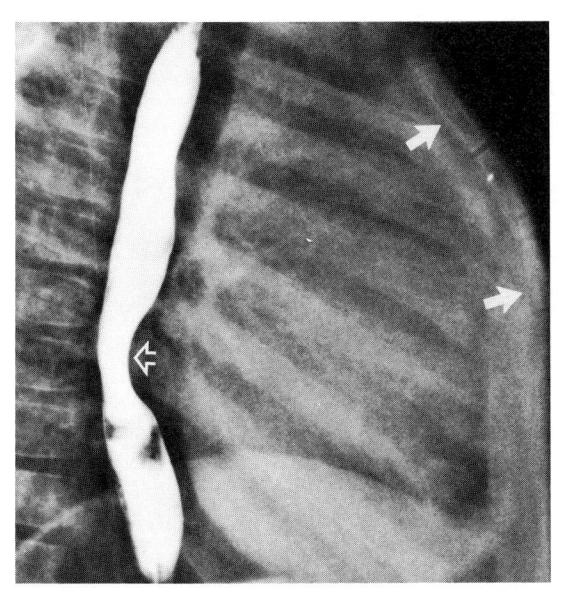

FIG 46–7.
Total anomalous pulmonary venous connection to coronary sinus. Thoracic roentgenogram. Lateral projection. Enlarged coronary sinus causes well-circumscribed indentation of barium-filled esophagus, allowing a specific diagnosis of total connection to coronary sinus. Unfortunately, this radiographic finding is not always present. Retrosternal space is obliterated by markedly enlarged right side of heart. Bowing of sternum by large right ventricle *(solid arrows)*.

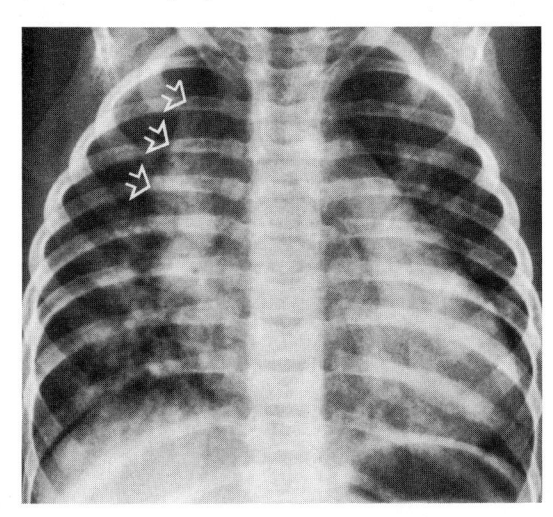

FIG 46–8.
Total anomalous pulmonary venous connection to right superior vena cava. Thoracic roentgenogram. Posteroanterior projection. Moderately enlarged heart. Markedly increased pulmonary arterial vasculature. Mass density in region of azygos vein just above right mainstem bronchus suggests specific diagnosis. Identical appearance may be seen in TAPVC to right superior vena cava.

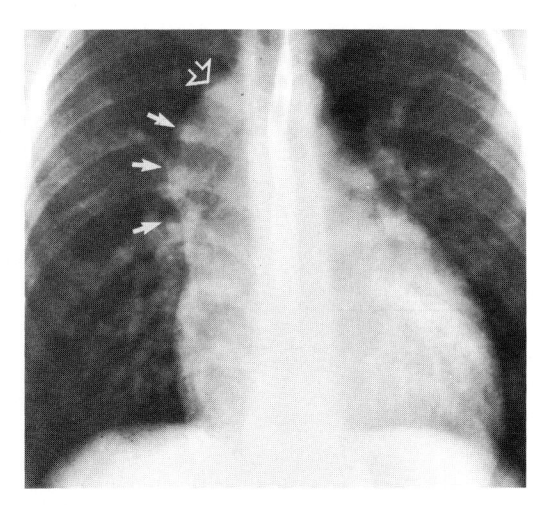

FIG 46–9.
Total anomalous pulmonary venous connection to azygos vein. Thoracic roentgenogram. Posteroanterior projection. Large round density *(open arrow)* in region of azygos vein. Dilatation of superior vena cava *(solid arrows)*. Cardiomegaly. Increased pulmonary arterial vasculature.

lateral film shows a midmediastinum mass and distinctly visualized venae cavae as linear densities (Fig 46–11). REASON: The anterior surfaces of both cavae seen on the lateral projection are bordered by lung. Mediastinal tumors, such as a lymphoma, almost invariably obliterate the retrosternal space without clear demonstration of the tumor edges on a lateral projection because the air-tumor interface is lateral and not seen in profile.

6. Total anomalous pulmonary venous connection to the left superior vena cava may not always result in

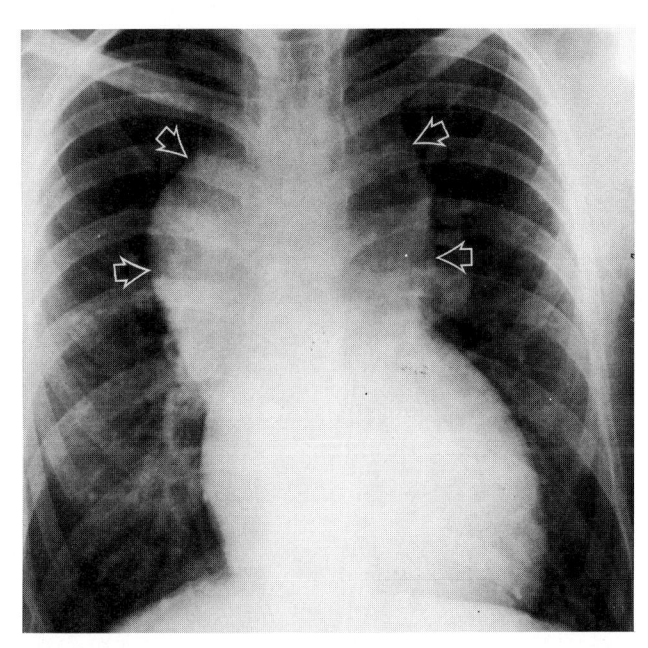

FIG 46–10.
Total anomalous pulmonary venous connection to left superior vena cava. Thoracic roentgenogram. Posteroanterior projection. Patient was referred for radiation therapy because of large superior mediastinal mass. Moderately enlarged heart. Pulmonary vasculature is normal because of venous obstruction (hemodynamic vise). Neoplasm should be seriously considered from this appearance without a lateral projection.

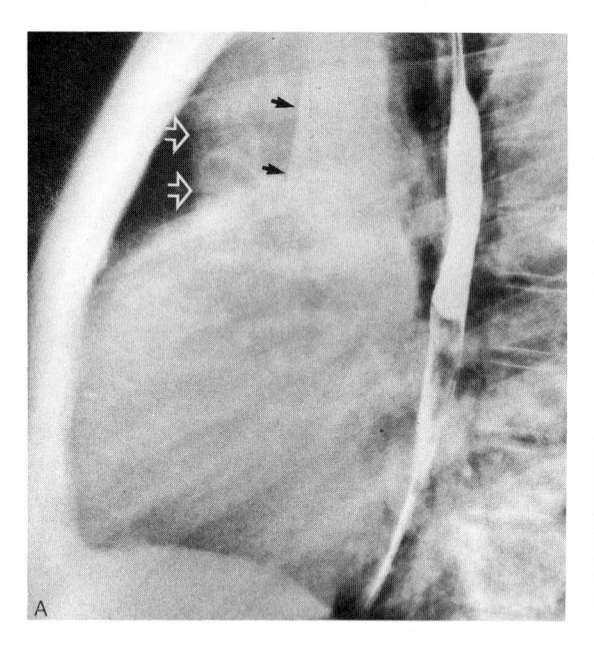

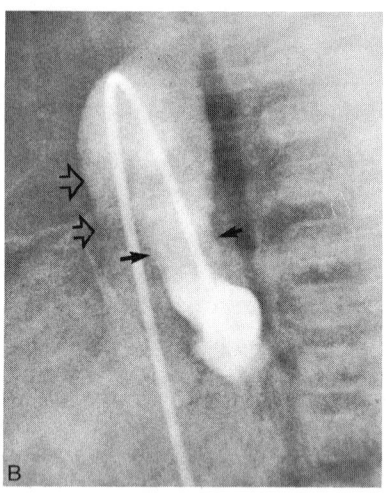

FIG 46–11.
Total anomalous pulmonary venous connection to left superior vena cava. **A,** thoracic roentgenogram. Lateral projection. Retrosternal space is free, and two linear densities corresponding to the cavae *(arrows)* are visualized. Anterior density *(open arrows)* is right superior vena cava. Posterior density is left superior vena cava. **B,** explanatory angiogram with catheter in left superior vena cava. Anterior density *(open arrow)* is border of right superior vena cava, and posterior density is persistent left superior vena cava.

marked enlargement of both superior vena cavae. Sometimes only the left superior vena cava is enlarged, and the right superior vena cava density is normal. In this instance, a typical snowman appearance is not present.

7. In infants with an enlarged thymus, only one linear density from the superior vena cava may be visible on a lateral projection.

8. In patients with total anomalous connection to the left superior vena cava but with obstruction, both superior vena cavae are normal in size. Sometimes poststenotic dilation of venous structures may result in aneurysmal dilatation, forming a mediastinal mass.

Elevated Pulmonary Arterial Pressure and Obstructed Venous Connections

The roentgenographic findings are very different in patients with TAPVC and severe pulmonary venous obstruction. REASON: The high resistance to flow through the pulmonary circulation limits the volume of pulmonary blood flow, which is usually less than normal. Consequently, the right ventricle is not dilated. Compensating right ventricular hypertrophy usually does not cause significant cardiomegaly on a posteroanterior roentgenogram.

Pulmonary venous obstruction may occur with supradiaphragmatic total connection because of either a narrow and long draining vein, extrinsic compression of the vein, or intimal proliferations causing intrinsic obstruction.

Total anomalous pulmonary venous connection to the portal venous system is associated with severe venous obstruction. In this instance the resistance to pulmonary venous blood flow is increased by (1) drainage occurring through a long connecting channel leading into the portal system, (2) the capillary resistance in the liver, which exceeds that in the lung, and (3) the constrictive effect of the diaphragm on the anomalous venous channel. Obstruction to pulmonary venous return can be suspected from a posteroanterior roentgenogram with a high degree of accuracy.

1. Depending on the degree of obstruction, the heart may be either normal or only slightly enlarged. Cardiac size is normal, whereas with less severe pulmonary venous obstruction or right ventricular decompensation, some cardiomegaly is found (Fig 46–12).

2. The most characteristic radiographic finding is a fine granular appearance in both lung fields (Fig 46–13). An air bronchogram is absent. The radiographic appearance may be indistinguishable from hyaline membrane disease, a much more common condition. In hyaline membrane disease, however, an air bronchogram is commonly seen, but this is the only differential radiographic feature. In most cases distinction cannot be made.

3. With supradiaphragmatic pulmonary venous connection and obstruction of the connecting venous channel, the degree of venous obstruction varies, but with infradia-

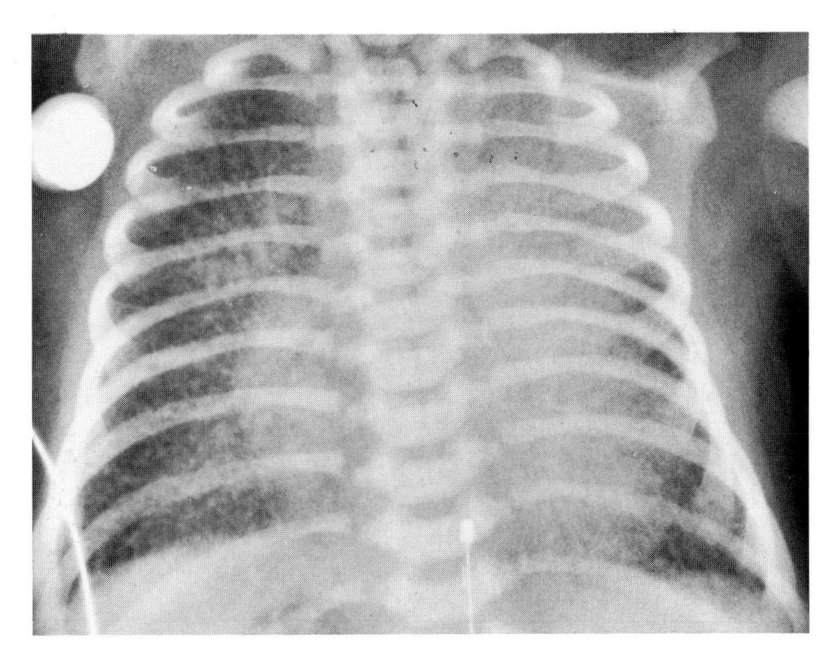

FIG 46–12.
Total anomalous pulmonary venous connection above diaphragm and moderate pulmonary venous obstruction. Thoracic roentgenogram. Posteroanterior projection. Markedly enlarged heart. Pulmonary vasculature has characteristic granular appearance of interstitial edema. Kerley B lines are absent. No air bronchogram.

phragmatic connection, pulmonary venous obstruction is usually severe (see Fig 46–13).

4. A rare exception of nonobstructing infradiaphragmatic connection is to the inferior vena cava above the level of the portal vein bypassing the liver or connections to a patent nonobstructive ductus venosus (the ductus venosus also bypasses the liver). Clinically such patients develop deep cyanosis after a few weeks of life when the ductus venosus closes.

5. The granular pattern in both lung fields is caused by interstitial edema. Kerley B lines are usually not seen in infants.

6. A slight pleural effusion may be seen on a thoracic roentgenogram (see Fig 46–13), a finding that is helpful in diagnosing increased pulmonary venous pressure. In many cases the differential diagnosis between TAPVC below the diaphragm and respiratory distress syndrome is otherwise difficult or impossible. An air bronchogram favors pulmonary disease, but exceptions exist (see Fig 46–13).

CARDIAC CATHETERIZATION

With the increasing accuracy of echocardiography, cardiac catheterization is unnecessary for the diagnosis of many instances of TAPVC. It may be used to answer spe-

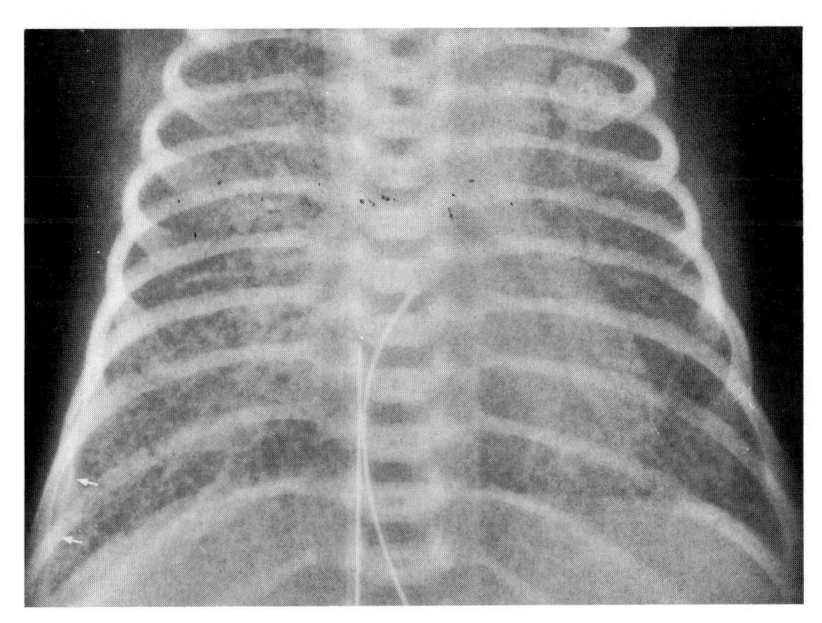

FIG 46–13.
Total anomalous pulmonary venous connection below diaphragm. Thoracic roentgenogram. Posteroanterior projection. Normal cardiac size. Both lung fields show diffuse granular pattern of interstitial edema. Small pleural effusion *(arrows)* at right base.

cific questions, such as the pulmonary arterial pressure, site of venous obstruction, and the size of the atrial communication.

The catheter can be passed from right to left at the atrial level. It is often possible to pass the catheter into the anomalously connecting venous channel. The catheter course is often diagnostic (see Chapter 6). The location of the catheter tip in the pulmonary venous system can be confirmed by obtaining a blood sample that is fully saturated. Pressures should be recorded on withdrawal of the catheter tip from the anomalous vein to the right atrium to detect sites of obstruction. Angiography should also be performed from this site, because it will visualize the pulmonary venous system and its anomalously connecting channel.

It is much easier to pass the catheter into a supracardiac connection than either a cardiac connection or an infradiaphragmatic connection. Catheterization of an infradiaphragmatic connection is particularly difficult when the umbilical vein is used, but the catheter may be passed through the ductus venosus into the anomalously connecting vein.

Serial sampling for oxygen saturations through the systemic venous system can localize the site of anomalous connection by identifying a left-to-right shunt. Oxygen saturations are elevated beyond this location. Blood from the left atrium, left ventricle, aorta, right ventricle, and pulmonary artery show approximately the same oxygen saturation value.

Pulmonary arterial and pulmonary wedge pressures should be measured as part of the catheterization. Pulmonary hypertension may be found.[2] If the pulmonary wedge pressure is elevated, obstruction to pulmonary venous connection is probably present and the cause of pulmonary hypertension. If the wedge pressure is normal, the elevation of pulmonary arterial pressure is related to either increased pulmonary blood flow or vascular resistance.

A balloon catheter inflated in the left atrium and withdrawn across the atrial septum helps determine the size of the atrial communication.

ANGIOGRAPHIC FEATURES

Careful angiography plays an important role in the preoperative assessment of patients with TAPVC, although

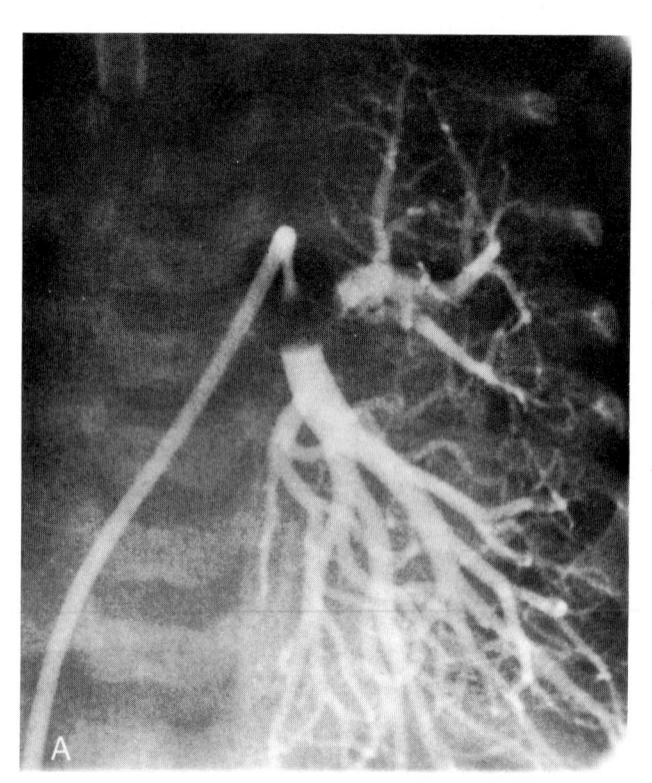

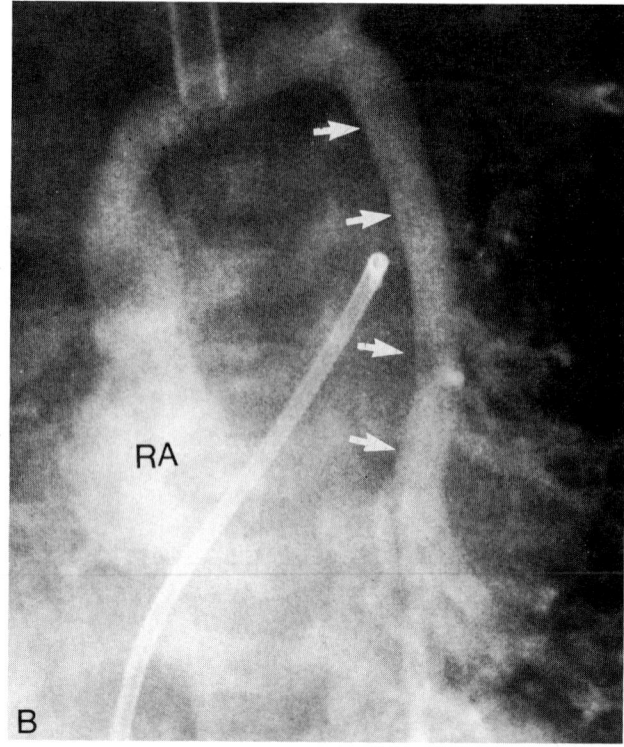

FIG 46–14.
Total anomalous pulmonary venous connection. Balloon occlusion pulmonary arteriogram. Anteroposterior projection. **A,** left pulmonary artery. Lack of enlargement of pulmonary arteries suggests venous obstruction. **B,** after deflation of balloon, there is excellent opacification of long and narrow persistent left superior vena cava, suggesting associated venous obstruction *(arrows)*. Without obstruction, left superior vena cava tends to be huge. No localized narrowing is demonstrated. Therefore, point of obstruction is probably located at level of foramen ovale. *RA* = right atrium.

some types of anomalous connections can now also be demonstrated by ultrasonography.

Each pulmonary vein should be demonstrated angiographically. REASON: Total anomalous pulmonary venous connection does not always occur to a common pulmonary vein, but there may be more than one site of anomalous connection (mixed type). Identification of each vein is therefore important to the surgeon.

Angiographic assessment can be made by pulmonary angiography or by direct injection into a pulmonary vein or the connecting venous channel. If pulmonary arterial injections are made, the right and the left pulmonary arteries should be injected separately, rapidly, and with a large amount of contrast medium or preferably with a balloon occlusive technique. REASON: Without venous obstruction, pulmonary blood flow is very rapid, and consequently the contrast medium is markedly diluted. Best results are obtained with balloon occlusion pulmonary arteriography (Fig 46–14).

If the anomalously connecting venous channel is entered during cardiac catheterization, it should always be injected selectively, and an attempt should be made to pass the catheter selectively into the individual pulmonary veins (Fig 46–15).

The spatial relationship between right and left superior vena cava causing the characteristic radiographic densities of TAPVC to the left superior vena cava is clearly visualized by angiography. The right superior vena cava projects slightly anterior to the left superior vena cava (see Figs 46–11,B).

Anomalous connection can also be suspected by dilution of contrast material by inflow of unopacified blood ("wash-in") (Fig 46–16).

With total connection to the coronary sinus, the coronary sinus is markedly dilated (Fig 46–17). A mixed type of supradiaphragmatic connection requires careful angiography, preferably using balloon occlusion (Figs 46–14 and 46–18) or by direct catheterization of the anomalous connecting channels (see Fig 46–15). Coexistent supradiaphragmatic and infradiaphragmatic connection may occur (see Fig 46–18).

Demonstration of venous obstruction is very important (Fig 46–19). The most common site of obstruction in TAPVC to the left vertical vein is located at the level of the left mainstem bronchus. The draining vein may be

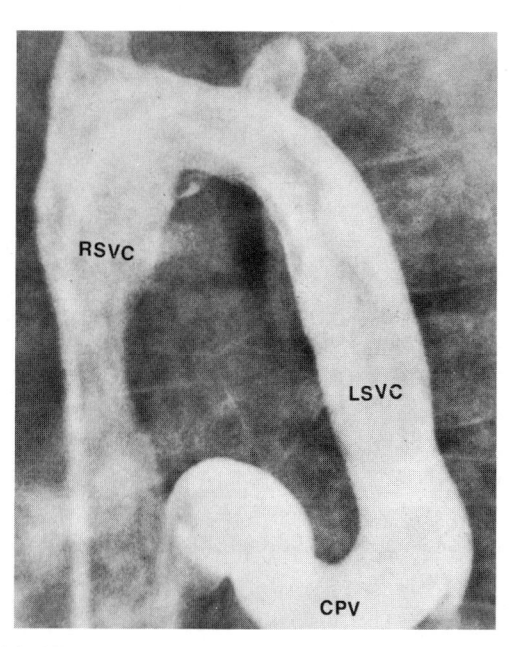

FIG 46–15.
Total anomalous pulmonary venous connection to left superior vena cava. Venous angiogram. Left anterior oblique projection. Catheter course from right superior vena cava *(RSVC)* into left innominate vein and persistent left superior vena cava. Nonobstructed left superior vena cava *(LSVC)* is huge because it passes in front of pulmonary artery rather than between pulmonary artery and bronchus as a left ventricle vein. Common pulmonary vein *(CPV)* is well seen.

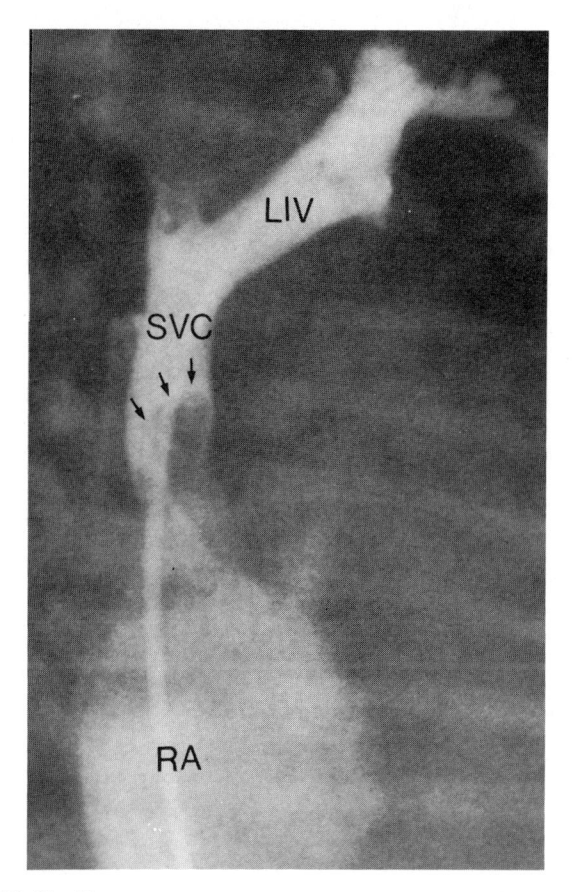

FIG 46–16.
Total anomalous pulmonary venous connection to right superior vena cava. Right superior vena cavogram. Anteroposterior projection. Anomalous venous connection is evident indirectly by marked dilution of contrast medium *(arrows)*. *LV* = left innominate vein; *RA* = right atrium; *SVC* = superior vena cava.

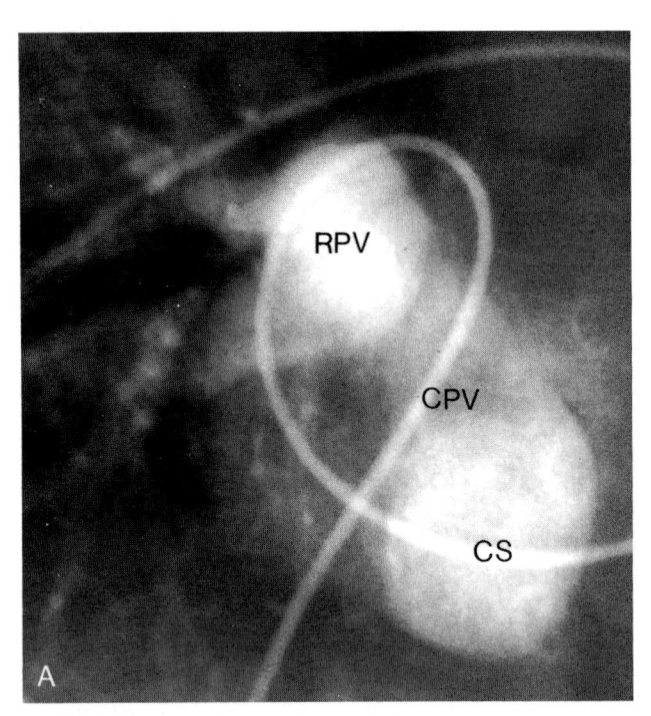

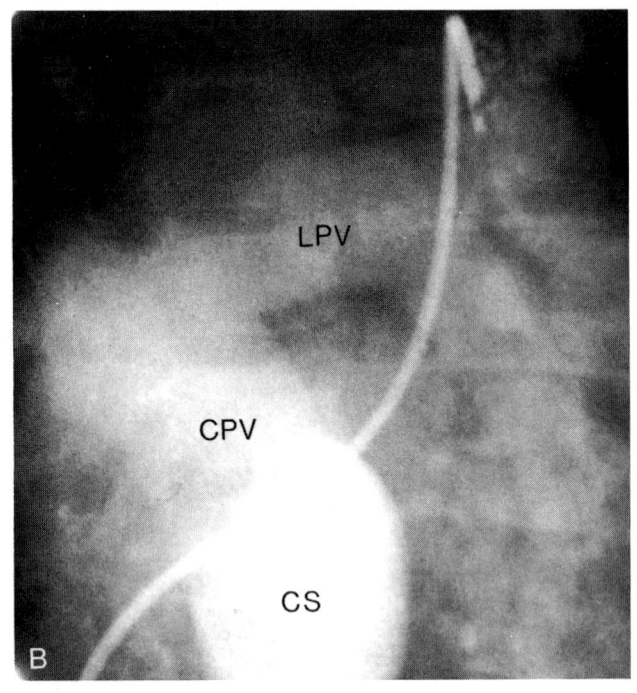

818 *Cyanosis and Increased Pulmonary Arterial Vasculature*

FIG 46–17.
Total anomalous pulmonary venous connection to coronary sinus. Angiograms. Late phase. **A,** anterposterior projection. Right pulmonary arteriogram. Right pulmonary vein *(RPV),* common pulmonary vein *(CPV),* and huge coronary sinus *(CS)* are opacified. **B,** left pulmonary arteriogram. Left pulmonary vein *(LPV),* common pulmonary vein and huge coronary sinus are outlined.

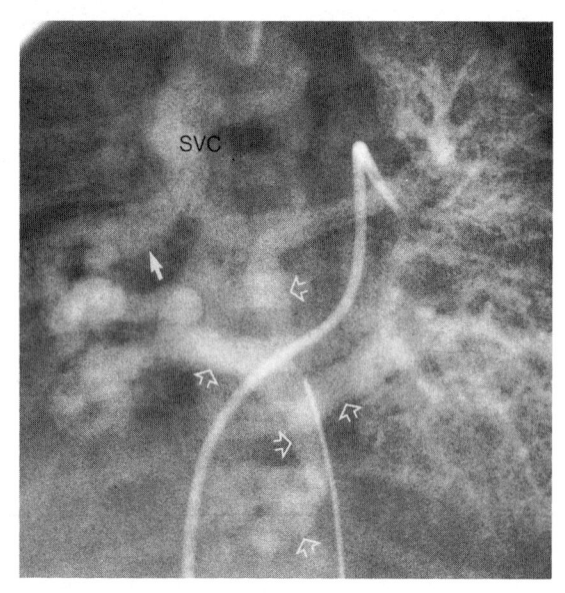

FIG 46–18.
Total anomalous pulmonary venous connection. Mixed type with supradiaphragmatic and infradiaphragmatic connection. Pulmonary arteriogram. Late phase. Anteroposterior projection. Right upper lobe pulmonary vein connects anomalously to superior vena cava *(SVC) (solid arrow).* Pulmonary veins from right lower lobe, left upper lobe, and left lower lobe connect anomalously *(open arrows)* into a connecting vein that empties into portal vein.

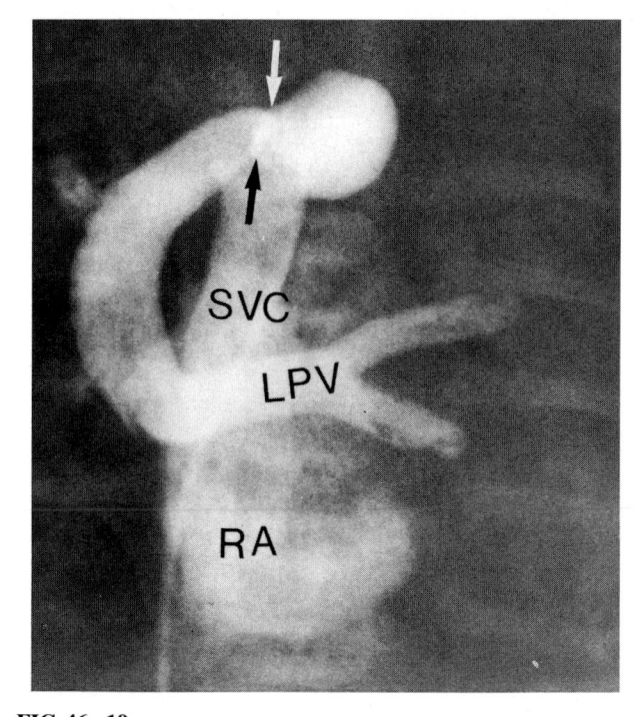

FIG 46–19.
Total anomalous pulmonary venous connection to right superior vena cava. Superior vena cavogram. Anteroposterior projection. Aneurysmal dilatation of left innominate vein. Distinct venous stenosis *(arrows)*. *LPV* = left pulmonary vein; *RA* = right atrium; *SVC* = superior vena cava.

pinched between the left pulmonary artery and left mainstem bronchus (hemodynamic vise) (Fig 46–20). Sometimes areas of narrowing, particularly intrinsic, may not be demonstrated by angiography, and, consequently, careful pressure measurements are very useful.

Total anomalous venous connection to the right atrium occurring typically with polysplenic syndrome (Fig 46–21) or right superior vena cava (Fig 46–22) is rare.

Right atrial injection shows the obligatory right-to-left shunt at the atrial level. On the late phase of a pulmonary arteriogram, as opaque material returns to the right atrium, the shunt is also seen as the left atrium becomes reopacified.

Selective left atrial injection demonstrates a small left atrium that appears to empty completely during atrial systole (Fig 46–23). The left ventricle seems small and empties almost completely. The size of the left ventricle appears relatively small compared with the dilated right ventricle. It is displaced posteriorly and superiorly by the enlarged right ventricle.

In patients with pulmonary venous obstruction from a stenotic but probe patent foramen ovale, herniation of the

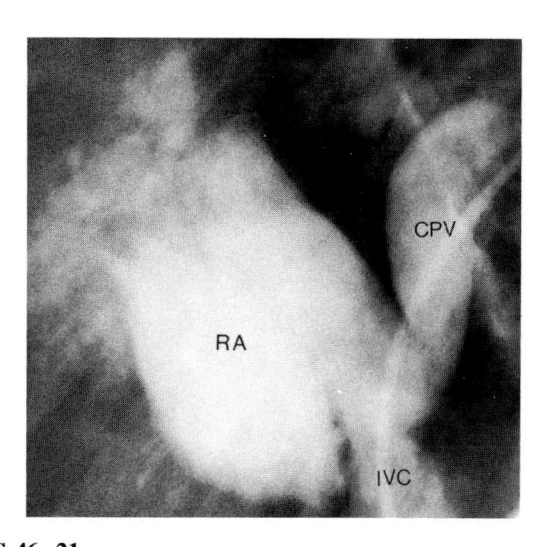

FIG 46–21.
Total anomalous pulmonary venous connection to supradiaphragmatic portion of inferior vena cava. Pulmonary venous angiogram. Lateral projection. Catheter has entered directly common pulmonary vein *(CPV)*. Right atrium is opacified. Common pulmonary vein joins right atrium *(RA)* at junction with inferior vena cava *(IVC)*.

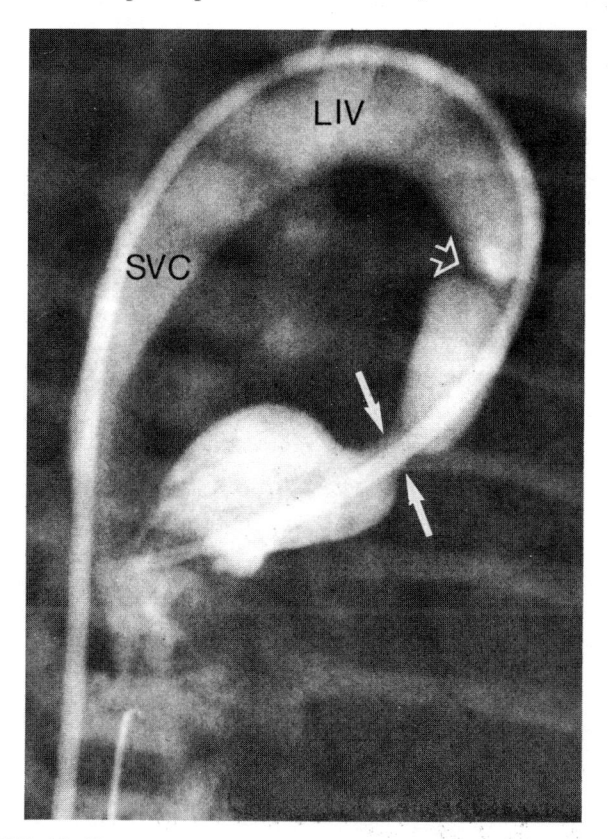

FIG 46–20.
Total anomalous venous connection to left ventrical vein with pulmonary venous obstruction. Principal obstruction *(solid arrows)* is at level of left mainstem bronchus (hemodynamic vise). Another, intrinsic stenosis *(open arrow)*, is caused by intimal proliferation. *LIV* = left innominate vein; *SVC* = superior vena cava.

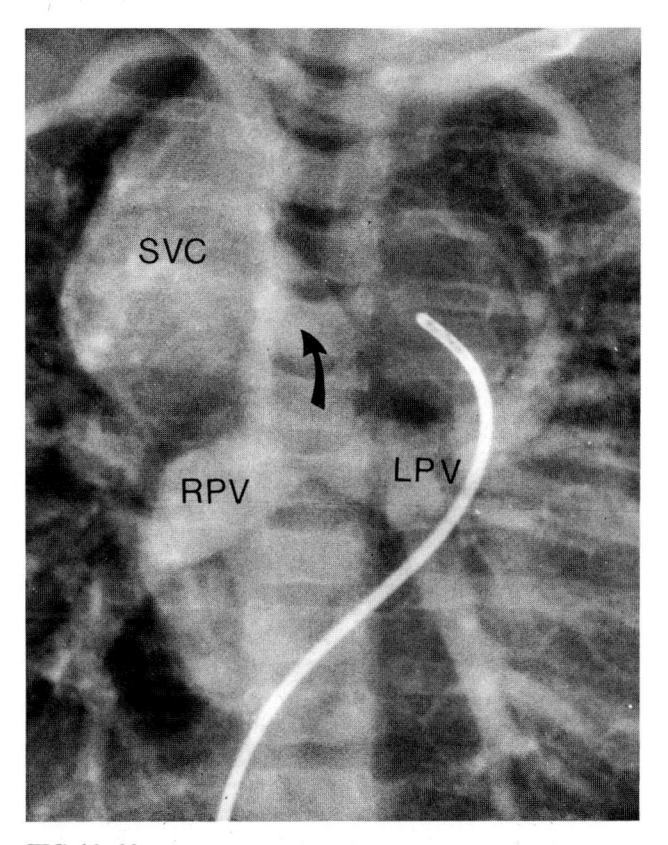

FIG 46–22.
Total anomalous pulmonary venous connection to right superior vena cava *(SVC)*. Pulmonary arteriogram. Late phase. Anteroposterior projection. Pulmonary veins join to form common pulmonary vein, which drains anomalously *(curved arrow)* into markedly dilated right superior vena cava. *RPV* = right pulmonary vein; *LPV* = left pulmonary vein.

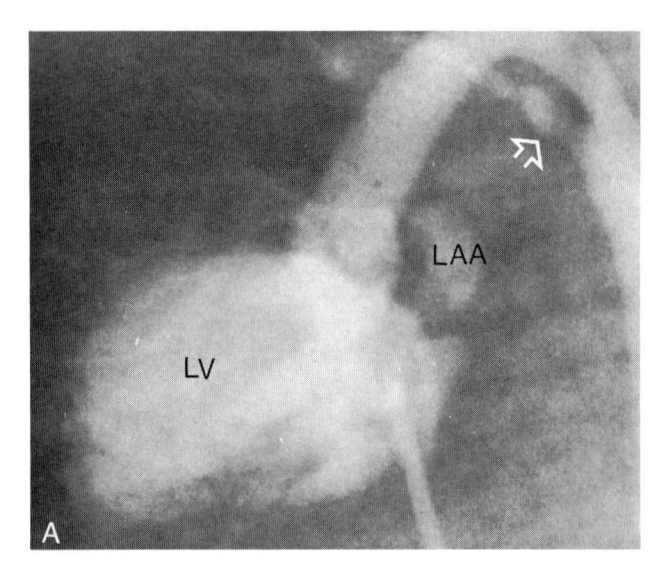

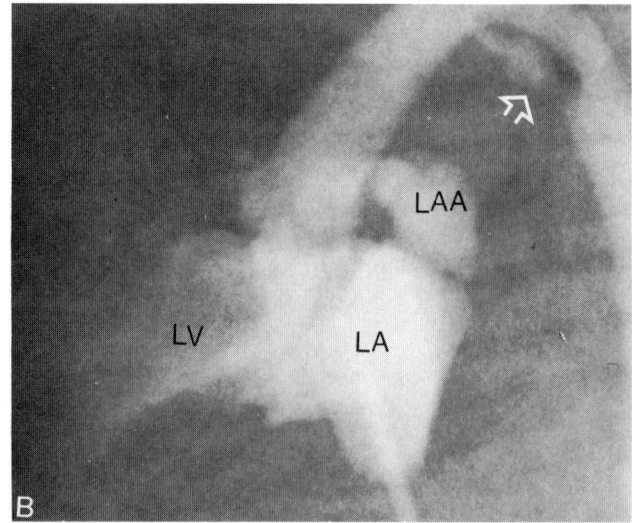

FIG 46–23.
Total anomalous pulmonary venous connection. Left atriogram. Lateral projection. **A,** diastole. Left atrium *(LA)* is completely contracted except for left atrial appendage *(LAA)*. **B,** systole. Left ventricle *(LV)* is almost completely empty. Small left atrium is opacified. Incidental patent ductus *(open arrow)*.

fossa ovalis may occur (Fig 46–24) and cause a large filling defect in the left atrium, which may be confused with a left atrial myxoma or cor triatriatum.

Total anomalous pulmonary venous connection below the diaphragm can be diagnosed either on the late phase of a pulmonary arteriogram or occasionally by direct catheterization of the anomalously connecting vein through the ductus venosus (Fig 46–25). The latter is the most definitive and the fastest way to diagnose this cardiac abnormality.

Connection below the diaphragm may occur directly to the portal vein or to the ductus venosus. Angiographically it is almost impossible to differentiate one from the other. Aneurysmal dilatation of the portal vein may occur (Fig 46–26).

Total connection directly to the right atrium occurs al-

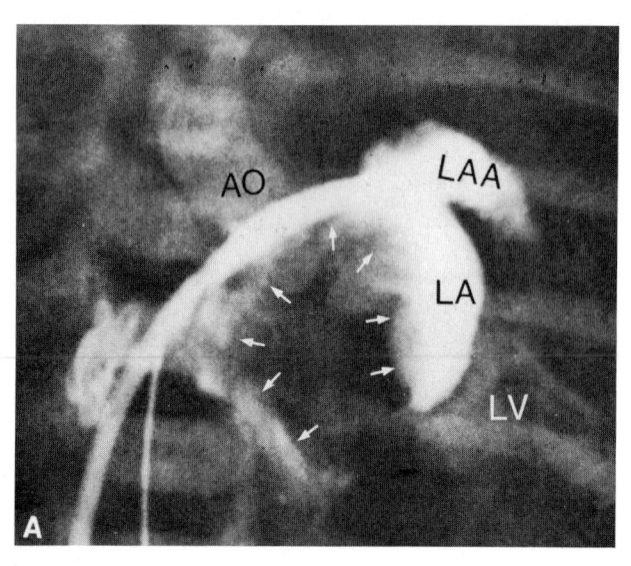

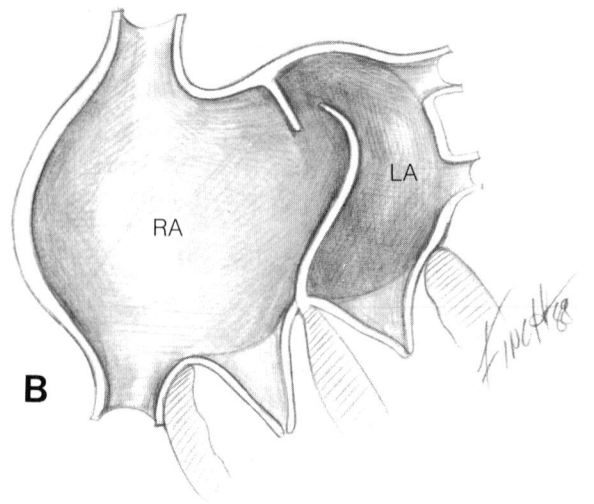

FIG 46–24.
Total anomalous pulmonary venous connection with stenotic foramen ovale **(A)**. Left atriogram. Anteroposterior projection. Marked herniation of foramen ovale *(arrows)*, causing huge filling defect in left atrium *(LA)* simulating left atrial myxoma. *AO* = aorta; *LAA* = left atrium appendage; *LV* = left ventricle; *RA* = right atrium. **B,** explanatory diagram.

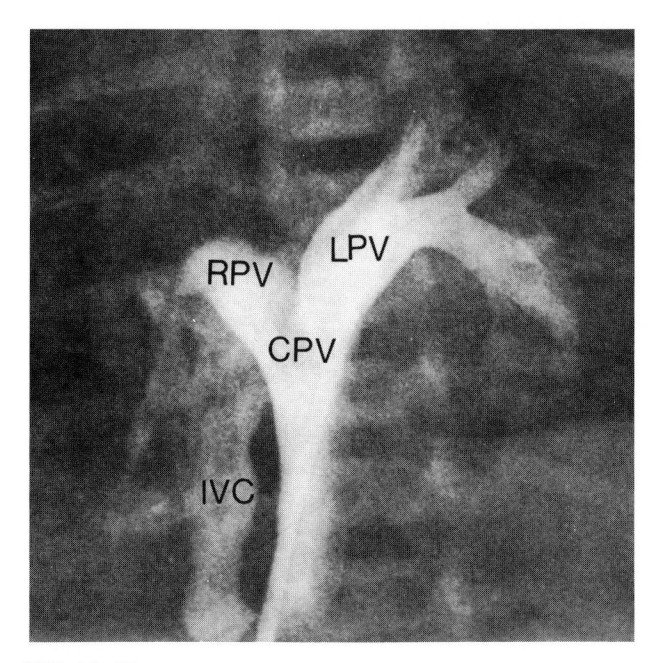

FIG 46-25.
Total anomalous pulmonary venous connection below diaphragm. Anteroposterior projection. Connection to ductus venosus. Catheter is passed from umbilical vein through ductus venosus into common pulmonary vein *(CPV)*. Junction of right pulmonary vein *(RPV)* and left pulmonary vein *(LPV)* is well demonstrated. Opacification of inferior vena cava *(IVC)*.

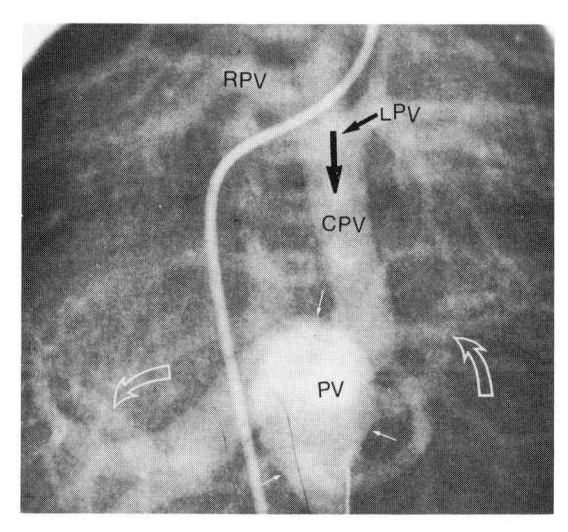

most exclusively with splenic anomalies (Fig 46-27) (see Chapter 58).

OPERATIVE CONSIDERATIONS

The survival of neonates and infants is improved by prompt recognition of the condition and referral of the patient for definitive diagnosis and operation. Recognition may be difficult in neonates with obstructed pulmonary venous connection, because they may be misdiagnosed as pulmonary parenchymal disease. Once the infant is referred, appropriate diagnostic tests should be immediately instituted and the infant treated vigorously. In patients with pulmonary venous obstruction, treatment includes correction of acidosis and reduction of oxygen requirements by placing the infant on a mechanical ventilator. Those without obstruction may require digitalis and diuretics.

Operation is usually performed when the diagnosis is made. Under conditions of cardiopulmonary bypass, the anterior wall of the confluence of pulmonary veins is opened and sutured to the posterior wall of the left atrium, the connecting vein ligated, and the foramen ovale closed (Fig 46-28). When the connection occurs to the coronary sinus, the anterior wall of the coronary sinus is opened

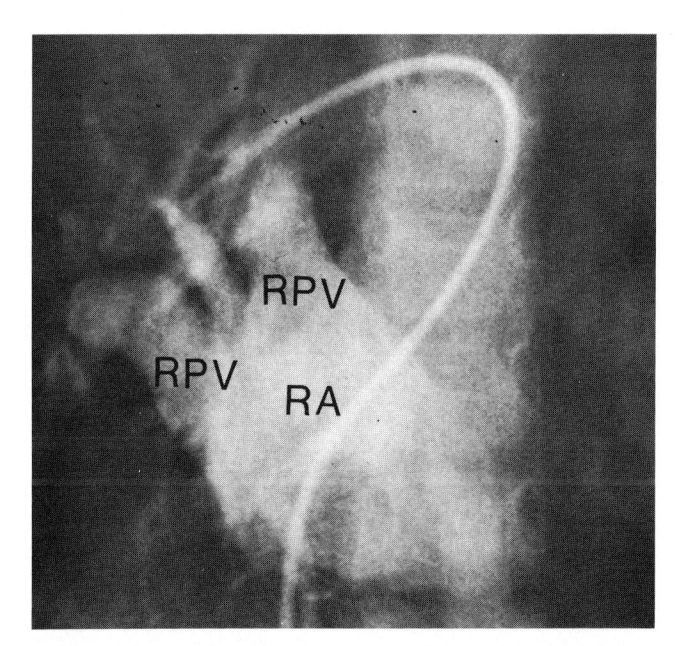

FIG 46-26.
Total anomalous pulmonary venous connection below diaphragm. Pulmonary arteriogram. Late phase. Anteroposterior projection. Right pulmonary vein *(RPV)* and left pulmonary vein *(LPV)* join together and form large common pulmonary vein *(CPV)* *(small arrows)*. Common pulmonary vein connects to venous aneurysm *(white arrows)*, which is part of portal vein *(PV)*. Right and left portal veins are opacified *(curved arrows)*.

FIG 46-27.
Total anomalous pulmonary venous connection to right atrium *(RA)*. Polysplenia syndrome. Right pulmonary arteriogram. Late phase. Anteroposterior projection. Right pulmonary veins *(RPV)* connect directly to right atrium. Injection of left pulmonary artery showed identical anomalous connection of left pulmonary veins to right atrium, indicating total venous drainage to right atrium.

SURGICAL CORRECTION OF TOTAL ANOMALOUS PULMONARY VENOUS CONNECTION TO THE LEFT SUPERIOR VENA CAVA

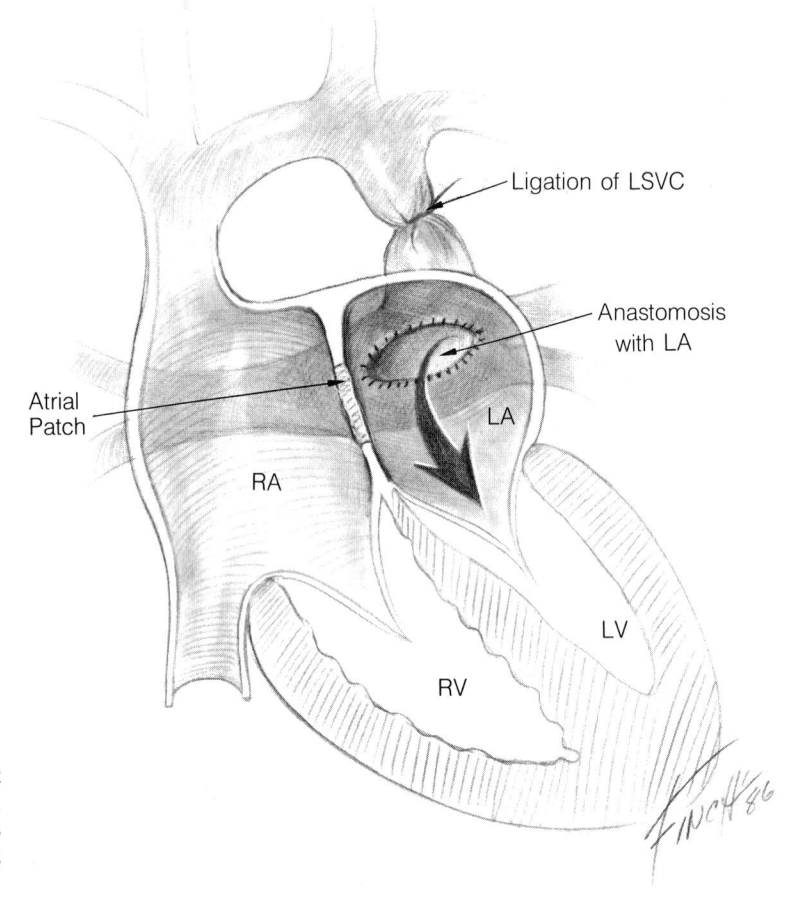

FIG 46–28.
Total anomalous pulmonary venous connection to left superior vena cava *(LSVC)*. Operative correction. *LSVC* is ligated. Confluence of pulmonary veins opened into left atrium *(LA)*. *LV* = left ventricle; *RA* = right atrium; *RV* = right ventricle.

SURGICAL CORRECTION OF TOTAL ANOMALOUS PULMONARY VENOUS CONNECTION TO THE CORONARY SINUS

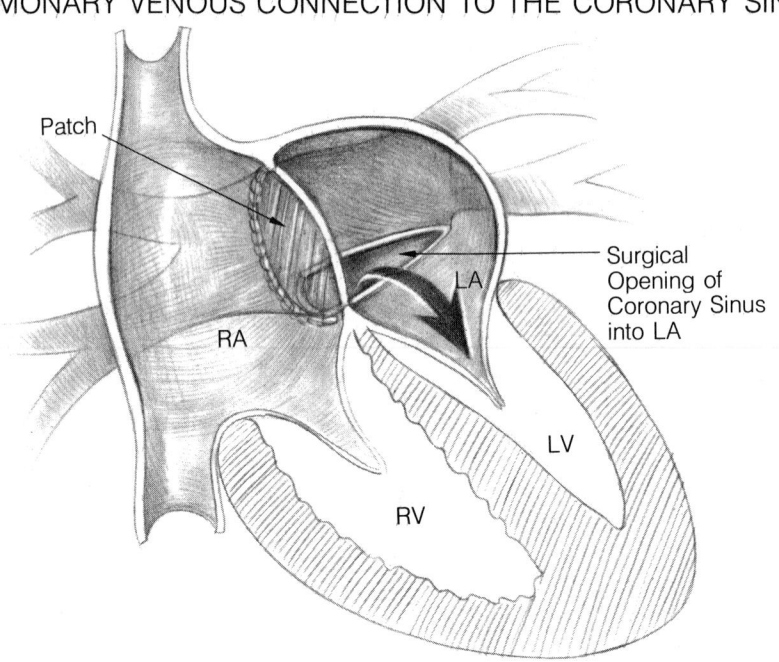

FIG 46–29.
Total anomalous pulmonary venous connection to coronary sinus. Operative correction. Atrial septal defect and mouth of coronary sinus are closed by patch. Anterior wall of coronary sinus is opened into left atrium *(LA)*. *LV* = left ventricle; *RA* = right atrium; *RV* = right ventricle.

SURGICAL REPAIR OF TOTAL DRAINAGE INTO AZYGOS VEIN

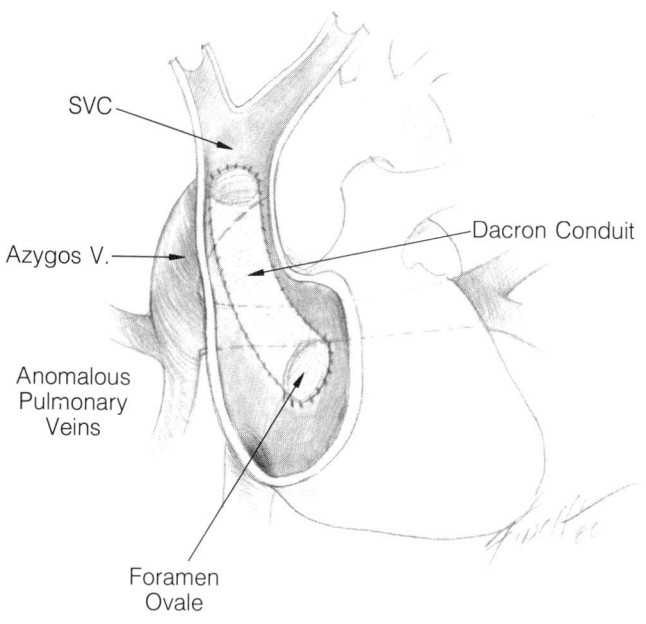

FIG 46–30.
Total anomalous pulmonary venous connection to azygos vein. Operative correction. Baffle is constructed in posterior aspect of superior vena cava *(SVC)* and directed to foramen ovale.

into the left atrium (Fig 46–29). This is possible because the coronary sinus lies immediately behind the left atrium. Then the atrial septal defect and orifice of the coronary sinus are patched closed. One operative approach to total anomalous pulmonary venous connection to the azygos vein is placement of a baffle over the orifice of the azygos vein and suturing this along the posterior atrial wall to the atrial septal defect (Fig 46–30). In total anomalous connection to the right atrium, a patch is sewn posteriorly into the right atrium. The posterior atrial septum is partially excised and the patch sewn to the septum (Fig 46–31). Operative correction of total venous connection below the diaphragm (Fig 46–32) carries the highest risk.

The operative mortality is greatest for those with infradiaphragmatic connection. It is higher in patients with connection to the superior vena cava than in those with connection either to coronary sinus or directly to the right atrium.[14] There has been concern whether the size of the left atrium influences operative outcome. Left atrial size is adequate,[15] particularly when the confluence of pulmonary veins is sutured to its posterior wall of the left atrium, thereby increasing the capacity of the left atrium. The long-term survivals after operation has been good.

POSTOPERATIVE RADIOGRAPHIC FEATURES

After the successful correction of total anomalous pulmonary venous connection there is a rapid and dramatic

SURGICAL CORRECTION OF TOTAL ANOMALOUS PULMONARY VENOUS CONNECTION TO RIGHT ATRIUM

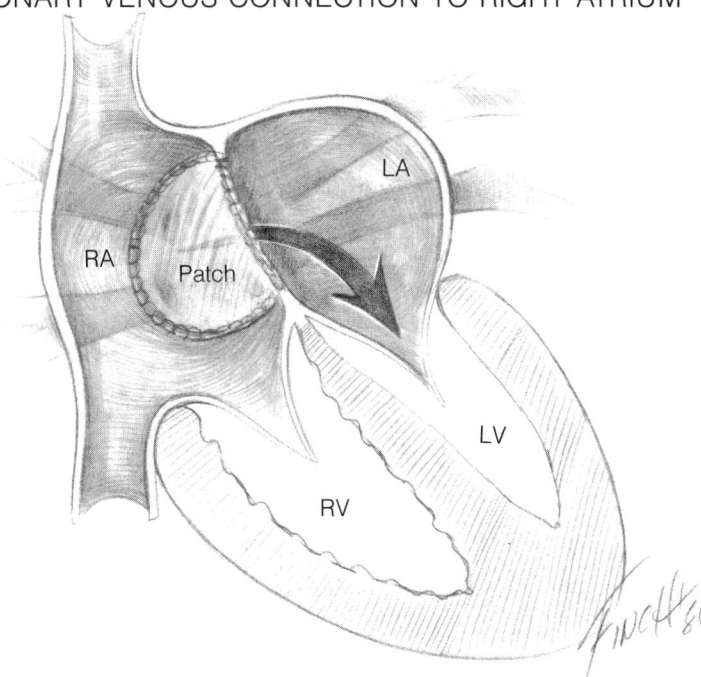

FIG 46–31.
Total anomalous pulmonary venous connection to right atrium *(RA)*. Operative correction. Large posterior atrial communication is created by partial excision of atrial septum. Patch is sewn to edges of defect and posterior right atrial wall to guide pulmonary venous blood through defect into left atrium *(LA)*. *RV* = right ventricle; *LV* = left ventricle.

SURGICAL CORRECTION OF TOTAL ANOMALOUS PULMONARY VENOUS CONNECTION OF THE INFRADIAPHRAGMATIC TYPE

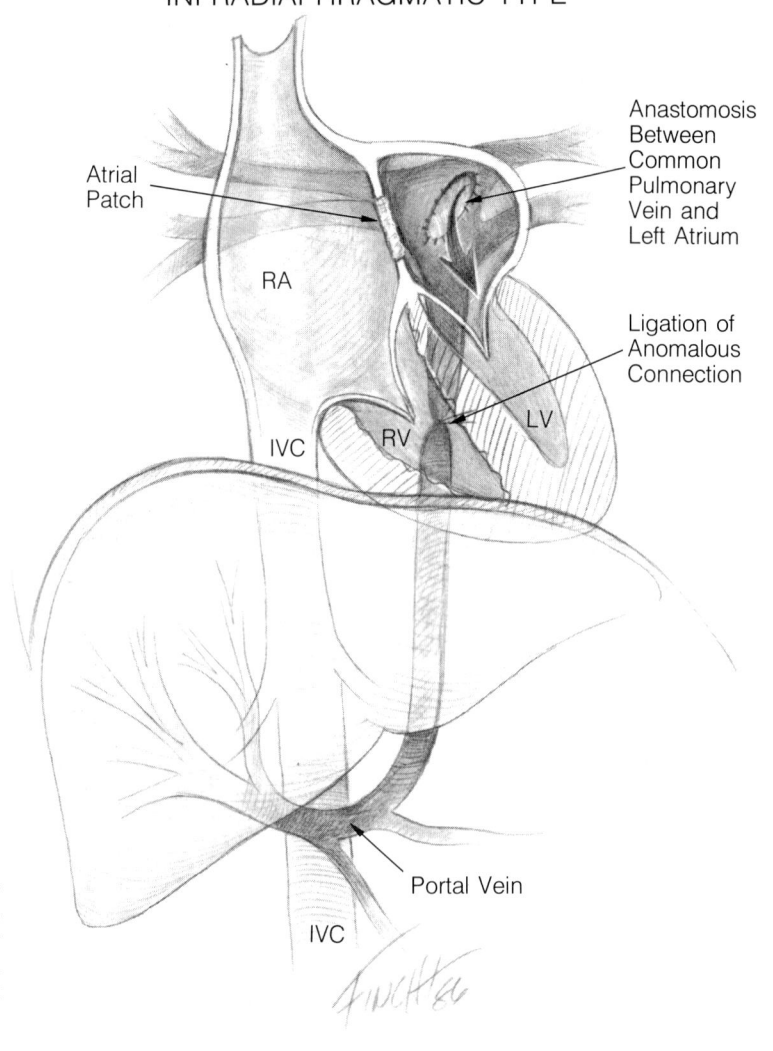

FIG 46–32.
Total anomalous pulmonary venous connection. Infradiaphragmatic type. Operative correction. Anomalous connecting channel ligated. Confluence of pulmonary veins is opened into left atrium. Atrial communication is closed by patch. *IVC* = inferior vena cava; *LV* = left ventricle; *RA* = right atrium. *RV* = right ventricle.

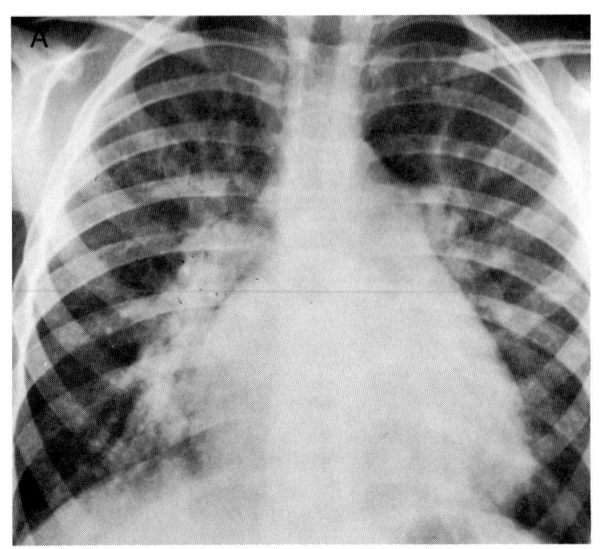

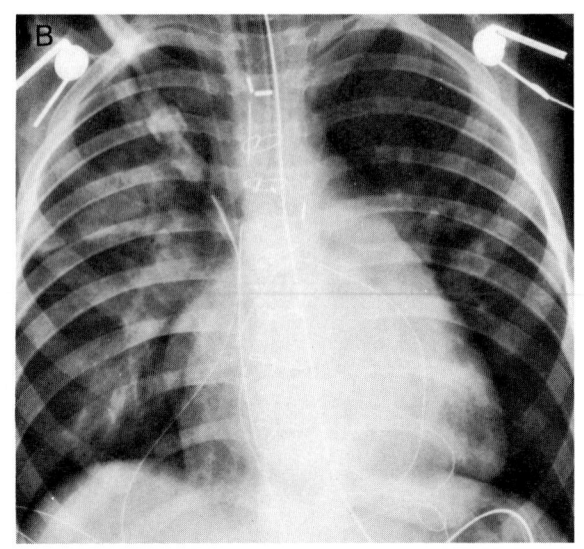

FIG 46–33.
Total anomalous connection to coronary sinus. Thoracic roentgenogram. Posteroanterior projection. **A,** preoperative view. Marked cardiomegaly and increased pulmonary flow. **B,** view several days postoperatively. Marked diminution in cardiac size and pulmonary blood flow.

decrease in pulmonary blood flow and cardiac size similar to that after correction of atrial septal defect. The enlarged heart and increased pulmonary vasculature caused by anomalous connection assume a normal appearance after operation (Fig 46–33).

REFERENCES

1. Edwards JE, Helmholz HF Jr: A classification of total anomalous pulmonary venous connection based on developmental considerations, *Mayo Clin Proc* 31:151, 1956.
2. Delisle G, Ando M, Calder AL, et al: Total anomalous pulmonary venous connection: report of 93 autopsied cases with emphasis on diagnostic and surgical considerations, *Am Heart J* 91:99, 1976.
3. Nakib A, Moller JH, Kanjuh VI, et al: Anomalies of the pulmonary veins, *Am J Cardiol* 20:77, 1967.
4. Kauffman SL, Ores CN, Andersen DH: Two cases of total anomalous pulmonary venous return of the supracardiac type with stenosis simulating infradiaphragmatic drainage, *Circulation* 25:376, 1962.
5. Carey LS, Edwards JE: Severe pulmonary venous obstruction in total anomalous pulmonary venous connection to the left innominate vein: report of case, *Am J Roentgenol Radium Ther Nucl Med* 90:593, 1963.
6. Duff DF, Nihill MR, McNamara DG: Infradiaphragmatic total anomalous pulmonary venous return: review of clinical and pathological findings and results of operation in 28 cases, *Br Heart J* 39:619, 1977.
7. Newfeld EA, Wilson A, Paul MH, et al: Pulmonary vascular disease in total anomalous pulmonary venous drainage, *Circulation* 61:103, 1980.
8. Tajik AJ, Gau GT, Schattenberg TT: Echocardiogram in total anomalous pulmonary venous drainage: report of case, *Mayo Clin Proc* 47:247, 1972.
9. Orsmond GS, Ruttenberg HD, Bessinger JB, et al: Echocardiographic features of total anomalous pulmonary venous connection to the coronary sinus, *Am J Cardiol* 41:597, 1978.
10. Aziz K, Paul MH, Bharati S, et al: Echocardiographic features of total anomalous pulmonary venous drainage into the coronary sinus, *Am J Cardiol* 42:108, 1978.
11. Sahn DJ, Allen HD, Lange LW, et al: Cross-sectional echocardiographic diagnosis of the sites of total anomalous pulmonary venous drainage, *Circulation* 60:1317, 1979.
12. Paquet M, Gutgesell H: Echocardiographic features of total anomalous pulmonary venous connection, *Circulation* 51:599, 1975.
13. Smallhorn JF, Sutherland GR, Tommasini G, et al: Assessment of total anomalous pulmonary venous connection by two-dimensional echocardiography, *Br Heart J* 46:613, 1981.
14. Turley K, Tucker WY, Ullyot DJ, et al: Total anomalous pulmonary venous connection in infancy: influence of age and type of lesion, *Am J Cardiol* 45:92, 1980.
15. Mathew R, Thilenius OG, Replogle RL, et al: Cardiac function in total anomalous pulmonary venous return before and after surgery, *Circulation* 55:361, 1977.

CHAPTER 47

Single Atrium (Common Atrium)

Single atrium without a coexistent defect in the ventricular septum is rare, and there are few clinical reports.[1,2] Most instances probably represent a form of endocardial cushion defect. As will be indicated, single atrium is a frequent component of the cardiac malformations associated with the asplenia and the polysplenia syndromes.

PATHOLOGIC ANATOMY

The atrial chamber is a single cavity usually with a minimal atrial septal remnant, although one or two strands of muscular tissue composed of myocardium may cross the upper portion in the anticipated plane of the septum. Complete absence of the septum is rare. The anterior mitral leaflet of the mitral valve is usually cleft and the superior aspect of the ventricular septum deficient as in endocardial cushion defect. There is, however, no ventricular communication.

A persistent left superior vena cava is present in one half of the patients, connecting either to the coronary sinus or directly to the superior and posterior aspect of the left side of the common atrium. In the latter instance, the coronary sinus is absent. Because in some instances single atrium is associated with the polysplenia syndrome, the right pulmonary veins may be anomalously connected and directly enter the posterior aspect of the right side of the common atrium. Also, infrahepatic interruption of the inferior vena cava with azygos continuation is common.

Single atrium is also a common component of the heart in asplenia syndrome, where it usually coexists with single ventricle (see Chapter 58).

HEMODYNAMICS

The basic hemodynamic features of single atrium resemble those of atrial septal defect. Because of the atrial communication, a shunt can occur, the direction and magnitude of which depend on the the relative ventricular compliances. Usually the shunt is left to right, because pulmonary vascular resistance is low. Pulmonary vascular disease may develop but is usually not severe. As it progresses, the shunt becomes less left to right and may eventually become right to left.

Systemic arterial desaturation may exist in these patients even without pulmonary vascular disease because of a persistent left superior vena cava connecting directly to the left side of the common atrium.

Mitral regurgitation may occur through the cleft in the anterior leaflet of the mitral valve and increase left ventricular volume.

CLINICAL FEATURES

A cardiac anomaly is usually suspected in early childhood because of slow growth and frequent respiratory tract infections. Mild cyanosis may be evident, which is accentuated on exercise. There is often a precordial bulge, and the cardiac apex may be located lateral to the midclavicular line. The auscultatory findings resemble those of an atrial septal defect. A soft pulmonary systolic ejection murmur, a middiastolic murmur in the tricuspid area, and a wide fixed splitting of the second heart sound are heard. An apical pansystolic murmur may be present, reflecting coexistent mitral regurgitation.

There may be findings of abnormal situs with dextrocardia, or abnormal placement of the liver in patients with coexistent polysplenia, or other positional abnormalities. Ellis–van Creveld syndrome has a high incidence of single atrium.

ELECTROCARDIOGRAPHIC FEATURES

The electrocardiograms typically resemble those of an endocardial cushion defect.[1,2] There is left-axis deviation, which may range as far as −120 degrees. A pattern of incomplete right bundle branch block with an rSR' pattern in lead V_1 is present.

The P-wave axis may be directed toward the left, which is not necessarily associated with a short P-R interval.

ECHOCARDIOGRAPHIC FEATURES

An atrial septum cannot be demonstrated in an apical or subcostal projection. As in other instances of endocardial cushion defect, the atrioventricular valves are located in the same plane, in contrast to normal, wherein the mitral valve is more cephalad than the tricuspid valve. Both the pulmonary and major systemic veins should be identified to determine if bilateral superior vena cava are present, their site of connection, and the site of entry of each pulmonary vein into the single atrium.

RADIOGRAPHIC FEATURES

The radiographic findings are indistinguishable from atrial septal defect (see Chapter 19).

1. The cardiac silhouette is enlarged. REASON: The atrial shunt is invariably large unless elevated pulmonary vascular resistance is present. Furthermore, cardiomegaly may be accentuated by the commonly associated mitral and occasionally tricuspid valve incompetence, secondary to the endocardial cushion defect.

2. The pulmonary arterial vasculature is greatly increased. Radiographic signs of pulmonary hypertension may be present, as indicated by peripheral vascular "pruning" (see Chapter 5).

3. The superior vena cava and ascending aorta are inconspicuous. REASON: The large left-to-right shunt results in dilation of the right ventricle and consequent clockwise rotation of the heart, as found in instances of atrial septal defect (see Chapter 19).

4. Radiographic evidence of left atrial enlargement is absent. REASON: The pressure in the common atrium tends to be low.

5. The pulmonary arterial segment is markedly enlarged. REASON: Large left-to-right shunt.

CARDIAC CATHETERIZATION

The catheter course may be abnormal. From an inguinal approach the catheter may pass from the inferior vena cava through an azygos continuation into the superior vena cava before reaching the atrial chamber. From the left arm the catheter may be passed through a persistent left superior vena cava either directly into the left side of the single atrium or through the coronary sinus.

Common atrium can also be suspected during cardiac catheterization. Characteristically the catheter forms a large loop across the cardiac silhouette from border to border, hugging the walls of the common atrium. This catheter course is diagnostic only if the catheter tip can be freely advanced along the roof of the common atrium to the right cardiac border (Fig 47–1). A passage of the catheter from the low right atrium to the low left atrium may also occur through a Raghib-type atrial septal defect, an ostium primum defect, into the coronary sinus, and through a coronary sinus fenestration into the left atrium. Characteristically the catheter course into the left ventricle from the atrium is low, as in an endocardial cushion defect.

Oxygen data show an increase in saturation from the vena cava into the atrium. A slight further increase may be found in the right ventricle because of streaming of blood or an associated ventricular shunt. Blood from the left ventricle or aorta may be slightly desaturated because of the site of entry of the left superior vena cava into the single atrium or an atrial level right-to-left shunt. Frequently oxygen saturation in the pulmonary artery and aorta are identical, indicating complete mixing.

Atrial pressures are low. If a pressure difference exists between the left atrium and the right atrium, a common atrium is excluded. Right ventricular and pulmonary artery systolic pressures may be normal but are frequently elevated to some degree. Elevation results from increased

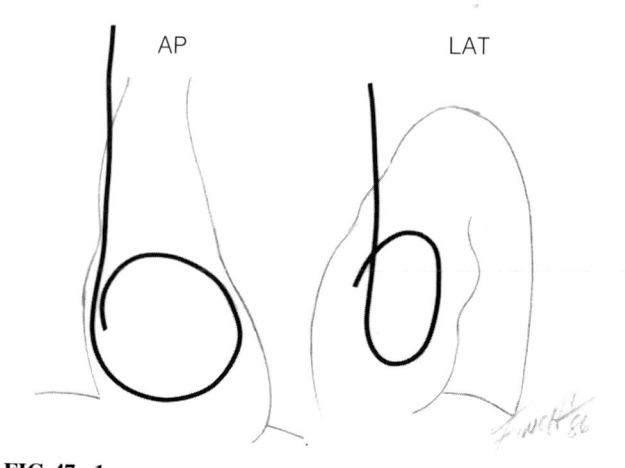

FIG 47–1.
Characteristic catheter course in common atrium. Anteroposterior *(AP)* and lateral *(LAT)* projections. Catherer hugs free wall of common atrium. This catheter position is diagnostic only if a complete circle can be formed with catheter.

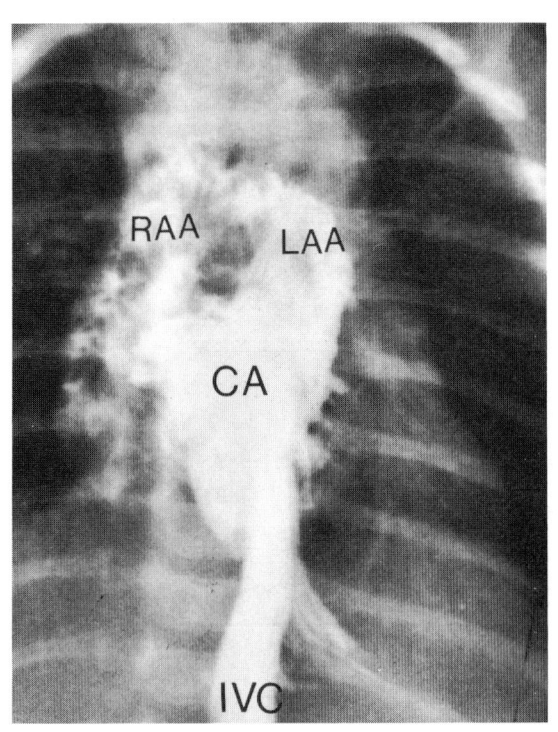

FIG 47–2.
Single atrium. Asplenia syndrome and abdominal heterotaxia. Venous angiogram. Inferior vena cava *(IVC)* is on the left. Reflux into hepatic veins. Common atrium *(CA)* is outlined. Both atrial appendages are opacified simultaneously. *RAA* = right atrial appendage; *LAA* = left atrial appendage. Note that left atrial appendage has a triangular shape and is broad based, as an anatomic right atrial appendage.

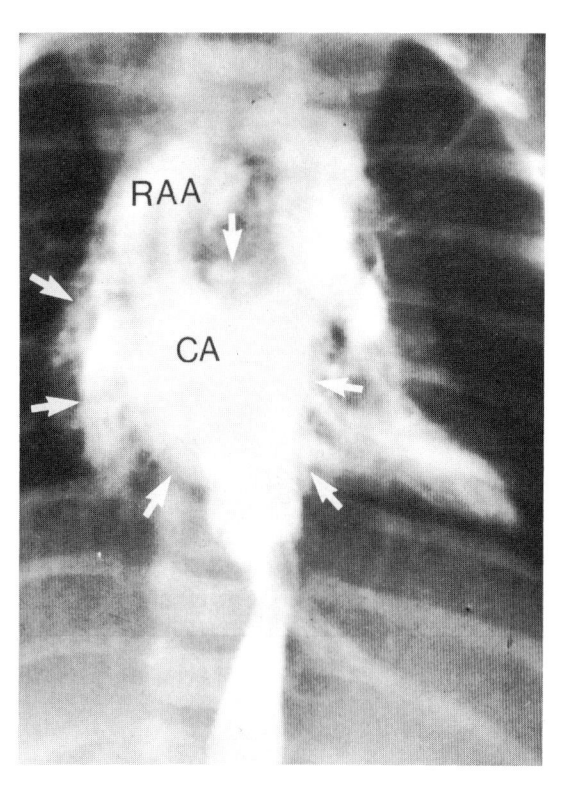

FIG 47–3.
Single atrium. Asplenia syndrome and abdominal heterotaxia. Venous angiogram. Contrast medium outlines single large atrial chamber *(arrows)*. Communication occupies location of both atria together. *CA* = common atrium; *RAA* = right atrial appendage.

pulmonary blood flow and in some patients from pulmonary vascular disease.

ANGIOGRAPHIC FEATURES

Angiography plays an important role for the preoperative assessment. Most patients have either asplenic or polysplenic syndrome. The entry site of each pulmonary vein into common atrium and the location of both vena cavae must be determined before operative partitioning of the atria can be considered. Particularly in common atrium and polysplenia, the pulmonary veins may connect to the right half of the common atrium (partial or total anomalous pulmonary venous connection). This anatomic variation makes operative repair more difficult. The anatomy may be even more complex in asplenic syndrome (see Chapter 58).

The common atrium can be demonstrated by a very rapid injection of a large amount of contrast medium into either the main pulmonary artery or preferably directly into the common atrium.[2] With injection into the atrium, the pulmonary veins are usually not demonstrated. Selective injection into each pulmonary artery may be required to demonstrate the connection of the pulmonary veins.

1. Both atrial appendages may be opacified (Fig 47–2).
2. Opacification of a large atrial chamber occurs. This chamber occupies the location normally occupied by both the right and the left atria (Fig 47–3).
3. In a left anterior oblique angled projection, an atrial septum cannot be demonstrated.
4. The inferior margin of the common atrium forms a smooth continuous curve from one lateral margin of the heart toward the other.

OPERATIVE CONSIDERATIONS

Operation involves placement of a large patch in the atrium, dividing it into two relatively equal-sized chambers (Fig 47–4). If mitral incompetence coexists, a mitral valvuloplasty is performed concomitantly. Difficulties can be encountered if the left superior vena cava connects directly to the left side of the single atrium. Usually the left

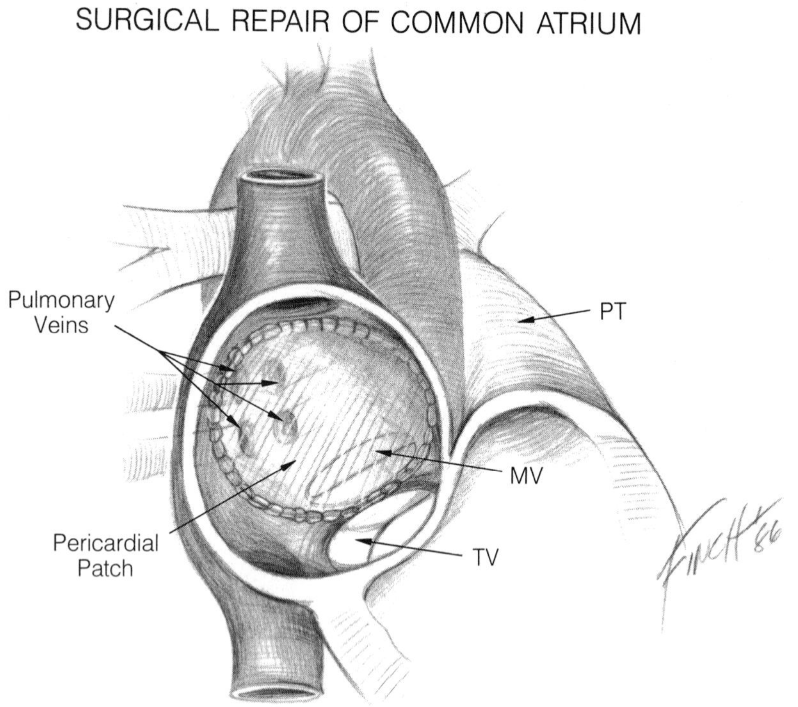

SURGICAL REPAIR OF COMMON ATRIUM

FIG 47–4.
Uncomplicated common atrium. Operative correction. Large patch is sewn into common chamber so atrioventricular valves are separated and pulmonary veins empty into left half of divided common atrium. PT = pulmonary trunk; MV = mitral valve; TV = tricuspid valve.

superior vena cava cannot be ligated because there are insufficient venous channels between the two vena caval systems to decompress the left caval system if it is ligated. It may be possible to tunnel it across into the right atrium, but if it remains connected to the left atrium, there is a potential for mild cyanosis and systemic embolization. Another technical difficulty for correction is entry of the hepatic veins into the left side of the common atrium (see Fig 47–2).

REFERENCES

1. Munoz-Armas S, Diaz Gorrin JR, Anselmi G, et al: Single atrium: embryologic, anatomic, electrocardiographic and other diagnostic features, *Am J Cardiol* 21:639, 1968.
2. Hung JS, Ritter DG, Feldt RH, et al: Electrocardiographic and angiographic features of common atrium, *Chest* 63:970, 1973.

PART SIX

Cyanosis and Normal Pulmonary Blood Flow

Cyanosis and normal pulmonary blood flow is a very rare combination. Pulmonary arteriovenous fistulas, direct connection of a major systemic vein to the left atrium, and connection of right pulmonary artery to the left atrium are the related conditions. Because the abnormal connection occurs at a low pressure, usually no murmur is present, except in exceptional cases of a large isolated pulmonary arteriovenous fistula. The diagnosis is usually discovered during the investigation of cyanosis without evident cardiac cause. Electrocardiography and thoracic roentgenograms are often normal, whereas echocardiography may reveal an abnormal systemic venous connection.

CHAPTER 48

Pulmonary Arteriovenous Fistula

Pulmonary arteriovenous fistulas are an uncommon cause of cyanosis. They may be either congenital or acquired. On a thoracic roentgenogram they may be large, single, or multiple nodules or microscopic, diffuse, and inapparent on a roentgenogram. The latter situation, namely, the presence of cyanosis with a normal thoracic radiograph and absence of abnormal clinical findings, is confusing to the cardiologist.

PATHOLOGIC ANATOMY

The basic problem is a direct connection between a branch of the pulmonary artery and the pulmonary venous system without the intervening pulmonary capillary system. The size, number, and distribution of these connections are extremely variable. They may be single or multiple, unilateral or bilateral. Small lesions tend to be widespread throughout both lungs; large fistulas are fewer in number, located subpleurally, and more common in the lower lobes. The afferent artery and efferent veins are dilated and tortuous, with the artery having a thinner wall and the vein a thicker wall than normal. The fistula may have a saccular appearance with a tendency for thrombosis or rupture, which could cause hemosiderosis (Fig 48–1).

Occasionally systemic arterial branches may also communicate with the fistula and may arise from the internal mammary, intercostal, or phrenic arteries.

Pulmonary arteriovenous fistulas occur most frequently (60% of cases) as part of the hereditary hemorrhagic telangiectasia syndrome (Rendu-Osler-Weber syndrome). In this syndrome, the number and size of fistulas increase with age.

Pulmonary arteriovenous fistulas also develop in individuals with chronic hepatic disease by an unknown mechanism. The cyanosis in these patients is accentuated because of direct communications between the portal system and the pulmonary veins. Direct communication of large size between the portal venous system and the pulmonary veins are known to occur on congenital basis. These venous anastomoses have been demonstrated pathologically but not angiographically. In chronic hepatic disease, innumerable diffuse fistulas develop in both lungs. The arteriovenous connections responsible for cyanosis are located at the precapillary level. They are too small to be visualized angiographically but allow the passage of microbubbles detected by ultrasonography (see Fig 48–10).

In patients with portal hypertension, the injection of contrast media into the portal system may demonstrate a portopulmonary communication. Portal hypertension results in direct blood flow from the portal venous system to a pulmonary vein. The existence of valves in these veins probably does not influence the direction of blood flow when the vessels are dilated and tortuous.

HEMODYNAMICS

Because of the fistulous communication between the pulmonary arterial and venous systems bypassing the capillaries, blood in the draining pulmonary vein is desaturated.

Systemic arterial oxygen saturation is reduced in direct proportion to the number and size of the fistulas. The size of the shunt through the fistulas may be as large as 80%. The hypoxemia is compensated by polycythemia, which maintains the oxygen-carrying capacity. Cardiac output is normal, unlike systemic arteriovenous fistulas.

While the blood flow through the pulmonary arteriovenous fistulas is rapid, pulmonary arterial pressure is normal because of great distensibility of the pulmonary vascular bed and small pressure gradient between pulmonary artery and pulmonary vein.

As in any right-to-left shunt, systemic embolism or brain abscess may occur. Bacterial endocarditis may also develop.

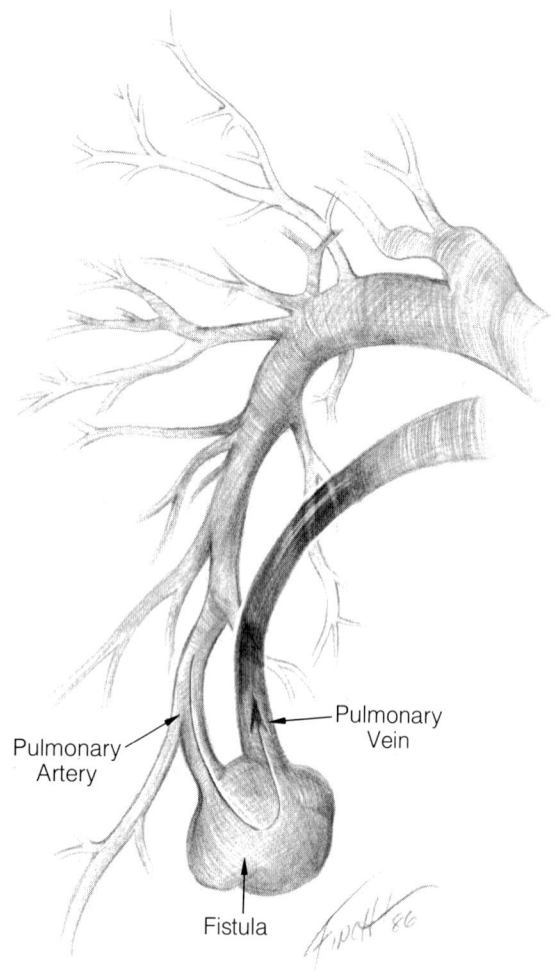

FIG 48-1.
Saccular pulmonary arteriovenous malformation. Afferent artery is enlarged, forming an aneurysm at junction with enlarged draining pulmonary vein. Because capillary bed is bypassed, desaturated blood enters left atrium. Speed of blood flow through fistula is only slightly faster than through normal pulmonary arteries.

CLINICAL FEATURES

The sex incidence is equal. Cyanosis without a cardiac murmur is the hallmark. Cyanosis is usually present during childhood and may be evident at birth. The degree of cyanosis is related to the size and number of arteriovenous fistulas. One third of patients are asymptomatic. The most frequent symptoms are dyspnea and easy fatiguability. Hemoptysis may develop from rupture of a fistula and may be recurrent and fatal. Central nervous symptoms such as diplopia and transient numbness are described in 20% of patients from associated brain abscess, paradoxical embolus, hypoxemia, or thrombosis of small vessels.

There may be a family history of hereditary hemorrhagic telangiectasis, or a personal history of excessive alcohol intake.

On physical examination cyanosis and clubbing are found. There may be telangiectasis on the skin or mucous membranes. In those patients with chronic hepatic disease, there may be cyanosis and spider-telangiectasis. The peripheral arterial pulses are normal. Cardiac size and heart sounds are normal. There may be a faint systolic or continuous murmur over the area of the lung in which the fistulas are located.

Patients with hereditary hemorrhagic telangiectasis may have anemia and perhaps melena or hematemesis from gastrointestinal bleeding.

ELECTROCARDIOGRAPHIC FEATURES

The electrocardiogram is normal in most patients, but rarely there may be a pattern of left ventricular hypertrophy.

RADIOGRAPHIC FEATURES

The most important and reliable radiographic finding is enlarged vascular structures supplying the fistula. These can sometimes be seen on a thoracic roentgenogram but are better visualized by laminagraphy, computed tomography (CT) scanning, or nuclear magnetic resonance imaging. During a Valsalva maneuver, because of increased intrathoracic pressure, the soft vascular lesion becomes smaller, and during a Mueller maneuver with decreased in-

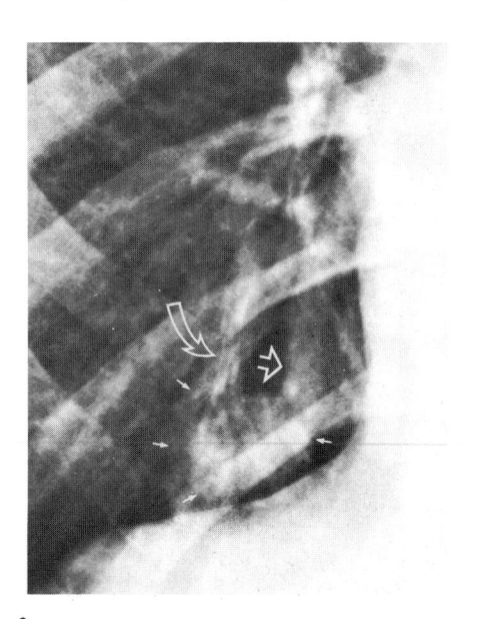

FIG 48-2.
Pulmonary arteriovenous malformation. Right lower lobe. Thoracic roentgenogram. Posteroanterior projection. Magnified view. Large mass (*small arrows*) connected to two vascular structures. One (*curved open arrow*) represents afferent pulmonary artery, and the other (*straight open arrow*) represents draining vein.

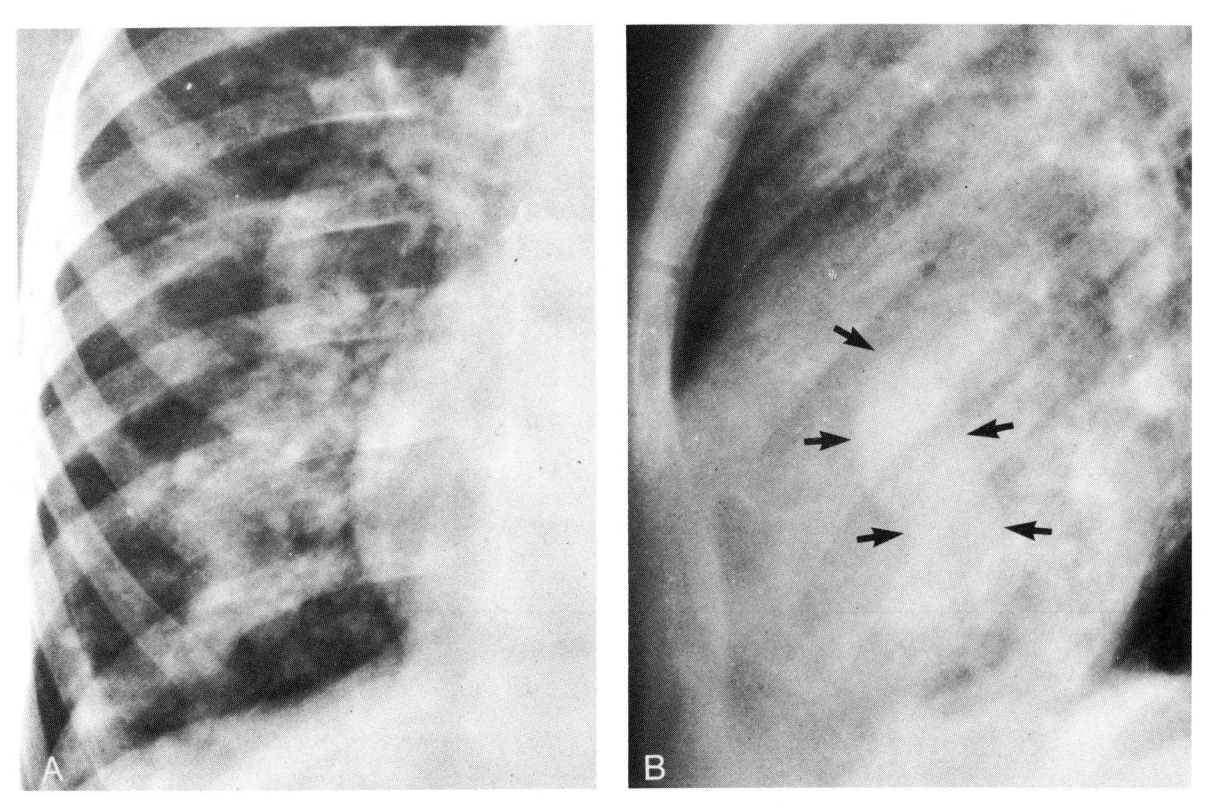

FIG 48–3.
Diffuse arteriovenous malformation in right lower lobe. Thoracic roentgenogram. Magnified views. **A,** posteroanterior projection. Appearance of consolidation. Vascular nature of lesion is not apparent. **B,** lateral projection. Elongated vascular structure *(arrows)* suggests arteriovenous pulmonary malformation rather than tumor.

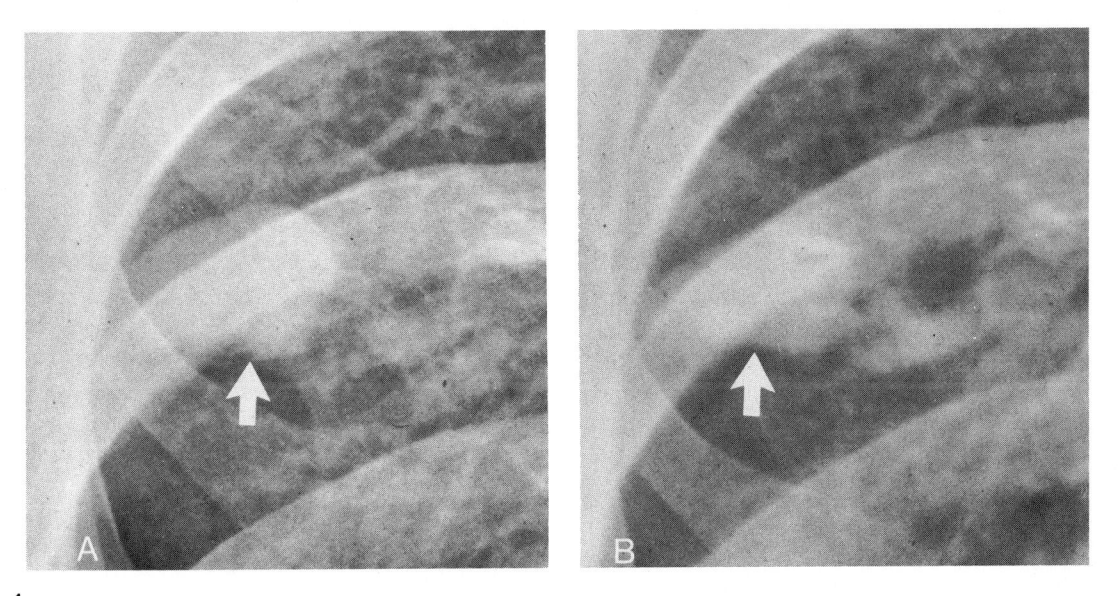

FIG 48–4.
Pulmonary arteriovenous malformation. Thoracic roentgenogram. Posteroanterior projection. Magnified views. **A,** during normal respiration. **B,** during Valsalva maneuver. Marked decrease in size, indicating soft collapsible structure such as vascular malformation.

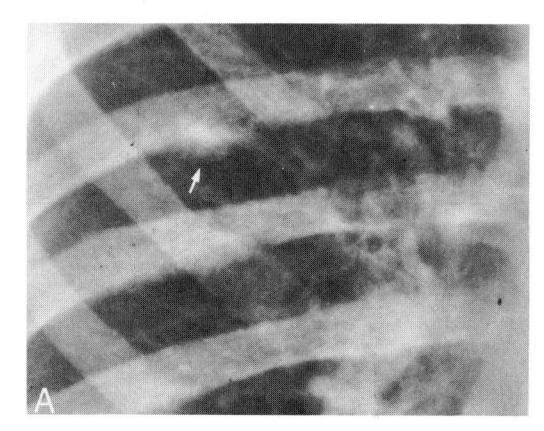

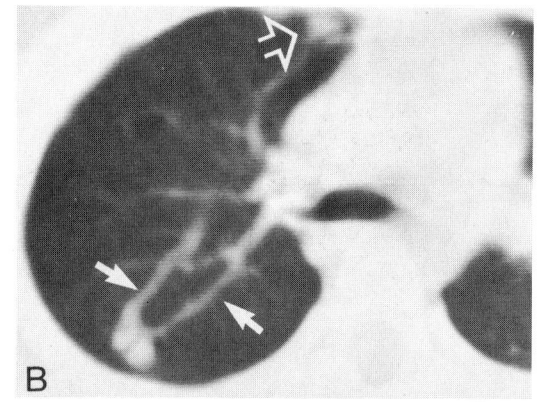

FIG 48–5.
Arteriovenous fistula in right lung. **A,** thoracic roentgenogram. Posteroanterior projection. Right upper lobe. Magnified view. Nodular density *(arrow)*. Vascular nature of lesion not apparent. **B,** contrast-enhanced CT scan. Visualization of supplying artery and draining vein *(arrows)*. Additional lesion, not seen on thoracic roentgenogram is present anteriorly *(open arrow)*.

trathoracic pressure, the lesion becomes larger. Neoplastic lesions that must be considered in the differential diagnosis of a pulmonary mass do not change in size with these maneuvers. Suspected arteriovenous fistulas in the lung were previously fluoroscoped during both a Valsalva and a Mueller maneuver. Experience, however, showed that the change in size may be minimal and that fluoroscopic observations were too subjective to be useful.

1. Typically, an arteriovenous fistula is a round or lobulated mass. The supplying artery and draining vein may be seen on a thoracic roentgenogram (Fig 48–2). The lesions occur more frequently at the base of the lung.

2. Sometimes the vascular nature of the lesion may not be evident on a single projection but is evident on oblique or lateral views (Fig 48–3).

3. Classically the lesion decreases in size during the Valsalva maneuver (Fig 48–4). Rarely a pulmonary arte-

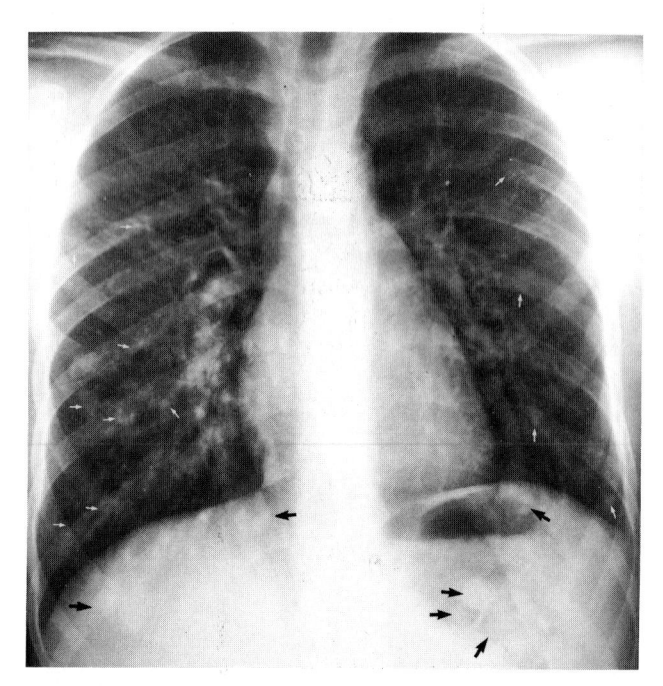

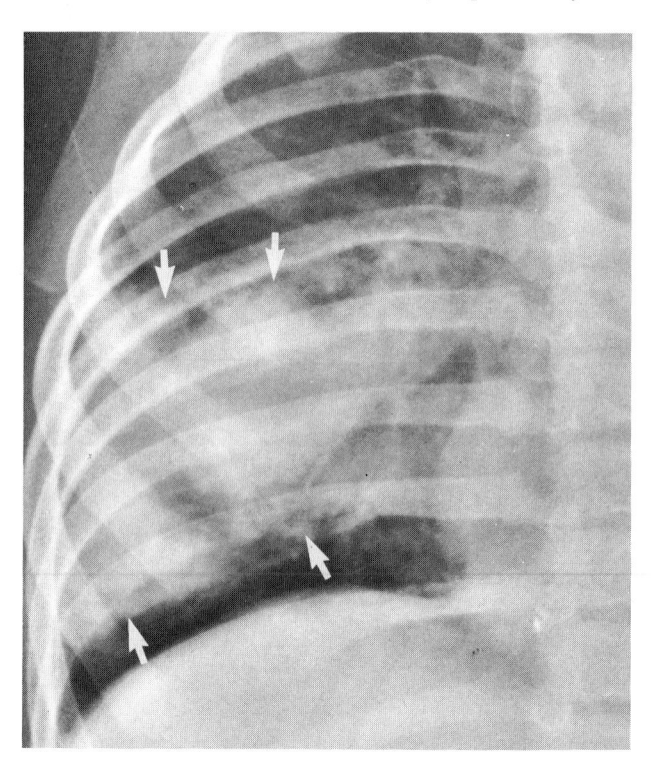

FIG 48–6.
Hereditary hemorrhagic telangiectasis. Thoracic roentgenogram. Posteroanterior projection. Diffuse lesions *(arrows)*. Largest in lower lobes.

FIG 48–7.
Large pulmonary arteriovenous malformation. Thoracic roentgenogram. Posteroanterior projection. Magnified view of right lower lobe. Radiographic appearance is suggestive of mass or pulmonary consolidation *(arrows)*, which proved to be huge arteriovenous malformation.

riovenous malformation manifests as a mass without apparent vascular supply. Under those circumstances, fluoroscopic or cine fluoroscopic examination is helpful.

4. If the afferent artery and efferent vein are not seen, laminography or CT scanning may establish the vascular nature of the lesion (Fig 48–5).

5. In spite of considerable hypoxemia and cyanosis, cardiac size is typically normal. REASON: The small pressure gradient between pulmonary artery and pulmonary vein does not cause a hemodynamic burden on the right side of the heart. The flow through an arteriovenous fistula is therefore only slightly faster than the flow through the normal pulmonary parenchyma. There is no extra volume load on the heart as in a systemic arteriovenous fistula.

6. Commonly, arteriovenous fistulas are multiple and large, being part of hereditary telangiectasia syndrome. In patients with hereditary hemorrhagic telangiectasis, the arteriovenous malformations tend to be diffuse and progress rapidly (Fig 48–6). The lesions tend to be larger at the lung bases. REASON: Probably hydrostatic pressure.

7. Rarely an extensive arteriovenous fistula may involve a large portion of a lung and mimic radiographically a pneumonic process (Fig 48–7).

8. In patients with cyanosis associated with chronic hepatic disease, cardiac size and pulmonary vasculature are normal. REASON: The small diffuse shunts in the lungs are not visible radiographically. Barium swallow may demonstrate varices. Depending on the stage of hepatic disease, there may be evidence for enlargement of the liver on abdominal films or CT scans. With the commonly present portal hypertension, enlargement of the spleen is present on thoracic or abdominal radiographs, CT scanning, or radioisotope studies.

CARDIAC CATHETERIZATION

The catheter course and cardiac pressures are normal. Oximetry data show no evidence of a left-to-right shunt, but the oxygen values on the left side of the heart are

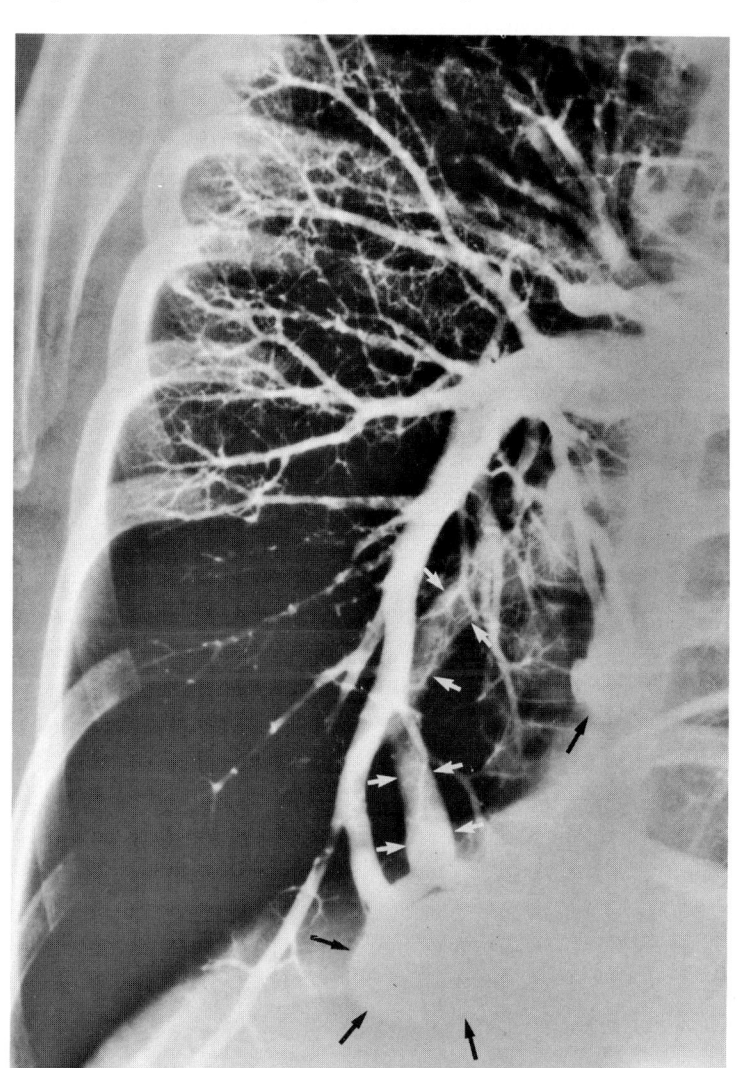

FIG 48–8.
Pulmonary arteriovenous malformations. Right pulmonary arteriogram. Anteroposterior projection. Two arteriovenous malformations *(black arrows)*. Malformation in right lower lobe. Afferent artery slightly enlarged. Early filling of large efferent vein *(white arrows)*. Beginning venous filling of right upper pulmonary veins. REASON: Decreased resistance. Branches to remaining right lower lobe are contracted. Hypoperfusion of right lung base because of steal phenomenon from arteriovenous malformation.

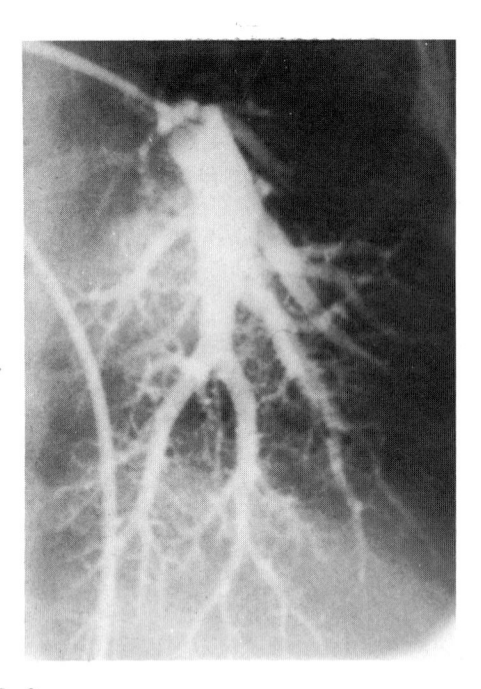

FIG 48-9.
Cyanosis in chronic hepatic disease. Balloon occlusion pulmonary arteriogram. Left lower lobe. Anteroposterior projection. Normal-sized pulmonary artery. Tiny arteriovenous communications located at precapillary level are not definitely demonstrable by angiography. However, a luzarri abundance of small vessels is consistent with the diagnosis.

ANGIOGRAPHIC FEATURES

If a patient has one or more nodular pulmonary densities and is cyanotic, the diagnosis is evident and angiography is indicated. Laminography, CT scanning, or nuclear magnetic resonance are usually not needed because angiography has the advantage of establishing a firm diagnosis, and treatment can be provided at the same time. Noninvasive tests are useful in noncyanotic patients with isolated nodules.

Contrast medium can be injected into the main pulmonary artery to demonstrate both lungs simultaneously. Preferably each pulmonary artery should be injected separately to demonstrate each vascular bed more clearly. The most brilliant results are obtained by balloon occlusion angiography. Biplane projections are valuable particularly if subsequent embolization of the fistulae is contemplated. Contrast medium is injected as with pulmonary angiography for other reasons. REASON: The speed of blood flow through the arteriovenous fistula is not markedly increased over the normal pulmonary blood flow. This is very different from systemic arteriovenous fistulas in which blood flow is very rapid requiring very rapid contrast injections.

1. The arteriovenous communication opacifies densely (Fig 48-8).
2. The afferent artery and efferent vein are clearly demonstrated. The artery is smaller than the vein.
3. In a lower lobe, the artery projects laterally to the vein (see Fig 48-8). In an upper lobe the vein projects laterally to the artery. The draining vein is slightly larger than the artery.
4. Opacification of the arteriovenous malformation occurs before the normal pulmonary venous system. REASON: The resistance in the malformation is less than through the pulmonary parenchyma.
5. The arteries in the surrounding normal lung show

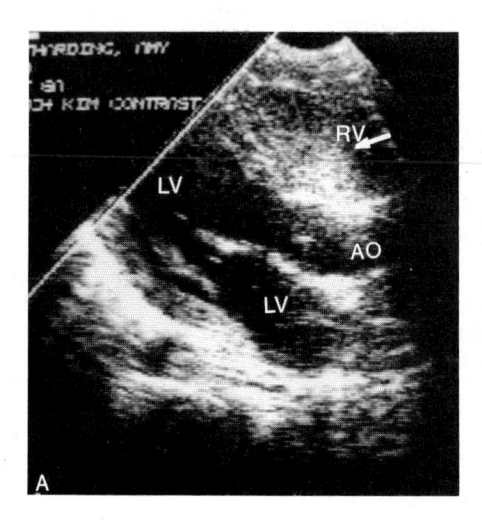

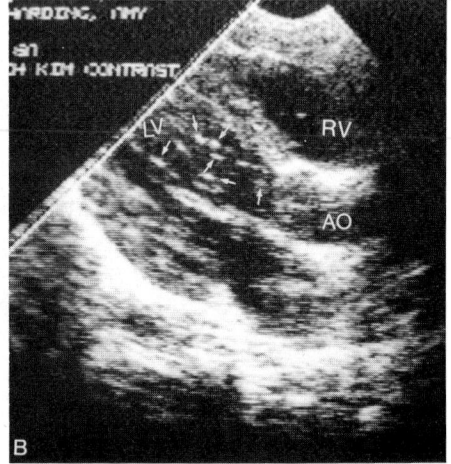

lower than normal because of the fistulas that allow blood to bypass the alveoli.

Oxygen saturations obtained in the left side of the heart are reduced in proportion to the size and number of arteriovenous fistulas.

The cardiac output is normal. Indicator dilution curves often do not show early appearance because the transit times through the fistula and normal pulmonary vascular bed are nearly the same.

FIG 48-10.
Cyanosis in chronic hepatic disease. Echocardiogram. Long-axial view. Patient with cyanosis, chronic hepatic disease, and a normal selective pulmonary arteriogram. Same patient as in Figure 48-8. **A,** saline solution is injected into peripheral vein. Cloud of echoes from microbubbles in right ventricle *(RV)* *(arrow).* **B,** late phase. Microbubbles have cleared from right ventricle. Echoes in left ventricle *(LV)* *(white arrows)* indicate bubbles have passed through capillary beds. Pulmonary arteriovenous shunting is proved. *AO* = aorta.

delayed opacification (vascular steal phenomenon) (see Fig 48–8).
6. Occasionally the speed of blood flow is only minimally increased through the arteriovenous malformation, but some early opacification of the draining vein invariably occurs.
7. The remainder of the pulmonary arterial tree is not enlarged.
8. In patients with chronic hepatic disease:
   a. Pulmonary arteries are not enlarged (Fig 48–9).
   b. Transit of contrast medium through both lungs is normal. Early opacification of pulmonary veins does not occur. REASON: The fistulous connections occur at a precapillary level and are so small that the speed of blood flow through the shunts is not significantly different from the speed of blood flow through normal capillaries. Furthermore, the shunts are so diffuse in both lungs that no comparison is available between normal transit time through the capillaries and abnormal transit time through the precapillary shunts.
   c. The capillary pattern is suspicious even with balloon occlusion angiography. REASON: The size of the communications is beyond the resolving power of standard radiography (see Fig 48–9).
   d. The capillary shunts can be detected by an echocardiogram. If a liquid such as saline solution is injected rapidly intravenously, microbubbles are produced by cavitation. These bubbles are strongly ectogenic, serving as a venous contrast medium. Microbubbles normally do not pass through the capillary bed of the lung. In the case of capillary shunting, as in chronic hepatic disease, bubbles are detected in the left side of the heart (Fig 48–10) indicating pulmonary shunting bypassing the alveoli causing cyanosis.

TREATMENT

Previously treatment was either partial or complete lobectomy when the arteriovenous fistulas were confined to a single lobe. Patients with diffuse pulmonary involvement were inoperable.

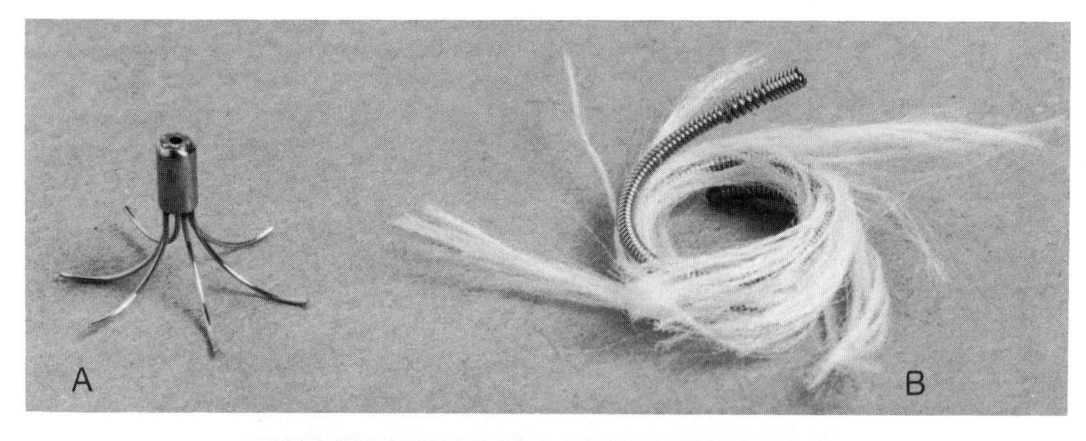

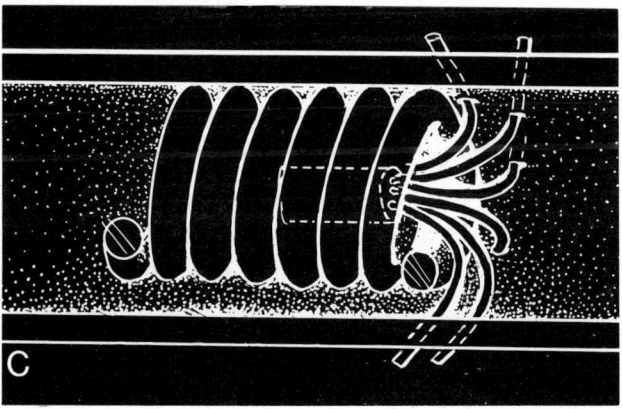

FIG 48–11.
Devices to occlude pulmonary arteriovenous fistulas. **A,** stainless steel spider. Magnified view. Used as baffle with huge fistulas. **B,** stainless steel coil. Close-up view. Attached Dacron fibers promote thrombosis. **C,** drawing. Action of steel spider, which penetrates vessel wall, providing firm baffle for back-loaded stainless steel coil, avoiding embolization into efferent vein.

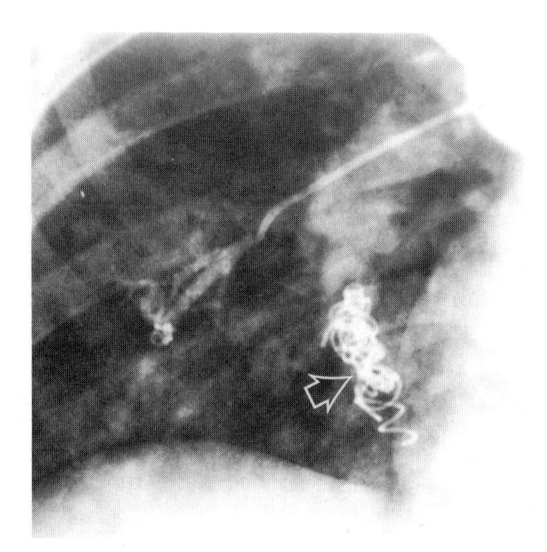

FIG 48–12.
Arteriovenous fistula after embolization. Right lower lobe. Magnified view. Large number of steel coils were used to completely occlude afferent artery. Several normal pulmonary branches were occluded as well.

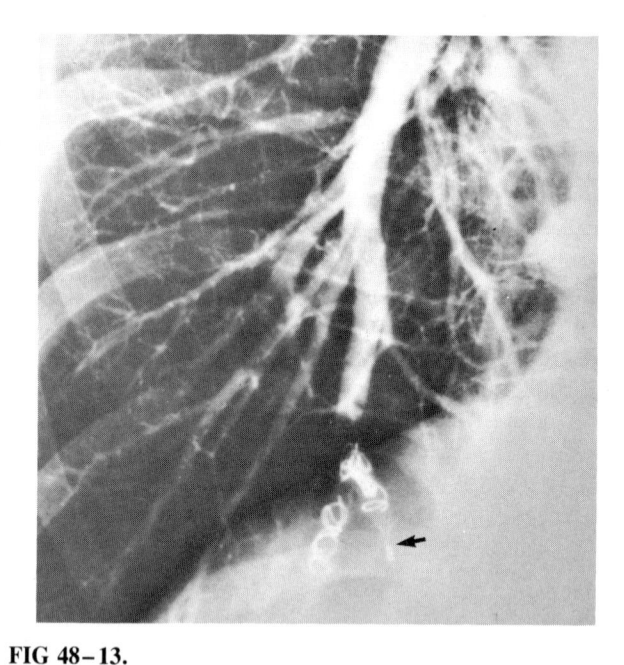

FIG 48–13.
Pulmonary arteriovenous fistula after embolization. Angiogram. Same patient as Figure 48–8. Thoracic roentgenogram. Posteroanterior projection. Magnified view. Coils and a spider *(arrow)* were used because of large size of communication. Perfusion of remaining right lower lobe is now normal (compare with Fig 48–8), and efferent vein no longer opacifies.

Recent advances in interventional techniques have made operation obsolete except for rare exceptions. Many fistulas, including those that are diffuse, can be managed by embolization. Whereas a discrete arteriovenous fistula can be cured by embolization, patients with diffuse involvement can only be palliated. Cyanosis improves after embolization but increases again because of growth of the remaining lesions.

Mainly two devices have been used to occlude pulmonary arteriovenous fistulas:

1. Stainless steel coils (Fig 48–11). Steel coils are relatively inexpensive and effective in obliterating the fistulas, particularly if more than one coil is introduced. Vascular occlusion usually does not occur immediately. A potential of peripheral embolization from fibrin forming on coils exists until complete occlusion of the afferent pulmo-

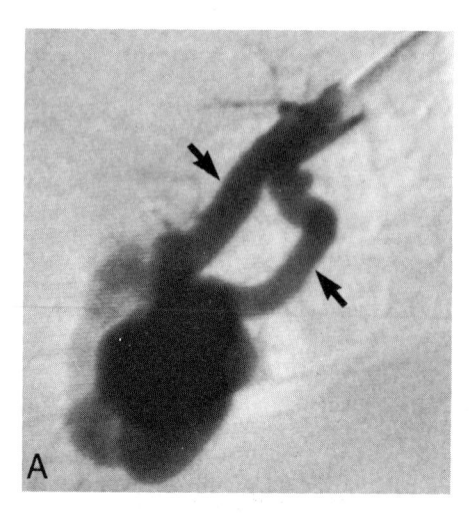

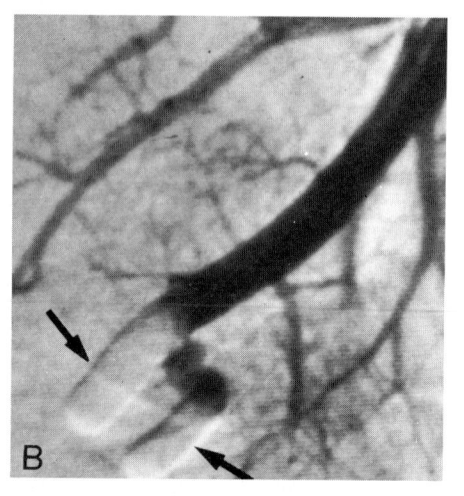

FIG 48–14.
Pulmonary arteriovenous fistula in right lower lobe. Selective angiogram. **A,** magnified view. Malformation has two feeding arteries *(arrows)*. **B,** after balloon occlusion. Obliteration of arteriovenous fistulas with two balloons *(arrows)*. (Courtesy of Dr. Robert White.)

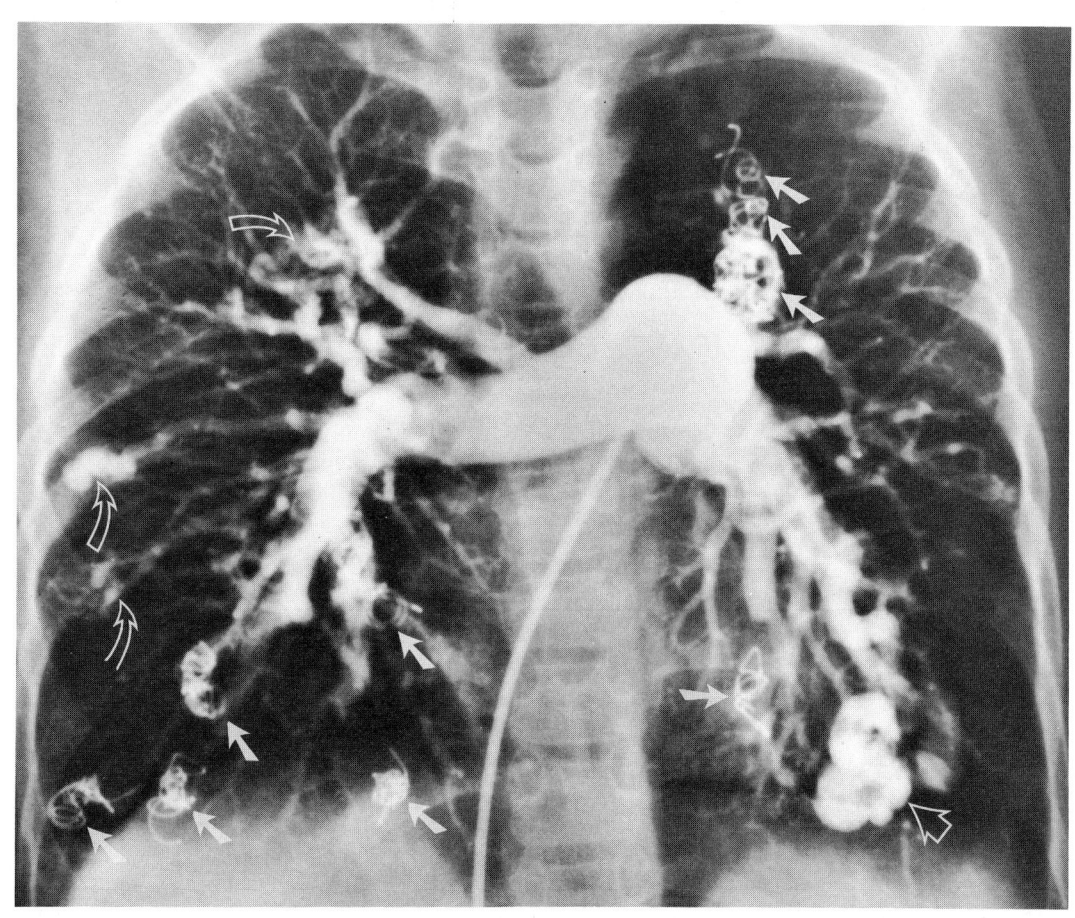

FIG 48–15.
Hereditary hemorrhagic telangiectasis and multiple pulmonary arteriovenous fistulas. Pulmonary arteriogram. Anteroposterior projection. Numerous arteriovenous malformations are closed by steel coils *(arrows)*. Larger communication *(open arrow)* at left base is occluded at subsequent catheterization. Patient became asymptomatic. Recurrence of smaller remaining communications *(curved arrows)* is expected with time, requiring retreatment.

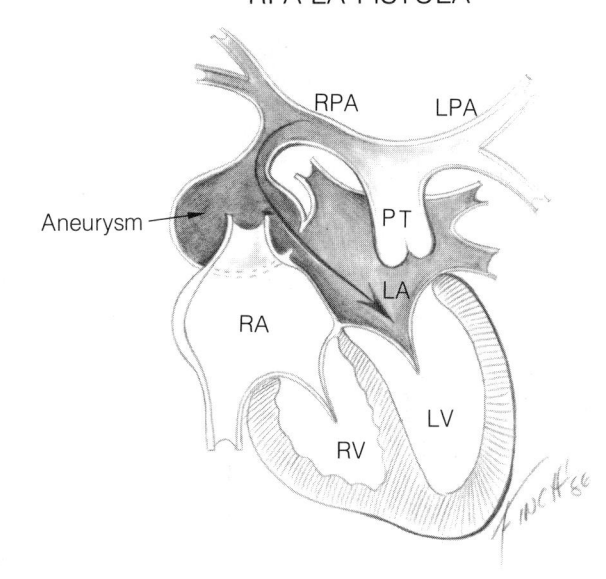

FIG 48–16.
Fistulous communication between right pulmonary artery *(RPA)* and left atrium *(LA)*. For unknown reasons, aneurysmal dilatation of right pulmonary artery at junction with left atrium occurs. *LPA* = left pulmonary artery; *LV* = left ventricle; *PT* = pulmonary trunk; *RA* = right atrium; *RV* = right ventricle.

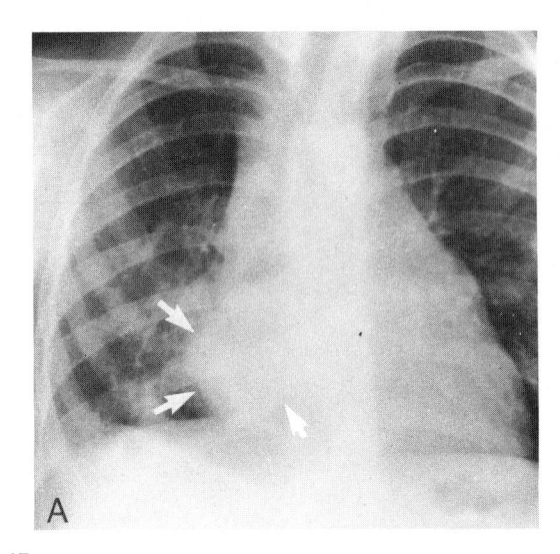

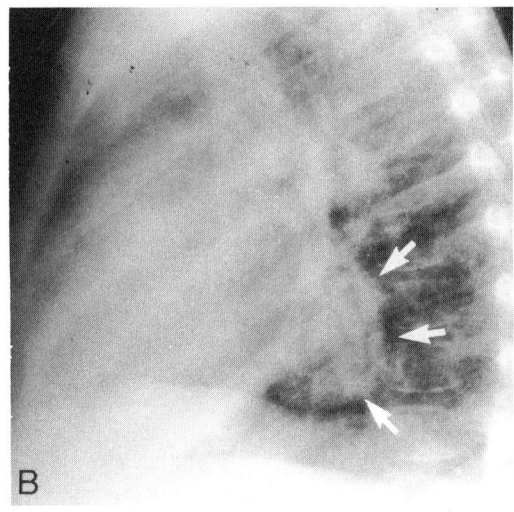

FIG 48–17.
Communication of right pulmonary artery to left atrium. Thoracic roentgenogram. **A,** posteroanterior projection. Mass *(arrows)* present at right base. **B,** lateral projection. Mass *(arrows)* posteriorly in region of left atrium. (Courtesy of Dr. Duane W. Krause.) This radiographic appearance in cyanotic patient should suggest diagnosis. Confirmation is required by enhanced CT scanning, nuclear magnetic imaging, or angiography.

nary artery occurs. In our experience, however, this has not happened. Many coils may be required to effectively occlude the afferent artery, and normal arterial branches may be inadvertently occluded, leading to loss of uninvolved pulmonary parenchyma (Fig 48–12). However, the volume of pulmonary parenchyma lost in this manner is much smaller than with operative lobectomy and is clinically unimportant.

Because the afferent arteries may be very large, steel coils may pass through the arteriovenous malformation and embolize into the systemic circulation. Systemic embolization can be prevented by prior placement of spiders (Fig 48–10,A,C). The combination of coils and spiders effectively occludes large pulmonary arteriovenous malformations (Fig 48–13).

2. A detachable balloon (Fig 48–14). Once the balloon is inflated, the parent vessel is immediately occluded, and systemic embolization of fibrin deposits is prevented. Only one balloon is required for each afferent artery. If the balloon is properly placed, normal pulmonary branches are not occluded.

The balloon deflates with time, but immediate deflation rarely occurs. In experienced hands, however, detachable balloons provide very effective, expedient occlusion of arteriovenous fistulas (see Fig 48–14). Patients with hereditary hemorrhagic telangiectasis previously considered inoperable can be successfully palliated by vascular occlusion devices (Fig 48–15). The procedure is carried out in stages and may have to be repeated if cyanosis recurs by enlargement of additional smaller malformations.

UNIQUE FORMS OF PULMONARY ARTERIOVENOUS FISTULAE

In addition to arteriovenous malformations in the lung, an aberrant connection between the pulmonary arterial tree and left atrium (Fig 48–16) may produce identical findings as an arteriovenous communication. A mass may be present on thoracic roentgenogram (Fig 48–17). The diagnosis is established by ultrasonography or angiography. This vascular malformation is a distinct but extremely rare entity. Twelve cases have been reported. Lucas et al.[1] reported a case of agenesis of a lobe of the lung with re-

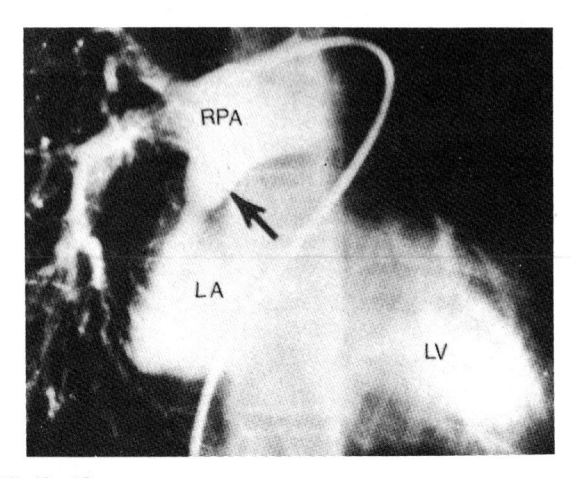

FIG 48–18.
Right pulmonary arteriogram. Same patient as Fig 48–17. Anterior-posterior projection. Fistulous communication with left atrium is well demonstrated *(arrow)*. Left atrium *(LA)* and left ventricle are opacified. *RPA* = right pulmonary artery.

sultant communication between that lobar pulmonary artery and the pulmonary vein.[2]

Pulmonary angiography demonstrates the fistulous communication with the left atrium (Fig 48–18).

REFERENCES

1. Lucas RV Jr, Lund GW, Edwards JE: Direct communication of a pulmonary artery with the left atrium: an unusual variant of pulmonary arteriovenous fistula, *Circulation* 24:1409, 1961.
2. Krause DW, Kuehn HD, Sellers RD, et al: Roentgen sign associated with an aberrant vessel connecting right main pulmonary artery to left atrium, *Radiology* 3:177, 1974.

PART SEVEN

Cyanosis and Increased Pulmonary Venous Vasculature

Conditions causing cyanosis and increased pulmonary venous obstruction have in common two features: a right-to-left shunt and an anatomic lesion that obstructs the pulmonary venous return. These conditions can be divided into two groups, depending on the connection of the pulmonary veins: (1) with normal pulmonary venous connection, and (2) with anomalous pulmonary venous connection. The hemodynamics, clinical features, and laboratory findings differ between these two groups.

In the group with normal pulmonary venous connection, the pulmonary veins connect to the left atrium. Elevation of pulmonary venous pressure results from anatomic obstruction at the mitral valve, such as mitral atresia, or within the left ventricle, such as hypoplastic left ventricle. Because of the obstruction, left atrial and therefore pulmonary venous pressures are elevated. In these conditions, bidirectional shunting is present. A left-to-right shunt occurs at the atrial level, usually through a restrictive foramen ovale. A right-to-left shunt is present at either the ventricular or great vessel level and represents the major source of systemic blood flow. In this group of patients the degree of cyanosis is usually mild, signs of congestive cardiac failure are common, and cardiomegaly is present.

In the group with anomalous pulmonary venous connection, all of the pulmonary veins connect abnormally to the right side of the heart (see Chapter 46). In this form of total anomalous pulmonary venous connection, the pulmonary veins connect to a systemic venous channel, but the connection or channel may be narrowed and obstructs pulmonary venous return. A right-to-left shunt is present at the atrial level through an atrial septal defect and represents the sole source of blood for the left side of the heart and the systemic circulation. Cyanosis is intense, signs of congestive cardiac failure are absent, and cardiac size is normal.

Therefore, clinically and radiographically these two groups can be distinguished, but additional investigations are required to diagnose the specific lesion within each group.

The conditions that must be considered in the differential diagnosis of cyanosis and increased pulmonary venous markings include the following:

1. Normal cardiac size.
   a. Total anomalous pulmonary venous connection with obstruction (see Chapter 46).
   b. Atresia of common pulmonary vein (Chapter 49).
2. Cardiomegaly
   a. Aortic atresia (Chapter 50).
   b. Mitral atresia (Chapter 51).
   c. Aortic stenosis with hypoplastic left ventricle (see Chapter 50).

CHAPTER 49

Atresia of the Common Pulmonary Vein

Atresia of the common pulmonary vein is rare, with only a few cases being recognized before death.[1-5] Developmentally it is considered closely related to total anomalous pulmonary venous connection, and, indeed, its clinical picture resembles that condition when pulmonary venous obstruction exists. An obligatory right-to-left shunt is present at the atrial level. In contrast to stenosis of the individual pulmonary veins, atresia of the common vein is a cyanotic condition.

PATHOLOGIC ANATOMY

Like total anomalous pulmonary venous connection, the pulmonary veins do not connect to the left atrium but join together into a venous confluence close to the posterior aspect of the left atrium. From this confluence a fibrous strand may pass to the left atrium, or a fibrous connection may be absent. This condition probably results late in the development of the heart when the pulmonary veins are being incorporated into the left atrium, at a stage after the common pulmonary vein has made contact with the pulmonary venous system but after the channels to the cardinal or umbilical-vitelline systems have disappeared (see Chapter 1). If at this stage the common pulmonary vein involutes, only a fibrous connection is left between the pulmonary veins and the left atrium, and there are no other connections to major systemic veins (Fig 49-1). Atresia of the individual pulmonary veins may occur bilaterally or unilaterally.

The only exit of blood from the pulmonary venous system is through intrapulmonary connections with the bronchial venous systems. The bronchial veins, in turn, may connect with esophageal veins. These enlarge with time and become an exit for the pulmonary venous system (see Fig 49-1). Because of the small caliber of the bronchial and esophageal veins, a high grade of pulmonary venous obstruction exists. If the pleural space has been entered during a thoracotomy or by chest tube placement and adhesions have developed, egress of blood occurs also through systemic veins (see Fig 49-5). A prominent accompaniment of atresia of the common pulmonary vein is marked enlargement of pulmonary lymphatics. Cases of this condition have been considered to have pulmonary lymphangiectasis.

The right ventricle is hypertrophied because pulmonary hypertension is present. The foramen ovale is patent, and in neonates the ductus arteriosus may be patent as well.

HEMODYNAMICS

The hemodynamics are identical to total anomalous pulmonary venous connection with severe pulmonary obstruction (see Chapter 46). There is marked pulmonary venous obstruction, with resultant elevation of pulmonary arterial and right ventricular systolic pressures. A right-to-left shunt is present at the atrial level, which represents the only source of blood into the left side of the heart. The degree of arterial desaturation is marked, because the volume of pulmonary venous blood return is very limited and the associated pulmonary edema interferes with oxygenation.

The pulmonary vascular resistance is elevated, and if the ductus arteriosus is patent, the shunt occurs in a right-to-left direction because of severe pulmonary hypertension.

CLINICAL FEATURES

Marked cyanosis is present from the neonatal period, and death usually occurs by 3 weeks. The prominent

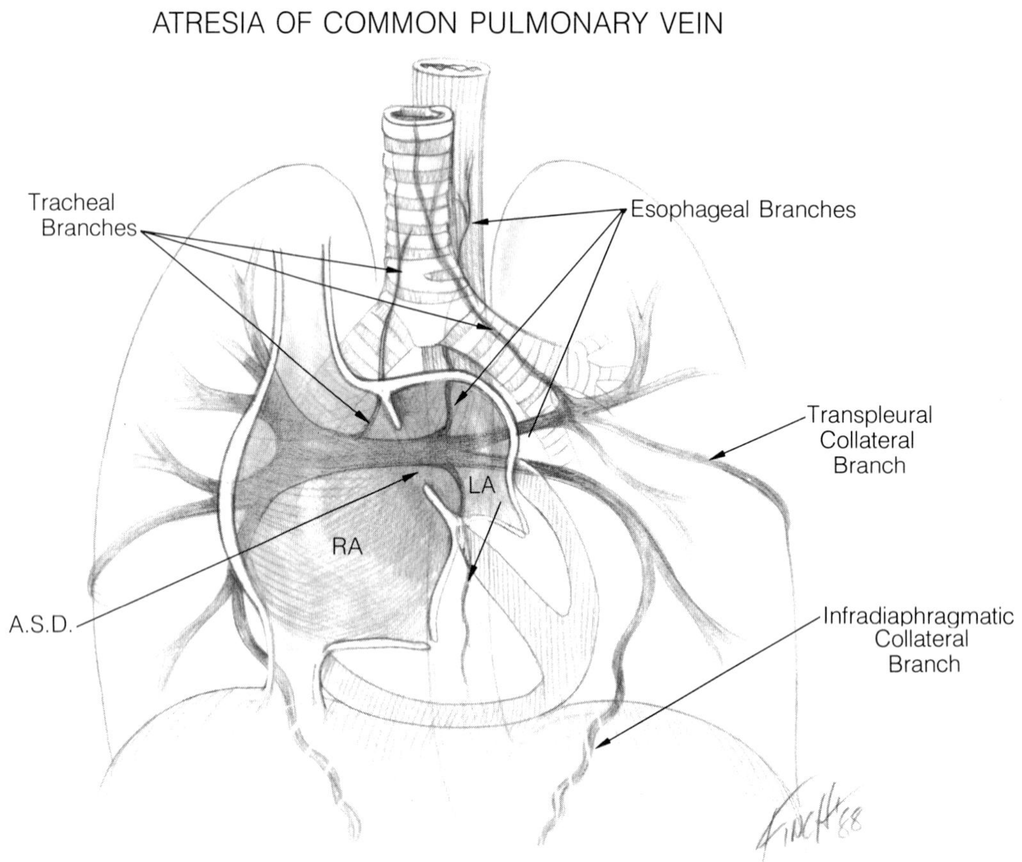

ATRESIA OF COMMON PULMONARY VEIN

FIG 49–1.
Atresia of common pulmonary veins with collateral flow to mediastinal veins. A.S.D. = atrial septal defect; LA = left atrium; RA = right atrium.

symptoms are respiratory, being tachypnea and dyspnea. There are no abnormal cardiac findings other than an accentuated pulmonary component of the second heart sound because of pulmonary hypertension. Either no murmur or a soft nonspecific murmur is found. Cardiac disease is generally not suspected from physical examination.

ELECTROCARDIOGRAPHIC FEATURES

In the neonate, the electrocardiogram is indistinguishable from normal. Later right ventricular hypertrophy is found.

ECHOCARDIOGRAPHIC FEATURES

We are unaware of a report describing an echocardiogram in this condition. We assume it would show the following features similar to total anomalous pulmonary venous connection: no pulmonary veins enter the left atrium, and an accessory chamber is located behind the left atrium. But unlike total anomalous pulmonary venous connection, no connecting channel extends from this confluence to a major systemic vein.

RADIOGRAPHIC FEATURES

The radiographic features are identical to other pulmonary venous obstructive conditions located proximal to the mitral valve, particularly infradiaphragmatic total anomalous pulmonary venous connection (discussed in Chapter 46). There are no distinctive features. Evidence of dilated subpleural lymphatics (Kerley B lines) might be found, but these have not been described in infancy.

1. The cardiac silhouette is not enlarged (Fig 49–2). REASON: The volume of blood within the heart is not increased. The only anatomic change is right ventricular hypertrophy from pulmonary hypertension. Right ventricular hypertrophy does not cause cardiomegaly on a posteroanterior projection as long as the right ventricle remains compensated.

2. The left atrium is not enlarged.

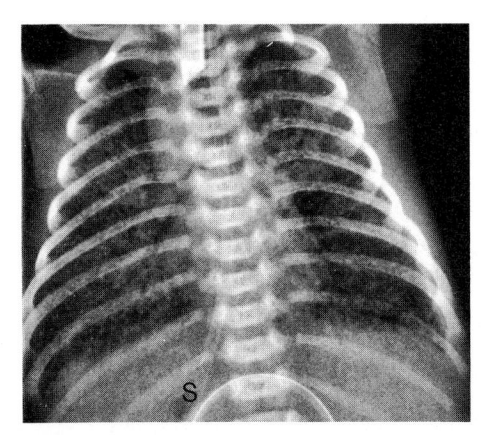

FIG 49–2.
Atresia of common pulmonary vein. Thoracic roentgenogram. Posteroanterior projection. Abdominal heterotaxia with stomach (S) on left side. Normal cardiac size. Lung fields show diffuse granular pattern without air bronchogram, as may occur in hyaline membrane disease. Radiographic appearance is indistinguishable from other lesions with severe pulmonary venous obstruction. Incidental right aortic arch.

3. A diffuse, granular pattern exists throughout both lung fields, resembling hyaline membrane disease (see Fig 49–2), but an air bronchogram is usually not present.

4. The differential diagnosis between hyaline membrane disease and atresia of the pulmonary veins becomes easier if a pleural effusion is present (Fig 49–3). This condition represents the most severe form of venous obstruction, leading to pulmonary edema and pleural effusion.

5. The differential diagnosis between respiratory distress syndrome and pulmonary venous obstruction on thoracic roentgenograms may be extremely difficult, and sometimes it is indeed impossible.

6. Unilateral atresia of pulmonary veins can be suspected by finding a smaller hemithorax, shift of the mediastinal structures (not uniformly present), and a unilateral pattern of pulmonary venous obstruction (Fig 49–4).

7. The typical granular pattern of pulmonary venous obstruction is observed in the involved lung. Kerley B lines and a pleural effusion may be present (see Fig 49–4).

CARDIAC CATHETERIZATION

As in total anomalous pulmonary venous connection, the oxygen saturation in each cardiac chamber is the same. All oxygen values are very low, and a site of entry of fully saturated pulmonary venous blood into the systemic venous system cannot be identified.

Marked pulmonary hypertension is present, and the wedge pressure is elevated. It may reflect pulmonary arterial pressure rather than pulmonary venous pressure, be-

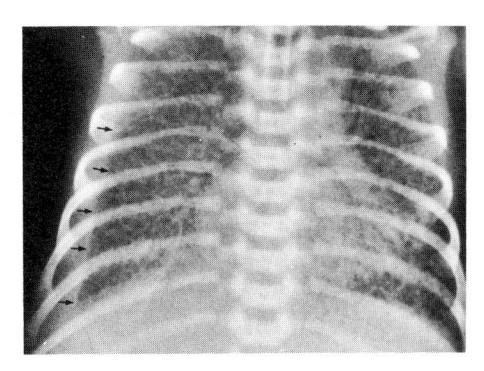

FIG 49–3.
Atresia of common pulmonary vein. Thoracic roentgenogram. Posteroanterior projection. Characteristic granular pattern throughout both lung fields. Normal cardiac size. Right pleural effusion (arrows) suggests cardiac nature of pulmonary pattern rather than a pulmonary problem.

cause there is so little flow through the pulmonary venous system.

ANGIOGRAPHIC FEATURES

There are angiographic features that are highly suggestive or even diagnostic of this condition. Selective injection of the right or left pulmonary arteries is mandatory, but even so, the atretic common pulmonary vein may never opacify. REASON: (1) there is virtually no flow in the atretic common pulmonary vein, and egress of contrast

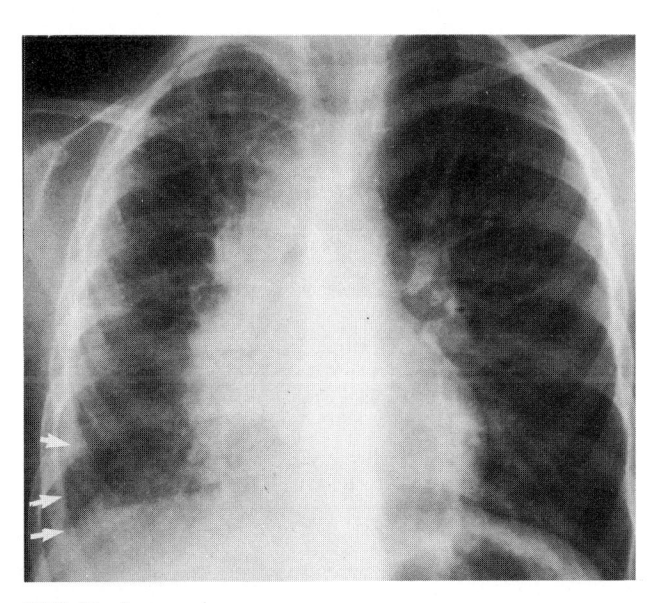

FIG 49–4.
Right pulmonary vein atresia. Thoracic roentgenogram. Posteroanterior projection. Right hemithorax is smaller than left. Mediastinum is slightly shifted toward right. Accentuated venous pattern in right lung. Right pleural effusion (arrows) and Kerley B lines at right base.

medium occurs only through mediastinal collateral veins which are usually very small; (2) most injected contrast medium may escape the pulmonary vascular bed through a reversing patent ductus arteriosus, if present; and (3) with unilateral atresia of the pulmonary veins, the pulmonary artery on the involved side may not opacify. REASON: Retrograde flow from bronchial inflow; oxygen saturations are elevated in that pulmonary artery blood which may be fully saturated. Best results are obtained with selective balloon occlusion pulmonary angiography, forcing the contrast medium through the pulmonary capillary bed into the pulmonary veins, which have little flow.

1. On pulmonary angiography, there is an extremely prolonged transit of contrast material through the lungs similar to other conditions causing pulmonary venous obstruction. Therefore, a large volume of contrast medium should be used, and filming has to be prolonged to visualize the pulmonary venous system.

2. The pulmonary veins may be visualized, or there may not be distinct opacification of the pulmonary veins. REASON: Inflow through bronchial collaterals. In either case, there is no opacification of the left atrium.

3. On pulmonary angiography the central pulmonary veins are usually not opacified. REASON: There is minimal flow in the pulmonary veins, because egress of blood occurs primarily via esophageal, mediastinal, and bronchial veins, and there is inflow from bronchial collaterals. If the pleural space has previously been entered by an operation and adhesions are present, blood flow may occur through transpleural collaterals (Fig 49–5).

4. Aortography or selective bronchial or intercostal angiography opacifies the pulmonary artery by retrograde flow (Figs 49–5 and 49–6).

5. Intrapulmonary collateral flow may develop, which

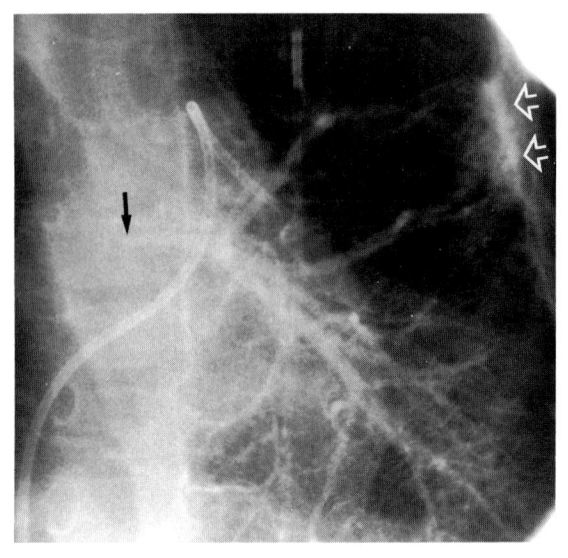

FIG 49–5.
Atresia of common pulmonary vein. Left pulmonary balloon occlusion arteriogram. Late phase. Anteroposterior projection. Pulmonary veins are very small (characteristic of hypoplasia). Atretic small left main pulmonary vein *(black arrow)*. Well-developed transpleural collaterals *(open arrows)* return pulmonary venous blood to systemic venous circulation. Transpleural collaterals are developed because pleural space had been previously entered during an operation and adhesions created. Otherwise, pulmonary venous return occurs primarily through bronchial, mediastinal, and esophageal veins.

can be demonstrated by balloon occlusion pulmonary arteriography (Fig 49–7). Normally there are no interpulmonary collateral channels, but they may develop in this condition. REASON: Connecting bronchial arterial collateral branches.

6. Left atrial injection does not opacify the pulmonary veins. Normally reflux of contrast material into pulmonary

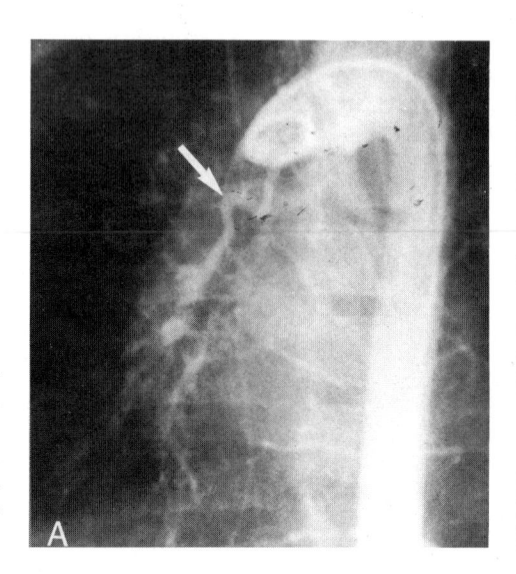

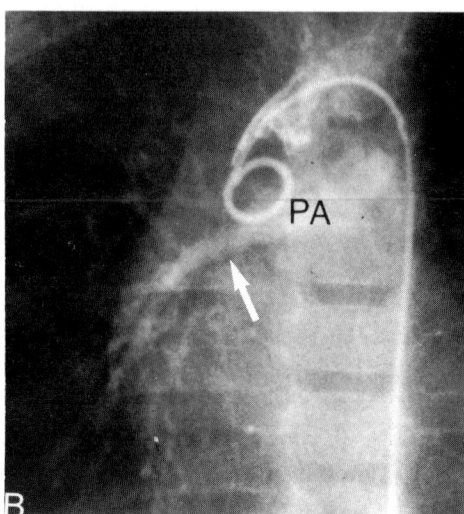

FIG 49–6.
Aortogram. Anteroposterior projection. Atresia of right pulmonary veins. **A,** early phase. Enlarged bronchial artery *(arrow)*. **B,** late phase. Opacification of pulmonary artery *(PA)* by retrograde flow.

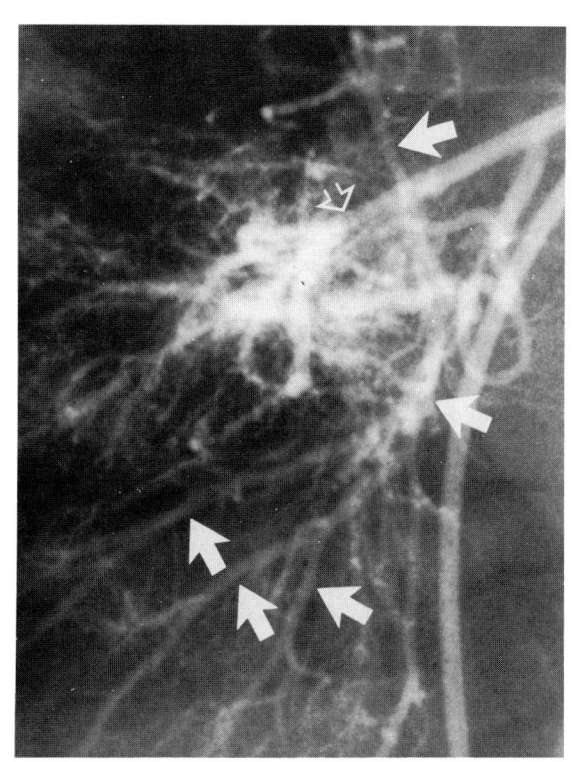

FIG 49–7.
Unilateral pulmonary vein atresia. Balloon occlusion pulmonary arteriogram. Right upper lobe pulmonary artery *(open arrow)*. Anteroposterior projection. Opacification of remaining right pulmonary artery *(arrows)* by interconnecting bronchial arteries.

veins occurs after left atrial angiography. Although the absence of pulmonary venous opacification is highly suggestive, it is not diagnostic, because this phenomenon may be present in some patients with normally connecting pulmonary veins.

7. A right-to-left shunt is demonstrated angiographically at the atrial level. This reflects an obligatory shunt and the sole source of systemic blood flow.

8. After pulmonary angiography, there may be visualization of a patent ductus arteriosus and opacification of the descending aorta, indicating a right-to-left shunt. This shunt complicates the angiographic demonstration of the pulmonary veins on the late phase, because the contrast medium escapes into the systemic circulation. Balloon occlusion angiography may be necessary.

OPERATIVE CONSIDERATIONS

The diagnosis should be considered in a neonate with findings of pulmonary parenchymal disease: cyanosis, respiratory distress, lack of a murmur, normal cardiac size, and radiographic appearance of the lung fields identical to pulmonary disease. If echocardiography is performed, the diagnosis may be suggested. If the diagnosis is made by echocardiography or angiography, an operation should be performed in an attempt to anastomose the pulmonary venous confluence to the left atrium. We are unaware that this has been successfully performed to date.

REFERENCES

1. Hawker RE, Celermajer JM, Gengos DC, et al: Common pulmonary vein atresia: premortem diagnosis in two infants, *Circulation* 46:368, 1972.
2. Levine MA, Moller JH, Amplatz K, et al: Atresia of the common pulmonary vein: case report and differential diagnosis, *Am J Roentgenol Radium Ther Nucl Med* 100:322, 1967.
3. Mody GT, Folger GM Jr: Atresia of the common pulmonary vein: report of one case, *Pediatrics* 54:62, 1974.
4. Lucas RV Jr, Woolfrey BF, Anderson RC, et al: Atresia of the common pulmonary vein, *Pediatrics* 29:729, 1962.
5. Rywlin AM, Fojaco RM: Congenital pulmonary lymphangiectasis associated with a blind common pulmonary vein, *Pediatrics* 41:931, 1968.

CHAPTER 50

Hypoplastic Left Ventricle Syndrome

Hypoplastic left ventricle syndrome is a term applied to conditions in which the left ventricle is diminutive. Usually the ascending aorta, aortic valve, mitral valve, and left atrium are also underdeveloped. Cardiac anomalies with these pathologic features account for 8% of instances of congenital cardiac anomalies, and are the most common cause of cardiac death in the first week of life, and represent one of the last frontiers for operative therapy.

PATHOLOGIC ANATOMY (FIG 50–1)

In most patients with a hypoplastic left ventricle, the aortic valve is either atretic or severely stenotic, and the mitral valve frequently shows either stenosis or atresia as well. Isolated mitral valve atresia has also been classified in this category, but because the anatomic, hemodynamic, and clinical features are so variable, it is discussed in Chapter 51.

The principal anatomic feature is the left ventricle, which almost always has a reduced chamber size, and is often minute.[1,2] When aortic and mitral atresia coexist, the left ventricle is only an endothelial-lined slit in the ventricular mass. If a left ventricle exists, its wall is quite hypertrophied, and its endocardial surface is lined by thickened, white endocardial fibroelastosis. Myocardial sinusoids may be enlarged, leading into the coronary arterial branches,[3,4] particularly over the left ventricular apex. They are analogous to similar vascular structures in pulmonary atresia with intact ventricular septum. Unlike pulmonary atresia, left ventricular sinusoids cannot be demonstrated angiographically because of the commonly associated mitral atresia, making injection of the left ventricle impossible (see Chapter 34).

If the mitral valve is patent, it is stenotic. The mitral annulus is narrow, and the papillary muscles are hypoplastic. Despite mitral obstruction, the left atrium is hypoplastic as well.

Usually the aortic valve is atretic, but there may be severe aortic stenosis from a unicommissural valve. In our experience, the left ventricle seems to be larger, although still diminutive, among the patients with aortic stenosis compared with aortic atresia. The aortic annulus and ascending aorta are narrow, usually in proportion to the volume of blood flow through the ascending aorta. In aortic atresia, the aortic diameter is only about 2 mm in diameter,[2] because the only flow is retrograde into the coronary arteries. The small ascending aorta in aortic atresia has therefore been termed "common coronary artery."

Compared with the left side of the heart, the right atrium, right ventricle, and pulmonary arteries are enlarged. The ductus arteriosus, although playing an integral role in the fetal circulation, is often restricted or occluded in postmortem specimens. A coarctation of the aorta may be found opposite the site of the ductus entering the aorta.[5,6] The caliber of the aortic arch successively increases as each successive brachiocephalic artery arises from it. This anatomic feature supports the theory that the size of a blood vessel is determined by blood flow through it. In 50% of the patients, a coarctation of the aorta coexists proximally to the patent ductus arteriosus. This anatomic

HERNIATION OF FORAMEN OVALE

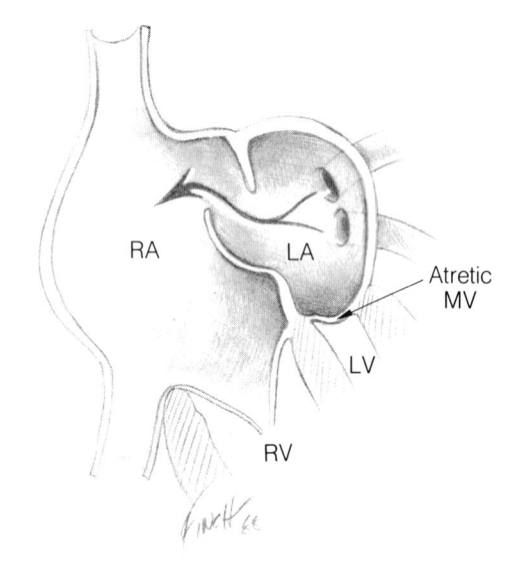

FIG 50–1.
Aortic and mitral atresia. Herniation of fossa ovalis, allowing egress of blood from left atrium *(LA)*. Communication remains small, and, consequently, left atrial pressure exceeds right atrial *(RA)* pressure. *LV* = left ventricle; *MV* = mitral valve; *RV* = right ventricle.

HEMODYNAMICS OF LEVO—ATRIO—CARDINAL VEIN

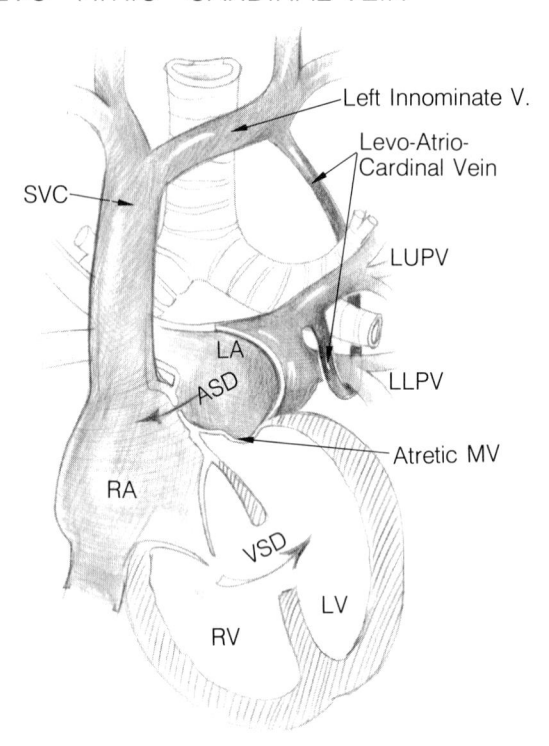

FIG 50–2.
Aortic and mitral atresia without atrial communication. Levoatrial-cardinal vein connecting left atrium (occasionally from left upper pulmonary vein), with left innominate vein providing egress of blood from left atrium. *ASD* = atrial septal defect; *LA* = left atrium; *LLPV* = left lower pulmonary vein; *LUPV* = left upper pulmonary vein; *LV* = left ventricle; *MV* = mitral valve; *RA* = right atrium; *RV* = right ventricle; *SVC* = superior vena cava; *VSD* = ventricle septal defect.

feature is important if a palliative operation is contemplated.

The status of the atrial septum is variable and an important determinant of the hemodynamics. A defect is usually present in the atrial septum at the fossa ovalis, which allows free communication between the atria. In 10%, premature closure of the foramen ovale is present, being considered a variant of left ventricular hypoplasia. A communication between the atria may be restrictive, causing herniation of the septum primum through the ostium secundum. In the presence of herniation, left atrial pressure greatly exceeds right atrial pressure (see Fig 50–1). If the communication is not restrictive, pressures are equal.

If no communication exists in the atrial septum, alternative pathways may be present for blood to leave the left atrium. When the pulmonary veins connect normally to the left atrium, a venous channel may leave the left atrium or upper lobe pulmonary vein and pass superiorly to the subclavian vein. This structure is called the "levoatrial cardinal vein" (Fig 50–2).[7] A rare alternative is a communication (or fenestration) between the left atrium and the coronary sinus (see Chapter 20).

Occasionally partial anomalous pulmonary venous connection allows an exit of blood from the lungs, and there may be intralobar pulmonary venous communications as well, which facilitate pulmonary venous return to the anomalous connection.[8]

The pulmonary vasculature may show changes of pulmonary venous obstruction, with dilated pulmonary veins and pulmonary lymphangiectasis. REASON: Depending on the size of the atrial communication, significant pulmonary venous obstruction may be present. Pulmonary arterial musculature is increased in thickness and extends distally into the pulmonary arterial tree.[9]

HEMODYNAMICS

The hemodynamics vary, depending on the status of the ductus arteriosus, atrial septum, and pulmonary arterial bed, although most individuals follow a similar course. In most neonates the atrial communication is restricted and the ductus arteriosus patent. The right ventricle, through

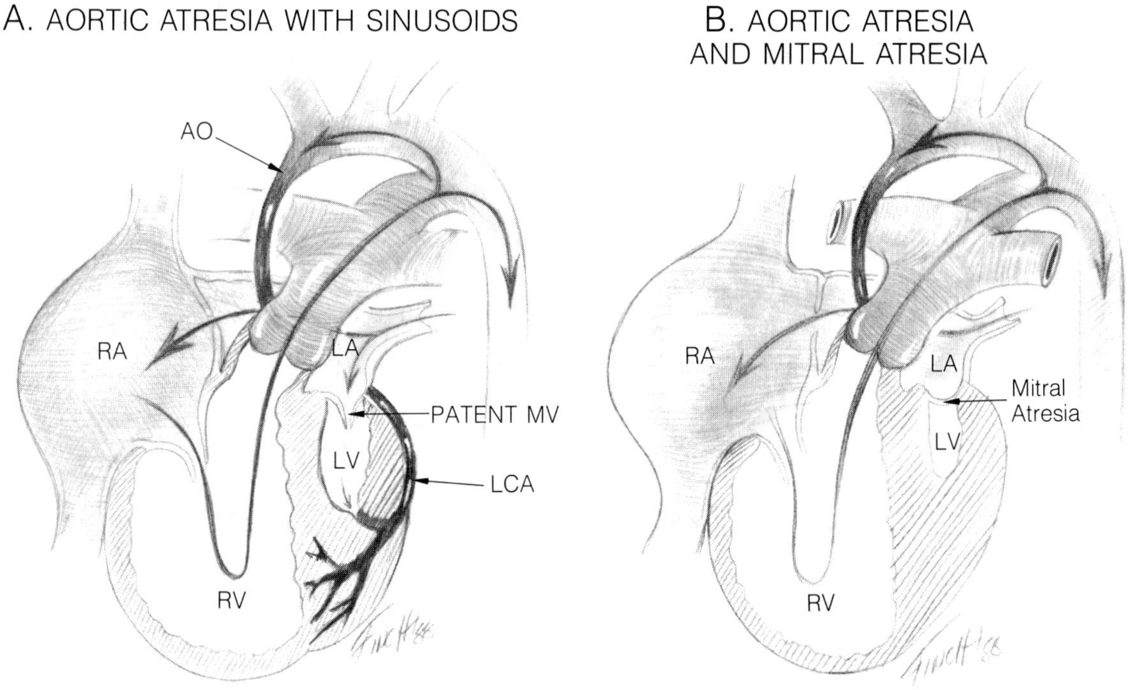

A. AORTIC ATRESIA WITH SINUSOIDS

B. AORTIC ATRESIA AND MITRAL ATRESIA

FIG 50-3.
Aortic atresia. Central circulation. **A,** patent mitral valve and, **B,** mitral atresia. Because of obstruction in left side of heart, a left-to-right shunt exists at atrial level. The entire systemic and pulmonary venous returns enter right atrium *(RA)* and right ventricle *(RV)*. Blood is ejected into pulmonary artery and through ductus arteriosus to supply systemic circulation. Blood flows in a retrograde direction through aortic arch into ascending aorta and coronary arteries. With a patent mitral valve some blood enters the left ventricle ejected during systole into coronary arteries *(LCA)* via sinusoids. If the mitral valve is incompetent, sinusoids are absent. REASON: Pressure in left ventricle is not suprasystemic. **B,** aortic atresia with mitral atresia. Left ventricle is a diminutive blind chamber. *AO* = aorta; *ASD* = atrial septal defect; *LA* = left atrium; *LV* = left ventricle; *RA* = right atrium; *RV* = right ventricle.

the pulmonary artery and patent ductus arteriosus, delivers blood into the aorta, where blood flows into the descending aorta and in a retrograde direction around the arch to supply the brachiocephalic and coronary arteries of the mitral valve is competent egress of blood from the left occurs via sinusoids (Fig 50–3).[10] Pulmonary arterial pressure is maintained by elevated pulmonary vascular resistance from the thickened media of the pulmonary arterioles, the vasoconstrictive effect of mild hypoxemia, and pulmonary venous obstruction. Thus, both the systemic and pulmonary arterial circulations are perfused by the ductus arteriosus. The oxygen saturation of blood reaching the systemic circulation is usually close to normal,[11] so that complications and symptoms of hypoxemia are uncommon at this stage.

Normally the ductus arteriosus begins to close functionally by 48 hours of age, and the rate of closure may be accelerated by the administration of an oxygen-rich environment to the neonate. As the ductus arteriosus closes, the sole source of systemic circulation is obliterated, and systemic arterial pressure falls. Inadequate renal, gastrointestinal, and cutaneous perfusion leads to renal shutdown, oliguria or anuria, necrotizing enterocolitis, a mottled color to the skin, and hypothermia. Death ensues.

In the 25% of patients with an unrestrictive atrial septal communication, as long as the ductus arteriosus is patent, there may be difficulty in maintaining an adequate systemic perfusion pressure. Because of the atrial communication, left atrial pressure is low, so that the passive and reflex effect of elevated pulmonary venous pressure on pulmonary arterioles is not present, and pulmonary vascular resistance is low. Therefore, as pulmonary vascular resistance decreases postnatally, systemic arterial pressure falls, even though the ductus arteriosus is widely patent. The inadequate systemic perfusion may be accentuated as the ductus closes.

CLINICAL FEATURES

Aortic atresia with a patent mitral valve is a disorder occurring predominantly in males, although the incidence is equal in males and females for coexistent aortic and mitral atresia. In patients with aortic atresia, the presence of a cardiac malformation is recognized during the first week of life. The initial feature is not cyanosis but usually tachypnea and poor color from inadequate peripheral perfusion. The neonate often appears mottled, cool, and dyspneic. The peripheral pulses are weak or nonpalpable. Cardiomegaly is present, and sharp heart sounds are heard. There may be no murmur or only a soft nonspecific murmur. A third heart sound (gallop) is present. The liver is usually enlarged, and the hepatic margin may be located at the level of the umbilicus.

With cardiotonic agents, peripheral perfusion, pulses, and blood pressure may initially improve but then deteriorate as the ductus arteriosus closes. The clinical picture and course are usually very characteristic. Most infants die during the first week of life.

ELECTROCARDIOGRAPHIC FEATURES

The electrocardiogram is often indistinguishable from the normal for a neonate. There is right-axis deviation and tall R waves in the right precordial leads. In our experience, a q wave is not present in lead V_6, but a q wave is not found in this lead among one half of normal neonates.[12] Thus, the presence of a q wave in lead V_6 excludes hypoplastic left ventricle syndrome. Right atrial enlargement or ST-wave changes, the latter from inadequate myocardial perfusion, may be the only electrocardiographic evidence of a cardiac malformation.

ECHOCARDIOGRAPHIC FEATURES

The echocardiogram is usually diagnostic and permits evaluation of the status of aortic and mitral valves and the size of the ascending aorta and left ventricle.[13-15] Diameters of the ascending aorta and the left ventricular cavity are reduced. A diameter of the ascending aorta less than 5 mm is diagnostic of aortic atresia. In contrast, the right ventricle and pulmonary artery are enlarged.

Subcostal, apical four-chamber, and parasternal long-axis projection shows the large right ventricle and small left ventricle. The movement and patency of the aortic and mitral valves can be assessed. Doppler studies are helpful in assessing coexistent tricuspid insufficiency. The atrial septum can be evaluated for the presence and size of the foramen ovale. The aortic arch can be assessed for size. The anatomic and functional status of the ductus arteriosus can be evaluated. Blood flow in the ascending aorta is usually retrograde.

RADIOGRAPHIC FEATURES

In aortic atresia, the radiographic findings vary considerably. REASON: The hemodynamics of this malformation vary, depending on the degree of obstruction at the level of the foramen ovale and the status of the patent ductus arteriosus. If an atrial septal defect is present, a large left-to-right shunt occurs at the atrial level, and the pulmonary arterial vasculature is greatly increased. In most patients, however, only a probe patent foramen ovale is present, offering resistance to the left-to-right shunt. The fossa ovalis may herniate into the right atrium, allowing a relatively small left-to-right shunt to occur (see Fig 50–1). If the resistance to flow across the foramen ovale is very high, pulmonary venous obstruction is present, causing a typical radiographic pattern in the lung fields (see Fig 50–7). In most cases, a mixture of arterial and venous pulmonary vasculature is present.

In the differential diagnosis of the radiograph, knowledge of the age of the patient is very important, because most patients do not survive beyond 1 week of life. Other conditions that may cause a similar radiographic appearance usually manifest later than 1 week of age:

1. The cardiac silhouette is most commonly very large (Fig 50–4). Aortic atresia is one of the conditions causing a very large heart and increased pulmonary vasculature in the first day of life.

2. Left atrial enlargement is absent (Fig 50–5). REASON: The left-sided hypoplasia also involves the left

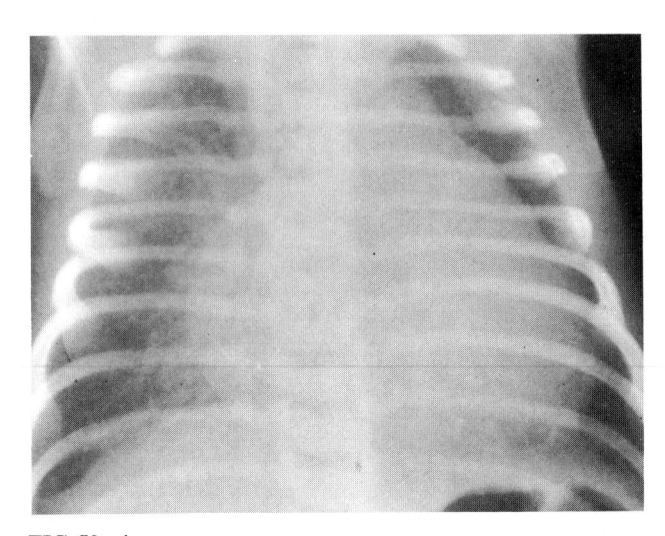

FIG 50–4.
Aortic atresia. Thoracic roentgenogram. Posteroanterior projection. Massive cardiomegaly. Increased pulmonary vasculature. Differentiation between arterial and venous pulmonary vasculature is not possible.

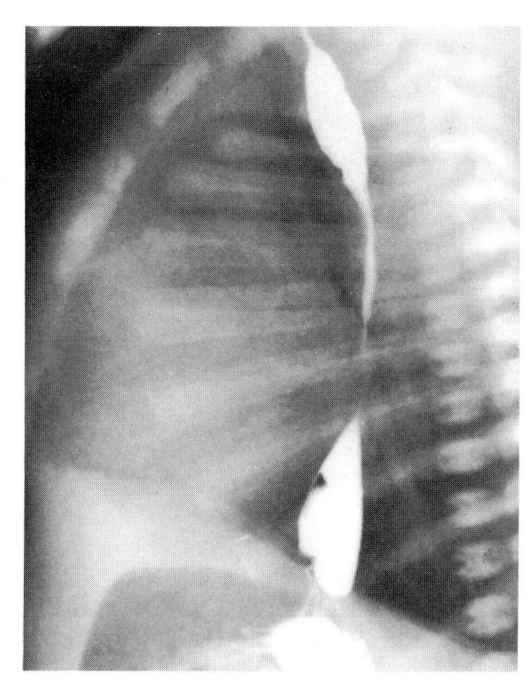

FIG 50-5.
Aortic atresia. Thoracic roentgenogram. Lateral projection. Barium swallow. Normal-sized left atrium because of left-sided hypoplasia.

atrium. If pulmonary blood flow is increased and the atrial defect obstructive, left atrial enlargement to some degree may occur.

3. Usually the pulmonary vasculature is a mixture of increased arterial markings from the left-to-right shunt, increased pulmonary venous markings from the obstruction, and cardiac failure.

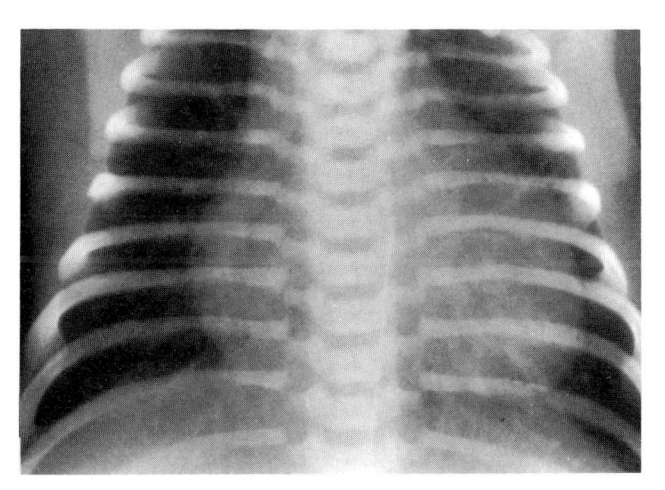

FIG 50-6.
Aortic atresia. Thoracic roentgenogram. Posteroanterior projection. Marked cardiomegaly. Increased pulmonary arterial vasculature as in left-to-right shunt. Cardiac size is increased out of proportion to degree of increased pulmonary vasculature.

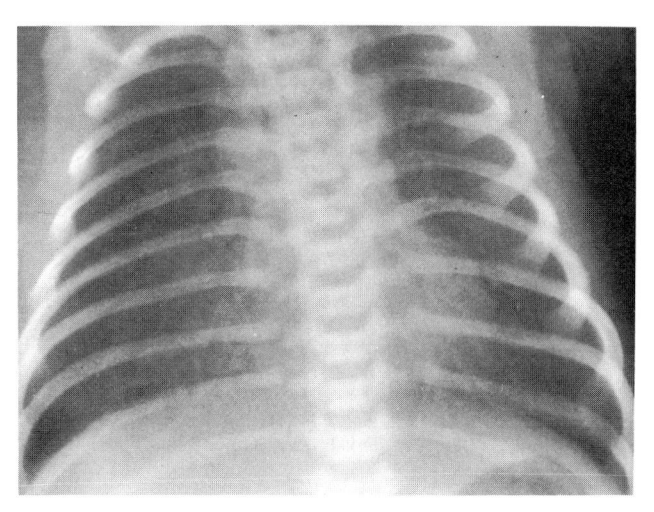

FIG 50-7.
Aortic atresia with severe obstruction at level of foramen ovale. Thoracic roentgenogram. Posteroanterior projection. Normal cardiac size. Accentuation of pulmonary venous vasculature. This radiograph of aortic atresia is unusual and indistinguishable from total anomalous venous return below the diaphragm.

4. Occasionally a pattern of pulmonary edema may be present.

5. If a large shunt occurs through the atrial communication, the accentuated pulmonary vascular markings are well defined, and the picture is indistinguishable from other conditions with a left-to-right shunt (Fig 50-6). The heart, however, tends to be larger than in uncomplicated left-to-right shunts. REASON: Massive right ventricular dilatation.

6. With severe obstruction at the atrial septum, the cardiac silhouette may not be enlarged (Fig 50-7). In this situation the pulmonary vasculature shows pulmonary venous obstruction indistinguishable from other pulmonary venous obstructive lesions.

CARDIAC CATHETERIZATION

With the accuracy of echocardiography in making a diagnosis of hypoplastic left ventricle and aortic atresia, cardiac catheterization and angiography are often unnecessary to establish a diagnosis. Catheterization may be used to obtain specific information needed for operative considerations. Often the neonates are very ill, their airways are electively intubated, and they are placed on a mechanical ventilator before catheterization.

The catheter tip can be passed through the ductus arteriosus and at times through the foramen ovale, but it is difficult to advance it into the left ventricle.

Oximetry data show a left-to-right shunt at the atrial level and a right-to-left shunt through the ductus arteriosus.[11] Systemic venous oxygen saturations are low, reflecting the low cardiac output. Pulmonary edema may interfere with oxygenation and lower pulmonary venous oxygen saturation, thus contributing to cyanosis.

Right ventricular and pulmonary arterial systolic pressures are elevated, and as the ductus arteriosus closes, a gradient is found between the pulmonary artery and aorta as systemic pressure falls often to the range of 30 to 45 mm Hg. Right atrial pressure is often elevated to 10 mm Hg. Left atrial and pulmonary capillary pressures likewise are elevated, perhaps to 35 mm Hg. If the aortic valve is patent but stenotic, a systolic pressure gradient is found.

A balloon atrioseptostomy may be performed to relieve pulmonary venous hypertension in patients who are being considered for operation.

ANGIOGRAPHIC FEATURES

The amount of contrast material used for angiography should be limited because it lowers systemic arterial pressure and reduces renal perfusion, increasing the risk of angiography.

An angiographic diagnosis may be necessary because some forms of hypoplastic left heart syndrome, such as critical aortic stenosis with a hypoplastic left ventricle, require a different operative procedure than aortic atresia. If the aortic valve is atretic, the diagnosis can be established by aortography.[16] REASON: Because there is no forward flow in the ascending aorta, the coronary arteries are supplied by retrograde flow of blood through the ascending aorta. Consequently, on aortography the hypoplastic ascending aorta and coronary arteries opacify. For aortography, contrast medium can be injected into the descending aorta through an umbilical catheter or, in retrograde fashion, through either brachial artery. The identification of coarctation of the aorta is important before cardiac operation.

Although aortography establishes the status of the aortic valve, the status of the mitral valve can be assessed only by selective injection into the left atrium.

1. The descending aorta is less densely opacified than the ascending aorta (Fig 50–8). REASON: The contrast medium in the descending aorta is diluted by blood flow through the reversing patent ductus arteriosus.

2. The ascending aorta is severely hypoplastic (see

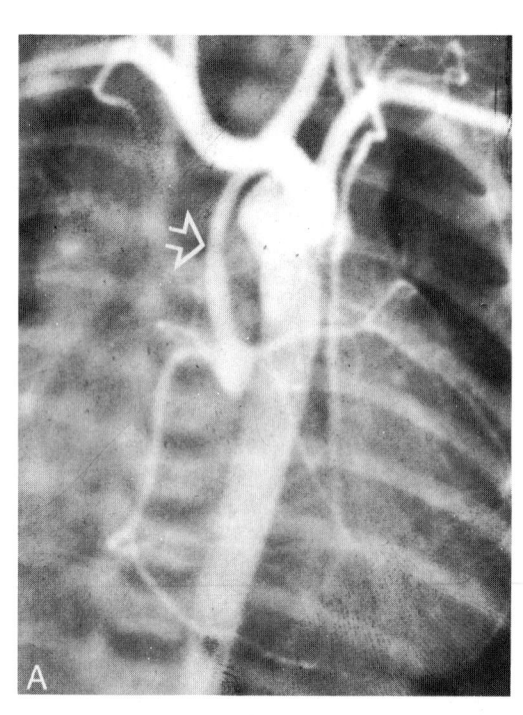

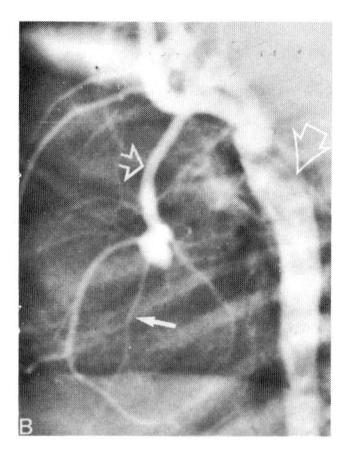

FIG 50–8.
Aortic atresia. Retrograde aortogram via left subclavian artery. **A,** anteroposterior projection. Descending aorta is larger than aortic arch. Dilution of contrast medium because of reversing patent ductus arteriosus. Brachiocephalic vessels are densely opacified because there is no dilution by forward flow through ascending aorta. Severely hypoplastic ascending aorta *(open arrow)*. Opacification of coronary arteries occurs densely by retrograde flow through the hypoplastic ascending aorta. REASON: No dilution by contrast medium by antegrade flow through aortic valve. **B,** lateral projection. Well-developed aortic sinuses. Severely hypoplastic aortic annulus. Left anterior descending coronary artery projects posteriorly to right coronary artery *(solid arrow)* because small size of left ventricular mass. Dilution of contrast medium in descending aorta by reversing patent ductus *(open arrow)*.

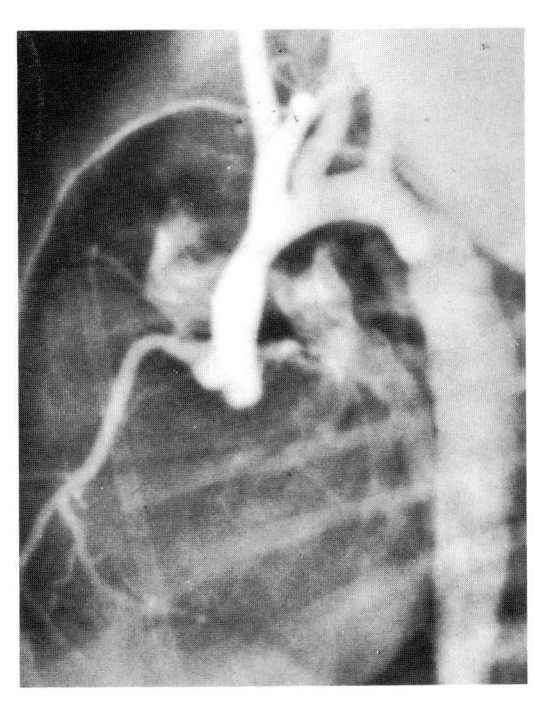

FIG 50–9.
Aortic atresia. Retrograde aortogram. Lateral projection. Ascending aorta shows only moderate hypoplasia. Aortic sinuses are well developed. This angiographic appearance is rare.

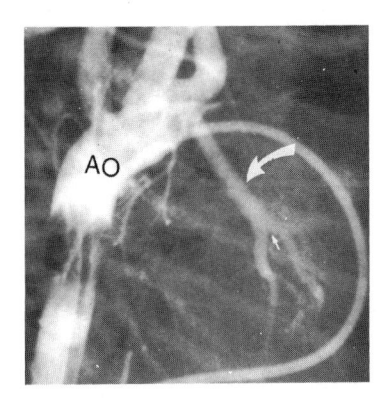

FIG 50–10.
Aortic atresia. Balloon occlusion aortography. Right anterior oblique projection. Ascending aorta *(AO)* is well opacified *(curved arrow)*. Coronary arteries are a direct continuation of ascending aorta because of the absence of sinuses of Valsalva *(small arrow)*.

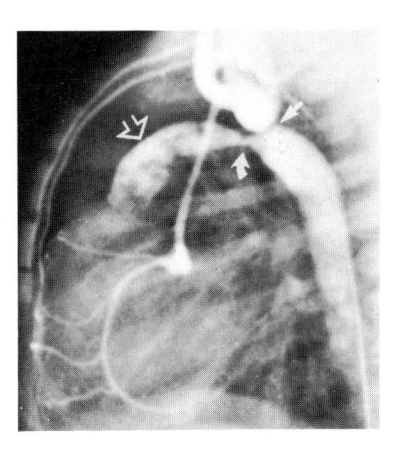

FIG 50–11.
Aortic atresia and coarctation of aorta *(arrows)*. Aortogram. Lateral projection. Pulmonary artery *(open arrow)* is partially opacified by small closing patent ductus arteriosus *(curved arrow)*. Severe coarctation of aorta *(solid arrow)* with unusually severe hypoplasia of ascending aorta.

Fig 50–8). REASON: The ascending aorta carries only the blood supply to the coronary arteries. In aortic atresia, the ascending aorta has also been called "common coronary artery," because its size corresponds to the combined caliber of right and left coronary arteries.

3. The right coronary artery and its branches to the right ventricle follow a sweeping and stretched course, indicating marked right ventricular enlargement. On a lateral projection the left anterior descending coronary artery is projected far posterior to the right coronary artery (see Fig 50–8). REASON: Small left ventricle.

4. The degree of hypoplasia of the sinuses of Valsalva (Fig 50–9) and of the ascending aorta is variable.

5. Rarely, there is only mild hypoplasia of the ascending aorta and a normal development of the sinuses of Valsalva (see Fig 50–9).

6. The sinuses of Valsalva may be completely absent (Fig 50–10).

7. If coarctation of the aorta coexists (Fig 50–11), perfusion of the coronary arteries and brachiocephalic vessels may be at risk.

8. There is a spectrum from clinical aortic atresia with severe hypoplasia of the ascending aorta to critical aortic stenosis with well-developed ascending aorta and hypoplasia of the left ventricle. Angiographic visualization of the left ventricle (Fig 50–12) is essential to determine the type of operative procedure.

9. The right ventricle is invariably enlarged and hypertrophied. REASON: The right ventricle carries the entire pulmonary and systemic blood flow, and, in addition, there is usually increased pulmonary blood flow because of a left-to-right shunt (Fig 50–13) at the atrial level. Furthermore, pulmonary hypertension is present.

10. The descending aorta opacifies through a reversing patent ductus arteriosus after injection into either the right ventricle or pulmonary artery (see Fig 50–13). The angiographic appearance could be misinterpreted as truncus arteriosus, but the ascending aorta opacifies.

11. The left ventricle is almost never opacified. REASON: Aortic atresia is commonly associated with mitral atresia, and the left ventricle is diminutive in size. Even if the mitral valve is patent, there is no significant inflow of

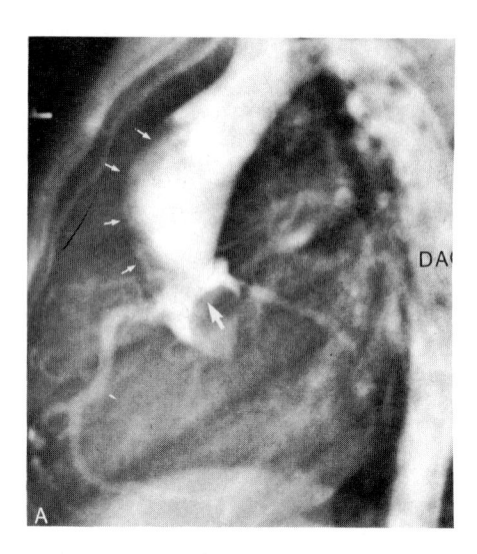

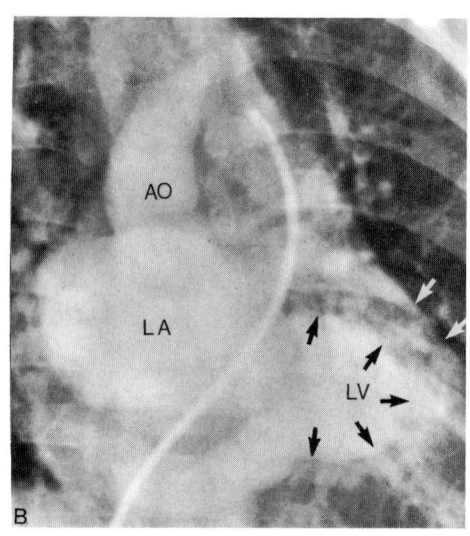

FIG 50-12.
Critical aortic stenosis and reversing patent ductus arteriosus. **A,** retrograde aortogram. Lateral projection. Aortic valve domes *(arrow)* and some dilution in ascending aorta *(small arrows),* indicating critical aortic stenosis. Dilution of contrast medium in descending aorta *(DAO)* from reversing patent ductus arteriosus. Poststenotic dilatation of ascending aorta. **B,** pulmonary arteriogram. Late phase. Anteroposterior projection. Enlarged left atrium *(LA)*. Severely hypoplastic and thick-walled left ventricle *(LV) (arrows)*. Contracted type of endocardial fibroelastosis. *AO* = aorta. (see Chapter 56).

blood. Rarely, a catheter can be passed through the mitral valve into the left ventricle. The selective injection of the left ventricle may demonstrate coronary arteries filling through myocardial sinusoids.

12. With a patent and hypoplastic mitral valve, left ventricular opacification may occur after a left atrial injection (Fig 50-14).

13. Rarely, with either severe hypoplasia or critical stenosis of the mitral and aortic valves, the left ventricle may be fairly well developed (Fig 50-15).

14. Endocardial fibroelastosis is present in most patients as evidenced by a smooth, round very thick-walled left ventricle (see Figs 50-12 and 50-15).

15. If the aortic valve is stenotic rather than atretic, the size of the left ventricle must be determined to make operative decisions.

16. Rarely, aortic atresia coexists with a ventricular septal defect. Under such circumstances, the left ventricle may be well developed and not hypoplastic (Fig 50-16) because of blood flows back and forth through ventricular communication.

OPERATIVE CONSIDERATIONS

Most forms of hypoplastic left ventricle syndrome are fatal within the first month of life, and the results of palliative operations have been dismal. There has been, however, renewed interest in operative palliation, and different approaches are being developed at a few centers.

These patients are extremely ill and require extensive treatment of their cardiac failure and complications of inadequate perfusion. Digitalis or other inotropic agents are given to improve myocardial contractility, and a diuretic is administered to treat edema and improve renal output. Acidosis, if present, is corrected. Efforts are made to maintain ductal patency by administering prostaglandin E_1[17] and limiting the oxygen concentration of inspired air. Usually the infant's airway is intubated and mechanically ventilated.

Two operative approaches have been used. In one, three features of the circulation are considered: (1) maintain systemic perfusion, (2) protect the pulmonary vascular bed, and (3) reduce pulmonary venous pressure. Systemic perfusion can be maintained by one of three operative approaches: (1) right ventricular to descending aortic conduit, (2) pulmonary arterial to descending aortic conduit, and (3) anastomosis of divided main pulmonary artery to ascending aorta and aortic arch (Norwood operation) (Fig 50-17). In the latter, pulmonary arterial perfusion is maintained through a Gortex graft from the aortic arch to the confluence of the pulmonary arteries. In the first two approaches, pulmonary arterial banding is applied to limit pulmonary blood flow and pulmonary arterial pressure. An atrial septal defect must be created during either cardiac catheterization or operation to decompress the pulmonary venous system. In a modification of the classic Norwood operation, the pulmonary artery and descending aorta are connected by a graft (Fig 50-18,A).

A second stage is eventually necessary to complete the

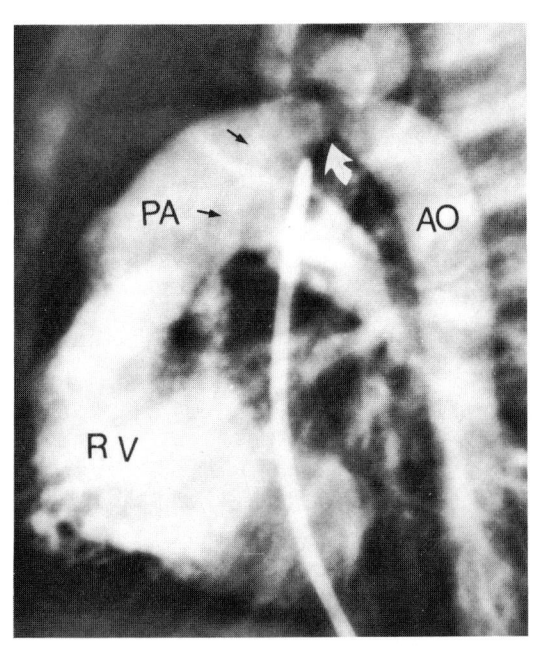

FIG 50–13.
Aortic atresia. Right superior vena cavogram. Lateral projection. Descending aorta opacifies via slightly stenotic patent ductus *(curved arrow)*. Angiographic appearance could be misinterpreted as truncus arteriosus, but diminutive aorta *(arrows)* is seen through pulmonary arterial *(PA)* density. *AO* = descending aorta; *RV* = right ventricle.

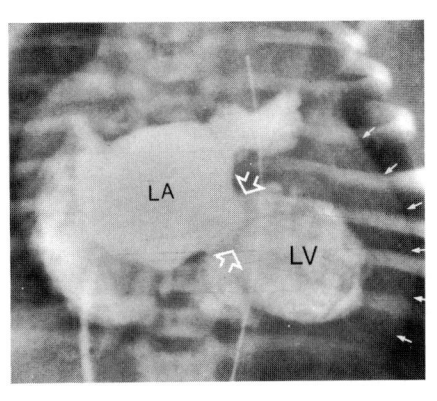

FIG 50–15.
Aortic atresia. Left atriogram. Anteroposterior projection. Left atrium *(LA)* and left ventricle *(LV)* fairly well developed. Mild hypoplasia of mitral annulus *(open arrows)*. Smooth rounded left ventricle and markedly increased wall thickness *(arrows)* indicate associated endocardial fibroelastosis.

palliation. A modified Fontan procedure is performed, diverting the systemic venous return to the pulmonary arteries and inserting an interatrial baffle to send pulmonary venous blood through the tricuspid valve. The second stage of the operation is performed after pulmonary resistance has declined to normal levels. These procedures carry a high operative risk,[18, 19] and few patients have survived both stages. Because of the exceedingly high risk separation of the circulation is carried out in steps. First, a modified Glenn operation is performed (see Fig 50–18), which is followed by an intra-atrial baffle (modified Fontan operation) (see Fig 50-18,C).

Another approach is neonatal cardiac transplantation. A limited number of neonates have been so treated, and both short- and long-term follow-up needs to be evaluated.

POSTOPERATIVE FEATURES

After a successful operation there may be considerable decrease in cardiac size (Fig 50–19). Angiography dem-

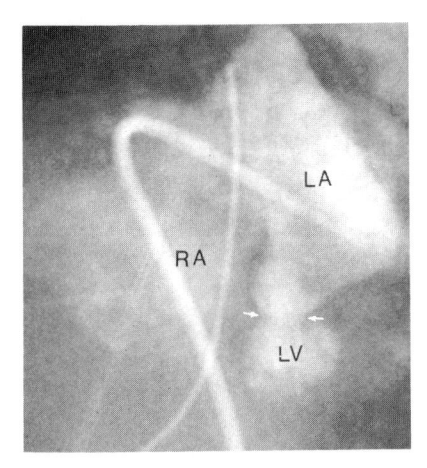

FIG 50–14.
Aortic atresia. Left atriogram. Left anterior oblique projection with cranial beam angulation. Large atrial communication. Left atrium *(LA)* is therefore well developed. Hypoplastic mitral annulus *(arrows)*. Diminutive left ventricle *(LV)*. Right atrium *(RA)* opacifies because of large left-to-right atrial shunt.

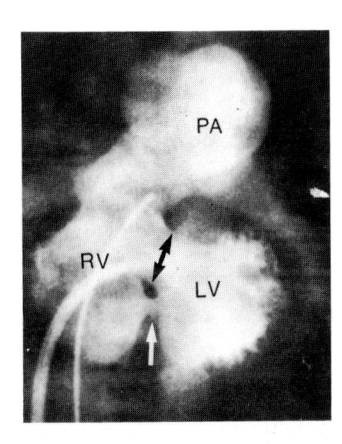

FIG 50–16.
Aortic atresia and ventricular septal defect. Left ventriculogram *(LV)* via cathether passed through a large, membranous ventricular septal defect *(black arrows)*. Left anterior oblique projection. Additional smaller communication *(white arrow)* in muscular septum. Normal-sized left ventricle. No angiographic features of endocardial fibroelastosis. *PA* = pulmonary artery; *RV* = right ventricle.

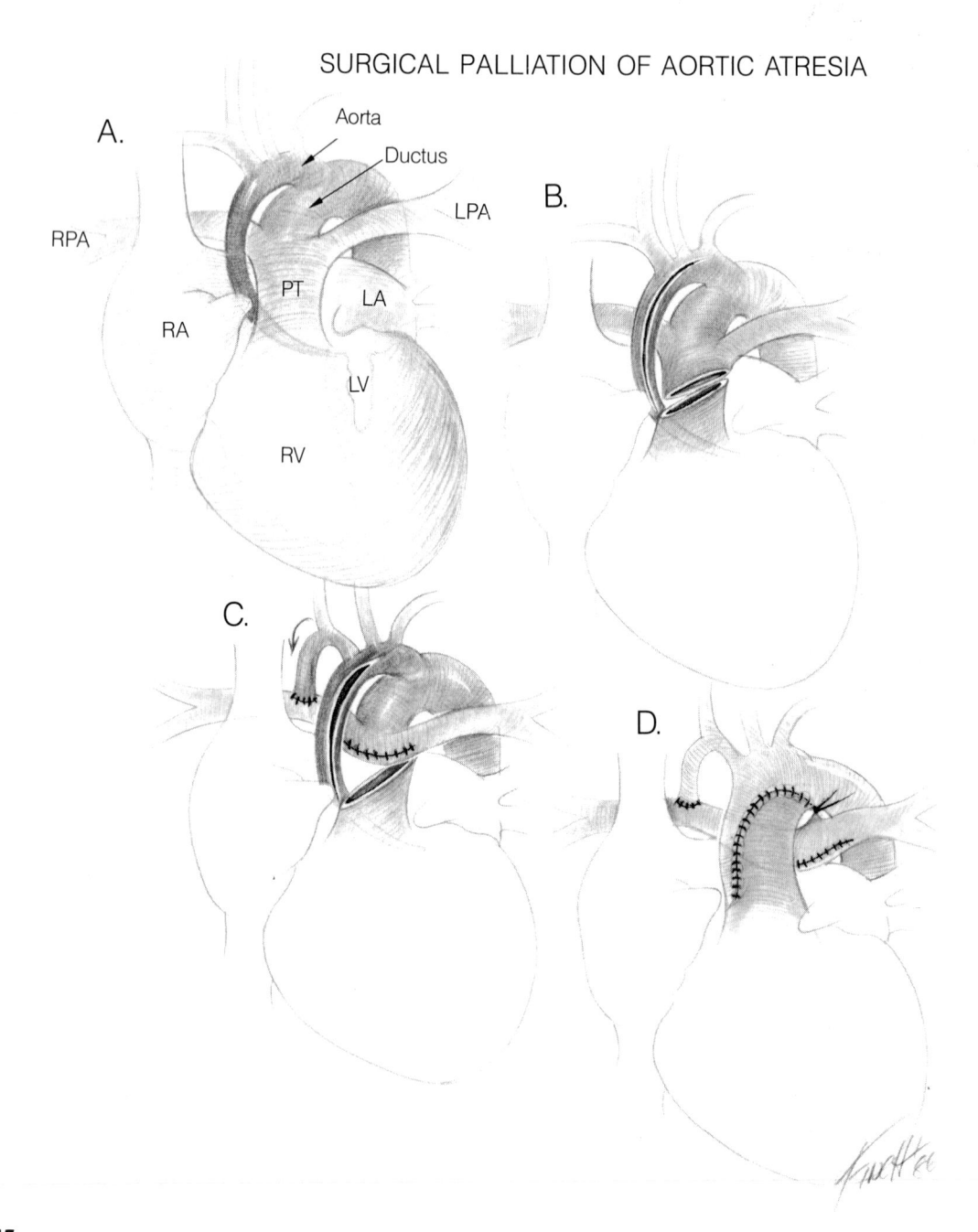

FIG 50-17.
Operative palliation of aortic atresia (Norwood procedure). **A,** external anatomy of aortic atresia. **B,** atrial septum has been excised. Longitudinal incision made in ascending aorta. Main pulmonary artery divided. **C,** distal end of pulmonary artery is oversewn. Right Blalock-Taussig shunt or Gortex shunt is performed. **D,** connection made between proximal pulmonary artery and ascending aorta. Ductus arteriosus ligated. *LA* = left atrium; *LPA* = left pulmonary artery; *LV* = left ventricle; *PT* = pulmonary trunk; *RA* = right atrium; *RPA* = right pulmonary artery; *RV* = right ventricle.

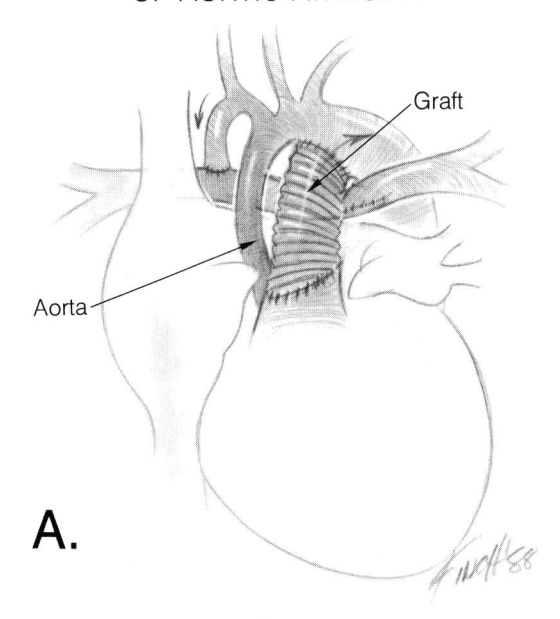

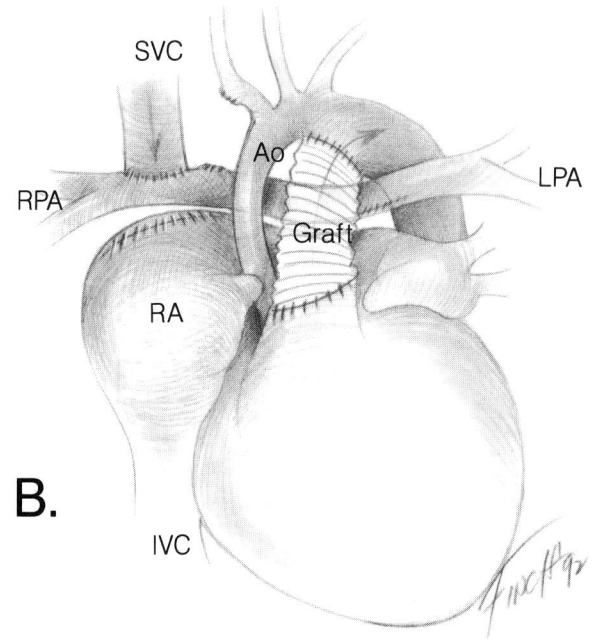

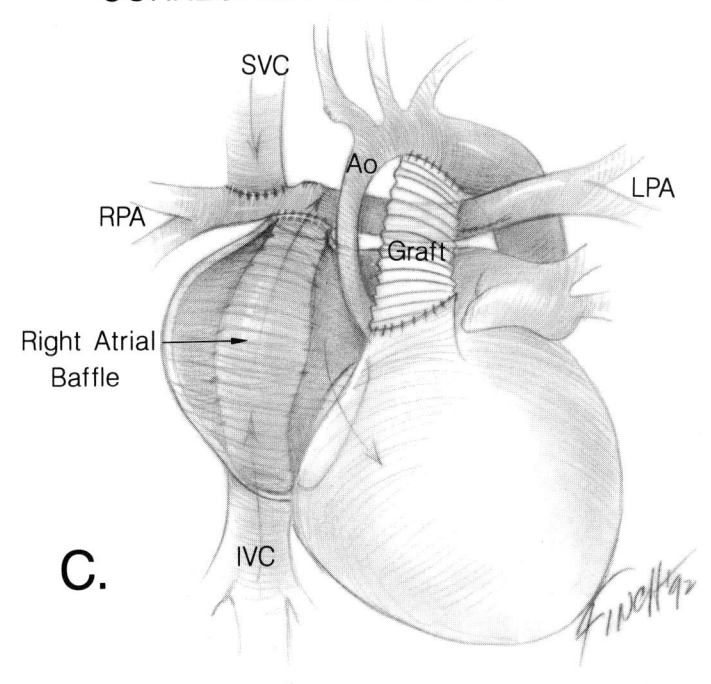

VARIATION OF SURGICAL CORRECTION OF AORTIC ATRESIA

A.

2nd STAGE OF SURGICAL CORRECTION OF AORTIC ATRESIA

B.

3rd STAGE OF SURGICAL CORRECTION OF AORTIC ATRESIA

C.

FIG 50–18.
A, modified Norwood operation. Hypoplastic ascending aorta is not used in repair because aortic size is adequate to carry coronary flow. Instead, pulmonary artery is connected to descending aorta by a graft. **B**, second stage of correction of aortic atresia: the Blalock anastomosis is taken down and the superior vena cava is anastomosed end-to-side to the right pulmonary artery (modified Glenn operation). **C**, third stage results in complete seperation of the circulation: an intraatrial baffle is sewn to the inferior vena cava and right pulmonary artery. Consequently, the patient is no longer cyanotic.

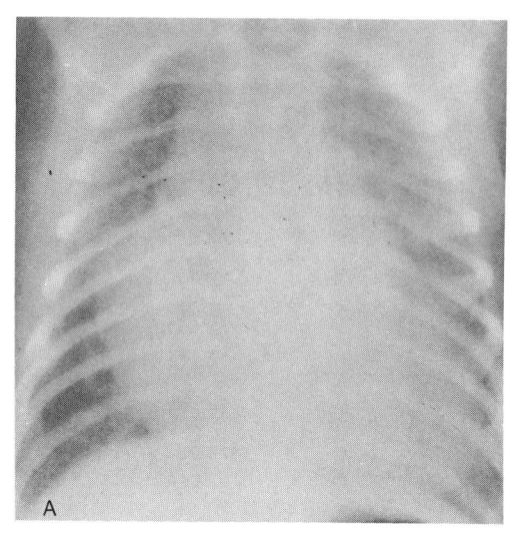

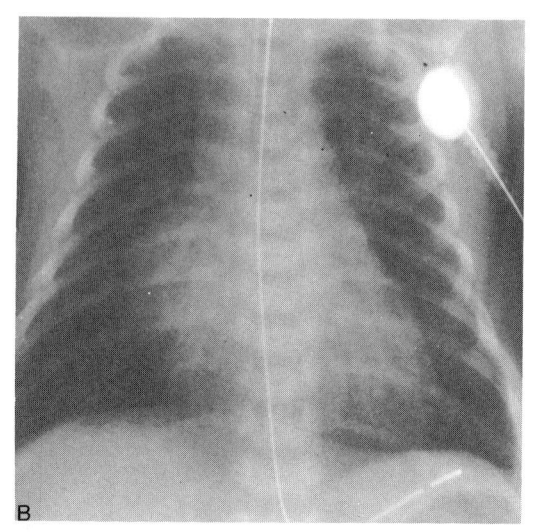

FIG 50-19.
Aortic atresia. Thoracic roentgenogram. Anteroposterior projections. **A,** before Norwood operation. Severe cardiomegaly and increased pulmonary arterial vasculature and congestion. **B,** 1 month after operation. Cardiac size has decreased. Pulmonary vasculature has improved.

onstrates the hemodynamic features of the Norwood operation (Fig 50-20).

PREMATURE CLOSURE OF LORAMEN

In 10% of patients with a hypoplastic left ventricle, the atrial septum is intact. This is called "premature closure of the foramen ovale." Presumably the underdevelopment of the left atrium and left ventricle has occurred from lack of blood flow from right-to-left atrium. Postnatally because the foramen ovale is closed, blood flow cannot occur from left to right. Such patients show striking pulmonary lymphangectasis and alternative routes for pulmonary venous return, such as levoatrial cardinal vein, left atrial-coronary sinus window, or partial anomalous pulmonary venous connection.

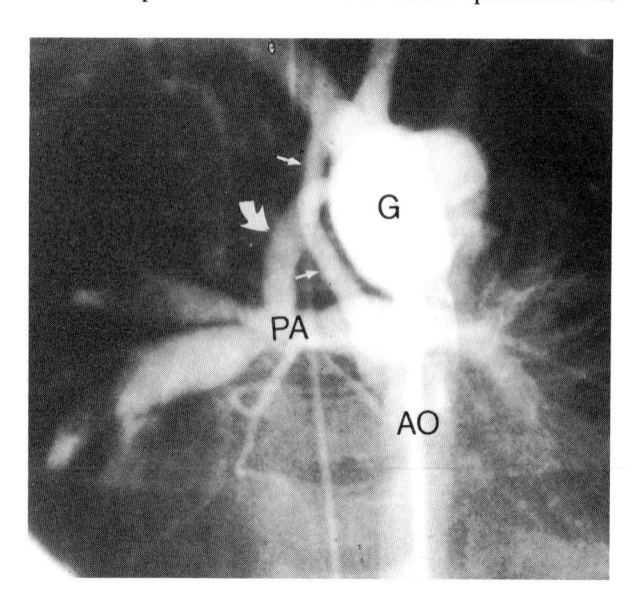

FIG 50-20.
Modified Norwood operation. Aortogram (AO). Anteroposterior projection. Catheter passed from descending aorta into main pulmonary artery via graft (G). Hypoplastic ascending aorta is not used in repair (small arrows). Pulmonary arteries (PA) opacify via central Gortex shunt (curved arrow) (Courtesy of Dr. H. Katkov). Graft is attached to descending aorta, bridging an area of coarctation, if present.

REFERENCES

1. Kanjuh VI, Eliot RS, Edwards JE: Coexistent mitral and aortic valvular atresia: a pathologic study of 14 cases, Am J Cardiol 15:611, 1965.
2. van der Horst RL, Hastreiter AR, DuBrow IW, et al: Pathologic measurements in aortic atresia, Am Heart J 106:1411, 1983.
3. Raghib G, Bloemendaal RD, Kanjuh VI, et al: Aortic atresia and premature closure of foramen ovale: myocardial sinusoids and coronary arteriovenous fistula serving as outflow channel, Am Heart J 70:476, 1965.
4. O'Connor WN, Cash JB, Cottrill CM, et al: Ventriculocoronary connections in hypoplastic left hearts: an autopsy microscopic study, Circulation 66:1078, 1982.
5. Von Rueden TJ, Knight L, Moller JH, et al: Coarctation of the aorta associated with aortic valvular atresia, Circulation 52:951, 1975.
6. Mahowald JM, Lucas RV Jr, Edwards JE: Aortic valvular atresia: associated cardiovascular anomalies, Pediatr Cardiol 2:99, 1982.
7. Lucas RV Jr, Lester RG, Lillehei CW, et al: Mitral atresia with levoatriocardinal vein: a form of congenital pulmonary venous obstruction, Am J Cardiol 9:607, 1962.

8. Shone JD, Edwards JE: Mitral atresia associated with pulmonary venous anomalies, *Br Heart J* 26:241, 1964.
9. Neumann MP, Heidelberger KP, Dick M II, et al: Pulmonary vascular changes associated with hypoplastic left ventricle syndrome, *Pediatr Cardiol* 1:301, 1980.
10. Bass JL, Berry JM, Einzig S: Flow in the aorta and patent ductus arteriosus in infants with aortic atresia or aortic stenosis: a pulsed Doppler ultrasound study, *Circulation* 74:315, 1986.
11. Krovetz LJ, Rowe RD, Scheibler GL: Hemodynamics of aortic valve atresia, *Circulation* 42:953, 1970.
12. Von Rueden TH, Moller JH: The electrocardiogram in aortic valvular atresia, *Chest* 73:66, 1978.
13. Farooki ZQ, Henry JG, Green EW: Echocardiographic spectrum of the hypoplastic left heart syndrome: a clinicopathologic correlation in 19 newborns, *Am J Cardiol* 38:337, 1976.
14. Covitz W, Rao PS, Strong WR, et al: Echocardiographic assessment of the aortic root in syndromes with left ventricular hypoplasia, *Pediatr Cardiol* 2:19, 1982.
15. Hastreiter AR, van der Horst RL, DuBrow IW, et al: Quantitative angiographic and morphologic aspects of aortic valve atresia, *Am J Cardiol* 51:1705, 1983.
16. Rosengart R, Jarmakani JM, Emmanouilides GC: Single film retrograde umbilical aortography in the diagnosis of hypoplastic left heart syndrome with aortic atresia, *Circulation* 54:345, 1976.
17. Hastreiter AR, van der Horst RL, Sepehri B, et al: Prostaglandin E_1 infusion in newborns with hypoplastic left ventricle and aortic atresia, *Pediatr Cardiol* 2:95, 1982.
18. Norwood WI, Lang P, Hansen DD: Physiologic repair of aortic atresia–hypoplastic left heart syndrome, *N Engl J Med* 308:23, 1983.
19. Lang P, Norwood WI: Hemodynamic assessment after palliative surgery for hypoplastic left heart syndrome, *Circulation* 68:104, 1983.

CHAPTER 51

Mitral Atresia

In this chapter, mitral atresia with normal aortic root is discussed. This chapter distinguishes this anomaly from the more commonly occurring condition in which mitral atresia coexists with aortic atresia or stenosis. The hemodynamics and clinical and laboratory features differ significantly, depending on whether the aortic valve is patent or not. Mitral atresia coexisting with aortic atresia is discussed in Chapter 50.

PATHOLOGIC ANATOMY

The basic anatomic feature of mitral atresia is absence of mitral valvar structures on the floor of the left atrium.[1] The site of the mitral valve may be represented by a dimple. No blood flows directly from the left atrium into the left ventricle. The left atrium is small, is thick walled, and communicates with an enlarged right atrium through a foramen ovale (most often) or secundum atrial septal defect. In the former there may be an aneurysm of the septum primum that bulges toward the right atrium.[2] Rarely, other connections are present through which blood exits the left atrium. These include a levoatrial cardinal vein (see Chapter 50) from left atrium or pulmonary veins to the left subclavian vein,[3] a fenestration in the coronary sinus (see Chapter 20), or a coexistent partial anomalous pulmonary venous connection.[4, 5]

The anatomic details of the ventricles and great vessels show considerable variation.[1, 6] Mitral atresia may coexist with either two ventricles or a single ventricle. The great vessels may show various relationships: (1) normally related (concordant); (2) transposed (discordant); (3) both great vessels arising from the right ventricle (double outlet); or (4) a single arterial outlet, such as coexistent pulmonary atresia or truncus arteriosus. A right aortic arch may be present.

The tricuspid valve is large and enters a large and hypertrophied right ventricle. In one fourth of the cases, the ventricular septum is intact, and a left ventricle is not identifiable. In such cases both great vessels originate from the right ventricle. In the remaining cases, a ventricular septal defect is present through which the right ventricle communicates with a small or hypoplastic left ventricle. Mitral atresia may coexist with a straddling tricuspid valve, in which case the left ventricle is more fully developed.[1] Rarely, the left ventricle is normal size, and either the aortic or pulmonary artery arises from this chamber, resulting in either normally related (concordant) or transposed (discordant) great vessels. Subaortic stenosis or subpulmonary stenosis may be present, respectively, if narrowing of the ventricular defect or reduction in size of the outlet chamber develops.

Other forms of outflow obstruction may coexist. When the great vessels are normally related and the aorta arises from a hypoplastic left ventricle, coarctation of the aorta or interruption of the aortic arch may coexist. If the great vessels are transposed or both arise from the right ventricle, pulmonary stenosis or atresia may occur. Mitral atresia and pulmonary atresia rarely occur with normally related great vessels.

A hemodynamic pattern similar to mitral atresia may result in patients with congenitally corrected transposition of the great vessels and left (tricuspid) valve atresia (discordant atrioventricular and ventriculoarterial connections). The anatomic details of such an anomaly are more fully discussed in Chapter 39.

HEMODYNAMICS

The hemodynamics are much more variable than among patients with aortic atresia and depend on the ease with which blood can exit the left atrium and the presence and type of coexistent conditions.

Basically mitral atresia is an admixture lesion, because the entire pulmonary venous return passes into the right atrium and mixes with the entire systemic venous return. Thus, aortic and pulmonary arterial oxygen saturations are equal. Like other admixture lesions, the degree of arterial desaturation is inversely related to the volume of pulmonary blood flow. Pulmonary blood flow may be limited by either pulmonary venous obstruction or pulmonary stenosis; both may result from a variety of anomalies.

If the foramen ovale is widely patent and no pulmonary stenosis exists, the volume of pulmonary blood flow is greatly increased and the patient is minimally cyanotic. Because of the large volume of pulmonary blood flow, the volume overload of the ventricle may lead to congestive cardiac failure. When pulmonary stenosis coexists, pulmonary blood flow is limited, and on a thoracic radiograph the pulmonary vascular markings may appear decreased. Cyanosis is more intense in these patients.

Cyanosis is also more intense in those patients in whom the flow from the left atrium is limited because the foramen ovale is narrowed (Fig 51–1). Left atrial pressure is elevated, pulmonary venous obstruction exists, leading to pulmonary edema and pulmonary arterial hypertension. In this circumstance, blood may pass by alternative routes such as levoatrial cardinal vein, anomalous pulmonary venous connection, or left atrial–coronary sinus fenestration. These escape routes, except for coronary sinus fenestration, are usually ineffective in decompressing the left atrium and lowering its pressure.

The entire venous return to the heart enters the right ventricle or common ventricle. In this chamber a systemic level of pressure is generated, and aortic and pulmonary arterial pressures are equal unless outflow tract obstruction occurs. If subaortic stenosis is present, aortic pressure is normal, but systolic pressure is elevated above systemic levels in the ventricle proximal to the obstruction. If pulmonary stenosis or atresia coexists, pulmonary arterial pressure is normal and the volume of pulmonary blood flow is limited. If the pulmonary valve is normal, as pulmonary vascular resistance decreases in the neonatal period, pulmonary blood flow increases, and therefore the pulmonary venous return increases. This accentuates the pulmonary venous obstruction or causes congestive cardiac failure. Both are further accentuated if aortic obstruction coexists.

CLINICAL FEATURES

Mitral atresia occurs equally in males and females[7, 8] in contrast to a male predominance in aortic atresia. There

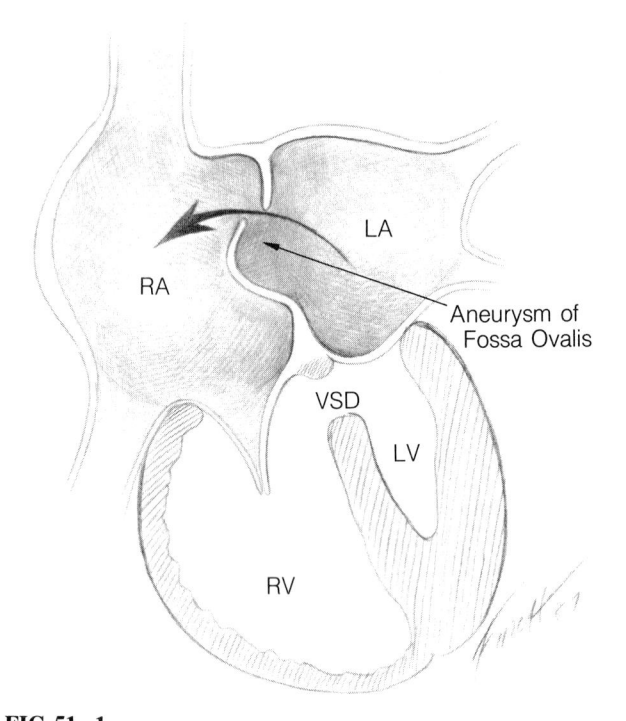

FIG 51–1.
Mitral atresia. Central circulation. Shunt occurs from left atrium *(LA)* to right atrium *(RA)* through foramen ovale or atrial septal defect. If foramen ovale represents only egress of blood from left atrium, an aneurysm of fossa ovalis may be present. Entire systemic and pulmonary blood flows pass into right ventricle *(RV)*. Blood enters left ventricle *(LV)* through a ventricular septal defect *(VSD)*. From ventricles blood is ejected into great vessels.

is also a broader age range and a longer life span on the average for mitral atresia compared with aortic atresia. Yet most patients die in infancy.

The initial symptom is cyanosis, which usually appears during the first week of life, but neither cyanosis or other symptoms may appear until several months of age.[7, 8] The presence of cardiac failure or a murmur may be the initial presenting symptom. The usual presenting symptoms are cyanosis, dyspnea, and low cardiac output. Patients who survive show growth failure and congestive cardiac failure. Definite cyanosis and cyanotic spells are found in patients with associated pulmonary stenosis.

The cardiac findings are nonspecific, and the auscultatory findings do not correlate well with the coexistent cardiac malformations. The second heart sound is often loud and single. Most patients have a murmur. In our experience, these have generally been loud (grade 3–4/6).

The pulse and blood pressure in the leg are decreased in infants with coexistent coarctation of the aorta. Hepatomegaly and other findings of cardiac failure are present in patients without pulmonary stenosis. The clinical findings vary so much that the correct diagnosis is not suspected on clinical grounds alone.

ELECTROCARDIOGRAPHIC FEATURES

There is usually right-axis deviation, right atrial enlargement, and right ventricular hypertrophy. The T waves are usually normal.

ECHOCARDIOGRAPHIC FEATURES

Several of the features resemble aortic atresia. The right atrium and right ventricle are enlarged, whereas the left atrium and left ventricle are small. The details of the mitral valve may be difficult to define because of the hypoplasia of the mitral structures. The atretic mitral valve tissue may move and appear to open. However, no flow is noted across the mitral valve by Doppler. The atrial septum bulges to the right and may show herniation of the valve of the foramen ovale. The origin and anatomy of both great vessels must be identified.

RADIOGRAPHIC FEATURES

The radiographic findings in mitral atresia are extremely variable because of the great variety of associated cardiac anomalies resulting in various hemodynamic states. Thus, the diagnosis cannot be suspected radiographically.

CARDIAC CATHETERIZATION

Although echocardiography can usually establish the diagnosis of mitral atresia, assess the status of the atrial septum, and identify the position of the great vessels and associated outflow obstruction, cardiac catheterization is useful in determining left atrial pressure and in performing balloon atrial septostomy.

The catheter may be passed into the left atrium but cannot be passed from that site into the left ventricle. Through the tricuspid valve, the catheter may be advanced from the right ventricle into both great vessels. The catheter position observed in the anteroposterior and lateral projections allows identification of coexistent transposition of the great vessels.

Oximetry data show an increase in oxygen saturation in the right atrium. This increase is usually large, and no further increase occurs in the ventricle or great vessel, because the pulmonary venous blood mixes in the right atrium. An increase in oxygen saturation may be found in the superior vena cava system from fully saturated pulmonary venous blood entering through an anomalously connecting pulmonary vein or a levoatrial cardinal vein. Pulmonary venous blood may be desaturated if pulmonary edema interferes with oxygenation.

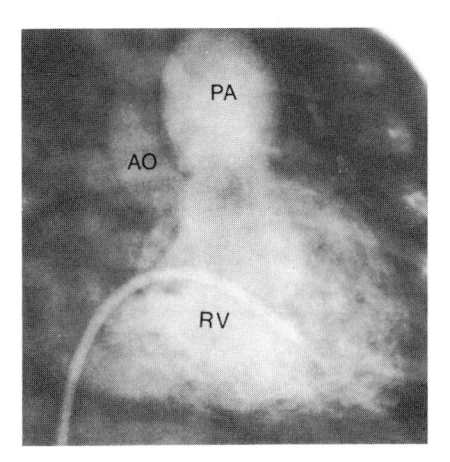

FIG 51–2.
Mitral atresia. Right ventriculogram. Anteroposterior projection. Markedly enlarged right ventricle *(RV)*. Both great vessels opacify simultaneously because pulmonary valve is patent. *AO* = aorta; *PA* = pulmonary artery.

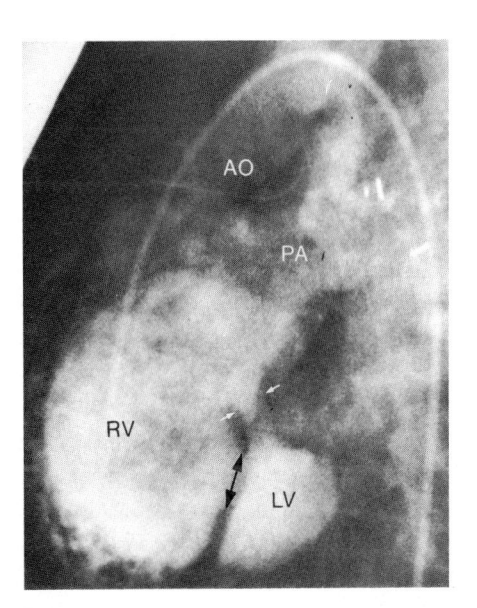

FIG 51–3.
Mitral atresia with transposition of great vessels. Right ventriculogram *(RV)*. Lateral projection. Catheter is passed in retrograde fashion through transposed aorta *(AO)*. Right ventricle is markedly enlarged. Hypoplastic left ventricle *(LV)* fills via ventricular septal defect *(white arrows)*. In spite of additional muscular ventricular communication *(black arrows)*, left ventricle shows significant hypoplasia. *PA* = pulmonary artery.

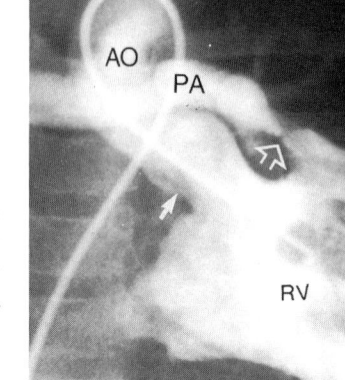

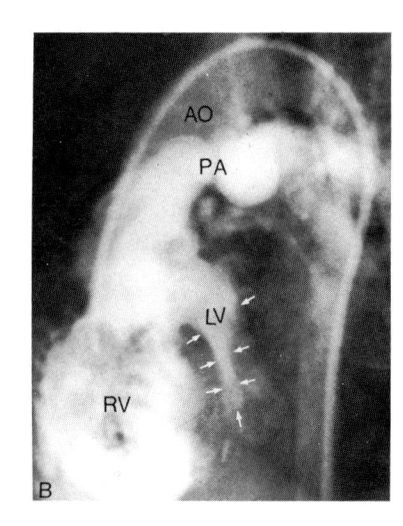

FIG 51–4.
Mitral atresia and infundibular *(open arrow)* pulmonary stenosis. Right ventriculogram *(RV)*. **A,** anteroposterior and, **B,** lateral projections. Aorta arises from an infundibulum as in double-outlet right ventricle *(arrow)*. **B,** large right ventricle and superimposition of aorta *(AO)* and pulmonary artery *(PA)*. Neither vessel is in continuity with atretic mitral valve. Diminutive left ventricle *(arrows)*.

Left atrial pressure is commonly elevated, often significantly to 25 to 30 mm Hg. The a wave may be prominent, indicating the restrictive nature of the foramen ovale. Right atrial pressure may be elevated.

Right ventricular systolic pressure equals aortic pressure unless there is subaortic stenosis from either a small ventricular septal defect or a hypoplastic left ventricle. Pulmonary arterial pressure is elevated unless pulmonary or subpulmonary stenosis is present, in which case pulmonary arterial pressure is low. A withdrawal pressure gradient is recorded.

During the cardiac catheterization, a balloon atrial septostomy should be performed. In the patients who become symptomatic beyond the neonatal period, the atrial septum is thickened, so a blade atrioseptostomy should be performed.

ANGIOGRAPHIC FEATURES

The complexity of congenital malformations associated with mitral atresia requires complete cardiac catheterization and selective angiography of various chambers. The diagnosis of mitral atresia is best established by selective injection into the left atrium. The levophase of a pulmonary arteriogram may be inadequate.

1. The right ventricle is markedly enlarged regardless of whether the great vessels are normally related or transposed (Fig 51–2). REASON: The hemodynamics resemble those of aortic atresia because the right ventricle ejects both the pulmonary and the systemic outputs. The entire cardiac output passes through right ventricle.

2. If the pulmonary valve is patent, as is common, both great vessels opacify simultaneously.

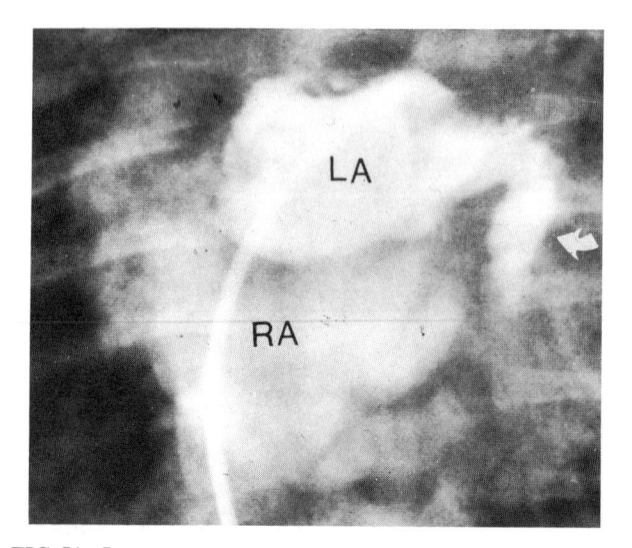

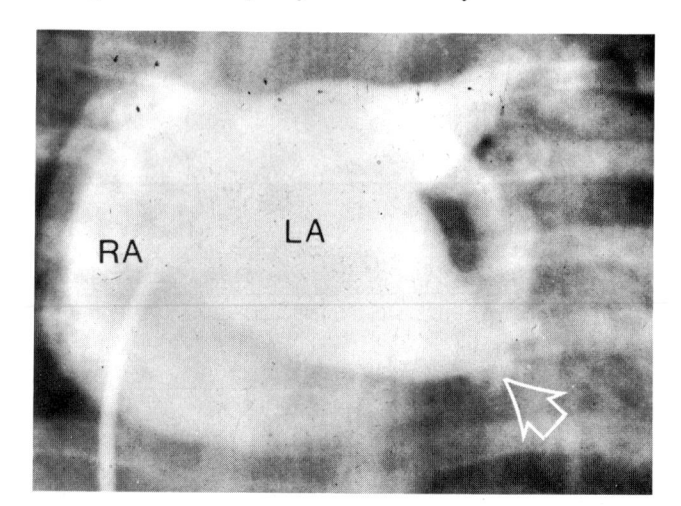

FIG 51–5.
Mitral atresia. Left atriogram. Anteroposterior projection. Left-to-right shunt at atrial level. Minimal hypoplasia left atrium *(LA)*. Atypical configuration of left atrial appendix *(arrow)*. RA = right atrium.

FIG 51–6.
Mitral atresia. Left atriogram *(LA)*. Anteroposterior projection. Dense obligatory left-to-right shunt at atrial level with opacification of right atrium *(RA)*. Because of nonobstructing atrial communication, left atrium is enlarged. Atretic mitral valve *(open arrow)*.

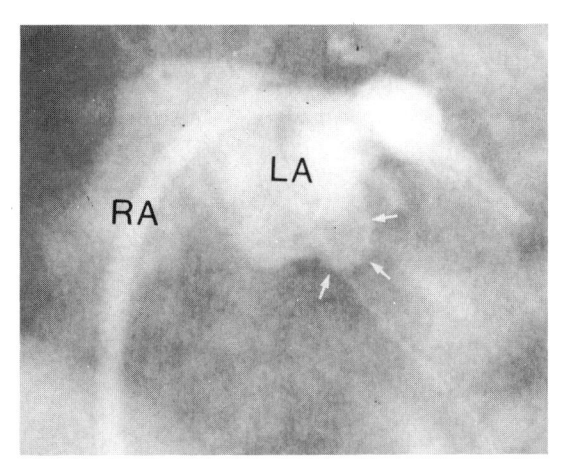

FIG 51-7.
Mitral atresia. Left atriogram *(LA)*. Anteroposterior projection. Catheter passed through atrial communication. Marked hypoplasia of left atrium. Catheter tip is in left atrial appendix. Atrial systole. Atretic mitral valve *(arrows)* bulges into left ventricle. RA = right atrium.

3. Typically the left ventricle is hypoplastic in spite of the presence of a ventricular septal defect (Fig 51-3).

4. The left ventricle may be diminutive in size, or it may not opacify at all (Fig 51-4).

5. Because of the small size of the left ventricle, both great vessels appear to arise from the right ventricle, and continuity between the aortic valve and mitral valve or pulmonary valve and mitral valve cannot be anatomically established. In most cases, therefore, a double-outlet right ventricle is present.

6. The diagnosis of double-outlet right ventricle becomes certain when double coni are present (see Fig 51-4).

7. Hypoplasia of the left side of the heart usually involves both the left atrium and the left ventricle (Fig 51-5).

8. Left atrial size largely depends on the volume of pulmonary flow and the degree of obstruction at the level of the atrial communication. If nonobstructive atrial septal defect is present, the left atrium may be of normal size or even enlarged (Fig 51-6).

9. The atretic mitral valve is best seen on a left anterior oblique projection after a left atrial injection. During diastole (atrial systole) the atretic mitral valve bulges into the left ventricle and forms a characteristic nipplelike density (Fig 51-7).

OPERATIVE CONSIDERATIONS

Intensive medical management is required. While the patient is being investigated, an atrial septal defect should be created by catheter techniques.[9, 10] If it is unsuccessful, a Blalock-Hanlon procedure can be carried out.

After this, patients without pulmonary stenosis should undergo pulmonary artery banding to reduce the volume of pulmonary blood flow and improve the congestive cardiac failure.[9, 10] If a coarctation of the aorta coexists, it should be treated by balloon angioplasty or surgically, because this decreases systemic impedance and also reduces pul-

SURGICAL CORRECTION OF MITRAL ATRESIA

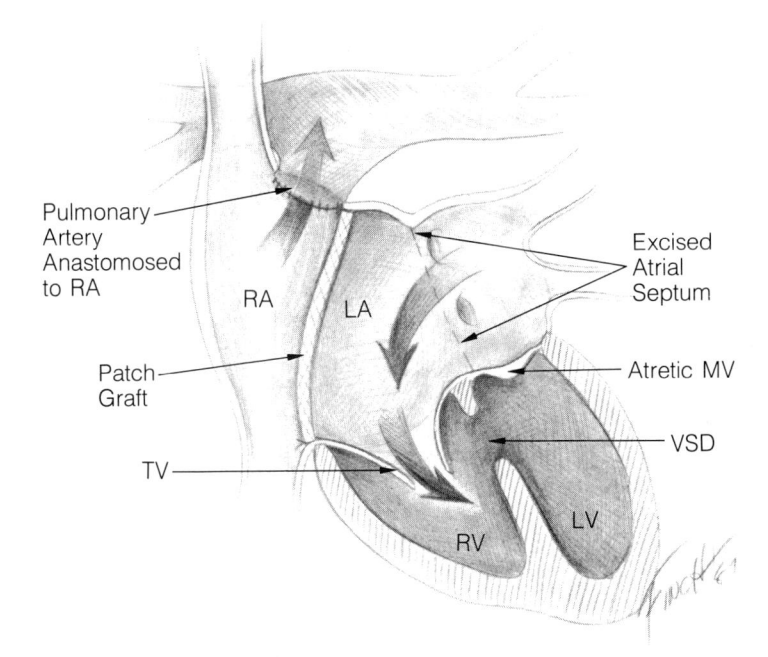

FIG 51-8.
Operative correction. Modified Fontan procedure. Atrial septum is excised. Patch is placed into atrium to separate atria, allowing pulmonary venous blood to flow through tricuspid valve *(TV)* into right ventricle *(RV)*. Right atrium *(RA)* anastomosed to pulmonary artery, allowing systemic blood flow into pulmonary circulation. LA = left atrium; LV = left ventricle; MV = mitral valve; VSD = ventricular septal defect.

monary blood flow. Patients with coexistent pulmonary stenosis may have few symptoms but may require an operatively created systemic-pulmonary arterial shunt.[9,10]

Ultimately these patients may be candidates for a modified Fontan procedure (right atrial–pulmonary arterial anastomosis). This is combined with partitioning of the right atrium with a patch so vena caval blood passes into the pulmonary arteries, and pulmonary venous blood passes through the tricuspid valve and ultimately to the aorta (Fig 51–8).

REFERENCES

1. Gittenberger-de Groot AC, Wenink ACG: Mitral atresia: morphological details, *Br Heart J* 51:252, 1984.
2. Eliot RS, Shone JD, Kanjuh VI, et al: Mitral atresia: a study of 32 cases, *Am Heart J* 70:6, 1965.
3. Lucas RV Jr, Lester RG, Lillehei CW, et al: Mitral atresia with levoatriocardinal vein: a form of congenital pulmonary venous obstruction, *Am J Cardiol* 9:607, 1962.
4. Shone JD, Edwards JE: Mitral atresia associated with pulmonary venous anomalies, *Br Heart J* 26:241, 1964.
5. Beckman CB, Moller JH, Edwards JE: CPC: alternate pathways to pulmonary venous flow in left-sided obstructive anomalies, *Circulation* 52:509, 1975.
6. Thiene G, Daliento L, Frescura C, et al: Atresia of left atrioventricular orifice: anatomical investigation in 62 cases, *Br Heart J* 45:393, 1981.
7. Moreno F, Quero M, Diaz LP: Mitral atresia with normal aortic valve: a study of eighteen cases and a review of the literature, *Circulation* 53:1004, 1976.
8. Watson DG, Rowe RD, Conen PE, et al: Mitral atresia with normal aortic valve: report of 11 cases and review of the literature, *Pediatrics* 25:450, 1960.
9. Mickell JJ, Mathews RA, Park SC, et al: Left atrioventricular valve atresia: clinical management, *Circulation* 61:123, 1980.
10. Shore D, Jones O, Rigby ML, et al: Atresia of left atrioventricular connection: surgical considerations, *Br Heart J* 47:35, 1982.

PART EIGHT

Cardiac Conditions Associated With Increased Pulmonary Venous Vasculature Without Cyanosis

Cardiac conditions in which the lung fields show a pattern of increased pulmonary venous vasculature can be divided into two categories: those producing cyanosis (discussed in Part VII) and those that do not show cyanosis. A difference between the two is that in the former, a communication, usually an atrial septal defect or, less commonly, a patent ductus arteriosus, is present that allows a right-to-left shunt. In conditions discussed in this section, such a communication is not present, and cyanosis does not develop unless pulmonary edema is superimposed.

Cardiac conditions with increased pulmonary venous vasculature without cyanosis can be divided into two categories depending on the site of the obstruction in relation to the mitral valve. Conditions located either at or proximal to the mitral valve are associated with normal cardiac size on a thoracic roentgenogram, and the electrocardiogram (ECG) shows isolated right ventricular hypertrophy. Conditions such as cardiomyopathy or left ventricular outflow obstruction located beyond the mitral valve cause pulmonary venous obstruction because of left ventricular failure. In these patients, cardiomegaly is present on a radiograph, and on the ECG left ventricular hypertrophy coexists with right ventricular hypertrophy.

Regardless of the anatomic cause or location of this obstruction, certain pathologic and clinical features are present because of the pressure elevation in each component of the pulmonary vascular system proximal to the obstruction.

In each of these conditions the pulmonary venous pressure is elevated. This is associated with thickening of the intima and media of the pulmonary veins for some distance into the lungs. With the elevation of pulmonary venous pressure, there is redistribution of pulmonary blood flow. In individuals without pulmonary venous obstruction, the major portion of the pulmonary blood flow is through the lower lobes, principally because of gravitational effects. Once pulmonary venous pressure exceeds 20 mm Hg, blood flow is redistributed toward the upper lobes. This is particularly related to changes in the relationship between pulmonary venous pressure and gravitational effects and perhaps by vasoconstriction of lower lobe vessels. The redistribution causes the upper lobe pulmonary veins to enlarge, which is manifested radiographically as cephalization (see Chapter 5).

Normally communications exist between the pulmonary and bronchial venous systems through which little flow occurs ordinarily. As a large pressure difference develops between the two, however, the communications enlarge. The bronchial veins enlarge and become tortuous because of the increased blood flow. If these become greatly enlarged, they may rupture into the bronchi and cause hemoptysis.

As a result of elevated pulmonary venous pressure, pulmonary capillary pressure is elevated. When capillary pressure exceeds the intravascular osmotic pressure, fluid and erythrocytes move into the alveoli. This gives a pattern of pulmonary edema on radiographs and clinical features of dyspnea and rales. Subpleural and intralobar lymphatics are dilated, and lymphatic flow may be several times normal. These dilated lymphatics may be evident radiographically as Kerley B lines.

Pulmonary arterial pressure is elevated by two mechanisms. The first occurs merely because pressure in the pulmonary artery has to increase to overcome pulmonary venous pressure. The second occurs through reflex pulmonary vasoconstriction. As a result, the pulmonary arterial segment is enlarged on a radiograph, and after a long duration of increased venous pressure, the proximal pulmonary arteries become tortuous and pruned. Elevated pulmonary arterial pressure results in a loud pulmonary component of the second heart sound.

Right ventricular systolic pressure is elevated, and, consequently, right ventricular hypertrophy is present, which can be recognized electrocardiographically and echocardiographically. If the pulmonary venous obstruction has been present from birth, congestive cardiac failure does not develop. Right atrial pressure may be elevated because of decreased right ventricular compliance secondary to hypertrophy. This may cause the foramen ovale to be stretched open and result in a right-to-left shunt.

Radiographically pulmonary venous obstruction can be recognized and its site in relation to the mitral valve identified according to cardiac size: cardiomegaly if beyond the mitral valve and normal cardiac size at or proximal to the mitral valve. Generally a specific anatomic cause cannot be identified radiographically. Usually echocardiography or angiography is required to establish the anatomic diagnosis.

In Part Eight the following conditions are discussed:

1. Normal cardiac size.
    a. Mitral stenosis (see Chapter 53).
    b. Supravalvar stenosing ring (see Chapter 53).
    c. Cor triatriatum (see Chapter 54).
    d. Stenosis of individual pulmonary veins (see Chapter 55).
2. Cardiomegaly.
    a. Anomalous left coronary artery (see Chapter 57).
    b. Cardiomyopathy (see Chapter 56).
    c. Left ventricular failure.

CHAPTER 52

Mitral Stenosis

After total anomalous pulmonary venous connection, mitral stenosis is the most common cause of pulmonary venous obstruction in children. It can usually be correctly diagnosed and distinguished from other causes of pulmonary venous obstruction, although its operative repair is more difficult and at a higher risk than several of the other obstructive lesions.

PATHOLOGIC ANATOMY

Mitral stenosis results from several anatomic entities,[1, 2] which blend with one another and can be understood by reviewing the features of the normal mitral valve (Figs 52–1 and 52–2). In a normal mitral valve, the distance between the anterolateral and posteromedial papillary muscles is wide. The chordae tendineae are relatively long, and the interchordal spaces are well formed. Chordal insertion into the free wall of the left ventricle does not occur. The leaflets are thin, mobile, and unfused (Fig 52–3). Many instances of mitral stenosis show significant variation of these features. In typical congenital mitral stenosis the margins of the leaflets are thickened and rolled (Fig 52–4). The chordae tendineae are short and thickened, intrachordal spaces are partially obliterated by fibrous tissue, the papillary muscles are underdeveloped, and the intrapapillary distance is reduced. The valve leaflets are fused (Fig 52–5), causing the stenotic mitral valve to dome during diastole.

Parachute mitral valve is a common cause of mitral stenosis (Fig 52–6). The loss of distance between papillary muscles is a variation of parachute mitral valve (see Fig 52–4). There is a continuous spectrum from classical dome-shaped mitral stenosis to classical parachute mitral valve with a single papillary muscle. In this classical form, a single papillary muscle is present in the left ventricle into which all chordae tendineae insert like shrouds of a parachute. Transitional forms show reduced interpapillary distance or partially or completely fused papillary muscles. The valve leaflets are fused into a funnel, and the intrachordal spaces are narrowed. This form of mitral stenosis is often associated with the Shone syndrome,[3] consisting of coarctation of the aorta, subaortic stenosis, supravalvar mitral ring, and parachute mitral valve (Fig 52–7). Not all features are universally present.

Mitral stenosis can also result from hypoplasia of all components of the mitral valve apparatus, including the mitral annulus (Fig 52–8). This form is usually associated with outflow obstruction and hypoplasia of the left ventricle, being a part of the spectrum of hypoplastic left heart syndrome. Many patients with this particular form of mitral stenosis develop symptoms during the neonatal period.

Mitral stenosis also can result from greatly enlarged papillary muscles, the bulk of papillary muscle causing submitral valve stenosis. This can occur with a mitral arcade (Fig 52–9) and also with otherwise normal mitral valve leaflets.

In a few instances, the anatomic details of the mitral valve resemble those of rheumatic mitral stenosis with commissural fusion. In such instances, the chordae tendineae are shortened and the papillary muscles small and underdeveloped. Often the stenotic valve shows features of several of these pathologic entities, and a precise pathologic classification may be difficult.

Regardless of its anatomic form, mitral stenosis has several consequences. Left atrial enlargement occurs, and the left atrium may be lined with endocardial fibroelastosis. Pulmonary parenchymal findings of pulmonary venous

THE NORMAL MITRAL VALVE (Opened)

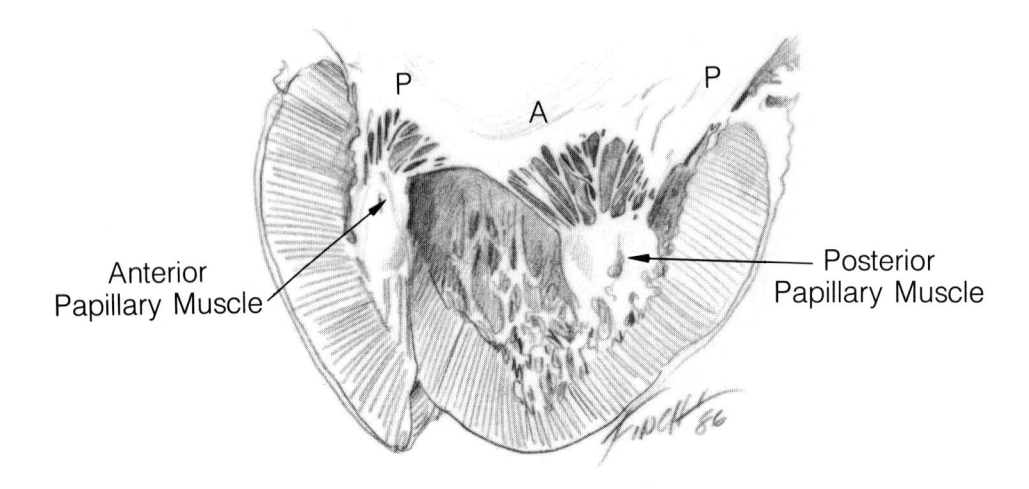

FIG 52-1.
Normal mitral valve. Anterior and posterior papillary muscles; each send chordae tendineae to anterior *(A)* and posterior *(P)* mitral valve leaflets. Commissures of anterior and posterior valve leaflets are not fused, and the papillary muscles are separated (normal interpapillary distance).

obstruction include pulmonary edema, dilated lymphatics, and enlarged tortuous bronchial arteries. The pulmonary trunk is dilated and the right ventricle hypertrophied. Pulmonary vascular disease can develop.

Mitral stenosis of any anatomic form may occur as an isolated condition or coexist with other cardiac malformations. In the latter circumstance, the features of the mitral stenosis are often overshadowed by the coexistent cardiac condition. Subaortic stenosis occurs with other forms of mitral stenosis than that associated with Shone's syndrome. Subaortic stenosis can occur with mitral arcade accompanying bulky papillary muscles. In other cases, accessory valve tissue of the anterior leaflet of a stenotic mitral valve (Fig 52–10) may obstruct abnormal chordae tendineae to the ventricular septum or can narrow the subaortic area (Fig 52–11).

THE NORMAL ANATOMY OF THE MITRAL VALVE
(Open Left Ventricle)

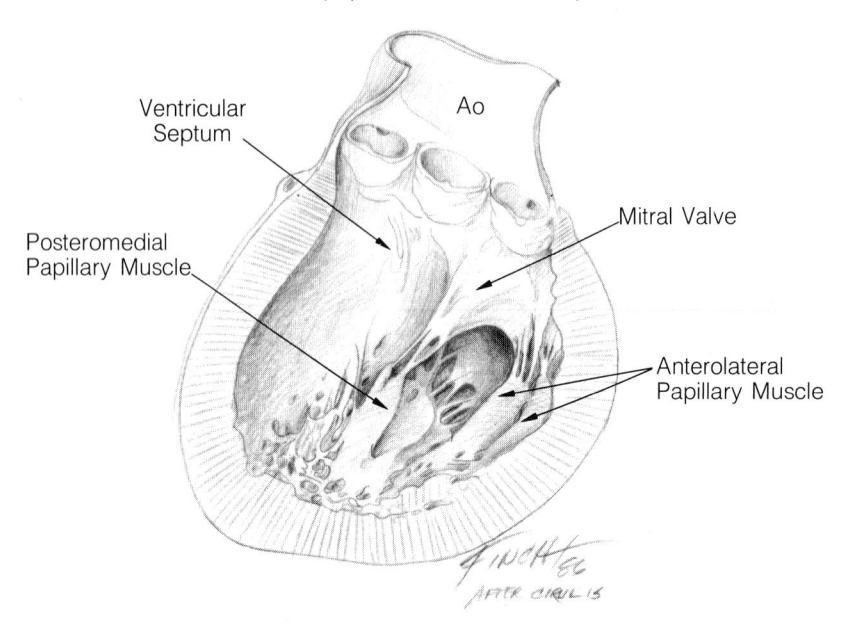

FIG 52-2.
Normal mitral valve. Left ventricle is opened. Distance between papillary muscles is shown. Papillary muscles are widely separated. *Ao* = aorta.

THE NORMAL MITRAL VALVE
(Viewed From Left Ventricle)

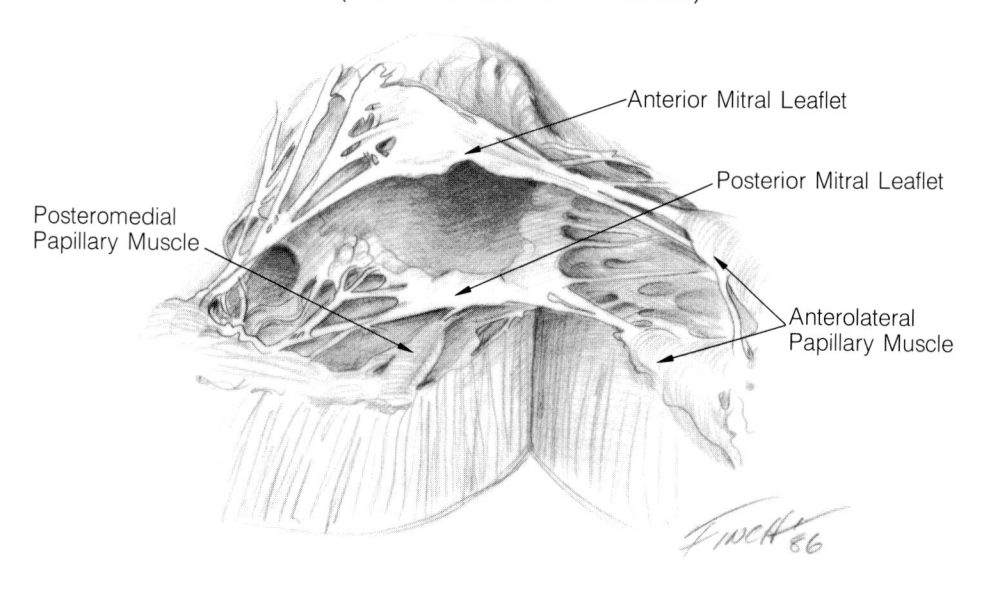

FIG 52–3.
Normal mitral valve is viewed from left ventricle. Relationship between papillary muscles and leaflets is shown.

HEMODYNAMICS

Across the stenotic orifice of the mitral valve, a gradient is present during diastole, being largest late in diastole with atrial contraction. The flow through the valve may be limited during exercise, so that the cardiac output does not increase appropriately, producing the symptom of exercise intolerance. With severe stenosis, cardiac output may be decreased even at rest.

Pressure is elevated in each portion of the vascular system proximal to the mitral valve. Specific clinical or laboratory features result. Left atrial pressure is elevated, which produces left atrial enlargement, evident by a thoracic roentgenogram with barium swallow, echocardio-

CONGENITAL MITRAL STENOSIS
(Mildy Reduced Interpapillary Distance and Short Chordae)

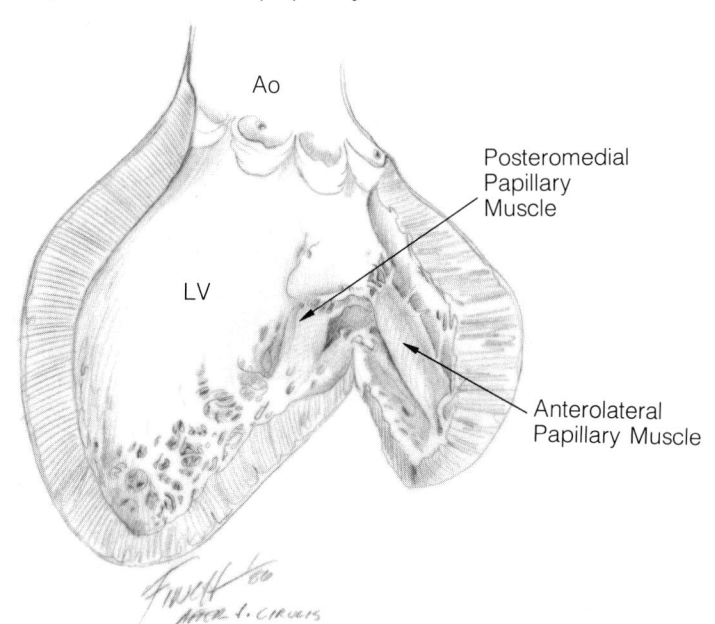

FIG 52–4.
Congenital mitral stenosis. Thickened valve leaflets. Shortened chordae tendineae. Underdeveloped papillary muscles. Interpapillary distance is reduced. *Ao* = aorta; *LV* = left ventricle.

CONGENITAL MITRAL STENOSIS
(Marked Reduction of Interpapillary Distance)

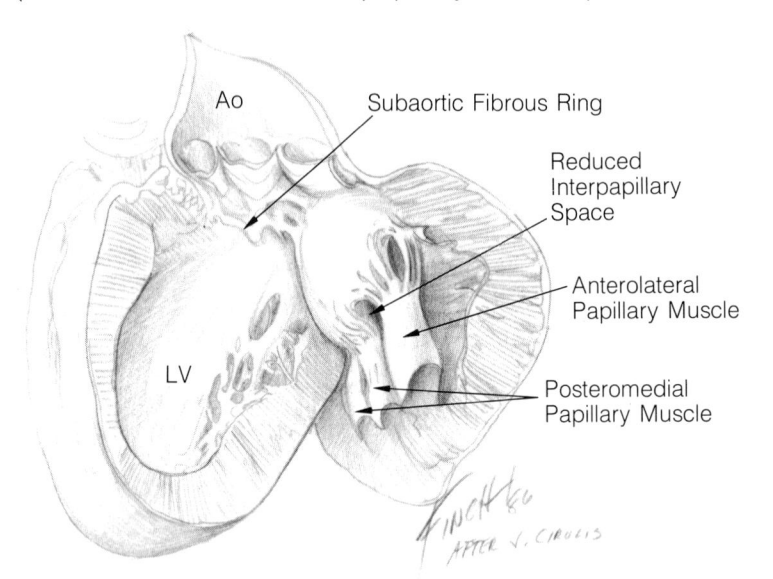

FIG 52–5.
Congenital mitral stenosis. Valve leaflets are thickened and fused. Reduced interpapillary space. Ao = aorta; LV = left ventricle. Appearance similar to parachute mitral valve, indicating a continuous spectrum from classical mitral stenosis to classical parachute mitral valve.

gram, or perhaps electrocardiogram (ECG). Pulmonary venous pressure is increased, which causes redistribution of pulmonary blood flow to the upper lobes of the lungs. This change is partially attributable to the increased vascular pressure overcoming gravitational effects on the pulmonary circulation in an upright individual. The upper lobe pulmonary veins become dilated, which may be apparent on a thoracic radiograph as "cephalization." With chronic elevation of pulmonary venous pressure, collaterals de-

CLASSICAL PARACHUTE MITRAL VALVE

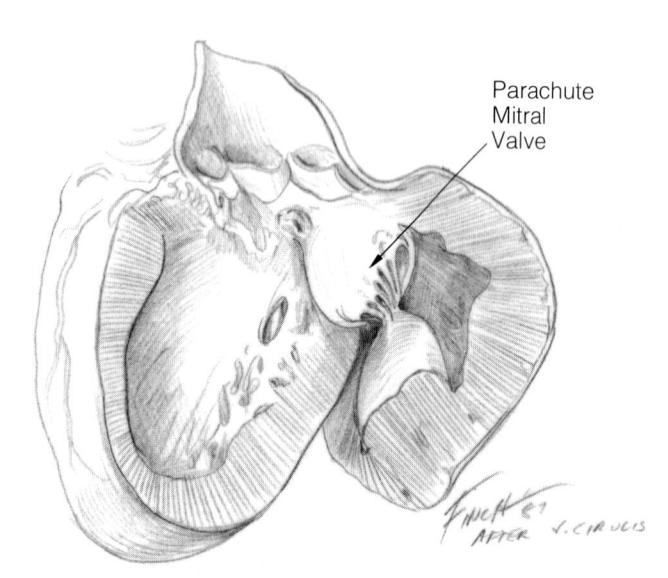

FIG 52–6.
Congenital mitral stenosis. Parachute mitral valve. All chordae tendineae insert into a single large papillary muscle.

velop with the bronchial venous system. The bronchial veins became dilated and tortuous. They may rupture and, because of their location in the bronchial submucosa, produce hemoptysis. Pulmonary capillary pressure is increased, and because of Starling's law affecting transcapillary movement of fluid, pulmonary edema results. Pulmonary arterial pressure increases, in part from pulmonary vasoconstriction. The pulmonary artery dilates, and the pulmonary component of the second heart sound is accentuated as a manifestation of pulmonary hypertension. Finally, because of increased right ventricular systolic pressure, right ventricular hypertrophy develops (evident on an echocardiogram, ECG, and lateral thoracic roentgenogram).

CLINICAL FEATURES

Although evidence of cardiac disease may be present during the neonatal period, usually mitral stenosis is initially recognized at a later age.[4–10] The delay in recognition is related to the fact that the major symptoms are respiratory and perhaps from pneumonia. Slow growth, irritability, chronic cough, and congestive cardiac failure are also common. Episodes of pulmonary edema may occur.

On physical examination, the infants may appear scrawny and in respiratory distress. There is a precordial bulge. In about one half of patients the first heart sound and pulmonary component of the second heart sound are accentuated. An opening snap is uncommon. A murmur is present in most patients and may be heard initially during the neonatal period. The murmur is soft, occurring in mid-diastole and late diastole, sometimes with presystolic ac-

SHONE'S SYNDROME

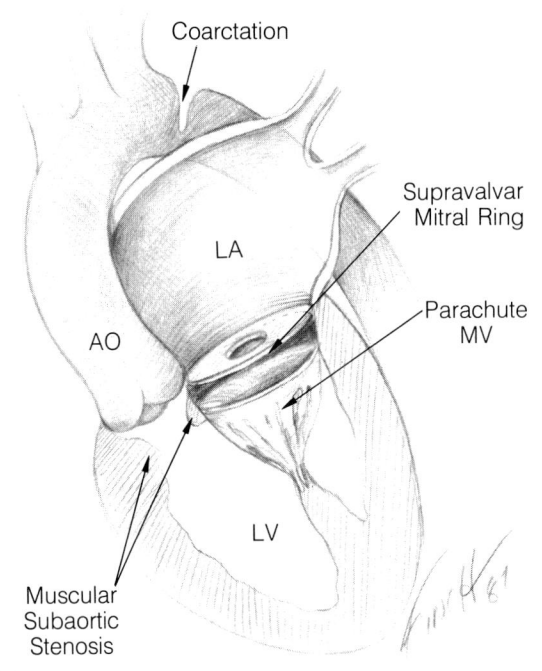

FIG 52-7.
Shone's syndrome. Anatomic features. Supravalvar mitral ring. Parachute mitral valve *(MV)*. Subaortic stenosis. Coarctation of aorta. A series of left-sided obstructions. *Ao* = aorta; *LA* = left atrium; *LV* = left ventricle.

centuation. Hepatomegaly is found. A systolic murmur may be heard as well, representing either coexistent mitral insufficiency or tricuspid insufficiency secondary to pulmonary hypertension.

ELECTROCARDIOGRAPHIC FEATURES

There is right-axis deviation and right ventricular hypertrophy. Left atrial enlargement, manifested by broad, notched P waves in lead I, aVL, V_5, and V_6 may be found.

ECHOCARDIOGRAPHIC FEATURES

Cross-sectional echocardiography provides more information about mitral stenosis by offering assessment of mitral valve mobility and information about chordal attachments. Abnormalities of the papillary muscle can be observed. Normally both papillary muscles are well identified. Parachute mitral valve may be diagnosed by identifying a single or fused papillary muscle. Mitral stenosis resulting from bulky papillary muscles can also be diagnosed by observing their size. Doppler recording shows high-velocity diastolic flow velocities across the valve. Measurements allow estimation of the diastolic gradient across the mitral valve. On M-mode the valve shows decreased E-F

HYPOPLASTIC TYPE MITRAL STENOSIS

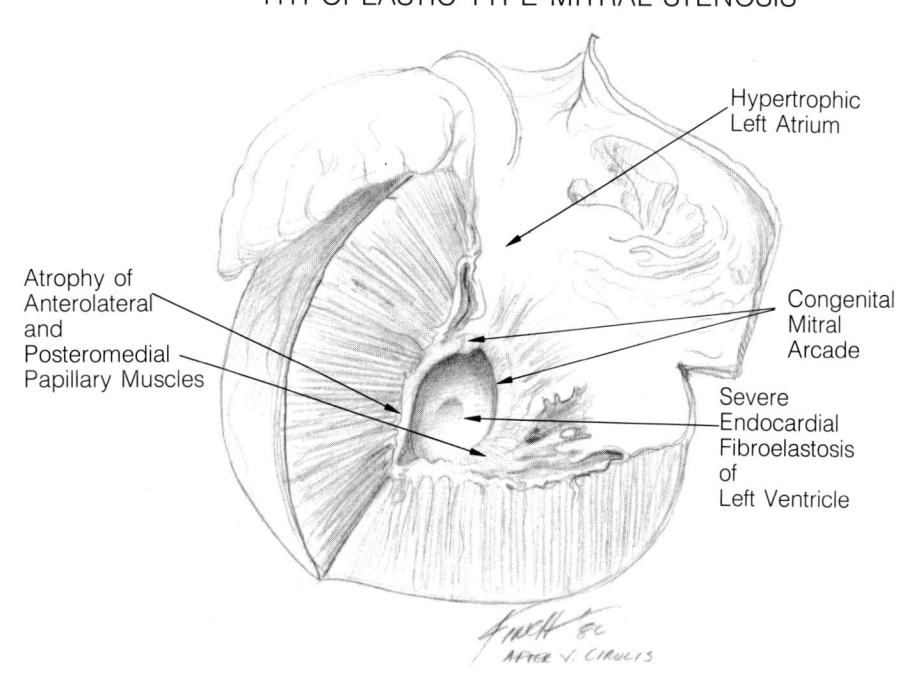

FIG 52-8.
Congenital mitral stenosis. Hypoplasia of all components of mitral valve. Mitral valve shows features of mitral arcade. Hypoplasia of left ventricle. Endocardial fibroelastosis coexists.

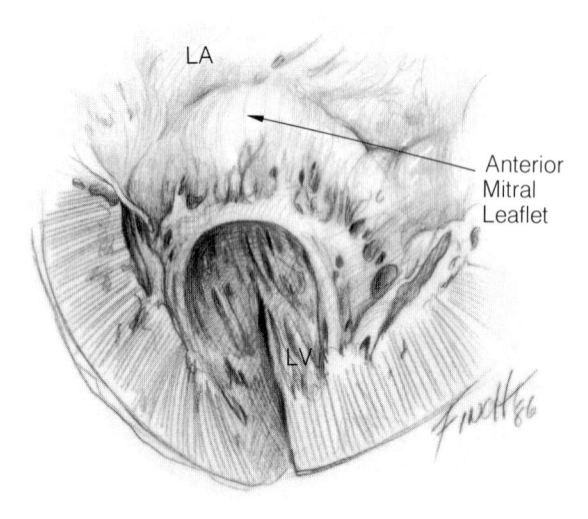

ANOMALOUS MITRAL ARCADE

FIG 52-9.
Congenital mitral stenosis. Anomalous mitral arcade. From each papillary muscle, a muscular band extends onto anterior mitral valve leaflet, forming an arch. LA = left atrium; LV = left ventricle.

slope, anterior movement of the posterior leaflet of the mitral valve, reduced D-E excursion, and multiple echoes from the leaflets.[11, 12] Left atrial enlargement, reduced left ventricular dimensions, and features of pulmonary hypertension can be detected as well.

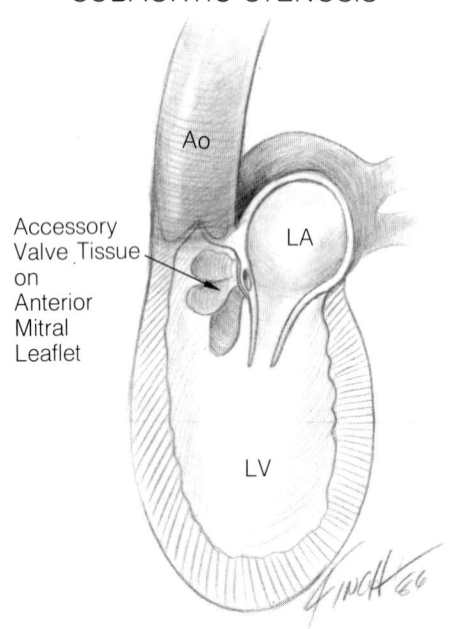

SUBAORTIC STENOSIS

FIG 52-10.
Subaortic stenosis resulting from accessory mitral valve tissue obstructing subaortic area. Ao = aorta; LA = left atrium; LV = left ventricle.

SUBAORTIC STENOSIS

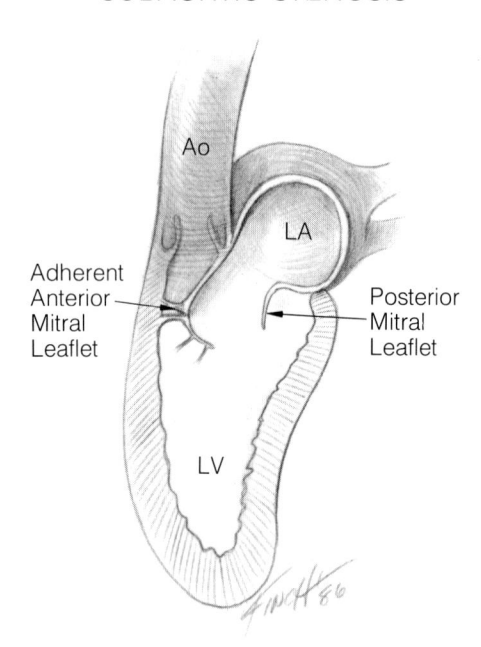

FIG 52-11.
Subaortic stenosis resulting from abnormal chordae tendinae passing from anterior mitral valve leaflet to ventricular septum. Abnormal attachment fixes anterior mitral leaflet during systole, resulting in outflow tract obstruction. Ao = aorta; LA = left atrium; LV = left ventricle.

RADIOGRAPHIC FEATURES

Congenital mitral stenosis elevates left atrial pressure and, in turn, pulmonary arterial pressure. The resultant right ventricular hypertrophy is difficult to determine on posteroanterior roentgenograms, but if decompensation of the right ventricle occurs, right ventricular dilatation develops and cardiomegaly appears radiographically.

1. As long as the right ventricle is compensated, cardiac size is normal or only minimally increased, which may make the radiographic diagnosis difficult or impossible. The pulmonary venous vasculature is accentuated (Fig 52-12) and shows various signs such as cephalization, pleural effusion, and pulmonary edema. Kerley B lines are very rare in infants and children.

2. Left atrial enlargement is demonstrated by posterior displacement of the esophagus on a barium swallow. The left atrial enlargement is always out of proportion to the degree of the accentuation of the pulmonary vasculature (see Fig 52-12,B). This discrepancy on the radiograph helps differentiate mitral stenosis from conditions with a left-to-right shunt and left atrial enlargement.

3. As with acquired mitral disease, there may be enlargement of the left atrial appendage, although in child-

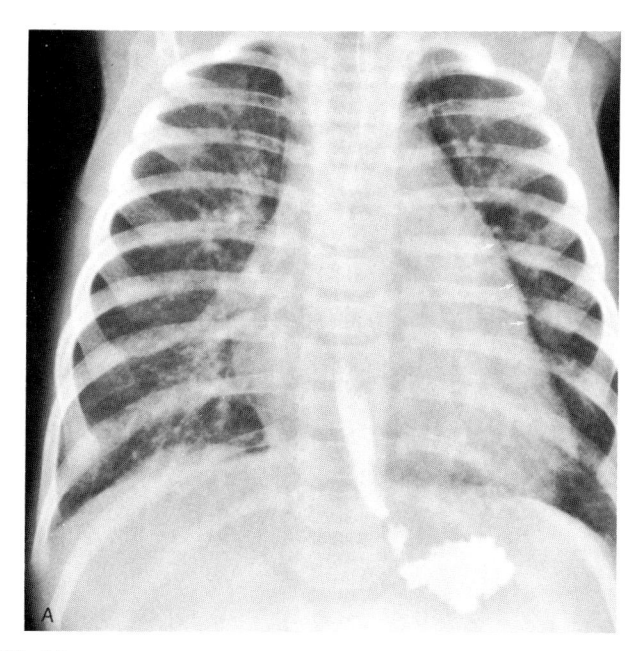

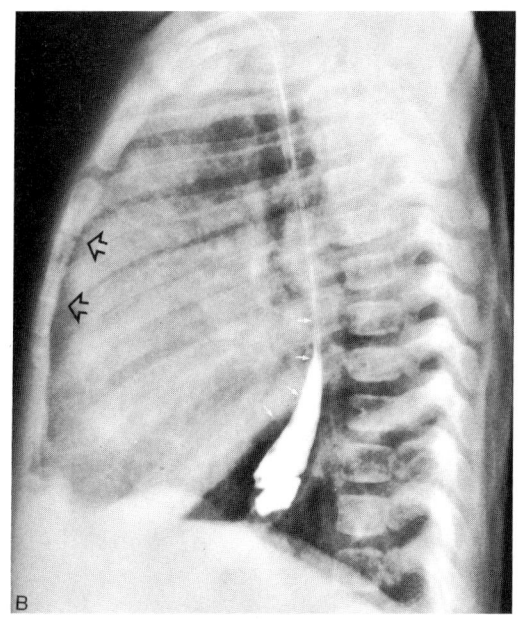

FIG 52–12.
Mitral stenosis from mitral arcade. Thoracic roentgenogram. **A,** posteroanterior projection. Minimal cardiomegaly. Slight bulge in region of left atrial appendage *(arrows)* could be dilated left atrial appendage, but differentiation from residual thymus is impossible at this age. Slight accentuation of venous pulmonary vasculature. Kerley B lines are not present. **B,** lateral projection. Retrosternal space is obliterated by enlarged right ventricle *(open arrows)*. Slight left atrial enlargement consistent with mild mitral stenosis. *(solid arrows)*.

hood, this area of the cardiac silhouette may be obscured by thymic tissue (see Fig 52–12,A).

4. In patients with severe mitral stenosis, the right ventricle decompensates, and marked cardiomegaly results (Fig 52–13).

5. With severe obstruction at the mitral valve level, pulmonary arterial pressure is elevated, and consequently the pulmonary arteries are dilated, which may make differentiation from a left-to-right shunt difficult. The extreme left atrial enlargement of mitral stenosis is a useful point in the differential diagnosis.

6. The pulmonary vasculature tends to be indistinct

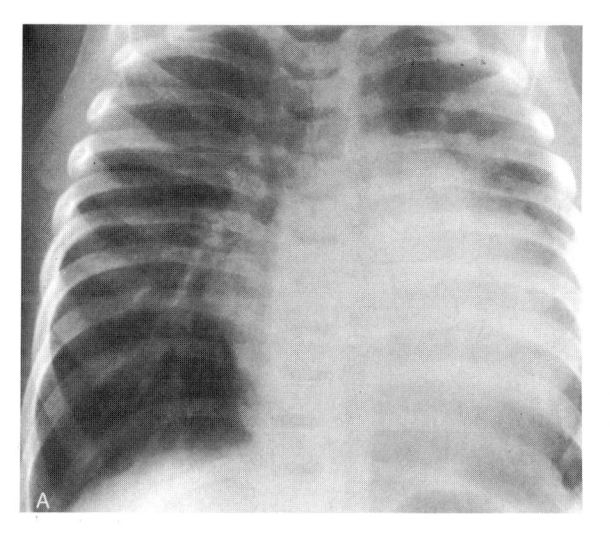

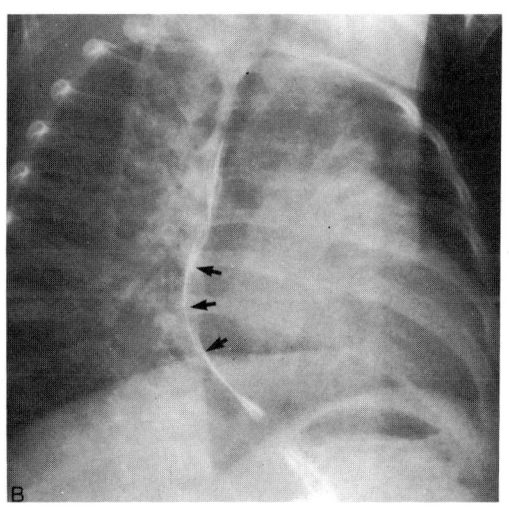

FIG 52–13.
Long-standing severe mitral stenosis and right ventricular decompensation. Thoracic roentgenogram. **A,** posteroanterior and, **B,** right anterior oblique projections. Markedly enlarged heart. Accentuation of pulmonary venous vasculature. Severe left atrial enlargement *(arrows)* helps differentiate mitral stenosis from left-to-right shunt. Radiographically it would be impossible to distinguish this appearance from obstruction distal to mitral valve (aortic stenosis or coarctation of aorta) which also causes marked cardiomegaly and left atrial enlargement in this age group.

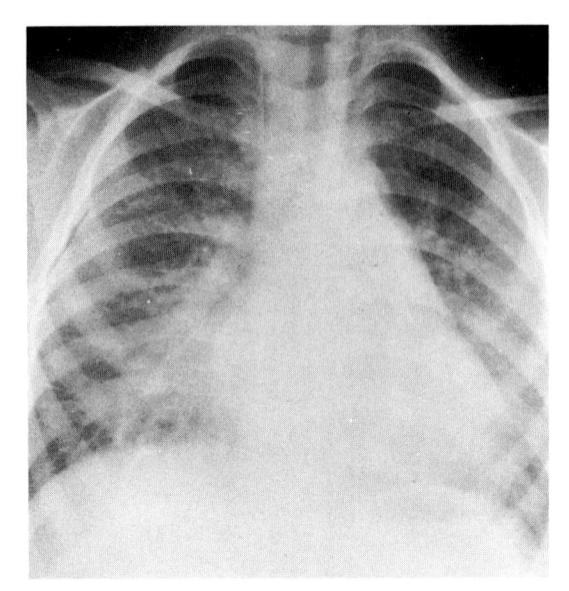

FIG 52-14.
Mitral stenosis from parachute mitral valve. Thoracic roentgenogram. Posteroanterior projection. Minimally enlarged heart (compensated right ventricle). Indistinct pulmonary vasculature as in pulmonary edema.

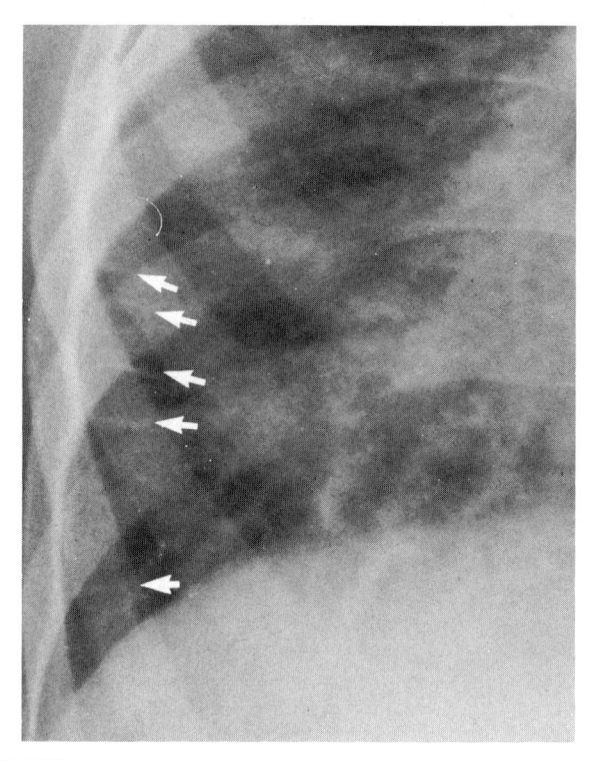

FIG 52-15.
Mitral stenosis in a 10-year-old child. Thoracic roentgenogram. Posteroanterior projection. Right base of lung. Kerley B lines *(arrows)*.

because of transudation of fluid or from episodes of pulmonary edema (Fig 52-14) (see also Chapter 5).

7. Kerley B lines can be encountered in individuals with long-standing mitral obstruction (Fig 52-15). Thus, they are seen only in older children and are exceedingly rare below the age of 6 years.

CARDIAC CATHETERIZATION

Cardiac catheterization is performed to determine the site and severity of pulmonary venous obstruction. Simultaneous measurement of pulmonary arterial wedge and left ventricular end-diastolic pressures shows a pressure difference between these two sites, localizing the obstruction at the mitral valve, in the left atrium or pulmonary veins. If the catheter can be advanced into the left atrium, the site of obstruction can be more precisely identified. Usually echocardiography performed before the catheterization has defined the location, and catheterization provides substantiating data. The left atrial or wedge pressure is elevated, often to 30 to 35 mm Hg. Pulmonary arterial pressure is elevated, with a great variability among patients. The value is higher in those with additional left-sided obstructive conditions or a left-to-right shunt. With long-standing mitral obstruction, pulmonary arterial systolic pressure may exceed 100 mm Hg.

The oxygen saturation data are usually normal in those patients without a coexistent shunt lesion (either left-to-right or right-to-left). At rest, cardiac output may be normal or decreased, depending on the severity of mitral obstruction.

ANGIOGRAPHIC FEATURES

Angiography is helpful in the diagnosis of the specific forms of mitral stenosis, but often a precise pathologic diagnosis cannot be made. Echocardiography is an important adjunct in defining the type of mitral valvular abnormality.

The late phase of a pulmonary arteriogram demonstrates an enlarged left atrium and delayed clearing of contrast material from this chamber. A specific anatomic diagnosis usually cannot be made by pulmonary arteriography (Fig 52-16). The mitral valve can be defined better by a direct left atrial injection. Left ventriculography is also indicated in these patients to demonstrate coexistent mitral regurgitation, because some obstructive lesions such as arcade mitral valve are usually associated with mitral regurgitation. Furthermore, the demonstration of the papillary muscles by left ventriculography provides a clue to the type of mitral abnormality, particularly mitral arcade or parachute mitral valve. The difficulty diagnosing the specific type of mitral valve anomaly is not surprising because

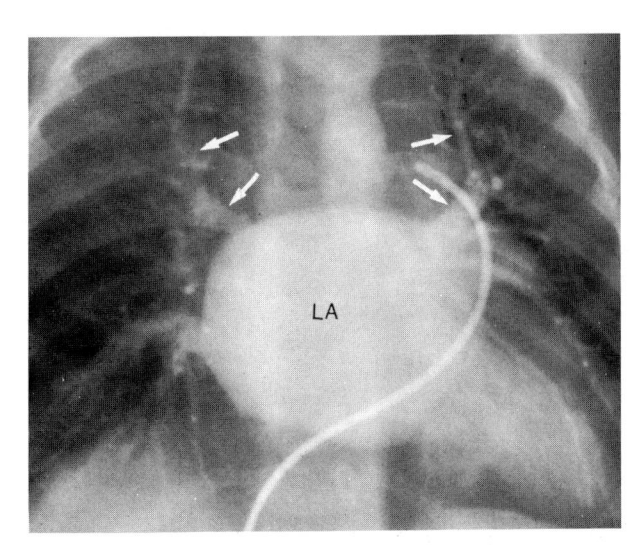

FIG 52-16.
Severe mitral stenosis. Pulmonary arteriogram. Anteroposterior projection. Late phase. Huge left atrium *(LA)* is densely opacified. Distention of upper lobe pulmonary veins (cephalization) *(arrows)*. Delayed clearing of contrast medium. Both are indirect findings consistent with mitral obstruction. Anatomic type of mitral abnormality is not apparent.

even pathologists sometimes find it challenging to define and classify cases of congenital mitral stenosis into a specific anatomic type. A right anterior oblique and angled steep left anterior oblique left ventriculograms provide excellent visualization of the mitral valvular apparatus.

1. In mitral stenosis with fused commissures, the mitral valve domes and is well outlined in both the right anterior oblique and left anterior oblique projections (Fig 52–17).
2. The stenotic mitral valve may markedly prolapse into the left ventricle during diastole, causing a large negative filling defect. This appearance of a stenotic mitral valve can be best demonstrated by direct left atrial injection outlining the valve leaflets on both sides (Fig 52–18). On such studies, a jet may be identified in addition to doming of the valve.
3. Typically the interpapillary distance is decreased in classic congenital mitral stenosis. The papillary muscles may be so close together that a single papillary muscle is simulated, thereby suggesting a diagnosis of parachute mitral valve (Fig 52–19). A continuous spectrum exists from classical mitral stenosis with a normal interpapillary distance, lesions with decreased interpapillary distance, to partially or completely fused papillary muscles. The last variation can also be considered a variation of parachute mitral valve. The classical parachute mitral valve, as originally described, however, had only a single papillary muscle, which can be identified angiographically (Fig 52–20).
4. Typically a stenotic mitral valve with fused commissures has a diaphragm-like configuration in systole and diastole. There may be slight systolic prolapse of the stenotic valve into the left atrium (Fig 52–21).
5. Classically, two well-defined papillary muscles can be identified, but commonly the interpapillary distance is decreased (see Fig 52–19). The papillary muscles are closer to the mitral valve because of shortened chordae tendineae (Fig 52–22).
6. A classic parachute mitral valve can be suggested if a single papillary muscle is demonstrated in the left ventricle, the mitral valve has a funnel-shaped appearance (Fig 52–23), and the mitral annulus may be small.
7. By a left atrial injection, the inflow of contrast medium is stopped by numerous chordae tendineae and

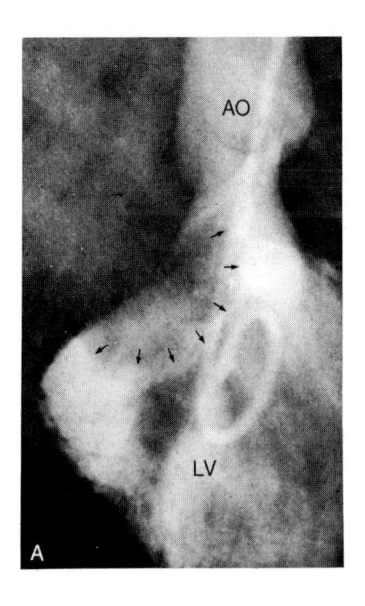

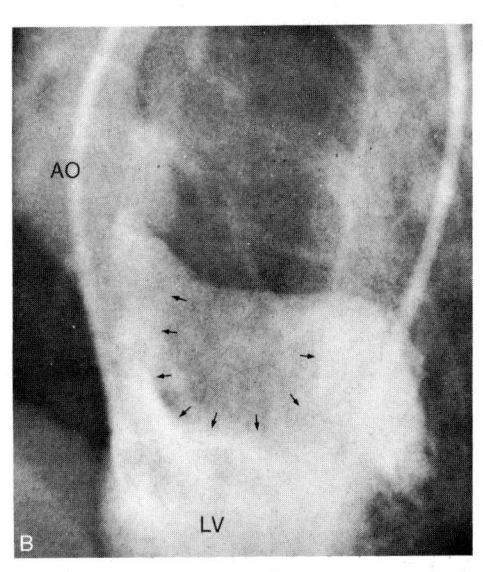

FIG 52-17.
Mitral stenosis from fused domed-shaped valve. Left ventriculogram *(LV)* **A,** right anterior oblique projection. Diastole. Stenotic mitral valve forms distinct dome-shaped filling defect *(arrows)* in left ventricle. **B,** left anterior oblique projection. Diastole. Fused doming mitral valve *(arrows)*. Normally leaflets of valve are straight and do not dome. Occasionally prolapsing left atrial myxoma may cause similar angiographic appearance on a left venticulogram. *AO* = aorta.

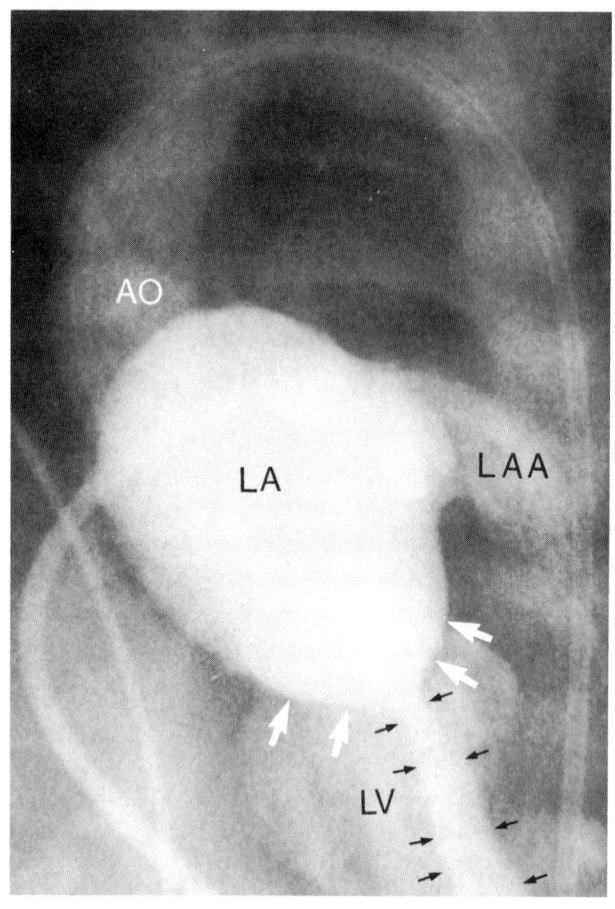

FIG 52–18.
Congenital mitral stenosis. Left atriogram *(LA)*. Left anterior oblique projection. Diastole. Fused stenotic valve domes *(white arrows)*. Stenotic orifice produces narrow jet *(black arrows)*. Normally in this projection both valve leaflets are straight. *Ao* = aorta; *LAA* = left atrial appendage; *LV* = left ventricle.

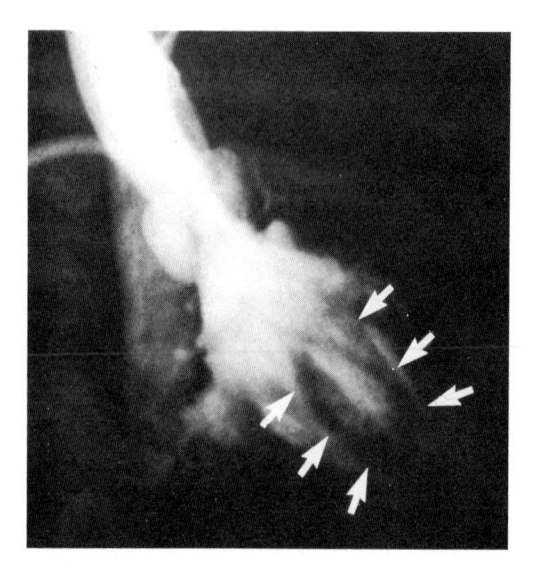

FIG 52–19.
Mitral stenosis. Left ventriculogram. Right anterior oblique projection. Interpapillary distance between papillary muscles *(arrows)* is approaching appearance of a parachute mitral valve.

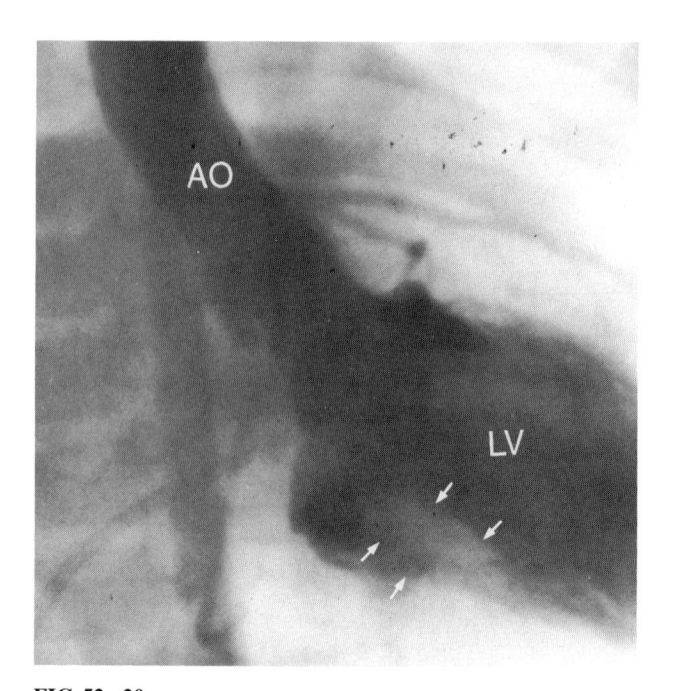

FIG 52–20.
Mitral stenosis caused by parachute valve. Left ventriculogram *(LV)*. Right anterior oblique projection. Single large papillary muscle *(arrows)*. Papillary muscle is close to mitral valve, indicating short chordae tendineae being part of parachute mitral valve or classic dome-shaped mitral stenosis, which typically has two papillary muscles. *Ao* = aorta.

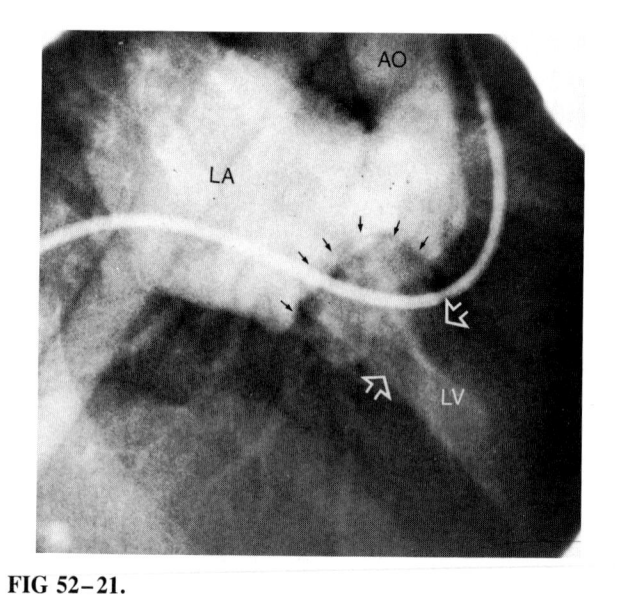

FIG 52–21.
Mitral stenosis. Pulmonary arteriogram. Late phase. End-systole. Enlarged densely opacified left atrium *(LA)*. Minimal left ventricular and systolic volume because amount of blood that enters left ventricle *(LV)* is ejected completely. Two well-defined, separated papillary muscles *(open arrows)*, excluding parachute mitral valve. Papillary muscles are situated close to mitral valve consistent with shortened chordae tendineae. Fused mitral valve shows slight systolic prolapse *(black arrows)* into left atrium. *Ao* = aorta.

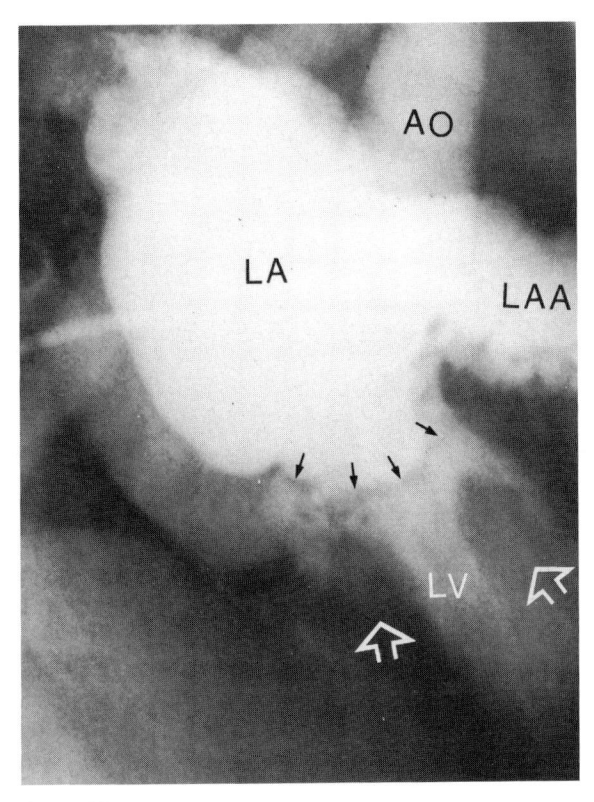

FIG 52–22.
Mitral stenosis caused by domed-shaped valve. Left atriogram. Right anterior oblique projection. Enlarged left atrium *(LA)*. Enlarged left atrial appendage *(LAA)*, characteristic of mitral disease. Mitral valve domes *(black arrows)* and bulges into left ventricle *(LV)*. Two large well-defined papillary muscles *(open arrows)* are positioned abnormally close to mitral valve because of shortened chordae tendineae. *Ao* = aorta.

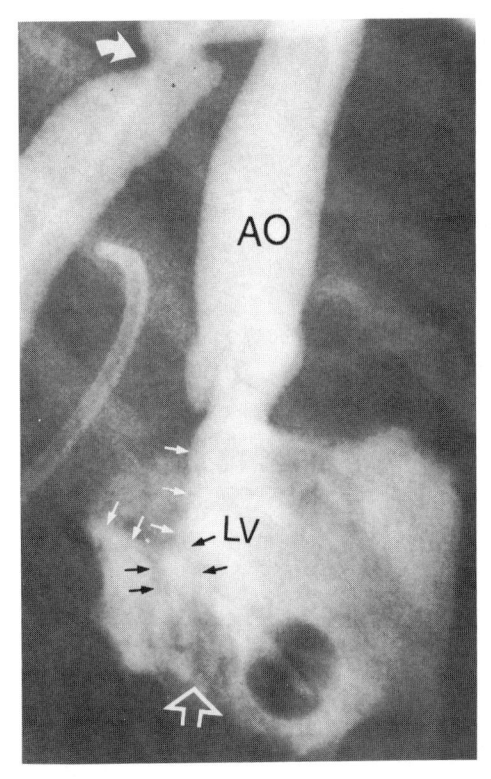

FIG 52–23.
Mitral stenosis. Left ventriculogram *(LV)*. Right anterior oblique projection. Small mitral annulus and funnel-shaped deformity of mitral valve *(white arrows)*. Large single papillary muscle is in close proximity to abnormal mitral valve. Characteristic findings for parachute mitral valve. Coarctation of aorta *(curved white arrow)* is commonly associated with parachute mitral valve (Shone's syndrome). From high-lying large single papillary muscle *(open arrow)*, stringy filling defects *(black arrows)* extend to funnel-shaped mitral valve and represent markedly thickened chordae tendineae which are normally not seen. *Ao* = aorta.

the single papillary muscle. Consequently, lateral jets can be observed (Fig 52–24). Normally the contrast medium enters the left ventricle along its long axis toward the apex.

8. Once the left ventricle is opacified, the funnel-shaped configuration of the valve can be identified (Fig 52–25).

9. Occasionally the papillary muscles are not identifiable, and the angiographic appearance is so atypical (Fig 52–24) that the type of mitral stenosis cannot be classified.

10. A redundant stenotic mitral valve may form an irregular filling defect in the left ventricular outflow tract during diastole (Fig 52–26). REASON: The redundant valve makes contact with the ventricular septum, displacing the contrast medium. If there are abnormal chordal attachments to the septum, subaortic obstruction may coexist, and the aortic valve may become thickened (Fig 52–27), as occurs from the subvalvar jet in instances of subaortic membrane.

11. The angiographic diagnosis of arcade mitral valve is virtually impossible. It can be suggested by the appearance of an abnormal mitral valve and the absence of papillary muscles. Many times even normal papillary muscles are not demonstrated on a left ventriculogram. Arcade mitral valve can be suspected only by exclusion. If either two well-defined or a large single papillary muscle is demonstrated, arcade mitral valve can be excluded. If a patient has significant mitral regurgitation (Fig 52–28), the diagnosis of arcade mitral valve is likely. REASON: Dome-shaped mitral valve and parachute mitral valve typically do not have significant mitral regurgitation.

12. Normally chordae tendineae are not seen angiographically, but they may be visualized in parachute mitral valve. REASON: The chordae tendineae are crowded together and markedly thickened (Fig 52–29).

13. Although these angiographic findings are characteristic for parachute mitral valve, differentiation from classical mitral stenosis with short chordae tendineae and closely spaced papillary muscles may not be possible.

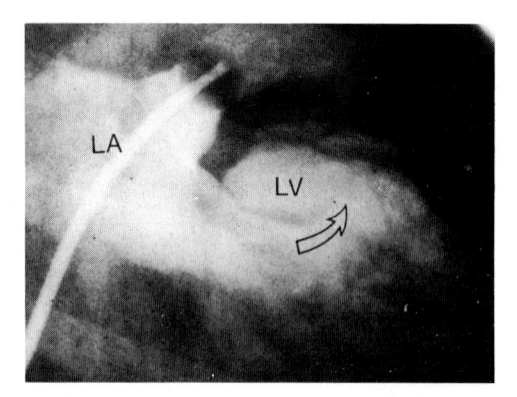

FIG 52-24.
Parachute mitral valve. Left atriogram *(LA)*. Right anterior oblique projection. Diastole. Contrast medium enters left ventricle laterally *(arrow)* through interchordal spaces instead toward apex of left ventricle *(LV)* as in normal mitral valve.

14. Rarely, mitral stenosis may be caused by a small mitral annulus that has an anatomically normal mitral valve. Such patients have a left-to-right shunt at the atrial level, which accounts for decreased blood flow through the mitral valve. Such hypoplasia of the mitral valve is an important consideration for operative repair.

15. Supravalvar stenosing ring of the left atrium may be confused with mitral stenosis, because it forms a membrane low in the left atrium and is sometimes attached to the mitral valve. Typically the membrane forms only a ringlike density but does not cause severe obstruction. It usually occurs as part of the Shone syndrome but may be an isolated condition. This condition is discussed more fully in Chapter 53.

OPERATIVE CONSIDERATIONS

For patients with mild or moderate mitral stenosis, management is medical and may incorporate the use of digitalis or diuretics. When congestive cardiac failure is intractable, episodes of pulmonary edema recur, or pulmonary arterial pressure is markedly elevated, operation on the mitral valve is indicated. In some patients, mitral valvulotomy or creation of fenestrations in the leaflets is performed, but this does not cause a significant decrease in gradient, but the short- and long-term mortality is 50%. In others, particularly with parachute mitral valve or from bulky papillary muscles, the mitral valve is replaced.[13, 14] The short- and long-term survival is better, but it is complicated by the need for anticoagulation.

Recently balloon valvuloplasty has been introduced as a new treatment method. A transseptal catheterization is performed, and a guidewire is manipulated into the aorta or coiled in the left ventricle. One or two balloons are inflated in the stenotic mitral valve (Fig 52–30). The technique has shown promising results in dome-shaped mitral stenosis with fused commissures and particularly in rheumatic mitral stenosis. Mitral arcade and parachute mitral valve probably cannot be treated by balloon dilatation. Whether a hypoplastic annulus can be significantly dilated is unlikely.

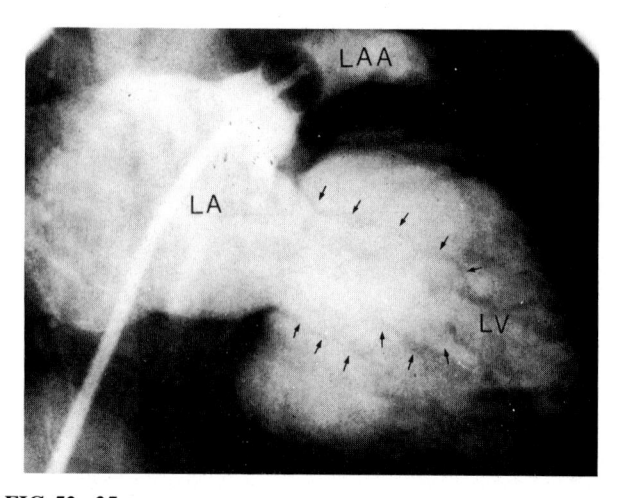

FIG 52-25.
Parachute mitral valve. Same patient as in Figure 52–24. Funnel-shaped mitral valve *(arrows)* is seen in profile. Normally mitral valve leaflets are not seen in this projection. LA = left atrium; LAA = left atrial appendage; LV = left ventricle.

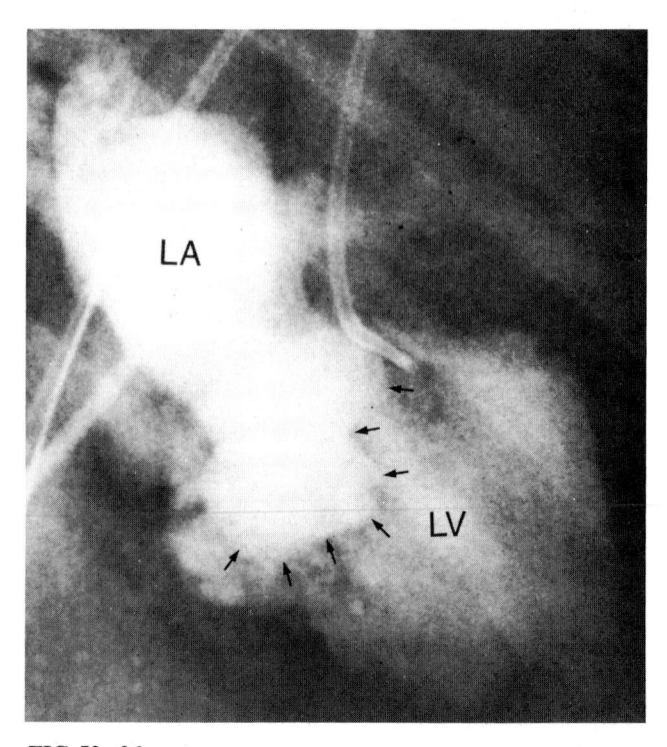

FIG 52-26.
Mitral stenosis. Left atriogram *(LA)*. Right anterior oblique projection. Diastole. Markedly redundant mitral valve *(arrows)* prolapses into left ventricle *(LV)* and forms an irregular dome.

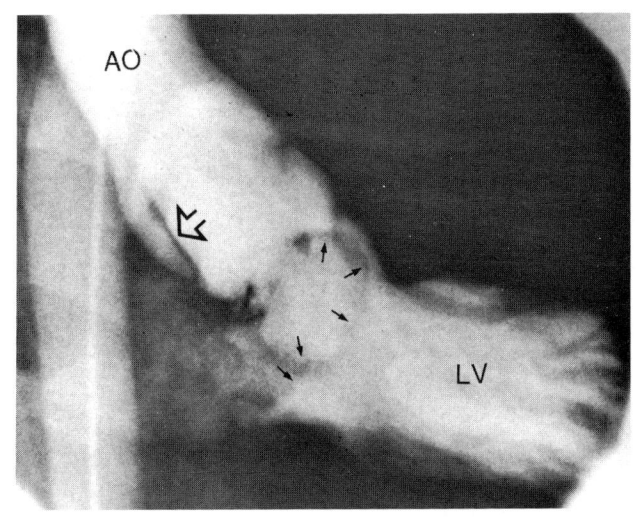

FIG 52–27.
Atypical redundant mitral valve. Left ventriculogram (LV). Right anterior oblique projection. Diastolic filling defect (arrows) in outflow tract. Thickening of posterior leaflet of aortic valve. Patient had mild left ventricular outflow obstruction and mild aortic insufficiency because of abnormal chordal attachment of anterior mitral leaflet to left ventricular septum. Ao = aorta.

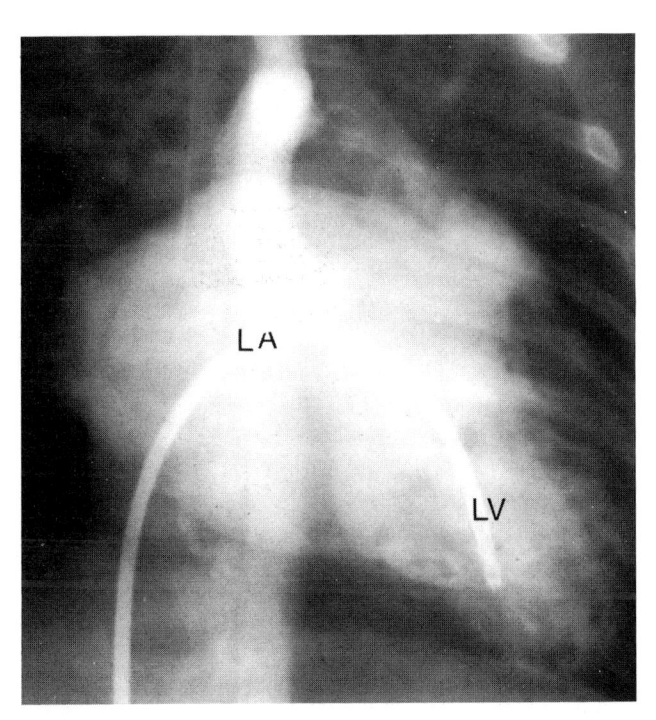

FIG 52–28.
Mitral valve arcade. Left ventriculogram (LV). Anteroposterior projection. Marked mitral reflux. No papillary muscle is seen. Type of mitral abnormality is not apparent angiographically. LA = left atrium.

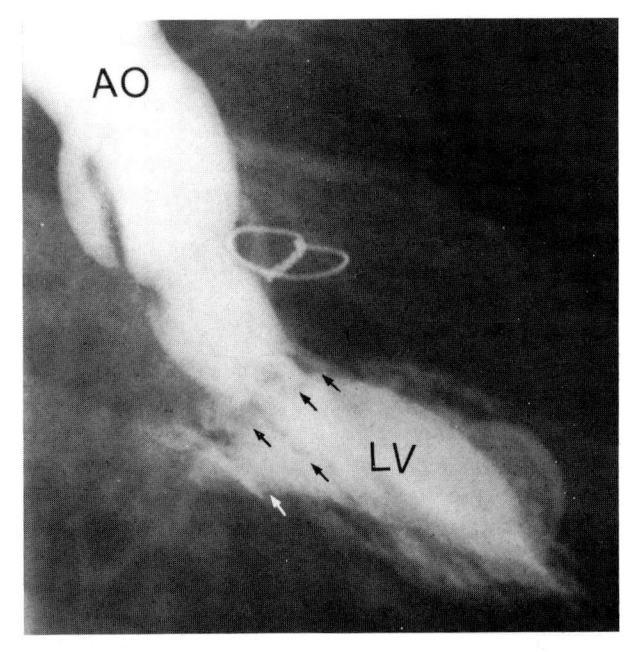

FIG 52–29.
Mitral valve arcade. Left ventriculogram (LV). Right anterior oblique projection. Systole. Numerous chordae tendineae (arrows) are visualized without papillary muscles. No mitral regurgitation in this patient. Thickened aortic valve leaflet. Ao = aorta.

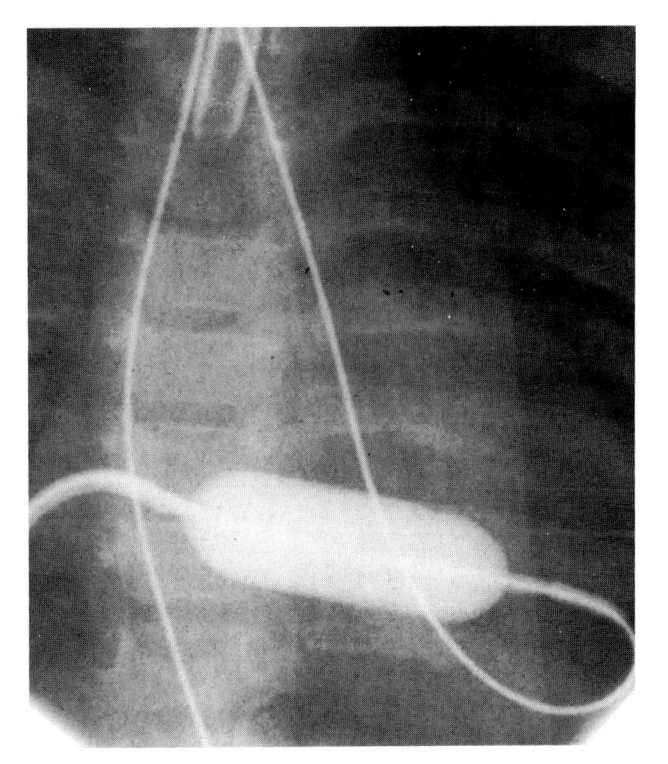

FIG 52–30.
Balloon angioplasty of mitral valve. Thoracic roentgenogram. Anteroposterior projection. Guidewire has been passed into aorta. Balloon is inflated in stenotic mitral valve.

FEATURES

After successful operation there is improvement of the pulmonary vasculature and decrease in cardiac size and left atrial enlargement.

REFERENCES

1. Lucas RV Jr, Anderson RC, Amplatz K, et al: Congenital causes of pulmonary venous obstruction, *Pediatr Clin North Am* 10:781, 1963.
2. Davachi F, Moller JH, Edwards JE: Diseases of the mitral valve in infancy: an anatomic analysis of 55 cases, *Circulation* 43:565, 1971.
3. Shone JD, Sellers RD, Anderson RC, et al: The developmental complex of "parachute mitral valve" supravalvular ring of left atrium, subaortic stenosis, and coarctation of aorta, *Am J Cardiol* 11:714, 1963.
4. Van der Horst RL, Hastreiter AR: Congenital mitral stenosis, *Am J Cardiol* 20:773, 1967.
5. Ferencz C, Johnson AL, Wiglesworth FW: Congenital mitral stenosis, *Circulation* 9:161, 1954.
6. Khalil KG, Shapiro I, Kilman JW: Congenital mitral stenosis, *J Thorac Cardiovasc Surg* 70:40, 1975.
7. Daoud G, Kaplan S, Perrin EV, et al: Congenital mitral stenosis, *Circulation* 27:185, 1963.
8. Elliott LP, Anderson RC, Amplatz K, et al: Congenital mitral stenosis, *Pediatrics* 30:552, 1962.
9. Glancy DL, Chang MY, Dorney ER, et al: Parachute mitral valve. Further observations and associated lesions, *Am J Cardiol* 27:309, 1971.
10. Collins-Nakai RL, Rosenthal A, Castaneda AR, et al: Congenital mitral stenosis: a review of 20 years' experience, *Circulation* 56:1039, 1977.
11. Cooperberg P, Hazell S, Ashmore PG: Parachute accessory anterior mitral valve leaflet causing left ventricular outflow tract obstruction: report of a case with emphasis on the echocardiographic findings, *Circulation* 53:908, 1976.
12. Driscoll DJ, Gutgesell HP, McNamara DG: Echocardiographic features of congenital mitral stenosis, *Am J Cardiol* 42:259, 1978.
13. Prado S, Levy M, Varco RL: Successful replacement of "parachute" mitral valve in a child, *Circulation* 32:130, 1965.
14. Castaneda AR, Anderson RC, Edwards JE: Congenital mitral stenosis resulting from anomalous arcade and obstructing papillary muscles: report of correction by use of ball valve prosthesis, *Am J Cardiol* 24:237, 1969.

CHAPTER 53

Supravalvar Stenosing Ring of Left Atrium

Supravalvar stenosing ring of the left atrium is a rare condition that occurs infrequently as an isolated lesion. A circumferential ring of connective tissue is attached to the base of the atrial surfaces of the mitral valve leaflets and protrudes into the orifice of the mitral valve.[1] Usually this is an incidental finding and is nonobstructive. If fully developed, however, it acts like a stenosing diaphragm and obstructs blood flow from the left atrium. It is most often a component of Shone's syndrome,[2] the coexistence of various left-sided obstructive conditions: parachute mitral valve, subaortic stenosis, coarctation of the aorta, and supravalvar ring (Fig 53–1). It has also been described in instances of tetralogy of Fallot,[3, 4] ventricular septal defect, and corrected transposition of the great vessels.[5] In contrast to cor triatriatum, the ring is located below the atrial appendage and fossa ovalis. If obstructive, the left atrium is enlarged, and the lungs show changes of pulmonary venous hypertension.

The hemodynamics resemble mitral stenosis. Because it usually coexists with other cardiac malformations, it is difficult to develop a specific clinical picture for the isolated cardiac malformation.[6, 7] Symptoms are related to pulmonary congestion and congestive cardiac failure. The pulmonary component of the second heart sound is accentuated, and no murmur is present. If a murmur is present, it results from an associated condition. The electrocardiogram shows right-axis deviation and right ventricular hypertrophy.

The echocardiogram can show the membrane and is very helpful in distinguishing this condition from other causes of pulmonary venous obstruction.[8] In either a long-axis or an apical view, the membrane can be observed; it moves toward the mitral valve during diastole and away during systole, passing as a thin membrane parallel to the mitral valve. The left atrium may be enlarged. The mitral valve appears thickened and to have decreased excursion.

RADIOGRAPHIC FEATURES

Basically the radiographic appearance is identical to other causes of pulmonary venous obstruction. The spe-

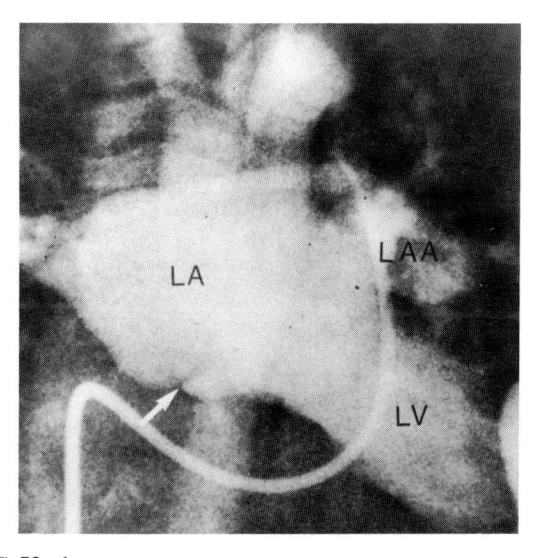

FIG 53–1.
Features of Shone's syndrome. Not all left-sided malformations are uniformly present. *Ao* = aorta; *LA* = left atrium; *LPV's* = left pulmonary veins, *LV* = left ventricle, *RPV's* = right pulmonary veins.

SHONE'S SYNDROME

1. Coarctation of the Aorta
2. Supravalvar Ring of Left Atrium
3. Parachute Mitral Valve
4. Subaortic Stenosis

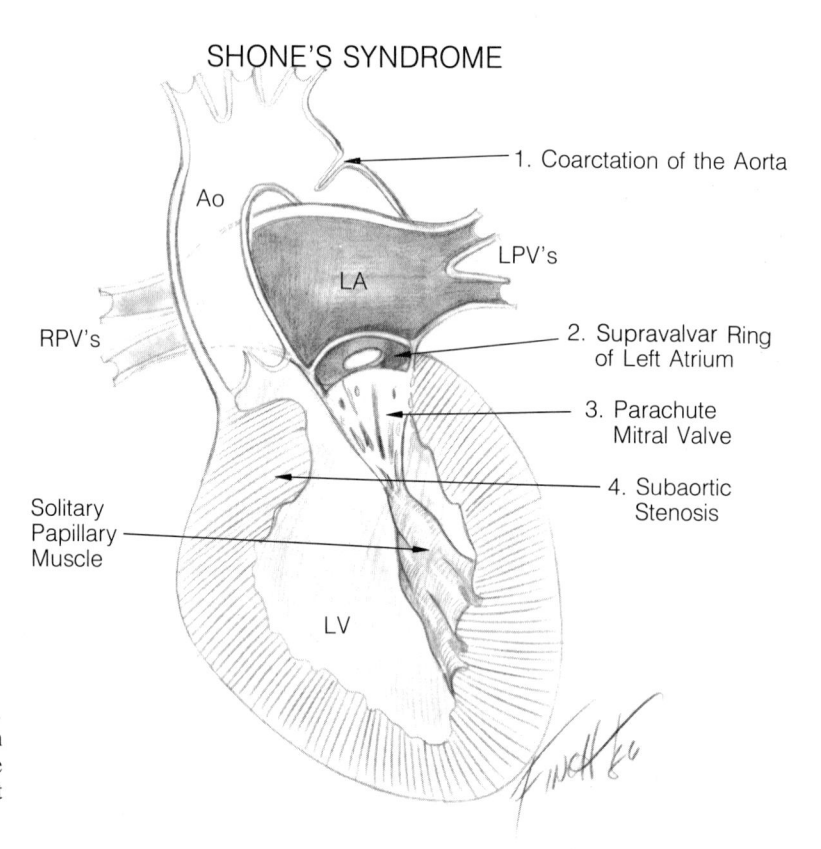

FIG 53–2.
Supravalvar stenosing ring. Pulmonary arteriogram. Levophase. Anteroposterior projection. Ring is seen as small radiolucency *(arrow)* immediately above level of mitral valve. LA = left atrium; LAA = left atrial appendage; LV = left ventricle.

cific diagnosis of supravalvar ring can therefore not be suspected. In most instances supravalvar mitral stenosing ring does not cause significant obstruction.

ANGIOGRAPHIC FEATURES

Opacification of the left atrium can be accomplished by the late phase of a pulmonary arteriogram or preferably by direct injection of the left atrium. A shallow right anterior oblique projection and a steep (60–70 degrees) left anterior oblique projection with cranial angulation are the preferred angiographic positions.

The supravalvar mitral ring is in most cases small and does not cause hemodynamic stenosis. The ring is seen as a membrane located immediately above the level of the mitral valve (Fig 53–2).

OPERATIVE CONSIDERATIONS

When recognized, the mitral ring can be excised from the left atrium.

REFERENCES

1. Davachi F, Moller JH, Edwards JE: Diseases of the mitral valve in infancy: an anatomic analysis of 55 cases, *Circulation* 43:565, 1971.
2. Shone JD, Sellers RD, Anderson RC, et al: The developmental complex of "parachute mitral valve", supravalvular ring of left atrium, subaortic stenosis, and coarctation of aorta, *Am J Cardiol* 11:714, 1963.
3. Benrey J, Leachman RD, Cooley DA, et al: Supravalvular mitral stenosis associated with tetralogy of Fallot, *Am J Cardiol* 37:111, 1976.
4. Hohn AR, Jain KK, Tamer DM: Supravalvular mitral stenosis in a patient with tetralogy of Fallot, *Am J Cardiol* 22:733, 1968.
5. Chesler E, Beck W, Barnard CN, et al: Supravalvular stenosing ring of the left atrium associated with corrected transposition of the great vessels, *Am J Cardiol* 31:84, 1973.
6. Mehrizi A, Hutchins GM, Wilson EF, et al: Supravalvular mitral stenosis, *J Pediatr* 67:1141, 1965.
7. Rao S, Anderson RC, Lucas RV Jr, et al: Clinical pathologic conference, *Am Heart J* 77:538, 1969.
8. Snider AR, Roge CL, Schiller NB, et al: Congenital left ventricular inflow obstruction evaluated by two-dimensional echocardiography, *Circulation* 61:848, 1980.

CHAPTER 54

Cor Triatriatum

Cor triatriatum, a rare condition causing pulmonary venous obstruction, is also called "stenosis of the common pulmonary vein." In this anomaly, the pulmonary veins enter a chamber that communicates with the left atrium. Its clinical identification is important because it can be operatively corrected with excellent results.

PATHOLOGIC ANATOMY

The condition represents faulty incorporation of the embryonic pulmonary venous confluence into the left atrium. The process of incorporation is incomplete and occurs after the primitive connections of the pulmonary venous system to the anterior cardinal or umbilical vitelline system have disappeared (Fig 54–1). Therefore, each pulmonary vein connects into the pulmonary venous confluence, which is an accessory chamber. The accessory chamber communicates through a single or occasionally several orifices with the left atrium. The size of the orifice varies from 2 mm to more than 1 cm. Rarely there may be atresia without a communication. Several pathologic variations of cor triatriatum exist.[1,2] The anatomic form of cor triatriatum has been divided into three groups:[1]

1. Diaphragmatic type (Fig 54–2). A fibromuscular diaphragm divides the left atrium from the accessory chamber. No external evidence of two distinct chambers is evident.
2. Hourglass type (Fig 54–3). A constriction between the accessory chamber and left atrium is evident externally.
3. Tubular type (Fig 54–4). A tubular channel is evident externally between the accessory chamber and the left atrium.

The left atrial appendage and fossa ovalis are located in the left atrium below the cor triatriatum (Fig 54–5), distinguishing this condition from supravalvar stenosing mitral ring, where both structures lie above the obstructing ring. Rarely, an atrial septal defect may be present below the cor triatriatum; the shunt through the defect in this instance is right to left (Fig 54–6,B). Rarely, a communication exists between the accessory chamber and the right atrium. In this case the shunt is from left to right (Fig 54–6,A).

In some instances of cor triatriatum, the primitive connections between the pulmonary venous system and the cardinal or umbilical-vitelline systems may persist and remain functional, forming coexistent anomalous pulmonary venous connection. Thus cor triatriatum may be associated with partial anomalous pulmonary venous connection,[3–5] with some pulmonary veins connecting to the accessory chamber and others connecting to a systemic vein (Fig 54–7). Cor triatriatum may also be partial, receiving only one or two pulmonary veins, whereas the remaining pulmonary veins connect to the left atrium directly (Fig 54–8).

The accessory atrial chamber normally joins the left atrium but may join the right atrium (cor triatriatum dextrum).[6] This may be caused by a faulty position of the atrial septum, which lies more to the left than normal. The cor triatriatum dextrum may be either complete (Fig 54–9,A) or incomplete (Fig 54–9,B). The complete form mimics total anomalous pulmonary venous connection directly to the right atrium. An obligatory right-to-left shunt is present at the atrial level (Fig 54–10). In another anatomic variation, the cor triatriatum is an imperforate membrane, blood exits the accessory chamber through a persistent left superior vena cava (Fig 54–11), and a right-to-left shunt is present at the atrial level.

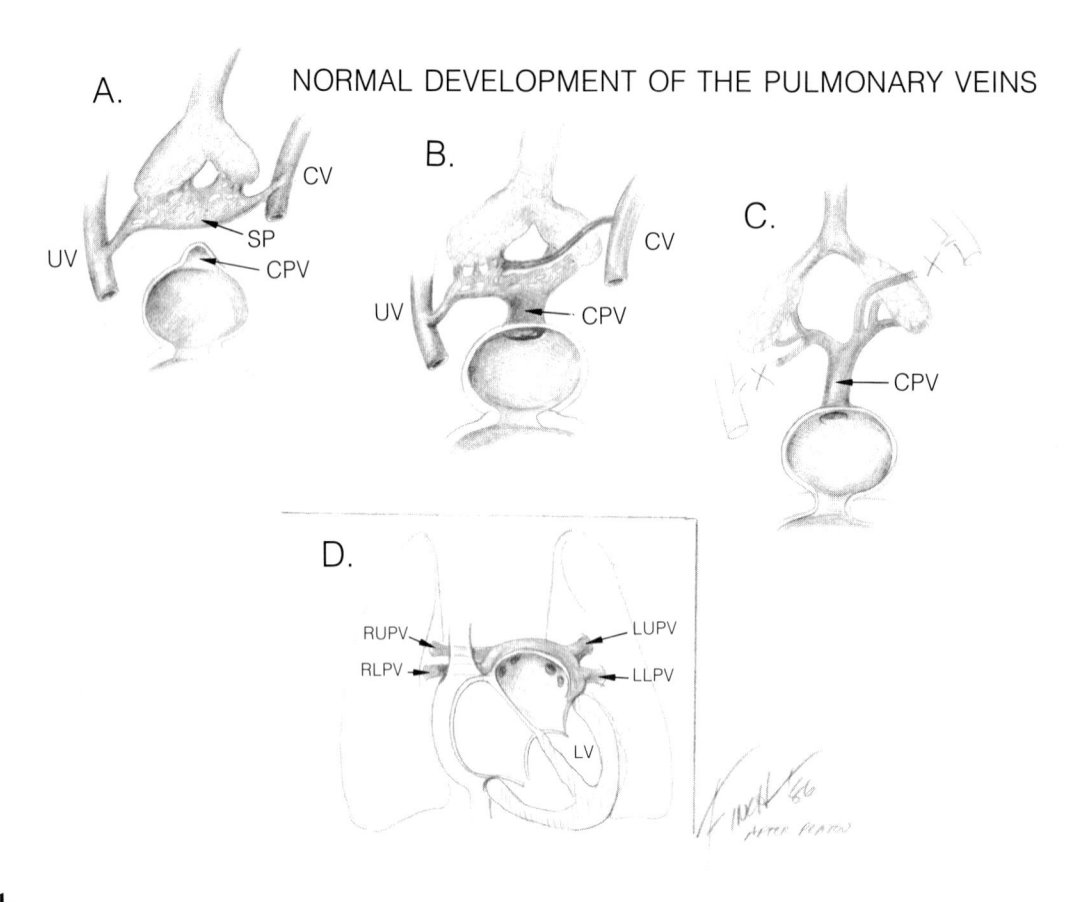

FIG 54–1.
Normal development of pulmonary veins. **A,** lung buds develop from foregut, and early venous return is to splanchnic bed *(SP),* which returns to cardinal veins *(CV)* and umbilical vitelline *(UV)* systems. Common pulmonary vein *(CPV)* forms from left atrium. **B,** common pulmonary vein makes contact with pulmonary venous system. **C,** connections between pulmonary venous system and cardinal and umbilical venous system have disappeared. **D,** common pulmonary vein and individual pulmonary veins have been incorporated into left atrium. *LLPV* = left lower pulmonary vein; *LUPV* = left upper pulmonary vein; *LV* = left ventricle, *RLPV* = right lower pulmonary vein; *RUPV* = right upper pulmonary vein.

Coexistent cardiac conditions are common with cor triatriatum, including ventricular septal defect, atrioventricular canal,[7] and coarctation of the aorta. In the first two, the physiologic effects of cor triatriatum may be accentuated by the increased pulmonary blood flow. Unusual associated conditions are the asplenia syndrome, tetralogy of Fallot, and Ebstein's malformation. In these situations the cor triatriatum may be inapparent because the volume of pulmonary blood flow is limited by the obstruction to right ventricular outflow. In the latter patients, if an aorticpulmonary artery shunt is operatively placed, the increased pulmonary blood flow causes the cor triatriatum to become apparent.

Cor triatriatum has certain predictable effects on the lungs. There may be pulmonary edema. Intralobar and subpleural lymphatics are dilated, and medial hypertrophy develops in pulmonary arterioles. The right ventricle is hypertrophied, whereas the left ventricular chamber may be smaller than normal, in part because the ventricular septum is displaced to the left by the dilated and hypertrophied right ventricle.

HEMODYNAMICS

Hemodynamic effects result from the obstruction to pulmonary venous return and are directly related to the size of the opening between the accessory chamber and left atrium. Pulmonary venous pressure is elevated, resulting in redistribution of pulmonary blood flow. More flow occurs through the upper lobes of the lungs. Pulmonary capillary pressure is elevated, and pulmonary edema results. Pulmonary hypertension is a constant feature, occurring not only as a passive phenomenon but also because of reflex pulmonary vasoconstriction. Right ventricular systolic pressure is elevated, and cardiac failure may occur. The cardiac output is in the low normal range.

Blood flow through the orifice between the accessory

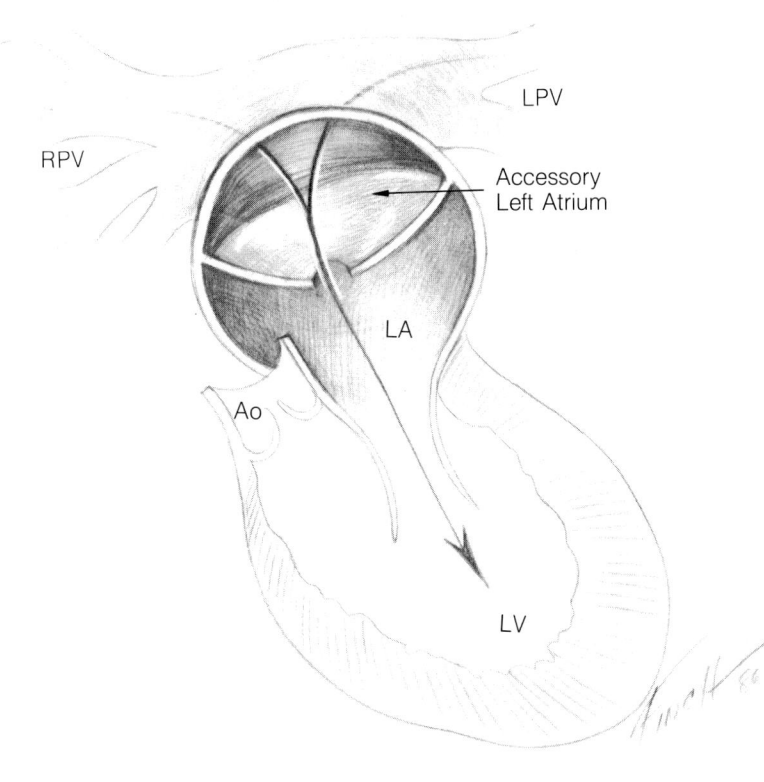

COR TRIATRIATUM DIAPHRAGMATIC TYPE

FIG 54–2.
Cor triatriatum. Diaphragmatic type. Fibromuscular diaphragm divides left atrium *(LA)*. No external evidence of two distinct chambers. *Ao* = aorta; *LPV* = left pulmonary veins; *LV* = left ventricle; *RPV* = right pulmonary veins.

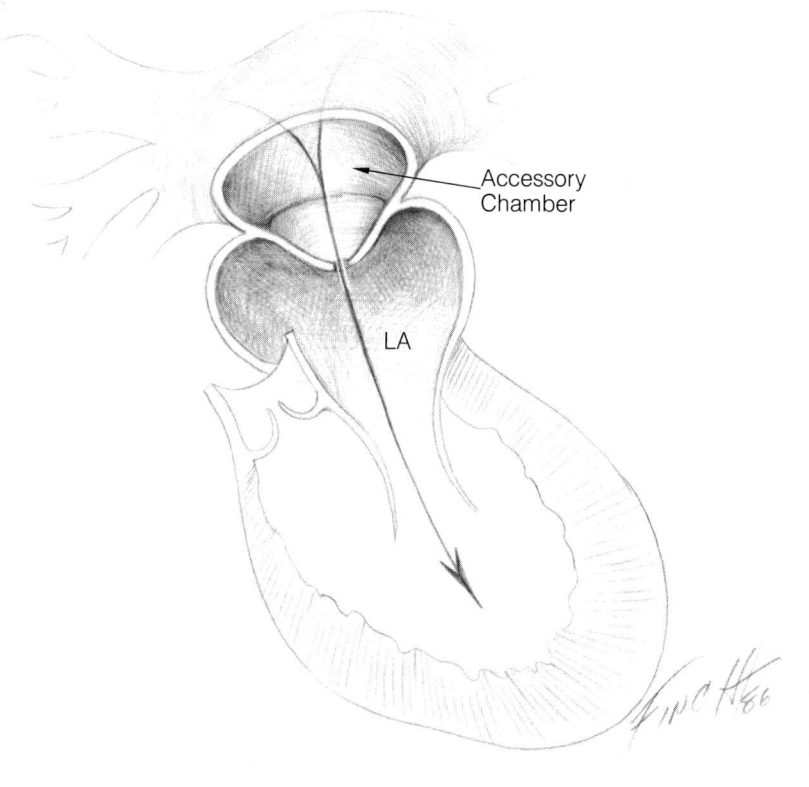

COR TRIATRIATUM HOUR GLASS TYPE

FIG 54–3.
Cor triatriatum. Hourglass type. Accessory chamber joins left atrium *(LA)* through a narrowed area evident externally.

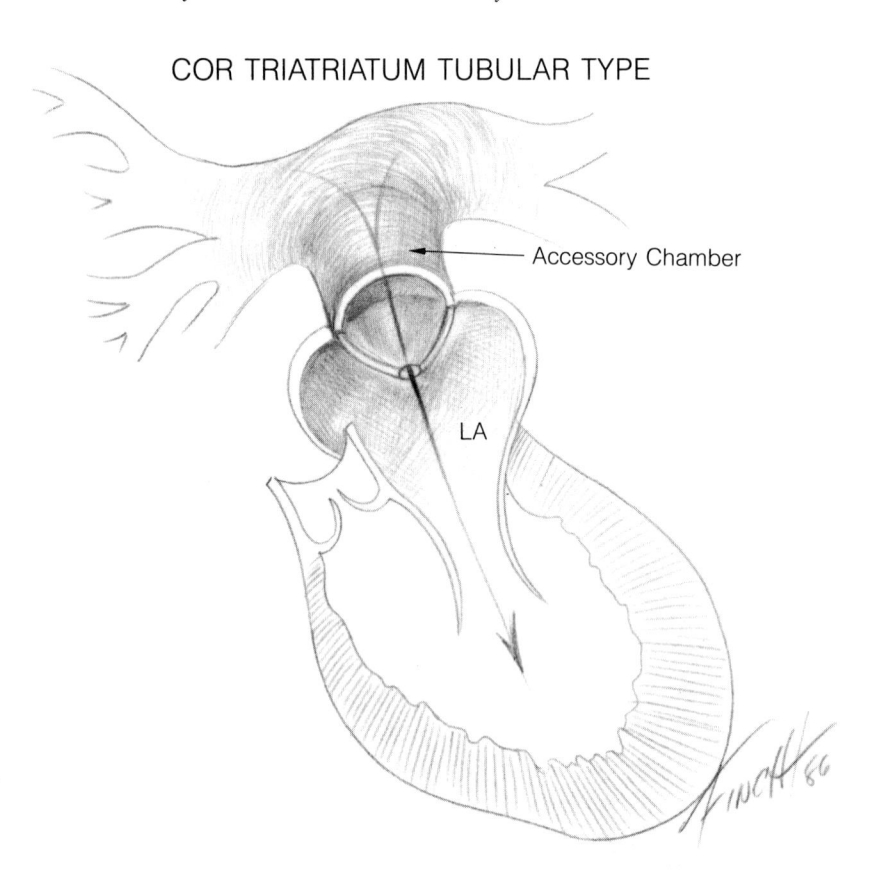

FIG 54–4.
Cor triatriatum. Tubular type. Accessory chamber joins left atrium (LA) through a tubular channel.

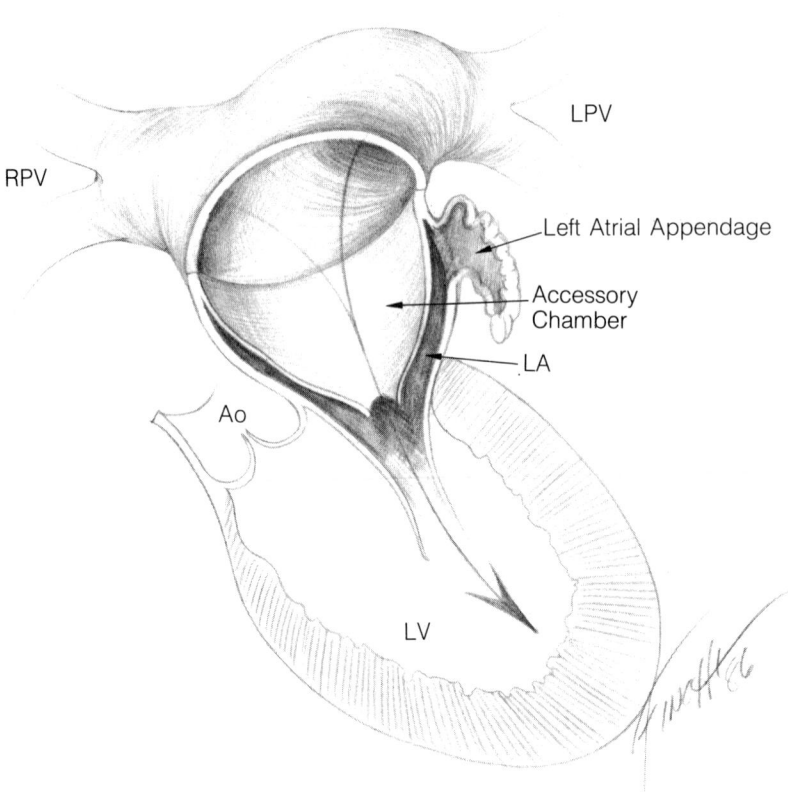

FIG 54–5.
Cor triatriatum. Left atrial appendage is located below accessory chamber. *Ao* = aorta; *LA* = left atrium; *LPV* = left pulmonary vein; *LV* = left ventricle; *RPV* = right pulmonary vein.

COR TRIATRIATUM WITH ATRIAL SEPTAL DEFECT

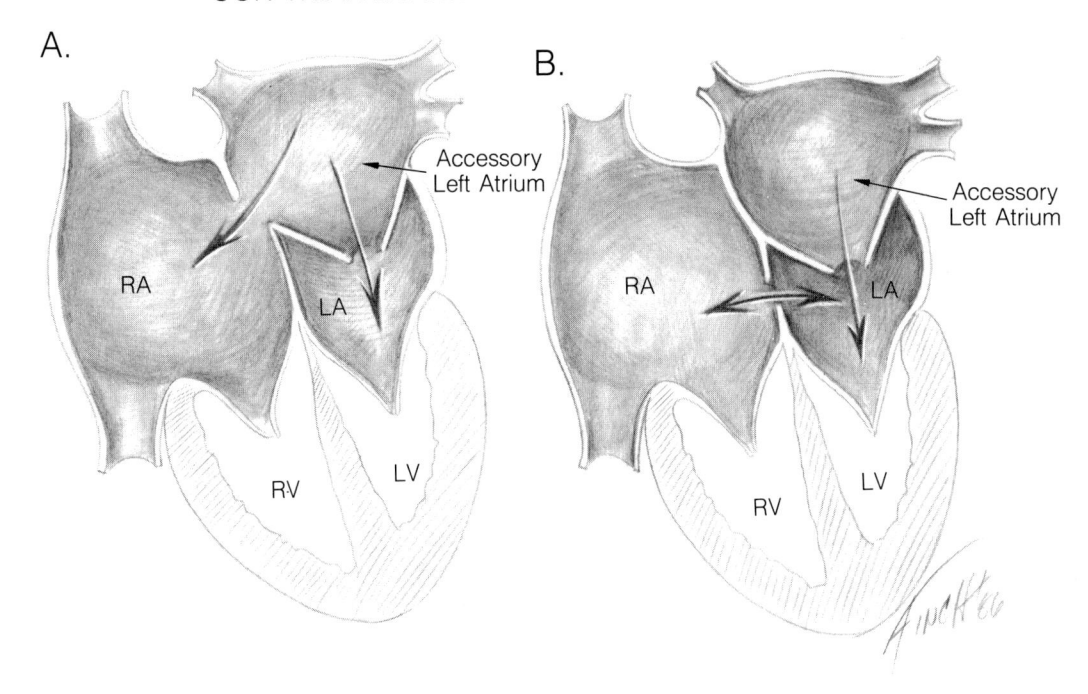

FIG 54–6.
Cor triatriatum with atrial septal defect. **A,** communication between accessory chamber and right atrium *(RA)*. **B,** coexistent atrial septal defect. *LA* = left atrium; *LV* = left ventricle; *RV* = right ventricle.

PARTIAL COR TRIATRIATUM AND PARTIAL ANOMALOUS PULMONARY VENOUS CONNECTION

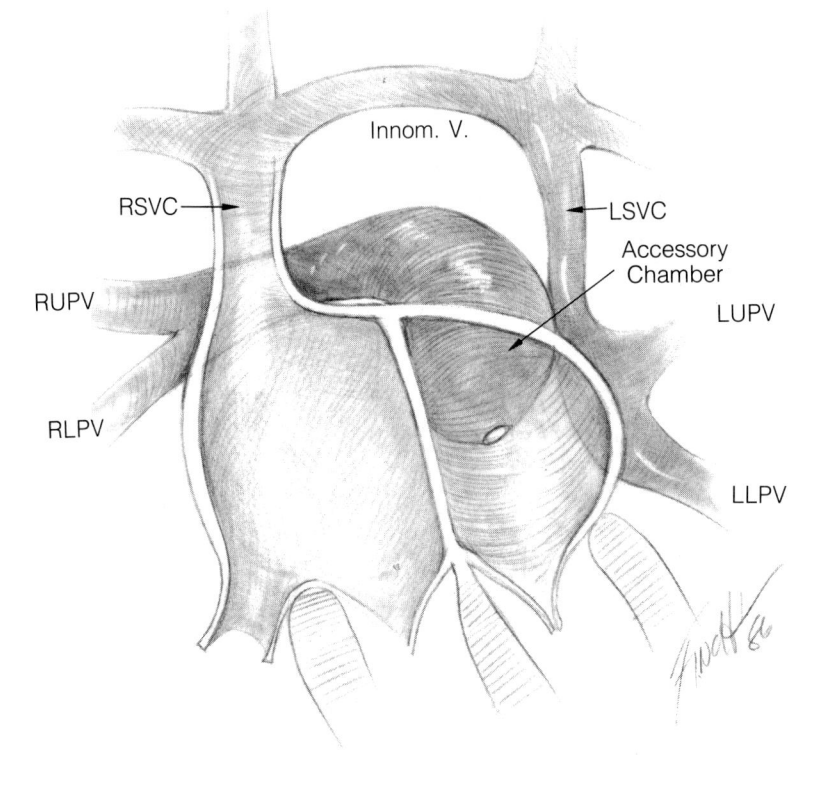

FIG 54–7.
Partial cor triatriatum involving right pulmonary veins *(RLPV and RUPV)*. Partial anomalous pulmonary venous connection of left pulmonary veins *(LLPV and LUPV)* to innominate vein *(Innom. V.)*, through left superior vena cava *(LSVC)*. RSVC = right superior vena cava.

PARTIAL COR TRIATRIATUM

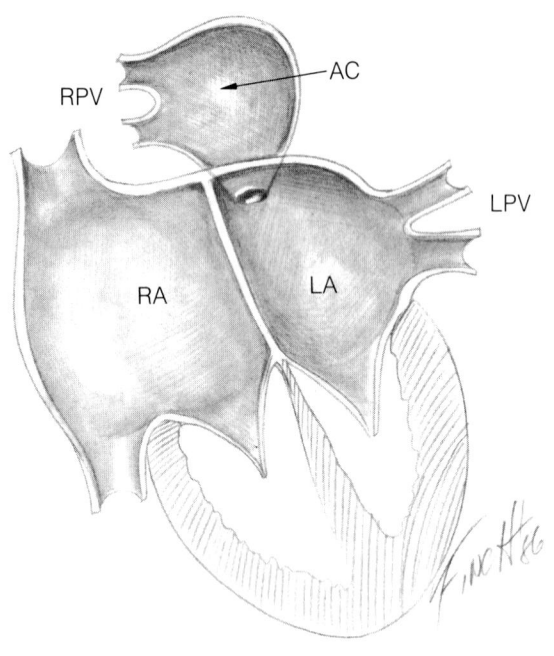

FIG 54-8.
Partial cor triatriatum involving right pulmonary veins *(RPV)* forming accessory chamber *(AC)*. Diagram. Left pulmonary veins *(LPV)* connect normally. *LA* = left atrium; *RA* = right atrium.

chamber and left atrium occurs throughout the cardiac cycle, in contrast to mitral stenosis, where blood flow occurs only during diastole. Thus, cor triatriatum tends to be tolerated better than mitral stenosis. Patients with an associated atrial septal defect have variable findings. If the defect or patent foramen ovale is located between the accessory chamber and right atrium, a left-to-right shunt occurs. A widely patent foramen ovale between the left atrium below the accessory chamber and the right atrium permits a right-to-left shunt, resulting in cyanosis. Cor triatriatum in combination with other cardiac malformations has variable hemodynamic effects.

CLINICAL FEATURES

Most patients develop symptoms within the first years of life, although an occasional patient remains asymptomatic until the second or third decade. The age of onset and severity of symptoms are directly related to the size of the orifice between the accessory atrial chamber and the left atrium. Symptoms are caused largely by the effects of pulmonary venous and arterial hypertension. The major symptoms are respiratory and not cardiac. Dyspnea, tachypnea, chronic cough, and episodes of pneumonia are prominent. There may be intermittent bouts of acute pul-

COR TRIATRIATUM WITH ACCESSORY CHAMBER JOINING RA
(Cor Triatriatum Dextrum)

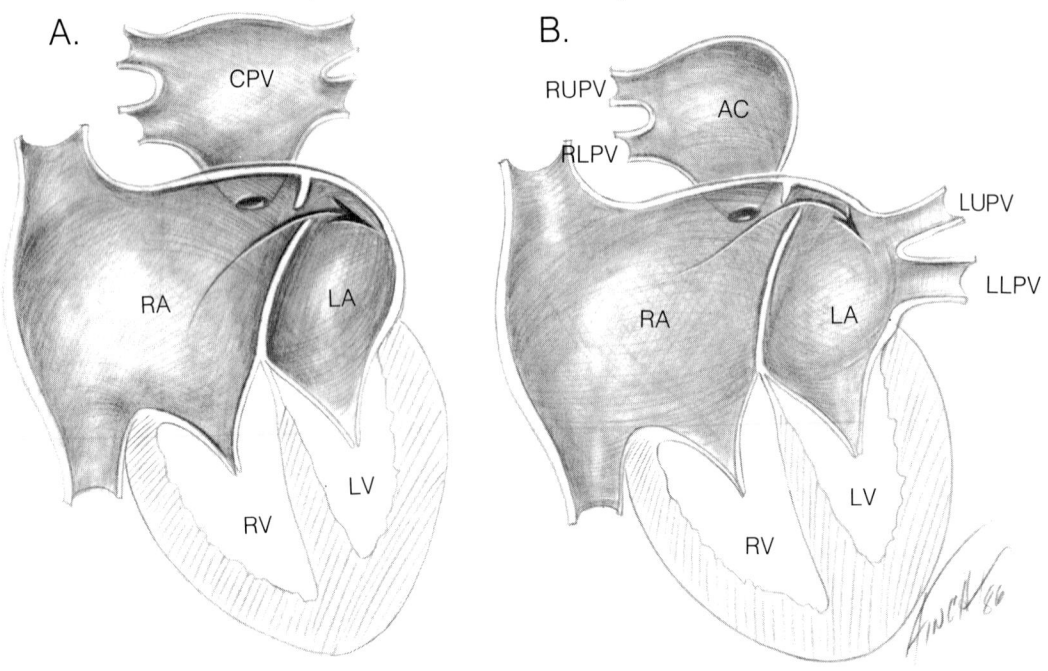

FIG 54-9.
Cor triatriatum dextrum. **A**, total. Accessory chamber *(CPV)* connects to right atrium *(RA)*. Right-to-left atrial shunt. **B**, partial. Left pulmonary veins *(LLPV* and *LUPV)* connect normally to left atrium *(LA)*. Right pulmonary veins *(RLPV* and *RUPV)* connect to accessory chamber *(AC)*. *LV* = left ventricle; *RV* = right ventricle.

COR TRIATRIATUM WITH LEFT TO RIGHT AND RIGHT TO LEFT SHUNTS

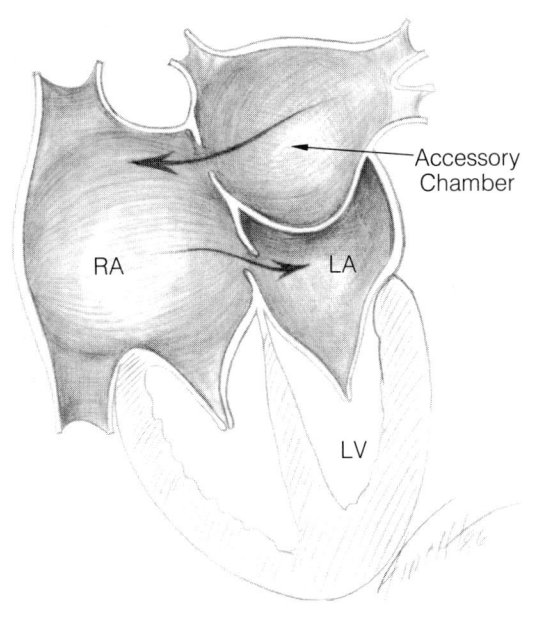

FIG 54–10.
Cor triatriatum. Hemodynamically identical to total anomalous connection to right atrium. Left-to-right shunt through atrial septal defect, right-to-left shunt through foramen ovale. *LA* = left atrium; *LV* = left ventricle; *RA* = right atrium.

monary edema and congestive cardiac failure. Often infants are irritable and have slow growth.

The infants appear chronically ill and in respiratory distress. There is a left precordial bulge and an accentuated pulmonary component, reflecting the pulmonary hypertension. Murmurs are not consistently found, and when they do occur, they are soft and nonspecific. A murmur of tricuspid regurgitation may be found. Pulmonary rales and hepatomegaly are usually present.

ELECTROCARDIOGRAPHIC FEATURES

As in other obstructive conditions located proximal to the mitral valve and causing pulmonary venous obstruction, the electrocardiogram shows right axis deviation, right atrial enlargement, and right ventricular hypertrophy. These are manifestations of the effects of pulmonary hypertension on the right side of the heart.

ECHOCARDIOGRAPHIC FEATURES[8-10]

A dense linear echo is found behind the anterior mitral valve leaflet or the posterior wall of the aortic root. The linear density of the cor triatriatum is seen crossing the left atrium and attaching to its opposite walls. Diastolic flutter

COR TRIATRIATUM WITHOUT COMMUNICATION WITH LEFT ATRIUM

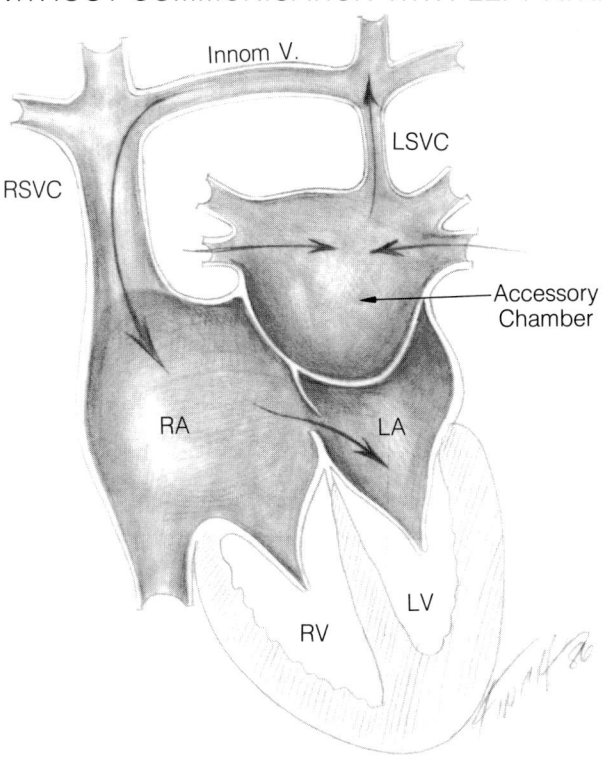

FIG 54–11.
Cor triatriatum. Imperforate membrane. Persistent left superior vena cava *(LSVC)*. *LA* = left atrium; *LV* = left ventricle; *RA* = right atrium; *RSVC* = right superior vena cava; *RV* = right ventricle. *Innominate vein = Innom V.*

of the posterior mitral leaflets is often found. The right ventricle is dilated, and hypertrophied and echoes from the pulmonary valve may suggest pulmonary hypertension. Doppler velocities in the pulmonary artery also reflect the pulmonary hypertension.

RADIOGRAPHIC FEATURES

The radiographic findings of cor triatriatum are often identical to other types of pulmonary venous obstruction. A posteroanterior and a lateral roentgenogram with barium swallow should be made because the presence of left atrial enlargement aids in the differential diagnosis among the possible causes of pulmonary venous obstruction. With the more common obstructive lesions at the level of the mitral valve (e.g., mitral stenosis), the left atrium is definitely enlarged. In cor triatriatum only slight displacement of the barium-filled esophagus is present. In mitral stenosis, the entire left atrium enlarges, whereas in cor triatriatum only the comparatively small accessory chamber enlarges, and the left atrium itself is actually smaller than normal. Cor triatriatum therefore shows only slight or no displacement of the barium-filled esophagus because the accessory chamber commonly lies to the right of the esophagus.

In other lesions causing pulmonary venous obstruction, such as stenosis of the individual pulmonary veins, atresia of the common pulmonary vein, and total anomalous pulmonary venous connection with obstruction, left atrial enlargement never occurs.

Because there are many anatomic variations and hemodynamic consequences of cor triatriatum, the radiographic appearance is variable. Five major variants of pulmonary vasculature pattern and cardiac size may occur:

1. In an individual with severe cor triatriatum, a reticular pattern, a ground glass appearance, or frank pulmonary edema are the expected findings in the lung fields.

2. The opening between the accessory chamber and the left atrium may offer minimal or no obstruction (incomplete cor triatriatum). Under those circumstances, cardiac size and pulmonary vasculature are normal.

3. The cor triatriatum may be partial, receiving the veins of only one lung. Under those circumstances, the vascular pattern between the lungs may be unequal, with evidence of pulmonary venous obstruction in only one lung or lobe. The other lung appears normal.

4. Cor triatriatum may be partial and associated with subtotal anomalous pulmonary venous connection. Under those circumstances, the pulmonary vasculature may be unequal or even increased in one lung field.

5. The venous obstruction may be masked by the presence of an associated anomaly such as ventricular or atrial septal defect. The pulmonary vasculature may be increased without signs of pulmonary venous obstruction.

The radiographic appearance of venous obstruction, like the clinical features, is directly related to the degree of obstruction between the accessory chamber and the left atrium. The obstruction may, however, be very severe, and the radiographic features may be surprisingly minor. REASON: Blood flow through the stenotic opening occurs during both systole and diastole, allowing greater passage of blood than through a stenotic mitral valve, wherein blood flow occurs only during diastole.

Specific Radiographic Features

1. The heart is usually normal sized or only minimally enlarged (Fig 54–12). REASON: A cor triatriatum obstructs blood flow into the left ventricle and causes right ventricular hypertrophy. Right ventricular hypertrophy is not well demonstrated radiographically, particularly on posteroanterior films. Only if the right ventricle decompensates does cardiac size increase significantly.

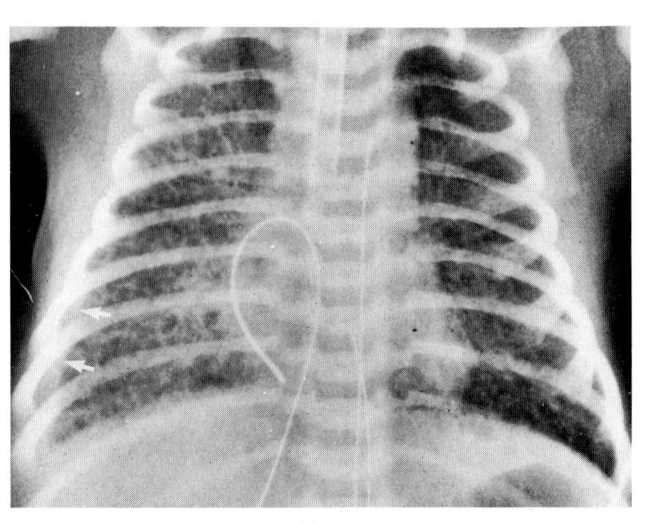

FIG 54–12.
Cor triatriatum. Severe obstruction. Thoracic roentgenogram. Posteroanterior projection. Normal cardiac size. Both lung fields show diffuse reticular pattern, more in right lung. Radiographic pattern is identical to other obstructive lesions such as total anomalous pulmonary venous connection below diaphragm. Small right pleural effusion *(arrows)* is helpful in suggesting cardiac cause for pulmonary pattern.

2. In infancy a diffuse reticular pattern is seen identical to other left-sided obstructive lesions and mimics closely respiratory distress syndrome. An air bronchogram is commonly found in respiratory distress syndrome and is helpful in the differential radiographic diagnosis. Furthermore, pulmonary changes in respiratory distress syndrome are seen at birth, whereas they develop after 24 hours of age in pulmonary venous obstruction. REASON: In utero the pulmonary blood flow is normally limited by the elevated pulmonary vascular resistance, and blood flows preferentially through the patent ductus arteriosus from right to left. After birth with closure of the ductus arteriosus, pulmonary blood flow increases, and the radiographic pulmonary changes develop. Still, in most neonates, respiratory distress syndrome cannot be differentiated radiographically from pulmonary venous obstruction. Typically an air bronchogram is not present, but there may be minimal pleural effusion (Fig 54–12).

3. In older patients the pulmonary vasculature is indistinct, giving a ground-glass appearance of the lungs. The upper lobe pulmonary veins (cephalization) are distended because of redistribution of blood flow within the lungs. The upper lobes receive a greater volume of blood than the lower lobes (Fig 54–13), identical to mitral obstruction.

4. In severe cases, frank pulmonary edema occurs (Fig 54–14).

5. There may be slight displacement of the barium-filled esophagus, but this is never as severe as in mitral

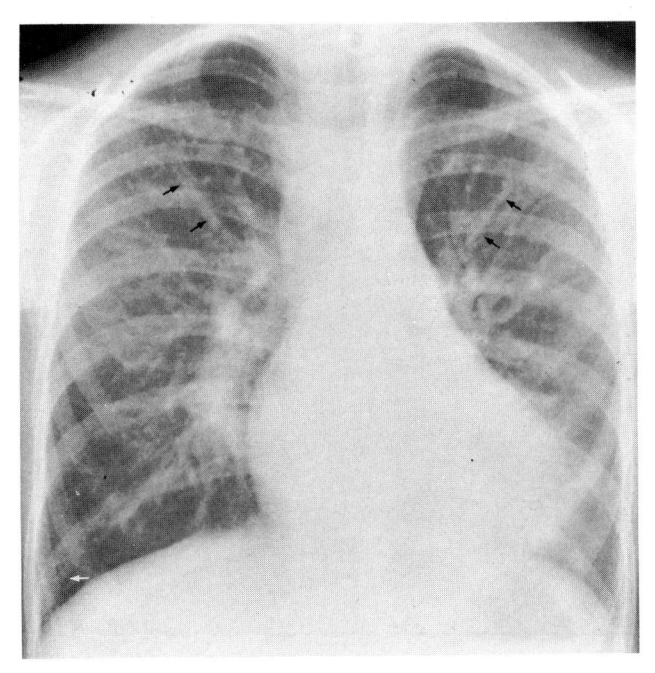

FIG 54–13.
Cor triatriatum. Older patient. Thoracic roentgenogram. Posteroanterior projection. Cardiac size at upper limits of normal. Nonspecific configuration. Redistribution of pulmonary blood flow with prominent upper lobe pulmonary veins and relatively underperfused lower lobes. Kerley B lines at right costophrenic angle *(white arrow)* are consistent with pulmonary venous hypertension.

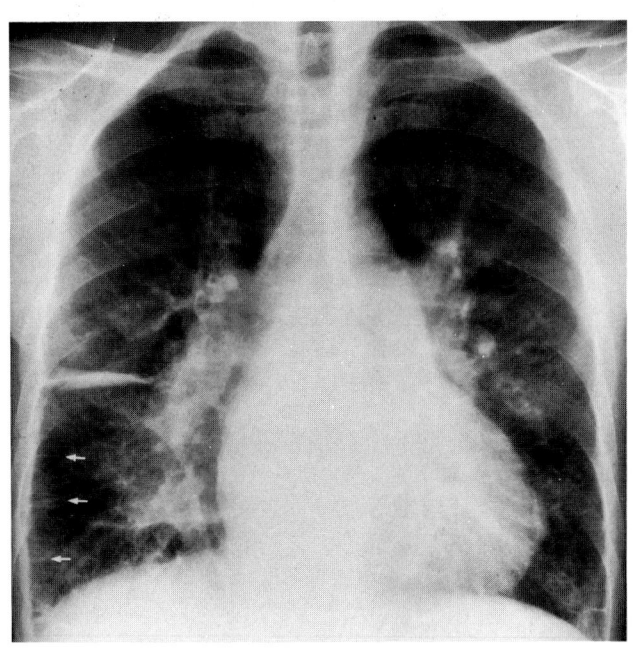

FIG 54–15.
Cor triatriatum in adult. Thoracic roentgenogram. Posteroanterior projection. Cardiomegaly is caused by right ventricular decompensation. Prominent pulmonary arterial segment and peripheral "pruning" are caused by secondary pulmonary hypertension. Right pleural effusion and Kerley B lines *(arrows)* are the result of long-standing increased pulmonary venous pressure.

valvular disease. REASON: The left atrium is relatively small because its pressure is normal and the accessory chamber usually does not show marked dilatation and typically lies to the right of the esophagus.

6. With long-standing obstruction, the pulmonary arterial pressure increases and right ventricular enlargement causes increased cardiac size (see Fig 54–14).

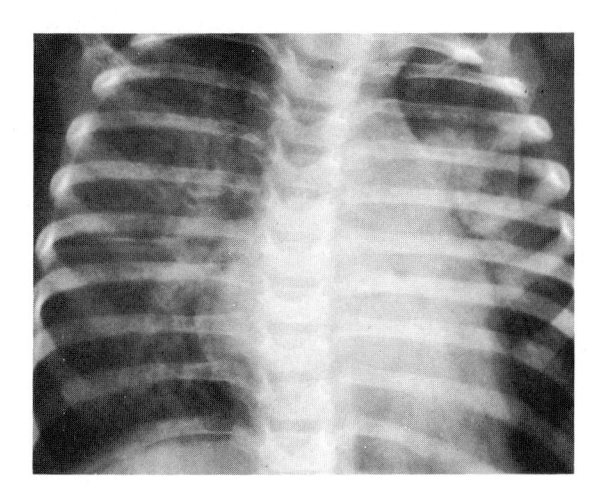

7. If the patient survives into adulthood, obvious radiographic findings of long-standing pulmonary venous obstruction and pulmonary hypertension are found (Fig 54–15).

8. The cor triatriatum may cause a double density along the right cardiac border (Fig 54–16). REASON: Typically the chamber is located above and to the right of the left atrium proper. This appearance is virtually identical to the normally observed left atrial density in infants and young children or a prominent confluence of the right pulmonary veins. Rarely, the third chamber in the hourglass-type cor triatriatum is distinctly seen on radiographs.

FIG 54–14.
Cor triatriatum. Severe obstruction. Thoracic roentgenogram. Posteroanterior projection. Slightly enlarged heart. Pulmonary edema. Appearance is indistinguishable from mitral stenosis and pulmonary edema. Accessory chamber is not visible.

CARDIAC CATHETERIZATION[11, 12]

The catheter course is normal. As in patients with pulmonary hypertension, it may be difficult to wedge the catheter in the pulmonary vasculature, but with a balloon catheter it is possible to obtain a wedge pressure recording. The wedge pressure is elevated, being as high as 30 or 35 mm Hg. When the wedge pressure is elevated, left ventricular end-diastolic pressure should also be measured to help localize the site of obstruction. Pulmonary arterial and right ventricular systolic pressures are elevated.

COR TRIATRIATUM

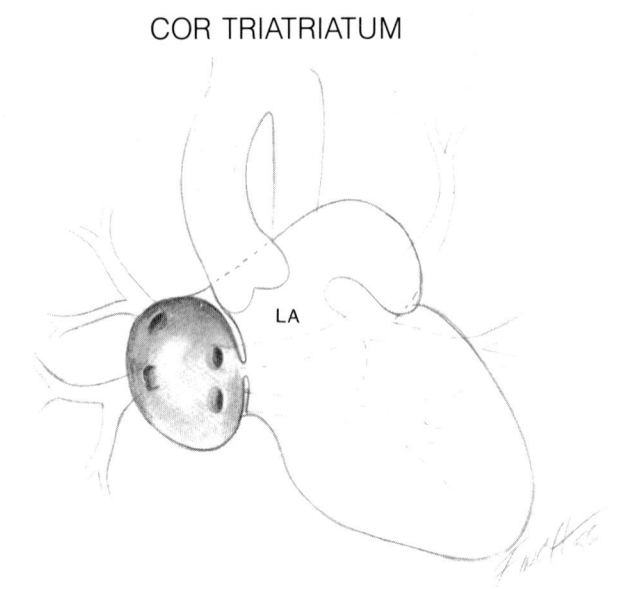

FIG 54–16.
Cor triatriatum. Typical location of accessory chamber in situ. *LA* = left atrium.

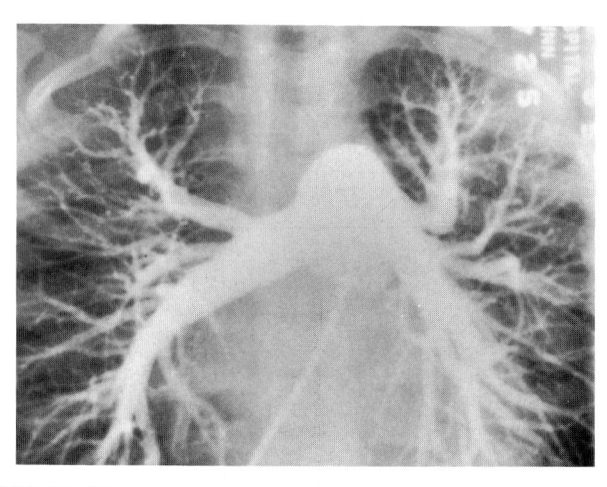

FIG 54–17.
Cor triatriatum. Pulmonary arteriogram. Anteroposterior projection. Mild enlargement of pulmonary artery because of increased pulmonary arterial pressure.

The values of oxygen saturation in the right-sided cardiac chambers may be lower than normal, reflecting low cardiac output. Systemic arterial oxygen saturation may also be less than normal if pulmonary edema is present. Sampling in the atria may show a left-to-right or right-to-left shunt, depending on the anatomy discussed above.

ANGIOGRAPHIC FEATURES

Angiography is important to identify the anatomy of the accessory chamber and left atrium and to determine the connection of each pulmonary vein, because anatomic variations exist. To demonstrate the pulmonary veins, pulmonary angiography with the injection of a large amount of contrast medium and prolonged filming is necessary. Reason: Because of the obstruction to pulmonary blood flow, the circulation time through the lungs is markedly prolonged. Because of the increased blood volume in the pulmonary artery and veins, considerable dilution of the contrast medium occurs, resulting in suboptimal opacification. Rarely, a communication to the right atrium exists, allowing selective injection of the accessory chamber.

The hourglass type of cor triatriatum is usually easily identified, but the membranous type requires an end-on visualization of the membrane. This is usually accomplished in an anteroposterior or slight right anterior oblique projection, but the membranes may be oriented in a different direction and may not be seen on end. Under the latter circumstances, the correct diagnosis cannot be made angiographically, but echocardiography usually provides additional diagnostic clues. The other useful angiographic technique is the injection of the left atrium below the accessory chamber through a catheter advanced into the left atrium through the foramen ovale. On opacification of the left atrium, contrast material does not reflux into pulmonary veins. A filling defect is present, which is caused by

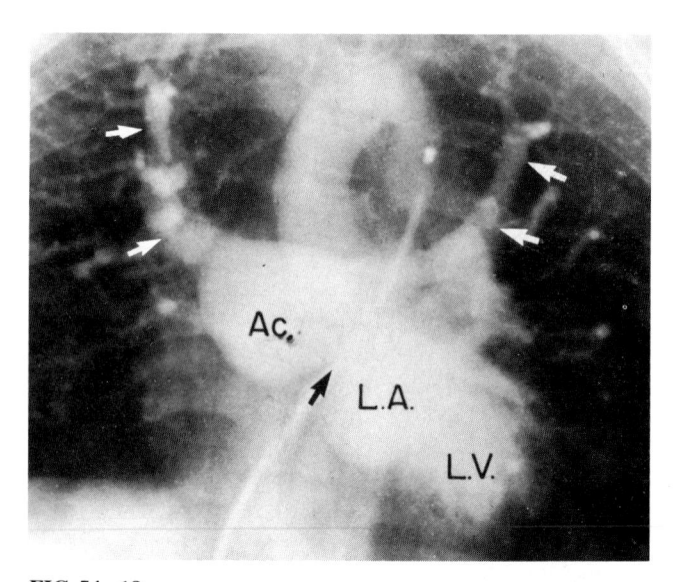

FIG 54–18.
Cor triatriatum. Hourglass type. Pulmonary arteriogram. Late phase. Anteroposterior projection. Distended upper lobe pulmonary veins caused by redistribution of pulmonary blood flow *(arrows)*. Contracted lower lobe veins. Small notch *(arrow)* at junction of accessory chamber *(Ac)* with atrium *LA*). Accessory chamber projects typically to right of spine and therefore is not in contact with barium-filled esophagus. Accessory chamber is unusually large. *LV* = left ventricle.

the accessory chamber bulging into the left atrium. The left atrium proper is smaller than normal.

1. The pulmonary artery is slightly or moderately enlarged (Fig 54–17). REASON: The venous obstruction caused by the cor triatriatum induces an increased pulmonary arterial pressure, which causes dilation of the pulmonary arterial tree.

2. The late phase of the pulmonary arteriogram demonstrates distention of upper lobe pulmonary veins because of redistribution of pulmonary blood flow. The lower lobe pulmonary veins showed a delayed circulation time and are narrowed (Fig 54–18).

3. The accessory chamber is usually located along the right cardiac border, and its size is variable (see Fig 54–18).

4. With the hourglass type, two distinct atrial chambers are visualized. If the chamber is large, it may be mistaken for the left atrium proper (see Fig 54–18).

5. Because of the side-by-side relationship of the left atrium and accessory chamber, these structures are superimposed on a lateral projection (Fig 54–19).

6. Whereas the angiographic diagnosis of the hourglass type is easily made, the diaphragmatic type is much more difficult to recognize. REASON: With the diaphragmatic type of cor triatriatum, the left atrium is divided into two chambers by a thin membrane that has to be seen on end to be recognized radiographically (Fig 54–20).

7. If the angiogram is slightly underexposed or the membrane is not seen on end, recognition may be extremely difficult. Commonly, however, a small notch is present at the junction between the cor triatriatum and left atrium (Fig 54–21).

8. If mitral insufficiency is present or can be induced by ventricular extrasystoles, the diagnosis can be made by left ventriculography (Fig 54–22). Contrast material refluxes into the left atrium and outlines the undersurface of the membrane.

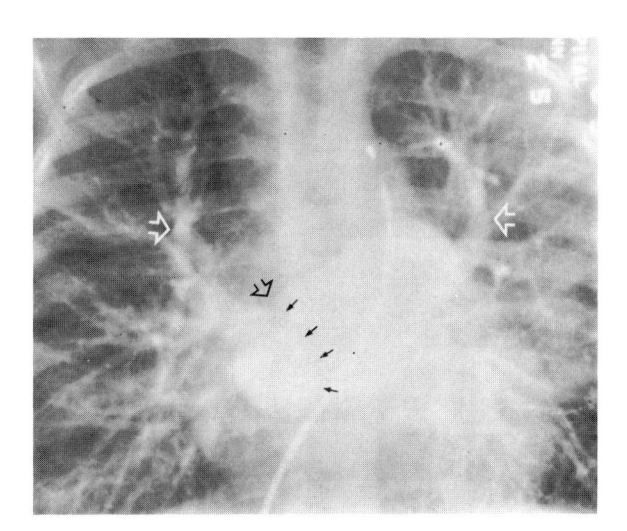

FIG 54–20.
Cor triatriatum. Diaphragmatic type. Pulmonary arteriogram. Late phase. Anteroposterior projection. Left atrium is divided by very thin membrane *(black arrows)* into left atrium *(LA)* and accessory chamber *(Ac)*. AO = aorta; LAA = left atrial appendage; LV = left ventricle.

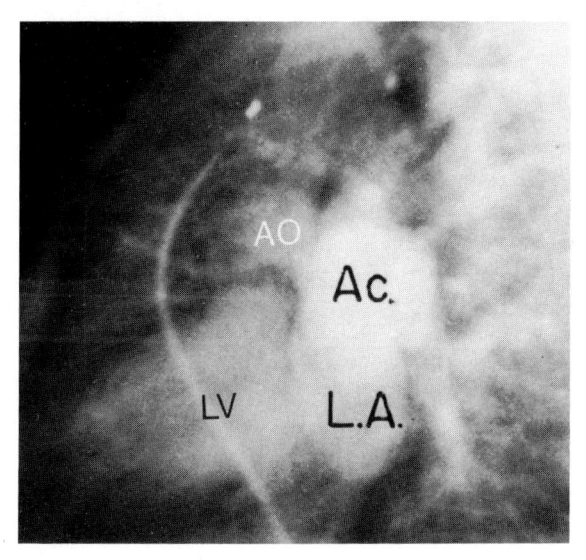

FIG 54–19.
Cor triatriatum. Pulmonary arteriogram. Late phase. Lateral projection. Accessory chamber *(Ac)* and left atrium *(LA)* are superimposed. Accessory chamber is located higher than left atrium. AO = aorta; LV = left ventricle.

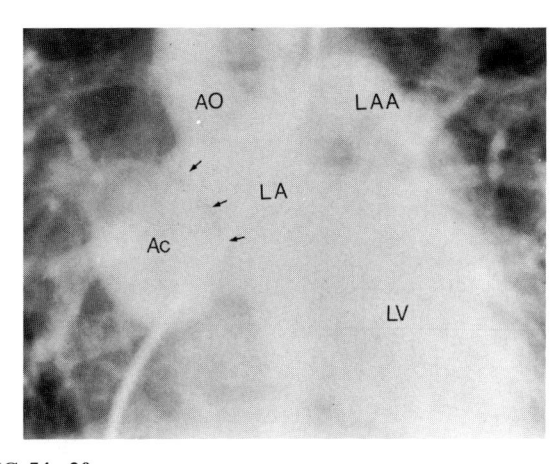

FIG 54–21.
Cor triatriatum. Diaphragmatic type. Pulmonary arteriogram. Late phase. Anteroposterior projection. Dilated upper lobe pulmonary veins because of redistribution of blood flow *(open arrows)*. Angiogram is slightly underexposed, making recognition of the membrane very difficult *(black arrows)*. Tiny notch at junction of third chamber with left atrium proper facilitates recognition of third chamber and thin membrane *(open black arrow)*.

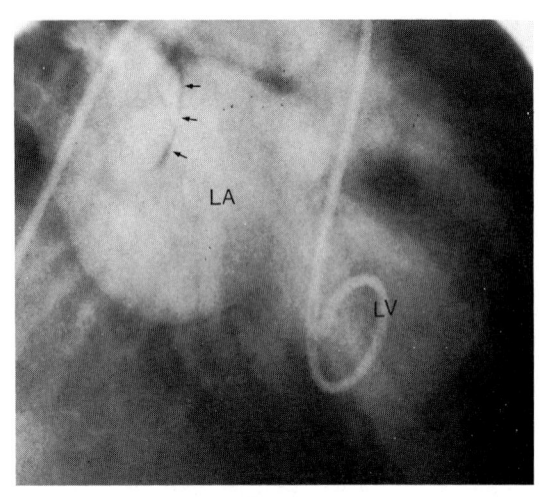

FIG 54–22.
Cor triatriatum. Left ventriculogram (LV). Right anterior oblique projection. Mitral insufficiency outlines an enlarged left atrium (LA). Incomplete nonobstructing cor triatriatum (arrows).

9. The cor triatriatum may be partial and may not cause obstruction (incomplete cor triatriatum) (see Fig 54–22).

10. If the catheter can be advanced through the foramen ovale, the left atrium proper can be injected (Fig 54–23). The left atrium proper can be recognized by opacification of the left atrial appendage. The pulmonary veins do not opacify.

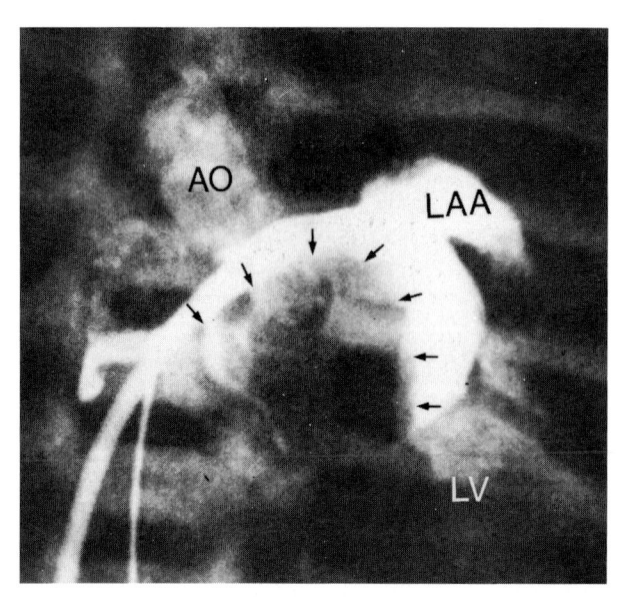

FIG 54–23.
Cor triatriatum. Diaphragmatic type. Catheter is passed through patent foramen ovale into left atrium, which is very small. Opacification of left atrial appendage (LAA). Unopacified cor triatriatum forms huge filling defect (arrows) in left atrium. AO = aorta; LV = left ventricle.

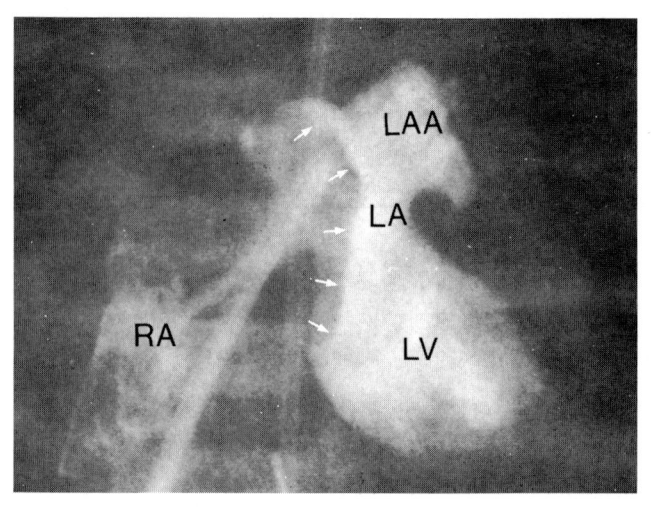

FIG 54–24.
Cor triatriatum. Diaphragmatic type. Left atriogram. Anteroposterior projection. Catheter is passed into left atrium (LA) via patent foramen ovale. Left atrium consists only of left atrial appendage. Typical wing-shaped appendage (LAA) is helpful in identifying left atrium proper. Some reflux of contrast medium along catheter into right atrium (RA). Membrane of cor triatriatum (arrows). LV = left ventricle.

11. On a left atrial injection, the unopacified cor triatriatum may form a huge filling defect indistinguishable from a left atrial mass (see Fig 54–23).

12. The left atrial appendage and fossa ovalis are typically part of the left atrium proper, allowing recognition of this chamber, which may be diminutive (Fig 54–24).

13. In patients without a communication between the accessory chamber and the left atrium or with only a pinpoint opening between the two chambers, egress of blood may be provided through a left vertical vein to the innominate vein (Fig 54–25). The condition is therefore hemodynamically identical to total anomalous pulmonary venous connection to the left vertical vein (persistent left superior vena cava).

14. Cor triatriatum can be recognized angiographically by pulmonary arteriography or preferably by direct injection into the accessory chamber. In the latter situation, pressure recordings can be made to demonstrate commonly associated areas of stenoses ("hemodynamic vise"; see Chapter 46).

15. In patients with only a pinpoint opening or only a fibrous connection between the accessory chamber and left atrium, the ultrasonographic pattern is usually mistaken as total anomalous pulmonary venous connection. Differentiation between these two conditions, however, is important because of the operative approach. Cor triatriatum is an intrapericardial structure, and the common pulmonary vein lies outside the pericardium.

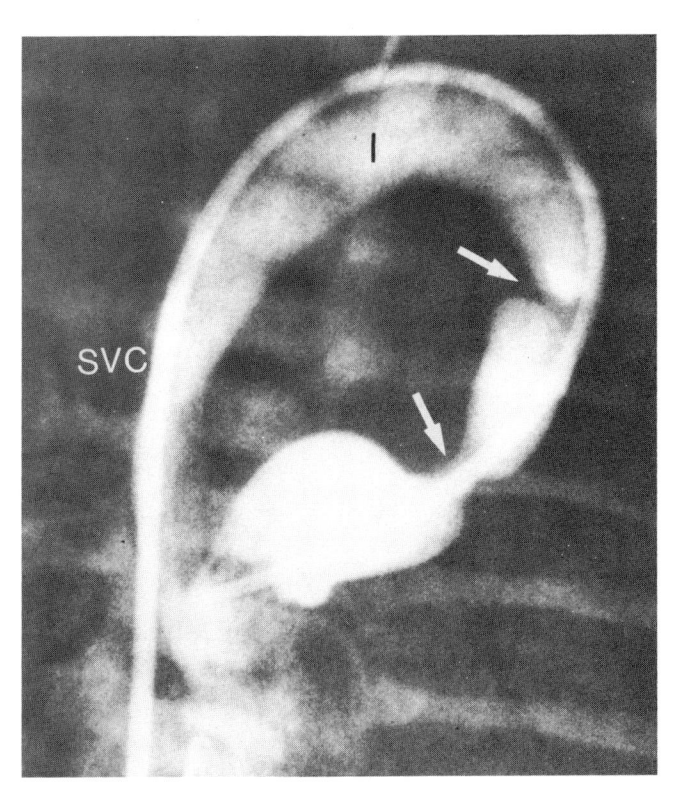

FIG 54–25.
Cor triatriatum and pinpoint connection between accessory chamber and left atrium. Egress of blood from accessory chamber occurs through persistent left vertical vein, which was selectively injected. Vertical vein connects to left innominate vein *(I)* and to right superior vena cava *(SVC)*. Condition is hemodynamically identical to total anomalous pulmonary venous connection. Venous obstructions are present as a result of two well-demonstrated areas of venous stenoses *(arrows)*. Hemodynamic vise (see Chapter 46).

OPERATIVE CONSIDERATIONS

The infant is treated with digitalis and diuretics as for congestive cardiac failure. Prompt diagnosis is necessary so that an operation can be planned. Operation is performed with cardiopulmonary bypass, and the membrane between the accessory chamber and left atria is excised.

Success of the operation depends on the age of the patient and the status of the pulmonary vasculature. In younger children, the elevated pulmonary vascular resistance usually declines to a normal level postoperatively.[13–15]

POSTOPERATIVE RADIOGRAPHIC FEATURES

After resection of the membrane, pulmonary venous congestion improves, and there may be some decrease in cardiac size. Resection of the membrane is usually complete, relieving the pulmonary venous obstruction.

REFERENCES

1. Marin-Garcia J, Tandon R, Lucas RV Jr, et al: Cor triatriatum: study of 20 cases, *Am J Cardiol* 35:59, 1975.
2. Niwayama G: Cor triatriatum, *Am Heart J* 59:291, 1960.
3. Shone JD, Anderson RC, Amplatz K, et al: Pulmonary venous obstruction from two separate coexistent anomalies: subtotal pulmonary venous connection to cor triatriatum and subtotal pulmonary venous connection to left innominate vein, *Am J Cardiol* 11:525, 1963.
4. Jennings RB Jr, Innes BJ: Subtotal cor triatriatum with left partial anomalous pulmonary venous return: successful surgical repair in an infant, *J Thorac Cardiovasc Surg* 74:461, 1977.
5. Wilson JW, Graham TP, Gehweiler JA, et al: Cor triatriatum with intact subdividing diaphragm and partial anomalous pulmonary venous connection to the proximal left atrial chamber (an unreported type), *Pediatrics* 47:745, 1971.
6. Hansing CE, Young WP, Rowe GG: Cor triatriatum dexter: persistent right sinus venosus valve, *Am J Cardiol* 30:559, 1972.
7. Thilenius OG, Vitullo D, Bharati S, et al: Endocardial cushion defect associated with cor triatriatum sinistrum or supravalve mitral ring, *Am J Cardiol* 44:1339, 1979.
8. Moodie DS, Hagler DJ, Ritter DG: Cor triatriatum: echocardiographic findings, *Mayo Clin Proc* 51:289, 1976.
9. LaCorte M, Harada K, Williams RG: Echocardiographic features of congenital left ventricular inflow obstruction, *Circulation* 54:562, 1976.
10. Canedo MI, Stefadouros MA, Frank MJ, et al: Echocardiographic features of cor triatriatum, *Am J Cardiol* 40:615, 1977.
11. Jegier W, Gibbons JE, Wiglesworth FW: Cor triatriatum: clinical, hemodynamic and pathological studies: surgical correction in early life, *Pediatrics* 31:255, 1963.
12. Miller GAH, Ongley PA, Anderson MW, et al: Cor triatriatum: hemodynamic and angiocardiographic diagnosis, *Am Heart J* 68:298, 1964.
13. Jorgensen CR, Ferlic RM, Varco RL, et al: Cor triatriatum: review of the surgical aspects with a follow-up report on the first patient successfully treated with surgery, *Circulation* 36:101, 1967.
14. Perry LW, Scott LP III, McClenathan JE: Cor triatriatum: preoperative diagnosis and successful surgical repair in a small infant, *J Pediatr* 71:840, 1967.
15. Anderson RC, Varco RL: Cor triatriatum: successful diagnosis and surgical correction in a three year old girl, *Am J Cardiol* 7:436, 1961.

CHAPTER 55

Stenosis of the Individual Pulmonary Veins

Stenosis of individual pulmonary veins is a very rare condition that must be considered in the differential diagnosis of pulmonary venous obstruction.

PATHOLOGIC ANATOMY

There are two types of stenosis of individual pulmonary veins. In one type, narrowing of the pulmonary veins extends for a variable distance from the left atrium into the lung.[1] This may be caused by either hypoplasia of the pulmonary veins (Fig 55–1) or hyperplasia of the wall of the pulmonary veins (Fig 55–2). In the third type, "localized pulmonary venous stenosis," the junction of of the pulmonary vein with the left atrium is stenotic (Fig 55–3) or atretic.[2-4] One or more veins may be stenotic, and this can affect one (Fig 55–4) or both lungs.

When only one vein is stenotic, no clinical manifestations results. When several are involved, pathologic features and clinical findings of pulmonary venous obstruction occur. Proximal to the obstruction the pulmonary vein may be dilated. Pulmonary parenchymal changes of edema and increased caliber of lymphatics are found. The pulmonary trunk is dilated, and the right ventricle is hypertrophied. There may be an atrial communication. With longstanding pulmonary venous obstruction, interstitial fibrosis may develop.

This condition may result from imperfect incorporation of the common pulmonary vein into the left atrial wall at a late developmental stage.

HEMODYNAMICS

Pulmonary capillary and pulmonary arterial pressures are elevated, usually markedly. Left atrial pressure is normal. Generally cardiac output is low because of the obstruction to blood flow through the lungs. There is usually no intracardiac shunt, and the patient is fully saturated unless pulmonary edema is marked.

CLINICAL FEATURES

Most patients are asymptomatic during the neonatal period and develop symptoms during infancy or early childhood. The patient has inadequate weight gain, dyspnea, and recurrent respiratory illness or symptoms.[1-4] Mild cyanosis may be present. The only abnormal auscultatory finding is an accentuated pulmonary component of the second heart sound. A murmur may be heard but is not specific.

ELECTROCARDIOGRAPHIC FEATURES

Right-axis deviation and right ventricular hypertrophy are present. A pattern of right atrial enlargement may be found.

ECHOCARDIOGRAPHIC FEATURES

No abnormalities of the left side of the heart are found, although excursion of the mitral valve leaflets may be less than normal because of low blood flow. The right ventricle is dilated and hypertrophied. Doppler flow signals demonstrate high velocity jets entering the posterior aspect of the left atrium as blood flows through the stenotic veins.

RADIOGRAPHIC FEATURES

The radiographic findings of severe stenosis of the individual pulmonary veins are identical to atresia of the

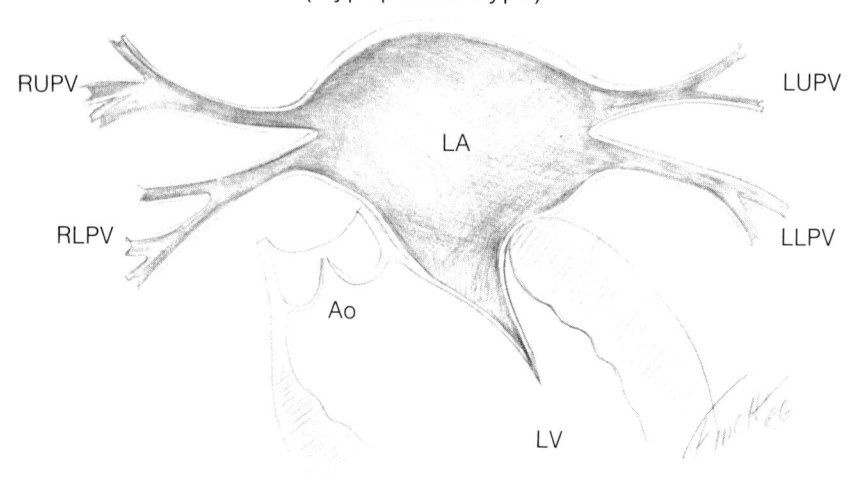

STENOSIS OF INDIVIDUAL PULMONARY VEINS
(Hypoplastic Type)

FIG 55–1.
Stenosis of individual pulmonary veins. Hypoplastic type. Each pulmonary vein shows tubular hypoplasia. *Ao* = aorta; *LA* = left atrium; *LLPV* = left lower pulmonary vein; *LUPV* = left upper pulmonary vein; *LV* = left ventricle; *RLPV* = right lower pulmonary vein; *RUPV* = right upper pulmonary vein.

STENOSIS OF INDIVIDUAL PULMONARY VEINS
(Hyperplastic Type)

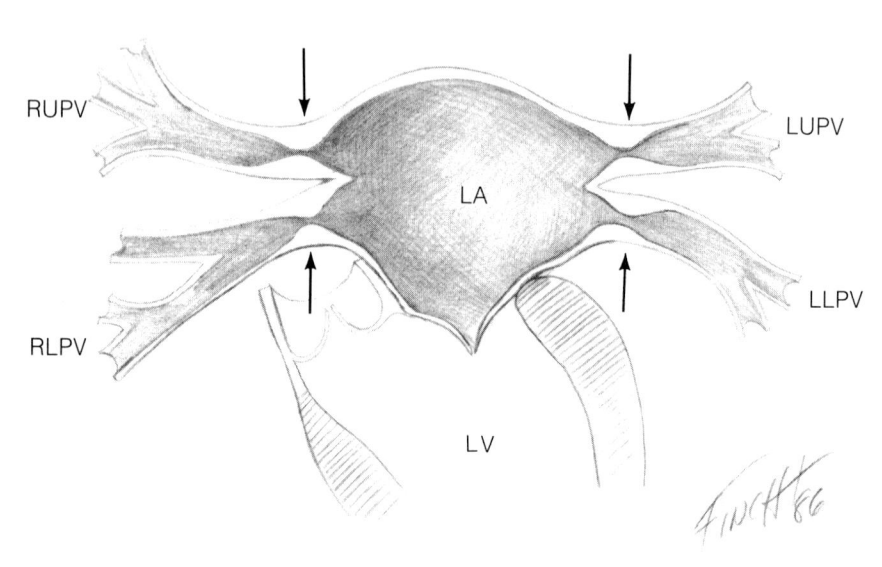

FIG 55–2.
Stenosis of individual pulmonary veins. Hyperplastic type. Stenosis occurs from thickened vein wall *(arrows)*. *LV* = left ventricle; *RLPV* = right lower pulmonary vein; *RUPV* = right upper pulmonary vein; *LA* = left atrium; *LLPV* = left lower pulmonary vein; *LUPV* = left upper pulmonary vein.

OSTIAL STENOSIS OF INDIVIDUAL PULMONARY VEINS

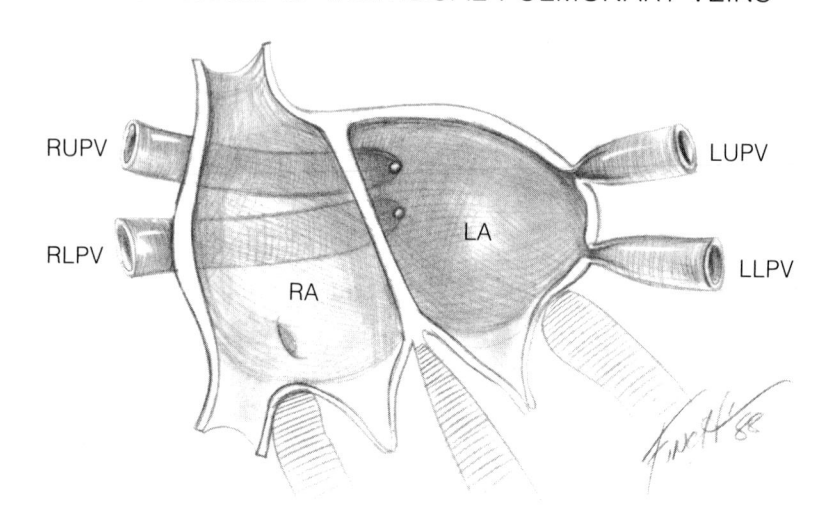

FIG 55–3.
Osteal stenosis of individual pulmonary veins involving orifice of each pulmonary vein. *RUPV* = right upper pulmonary vein; *RA* = right atrium; *LA* = left atrium; *RLPV* = right lower pulmonary vein; *LUPV* = left upper pulmonary vein; *LLPV* = left lower pulmonary vein.

UNILATERAL STENOSIS OF INDIVIDUAL PULMONARY VEINS

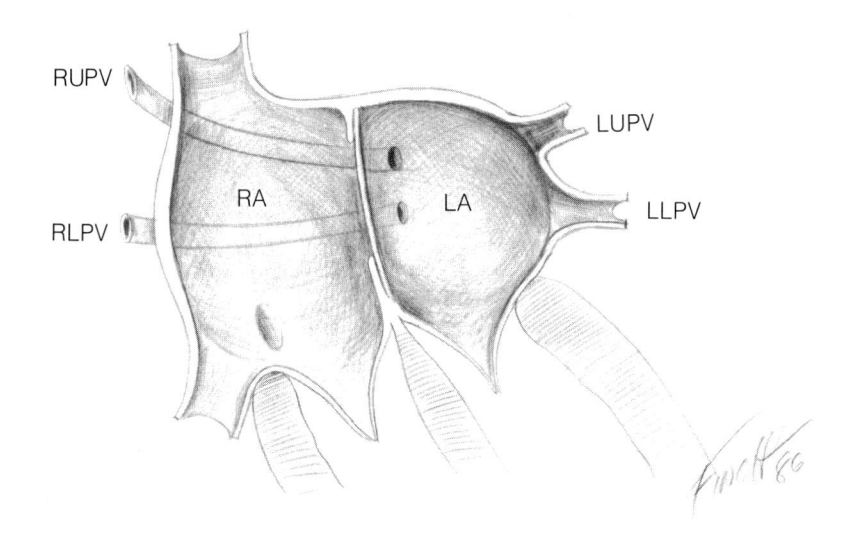

FIG 55–4.
Unilateral stenosis of pulmonary veins. Right pulmonary vein stenosis. Left pulmonary veins normal. *RUPV* = right upper pulmonary vein; *RLPV* = right lower pulmonary vein; *RA* = right atrium; *LA* = left atrium; *LUPV* = left upper pulmonary vein; *LLPV* = left lower pulmonary vein.

common pulmonary vein. In most cases, however, the degree of stenosis is not the same in each pulmonary vein, and, consequently, uneven perfusion occurs in the lung fields. The lung or pulmonary lobe with the most severe stenosis of the pulmonary vein is underperfused compared with areas with less stenotic veins. The difference is obvious if one lung or lobe is drained by a nonstenotic pulmonary vein. Under this latter circumstance, most of the pulmonary blood flow occurs through the lung connected to the nonstenotic venous system. REASON: The pulmonary capillary system of one lung can accept total cardiac output without increasing pulmonary arterial pressure.

1. With severe and equal stenosis of the individual pulmonary veins, radiographic signs of venous pulmonary obstruction are present. Granular lung fields are found in neonates. Cephalization of blood flow, accentuation of the pulmonary venous vasculature, Kerley B lines, and pleural effusion in older patients may occur.

2. With unilateral or lobar stenosis of the individual pulmonary veins, unequal pulmonary arterial perfusion is seen (Fig 55–5). The radiographic findings are indistinguishable from proximal interruption of a pulmonary artery. Although, in view of a left aortic arch, this diagnosis would be very unlikely. Lack or underperfusion of one lung can also be demonstrated by radioisotopic perfusion scans (Fig 55–6).

3. The cardiac silhouette is not enlarged. REASON: Stenosis of the individual pulmonary veins increases pulmonary arterial pressure, which, in turn, causes only right

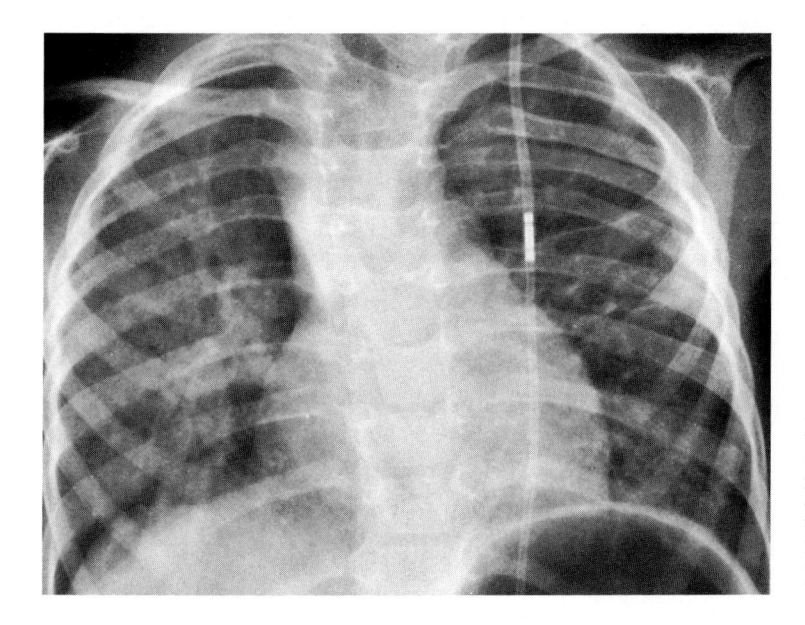

FIG 55–5.
Stenosis of individual left pulmonary veins. Thoracic roentgenogram. Posteroanterior projection. Normal pulmonary veins on right. Increased pulmonary vasculature on right. Decreased pulmonary vasculature on left because of unilateral stenosis of left pulmonary veins.

FIG 55–6.
Stenosis of individual pulmonary veins. Perfusion scan. Same patient as Figure 55–5. Normal perfusion of right lung. Absence of perfusion in left lung. REASON: Because of higher resistance in left lung from severe stenosis of individual pulmonary veins, entire pulmonary blood flow is through right lung.

ventricular hypertrophy. Right ventricular hypertrophy is not well seen on a posteroanterior roentgenogram. The volume of blood in the heart is normal. The left atrium is not enlarged.

CARDIAC CATHETERIZATION

Pulmonary hypertension is present, which may be extreme (170/80 mm Hg). It may be difficult to obtain a pul-

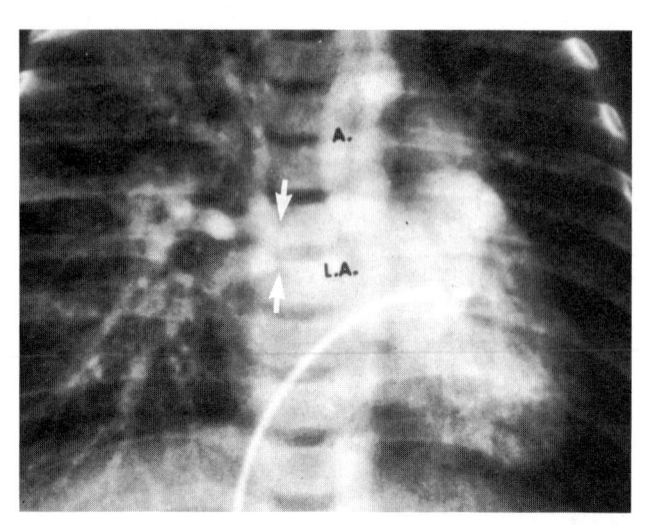

FIG 55–7.
Stenosis of individual pulmonary veins. Pulmonary arteriogram. Late phase. Anteroposterior projection. Normal left pulmonary veins have cleared. Right pulmonary veins are still well opacified. Localized stenosis (arrows) at junction with left atrium (L.A.). Ao = aorta.

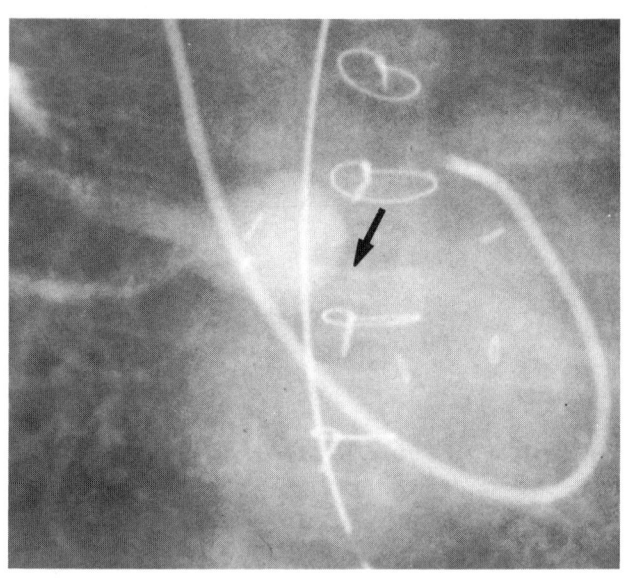

FIG 55–8.
Very severe stenosis of right upper lobe pulmonary vein. Pulmonary arteriogram. Late phase. Anteroposterior projection. All other pulmonary veins are cleared of contrast medium. Stenotic vein is opacified for longer time. REASON: Speed of blood flow is greatly delayed because of stenosis. Small jet of contrast medium (arrow) enters left atrium. Obstructed vein is well seen because it is dilated. REASON: Radiographic contrast density depends not only on concentration but also on diameter of opacified structure.

monary capillary wedge pressure without a balloon catheter. Oxygen saturations on the right side of the heart are low, reflecting a low cardiac output.

ANGIOGRAPHIC FEATURES

1. In contrast to atresia of the individual pulmonary veins, opacification of pulmonary veins can be obtained by selective right and left pulmonary arteriography. REASON: The stenotic pulmonary veins tend to be of normal caliber, and the blood flow is slow, which allows good opacification (Fig 55–7).

2. Opacification of the right and left pulmonary veins is rarely equal (Fig 55–7). REASON: The degree of stenosis is not identical between the veins. Consequently, a shift of pulmonary blood flow occurs within the lung.

3. The diagnosis becomes particularly obvious if only one lobe is involved or there is dilatation of the stenotic pulmonary vein (Fig 55–8).

4. The stenotic pulmonary veins remain opacified longer than the nonstenotic veins (see Fig 55–8).

5. If the diagnosis is suspected, an attempt should be made to enter the left atrium and catheterize the individual pulmonary veins. This has the advantage of better contrast visualization and confirmation by pressure measurements (Fig 55–9). However, if only one or two veins are

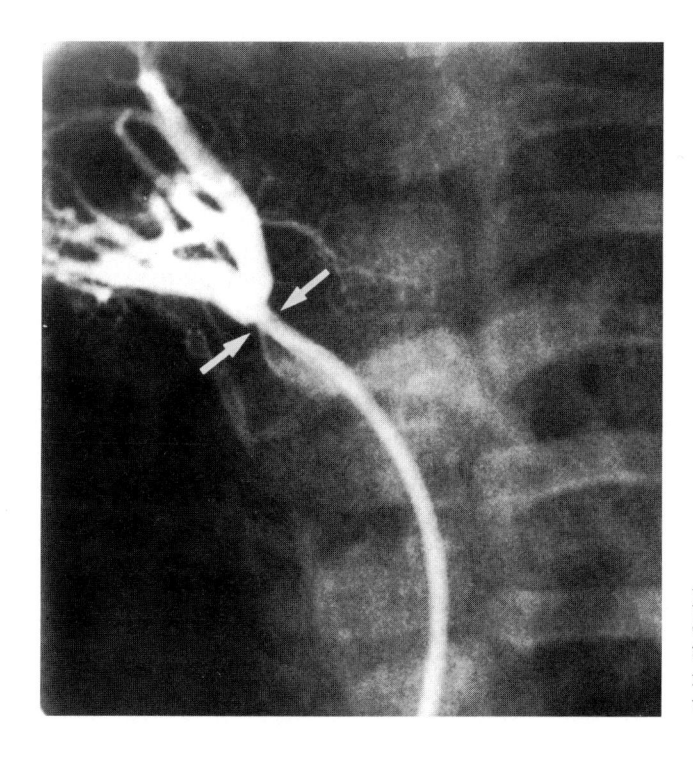

FIG 55–9.
Stenosis of individual pulmonary veins. Pulmonary venogram. Anteroposterior projection. Left atrium is catheterized through foramen ovale. Catheter is passed into right upper lobe pulmonary vein. Severe stenosis *(arrows)* of hyperplastic type.

STENOSIS OF PULMONARY VEINS

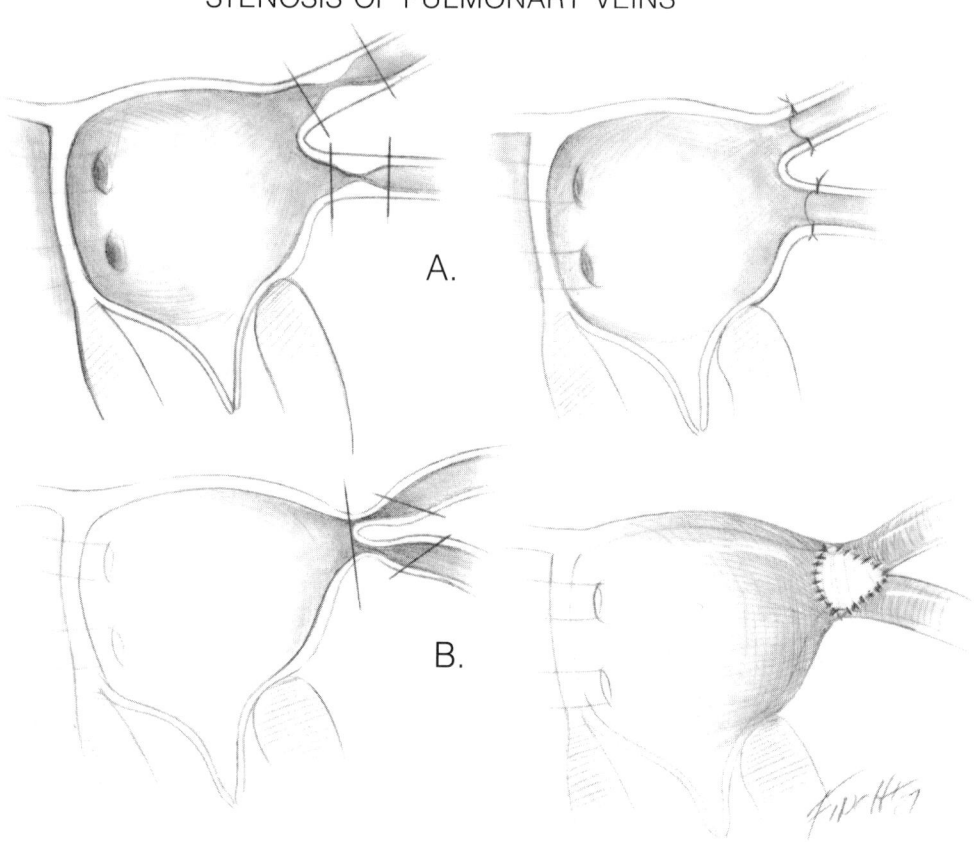

FIG 55–10.
Stenosis of individual pulmonary veins. Operations. **A,** resection of proximal portion of stenotic veins and reanastomosis to left atrium. **B,** resection of proximal portion of veins and patch placement.

stenotic, no gradient may be recorded. REASON: Flow through this lung segment is decreased, and pressure is related to flow. Gradients are present only if all veins are stenotic and the entire cardiac output has to pass through all lung segments.

6. In patients with very severe stenosis of the individual pulmonary veins, retrograde catheterization may not be possible.

OPERATIVE CONSIDERATIONS

After medical management, balloon dilatation of the pulmonary veins has been performed.[5] Although the initial response is favorable and the wedge pressure reduced, the stenosis redevelops within 1 year. Two operative approaches (Fig 55–10) have been proposed. The veins reattached to the left atrium (see Fig 55–10,A). An alternative is resecting the proximal pulmonary veins and widening the anastomosis by a patch (see Fig 55–10,B).

REFERENCES

1. Moller JH, Noren GR, David PR, et al: Congenital stenosis of individual pulmonary veins, *Am Heart J* 72:530, 1966.
2. Shone JD, Amplatz K, Anderson RC, et al: Congenital stenosis of individual pulmonary veins, *Circulation* 26:574, 1962.
3. Nasrallah AT, Mullins CE, Singer D, et al: Unilateral pulmonary vein atresia: diagnosis and treatment, *Am J Cardiol* 36:969, 1975.
4. Anderson JL, Durnin RE, Ledbetter MK, et al: Clinical pathologic conference, *Am Heart J* 97:233, 1979.
5. Driscoll DJ, Hesslein PS, Mullins CE: Congenital stenosis of individual pulmonary veins. clinical spectrum and successful treatment by transvenous balloon dilation, *Am J Cardiol* 49:1767, 1982.

CHAPTER 56

Cardiomyopathy

The term cardiomyopathy is applied to cardiac diseases in which the myocardium is principally involved without an identified cardiovascular anomaly. Such conditions are not associated with diseases that may cause myocardial abnormalities themselves, such as (1) systemic hypertension, (2) coronary arterial anomalies, (3) primary valvar anomalies, or (4) congenital cardiac anomalies. Cardiomyopathy is a broad and general term referring to a category of cardiac diseases in which the etiology has been identified in some instances, but usually the cardiomyopathy is idiopathic. Cardiomyopathy almost always involves the left ventricle and, rarely, the right ventricle.

Cardiomyopathy has been divided into three forms reflecting pathologic and hemodynamic features[1-3]: hypertrophic, dilated, and restrictive (Fig 56–1). Each form has different and generally distinctive clinical, radiographic, and angiographic features.

PATHOLOGIC ANATOMY

Among the three forms, one idiopathic hypertrophic cardiomyopathy was discussed in Chapter 26, because many features mimic aortic valvar stenosis. Idiopathic hypertrophic cardiomyopathy has been called "asymmetric septal hypertrophy," but this term is misleading because the entire myocardium is involved, not merely the septum. The term "hypertrophic obstructive cardiomyopathy," has also been applied, but this term tends to stress the obstructive element and not the cardiomyopathy.

The degree of hypertrophy ranges from mild to massive and generally involves the septum more than the free ventricular wall. The left ventricular papillary muscles may be hypertrophied as well. Often on the left ventricular side of the septum, a thickened ridge of fibrous tissue develops at the site where the anterior leaflet of the mitral valve strikes the septum during systole. The basis of left ventricular outflow obstruction is systolic anterior motion (SAM) of the mitral valve. This abnormal motion of the mitral valve can be readily seen angiographically and by ultrasonography. Histologically, several features are present, which, although also found in normal hearts and in patients with congenital cardiac malformations, are present to a greater extent in patients with hypertrophic cardiomyopathy.[4,5] These changes are (1) disorganization of myocardial bundles, (2) variation in myocardial cell to cell arrangement, and (3) disorganization of myofibrillary arrangement. Idiopathic hypertrophic cardiomyopathy is inherited as an autosomal dominant condition, or it may occur sporadically. Similar gross anatomic features may be found in the hearts of infants of diabetic mothers and in individuals with Friedreich's ataxia.

In dilated cardiomyopathy, the left ventricle is dilated but not hypertrophied.[6] Cardiac weight is increased, perhaps doubled (see Fig 56–1,C). Often each cardiac chamber is dilated, and mural thrombi may be present. Histologically nonspecific changes are found, such as alternating areas of hypertrophied and atrophied cells. Inflammatory cells are not found.

A variety of conditions have been identified as etiologic factors of dilated cardiomyopathy, including long-term increased alcohol intake, late sequelae of viral myocarditis, familial tendency, and administration of cytotoxic drugs for malignancies.

In the third form, restrictive cardiomyopathy, the cardiac mass is normal or slightly increased (see Fig 56–1,D). Unlike the other two forms, left ventricular cavity size is normal or slightly reduced, and usually left ventricular wall thickness is normal. The atria are dilated. Usually the histologic appearance of the myocardium is

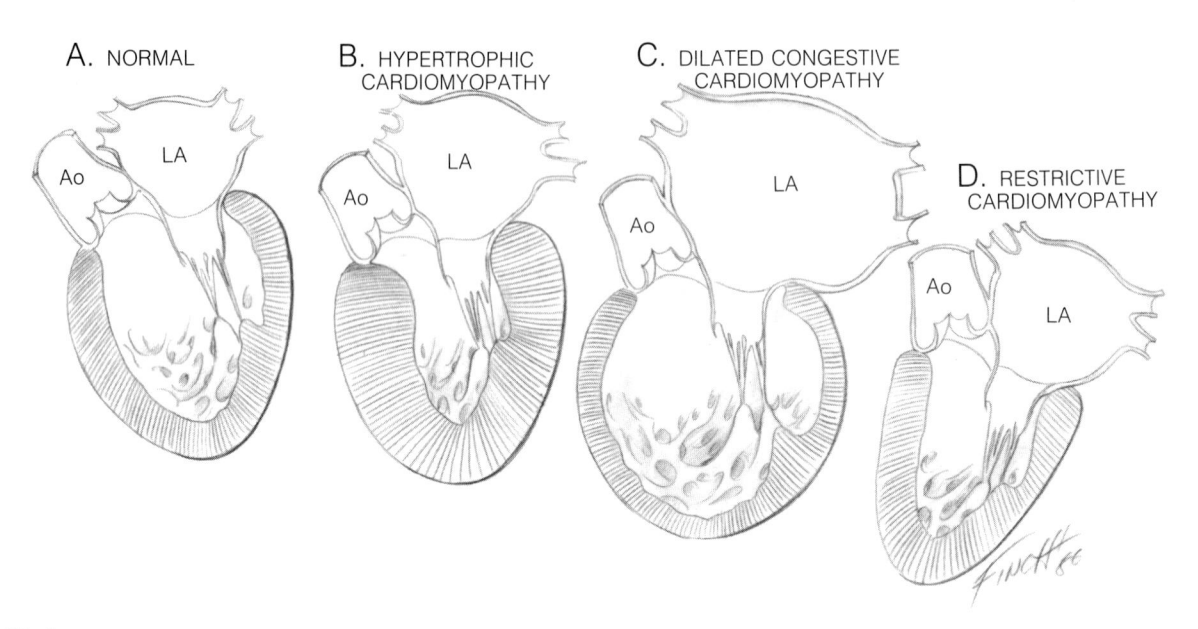

FIG 56–1.
Basic features of the three types of cardiomyopathy and comparison with normal. **A,** normal heart. Normal left ventricular cavity and thickness of musculature. **B,** hypertrophic cardiomyopathy. Marked thickening of left ventricular myocardium. End-systolic volume commonly decreased. Ejection fraction is increased. **C,** dilated cardiomyopathy. Thinning of myocardium. Increased end-diastolic and end-systolic volumes. Decreased ejection fraction. In spite of decreased ejection fraction, stroke volume and cardiac output may be normal at rest. REASON: Because of enlargement of left ventricular cavity, even a small contraction produces a normal systolic stroke volume. **D,** restrictive cardiomyopathy. Normal or slightly decreased left ventricular volume. Normal thickness of left ventricular musculature. *Ao* = aorta; *LA* = left atrium.

normal. In most instances an etiologic factor cannot be identified. It may occur with the unusual contracted form of endocardial fibroelastosis and various myocardial storage diseases, such as glycogen storage disease type II. Cardiac tumors may simulate the hemodynamic features of restrictive cardiomyopathy.

HEMODYNAMICS

The principal hemodynamic features also vary among the three forms of cardiomyopathy[1,2]:

Hypertrophic

In the hypertrophic form, the contractile function of the left ventricle is often increased, resulting in a small end-systolic volume seen on angiography. A pressure gradient may be found across the left ventricular outflow tract. The myocardial changes may reduce left ventricular compliance, resulting in elevation of left ventricular end-diastolic pressure. Mitral insufficiency is present in some patients (see Fig 56–1,B).

Dilated

The contractile function of the left ventricle is decreased, often markedly. Left ventricular volume is increased in both systole and diastole. Cardiac output is low. Left ventricular end-diastolic pressure is often elevated, not only because of reduced compliance but because of increased left ventricular volume, which may lead to pulmonary edema (see Fig 56–1,C).

Restrictive

Contractile function is normal. Left ventricular volume is normal or slightly decreased (See Fig 56–1,D). Ventricular compliances are reduced, so atrial pressures are elevated. The principal clinical features result from elevation of venous pressure in the pulmonary and systemic venous systems. Cardiac output may be reduced. The hemodynamics caused by impeded ventricular inflow resemble constrictive pericarditis.

CLINICAL FEATURES

In each of the three forms there may be clinical features that suggest the underlying etiology of the cardiomyopathy. A list is given in Table 56–1.

Hypertrophic

Many patients are asymptomatic, and the cardiac disease is detected by a murmur. Angina pectoris, arrhyth-

TABLE 56–1.
Conditions Showing Cardiomyopathy

Condition	Genetic Association or Mode of Inheritance
1. Inflammatory	
Lyme disease	HLA-DR2
Systemic lupus erythematosus	HLA associated (hydralazine and HLA-DR4)
2. Infiltrative	
Amyloidosis III	Autosomal dominant
Phytanic acid storage disease (Refsum disease)	Autosomal dominant
Hemochromatosis	Autosomal Recessive (HLA + transferrin saturation)
Glycogenoses	Autosomal recessive
Mucopolysaccharidoses	Autosomal Recessive and X-linked
Fabry's disease	X-linked
Sandhoff disease	Autosomal recessive
3. Defects in energy supply	
Endocardial fibroelastosis	Autosomal recessive
Carnitine deficiency	Autosomal recessive
4. Cardioneurologic associations	
Friedreich's ataxia	Autosomal recessive
Leigh disease	Autosomal recessive
Kearns-Sayre syndrome	Autosomal recessive
5. Structural and miscellaneous	
Noonan's syndrome	Autosomal dominant
Leopard syndrome	Autosomal dominant
Muscular dystrophies	X-linked
Mulibrey nanism	Autosomal recessive
Hyperthyroidism	Autosomal dominant
6. Environmental	
Keshan disease	Unknown
7. Conduction abnormalities	
Dysrhythmias	Unknown
Sudden death	Autosomal recessive

mia, or dyspnea may be the presenting features or may develop during the course of the disease.[1, 2, 7] Sudden death may occur.

Physical examination during infancy may be normal, with a murmur developing subsequently. There is a long systolic murmur along the lower left sternal border, which increases in intensity during the Valsalva maneuver. The peripheral arterial pulses are brisk. Third and fourth heart sounds are present.

Dilated

The pertinent clinical features are usually those of reduced cardiac output and congestive cardiac failure.[8, 9] Less often, clinical findings may be related to cardiac arrhythmia or embolic phenomena, either pulmonary or systemic. Many times no murmur is present, but there is tachycardia and a gallop rhythm. Cardiomegaly is evident by a laterally displaced cardiac apex. Tachypnea, rales, and hepatomegaly, features of congestive cardiac failure, may be prominent.

Restrictive

The clinical features are related to elevated systemic and pulmonary venous pressures. Elevated systemic venous pressure is reflected by increased jugular venous pressure, hepatomegaly, peripheral edema, ascites, and increased pulmonary venous pressure by tachypnea, dyspnea, and rales, reflecting pulmonary edema. Usually no murmurs are present. A fourth heart sound may be found.

ELECTROCARDIOGRAPHIC FEATURES

The electrocardiogram (ECG) may be normal in each form, but there are specific patterns associated with each type of cardiomyopathy.

Hypertrophic

Usually a pattern of left ventricular hypertrophy is found, and left atrial enlargement may be associated. ST- and T-wave changes in the left precordial leads may coexist. Deep Q waves may be found in left precordial leads, which may be misinterpreted as anterior or anteroseptal myocardial infarction.

Dilated

There is left ventricular hypertrophy, and inverted T waves in the left precordial leads are the rule. Left bundle branch block may be found.

Restrictive

The QRS complex is usually normal, but patterns of left or right (or both) atrial enlargement may be present.

ECHOCARDIOGRAPHIC FEATURES

The echocardiogram is extremely helpful in the differential diagnosis of cardiomyopathies. In the hypertrophic form, echocardiography has clarified the pathophysiologic mechanisms of the obstructive type, namely, systolic anterior motion of the mitral valve, which was often missed by angiocardiography. In these patients Doppler echocardiography can help identify obstruction and valvar regurgitation.

Hypertrophic

There is increase in left ventricular wall thickness, with the ventricular septum being thickened more than the posterior wall.[10, 11] Left ventricular cavity dimensions are usually decreased. The anterior leaflet of the mitral valve moves anteriorly during systole and coapts with the interventricular septum. There is midsystolic closure of the aortic valve. Doppler allows location of the obstructive flow disturbance, which can be estimated as to gradient by continuous wave analysis.

Dilated

Left ventricular diastolic volume is increased, often markedly.[12] Systolic ventricular wall motion and ejection fraction are reduced. Areas of dyskinesia may be noted. Doppler shows mitral regurgitation and, in extreme cases, aortic regurgitation. Mitral valve motion is reduced. In patients with severe myopathy, swirling motion can be seen in the left ventricular cavity. Apical clots may be noted. Mitral valve motion is reduced.

Restrictive

Left ventricular cavity dimensions and wall thickness are normal, whereas left and right atrial dimensions are increased. The left ventricular wall shows impaired motion and the posterior mitral valve leaflet motion shows reduced rate of opening. Doppler velocities reflect the altered ventricular compliance by tall waves during atrial contraction. Retrograde filling of the venae cavae may be observed.

RADIOGRAPHIC FEATURES

Among the cardiomyopathies, the radiographic features vary depending on the specific type. Rarely, radiographic findings allow a roentgenographic diagnosis of the cause of the cardiomyopathy, as in the mucopolysaccharidoses, in which characteristic bony changes are present (Fig 56–2).

Dilated

Dilated cardiomyopathies are characterized by generalized cardiomegaly, because both ventricles are usually dilated. In some types of dilated cardiomyopathy, such as endocardial fibroelastosis, only the left ventricle is involved. In these instances, radiographic evidence of cardiac enlargement is confined to the left ventricle. Although the right ventricle may be secondarily hypertrophied, this is not visible on a thoracic roentgenogram.

Both atria tend to be enlarged and contribute to the generalized cardiomegaly observed on a roentgenogram. REASON: First, the increased end-diastolic pressures of the failing right and left ventricles elevate right atrial and left atrial pressures, respectively. Second, with dilatation of the ventricles, one or both atrioventricular valves may become insufficient. Atrioventricular valve insufficiency occurring secondary to ventricular dilatation is termed "relative atrioventricular valve insufficiency," because anatomically the valves are normal.

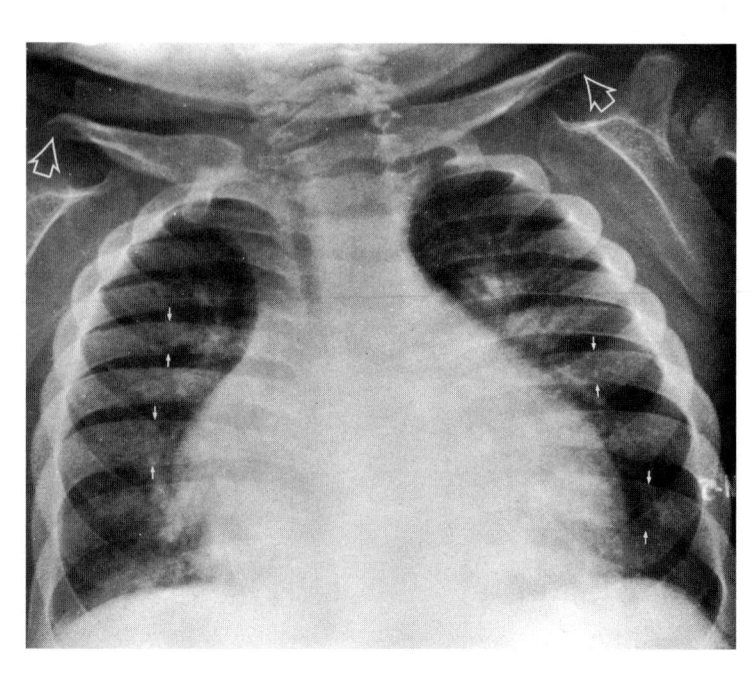

FIG 56–2.
Mucopolysaccharidosis. Hurler's syndrome. Thoracic roentgenogram. Posteroanterior projection. Pulmonary vasculature at upper limit of normal. Markedly enlarged heart, consistent with cardiomyopathy. Specific radiographic diagnosis of Hurler's syndrome can be made because of characteristic bony changes such as broad ribs *(arrows),* tapered, truncated clavicles *(open arrows),* and deformed scapulae. Cardiomyopathy is caused by deposition of mucopolysaccharide throughout myocardium.

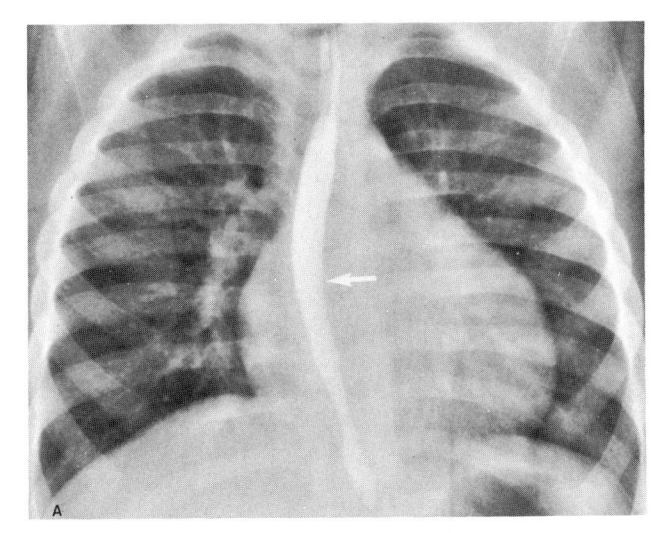

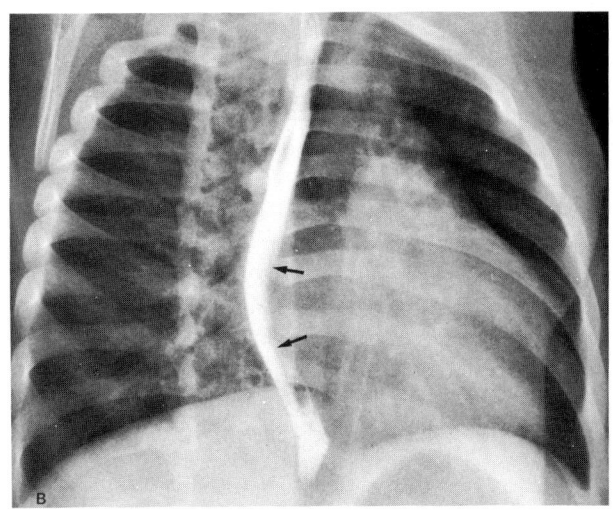

FIG 56–3.
Early cardiomyopathy. Thoracic roentgenogram. **A,** posteroanterior projection. Only minimal enlargement of heart. Normal pulmonary vasculature. Barium-filled esophagus is slightly displaced toward left *(arrow).* Findings are consistent with cardiomyopathy, although differentiation from other left ventricular obstructive lesions or other congenital conditions such as tricuspid atresia, pulmonary atresia, and left-sided lesion is impossible. **B,** right anterior oblique projection. Considerable displacement of barium-filled esophagus from enlarged left atrium *(arrows).* This finding is very helpful in the differential diagnosis. Specific diagnosis of cardiomyopathy cannot be made.

Pulmonary venous vasculature is accentuated (pulmonary congestion, pulmonary edema), or other radiographic signs of pulmonary venous hypertension occur. REASON: The failing left ventricle increases end-diastolic pressure with left atrial and pulmonary venous pressure resulting in venous pulmonary hypertension (see Chapter 5).

Radiographically, the differential diagnosis may be difficult. Other conditions causing a greatly enlarged cardiac silhouette with near-normal pulmonary vascular markings have to be considered, such as (1) left ventricular obstruction, (2) pericardial effusion, (3) Ebstein's malformation, (4) trilogy of Fallot (pulmonary stenosis and right-to-left atrial shunt), and (5) mediastinal tumor simulating an enlarged heart. Sometimes the differential diagnosis may be impossible, and other techniques, particularly ultrasonography and magnetic resonance scanning, can be extremely helpful in establishing the correct diagnosis.

Decompensated left ventricular obstructive lesions give the typical radiographic features of cardiomyopathy, because they also have a dilated left ventricle.

Pericardial effusion causes an enlarged cardiac silhou-

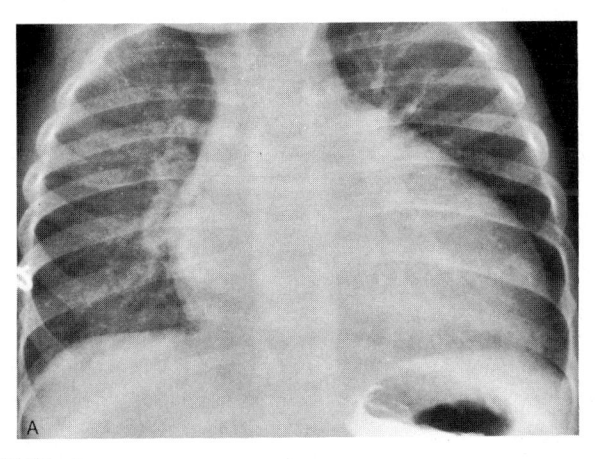

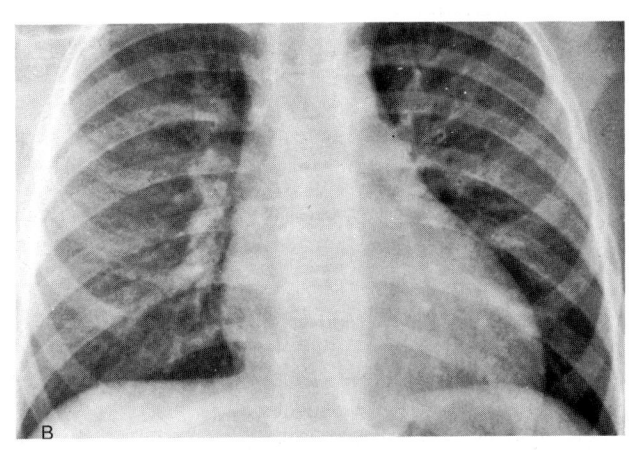

FIG 56–4.
Cardiomyopathy because of myocarditis. Thoracic roentgenogram. Posteroanterior projection. **A,** diffusely enlarged heart. Accentuation of pulmonary venous vasculature. **B,** 2 years later. Marked decrease in cardiac size. Normal pulmonary vasculature. Contrary to congenital cardiomyopathies, myocarditis has a diffusely dilated heart, because both ventricles undergo considerable dilatation. Decrease in cardiac size is most commonly seen in myocarditis, but it may also rarely occur in lipid storage diseases.

ette identical to cardiomyopathy, but the pulmonary vasculature is normal.

Ebstein's malformation and trilogy of Fallot may have an identical cardiac configuration as cardiomyopathy, but left atrial enlargement is absent, and the usually decreased pulmonary vasculature help distinguish these conditions.

A mediastinal tumor such as a lymphoma may closely simulate cardiomegaly with normal pulmonary vasculature. Oblique or lateral projections usually demonstrate an anterior (retrosternal) or midmediastinal density and a normal posterior cardiac contour, features that help to distinguish the conditions. Of course, additional information can be gained by ultrasonography, computed tomography, or nuclear magnetic resonance imaging.

Specific Radiographic Features

1. The cardiac silhouette is enlarged to a variable degree. In the early stages of a cardiomyopathy, cardiac enlargement may be minimal (Fig 56–3,A), and the pulmonary vasculature is normal.

2. The left atrium is enlarged to a variable degree. REASON: Increased left ventricular end-diastolic pressure causes an increased left atrial pressure (Fig 56–3,B). In the advanced stages of cardiomyopathy, the mitral annulus becomes dilated, resulting in relative mitral insufficiency.

3. During the early stages of cardiomyopathy and relative compensation of the left ventricle, the pulmonary vasculature is normal (see Fig 56–3).

4. Although typically cardiomyopathy involves both the right ventricular and the left ventricular myocardium, left ventricular enlargement is more marked. REASON: Myocardial damage is better tolerated by the low-pressure right ventricle than the high-pressure left ventricle. A left anterior oblique projection is helpful in showing an abnormal left ventricular contour.

5. A hallmark of cardiomyopathies is gradual increase in cardiac size. Exceptions exist, however. A significant decrease in cardiac size with return to normal is confirmatory of myocarditis (Fig 56–4). Congenital cardiomyopathies and endocardial fibroelastosis are generally not reversible.

6. In patients with rapidly developing cardiomegaly, as in myocarditis, the left atrium may be enlarged out of proportion because of the development of relative mitral insufficiency (Fig 56–5).

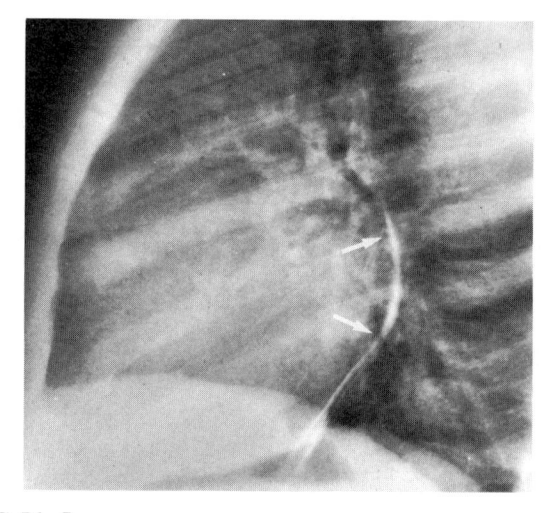

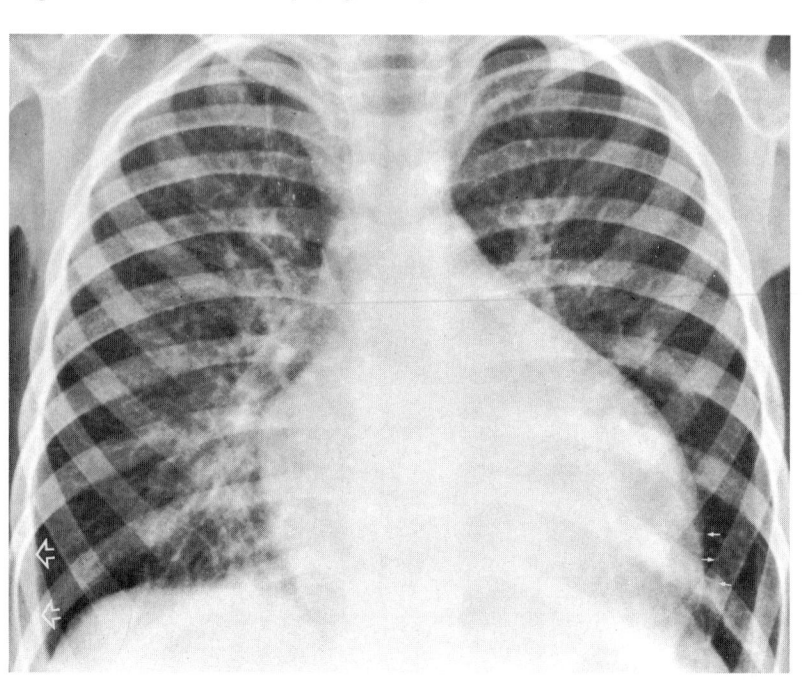

FIG 56–5.
Myocarditis. Thoracic roentgenogram. Lateral projection. Severe left atrial enlargement caused by relative mitral insufficiency, out of proportion of cardiomegaly.

FIG 56–6.
Cardiomyopathy and marked decompensation of left ventricle. Thoracic roentgenogram. Posteroanterior projection. Cardiomegaly. Left ventricular contour. Diffuse accentuation of pulmonary venous vasculature. Interstitial edema. Small pleural effusion *(open arrows)*. Kerley B lines *(solid arrow)* indicate venous pulmonary hypertension.

7. In spite of considerable generalized cardiomegaly, the pulmonary vasculature may remain normal, making differentiation from pericardial effusion and other conditions with large cardiac silhouettes impossible. The cardiac configuration of pericardial effusion is nonspecific and usually identical to cardiomyopathy.

8. Return of the cardiac size to normal is consistent with myocarditis. Some myocardial storage diseases may also show decrease in cardiac size under medical management.

9. With left ventricular decompensation and increase in end-diastolic pressure, radiographic findings of pulmonary venous hypertension develop. These changes vary from increased venous pulmonary vasculature, cephalization and Kerley B lines, to pleural effusion and diffuse pulmonary edema (Fig 56–6).

In hypertrophic cardiomyopathy, the left ventricle is exclusively involved. Rarely, the thickened ventricular septum also causes right ventricular outflow obstruction ("Bernheim phenomenon"). A typical left ventricular configuration of the heart results. This appearance is indistinguishable from left ventricular hypertrophy secondary to aortic stenosis or coarctation of the aorta. The radiographic features are discussed in greater detail in Chapter 26.

Restrictive

1. The thoracic roentgenogram may be within normal limits. REASON: The left ventricular and right ventricular cavities are hypertrophied but of normal size. Hypertrophy may not be evident on a thoracic roentgenogram.

2. In a patient with significant mitral or relative tricuspid regurgitation, commonly seen in restrictive myopathy, significant enlargement of the cardiac silhouette, specifically of the left or right atrium, occurs. The cardiac configuration is nonspecific, and a correct diagnosis cannot be made from thoracic roentgenograms.

3. Pulmonary venous vasculature may be accentuated with signs of pulmonary congestion, increased pulmonary venous pressure, and pleural effusion. REASON: In restrictive cardiomyopathy of the left ventricle, end-diastolic pressure increases. Left atrial and pulmonary venous pressures are elevated, as in the much more common congestive cardiomyopathies.

CARDIAC CATHETERIZATION

In each form of cardiomyopathy, both the left and right ventricles should be catheterized and appropriate angiography performed. The purposes of catheterization are (1) to exclude primary valvar anomalies; (2) to exclude coronary arterial anomalies; (3) to define ventricular anatomy; (4) to measure hemodynamics, especially left ventricular function and the effect on pulmonary circulation; (5) to assess hemodynamic effects of acute pharmacologic interventions; and (6) to perform myocardial biopsy.

In each form of myopathy, the catheter course is normal, no gradients are found across cardiac valves, and oximetry data are normal. The arteriovenous oxygen difference may be increased if the cardiac output is low, a feature indicating congestive cardiac failure.

Hypertrophic

The unique catheterization data of this form of cardiomyopathy are discussed in Chapter 26. In this form left ventricular end-systolic pressure is elevated, and there may be a gradient within the left ventricle, which can be reduced by decreasing left ventricular contractility. The gradient may be increased by drugs that increase left ventricular contractility, such as isoproterenol (Isuprel). The aortic pulse tracing shows a sharp upstroke.

Myocardial biopsy from the right ventricular septum may reveal areas of myocardial disarray.

Dilated

The only abnormality is related to increased left ventricular end-diastolic pressure. Myocardial biopsy may reveal areas of inflammatory cells, suggesting that the cardiomyopathy has resulted from myocarditis.

Restrictive

In both the right and left ventricles, the pressure contours are similar to those in constrictive pericarditis. There is an early diastolic dip and subsequent plateau. Diastolic

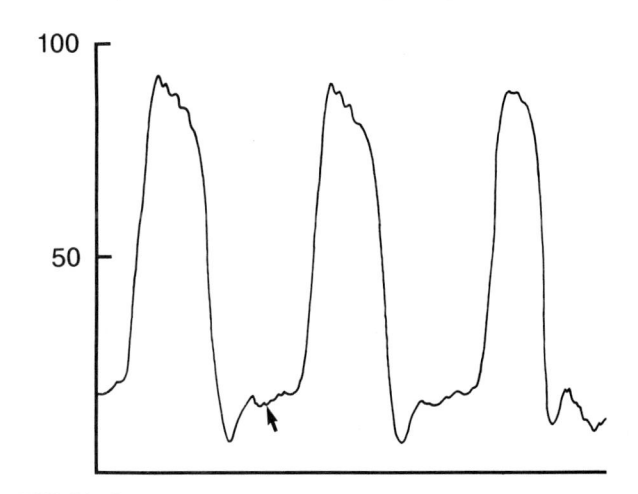

FIG 56–7.
Restrictive cardiomyopathy. Left ventricular pressure tracing. Early diastolic dip and subsequent plateau (*square root sign*). End-diastolic pressure is elevated. Pressure tracing is identical to constrictive pericarditis.

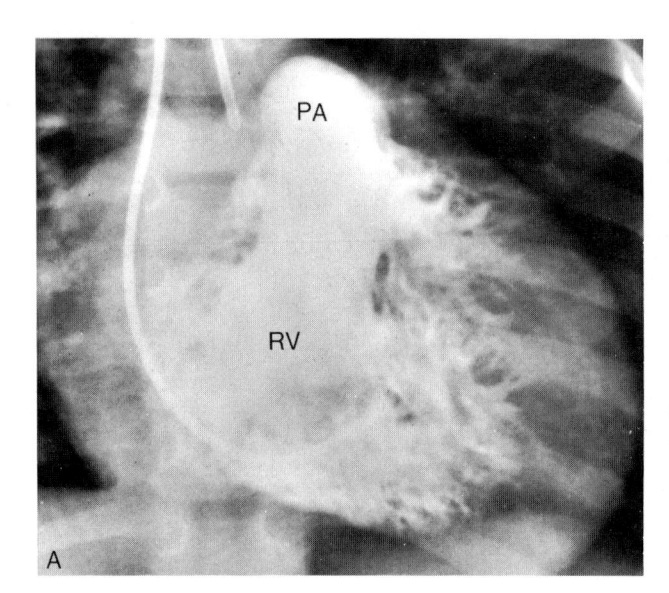

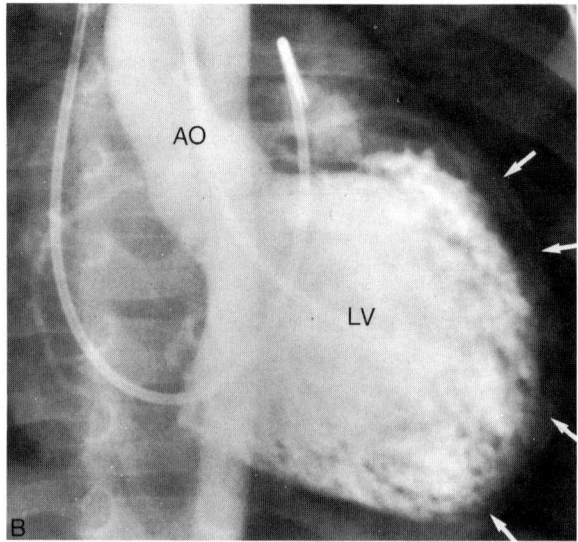

FIG 56-8.
Dilated cardiomyopathy. **A,** right ventriculogram *(RV).* Anteroposterior projection. Diffusely dilated right ventricle. Competent tricuspid valve. *PA* = pulmonary artery. **B,** left ventriculogram. Anteroposterior projection. Diastole. Diffusely dilated left ventricle *(LV).* Ventricle is thin walled *(arrows).* End-diastolic volume is markedly increased. Competent mitral valve. *AO* = aorta.

pressure may reach 25 to 35 mm Hg. Pressures may be identical in both ventricles, thus making a distinction from constrictive pericarditis virtually impossible (Fig 56-7). Because of elevated end-diastolic pressure, atrial pressures also show marked elevation. Myocardial biopsy specimen may reveal stored material, such as amyloid, glycogen, or eosinophils, reflecting Löffler's eosinophilic cardiomyopathy.

Propranolol, verapamil, or other medications may be administered and hemodynamic measurements made to detect improvement in diastolic function in effort to identify a mechanism for treatment.

ANGIOGRAPHIC FEATURES

Angiography is indicated to determine the size and contractility of right and left ventricles. Left ventriculography is particularly helpful to visualize the degree of mitral regurgitation, because patients with severe mitral regurgitation may be treated by replacement of the valve.

Aortography is indicated to exclude anomalous left coronary artery, aortic stenosis, or coarctation of the aorta, which in infants produces an angiographic appearance left ventricular cardiomyopathy.

Dilated

1. Typically right ventriculography and left ventriculography show enlarged ventricular chambers (Fig 56-8).
2. The thickness of the right and left ventricular walls vary from increased to thinned. Characteristically myocarditis has a normal or thin ventricular wall thickness (see Fig 56-8).
3. The volume change of the ventricles between systole and diastole is decreased. REASON: Although the cardiac output is normal in most patients, an enlarged ventricle can deliver a normal stroke volume with little shortening of the myocardial fibers compared with a normal-sized ventricle. The decreased systolic-diastolic excursion of an enlarged left ventricle is fluoroscopically apparent by decreased pulsations.
4. The end-systolic volume is increased, which is a consistent angiographic finding for ventricular failure.
5. As ventricular dilatation progresses, relative tricuspid and mitral insufficiency may occur (Fig 56-9).
6. Cardiomyopathy may involve predominantly the right ventricle and show relative tricuspid insufficiency and markedly increased right ventricular end-diastolic pressures. Under such circumstances, right atrial pressure may exceed left atrial pressure, resulting in the herniation of a sealed foramen ovale into the left atrium (Fig 56-10).

Restrictive

Right and left ventriculography are indicated to demonstrate the size of the ventricles and the degree of the commonly associated mitral and tricuspid regurgitation. The radiographic diagnosis of restrictive cardiomyopathy is very difficult and possible only with knowledge of the hemodynamic data. REASON: Left ventricular chamber size and global function of the left ventricle are normal. The only clue of the presence of restrictive cardiomyopathy is an increased left ventricular wall thickness.

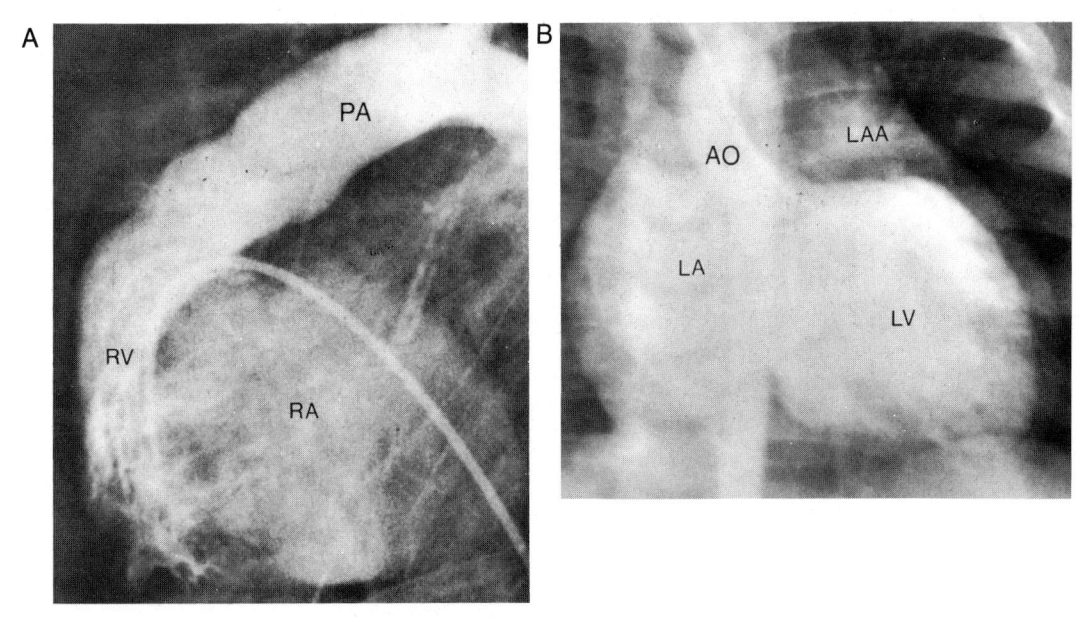

FIG 56–9.
Dilated cardiomyopathy. **A,** right ventriculogram. Lateral projection. Enlarged right ventricle *(RV)*. Opacification of right atrium *(RA)* is caused by relative tricuspid insufficiency. *PA* = pulmonary artery. **B,** Left ventriculogram. Anteroposterior projection. Dilated left ventricle *(LV)* with normal wall thickness. Opacification of left atrium *(LA)* is caused by relative mitral regurgitation. *AO* = aorta; *LAA* = left atrial appendage.

1. Left ventriculography demonstrates a normal-sized left ventricle and normal end-diastolic volume (Fig 56–11).

2. The left ventricular wall thickness is increased (see Fig 56–11).

3. There are various degrees of mitral regurgitation (see Fig 56–11).

4. During systole, the left ventricle contracts well and the end-systolic volume is relatively small (see Fig 56–11).
REASON: The contractility of the left ventricle is normal.

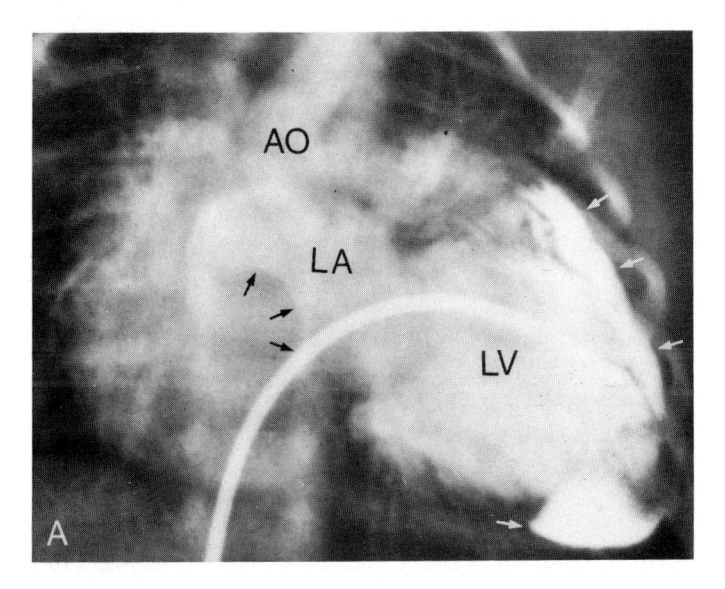

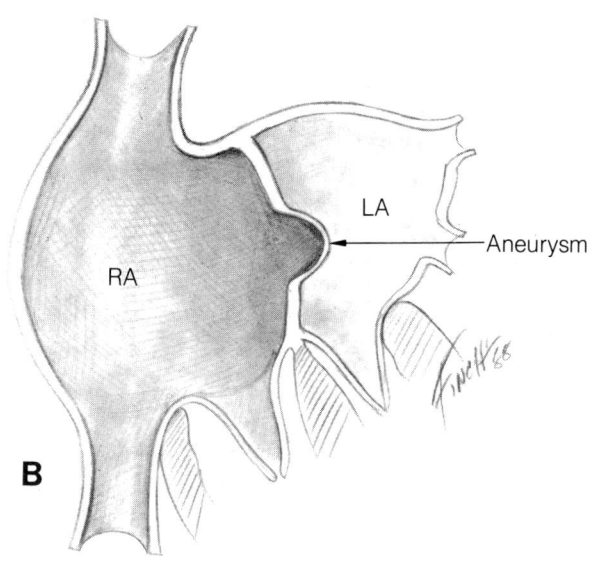

FIG 56–10.
Dilated cardiomyopathy. **A,** left ventriculogram *(LV)*. Anteroposterior projection. Transmural injection with deposition of contrast medium beneath epicardium *(white arrows)*. Left ventricle is markedly dilated. Marked mitral regurgitation outlines mildly enlarged left atrium *(LA)*. Distinct bulge *(black arrows)* along atrial septum indicates elevated right atrial pressure with herniation of fossa ovalis into left atrium. Elevation of right atrial pressure is caused by marked relative tricuspid insufficiency. *AO* = aorta. **B,** dilatation of right atrium *(RA)* because of elevated pressure causes fossa ovalis to herniate into left atrium, forming an aneurysm.

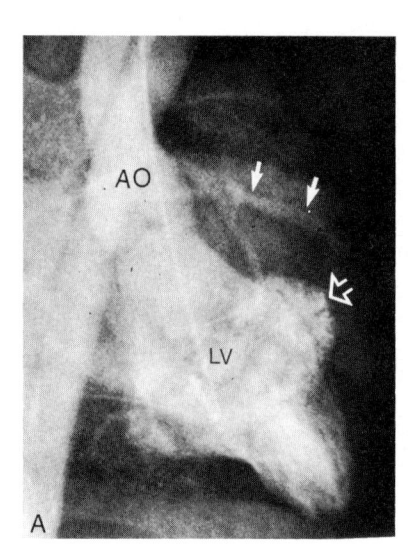

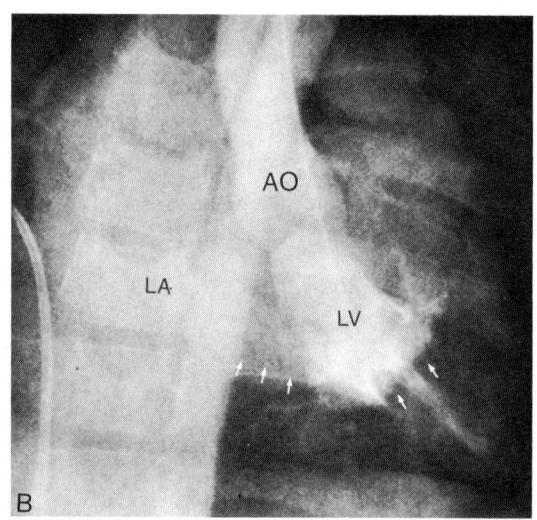

FIG 56-11.
Restrictive cardiomyopathy. **A,** left ventriculogram *(LV)*. Right anterior oblique projection. Diastole. Normal left ventricular end-diastolic volume. Increased wall thickness of left ventricle as indicated by distance between the opacified left ventricular chamber and left coronary artery *(arrows)*. Incidental left ventricular diverticulum *(open arrow)*. AO = aorta **B,** systole. Relatively small end-systolic volume. Two papillary muscles *(arrows)*. Mild mitral regurgitation *(arrows)* outlines enlarged left atrium *(LA)*. Left ventricular diverticulum is no longer seen, indicating contractile myocardium in diverticulum (see Chapter 70).

5. A right ventriculogram demonstrates a normal or enlarged right ventricular cavity and normal contraction. Significant tricuspid reflux may be present.

OPERATIVE CONSIDERATIONS

The initial treatment is primarily medical. For hypertrophic forms, efforts are directed to decrease the left ventricular outflow tract gradient and thereby reduce symptoms by β-adrenergic or calcium channel blockade. In the dilated form, medical treatment can increase myocardial contractility, promote diuresis, and reduce systemic vascular resistance, but these measures are only temporizing. In those patients with restrictive cardiomyopathy, diuretics are indicated to treat pulmonary edema and symptoms related to systemic venous congestion. Specific medications that improve diastolic relaxation significantly are currently unavailable.

If major atrioventricular valvar insufficiency develops, valve replacement may be undertaken. Currently both the dilated and restrictive forms are considered for cardiac transplantation. Patients with normal pulmonary vascular resistance, no prior thoracic surgery, or involvement of other organ systems have an excellent survival rate after cardiac transplantation, particularly with the use of cyclosporin A.

SPECIFIC FORMS OF CARDIOMYOPATHY

Two forms of cardiomyopathy present signs and symptoms in infants that are relatively characteristic and allow an accurate clinical diagnosis in most instances. These conditions are endocardial fibroelastosis and glycogen storage disease of the heart.

Endocardial Fibroelastosis

In endocardial fibroelastosis, the left ventricular endocardium is diffusely thickened and has a white appearance. The endocardium may be 1 mm thick and is composed of fibrous and elastic tissue (Fig 56-12), therefore, "endocardial fibroelastosis." The left atrium and occasionally right-sided cardiac chambers may be involved as well. The left ventricle is greatly dilated, and the cardiac weight is several times normal. Mitral insufficiency is regularly present, resulting from high position of the papillary muscles on the left ventricular wall, shortened chordae tendineae, and abnormal orientation of the papillary muscle-chordal mechanism (Fig 56-13).

Endocardial fibroblastosis has been subdivided into primary and secondary forms.[13] In the latter, the endocardial thickening is associated with a left-sided cardiac condition, such as aortic stenosis, coarctation of the aorta, or anomalous left coronary artery. In the primary form, an associated cardiac malformation is absent. In most instances the left ventricle is dilated, but in a few instances the left ventricle is small. The latter is called the contracted type (see Fig 56-13,B).

The hemodynamics are those of a dilated cardiomyopathy, with decreased cardiac output, elevated left ventricular end-diastolic pressure, and perhaps pulmonary edema. Mitral insufficiency may complicate the hemodynamics, augmenting left ventricular and left atrial dilatation.

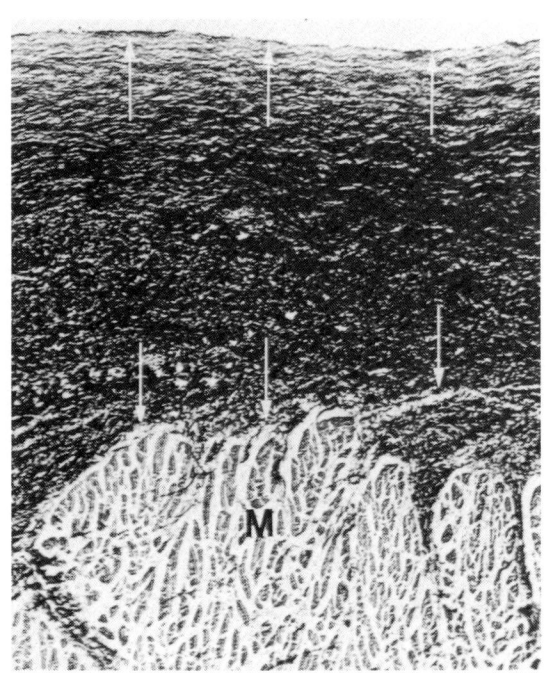

FIG 56–12.
Endocardial fibroelastosis. Photomicrograph. Endocardium is several millimeters thick and consists of dense fibrous layer containing excessive elastic tissue *(arrows)*. Hypertrophied muscle fibers *(M)*.

Congestive cardiac failure, which may be profound, develops in infancy but typically responds well to digitalis. Growth may be delayed. Although widely held that a cardiac murmur is not present, we have been impressed by the number of patients with an apical systolic murmur representing mitral insufficiency.[13] A gallop rhythm and accentuated pulmonary second sound may be heard.

The ECG usually shows left ventricular hypertrophy and strain, with left atrial enlargement being found as well in older patients. Echocardiographic, radiographic, and angiographic features are those of a congestive cardiomyopathy. Although initially responding to digitalis, chronic medications are required, and death ultimately ensues, although perhaps not until the teenage years.

Radiographic Features

The common radiographic feature of both the dilated and constricted type of primary endocardial fibroelastosis is severe cardiomegaly. REASON: With the dilated type the left ventricle is markedly enlarged, and with the constricted type, which has a smaller than normal left ventricular cavity, marked secondary enlargement of the right ventricle occurs. Venous congestive changes are commonly present because of the associated mitral regurgita-

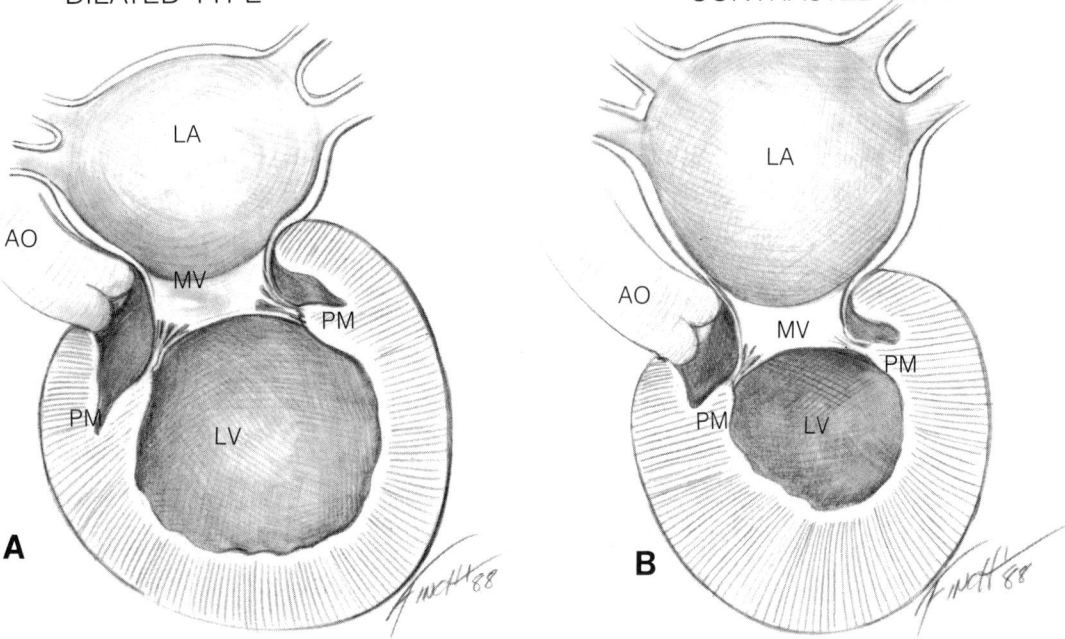

FIG 56–13.
Endocardial fibroelastosis. **A,** dilated form. Round and markedly dilated left ventricle *(LV)*. Myocardium has increased thickness because of hypertrophy. Endocardium is markedly thickened. Papillary muscles *(PM)* insert high on left ventricular wall. Chordal attachment is unusually short, which contributes to associated mitral regurgitation. **B,** contracted form of endocardial fibroelastosis (rare). Identical anatomic features as **A** except for smaller than normal left ventricular cavity. In either form, mural thrombi may be present and a source of peripheral embolism. *AO* = aorta; *LA* = left atrium; *MV* = anterior leaflet of mitral valve.

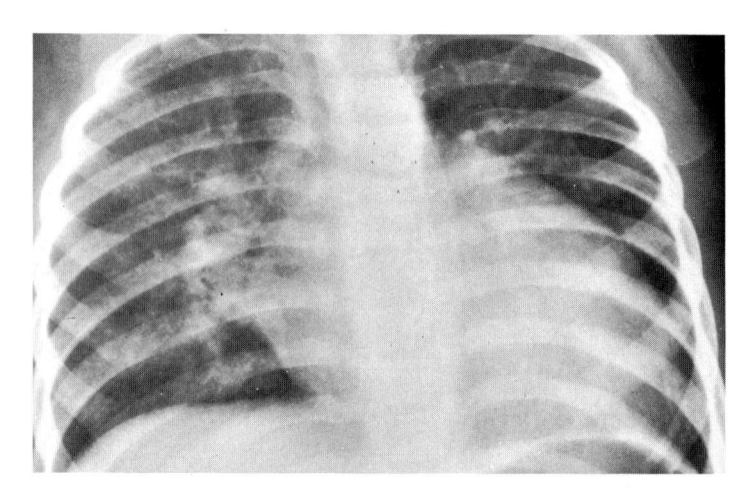

FIG 56–14.
Endocardial fibroelastosis. Thoracic roentgenogram. Anteroposterior projection. Marked left ventricular cardiomegaly. Mild congestive changes. Findings are indistinguishable from other left-sided lesions.

tion and left ventricular failure. Pulmonary edema may occur.

1. The heart is markedly enlarged and has a left ventricular contour (Fig 56–14). The cardiac configuration is therefore indistinguishable from a left-sided obstructive lesion.
2. The pulmonary venous vasculature is diffusely accentuated because of left ventricular failure or associated mitral regurgitation (see Fig 56–14).
3. The right anterior oblique view shows distinct left atrial enlargement. REASON: The end-diastolic pressure in the left ventricle is uniformly increased, and there is commonly associated mitral regurgitation.
4. Late in the disease, cardiomegaly becomes unusually severe, displacing the esophagus laterally (Fig 56–15) and posteriorly.

5. As the disease process progresses, cardiomegaly increases (Fig 56–16). REASON: The left ventricle becomes more and more dilated, and mitral reflux is commonly a complicating factor.

Angiographic Features

Left ventriculography is indicated to demonstrate left ventricular size and the degree of associated mitral regurgitation. It should also be performed to exclude endocardial fibroelastosis secondary to conditions such as aortic stenosis, hypoplastic left heart syndrome, coarctation of aorta, and aberrant left coronary artery.

1. The left ventricular cavity is smooth-walled and markedly enlarged, with the much more common dilated type of the disease (Fig 56–17).
2. If the mitral valve is competent, the end-systolic

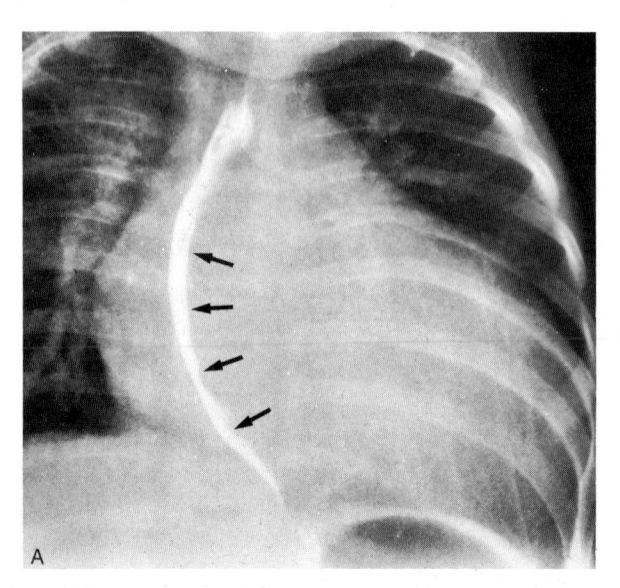

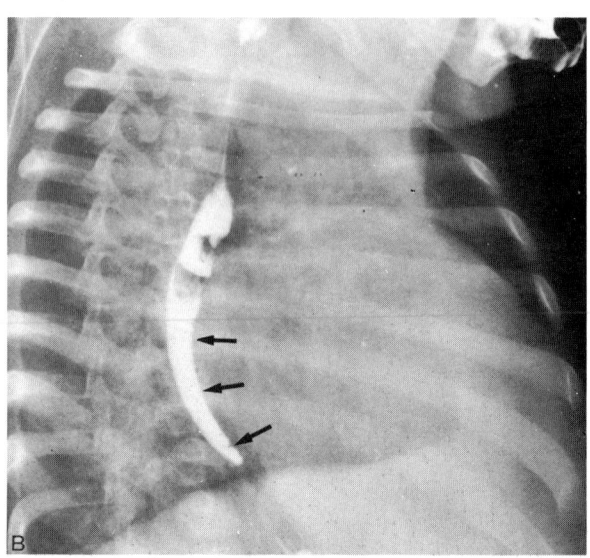

FIG 56–15.
Endocardial fibroelastosis. Thoracic roentgenogram. **A,** posteroanterior projection. Markedly enlarged heart. Characteristic left ventricular contour indicates a "left-sided lesion." Diffuse pulmonary congestion is caused by left ventricular failure. Esophagus is displaced to right *(arrows)*. **B,** right anterior oblique projection. Marked left atrial enlargement *(arrows)*.

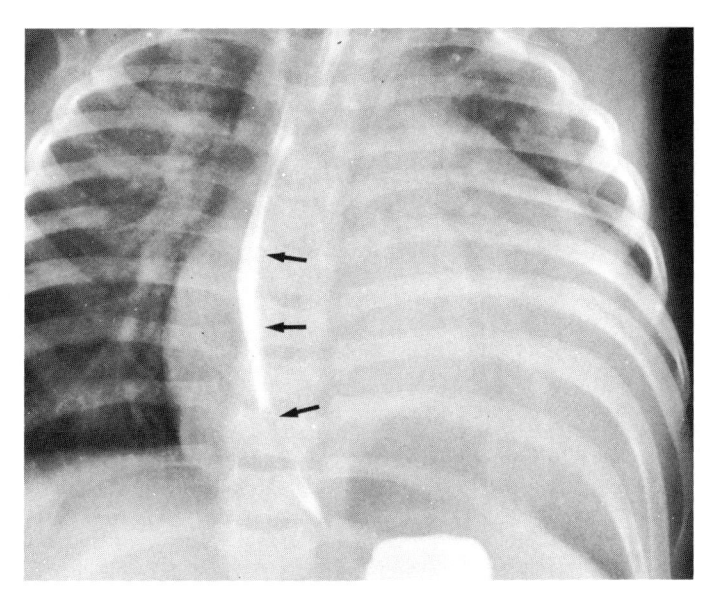

FIG 56–16.
Endocardial fibroelastosis. Late stage. Thoracic roentgenogram. Posteroanterior projection. Massively enlarged cardiac silhouette. Barium-filled esophagus (arrows) is displaced toward right by huge left atrium. Bilateral pulmonary congestion in end stages of disease; left atrial enlargement may be so marked that left mainstem bronchus is compressed, resulting in atelectasis of left lung.

volume is markedly increased and similar to end-diastolic volume. Thus, left ventricular contractions appear minimal and give the radiographic appearance of a noncontractile left ventricle (See Fig 56–17).

3. In spite of the apparent "noncontractile" left ventricle, the systolic stroke volume and cardiac output, at least at rest, can be normal. REASON: An enlarged left ventricle requires only minimal systolic fiber shortening to produce a normal stroke volume.

4. The myocardium shows varying degrees of hypertrophy, which combined with the endocardial thickening yields a characteristic massively thickened left ventricle (Fig 56–18).

5. The degree of mitral insufficiency varies from none to severe (Fig 56–19).

6. With severe mitral regurgitation, the left ventricle may show a normal stroke volume (Fig 56–19), giving the angiographic appearance of a normally contractile left ventricle.

7. With the contracted type of endocardial fibroelastosis, the left ventricular cavity is comparatively small. Inflow of blood into the left ventricle is impaired, and herniation of the foramen ovale similar to left-sided hypoplastic syndrome may occur, decompressing the left side of the heart (Fig 56–20).

8. Aortograms show very dense opacification of the

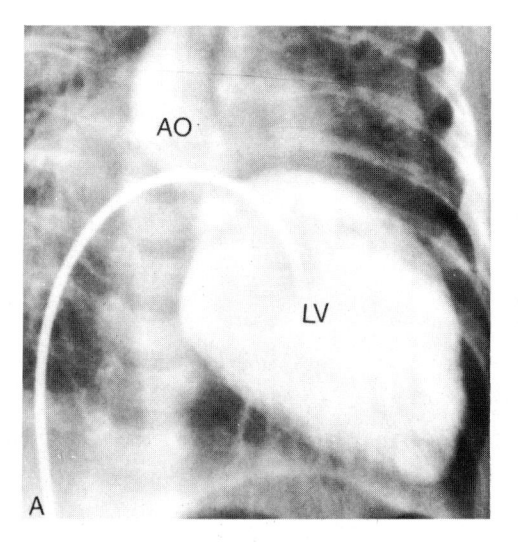

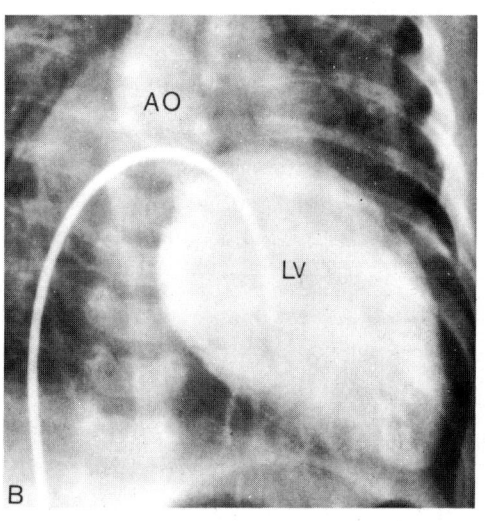

FIG 56–17.
Endocardial fibroelastosis. Transatrial catheterization. Left ventriculogram (LV). Anteroposterior projection. Markedly dilated and smooth-walled left ventricle. **A,** diastole. **B,** systole. Change of left ventricular size between systole and diastole is hardly noticeable, giving angiographic appearance of noncontractile rigid left ventricle. In spite of angiographic appearance, stroke volume is normal at rest. No mitral regurgitation. AO = aorta.

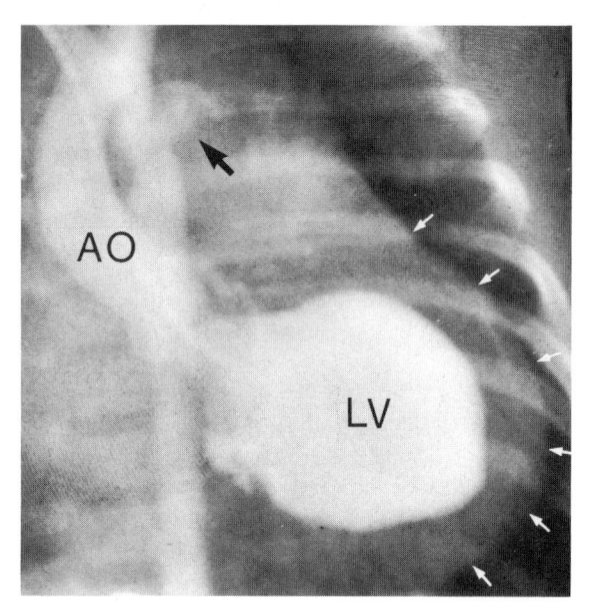

FIG 56–18.
Endocardial fibroelastosis. Left ventriculogram *(LV)*. Anteroposterior projection. Smooth-walled somewhat enlarged left ventricular cavity. Massively thickened endocardium and myocardium *(white arrows)*. Incidental small patent ductus arteriosus *(black arrow)*. No mitral regurgitation. *AO* = aorta.

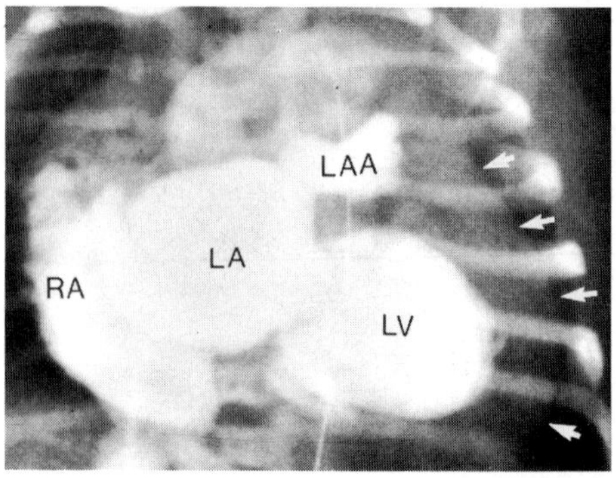

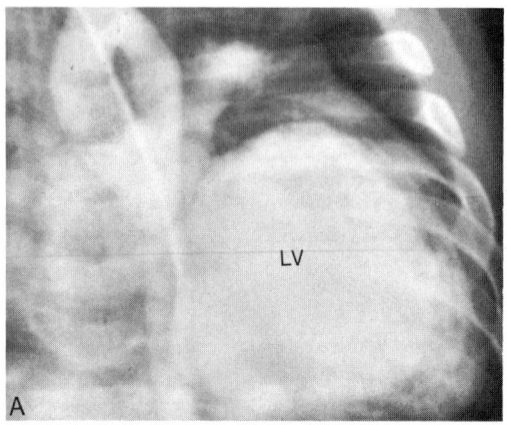

FIG 56–20.
Contracted type of endocardial fibroelastosis. Left atriogram. Anteroposterior projection. Relatively small left ventricular cavity. Massive thickening of endocardium and myocardium *(arrows)*. Enlarged left atrium *(LA)*. Dense left-to-right shunt at atrial level because of stretching of fossa ovalis similar to hypoplastic left heart syndrome (see Chapter 50). *LAA* = atrial appendage; *LV* = left ventricle; *RA* = right atrium.

aorta. REASON: Decreased cardiac output. The thoracic aorta may be displaced toward the right by the huge left ventricle and left atrium. The displaced aorta may give a right paramediastinal density on thoracic roentgenograms (Fig 56–21).

Glycogen Storage Disease

In this condition a lysosomal enzyme, acid maltase, is deficient. As a result, glycogen accumulates in the myocardium, as well as other organs, particularly in skeletal muscle and liver (Fig 56–22). As glycogen accumulates in myocardial cells, the contractile elements are displaced, and cells appear vacuolated because of the central glycogen accumulation. As a result, ventricular free wall and septum become thickened, perhaps to two or three times normal. The left ventricular cavity is normal sized or reduced (Fig 56–23).

Because of the myocardial infiltration, ventricular contractility and compliance are decreased. Cardiac output is reduced, and both systemic and pulmonary venous pressures are elevated.

Because of skeletal muscular involvement, hypotonia is a striking clinical feature, along with congestive cardiac failure, which appears by 2 months of age. Hepatomegaly,

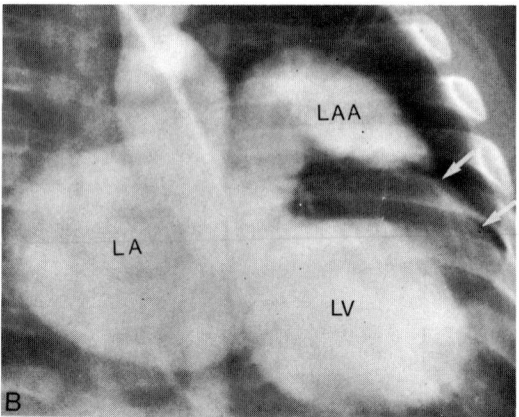

FIG 56–19.
Endocardial fibroelastosis and massive mitral regurgitation. Left ventriculogram *(LV)*. Anteroposterior projection. **A,** diastole. Markedly increased left ventricular end-diastolic volume. **B,** systole. Dense opacification of enlarged left atrium and distended left atrial appendage *(LAA)*. Left ventricular cavity is much smaller than **A** because of increased ventricular stroke volume consisting of cardiac output and regurgitant volume. Marked systolic myocardial thickening *(arrows)*. Angiographically, left ventricle appears to have excellent contractility.

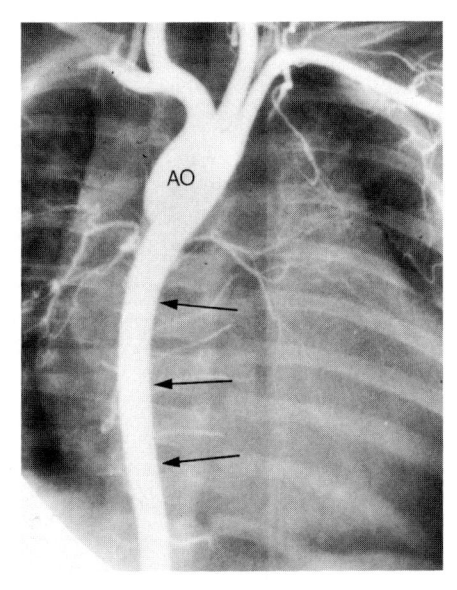

FIG 56–21.
Endocardial fibroelastosis. Retrograde aortogram. Anteroposterior projection. Opacification of aorta is unusually dense because of decreased cardiac output. Descending aorta *(AO)* is displaced to right of spine *(arrows)* because of enlarged heart and left atrium.

caused by infiltration of the liver out of proportion to cardiac failure, is present. No murmur is evident.

The type II glycogenosis (Pompe's disease) causes massive cardiac enlargement (Fig 56–24). Because of the striking infiltration of the myocardium, there may be en-

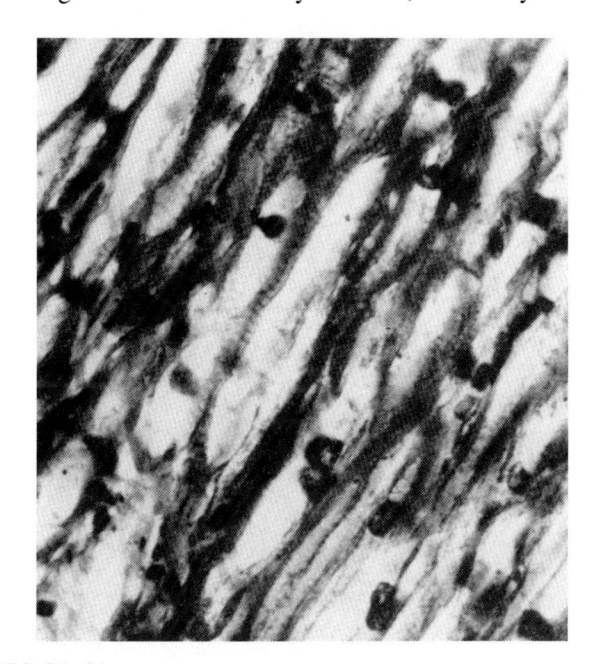

FIG 56–22.
Glycogen storage disease of heart. Photomicrograph of myocardium. Extensive deposition of glycogen in myocardial fibers, resulting in characteristic vacuolization. (Courtesy of Dr. Jesse Edwards.)

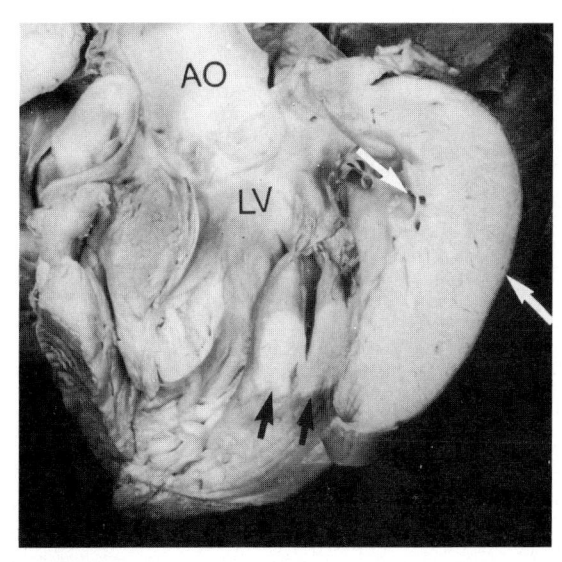

FIG 56–23.
Glycogen storage disease of heart. Left ventricle *(LV)*. Thickened wall *(white arrows)*. Involvement of papillary muscles *(black arrows)*. AO = aorta. (Courtesy of Dr. Jesse Edwards.)

croachment of the right and left ventricular cavities (Fig 56–25). Right and left ventricular outflow tract obstruction may occur.[14, 15] There may be enlargement of the left ventricular cavity and the association with endocardial fibroelastosis. Filling of the ventricles is impaired similar to idiopathic myocardial hypertrophy.

Angiographic Features

Bilateral ventriculography demonstrates the massive thickening of the myocardium, which is more severe than in any other condition except for myocardial tumor. Tumor infiltration, however, does not tend to be so diffuse.

1. The right ventricular cavity may be encroached upon by the massively thickened septum and infiltrated muscle (see Fig 56–25).

2. The right atrioventricular valve tends to be competent.

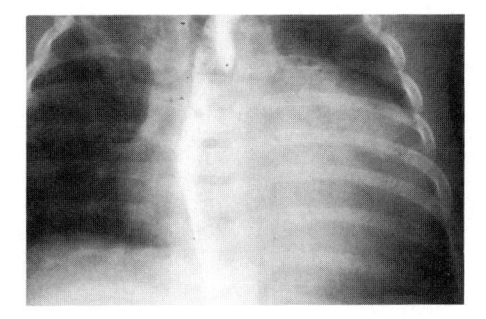

FIG 56–24.
Glycogen storage disease of heart. Thoracic roentgenogram. Posteroanterior projection. Massive cardiac enlargement.

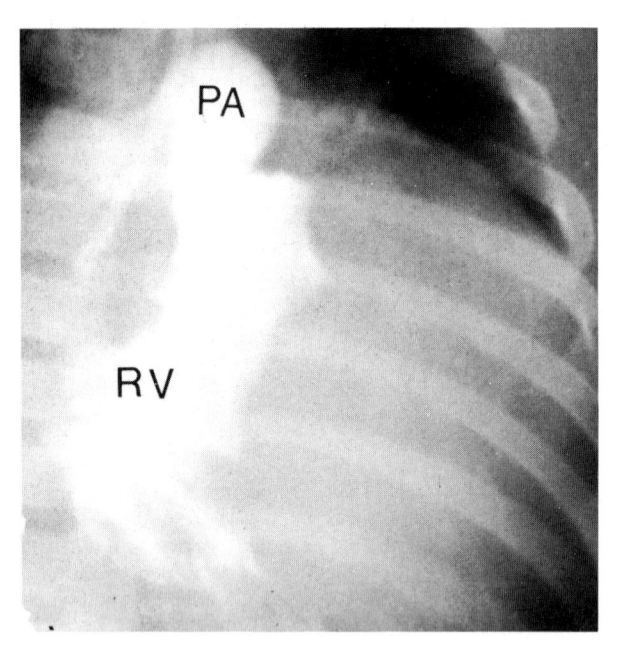

FIG 56–25.
Glycogen storage disease of heart. Right ventriculogram. Anteroposterior projection. Right ventricular cavity *(RV)* is encroached on by thickened muscle. Competent tricuspid valve. *PA* = pulmonary artery.

3. Left ventriculography demonstrates encroachment of the left ventricular cavity by the thickened ventricular septum and left ventricular wall.

4. Left ventricular outflow tract obstruction may be demonstrated.

5. If glycogen storage disease is associated with endocardial fibroelastosis, the left ventricular cavity may be enlarged, at least in diastole (Fig 56–26,A).

6. The end-systolic volume tends to be small (Fig 56–26,B).

7. Typically the mitral valve is competent.

8. Infiltration of the aortic wall may cause narrowing simulating coarctation.

This chapter is not meant to be a complete outline of the vast field of cardiac myopathies. A basic classification is given in Table 56–1.

REFERENCES

1. Bulkley BH: The cardiomyopathies, *Hosp Pract* 19:59, 1984.
2. Oakley CM: Clinical decisions in the cardiomyopathies, *Hosp Pract* 20:41, 1985.
3. Goodwin JF: The frontiers of cardiomyopathy, *Br Heart J* 48:1, 1982.
4. Maron BJ: Myocardial disorganisation in hypertrophic cardiomyopathy, another point of view, *Br Heart J* 50:1, 1983.
5. Davies MJ: The current status of myocardial disarray in hypertrophic cardiomyopathy, *Br Heart J* 51:361, 1984.
6. Johnson RA, Palacios I: Dilated cardiomyopathies of the adult [first of two parts], *N Engl J Med* 307:1051, 1982.
7. Maron BJ, Tajik AJ, Ruttenberg HD, et al: Hypertrophic cardiomyopathy in infants: clinical features and natural history, *Circulation* 65:7, 1982.

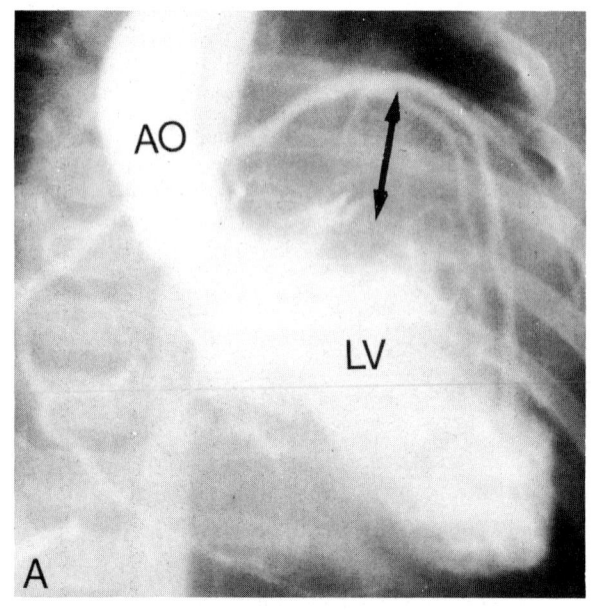

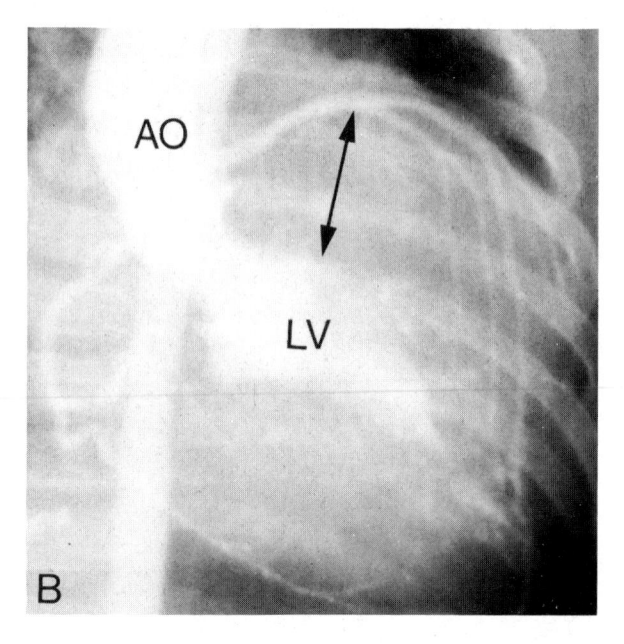

FIG 56–26.
Glycogen storage disease of heart. Left ventriculogram *(LV)*. Anteroposterior projection. **A,** diastole. Enlarged left ventricular cavity and massive thickening of the myocardium *(arrows)*. Associated endocardial fibroelastosis. **B,** systole. Excellent contraction of left ventricle. Myocardium further thickened *(arrows)*. Small end-systolic volume. Competent mitral valve *AO* = aorta.

8. Taliercio CP, Seward JB, Driscoll DJ, et al: Idiopathic dilated cardiomyopathy in the young: clinical profile and natural history, *J Am Coll Cardiol* 6:1126, 1985.
9. Fuster V, Gersh BJ, Giuliani ER, et al: The natural history of idiopathic dilated cardiomyopathy, *Am J Cardiol* 47:525, 1981.
10. Maron BJ, Gottdiener JS, Epstein SE: Patterns and significance of distribution of left ventricular hypertrophy in hypertrophic cardiomyopathy: a wide angle, two dimensional echocardiographic study of 125 patients, *Am J Cardiol* 48:418, 1981.
11. Maron BJ, Wolfson JK, Ciro E, et al: Relation of electrocardiographic abnormalities and patterns of left ventricular hypertrophy identified by 2-dimensional echocardiography in patients with hypertrophic cardiomyopathy, *Am J Cardiol* 51:189, 1983.
12. Van der Hauwaert LG, Denef B, Dumoulin M: Long-term echocardiographic assessment of dilated cardiomyopathy in children, *Am J Cardiol* 52:1066, 1983.
13. Moller JH, Lucas RV Jr, Adams P Jr, et al: Endocardial fibroelastosis: a clinical and anatomic study of 47 patients with emphasis on its relationship to mitral insufficiency, *Circulation* 30:759, 1964.
14. Ehlers KH, Hagstrom JWC, Lukas DS, et al: Glycogen-storage disease of the myocardium with obstruction to left ventricular outflow, *Circulation* 25:96, 1962.
15. Hernandez A Jr, Marchesi V, Goldring D, et al: Cardiac glycogenosis: hemodynamic, angiocardiographic, and electron microscopic findings—report of a case, *J Pediatr* 68:400, 1966.

CHAPTER 57

Anomalous Origin of Coronary Arteries From the Pulmonary Trunk

The condition, anomalous origin of a coronary artery from the pulmonary trunk, represents 0.5% of cases of congenital heart disease. It usually occurs as an isolated cardiac anomaly, although it has been described as coexisting with patent ductus arteriosus, ventricular septal defect, truncus arteriosus, or tetralogy of Fallot. In this chapter, emphasis is placed on anomalous left coronary artery, because it is the most common congenital anomaly of the coronary arteries. Other types of anomalous coronary arterial anomalies are presented briefly in this chapter and in Chapter 64.

PATHOLOGIC ANATOMY

Various anatomic types of anomalous origin of coronary arteries from the pulmonary artery are demonstrated in Figure 57–1.

In instances of anomalous origin of the left coronary artery, the right coronary artery arises normally above the right aortic sinus (see Fig 57–1,A), whereas the left coronary artery arises from the left and posterior aspect of the pulmonary trunk immediately above a pulmonary sinus of Valsalva. If collaterals are well developed, the right coronary artery and its major branches are dilated and tortuous, and the left coronary artery has a thin, veinlike wall because of the low-perfusion pressure.

The heart, primarily the left ventricle, and left atrium are greatly enlarged.[1] The left ventricular wall may be slightly hypertrophied, and the dilated chamber is lined by endocardial fibroelastosis. Subendocardial scarring may be visible. The papillary muscles of the mitral valve arise higher from the left ventricular wall than normal because left ventricular dilatation occurs primarily in the apical region. The papillary muscles, particularly the anterolateral, may be scarred and thinned from myocardial infarction.[1] The chordae tendineae are shortened. The papillary muscles seem to attach directly to the mitral valve leaflets.

The area most vulnerable to ischemia from inadequate coronary perfusion is the anterolateral papillary muscle, which is the most distant point from the anterior descending coronary artery. There is resultant fibrosis, shortening, and retraction of chordae tendineae. Mitral insufficiency may be a major hemodynamic consequence of the papillary muscle changes. Pathologic evidence of mitral insufficiency includes enlargement of the left atrium and thickening of the free margin of the anterior mitral valve leaflet. The reason for myocardial ischemia is not the desaturation of pulmonary artery blood but the low-perfusion pressure in the left coronary arterial system.

Two factors prolong survival into adult life: (1) the development of interarterial collaterals and (2) right coronary artery preponderance.

Histologic examination of the left ventricular myocardium shows a thickened endocardium with changes of endocardial fibroelastosis. The underlying myocardium may show evidence of acute or healed myocardial infarction. Myocardial calcification may be present, particularly in the papillary muscles of the left ventricle.

Rarely, the right coronary artery may arise anomalously from the pulmonary trunk (see Fig 57–1,B) and the

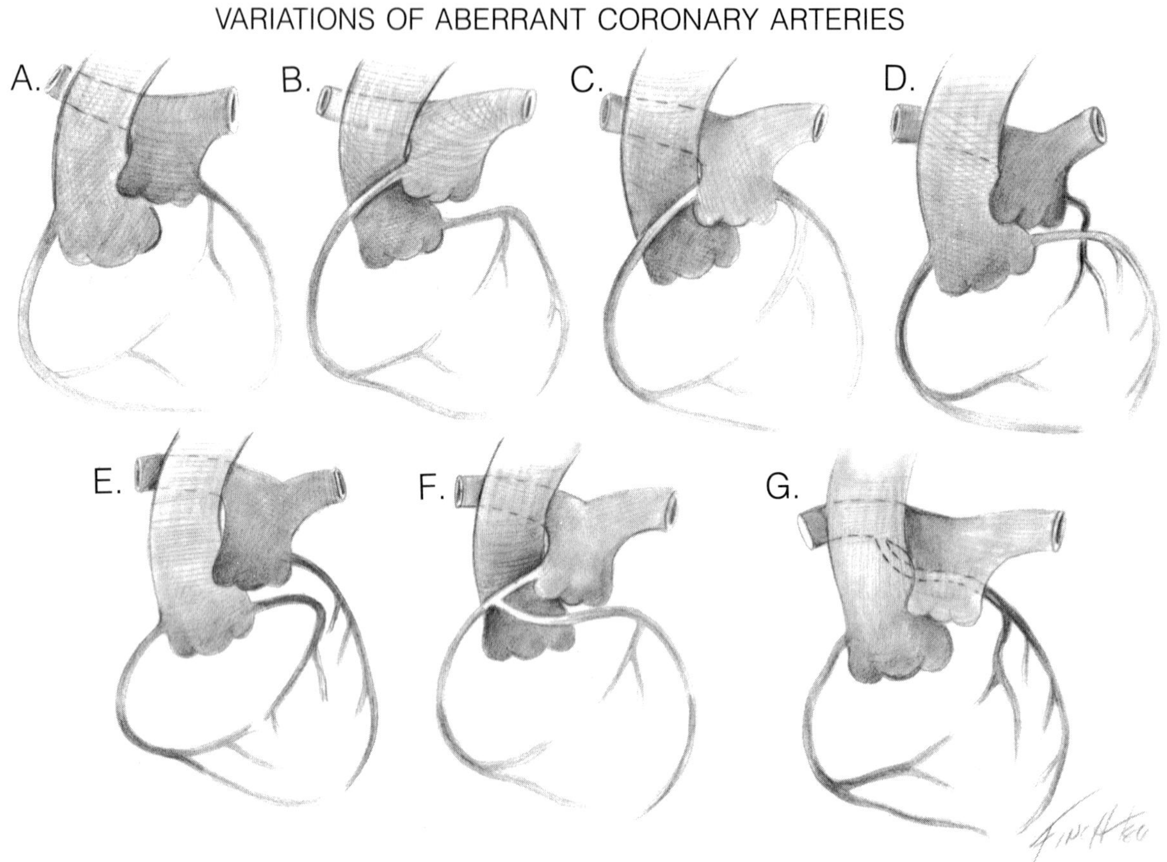

VARIATIONS OF ABERRANT CORONARY ARTERIES

FIG 57–1.
Anomalous origin of coronary arteries from pulmonary artery. **A**, left coronary artery. **B**, right coronary artery. **C**, both coronary arteries. **D**, Left circumflex or diagonal branch. **E**, left anterior descending branch. **F**, single coronary artery. **G**, left coronary artery from right pulmonary artery.

left coronary artery normally from the aorta.[2–4] This condition is recognized in adulthood and has few ischemic complications.

Anomalous origin of the left anterior descending (see Fig 57–1,E), circumflex (see Fig 57–1,D), or marginal branches have been described and also have few ischemic complications.

When a single artery (see Fig 57–1,F) or both coronary arteries arise from the pulmonary artery (Fig 57–1,C),[5, 6] blood flow is from the pulmonary artery into the coronary arterial system. As pulmonary vascular resistance falls in the neonatal period, coronary perfusion decreases, and myocardial infarction occurs. Anomalous origin of both coronary arteries has been rarely described in association with ventricular septal defect.[7–9] As long as pulmonary hypertension is present, the coronary arteries are perfused, and symptoms do not occur. Closure of the ventricular septal defect is lethal, because pulmonary arterial pressure falls as a result, and therefore coronary arterial perfusion decreases. Because coronary arteriography is not performed routinely in ventricular septal defect preoperatively, there is a high mortality rate after operative closure of the ventricular septal defect in patients with coexistent anomalous origin of the coronary arteries.

Associated intracardiac malformations may mask the hemodynamics of an anomalous coronary artery. Whenever a patient with a congenital cardiac anomaly is being evaluated whose left ventricular function is depressed or in whom mitral insufficiency coexists, particularly after operation, anomalous coronary artery should be suspected. Anomalous coronary artery in tetralogy of Fallot is rare, but when present, it may represent an important source of pulmonary blood flow. In pulmonary atresia with intact septum, an aberrant coronary artery may provide pulmonary flow through myocardial sinusoids.

HEMODYNAMICS

There are two important considerations about the hemodynamics of anomalous left coronary artery: those related to the abnormal coronary arterial circulation and those reflecting the effect of myocardial ischemia on the structures of the left side of the heart.

Considerable interest has been directed to the pattern of blood flow through a coronary artery with an anomalous origin from the pulmonary artery. Brooks in 1886 and Abbott in 1908 suggested that blood flow in the anomalous coronary artery was toward the pulmonary artery. Edwards[10] reestablished this viewpoint in 1958, and Sabiston et al.[11] in 1960 during an operation of a patient with anomalous left coronary artery sampled blood from that artery. The blood was fully saturated, indicating that blood flow was from the aorta into the pulmonary artery.

The pattern of blood flow through the coronary arterial system changes with age, and a third[12] and possibly a fourth stage[13] of this process have been described (Fig 57–2). The first stage is present at birth and during the immediate neonatal period (see Fig 57–2,A). At this age aortic and pulmonary arterial pressures are equal. Blood flows from the aorta into the right coronary artery and from the pulmonary trunk into the left coronary arteries. During the second stage (see Fig 57–2,B), with the postnatal decrease in pulmonary vascular resistance and pressure, the left coronary artery is perfused at a low pressure. This stage of low perfusion is critical for the myocardium, which is supplied by the left coronary artery. The potential for ischemia and infarction is maximal at this stage. The left and right coronary arterial systems have small interconnections. Because of the arterial pressure difference between the two systems, these connections progressively enlarge. This development of collaterals has two potential effects: (1) an increase of blood flow into the left coronary arterial system from the right coronary artery and improved potential myocardial perfusion, and (2) runoff of blood from the left coronary arterial system into the pulmonary artery away from the left ventricular myocardium. At this third stage (see Fig 57–2,C), blood flows in a retrograde direction in the left coronary artery in the pulmonary trunk. This pattern of coronary arterial blood flow has been amply shown angiographically.

A fourth stage has been found in adults in which the collateral development is so extensive that hemodynamically the condition becomes an arteriovenous fistula. The large blood flow from the right to the left coronary arterial system may cause a continuous murmur and rarely congestive cardiac failure because of left ventricular volume overload.

Because of inadequate myocardial perfusion early in infancy from low pulmonary arterial pressure or subse-

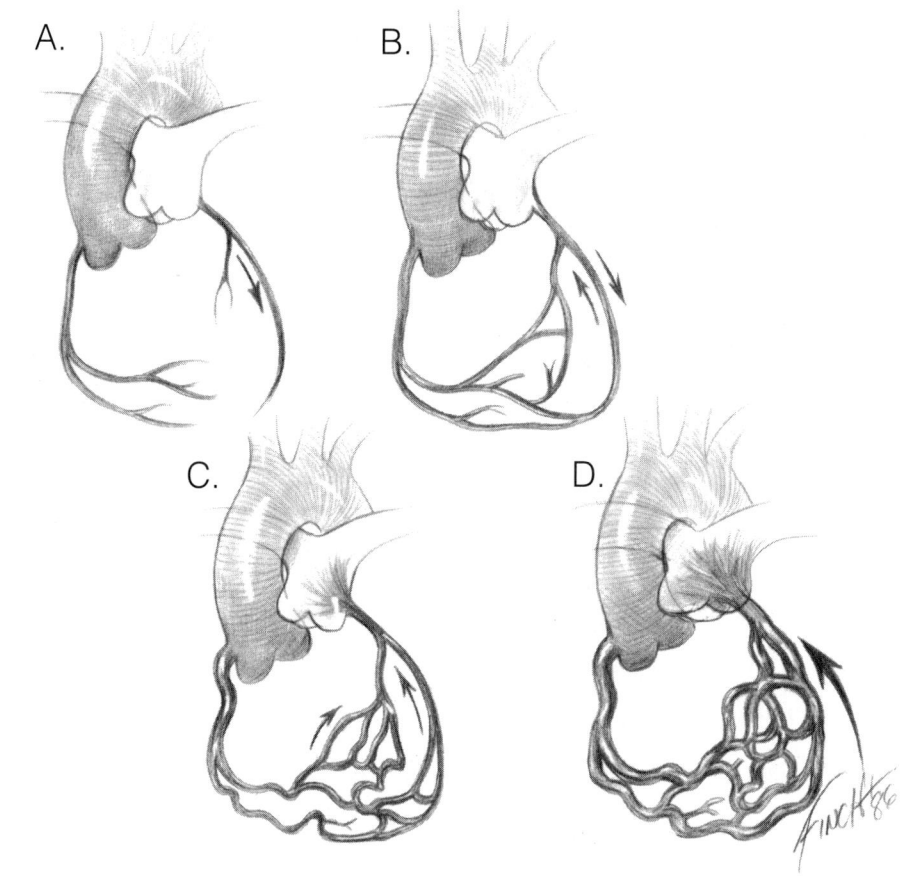

FIG 57–2.
Pattern of blood flow in anomalous left coronary artery. **A,** blood flow from pulmonary artery into aberrant left coronary artery because of high pulmonary vascular resistance. **B,** bidirectional flow in anomalous left coronary artery after decrease of pulmonary vascular resistance. **C,** reversal of blood flow from right coronary artery into anomalous left coronary artery via anastomotic connections. **D,** massive blood flow through anastomotic channels from right coronary artery into pulmonary artery.

quently from runoff into the pulmonary artery, infarction occurs. The normal decline of total and fetal hemoglobin levels during the first 6 months of life may accentuate these pathologic changes.

Myocardial fibrosis of the left ventricular free wall decreases contractility of this chamber and limits cardiac output. The scarring of the papillary muscles, their high location on the left ventricular wall, left ventricular dilatation, dilatation of the mitral annulus cause mitral regurgitation. The degree of regurgitation varies considerably among cases. It may be massive,[14] leading to congestive cardiac failure.

The left mainstem bronchus may be compressed by the greatly enlarged left atrium and may cause cough or atelectasis of the left lower lobe.

CLINICAL FEATURES

The clinical presentation may be (1) angina-like symptoms, (2) features of cardiomyopathy, (3) a left-to-right shunt, or (4) sudden death.[1, 15, 16]

Symptoms usually develop early in infancy; they may be nonspecific. Often there are episodes of respiratory distress, wheezing, coughing, and cyanosis. These may be associated with irritability and crying, possibly caused by angina. We have noted in hospitalized infants with this condition episodes of pallor, distress, dyspnea, and excessive perspiration. Usually the history and physical findings suggest congestive cardiac failure associated with the cardiomyopathy. There is often growth retardation. In a few instances, anomalous left coronary artery is asymptomatic in infancy and childhood and presents in adulthood as angina or sudden death.

In the usual case, the child is small for age, is irritable, and has a cough. Pulmonary auscultation may show fine rales. There is a left precordial bulge, and the cardiac apex is displaced laterally and downward. On auscultation a gallop rhythm is heard. A systolic murmur is often present at the cardiac apex. The murmur may be faint and nonspecific or moderately loud and more typical of mitral insufficiency. In infants, hepatomegaly is found.

Among older children and adults with anomalous left coronary artery, the initial indication of a cardiac problem may be a murmur of mitral insufficiency[17] or a continuous murmur (of large coronary arterial collaterals),[15] which may mimic patent ductus arteriosus.

ELECTROCARDIOGRAPHIC FEATURES

In 80% of instances, the electrocardiogram is highly suggestive of the diagnosis. A pattern of anterolateral myocardial infarction and left ventricular hypertrophy is typical.[1, 15, 16] The QRS axis tends to be located between 0 and −30 degrees. Deep and broad Q waves are found in leads I, aVL, V_5, and V_6. The T waves are inverted in these leads.[18] Usually the S waves in the right precordial leads and R waves in left precordial leads are prominent. The P waves may be broad and notched, indicating left atrial enlargement.

ECHOCARDIOGRAPHIC FEATURES

Two-dimensional echocardiography can demonstrate the abnormality. On a long-axis cross-sectional view across the aortic root, an enlarged right coronary artery is identified, but the origin of the left coronary artery cannot be seen. The left ventricle and left atrium are dilated, and the left ventricle shows reduced contractility. Doppler recording identifies coexistent mitral insufficiency.

RADIOGRAPHIC FEATURES

In most patients the roentgenographic appearance of the heart is indistinguishable from other cardiac conditions affecting principally the left ventricle, such as endocardial fibroelastosis, coarctation of the aorta, aortic stenosis, myocarditis, and various cardiomyopathies.[19]

1. In infancy the heart is invariably enlarged and has a left ventricular configuration (Fig 57–3), with a broad round left cardiac border.

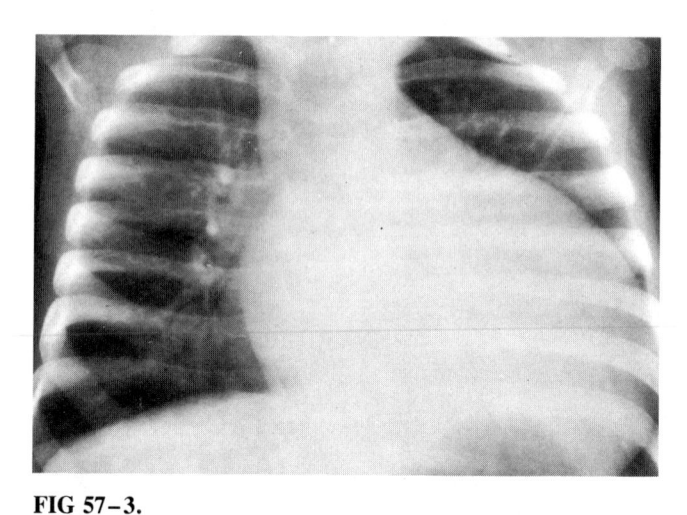

FIG 57–3.
Anomalous left coronary artery. Thoracic roentgenogram. Posteroanterior projection. Huge cardiac silhouette. Distinct left ventricular contour. Pulmonary vasculature is slightly accentuated. Radiographic appearance resembles other left-sided cardiac conditions in infancy.

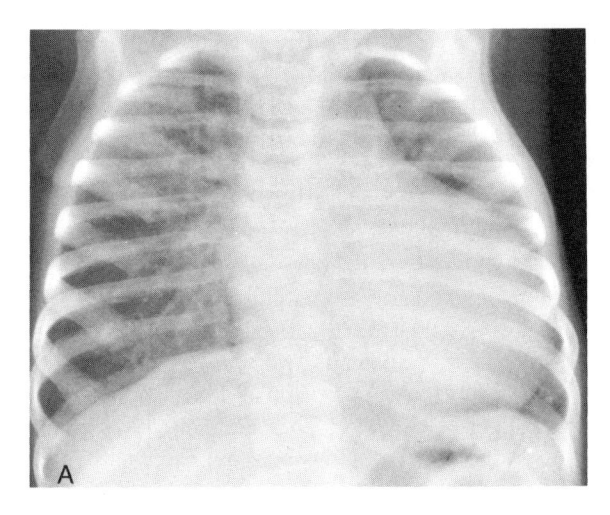

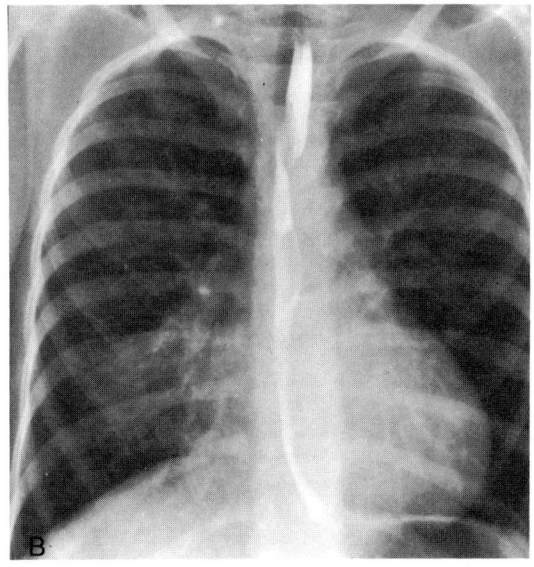

FIG 57-4.
Anomalous left coronary artery. Thoracic roentgenogram. Posteroanterior projection. **A,** age 1 month. Markedly enlarged heart. Left ventricular contour. Slightly accentuated pulmonary vasculature. **B,** age 6 years. Normal-sized heart from development of collaterals. Incidental aberrant left subclavian artery indenting esophagus.

2. The pulmonary vasculature may be slightly accentuated. The accentuated markings are venous. REASON: Pulmonary venous congestion occurs from elevated end-diastolic pressure in the dilated left ventricle and from mitral regurgitation. A discrepancy exists between cardiac size and the appearance of the pulmonary vasculature. Cardiac size is increased out of proportion to the degree to which pulmonary vasculature is accentuated. This discrepancy suggests pulmonary venous congestion rather than a left-to-right shunt.
3. In adults, the intracoronary collaterals increase in size. A large left-to-right shunt develops, and the pulmonary arterial vasculature becomes increased. Such patients may also develop left ventricular failure from a high-output state.
4. As the child grows, cardiac size may diminish even without a cardiac operation. REASON: Left ventricular ischemia improves because of the development of intercoronary collateral vessels (Fig 57–4).
5. Typically cardiac enlargement involves only the left ventricle. This chamber is best demonstrated on a left anterior oblique projection (Fig 57–5).
6. Typically the left atrium is enlarged. REASONS:
   a. Fibrosis in the left ventricular myocardium causes left ventricular dysfunction and dilation. Left ventricular end-diastolic pressure increases, and therefore a higher left atrial filling pressure is present.
   b. Infarction of the papillary muscles, resulting in scarring and fibrosis and consequent shortening of chordae tendineae, causes mitral regurgitation, which may be the presenting clinical sign.
   c. The almost invariably associated endocardial fibroelastosis results in marked dilatation of the left ventricle, particularly the apical area. The papillary muscles arise high on the left ventricular wall (see Chapter 56).
   d. Dilation of the left ventricle may induce dilatation

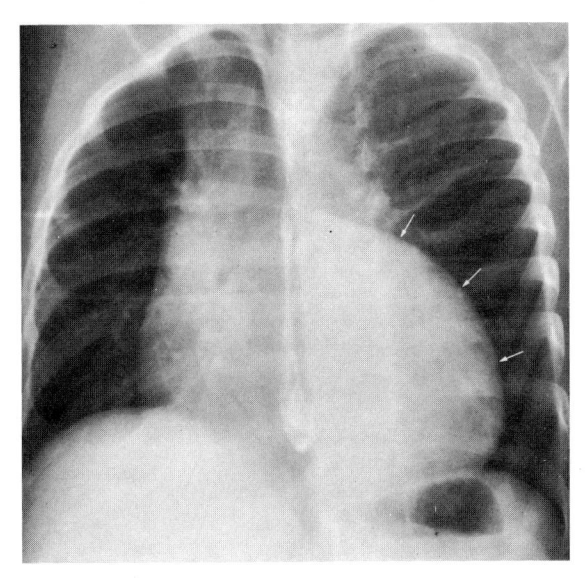

FIG 57-5.
Anomalous left coronary artery. Thoracic roentgenogram. Left anterior oblique projection. Huge left ventricle *(arrows)*.

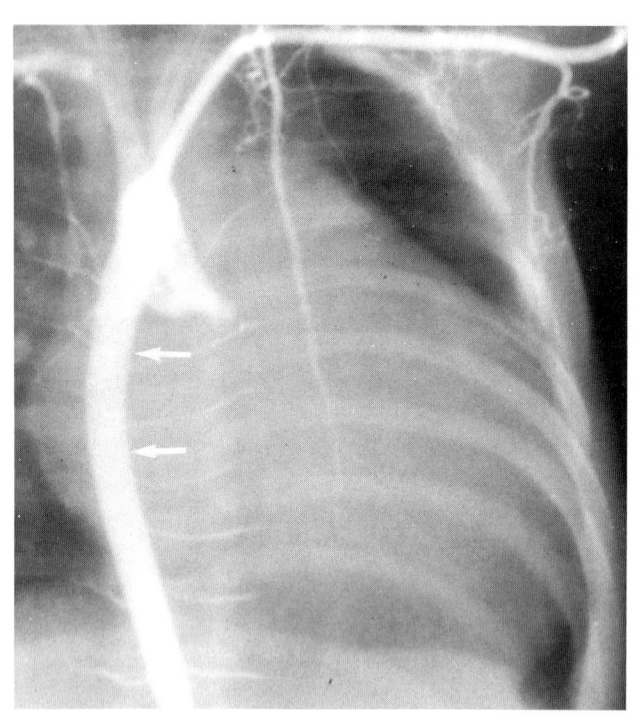

FIG 57-6.
Anomalous left coronary artery. Aortogram. Anteroposterior projection. Displacement of thoracic aorta *(arrows)* by huge left ventricle and left atrium.

of the mitral annulus, increasing mitral regurgitation (relative mitral insufficiency).
7. Left ventricular and left atrial enlargement may be so severe that the thoracic aorta is displaced toward the right (Fig 57-6), causing a paramediastinal mass on a thoracic roentgenogram.
8. Rarely, an infant with an anomalous left coronary artery may have a normal cardiac size and be asymptomatic (Fig 57-7). The correct diagnosis is usually suspected by echocardiography. The absence of left ventricular enlargement may occur under the following circumstances:
   a. Aberrant right coronary artery and normal origin of the left coronary artery.
   b. Origin of the circumflex or part of the circumflex circulation only. REASON: With a right preponderant coronary arterial pattern, the posterior and anterior ventricular septum, as well as a large portion of the left ventricle by diagonal branches, are normally perfused. Only a comparatively small segment of the left ventricle is ischemic (see Fig 57-7). A normal thoracic roentgenogram does therefore not exclude this condition.
   c. Aberrant coronary artery with stenosis of its origin. These patients are hemodynamically identical to patients with a single coronary artery and are asymptomatic.
9. The enlarged left ventricle and left atrium may cause atelectasis of the left lung because of bronchomalacia of the left mainstem bronchus (Fig 57-8). The left mainstem bronchus becomes compressed from above by the left pulmonary artery and from below by the large left atrium.

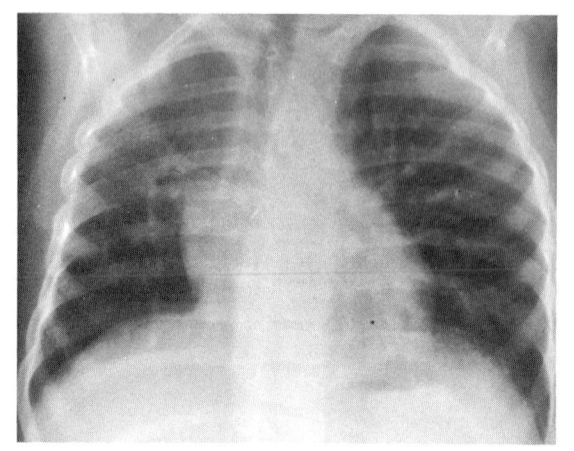

FIG 57-7.
Anomalous circumflex coronary artery from pulmonary artery. Thoracic roentgenogram. Posteroanterior projection. Normal cardiac size and pulmonary vasculature. Correct diagnosis is suggested by echocardiography in this case.

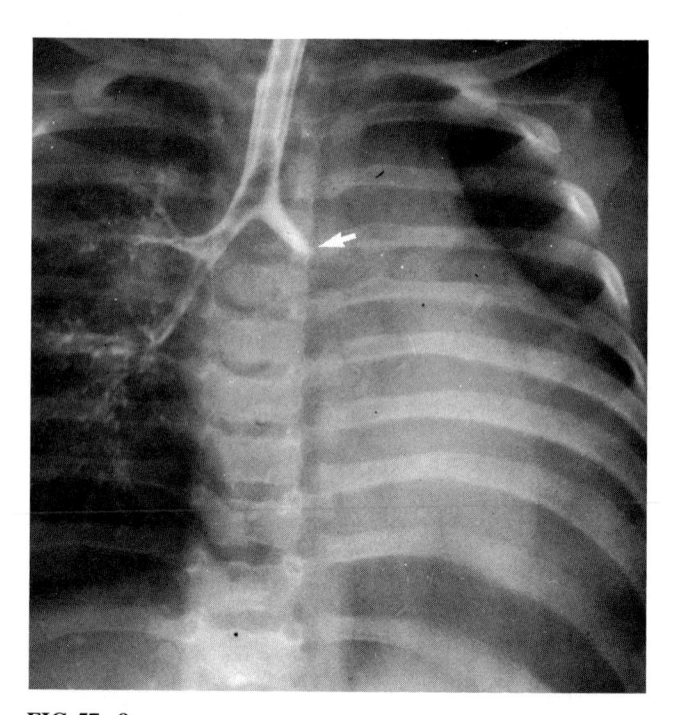

FIG 57-8.
Anomalous left coronary artery. Recurrent pneumonitis in left lung. Bronchogram. Posteroanterior projection. Bronchomalacia and obstruction of left mainstem bronchus *(arrow)* by huge left atrium and ventricle.

CARDIAC CATHETERIZATION

Cardiac catheterization should be undertaken carefully. Myocardial ischemia may induce ventricular arrhythmias. The venous catheter course is normal. Rarely oxygen data show evidence of a left-to-right shunt, but sensitive indicators may show evidence of a shunt into the pulmonary artery. Right-sided cardiac pressures are normal, but left ventricular end-diastolic pressure is elevated. If associated mitral insufficiency is present, left atrial pressures are elevated.

ANGIOGRAPHIC FEATURES

If an anomalous left coronary artery is suspected on clinical or echocardiographic grounds, careful angiography is indicated for the demonstration of the exact anatomy of the coronary arterial system. An aortogram should be performed with the catheter tip immediately above the aortic valve using a large amount of contrast medium. If collateral arterial branches between the right and left coronary arterial system are not well developed, filling of the anomalous left coronary artery may be minimal, and opacification of the pulmonary artery may not be seen. Furthermore, the transit time from right to left coronary artery through collaterals may be as rapid as 0.3 second, and the erroneous impression may be gained that both coronary arteries fill simultaneously from the aorta. This was particularly true when cut-film angiography was performed at a rate of only six frames per second. A filming rate of 60 frames per second is mandatory.

The best angiographic results for determination of the

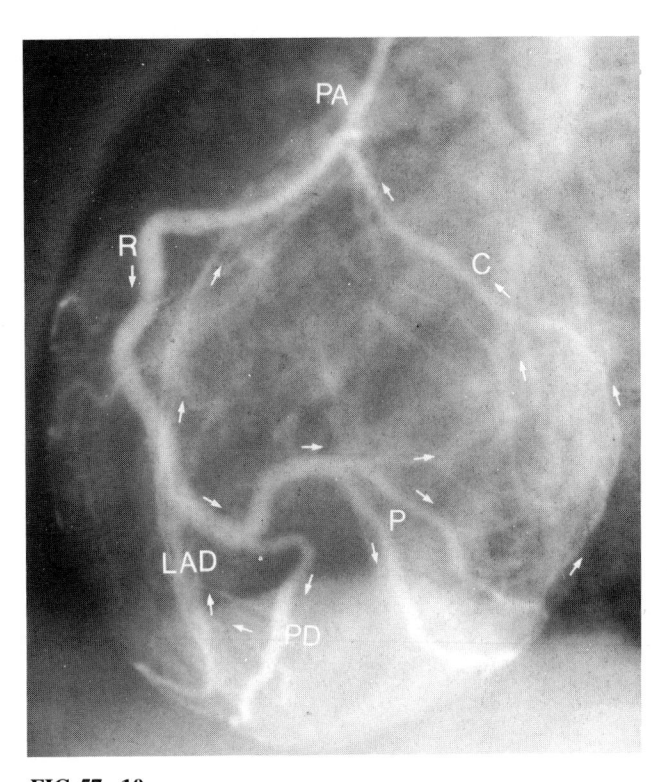

FIG 57-10.
Anomalous left coronary artery. Selective right coronary arteriogram. Lateral projection. Enlarged and dominant right coronary artery *(R)*. Retrograde opacification of left anterior descending branch *(LAD)*. Reversal of flow *(arrows)* in LAD. Collateral flow occurs through posterior descending *(PD)* and septal branches. Posterolateral branches of right coronary artery *(P)* are huge because of large collaterals through circumflex *(C)* circulation. Retrograde flow *(arrows)* through circumflex circulation into pulmonary artery *(PA)*.

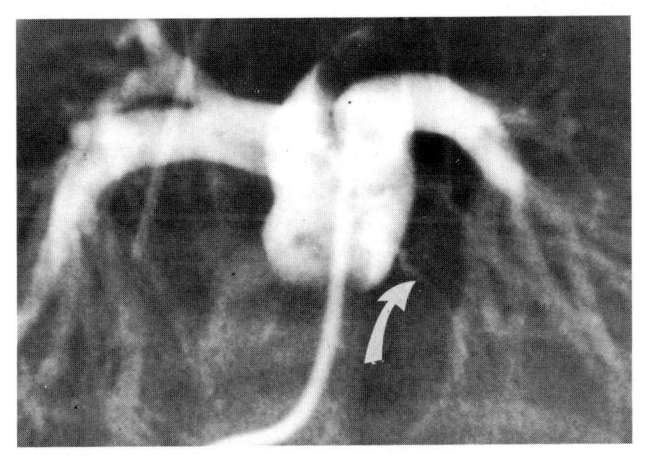

FIG 57-9.
Anomalous origin of left coronary artery. Neonate. Balloon occlusion pulmonary arteriogram. Left coronary artery *(arrow)* is perfused from pulmonary trunk because of fetal pulmonary hypertension.

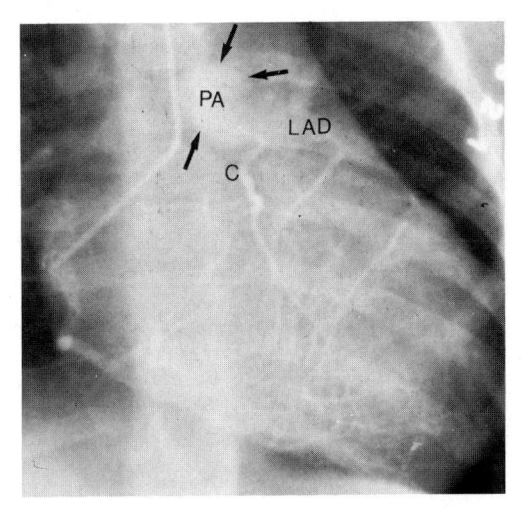

FIG 57-11.
Anomalous left coronary artery. Right coronary arteriogram. Anteroposterior projection. Late phase. Opacification of left coronary septal branches, circumflex *(C)*, anterior descending *(LAD)*, and pulmonary artery *(PA)* *(arrows)*.

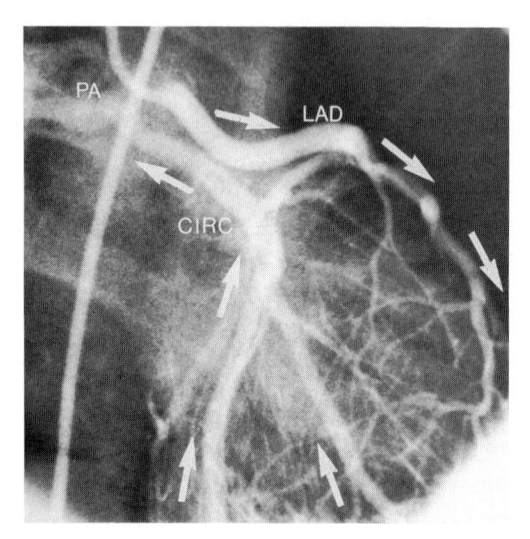

FIG 57–12.
Anomalous circumflex coronary artery. Left coronary arteriogram. Right anterior oblique projection. Large left anterior descending artery *(LAD)* and retrograde filling of the circumflex branch *(CIRC)*, which arises from pulmonary artery *(PA)*.

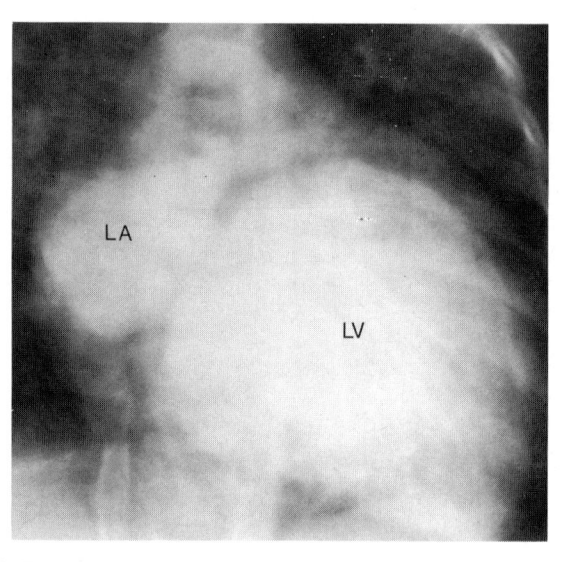

FIG 57–14.
Anomalous left coronary artery. Pulmonary arteriogram. Late phase. Anteroposterior projection. Enormous enlargement of left ventricle *(LV)*. Almost normal-sized left atrium *(LA)* displaced toward right.

exact anatomy are obtained by selective coronary arterial injection. Proper angiograms are important because:

1. Collateral arterial branches between the right and left coronary arterial systems may be underdeveloped.

This represents a contraindication for operative ligation of the anomalous left coronary artery.

2. The left main coronary artery may be very short, making ligation proximal to the division into the circumflex and left anterior descending branches difficult.

3. Only one branch of the left coronary arterial system, either the left anterior descending or circumflex, may arise from the pulmonary artery.

In a neonate the anomalous left coronary artery may not opacify after aortography. REASON: The pulmonary hypertension in a neonate favors flow from the pulmonary artery into the anomalous left coronary artery. Intercoronary collaterals have not yet developed, so antegrade perfusion of the left coronary arterial system occurs from the pulmonary artery. Under such circumstances a pulmonary arteriogram demonstrates the anomalous left coronary artery (Fig 57–9).

Even in children, pulmonary arteriography is indicated when the aberrant left coronary artery does not visualize after aortography or selective right coronary arteriography. There are patients without collateral branches between right and left coronary arterial systems and patients with pulmonary hypertension and antegrade perfusion of the aberrant coronary artery from the pulmonary artery.

Left ventriculography is indicated to determine the size and contractility of the left ventricle and the degree of mitral regurgitation.[8] REASON: Mitral regurgitation may be the patient's major clinical manifestation and the initial presenting feature of anomalous left coronary artery.

The angiographic findings vary.

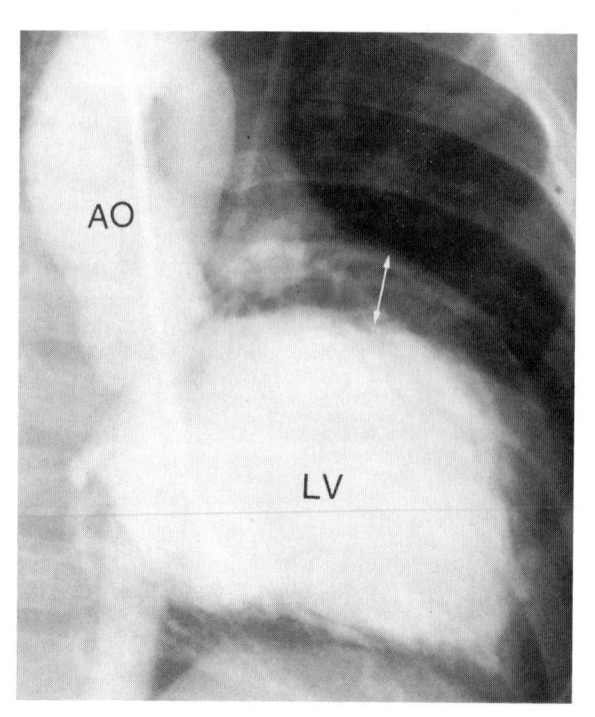

FIG 57–13.
Anomalous left coronary artery. Left ventriculogram. Diastole. Anteroposterior projection. Enlarged left ventricle *(LV)*. Increased wall thickness *(arrow)* from endocardial fibroelastosis. *AO* = aorta.

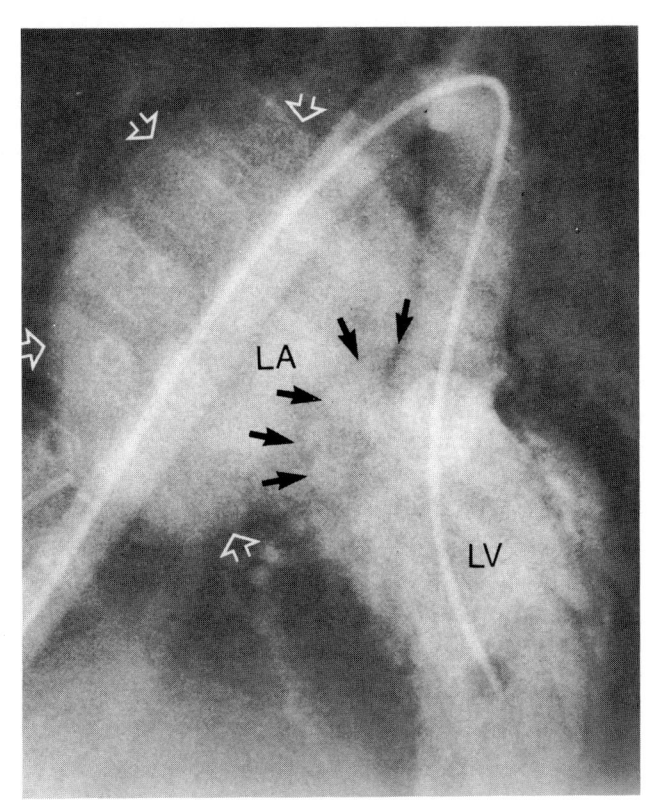

FIG 57-15.
Anomalous left coronary artery. Left ventriculogram *(LV)*. Right anterior oblique projection. Marked mitral insufficiency from infarction of posteromedial papillary muscle. Greatly enlarged left atrium *(LA) (open arrows)*. Prolapsing posterior leaflet faintly seen *(arrows)*.

1. The right coronary artery is enlarged (Fig 57-10). REASON: The right coronary artery carries blood flow for both the right and the left coronary arterial circulations. Its size depends largely on the size and number of collateral arteries.

2. Collateral arterial branches enlarge with age. Consequently, the size of the right coronary artery progressively increases. Finally, a huge left-to-right shunt may develop.

3. After selective injection of the right coronary artery, which should be performed rapidly with a large amount of contrast medium, there is sequential and retrograde filling of the left coronary arterial circulation (see Fig 57-10). Filming rate should be 60 frames per second.

4. Opacification of the pulmonary artery from retrograde flow through the left coronary artery is seen best on either an anteroposterior or a right anterior oblique projection (Fig 57-11).

5. Although the most common malformation is origin of the left coronary artery from the pulmonary artery, isolated origin of the left anterior descending or circumflex arterial branch may occur (Fig 57-12).

6. If only the circumflex branch arises anomalously, the heart may remain normal in size, the patient is asymptomatic, and left ventricular function is preserved, particularly when a right preponderant coronary artery pattern preserves normal perfusion of the entire ventricular septum.

7. If a selective right coronary arteriogram does not demonstrate the aberrant left coronary artery, perfusion from the pulmonary artery is present. This is most commonly seen in neonates with pulmonary hypertension. A balloon occlusion pulmonary arteriogram demonstrates the aberrant left coronary artery (see Fig 57-10).

8. With aberrant origin of the entire left coronary arterial circulation from the pulmonary artery, left ventricular impairment and enlargement of the left ventricular cavity are the rule (Fig 57-13). REASON: Diffuse myocardial fibrosis from infarction and secondary endocardial fibroelastosis.

9. The left ventricle is enlarged (see Fig 57-13). End-systolic volume is increased as in left ventricular failure. The larger the size of the left ventricle, the more apparent the decrease of the left ventricular contractility on cine angiograms. REASON: To eject the same stroke volume, an enlarged ventricle changes its dimension less than

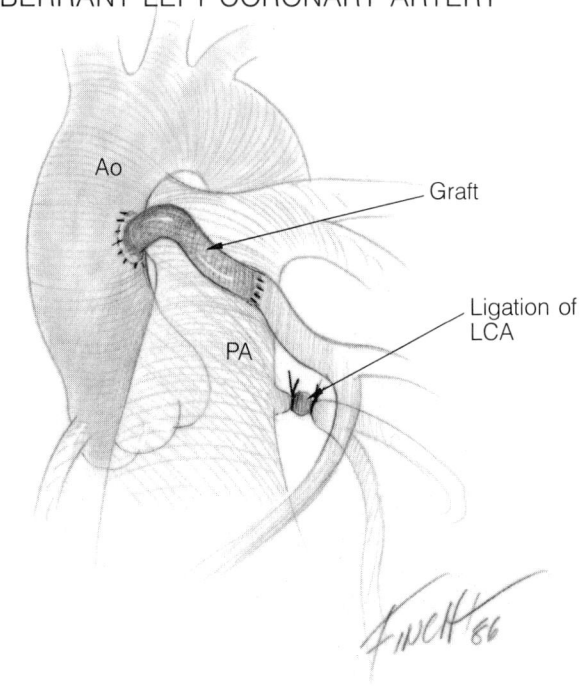

FIG 57-16.
Anomalous left coronary artery. End-to-end anastomosis with left subclavian artery. Left coronary artery *(LCA)* is ligated at origin from pulmonary artery *(PA)* and anastomosed end-to-end either using graft or left subclavian artery. *Ao* = aorta.

938 Cardiac Conditions Associated With Increased Pulmonary Venous Vasculature Without Cyanosis

a small ventricle. Therefore, an enlarged ventricle that does not show significant change in dimensions is usually interpreted as showing "poor contractility." However, cardiac output may be normal at rest.

10. The wall thickness of the left ventricle varies. Although myocardial fibrosis and scarring thin the left ventricle, there is almost invariably associated endocardial fibroelastosis of varying degrees. If endocardial fibroelastosis is pronounced, the wall thickness of the ventricle may be increased (see Fig 57–13).

11. In infants the left ventricle may be huge (Fig 57–14).

12. There may be massive mitral regurgitation (Fig 57–15). REASON: Infarction of the papillary muscles.

OPERATIVE CONSIDERATIONS

Infants with anomalous left coronary artery are at risk of sudden death, presumably from ventricular arrhythmia secondary to myocardial ischemia. Prompt angiography and operative treatment are needed. Morphine may be given to relieve pain and restlessness. The infant with congestive cardiac failure should be treated with diuretics and an inotropic agent, either digitalis or a combination of dopamine and dobutamine. The latter has an advantage, the effects are transient, and fewer arrhythmias are caused.

Several types of operations are available, reflecting that each has advantages and disadvantages. No center has a sufficient number of cases and long-term follow-up studies to assess the effectiveness of various operations.

1. Ligation of left coronary artery.[20, 21] This operation was originally proposed because it eliminated the fistulous communication through the coronary arterial system. It has an advantage of being quick, and cardiopulmonary bypass is unnecessary. It does require, however, sufficient collaterals between the right and left coronary arterial systems, so that the myocardium supplied by the left coronary arterial system be adequately perfused after operation. Pressure measurements in the left coronary artery show prompt pressure increase after ligation.

Nevertheless, the left coronary arterial system is particularly vulnerable to development of atherosclerosis, and the long-term follow-up may show problems in this regard. We have four 20-year survivors of ligation, and in each patient cardiac size has returned to normal and no symptoms are present, although two have a positive exer-

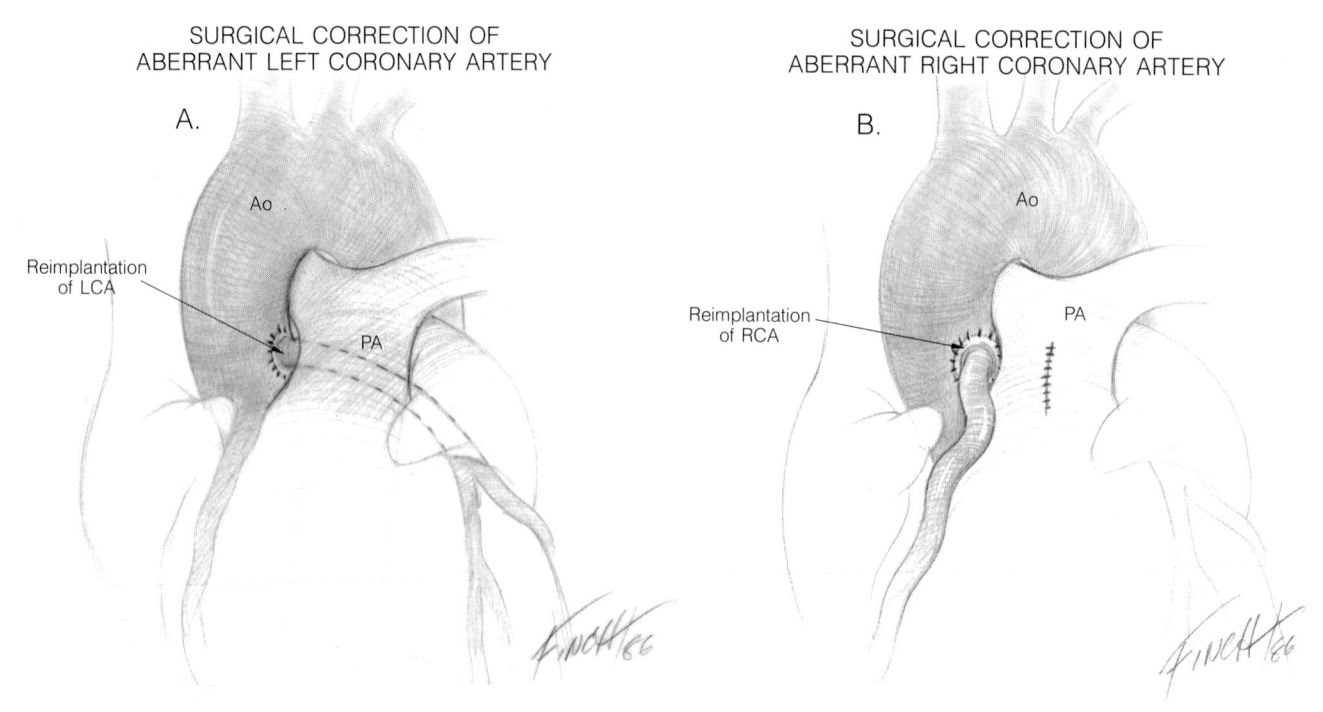

FIG 57–17.
Anomalous coronary artery. Reimplantation of anomalous left coronary artery *(LCA)* into aorta *(Ao)*. **A,** origin of anomalous coronary artery is excised from pulmonary artery *(PA)*, together with a small tissue button, and reimplanted behind pulmonary artery into aorta. **B,** reimplantation of anomalous right coronary artery *(RCA)* into aorta. Origin of anomalous coronary artery is excised from pulmonary artery with tissue button and reimplanted into aorta. Because anomalous right coronary artery usually arises from anterior aspect of aorta, operation is easier than reimplantation of anomalous left coronary artery.

TUNNEL REPAIR

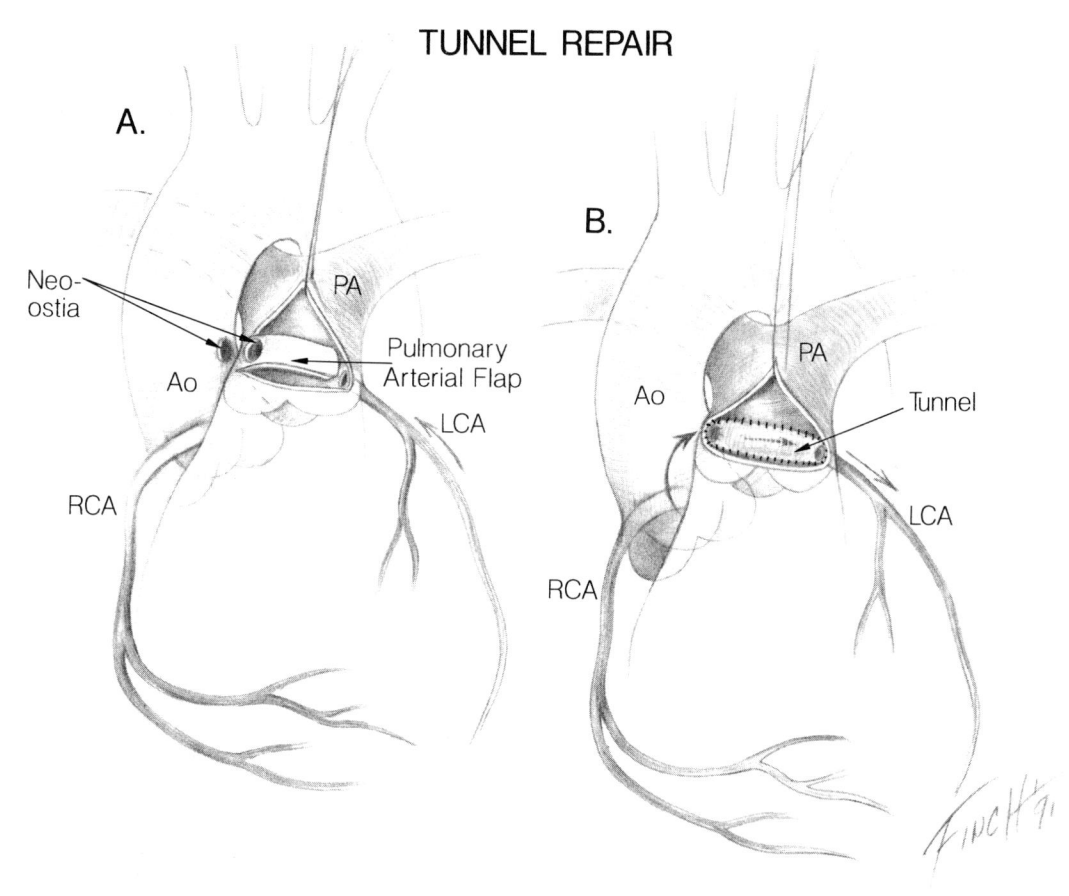

FIG 57–18.
Anomalous left coronary artery. Tunnel repair. **A,** pulmonary artery *(PA)* is opened. Opening (neo-ostia) are created between aorta *(Ao)* and pulmonary artery. **B,** pulmonary artery flap is sutured to posterior wall of pulmonary artery, creating a tunnel between neo-ostium and left coronary artery *(LCA)*. RCA = right coronary artery.

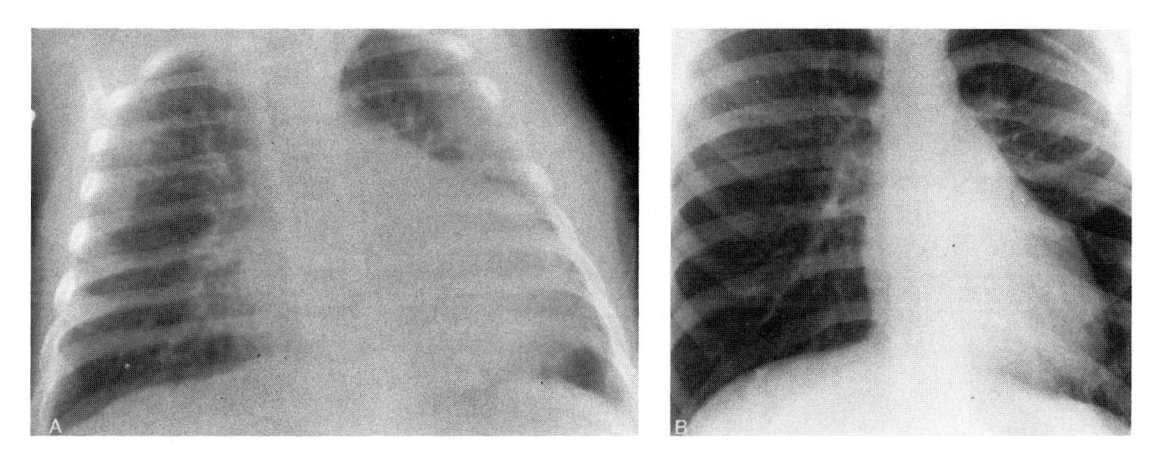

FIG 57–19.
Anomalous left coronary artery. Postoperative view. Thoracic roentgenogram. Posteroanterior projection. **A,** immediately after operation. Marked cardiac enlargement and pulmonary congestion. Resection of fourth left rib for operative approach. **B,** 15 years later. Regression of cardiac size to normal. Normal pulmonary vasculature.

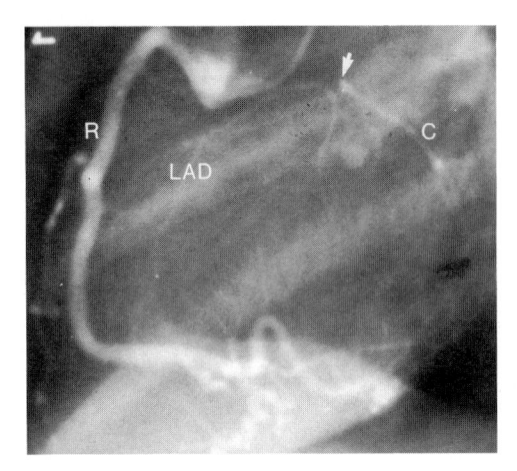

FIG 57-20.
Anomalous left coronary artery after ligation. Right coronary arteriogram. Lateral projection. Enlarged right coronary artery *(R)*. Opacification of left anterior descending *(LAD)* and circumflex *(C)* branches through poorly developed collaterals. Pulmonary artery no longer opacifies because of coronary artery ligation *(arrow)*. With poorly established collaterals, symptoms of angina may persist and stress test results remain positive.

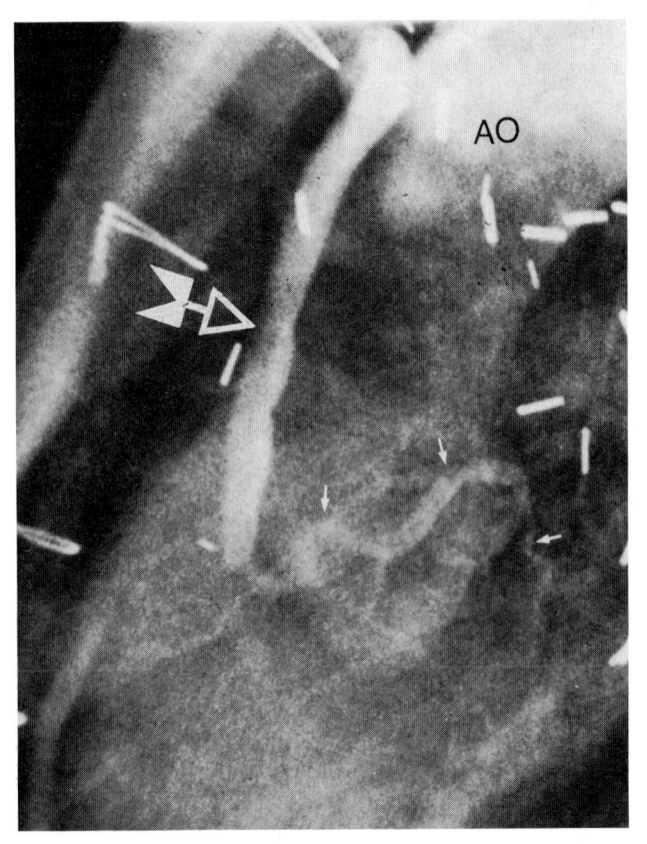

FIG 57-21.
Anomalous left coronary artery. Postoperative view. Saphenous vein graft to left anterior descending coronary artery *(open arrow)*. Selective injection of graft. Lateral projection. Left anterior descending and circumflex branches are opacified *(small white arrows)*. *AO* = aorta.

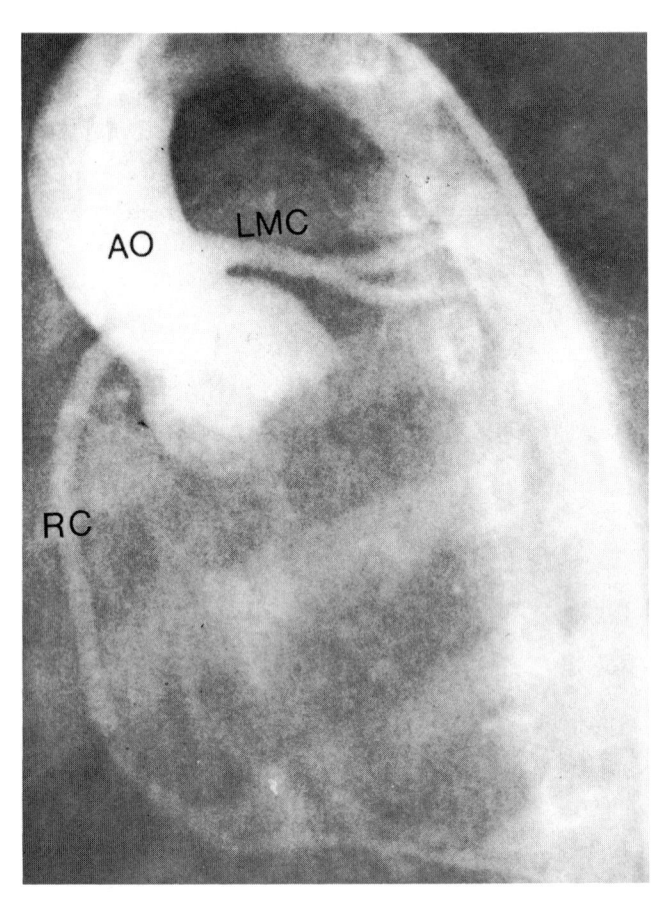

FIG 57-22.
Coronary arteriogram. Left anterior oblique projection. Left main coronary *(LMC)* is relatively long, which made this operation possible. Reimplantation into aorta *(AO)* was made slightly higher than seen in the normal left coronary artery. *RC* = right coronary artery.

cise stress test. Another study reported late deaths after ligation alone.

2. Ligation plus end-to-end anastomosis of the left subclavian artery or a graft to the left coronary artery (Fig 57–16).[22] This procedure allows antegrade flow into the left coronary arterial system at systemic level of pressure. This procedure does not require cardiopulmonary bypass. However, if the heart fibrillates during the operation, as happened in one of our patients, the problem is difficult to manage. The other problem is clotting or narrowing of the graft, but this has a similar effect to ligation unless it occurs late at a time when collaterals have regressed.

3. Ligation and saphenous vein bypass.[23–25] A saphenous vein is connected to the left coronary artery end-to-side and to the aorta, as for treatment of atherosclerotic heart disease. This is not an ideal procedure, because there are long-term problems with patency of saphenous vein grafts. Indeed, this has also been found in patients with anomalous left coronary artery. At the time the graft narrows, the collaterals have regressed. However, an angio-

gram of the anomalous coronary artery repaired by saphenous vein bypass graft showed persistent patency of the graft 8 years later.[24]

4. Reimplantation of the left coronary artery to aorta (Fig 57–17,A).[26, 27] Transplanting the orifice of the left coronary artery to the aorta has the greatest potential because it creates a two-coronary artery system. The major problem in performing this operation is the distance between the aorta and the site at which the anomalous coronary artery arises from the pulmonary trunk. Particularly if the anomalous coronary artery arises more anteriorly, the distance to the posteriorly positioned aorta is too great, making this operation impossible. Transplantation of the right coronary artery is easier than of the left coronary artery (Fig 57–17,B).

In this procedure, a button of tissue surrounding the coronary artery is removed, and this button is sewn into an operatively created circular opening in the aortic wall. An alternative involves using a portion of the wall of the pulmonary trunk to create a tube to connect to the aorta.[28]

5. Creation of an aorticopulmonary window.[29] In this procedure an aorticopulmonary window is created, and a pericardial baffle is inserted into the pulmonary artery so that blood is directed from the aorta though the window behind the baffle into the orifice of the anomalous left coronary artery. This creates a two-coronary arterial system but is a more complicated procedure. Little information is available regarding long-term results.

6. Tunnel repair. The pulmonary artery is incised, and a flap is made from the anterior arterial wall of the pulmonary artery. A hole is cut in the flap and the ascending aorta (Fig 57–18,A). The flap is sewn to the posterior wall of the pulmonary artery and around the anomalous coronary artery, directing blood flow through the tunnel into the left coronary artery (Fig 57–18,B). Because the flap consists of the native pulmonary arterial wall, it is postulated that it will show normal growth.

POSTOPERATIVE RADIOGRAPHIC FEATURES

1. After ligation of the aberrant coronary artery or a revascularization procedure, there is striking decrease in cardiac size (Fig 57–19).

2. After ligation of the left main coronary artery, the entire coronary arterial system is perfused from the right coronary artery (Fig 57–20). Flow into left coronary arterial system is still in a retrograde direction. The proximal left coronary artery is smaller than before operation.

3. With a saphenous venous graft, the graft can be selectively injected. Collateral flow from the right coronary artery no longer occurs, and the entire left coronary tree opacifies via saphenous vein graft (Fig 57–21).

4. If the left main coronary artery has some length, it can be reimplanted into the aorta (Figs 57–17,A and 57–22). Probably this represents the best operative correction.

REFERENCES

1. Noren GR, Raghib G, Moller JH, et al: Anomalous origin of the left coronary artery from the pulmonary trunk with special reference to the occurrence of mitral insufficiency, *Circulation* 30:171, 1964.
2. Wald S, Stonecipher K, Baldwin BJ, et al: Anomalous origin of the right coronary artery from the pulmonary artery, *Am J Cardiol* 27:677, 1971.
3. Tingelstad JB, Lower RR, Eldredge WJ: Anomalous origin of the right coronary artery from the main pulmonary artery, *Am J Cardiol* 30:670, 1972.
4. Bergman D, Brennan FJ, Singer A, et al: Anomalous origin of the right coronary artery from the pulmonary artery, *J Thorac Cardiovasc Surg* 72:626, 1976.
5. Roberts WC: Anomalous origin of both coronary arteries from the pulmonary artery, *Am J Cardiol* 10:595, 1962.
6. Tedeschi CG, Helpern MM: Heterotopic origin of both coronary arteries from the pulmonary artery: review of literature and report of a case not complicated by associated defects, *Pediatrics* 14:53, 1954.
7. Wilcox WD, Hagler DJ, Lie JT, et al: Anomalous origin of left coronary artery from pulmonary artery in association with intracardiac lesions: report of two cases, *J Thorac Cardiovasc Surg* 78:12, 1979.
8. Pinsky WW, Gillette PC, Duff DF, et al: Anomalous origin of left coronary artery from the pulmonary artery with ventricular septal defect, *Circulation* 57:1026, 1978.
9. Feldt RH, Ongley PA, Titus JL: Total coronary arterial circulation from pulmonary artery with survival to age seven: report of case, *Mayo Clin Proc* 40:539, 1965.
10. Edwards JE: Anomalous coronary arteries with special reference to arteriovenous-like communications, *Circulation* 17:1001, 1958.
11. Sabiston DC Jr, Neill CA, Taussig HB: The direction of blood flow in anomalous left coronary artery arising from the pulmonary artery, *Circulation* 22:591, 1960.
12. Edwards JE: Editorial: the direction of blood flow in coronary arteries arising from the pulmonary trunk, *Circulation* 29:163, 1964.
13. Baue AE, Baum S, Blakemore WS, et al: A later stage of anomalous coronary circulation with origin of the left coronary artery from the pulmonary artery: coronary artery steal, *Circulation* 36:878, 1967.
14. Graham TP Jr, Volberg FM Jr, Cline RF, et al: Severe mitral insufficiency in early infancy: associated with anomalous origin of the left coronary artery from the pulmonary artery, *Am J Cardiol* 23:858, 1969.
15. Wesselhoeft H, Fawcett JS, Johnson AL: Anomalous origin

of the left coronary artery from the pulmonary trunk: its clinical spectrum, pathology, and pathophysiology, based on a review of 140 cases with seven further cases, *Circulation* 38:403, 1968.
16. Askenazi J, Nadas AS: Anomalous left coronary artery originating from pulmonary artery: report on 15 cases, *Circulation* 51:976, 1975.
17. Burchell HB, Brown AL Jr: Anomalous origin of coronary artery from pulmonary artery masquerading as mitral insufficiency, *Am Heart J* 63:388, 1962.
18. Flaherty JT, Spach MS, Boineau JP, et al: Cardiac potentials on body surface of infants with anomalous left coronary artery (myocardial infarction), *Circulation* 36:345, 1967.
19. Lundquist C, Amplatz K: Anomalous origin of the left coronary artery from the pulmonary artery, *Am J Roentgenol Radium Ther Nucl Med* 95:611, 1965.
20. Likar I, Criley JM, Lewis KB: Anomalous left coronary artery arising from the pulmonary artery in an adult: a review of the therapeutic problem, *Circulation* 33:727, 1966.
21. Castaneda AR, Indeglia RA, Varco RL: Anomalous origin of the left coronary artery from the pulmonary artery: certain therapeutic considerations, *Circulation* 33, 34(suppl I):52, 1966.
22. Monro JL, Sharratt GP, Conway N: Correction of anomalous origin of left coronary artery using left subclavian artery, *Br Heart J* 40:79, 1978.
23. Gasior RM, Winters WL, Glick H, et al: Anomalous origin of left coronary artery from pulmonary artery: treatment by aorto-left coronary saphenous vein bypass, *Am J Cardiol* 27:215, 1971.
24. Chaitman BR, Bourassa MG, Lesperance J, et al: Anomalous left coronary artery from pulmonary artery: an eight year angiographic follow-up after saphenous vein bypass graft, *Circulation* 51:552, 1975.
25. El-Said GM, Ruzyllo W, Williams RL, et al: Early and late result of saphenous vein graft for anomalous origin of left coronary artery from pulmonary artery, *Circulation* 47, 48(suppl III):2, 1973.
26. Richardson JV, Doty DB: Correction of anomalous origin of the left coronary artery, *J Thorac Cardiovasc Surg* 77:699, 1979.
27. Neches WH, Mathews RA, Park SC, et al: Anomalous origin of the left coronary artery from the pulmonary artery: a new method of surgical repair, *Circulation* 50:582, 1974.
28. Armer RM, Shumacker HB Jr, Lurie PR, et al: Origin of the left coronary artery from the pulmonary artery without collateral circulation: report of a case with a suggested surgical correction, *Pediatrics* 32:588, 1963.
29. Hamilton DI, Ghosh PK, Donnelly RJ: An operation for anomalous origin of left coronary artery, *Br Heart J* 41:121, 1979.
30. Takeuchi S, Imamura H, Katsumoto K, et al: New surgical method for repair of anomalous left coronary artery from pulmonary artery, *J Thorac Cardiovasc Surg* 78(1):7–11, 1979.

PART NINE

Cardiac Malposition

Each thoracic roentgenogram must be assessed for the presence of a cardiac malposition, even if the cardiac silhouette is in the left hemithorax. A variety of different anatomic arrangements may be present with either levocardia or dextrocardia. The type of malposition can often be defined by carefully analyzing the roentgenogram. Because certain types of cardiac anomalies coexist with specific types of malposition, these can be predicted as well.

CHAPTER 58

Malposition of the Heart

Malposition of the heart represents an abnormality of position of the heart either in the thorax or in relation to other organs. Thus, the heart may be malposed in either the right or left side of the thorax. Usually malposition of the heart coexists with other cardiac anomalies, often complicated. As a result, the interpretation of clinical, radiographic, and angiographic data in such patients is difficult. This difficulty has been compounded by a variety of classifications, approaches, and terms that have been used to describe these conditions.[1-12] In this chapter we describe a radiographic approach to cardiac malposition that we have found useful.

To fully understand cardiac malpositions, one must understand the following concepts: visceroatrial situs, anatomic characteristics of cardiac chambers, ventricular inversion, and transposition of the great vessels.

VISCEROATRIAL SITUS

In almost all individuals, whether the heart is located in right or left hemithorax, certain basic anatomic relationships exist between the atria and viscera.

These basic relationships are used to determine if an individual has situs solitus, situs inversus, or situs ambiguus. In most individuals, regardless of the position of the cardiac apex, constant relationships exist between particular organs. Thus, on one side of the body, the four following structures are located: right atrium; inferior vena cava; liver; and trilobed lung, which has an epiarterial bronchus. On the opposite side of the body are located the left atrium, descending aorta, stomach, and bilobed lung, which has a hyparterial bronchus. When these interrelationships between organs exist, they are described as concordant. In virtually all individuals, concordance is found.

Rarely, these relationships do not exist, and this state is called "discordant." Such patients are considered to have ambiguous situs, a condition almost always associated with anomalies of a number of organs, including the spleen. The conditions with discordance are often named after the associated splenic anomaly, either the asplenia or the polysplenia syndrome, or after features of the atria, either right atrial or left atrial isomerism.

There are three types of visceroatrial situs, two of which are concordant, and the third of which is discordant.

Situs Solitus

Situs solitus is the pattern present in normal individuals and even in many individuals with dextrocardia.

1. The right atrium, major lobe of liver, inferior vena cava, and trilobed lung are located on the *right* side of the body.
2. The left atrium, stomach, descending aorta, and bilobed liver are located on the *left* side of the body (Fig 58-1,A). The aortic arch is an unreliable indicator of situs, because it may be on either side of the trachea.

Situs Inversus

Situs inversus can be considered the mirror image of situs solitus. The heart is usually located in the right hemithorax but may be present in the left side as well.

1. The anatomic right atrium, major lobe of liver, inferior vena cava, and trilobed lung are located on the *left* side of the body.
2. The anatomic left atrium, stomach, descending aorta, and bilobed lung are located on the *right* side of the body (Fig 58-1,B).

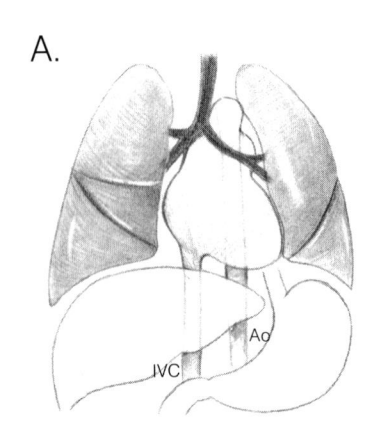

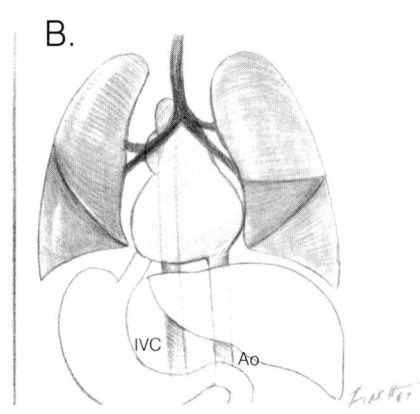

FIG 58–1.
Anatomic relationships. **A,** situs solitus: liver, inferior vena cava *(IVC)*, and trilobed lung on right; stomach, descending aorta *(Ao)*, and bilobed lung on left side of body. **B,** Situs inversus. Mirror-image of situs solitus. Liver, inferior vena cava, and trilobed lung on left; stomach, descending aorta, and bilobed lung on right side of body. Bronchus of bilobed lung is longer than bronchus of trilobed lung.

Situs Ambiguous

There are rare anatomic situations in which the normal relationships between major organs are not present and visceroatrial discordance exists. In most of these individuals, either the asplenia or polysplenia syndrome is found. The heart is located in the left or right hemithorax with equal frequency.

ANATOMIC FEATURES OF CARDIAC CHAMBERS

When a cardiac malposition exists, it may be difficult to properly identify and name the individual cardiac chambers. Furthermore, even if the anatomic features of the chamber are identified, there may be a tendency to name it primarily for the side of the body, for instance, an atrium with anatomic features of a right atrium; receiving systemic venous blood may be described improperly as a left atrium in a patient with situs inversus. Atria have also been described according to the type of blood they receive, such as pulmonary atrium or venous atrium, but this system also has problems in individuals with associated anomalies, such as single atrium, total anomalous pulmonary venous connection, or mitral atresia, in whom it is difficult to ascribe one atrium to a particular type of venous return.

Similarly, ventricles may be described on the basis of their position in the body or according to the vascular bed, either pulmonary or systemic, into which they eject. This nomenclature also causes confusion.

Therefore, it is preferable to describe atria and ventricles on the basis of their anatomic features. These particular anatomic features often can be determined during the angiographic study of a patient.

Right Atrium

The anatomic right atrium may be located on either the right side (situs solitus) or the left side (situs inversus) of the body. It receives a superior vena cava and the inferior vena cava. Its shape is irregular and elongated. The atrial appendage is broad and pyramidal (see Fig 2–15).

Left Atrium

The anatomic left atrium may be located on either the left side (situs solitus) or the right side (situs inversus) of the body. It receives pulmonary veins (except in anomalous pulmonary venous connection). The major portion of the left atrium has very regular, nearly geometric form. In an anteroposterior projection it forms a circle, and on a lateral projection, an ellipse. The atrial appendage is long and narrow. Its shape has been compared with a finger or birdwing (see Fig. 2–15).

Right Ventricle

The anatomic right ventricle may connect to the right atrium (atrioventricular concordance) or to the left atrium (atrioventricular discordance). The right ventricle receives the tricuspid valve. The tricuspid and semilunar valve of this ventricle are not in continuity because of the interposition of the infundibulum. This muscular outflow tract, formed by crista supraventricularis and its septal and parietal bands, separates these two valves. The right ventricle has coarse trabeculations over the lower two thirds of the ventricular septum.

Left Ventricle

The anatomic left ventricle may connect to the left atrium (atrioventricular concordance) or to the right atrium (atrioventricular discordance). It receives the mitral valve, which is in fibrous continuity with the semilunar valve. The mitral valve has two distinct papillary muscles, the anterior and posterior, which are usually seen angiographically. The trabeculations of the left ventricle are regular and fine, and the septum is generally smooth.

VENTRICULAR INVERSION

In cardiac malpositions, the formation of the bulboventricular loop is important for two reasons. First, some malpositions are related to intrinsic movements of the primitive loop during the early developmental stages, and, second, some forms of malposition are associated with specific abnormalities associated with the type of ventricular loop. The embryology of the formation of the ventricular loop is briefly reviewed.

Early in the embryo, the right and left cardiac primordia fuse, forming a single tubular organ that has primitive demarcation into the atrium, ventricle, and bulbus cordis (Fig 58–2,A). Normally the primitive cardiac tube protrudes initially to the right, forming a right or D-ventricular loop. From this loop (bulboventricular loop), the two future ventricles develop. In the D-loop the right ventricle forms from the rostral segment and the left ventricle from its caudal segment. Therefore, the anatomic right ventricle in D-loop is located on the right side. In most hearts the D-ventricular loop rotates in a leftward direction so that the cardiac apex ultimately occupies a position in the left hemithorax. In D-loop the relationship of the atria and ventricles is concordant (i.e., the right ventricle connects to the right atrium and the left ventricle to the left atrium). This relationship is also termed "noninversion of the ventricles."

On the other hand, if the primitive cardiac tube initially bends toward the left, an L-ventricular loop and ventricular inversion results (Fig 58–2,B). When the cardiac loop swings to the left (L-loop), the developing anatomic right ventricle is shifted leftward also; hence, it will be located on the left side, whereas the anatomic left ventricle is located relatively on the right side. In most hearts with an L-ventricular loop, the cardiac mass does not migrate to the right, so that the heart remains positioned in the left hemithorax. With L-loop the atrioventricular relationship is discordant, the right ventricle connects with the left atrium, and the left ventricle connects with the right atrium. This condition is called "ventricular inversion," or atrioventricular discordance, because the ventricles are inverted with respect to the atria.

The concordance of the atrial and the visceral situs is explained by the fact that the visceral (vitelline) veins terminate in the sinoatrium from which the future right atrium is differentiated, and the vestibule of the left atrium is an expansion of the pulmonary veins.

TRANSPOSITION OF GREAT VESSELS

Because transposition of the great vessels commonly coexists with cardiac malposition, this term is also defined again. Transposition literally means carried across (from the Latin word transponere, meaning to place across). When applied to the great vessels, the term indicates that the great vessels are placed across the ventricular septum and originate from the opposite ventricle. Another term that describes the situation of transposition of the great vessels is ventriculoarterial discordance, indicating that the connection between ventricles and great vessels is incorrect, with the aorta arising from an anatomic right ventricle and pulmonary artery from an anatomic left ventricle. This definition is preferable to one that defines transposition as a state in which the aorta is located anteriorly to the pulmonary artery; although this anatomic relationship of the great vessels exists almost invariably in transposition, it is not always present (see Chapter 38). The circulatory pattern associated with complete transposition of the great vessels may exist with the great vessels in a side-to-side relationship or even with the aorta located posteriorly ("posterior transposition").

Fundamentally there are two types of transposition of the great vessels:

1. Complete transposition, D-transposition, or atrioventricular concordance with ventriculoarterial discordance. In this condition the right atrium, right ventricle, and aorta are in continuity, as are the left atrium, left ventricle, and pulmonary artery.

2. Corrected transposition, L-transposition, or atrioventricular discordance with ventriculoarterial discordance. The right atrium, left ventricle, and pulmonary artery are in continuity, as are the left atrium, right ventricle, and pulmonary artery.

SUMMARY

I. Three types of visceroarterial situs.
   A. Situs solitus.
   B. Situs inversus.
   C. Situs ambiguus ("indeterminate situs").
II. Two types of bulboventricular loops.
   A. L-ventricular loop (inversion of ventricles).
   B. D-Ventricular loop (noninversion of ventricles).
III. Position of great vessels.
   A. Normal.
   B. Transposed.
      1. L-Transposition of great vessels (corrected transposition).
      2. D-Transposition of great vessels (complete transposition).
IV. Position of heart.
   A. Left hemithorax.
   B. Right hemithorax.

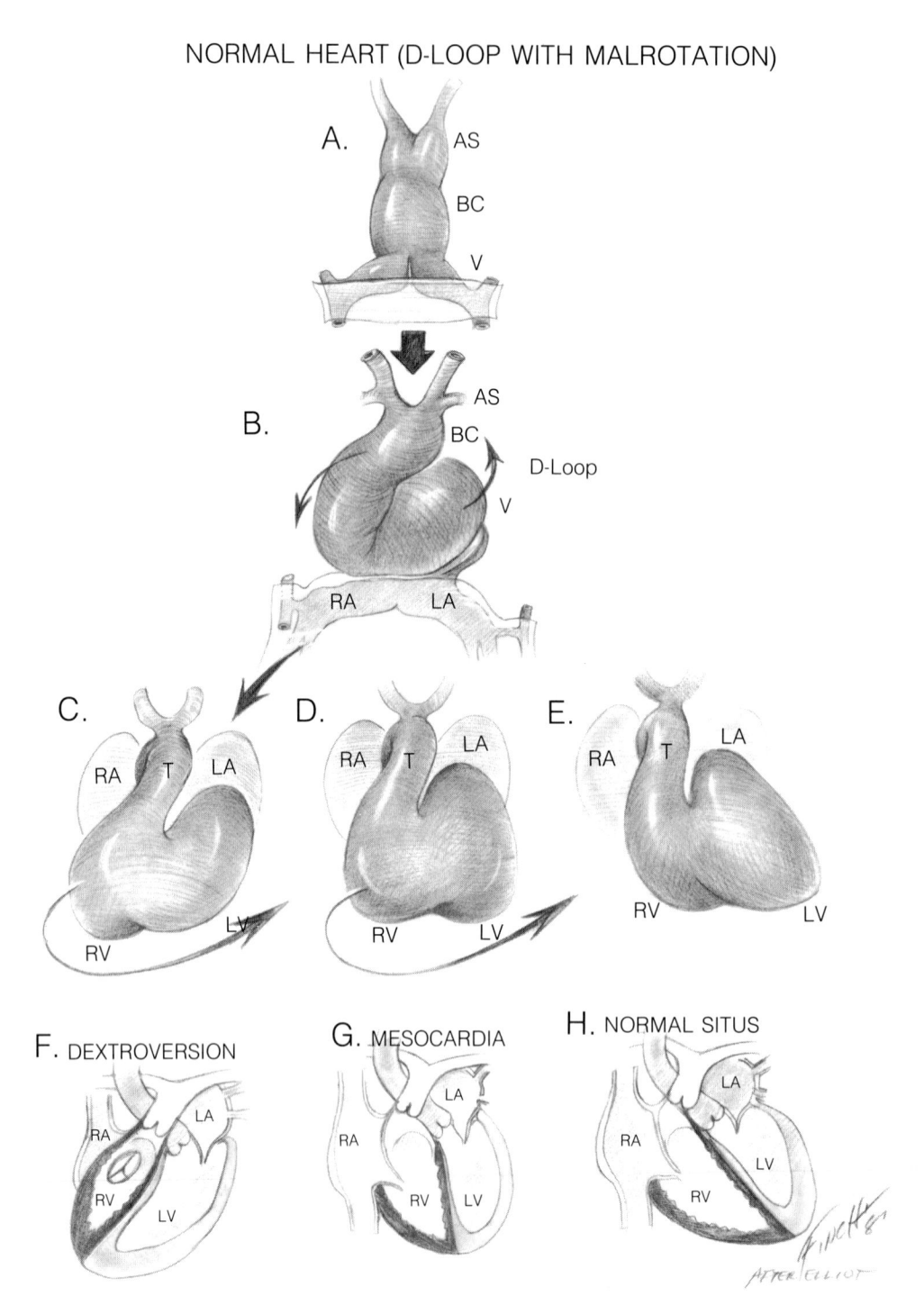

FIG 58–2.
Embryology of ventricular loops in malposition of heart. D-ventricular loop. **A,** primitive cardiac tube. **B,** cardiac tube loops toward right. **C–E,** primitive loop migrates into left hemithorax. If rotation does not occur from **C**, dextroversion of the heart results **(F)**. If partial rotation occurs, mesocardia is present **(G)**. A normally positioned heart results from complete rotation **(H)**. *(Continued.)*

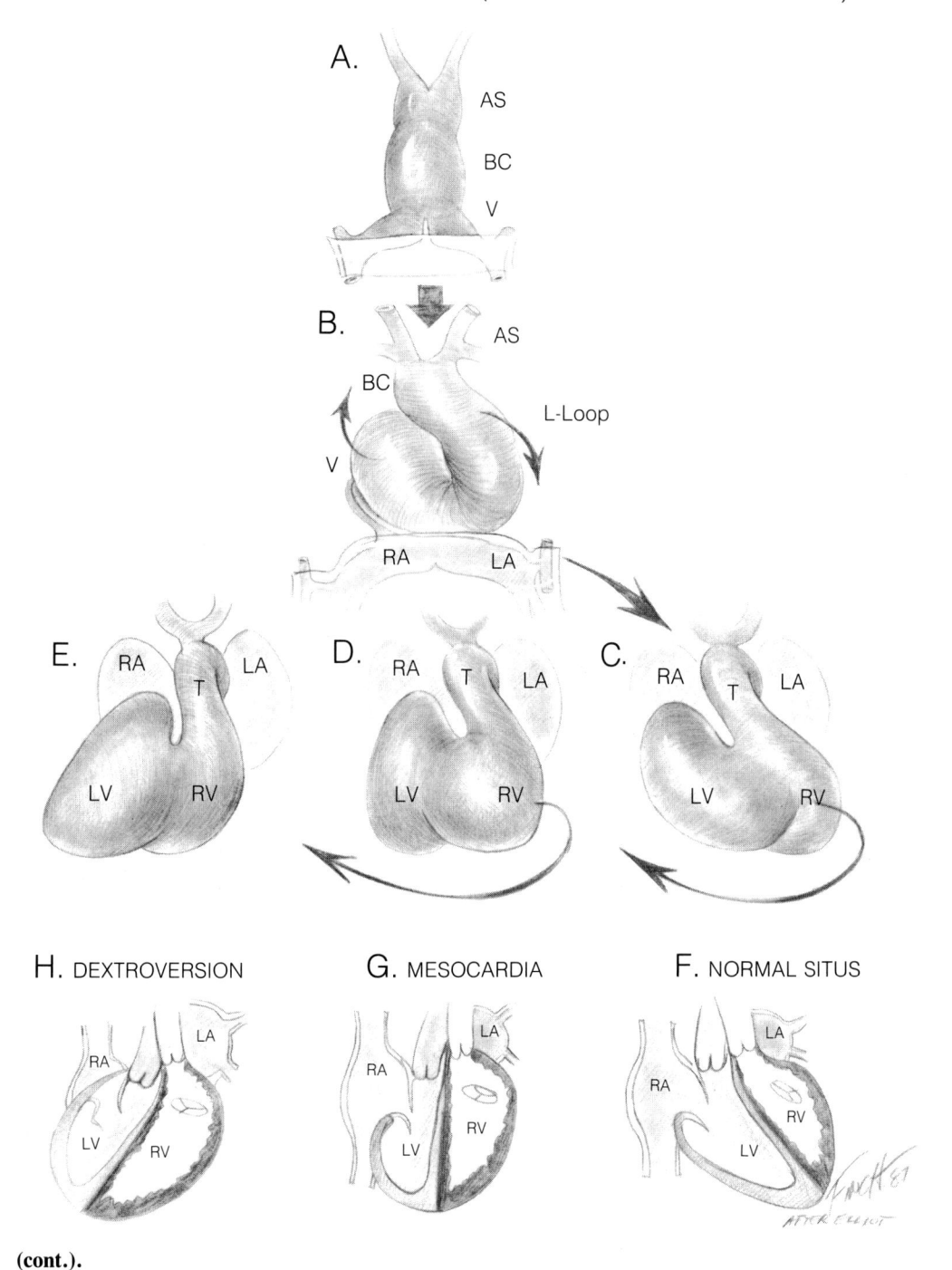

FIG 58–2 (cont.).
L-Ventricular loop. **A,** primitive cardiac tube. **B,** cardiac tube loops toward the left. The cardiac loop may migrate into right hemithorax from **C** to **E.** If rotation does not occur from **C,** corrected transposition with normal situs is present **(F).** If partial rotation occurs **(D),** mesocardia with corrected transposition results **(G).** If complete rotation occurs **(E),** dextroversion with situs solitus and corrected transposition results **(H).** AS = aortic sac; BC = bulbus cordis; V = ventricle; LA = left atrium; LV = left ventricle; RA = right atrium; RV = right ventricle; T = truncus; V = ventricularis.

Thus, a number of combinations exist among instances of cardiac malposition. Careful and systemic analysis of radiographic findings should allow the identification of the varieties of cardiac malposition and associated malformations, even if complicated.

DEXTROCARDIA

Dextrocardia occurs in five situations: two with situs solitus, one with situs inversus, and the remaining two with ambiguous situs, one being with asplenia and the other with polysplenia.

Situs Solitus

The visceroatrial situs is normal, and there is concordance. The liver, inferior vena cava, and right atrium are on the right side of the body. The cardiac mass, however, is located predominantly in the right hemithorax.

Dextroposition of the Heart

In this form of dextrocardia, the heart is displaced into the right hemithorax because of extrinsic factors, usually hypoplasia or agenesis of the right lung (Fig 58–3). Cardiac abnormalities, particularly those associated with a left-to-right shunt, frequently coexist. Pulmonary hypertension may ensue because of the reduced size of the total pulmonary vascular bed.

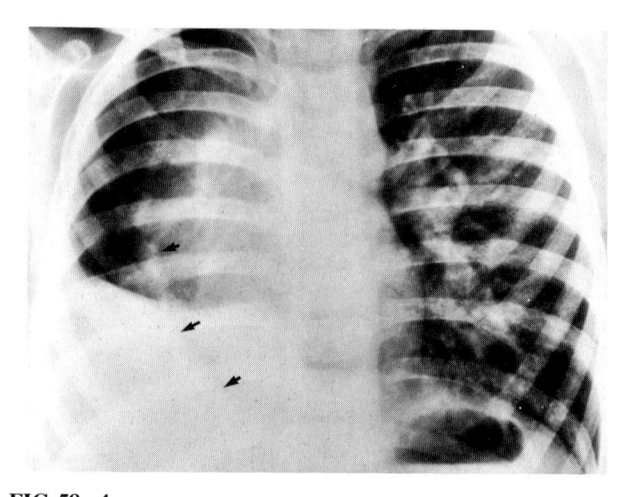

FIG 58–4.
Dextroposition of heart. Scimitar syndrome. Thoracic roentgenogram. Posteroanterior projection. Right hemithorax is smaller than left. Sparse pulmonary vasculature in right lung (hypoplasia of right pulmonary artery). Gently curved scimitar vein *(arrows)* is faintly visible. Marked elevation right hemidiaphragm.

A unique form of dextroposition of the heart is the scimitar syndrome (Chapter 22). The basic components of the syndrome (Figs 58–4 and 58–5) are as follows:

1. Hypoplastic right lung.
2. Anomalous right bronchial system, particularly in the right middle and lower lobes. Bronchi to these two

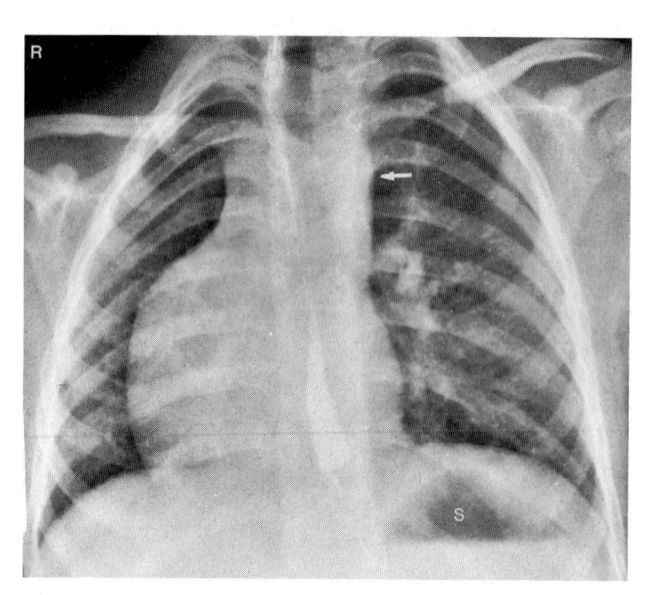

FIG 58–3.
Dextroposition of heart. Thoracic roentgenogram. Posteroanterior projection. Small right hemithorax. Hypovascularity of right lung. Aortic arch *(arrow)* and stomach *(S)* on left, indicating situs solitus. Trachea, esophagus, and heart are displaced toward right. R = right.

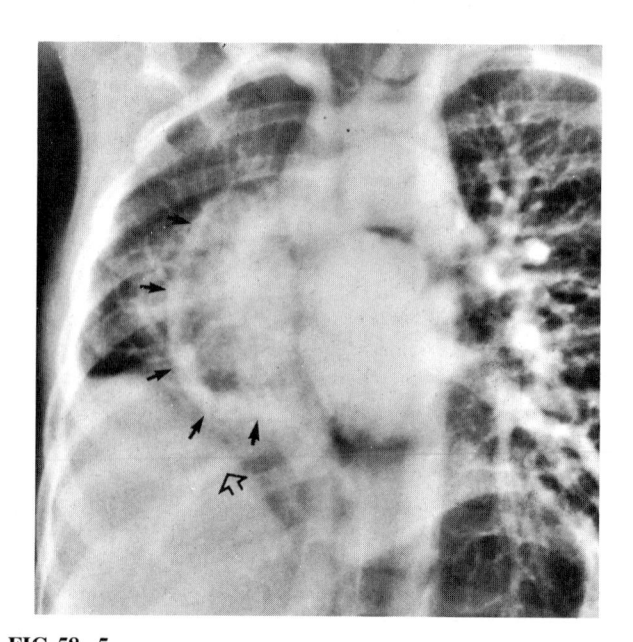

FIG 58–5.
Dextroposition of heart. Scimitar syndrome. Same patient as in Figure 58–4. Venous angiogram. Anteroposterior projection. Late phase. Scimitar vein *(arrows)* drains into junction of supradiaphragmatic portion of inferior vena cava and right atrium. Reflux into hepatic veins *(open arrow)*.

lobes may be hypoplastic or absent. The bronchi show cystic changes or diverticula.

3. Anomalous right pulmonary arterial system, in which the pulmonary arterial branches are smaller and show less arborization than in the left lung.

4. Total or partial anomalous connection of the right pulmonary veins into the suprahepatic portion of the inferior vena cava or the right atrium. The main trunk of the right pulmonary veins runs aberrantly in craniocaudal direction, and because of its larger size in the supradiaphragmatic portion, it resembles a scimitar (a curved sword from the Middle East).

5. Systemic blood supply to the hypoplastic lung from the abdominal aorta, but this is variable.

Often no intrinsic cardiac anomalies coexist, but if present, they are usually atrial septal defect, pulmonary stenosis, or tetralogy of Fallot.

Radiographic Features.—The right hemithorax is smaller than the left (see Figs 58–3 and 58–4). The intercostal spaces are narrowed, and the right hemidiaphragm is elevated. On a lateral projection, a homogeneous, low density shadow is seen along the thoracic wall and represents a fat layer around the hypoplastic lung. The heart is displaced to a variable degree into the right hemithorax.

A discrepancy in pulmonary vascularity is found between the two lungs. The pulmonary vasculature of the left lung is accentuated, reflecting the increased blood flow to the left lung because of the hypoplastic right pulmonary arterial tree. If the scimitar syndrome is present, the scimitar vein gently curves toward the medial aspect of the right hemidiaphragm. The vein becomes larger as it approaches the diaphragm (see Figs 58–4 and 58–5).

Angiographic Features.—Pulmonary arteriography shows a normal position of the right pulmonary artery but reduced caliber and number of pulmonary arterial branches in the right lung.

In scimitar syndrome, the anomalously connecting vein can be seen on the late phase of the pulmonary angiogram (see Fig 58–5). Also, abdominal arteriography may demonstrate abnormal arteries that pierce the diaphragm to reach the right lower lobe in this syndrome.

Dextroversion of the Heart

Dextroversion of the heart (actually, lack of levorotation (see Fig 58–2,C) occurs in situs solitus (Fig 58–6). In this form of dextrocardia, the cardiac apex points to the right, but the basic features are those of situs solitus. This malposition occurs once in each 29,000 individuals in the general population.

There are two basic forms of dextroversion, each of which can be related to embryologic events:

1. Dextroversion with D-ventricular loop. In the developing heart, after the primitive bulboventricular loop has formed and is oriented toward the right (see Fig 58–2,C), it fails to migrate into the left hemithorax. Therefore, the anatomic right ventricle remains along the right cardiac border and forms the cardiac apex (see Fig 58–6). There is atrioventricular and usually ventriculoarterial concordance. Often the great vessels are normally related but may show double-outlet right ventricle or ventriculoarterial discordance, resulting in a circulatory pattern of complete transposition of the great vessels.

2. Dextroversion with L-ventricular loop (see Fig 58–2,E). In the primitive heart, and L-bulboventricular loop forms, and if it rotates into the right hemithorax, the second variety of dextroversion results. There is both atrioventricular and ventriculoarterial discordance and ventricular inversion. The anatomic left ventricle forms the right cardiac border and the cardiac apex. The anatomic right ventricle is located medially. Because ventriculoarterial discordance is almost always present, the circulatory pattern is that of congenitally corrected transposition of the great vessels.

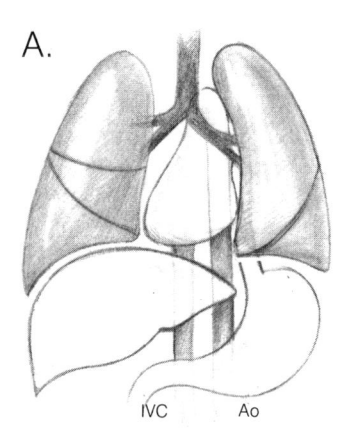

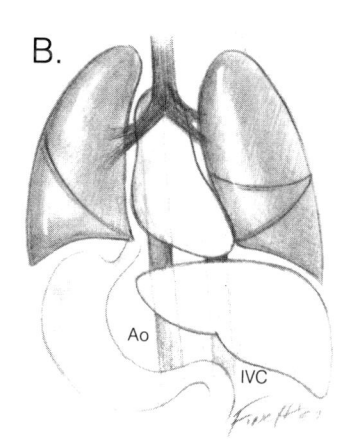

FIG 58–6.
Version of heart. **A,** dextroversion with situs solitus. Liver, inferior vena cava *(IVC),* trilobed lung, and cardiac apex on right; descending aorta *(Ao)* and stomach on left. **B,** levoversion with situs inversus. Liver, inferior vena cava, and trilobed lung on left; stomach, descending aorta, and bilobed lung on right, as in situs inversus. Cardiac apex on left indicates situs inversus with levoversion (a very rare condition).

Associated Anomalies.—With a D-ventricular loop, associated congenital cardiac malformations occur. A specific type of malposition is not prevalent, but the anomalies are often complex. There is one distinct form, described by Cantrell, in which there is a left ventricular diverticulum that passes through an anterior diaphragmatic hernia and projects as a pulsating mass in an epigastric hernia.

If an L-ventricular loop is present, corrected transposition of the great vessels occurs, and there is a very high incidence of associated ventricular defect and pulmonary stenosis. Tricuspid atresia and less commonly isolated ventricular septal defect or pulmonary valvar stenosis occur.

Radiographic Features.—Generally the radiographic diagnosis of dextroversion can be made with a high degree of certainty, but the associated type of ventricular looping cannot be identified. The cardiac configuration is identical to dextroposition, but no external cause can be identified to account for the cardiac malposition, thereby excluding dextroposition of the heart.

1. The abdomen shows features of situs solitus, with the liver located on the right and the stomach bubble on the left side of the abdomen (Fig 58–7).
2. The aortic arch usually is on the left, as is the descending aorta, as expected in situs solitus. A right aortic arch, however, may be found in dextroversion.
3. The interlobar fissures are normal, with a minor fissure appearing in the right lung. If the bronchi can be clearly visualized, the hyparterial (long) bronchus is located on the left.
4. The cardiac apex is located on the right. The degree of shift of the cardiac apex varies and ranges from mesocardia to dextroversion.
5. The pulmonary arterial segment is usually not seen (central position of the pulmonary artery).
6. In dextroversion, it is difficult to distinguish L-loop from D-loop. Dextroversion is most commonly associated with an L-loop (corrected transposition of the great vessels). Typically with L-loop the ascending aorta forms a bulge along the upper left cardiac border, whereas with D-loop the bulge is formed along the right cardiac border, but exceptions occur. Angiography is required for the diagnosis of the cardiac anatomy.

Angiographic Features.—Angiography allows distinction between the forms of dextroversion and identifies associated cardiac conditions. By observing the catheter course and angiographic features, one can observe the location of the inferior vena cava and descending aorta at the level of the diaphragm, which together with the position of

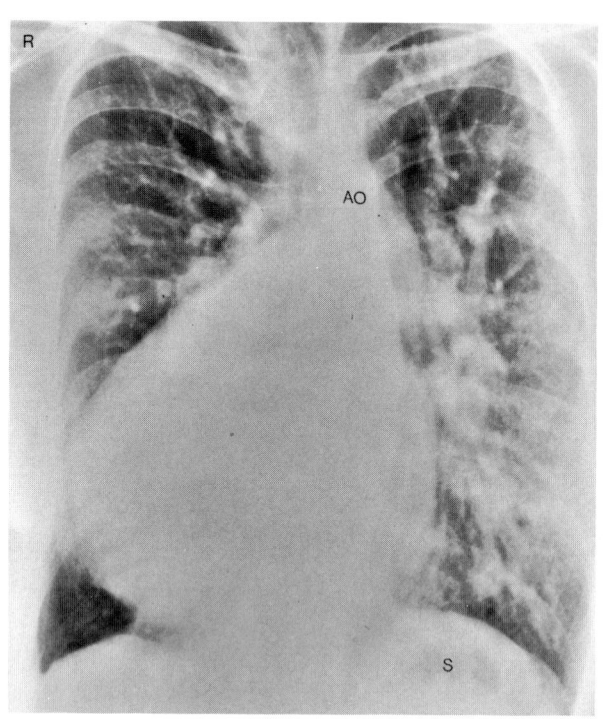

FIG 58–7.
Dextroversion with situs solitus. Thoracic roentgenogram. Posteroanterior projection. Symmetric thorax; therefore, dextroposition is excluded. Markedly increased pulmonary vasculature bilaterally. Cardiac apex is on right. Stomach *(S)* and aortic arch *(AO)* are on left. Concordant relationships. Most likely diagnosis is corrected transposition with left-to-right shunt. *R* = right.

the stomach help define the type of situs. These relationships are much more reliable for determination of situs than the position of the aortic arch, which may occur on either side regardless of situs. For the angiographic diagnosis of the cardiac malformation, the atrioventricular and ventriculoarterial connection must be determined by sequential analysis, because the relative position of the ventricles and great vessels may be distorted. The knowledge of the oxygen saturation in the injected ventricle is most helpful in the interpretation of angiograms.

1. D-Dextroversion with D-ventricular loop.
    a. Atrioventricular concordance is present.
    b. There is a side-by-side position rather than normal anteroposterior relationship between the ventricles. The right ventricle is positioned to the right, and the left ventricle is medially placed.
    c. The cardiac apex is formed by the right ventricle.
2. Dextroversion with L-ventricular loop (see Chapter 39).
    a. The right atrium connects to a morphologic left ventricle, which is smooth walled and often tail shaped.
    b. The pulmonary artery arises posteriorly and to the

right of aorta, and from the medially placed, inverted left ventricle.
c. Continuity exists between the right atrioventricular valve and the pulmonary valve.
d. The left atrium connects to a morphologic right ventricle, which is heavily trabeculated and has an infundibulum. Thus, the right atrioventricular and semilunar valves are not in continuity.
e. From the infundibulum, the aorta arises anteriorly and to left.
f. The level of aortic valve is higher than that of the pulmonary valve, as in individuals with transposition of the great vessels.
g. The aorta ascends medially along the upper left cardiac border, causing bulge in this area of the cardiac contour.
h. Associated malformations may modify the hemodynamics and the passage of contrast material.

Situs Inversus

A third type of dextrocardia occurs in situs inversus and has also been called "mirror-image dextrocardia." Concordance exists between abdominal and cardiac structures; however, the right atrium, major lobe of the liver, and inferior vena cava are located on the left side of the body, whereas the left atrium, stomach and aorta are on the right. The left lung is trilobed and right lung bilobed (see Fig 58–1,B). Situs inversus occurs in slightly more than 1 in 10,000 individuals.

The incidence of associated malformations in situs inversus is unknown. It may be as great as 50% in infants and young children with situs inversus but less than 10% in older children or adults with this type of situs. The cardiac anomalies are often complex and may cause death at an early age. There is no characteristic cardiac anomaly.

In a unique form of situs inversus, Kartagener's syndrome, situs inversus is associated with bronchiectasis and sinusitis. In most of the involved individuals, associated cardiac malformations do not coexist. This syndrome has also been called the "immotile cilia syndrome," because abnormalities present in cilia affect their function. These abnormalities account for the respiratory symptoms and probably also the situs inversus, because ciliary action plays an important role during embryogenesis.

Radiographic Features

The posteroanterior projection of thoracic roentgenograms is the mirror image of situs solitus (Fig 58–8). The lateral projection shows no difference from situs solitus.

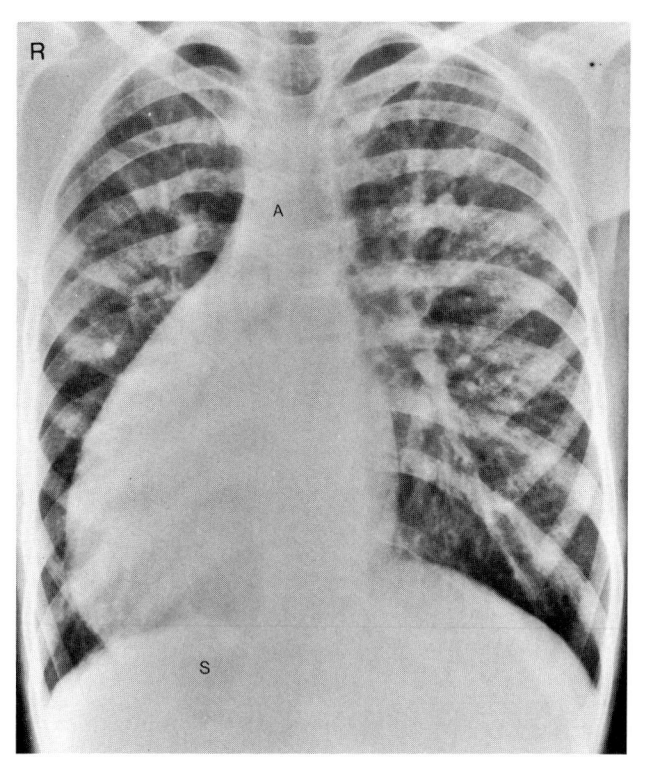

FIG 58–8.
Situs inversus. Thoracic roentgenogram. Posteroanterior projection. Stomach *(S)*, aortic arch *(A)*, and cardiac silhouette on right. Concordant relationship of stomach, aorta, and cardiac silhouette indicates situs inversus. Left hemidiaphragm is higher than right. If this radiograph were turned around, thorax and abdomen would appear normal. Therefore, "mirror-image" dextrocardia. *R* = right.

A symptom complex occurring with complete situs inversus is Kartagener's syndrome, consisting of situs inversus, chronic sinusitis, and cough secondary to bronchiectases (Fig 58–9).

Situs Ambiguus

Dextrocardia may also occur with an ambiguus situs. In the two other forms of visceroatrial situs, situs solitus and situs inversus, a concordant relationship exist between organs, indicating, for instance, that the anatomic right atrium, major hepatic lobe, and inferior vena cava lie on one side of the body and the left atrium, stomach, and descending aorta lie on the opposite side (Fig 58–10,A and B).

In situs ambiguus, visceroatrial discordance occurs, and it is frequently difficult to distinguish the anatomic right or left side of the viscera or atria (Fig 58–10,C and D).

Most instances of situs ambiguus can be classified into one of two syndromes, asplenia or polysplenia, according to major anatomic findings.

954 *Cardiac Malposition*

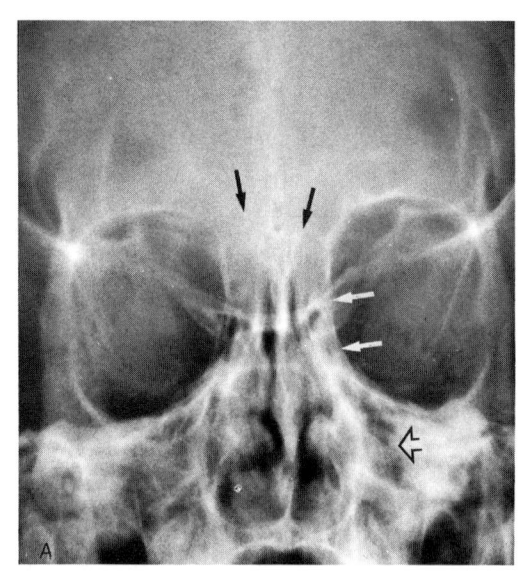

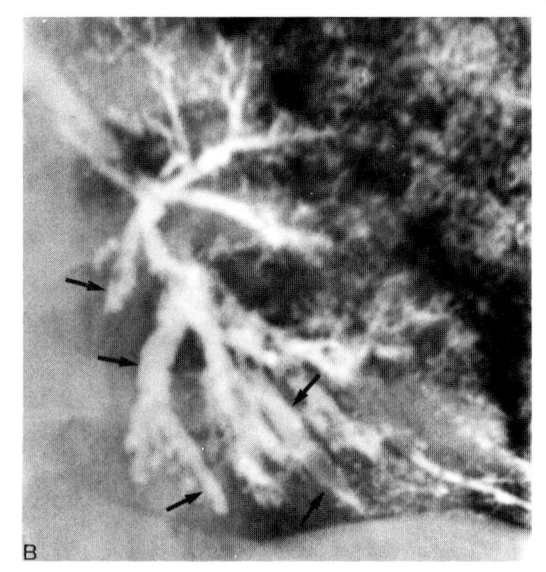

FIG 58–9.
Situs inversus. Kartagener's syndrome. **A,** sinus films. Opacification of left maxillary *(open arrow)*, left ethmoid *(white arrows)*, and frontal sinuses *(black arrows)*. **B,** bronchogram. Left lower lobe. Cylindrical bronchiectases *(arrows)*.

Because the cardiac apex may be located in either the right or left hemithorax and there may be malposition of abdominal contents, these two conditions must be considered in the differential diagnosis of dextrocardia and unusual forms of levocardia. Asplenia and polysplenia are discussed in greater detail later in this chapter.

LEVOCARDIA

The heart can also be located abnormally in the left hemithorax. There are five types of levocardia: two associated with situs solitus, one with situs inversus, and two with ambiguus situs.

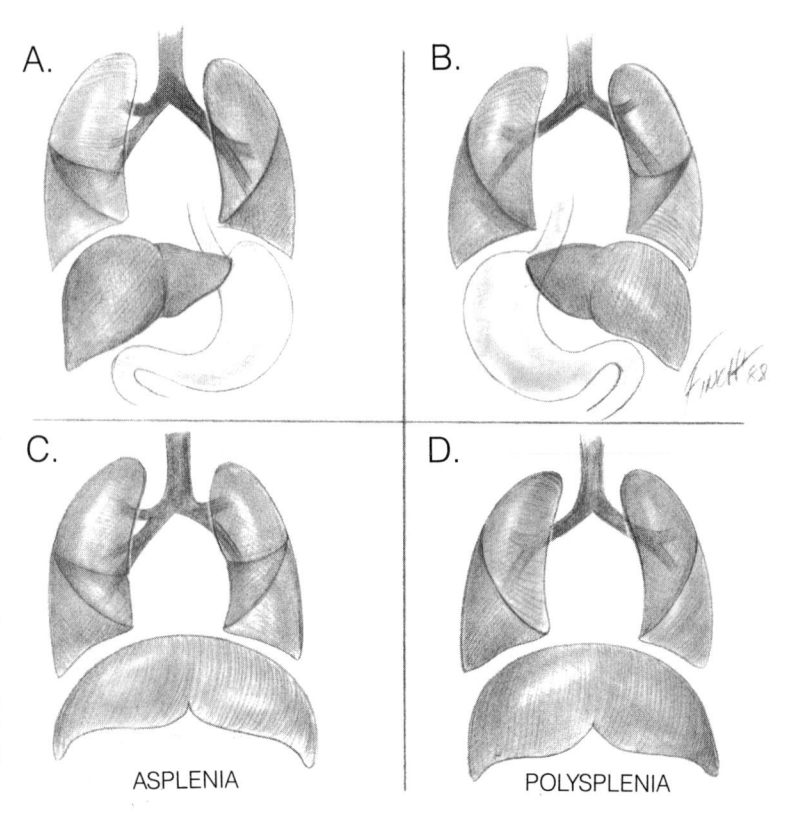

FIG 58–10.
Four basic types of situs. **A,** situs solitus. Liver and trilobed lung on right; stomach and bilobed lung on left. Long *(left)* bronchus to bilobed lung. Short bronchus on right. Either D- or L-loop may be present. **B,** situs inversus. Liver and trilobed lung on left; stomach and bilobed lung on right. Longer bronchus on right, short bronchus on left (mirror image). Either D- or L-loop may be present. **C,** situs ambiguus (indeterminate situs). Asplenia. Bilateral right-sidedness. Variable position of viscera. Midline liver, bilateral trilobed lung with short bronchi. Neither lung has long bronchus. **D,** situs ambiguus polysplenia. Bilateral left-sidedness. Bilateral bilobed lungs and long bronchi, midline liver.

Situs Solitus Heart

Almost all individuals show the visceroatrial relationship of situs solitus, D-ventricular loop, and normally related great vessels. Furthermore, most individuals with congenital cardiac malformations show this pattern of situs.

There are individuals with situs solitus with an L-ventricular loop (congenitally corrected transposition of the great vessels). These patients were discussed in the section on congenitally corrected transposition of the great vessels (see Chapter 39).

Levoposition in Situs Solitus

In this situation, situs solitus is present and the cardiac apex is located in the left hemithorax but displaced further laterally because of an extrinsic factor, particularly hypoplasia or agenesis of the left lung.

Cardiac malformations may coexist, which if associated with increased pulmonary blood flow lead to pulmonary hypertension because of the reduction in the cross-sectional area of the pulmonary vascular bed.

Hypoplasia of the left lung may occur from proximal interruption of the left sixth aortic arch (Chapter 62, "Anomalies of the Aortic Arch System"). Occasionally absence of the left pericardium is associated with displacement of the heart into the left hemithorax (Chapter 72, "Pericardial Defect").

Radiographic Features

The radiographic appearance is the opposite of Figure 58–3. The intercostal spaces of the left side of the thorax are narrowed and the left hemidiaphragm is elevated. Discrepancy exists between the pulmonary vascularity of the two lungs. The vasculature is increased in the right lung and stringy in the left lung.

Angiographic Appearance

Pulmonary arteriograms show normal distribution of the right and left pulmonary arteries, but the number and caliber of the pulmonary arteries in the left lung may be reduced.

Levoversion With Situs Inversus

In this rare anomaly, there is situs inversus, but the cardiac apex is directed to the left (Fig 58–6,B). In most individuals there is atrioventricular and ventriculo-arterial discordance, forming the pattern of corrected transposition of the great vessels. This represents the mirror-image of dextroversion of situs solitus, and has the same anatomic and angiographic features.

Situs Ambiguus

In half of patients with ambiguus situs, the heart is located in the left hemithorax. These individuals have either asplenia or polysplenia (Fig 58–10,C,D). This represents the largest group of patients with malposition associated with a left-sided heart and is discussed in more detail below.

Radiographic Approach

By careful analysis of thoracic roentgenograms, the type of cardiac malposition can be identified with a high degree of accuracy. If certain anatomic facts and steps are carefully followed, the position of the viscera and aorta and consequently the type of situs can be diagnosed without angiography. Anatomic variations exist, so these steps are not infallible, and angiography is often indicated for definitive diagnosis.

Radiographic Features of Cardiac Malpositions

In the following examples of roentgenograms, the steps leading to the identification of the situs are described:

1. External causes such as pneumothorax, atelectasis, or thoracoplasty may be responsible for an abnormally placed heart (see Fig 58–3). In addition, the size of each hemithorax and the vascularity in each lung should be compared for discrepancies that would indicate a hypoplastic lung (see Fig 58–3). External factors are the most common cause of cardiac malposition.

2. The presence of a catheter on an abdominal roentgenogram helps determine the situs with certainty. Depending on its site of insertion, the catheter identifies the course of the inferior vena cava or aorta. In situs solitus, the inferior vena cava lies on the right side and the aorta on the left of the abdomen. In situs inversus, the inferior vena cava lies on the left side and the descending aorta on the right. In ambiguous situs, the aorta and inferior vena cava may be on the same side of the abdomen or may cross one another as in asplenia, or the venous catheter may show a course of interrupted inferior vena cava as in polysplenia.

3. If gastric air bubble and aortic arch both lie on the right side (concordant), situs inversus is very likely (Fig 58–11).

4. In a patient with situs inversus who has sinusitis and bronchiectasis, Kartagener's syndrome should be considered (see Fig 58–9). In these patients, radiographic views of the nasal sinuses and bronchography are indicated to identify the associated sinusitis and bronchiectasis.

5. When the gastric air bubble and aorta are located on the left side (concordant) but the cardiac silhouette is located in the right hemithorax and there are no evident

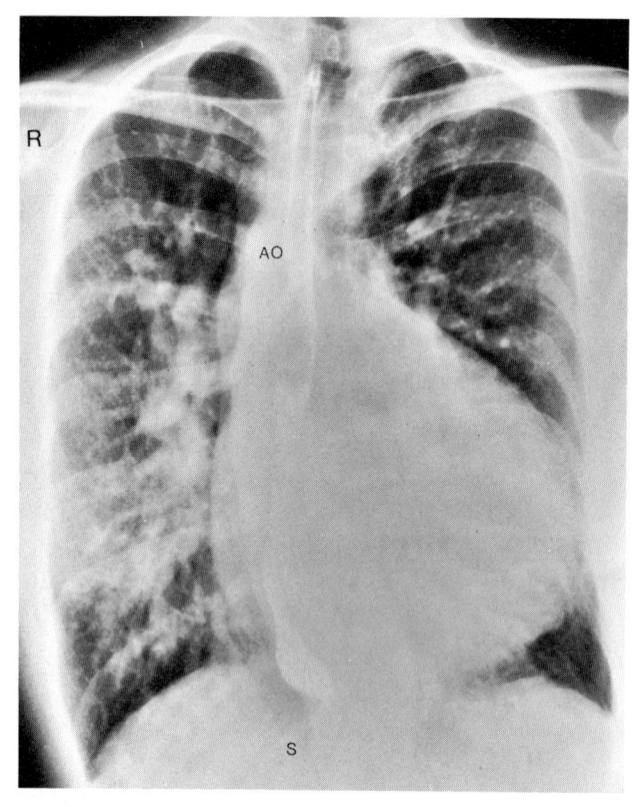

FIG 58–11.
Levoversion with situs inversus. Thoracic roentgenogram. Posteroanterior projection. Aortic arch *(AO)* and stomach *(S)* concordant on right. Cardiac apex on left. This combination is exceedingly rare. Most likely diagnosis is situs ambiguous (abdominal heterotaxia). R = right.

extrinsic factors, the most likely diagnosis is dextroversion of the heart (see Fig 58–7).

6. If the gastric air bubble and aorta are concordant and on the right and the cardiac apex is on the left, the diagnosis is situs inversus and levoversion (Fig 58–11). With this radiographic combination, however, abdominal heterotaxia (ambiguous situs) is most likely, because situs inversus with levoversion is exceedingly rare.

7. Whereas a left-sided stomach and right aortic arch most likely occur in situs solitus with right aortic arch, a right-sided gastric air bubble and left aortic arch strongly suggest abdominal heterotaxia (situs ambiguus) (Fig 58–12).

8. The pitfall of this radiographic approach using the aortic arch occurs in patients with situs solitus and right aortic arch or situs inversus and left aortic arch. REASON: The descending aorta normally lies on the left and same side as the stomach at the level of the diaphragm, but in children only the position of the aortic arch can be identified. Therefore, patients with a right aortic arch do not necessarily have situs ambiguus because of discordance of aortic arch and stomach air bubble. Situs solitus with a right aortic arch is so common that the question of cardiac malposition is usually not raised in this situation (Fig 58–13).

9. Ambiguus situs (abdominal heterotaxia) can be diagnosed with certainty if a midline liver (Fig 58–14) or an enlarged azygos vein is demonstrated (Fig 58–15).

Angiography provides a definitive diagnosis by demonstrating the relationship between the inferior vena cava

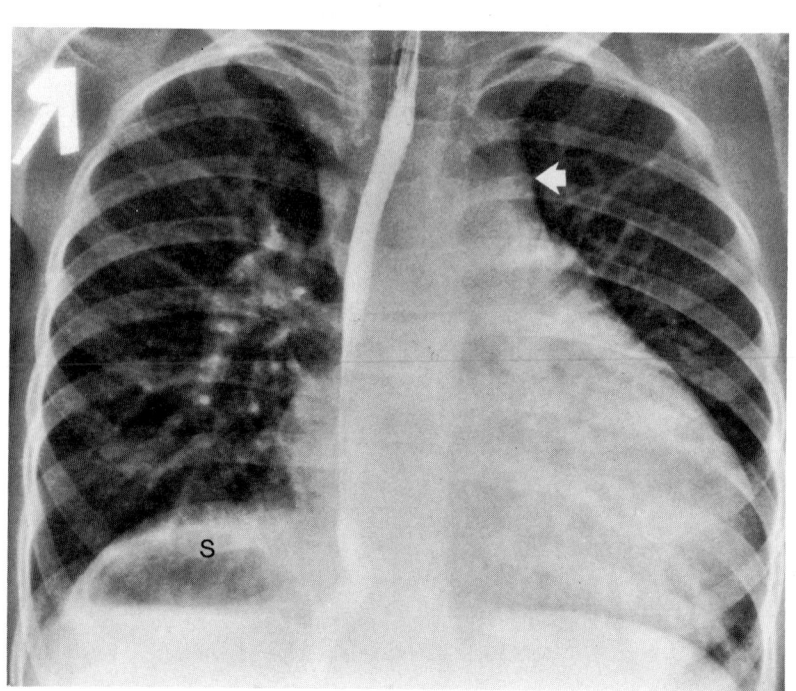

FIG 58–12.
Situs ambiguous. Thoracic roentgenogram. Posteroanterior projection. Stomach *(S)* on right; aortic arch *(arrow)* and cardiac apex on left. Theoretically this roentgenogram could represent situs inversus with levoversion and left aortic arch, a virtually unheard combination. Discordant relationship of aortic arch, apex, and stomach is diagnostic of abdominal heterotaxia (ambiguous situs). This topographic relationship has also been called "transposition of the stomach."

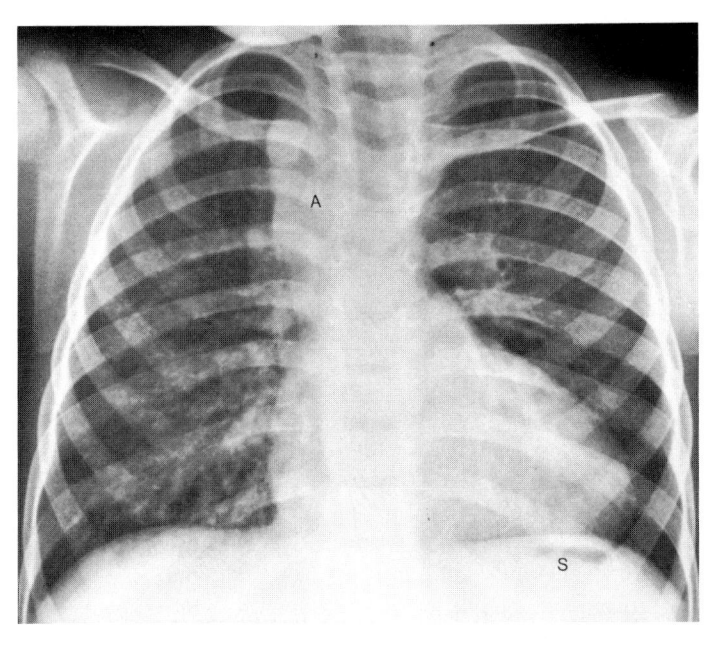

FIG 58–13.
Situs solitus. Tetralogy of Fallot and right aortic arch. Thoracic roentgenogram. Posteroanterior projection. Discordant relationship between aortic arch *(A)* and stomach *(S)*, as in situs ambiguus. However, aorta pierces diaphragm to left of inferior vena cava, which is seen only by angiography and echocardiography. Therefore, concordant relationship exists.

and descending aorta below the level of the diaphragm, which for all practical purposes determines the situs with certainty. Almost invariably the right atrium is an extension of the inferior vena cava, although very rare exceptions exist in which the inferior vena cava empties into the left atrium. Another exception of an abnormal right-left relationship of abdominal aorta and inferior vena cava is a persistent left inferior vena cava.

ASPLENIA SYNDROME

The asplenia syndrome is a serious condition with complex cardiac and visceral anomalies.[13] In this syndrome, there is symmetry of several organs: the atria, each having features of a right atrium; the lungs, each being trilobed and having an epiarterial bronchus; the liver; and absence of the spleen, normally a left-sided structure. Because of these characteristics, the asplenia syndrome has also been called "bilateral right-sidedness," "bilateral dextroisomerism," or "right atrial isomerism." The condition is highly lethal, with 80% to 90% of patients dying by 1 year of age, usually from the cardiac condition, often related to a cardiac operation. Perhaps 75% of cases occur in males. Overwhelming infection is an uncommon cause of death.

Pulmonary and Cardiac Anomalies

Almost invariably there are two right (trilobed) lungs (Fig 58–16). Both bronchi are anatomically right (short), epiarterial in position, and symmetric. At each level of the heart, cardiac anomalies may be found. The cardiac apex is located in the right hemithorax in roughly 40% and in the left hemithorax in roughly 60%.

Bilateral superior venae cavae are present in two thirds of the cases. In the remaining cases there is an equal proportion of a single superior vena cava on the left or on the right. Generally the superior vena cava joins directly the superior posterior wall of the atrium, and the second superior vena cava connects also to the atrium and not to the coronary sinus because of characteristic features of the atrial septum. The location of the inferior vena cava is

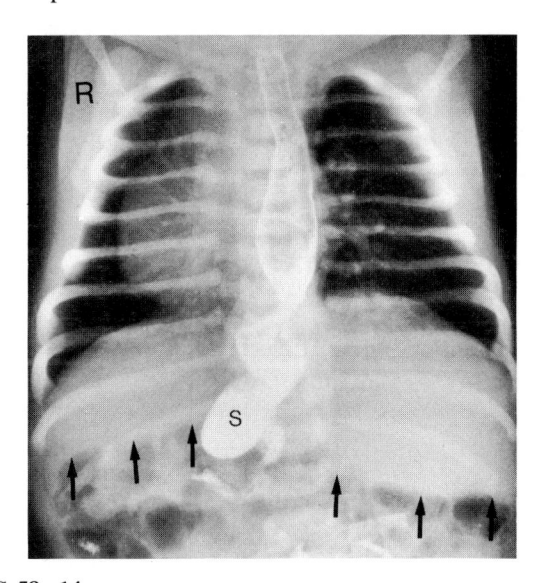

FIG 58–14.
Dextrocardia in asplenia. Thoracic roentgenogram. Posteroanterior projection. Right-sided stomach *(S)*. Right aortic arch. Concordant relationship. Cardiac apex on right. Roentgen picture is consistent with situs inversus. Transverse position of liver is virtually diagnostic for ambiguous situs. *R* = right.

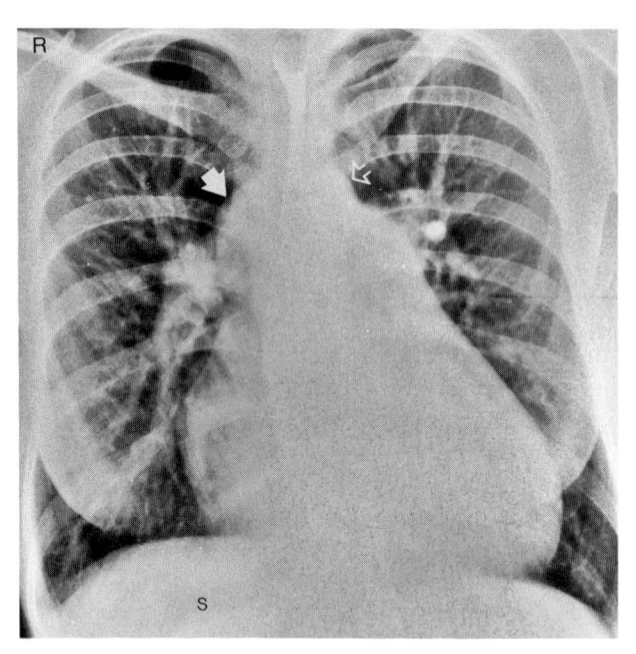

958 *Cardiac Malposition*

FIG 58–15.
Levocardia in polysplenia. Thoracic roentgenogram. Posteroanterior projection. Right-sided stomach *(S)*. Aortic arch *(open arrow)*, cardiac apex, and arch are concordant on left; therefore, discordant relationship. Density *(solid arrow)* (enlarged azygos vein) opposite aortic arch indicates interruption of inferior vena cava with azygos continuation, strongly suggesting polysplenia syndrome and abdominal heterotaxia. *R* = right.

variable; it frequently lies in the midline and crosses the aorta in the abdomen.

Anomalous pulmonary venous connection occurs in more than 80% of patients and is almost always total. The total connection may be to either a supracardiac or an infradiaphragmatic location. We have been impressed by the number of instances with connection to the portal venous system. If the assumption is made that each atrium has basic features of a right atrium, then developmentally a common pulmonary vein would not form. As a consequence, total anomalous pulmonary venous connection results.

Defects of the atrial and ventricular septae are present in almost all cases. Usually there is at least a complete endocardial cushion defect with a common atrioventricular valve (Fig 58–17). Often the atrial septum is entirely absent except for a narrow band of myocardium that passes in an anteroposterior direction across the midportion of the atrium in the plane where an atrial septum should be. There may be a single ventricle (50%), which is generally of an indeterminate morphology. The common ventricle usually does not have a rudimentary chamber for the aorta. Furthermore, the ventricular communications are unusually large, with only a remnant of ventricular septum approaching a true common ventricle. Both atria show a broad-based triangular atrial appendage, and have pectinate muscles like a right atrial appendage. The coronary

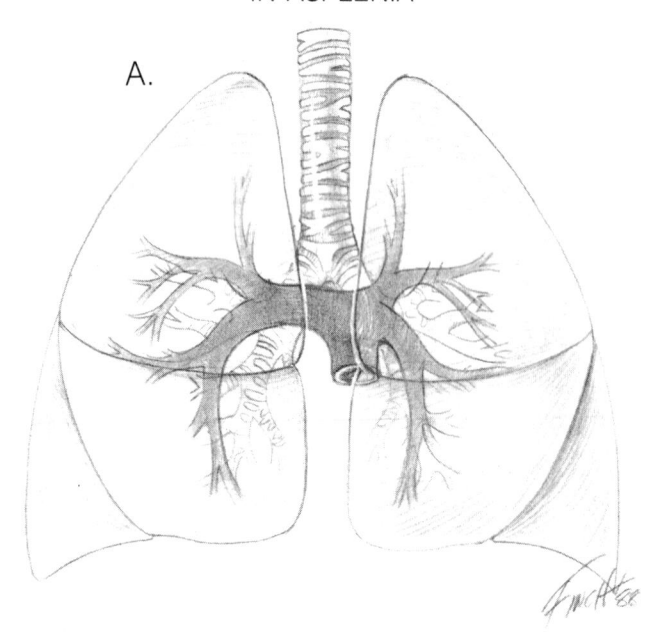

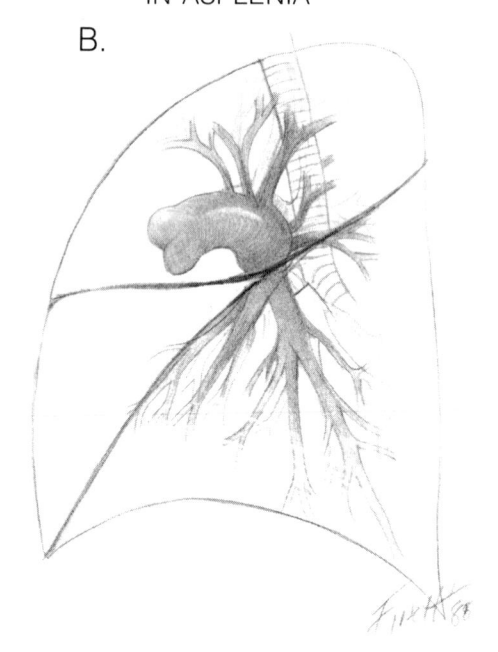

FIG 58–16.
Basic pulmonary features of asplenia syndrome. **A**, anteroposterior and **B**, lateral projections. Both lungs are trilobed. Major bronchi are symmetric and short. Pulmonary arteries are symmetric and do not cross over mainstem bronchi. Bilateral epiarterial bronchi.

THE COMMON VENTRICLES IN ASPLENIA

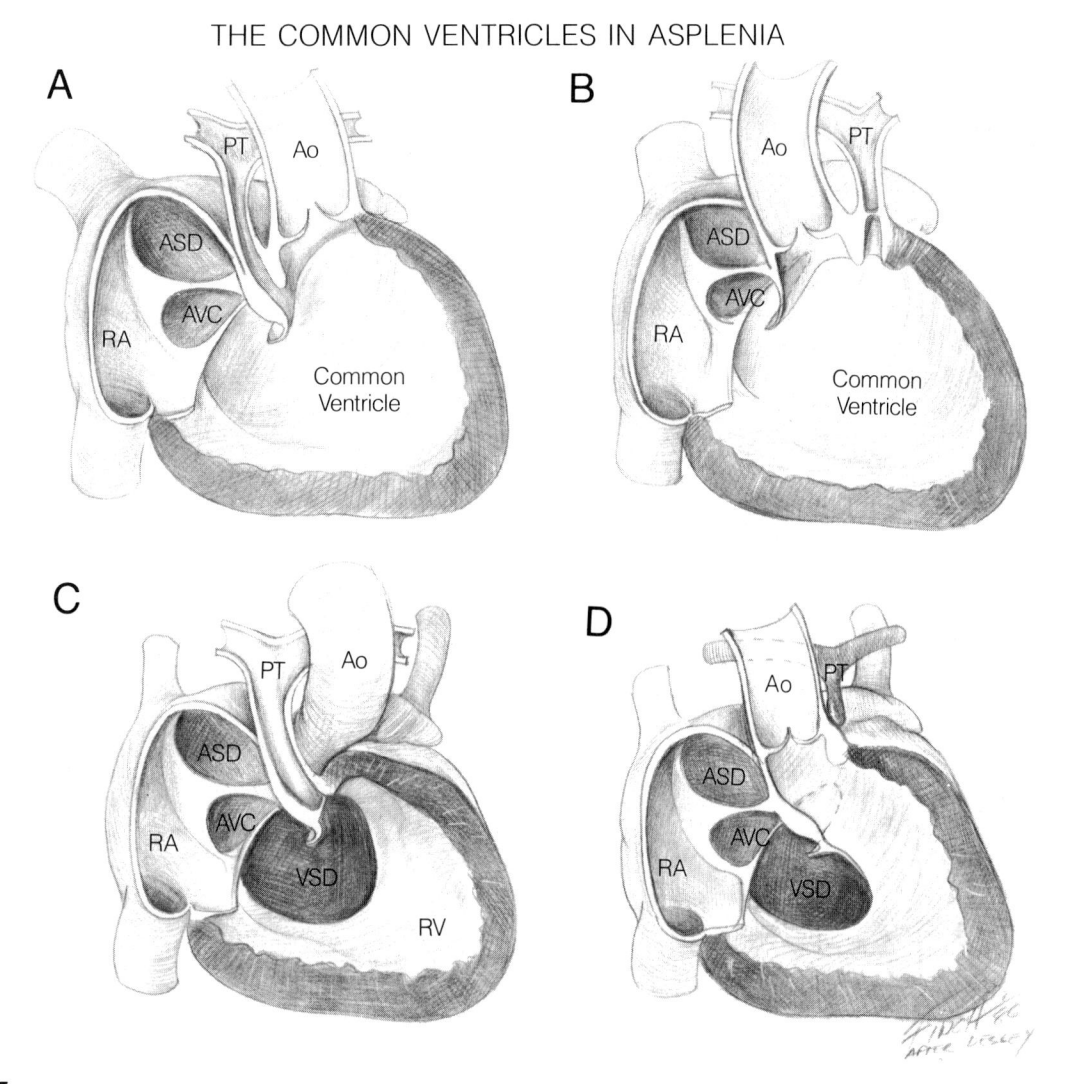

FIG 58–17.
Asplenia. Pattern of atria, ventricle, and great vessels. The atrial septum may be completely absent except for a narrow band separating a large secundum and primum defect. **A,** common ventricle, L-malposition with pulmonary stenosis. **B,** common ventricle, D-malposition with pulmonary atresia. **C** and **D,** large ventricular septal defect *(VSD)* as part of atrioventricular canal *(AVC)*. **C,** L-malposition with pulmonary stenosis and, **D,** D-malposition with pulmonary atresia. *Ao* = aorta; *ASD* = atrial septal defect; *PT* = pulmonary trunk; *RA* = right atrium; *RV* = right ventricle.

sinus, a structure formed from the left sinus horn, is usually absent.

In two thirds of the cases the aorta lies anterior to the pulmonary artery, as in transposition of the great vessels. Pulmonary stenosis or atresia is present in three fourths of the patients, with atresia occurring more frequently than stenosis.

Visceral Anomalies

The spleen is absent. One patient with this syndrome was reported with an accessory spleen. The lungs each are trilobed and show an epiarterial bronchus. At times this relationship is difficult to demonstrate, because with pulmonary atresia, the main pulmonary artery is commonly absent. In this case the pulmonary arterial systems are small and supplied by systemic arterial vessels. Because of the size and the unusual course of the systemic arteries, the relationship to the bronchus may be difficult to establish.

The liver tends to be symmetric (50%) and occupies the entire upper abdomen. The gallbladder is located more commonly on the right side even when the liver is symmetric. The exact incidence of malrotation of the bowel is difficult to determine from autopsy series because detailed study of the gastrointestinal system often has not been performed. In our radiographic study, malrotation, either nonrotation or reversed rotation of the midgut loop, was found in each case.

Abnormalities of the genitourinary tract, seen as horseshoe kidney, double collecting system, and hydroureter, were found in 15%. Fused adrenal glands have also been described.

Diagnosis

The diagnosis of cardiac anomaly associated with asplenia is usually suspected in a cyanotic neonate or infant, whose thoracic radiograph shows reduced vascularity and features suggesting an abnormal situs. These radiographic features include the presence of a bilateral middle lobe fissure, a horizontal lower margin of the liver, as outlined by colonic gas, or, most important, a cardiac malposition with ambiguous situs.

A blood smear can be evaluated for Howell-Jolly bodies or for pitting of erythrocytes. Although these abnormalities may be found during the first 10 days of life in normal neonates, their presence beyond that time indicates reduced splenic function.

Radioactive nuclear scan fails to demonstrate a spleen.

Electrocardiograms reflect the underlying type of cardiac anomaly. In asplenia there is a tendency of the P wave to be directed rightward (+90 to +120 degrees) in patients with levocardia and in dextrocardia slightly to the left (+75 to +90 degrees).

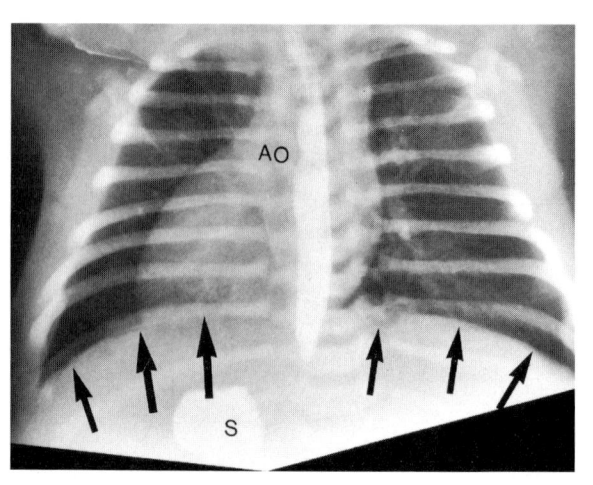

Specific Radiographic Features of Splenic Syndrome

The radiographic diagnosis of a splenic abnormality in a patient with a congenital cardiac malformation can be made with a high degree of accuracy. REASON: Splenic abnormalities such as asplenia, polysplenia, and rudimentary spleen have a high incidence of congenital cardiac malformation associated with abdominal heterotaxia (synonyms: transposition of the stomach, indeterminate situs, and situs ambiguus). Once a diagnosis of indeterminate situs is made in a patient with congenital heart disease, the diagnosis of "splenic cardiac syndrome" is almost certain.

Differentiation Between Asplenia Syndrome and Polysplenia Syndrome

Differentiation between asplenia and polysplenia is possible by taking into consideration the following facts:

1. Age. Cardiac abnormalities in asplenia are severe, and most patients die in early childhood. Asplenia occurring beyond the age of 2 years is rare. The patients come to examination in infancy.

2. Pulmonary vasculature: Asplenia is commonly associated with cardiac conditions in which pulmonary stenosis or pulmonary atresia is a component, and therefore the pulmonary vasculature is decreased. In contrast, the cardiac anomalies in polysplenia generally have increased pulmonary blood flow.

3. Visualization of bronchi. Asplenia has short bilateral epiarterial bronchi (bilateral right-sidedness), whereas polysplenia is characterized by bilateral left-sidedness and hyparterial bronchi.

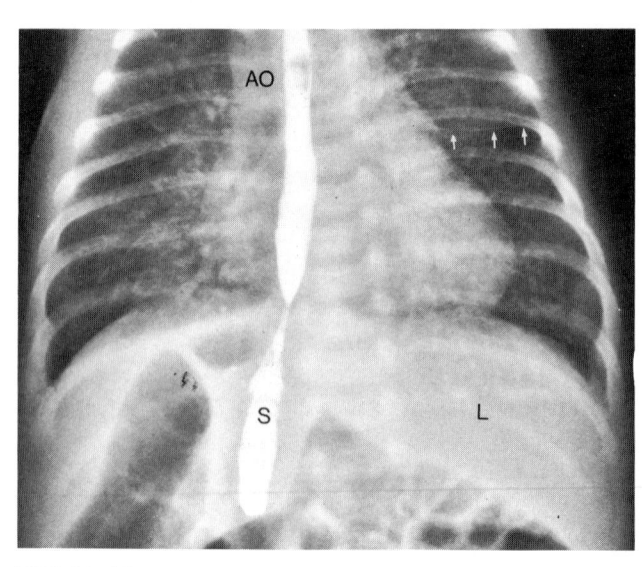

FIG 58–18.
Asplenia syndrome. Thoracic roentgenogram. Posteroanterior projection. Stomach (S), aorta (AO), and cardiac apex on right, as in situs inversus. Both hemidiaphragms (arrows) are at same level, suggesting midline liver with abdominal heterotaxia. Decreased pulmonary vasculatures.

FIG 58–19.
Asplenia syndrome. Thoracic roentgenogram. Posteroanterior projection. Liver (L) on left; stomach (S) and aortic arch (AO) on right. Stomach is in vertical position, is tubular, and lacks a well-developed fundus. Middle lobe fissure (arrows) in left lung. This combination could represent situs inversus with levoversion of heart (extremely rare); therefore, diagnosis of abdominal heterotaxia is statistically much more likely. Increased pulmonary vasculature is more consistent with polysplenia syndrome than asplenia syndrome. Middle lobe fissure indicates an anatomically trilobed lung; therefore, asplenia syndrome.

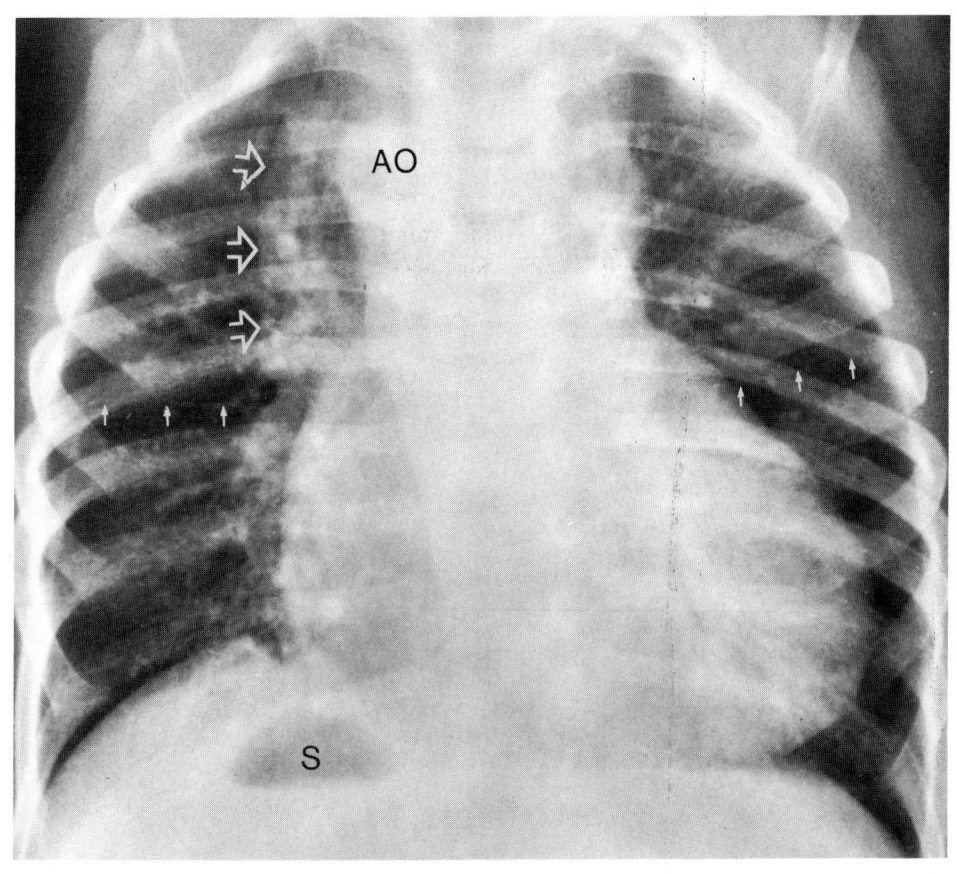

FIG 58-20.
Asplenia syndrome. Thoracic roentgenogram. Posteroanterior projection. Stomach *(S)* and aortic arch *(AO)* are concordant and on right side. Cardiac apex is discordant on left side. Increased pulmonary vasculature (atypical for asplenia). Marked enlargement of right superior vena cava *(open arrows)* suggests total anomalous pulmonary venous connection. Bilateral middle lobe fissures *(small white arrows)* establish diagnosis of asplenia syndrome.

The diagnosis of abdominal heterotaxia requires a careful observation of the aortic-gastric-cardiac apex position, as well as other radiographic features of the abdomen.

1. Abdominal heterotaxia can be diagnosed radiographically when there is a midline ("horizontal") position of the liver (see Figs 58-10,C and 58-14). With the midline position of the liver, both hemidiaphragms tend to be at the same level (Fig 58-18). Normally the liver elevates one hemidiaphragm, with the right hemidiaphragm being higher in situs solitus and the left hemidiaphragm in situs inversus. The position of the diaphragm, however, is not a reliable radiographic sign. Furthermore, the liver is not always midline among patients with asplenia (Fig 58-19).

2. Congenital absence of the spleen is associated with other visceral anomalies. The stomach is commonly malpositioned and located ipsilateral or contralateral to the liver or is in a midline position (see Fig 58-19). The stomach may be tubular and without the normal differentiation into a distinct fundus, body, and antrum. Microgastria may be part of the asplenic syndrome.

3. The diagnosis of asplenia becomes almost certain if bilateral right-sidedness can be diagnosed by visualization of a middle lobe in each lung (Fig 58-20). The demonstration of bilateral horizontal fissures in the lungs allows differentiation between asplenia and polysplenia in spite of increased pulmonary vasculature (see Fig 58-20). REASON: Asplenia is almost invariably associated with pulmonary stenosis, pulmonary atresia, or both, resulting in decreased pulmonary blood flow. Exceptions exist (see Fig 58-20).

4. Whenever the cardiac malposition suggests situs inversus and levoversion of the heart, the diagnosis of abdominal heterotaxia is almost certain (see Fig 58-20). REASON: Situs inversus with levoversion is an exceedingly rare combination.

5. In a patient with abdominal heterotaxia and enlargement of one right superior vena cava (see Fig 58-20) or both superior venae cavae, asplenia is the most likely diagnosis. REASON: Eighty percent of the patients with asplenia have total anomalous pulmonary venous connection.

6. If the inferior vena cava is outlined by a venous

FIG 58–21.
Asplenia syndrome. Common atrium, common ventricle, and total anomalous pulmonary venous connection. Thoracic roentgenogram. Posteroanterior projection. Aortic arch *(AO)* and cardiac apex are concordant and on left side. Gastric bubble *(S)* is on right side and liver *(L)* on left, indicating abdominal heterotaxia. Venous catheter *(arrows)* crosses from left side to right. Markedly increased pulmonary arterial vasculature. In spite of increased vasculature, patient proved to have asplenic syndrome.

catheter that crosses the midline of the abdomen, heterotaxia becomes almost certain (Fig 58–21).

7. In patients with asplenia and total anomalous pulmonary venous connection below the diaphragm, the vascular pattern is one of pulmonary venous obstruction (Fig 58–22). Although 80% of the patients with asplenia have total anomalous pulmonary venous connection, in only 20% does it occur below the diaphragm.

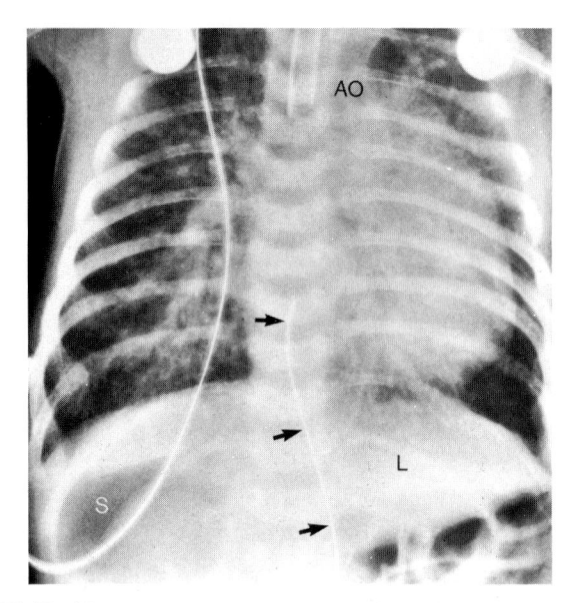

8. Identification of the location and form of the liver may be aided during angiography if contrast material refluxes into the hepatic veins. This may, for instance, show symmetric hepatic veins (Fig 58–23), indicating hepatic symmetry.

9. With asplenia syndrome, malrotation of the bowel occurs because of nonrotation of the midgut loop, reversed rotation of the midgut loop, or mobile cecum. In reversed rotation of the midgut loop, the bowel rotates 90 degrees counterclockwise about the superior mesenteric artery compared with 270-degree clockwise rotation in the normal patient. The identification of intestinal abnormalities by barium swallow has aided in the diagnosis of abdominal heterotaxia (Fig 58–24). The associated malrotation of the colon can be diagnosed by barium enema (Fig 58–25).

10. In addition to hematologic studies, radioactive sulfur can be used to prove absence of the spleen.

11. Abdominal heterotaxia can be diagnosed by catheter position. Whereas in situs solitus the descending aorta

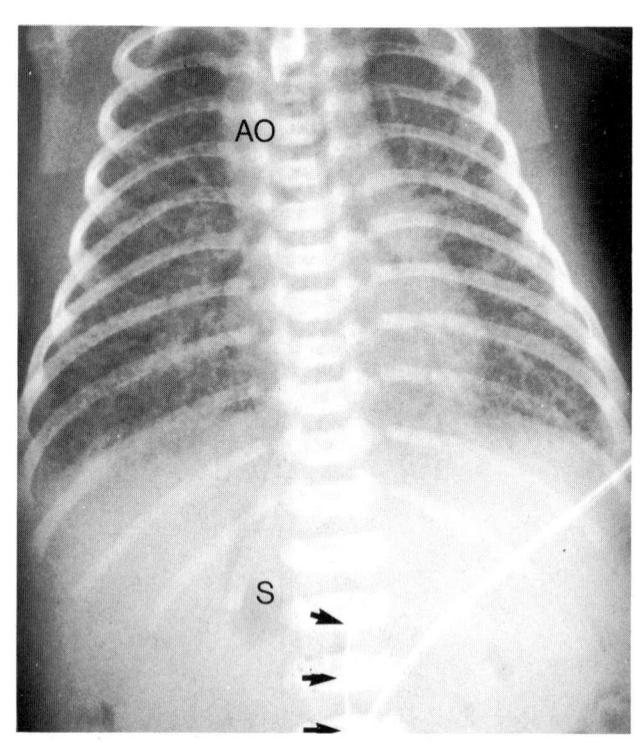

FIG 58–22.
Asplenia syndrome. Total anomalous pulmonary venous connection below diaphragm. Thoracic roentgenogram. Posteroanterior projection. Aortic arch *(AO)* and stomach *(S)* are concordant and on right. Cardiac apex is on left. Most likely diagnosis is abdominal heterotaxia. Hepatic position is not well seen, but equal levels of hemidiaphragm suggest midline liver. Catheter in inferior vena cava in midline position *(arrows)* is consistent with asplenia. Pulmonary vasculature is typical for pulmonary venous obstruction. Because 80% of cases of asplenia syndrome have total anomalous pulmonary venous connection, most likely diagnosis is asplenia syndrome with pulmonary venous obstruction.

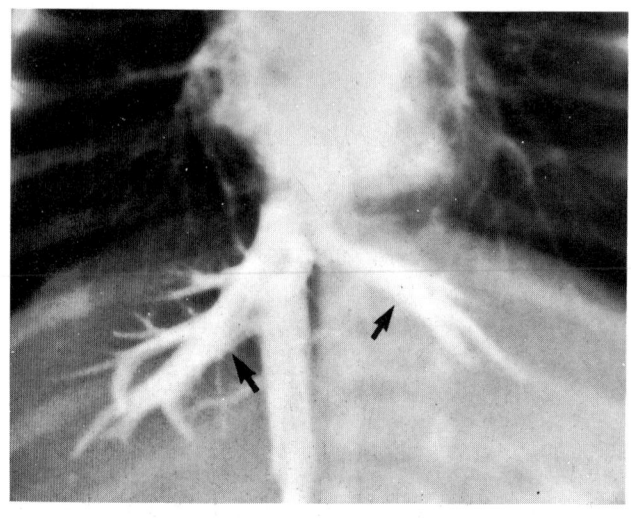

FIG 58–23.
Asplenia syndrome. Venous angiogram. Anteroposterior projection. Reflux of contrast medium from common atrium into hepatic veins. Symmetric distribution of hepatic veins *(arrows)* indicates midline liver, characteristic for ambiguous situs.

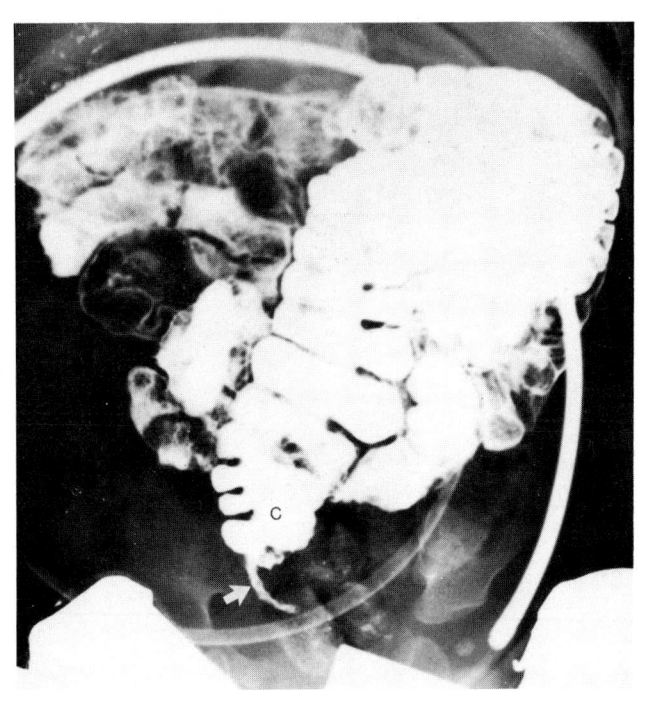

FIG 58–24.
Asplenia syndrome. Barium swallow. Anteroposterior projection. Malrotation of bowel. Upper small bowel is located on right side of abdomen. Large bowel is on left side of abdomen. Cecum *(C)* occupies low and abnormal position in pelvis. Appendix is well outlined *(arrow)*. Malrotation of bowel is common in both asplenia and polysplenia syndromes, but most patients with malrotation of bowel do not have one of these syndromes.

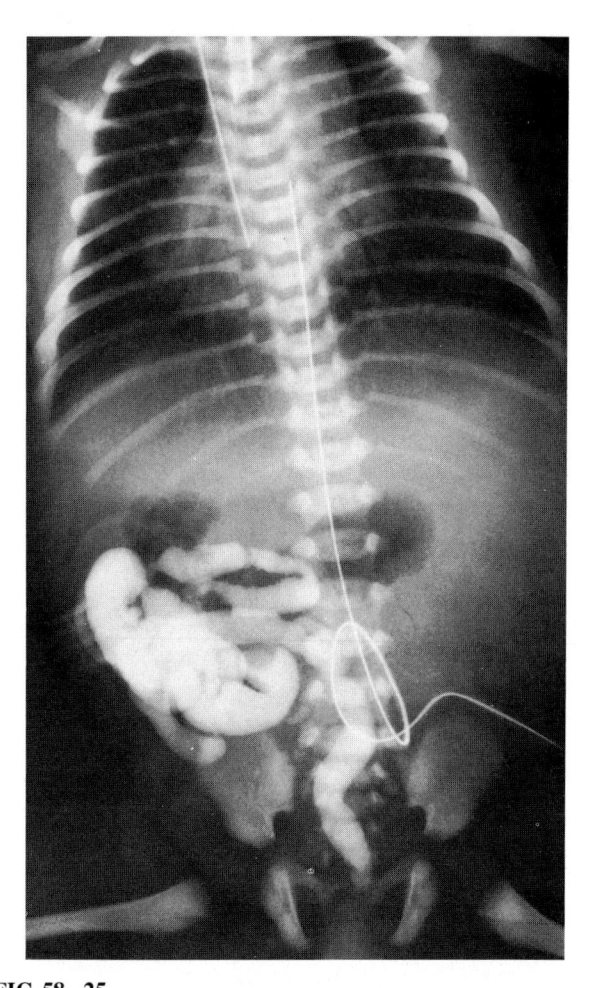

FIG 58–25.
Asplenia syndrome. Roentgenogram of thorax and abdomen. Anteroposterior projection. Cardiac apex is on right. Descending aorta (outlined by catheter) is midline. Entire colon occupies abnormal position in left upper quadrant. Density in upper midabdomen represents midline liver. Findings are characteristic for ambiguous situs.

is on the left and the inferior vena cava on the right in the abdomen (reversed in situs inversus), these two major vessels cross or are ipsilateral with asplenia (Fig 58–26). The phenomenon is best demonstrated by angiography. Crossing of the venous and arterial catheters is not always present. REASON: Patient may have a right inferior vena cava or interruption of the inferior vena cava with azygos or hemiazygos continuation.

Angiographic Features

Although the cardiac malformations in asplenia are invariably complex, not suitable for a corrective operation, palliative procedures may significantly prolong life. Angiography plays an important role in the preoperative assessment. The complex intracardiac anatomy, particularly of the pulmonary arteries, the pulmonary veins, the superior and inferior venae cavae, and the hepatic veins, must be demonstrated.

1. Angiography from the upper extremities or selective injection into the venae cavae should be performed. REASON: Approximately two thirds of patients have bilateral superior venae cavae without a connection between the two innominate veins (Fig 58–27).

2. The persistent left superior vena cava tends to empty directly into the atrium because the coronary sinus is absent in approximately 50% of the cases. REASON: Both atria are anatomically right atria.

3. The superior venae cavae receive the azygos and hemiazygos veins, respectively, in symmetric fashion (Fig 58–28).

4. Selective injection of contrast medium into the atrium is advisable because abnormalities of the atria are frequent. Almost two thirds of the cases show a common atrium. In the patients with asplenia without a common atrium, there is almost always a large or several atrial communications (Fig 58–29). The entrance of the pulmonary veins, inferior vena cava, and hepatic veins have to be demonstrated before correction if operative closure of the atrial communication is planned. REASON: The site of connection of inferior vena cava, pulmonary veins, and hepatic veins varies.

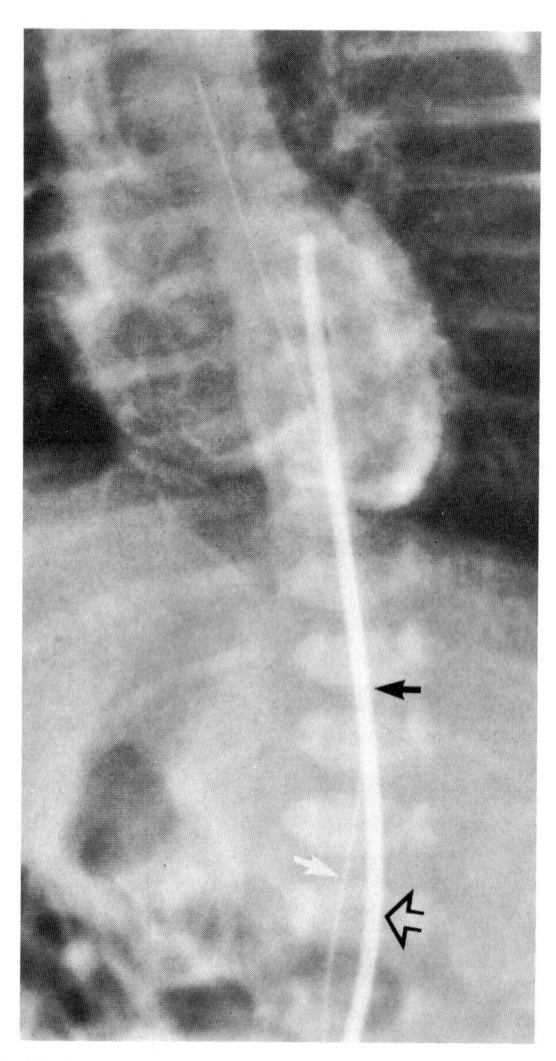

FIG 58–26.
Asplenia syndrome. Roentgenogram of thorax and abdomen. Anteroposterior projection. Venous catheter *(open arrow)* and umbilical arterial catheter *(white arrow)*. Aorta and inferior vena cava are superimposed *(black arrow)*. Normally, abdominal aorta and inferior vena cava are parallel. In asplenia syndrome, they cross and commonly occupy an ipsilateral position.

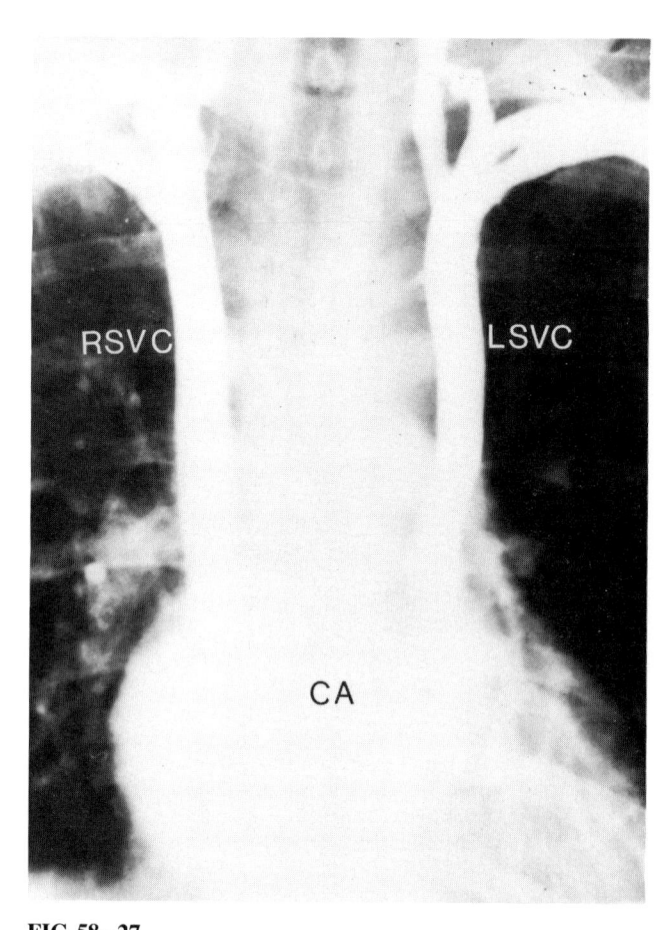

FIG 58–27.
Asplenia syndrome. Simultaneous injection of both antecubital veins. Anteroposterior projection. Bilateral symmetric superior vena cavae. No connection between right and left superior venae cavae. Persistent left superior vena cava *(LSVC)* empties directly into common atrium *(CA)* and not into coronary sinus. RSVC = right superior vena cava. Sometimes a connecting vein may be present (see Fig 58–36).

5. Common atrium (Fig 58–30) may be associated with a common atrioventricular valve (Fig 58–31).

6. Ventricular abnormalities are uniformly present. One half of the patients have a large ventricular septal defect of the atrioventricular canal type (see Fig 58–31). About one third of the patients have a common ventricle but without a rudimentary chamber (Fig 58–32), in contrast to most instances of single ventricle in which a rudimentary chamber is found. Rarely, the common ventricle of asplenia has a rudimentary chamber (Fig 58–33); although common ventricle with transposition is the rule, normally related great vessels or double outlet, both with and without pulmonary stenosis, may occur (rare).

7. In patients with pulmonary atresia, the pulmonary arteries usually fill through a patent ductus arteriosus (see Figs 58–32 and 58–33). In most patients the pulmonary arteries are symmetric; each shows the pattern of a right pulmonary artery (Fig 58–34), and epiarterial bronchi are found bilaterally.

8. Although most patients with asplenia have bilateral epiarterial bronchi, exceptions exist, with both showing hyparterial bronchi or a normal pattern (Fig 58–35).

9. Angiographic demonstration of the pulmonary veins is important, because total anomalous pulmonary venous connection occurs in 80% of patients with asplenia. Supradiaphragmatic connection to either the right atrium or the superior vena cava (Fig 58–36) is most common, but infradiaphragmatic connections also occur (Fig 58–37).

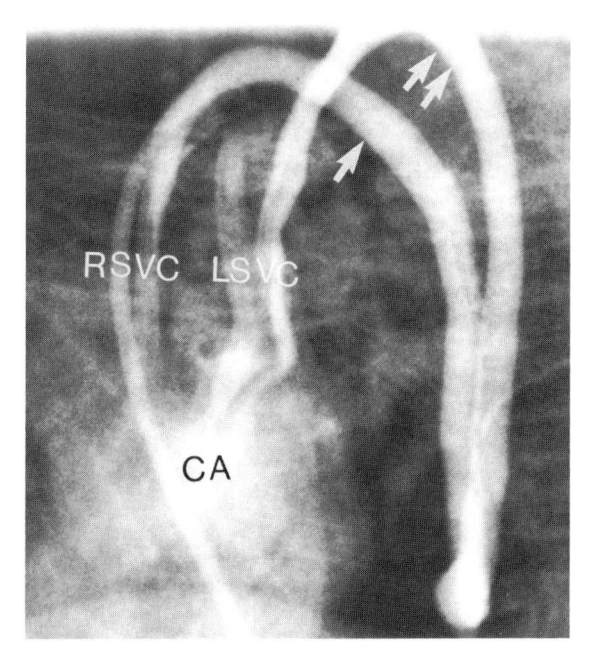

FIG 58–28.
Asplenia syndrome. Right superior vena cavogram *(RSVC)*. Lateral projection. Reflux into azygos vein *(single arrow)* with filling of hemiazygos *(double arrows)*, which connects to left superior vena cava *(LSVC)*. Both superior venae cavae empty into common atrium *(CA)*. Double candy-cane appearance.

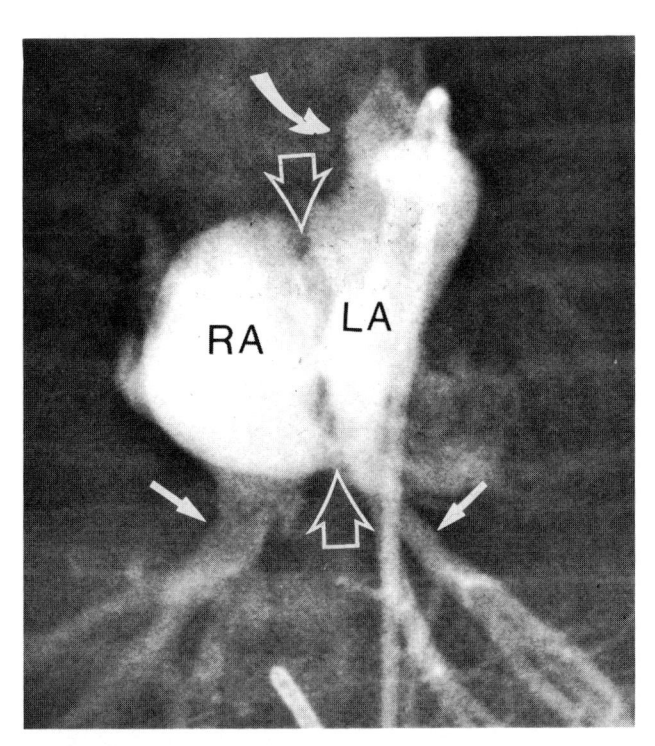

FIG 58–30.
Asplenia syndrome. Right superior vena cavogram *(RSVC)*. Anteroposterior projection. Common atrium *(CA)*. Reflux into left superior vena cava *(LSVC)* entering left side of common atrium. Inferior vena cava *(arrows)* with hepatic veins occupies midline position.

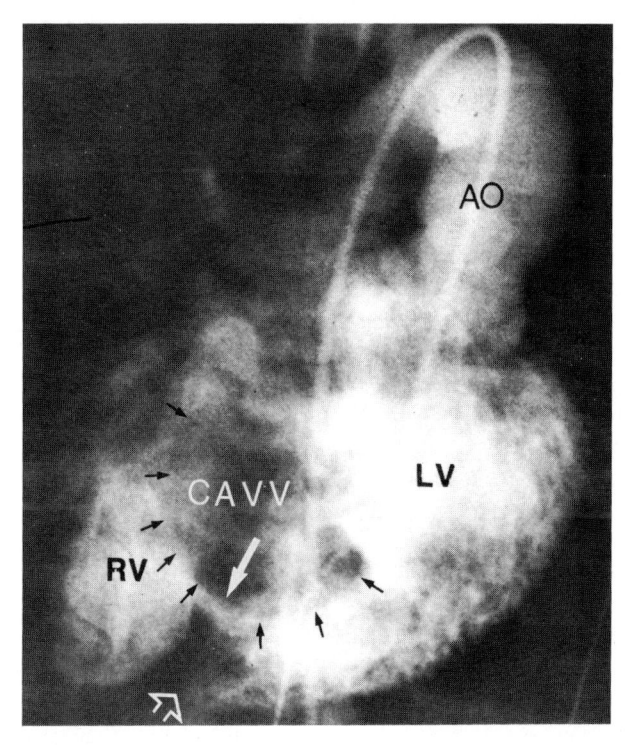

FIG 58–29.
Asplenia syndrome. Left atriogram. Anteroposterior projection. Left-sided inferior vena cava (outlined by catheter) empties into left atrium *(LA)*. Remnant of atrial septum *(open arrows)* divides atria. Right atrium *(RA)* and left atrium receive hepatic veins *(solid arrows)*. Reflux into left superior vena cava *(curved arrow)* entering left atrium.

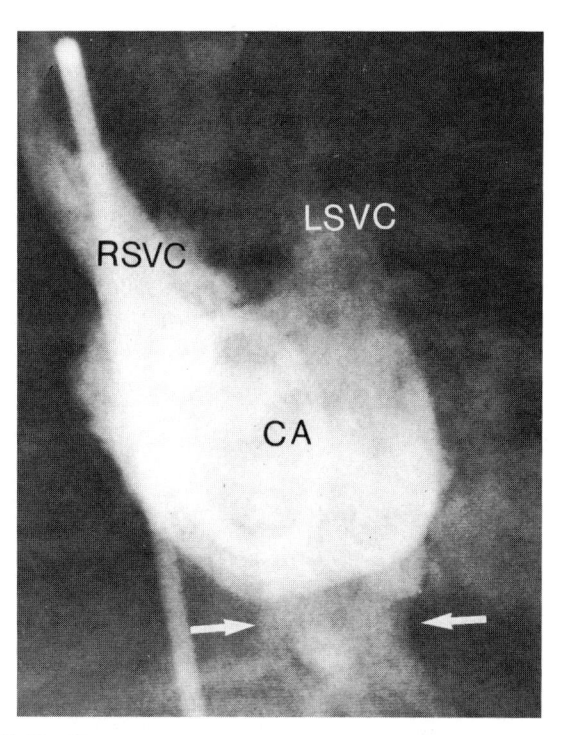

FIG 58–31.
Asplenia syndrome. Ventriculogram via transaortic catheter. Anteroposterior projection. Aorta *(AO)* transposed and in L-malposition. Huge ventricular communication with remnant of septum *(open arrow)*. Common atrioventricular valve *(CAVV)* overriding short septum *(arrows)*. Ventricular communication *(solid white arrow)* immediately beneath common valve, as in atrioventricular canal. *LV* = left ventricle; *RV* = right ventricle.

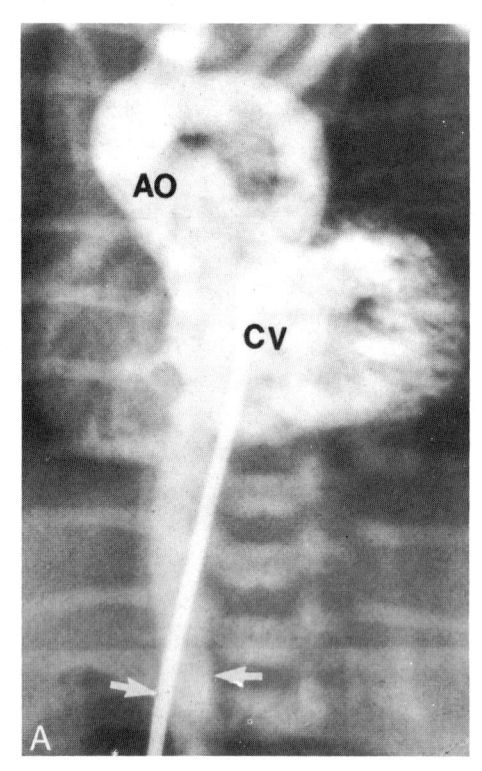

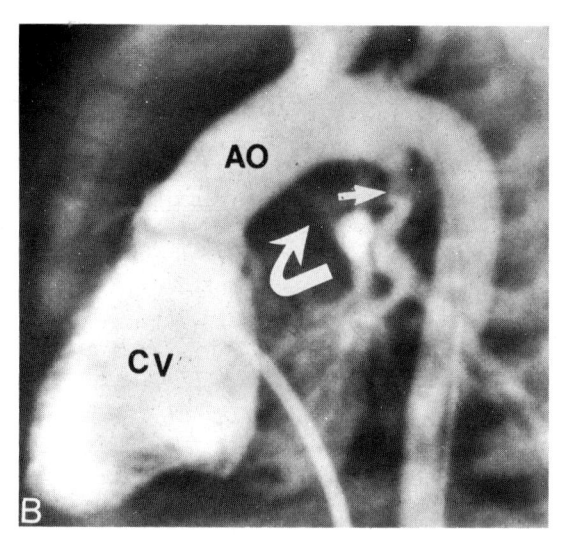

FIG 58-32.
Asplenia syndrome. **A,** ventriculogram. Anteroposterior projection. Venous and arterial catheters cross in abdomen, indicating abdominal heterotaxia *(arrows)*. Aorta arises from common ventricle. No rudimentary chamber. **B,** lateral projection. Common ventricle *(CV)* without rudimentary chamber. Dense opacification of aorta *(AO)*. Pulmonary arteries opacify via patent ductus *(arrow)*. Main pulmonary artery is absent *(curved arrow)*.

POLYSPLENIA SYNDROME

The polysplenia syndrome is the other major cause of situs ambiguus and is also associated with a variety of cardiac and visceral anomalies.[14] Because of the pattern of the anomalies, this syndrome has been called "bilateral left-sidedness" or "bilateral levoisomerism" because of the tendency for each lung to have hyparterial bronchi, the atria have features of a left atrium, the presence of multiple splenic masses, and interruption of the infrahepatic portion of the inferior vena cava. These are some of the important features that tend to distinguish this type of situs ambiguus from the asplenia syndrome.

The polysplenia syndrome occurs as commonly as asplenia syndrome, with equal frequency in males and females. Generally patients with polysplenia survive longer than those with asplenia syndrome. In one review, one half of the patients were dead by 4 months of age, and only one fourth were alive at 5 years of age. This study presents a pessimistic view, because it had a predominance of cases ascertained at autopsy. In clinical experience many patients do well throughout childhood, although many have severe cardiac malformations and symptoms during infancy. Deaths are generally related to the cardiac problem and not from immunologic problems secondary to the splenic anomaly.

Cardiac Anomaly

Virtually each segment of the heart can be abnormal in polysplenia syndrome. These anomalies are discussed in a segmental approach. The cardiac apex may be located in either the left or the right hemithorax in nearly equal proportions.

In one half of the cases, bilateral superior venae cavae are present, with the left superior vena cava connecting either to the coronary sinus or directly to the left atrium (equal proportions).

In two thirds of the cases, there is infrahepatic interruption of the inferior vena cava with azygos termination. Because of the tendency for atrial and visceral symmetry, it is difficult to distinguish azygos from hemiazygos termination. In these instances, the hepatic veins connect directly to an atrium. In the remaining instances, the inferior vena cava connects directly to the atria.

The pulmonary veins connect normally in one half of the patients. In the remaining half there is either partial or less commonly total anomalous pulmonary venous connec-

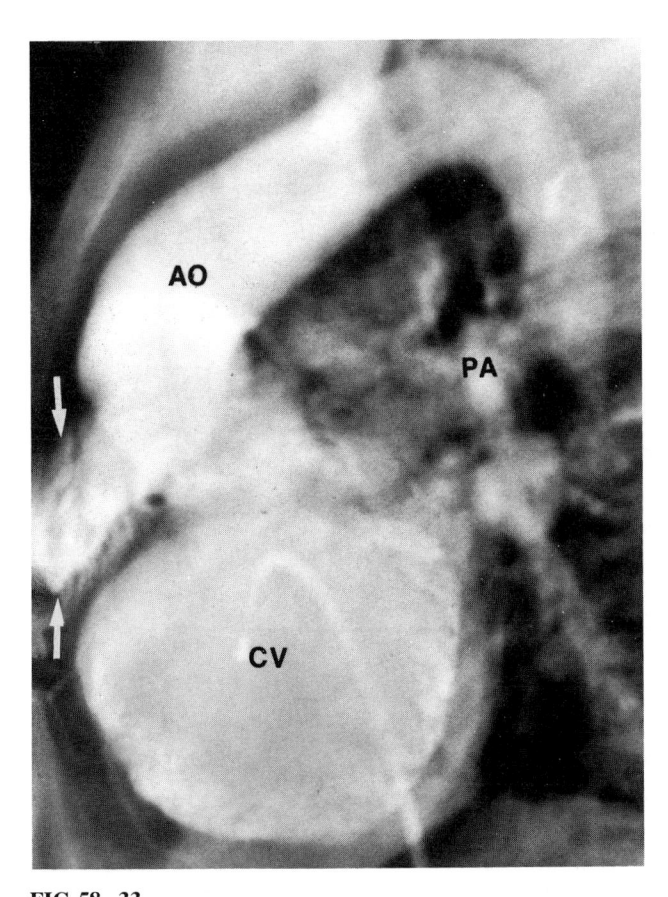

FIG 58-33.
Asplenia syndrome. Ventriculogram. Lateral projection. Common ventricle (CV). Large smooth-walled left ventricle. Opacification of rudimentary anterior right ventricle (arrows). Transposed aorta (AO) arises from rudimentary chamber. Small pulmonary arteries (PA) fill via ductus arteriosus. Obstruction to pulmonary flow by infundibular and valvar pulmonary stenosis or pulmonary atresia is almost invariably present. Absent main pulmonary artery.

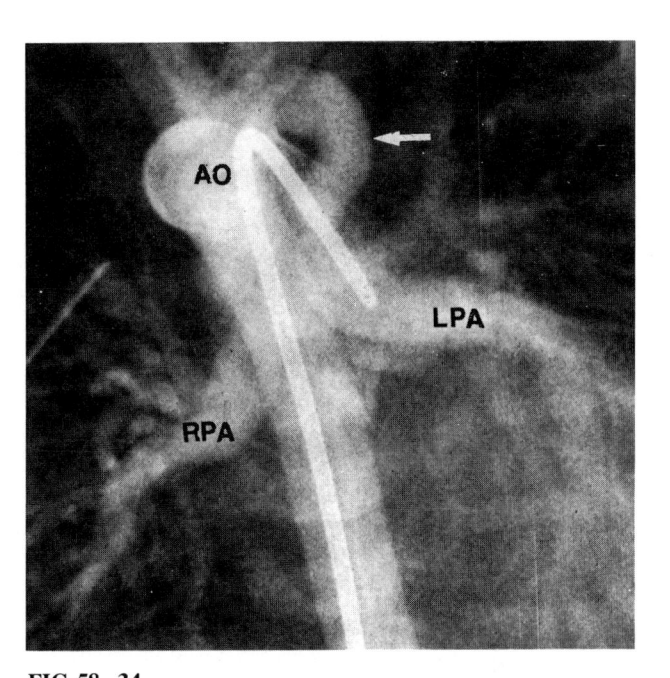

FIG 58-34.
Asplenia syndrome. Transposition of great vessels and pulmonary atresia. Aortogram (AO). Anteroposterior projection. Pulmonary arteries (RPA and LPA) fill through long large patent ductus arteriosus (arrow) from left subclavian artery (right aortic arch). Pattern of pulmonary arteries is symmetric, and each is characteristic of a right pulmonary arteries. Absent main pulmonary artery is commonly seen in asplenia.

tion. The form of anomalous pulmonary venous connection is unique, being seen rarely in other conditions. The anomalous pulmonary veins connect directly to the posterior wall of the right atrium.

In 80% of cases there is a defect in the atrial septum, two thirds being a form of endocardial cushion defect and one third showing an ostium secundum type of atrial septal defect. When the atrial septum is intact, frequently the septum secundum is absent, and the rim of the foramen ovale cannot be identified on either side of the atrial septum.

The ventricular septum is intact in one third of cases, and in the remaining cases there was a ventricular septal defect. In 5% there is a single ventricle.

The great vessels are normally related (70%) or malpositioned or transposed (30%). There is an equal proportion of double-outlet right ventricle or complete transposition, with an occasional instance of corrected transposition.

In distinction to asplenia, the pulmonary outflow area is normal in two thirds of cases. Valvar pulmonary stenosis is present in most of the remaining, with pulmonary atresia found in about 10% of cases.

In one half of our personally reviewed cases, obstructive lesions through the left side of the heart were found, including coarctation of the aorta, hypoplasia of the left ventricle, valvar and subvalvar aortic stenosis, and mitral stenosis.

Visceral and Pulmonary Anomalies

The polysplenia is manifested by the presence of 2 to 16 splenic masses, the masses being relatively equal in size. They are supplied by the splenic artery and located along the greater curvature of the stomach. Most commonly 6 to 12 spleens are present. Contrary to multiple spleen, the spleens in polysplenia remain clumped together, giving the spleen a diced appearance (Fig 58-38).

The lungs have been described as normal (20%) or as mirror image (20%). In most of the remaining cases, each lung had the appearance of a left lung, and in the remaining each lung had the appearance of a right lung. In those

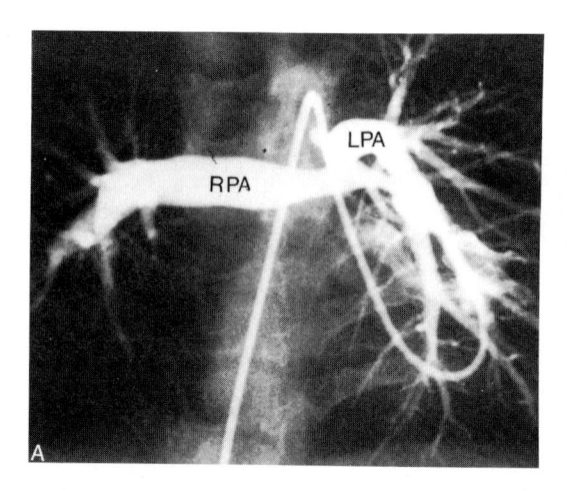

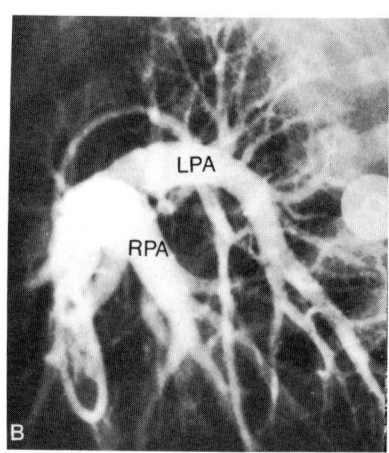

FIG 58-35.
Asplenia syndrome. Pulmonary arteriogram. **A,** anteroposterior and, **B,** lateral projections. Stenotic *(arrow)* right-sided pulmonary artery *(RPA)* has anatomic features of a right pulmonary artery. Left pulmonary artery *(LPA)* crosses over the left mainstem bronchus, indicating hyparterial bronchus and features of an anatomic left pulmonary artery. This is rare occurrence in asplenia syndrome.

with an appearance of bilateral left lungs, there are two lobes and hyparterial bronchi in each lung. If bilateral bilobed lungs are present, both bronchi are hyparterial. Both pulmonary arteries pass over the symmetric left bronchi, as with bilateral left pulmonary arteries (Fig 58-39).

As in asplenia, anomalies of abdominal organs are very common. In perhaps one half the cases, the liver is symmetric and occupies both sides of the upper half of the abdomen. In 10% of cases the gallbladder is hypoplastic, and biliary atresia may coexist with these cases. Rotational anomalies of the bowel are common, either nonrotation or reverse rotation of the midgut loop.

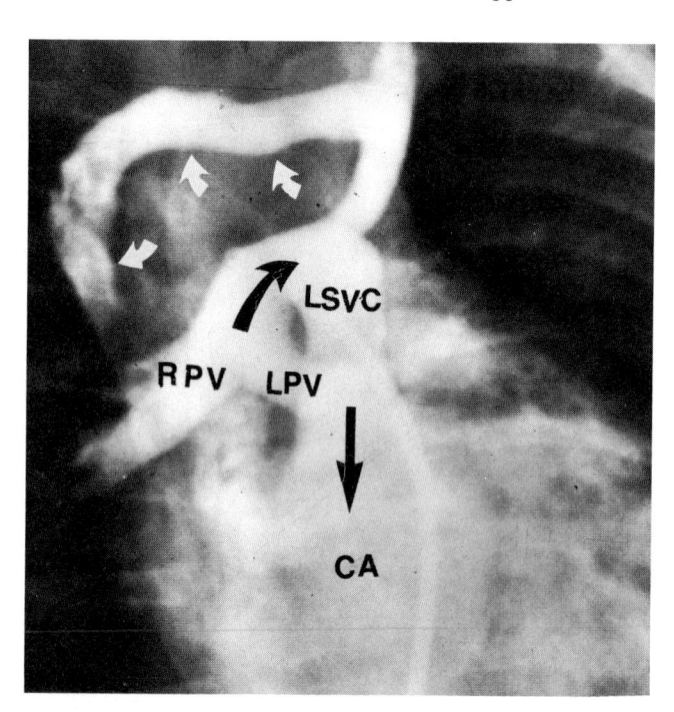

Diagnosis

The diagnosis of polysplenia can generally be made by interpretation of thoracic roentgenograms. Catheterization or angiographic findings of an interrupted inferior vena cava, unusual relationship between inferior vena cava and aorta, abnormal relationship of these major vessels and other organs, or the presence of bilateral hyparterial bronchi essentially establish the diagnosis.

The electrocardiogram generally reflects the underlying cardiac anomaly, although frequently there is a superiorly directed P-wave axis, between 0 and −60 degrees with levocardia and +180 and +240 degrees in dextrocardia.

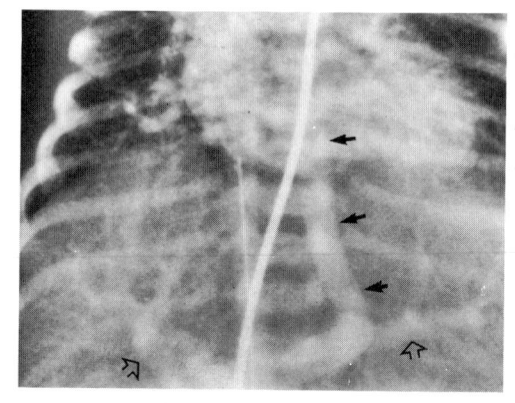

FIG 58-36.
Asplenia syndrome. Left superior vena cavogram. Anteroposterior projection. Catheter is passed through inferior vena cava and common atrium *(CA)* into left superior vena cava *(LSVC)*. Right *(RPV)* and left *(LPV)* pulmonary veins form common pulmonary vein, which joins left superior vena cava connecting to common atrium. Direction of blood flow is indicated by arrows. Right superior vena cava with connecting innominate vein *(white arrows)*.

FIG 58-37.
Asplenia syndrome. Infradiaphragmatic total anomalous pulmonary venous connection to portal vein. Pulmonary angiogram. Late phase. Anteroposterior projection. All pulmonary veins connect to venous channel *(arrows)*, which passes with esophagus through diaphragm connecting to portal system. Portal vein is well opacified *(open arrows)*. Midline liver.

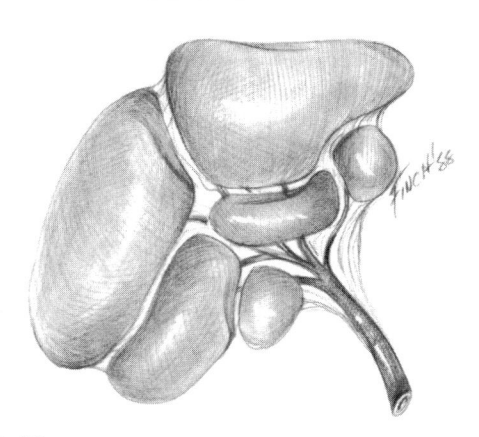

POLYSPLENIA

FIG 58-38.
Spleen in polysplenia. Shape of spleen is preserved. Spleen has a diced appearance.

Infants with polysplenia generally have the murmur and other clinical findings related to their cardiac disease. Infrequently, neonates with this condition have upper gastrointestinal obstruction. Splenic function must be normal, because frequent infections and the presence of Howell-Jolly bodies are rare.

The correct diagnosis of polysplenia can be made from thoracic roentgenograms in most cases. Although abdominal heterotaxia occurs with either asplenia or polysplenia, differentiation between these two conditions can be made fairly accurately.

1. Abdominal heterotaxia associated with a congenital cardiac malformation strongly suggests a coexistent splenic anomaly.
2. If abdominal heterotaxia occurs in a patient more than 2 years of age, polysplenia is much more likely than asplenia. REASON: The cardiac malformations in asplenia are much more severe than in polysplenia. Three fourths of patients with asplenia die before the age of 1 year.
3. If the pulmonary arteries are symmetric and each located above the associated bronchus (hyparterial bronchi), polysplenia syndrome is present, because in this condition there is bilateral left-sidedness.
4. If both bronchi are symmetric and long (bilateral left bronchi), the diagnosis of polysplenia is virtually certain (see Fig 58-39).
5. If the pulmonary vasculature is increased, the patient very likely has polysplenia. REASON: Most patients with asplenia have pulmonary stenosis or atresia and there-

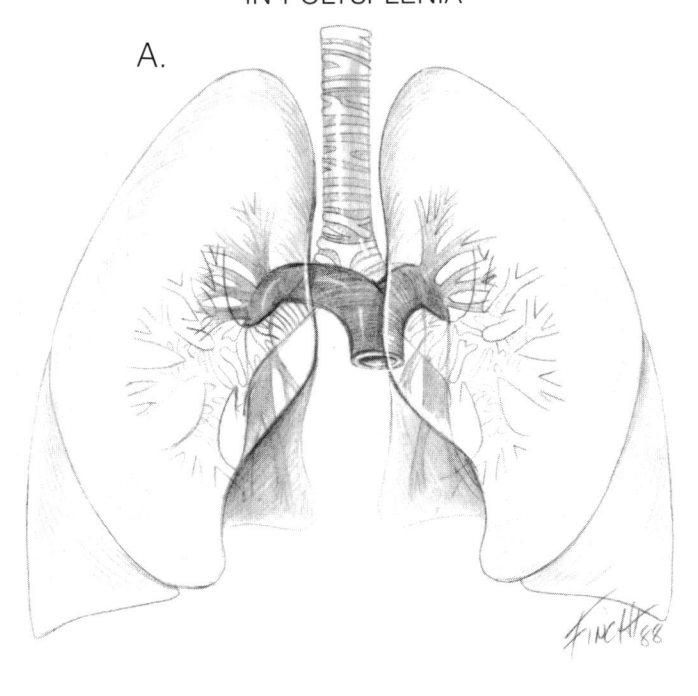

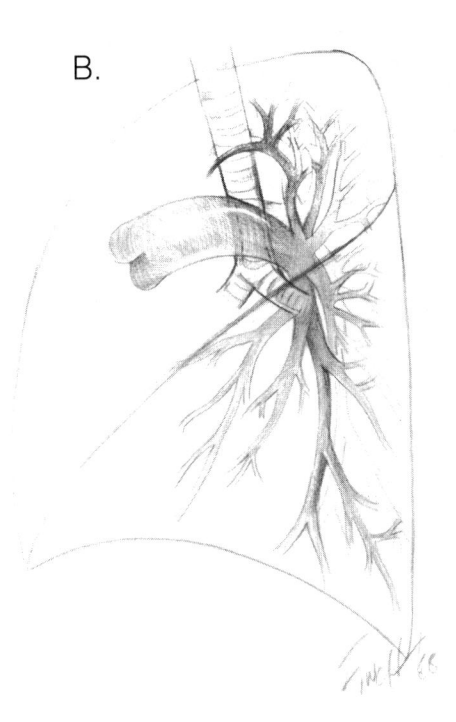

FIG 58-39.
Lungs, pulmonary arteries, and bronchi in polysplenia. **A,** anteroposterior and, **B,** lateral projections. Both lungs are bilobed. Both bronchi are symmetric, long, and hyparterial. Symmetric pulmonary arteries have appearance of left pulmonary arteries passing over bronchi.

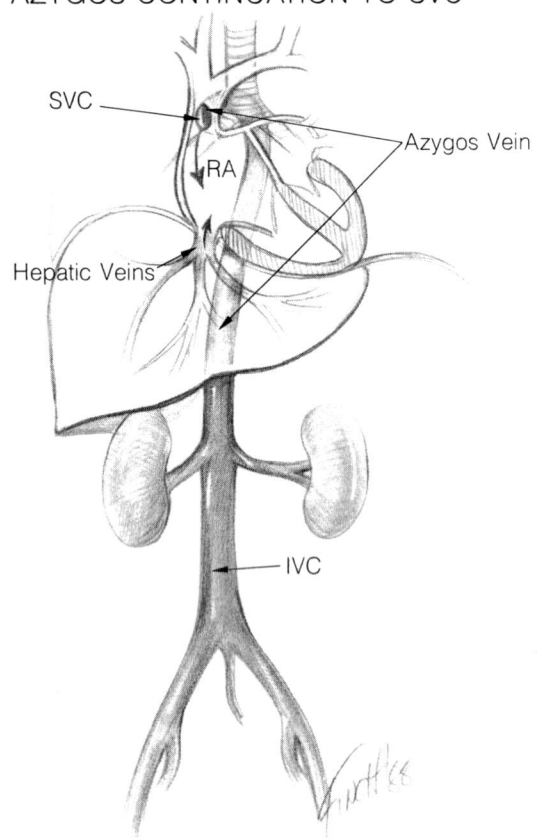

FIG 58–40.
Interruption of inferior vena cava *(IVC)* with azygos continuation to superior vena cava *(SVC)*. Infrahepatic portion of IVC is interrupted and continues in azygos system. Blood from kidneys and lower portion of body return to heart through this route. Hepatic veins connect directly to right atrium. *(RA)*.

fore decreased pulmonary vasculature, whereas the cardiac anomalies in polysplenia are often associated with increased pulmonary blood flow.

6. If a density representing an enlarged azygos or hemiazygos vein is identified on a thoracic roentgenogram, a diagnosis of polysplenia is almost certain. REASON: Interruption of the inferior vena cava with azygos continuation is uncommon in asplenia but occurs in one half of the patients with polysplenia (Fig 58–40).

7. A midline liver may occur in either asplenia or polysplenia.

Radiographic Features

1. Occasionally the abdominal situs appears normal radiographically (Figs 58–41 and 58–42). This occurs rarely in polysplenia syndrome and almost never in asple-

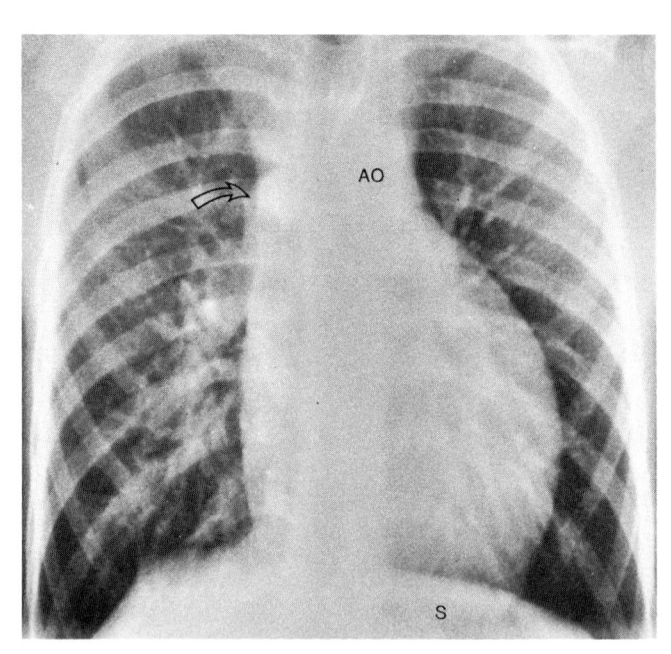

FIG 58–41.
Polysplenia syndrome. Thoracic roentgenogram. Posteroanterior projection. Aorta *(AO)*, cardiac apex, and gastric air bubble *(S)* are concordant on left side: therefore, no radiographic evidence for abdominal heterotaxia. Increased pulmonary arterial vasculature. Left cardiac border is suggestive of corrected transposition of great vessels. Enlarged azygos vein *(arrow)*. Combination of increased pulmonary blood flow, patient's older age, and enlarged azygos are consistent with interruption of hepatic segment of inferior vena cava, as in polysplenia syndrome.

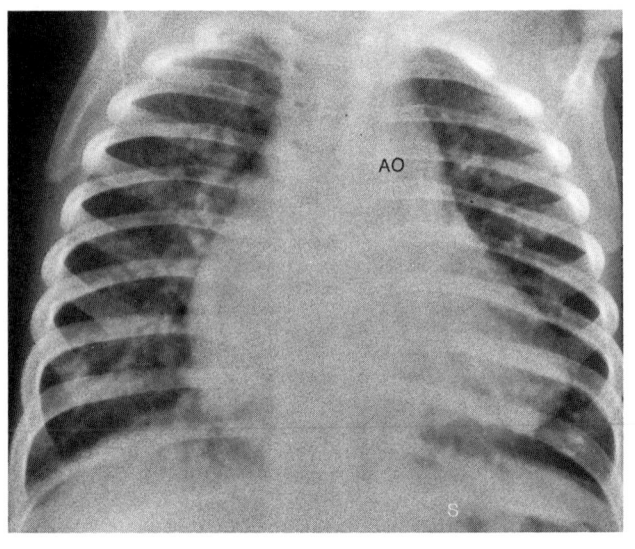

FIG 58–42.
Polysplenia syndrome and interruption of inferior vena cava. Thoracic roentgenogram. Posteroanterior projection. Aorta *(AO)*, cardiac apex, and stomach *(S)* are concordant on left. Enlarged heart. Increased pulmonary vasculature. No radiographic evidence of abdominal heterotaxia.

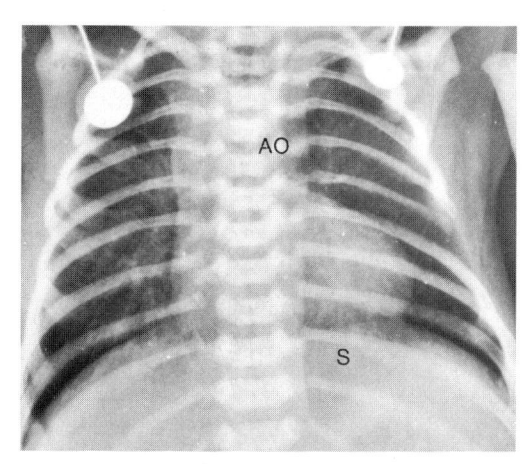

FIG 58–43.
Polysplenia syndrome. Thoracic roentgenogram. Posteroanterior projection. Concordant stomach bubble *(S)*, cardiac apex, and aorta *(AO)*. Decreased pulmonary blood flow. Diagnosis of polysplenia is not suggested from roentgenograms, because situs appears normal and pulmonary vasculature is decreased. Tetralogy of Fallot and polysplenia were found at postmortem examination.

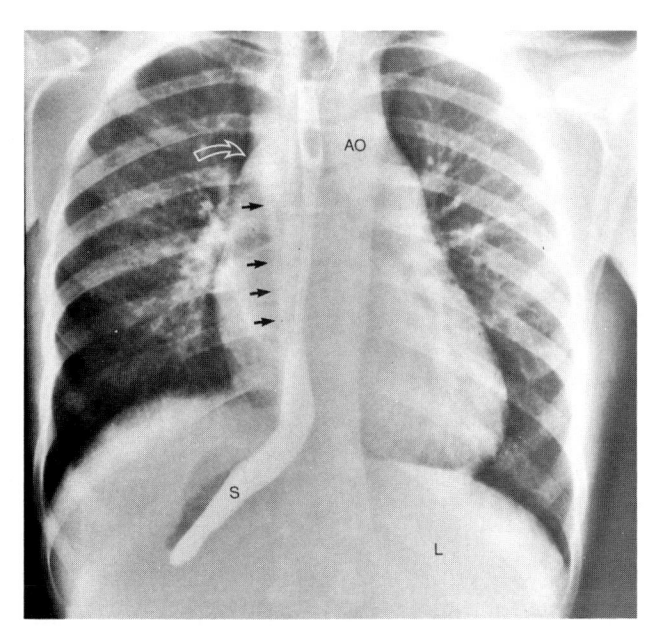

FIG 58–45.
Polysplenia syndrome in adult. Thoracic roentgenogram. Posteroanterior projection. Abdominal heterotaxia. Cardiac apex and aorta *(AO)* on right. Stomach *(S)* on left. Trachea is slightly deviated toward left, indicating right-sided aortic arch. Large bulge opposite aortic arch is huge hemiazygos vein *(curved arrow)*.

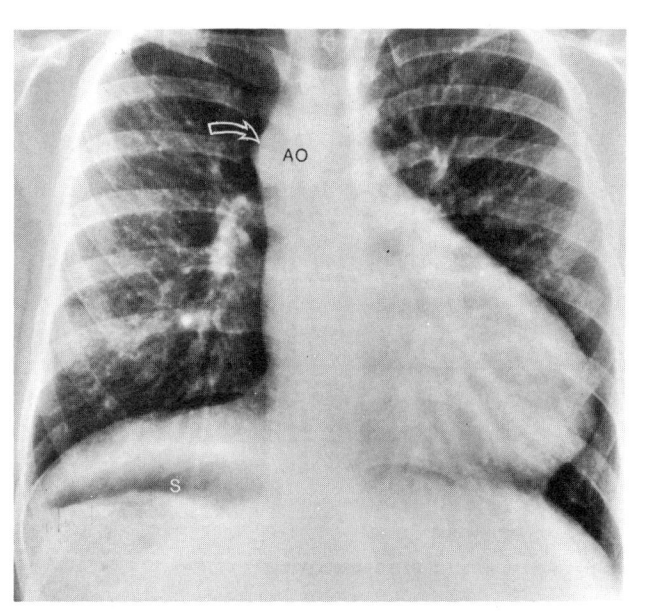

FIG 58–44.
Polysplenia syndrome. Thoracic roentgenogram. Posteroanterior projection. Aortic arch *(AO)*, cardiac apex and liver *(L)* on left; stomach bubble *(S)* on right. Discordant position. Pattern of abdominal heterotaxia. Density of enlarged azygos vein *(arrows)*. Round density *(open arrow)* azygos vein is seen on end above right bronchus. Symmetric left-sided bronchi. These features indicate polysplenia.

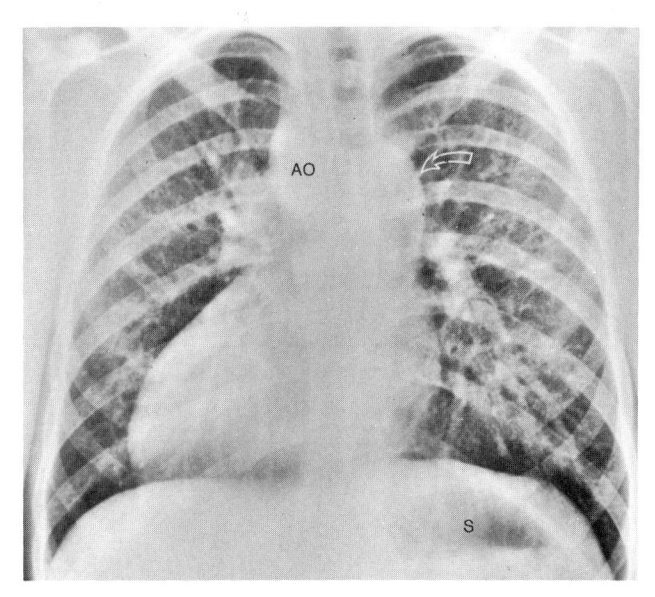

FIG 58–46.
Polysplenia syndrome. Atrioventricular canal and pulmonary stenosis. Thoracic roentgenogram. Posteroanterior projection. Normal pulmonary vasculature. Trachea is deviated slightly toward left, indicating right-sided aortic arch *(AO)*. Aortic arch and stomach bubble *(S)* concordant on right; cardiac apex on left. Although this pattern could indicate situs inversus with levoversion, abdominal heterotaxia is much more likely statistically. Enlarged azygos vein *(curved arrow)* is overshadowed by aortic arch and therefore difficult to recognize.

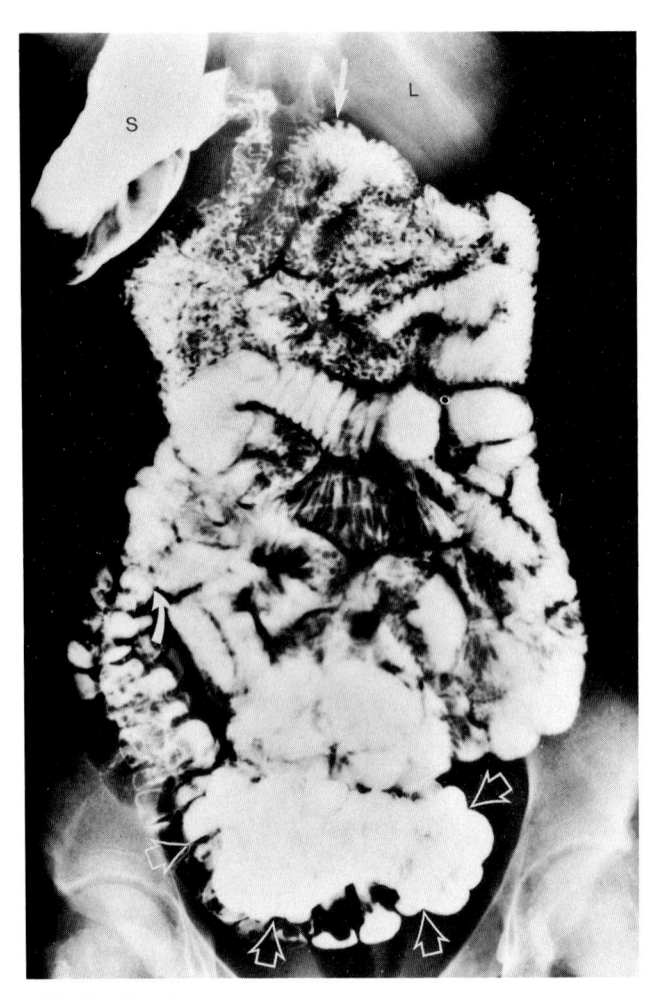

FIG 58–47.
Polysplenia syndrome. Abdominal roentgenogram after barium swallow. Posteroanterior projection. Abdominal heterotaxia. Stomach *(S)* on right side; liver *(L)* on left side. Ligament of Treitz *(white arrow)* has characteristic midline position. All large bowel loops *(open arrows)* are superimposed in pelvis. No ascending and transverse colon. Ileal cecal valve high *(curved arrow)*.

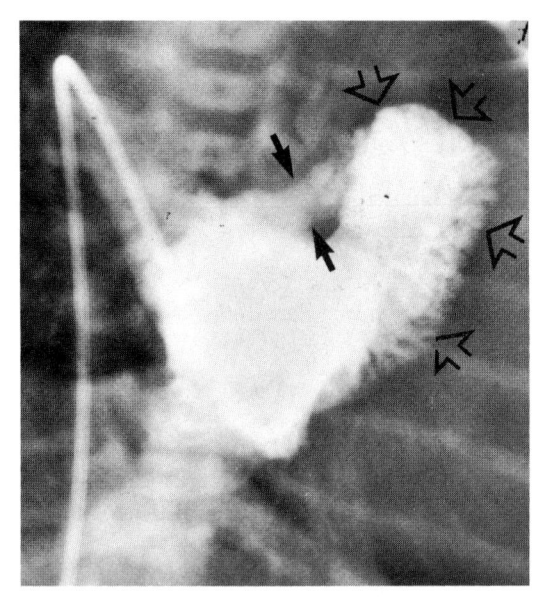

FIG 58–48.
Polysplenia syndrome and common atrium. Injection of common atrium. Anteroposterior projections. Catheter is passed through interrupted inferior vena cava and azygos vein into common atrium. One large atrial appendage *(open arrows)* and one small atrial appendage *(solid arrows)* are opacified. Both appendages are long and narrow, as a left appendage. At postmortem examination, three lobes were present in each lung, and multiple spleens were found.

nia syndrome. Despite the normal appearance, ambiguous situs is present.

2. If the situs is normal (rare) and the enlarged azygous vein cannot be seen on a thoracic roentgenogram (see Fig 58–42), a diagnosis cannot be made (only about 50% of the patients have interruption of the inferior vena cava and azygos continuation).

3. Pulmonary vasculature is increased (see Figs 58–41 and 58–42). REASON: Most patients with polysplenia have conditions such as partial anomalous pulmonary venous connection or atrial septal defect that are associated with increased pulmonary blood flow. Rarely, the pulmonary vasculature is decreased (Fig 58–43).

4. The azygos or hemiazygos vein is often markedly enlarged. REASON: At least one half of the patients with polysplenia have interruption of the hepatic segment of the inferior vena cava and azygos or hemiazygos continuation. The azygos venous system carries the entire venous return from below the diaphragm except for the hepatic venous blood flow, which returns directly into the atrium.

5. In most cases abdominal heterotaxia is present (Figs 58–41 and 58–44) and recognized by unusual relationships between the cardiac silhouette, liver, and stomach bubble.

6. In an adult the azygos vein may be so enlarged that it mimics an aortic arch, and the thoracic radiograph appears to show two aortic arches. The aortic arch is found on one side and the dilated azygos vein on the contralateral side, mimicking a double aortic arch (Fig 58–45). Differentiation between aorta and azygos vein is difficult because both structures cause an identical density. However, the aortic arch tends to shift the trachea away, whereas with double arches the trachea usually does not shift.

7. If the aortic arch and dilated azygos vein are on the same side of the mediastinum, the azygous vein may be difficult to see (Fig 58–46).

8. Polysplenia syndrome is usually associated with gastrointestinal abnormalities, such as nonrotation of midgut loop, reversed rotation of midgut loop, or mobile

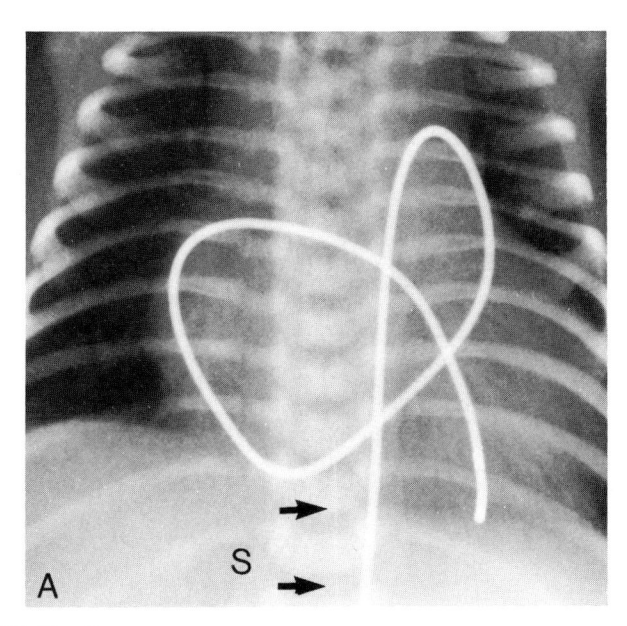

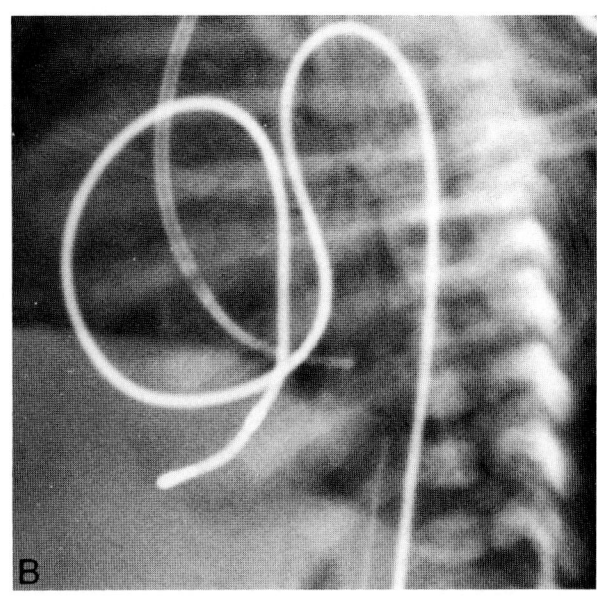

FIG 58–49.
Polysplenia syndrome. Thoracic roentgenogram. **A,** posteroanterior and, **B,** lateral projections. Abdominal heterotaxia. Right-sided stomach *(S)*. Left-sided inferior vena cava. Midline aorta (outlined by umbilical catheter) *(arrow)*. Interruption of right-sided inferior vena cava. Catheter is passed through hemiazygos vein, which enters left-sided superior vena cava. Catheter is coiled in common atrium and advanced into posterior ventricle.

cecum. Each can be diagnosed with more certainty by barium swallow (Fig 58–47).

9. Malrotation of the large bowel is better seen by a barium enema. Often the ascending colon is not a retroperitoneal structure and is attached by a mesentery. Frequently, as a result, the ascending and descending portions of the colon are adjacent and positioned entirely on one side of the abdomen.

Angiographic Features

The complexity and unpredictability of cardiac malformations in polysplenia in contrast to asplenia challenges

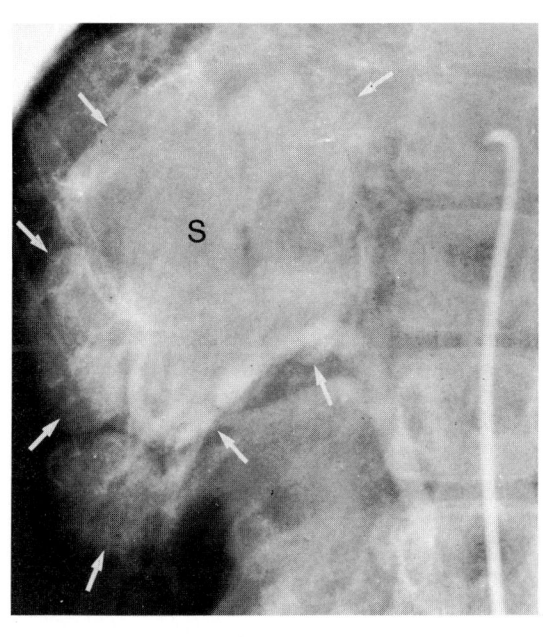

FIG 58–50.
Celiac axis arteriogram. Late phase. Spleen *(S)* is opacified in right upper quadrant. Overall configuration of spleen is preserved, but there are at least six separate spleens *(arrows)*.

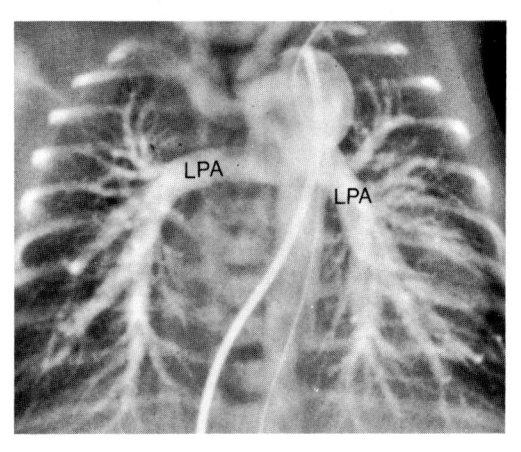

FIG 58–51.
Polysplenia syndrome and mitral atresia. Pulmonary arteriogram. Anteroposterior projection. Concordant aorta, cardiac apex, and stomach. Normal inferior vena cava on right side; aortic catheter on left side. Consequently, abdominal heterotaxia is not present. Pulmonary arteries *(LPA)* are symmetric, having appearance of left pulmonary arteries bilaterally. Bilateral hyparterial bronchi (see also Fig 58–39).

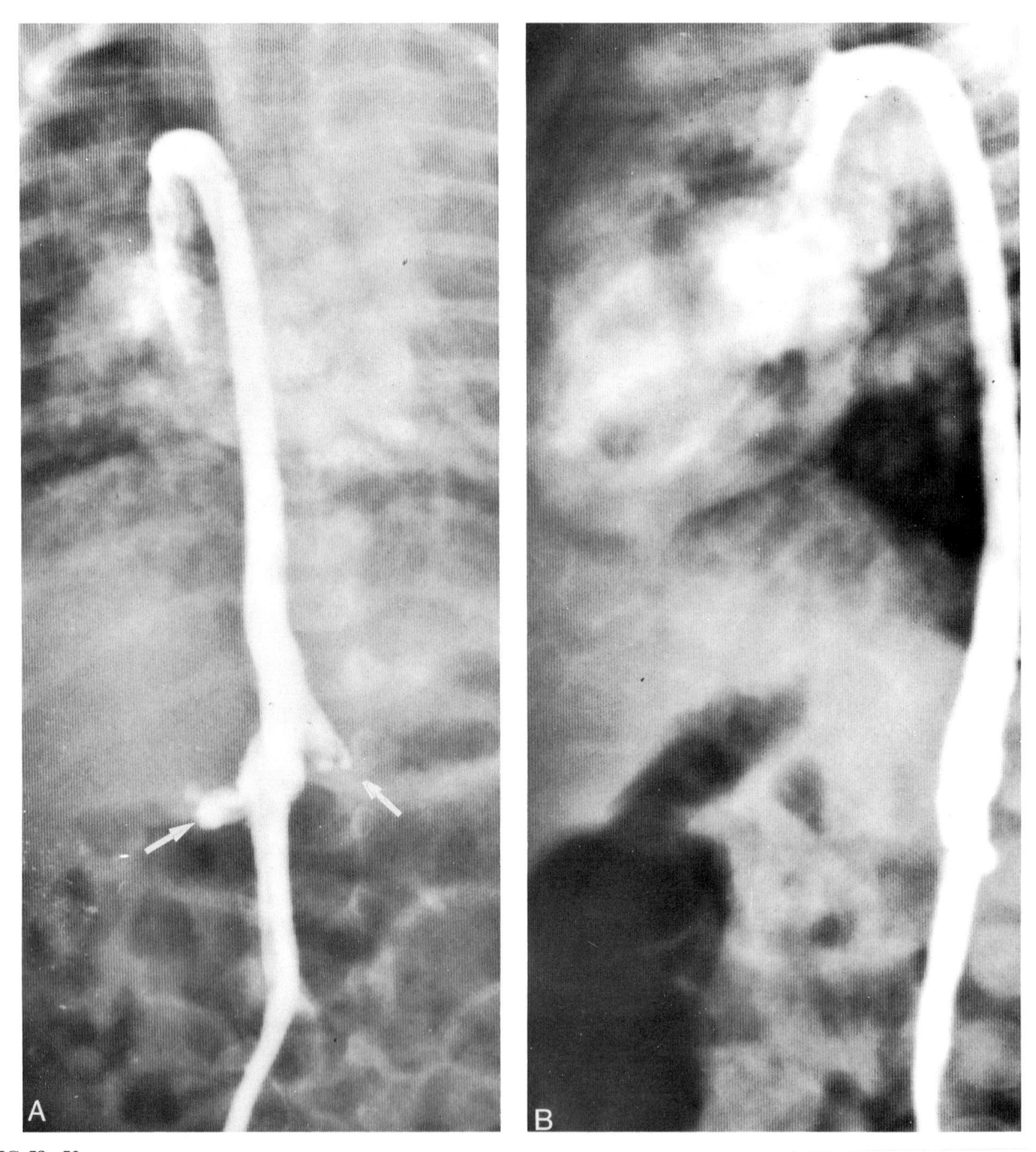

FIG 58–52.
Polysplenia syndrome. Interruption of inferior vena cava. Selective venography of right femoral vein. **A,** anteroposterior projection. Reflux into renal veins *(arrows)*. Interruption of inferior vena cava above level of renal veins, with azygos continuation. Therefore, interruption involves infrahepatic segment of inferior vena cava. **B,** lateral projection. Typical candy cane appearance of azygos continuation of inferior vena cava.

the cardiologist and requires careful angiographic studies. Venography must be performed because of the high incidence of bilateral superior venae cavae. Angiographic demonstration of atrial anatomy is necessary, particularly before an atrial septation operation, because of the frequent occurrence of atrial abnormalities, especially common atrium and anomalies of pulmonary or systemic venous connection. The hepatic veins may enter either the right-sided or left-sided atrium, which is very important to the surgeon. Most patients with polysplenia have bilateral left atrial appendages, each being long and narrow, reflecting that each atrium has anatomic features of a left atrium.

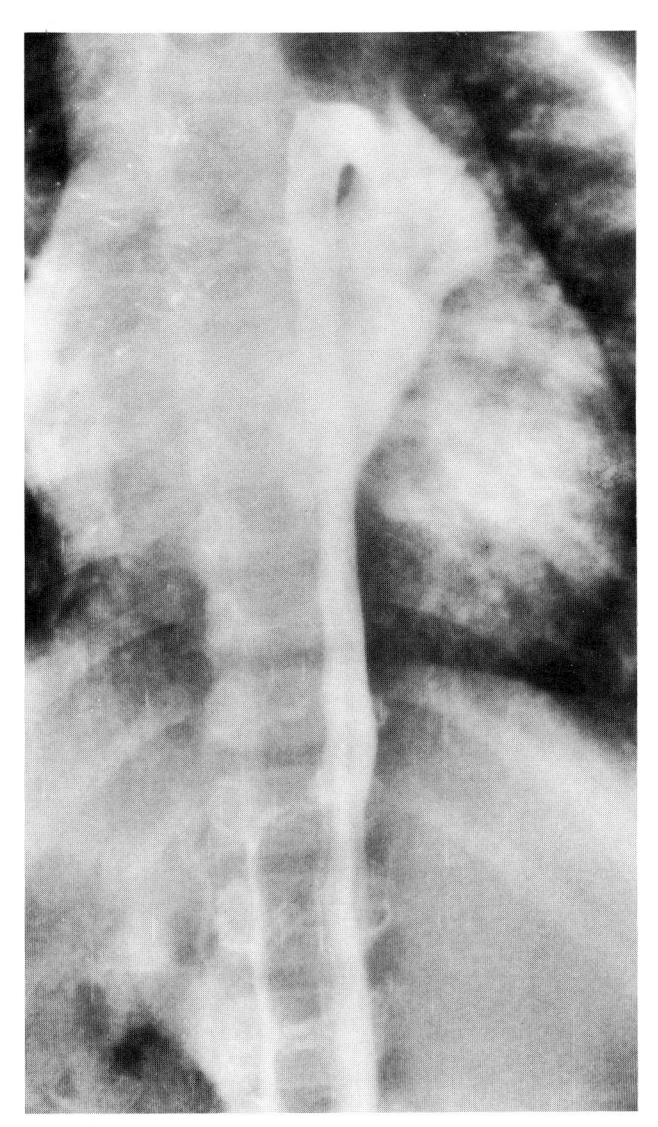

FIG 58–53.
Polysplenia syndrome. Venous angiogram. Anteroposterior projection. Interrupted left-sided inferior vena cava and hemiazygos continuation. Termination into left atrium rather than coronary sinus.

If an atrial appendage is entered with a catheter tip, it should be injected to identify its characteristics (Fig 58–48). The pulmonary venous connection must also be identified. REASON: The incidence of anomalous pulmonary venous connection is increased. Usually there is partial anomalous pulmonary venous connection directly to the right atrium rather than to either the coronary sinus or the superior vena cava. Occasionally total anomalous pulmonary venous connection is present and also occurs directly to the right atrium.

1. The catheter position may be diagnostic if interruption of the azygos or hemiazygos vein is present (Fig

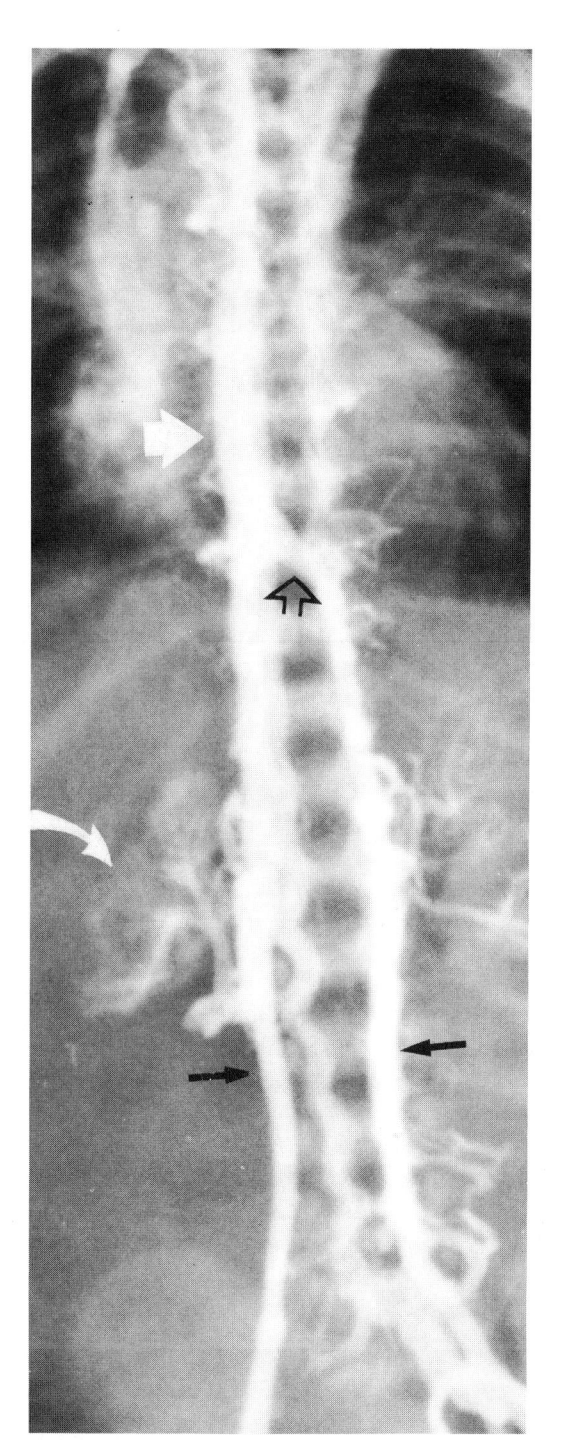

FIG 58–54.
Polysplenia syndrome. Duplication of inferior vena cava. Venogram. Anteroposterior projection. Both inferior vena cavae *(arrows)* show interruption of intrahepatic segment. They join *(open arrow)* and continue as a large azygos vein *(large white arrow)*. Reflux into right adrenal vein outlining large adrenal gland *(curved white arrow)* is normal for neonate.

58–49). On a posteroanterior projection, the catheter ascends on one side of the spine to a position above the cardiac silhouette and then loops back on itself and passes caudally toward the heart. On a lateral film of the thorax, the catheter is seen to pass posterior to the heart. Above the cardiac shadow, it curves anteriorly and inferiorly to enter the heart. This appearance on a lateral film has been called "candy-cane" or "shepherd's crook" inferior vena cava.

2. Not only the interruption of the inferior vena cava can be diagnosed by catheter position but also the presence of a common atrium (see Fig 58–49) if the catheter forms a broad loop from one cardiac border to the other at the atrial level.

3. The demonstration of the multiple spleens (usually 8–12, not to be confused with accessory spleens) can be made by ultrasound, radioisotope studies, or nuclear magnetic resonance. These studies are usually unnecessary because the diagnosis can be inferred from other radiographic findings.

4. The diagnosis can also be made angiographically with certainty. REASON: The normal division of the splenic artery in the region of the splenic hilum is lacking, and the individual spleens can be seen in the parenchymal phase (Fig 58–50). Commonly the spleens occupy an abnormal, sometimes midline position.

5. Bilateral left-sidedness can be proved by the visualization of anatomical symmetric left pulmonary arteries (Fig 58–51). On the lateral projection, both branch pulmonary arteries cross over the respective bronchi. Thus, there are bilateral hyparterial bronchi.

6. Bilateral left-sidedness can also be proved by the injection of the atrial appendages. REASON: Most patients with polysplenia have anatomic left atria and consequently anatomic left atrial appendages (see Fig 58–48). Exceedingly rare exceptions occur.

7. A selective injection of one of the femoral veins outlines the typical picture of interruption of the inferior vena cava with azygos continuation. The appearance has been compared to a candy cane (Fig 58–52). Interruption of the inferior vena cava may occur with hemiazygos continuation (Fig 58–53).

8. Other variations such as bilateral inferior venae cavae with bilateral interruption of their intrahepatic segments and azygos or hemiazygos venous continuation exist (Fig 58–54).

REFERENCES

1. Anselmi G, Munoz S, Blanco P, et al: Systematization and clinical study of dextroversion, mirror-image dextrocardia, and laevoversion, *Br Heart J* 34:1085, 1972.
2. Lev M, Liberthson RR, Eckner RAO, et al: Pathologic anatomy of dextrocardia and its clinical implications, *Circulation* 37:979, 1968.
3. Shinebourne EA, Macartney FJ, Anderson RH: Sequential chamber localization: the logical approach to diagnosis in congenital heart disease, *Br Heart J* 38:327, 1976.
4. Stanger P, Rudolph AM, Edwards JE: Cardiac malpositions: an overview based on study of 65 necropsy specimens, *Circulation* 56:159, 1977.
5. Tynan MJ, Becker AE, Macartney FJ, et al: Nomenclature and classification of congenital heart disease, *Br Heart J* 41:544, 1979.
6. VanPraagh R: Terminology of congenital heart disease: glossary and commentary, *Circulation* 56:139, 1977.
7. Van Praagh R, Van Praagh S, Vlad P, et al: Anatomic types of congenital dextrocardia: diagnostic and embryologic implications, *Am J Cardiol* 13:510, 1964.
8. Van Praagh R, Van Praagh S: Isolated ventricular inversion: a consideration of the morphogenesis, definition and diagnosis of nontransposed and transposed great arteries, *Am J Cardiol* 17:395, 1966.
9. Van Praagh R, Van Praagh S, Vlad P, et al: Diagnosis of anatomic congenital dextrocardia, *Am J Cardiol* 15:234, 1965.
10. Squarcia U, Ritter DG, Kincaid OW: Dextrocardia: angiocardiographic study and classification, *Am J Cardiol* 32:965, 1973.
11. Calcaterra G, Anderson RH, Lau KC, et al: Dextrocardia—value of segmental analysis in its categorisation, *Br Heart J* 42:497, 1979.
12. Elliott LP, Jue KL, Amplatz K: A roentgen classification of cardiac malposition, *Radiology* 1:17, 1966.
13. Ivemark B: Implications of agenesis of the spleen on the pathogenesis of conotruncus anomalies in childhood, *Acta Paediatr Scand* 44(suppl 104):1, 1955.
14. Moller JH, Nakib A, Anderson RC, et al: Congenital cardiac disease associated with polysplenia: a developmental complex of bilateral "left-sidedness," *Circulation* 36:789, 1967.

CHAPTER 59

Criss-Cross Heart

Criss-cross heart is a cardiac malformation caused by abnormal rotation of the ventricles early in embryonic development. It is also known as "superior inferior ventricles" or "upstairs-downstairs ventricle." The ventricular rotation displaces the atrioventricular and the semilunar valves and causes a different orientation of the ventricular septum.[1-7] Consequently, the angiographic interpretation of such cases is challenging.

Rotation of the ventricles may occur in either a clockwise or a counterclockwise direction when they are viewed from the cardiac apex. Either direction of rotation results in apparent crossing of the venous inflow tracts, displacement of the atrioventricular valves, the semilunar valves, and distortion of the ventricular septum. The direction of rotation is fairly constant among the type of positional anomalies of great vessels with which criss-cross heart is associated:

1. A normal heart (concordant atrioventricular and ventricular arterial connections)—clockwise rotation. With complete transposition of the great vessels (D-loop transposition, concordant atrioventricular connection, and discordant ventriculoarterial connection)—clockwise rotation.
2. With corrected transposition of the great vessels (discordant atrioventricular connection and discordant ventriculoarterial connection)—counterclockwise rotation.
3. Double-outlet right ventricle—clockwise rotation.

The most constant and characteristic feature of a criss-cross heart is displacement of the atrioventricular valves, and these may no longer be in fibrous continuity. When clockwise rotation of the ventricles occurs, the right atrioventricular valve is positioned higher and to the left of the left atrioventricular valve. The right atrioventricular valve empties into the venous ventricle, which is also located to the left, and forms the left cardiac border. The left atrioventricular valve, emptying the left atrium, lies medial and lower than the right atrioventricular valve. This position of the atrioventricular valves results in an apparent crossing of ventricular inflow paths, leading to the term criss-cross heart (Fig 59-1). When counterclockwise rotation occurs, the left atrioventricular valve is located higher and to the right, whereas the right atrioventricular valve is rotated and positioned posteriorly and to the left.

CLINICAL FEATURES AND HEMODYNAMICS

The clinical findings, electrocardiogram, radiographic features, and hemodynamics are not altered by the criss-cross anomaly and depend on the associated cardiac anomalies. The only clue of the criss-cross orientation obtained during cardiac catheterization is an unusual catheter course into the ventricles or the great vessels.

ANGIOGRAPHIC FEATURES

Because the angiographic appearance may be confusing, one has to proceed in an orderly fashion using a segmental and hemodynamic analysis. Because of the rotation of the heart, the ventricular septum is commonly perpendicular to the anterior thoracic wall and is seen on end on the anteroposterior projection. This appearance mimics closely the features of the ventricles in corrected transposition of the great vessels (L-loop transposition).

Identification of the venous and arterial atria by oximetry and angiography is important in the diagnostic process. After the right atrium is identified, the contrast material enters the venous ventricle, which occupies a high and leftward position leading to the term criss-cross heart. Then the artery arising from the ventricle is identified. If the pulmonary artery originates from this ventricle, the diagnosis is either a normal criss-cross heart or criss-cross heart with corrected transposition of the great vessels. If

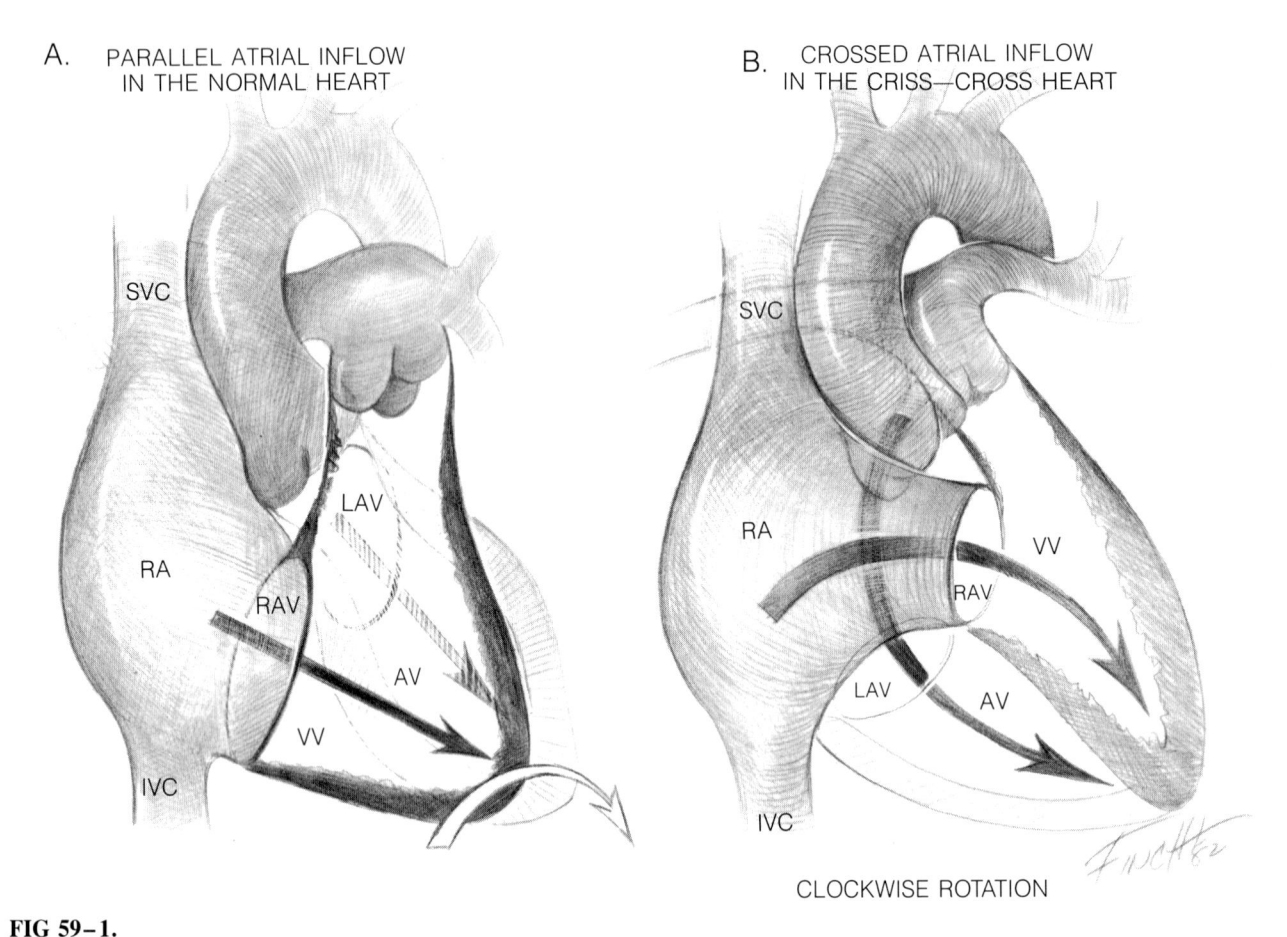

FIG 59–1.
Comparison of normal and criss-cross heart. **A,** normal heart. Inflow pathways of blood through right and left atrioventricular valves are parallel. Ventricular septum has oblique orientation. **B,** criss-cross heart. Clockwise rotation of heart along its long axis *(arrow)* causes apparent crossing but not mixing of venous inflow tracts. *AV* = arterial ventricle; *IVC* = inferior vena cava; *LAV* = left atrioventricular valve; *RA* = right atrium; *RAV* = right atrioventricular valve; *SVC* = superior vena cava; *VV* = venous ventricle.

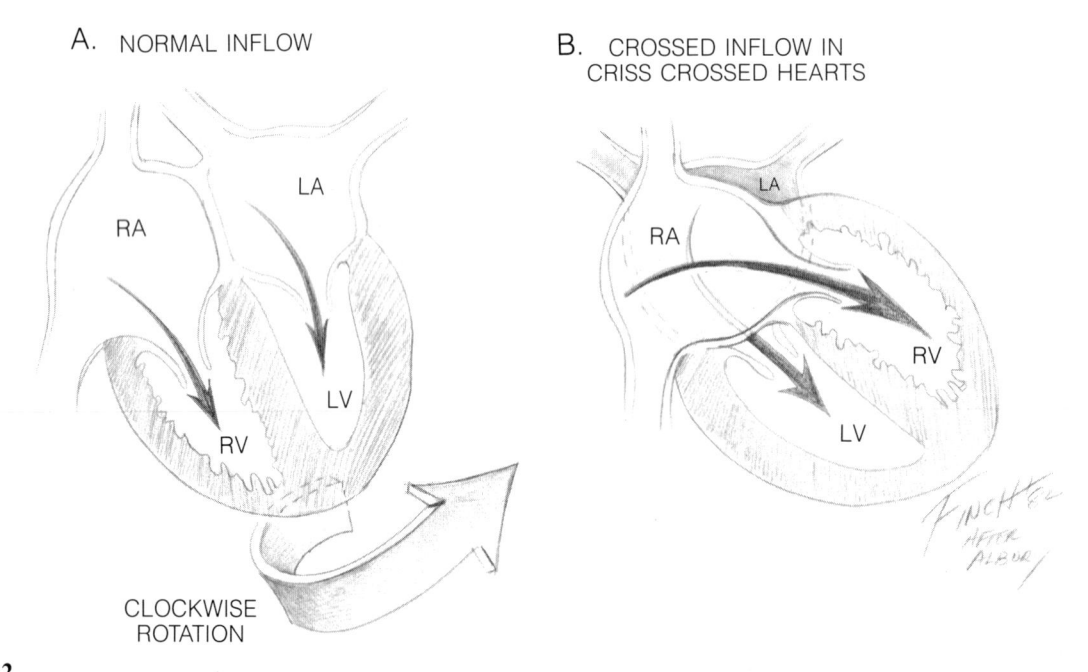

FIG 59–2.
Comparison of normal and criss-cross hearts. **A,** normal heart. Parallel venous inflow and oblique ventricular septum. **B,** criss-cross heart. Clockwise rotation. Displacement of atrioventricular valves with apparent crossing of venous inflows. Because of this rotation, ventricular septum seen on end on anteroposterior projection as in corrected transposition. Displacement of pulmonary artery. *RA* = right atrium; *LA* = left atrium; *LV* = left ventricle; *RV* = right ventricle.

the aorta arises from the venous ventricle, the diagnosis is complete transposition of the great vessels regardless of the position of the aorta on a lateral projection. As a last step the internal architecture of the venous ventricle is analyzed to determine concordance or discordance of atrioventricular connection. A similar process can be performed on the levophase or a left atrial injection to evaluate anatomic details of the left side of the heart.

The angiographic features vary, depending on the position of the great vessels. The abnormality has been described with a normal heart, with complete transposition of the great vessels, corrected transposition of the great vessels, or double-outlet ventricle.

THE NORMAL CRISS-CROSS HEART (CONCORDANCE ATRIOVENTRICULAR AND VENTRICULOARTERIAL CONNECTIONS)

Criss-cross heart without malposition of the great vessels is uncommon. The few reported cases with normally related great vessels have been associated with a ventricular septal defect.

The criss-cross arrangement is caused by a marked

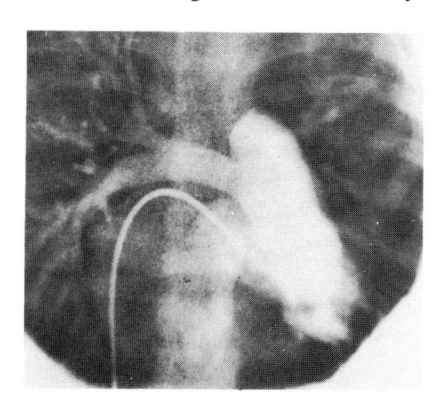

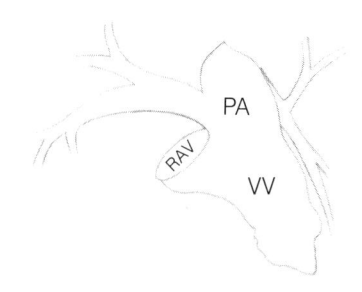

FIG 59–3.
Criss-cross heart without malposition of great vessels. Right ventriculogram. Anteroposterior projection. Abnormal catheter course through right atrioventricular valve *(RAV)* into venous ventricle *(VV)*, which lies along left cardiac border. Pulmonary artery *(PA)* arises from venous ventricle. Normal hemodynamics. (Courtesy of Dr. T. Ovitt.)

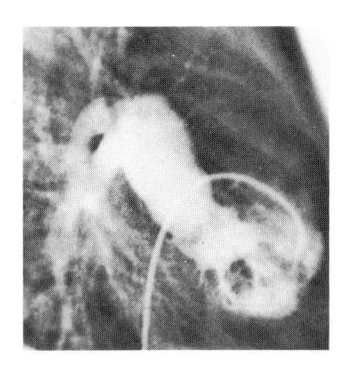

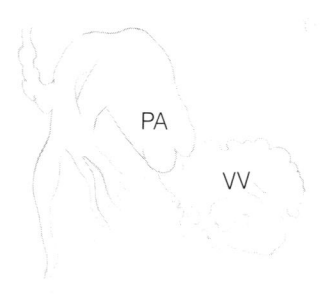

FIG 59–4.
Criss-cross heart without malposition of great vessels. Angiogram of venous ventricle *(VV)*. Lateral projection. Typical trabeculations of an anatomic right ventricle. Pulmonary artery *(PA)* is located posteriorly.

clockwise rotation of a normal heart (Fig 59–2). The following alterations result.

1. The right atrioventricular valve is displaced superiorly, anteriorly, and to the left of its normal position.
2. The venous (anatomic right) ventricle is located higher and to the left of its normal medial position, and forms the left cardiac border.
3. The clockwise rotation displaces the pulmonary artery posteriorly.
4. The left atrioventricular valve occupies a low and medial position.
5. The arterial (anatomic left) ventricle is also located in a more medial position.
6. The ventricular septum separating the trabeculated right ventricle above and to the left from the medially placed smooth right ventricle, lies perpendicular to the anterior chest wall.

Angiographic Features

1. The catheter passes from the venous atrium through the right atrioventricular valve, which is located leftward and leads into the venous ventricle (Fig 59–3).
2. The venous ventricle is a trabeculated anatomic right ventricle (normal atrioventricular connection). On the

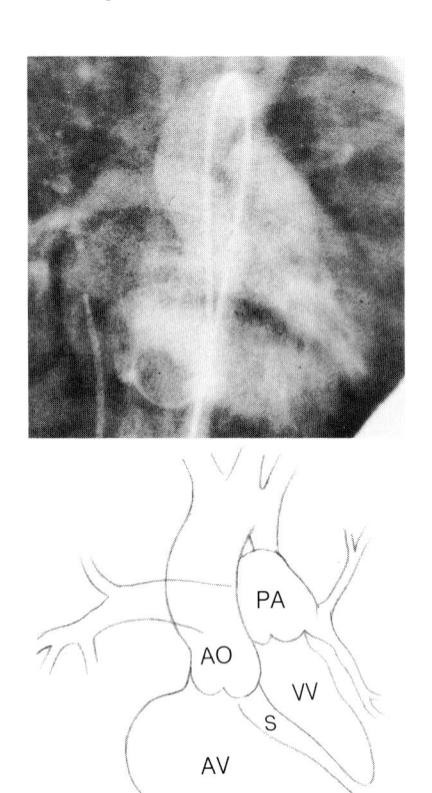

FIG 59–5.
Criss-cross heart without malposition of great vessels. Angiogram of arterial ventricle *(AV)*. Anteroposterior projection. Low medial position of anterior ventricle. Venous ventricle *(VV)* is opacified from a left-to-right shunt through ventricular septal defect. Horizontal ventricular septum *(S)* separates ventricles. *AO* = aorta; *PA* = pulmonary artery.

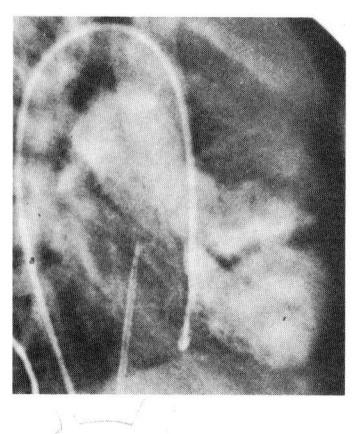

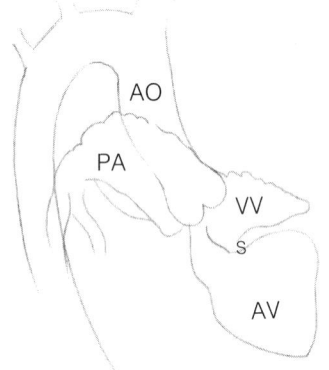

FIG 59–6.
Criss-cross heart. Same patient as in Figure 59–5. Arterial ventriculogram *(AV)*. Lateral projection. Horizontal interventricular septum *(S)*. "Upstairs-downstairs" position of ventricles, with venous ventricle *(VV)* above and arterial ventricle below. Pulmonary artery *(PA)* projects slightly posteriorly to aorta *(AO)* but is not transposed.

lateral projection, the pulmonary artery is located posteriorly (Fig 59–4). This position could lead to a mistaken diagnosis of transposition of the great vessels. If a segmental and hemodynamic approach is used, this mistake can be avoided.

3. Injection into the left ventricle demonstrates the position of the left atrioventricular valve to be low and medial. The ventricles are separated by a horizontally positioned ventricular septum, (Fig 59–5).

4. On a lateral projection (Fig 59–6) the aorta projects slightly anterior to the pulmonary artery, again simulating transposition of the great vessels. The great vessels, however, originate from concordant ventricles. On a lateral projection the right ventricle lies above the left ventricle. The ventricles are separated by the horizontally positioned septum. As mentioned earlier, because of the characteristic location of one ventricle above the other, this condition has also been called upstairs-downstairs heart.

5. The arterial ventricle, which is an anatomic left ventricle, shows a smooth internal architecture and mitral-aortic continuity (Fig 59–7).

CRISS-CROSS HEART WITH COMPLETE TRANSPOSITION OF THE GREAT VESSELS (D-LOOP TRANSPOSITION, CONCORDANT ATRIOVENTRICULAR-DISCORDANT VENTRICULOARTERIAL CONNECTION)

Criss-cross heart may occur with either complete transposition of the great vessels or double-outlet right ventricle. Marked, clockwise rotation of the heart occurs with this type of great vessel malposition (Fig 59–8). The clockwise rotation displaces the right ventricle and aorta toward the left cardiac border, simulating corrected transposition of the great vessels. The right ventricle is displaced not only toward the left but also superiorly. The pulmonary artery and left ventricle are displaced medially and slightly anteriorly. The rotation of the ventricles results in the ventricular septum being positioned horizontally, as in corrected transposition of the great vessels.

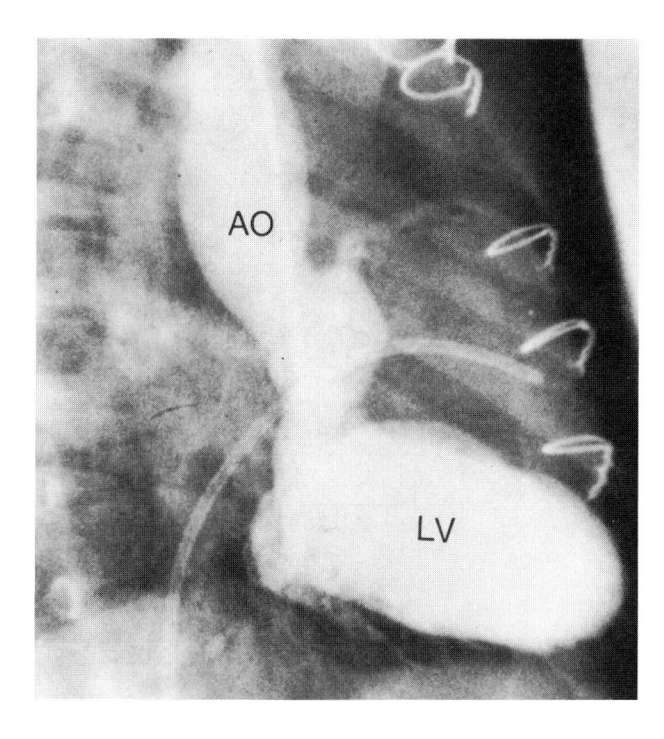

FIG 59-7.
Criss-cross heart. Same patient as Figure 59-5. Arterial ventriculogram *(LV)*. Lateral projection after closure of ventricular septal defect. Smooth internal architecture of ventricle and absence of an infundibulum indicate chamber is anatomic left ventricle. *AO* = aorta.

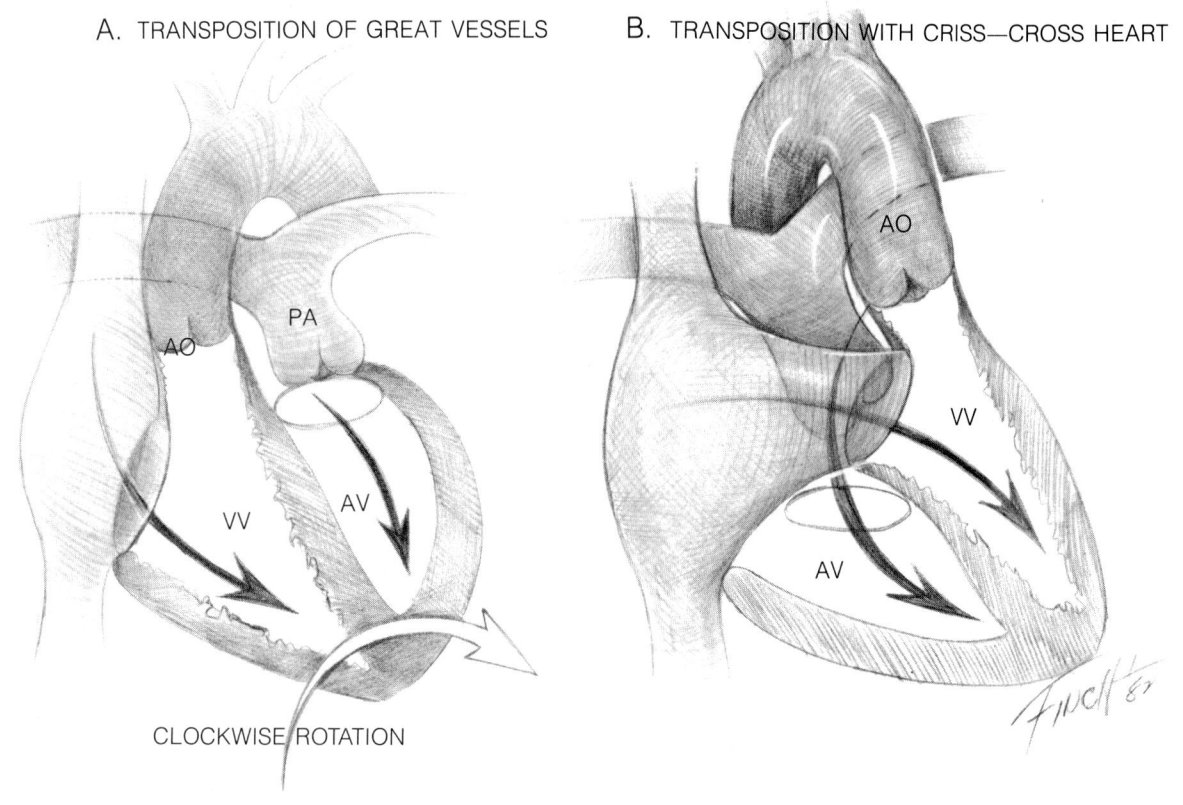

FIG 59-8.
Complete transposition of great vessels (D-loop transposition, concordant atrioventricular, and discordant ventriculoarterial connections). **A,** without criss-cross heart. **B,** with criss-cross heart. Clockwise rotation *(arrow)* around long axis of the heart results in: (1) superior displacement of right (tricuspid) atrioventricular valve and inferior displacement of left (mitral) atrioventricular valve, (2) horizontal position of ventricular septum, (3) superior displacement of right ventricle and inferior and medial displacement of left ventricle, and (4) displacement of the aorta *(AO)* to the left of the pulmonary artery *(PA)* simulating corrected transposition of great vessels. *VV* = venous ventricle; *AV* = arterial ventricle.

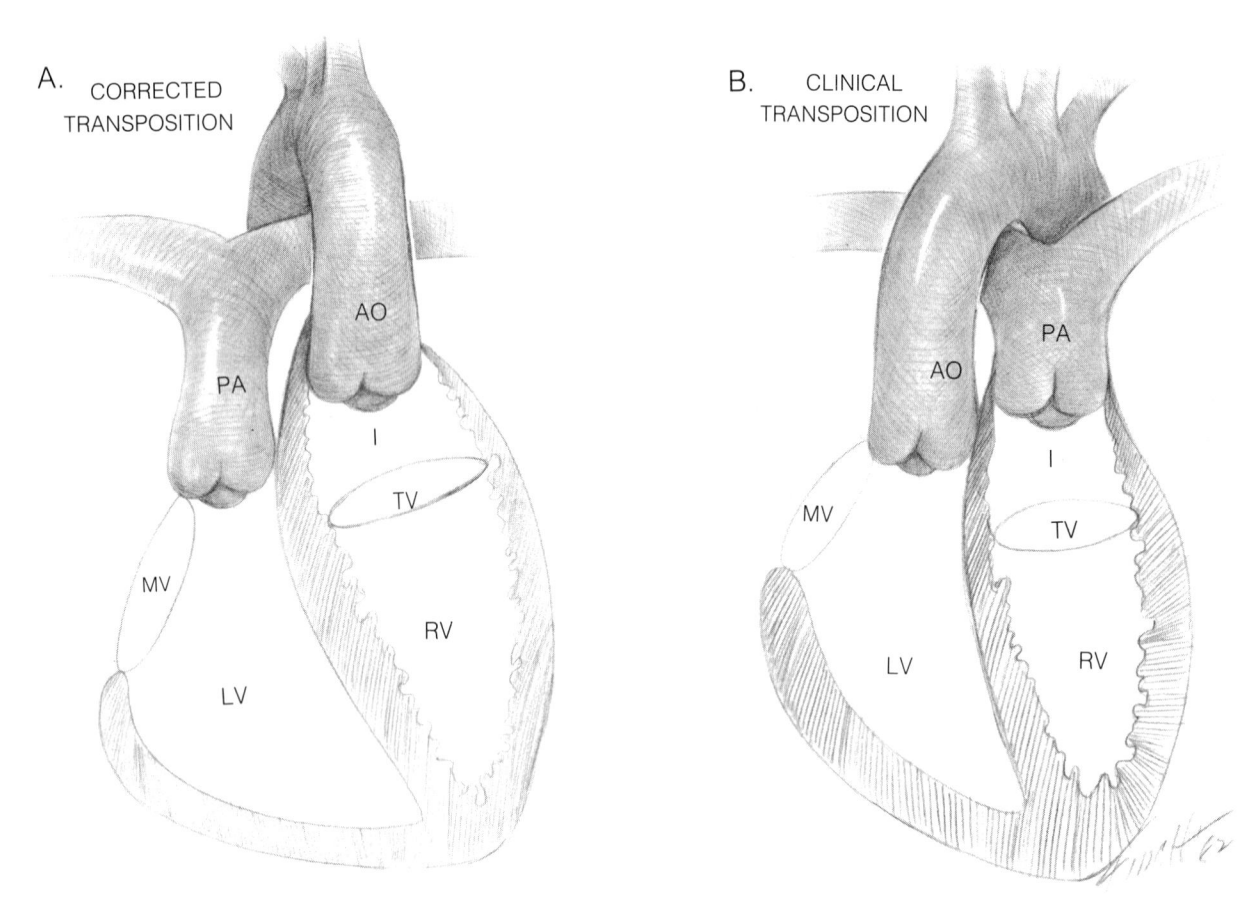

FIG 59–9.
Comparison of forms of transposition. **A,** corrected transposition of great vessels (atrioventricular and ventriculoarterial discordant), an acyanotic condition, and, **B,** clinical transposition (discordant atrioventricular and concordant ventriculoarterial connection). *AO* = aorta; *I* = infundibulum; *LV* = left ventricle; *MV* = mitral valve; *PA* = pulmonary artery; *TV* = tricuspid valve; *RV* = right ventricle.

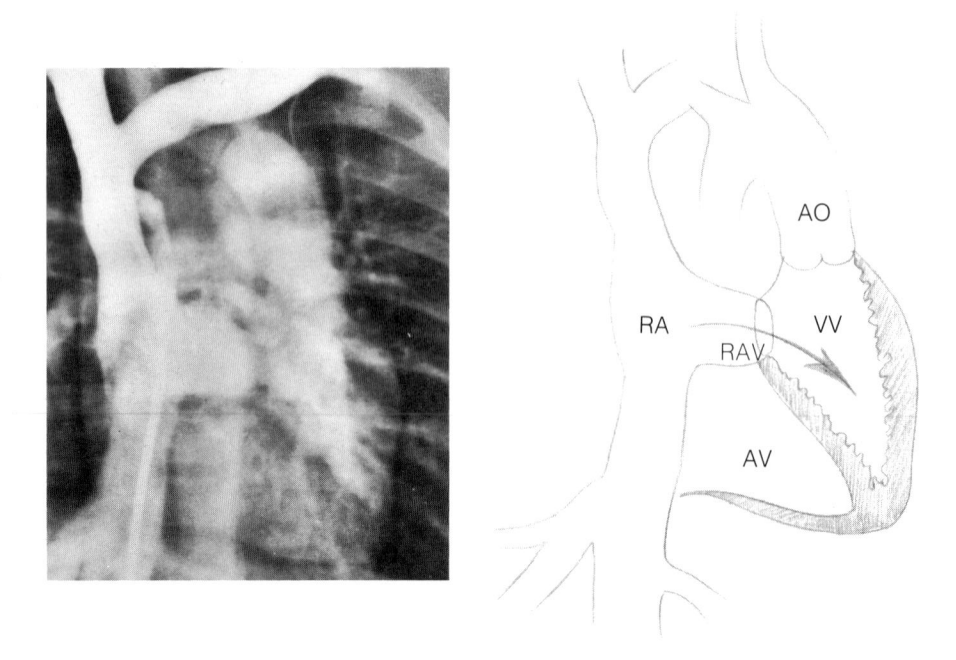

FIG 59–10.
Criss-cross heart and complete transposition of great vessels. Right atriogram. Anteroposterior projection. High and distorted right atrium *(RA)* and unusually long inferior vena cava. Right atrioventricular valve *(RAV) (arrow)* lies high and slightly to left of spine and leads into venous ventricle *(VV)*. Aorta *(AO)* arises from this ventricle and is displaced toward left. *AV* = arterial ventricle.

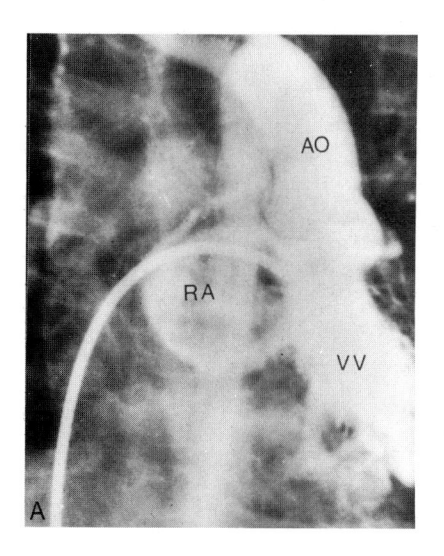

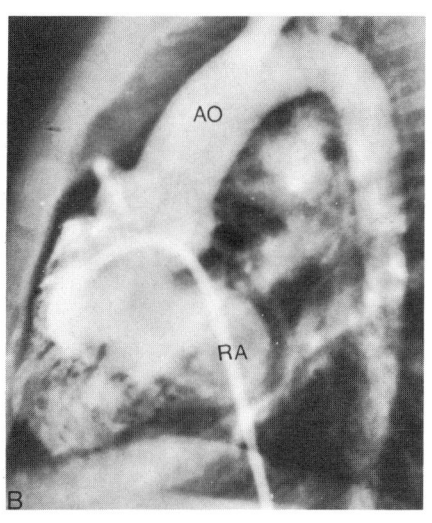

FIG 59–11.
Criss-cross heart and complete transposition of great vessels. **A,** anteroposterior projection. High and abnormal course of catheter through right atrioventricular valve into trabeculated right ventricle. Unusual right atrium *(RA)* is outlined by regurgitation of contrast material. Aorta *(AO)* ascends along left cardiac border. **B,** lateral projection. Anterior origin of aorta from trabeculated venous ventricle *(VV)*.

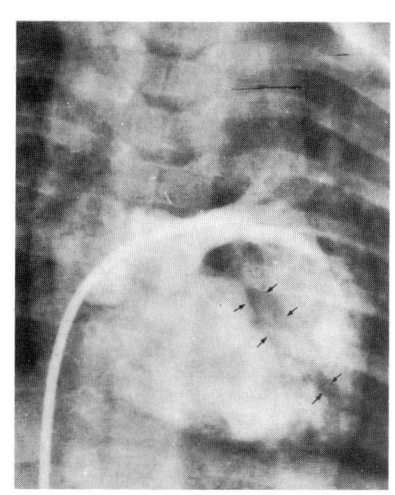

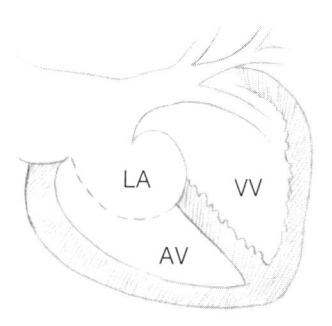

This condition should not be confused with clinical transposition ("isolated atrioventricular discordance," "isolated ventricular inversion"), which has a discordant atrioventricular connection and concordant arterial connection (Fig 59–9) (see Chapter 40).

Angiographic Features

1. A right atriogram demonstrates an unusually long supradiaphragmatic portion of the inferior vena cava. Displacement of the right atrioventricular valve superiorly is a feature common to many criss-cross hearts (Fig 59–10).
2. A selective injection of the anatomic right ventricle demonstrates the architecture of the venous right ventricle giving rise to the aorta (Fig 59–11).
3. The sequential opacification right atrium–right ventricle–aorta is hemodynamically and anatomically consistent with complete transposition of the great vessels despite the atypical location of the aorta, which is located posteriorly.
4. The atrial opacification, either by selective injection, levography, or reflux of contrast medium from the ventricles, is very helpful to identify the atrioventricular connection.
5. Injection into the left atrium demonstates opacification of the medially-placed arterial ventricle (Fig 59–12).

FIG 59–12.
Criss-cross heart and complete transposition of great vessels. Injection into left atrium *(LA)* and left pulmonary vein. Anteroposterior projection. Left atrium is opacified. Opacification of medially placed and low-lying anatomic left ventricle *(AV)*, which is smooth walled. Anatomic right ventricle *(VV)* is opacified through coexistent ventricular septal defect via left to right shunt. Horizontal interventricular septum *(black arrows)*.

CRISS-CROSS HEART WITH CORRECTED TRANSPOSITION OF THE GREAT VESSELS (L-LOOP TRANSPOSITION, DISCORDANT ATRIOVENTRICULAR, AND VENTRICULOARTERIAL CONNECTIONS)

Criss-cross heart may also be associated with corrected transposition of the great vessels (L-loop transposi-

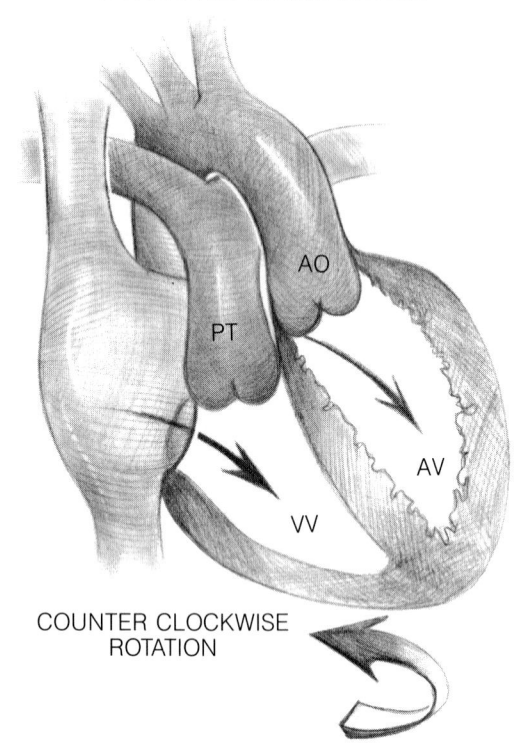

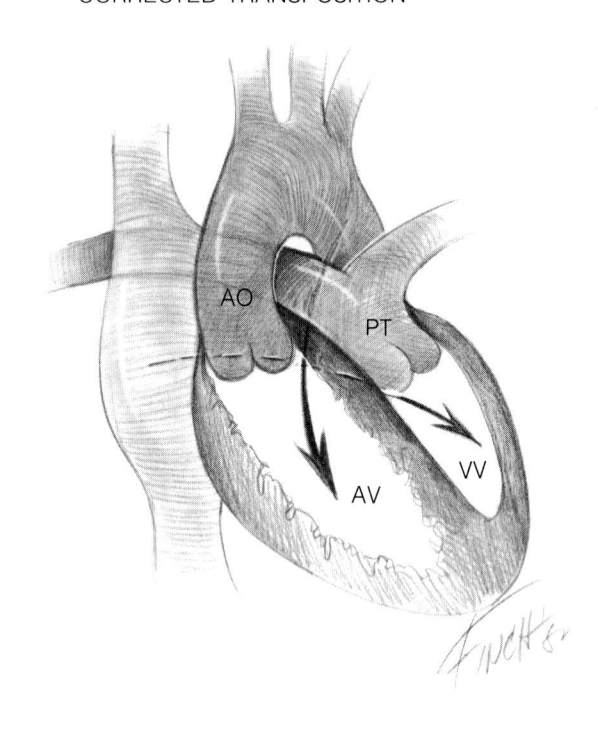

FIG 59–13.
Corrected transposition of great vessels (L-loop transposition). **A,** without criss-cross heart. Medially placed venous ventricle *(VV)* is an anatomic left ventricle. It lacks infundibulum and gives rise to pulmonary artery *(PT)*. Arterial ventricle *(AV)* lies to left and above venous ventricle, being separated by horizontal ventricular septum. Parallel venous inflow. **B,** with criss-cross heart. Counterclockwise rotation indicated by arrow. Therefore: (1) venous ventricle lies to left and slightly above arterial ventricle, (2) ventricular septum previously horizontal now positioned in an inclined frontal plane, (3) displaced aorta *(AO)* and pulmonary artery, and (4) aorta lies anterior to the right of pulmonary artery.

tion). In this situation the rotation of the heart is in a counterclockwise direction. Because of this rotation, the typical horizontal position of the ventricular septum and the characteristic position of the great arteries of the corrected transposition are not present (Fig 59–13).

The internal anatomic features are those of ventricular inversion. The right atrioventricular valve is bicuspid. The venous ventricle has features of an anatomic left ventricle but is displaced. The right atrioventricular valve and venous ventricle are rotated posteriorly. The left atrium is normal, and the left atrioventricular valve, which is tricuspid, leads into an anteriorly displaced anatomic right ventricle. The aorta arises from the infundibulum of this ventricle. The left atrioventricular valve and arterial ventricle are rotated anteriorly.

Angiographic Features

1. Injection of the venous ventricle demonstrates dense filling of the pulmonary artery consistent with the normal hemodynamics.

2. The venous ventricle has anatomic features of a left ventricle. It is smooth walled and does not have an infundibulum. The atrioventricular and semilunar valves are in continuity (Fig 59–14).

3. The venous ventricle lies posteriorly and toward the left of the cardiac silhouette.

4. A levogram of a pulmonary arteriogram demonstrates the pulmonary veins, left atrium, arterial ventricle, and aorta, indicating normal hemodynamics consistent with corrected transposition of the great vessels.

5. Selective injection of the arterial ventricle demonstrates a trabeculated, medially placed ventricle, with an infundibulum giving rise to the aorta (Fig 59–15). These angiographic features are those of an anatomic right ventricle.

SUMMARY

Criss-cross hearts are rotational anomalies that cause confusing angiograms, requiring a thorough hemodynamic

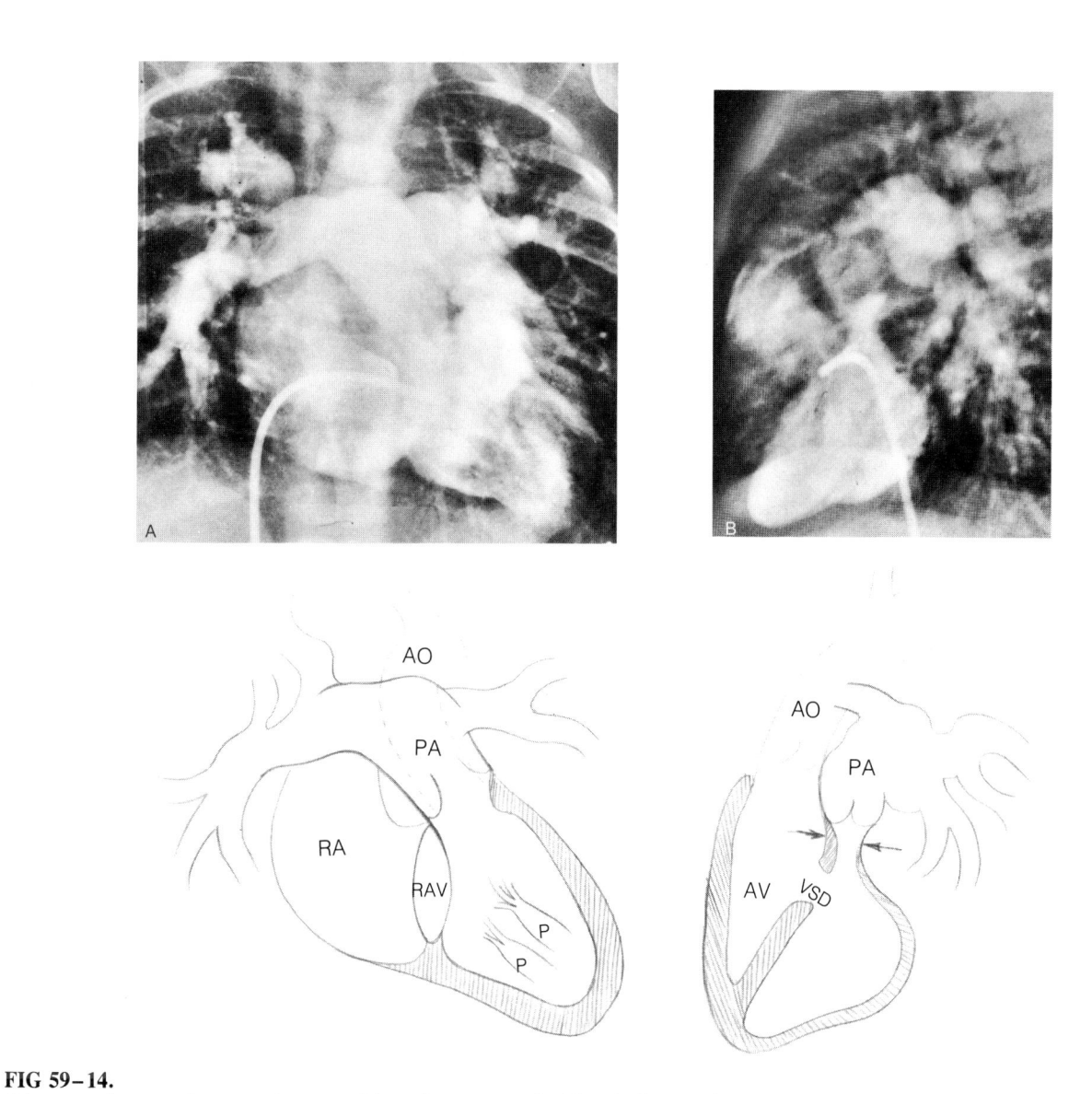

FIG 59–14.
Criss-cross heart and corrected transposition of great vessels. Ventriculogram from venous ventricle. **A,** anteroposterior projection. Right atrium *(RA)* is in normal position and connects to smooth-walled venous ventricle through right atrioventricular valve *(RAV)*. Because this ventricle contains papillary muscles *(P)* and lacks an infundibulum, it is an anatomic left ventricle. Pulmonary artery *(PA)* arises from this ventricle. **B,** lateral projection. Smooth-walled posteriorly positioned venous ventricle does not have an infundibulum. Arterial ventricle *(AV)* is faintly opacified through ventricular septal defect *(VSD)*. Subpulmonary stenosis *(arrows)* is present. Ventricular septum lies in an inclined frontal plane and is not horizontal, as in corrected transposition of great vessels without criss-cross heart. *AO* = aorta.

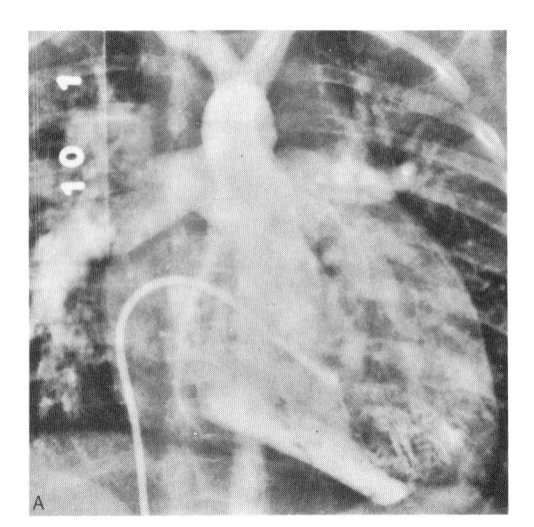

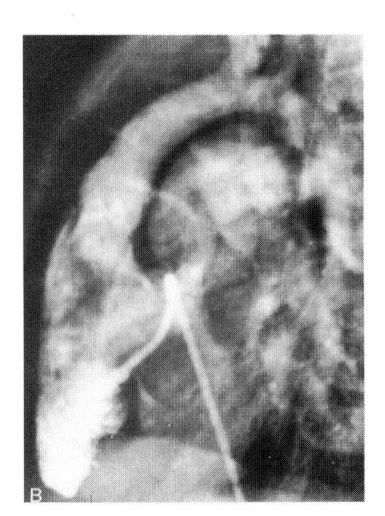

FIG 59–15.
Criss-cross heart and corrected transposition of great vessels. Ventriculogram of arterial ventricle *(AV)*. **A,** anteroposterior projection. Catheter from right atrium into venous ventricle and through ventricular septal defect into anteriorly positioned arterial ventricle. Arterial ventricle is displaced medially and has an infundibulum *(I)*. **B,** lateral projection. Aorta *(AO)* arises from infundibulum of a trabeculated (anatomic right) ventricle. Aortic valve located higher than pulmonary valve. Posterior venous ventricle *(VV)* and pulmonary artery *(PA)* are faintly opacified through ventricular septal defect *(VSD)*.

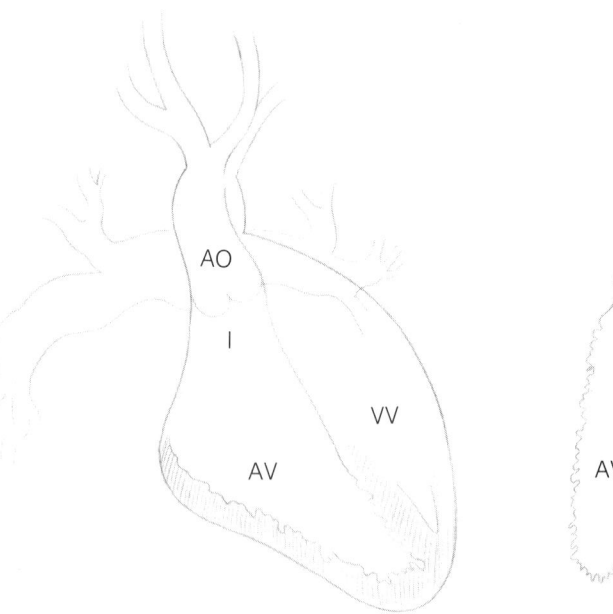

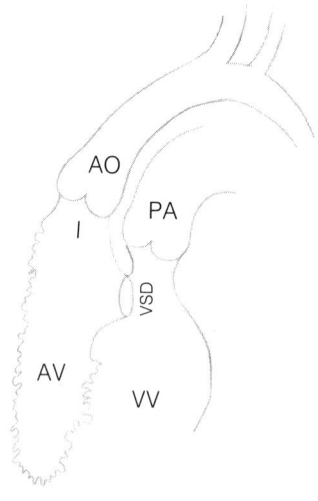

and anatomic analysis. Clockwise rotation of the heart occurs in:

1. The normal heart.
2. Complete transposition.
3. Double outlet ventricle.

and counterclockwise rotation occurs in corrected transposition of the great vessels. Either direction of rotation results in apparent crossing of the venous inflow tracts, displacement of the atrioventricular valves, the semilunar valves, and distortion of the ventricular septum.

REFERENCES

1. Anderson KR, Lie JT, Sieg K, et al: A criss-cross heart: detailed anatomic description and discussion of morphogenesis, *Mayo Clin Proc* 52:569, 1977.
2. Anderson RH, Shinebourne EA, Gerlis LM: Criss-cross atrioventricular relationships producing paradoxical atrioventricular concordance or discordance: their significance to nomenclature of congenital heart disease, *Circulation* 50:176, 1974.
3. Sato K, Ohara S, Tsukaguchi I, et al: A criss-cross heart with concordant atrioventriculoarterial connections: report of a case, *Circulation* 57:396, 1978.
4. Ruttenberg HD, Anderson RC, Elliott LP, et al: Origin of both great vessels from the arterial ventricle: a complex with ventricular inversion, *Br Heart J* 26:631, 1964.
5. Freedom RM, Culhan JAG, Rowe RD: The criss-cross and superio-inferior ventricular heart: an angiocardiographic study, *Am J Cardiol* 42:620, 1978.
6. Guthaner D, Higgins CB, Silverman JF, et al: An unusual form of transposition complex: uncorrected levo-transposition with horizontal ventricular septum: report of two cases, *Circulation* 53:190, 1976.
7. Tadavarthy SM, Formanek A, Castañeda-Zúñiga WR, et al: The three types of criss-cross heart: a simple rotational anomaly. *Br J Radiol* 54:736–743, 1981.

CHAPTER 60

Ectopia Cordis

Ectopia cordis is a congenital malposition of the heart, either partially or completely outside the thorax. Four types of ectopia cordis have been described in the literature: cervical, thoracic, thoracoabdominal, and abdominal.[1] The first type is not truly a form of ectopia cordis, because the skin is intact over the cardiovascular structures. This abnormality merely represented an instance of cleft sternum. Abdominal ectopia cordis was reported once and was associated with a diaphragmatic hernia. The proportion of thoracic and thoracoabdominal ectopia cordis is present in a ratio of 3:2. In each of these two forms, the parietal pericardium is absent and the thoracic cage is small.

In the thoracic type, there is a sternal defect through which the heart is displaced, and the cardiac apex is oriented anteriorly and superiorly. An epigastric omphalocele may coexist.

In the thoracoabdominal type, there is a cleft or absence of the lower sternum, and a defect is present in the lower anterior thoracic wall, epigastrium, and anterior portion of the diaphragm. The ventricular portion of the heart is displaced through the diaphragm into the abdominal cavity. An omphalocele always coexists.

Other noncardiac anomalies are common, particularly cleft lip and palate. Cardiac anomalies are present in almost all cases and represent a spectrum of malformations, usually serious.

Death appears related to complications of the exposed cardiac and abdominal contents rather than to the type of cardiac anomaly itself. Operative repair has been attempted[2-11] and has been successful in some cases. The limitation for successful operation is the small size of the thoracic and abdominal cavities. Experience has shown tamponade of the heart may ensue if attempts are made to close the sternum over the heart. A staged approach is attempted, with the initial phase being mobilization of skin to cover the exposed organs. Subsequently, the sternum is reconstructed with prosthetic material to widen it so a more spacious thorax can be provided.

RADIOGRAPHIC FEATURES

Ectopia cordis is not primarily a radiographic diagnosis, although it can be correctly suspected without clinical information.

1. The cardiac silhouette is highly atypical (Fig 60-1). REASON: The heart is twisted and displaced.
2. The outline of the heart is unusually sharp because of high contrast (see Fig 60-1). REASON: The heart lies outside the thoracic cavity and is not surrounded by lungs but by air.
3. There is usually an associated soft tissue mass in the abdomen also sharply outlined by air (see Fig 60-1). This represents the associated anterior abdominal wall defect and hernia.
4. The cardiac silhouette is sharply outlined by air in all projections (Fig 60-2).

ANGIOGRAPHIC FEATURES

Angiography is indicated because congenital cardiac malformations are usually present. Interpretation of the angiograms may be difficult because of marked distortion of the cardiac anatomy, which results in an "upside-down heart."

Selective angiography is difficult to interpret because of marked distortion of the anatomy (Fig 60-3).

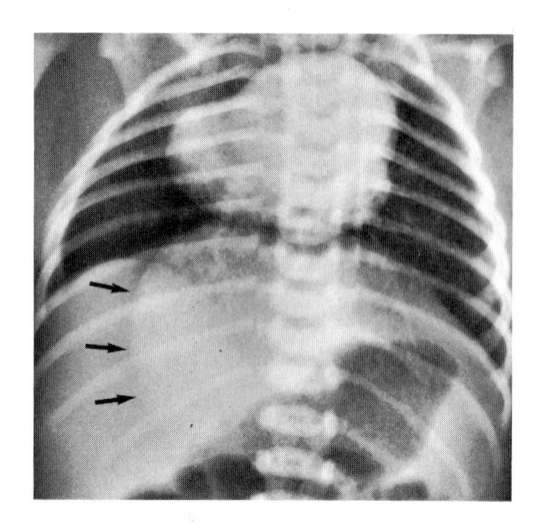

FIG 60-1.
Ectopia cordis. Thoracic roentgenogram. Posteroanterior projection. Normal situs. Right-sided liver. Stomach is on left. Sharply outlined large mass *(arrows)* in superior abdomen is characteristic of anterior wall abdominal defect with herniation. Cardiac contour is distorted. Right-sided apex. Large bulge in area of normal aortic arch and pulmonary arterial segment. Bulge is formed by right ventricle. Heart borders are abnormally sharp because heart is surrounded by air.

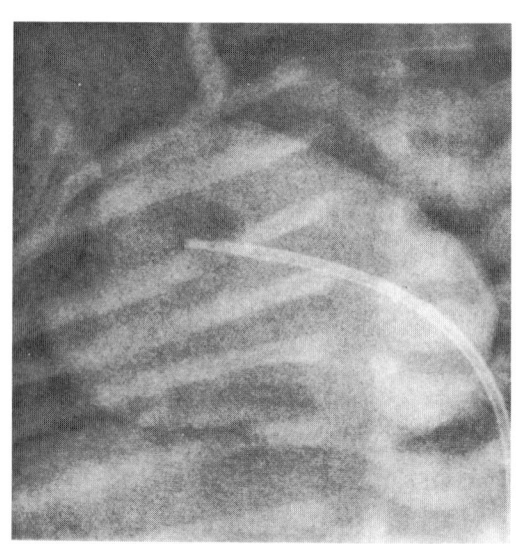

FIG 60-2.
Ectopia cordis. Cine frame before injection of contrast medium left anterior oblique projection. Outline of cardiac contour is sharp because heart is surrounded by air.

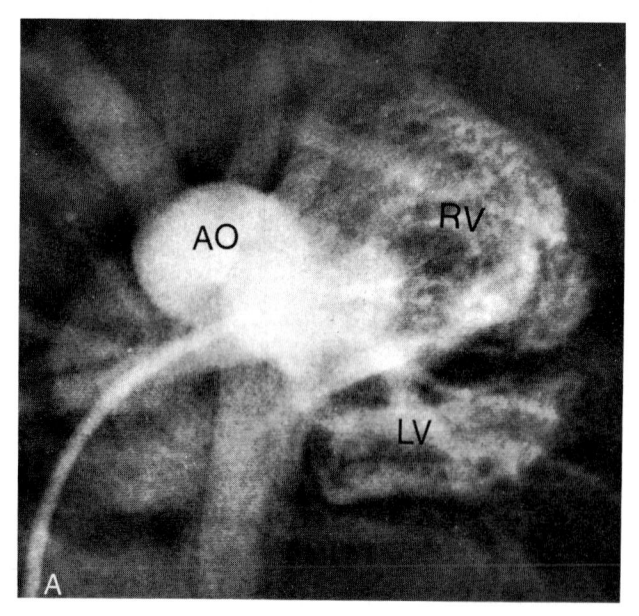

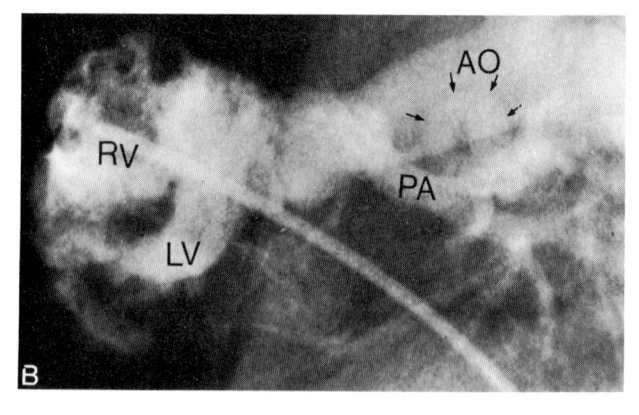

FIG 60-3.
Ectopia cordis. Right ventriculogram. **A,** anteroposterior projection. Trabeculated large right ventricle *(RV)*. Filling of left ventricle via ventricular septal defect. Marked distortion of ventricular chambers. Small left ventricle *(LV)* lies beneath right ventricle and fills through ventricular septal defect. Aorta arises from right ventricle. **B,** lateral projection. Extra thoracic location of entire heart. Aorta *(AO)* arises largely from superiorly located right ventricle. Pulmonary atresia with filling of pulmonary artery *(PA)* through long tortuous patent ductus arteriosus *(arrows)*.

POSTOPERATIVE FEATURES

Although previously most patients with ectopia cordis died within 48 hours, modern operative techniques and advances in neonatal care have permitted survival. After the repair of the anterior abdominal wall defect and hernia and relocation of the heart into the thorax, the radiographic findings are restored to normal.

REFERENCES

1. Kanagasuntheram R, Verzin JA: Ectopia cordis in man, *Thorax* 17:159, 1962.
2. Verska JJ: Surgical repair of total cleft sternum, *J Thorac Cardiovasc Surg* 69:301, 1975.
3. Major JW: Thoracoabdominal ectopia cordis: report of a case successfully treated by surgery, *J Thorac Surg* 26:309, 1953.
4. Byron F: Ectopia cordis: report of a case with attempted operative correction, *J Thorac Surg* 17:717, 1948.
5. Maier HC, Bortone F: Complete failure of sternal fusion with herniation of pericardium: report of a case corrected surgically in infancy, *J Thorac Surg* 18:851, 1949.
6. Jones AF, MacGrath RL, Edwards SM, et al: Immediate operation for ectopia cordis, *Ann Thorac Surg* 28:484, 1977.
7. Cywes S: Ectopia cordis: report of a case with attempted operative correction, *S Afr Med J* 41:37, 1967.
8. Van der Horst RL, Mitha AS, Chesler E: Ectopia cordis with single ventricle and a diverticulum: exsanguination from septic necrosis of the ductus arteriosus, *S Afr Med J* 49:109, 1975.
9. Sabiston DC Jr: The surgical management of congenital bifid sternum with partial ectopia cordis, *J Thorac Surg* 35:118, 1958.
10. Garson A Jr, Hawkins EP, Mullins CE, et al: Thoracoabdominal ectopia cordis with mosaic Turner's syndrome: report of a case, *Pediatrics* 62:218, 1978.
11. Aytac A, Saylam A: Successful surgical repair of congenital cleft sternum with partial ectopis cordis, *Thorax* 31:466, 1976.

CHAPTER 61

Thoracopagus (Conjoined Twins, Siamese Twins)

Conjoined twins is a rare condition, occurring once in every 50,000 births. There is a striking predilection for this to occur in females, many of whom are stillborn.

Conjoined twins are classified according to the site of their union. In the most common thoracopagus form, the anterior thoracic and upper abdominal wall are joined. Because the twins are joined at the thoracic wall, a high incidence of congenital cardiac malformations and shared cardiovascular structures is present. Seventy-five percent of thoracopagus conjoined twins also have conjoined cardiac structures. These cardiac connections may involve the pericardium, the atria, and the ventricles. Conjoined gastrointestinal tract occurs in 50%, pericardium in 90%, and liver in 100%.

If the hearts are not shared, the cardiac apices are directed in opposite directions. When atrial conjunction occurs, it may involve the posterior free wall of the atrium, as well as the coronary sinus. When the atria and ventricles are joined, a complex circulatory pattern occurs; often this is in the form of a shared common atrium and a single atrioventricular valve. Frequently a single ventricle or a large ventricular septal defect coexists as well. No case of fusion of the great arteries has been reported. Transposition of the great vessels or double-outlet right ventricle may be present. Truncus arteriosus and pulmonary atresia commonly occur in the individual twins.

Absence of the hepatic segment of the inferior vena cava with azygos continuation, total anomalous pulmonary venous connection to the coronary sinus, or partial anomalous pulmonary venous connection has been reported.

When different QRS complexes and different cardiac rates are present, only pericardial union is present.

Cardiac catheterization of twins is technically difficult and is mandatory before operative separation. Vascular access is awkward.

ANGIOGRAPHIC FEATURES

The great veins must be demonstrated, because venous anomalies such as interruption of the hepatic segment of the inferior vena cava may occur. The atria must be injected, because in some twins the atria are either conjoined or shared as a common atrium. Ventriculography is mandatory, because most patients have either a large ventricular septal defect or a single ventricular chamber shared by the two infants.

Ventriculography should be performed first, because opacification of the great arteries of both twins is diagnostic for ventricular conjunction. Filling of one aorta does not exclude the possibility of ventricular conjunction, because one twin may have aortic atresia and the other pulmonary atresia. Angiograms are difficult to interpret because of superposition of the hearts on the lateral projection.

Some conjoined twins can be separated by an operation. Therefore, preoperative radiographic examination of conjoined twins is very important, particularly of the gastrointestinal system, liver, and heart, because cardiac anomalies are almost always present.

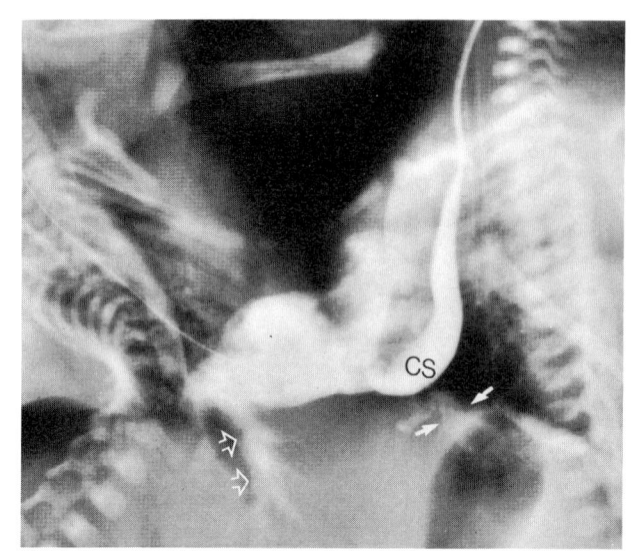

992 Cardiac Malposition

FIG 61-1.
Injection of superior vena cava of twin on right. Filling of coronary sinus *(CS)*, through persistent left superior vena cava, and right atrium, as evidenced by reflux into hepatic veins *(white arrows)*. Immediate opacification of atrium of other twin with reflux into hepatic veins *(open arrows)*. This pattern indicates free communication between the atria of right and left twin (conjoined atria).

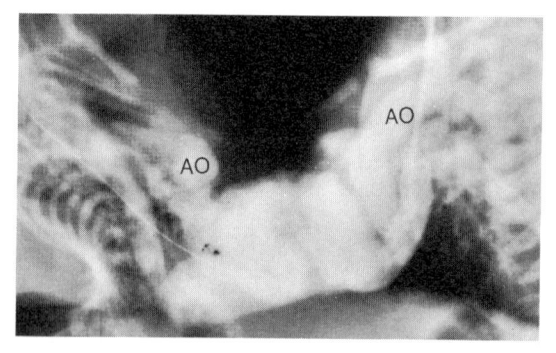

FIG 61-2.
Injection of superior vena cava of right twin. Later phase. Hearts and aortas *(AO)* of each twin opacify with approximately the same density. Free mixing as with a large communication between atria and ventricles. Coexistent pulmonary atresia in each twin. Operative separation is not feasible.

1. After the injection of the superior vena cava or right atrium of one twin, the atrium of the other twin should not opacify. When the atria are conjoined, both atria opacify (Fig 61–1).

2. After the injection of the atrium or ventricle of one twin, the degree of opacification of cardiac structures or great vessels of the contralateral twin reflects the size of the communication and degree of mixing (Fig 61–2).

3. In addition to the atrial status, ventriculography is mandatory to demonstrate the usually complex ventricular anatomy (Fig 61–3).

4. A conjoined common ventricle precludes operative separation (Fig 61–4).

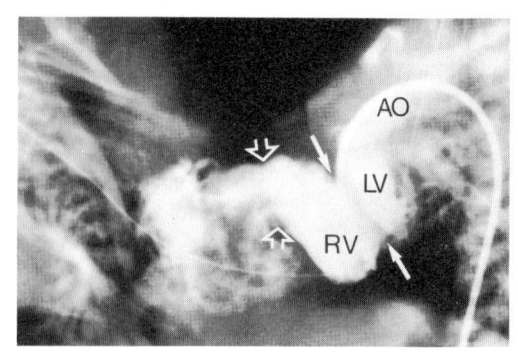

FIG 61-3.
Right ventriculography *(RV)* is performed via retrograde aortic catheterization. Large right ventricle and pulmonary atresia. Both ventricles of the right twin communicate via a large ventricular communication *(arrows)*, approaching a common ventricle. Right ventricles of both twins are conjoined by a large communication *(open arrows)*. *AO* = aorta; *LV* = left ventricle.

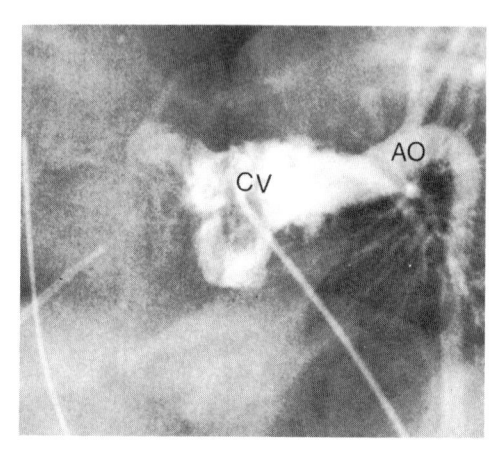

FIG 61-4.
Ventriculogram. Common conjoined ventricle *(CV)* shared by both twins. *AO* = aorta.

PART TEN

Anomalies of Major Blood Vessels

In this section congenital anomalies of major arteries and veins are discussed. Some of these conditions have major clinical significance, whereas others are incidental anomalies that do not alter cardiovascular function.

Aortic arch anomalies are discussed, some of which are merely anatomic variants, whereas others cause symptoms because of their anatomic proximity to the trachea and esophagus. Anomalies of the superior vena caval system are common among patients with certain forms of congenital cardiac malformations and generally cause no problems.

A variety of coronary anomalies, in addition to those described elsewhere in this text, are described. Some, such as origin of the anterior descending coronary artery from the right coronary artery, do not have significance unless they are present in a patient with a cardiac anomaly who requires an operation. Others, such as anomalous origin of a coronary artery from the aorta or an anomalous course of a coronary artery, may cause myocardial ischemia or associated with sudden death, but the frequency of the anomaly or the incidence of shunts is unknown.

Finally, systemic arteriovenous fistulas, particularly those causing symptoms in the neonatal period, are discussed.

CHAPTER 62

Anomalies of the Aortic Arch System

Several types of anomalies can occur in the development of the aortic arch system. Often no symptoms result, and the anomaly is evident only as radiographic finding, but on occasion the anomaly may lead to major cardiovascular or respiratory symptoms. Knowledge of the normal development of the aortic arch and its major branches helps to understand and classify the anatomic forms of the various anomalies that may exist.

DEVELOPMENT OF THE AORTIC ARCH SYSTEM[1, 2]

In the early embryo the first major arterial vessels, the paired dorsal aortae, form and lie on either side of the foregut. Because of the change in the relative position of the cardiogenic plate in the embryo, the proximal portion of these dorsal aortae form an arc and represent the primitive paired first aortic arches.

At the junction of the truncus arteriosus and the dorsal aortae lies the aortic sac, from which sequentially the proximal portion of each of the other five paired arches form and pass posteriorly into the dorsal aortae on the corresponding sides. In the human embryo, all of the six pairs of arches are never present simultaneously.

As the successive aortic arches are developing, the paired dorsal aortae fuse (Fig 62-1), and this fusion progresses cranially. The second arch forms as the first arch is regressing, and so forth through the sixth arch, although in the human, the fifth arch is never well formed.

Although remnants of the first, second, and third arches are present in humans, the major persistent arches in humans, and in which most abnormalities occur, are the fourth and sixth arches.

The normally present derivatives of these arches in humans (see Fig 62-1) are as follows:

First arches: The first arches are a component of maxillary arteries.

Second arches: The second arches are a component of stapedial arteries.

Third arches: The third arches form the common carotid arteries and a portion of the internal carotid arteries.

Fourth arches: The left fourth arch forms a portion of the aortic arch between the left common carotid and left subclavian arteries.

The right fourth arch largely regresses except the most ventral portion which becomes the proximal right subclavian artery.

Fifth arches: The fifth arches are transient, are poorly developed, and have no remnants. On rare occasions the fifth arch may persist, forming a double-lumen aortic arch (Fig 62-2).

Sixth arches: The proximal portion of the left sixth arch becomes part of the left pulmonary artery and the distal portion the ductus arteriosus.

Of the right sixth arch, the proximal portion becomes part of the right pulmonary artery, and the distal part almost always disappears. The distal portion of either the right- or left-sided sixth aortic arch can persist as a patent ductus arteriosus. If it persists

FETAL DEVELOPMENT OF THE ARTERIAL TRUNK AND BRACHIOCEPHALIC ARTERIES

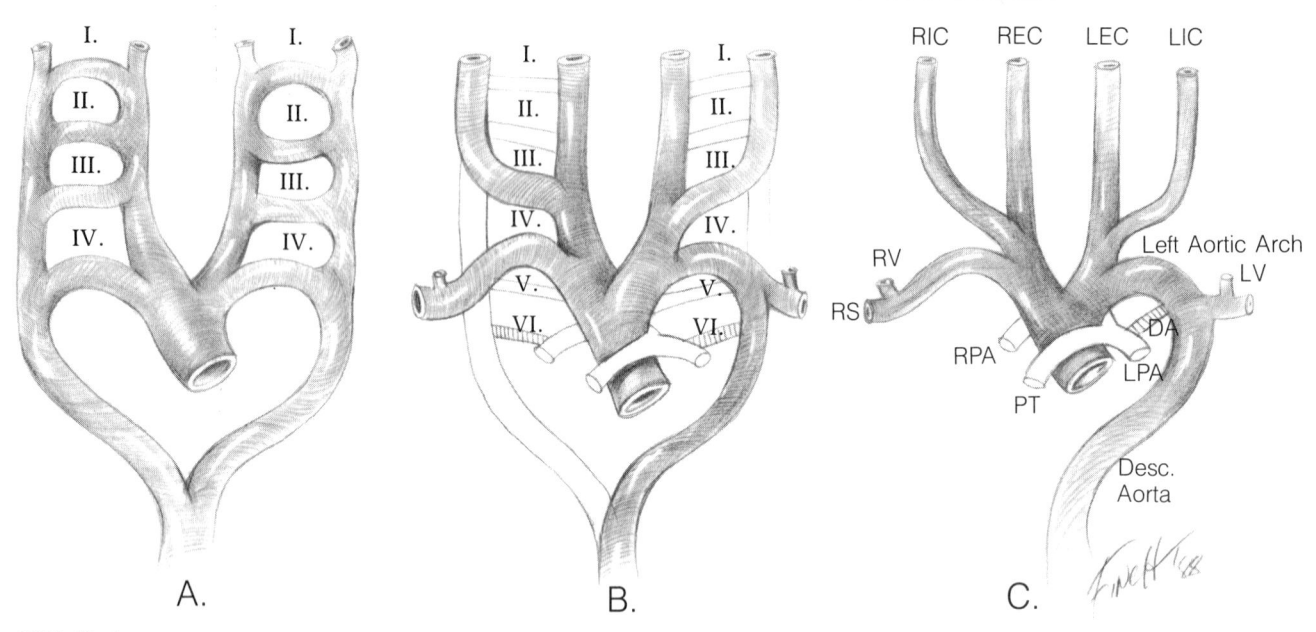

FIG 62–1.
Development of arterial trunks and brachiocephalic arteries. **A,** early developmental stage showing first *(I.)*, second *(II.)*, third *(III.)*, and fourth *(IV.)*, left and right arches, which join and form single dorsal aorta. **B,** later stage showing regression of first and second arches and subsequent development of the fifth *(V.)*, and sixth *(VI.)* arches. At this stage primitive truncus has divided into separate aorta and pulmonary artery. Right fourth arch has also regressed so that major aortic arch connecting ventral to dorsal aorta is on left. (NOTE: Dorsal right aortic arch has regressed, whereas proximal right arch has formed portions of right subclavian artery.) **C,** pattern of aortic arch and major brachiocephalic vessels at birth showing their derivations. *RV* = right vertebral artery; *RS* = right subclavian artery; *RPA* = right pulmonary artery; *PT* = pulmonary trunk; *LPA* = left pulmonary artery; *DA* = ductus arteriosus; *LV* = left vertebral artery; *Desc. aorta;* descending aorta; *RIC* = right internal carotid artery; *REC* = right external carotid artery; *LEC* = left external carotid artery; *LIC* = left internal carotid artery.

	on the side opposite the aortic arch, it passes from the subclavian artery to the ipsilateral pulmonary artery. Rarely, the ductus arteriosus persists bilaterally.
Seventh cervical intersegmental artery:	These arteries of the dorsal aortae migrate cranially to a position opposite the fourth arches and become part of the subclavian arteries. On the left, this artery arises directly from the left aortic arch, and on the right, because of the regression of the fourth aortic arch, the right subclavian artery meets with its most ventral portion.
Right dorsal aorta:	The right dorsal aorta usually regresses except for the proximal portion. The proximal portion forms part of the right subclavian artery. If the right distal aorta persists, it forms a right-sided descending aorta and is present in the condition left aortic arch and right-sided descending aorta (left circumflex aortic arch).
Left dorsal aorta:	The left dorsal aorta forms the distal left arch and the descending aorta. In this condition right aortic arch and left dorsal aorta (right circumflex aortic arch), the mirror image of the circumflex aorta described earlier is found.

ABNORMALITIES OF THE FOURTH AORTIC ARCH SYSTEM

Almost all anomalies of the aortic arch system can be explained by the hypothetical double-aortic arch system of Edwards (Fig 62–3).[3–15] The abnormalities of the fourth aortic arch system discussed in this section result from (1) failure of regression, (2) regression in an abnormal site in the fourth aortic arch system, or (3) more than one site of regression.

A list of the five major abnormalities of the fourth aortic arch system and their basic developmental anomalies follow. In each of these five abnormalities, several anatomic variations may exist, and each is also discussed in individual sections:

PERSISTENT FIFTH ARCH

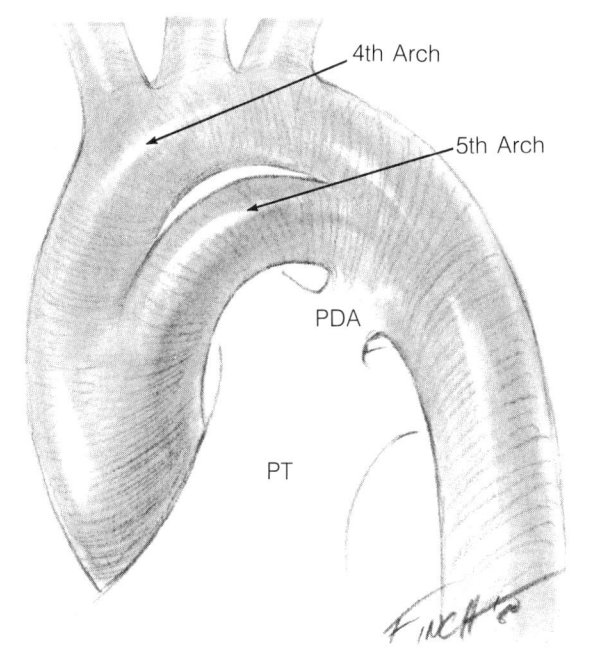

FIG 62–2.
Persistence of the fourth, fifth, and sixth (patent ductus arteriosus [PDA]) left aortic arches. *PT* = pulmonary trunk.

DOUBLE AORTIC ARCH

FIG 62–3.
Hypothetical double aortic arch proposed by Edwards.[4] This diagram showing two aortic arches is used in this chapter to illustrate where regressions occur in various portions of the two aortic arches to result in various abnormalities of aortic arches. *ES* = esophagus; *LCC* = left common carotid artery; *LPA* = left pulmonary artery; *LS* = left subclavian artery; *PT* = pulmonary trunk; *RCC* = right common carotid artery; *RPA* = right pulmonary artery; *RS* = right subclavian artery; *TR* = trachea.

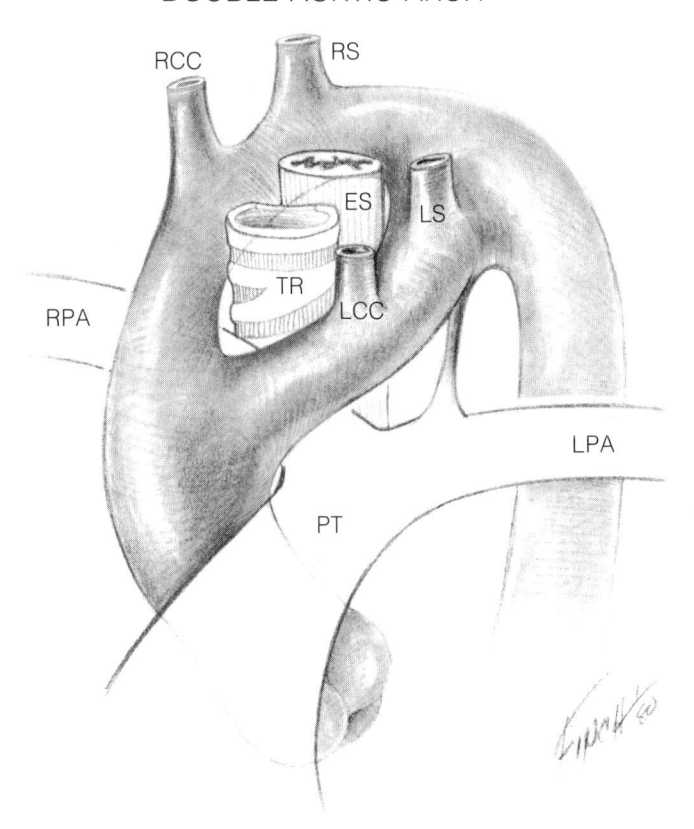

1. Left aortic arch—regression in right fourth arch.
2. Right aortic arch—regression in left fourth arch.
3. Double aortic arch—no regression in fourth aortic arch system.
4. Isolation of a subclavian artery—two sites of regression in fourth aortic arch system.
5. Interruption of the aortic arch—two or three sites of regression in fourth aortic arch system.

Before the individual anomalies of the fourth aortic arch are discussed, five terms need to be defined:

1. Left aortic arch: An aortic arch (fourth) that lies to the left of the trachea and arches over the left mainstem bronchus. The first major brachiocephalic artery passes to the right, being either the right innominate or right carotid artery.
2. Right aortic arch: An aortic arch (fourth) lies to the right of the trachea and arches over the right mainstem bronchus. The first major brachiocephalic artery passes to the left, being either a left carotid or left subclavian artery.
3. Vascular ring: An anomaly of aortic arch formation, in which the trachea and esophagus are surrounded and compressed by vascular structures or fibrous deriva-

998 Anomalies of Major Blood Vessels

tives of an aortic arch. Vascular rings may cause respiratory symptoms or dysphagia.

4. Left descending aorta: Persistence of left dorsal aorta as in normal individuals. This may coexist with a left, right, or double aortic arch.

5. Right descending aorta: Persistence of right dorsal aorta. This may coexist with a left, right, or double aortic arch.

Left Aortic Arch

The left aortic arch courses over the left mainstem bronchus and continues with the descending aorta, which almost always lies to the left of the spine. The types of left aortic arch can be divided into two broad categories: those without and those with a retroesophageal arterial vessel.

Left Aortic Arch Without Retroesophageal Arterial Vessel (Fig 62–4)

The left aortic arch without a retroesophageal arterial vessel is the normal aortic arch. It results from regression in the right fourth arch beyond the right subclavian artery and represents the persistence of the left aortic arch, left dorsal aorta, and left ductus (or ligamentous) arteriosus.

The left aortic arch courses obliquely from the right anterior to the left posterior, above the left main bronchus. The left ductus arteriosus (ligamentous or patent) passes from the anterior aspect of the distal arch obliquely to the proximal left pulmonary artery. The upper portion of the descending aorta is slightly to the left of the midline. The upper esophagus lies medially to the aorta, crosses anteriorly, and at the diaphragm lies on its left side.

The major arterial vessels originating from the arch in order of origin are the right innominate artery, giving rise to the respective common carotid and subclavian arteries, the left common carotid artery, and the left subclavian artery.

In approximately 10% of patients with left aortic arch the right brachiocephalic trunk and the left common carotid artery arise from a common trunk (Fig 62–5).[6] The left vertebral artery may originate separately from the aortic arch proximal to the left subclavian artery in 10% of individuals (see Fig 62–5).[5]

Other less common variations of normal[6] are illustrated in Figures 62–5,D and E and 62–6. These do not cause symptoms except when the innominate artery arises to the left of the trachea and crosses in front of it toward the right. In this situation, the anterior wall of the trachea may be compressed.[7–9]

Radiographic Features

1. In infants and young children the aortic arch itself may be obscured by the thymus. Therefore, the location of the aortic arch cannot be detected. The trachea is the most important indicator.

NORMAL CONFIGURATION OF AORTIC ARCH SYSTEM

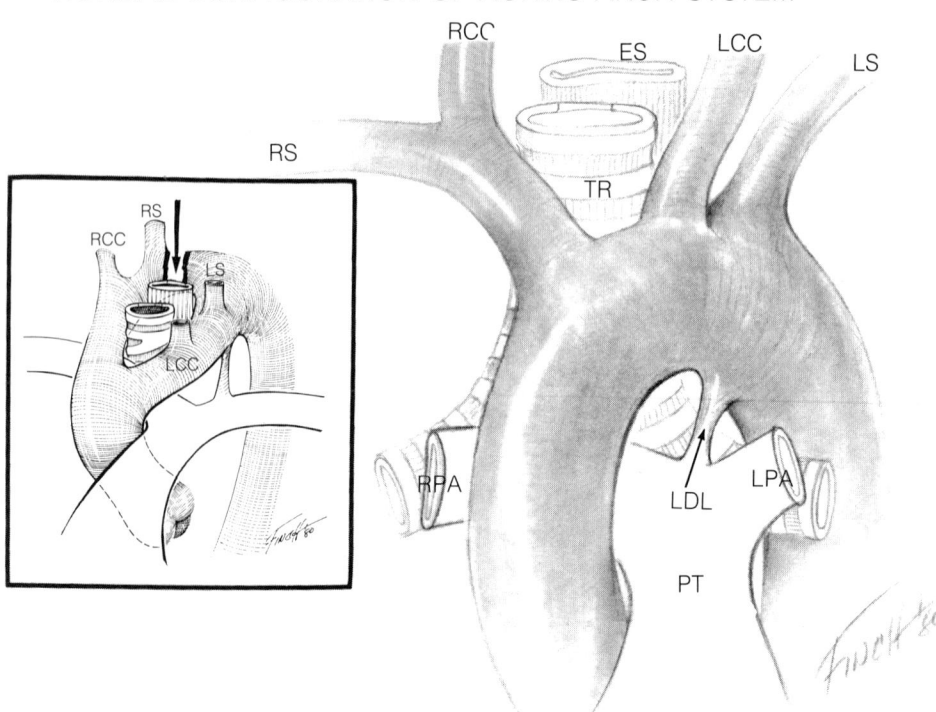

FIG 62–4.
Normal aortic arch. *Insert*, regression of primitive right aortic arch beyond origin of right subclavian artery. *RS* = right subclavian artery; *RCC* = right common carotid artery; *ES* = esophagus; *TR* = trachea; *LCC* = left common carotid artery; *LS* = left subclavian artery; *LDL* = left ductus ligament; *LPA* = left pulmonary artery; *RPA* = right pulmonary artery; *PT* = pulmonary trunk.

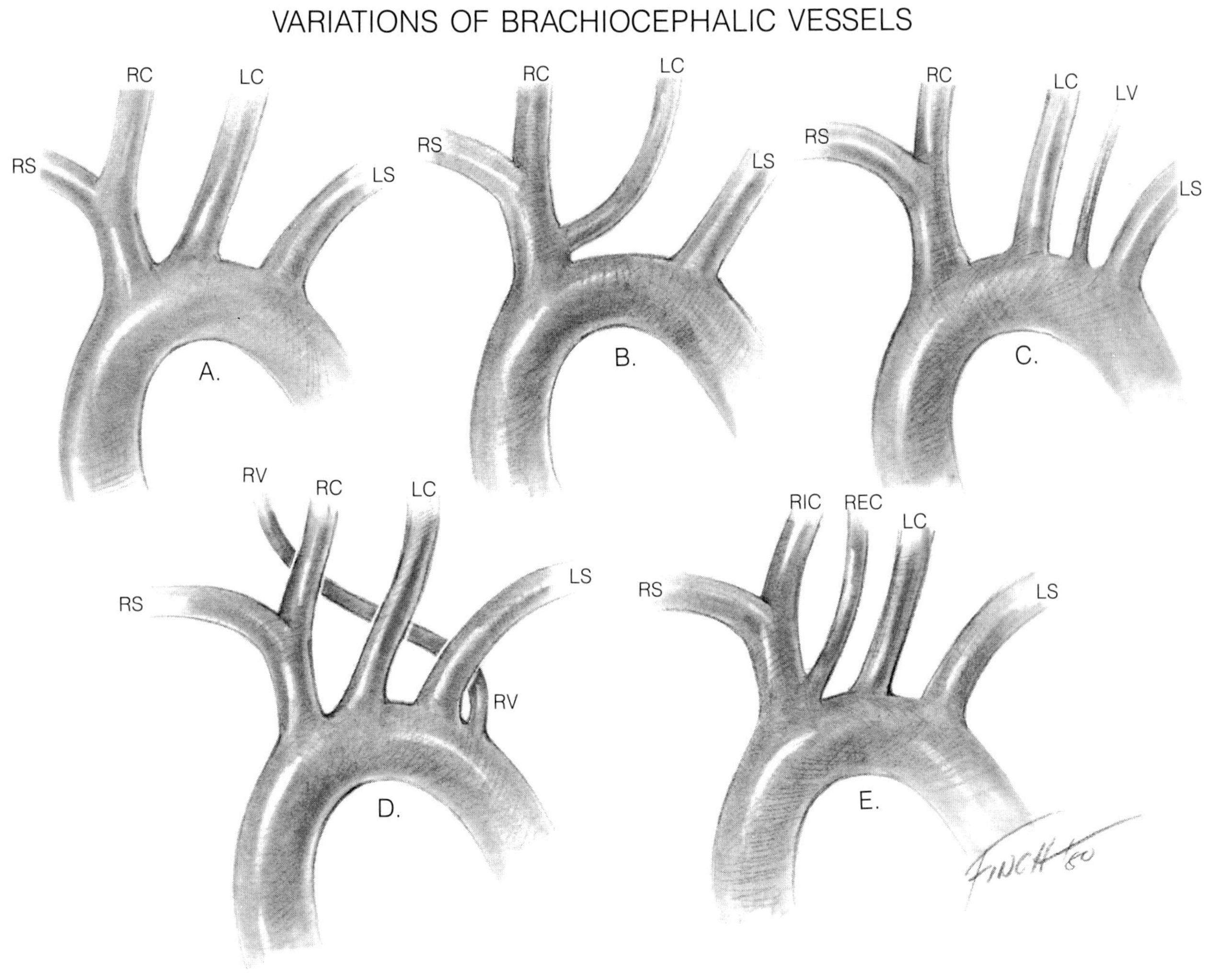

VARIATIONS OF BRACHIOCEPHALIC VESSELS

FIG 62–5.
Common variations of origin of major arterial vessels from left aortic arch. **A,** normal pattern. **B,** left carotid artery *(LC)* arises from common trunk with right subclavian artery *(RS)* and right carotid artery *(RC)*. **C,** separate origin of left vertebral artery *(LV)*. **D,** separate origin of right vertebral artery *(RV)* from arch beyond origin of left subclavian artery *(LS)*. **E,** separate origin of right external carotid artery *(REC)*. *RIC* = right internal carotid artery.

2. In infants the aortic arch does not indent the barium-filled esophagus as in older children and adults. Consequently, in this age group the aortic arch has to be located by the relative position of the trachea.

3. The tracheal air shadow is best visualized by high-kilovoltage technique (120–140 kVp with 1-mm copper filtration) (Fig 62–7).

4. The tracheal air column deviates away from the side of the aortic arch, particularly during expiration. During forceful expiration as from crying, the pliable mediastinal tissues buckle and the trachea deviates away from the aortic arch. A radiograph obtained at this time can visualize the displaced trachea.

5. On a posteroanterior thoracic roentgenogram, the barium-filled esophagus projects slightly to the left of the tracheal air column (Fig 62–8). REASON: The aortic arch crosses obliquely from anterior to posterior and from right to left. Because the trachea lies in front of the esophagus, it is pushed slightly more toward the right. In a right aortic arch this relationship is reversed. This radiographic finding is not infallible and requires a perfectly straight posteroanterior projection.

6. In neonates, tracheal shift becomes more obvious during expiration or crying, where the trachea buckles away from the aortic arch.

7. In a vascular ring or interruption of aortic arch, the trachea does not shift. REASON: With a vascular ring the trachea is fixed by the contralateral aortic arch, atretic arch, or ductus ligament. With interruption of the aortic arch, the segment of the arch that deviates the trachea is absent.

8. Although the descending aorta can usually be seen

VARIATION OF BRACHIOCEPHALIC VESSELS

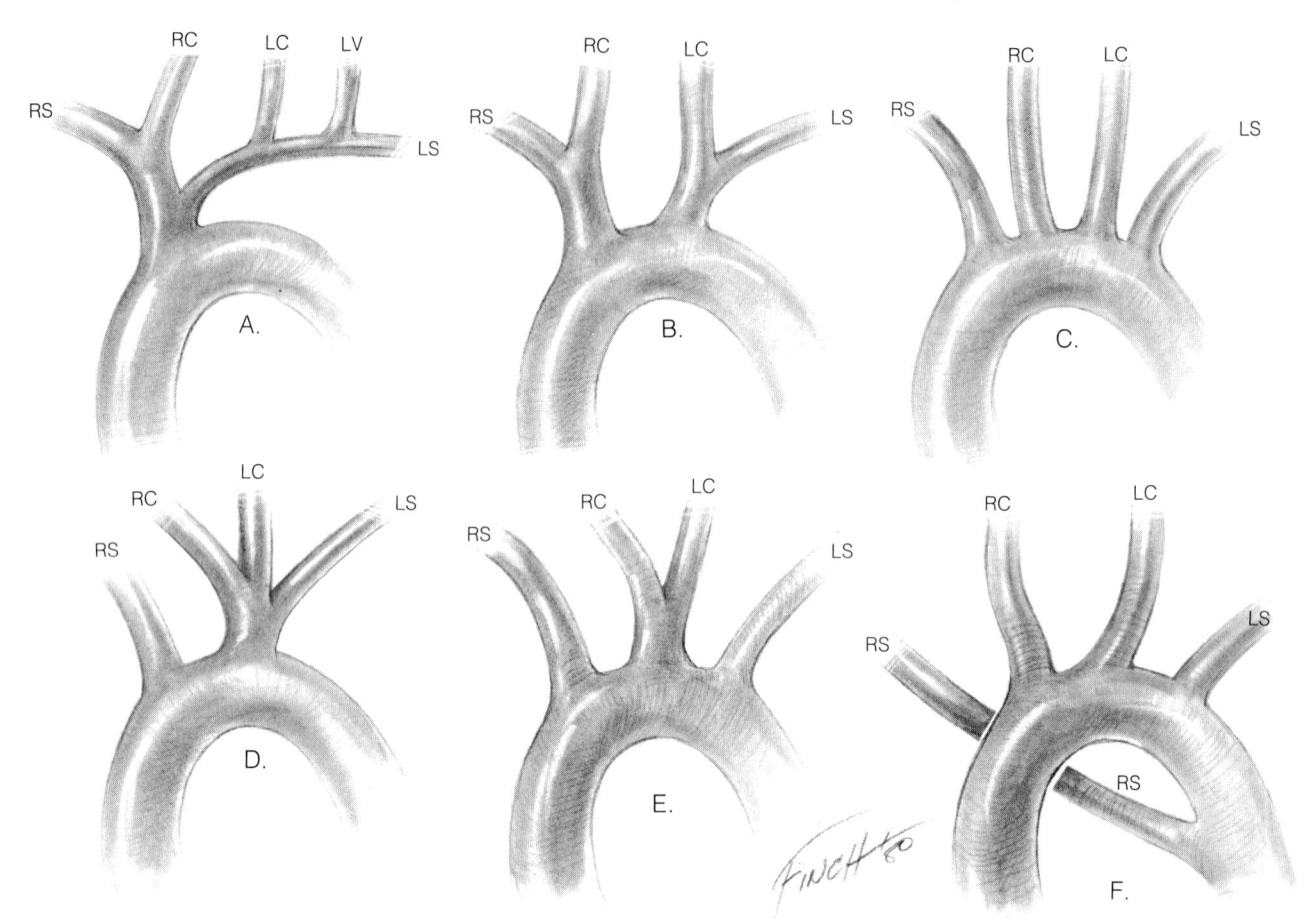

FIG 62–6.
Less common variations of major arterial vessels from left aortic arch. **A,** common trunk with origin of each major brachiocephalic artery. This may represent one form of persistent fifth aortic arch. **B,** two arterial trunks, each supplying a subclavian and carotid artery. **C,** separate origin of each of major brachiocephalic arterial vessels from aortic trunk. **D,** common origin of right carotid, left carotid, and left subclavian arteries. **E,** common origin of right carotid and left carotid arteries. **F,** aberrant right subclavian artery. *RS* = right subclavian artery; *RC* = right carotid artery; *LC* = left carotid artery; *LV* = left vertebral artery; *LS* = left subclavian artery.

in older children and adults, it is commonly not visible in infants. REASON: The descending aorta tends to have a slightly more medial position in infancy, projecting over the spine.

9. Normally a blood vessel does not pass behind the esophagus. Consequently, the barium-filled esophagus is not indented posteriorly by a vascular structure.

Left Aortic Arch With Retroesophageal Arterial Vessel

In two anatomic variations of left aortic arch, a retroesophageal arterial vessel is present. These two forms may cause symptoms and are recognized radiographically by having a left aortic arch and also a posterior indentation of the barium-filled esophagus.

Left Aortic Arch With Aberrant Right Subclavian Artery (Fig 62–9).

—In this form of left aortic arch the right subclavian artery arises as the last branch of the aortic arch and courses from the descending aorta to the right arm, passing behind the esophagus. It has been stated that the aberrant subclavian artery may pass between esophagus and trachea or in front of the trachea, and, indeed, sporadic cases have been described in the old literature. However, it always passes behind the esophagus. It is reported to occur in 1% of the population.[5] This anomaly of the fourth aortic arch system results from regression of the right aortic arch between the right carotid and subclavian arteries (see Fig 62–9, insert).

This is an isolated anomaly of the aortic arch, which is usually recognized radiographically on a barium esopha-

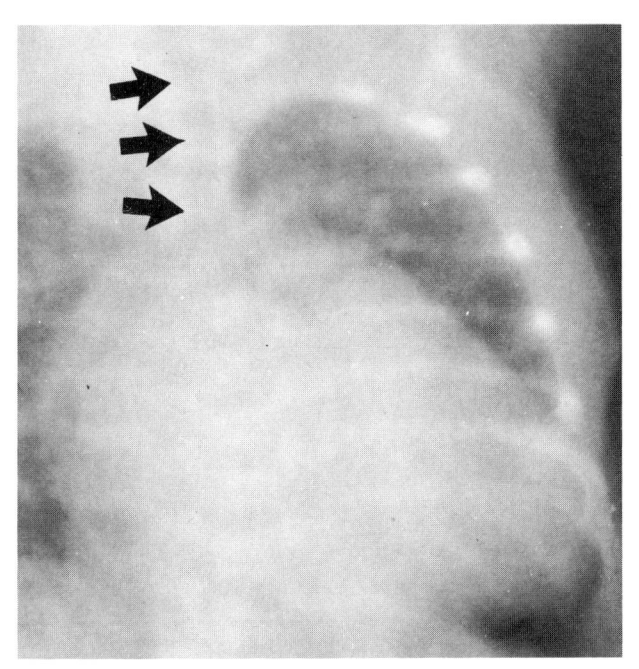

FIG 62–7.
Right aortic arch in patient with persistent truncus arteriosus. Thoracic roentgenogram. Posteroanterior projection. Deviation of trachea toward left indicates right aortic arch *(arrows)*. This subtle finding in cyanotic patient with increased pulmonary blood flow is virtually diagnostic of persistent truncus arteriosus.

gogram performed for other reasons. Rarely, symptoms occur from the vascular anomaly, because the trachea and esophagus are usually not encircled by vascular structures. If a right-sided ductus arteriosus is present between the right subclavian and right pulmonary arteries, a vascular ring is formed and may produce symptoms. In contrast to the mirror-image right arch and aberrant left subclavian artery, the aberrant right subclavian artery which typically does not arise from an aortic diverticulum. Interestingly, Kommerrell[50] described the aortic diverticulum (diverticulum of Kommerrell) in an asymptomatic patient with a left arch and aberrant right subclavian artery on barium swallow examination. The retroesophageal indentation was larger than the aberrant subclavian artery, and he postulated that the artery must arise from an aortic diverticulum. In most cases, however, the aberrant right subclavian artery does not arise from a diverticulum because the ductus is left sided and arises from the aorta.

The anomaly such as other congenital malformations were thought to be a "game of nature" (Lusus naturae, Ludere, Latin, meaning to play). Aberrant right subclavian artery became known as "arteria lusoria" and symptoms as "dysphagia lusoria," which do not exist unless an aneurysm is present.

The only significance of this condition relates to car-

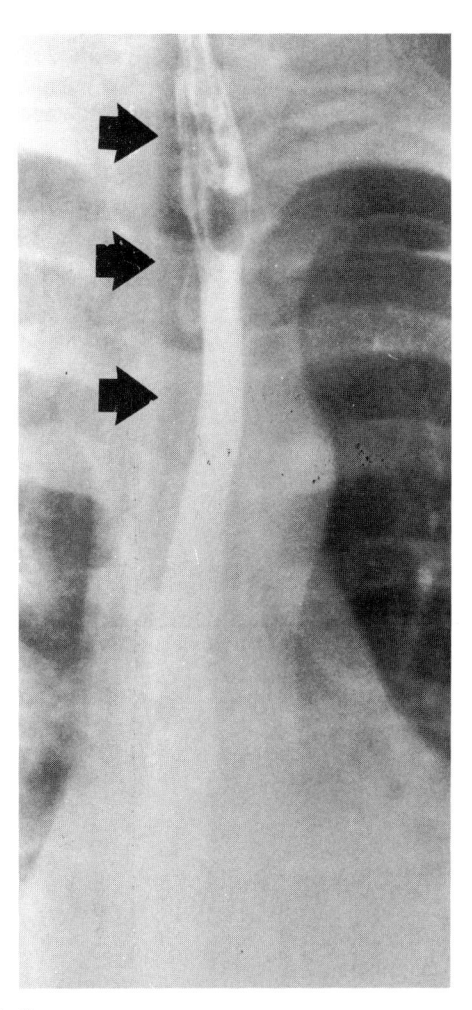

FIG 62–8.
Normal left arch. Thoracic roentgenogram. Barium swallow. Posteroanterior projection. Tracheal air column *(arrows)* projects to the right of the esophagus.

diac catheterization. If an arterial catheter is inserted in the right arm, it passes through the right subclavian artery and enters the descending aorta. From this site it is virtually impossible to advance the catheter into the ascending aorta. Therefore, in every patient undergoing cardiac catheterization, a barium swallow is useful to identify this variation.

Radiographic Features.—Without opacification of the esophagus, the anomaly cannot be diagnosed radiographically, but it may be seen by ultrasound.

1. A posteroanterior projection demonstrates a radiolucent band crossing the upper esophagus in an oblique direction upward toward the right shoulder (Fig 62–10,A). This finding may be subtle.
2. The posterior indentation of the upper esophagus is

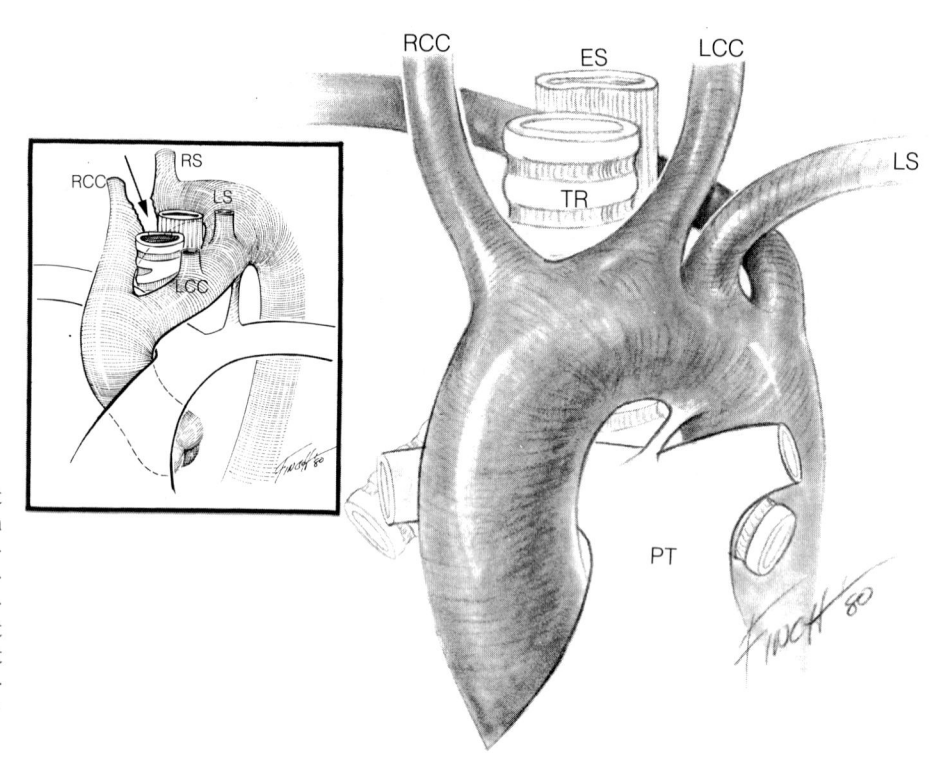

LEFT AORTIC ARCH WITH ABERRANT RIGHT SUBCLAVIAN ARTERY

FIG 62–9.
Left aortic arch with aberrant right subclavian artery. *Insert;* regression in primitive right aortic arch between right carotid and right subclavian arteries. *RCC* = right common carotid artery; *LCC* = left common carotid artery; *RS* = right subclavian artery; *LS* = left subclavian artery; *ES* = esophagus; *TR* = trachea.

usually evident on a lateral projection but is best seen on a left anterior oblique projection (Fig 62–10,B). The right anterior oblique projection is not helpful. Gastrointestinal radiologists commonly examine the esophagus only in the right anterior oblique projection and consequently overlook this anomaly.

Angiographic Features.—Aortography demonstrates the abnormality well (Fig 62–11). The right carotid artery is the first branch originating from the aorta, the left carotid artery is the second branch, and the left subclavian artery is the third branch. The right subclavian artery arises as the last branch from the medial aspect of the distal aortic arch. It passes obliquely upward toward the right arm. In contrast to the right arch and aberrant left subclavian artery (the mirror-image anomaly), an aortic diverticulum is not present.

Persistence of Right and Left Dorsal Aortae

Left Aortic Arch and Right Descending Aorta (Circumflex Aorta) (Fig 62–12).—In this anomaly there is a left aortic arch, but the distal part of the arch passes behind the esophagus and then descends to the right of the spine (persistence of right dorsal aorta). This is an extremely rare anomaly and is usually not associated with a congenital cardiac malformation. We have not encountered a case. In this form of left aortic arch, the embryonic proximal left aortic arch and the right dorsal aorta persists (see Fig 62–12). There are two anatomic variations according to the site of origin of the right subclavian artery:

1. Mirror-image branching (see Fig 62–12, A).
2. Right subclavian artery arising as a fourth branch from a diverticulum from the descending aorta (see Fig 62–12,B).

In either case, if a right-sided ductus arteriosus is present, a vascular ring is formed and may produce symptoms; otherwise, it may not be evident clinically.

The more common mirror-image form of circumflex aortic arch, right arch with left descending aorta (circumflex aortic arch), is discussed in the following section on right aortic arch.

Radiographic Features

1. The aortic knob is visualized on the left, but the descending aorta casts a shadow along the right side of the spine.
2. The barium-filled esophagus is indented from behind by a large structure, which is the circumflex aortic arch. The indentation is large and has a horizontal or slightly descending course toward the right.
3. The large size and direction of the indentation al-

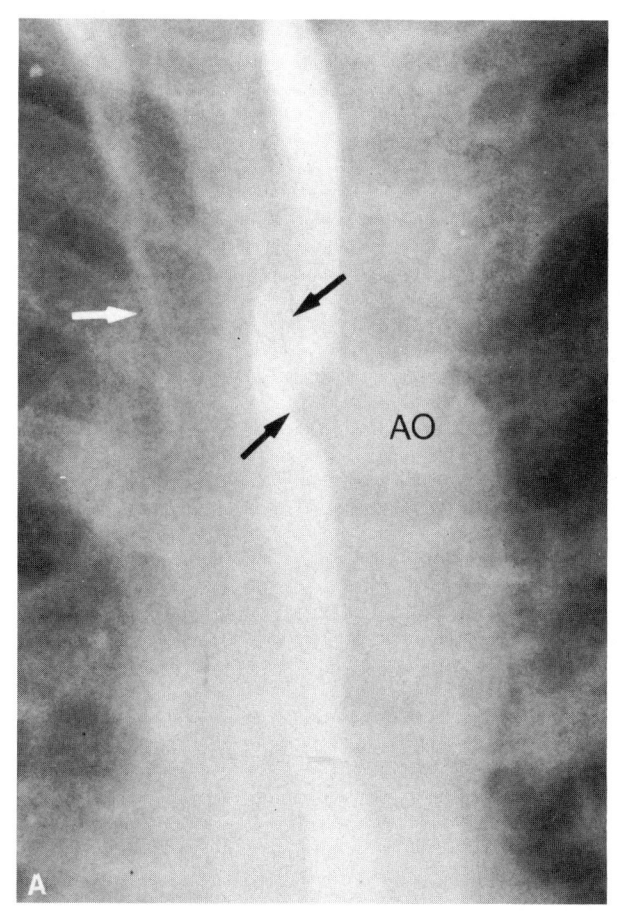

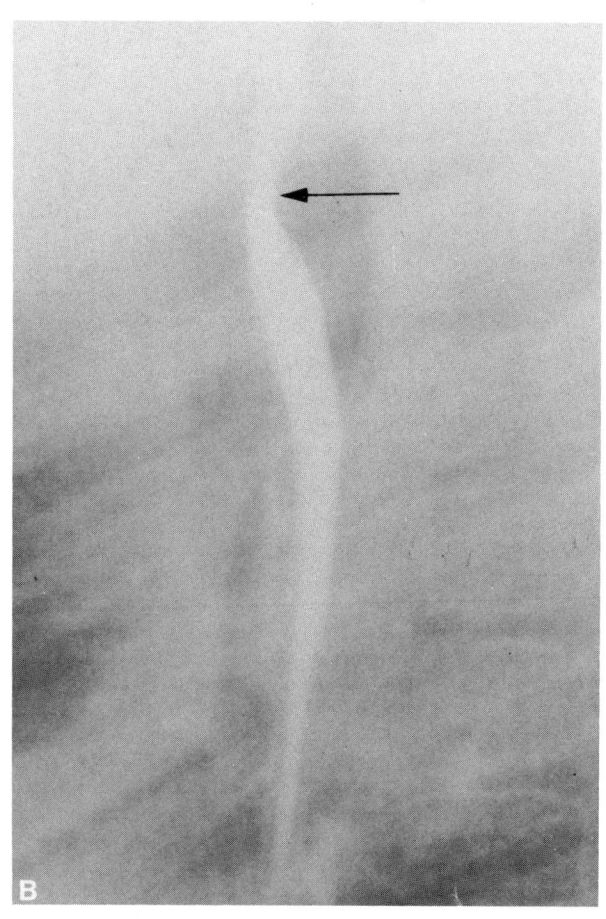

FIG 62–10.
Left aortic arch with aberrant right subclavian artery. Thoracic roentgenogram. **A,** posteroanterior projection. Characteristic oblique indentation of barium-filled esophagus *(black arrows)* toward right shoulder. Trachea *(white arrows)* projected to right of esophagus indicates that aortic arch is left sided. *AO* = aorta. **B,** lateral projection. Aberrant right subclavian artery typically causes small indentation *(arrow)* of barium-filled esophagus. *AO* = aorta.

low differentiation from the more common condition, left aortic arch and aberrant right subclavian artery. In the latter, the posterior indentation is smaller and passes obliquely and upward toward the right.

Angiographic Features.—In this condition, an aortogram shows the ascending aorta, and a left aortic arch, from which the brachiocephalic arteries arise. Beyond the arch the aorta continues downward and toward the right before turning caudally to descend along the right side of the spine.

Angiography allows differentiation from two other conditions causing similar radiographic findings, namely:

1. A double aortic arch with a right descending aorta (discussed subsequently). This condition has two arches, one lying anteriorly and the other posteriorly. If the anterior arch is atretic, differentiation from circumflex arch cannot be made.

2. A left arch with an aberrant right subclavian artery. The retroesophageal indentation is smaller and oblique as previously discussed.

Operative Consideration.—If patients need an operation for relief of the symptoms of a vascular ring, the right-sided ductus ligament should be divided. We have no operative experience with patients with left circumflex aortic arch and right descending aorta.

Persistence of both dorsal aortae

"Duplication of the thoracic aorta" is an exceedingly rare condition. Anatomically, two thoracic aortae are present, one of them giving rise to intercostal arteries. It represents a persistence of the two primitive thoracic aortae. If this fusion does not take place, two aortae persist. Agenesis of one kidney may occur. Angiography demonstrates one aorta without intercostal arteries (Fig 62–13,A). The duplicated aorta gives rise to intercostal arteries (Fig 62–13,B).

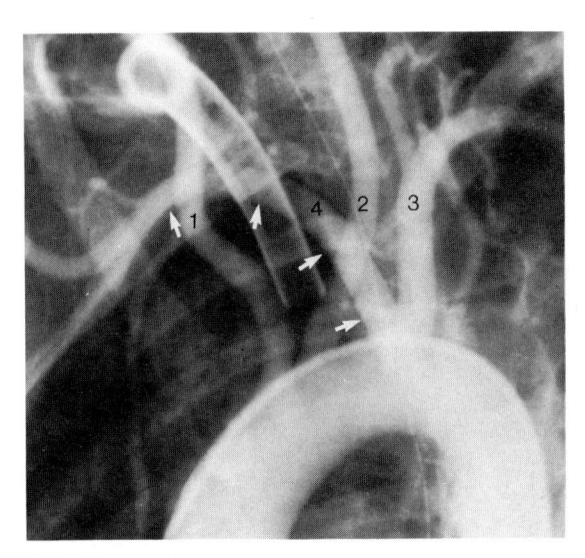

FIG 62-11.
Aortogram in patient with aberrant right subclavian artery. First branch from aortic arch is right carotid, the second is left carotid, the third is left subclavian, and the last branch is aberrant right subclavian artery. Contrary to the aberrant left subclavian artery, the aberrant right subclavian artery does not arise from a diverticulum (exceptions exist).

Both aortae join above the renal arteries to form a normal abdominal aorta.

Right Aortic Arch

In a right aortic arch, the arch courses to the right of the trachea and passes over the right mainstem bronchus. The incidence of right aortic arch is unknown. It is rare in normal individuals and common (1.4%) in patients with a congenital cardiac malformation.[10-12] As in left aortic arch, right aortic arch may occur either with or without a retroesophageal segment.

Right Aortic Arch Without a Retroesophageal Segment or Vessel (Mirror-Image Left Aortic Arch) (Fig 62-14)

In this form the aortic arch passes over the right mainstem bronchus and to the right of the trachea and esophagus. The arterial branches of the aortic arch in order are (1) the left innominate artery, (2) the right common carotid artery, and (3) the right subclavian artery. The proximal descending aorta is on the *right*.

This condition results from regression in the distal left aortic arch beyond the left subclavian artery (see Fig 62-14, insert). Either the left or right sixth aortic arch (ductus arteriosus) may persist.

Right aortic arch without retroesophageal segment is almost always associated with a congenital cardiac anomaly and (rarely) occurs as an isolated lesion.[12, 13] The most common cardiac malformation associated with this type of right aortic arch are tetralogy of Fallot, persistent truncus arteriosus, transposition with pulmonary stenosis, and ventricular septal defect with infundibular pulmonary stenosis; a less frequent anomaly is tricuspid atresia.

The clinical symptoms are dominated by the associated congenital cardiac malformations. By itself the right aortic arch does not cause symptoms.

The ductus arteriosus may show one of two patterns, neither of which causes a vascular ring:

1. Left ductus arteriosus. Passes from proximal left subclavian artery to left pulmonary artery (most common type).
2. Right ductus arteriosus. Mirror-image right aortic arch (very rare).

Radiographic Features.[12]—Identification of the mirror-image aortic arch in patients with a cardiac malformation is important, especially in those who require operative creation of a systemic to pulmonary arterial shunt.

1. The trachea deviates to the left (see Fig 62-7). REASON: The aortic arch is in direct contact with the trachea and pushes the trachea away from the aortic arch. This is particularly prominent in infants. During expiration, the pliable mediastinum buckles away from the aortic arch. This deviation does not occur with double aortic arch, where the trachea is fixed between the right and left aortic arches.
2. The trachea projects slightly to the left of the barium-filled esophagus. REASON: The aortic arch crosses obliquely from left anterior to right posterior, and the trachea lies in front and is displaced more to the left than the posteriorly positioned esophagus.
3. The barium-filled esophagus is indented from the right. This finding is seen only in older children and adults, in whom the aortic knob is well developed.

Right Aortic Arch With Retroesophageal Segment or Vessel

There are two anatomic variations of right aortic arch with retroesophageal segment or vessel:

1. Right aortic arch with aberrant left subclavian artery.
2. Right aortic arch With left descending aorta (circumflex aorta).

These forms may cause symptoms if a vascular ring is completed by a ductus ligament. They are suspected when

Anomalies of the Aortic Arch System **1005**

LEFT CIRCUMFLEX AORTIC ARCH

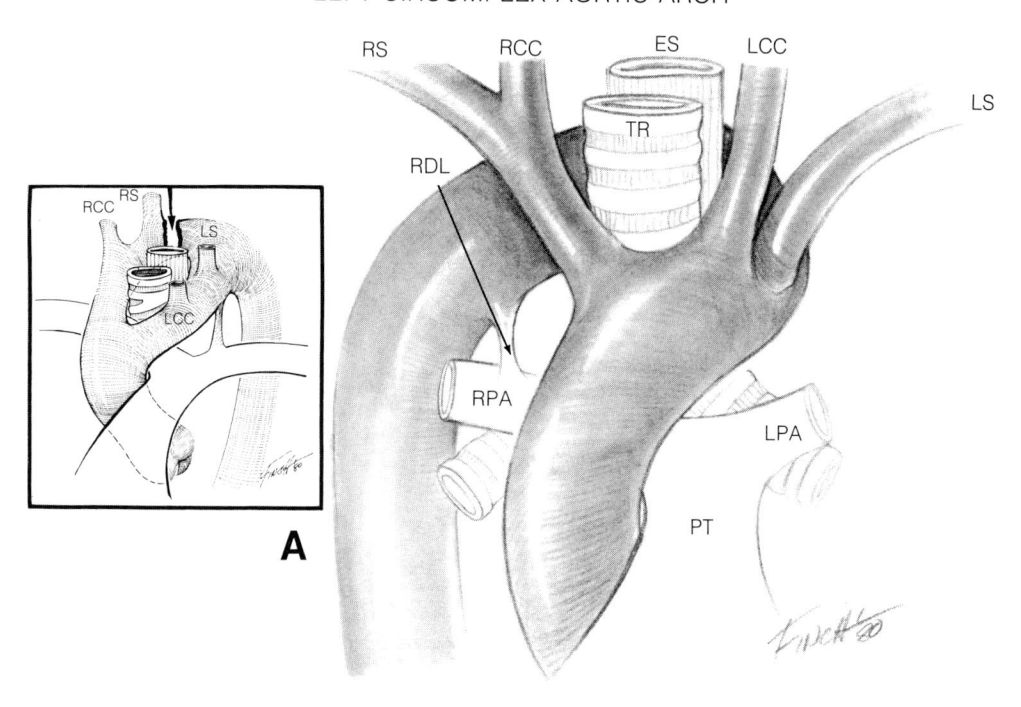

LEFT AORTIC ARCH WITH ABERRANT RIGHT SUBCLAVIAN ARTERY AND RIGHT DESCENDING AORTA

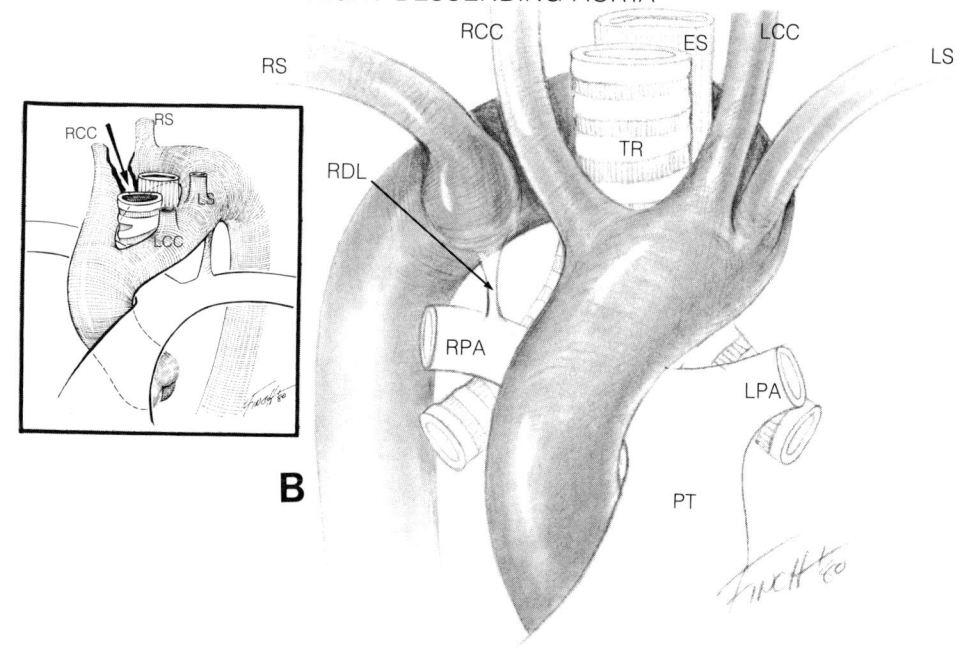

FIG 62–12.
Left aortic arch and right descending aorta (circumflex aorta). **A,** uncommon type of circumflex aortic arch. Right subclavian artery *(RS)* arises from diverticulum of right arch. *Insert,* regression of primitive right fourth arch between right common carotid *(RCC)* and right subclavian arteries and persistence of primitive right dorsal aorta. *LS* = left subclavian artery; *LCC* = left common carotid artery; *RPA* = right pulmonary artery; *LPA* = left pulmonary artery; *PT* = pulmonary trunk; *TR* = trachea; *ES* = esophagus; *RDL* = right ductus ligament. **B,** right subclavian artery originates from innominate artery. *Insert,* regression of primitive right aortic arch beyond right subclavian artery. In both Figures 62–12 and 62–13, right-sided ductus arteriosus completes a vascular ring.

1006   *Anomalies of Major Blood Vessels*

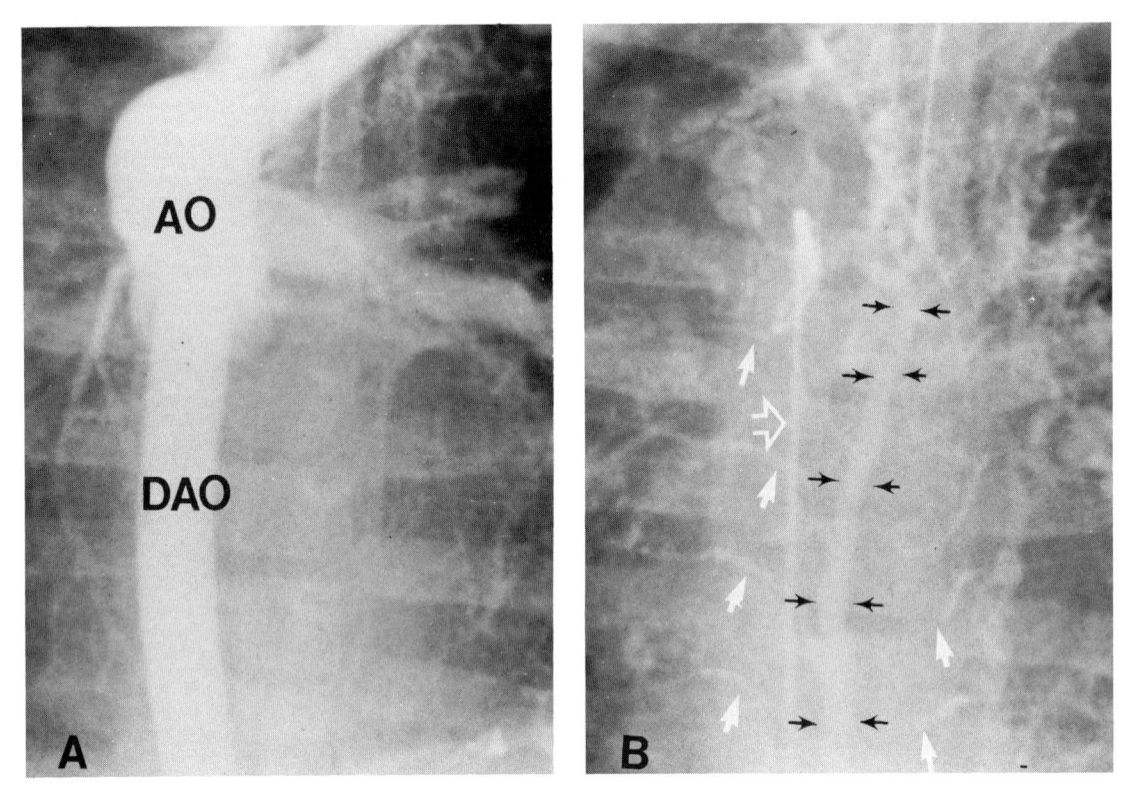

FIG 62-13.
Cyanotic congenital heart disease. **A,** aortogram. Anteroposterior projection. Right aortic arch *(AO)* with right descending aorta *(DAO)*. No intercostal arteries are opacified. **B,** after the contrast medium has cleared, the catheter is seen in the larger descending aorta *(open arrow)*. A much smaller additional descending aorta is visualized *(black arrow)*; giving rise to intercostal arteries *(white arrows)*. (Courtesy of Dr. A. Formanek.)

RIGHT AORTIC ARCH AND ABERRANT LEFT SUBCLAVIAN ARTERY

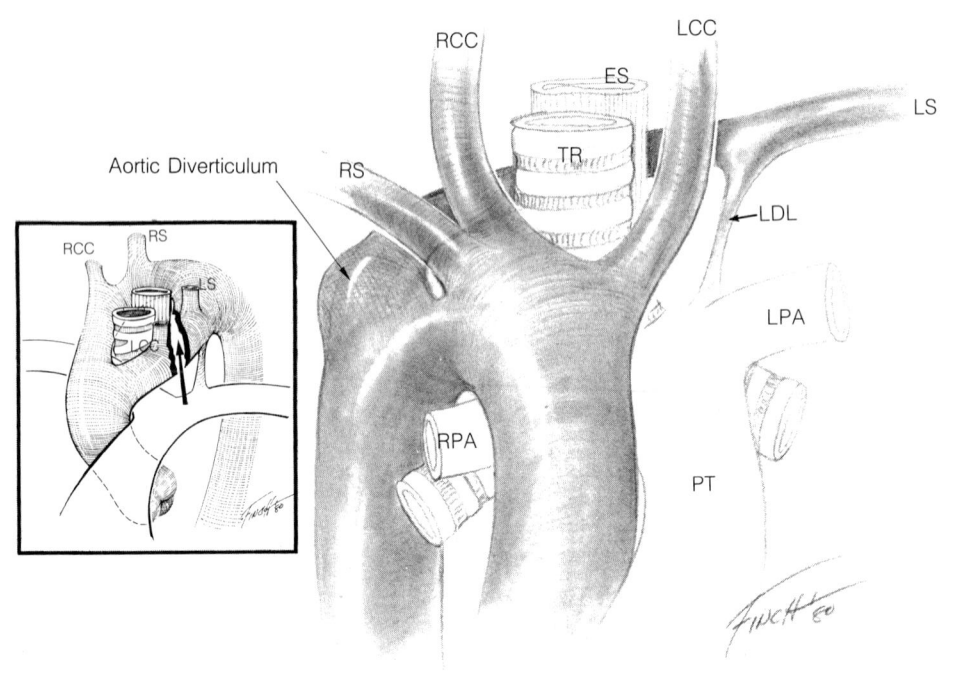

FIG 62-14.
Right aortic arch without retroesophageal segment or artery (mirror image of left aortic arch). Right-sided descending aorta. *Insert,* regression in left fourth aortic arch beyond origin of left subclavian artery *(LS)*. *RS* = right subclavian artery; *RCC* = right common carotid artery; *LCC* = left common carotid artery; *ES* = esophagus; *TR* = trachea; *RDL* = right ductus ligament; *RPA* = right pulmonary artery; *LPA* = left pulmonary artery; *PT* = pulmonary trunk.

a right aortic arch and a retroesophageal indentation are found on a radiograph.

Right Aortic Arch With Aberrant Left Subclavian Artery (Fig 62–15).—In this anomaly the aortic arch is right sided, and the left subclavian artery arises as the fourth branch and passes behind the esophagus to the left arm. Embryologically regression occurs in the fourth left aortic arch between the left carotid and left subclavian arteries. The left subclavian artery arises from the dorsal aorta.

There is a right aortic arch, and the left subclavian artery arises as the fourth branch from the aortic arch. The left subclavian artery arises from a diverticulum (diverticulum of Kommerrell) at the junction of the right arch and *right* descending aorta and passes obliquely upward behind the esophagus toward the left arm. The diverticulum is present because the large volume of blood flow through the fetal ductus arteriosus and also the retroesophageal segment is a remnant of the aortic arch. In contrast, among patients with tetralogy of Fallot and this aortic arch anomaly, the left subclavian artery does not arise from an aortic diverticulum. During fetal life the volume of ductal flow is small,[14] because the pulmonary stenosis limits the right-to-left flow normally present through the ductus.

There may be a ductus arteriosus between the left subclavian artery and left pulmonary artery, and in such patients a vascular ring results. The combination of right aortic arch, aberrant left subclavian artery, and left ductus arteriosus is the most common type of right aortic arch.[5] This type of aortic arch is usually not associated with a congenital cardiac malformation except by mere coincidence. Although a vascular ring is present in most of these patients, it is, however, a loose ring, and symptoms of tracheal or esophageal compression are absent or mild.

Radiographic Features.—The condition can be readily diagnosed on barium swallow.

1. Signs of right aortic arch are present. There is displacement of the trachea and indentation of the esophagus on the right (Fig 62–16) and posterior indentation of the esophagus. Depending on the position of the aortic diverticulum in relation to the esophagus, the retroesophageal indentation may be small (see Fig 62–16) or large (Fig 62–17).

2. With an aortic diverticulum, there is a large horizontal posterior indentation of the esophagus (see Fig 62–17). REASON: The indentation is caused by the aortic diverticulum and not the left subclavian artery itself.

3. If an aortic diverticulum is not present, the indentation of the esophagus is small and directed upward toward the left arm. This pattern is the mirror image of the much more common left aortic arch and aberrant right subclavian artery (see Fig 62–16).

4. If the diverticulum is very large, it may be seen on the posteroanterior thoracic roentgenogram as a round mass density projecting to the left of the trachea, mimick-

RIGHT AORTIC ARCH WITH RIGHT DUCTUS AND RIGHT DESCENDING AORTA

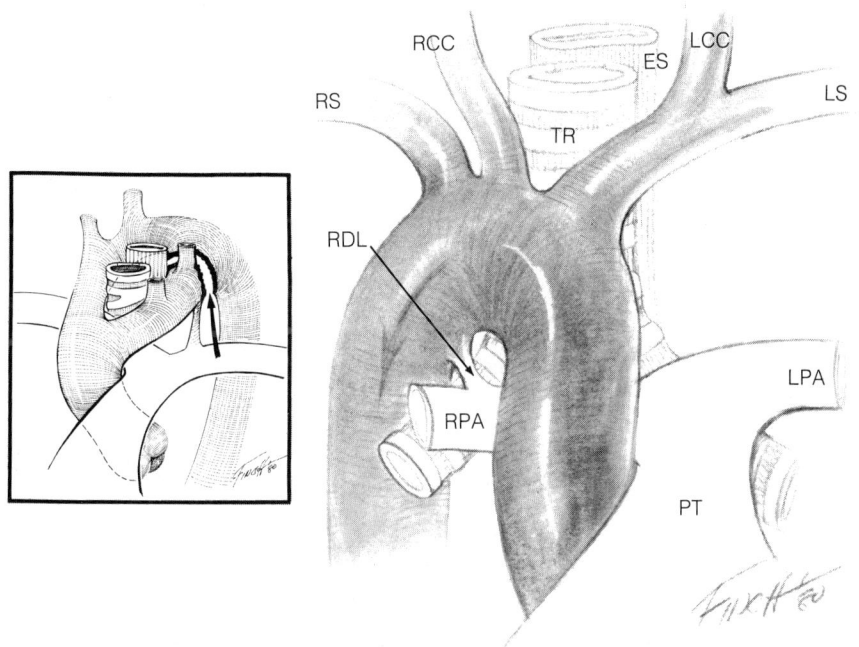

FIG 62–15.
Right aortic arch with aberrant origin of left subclavian artery from aortic diverticulum on proximal descending aorta. *Insert*, regression of left fourth aortic arch between left common carotid artery (*LCC*) and left subclavian artery (*LS*). *RS* = right subclavian artery; *RCC* = right common carotid artery; *ES* = esophagus; *TR* = trachea; *LDL* = left ductus ligament; *LPA* = left pulmonary artery; *RPA* = right pulmonary artery; *PT* = pulmonary trunk.

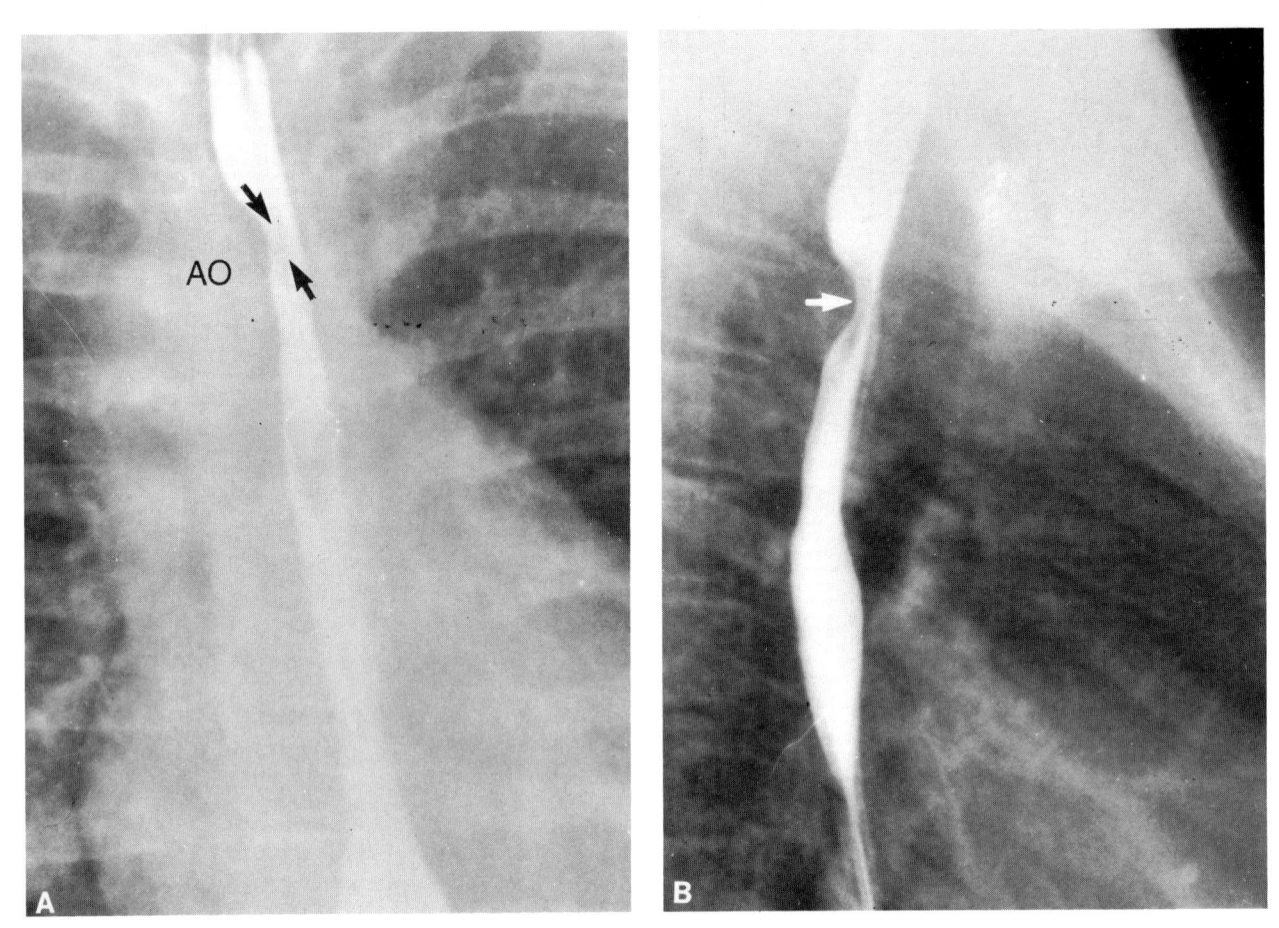

FIG 62–16.
Right aortic arch and aberrant left subclavian artery in tetralogy of Fallot. No aortic diverticulum. Thoracic roentgenogram. **A,** posteroanterior projection. Trachea displaced to left by right aortic arch *(heavy arrow)*. Indentation of esophagus *(small arrows)* directed toward left shoulder. This appearance is mirror image of left arch with aberrant right subclavian artery, which occurs in tetralogy of Fallot and ventricular septal defect. **B,** lateral projection. Small indentation *(arrow)* by aberrant left subclavian artery. *AO* = aorta.

FIG 62–17.
Right aortic arch and aberrant left subclavian artery and large aortic diveritulum. Thoracic roentgenogram. **A,** Posteroanterior projection. Indentation of trachea *(large arrow)* and indentation of esophagus *(small arrows)*. Indentation larger than caliber of subclavian artery, suggesting an aortic diverticulum. The descending aorta is on the right *(open arrows)* in distinction from right circumflex arch (see Fig 62–19). **B,** lateral projection. Large posterior indentation on esophagus *(white arrows)* indicate aortic diverticulum from which left subclavian artery arises. Tracheal air column *(black arrows)* is not narrowed, in distinction from double aortic arch.

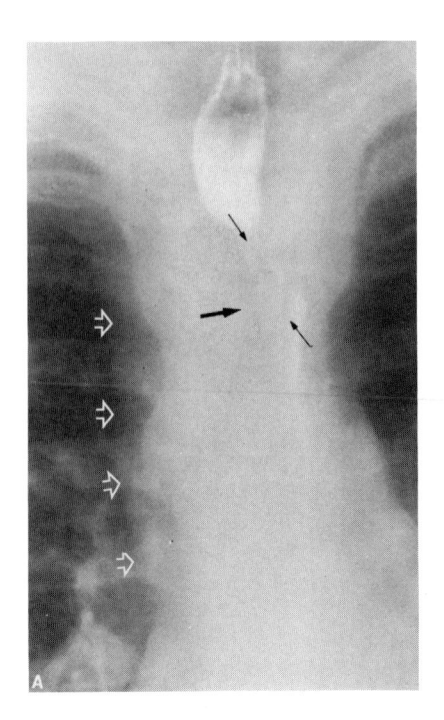

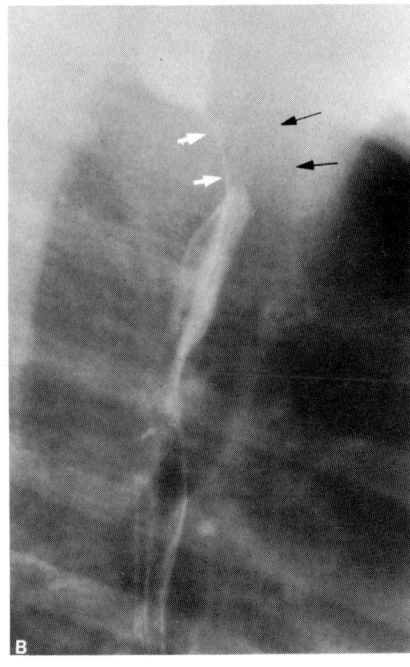

ing a double aortic arch. With double aortic arch, however, the barium-filled esophagus is compressed from three sides: a large posterior indentation and two lateral impressions are present. In contrast, right aortic arch with aberrant left subclavian artery and aortic diverticulum usually does not indent the esophagus on the left side unless a large left-sided ductus arteriosus is present.

5. The aortic diverticulum may be so huge that the patient may be referred for evaluation of a possible mass or aortic aneurysm.

6. A right circumflex aortic arch causes an identical large posterior indentation, but the aorta descends on the left (Fig 62–18).

Angiographic Features

1. There are features of a right aortic arch, with the arch giving rise to the left carotid, right carotid, and right subclavian arteries successively.

2. The aorta descends on the right (Fig 62–19).

3. The left subclavian artery arises as the last branch from an aortic diverticulum on the medial aspect of the proximal descending aorta and passes superiorly to the left arm.

Operative Considerations.—Because only a loose vascular ring is formed by the anomaly, usually no symptoms occur. Sometimes symptoms of tracheal or esophageal compression develop, primarily because the left carotid artery passes anteriorly to the trachea. Through a left thoracotomy, the left ductus arteriosus (usually ligamentous) is divided, and the left carotid artery may be sutured to the sternum.[15, 16]

Right Aortic Arch With Left Descending Aorta (Right Circumflex Arch).[17, 18]—The aorta, after passing over the right bronchus, crosses immediately, to the left behind the esophagus to form a *left* descending aorta (Fig 62–18 and 62–20). The ductus arteriosus is much more common on the left side than the right and arises from the descending aorta, forming a vascular ring. This represents an exception to the rule that the ductus arteriosus opposite the side of the aortic arch always arises from the subclavian artery. This rare anomaly may also occur with an aberrant left subclavian artery (see Fig 62–18).

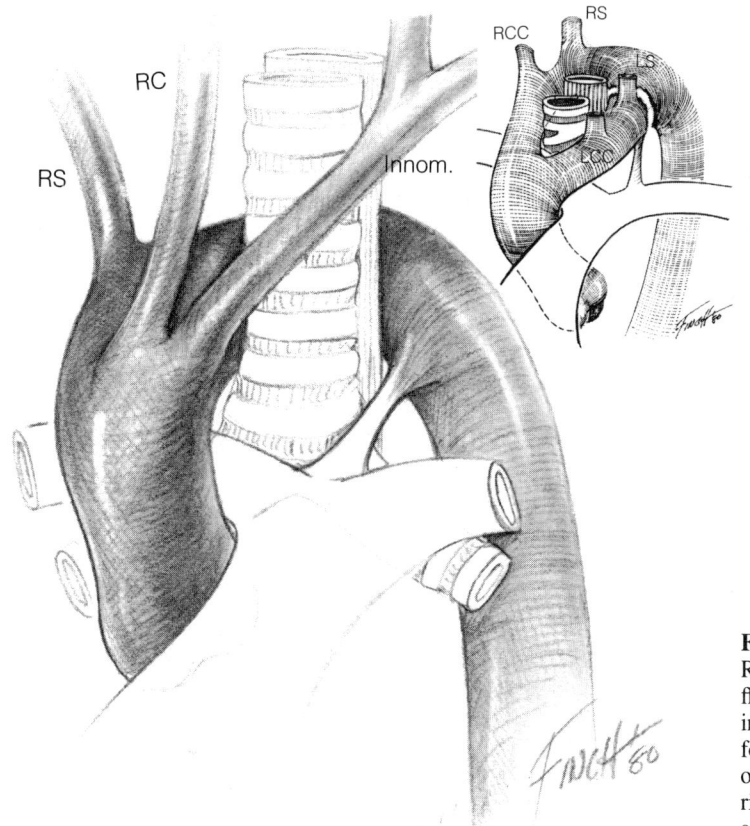

FIG 62–18.
Right aortic arch and left descending aorta (right circumflex aortic arch). Left subclavian artery *(LS)* arises from innominate artery *(Innom.)*. Insert, regression of left fourth arch beyond left subclavian artery and persistence of left dorsal aorta. *RS* = right subclavian artery; *RCC* = right common carotid artery; *LCC* = left common carotid artery; *RC* = right carotid artery.

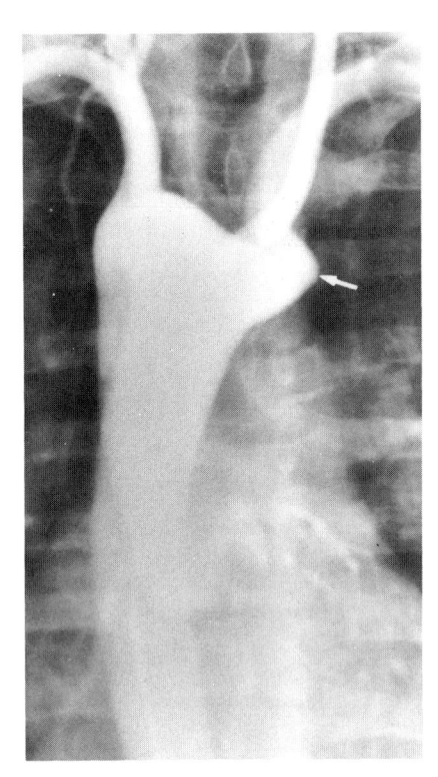

FIG 62–19.
Right aortic arch and aberrant left subclavian artery. Aortogram. Anteroposterior projection. Left subclavian artery arises from aortic diverticulum *(arrow)*. Descending aorta is on right.

Embryologically there is a right aortic arch, but the dorsal aortae fuse into a left descending aorta. The retroesophageal (circumflex) segment of the aorta is the distal part of the fourth right aortic arch and represents the most distal part of the fourth left arch (dorsal aortic root) (see Fig 62–18, insert).

The regression in the fourth left aortic arch may occur either between the left common carotid and left subclavian arteries or, less frequently, distal to the left subclavian artery, and only the ductus arises from the aortic diverticulum.

Thus, there are two anatomic subtypes. The left subclavian artery may arise from an aortic diverticulum as the fourth branch from the aorta (Fig 62–20).[12] There is a left-sided ductus. A loose vascular ring is present, which usually causes no symptoms. In the other subtype, the left subclavian artery arises normally from the innominate artery (see Fig 62–18). The left-sided ductus usually forms a symptomatic vascular ring.

Radiographic Features.—Several radiographic features allow a strong suspicion of this anomaly:

1. The trachea deviates to the left, indicating the presence of a right aortic arch (Fig 62–21).
2. The aortic arch is visualized on the right side.
3. The descending aorta is seen on the left side of the spine.
4. The barium-filled esophagus is indented from behind by a large vascular structure, crossing obliquely from the right to the left (Figs 62–21 and 62–22). The impression is directed either downward toward the left or horizontally as in an aortic diverticulum. Both conditions give such an impression and must be distinguished. In right arch with circumflex aorta, the descending aorta is on the left. In right arch with aberrant left subclavian artery, the descending aorta is on the right, but a right circumflex arch may coexist with an aberrant left subclavian artery (see Fig 62–20).
5. Right arch with circumflex aorta usually does not compress the trachea. Rare exceptions exist. It must be differentiated from double aortic arch with an atretic segment, which is a vascular ring and compresses the trachea circumferentially. Tracheal compression can be identified usually on a thoracic radiograph, and this finding is a helpful differential diagnostic sign (see Fig 62–21,B).
6. Each ductus arteriosus may persist. The ductus arises from the contralateral aberrant subclavian artery or from the aorta (see Figs 62–18 and 62–22).

Angiographic Features.—Angiography demonstrates this malformation well (see Fig 62–22), but angiograms cannot distinguish between circumflex arch and double aortic arch with atretic anterior segment (discussed subsequently).

Operative Considerations.—Symptoms of tracheoesophageal compression usually do not occur in a patient with a right aortic arch and a retroesophageal segment. If symptoms are present, a double aortic arch with atretic left segment is probably present. Fortunately, for therapeutic purposes, this differentiation is not essential. The compressing vascular ring of either type can be interrupted through a left thoracotomy.

Double Aortic Arch

Double aortic arch usually occurs as an isolated anomaly and without an associated congenital cardiac anomaly.[5, 19] Two aortic arches are present: one lying anterior to the trachea and the other posterior to the esophagus. Each arch crosses over the ipsilateral bronchus and fuses into a single descending aorta, which may be located on either the left or right side of the thorax. Because the trachea and esophagus are encircled, symptoms usually occur. The size of the aortic arches are rarely equal in size. Commonly the posterior arch is the larger of the two, and occasionally the anterior may be present only as a fibrous band,[5] but this cannot be demonstrated angiographically.

RIGHT AORTIC ARCH WITH ABERRANT LEFT SUBCLAVIAN ARTERY

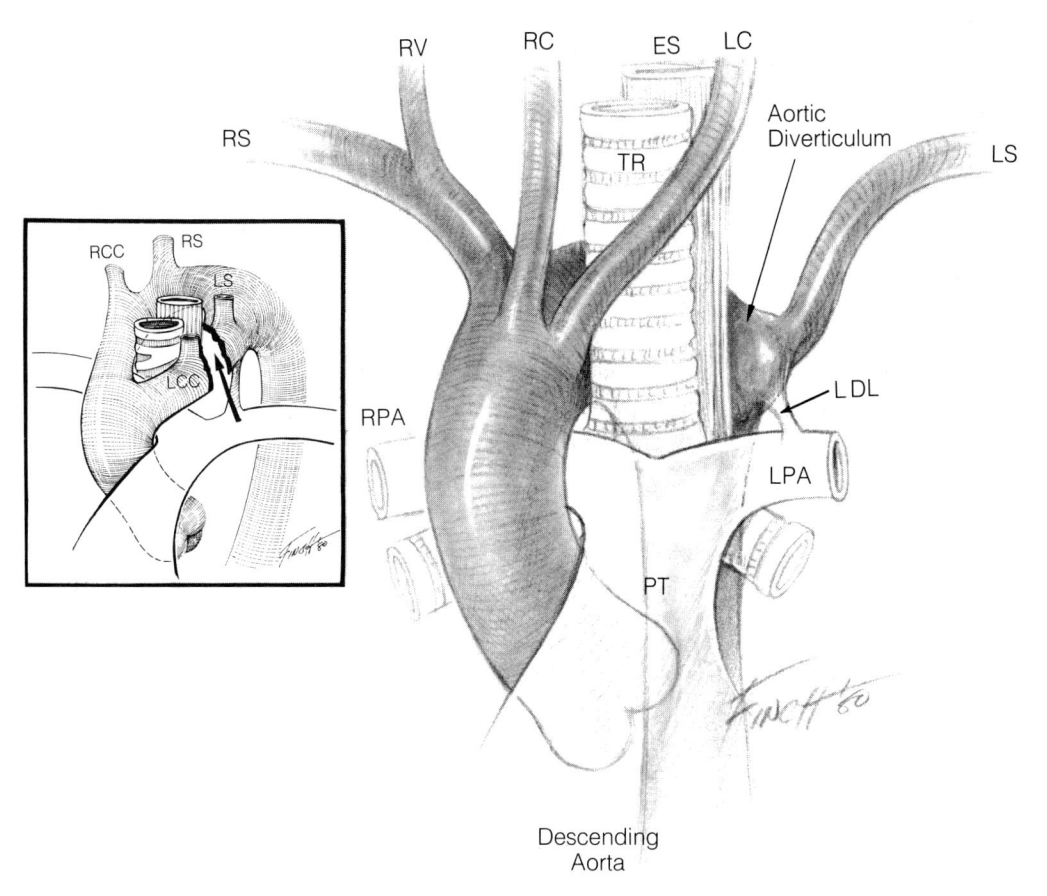

FIG 62–20.
Right aortic arch and left descending aorta (right circumflex aortic arch). Aberrant left subclavian artery *(LS)*. Insert, regression in left fourth and between left subclavian and persistent left dorsal aorta. Operation consists of dividing left ductus ligament and arteriopexy of left common carotid artery *(LCC)*. *RS* = right subclavian artery; *RCC* = right common carotid artery; *LC* = left carotid artery; *ES* = esophagus; *TR* = trachea; *LDL* = left ductus ligament; *LPA* = left pulmonary artery; *RPA* = right pulmonary artery; *PT* = pulmonary trunk; *RV* = right vertebral artery; *RC* = right carotid artery.

Double Aortic Arch With Both Arches Patent

Double aortic arch develops when regression in neither fourth aortic arch occurs (Fig 62–23). Usually the descending aorta is on the left (see Fig 62–23) but rarely on the right side of the thorax (Fig 62–24). The distal portion of either or both the left or right sixth aortic arch (ductus arteriosus) may be present.

The aortic arches are located over the right and left bronchi, respectively. Because the descending aorta is usually on the left, the left aortic arch is in front of the trachea and the right arch passes behind the esophagus.

The branches of the aortic arch are symmetrically arranged: the right common carotid artery and right subclavian artery originate from the right arch, and the left common carotid and left subclavian artery originate from the left aortic arch. The ductus arteriosus may connect to either pulmonary artery from the right or left aortic arch, respectively.

Symptoms are usually present[20] and caused by tracheal or esophageal compression when the vascular ring is tight.

Radiographic Features.—Several radiographic features strongly suggest the diagnosis:

1. Because of prominent thymic tissue, no abnormalities may be seen in infants and children.

2. If the trachea can be visualized, it is not shifted to either side. Therefore, it is impossible to determine the position of the aortic arch (Fig 62–25). REASON: Because the trachea is fixed between the two arches, it cannot deviate.

3. The aortic arch tends to be inconspicuous. REASON: Each of the individual double arches is smaller than a normal single arch.

4. An aortic knob may be present and visualized in

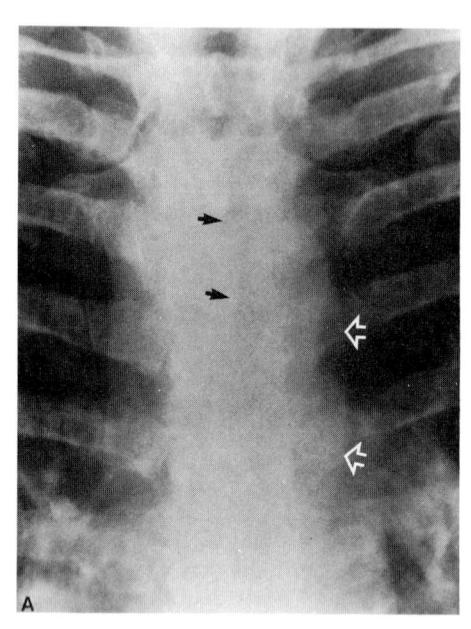

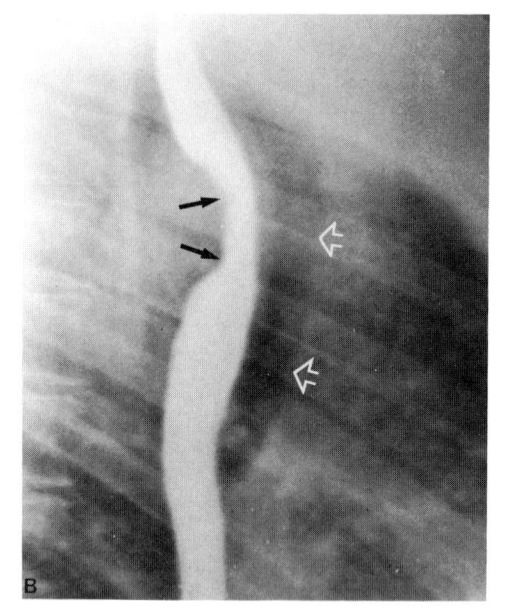

FIG 62–21.
Right aortic arch and left descending aorta (right circumflex aorta). Thoracic roentgenogram. **A,** posteroanterior projection. Trachea is displaced to left. Indentation *(black arrows)* of right aortic arch. **B,** lateral projection. Large indentation on esophagus *(black arrows)* caused by retroesophageal aorta. Tracheal air column *(open arrows)* is normal, in distinction from double aortic arch.

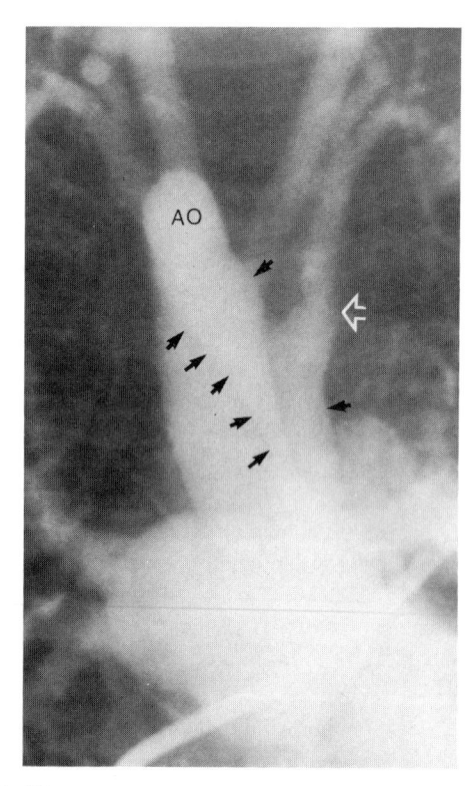

FIG 62–22.
Right aortic arch and left descending aorta (right circumflex aorta). Pulmonary arteriogram. Anteroposterior projection. Late phase. Right-sided aortic arch. Aorta *(AO)* crosses behind trachea and esophagus and descends on left side of thorax *(arrows)*. Aberrant left subclavian artery arises from aortic diverticulum *(open arrow)*.

each side. REASON: Both aortic arches may be equally well developed. Usually, however, the right aortic arch is larger and slightly higher and more prominent than the left aortic arch.

5. The esophagus is indented posteriorly and from both sides (see Fig 62–25,B). The bilateral compression represents the most diagnostic feature of double arch and does not occur in other arch anomalies.

Angiographic Features.—Angiography is important to identify the specific anatomic details. Then the proper operative approach can be selected.

1. On the anteroposterior projection, the arches may be superimposed and cause a confusing angiographic picture (Fig 62–26,A). Better visualization can be obtained by angulated views, particularly a cranial projection. REASON: Because the left aortic arch usually lies lower and more anterior, it projects downward with cranial angulation.

2. On a lateral projection, both arches are distinctly visualized. The right posterior arch is slightly higher than the lower anterior arch (Fig 62–26,B).

3. The right and posterior arch is usually larger.

4. Rarely, the anterior arch is larger. In such cases the surgeon divides the posterior arch.

5. Typically the posterior arch has a downward course and is well seen on the anteroposterior projection (Fig 62–27).

Anomalies of the Aortic Arch System **1013**

DOUBLE AORTIC ARCH

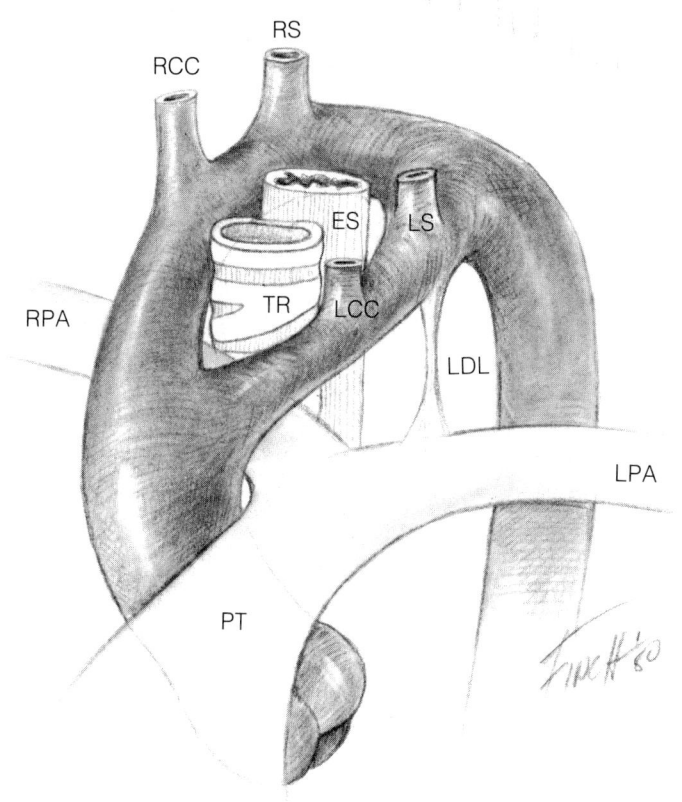

FIG 62–23.
Double left aortic arch and left descending aorta. Hypoplasia of anterior left arch. *Insert,* persistence of both aortic arches and left dorsal aorta. *RS – right subclavian artery; LS* = left subclavian artery; *RCC* = right common carotid artery; *LCC* = left common carotid artery; *ES* = esophagus; *TR* = trachea; *LDL* = left ductus ligament; *LPA* = left pulmonary artery; *RPA* = right pulmonary artery; *PT* = pulmonary trunk.

DOUBLE AORTIC ARCH WITH RIGHT DESCENDING AORTA AND RIGHT DUCTUS LIGAMENT

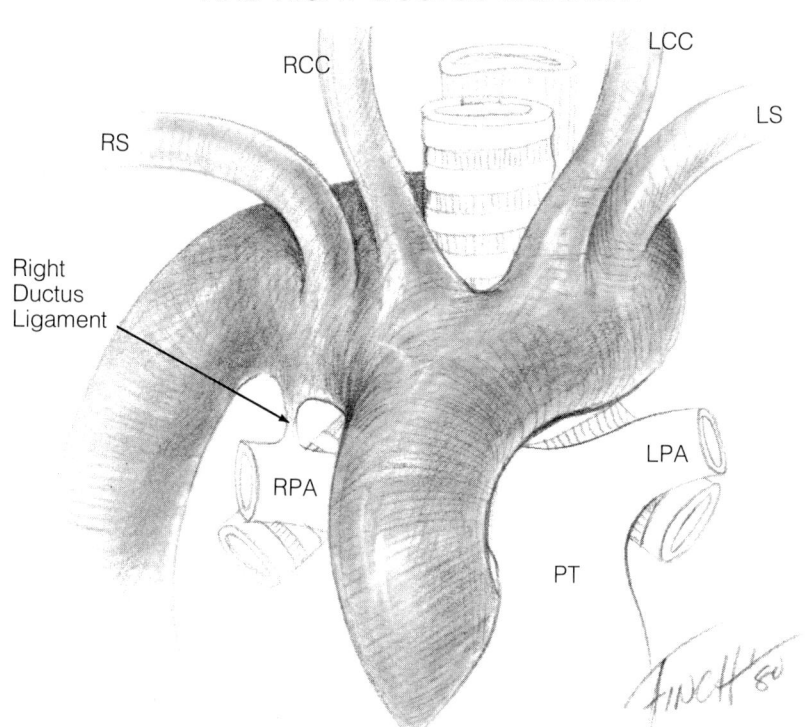

FIG 62–24.
Double right aortic arch with both arches patent. Persistence of both fourth aortic arches and right dorsal aorta. *RCC* = right common carotid artery; *LCC* = left common carotid artery; *RS* = right subclavian artery; *LS* = left subclavian artery; *RPA* = right pulmonary artery; *LPA* = left pulmonary artery; *PT* = pulmonary trunk.

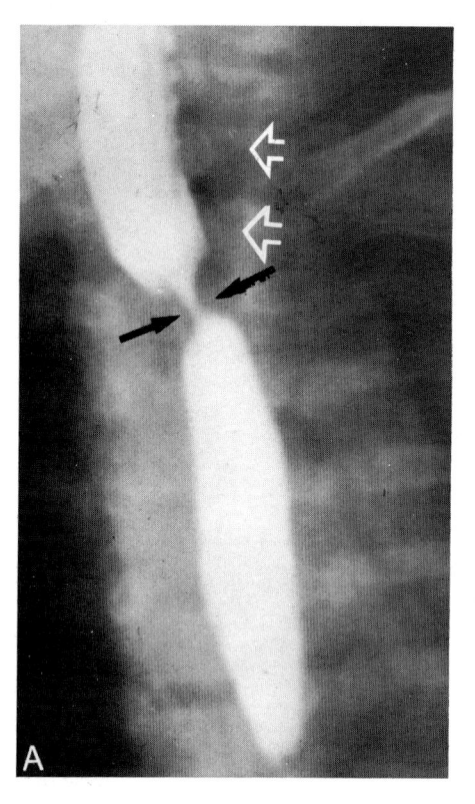

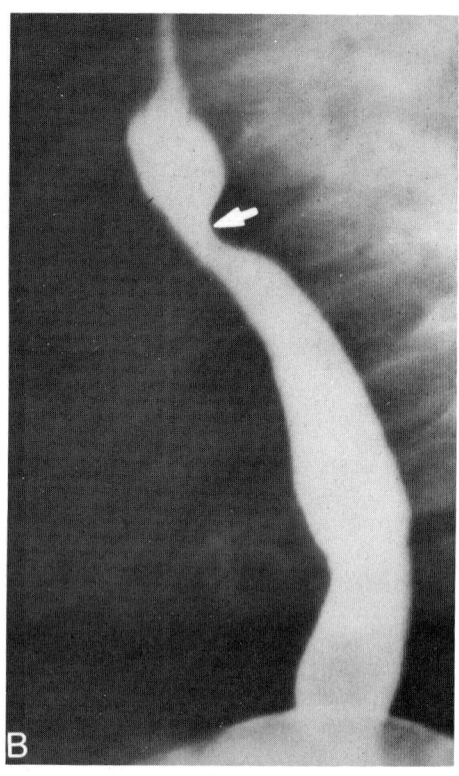

FIG 62–25.
Double left aortic arch. Thoracic roentgenogram. **A,** posteroanterior and **B,** lateral projections. Location of aortic arch cannot be determined because trachea is not displaced *(open arrows).* Esophagus is indented from behind *(white arrow)* and from both sides *(black arrows),* characteristic for double arch. Trachea is narrowed.

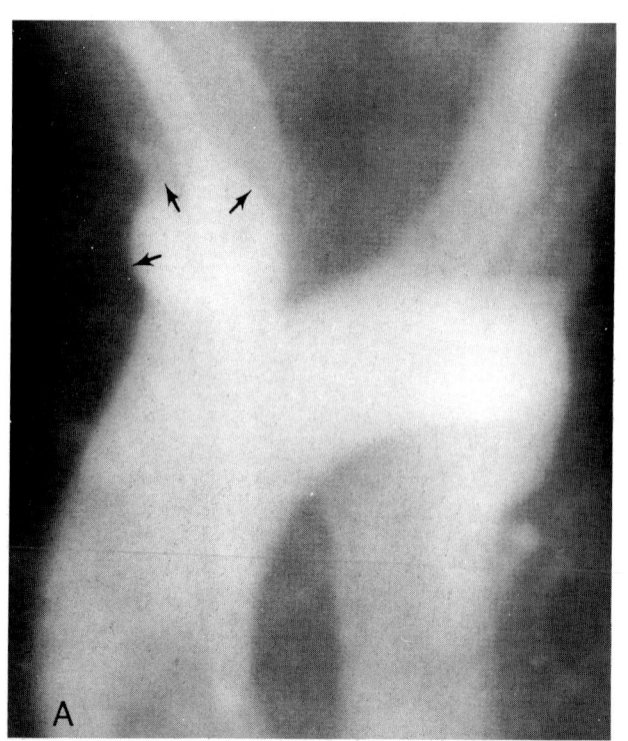

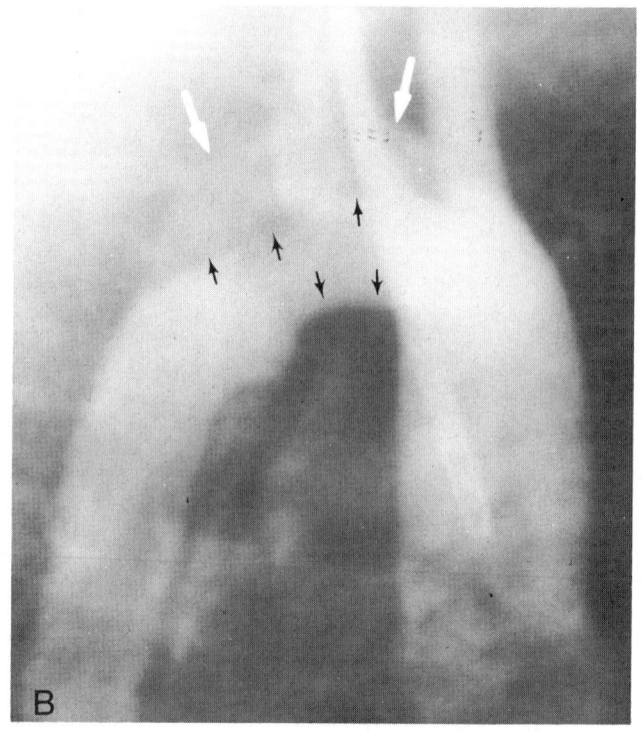

FIG 62–26.
Double left aortic arch. Aortogram. **A,** anteroposterior projection. Both aortic arches are superimposed and not distinctly visible. Right aortic arch is smaller, seen as round density *(arrows)* passing from right toward left. **B,** lateral projection. Both arches are visualized. Right arch *(white arrows)* is higher and larger than the left arch *(black arrows).*

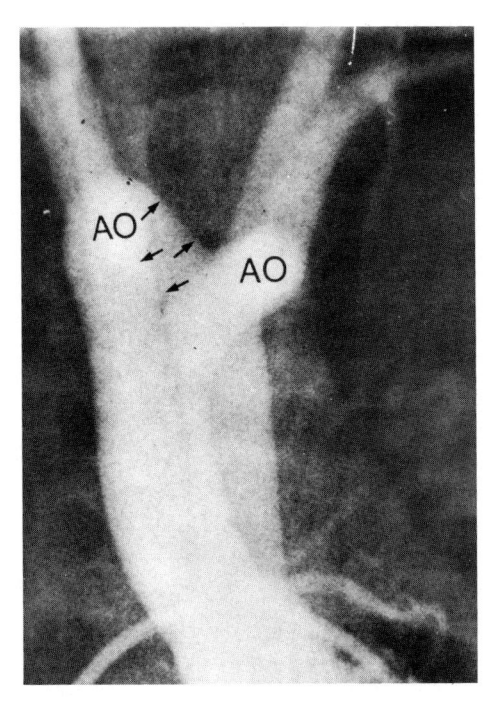

FIG 62-27.
Double aortic arch. Left ventriculogram. Anteroposterior projection. Retroesophageal portion of double arch is higher, is larger, and has a downward course *(arrows)*. Left descending aorta. Better angiographic visualization could be obtained by cranial angulation. *AO* = aorta.

Operative Considerations.—At operation the smaller aortic arch and ductus ligament are divided (Fig 62–28).[15, 16, 19] Therefore, angiography is important to demonstrate the size of the arches. With division of the anterior arch (most common), tracheal compression may be fully relieved, but the impression on the esophagus persists. If symptoms of tracheal compression persist because of compression by the left carotid artery and the posterior esophagus, the left carotid artery can be sutured to the sternum (Fig 62–29).[21]

Double Aortic Arch With Atresia of Part of the Left Arch

This is a variant of double aortic arch in which a portion of the left arch is present as an atretic strand. Double aortic arch with an atretic segment of the right arch has not been reported. Definitive proof of double aortic arch with an atretic segment can be obtained only at autopsy, but radiologic examinations are very suggestive of the diagnosis. Symptoms of vascular ring may be present in each subtype of double aortic arch with atresia of the left arch.

In this condition both fourth aortic arches persist, but a portion of the left fourth arch is atretic. Usually the aortic diverticulum of the left fourth arch persists because of the large blood flow through the fetal ductus arteriosus. Other structures of the left arch are the ductus (liagmentum arteriosus), and left subclavian artery. The atretic distal arch may be attached to this diverticulum, depending on the site of the atresia in the left fourth aortic arch (Fig 62–30).

Radiographic Features

1. The radiographic findings are identical to those of a right aortic arch and aberrant left subclavian artery arising from an aortic diverticulum and right circumflex arch. Right aortic arch with aberrant left subclavian artery forms a loose vascular ring that is completed by the ductus ligament. In double aortic arch with an atretic segment, a tight vascular ring is formed that compresses the trachea anteriorly. Tracheal compression is best seen on a lateral roentgenogram cinefluorography and MRI examination. This finding is highly suggestive of a double arch with atretic left segment.

2. In addition to the large posterior transverse indentation of the esophagus, two lateral impressions at the level of the aortic arch are present, suggesting the diagnosis of double aortic arch. Occasionally double aortic arch with atresia of the entire anterior arch cannot be diagnosed even by angiography.

Angiographic Features.—The angiographic diagnosis is much more difficult than in patients with a double aortic arch in which both arches are patent.

1. With the type of double arch demonstrated in Figure 62–30,A, the angiographic findings are identical to a right circumflex aortic arch with mirror-image branching and a left ductus ligament arising from an aortic diverticulum. Because the latter condition is extremely rare, such an angiogram is very suggestive of double arch with atretic left arch. Careful inspection of the tracheal air column is helpful in the differential diagnosis.

2. With the type of double arch demonstrated in Figure 62–30,B, the angiographic findings are identical to right arch with aberrant left subclavian artery and ductus diverticulum. Angiographic differentiation from this much more common anomaly is impossible. Tracheal compression suggests an additional anterior atretic segment.

3. Double arch with atretic segment cannot be diagnosed angiographically, but the pattern of tracheal compression may suggest the diagnosis and MRI examination.

Operative Considerations.—Each form can be corrected through a left thoracotomy. The atretic segment and ligamentous ductus are divided. Rarely, additional sutur-

SURGICAL CORRECTION OF DOUBLE AORTIC ARCH

A.

Anterior Division of Double Aortic Arch

B.

Posterior Division of Double Aortic Arch

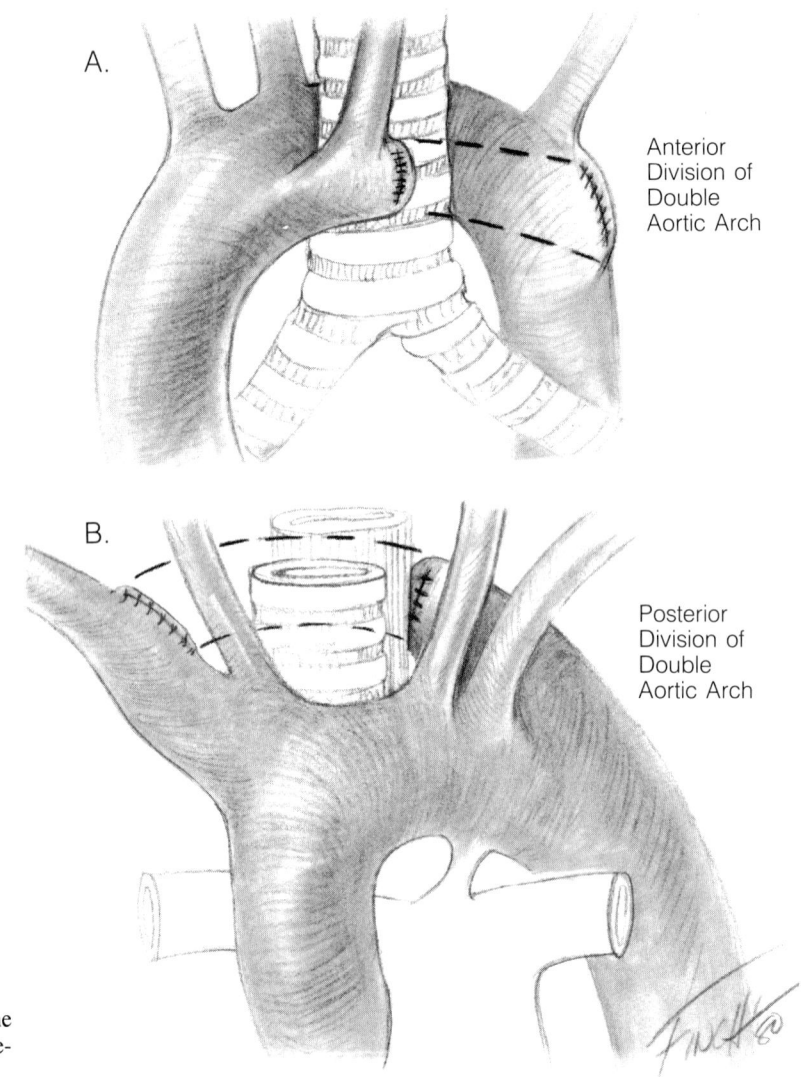

FIG 62–28.
Operative correction of double aortic arch. The smaller arch is divided. **A,** division of smaller anterior arch. **B,** division of posterior aortic arch.

ing of the carotid artery to the sternum is required to relieve anterior compression (see Fig 62–29).

Isolation of a Subclavian Artery

In this condition, one subclavian artery is not in continuity with the aortic arch but is attached to the ipsilateral pulmonary artery by a ductus arteriosus (usually ligamentous).[17] This is an uncommon anomaly, and in one third of cases, tetralogy of Fallot coexists.[12]

Developmentally two regressions occur in one fourth aortic arch, these regressions being located proximally and distally to the subclavian artery (Fig 62–31). The subclavian artery is attached to the ductus arteriosus. The ductus may be patent, which results in a subclavian steal and left-to-right shunt into the pulmonary artery (see Fig 62–31).

Isolation of the subclavian artery always occurs on the side opposite the aortic arch. In most cases there is a right aortic arch, and the left subclavian artery is isolated. Blood flow into the isolated subclavian artery is maintained by the vertebral artery (subclavian steal).

An extremely rare variant is isolation of the left brachiocephalic arteries (innominate arteries). Both the left common carotid and left subclavian arteries are isolated. This arch anomaly can be explained by regression of the left arch proximal to the left carotid and distal to the left subclavian artery (Fig 62–32).

A left aortic arch with isolation of the right subclavian artery is extremely rare (Fig 62–33).

The patient may be asymptomatic or may show signs of cerebrovascular insufficiency or signs of inadequate circulatory supply to the involved arm. In the latter, symp-

ANTERIOR SURGICAL CORRECTION OF DOUBLE AORTIC ARCH

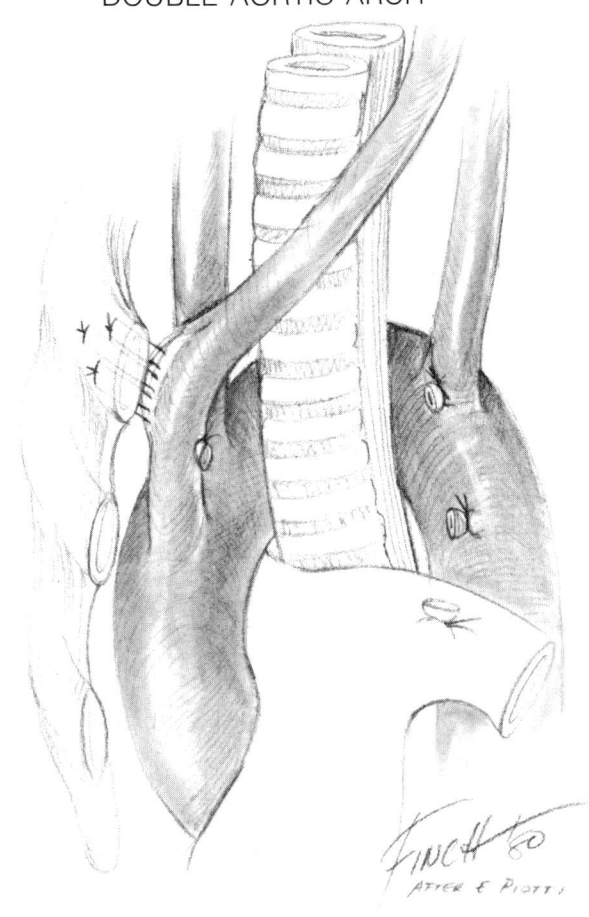

FIG 62–29.
Operative correction of double aortic arch. Smaller anterior arch and left ductus arteriosus have been divided. Left common carotid artery has been sutured anteriorly to sternum to relieve compression of anterior wall of trachea.

toms occur because the blood supply to the subclavian artery through collateral arterial vessels is inadequate. The pulse pressure in the involved arm is decreased, a feature allowing clinical recognition of this rare entity.

Radiographic Features

Isolation of the subclavian artery cannot be diagnosed by a thoracic roentgenogram. Because the isolation occurs on the opposite side of the aortic arch, the radiographic finding of a right-sided arch, combined with the clinical information of a decreased pulse in the left arm, suggests the correct diagnosis.

Angiographic Features

Isolation of a subclavian artery may exist either with or without a patent ductus arteriosus. Late angiographic films are essential in patients with a ligamentous ductus. If the ductus is patent, blood flow occurs from the isolated subclavian artery into the pulmonary artery, because the pulmonary resistance is lower than systemic resistance.

1. If the ductus arteriosus is patent, the pulmonary artery opacifies from a subclavian arteriogram or during the late phase of an aortogram (Fig 62–34).
2. Aortography demonstrates prompt opacification of each brachiocephalic vessel except the isolated subclavian artery. This artery opacifies late through collateral arteries (Fig 62–35), primarily from the vertebral artery (subclavian steal).

Operative Considerations

Because of the association with tetralogy of Fallot, the diagnosis of isolated subclavian artery must be made angiographically before consideration of a Blalock-Taussig shunt.[18] If isolation is present, such a shunt cannot be performed on the involved side. The Blalock-Taussig operation has to be performed on the same side as the aortic arch. Only in cases of cerebral or peripheral vascular insufficiency is bypass to the isolated subclavian artery warranted.

Interruption of the Aortic Arch

The clinical picture of interruption of the aortic arch is very different from other anomalies of the fourth aortic arch. Almost all patients with interruption of the aortic arch have congestive cardiac failure, and many die in infancy. Its clinical features usually resemble severe coarctation of the aorta. The condition is discussed here because it also results from abnormalities in regression of segments of the primitive aortic arches. It represents 1% of congenital cardiac disease.[22]

Interruption of the aortic arch results from regression in both the right and left aortic arches. The site of regression in each arch varies, and thus several anatomic forms exist. In interruption of the aorta, continuity between the ascending and descending aorta is lacking. The descending aorta is supplied by a patent ductus arteriosus or by collateral arteries if the ductus arteriosus is closed.

Interruption of the aortic arch is usually associated with a ventricular septal defect.[22-24] In many patients a muscular extension of the conus septum in the left ventricle produces subaortic stenosis.[22, 24] The location of the ventricular septal defect varies, but it is frequently supracristal.[23] Associated left ventricular outflow obstruction is frequent, and the major cause of subaortic obstruction is a muscular subaortic ridge.[22, 23] Rarely, there is neither a ventricular septal defect nor patent ductus arteriosus, and the prognosis in these few patients with isolated interrup-

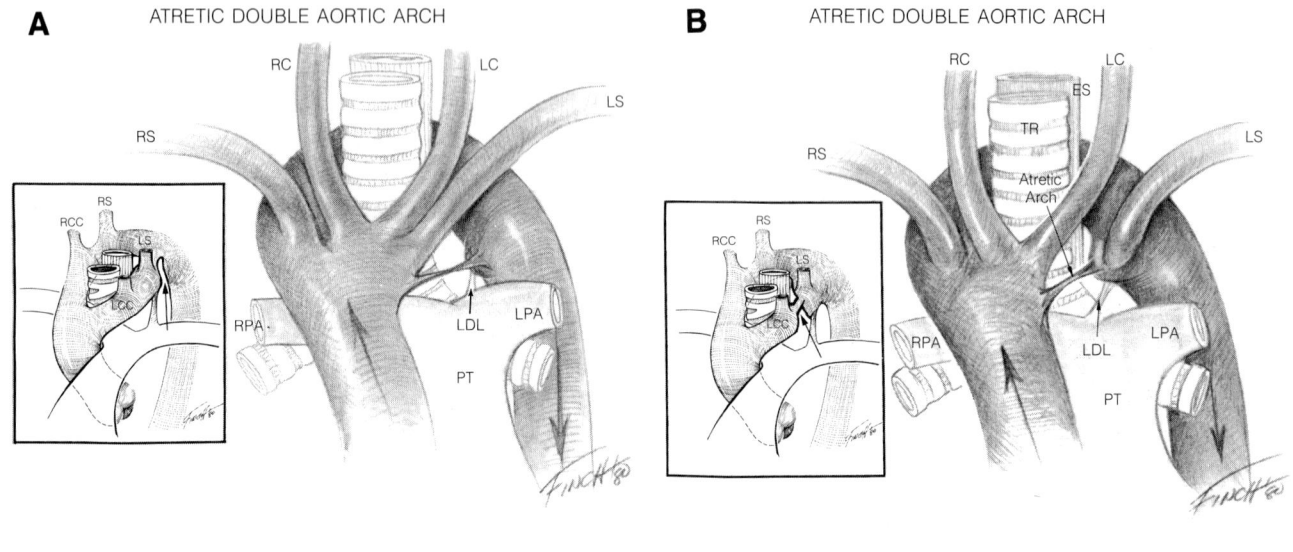

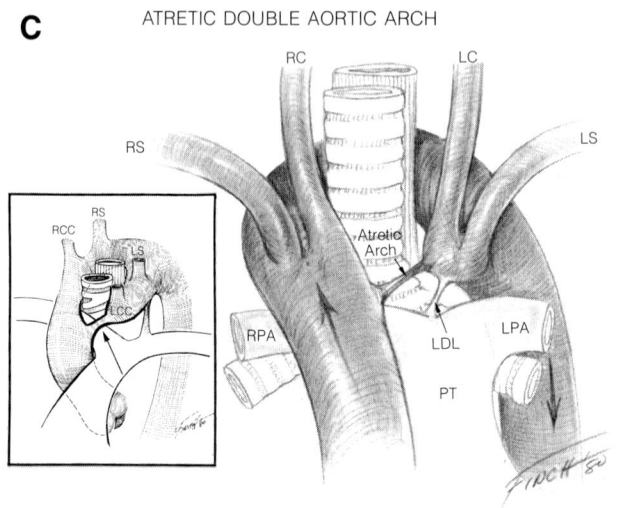

FIG 62–30.
Double aortic arch with atresia of part of left aortic arch. **A,** atresia of left arch beyond left subclavian artery. Innominate artery arises from ascending aorta. **B,** atresia between left carotid and left subclavian arteries. **C,** atresia of left aortic arch proximal to left carotid artery. Both left carotid and left subclavian arteries arise from descending aorta. Inserts illustrate site in left aortic arch that becomes atretic. *RS* = right subclavian artery; *LS* = left subclavian artery; *RCC* = right common carotid artery; *LCC* = left common carotid artery; *ES* = esophagus; *TR* = trachea; *LDL* = left ductus ligament; *LPA* = left pulmonary artery; *RPA* = right pulmonary artery; *PT* = pulmonary trunk; *RC* = right carotid artery; *LC* = left carotid artery.

tion of the aortic arch is good, because they may survive into adulthood.[24, 25]

Interruption of aortic arch can coexist with most congenital cardiac anomalies,[22] particularly complete transposition of the great vessels, persistent truncus arteriosus, double-outlet right ventricle, and aorticopulmonary window.[24]

Interruption of aortic arch usually occurs with a left aortic arch. Association with a right aortic arch is extremely rare. In the latter, the right ductus may lead to bronchial compression and pulmonary emphysema (see Fig 62–18; see also Chapter 16). Interruption is classified according to the site of interruption in the left aortic arch.[24] Each of the forms can occur as a mirror-image form with a right aortic arch.

Interruption Distal to Left Subclavian Artery

In this form, interruption distal to left subclavian artery (40%), the left aortic arch is interrupted (has regressed) beyond the left subclavian artery. Two subtypes are found, depending on location of the interruption (regression) in the right aortic arch:

1. Right arch interrupted beyond right subclavian artery. Therefore, each of the brachiocephalic vessels arises from the ascending aorta (Fig 62–36).

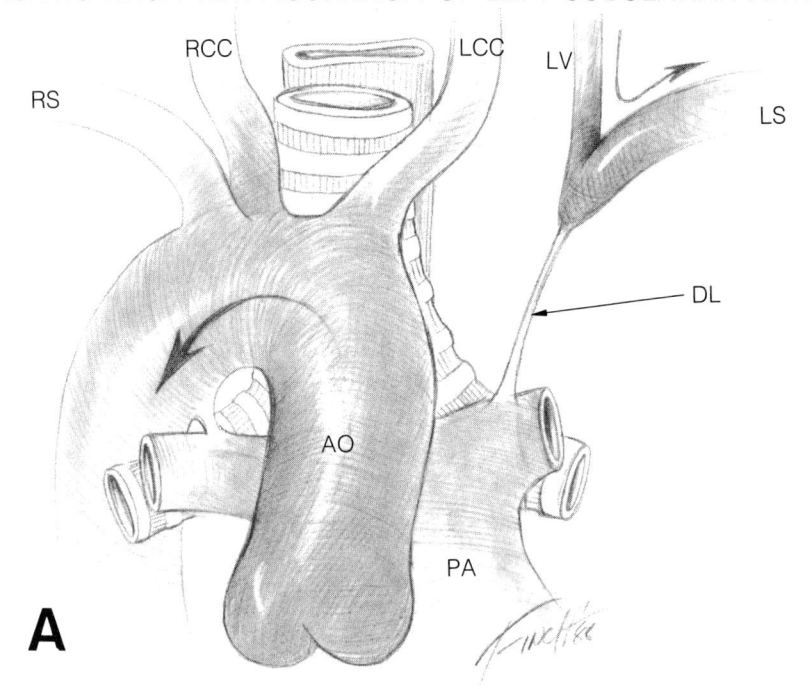

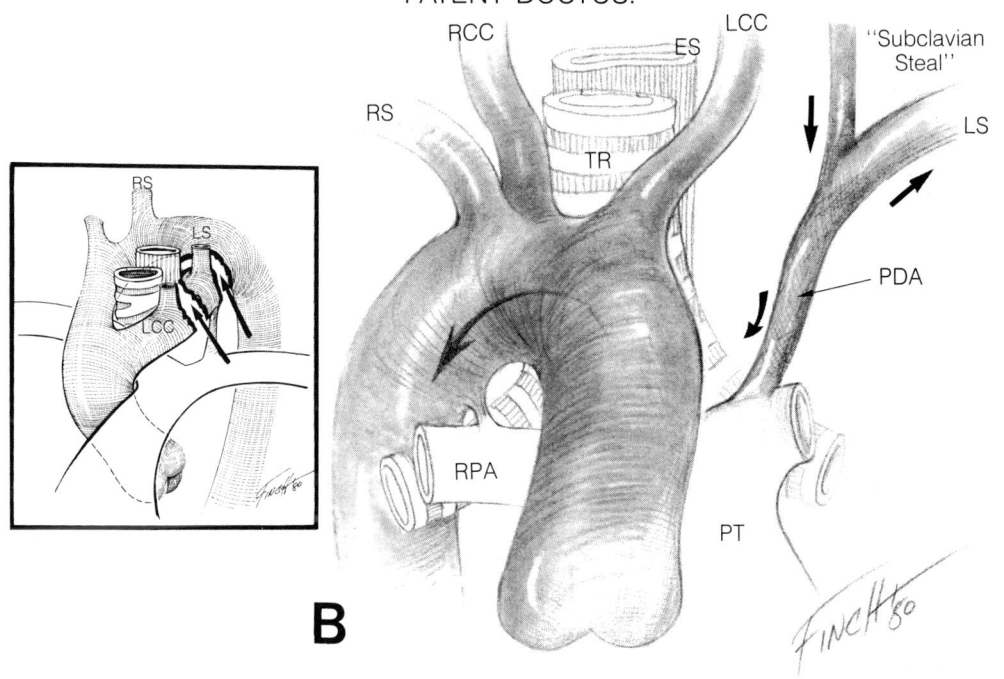

FIG 62–31.
Isolation of left subclavian artery *(LS)*. **A,** right aortic arch and ductus ligament. Left subclavian artery is attached to left pulmonary artery through ligamentous ductus *(DL)*. Blood flow occurs to left subclavian artery through subclavian steal from vertebral artery. **B,** Isolation of left subclavian artery and patent ductus arteriosus *(PDA)*. Blood flow occurs into pulmonary artery *(PA)* or in left-to-right shunt. *Insert,* regression in left fourth aortic arch proximal and distal to left subclavian artery. *RS* = right subclavian artery; *RCC* = right common carotid artery; *LCC* = left common carotid artery; *ES* = esophagus; *TR* = trachea; *RPA* = right pulmonary artery; *PT* = pulmonary trunk; *LV* = left vertebral artery; *AO* = aorta.

RIGHT AORTIC ARCH WITH ISOLATION OF LEFT INNOMINATE ARTERY

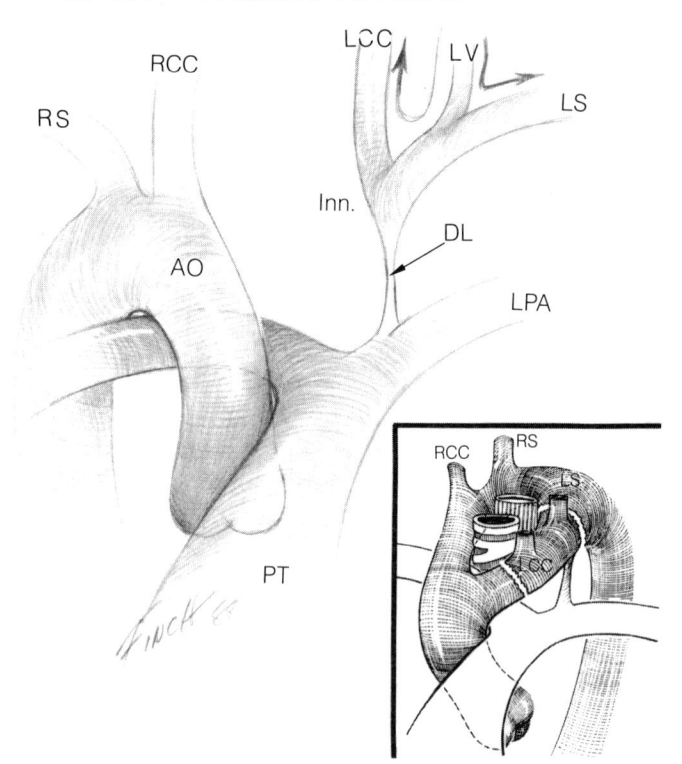

FIG 62–32.
Right aortic arch and isolation of left innominate artery *(Inn.)* Subclavian steal is present. *Insert,* two regressions occur in left aortic arch. *RS* = right subclavian artery; *LS* = left subclavian artery; *RCC* = right common carotid artery; *LCC* = left common carotid artery; *LV* = left vertebral artery; *DL* = ductus ligamentosis; *LPA* = left pulmonary artery; *PT* = pulmonary trunk; *AO* = aorta.

LEFT AORTIC ARCH WITH INTERRUPTION OF RIGHT SUBCLAVIAN ARTERY

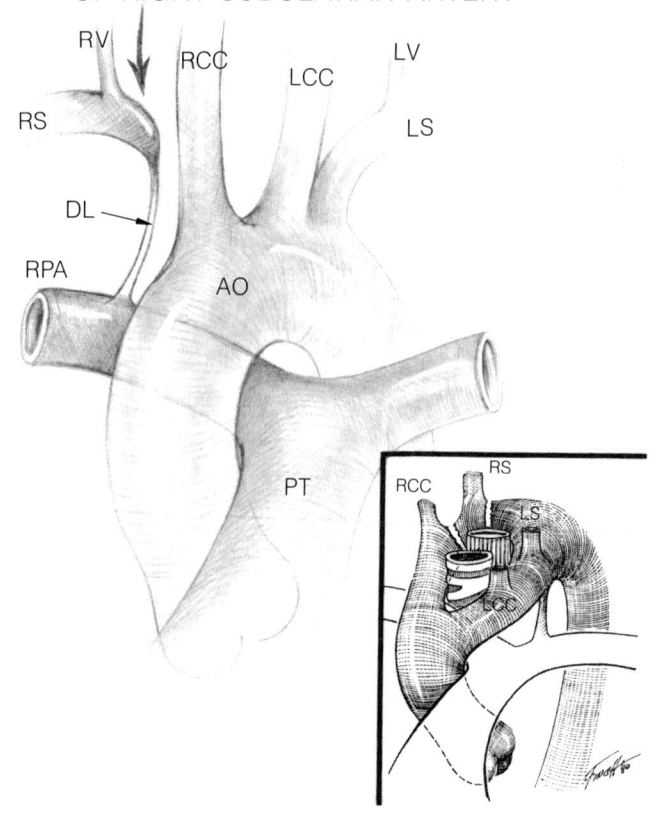

FIG 62–33.
Isolation of right subclavian artery *(RS)* and left aortic arch. Extremely rare condition. *RV* = right vertebral artery; *LV* = left vertebral artery; *RCC* = right common carotid artery; *LCC* = left common carotid artery; *LS* = left subclavian artery; *RS* = right subclavian artery; *DL* = ductus ligament; *AO* = aorta; *RPA* = right pulmonary artery; *PT* = pulmonary trunk.

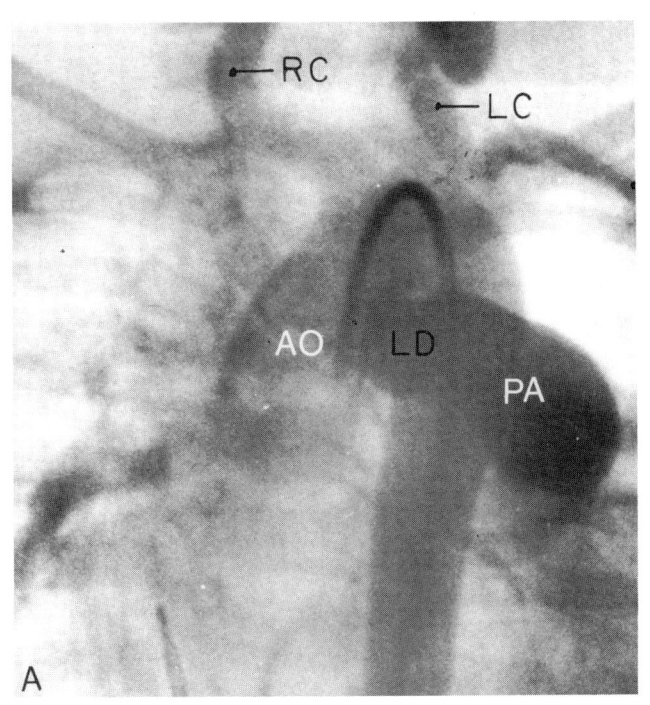

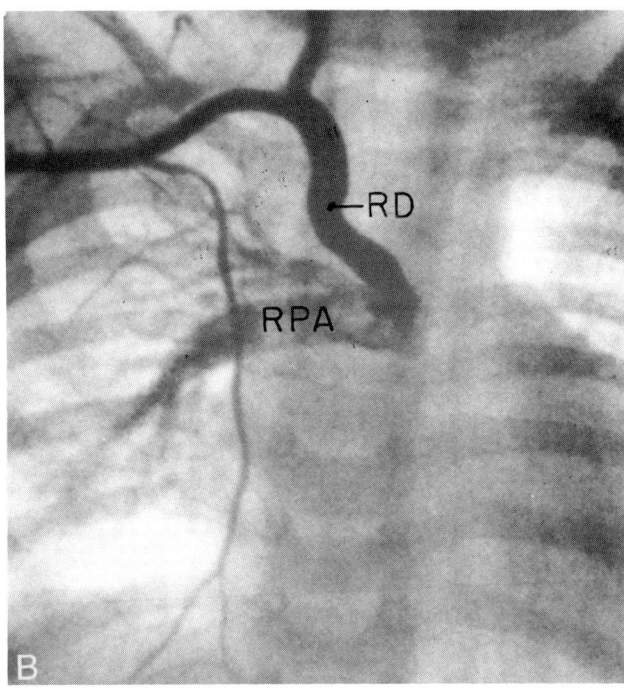

FIG 62-34.
Isolation of subclavian artery. Aortogram. Anteroposterior projection. **A,** isolation of right subclavian artery. Opacification of right carotid *(RC),* left carotid *(LC),* and left subclavian arteries. Right subclavian artery is not opacified. It is isolated and fills via collateral arteries. Through large left-sided ductus arteriosus *(LD),* pulmonary arteries *(PA)* opacify. *AO*= aorta. **B,** same patient; brachial arteriogram. Isolation of right subclavian artery and persistent right ductus arteriosus *(RD).* Opacification of right pulmonary artery *(RPA).*

2. Right arch interrupted between left subclavian and aberrant right subclavian arteries. Right carotid, left carotid, and left subclavian arteries originate from the ascending aorta (Fig 62-37). The right subclavian artery originates from the proximal descending aorta. The latter vessel then passes behind the esophagus to the right arm as in left aortic arch with aberrant right subclavian artery.

Interruption Between Left Carotid and Left Subclavian Arteries

Three anatomic subtypes of interruption between the left carotid and left subclavian arteries (60%) are found, depending on location of the interruption in the right arch:

1. Right arch interrupted beyond right subclavian artery (Fig 62-38). Carotid arteries and the right subclavian artery arise from the ascending aorta. The left subclavian artery arises from the descending aorta.

2. Right arch interrupted between right carotid and right subclavian arteries (Fig 62-39). The ascending aorta supplies only the carotid arteries. Both subclavian arteries originate from the descending aorta, with the right subclavian artery passing behind the esophagus to the right arm.*

3. Right arch interrupted proximally and distally to the right subclavian artery (Fig 62-40). The ascending aorta supplies both carotid arteries; the right subclavian artery is connected to the right pulmonary artery by a ligamentous ductus arteriosus (isolation of the right subclavian artery). The left subclavian artery arises from the descending aorta.

Interruption Distal to Innominate Artery

In this rare form, the left common carotid and left subclavian arteries originate from the descending aorta (Fig 62-41).[22-24] Regression occurs in the left aortic arch proximal to left common carotid artery and in the right arch beyond the right subclavian artery.

Clinical Features

Almost all patients with interruption of the aortic arch have clinical symptoms within the first month of life, often by the end of the first week. The onset of symptoms occur

---

*Theoretically this results in desaturation in all for extremities and normal saturation of the face ("pink face" syndrome). Clinically this is rarely evident because of the common coexistence of a ventricular septal defect.

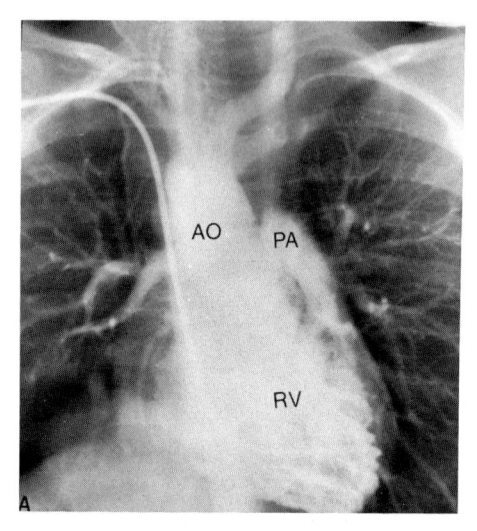

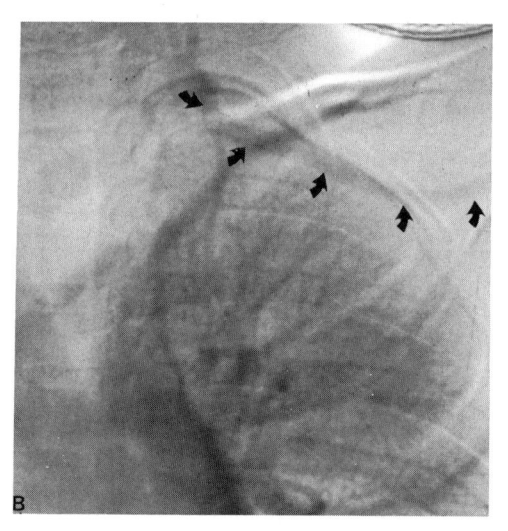

FIG 62–35.
Tetralogy of Fallot and interruption of left subclavian artery. **A,** right ventriculogram. Anteroposterior projection. Pulmonary arteries *(PA)* and aorta *(AO)* are opacified. Right aortic arch. Left subclavian and left vertebral arteries are not opacified. *RV* = right vertebral artery. **B,** late phase. Left vertebral and left subclavian arteries fill via subclavian steal *(arrows)*.

as the ductus arteriosus closes. The clinical picture resembles that of severe coarctation of the aorta,[24, 26] showing features of congestive cardiac failure and respiratory distress.

There are no diagnostic features on physical examination. As the ductus arteriosus closes, the pulses and blood pressure decrease in the legs and other arteries originating from the descending aorta. Although differential cyanosis would be expected, this is rarely seen because of a left-to-right shunt through the coexistent ventricular septal defect.

The murmurs are not specific. There is hepatomegaly because of congestive cardiac failure.

Electrocardiographic Features

The electrocardiogram shows right-axis deviation and right ventricular hypertrophy because of pulmonary hypertension.

INTERRUPTION OF AORTIC ARCH DISTAL TO LEFT SUBCLAVIAN

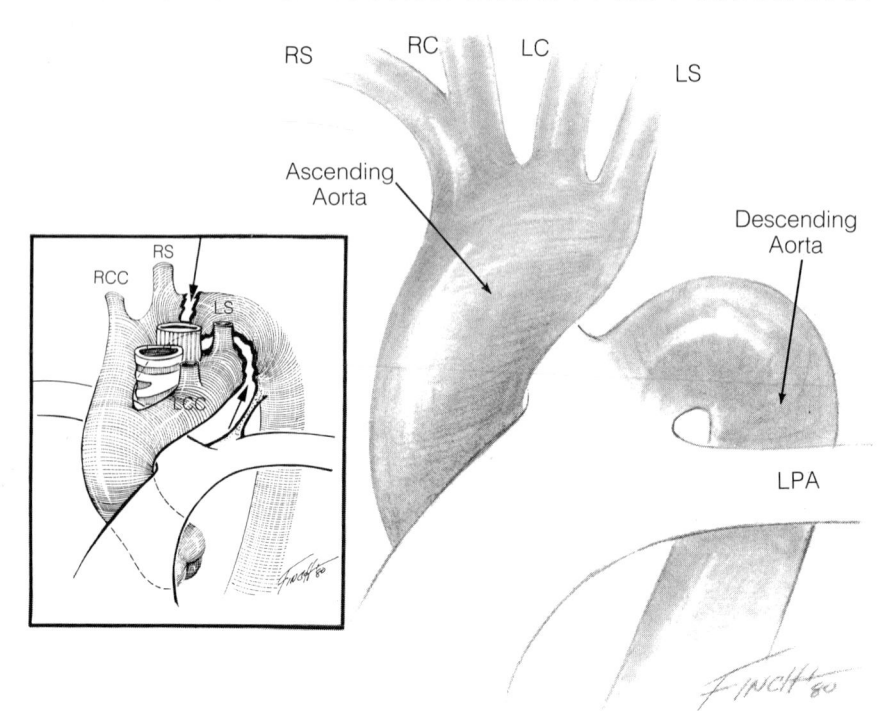

FIG 62–36.
Interruption of the aortic arch beyond left subclavian artery *(LS)*. Insert, regression of each aortic arch beyond subclavian arteries. *RS* = right subclavian artery; *RCC* = right common carotid artery; *LCC* = left common carotid artery; *LPA* = left pulmonary artery; *RC* = right carotid artery; *LC* = left carotid artery.

INTERRUPTION OF AORTIC ARCH BEYOND LEFT SUBCLAVIAN ARTERY
ORIGIN OF RIGHT SUBCLAVIAN ARTERY FROM DESCENDING AORTA

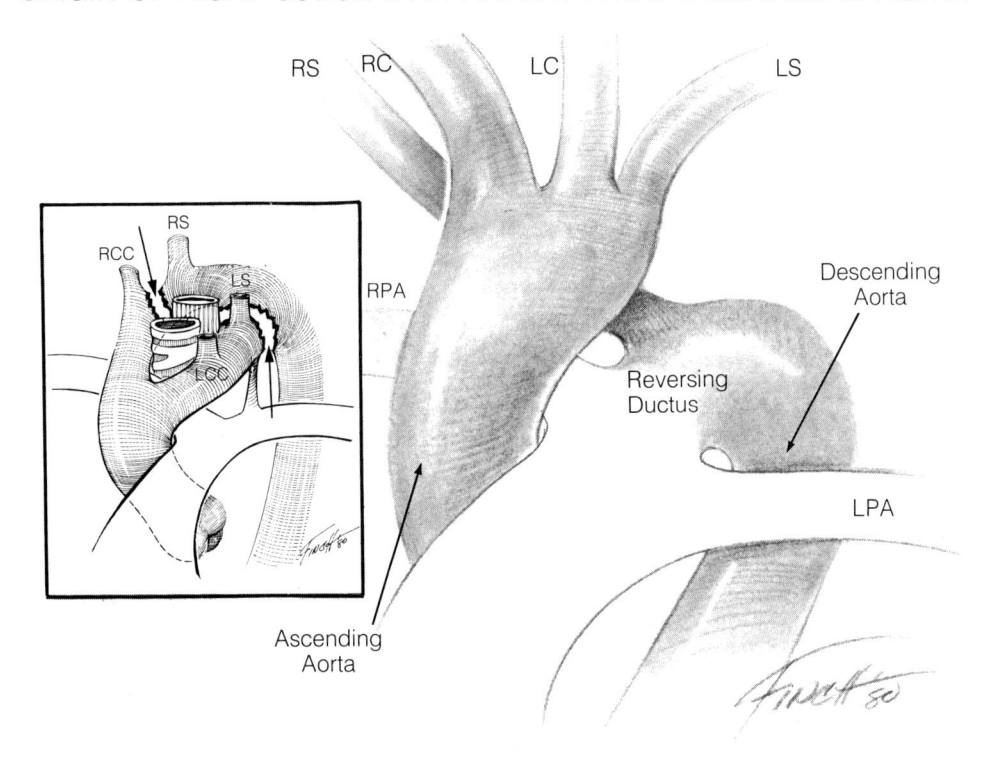

FIG 62–37.
Interruption of aortic arch distal to left subclavian artery *(LS)*. Right subclavian artery *(RS)* arises from descending aorta and crosses behind esophagus. *Insert*, regression of left arch beyond left subclavian artery and of right arch between right common carotid *(RCC)* and right subclavian arteries. *RC* = right carotid artery; *LCC* = left common carotid artery; *RPA* = right pulmonary artery; *LPA* = left pulmonary artery; *LC* = left carotid artery.

INTERRUPTION OF AORTIC ARCH BETWEEN
LEFT CAROTID AND LEFT SUBCLAVIAN ARTERY

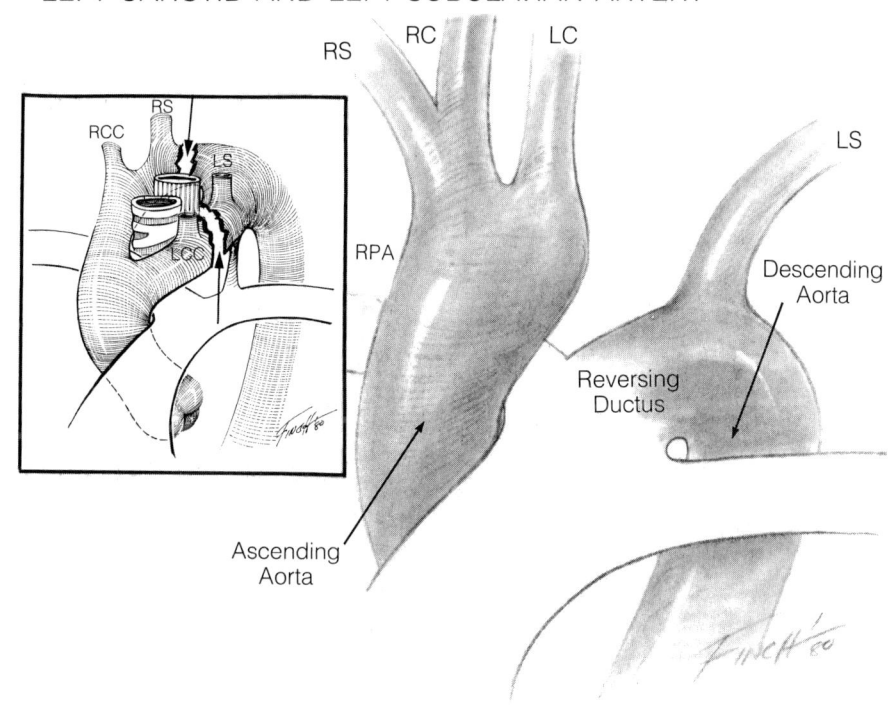

FIG 62–38.
Interruption of the aortic arch beyond left carotid artery *(LC)*. Left subclavian artery *(LS)* arises from descending aorta. *Insert;* regression of left arch between left common carotid *(LCC)* and left subclavian arteries and of the right arch beyond right subclavian artery *(RS)*. *RC* = right carotid artery; *RPA* = right pulmonary artery; *RCC* = right common carotid artery.

1024 Anomalies of Major Blood Vessels

INTERRUPTION OF LEFT AORTIC ARCH WITH ORIGIN OF LEFT CAROTID AND SUBCLAVIAN ARTERIES FROM DESCENDING AORTA

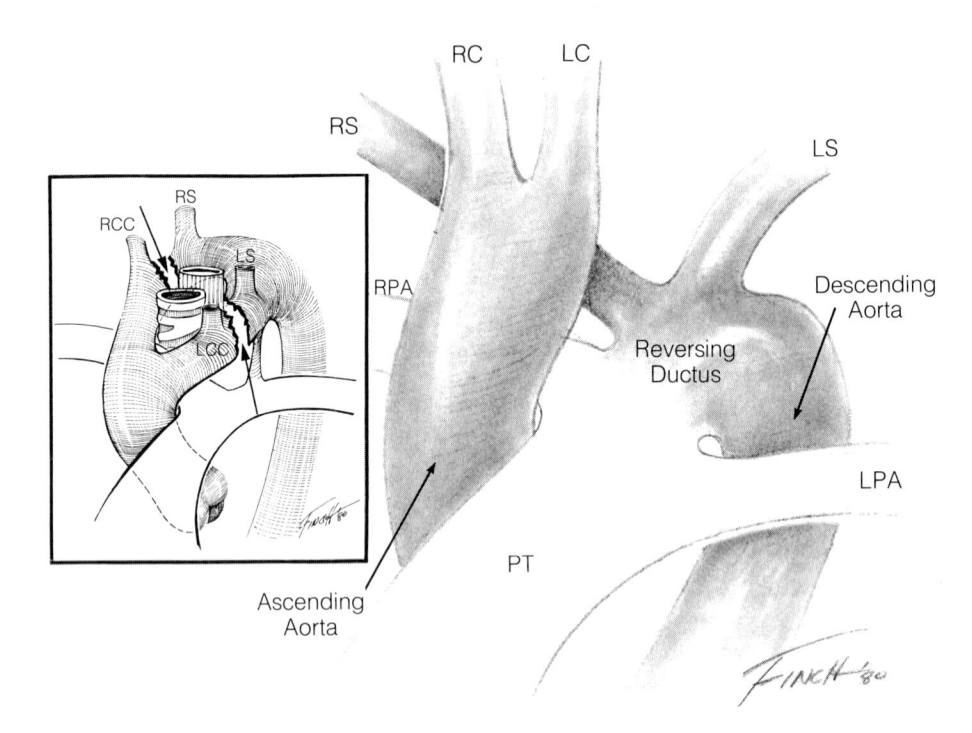

FIG 62–39.
Interruption of the aortic arch beyond left carotid artery (LC). Right subclavian artery (RS) arising from descending aorta. Insert; regression of each aortic arch between common carotid and subclavian arteries. RC = right carotid artery; LS = left subclavian artery; LPA = left pulmonary artery; PT = pulmonary trunk; RPA = right pulmonary artery; RCC = right common carotid artery; LCC = left common carotid arteries.

INTERRUPTION OF AORTIC ARCH ISOLATION OF RIGHT SUBCLAVIAN ARTERY

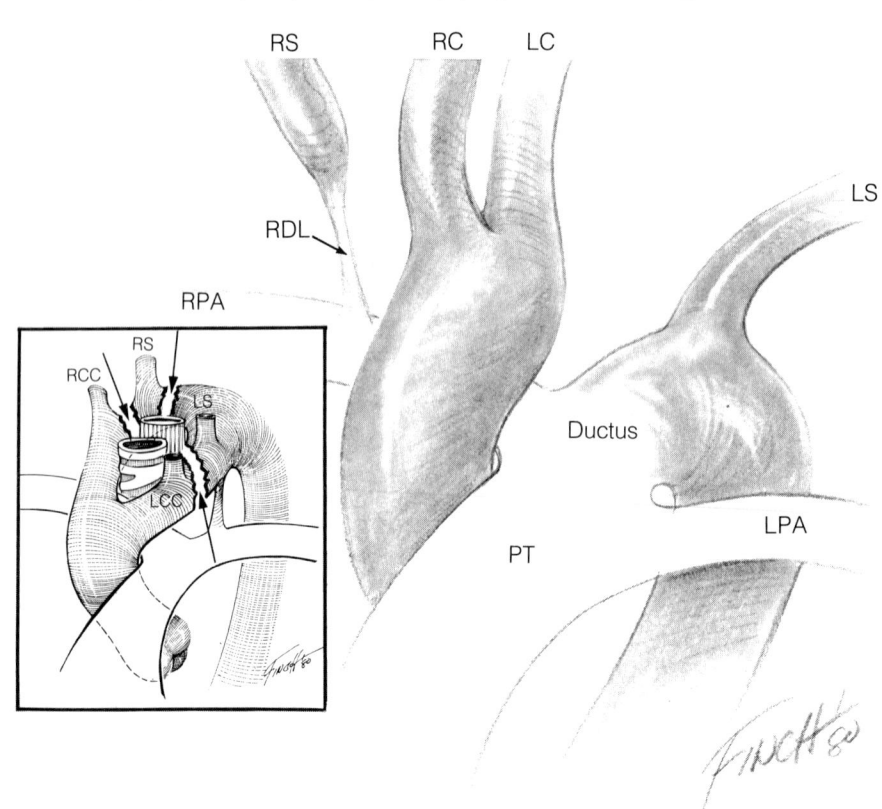

FIG 62–40.
Interruption of aortic arch beyond left carotid artery (LC). Right subclavian artery (RS) connects right pulmonary artery (RPA) through ligamentous ductus arteriosus. Insert; regression of primitive left arch between left common carotid (LCC) and left subclavian (LS) arteries and of the right arch proximal and distal to right subclavian artery (RS). RDL = right ductus ligament; RC = right carotid artery; LPA = left pulmonary artery; PT = pulmonary trunk; RCC = right common carotid artery.

INTERRUPTION OF AORTIC ARCH DISTAL TO INNOMINATE

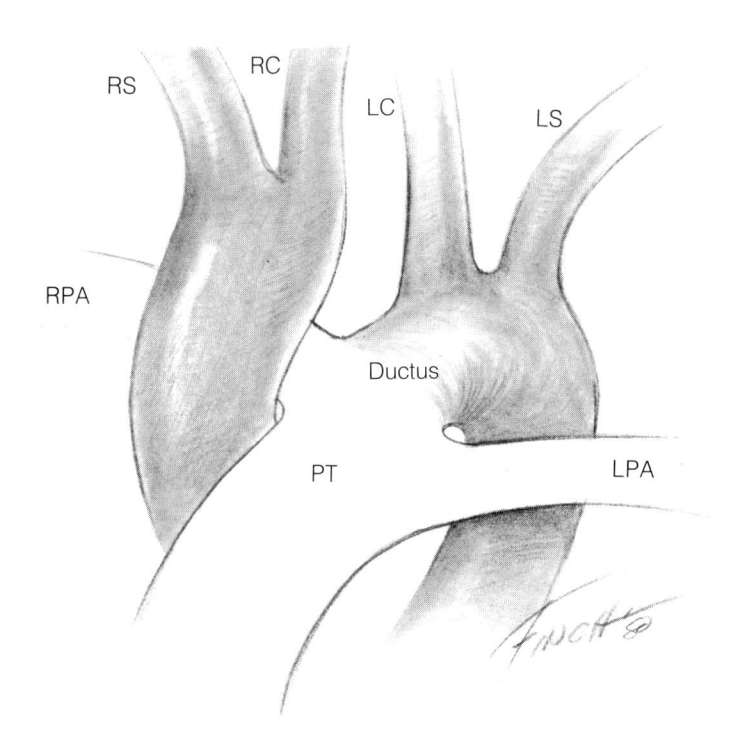

FIG 62–41.
Interruption of aortic arch beyond right carotid artery *(RC)*. Left carotid *(LC)* and left subclavian *(LS)* arteries arise from descending aorta. *RS* = right subclavian artery; *RPA* = right pulmonary artery; *LPA* = left pulmonary artery; *PT* = pulmonary trunk.

Echocardiographic Features

Echocardiography can demonstrate the abnormality of the aortic arch and shows the lack of continuity of the aortic arch and the site of origin of each brachiocephalic vessel. A ventricular septal defect can be identified and often other coexistent conditions. Retrograde filling through a patent ductus arteriosus is observed.

Radiographic Features

The diagnosis of interruption of the aortic arch by thoracic roentgenogram alone is very difficult, and the correct diagnosis is rarely suggested.[27] The hemodynamic consequences of interruption of the aortic arch vary so widely that the radiographic appearance is nonspecific. In infancy the radiographic diagnosis is virtually impossible. There are several nonspecific radiographic features, depending on the hemodynamics:

1. Interruption with large patent ductus arteriosus (common). Cardiomegaly, increased main pulmonary arterial segment, enlarged proximal pulmonary arteries as in pulmonary hypertension, and left atrial enlargement are present.
2. Interruption with small patent ductus arteriosus in older patients (rare). The findings are identical to coarctation of the aorta (Fig 62–42). REASON: Blood supply to the descending aorta occurs through collateral arteries and is evident by rib notching. Bilateral rib notching indicates origin of both subclavian arteries proximal to the interruption. Unilateral rib notching occurs if one subclavian artery arises from the proximal aorta.

Specific radiographic findings that allow a correct diagnosis are as follows:

1. An aortic "knob" is not visualized. REASON: In interruption of the aortic arch, the distal aortic arch does not develop.
2. The impression of the aortic arch on the trachea and barium-filled esophagus is absent. REASON: The portion of the arch adjacent to the trachea and esophagus is absent.
3. The trachea is in the midline. REASON: The slightly oblique course of the normal aortic arch causes a shift of the trachea away from the aortic arch. In interruption of the aortic arch, there is no pressure against the trachea because this portion of the arch does not develop (Fig 62–43).
4. The ascending aorta appears to be small on posteroanterior and left anterior oblique projections, in distinction from coarctation of the aorta. REASON: In interruption of the aortic arch, blood flow to the ascending aorta is always decreased because the lower body is supplied by the almost invariably present reversing patent ductus arteriosus.

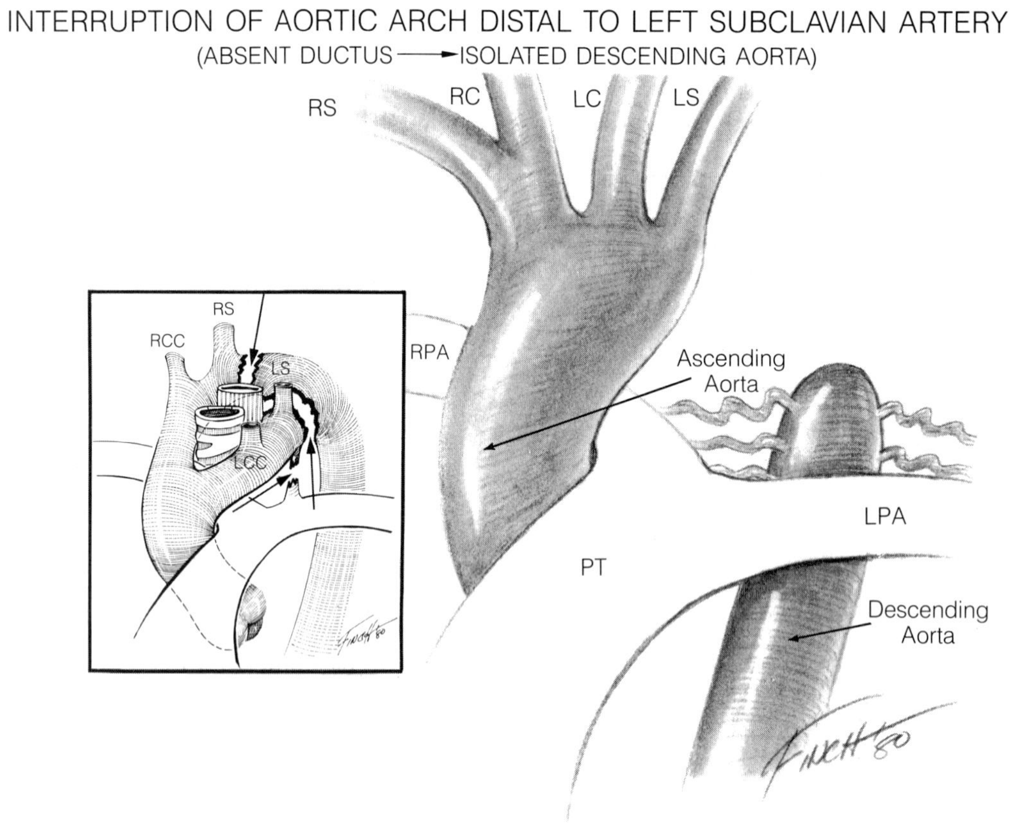

INTERRUPTION OF AORTIC ARCH DISTAL TO LEFT SUBCLAVIAN ARTERY
(ABSENT DUCTUS ⟶ ISOLATED DESCENDING AORTA)

FIG 62–42.
Interruption of aortic arch beyond left subclavian artery *(LS)*. Closed ductus. Descending aorta supplied through intercostal arteries. *RS* = right subclavian artery; *RC* = right carotid artery; *LC* = left carotid artery; *RPA* = right pulmonary artery; *LPA* = left pulmonary artery; *PT* = pulmonary trunk; *RCC* = right common carotid artery; *LCC* = left common carotid artery.

If both subclavian arteries arise distal to the interruption of the aortic arch, only coronary and cerebral blood flows through the ascending aorta.

5. The "aortic" arch may appear to have an unusually low position on posteroanterior and lateral projections (see Fig 62–43). REASON: The large patent ductus arteriosus is in direct communication with the large descending aorta simulating an aortic arch.

6. In patients with either a small or absent ductus arteriosus, the figure-of-3 sign seen in coarctation is incomplete. REASON: The proximal part of the figure-of-3 sign found in coarctation of the aorta is formed by the aortic arch but absent in interruption of the aortic arch (see Chapter 28).

The left upper mediastinum is not as prominent as in coarctation of the aorta. REASON: Even though the left subclavian artery commonly arises distal to the interruption of the aortic arch, it is not dilated as in coarctation of the aorta.

Angiographic Features[28]

Exact demonstration of the anatomy of the aortic arch is of paramount importance before operation. The origin of each of the brachiocephalic artery, the presence of the ventricular septal defect, and association of subaortic stenosis have to be demonstrated.

The descending aorta can be visualized by injecting the pulmonary artery, because patients with interruption of the aortic arch have a right-to-left shunt through a patent ductus arteriosus. A pulmonary arteriogram usually does not clearly demonstrate the brachiocephalic arteries arising from the descending aorta distal to the interruption. These arteries are best visualized by an aortogram performed from the descending aorta using balloon occlusion. In patients with a small patent ductus arteriosus, the brachiocephalic arteries act as collaterals and carry blood toward the descending aorta. Consequently, they may not opacify if a standard descending aortogram is performed.

Left ventriculography must be performed to demonstrate the ventricular septal defect and possibly subaortic stenosis. Because the ascending aorta is filled from the left ventricle and the descending aorta is opacified by the left-to-right shunt through a ventricular defect and reversing patent ductus arteriosus, the interruption may be overlooked. Thus, an aortogram from the ascending aorta may

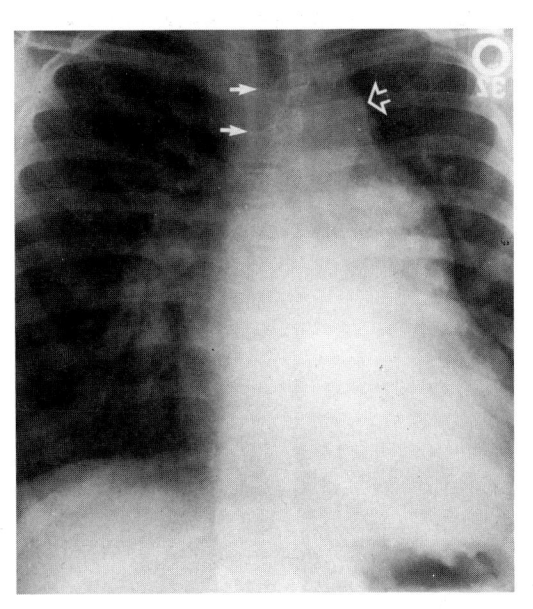

FIG 62-43.
Interruption of aortic arch. Thoracic roentgenogram. Posteroanterior projection. Cardiac size, pulmonary arterial segment, and pulmonary vasculature are increased. REASON: Many patients have an associated ventricular septal defect. What appears to be a prominent aorta *(open arrow)* is a large patent ductus arteriosus. Midline trachea in the presence of what appears to be a large aorta suggests interruption of aortic arch with large patent ductus simulating a prominent aortic arch.

be required to delineate the exact anatomy of the ascending aorta and its major arterial branches.

1. The ascending aorta tends to be small (Fig 62-44). REASON: Normally the ascending aorta carries the entire cardiac output. In interruption of the aortic arch, only the upper half of the body is supplied by the ascending aorta, and at times blood flow consists only of the coronary and cerebral circulation because the arteries to the arm may arise from the descending aorta, which is supplied through a reversing patent ductus arteriosus.

2. The ascending aorta is in a midline position and continues straight cephalad toward the neck. Normally the aortic arch has a slightly oblique course. Because the aortic arch is absent in instances of interruption, the ascending aorta tends to be more in the midline.

3. The origin of the brachiocephalic arteries appears symmetric, giving the typical staghorn configuration in cases with interruption beyond the left-carotid artery (see Fig 62-44).

4. After the origin of the last branch from the ascending aorta, the ascending aorta ends abruptly and the distal aortic arch is not visualized. This pattern is in distinction from coarctation of the aorta, where a segment of tubular hypoplasia is usually seen.

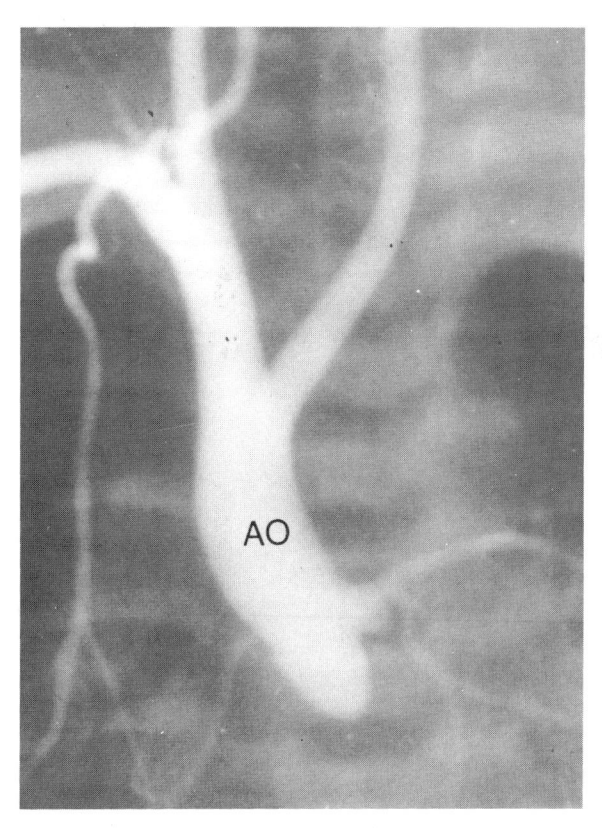

FIG 62-44.
Interruption of aortic arch beyond left carotid artery. Aortogram. Anteroposterior projection. Ascending aorta has staghorn appearance because it ends with left carotid artery. Left subclavian artery and descending aorta are unopacified because of interruption. Their blood supply is through a reversing ductus arteriosus from right ventricle. No collateral arteries are visualized, indicating that reversing patent ductus arteriosus is large. *AO* = aorta.

5. Patients with severe coarctation or atresia of the segment of the aortic arch beyond the last brachiocephalic artery cannot be differentiated from interruption of the aortic arch.

6. The ductus is a direct continuation of the pulmonary artery (Fig 62-45).

7. The descending aorta opacifies well by injecting the right ventricle or the pulmonary artery (see Fig 62-45). If the patent ductus arteriosus is small, the brachiocephalic arteries arising from the descending aorta may not opacify well. REASON: Blood flow may be reversed in these arteries, because they may serve as collaterals. Balloon occlusion descending aortography yields better results.

8. The right ventricle and pulmonary artery are enlarged. REASON: There is pulmonary hypertension.

9. With a small (pressure-limiting) patent ductus arteriosus, collateral arteries are visualized as in coarctation of the aorta. Collateral pathways vary, depending on the type of interruption of the aortic arch (Fig 62-46).

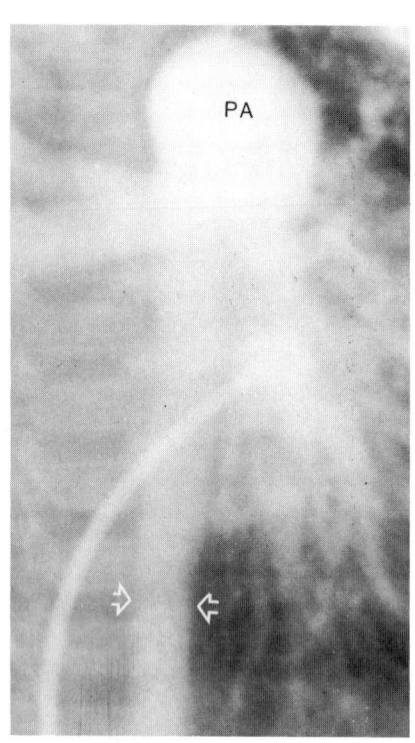

FIG 62–45.
Interruption of the aortic arch. Right ventriculogram. Anteroposterior projection. Dense opacification of descending aorta *(open arrow)* through large patent ductus arteriosus. *PA* = pulmonary artery.

10. A ventricular septal defect is almost always present. Subaortic stenosis may be found. The ventricular septal defect may be located at any site in the ventricular septum. The muscular subaortic stenosis forms a characteristic spurlike filling defect (Fig 62–47).

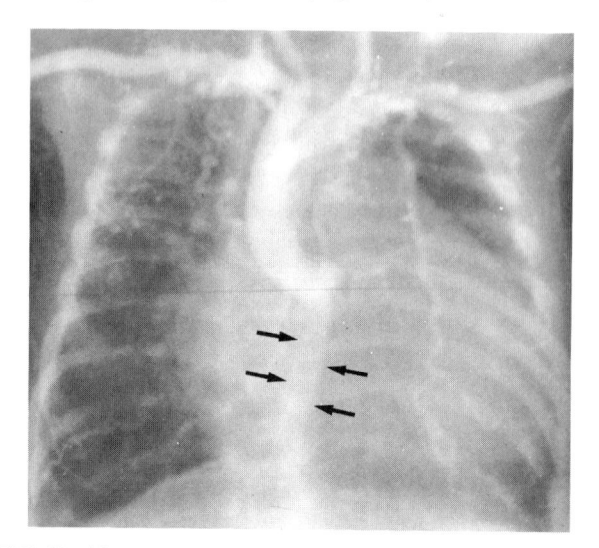

FIG 62–46.
Interruption of the aortic arch with narrowed ductus arteriosus. Aortogram. Anteroposterior projection. Descending aorta *(arrows)* is opacified through extensive collateral arteries.

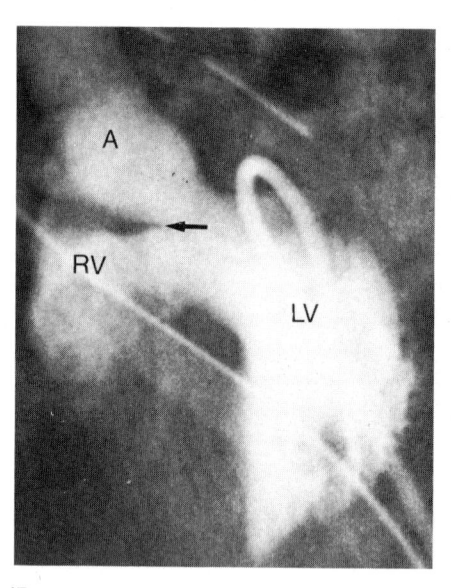

FIG 62–47.
Interruption of aortic arch. Ventricular septal defect and muscular subaortic stenosis (mild). Left ventriculogram. Anteroposterior projection. Ventricular septal defect does not involve membranous septum, and muscular subaortic stenosis forms a characteristic spur just above ventricular communication *(arrow)*. *A* = aorta; *RV* = right vertebral artery; *LV* = left ventricle.

11. Interruption of the aortic arch may coexist with truncus arteriosus or aorticopulmonary window (Fig 62–48).

Operative Considerations

Because of the very high mortality, 75% in the first month of life,[24] operative correction should be performed as an urgent procedure. Many patients become symptomatic as the ductus arteriosus closes. With the administration of prostaglandin E_1, systemic perfusion can be maintained in order to stabilize the infant's condition for operation.[29] Several techniques have been developed, depending on the anatomy, but commonly a conduit is placed from the ascending to the descending aorta (Fig 62–49) or an end-to-end anastomosis is made. The ductus is divided.[30] Pulmonary artery banding is often carried out. Usually at a second operation the ventricular septal defect is closed.

ABNORMALITY OF THE THIRD AORTIC ARCH SYSTEM

The only abnormality of the third aortic arch discussed in this chapter is cervical aortic arch.

Cervical Aortic Arch[31–33]

In this rare condition, the apex of the aortic arch is in either the apex of the thoracic cavity or base of the neck. In two thirds of the cases the arch is on the right side, and

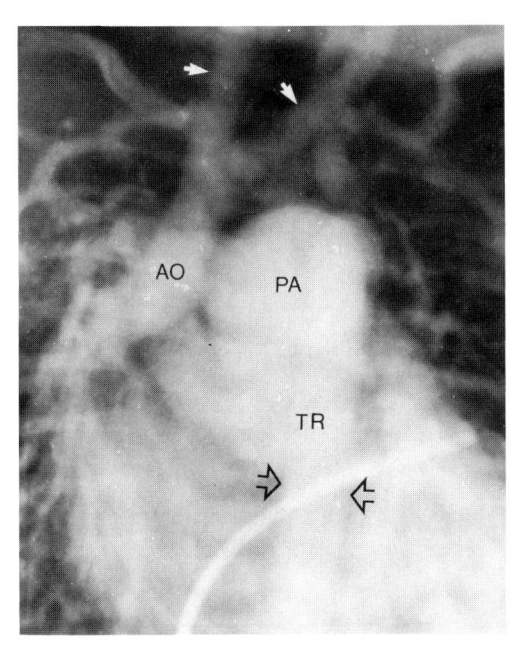

FIG 62-48.
Interruption of the aortic arch and persistent truncus arteriosus *(TR)*. Both subclavian arteries arise distal to the interruption of aortic arch. Right and left carotid arteries *(arrows)* arise from ascending aorta *(AO)* "staghorn" aorta *(open arrows)*. Descending aorta fills via patent ductus arteriosus. *PA* = pulmonary artery.

in one third is on the left side. It may be associated with a congenital cardiac anomaly but not with a specific type.

Cervical aortic arch is a distinct developmental and radiologic entity consisting of a persistence of the third arch and regression of the fourth arches. Simply, a high position of an otherwise normal aortic arch by itself should not be considered to be a cervical arch. Cases have been described as a cervical aortic arch, which have a high position of the aortic arch in the thorax, normal branching of the brachiocephalic vessels, and no retroesophageal segment. Such cases do not represent a true cervical aortic arch but should be termed "redundant aorta," buckling of the thoracic aorta, or "pseudocoarctation" (Fig 62–50).

Cervical aortic arch most likely represents persistence of the third aortic arch and regression of the fourth arches, because the internal and external carotid arteries originate separately from the aortic arch. Evidence supporting this view is the fact that normally the third arch forms the common carotid artery and the proximal portion of the internal carotid artery. Almost invariably the dorsal aorta on the side opposite the aortic arch persists, and therefore a retroesophageal segment is present.

Cervical aortic arch lies in the supraclavicular fossa. The arch may occur on either the right (Fig 62–51) or the left (Fig 62–52) side. The aorta is redundant and crosses behind the esophagus to the opposite side. There is an in-

SURGICAL CORRECTION OF INTERRUPTED AORTIC ARCH

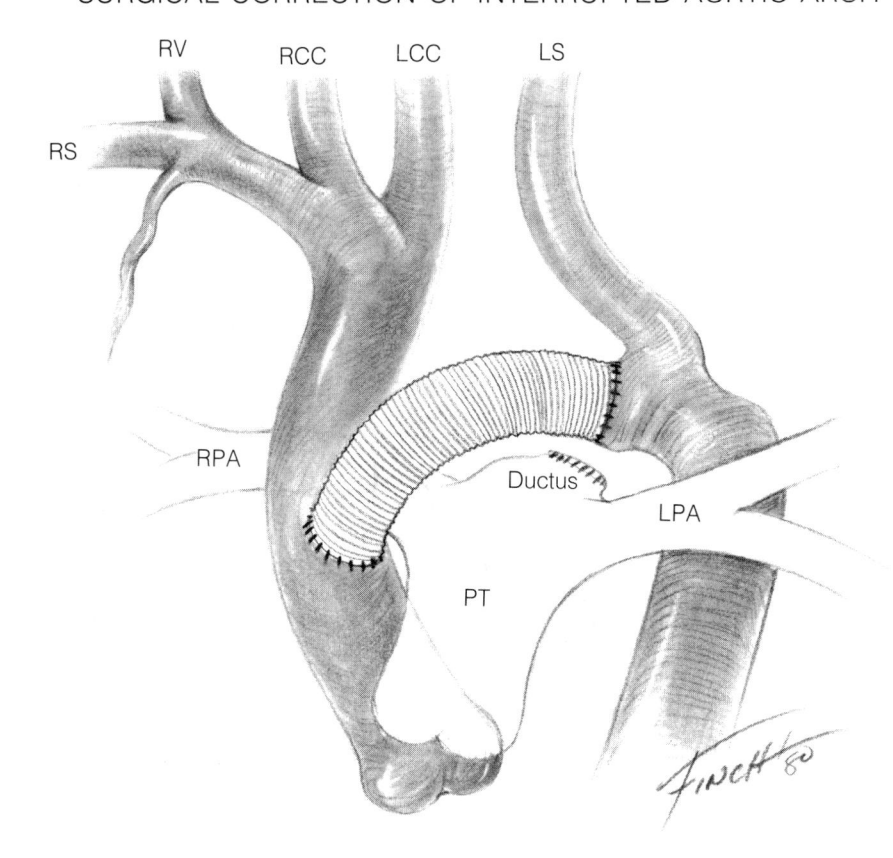

FIG 62-49.
Operation for interruption of aortic arch. Insertion of Gortex graft from ascending aorta to mouth of divided ductus arteriosus and descending aorta. *RV* = right vertebral artery; *RS* = right subclavian artery; *LS* = left subclavian artery; *RCC* = right common carotid artery; *LCC* = left common carotid artery; *RPA* = right pulmonary artery; *LPA* = left pulmonary artery; *PT* = pulmonary trunk.

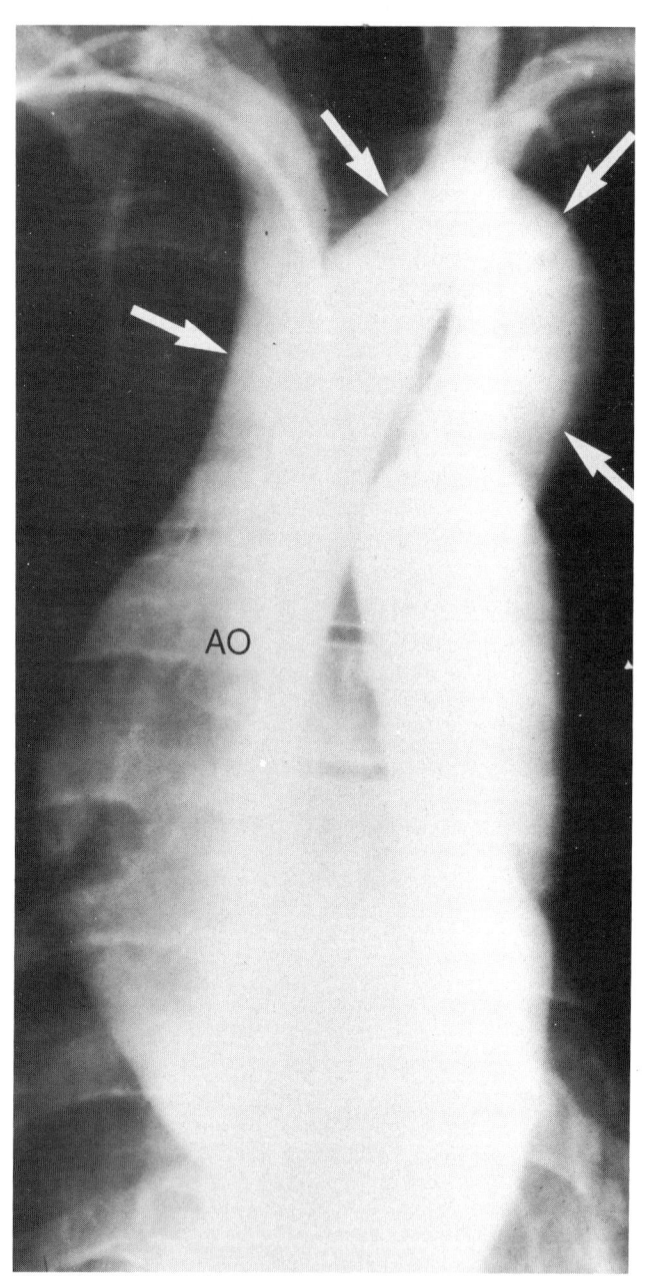

FIG 62-50.
Elongation of aorta *(AO)* (pseudocoarctation). Aortogram. Anteroposterior projection. Aortic arch *(arrows)* extending high into upper mediastinum, caused by elongation or buckling of the aorta. In distinction to true cervical arch, aortic arch and descending aorta are on same side, number of brachiocephalic vessels arising from aortic arch is normal, and subclavian artery does not arise aberrantly. Buckling of the descending aorta occurs at attachment of ductus arteriosus, mimicking coarctation of the aorta. However, true coarctation of aorta (with or without pressure gradient) may also have an elongation of aortic arch mimicking pseudocoarctation.

creased number of brachiocephalic vessels arising from the aortic arch because the internal and external carotid arteries arise separately on the same side of the aortic arch. In addition, there is usually an aberrant subclavian artery that arises from an aortic diverticulum and that may be atretic or stenotic at its origin.

A pulsating mass in the base of the neck is the most common physical finding. Additional symptoms may be respiratory distress or, less frequently, dysphagia. Symptoms occur much more frequently with a left cervical arch. When the mass is compressed, femoral pulses decrease in amplitude.

Radiographic Features

1. The aortic knob is not in its normal position.
2. A mass lesion is located in the superior mediastinum (Fig 62-53,A).
3. The barium-filled esophagus is indented posteriorly by a large vascular structure crossing behind the esophagus.
4. The direction of the indentation is obliquely downward toward the mass in the superior mediastinum. REASON: The aorta crosses obliquely behind the esophagus toward the opposite side of the thorax.
5. The descending aorta is visualized opposite the superior mediastinal mass. REASON: The aorta descends in the thorax on the side opposite the arch.
6. The trachea is displaced anteriorly (Fig 62-53,B) but not circumferentially, as with a vascular ring.

Angiographic Features

The diagnosis is confirmed by aortography, computerized tomography or best by nuclear magnetic resonance imaging.

1. The aortic arch lies high in the superior mediastinum and accounts for the mass seen on a thoracic roentgenogram. With a right arch, the major density is caused by a dilated right subclavian artery (Fig 62-54). With a left aortic arch, the major density is caused by the cervical arch itself.
2. The aorta crosses obliquely behind the esophagus to the opposite side of the thorax. This accounts for the oblique indentation of the esophagus (see Fig 62-53,A).
3. The subclavian artery arises as a last branch of the aortic arch from an aortic diverticulum (see Fig 62-54,A), but this is not always the case (see Fig 62-54,B).
4. The external and internal carotid arteries arise separately from the aortic arch, and commonly the vertebral artery does also (see Fig 62-54). Therefore, the number of brachiocephalic arteries arising from the arch is greater than normal.

RIGHT CERVICAL AORTIC ARCH

FIG 62–51.
Right cervical aortic arch. Aortic arch is located high and on right side. Right external *(REC)* and internal *(RIC)* carotid arteries arise as separate vessels from arch. Right subclavian artery *(RS)* arises from aortic diverticulum. Aorta crosses midline and descends in left side of thorax. Left subclavian artery *(LS)* arises aberrantly from diverticulum. *LCC* = left common carotid artery.

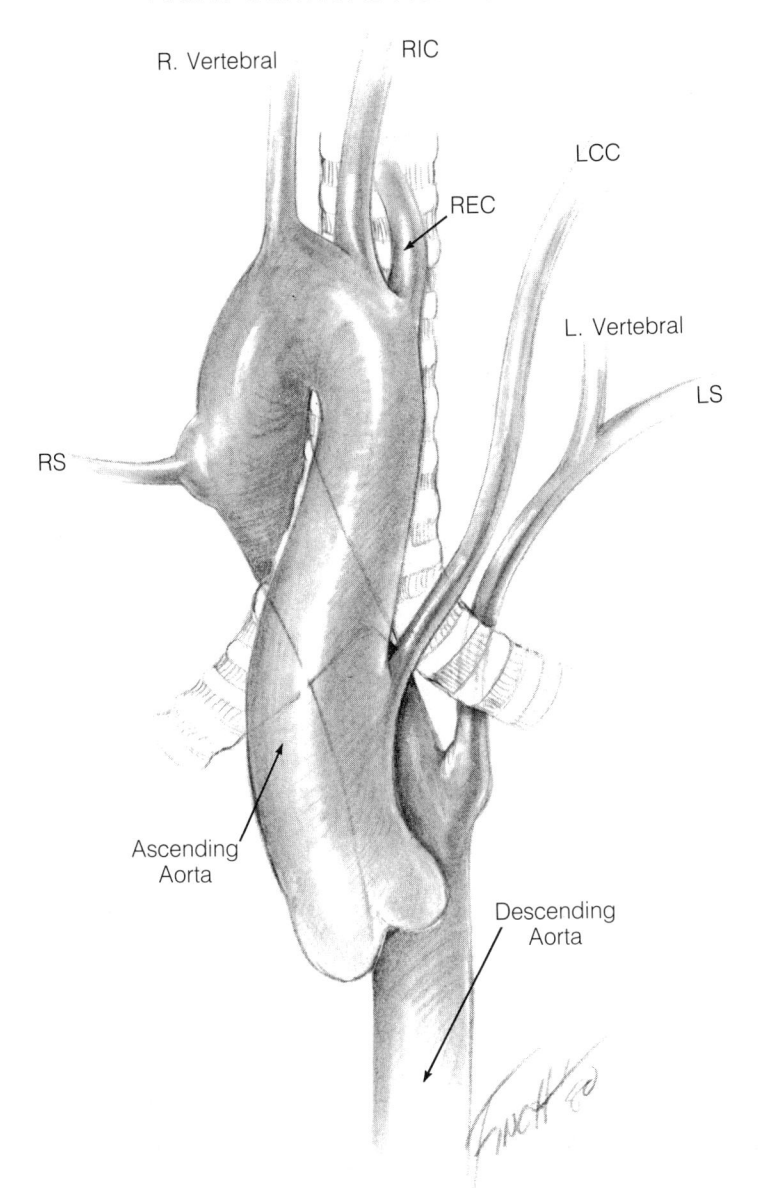

5. With a left cervical aortic arch the right subclavian artery is markedly dilated. REASON: Increased blood flows in utero through a right-sided ductus arteriosus (see Fig 62–54).

6. A small diverticulum-like outpouching can sometimes be seen in the ascending aorta. REASON: Developmentally the cervical aortic arch represents a persistence of the third arch and obliteration of the fourth arch. The small diverticulum represents a remnant of the fourth arch (Fig 62–55).

Operative Considerations

In patients with severe respiratory problems, operation is indicated to relieve the tracheal compression. If stenosis or atresia of the aberrant subclavian artery is present, the symptoms of cerebral ischemia caused by the subclavian steal can be relieved by placing a venous graft from either the aorta or from one of the carotid arteries. Most patients do not require operative treatment.

ABNORMALITY OF FIFTH AORTIC ARCH SYSTEM

Normally the fifth aortic arch is poorly developed in the human embryo, and instances of its persistence are rare.[34–36] Rarely the entire fifth aortic arch may persist and form what has been termed a "double-lumen aortic

1032 Anomalies of Major Blood Vessels

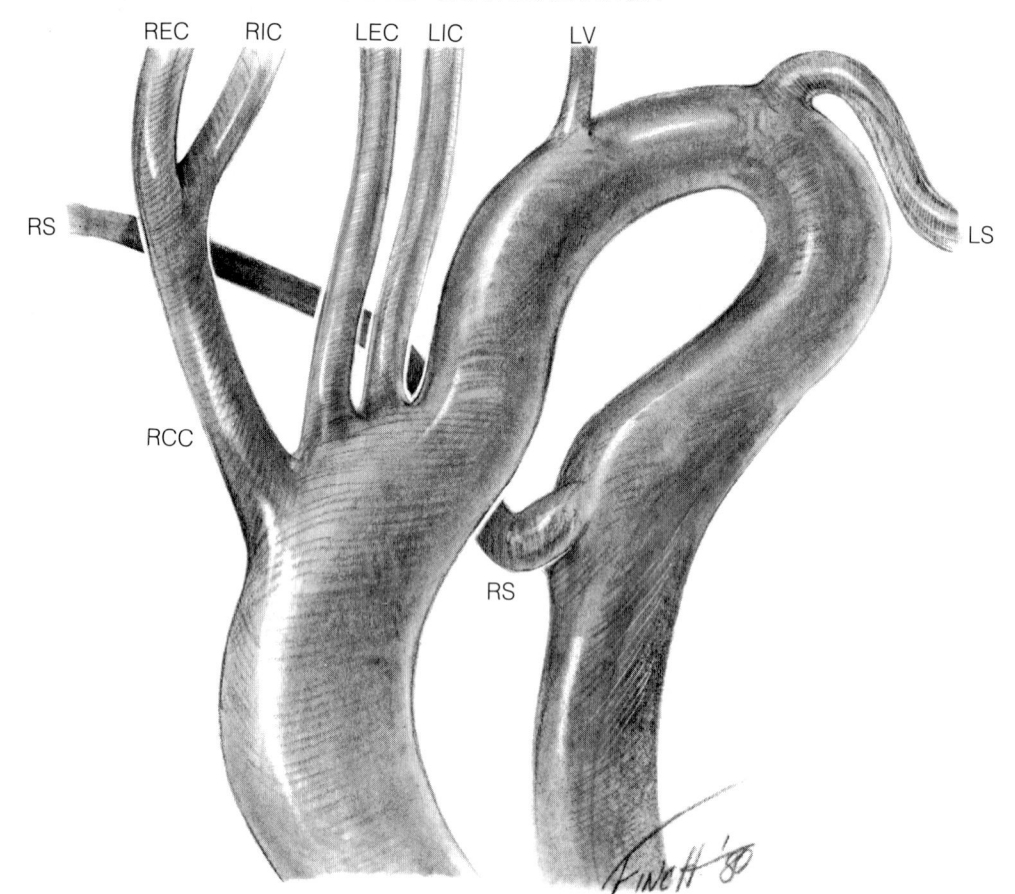

FIG 62–52.
Left cervical aortic arch. Aortic arch is located high and on left side. Left internal *(LIC)* and external *(LEC)* carotid arteries arise separately. Aorta crosses behind esophagus to descend on right side of thorax. Right subclavian artery *(RS)* arises from aortic diverticulum and passes behind esophagus to right arm. This is a mirror image of more common form (right cervical aortic arch; see Fig 62–51). *REC* = right external carotid artery; *RIC* = right internal carotid artery; *LV* = left vertebral artery; *LS* = left subclavian artery; *RCC* = right common carotid artery.

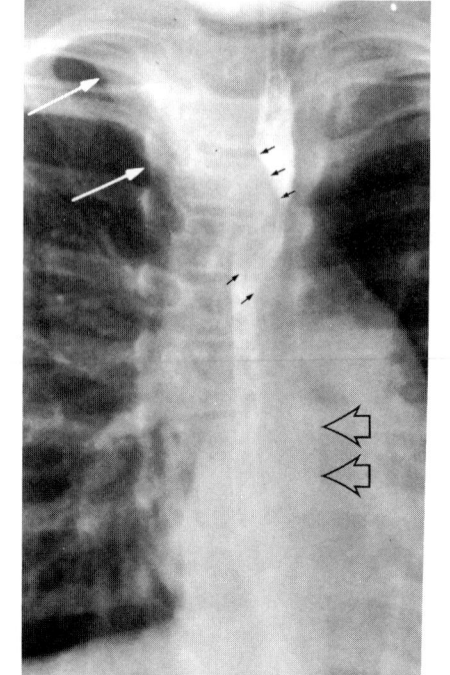

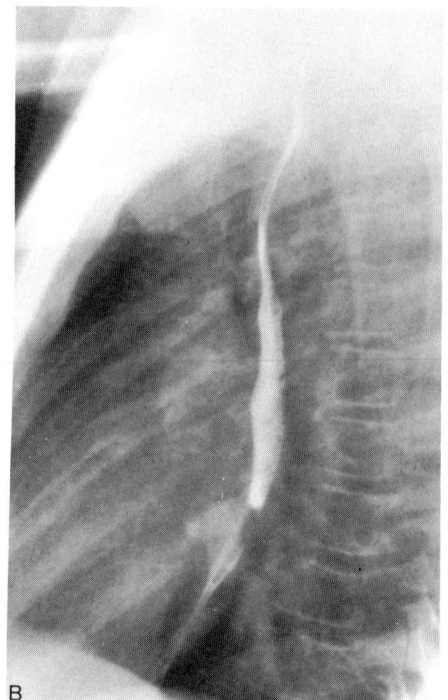

FIG 62–53.
Right cervical aortic arch. Thoracic roentgenograms. **A,** anteroposterior projection. Mass density in right upper mediastinum *(white arrows)*. Trachea is shifted to left. Oblique indentation *(black arrows)* of esophagus is caused by retroesophageal aorta. Descending aorta *(open arrows)* on left side of thorax. **B,** lateral projection. Long, shallow indentation of esophagus from behind is caused by aorta crossing behind esophagus.

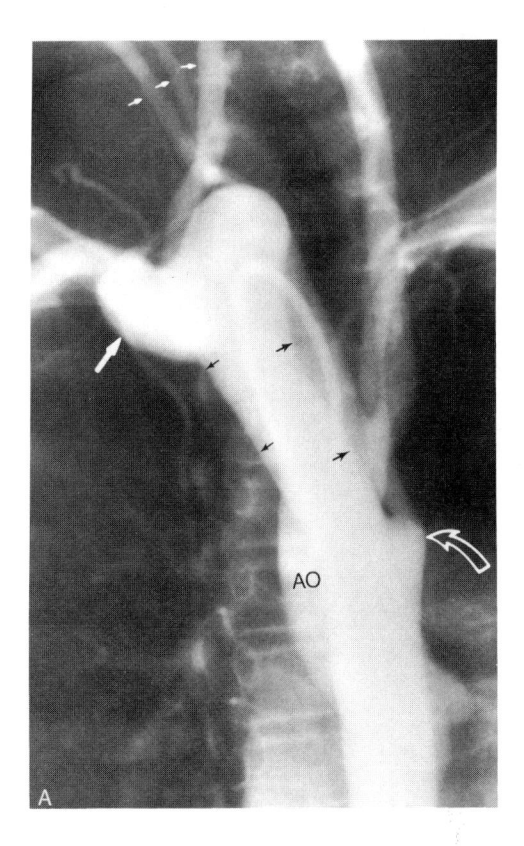

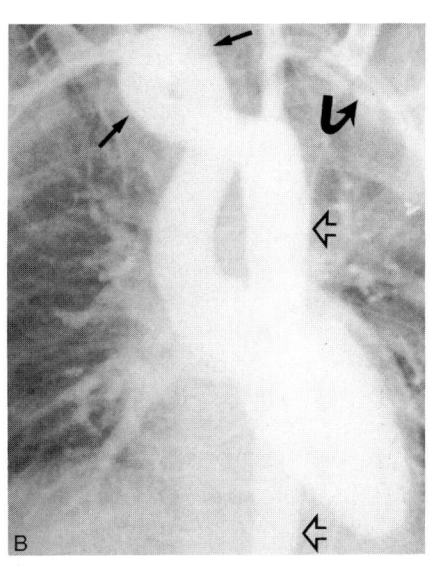

FIG 62–54.
Right cervical aortic arch. **A,** aortogram. Anteroposterior projection. Dilated origin of right subclavian artery *(white arrows)*, probably because it carried blood flow through fetal ductus arteriosus. Right external carotid, right internal carotid, and right vertebral arteries arise separately *(small white arrows)*. Aorta *(AO)* crosses obliquely behind esophagus *(black arrows)* to descend in left hemithorax. Left subclavian artery arises aberrantly from aortic diverticulum *(open arrow)*. **B,** pulmonary arteriogram. Late phase. Anteroposterior projection. Right cervical arch *(black arrows)*. Aorta descends on left *(open arrow)*. Right subclavian artery does not arise from diverticulum. Aberrant left subclavian artery *(curved arrow)*.

arch." This malformation is so rare that experienced cardiac pathologists doubt its existence. Nevertheless, isolated cases have been demonstrated angiographically (Fig 62–56).

In this anomaly the fourth arch persists and gives rise in normal fashion to the brachiocephalic arteries. In addition, another left arch (the fifth) connects the ascending and descending aorta. Proof that this second arch is not a variant of the sixth arch is by the identification of a ductus arteriosus. A possible variant of the fifth arch is the occurrence of a single arterial trunk giving rise to each of the brachiocephalic vessels. This arterial trunk perhaps represents the primitive fourth left aortic arch, which is interrupted distally. The aortic arch then represents the fifth arch.

ABNORMALITIES OF THE SIXTH AORTIC ARCH

There are three abnormalities of the sixth aortic arch: (1) patent ductus arteriosus, (2) proximal interruption of the sixth aortic arch, and (3) pulmonary arterial sling. Because it is so common and presents a different clinical picture, patent ductus arteriosus is discussed in Chapter 16.

Early in the embryo, primitive right and left pulmonary arteries join the respective sixth aortic arches (Fig 62–57).[37] Subsequently, the dorsal part of the right sixth aortic arch disappears, and that portion of the sixth left aortic arch persists as patent ductus arteriosus. The ventral portion of each sixth arch forms the proximal part of the right and left pulmonary arteries, respectively. After birth the distal part of the left sixth aortic arch, the patent ductus arteriosus, normally closes.

Proximal Interruption of the Sixth Aortic Arch

Proximal interruption of the sixth aortic arch has also been called "absence of the pulmonary artery" or "ductal origin of the pulmonary artery." It is an uncommon lesion that may occur either as an isolated condition (one half of the cases) or in association with other congenital cardiac abnormalities (one half of cases), particularly tetralogy of Fallot.[38]

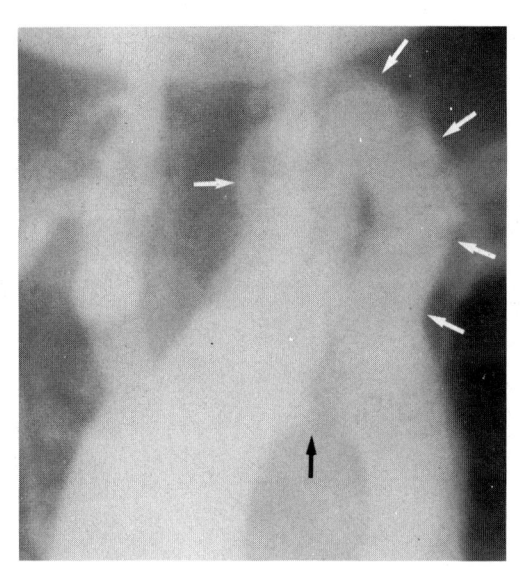

FIG 62-55.
Left cervical aortic arch *(white arrow)*. Aortogram. Anteroposterior projection. Remnant of obliterated fourth arch *(black arrow)* is evidenced by small diverticulum of aorta. This finding supports idea that cervical aortic arch represents persistence of third aortic arch.

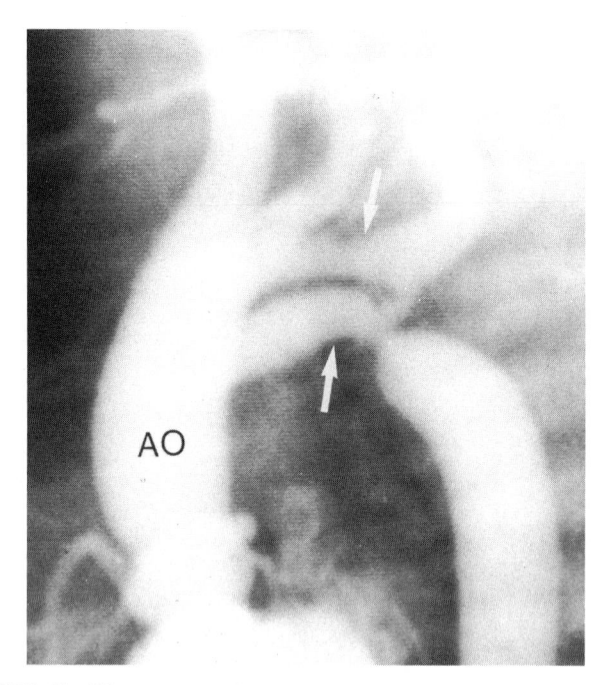

FIG 62-56.
Persistence of fifth aortic arch. Aortogram. Lateral projection. Double-lumen aortic arch *(arrows)* and coarctation of aorta *(AO)* are demonstrated. (Courtesy of Dr. Gordon Culham, M.D.)

The name of the condition describes the developmental problem, interruption of the proximal portion of a sixth aortic arch.[37] Normally the distal portion of the right sixth aortic arch disappears early in fetal life, whereas that of the left (the ductus arteriosus) persists to term and normally closes on the first day of life.

In proximal interruption of the sixth aortic arch, the ventral part of the sixth arch regresses and disappears, and the dorsal portion of a sixth arch persists. Therefore, the involved lung receives blood during fetal life through the ductus arteriosus and not from the pulmonary trunk.

After birth, the ductus arteriosus normally closes. If it closes before birth, the bronchial-segmental or intercostal arteries persist, eventually supplying blood to the pulmonary arterial system. If the ductus remains patent, this vessel provides the major source of pulmonary blood flow to the involved lung.

Anatomic Relationships

The left and the right pulmonary arteries are interrupted in equal frequency. Rarely, both pulmonary arteries are interrupted in the same patient. Usually the interrupted pulmonary artery occurs opposite the side of the aortic arch, except in instances of tetralogy of Fallot, where the left lung is involved regardless of the side of the aortic arch.[38]

The ductus arteriosus remains patent more frequently with interruption of the right pulmonary artery than with interruption of the left pulmonary artery. If the ductus arteriosus remains patent and is large, pulmonary vascular disease may develop in the involved lung, and the pulmonary arterioles appear normal in the opposite normally connected lung.

If the ductus is occluded, a complete pulmonary arterial tree originating from the hilus exists in the involved lung (Fig 62-58).[39] In this instance, the pulmonary arterial tree remains patent because it is perfused by the bronchial intercostal or other systemic arteries, which enter the lung and join the pulmonary arterial system at various levels within the pulmonary parenchyma (Fig 62-59).

The hemithorax and lung on the involved side are smaller than the opposite side. Bronchiectasis is common.

Clinical Features

The clinical features vary but are usually those of the major associated cardiac malformation. Without an associated cardiac malformation, the condition may be unrecognized until adolescence or early childhood, when pulmonary problems related to bronchiectasis, hemoptysis, or pulmonary hypertension become evident.[40] Patients may develop unilateral pulmonary edema, particularly when exposed to high altitude.[41]

On physical examination the thoracic cage on the involved side is smaller than the contralateral side, and the breath sounds may be distant. The heart may be shifted toward the involved side, so that the apex impulse is displaced.

EMBRYOLOGY OF THE AORTIC ARCH SYSTEM

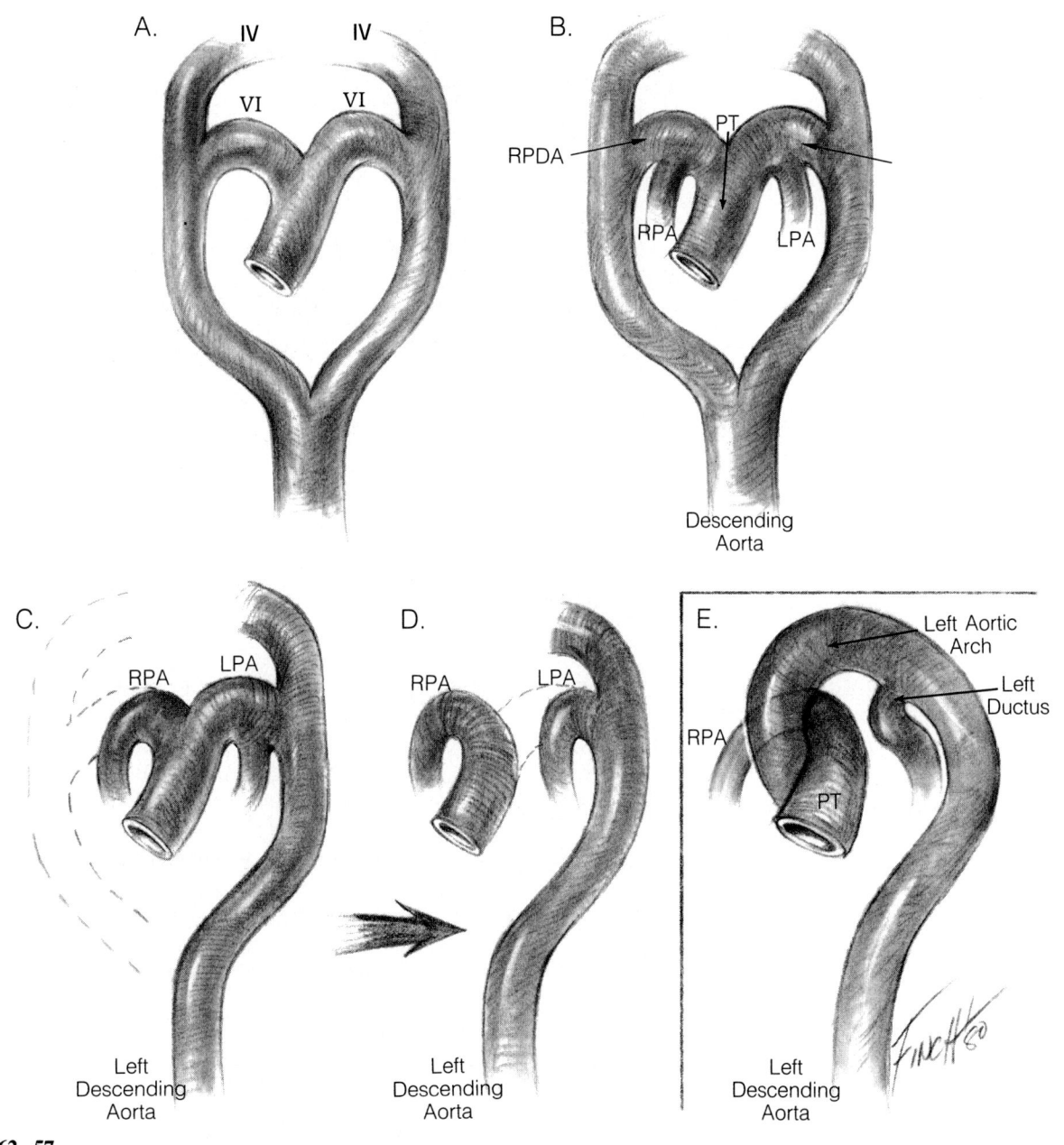

FIG 62–57.
Development of pulmonary arteries. *IV* = 4th arch; *VI* = 6th arch; *RPDA* = right patent ductus arteriosus; *PT* = pulmonary trunk; *RPA* = right pulmonary artery; *LPA* = left pulmonary artery.

PROXIMAL INTERRUPTION OF RIGHT PULMONARY ARTERY
"ABSENT RIGHT PULMONARY ARTERY"

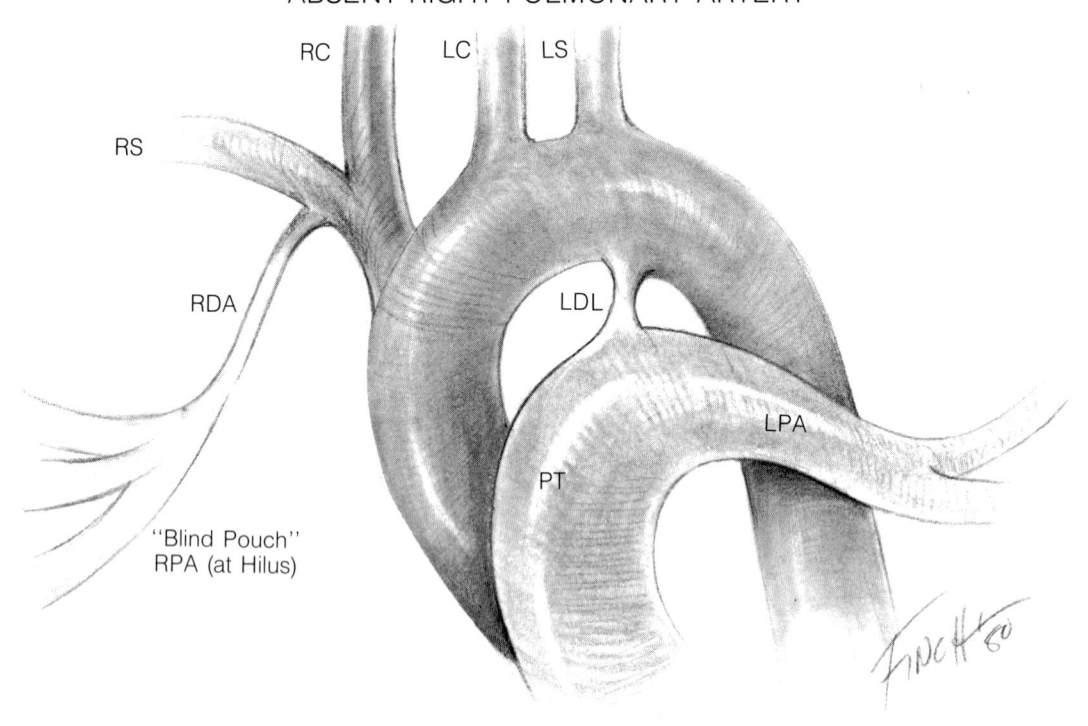

FIG 62–58.
Interruption of the right pulmonary artery *(RPA)* (absence of right pulmonary artery). Pulmonary trunk *(PT)* continues as left pulmonary *(LPA)*. Right pulmonary artery is connected to right subclavian artery *(RS)* by right-sided ductus arteriosus *(RDA)*. *RC* = right carotid artery; *LC* = left carotid artery; *LS* = left subclavian artery; *LDL* = left ductus ligament.

In patients with pulmonary hypertension, the pulmonary component of the second heart sound is accentuated, and there may be a pulmonary systolic ejection click, third heart sound, and a murmur of pulmonary insufficiency.

Electrocardiographic Features

The electrocardiogram (ECG) in isolated cases is normal or shows right ventricular hypertrophy if pulmonary hypertension develops. In instances with associated cardiac conditions, the ECG reflects the major cardiac anomaly.

Echocardiographic Features

There are no diagnostic features in M-mode echocardiography, but with sector scanning the diagnosis may be suggested by demonstration of discontinuity of the pulmonary trunk with the branch pulmonary arteries.

Radiographic Features

Although this condition has also been referred to as absence of the pulmonary artery, the pulmonary arterial system remains patent because it is supplied through collateral arteries.

1. The thoracic cage is usually asymmetric, with the involved side being smaller. The intercostal spaces may be narrowed and the diaphragm elevated on the affected side (Fig 62–60).
2. There may be only a slight mediastinal shift toward the affected side, and the unaffected lung is over expanded and may herniate to the opposite side (Fig 62–61).
3. The pulmonary vasculature is diminished on the affected side, and the normally seen comma shadow of the pulmonary artery may be absent or smaller than normal.
4. The vascular pattern on the affected side may be bizarre, with small round vascular densities seen in the peripheral lung fields. REASON: Bronchial collateral arteries are more tortuous than pulmonary arteries and are therefore much more frequently visualized on end, casting round densities (see Fig 62–61).
5. There may be rib notching on the affected side. REASON: Enlargement of intercostal collaterals that develop if the pleural space is obliterated (Fig 62–62).
6. There may be pleural thickening. REASON: Collateral arterial supply to the interrupted pulmonary artery occurs through transpleural collateral arteries.
7. The aortic arch is almost invariably opposite the site of interruption, but exceptions occur (Fig 62–63).

INTERRUPTION LEFT PROXIMAL PULMONARY ARTERY AND ITS COLLATERAL SUPPLY

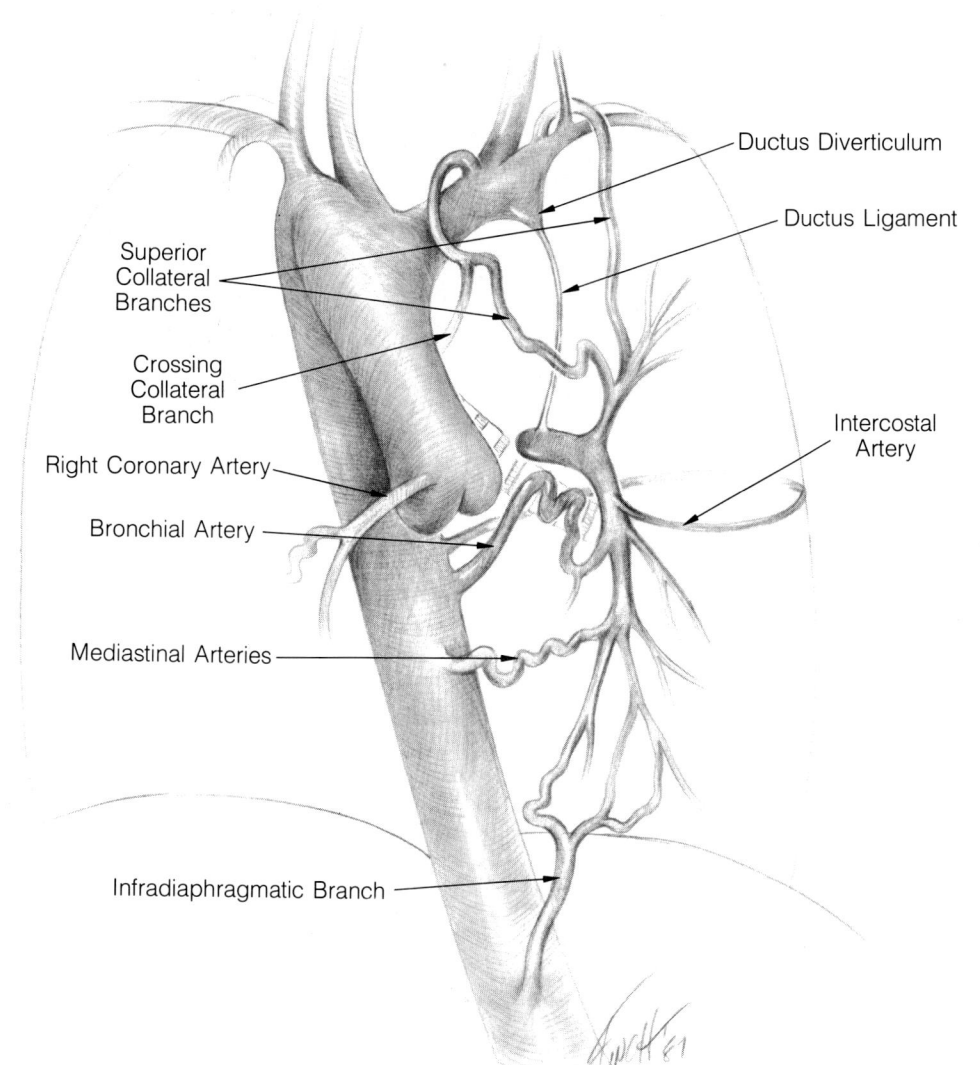

FIG 62–59.
Interruption of pulmonary artery. Diagram of the major collateral arterial supply to interrupted pulmonary artery through (1) bronchial arteries; (2) intercostal arteries, if the pleural space is obliterated; and (3) systemic arteries, such as inferior phrenic artery from below diaphragm. Aortic arch is on opposite side of interruption of pulmonary artery.

8. The pulmonary artery on the unaffected side is larger than normal. REASON: Most of the cardiac output passes through the unaffected pulmonary artery.

9. Transpleural collaterals occur only if the pleural space is obliterated.

Angiographic Features

Angiographic demonstration of an interrupted pulmonary artery may be difficult and require sophisticated angiographic techniques. The arterial supply to the involved pulmonary artery originates from either a patent ductus arteriosus, intercostal, bronchial, mediastinal arteries, or subdiaphragmatic arteries. Because of the various sources of collateral blood flow, opacification of any one of the collateral sources may be insufficient to opacify the pulmonary arterial tree because of dilution of unopacified blood from other sources. The following techniques are helpful to demonstrate the pulmonary arterial system, which is invariably patent:

1. Aortography during balloon occlusion. The descending aorta is temporarily occluded with a balloon catheter, and a thoracic aortogram is performed. The bronchial and intercostal arteries are usually filled excellently. This technique is only possible in younger patients in whom the small thoracic aorta can be readily occluded.

2. Wedge injection of pulmonary veins. The catheter is wedged in a peripheral pulmonary vein, and contrast

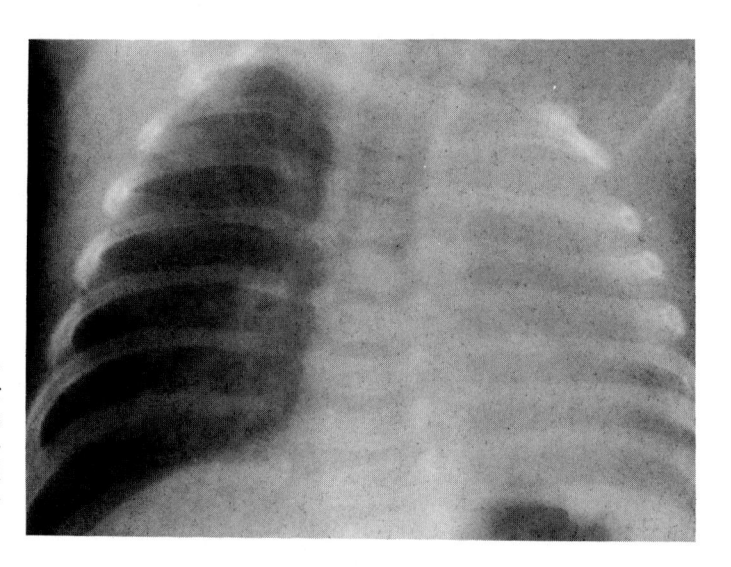

FIG 62–60.
Interruption of left pulmonary artery. Thoracic roentgenogram. Posteroanterior projection. Left hemithorax is smaller than right. Mediastinum is shifted to left. Pleura on left is thickened. Position of aortic arch cannot be determined. Patient should have right arch since interruption of the proximal pulmonary artery typically occurs opposite the aortic arch except for tetralogy.

medium is forced across the capillary bed into the pulmonary artery. This approach is rarely necessary.

3. Simultaneous selective injection of several intercostal arteries in patients with rib notching. Two or three catheters are introduced into intercostal arteries serving as collateral arteries and injected simultaneously, providing visualization of the pulmonary arterial tree (Fig 62–64).

4. Pulmonary arteriography, which demonstrates the normal pulmonary artery and no stump for the interrupted pulmonary artery (Fig 62–65).

5. There is a continuous spectrum from interruption of the pulmonary artery to hypoplasia (Fig 62–66) to agenesis and absence of the main pulmonary artery. Blood supply to the lungs occurs through either collateral arteries or a patent ductus arteriosus (Fig 62–67).

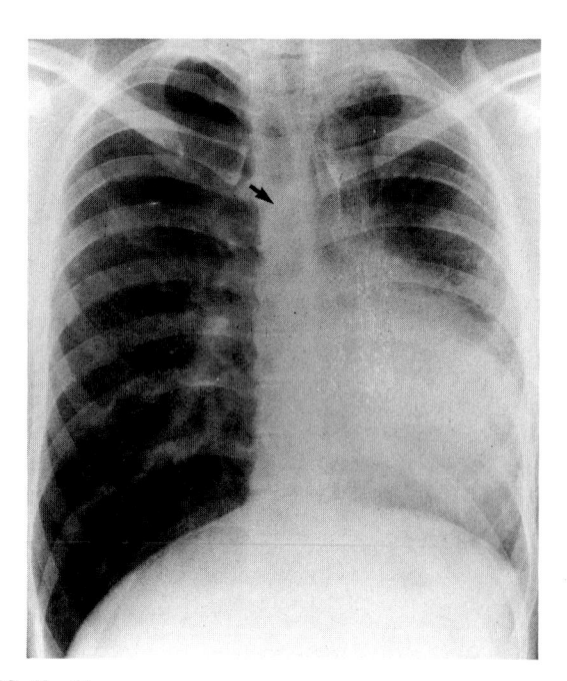

FIG 62–61.
Interruption of left pulmonary artery. Thoracic roentgenogram. Posteroanterior projection. Right aortic arch *(arrow)* is difficult to identify because of tracheal shift to left. Small left hemithorax. Narrowed left intercostal spaces. Elevated left hemidiaphragm. Overexpansion of right lung. Prominent right pulmonary artery. Bizarre and decreased left pulmonary vascular pattern. Left pulmonary artery is not evident in left hilum.

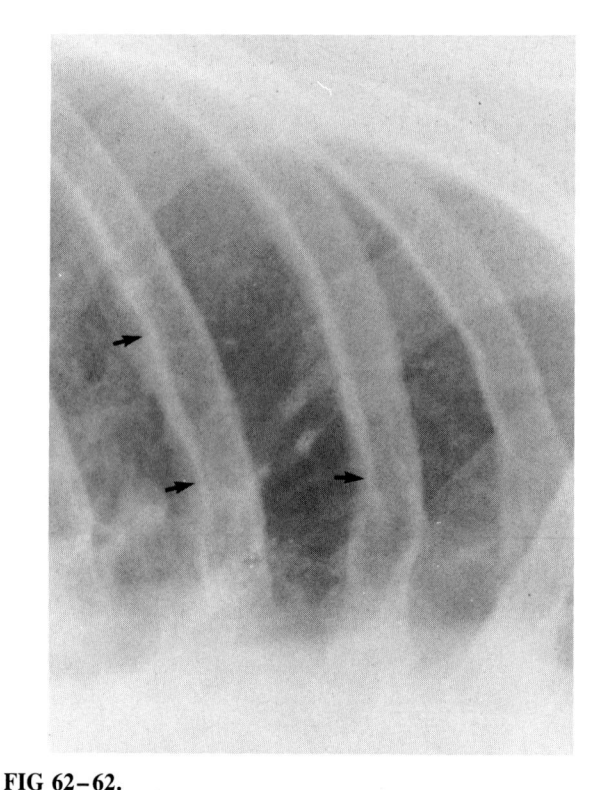

FIG 62–62.
Interruption of left pulmonary artery. Thoracic roentgenogram. Anteroposterior projection. Rib notching *(arrows)* because of enlarged intercostal collateral arteries bridging the pleural space.

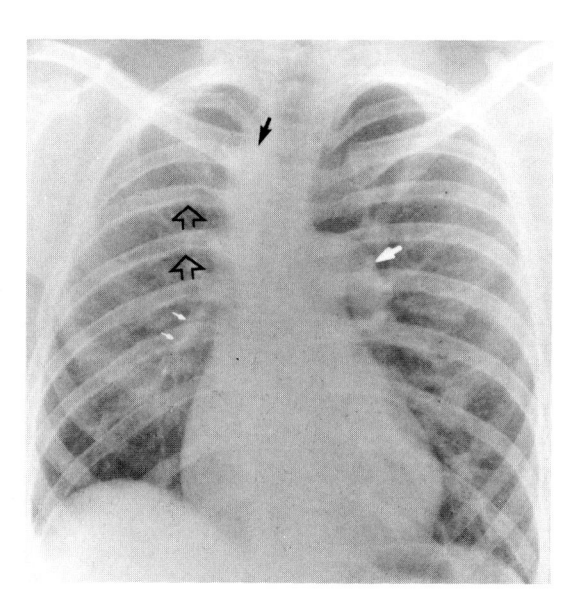

FIG 62-63.
Interruption of pulmonary artery on same side as aortic arch. Thoracic roentgenogram. Posteroanterior projection. Right aortic arch *(black arrow)*. Prominent left pulmonary artery *(white arrow)*. Elevated right hemidiaphragm. Smaller right hemithorax. Narrow right intercostal spaces. Rib notching *(open arrows)*, indicating intercostal collateral arteries. Right pulmonary artery is small but visualized *(small white arrows)*.

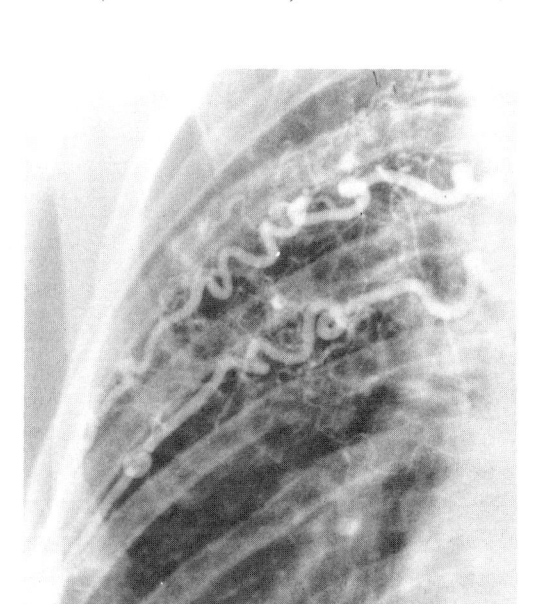

Operative Considerations

Because most infants have no pulmonary symptoms, treatment is not required. If there are severe pulmonary symptoms, pneumonectomy can be performed without affecting ventilatory function.

If a cardiac condition associated with increased pulmonary blood flow is present, it should be corrected at an early age to reduce the progression of major pulmonary vascular changes in the normal lung. The operation to correct the underlying anomaly may be combined with an attempt to reconnect the pulmonary artery,[42] but because the pulmonary artery at the hilus is frequently small, it may be difficult to maintain a patent communication. If the interrupted pulmonary artery is of fair size, it can be connected to the main pulmonary artery by a graft (Fig 62-68).

In patients with tetralogy of Fallot, because of cyanosis, it may be possible to place a shunt, such as a Blalock-Taussig, into the pulmonary artery and increase pulmonary blood flow.

PULMONARY ARTERY SLING[43-49]

Pulmonary artery sling has also been called origin of the left pulmonary artery from the right pulmonary artery.

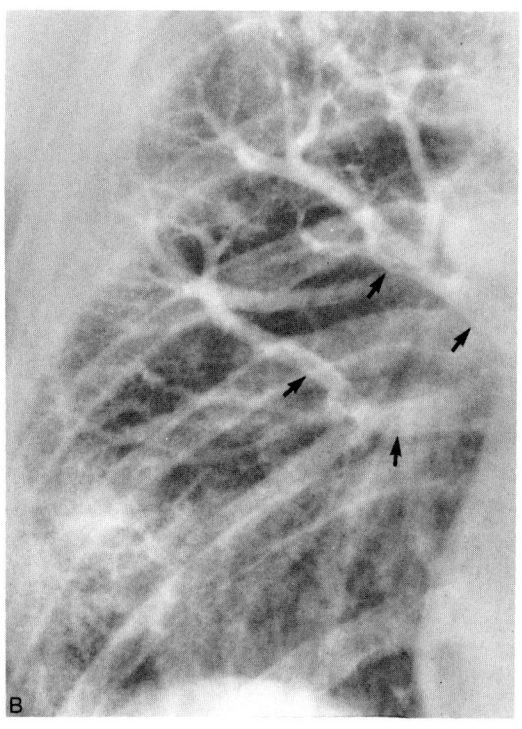

FIG 62-64.
Interruption of right pulmonary artery. Simultaneous selective injection of two intercostal arteries. **A,** opacification of two tortuous intercostal arteries serving as collateral arteries. **B,** late phase. Through transpleural collateral arteries, smaller right pulmonary artery opacifies *(arrows)*.

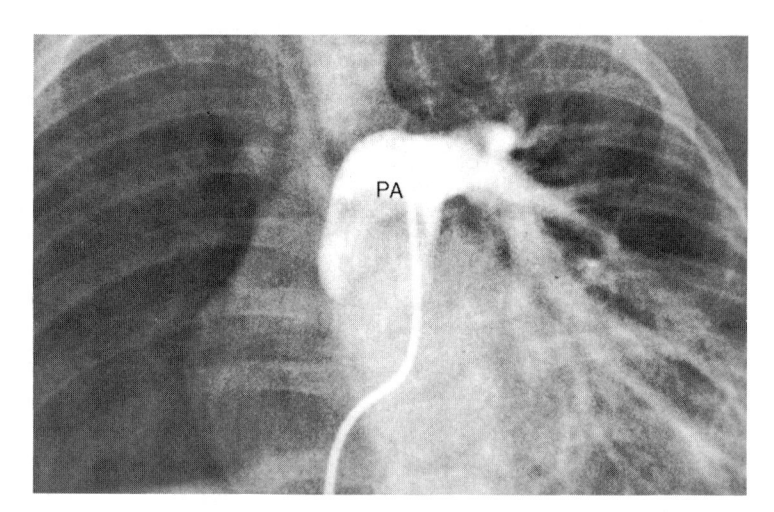

FIG 62–65.
Interrupted right pulmonary artery. Left aortic arch. Pulmonary arteriogram. Anteroposterior projection. Only left pulmonary artery is opacified. No stump for interrupted right pulmonary artery.

Although uncommon, it is important because, if unoperated, it leads to death in 50% of involved infants.

The abnormality probably develops early in embryonic life when the lungs are still a single mass. Left and right pulmonary arteries form on each side of this common pulmonary mass and make contact with the respective sixth aortic arches. At an early stage in pulmonary artery sling, this connection fails to take place on the left side. Because the lungs are still a single mass and have a common vascular supply, that portion that eventually becomes the left lung retains a vascular connection with the portion of the pulmonary mass that will become the right lung. As the lung buds separate, the vascular connection persists between the left lung and the right pulmonary artery.

The left pulmonary artery arises from the right pulmonary artery and passes to the right of the trachea, above the right mainstem bronchus, and then between the trachea and esophagus to the left lung (Fig 62–69,A). A rare variation is a pulmonary sling formed by only the left lower lobe artery (Fig 62–69,B). Because the tracheal rings of neonates are soft, they are compressed by the left pulmonary artery, which may lead to obstructive emphysema or atelectasis of the right lung. Associated tracheobronchial malformations are common, particularly bronchus suis (i.e., origin of the right upper lobe bronchus from the trachea). The surgeon should be forewarned of this possibility so as not to mistake a bronchus suis for the tracheal bifurcation.

Usually pulmonary artery sling is an isolated abnor-

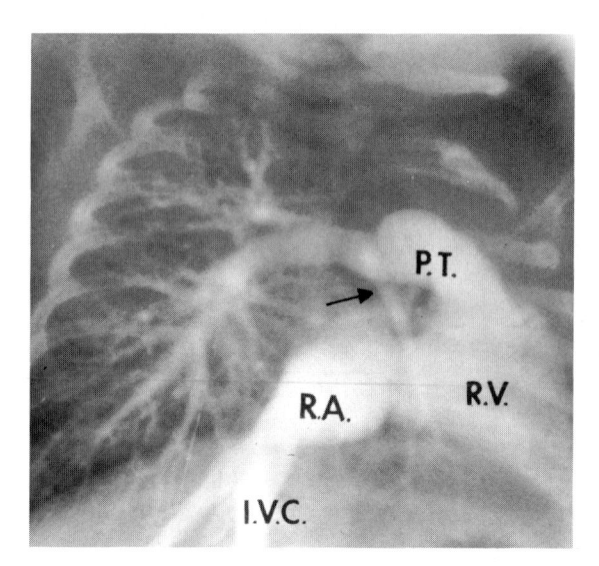

FIG 62–66.
Hypoplasia of left pulmonary artery *(arrow)*. Venous angiogram. Anteroposterior projection. Associated hypoplasia of left lung. Right pulmonary artery is normal. *I.V.C.* = inferior vena cava; *P.T.* = pulmonary trunk; *R.A.* = right atrium; *R.V.* = right ventricle.

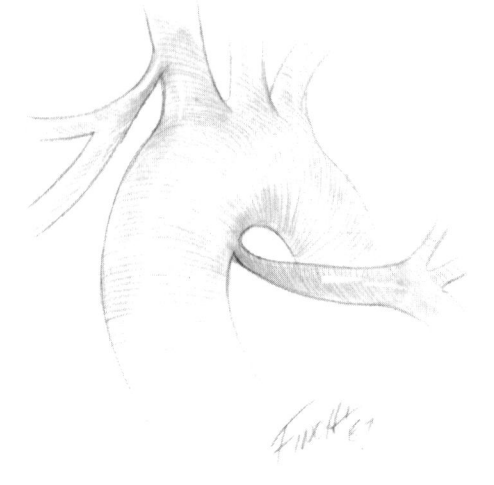

FIG 62–67.
Atresia of main pulmonary artery. Blood supply to lungs occurs through bilateral patent ductus arteriosus or collaterals.

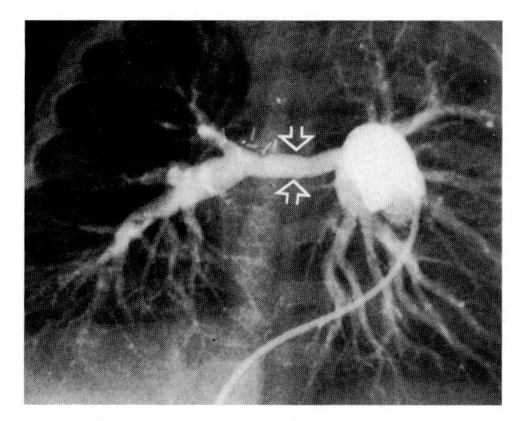

FIG 62–68.
Interruption right pulmonary artery. Pulmonary arteriogram. Anteroposterior projection. Right pulmonary artery is reconnected to pulmonary trunk via graft *(open arrows)* placed behind aorta.

mality, but cardiac anomalies commonly coexist—the most frequent being persistent left superior vena cava (20%), atrial septal defect (20%), ventricular septal defect (10%), and patent ductus arteriosus (25%).

Clinical Features

The major clinical manifestations are respiratory, particularly stridor, and are accentuated by respiratory tract infections. There is an increased incidence of respiratory tract infections and also symptoms of dyspnea and intermittent cyanosis. There are no unique findings on physical examination. There may be rales or stridor.

Radiographic Features

The diagnosis of pulmonary artery sling can be readily made on thoracic roentgenograms with barium in the esophagus.

1. The barium-filled esophagus is indented anteriorly and the trachea pushed anteriorly by a mass that lies between the esophagus and the trachea (Fig 62–70).
2. Pneumonitis, atelectasis, or emphysema of the right lung may be present. REASON: Compression of the right mainstem bronchus (Fig 62–71).
3. The mass shows pulsations on fluoroscopy or cine fluorography.
4. Demonstration of a pulsatile mass between the trachea and esophagus is virtually diagnostic of a pulmonary sling. An aberrant subclavian artery *never* passes between the trachea and esophagus. Rarely, a bronchial artery in coexistent ventricular septal defect and pulmonary atresia passes between the trachea and esophagus, but almost invariably bronchial arteries also cross *behind* the esophagus.

5. In adult patients this diagnosis is usually not suspected. The left pulmonary artery arising from the right pulmonary artery may mimic a mediastinal mass. Laminography (Fig 62–72) demonstrates the mass well. The diagnosis of pulmonary sling can be established firmly by barium swallow (Fig 62–73).
6. Rarely, the esophagogram is normal. Therefore, pulmonary artery sling cannot be absolutely excluded by a normal esophagogram.

Angiographic Features

Angiographic demonstration of pulmonary sling may be difficult, and the findings may be less obvious than with barium swallow.

1. If the catheter passes from the main pulmonary artery into the left pulmonary artery, its course is always to the *right* of the trachea. Normally the catheter passes into the left pulmonary artery by a course to the left of the trachea.
2. The anomalous origin of the left pulmonary artery from the right pulmonary artery can sometimes be well demonstrated by angiography in anteroposterior projection with the beam angle toward the feet (cranial angulation).
3. Because the left pulmonary artery tends to cross transversely behind the esophagus, cranial angulation of the beam is useful on the lateral projection as well.
4. On an anteroposterior projection, an abnormal round density can be seen to the left and behind the trachea (Fig 62–74,A and B). REASON: The left pulmonary artery is no longer a direct extension of the main pulmonary artery but crosses transversely behind the trachea, thus being seen on end.
5. If there is no beam angulation, the finding may not be obvious (see Fig 62–74). With cranial angulation (looking down), the abnormal origin of the left pulmonary artery from the right pulmonary artery is obvious (Fig 62–74,C).

Operative Considerations

Diagnosis is made radiographically. Bronchoscopy should not be performed. If left untreated, most patients with pulmonary artery sling die because of pulmonary complications. Even with operation a high mortality has been reported, but recent experience is more favorable.

Through a left thoracotomy, the left hilum and the trachea and esophagus are dissected free.[43, 45, 49] The left pulmonary artery is divided from the right pulmonary artery and then anastomosed directly to the pulmonary trunk (Fig 62–75,B).

In the immediate postoperative period, respiratory

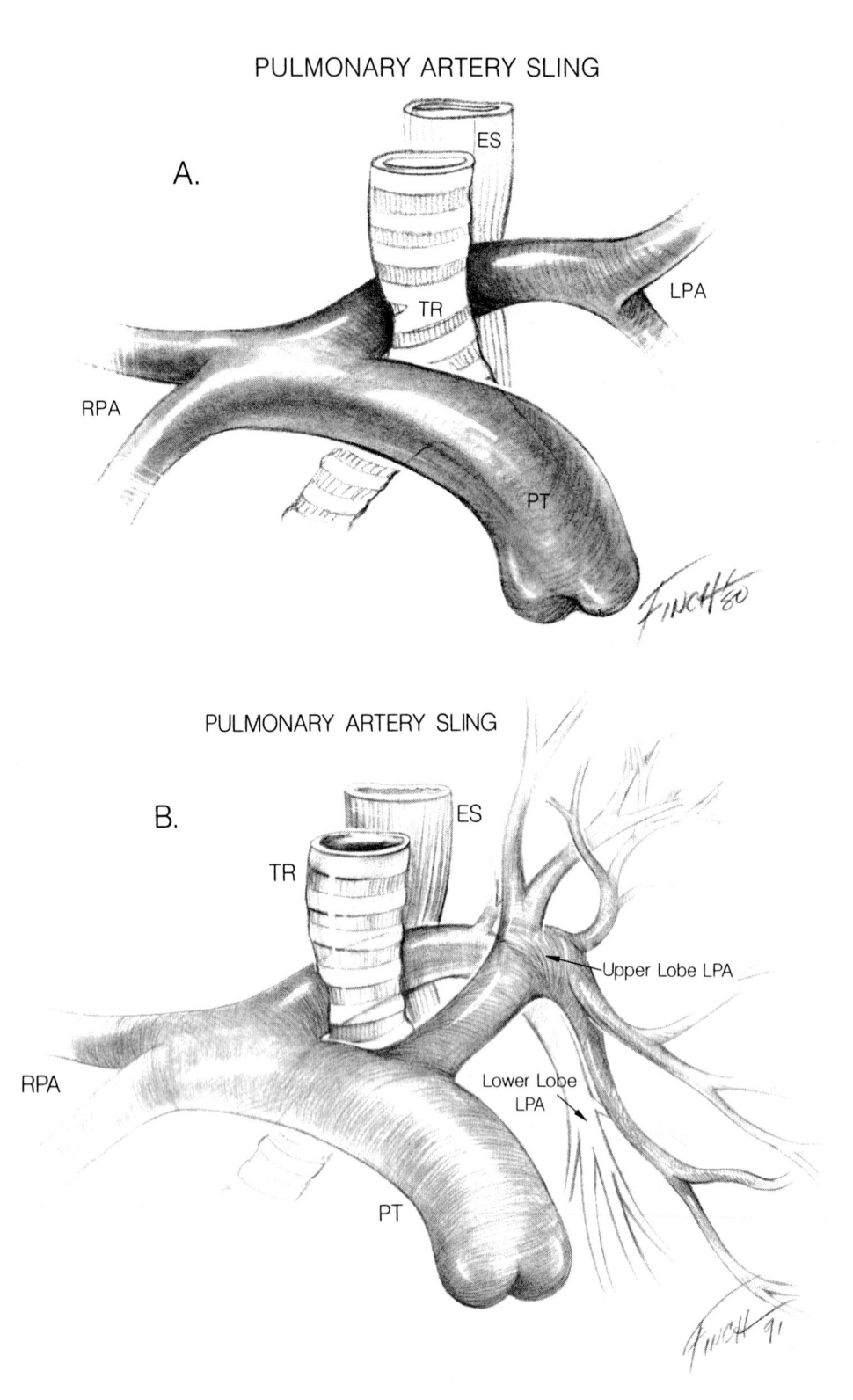

FIG 62–69.
A, pulmonary artery sling. Left pulmonary artery *(LPA)* arises from right pulmonary artery *(RPA)* and passes between trachea *(TR)* and esophagus *(ES)* to left lung. **B,** pulmonary artery sling. Rare variation. Artery to left lower lobe arises from right pulmonary artery. Artery to left upper lobe arises from pulmonary trunk *(PT)*.

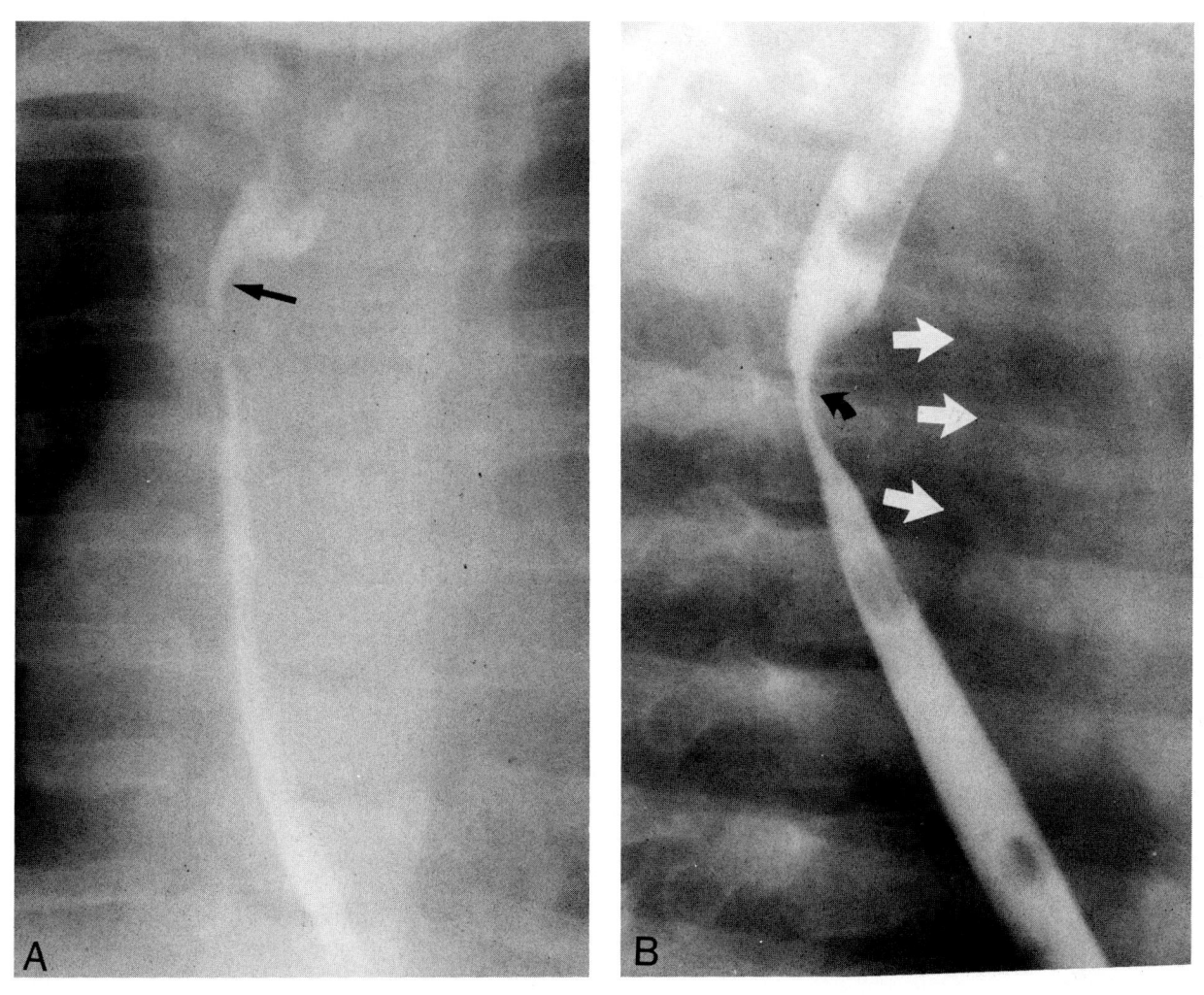

FIG 62–70.
Pulmonary artery sling (origin of left pulmonary artery from right pulmonary artery). Thoracic roentgenogram. **A,** Posteroanterior and, **B,** lateral projections. Round mass present between esophagus and trachea, displacing esophagus posteriorly and right *(black arrows)* and trachea *(white arrows)* anteriorly. This appearance is diagnostic.

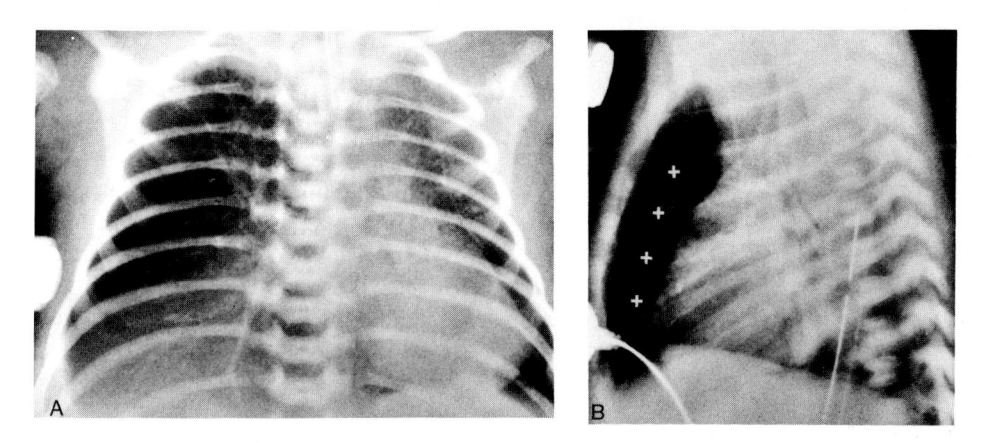

FIG 62–71.
Thoracic roentgenogram pulmonary sling. **A,** obstructive emphysema of the right lung with marked mediastinal shift to the left. **B,** anterior herniation of the right lung because of obstructive emphysema caused by pulmonary sling *(four crosses)*.

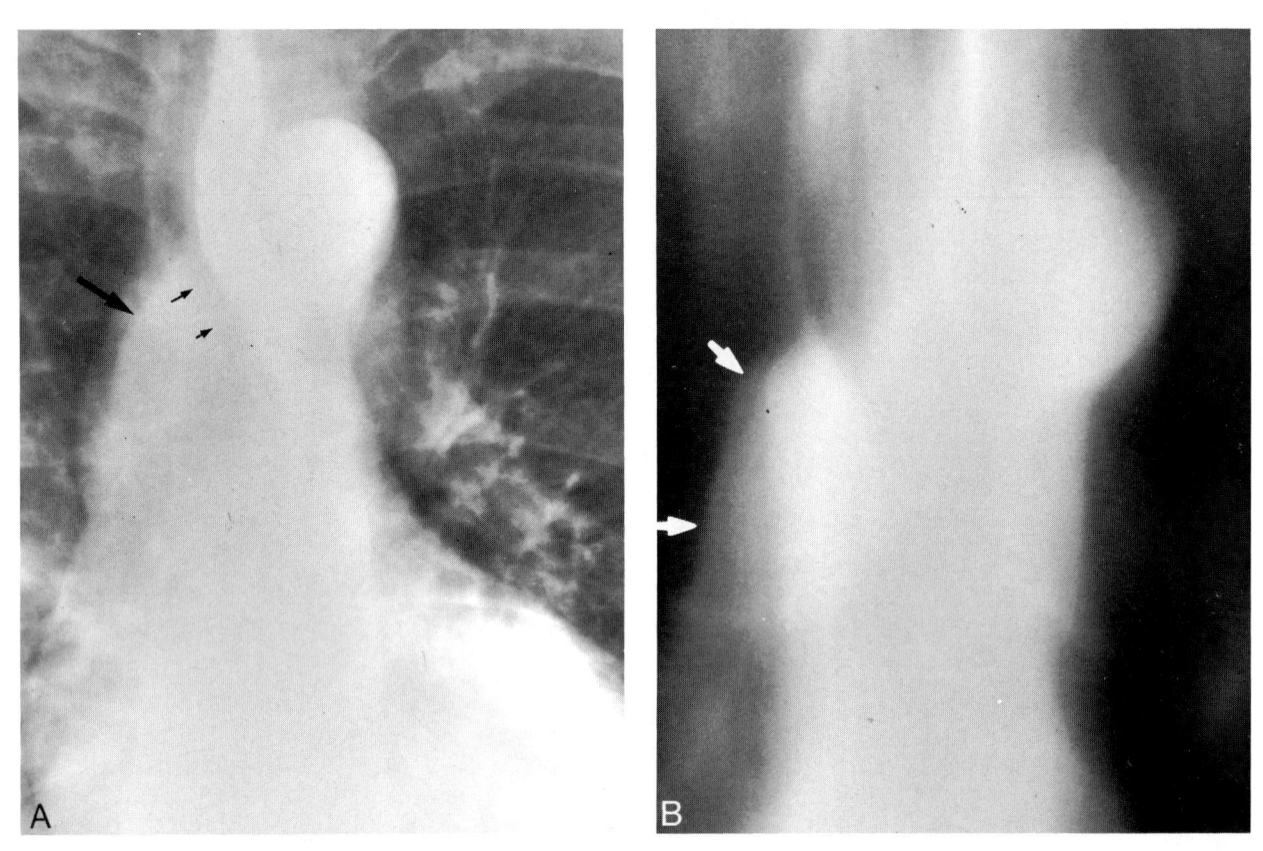

FIG 62–72.
Pulmonary artery sling. **A,** thoracic roentgenogram. Posteroanterior projection. Mediastinal mass *(arrow)* displaces trachea to left *(small arrows).* **B,** laminography demonstrates mediastinal mass *(arrows)* to better advantage.

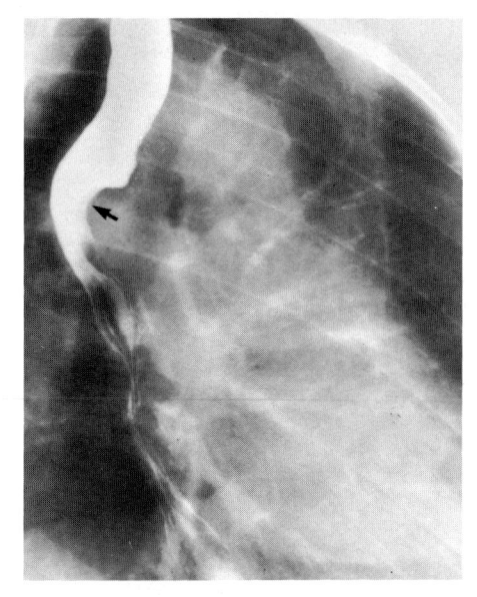

FIG 62–73.
Pulmonary artery sling. Same patient as Figure 62–69. Thoracic roentgenogram. Right anterior oblique projection. Mediastinal mass *(arrow)* lies between esophagus and trachea, suggesting a pulmonary sling rather than neoplasm. Fluoroscopy or cine fluorography is helpful to demonstrate vascular nature of mass.

symptoms and stridor may persist a few months until the deformed tracheal cartilages return to a more normal shape. Pulmonary arteriography or radioisotopic pulmonary scan should be performed after operation to demonstrate patency of the anastomosis.

ECTOPIC ORIGIN OF BRACHIOCEPHALIC VESSELS

Whereas tracheal compression is commonly caused by abnormalities of the aortic arch system, such as double aortic arch, vascular ring, or pulmonary sling, rarely an artery from a normal aortic arch may compress the trachea. In this circumstance a brachiocephalic artery has an ectopic origin and compresses the trachea anteriorly, in contrast to a double aortic arch or vascular ring, wherein the trachea and esophagus are surrounded.

If a brachiocephalic artery arises either more toward the right or more toward the left of the midline, it crosses in front of the trachea to pass to the opposite side. Tracheal compression and tracheomalacia may occur as a consequence. Usually ectopic origin of a brachiocephalic artery is an asymptomatic and incidental finding. Its clinical

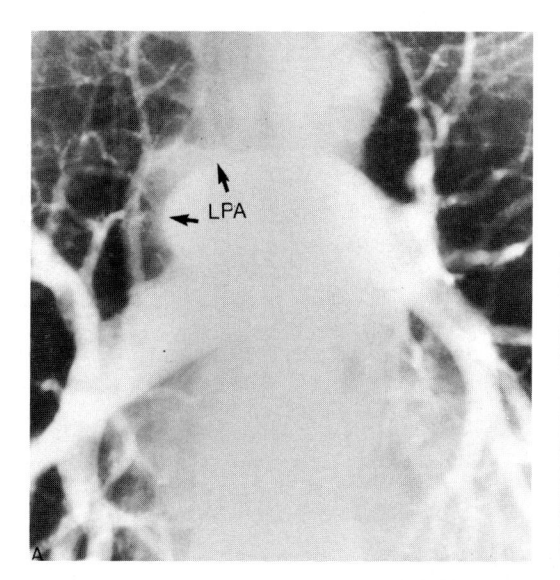

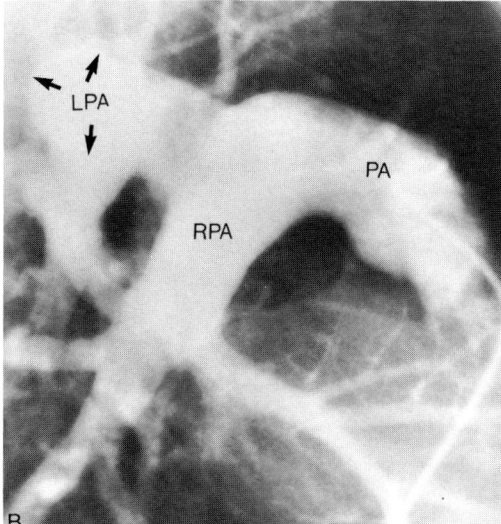

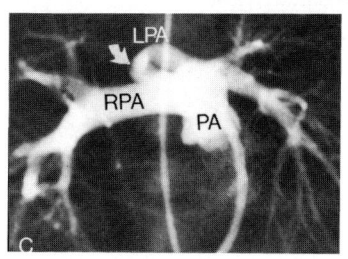

FIG 62-74.
Pulmonary artery sling. Pulmonary arteriogram. (No angulation.) **A,** anteroposterior projection. Round density *(arrow)* to right of trachea represents origin of left pulmonary artery *(LPA)* from right pulmonary artery *(RPA).* **B,** lateral projection. Abnormal course *(arrows)* of left pulmonary artery behind trachea. **C,** anteroposition projection. Cranial beam angulation. Abnormal origin of left pulmonary artery from right pulmonary artery *(arrow). PA* = pulmonary artery.

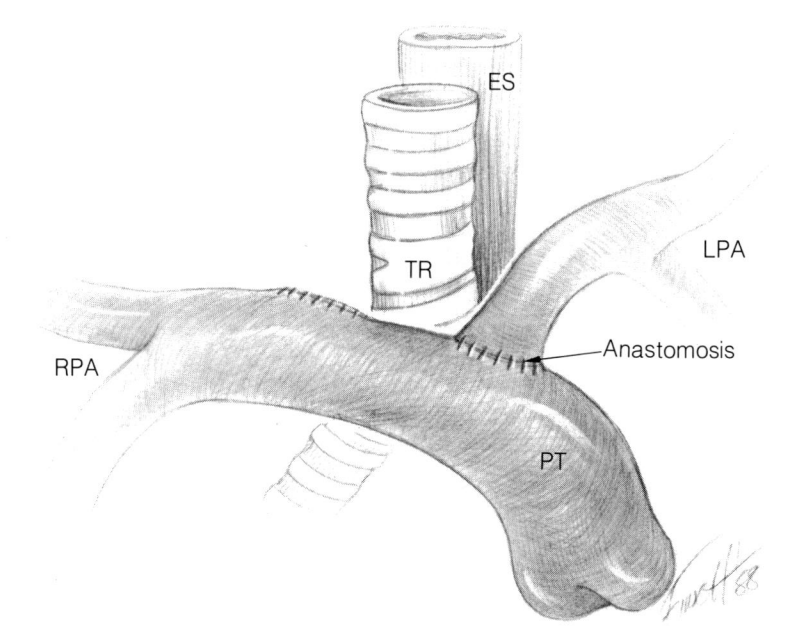

FIG 62-75.
Operative correction of pulmonary sling. The left pulmonary artery is disconnected and anastomosed to pulmonary trunk *(PT). LPA* = left pulmonary artery.

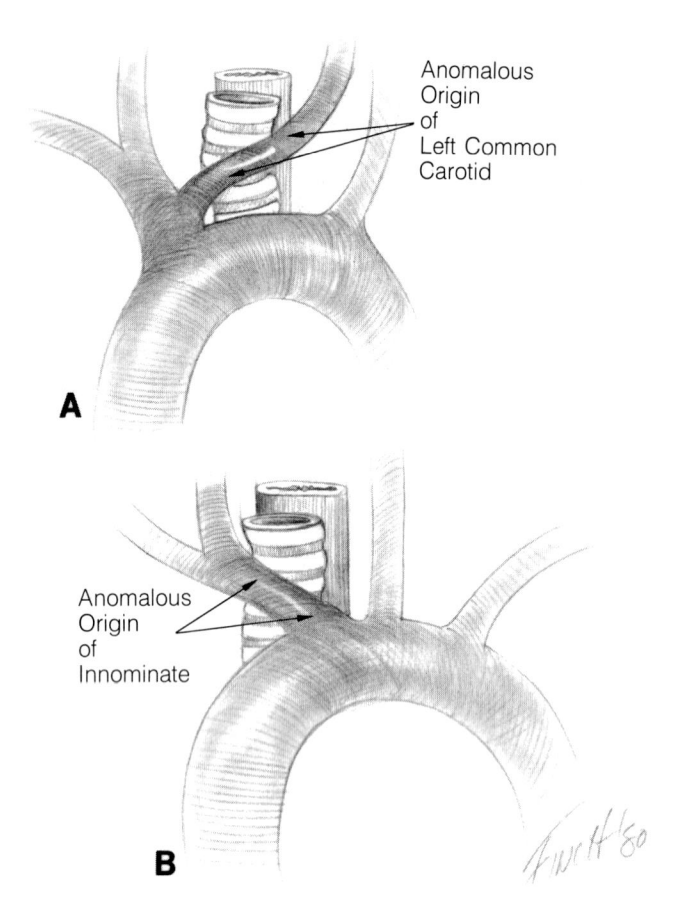

FIG 62–76.
Anomalous origin of brachiocephalic vessels. **A,** anomalous origin of left carotid artery from right innominate artery. Left carotid artery passes in front of trachea and compresses trachea. **B,** anomalous origin of right innominate artery. Right innominate artery arises from left of midline and passes in front of trachea and causes tracheal compression.

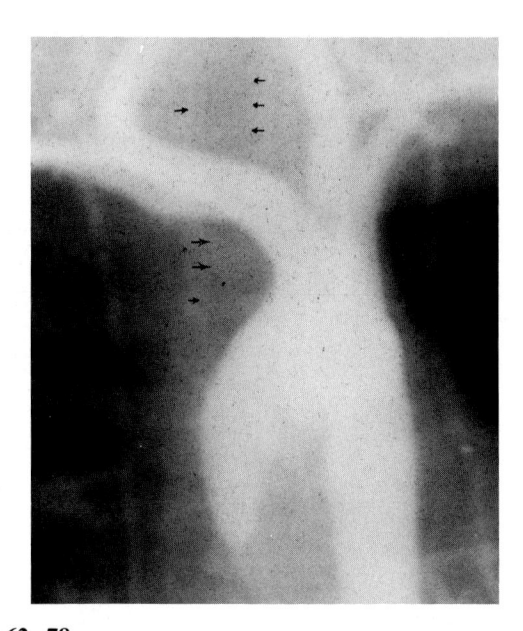

FIG 62–78.
Aberrant origin of right innominate artery. Aortogram. Anteroposterior projection. Innominate artery arises from left of midline and displaces trachea *(arrows)* toward right.

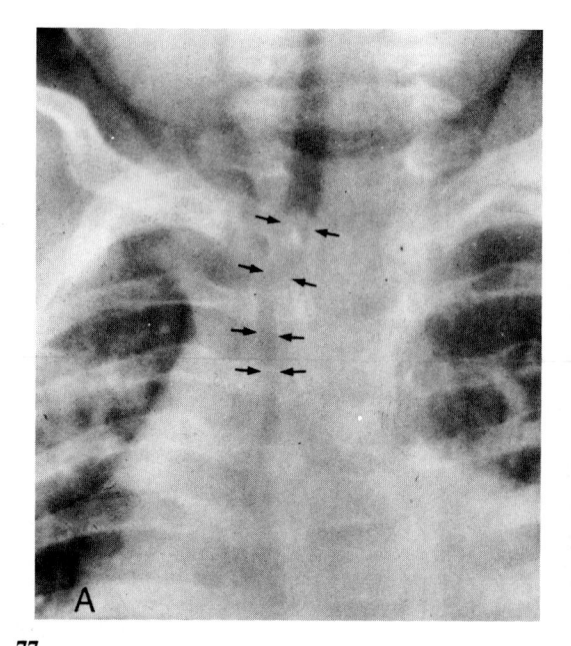

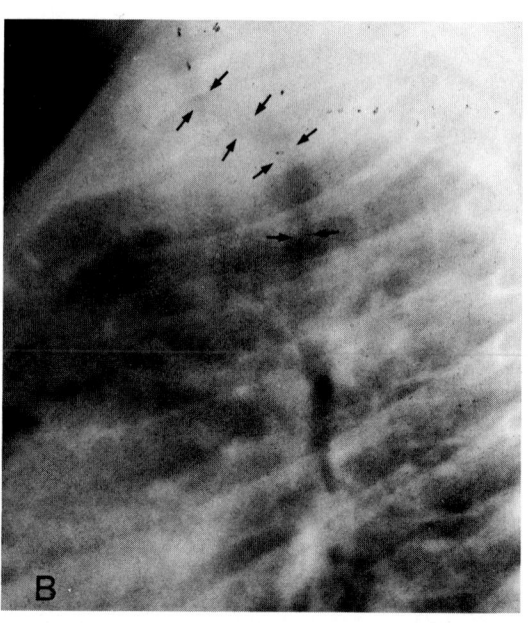

FIG 62–77.
Aberrant origin or right innominate artery. Thoracic roentgenogram. **A,** posteroanterior projection. Tracheal air column, somewhat narrowed *(arrows),* is displaced toward right. **B,** lateral projection. Posterior displacement of trachea is consistent with aberrant origin of right innominate artery.

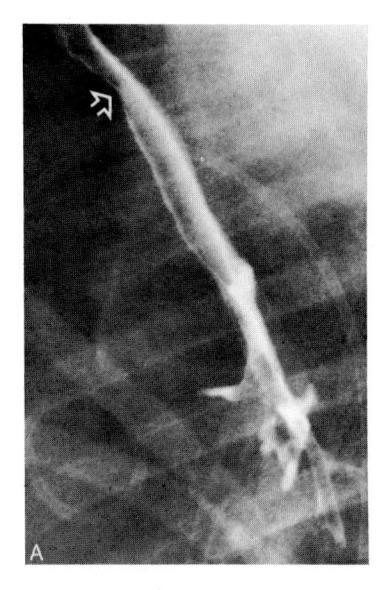

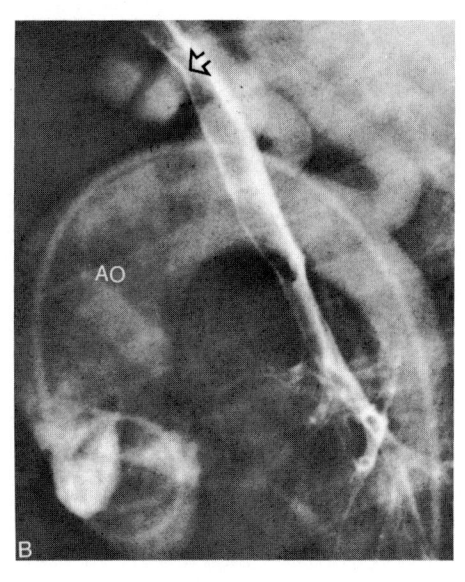

FIG 62–79.
Aberrant origin of right innominate artery. **A,** bronchogram. Lateral projection. Anterior indentation of trachea *(open arrow).* **B,** aortogram. Anteroposterior projection. Innominate artery crosses midline in front of trachea *(arrow).* Slight indentation of trachea *(open arrow)* is caused by right innominate artery. *AO* = aorta. This minor compression is likely not the cause of symptoms.

significance is controversial. Endoscopy reveals a pulsatile indentation of the anterior wall of the trachea. The most common variations are an anomalous origin of the left carotid artery from the innominate artery and aberrant origin of the right innominate artery from the left side of the aortic arch (Fig 62–76). Both anomalies can also occur with situs inversus.

The trachea may be compressed anteriorly by an innominate vein that arises from the aortic arch to the left of the midline or a left carotid artery to the right of the midline (see Fig 62–76). The artery then crosses the midline to its normal location. In its course it may indent the trachea anteriorly and cause respiratory symptoms. In a right aortic arch, the mirror-image pattern may also cause indentation.

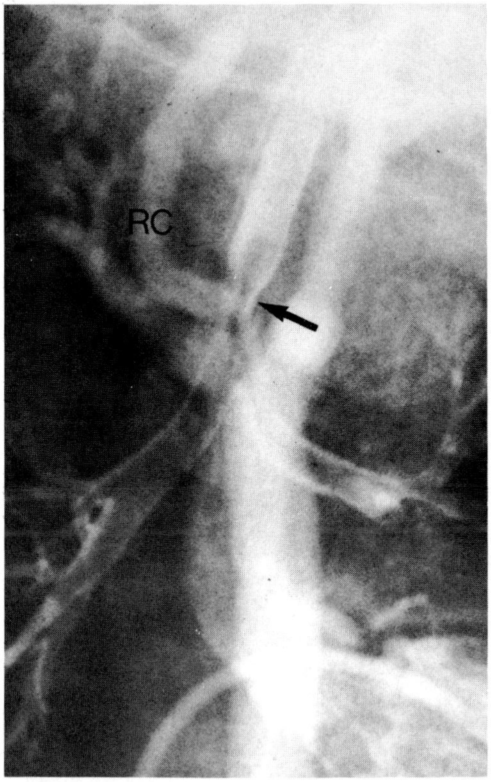

Radiographic Features

Careful inspection of the tracheal air column can reveal narrowing related to aberrant brachiocephalic vessels crossing in front of the trachea. Better visualization of the tracheal air column is accomplished by laminography. The pulsatile nature of the brachial compression is well demonstrated by magnification cine radiography:

1. Typically the tracheal air column is narrowed at the level of the brachiocephalic vessels (Fig 62–77). This may be seen on the anteroposterior projection but is best visualized on the lateral view.
2. The tracheal air column is not only narrowed but commonly displaced to the right side if the more common ectopic origin of the right innominate artery is present.
3. On the lateral view the trachea is seen to be displaced posteriorly but not invariably.
4. The spatial relationship of the innominate artery and the tracheal air column is best demonstrated by ascending aortography (Fig 62–78).
5. Combined aortography and bronchography allow excellent demonstration of the causal relationship of the tracheal compression by ectopic origin of brachiocephalic vessels (Fig 62–79).

FIG 62–80.
Anterior vascular compression of trachea. Simultaneous aortogram and bronchogram. Separate origin for right subclavian and right carotid arteries. Right carotid artery arises aberrantly from left side of aortic arch and crosses midline, causing compression of trachea *(arrow).*

6. A very rare cause of anterior tracheal compression is an ectopic origin of the right carotid artery (Fig 62–80).

Operative correction of these anomalies is accomplished by a pexy of the aberrant artery to the sternum similar to correction of a double aortic arch (see Fig 62–29).

REFERENCES

1. Congdon ED: Transformation of the aortic arch system during the development of the human embryo, *Carnegie Contrib Embryol* 14:47, 1922.
2. Barry A: The aortic derivatives in the human adult, *Anat Rec* 111:221, 1951.
3. Edwards JE: Anomalies of the aortic arch system, *Birth Defects* 47:63, 1977.
4. Edwards JE: Malformations of the aortic arch system manifested as "vascular rings," *Lab Invest* 2:56, 1953.
5. Stewart JR, Kincaid OW, Edwards JE: *An atlas of vascular rings and related malformations of the aortic arch system*, Springfield, Ill, 1964, Charles C Thomas, p 171.
6. Bosniak MA: Aortic arch variations in arteriography, *AJR* 91:1222, 1964.
7. Ericsson NO, Goderlund S: Compression of trachea by anomalous innominate artery, *J Pediatr Surg* 4:424, 1969.
8. Beardon ME, Baker DH, Bordick J, et al: Innominate artery compression of the trachea in infants with stridor and apnea, *Radiology* 92:272, 1969.
9. Moes CAF, Izukawa T, Trusler GA: Innominate artery compression of the trachea, *Arch Otolaryngol* 101:733, 1975.
10. Keats TE, Martt JM: Tracheoesophageal constriction produced by an unusual combination of anomalies of the great vessels: a case report, *Am Heart J* 63:265, 1962.
11. D'Cruz IA, Cantez T, Namm EP, et al: Right sided aorta: part II, right aortic arch, right descending aorta, and associated anomalies, *Br Heart J* 28:725, 1966.
12. Knight L, Edwards JE: Right aortic arch: types and associated cardiac anomalies, *Circulation* 50:1047, 1974.
13. Baron MG: Right aortic arch, *Circulation* 44:1137, 1971.
14. Velasquez G, Nath PH, Castaneda-Zuniga WR, et al: Aberrant left subclavian artery in tetralogy of Fallot, *Am J Cardiol* 45:811, 1980.
15. Arciniegas E, Hakimi M, Hertzler JH, et al: Surgical management of congenital vascular rings, *J Thorac Cardiovasc Surg* 77:721, 1979.
16. Wychulis AR, Kincaid OW, Weidman WH, et al: Congenital vascular ring: surgical considerations and results of operation, *Mayo Clin Proc* 46:182, 1971.
17. Shuford WH, Sybers RG, Schlant RC: Right aortic arch with isolation of the left subclavian artery, *AJR* 109:75, 1970.
18. Rodriguez L, Izukawa T, Moes CAF, et al: Surgical implications of right aortic arch with isolation of left subclavian artery, *Br Heart J* 37:931, 1975.
19. Bernatz PE, Lewis DR, Edwards JE: Division of the posterior arch of a double aortic arch for relief of tracheal and esophageal obstruction, *Mayo Clin Proc* 34:173, 1959.
20. Ekstrom G, Sandblom P: Double aortic arch, *Acta Chir Scand* 102:183, 1951.
21. Gross RE: Arterial malformations which cause compression of the trachea or esophagus, *Circulation* 11:124, 1955.
22. Van Praagh P, Bernhard WF, Rosenthal A, et al: Interrupted aortic arch: Surgical treatment, *Am J Cardiol* 27:200, 1971.
23. Freedom RM, Bain HH, Esplugas E, et al: Ventricular septal defect in interruption of aortic arch, *Am J Cardiol* 39:572, 1977.
24. Moller JH, Edwards JE: Interruption of aortic arch: anatomic patterns and associated cardiac malformations, *AJR* 95:557, 1965.
25. Dische MR, Tsai M, Baltaxe HA: Solitary interruption of the arch of the aorta: clinicopathologic review of eight cases, *Am J Cardiol* 35:271, 1975.
26. Higgins CB, French JW, Silverman JF, et al: Interruption of the aortic arch: preoperative and postoperative clinical, hemodynamic and angiographic features, *Am J Cardiol* 39:563, 1977.
27. Jaffe RB: Complete interruption of the aortic arch: I, characteristic radiologic findings in 21 patients, *Circulation* 52:714, 1975.
28. Jaffe RB: Complete interruption of the aortic arch: 2, characteristic angiographic features with emphasis on collateral circulation to the descending aorta, *Circulation* 53:161, 1976.
29. Lang P, Freed MD, Rosenthal A, et al: The use of prostaglandin E_1 in an infant with interruption of the aortic arch, *J Pediatr* 91:805, 1977.
30. Collins-Nakai RL, Dick M, Parisi-Buckley L, et al: Interrupted aortic arch in infancy, *J Pediatr* 88:959, 1976.
31. Mullins CE, Gillette PC, McNamara DG: The complex of cervical aortic arch, *Pediatrics* 51:210, 1973.
32. DeJong IH, Klinkhamer AC: Left-sided cervical aortic arch, *Am J Cardiol* 23:285, 1969.
33. Shuford WH, Sybers RG, Milledge RD, et al: The cervical aortic arch, *AJR* 116:519, 1972.
34. Van Praagh R, Van Praagh S: Persistent fifth arterial arch in man: congenital double-lumen aortic arch, *Am J Cardiol* 24:279, 1969.
35. Izukawa T, Scott ME, Durrani F, et al: Persistent left fifth aortic arch in man: report of two cases, *Br Heart J* 35:1190, 1973.
36. Lawrence TYK, Stiles QR: Persistent fifth aortic arch in man, *Am J Dis Child* 129:1229, 1975.
37. Anderson RC, Char F, Adams P Jr: Proximal interruption of a pulmonary arch (absence of one pulmonary artery): case report and a new embryologic interpretation, *Dis Chest* 34:73, 1958.
38. Pool PE, Vogel JHK, Blount SG Jr: Congenital unilateral absence of a pulmonary artery: the importance of flow in pulmonary hypertension, *Am J Cardiol* 10:706, 1962.
39. Sotomora RF, Edwards JE: Anatomic identification of so-called absent pulmonary artery, *Circulation* 57:624, 1978.
40. Green GE, Reppert EH, Cohlan SQ, et al: Surgical correc-

tion of absence of proximal segment of left pulmonary artery, *Circulation* 37:62, 1968.
41. Hackett PH, Creagh CE, Grover RF, et al: High-altitude pulmonary edema in persons without the right pulmonary artery, *N Engl J Med* 302:1070, 1980.
42. Kieffer SA, Amplatz K, Anderson RC, et al: Proximal interruption of a pulmonary artery: roentgen features and surgical correction, *AJR* 95:592, 1965.
43. Sade RM, Rosenthal A, Fellows K, et al: Pulmonary artery sling, *J Thorac Cardiovasc Surg* 69:33, 1975.
44. Koopot R, Nikaidoh H, Idriss FS: Surgical management of anomalous left pulmonary artery causing tracheobronchial obstruction: pulmonary artery sling, *J Thorac Cardiovasc Surg* 69:239, 1975.
45. Grover FL, Norton JB Jr, Webb GE, et al: Pulmonary sling: case report and collective review, *J Thorac Cardiovasc Surg* 69:295, 1975.
46. Contro S, Miller RA, White H, et al: Bronchial obstruction due to pulmonary artery anomalies: I, vascular sling. *Circulation* 17:418, 1958.
47. Jue KL, Raghib G, Amplatz K, et al: Anomalous origin of the left pulmonary artery from the right pulmonary artery: report of 2 cases and review of the literature, *AJR* 95:598, 1965.
48. Gumbiner CH, Mullins CE, McNamara DG: Pulmonary artery sling, *Am J Cardiol* 45:311, 1980.
49. Lenox CC, Crisler C, Zuberbuhler JR, et al: Anomalous left pulmonary artery: successful management, *J Thorac Cradiovasc Surg* 77:748, 1979.
50. Kommerell B: Verlagrung des oesophagus durch eine abnorm verlaufende a. subclavia dextra (arteria lusoria). *Fortschur Geb Rontgenstr* 54:590–595, 1936.

CHAPTER 63

Abnormalities of the Venae Cavae

Several types of anomalies may occur in the superior vena caval or inferior vena caval system. The importance of these anomalies lies in the fact that they may complicate passage of a catheter during catheterization, and the abnormality may help identify the type of associated cardiac malformation. This chapter deals only with venous anomalies in the thorax and upper half of the abdomen.

SUPERIOR VENA CAVA

The anomalies of the superior vena caval system include the following:

1. Persistent left superior vena cava, with the left superior vena cava connecting to either the coronary sinus or left atrium.
2. Absence of right superior vena cava.
3. Idiopathic dilatation of the superior vena cava.
4. Connection of right superior vena cava to left atrium.

Persistent Left Superior Vena Cava

If the embryonic formation of the coronary sinus proceeds normally but the left anterior cardinal vein does not obliterate, the left jugular and subclavian veins drain through the left superior vena cava into the coronary sinus to empty into the right atrium or directly into the left atrium.

The incidence in the general population has been reported as 0.3% but is higher, perhaps 3%, in individuals with other congenital cardiac anomalies.[1] This anomaly occurs in 10% of patients with atrial septal defect and with tetralogy of Fallot. It is also a common feature of patients with cardiac malposition, particularly those associated with either the asplenia or polysplenia syndrome.

Pathologic Anatomy

In most cases of persistent left superior vena cava, both superior vena caval systems are present. Venous communications at the site of innominate vein are present between the two superior venae cavae. There are, of course, more remote communications between the two venous systems, such as the cerebral sinuses and other mediastinal veins.

The left innominate and left jugular veins join to form the left superior vena cava, which descends vertically in front of the aortic arch and left pumonary artery. Below the hilum of the lung, it usually receives the hemiazygos vein and then courses posteriorly and medially to the posterior atrioventricular groove to become continuous with the coronary sinus (Fig 63–1). The coronary sinus is enlarged, because it carries a greater than normal volume of blood. Injection of contrast medium into the left innominate vein fills the persistent left superior vena cava and coronary sinus because drainage occurs into the right atrium. With stenosis or atresia of the coronary sinus, blood flow occurs retrograde into the left innominate vein, evidenced as dilution (Fig 63–2,A). Selective injection of the persistent left superior vena cava is required for opacification (Fig 63–2,B).

The site of connection of the left superior vena cava varies. In most patients it connects to the coronary sinus; thus, systemic venous blood is delivered to the right atrium.[1] A communicating left innominate vein is usually present, but it may be absent (Fig 63–3). Uncommonly the left supeior cava connects to the left atrium directly or to the left side of a common atrium (see Fig 63–3).[1-3] (See also Chapter 20.)

Variations result if the coronary sinus orifice is atretic or narrowed (Fig 63–4). In the first instance, blood flow may occur from the coronary sinus, superiorly toward the innominate vein, which, in the second instance, coronary

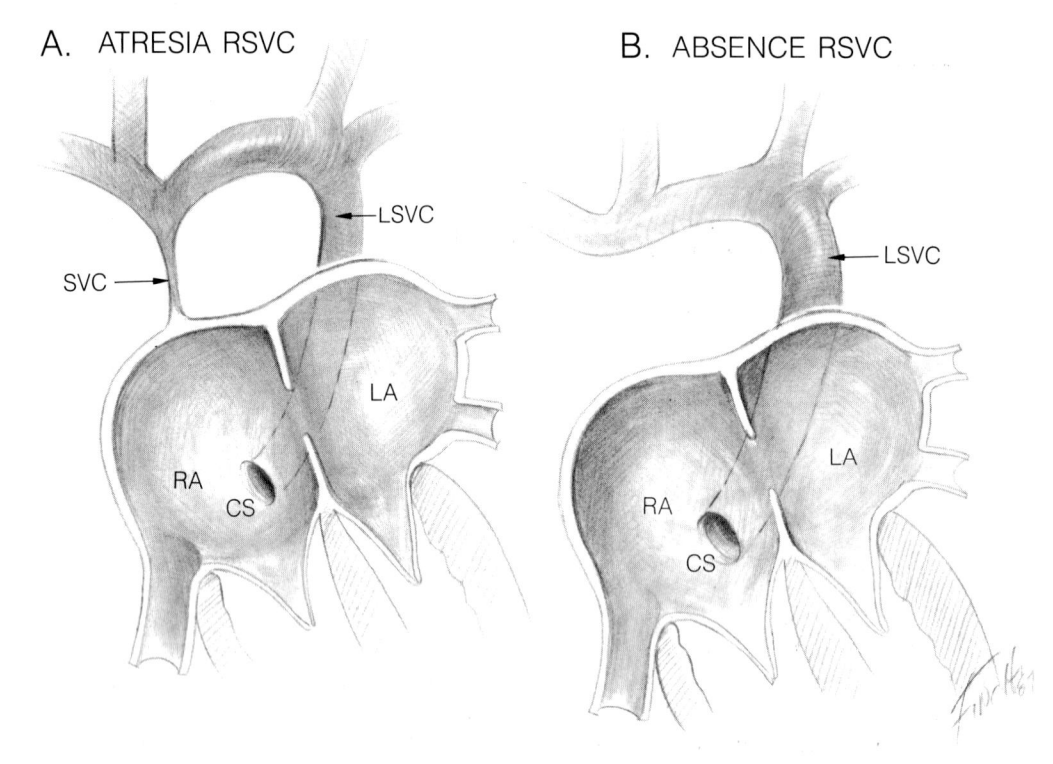

FIG 63–1.
Persistent left superior vena cava *(LSVC)* to coronary sinus *(CS)*. Right superior vena cava *(RSVC)*. **A,** with atresia of right superior vena cava. **B,** with absence of right superior vena cava. *SVC* = superior vena cava; *LA* = left atrium; *RA* = right atrium.

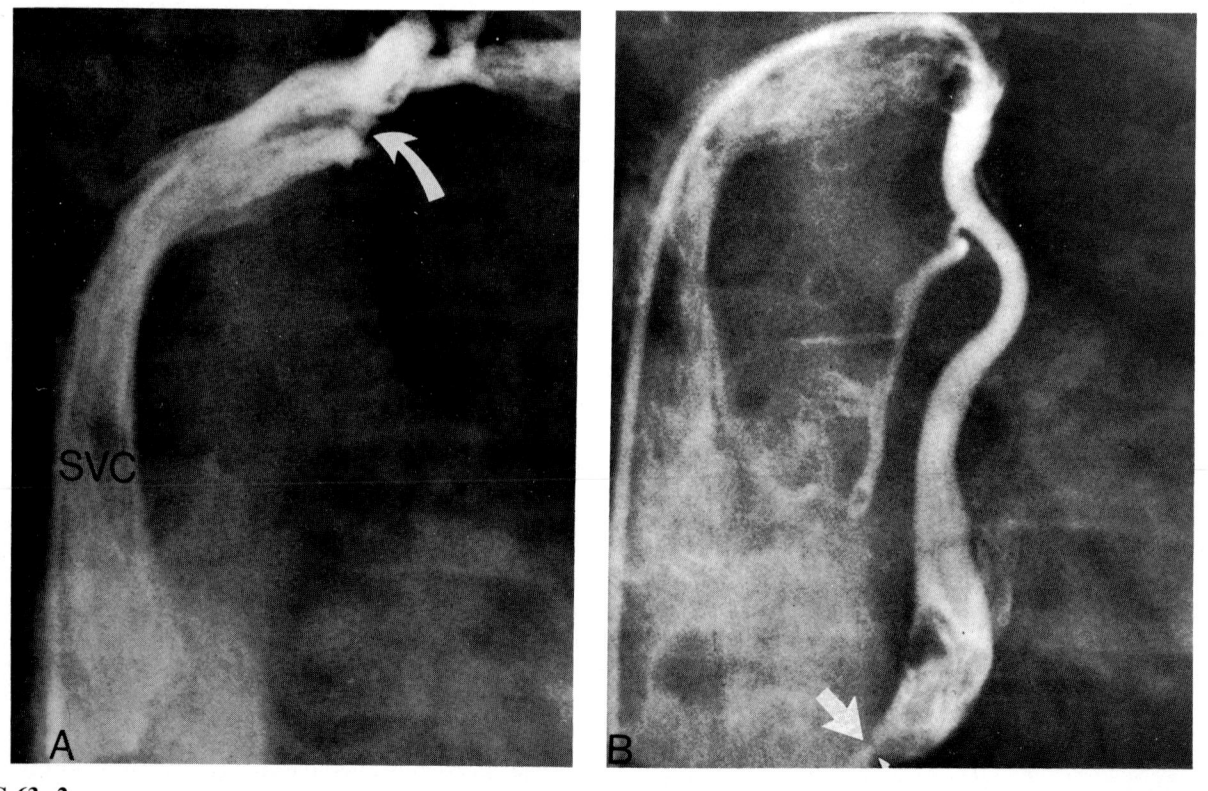

FIG 63–2.
Persistent left superior vena cava *(SVC)*. **A,** injection in left innominate vein. Anteroposterior projection. Dilution of contrast medium *(arrow)* from retrograde flow in persistent left superior vena cava. **B,** selective injection. Severe stenosis *(arrows)* of coronary sinus.

DOUBLE SVC - NO COMMUNICATING VEIN

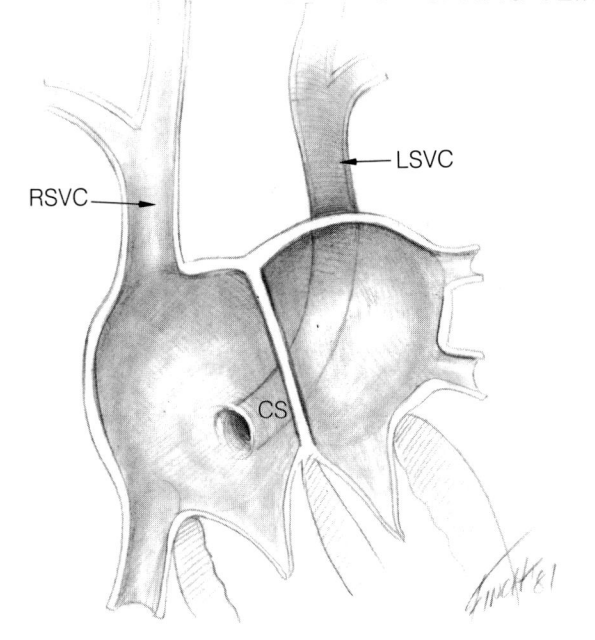

FIG 63-3.
Persistent left superior vena cava *(LSVC)* into coronary sinus. No connecting left innominate vein. *RSVC* = right superior vena cava; *CS* = coronary sinus.

DOUBLE SUPERIOR VENAE CAVAE IN ASPLENIA

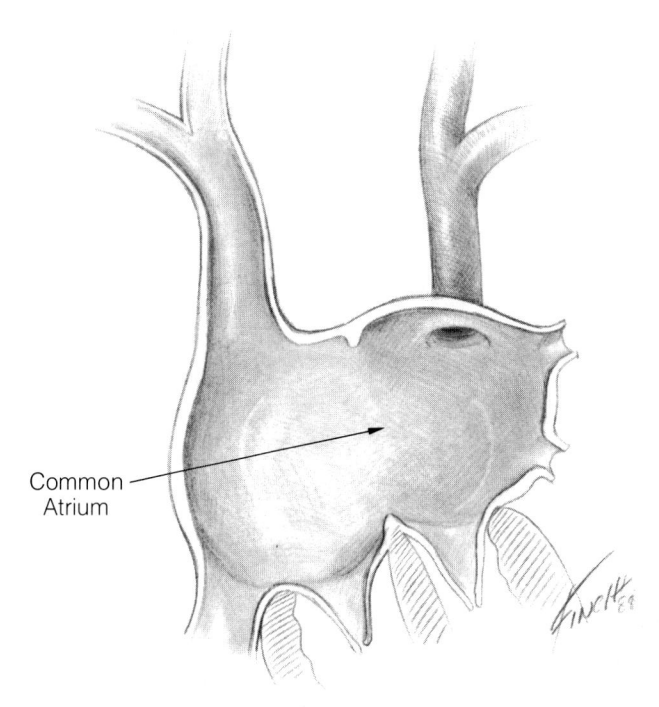

FIG 63-4.
Persistent left superior vena cava with connection to common atrium. No innominate vein.

STENOSIS OR ATRESIA OF CORONARY SINUS WITH FENESTRATION

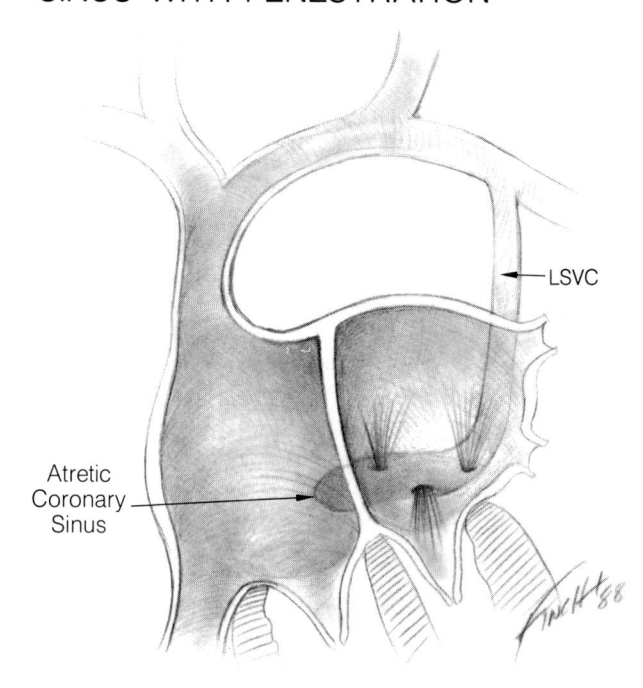

FIG 63-5.
Atresia of coronary sinus ostium with fenestration. Rare form of right-to-left shunt. *LSVC* = left superior vena cava.

RHAGIB SYNDROME
(Absent Coronary Sinus)

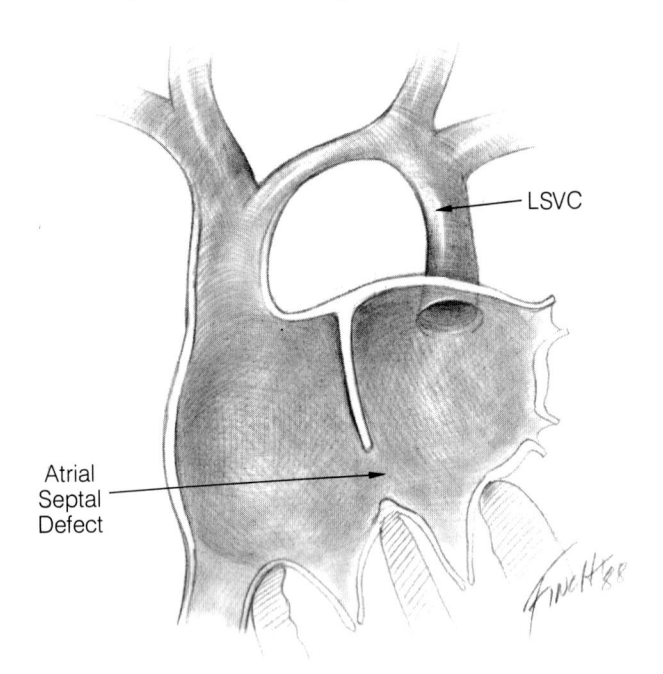

FIG 63–6.
Raghib syndrome with absence of coronary sinus. Atrial septal defect in position of coronary ostium. Hemodynamically a right-to-left (left superior vena cava *[LSVC]* connecting to left atrium) and left-to-right (atrial defect) shunt exists.

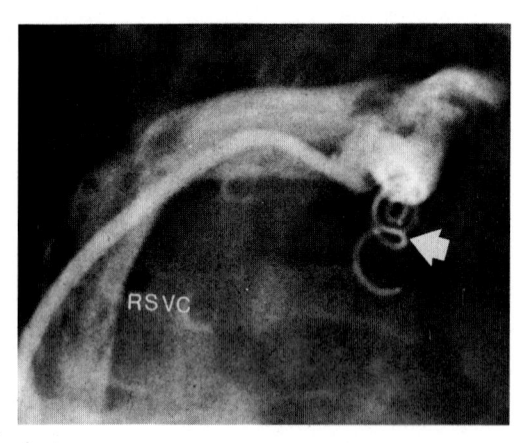

FIG 63–7.
Left innominate venogram. Persistent left superior vena cava after obliteration by coils *(arrow)*. Left innominate vein injection shows occlusion of left superior vena cava. *RSVC* = right superior vena cava.

ISOLATED DRAINAGE RSVC INTO LA

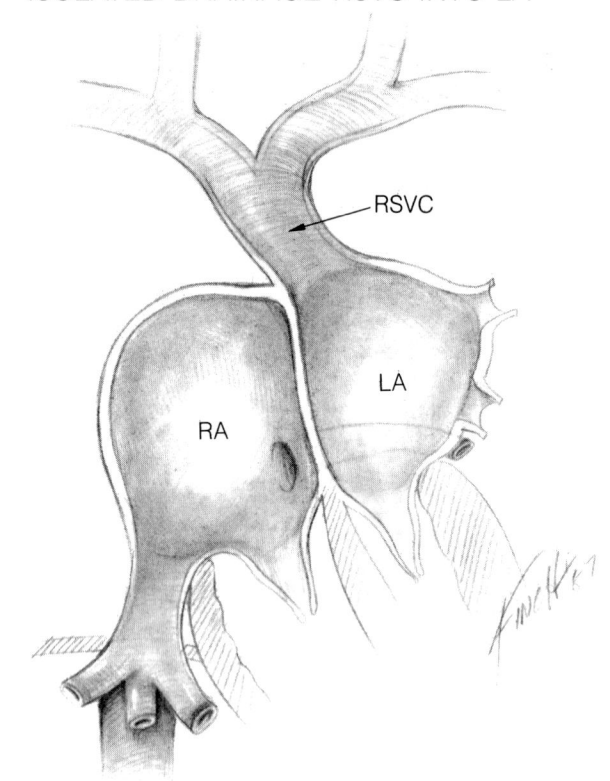

FIG 63–8.
Right superior vena cava *(RSVC)* connecting to left atrium *(LA)*. Cyanosis results. *RA* = right atrium.

IDIOPATHIC DILATION OF SVC (ANEURYSM)

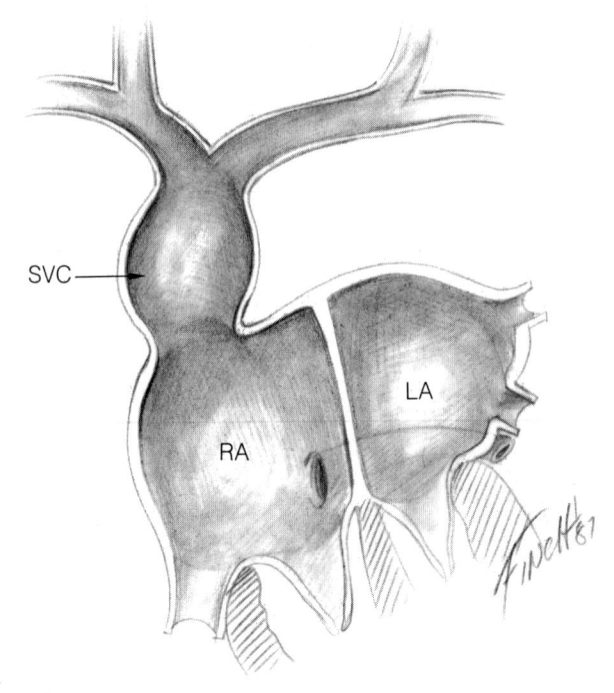

FIG 63–9.
Idiopathic dilatation of superior vena cava *(SVC)*. *LA* = left atrium; *RA* = right atrium.

Abnormalities of the Venae Cavae **1055**

LOW INSERTION OF SVC INTO RA

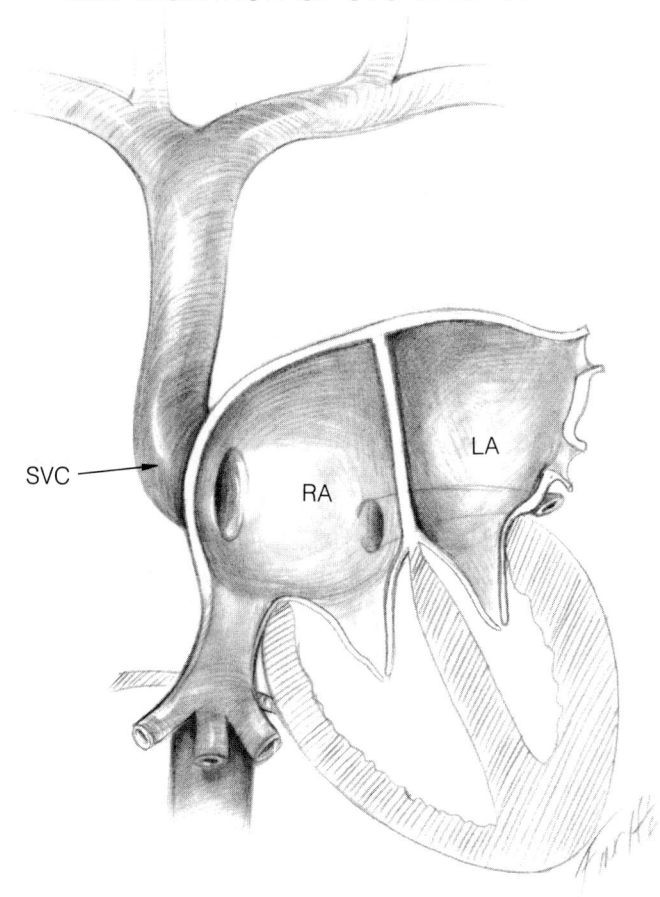

FIG 63–10.
Low insertion of superior vena cava *(SVC)* into right atrium *(RA)*. *LA* = left atrium.

DIAPHRAGM IN LEFT SUBCLAVIAN V.

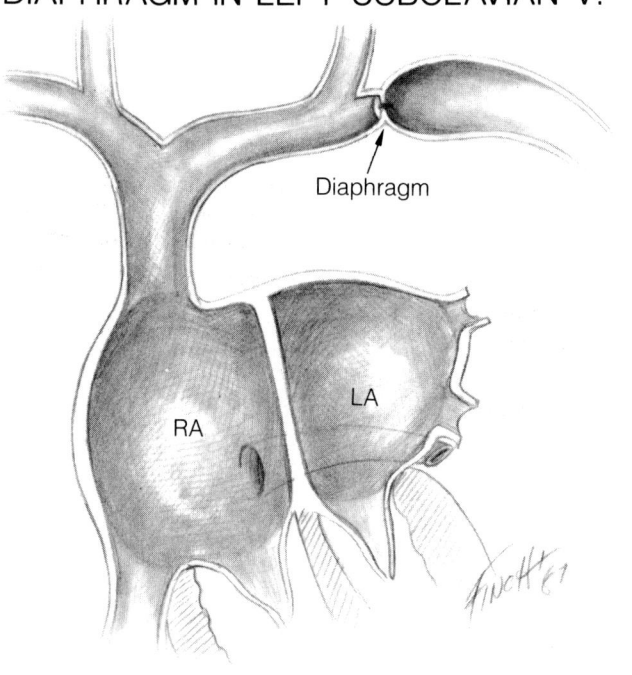

FIG 63–11.
Diaphragm in right subclavian vein. *LA* = left atrium; *RA* = right atrium.

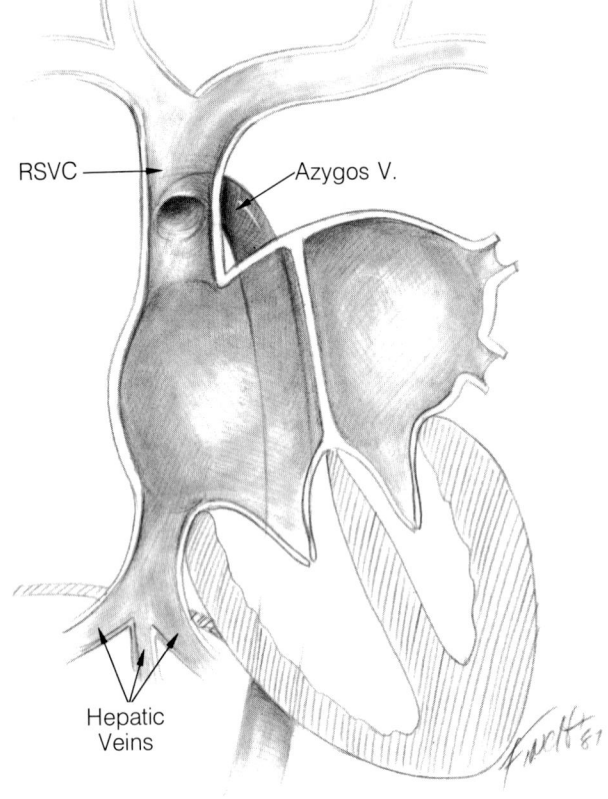

FIG 63-12.
Interruption of inferior vena cava *(IVC)* with azygos continuation to right superior vena cava *(RSVC)*.

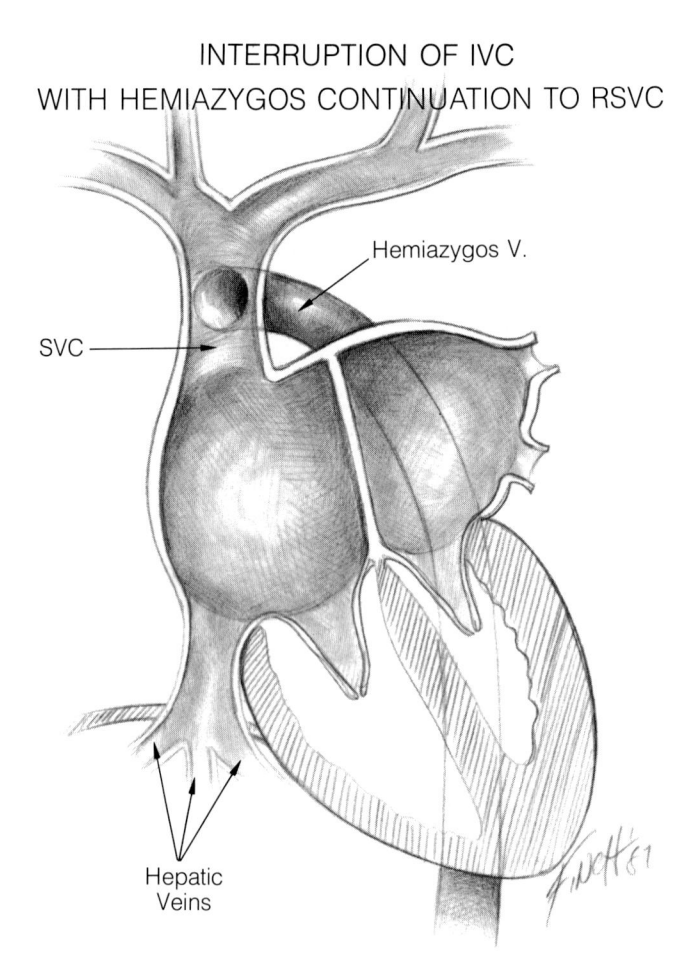

FIG 63-13.
Interruption of inferior vena cava *(IVC)* with hemiazygos connection to right superior vena cava *(SVC)*. RSVC = right superior vena cava.

sinus blood flow is impeded. In either instance, a fenestration may be present between the coronary sinus and left atrium (Fig 63-5) (see Chapter 20) permitting blood flow into the left atrium. In the rhagib syndrome the left superior cava connects directly to the left atrium, the coronary sinus is absent and an atrial communication exists at the location of the coronary sinus ostium (Fig 63-6). Thus, a right-to-left and a left-to-right shunt are present. (See Chapter 20.)

When the connection is directly to the left atrium, severe and multiple cardiac malformations may coexist.[1] These include common atrium, complete atrioventricular canal, single ventricle, and the heart associated with either the asplenia or polysplenia syndrome.

Left superior vena cava may also coexist with anomalous pulmonary venous connection, either partial (see Chapter 21) or total (see Chapter 46).

Hemodynamics and Clinical Features

When the left superior vena cava connects to the coronary sinus, there are no hemodynamic or clinical anomalies. On echocardiography the presence of this anomaly may be suspected by finding an enlarged coronary sinus, which may appear as an abnormal echo within the left atrium.

The presence of a left superior vena cava connecting to the coronary sinus makes cardiac catheterization from the left arm more difficult. Even with flow-directed catheters, the catheter must take a sharp curve in the right atrium to be advanced into the right ventricle.

The pressures in the coronary sinus are normal. The oximetry samples are usually 65% to 75%, greater than the expected 45% normally found in the coronary sinus, reflecting the systemic venous return from the left arm and left side of head.

If the left superior vena cava connects directly to the left atrium, desaturated blood is delivered to the left ventricle and aorta. Cyanosis may result, and desaturation of blood in left-sided cardiac chambers is found.[2,3] Because in most instances a left-to-right shunt usually coexists at the atrial level, the large volume of pulmonary venous blood entering the left atrium dilutes the blood returning

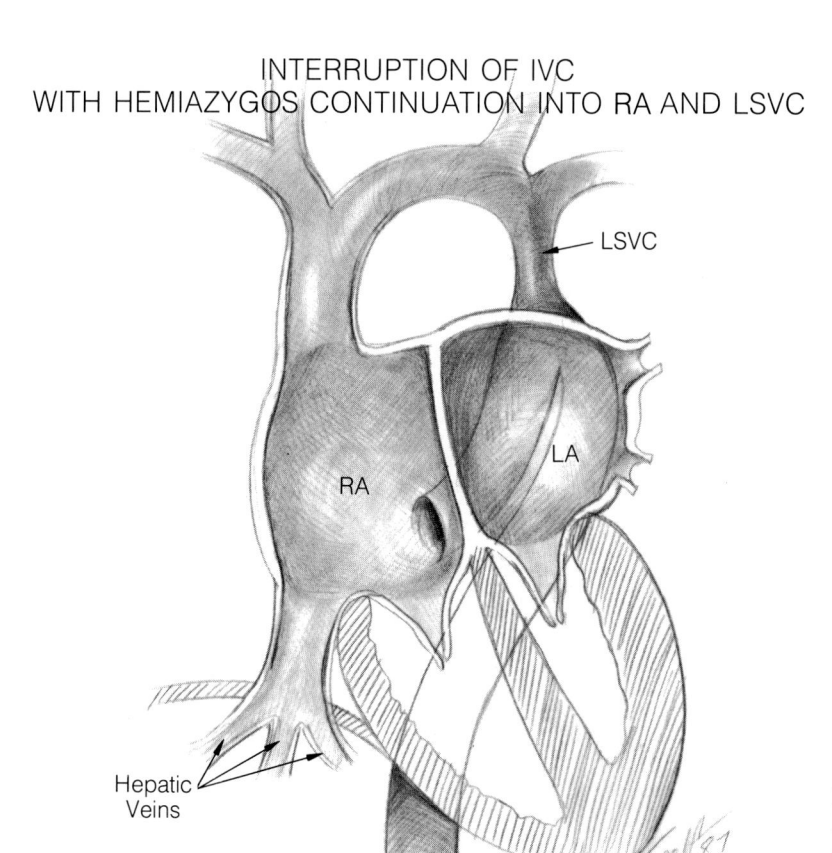

FIG 63-14.
Interruption of inferior vena cava with hemiazygos connection to left superior vena cava *(LSVC)*. LSVC connects to coronary sinus. *LA* = left atrium; *RA* = right atrium.

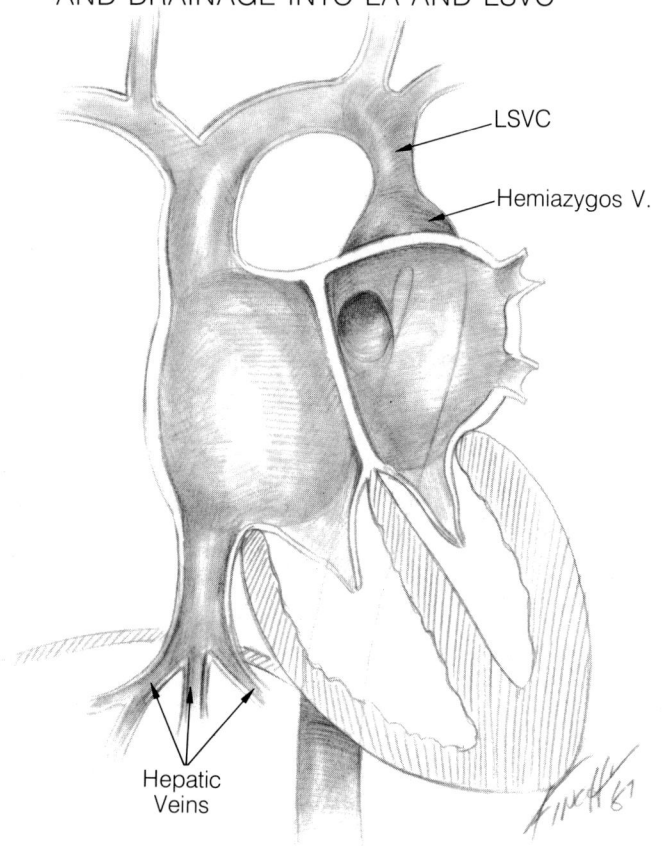

FIG 63-15.
Interruption of inferior vena cava *(IVC)* with hemiazygos connection to left superior vena cava *(LSVC)*. LSVC connects to left atrium *(LA)*.

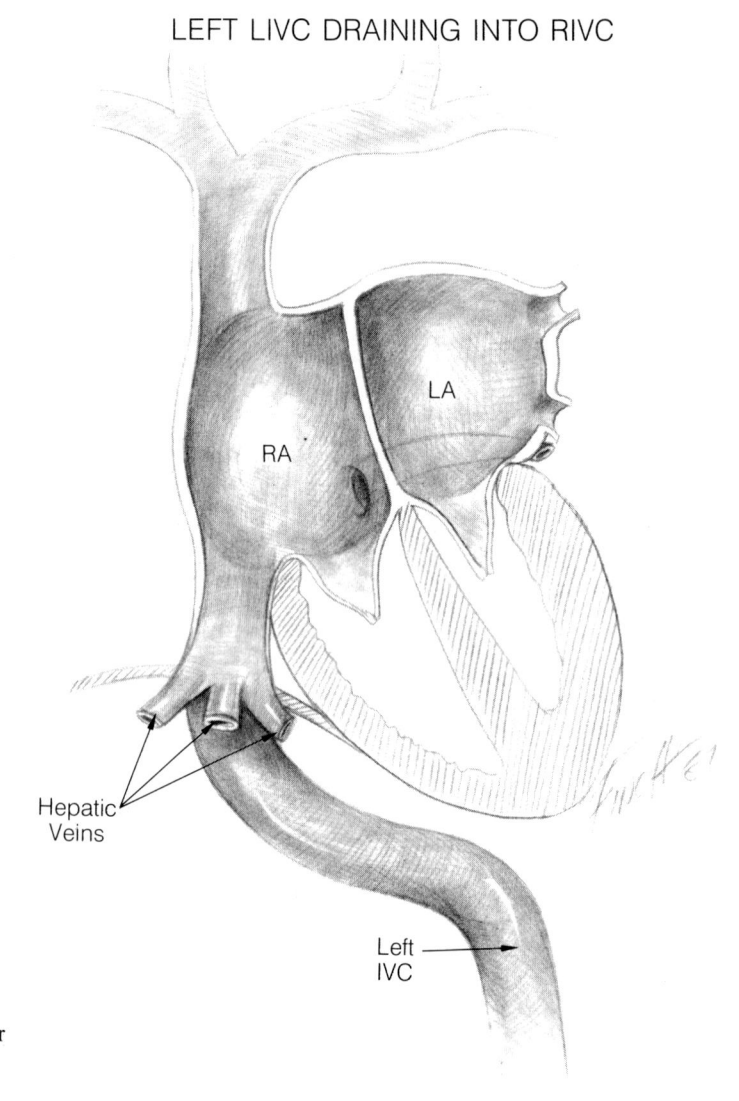

FIG 63–16.
Left inferior vena cava *(LIVC)* connecting to right inferior vena cava *(RIVC)*. *LA* = left atrium; *RA* = right atrium.

from the left superior vena cava and minimizes the degree of desaturation.

Selected drainage of the left superior vena cava into left or common atrium can also be treated nonoperatively by occlusion with coils or detachable balloons (Fig 63–7).

Persistent Left Superior Vena Cava With Absence of Right Superior Vena Cava

In a rare patient with situs solitus, there is atresia or absence of the right superior vena cava and persistence of the left superior vena cava to the coronary sinus (see Fig 63–1).[4, 5] This has been described only in patients with other forms of congenital cardiac anomalies. Although of no physiologic significance, it complicates cardiac catheterization performed from the arm. It may be difficult to advance the catheter from the right atrium into the pulmonary trunk because of the hairpin curve the catheter must take in the right atrium. Absence of the right superior vena cava may also be important at time of cardiac surgery. Therefore, if a left superior vena cava is found, it is mandatory to demonstrate the presence of a right superior cava. In one case the persistent left superior vena cava connected directly to the left atrium and caused cyanosis (Fig 63–8).[6]

With absence and hypoplasia of right superior vena cava, the left superior vena cava may empty into either the azygos vein or directly into the left atrium. This can be approached surgically by ligation of the left superior vena cava and anastomosis of the innominate vein to the right atrium.

Other Anomalies

Idiopathic dilatation of the superior vena cava may manifest itself as a mass in the right superior mediastinum (Fig 63–9).[7] Nuclear magnetic resonance imaging is the preferred method to identify this lesion.

DRAINAGE OF IVC INTO LA

HIGH INSERTION OF IVC INTO RA

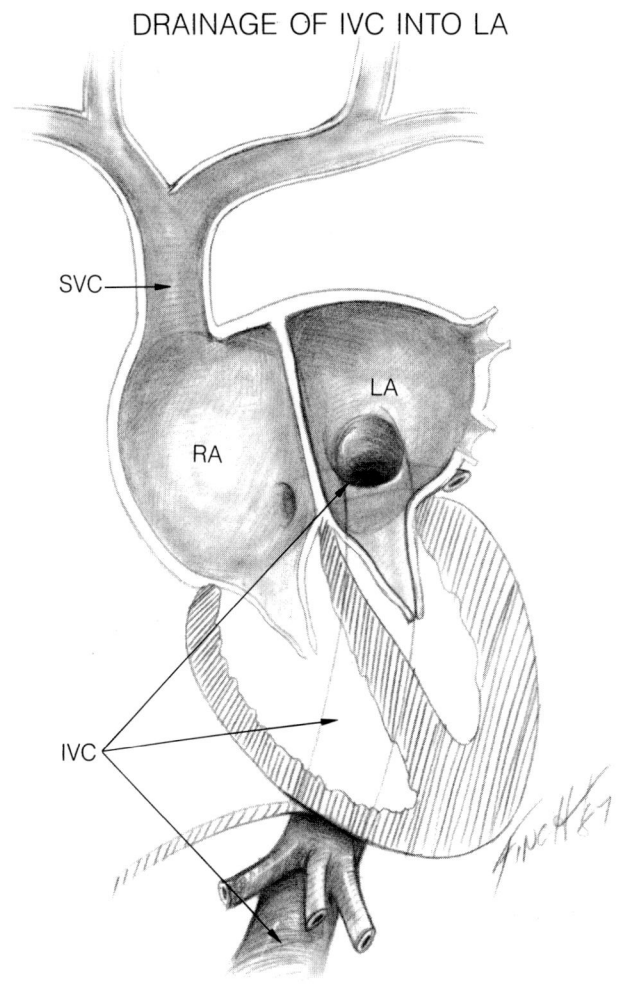

FIG 63–17.
Connection of inferior vena cava *(IVC)* into left atrium *(LA)*. Rare condition with intact atrial septum. Fairly common with common atrium in asplenic syndrome. *RA* = right atrium; *SVC* = superior vena cava.

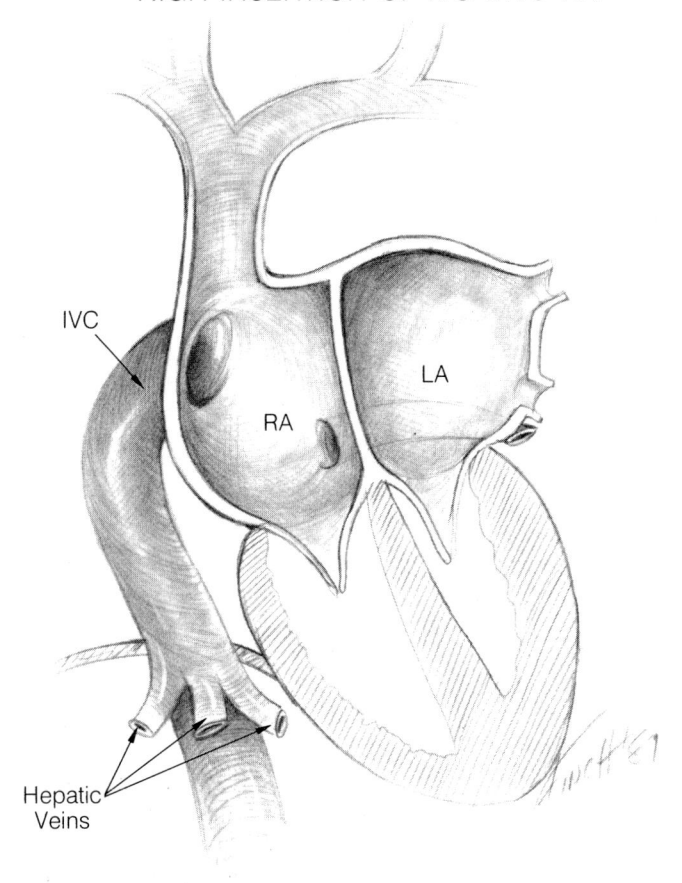

FIG 63–18.
High insertion of inferior vena cava *(IVC)* into right atrium *(RA)*. *LA* = left atrium.

Another rare anomaly is low insertion of the right superior vena cava into the right atrium (Fig 63–10).[8] The anomalous superior vena cava may be seen on a thoracic roentgenogram as a vertically oriented linear density surrounded by air in the right lung.

Rarely, the right superior vena cava may connect to the left atrium and cause cyanosis (see Fig 63–8).[9] Another rare anomaly is a diaphragm in the subclavian vein (Fig 63–11). Another very rare variation is passage of the left innominate vein behind the aortic arch.

Inferior Vena Cava

Inferior vena caval anomalies are rare, except in individuals with either asplenia or polysplenia. The most frequently occurring anomaly is intrahepatic interruption with azygos continuation (also called "interruption of the inferior vena cava") (Fig 63–12). This is present almost invariably with the polysplenia syndrome (see Chapter 58.)[10] Interruption of the inferior vena cava with hemiazygos continuation has also been described (Fig 63–13), but we do not believe it is possible to distinguish the azygous from the hemiazygos vein in patients with splenic anomalies. The interrupted inferior vena cava may also connect to the left superior vena cava, which, in turn, may connect to the coronary sinus (Fig 63–14) or left atrium (Fig 63–15).

In patients with asplenia, the relationship between the inferior vena cava and descending aorta is abnormal, because they lie on the same side of the abdomen, either left or right, rather than normally on opposite sides of the spine.[11]

Rarely, in situs solitus, the inferior vena cava may lie on the left side of the abdomen, in which case it connects to the right inferior vena cava (Fig 63–16).

A rare anomaly[12, 13] is isolated connection of the inferior vena cava to the left atrium (Fig 63–17). A hemodynamically similar condition may result in a normally con-

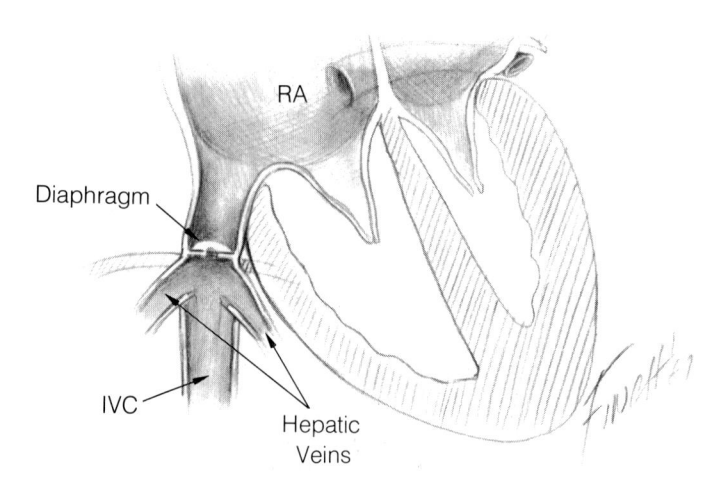

FIG 63–19.
Diaphragm in inferior vena cava *(IVC)*. RA = right atrium.

necting inferior vena cava with a long septum secundum that adheres to the eustachian valve. As a result, a right-to-left shunt with cyanosis occurs. The pulmonary vasculature is diminished in both instances.

An anomaly of no hemodynamic consequence is high insertion of the inferior vena cava into the right atrium (Fig 63–18). The anomalous vein may cause a confusing density on a chest x-ray film.

A diaphragm may occur in the inferior vena cava (Fig 63–19). There are perhaps many unrecognized cases with membranous obstruction of the hepatic portion of the inferior vena cava. Therefore, in a patient with a history of edema and abdominal ascites, diagnosis is made by careful pressure measurements and angiography.

A very rare anomaly is congenital absence of the portal vein.[14] Under those circumstances, venous return from the gastrointestinal tract, spleen, and pancreas occurrs through the left renal vein into the inferior vena cava.

The inferior vena cava may be hypoplastic with partial azygos or hemiazygos drainage (very rare). There may be duplication of the inferior vena cava and there are other variations not associated with congenital heart disease.

REFERENCES

1. DeLeval MR, Ritter DG, McGoon DC, et al: Anomalous systemic venous connection: surgical considerations, *Mayo Clin Proc* 50:599, 1975.
2. Konstam MA, Levine BW, Strauss HW, et al: Left superior vena cava to left atrial communication diagnosed with radionuclide angiocardiography and with differential right to left shunting, *Am J Cardiol* 43:149, 1979.
3. Ezekowitz MD, Alderson PO, Bulkley BH, et al: Isolated drainage of the superior vena cava into the left atrium in a 52-year-old man: a rare congenital malformation in the adult presenting with cyanosis, polycythemia, and an unsuccessful lung scan, *Circulation* 58:751, 1978.
4. Karnegis JN, Wang Y, Winchell P, et al: Persistent left superior vena cava, fibrous remnant of the right superior vena cava and ventricular septal defect, *Am J Cardiol* 14:573, 1964.
5. Lenox CC, Zuberbuhler JR, Park SC, et al: Absent right superior vena cava with persistent left superior vena cava: implications and management, *Am J Cardiol* 45:117, 1980.
6. Sibley YDL, Roberts KD, Silove ED: Surgical correction of isolated persistent left superior vena cava to left atrium in a neonate, *Br Heart J* 55:605, 1986.
7. Franken EA Jr: Idiopathic dilatation of the superior vena cava (superior vena cava dilatation), *Pediatrics* 49:297, 1972.
8. Freedom RM, Schaffer MS, Rowe RD: Anomalous low insertion of right superior vena cava, *Br Heart J* 48:601, 1982.
9. Vazquez-Perez J, Frontera-Izquierdo P: Anomalous drainage of the right superior vena cava into the left atrium as an isolated anomaly: rare case report, *Am Heart J* 97:89, 1979.
10. Moller JH, Nakib A, Anderson RC, et al: Congenital cardiac disease associated with polysplenia: a developmental complex of bilateral "left-sidedness," *Circulation* 36:789, 1967.
11. Randall PA, Moller JH, Amplatz K: The spleen and congenital heart disease, *Am J Roentgenol Radium Ther Nucl Med* 11:551, 1973.
12. Singh A, Doyle EF, Danilowicz D, et al: Masked abnormal drainage of the inferior vena cava into the left atrium, *Am J Cardiol* 38:261, 1976.
13. Meadows WR, Bergstrand I, Sharp JT: Isolated anomalous connection of a great vein to the left atrium: the syndrome of cyanosis and clubbing, "normal" heart, and left ventricular hypertrophy on electrocardiogram, *Circulation* 24:669, 1961.
14. Marois D, vanHeerden JA, Carpenter HA, et al: Congenital absence of the portal vein, *Mayo Clin Proc* 54:55, 1979.

CHAPTER 64

Coronary Artery Anomalies

Congenital anomalies of the coronary arteries occur much more frequently in association with congenital cardiac malformations than as an isolated anomaly.[1-3] Whereas many coronary anomalies are without hemodynamic consequence and compatible with a normal life span, some are life-threatening.[4,5] Some coronary anomalies may prevent a ventriculotomy during a planned corrective operation of the associated congenital cardiac malformations.

Knowledge of the various coronary anomalies is important for the physician performing coronary arteriograms, for the radiologist interpreting coronary angiograms, and particularly for the pediatric cardiologist giving advice to the cardiac surgeon.

Although the coronary arteries are best visualized by selective injection, in infants and young children a balloon occlusion aortogram is sufficient to identify an anomalous course of a coronary artery before a cardiac operation. With an anomalous origin of a coronary artery, a balloon occlusion aortogram is advisable before selective coronary angiography to clarify the anatomic variation.

Variations of coronary artery anatomy are numerous, and only the common ones are described in this text.

Anomalies of coronary arteries can be divided into three groups: (1) variations in number, (2) variations in position, and (3) variations in both origin and distribution.

VARIATIONS IN THE NUMBER OF CORONARY ARTERIES

Normally two coronary arteries, the left and right, supply the myocardium. Frequently three coronary arteries, the left coronary artery, right coronary artery, and the right conal branch, are present (Fig 64–1). Separate origin of a conus artery is considered a normal variant. The incidence of a separate conal branch in infancy is perhaps 20%, whereas approximately 40% of the adult hearts demonstrate a separate origin for the right conal branch. The increased incidence is likely caused by aortic growth and resultant separation of the orifices of the conal branch from of the right coronary artery. This variation has no hemodynamic consequence but is important, because after selective injection of the conal branch with contrast material, a dense myocardial stain and sometimes ventricular fibrillation may develop.

Another variation is an unusually large conus branch supplying not only the right ventricular outflow tract but also most of the remaining right ventricular myocardium (Fig 64–2). This variation may be important in case of a right ventriculotomy.

Rarely, four separate coronary ostia are present (Fig 64–3). In addition to separate origin of the right conal branch, the left circumflex artery and left anterior descending artery may have separate orifices, but both arise above the left coronary cusp (Fig 64–4). This anomaly is considered a variant without clinical significance. It is important for the angiographer, who must catheterize each coronary ostium separately to visualize their course.

Single Coronary Artery

Instead of two coronary arteries a single coronary artery may be present, supplying the myocardium of both left and right ventricles. This anomaly may be a coincidental finding at the time of coronary angiography or postmortem examination. The incidence of a single coronary artery is much higher in patients with a congenital cardiac malformation. Whereas the overall incidence of a single coronary artery is only 0.04%, 40% of the patients with this anomaly have an associated congenital cardiac malformation such as tetralogy of Fallot, transposition of the great vessels, truncus arteriosus, bicuspid aortic valve, or coronary arterial fistula.

There are three major complications of a single coronary artery. Depending on the type of single coronary artery, myocardial ischemia with myocardial infarction and

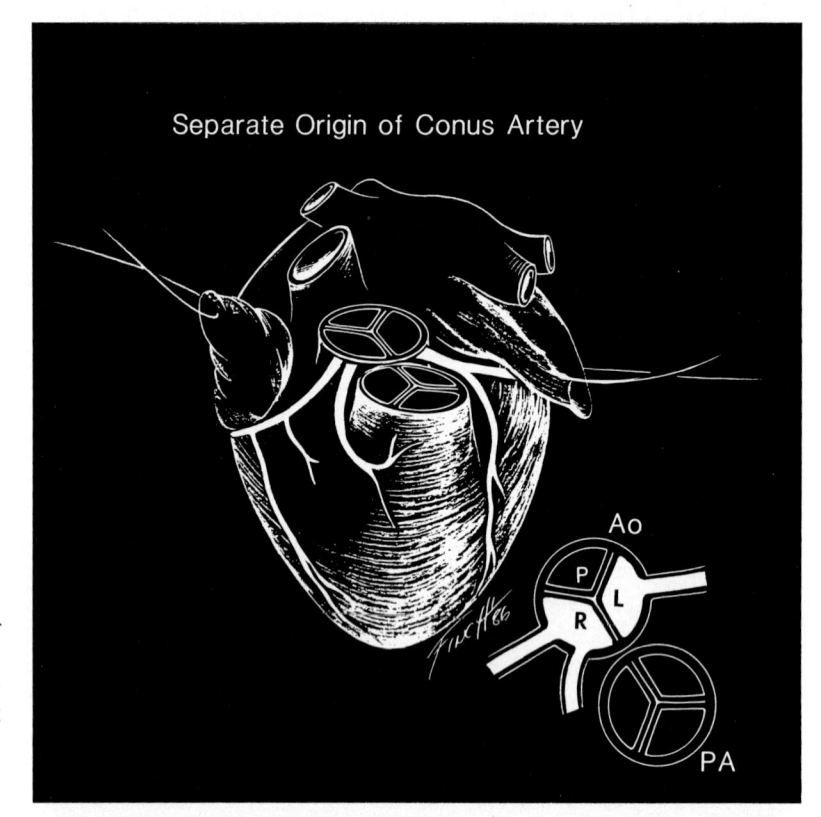

FIG 64–1.
Separate origin of conal artery. Variation of normal coronary artery pattern. Occurs in 40% of normal adults. Left coronary artery passes normally behind right ventricular outflow tract, giving rise to circumflex and left anterior descending arteries. Right coronary artery has normal course, but conal branch has separate origin from aorta. *Ao* = aorta; *PA* = pulmonary artery.

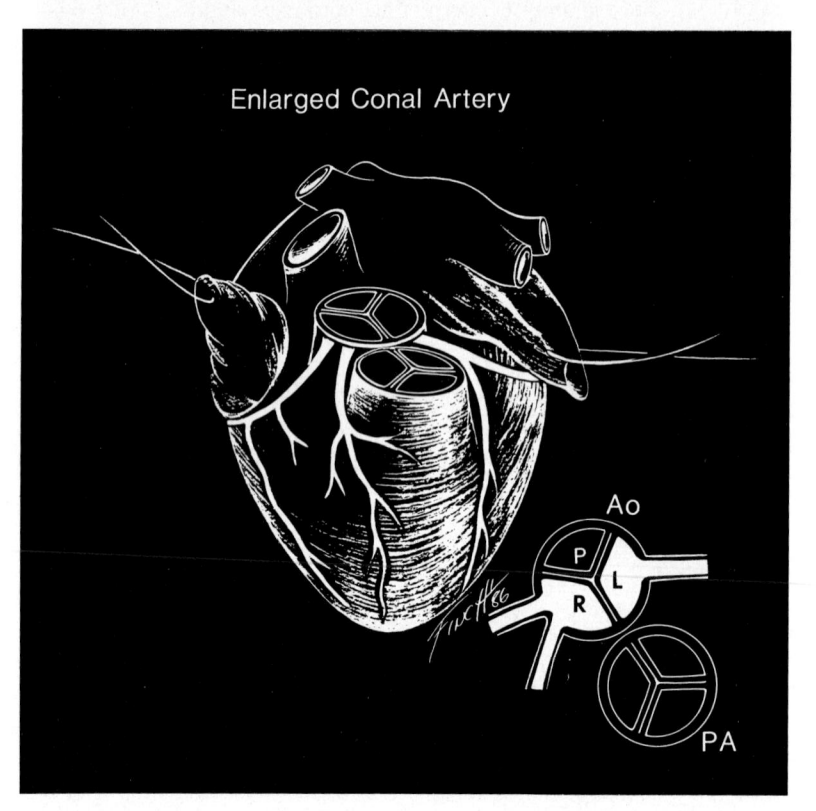

FIG 64–2.
Separate origin of large right conal branch, which may interfere with right ventriculotomy. *Ao* = aorta; *PA* = pulmonary artery.

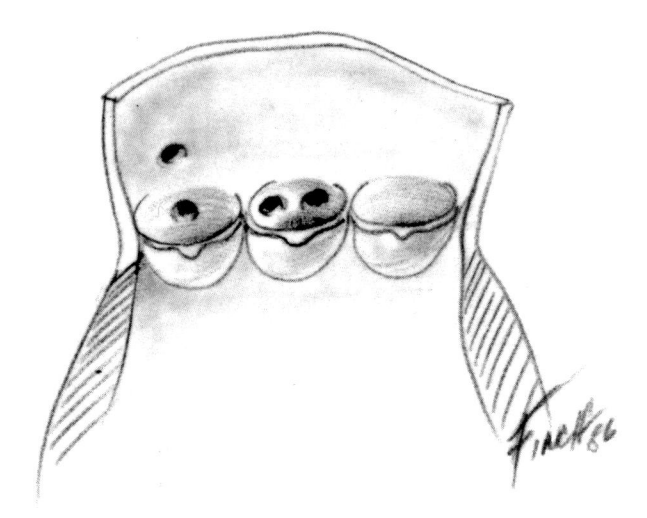

FIG 64–3.
Four separate coronary ostia. Aorta is opened. Right coronary artery arises above right cusp, conal branch arises above right cusp, circumflex, and left anterior descending artery above left aortic cusp.

erosclerosis develops. Obstructive atherosclerotic disease involving the origin of the circumflex and left anterior descending arteries in patients with two coronary arteries represents two vessel disease, but a similar obstructive process in a patient with the single coronary artery is equivalent to triple-vessel disease. Of course, obstructive atherosclerotic disease in the main single coronary artery has much more severe consequences than when two separate coronary arteries are present and connected by collaterals.

The undivided portion of a single coronary artery carries the entire blood flow to both the left and right ventricles. This volume is normally carried by two coronary arteries, which together have a larger cross-sectional area. Therefore, a stenotic lesion is much more significant hemodynamically because of the increased volume of blood flow through the main single coronary artery.

sudden death may result. Second, a single coronary artery may also preclude a ventriculotomy required for correction of a congenital cardiac malformation.

Finally, whereas some patterns and distribution are compatible with a normal life span without cardiac symptoms, the anomaly may have severe consequences if ath-

A single coronary artery may arise above either the right or left aortic cusp. To our knowledge, origin of a single coronary artery above the posterior aortic cusp has not been described. In the analysis of coronary arteriograms with this anomaly, it is essential to realize that the left circumflex artery lies in the posterior atrioventricular groove, whereas the right coronary artery courses toward the right in the anterior atrioventricular groove. The left anterior and posterior descending arteries outline the anterior and posterior interventricular grooves. Regardless of the origin

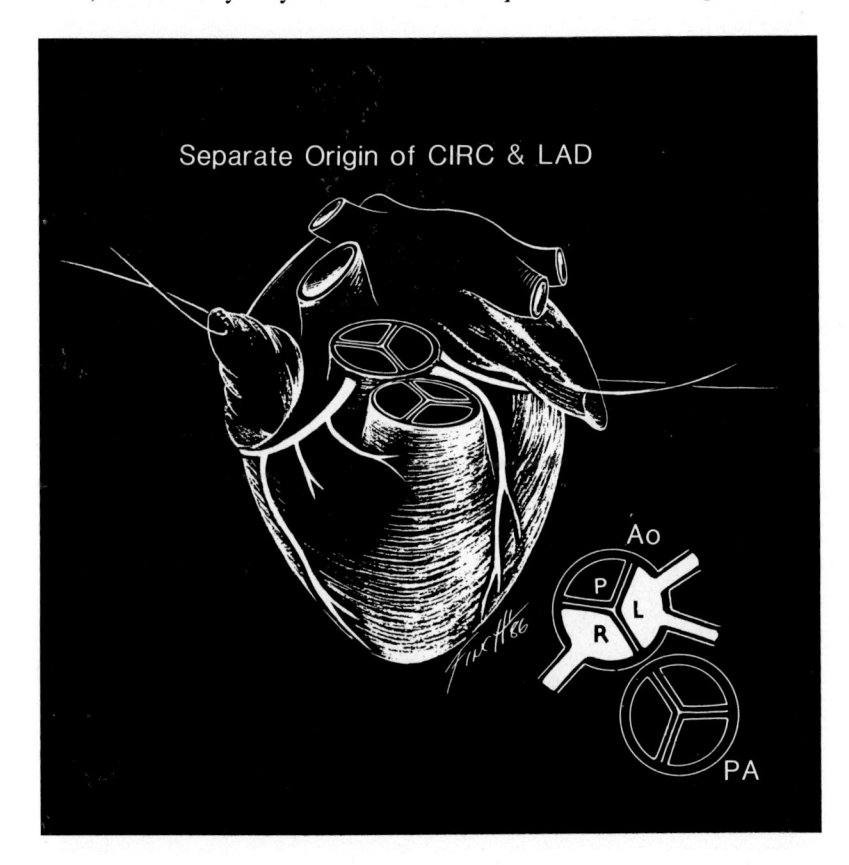

FIG 64–4.
Separate origin of circumflex *(CIRC)* and left anterior descending *(LAD)* arteries above left aortic cusp. Common variation without clinical significance except for technical difficulties to selectively catheterize both coronary ostia. Sometime it is misdiagnosed as congenital absence of circumflex artery. *Ao* = aorta; *PA* = pulmonary arter.

of the single coronary artery above the right or left aortic cusp, some branches must take an abnormal course to reach their site of distribution. The spatial relationships between the aorta and pulmonary artery and the atrial and ventricular grooves have to be clearly understood.

Single Coronary Artery Without Hemodynamic Consequences or Operative Implications

Several variations of a single coronary artery do not cause symptoms or interfere with a ventriculotomy.

Single Coronary Artery Arising Above Right Aortic Cusp.—The single coronary artery arises above the right aortic cusp and takes a course in the anterior atrioventricular groove, continues in the posterior interventricular groove as a circumflex artery, and finally gives rise to the left anterior descending artery (Fig 64–5). This condition is essentially absence of the left coronary artery. None of the arteries cross between the aorta and pulmonary arteries and no major artery crosses the right ventricular outflow tract. Consequently, there is no danger of sudden death, and a right ventriculotomy can be performed without difficulty.

Atherosclerotic disease of the main coronary artery, however, may prove fatal.

A variation of this type of single coronary artery is congenital atresia of either the right or left coronary ostium.[4] In this instance, the coronary system functions as a single coronary artery similar to a congenital single coronary artery. With this anomaly, collaterals exist between the right and left coronary arteries, particularly if the atresia is acquired later in life (Fig 64–6). At postmortem examination, a dimple is present at the site of the atretic coronary ostium. Congenital atresia of a coronary artery occurring at an early stage of development may result in an identical pattern as single coronary artery, but a dimple is found for the atretic coronary ostium at postmortem examination (see Fig 64–6). One of the coronary arteries, most commonly the right or circumflex, may be hypoplastic (Fig 64–7).

In another variation, the single coronary artery gives rise to the left common coronary artery, which has a retroaortic course (Fig 64–8). This anomaly has no hemodynamic significance.

Single Coronary Artery Arising Above the Left Aortic Cusp.—A single coronary artery may arise above the left aortic cusp and divide into left anterior descending and circumflex arteries, the latter continuing in the atrioventricular groove as a right coronary artery. This condition is essentially absence of the right coronary artery (Fig 64–9). If a dimple is found above the right cusp at the time of postmortem examination, this coronary pattern is considered as atresia of the right coronary ostium. Neither

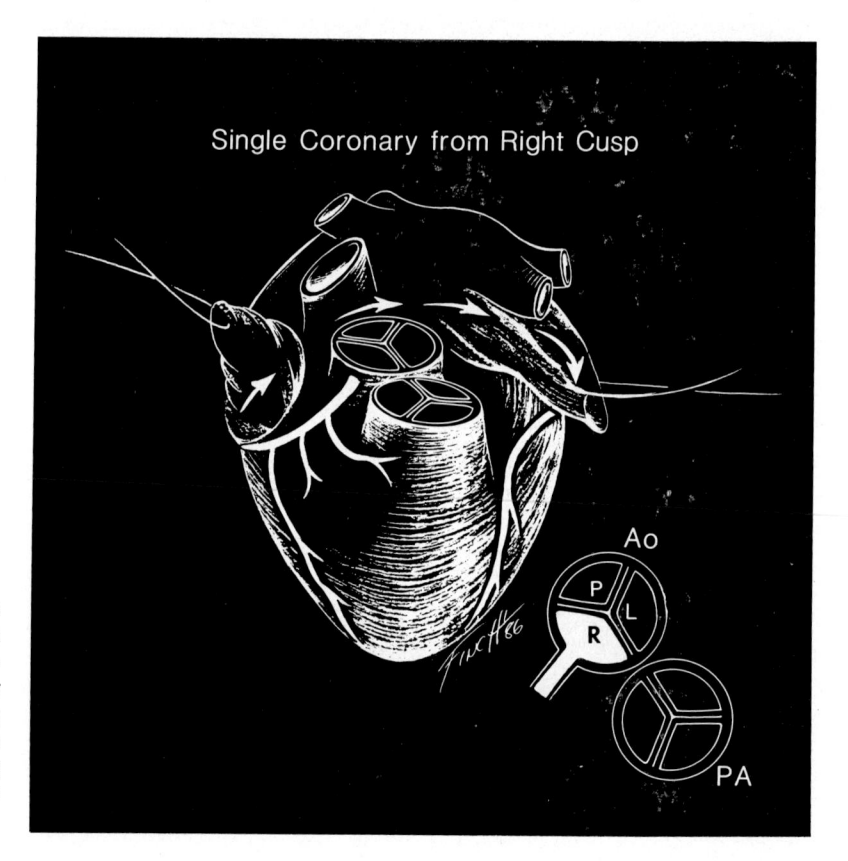

FIG 64–5.
Single coronary artery arising above right aortic cusp. Right coronary artery courses normally in anterior atrioventricular groove, continues as circumflex artery in posterior atrioventricular groove, and gives rise to left anterior descending artery. At postmortem examination, no dimple was found in left aortic sinus, thereby excluding atresia of left coronary artery. Ao = aorta; PA = pulmonary artery.

CONGENITAL STENOSIS & ATRESIA OF CORONARY ARTERIES

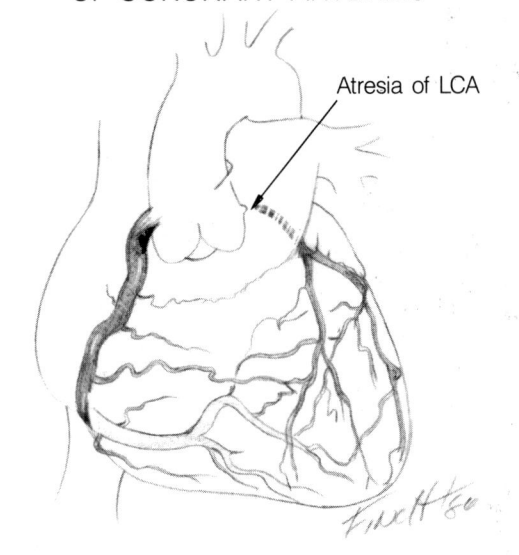

FIG 64-6.
Left coronary artery *(LCA)* atresia. Same pattern as a single right coronary artery. Dimple present in left aortic cusp indicates atresia rather than congenitally single coronary artery.

condition is important to the pediatric cardiologist and is an incidental finding on coronary angiography or postmortem examination. The anomaly is important, however, in older patients with atherosclerosis.

In a variant, the single coronary artery arises above the left aortic cusp and divides normally into the circumflex and left anterior descending arteries. In contrast to Figure 64-9, the right coronary artery has a retroaortic course to reach the anterior atrioventricular grooves (Fig 64-10). This variation has no hemodynamic consequences.

Single Coronary Artery With Hemodynamic Consequences or Operative Implications.—Several variations must be identified because of important clinical consequences. Some lead to angina pectoris, myocardial infarction, or sudden death presumably from their course between the aorta and pulmonary artery (5-7) and others interfere with ventriculotomy to correct a cardiac malformation.

Single Coronary Artery Arising Above the Right Aortic Cusp.—The single coronary artery arises above the right aortic cusp and gives rise to the left coronary artery, which passes between the aorta and pulmonary artery and then bifurcates into left anterior descending and circumflex arteries (Fig 64-11). A variation of this pattern (Fig 64-12) is retroaortic course of the circumflex artery and an anomalous course of the left anterior descending artery between the pulmonary artery and aorta. The course of a coronary artery between the two great arteries may result in serious hemodynamic consequences discussed later on in the chapter.

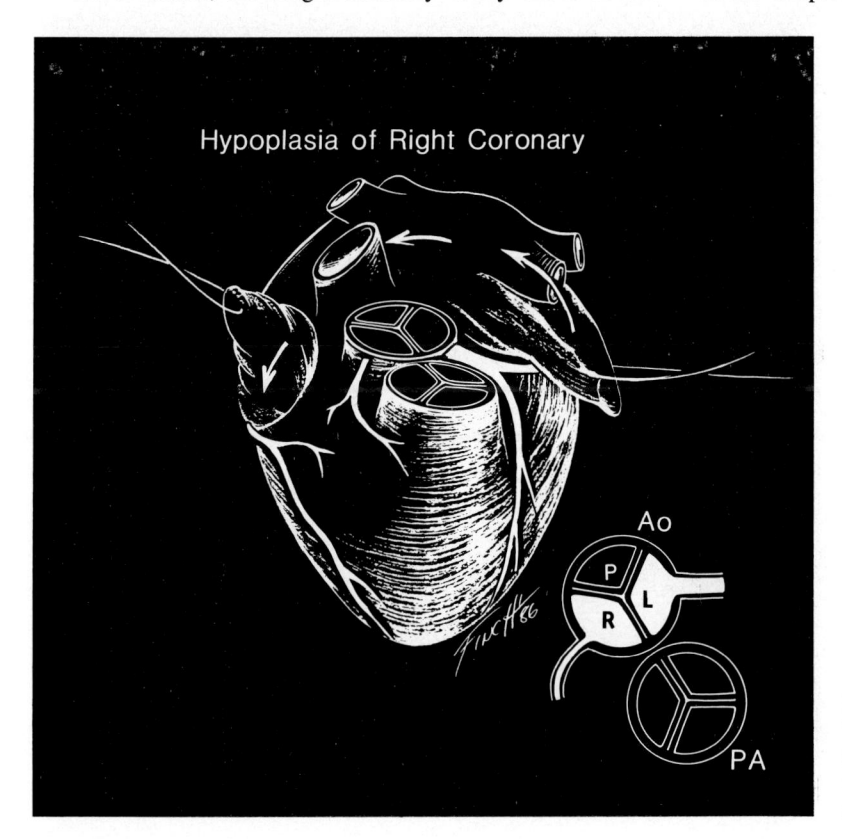

FIG 64-7.
Variation of single left coronary artery demonstrating severe hypoplasia of right coronary artery. Circulatory pattern resembles single left coronary artery. *Ao* = aorta; *PA* = pulmonary artery.

1066 *Anomalies of Major Blood Vessels*

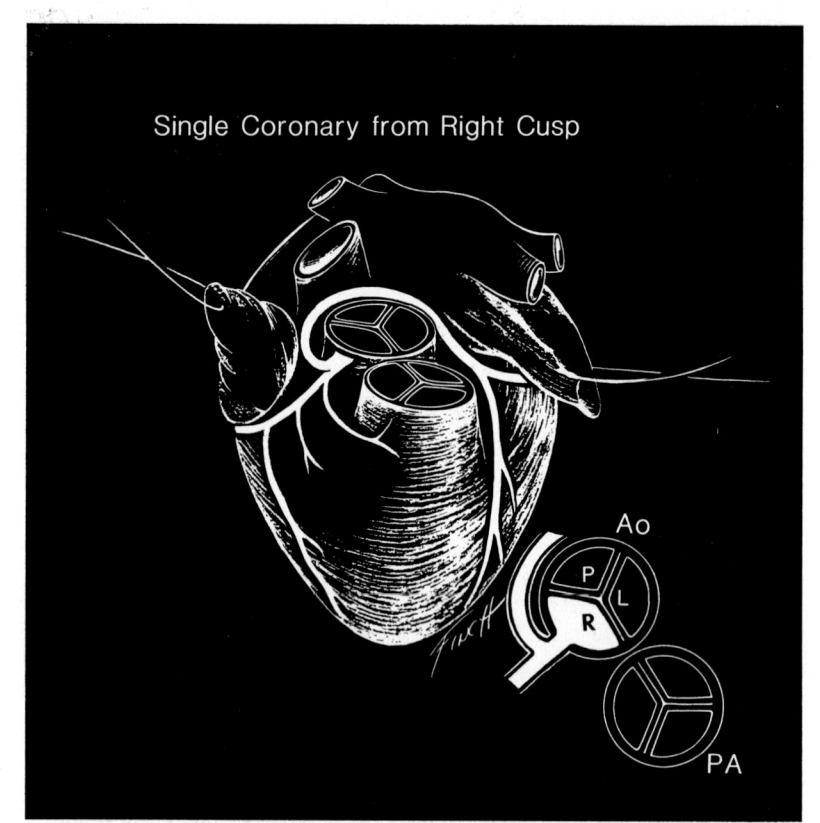

FIG 64-8.
Pattern of single coronary artery arising above right aortic cusp. Right coronary artery has normal course in anterior atrioventricular groove. It gives rise to left common coronary artery, which crosses behind aorta (retroaortic), giving rise to circumflex and left anterior descending arteries. *Ao* = aorta; *PA* = pulmonary artery.

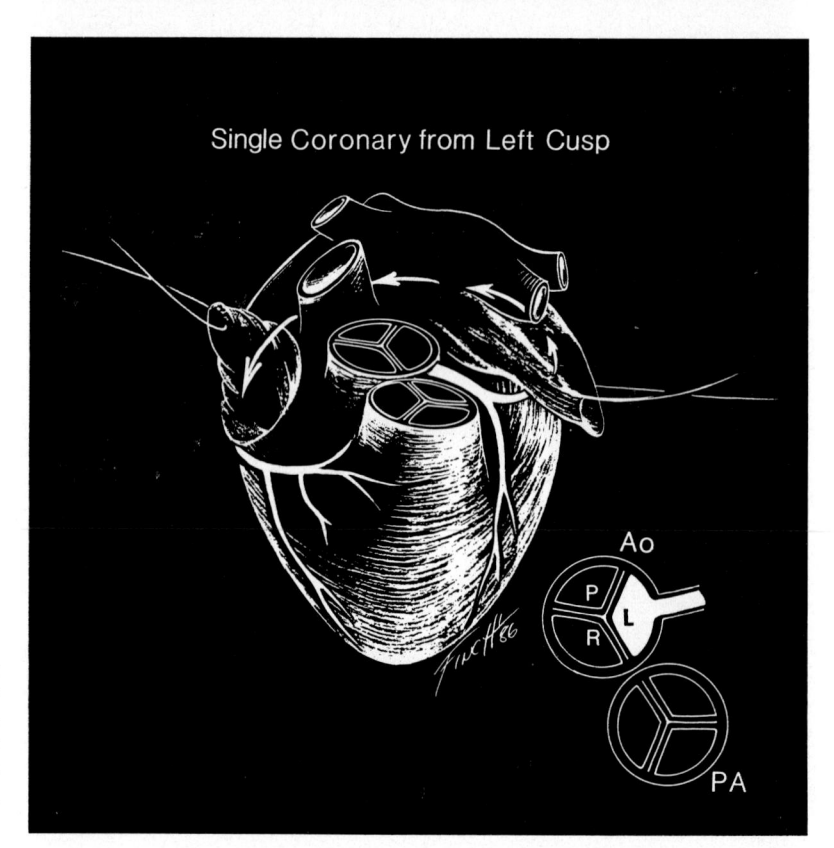

FIG 64-9.
Single coronary artery arising above left aortic cusp. Single coronary artery divides normally into left anterior descending and circumflex arteries. Latter continues in posterior atrioventricular groove as a right coronary artery. Right coronary artery is absent. *Ao* = aorta; *PA* = pulmonary artery.

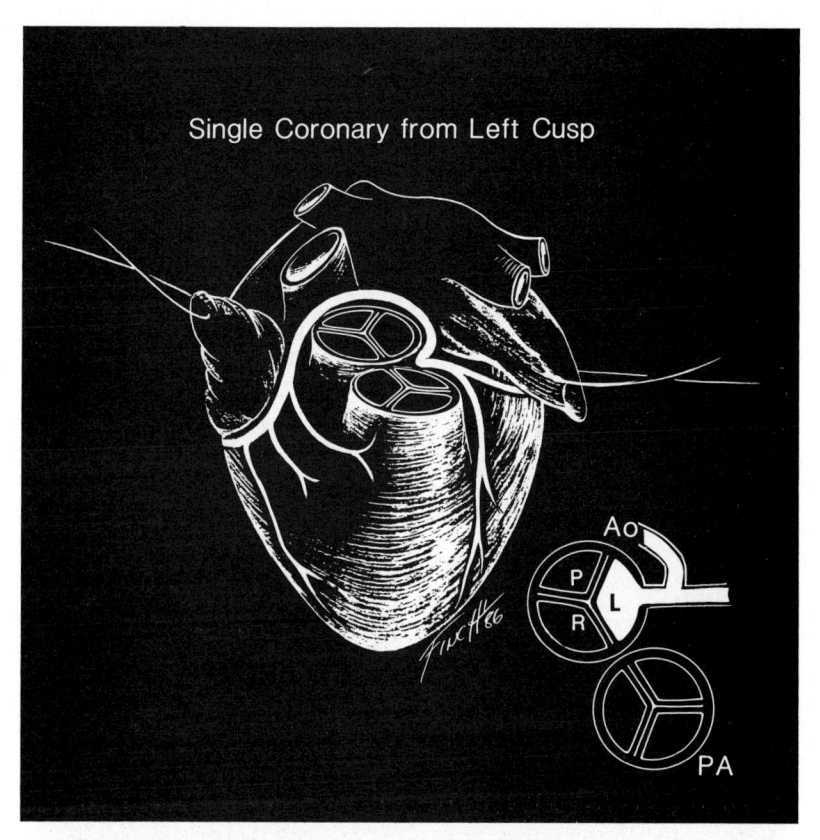

FIG 64–10.
Variation of single coronary artery arising above left aortic cusp. Division into circumflex and left anterior descending arteries is normal, but right coronary artery has retroaortic course to anterior atrioventricular groove. *Ao* = aorta; *PA* = pulmonary artery.

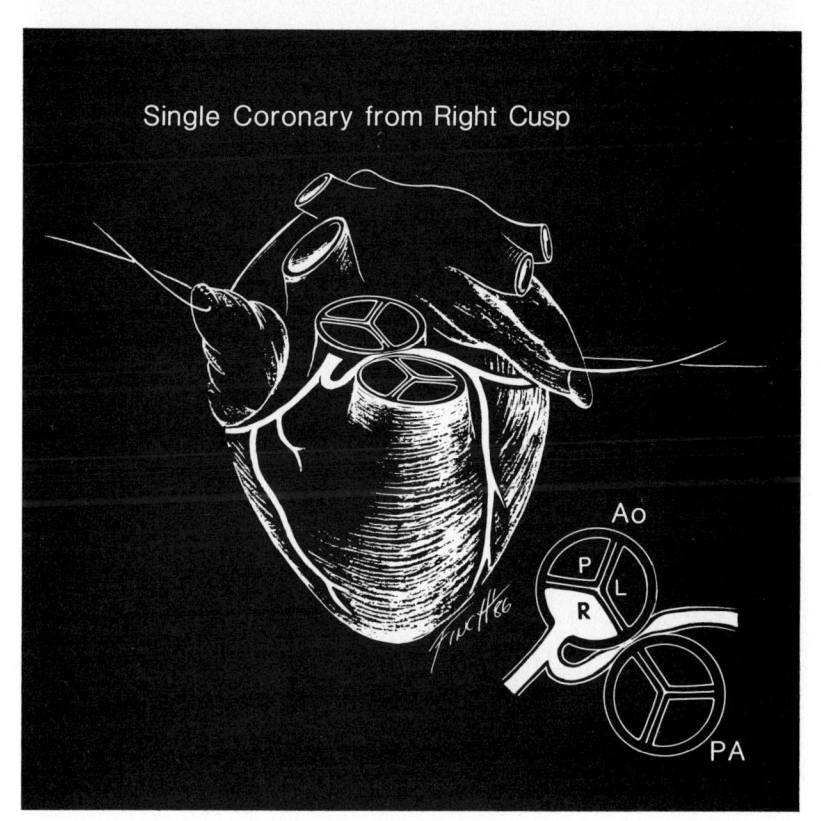

FIG 64–11.
Variation of single coronary artery arising above right aortic cusp. Left common coronary artery passes between aorta and pulmonary outflow tract and divides into circumflex and left anterior descending arteries. *Ao* = aorta; *PA* = pulmonary artery.

FIG 64–12.
Single coronary artery arising above right aortic cusp. Retroaortic circumflex and anomalous course of left anterior descending artery between aorta and right ventricular outflow tract. Compression of left anterior descending artery may occur. *Ao* = aorta; *PA* = pulmonary artery.

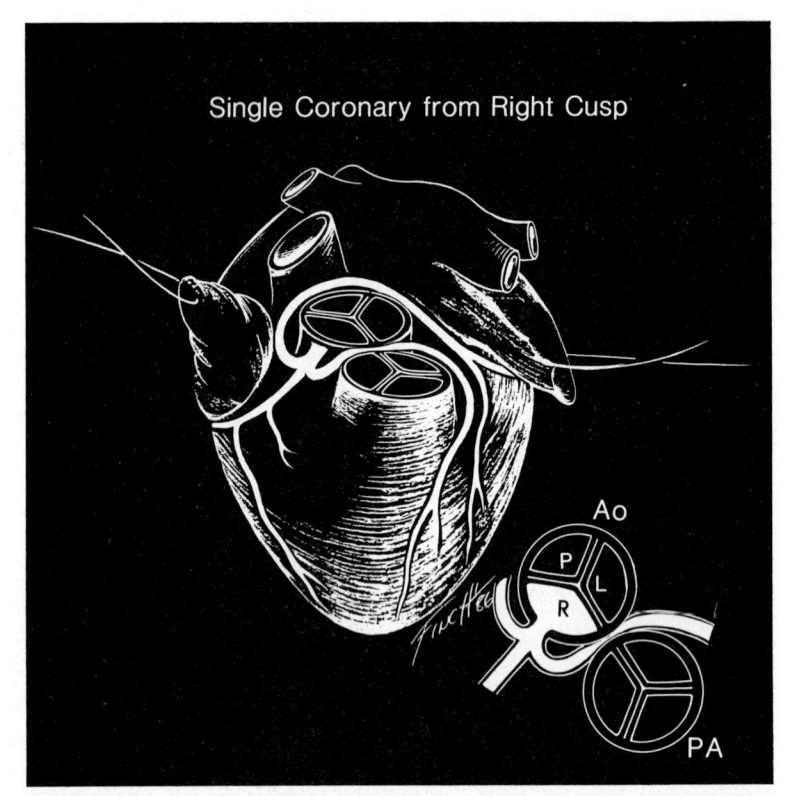

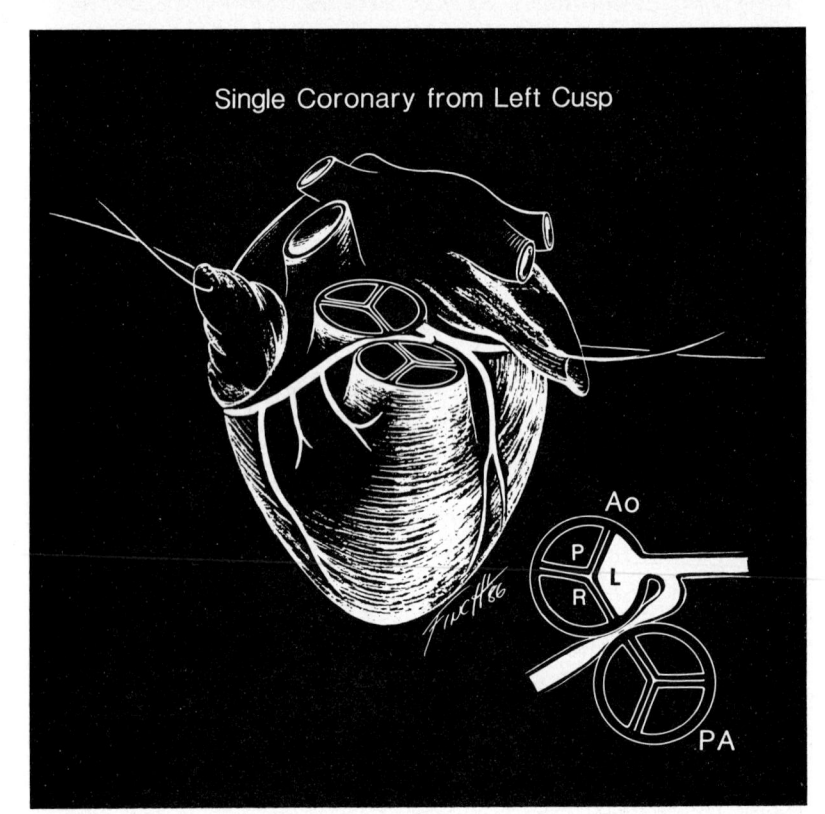

FIG 64–13.
Single coronary artery arising above left aortic cusp, giving rise to right coronary artery, which passes between aorta and right ventricular outflow tract. *Ao* = aorta; *PA* = pulmonary artery.

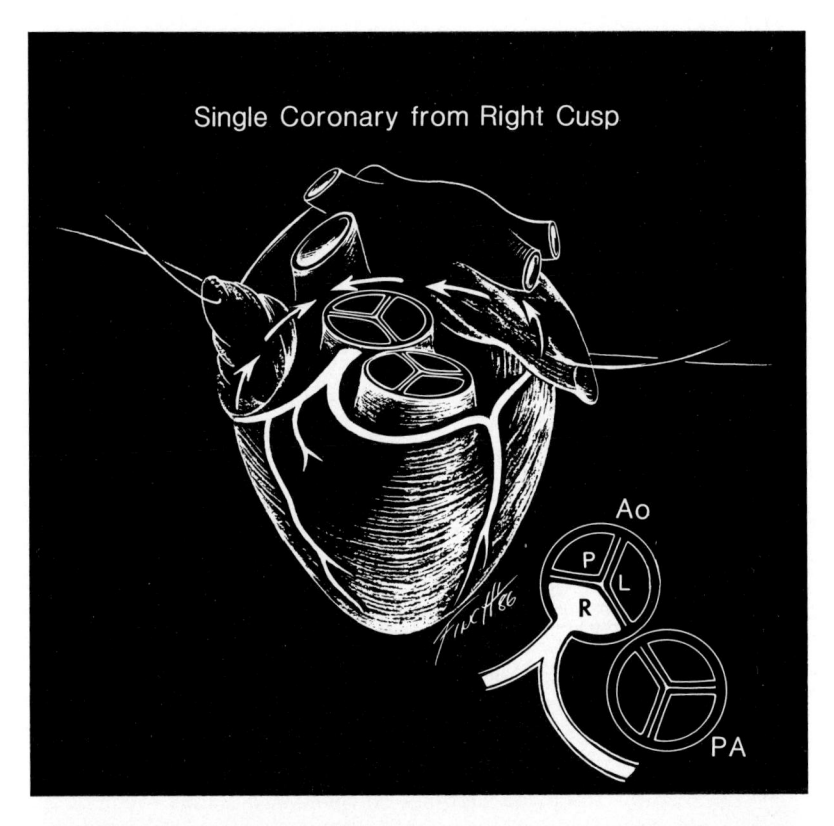

FIG 64-14.
Single coronary artery arising above right aortic cusp. Left main coronary artery passes in front of right ventricular outflow tract and divides normally into left anterior descending and circumflex arteries. Its course interferes with right ventriculotomy. Ao = aorta; PA = pulmonary artery.

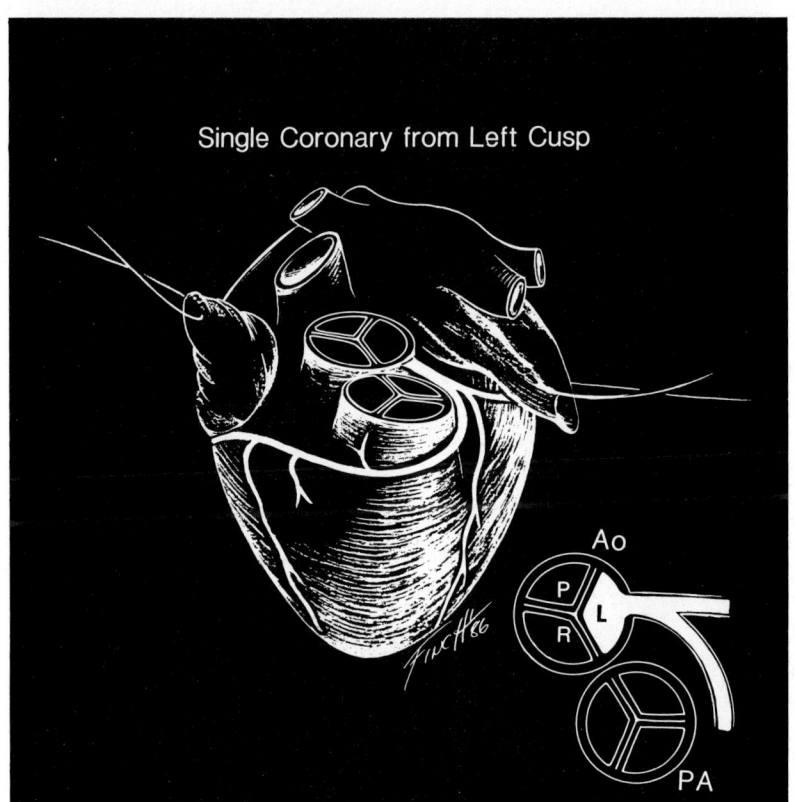

FIG 64-15.
Single coronary artery arising above left aortic cusp. Right coronary artery courses anteriorly across right ventricular outflow tract, preventing right ventriculotomy. Ao = aorta; PA = pulmonary artery.

HIGH ORIGIN OF RCA

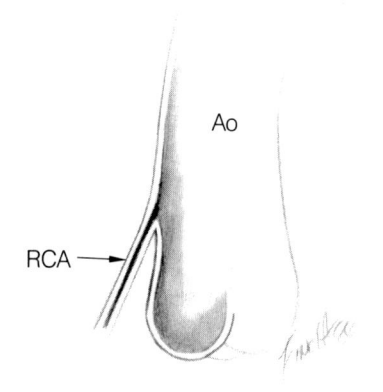

FIG 64-16.
High and ectopic origin of right coronary artery *(RCA)*. Three major problems: difficulty in selective catheterization, decreased coronary flow by acute angled origin, and potential complications at operation. *Ao* = aorta.

Single Coronary Artery Arising Above Left Aortic Cusp.—The single left coronary artery arises above the left aortic cusp and the right coronary artery may pass between the aorta and pulmonary artery (Fig 64–13). Similar to the pattern in Figures 64–11 and 64–12, compression of the coronary artery passing between the right ventricular outflow tract and aorta may occur.

Single Coronary Artery Interfering With a Ventriculotomy.—Two anomalies can interfere with a ventriculotomy. The single coronary artery arises above the right cusp and gives rise to the left coronary artery, which crosses the ventricular outflow tract anteriorly before dividing into the circumflex and left anterior descending arteries (Fig 64–14). This pattern is common in various congenital cardiac malformations, particularly transposition of the great vessels and tetralogy of Fallot and its variants.

Such an anterior course across the outflow tract is normally present in patients with corrected transposition of the great vessels and also prevents ventriculotomy. In either situation the ventricular outflow tract cannot be incised, and a conduit may be required for correction of ventricular outflow obstruction (see Chapter 39).

The single left coronary artery can also arise above the left aortic cusp and give rise to the right coronary artery, which crosses the right ventricular outflow tract to reach the right atrioventricular groove (Fig 64–15). This anomaly also precludes ventriculotomy.

VARIATION IN THE POSITION OF THE CORONARY OSTIA

In most cases the coronary arteries arise immediately below the sinotubular ridge, but they may also arise from either the sinus of Valsalva or above the sinotubular ridge (Fig 64–16). The latter origin of the coronary arteries may involve the left, right, or both coronary arteries (Fig 64–17). Origin of a coronary artery above the sinotubular ridge may be clinically significant because of the possibility of myocardial ischemia from the acute angle of its origin (discussed later on). An anomalously high origin of the right coronary artery is also important at the time of a cardiac operation, because the coronary artery may not be identified because it is covered by pericardial fat (Fig 64–18). Thus, these complications may occur during a cardiac operation:

1. The right coronary artery may be accidentally divided during aortotomy.
2. Low cross-clamping of the aorta may occlude the right coronary artery.
3. The artery may be divided when the aortic root is dissected free for valve replacement.

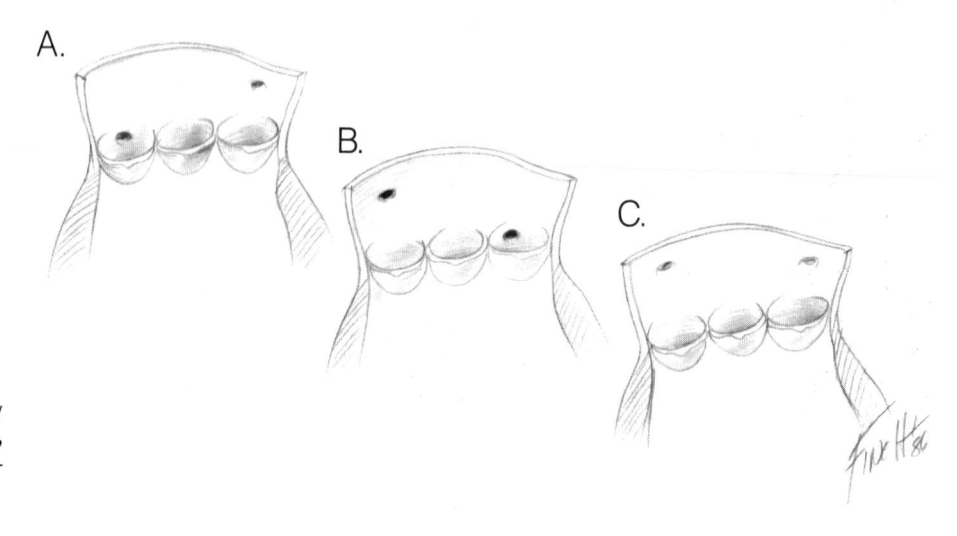

FIG 64-17.
High and ectopic origin of coronary arteries. **A**, left coronary artery. **B**, right coronary artery. **C**, both coronary arteries.

HIGH ETOPIC ORIGIN OF RCA

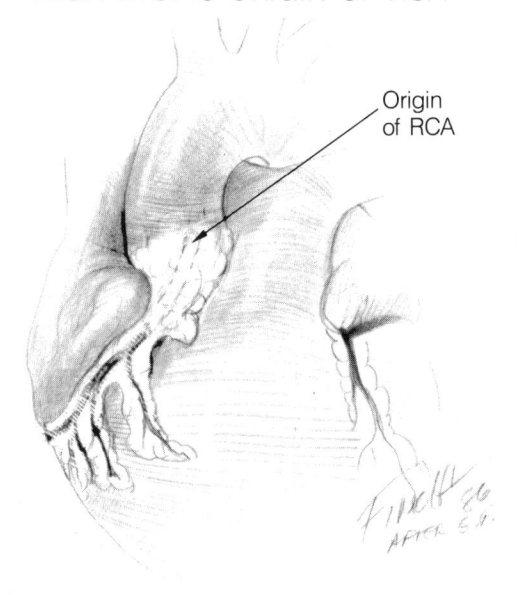

FIG 64–18.
High and ectopic origin of right coronary artery *(RCA)* may not be apparent to surgeon at time of aortotomy, because pericardial fat obscures origin of right coronary artery.

Furthermore, selective coronary arteriography is usually more difficult.

VARIATION IN ORIGIN AND DISTRIBUTION OF CORONARY ARTERIES

Several variations exist in which both the origin and distribution of the coronary arteries are abnormal. These may have clinical significance.

Without Hemodynamic Consequences

Several variations characterized by an abnormal origin or course of a coronary artery may occur:

1. The left coronary artery originates above the right aortic cusp. If either the left coronary artery or the left anterior descending artery arise from the right coronary artery or above the right aortic cusp, it usually crosses in front of the right ventricular outflow tract. This anomaly is common in tetralogy of Fallot and makes right ventriculotomy difficult in such infants. There are two variations of this anomaly:
    a. The left coronary artery may arise above the right aortic cusp (Fig 64–19).[8, 9]
    b. The left anterior descending artery may arise from the right coronary artery. This is the more common variation in tetralogy of Fallot (Fig 64–20).
2. The circumflex coronary artery may arise from the right coronary artery and pass behind the aorta to reach the posterior atrioventricular groove (Fig 64–21).[10] This represents one of the most common coronary arterial anomalies without significance.
3. Both coronary arteries may arise above the right aortic cusp. The left main coronary artery has a retroaortic course and subsequently divides into the left anterior descending and the left circumflex arteries (Fig 64–22). This is similar to single coronary artery from right aortic cusp.
4. The left circumflex artery has a separate origin above the right aortic cusp and passes behind the aorta. In this instance the left anterior descending artery arises normally above the left aortic cusp (Fig 64–23).
5. All major coronary arteries may arise above the right aortic cusp as in a single coronary artery, but a diagonal branch may arise separately above the left aortic cusp (Fig 64–24).
6. The right coronary artery may arise above the left aortic cusp and may have a retroaortic course (extremely rare) (Fig 64–25).
7. The right coronary artery arises above the posterior cusp (extremely rare), the usual pattern in transposition (Fig 64–26).

With Hemodynamic Consequences

Whereas anomalous origin of a coronary artery from the pulmonary artery (see Chapter 57) is the major congenital coronary artery anomaly causing myocardial ischemia in children whenever a coronary artery passes between the aorta and pulmonary outflow tract, myocardial ischemia may also occur. In a young patient with exertional chest pain, syncope, or sudden death, anomalous coronary arterial origin and distribution must be considered. Myocardial perfusion may be compromised because of the anomalous coronary artery branch passing between the aorta and right ventricular infundibulum.

Although such an anomaly is not uniformly fatal, sudden death may occur in about 18% of the cases. In 5% of all patients with angina pectoris or myocardial infarction, coronary atherosclerosis cannot be demonstrated by coronary arteriography. A very small percentage of these patients have an aberrant origin of a coronary artery as a cause of myocardial ischemia. In several variations, in addition to those discussed earlier, a coronary artery follows an anomalous course between the aorta and right ventricular outflow tract.

1. The right coronary artery originates above the left aortic cusp. If the right coronary artery arises above the left aortic cusp, it almost invariably crosses between the right ventricular outflow tract and the aorta as it passes to the right atrioventricular groove (Fig 64–27).[11] Rarely, it may pass in front of the right ventricular outflow tract.

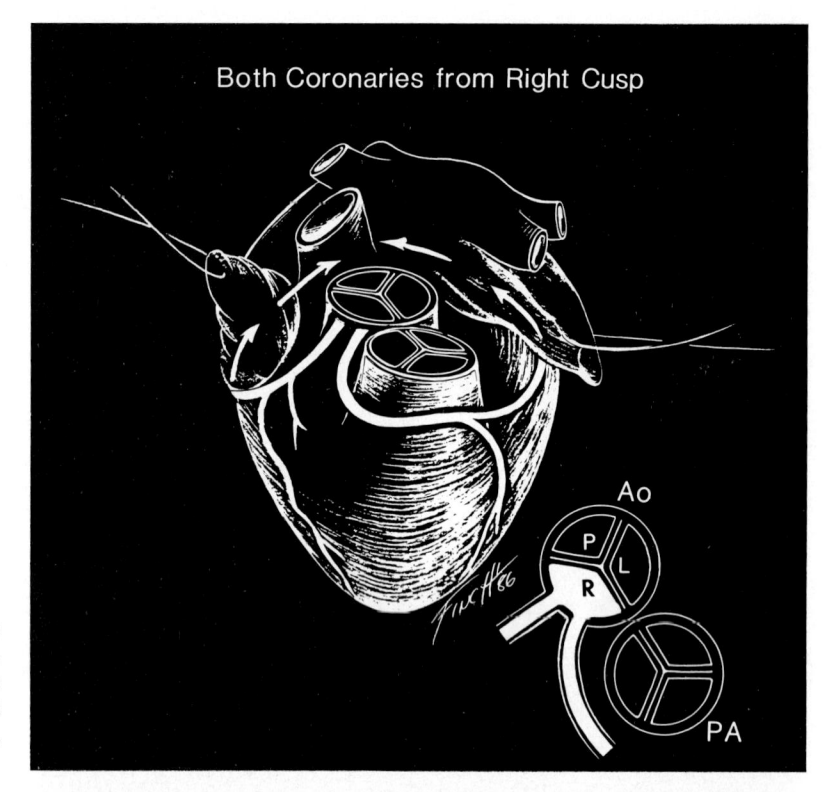

1072 Anomalies of Major Blood Vessels

FIG 64–19.
Origin of both coronary arteries above right aortic cusp. Right coronary artery has normal course. Left coronary artery courses anteriorly across right ventricular outflow tract, giving rise to left anterior descending and left circumflex arteries. *Ao* = aorta; *PA* = pulmonary artery.

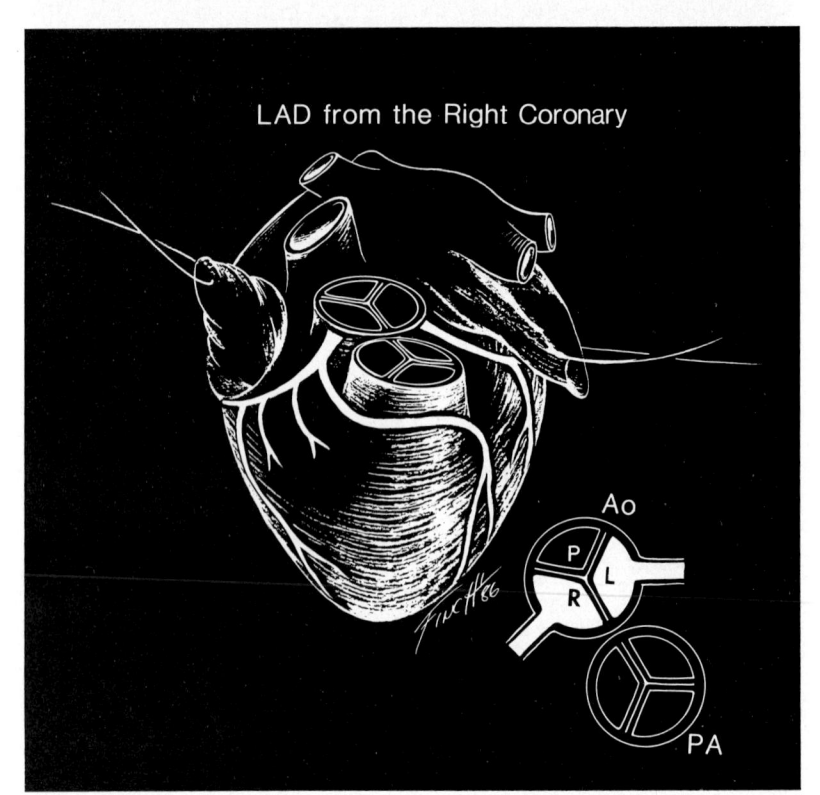

FIG 64–20.
Variation of pattern in Figure 64–19. Origin of left anterior descending *(LAD)* from right coronary artery. Left anterior descending artery crosses right ventricular outflow tract, but circumflex has normal origin about left aortic cusp. *Ao* = aorta; *PA* = pulmonary artery.

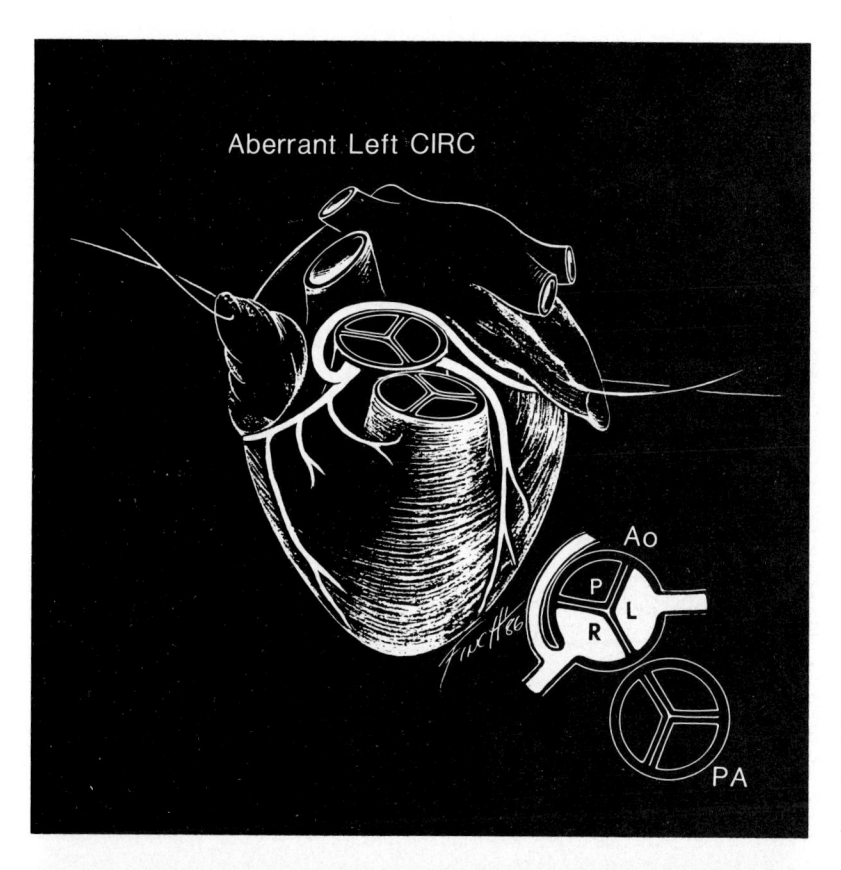

FIG 64–21.
Aberrant left circumflex *(CIRC)* arising from right coronary artery. Left coronary artery originates normally above left aortic cusp. A common variation without clinical significance. *Ao* = aorta; *PA* = pulmonary artery.

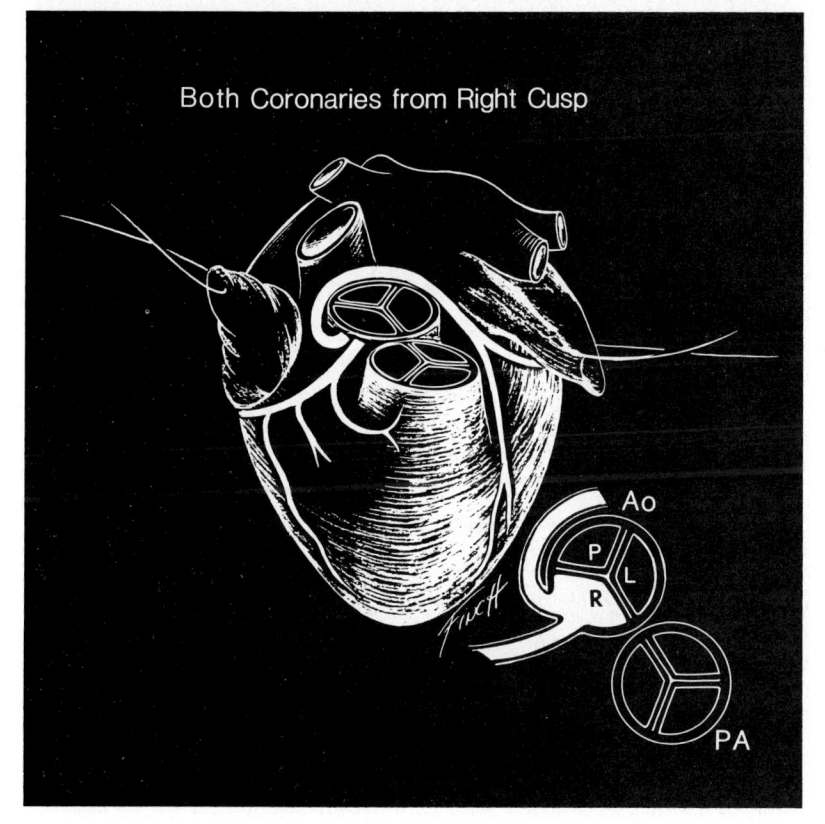

FIG 64–22.
Variation of pattern shown in Figure 64–19. Both coronary arteries arise above right aortic cusp. Retroaortic course of left coronary artery, which divides into left anterior descending and circumflex arteries. *Ao* = aorta; *PA* = pulmonary artery.

1074 Anomalies of Major Blood Vessels

FIG 64–23.
Variation of patterns in Figures 64–21 and 64–22. Circumflex (CIRC) artery arises separately above right aortic cusp and has a retroaortic course. Right coronary artery rises normally above right aortic cusp. Left anterior descending artery arises above left aortic cusp. Ao = aorta; PA = pulmonary artery.

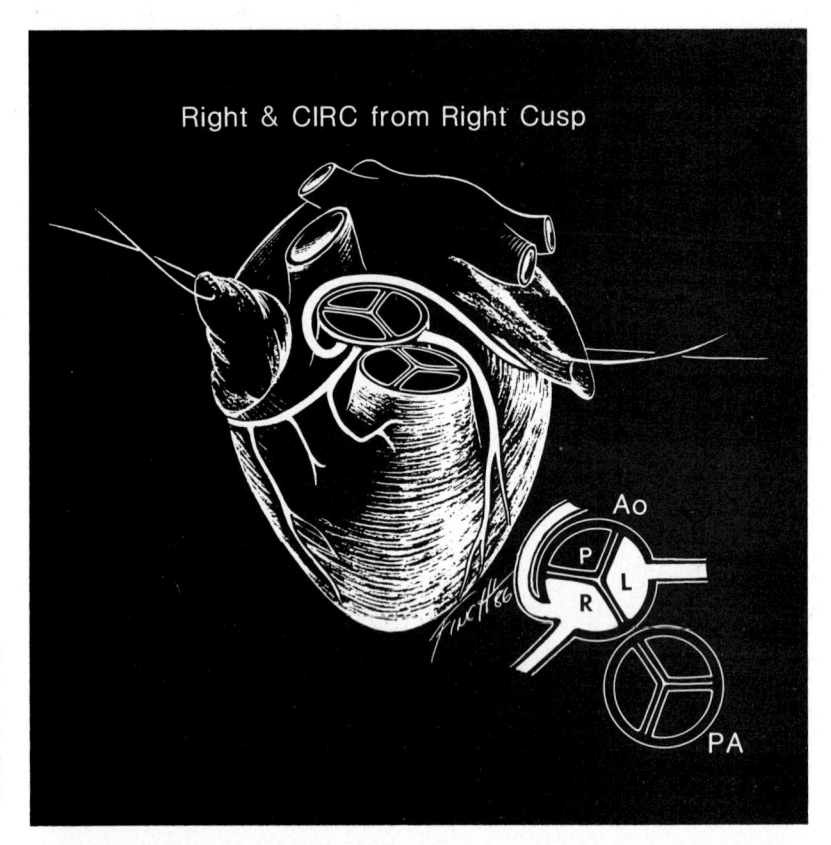

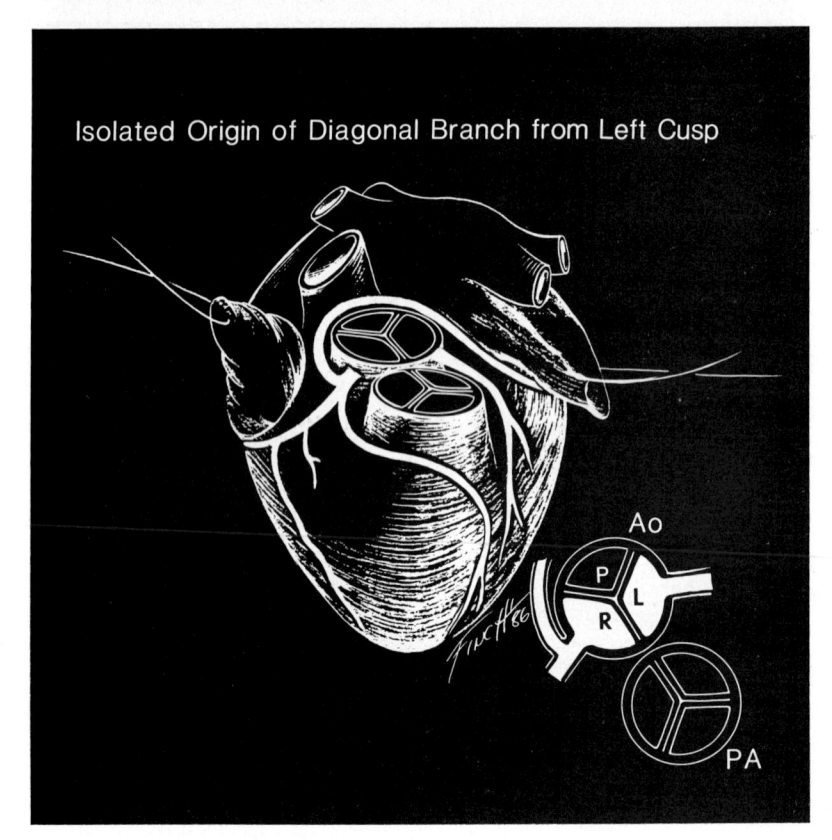

FIG 64–24.
Rare variation of patterns shown in Figure 64–23. Origin of left anterior descending and retroaortic circumflex arteries above right coronary artery. Isolated origin of diagonal brach above left aortic cusp. Ao = aorta; PA = pulmonary artery;

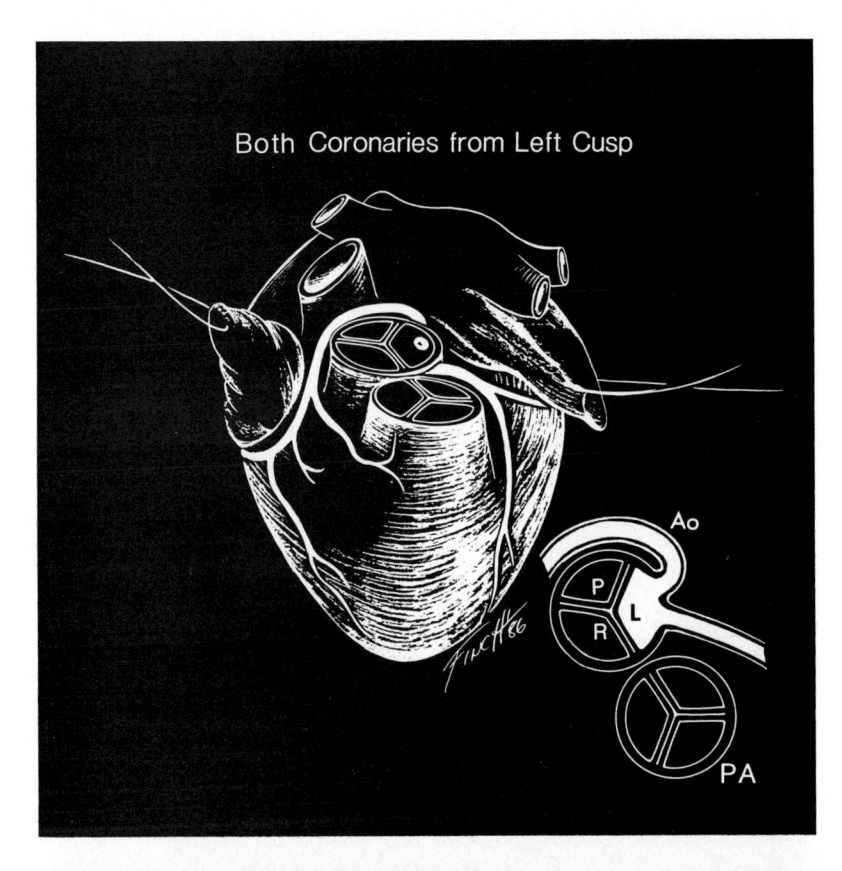

FIG 64–25.
Rare occurrence of right coronary artery and left coronary artery arising above left aortic cusp. Right coronary artery has retroaortic course. Left coronary artery has normal pattern. *Ao* = aorta; *PA* = pulmonary artery.

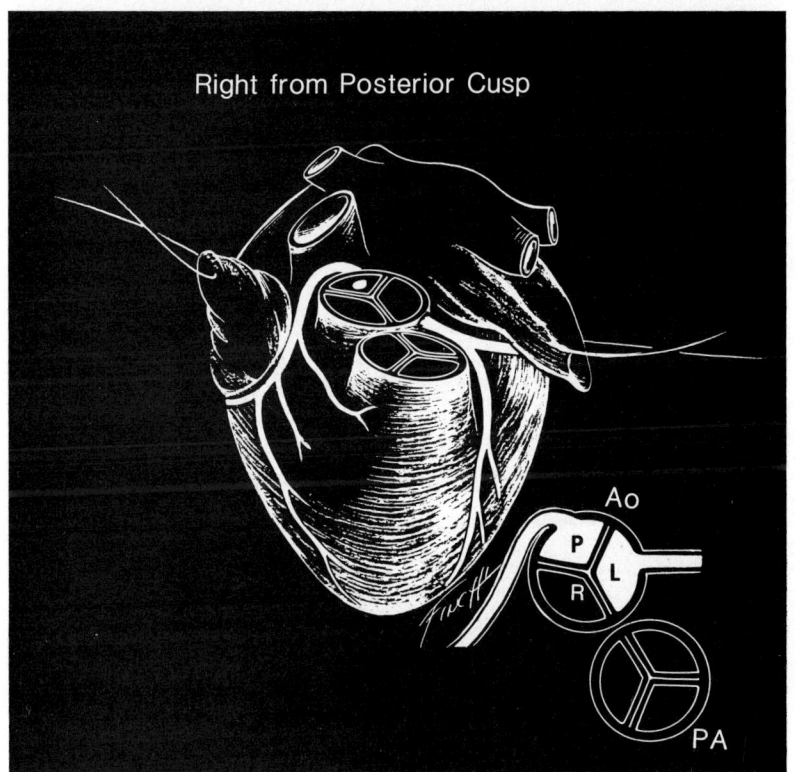

FIG 64–26.
Extremely rare anomaly. Anomalous origin of right coronary artery above posterior (noncoronary cusp). *Ao* = aorta; *PA* = pulmonary artery.

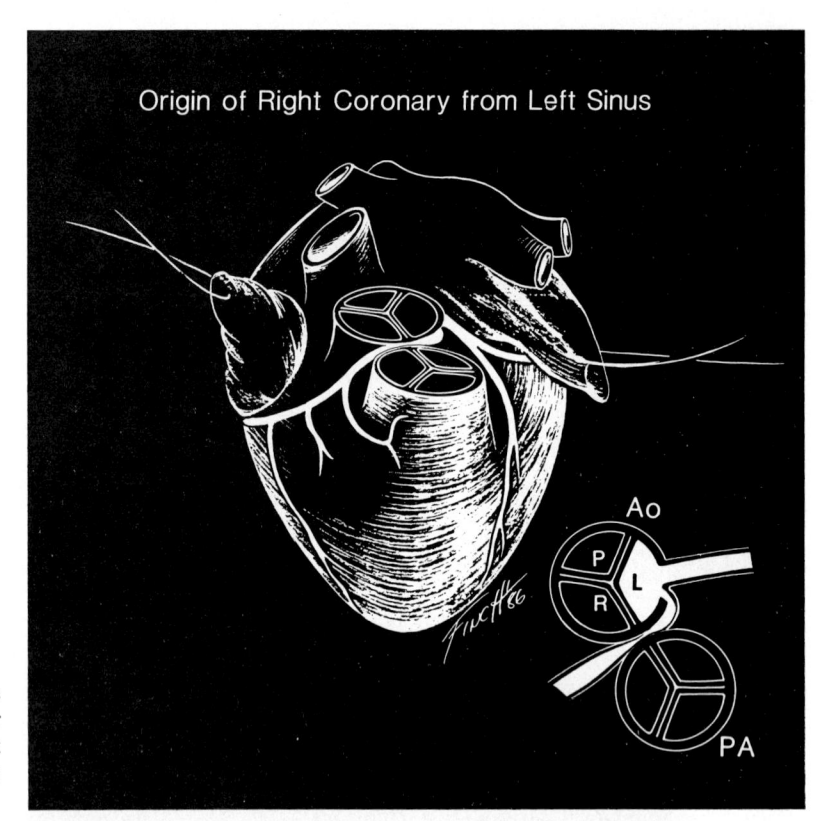

FIG 64–27.
Anomalous origin of right coronary artery above left cusp and passing between right ventricular outflow tract and aorta. This variation may result in severe hemodynamic consequence. *Ao* = aorta; *PA* = pulmonary artery.

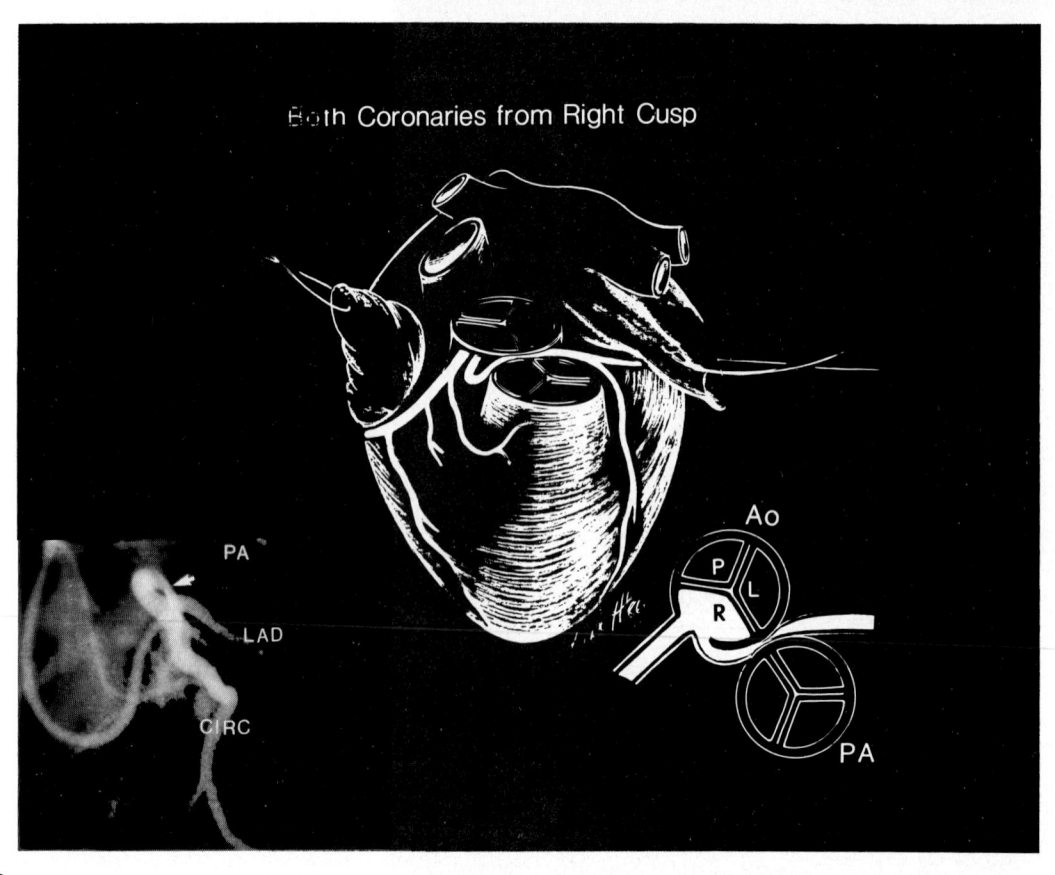

FIG 64–28.
Separate origin of left coronary artery above right aortic cusp passing between right ventricular outflow tract and aorta. *Insert*, selective coronary arteriogram. Right anterior oblique projection. Aberrant origin of left main coronary artery from right aortic cusp. Left main coronary arises anteriorly and passes acutely posteriorly between aorta and right ventricular outflow tract, where it is narrowed *(arrow)*. *LAD* = left anterior descending artery; *CIRC* = circumflex branch; *PA* site of pulmonary artery; *Ao* = aorta.

2. Both coronary arteries may arise above the right aortic cusp, and the left main coronary artery passes between the aorta and right ventricular outflow tract (Fig 64–28).

3. The left main coronary artery arises above the right aortic cusp and gives rise to the circumflex artery, which passes between the aorta and right ventricular outflow tract.[12] In this instance, the left anterior descending artery courses in front of the right ventricular outflow tract (Fig 64–29).

4. All three coronary arteries arise separately above the right aortic cusp. The right has a normal course, the circumflex artery has a retroaortic course, and the left anterior descending artery passes between the aorta and right ventricular outflow tract (Fig 64–30).

5. The right coronary artery may arise separately above the left aortic cusp and pass between the aorta and right ventricular outflow tract (Fig 64–31).

Ectopic Origin of the Coronary Arteries

1. Origin of the coronary arteries from the pulmonary artery. This anomaly is discussed in detail in Chapter 57.

2. Origin of coronary arteries from systemic vessels. These extremely rare anomalies are of no hemodynamic consequence. They are, however, important to the angiographer who may not be able to visualize the coronary artery by standard coronary arteriography or even aortography.

3. A single coronary artery may arise ectopically from the innominate (Fig 64–32) or carotid artery (Fig 64–33). Ectopic origin of a coronary artery from bronchial branches or from the internal mammary artery is exceedingly rare (Fig 64–34).

Mechanism of Myocardial Ischemia in Aberrant Origin of a Coronary Artery

Anomalous origin of a coronary artery should be suspected in a young male who has ischemic symptoms and a positive stress electrocardiogram. The mechanism of angina pectoris, syncope, or sudden death in these patients is obscure. Definitive diagnosis is made by selective coronary angiography, which may be difficult because of the anterior origin of the left coronary artery. The Amplatz-type left coronary catheter is most successful for selective cannulization of the aberrant coronary artery.

The etiology of myocardial ischemia and sudden death is unclear. Several theories have been advanced. The first is compression of the left coronary artery between aorta and right ventricular outflow tract during exercise because of the increased blood volume in both great arteries. This theory is disputed because of the normally low pulmonary artery pressure, which should not compromise the lumen

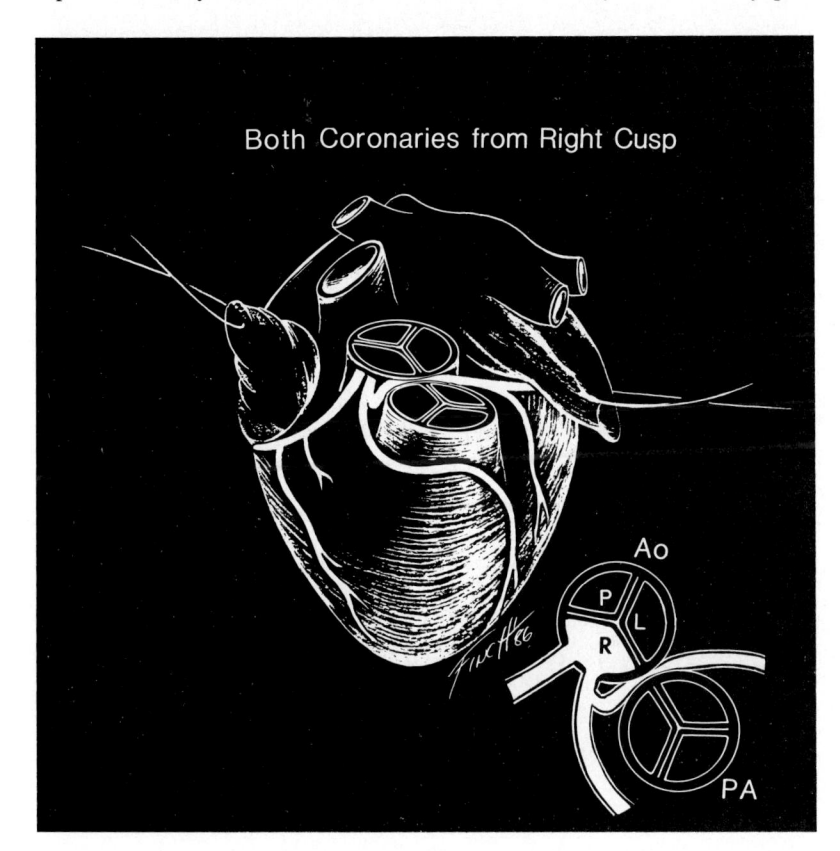

FIG 64–29.
Anomalous origin of left coronary artery above right aortic cusp. Rare variation of pattern in Figure 64–28. Left anterior descending artery crosses abnormally in front of right ventricular outflow tract. Circumflex artery passes between right ventricular outflow tract and aorta, making it vulnerable to compression. Ao = aorta; PA = pulmonary artery.

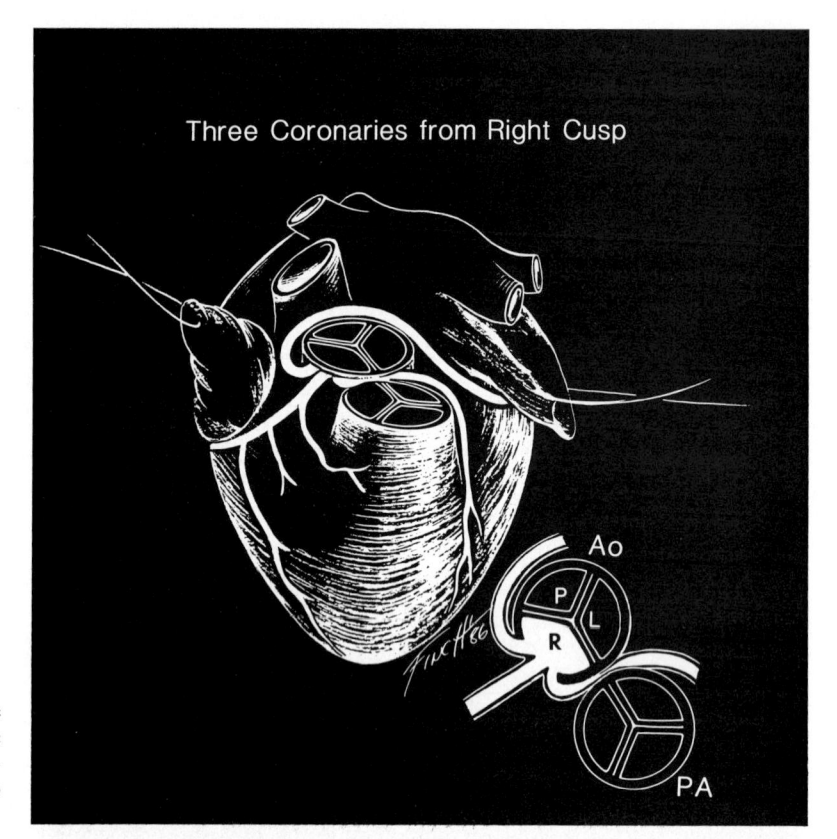

1078 *Anomalies of Major Blood Vessels*

FIG 64–30.
All three coronary arteries arise separately above right aortic cusp. Circumflex artery has retroaortic course. Left anterior descending artery passes between aorta and right ventricular outflow tract. *Ao* = aorta; *PA* = pulmonary artery.

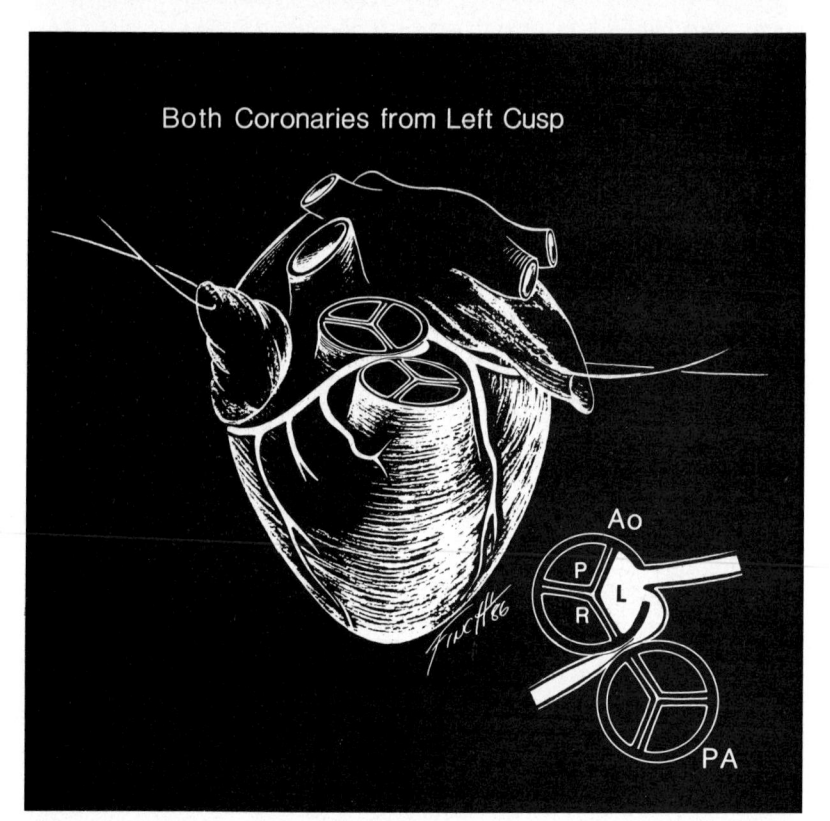

FIG 64–31.
Origin of right coronary artery above left aortic sinus. Right coronary artery passes between aorta and right ventricular outflow tract. *Ao* = aorta; *PA* = pulmonary artery.

SINGLE CORONARY ARTERY FROM R. INNOMINATE ARTERY

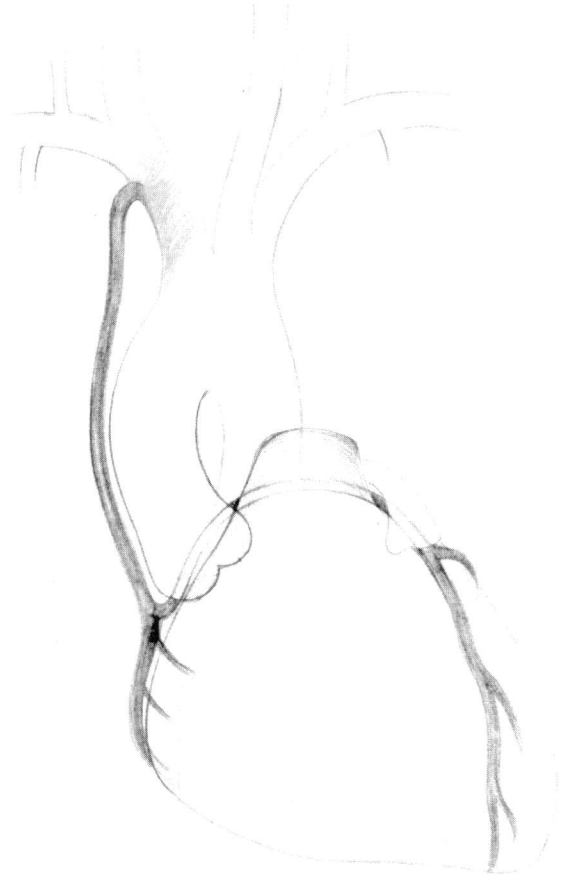

FIG 64–32.
Ectopic origin of single coronary artery from right *(R)* innominate artery.

of the coronary artery, which is under a much higher pressure. Second is stretching of the long main left coronary artery. With expansion of the aorta during exercise, stretching and compression of the artery may occur because it passes acutely posteriorly in intimate contract with the aortic wall. With growth of the aorta, angulation and stretching and consequent narrowing of the long left main coronary artery may occur. Third is kinking of the acutely angled left main coronary artery, particularly during exercise, resulting from increased blood volume in the aorta. Fourth is occlusion of the coronary ostium because of its slitlike orifice through the intramural portion of the aorta[13] (Fig 64–35). The fifth theory is hypoplasia of the left coronary arterial tree, which appears to be part of this syndrome, probably related to impaired myocardial flow.

Summary.—In anomalous origin of a coronary artery from the contralateral aortic cusp it has to cross from right to left or left to right respectively. This can occur in four ways:

1. Retroaortic (not significant).
2. Between aorta and pulmonary artery (significant).
3. Across the right ventricular outflow tract (significant).
4. Intramyocardia (significant).

SINGLE CORONARY ARTERY FROM R. CAROTID ARTERY

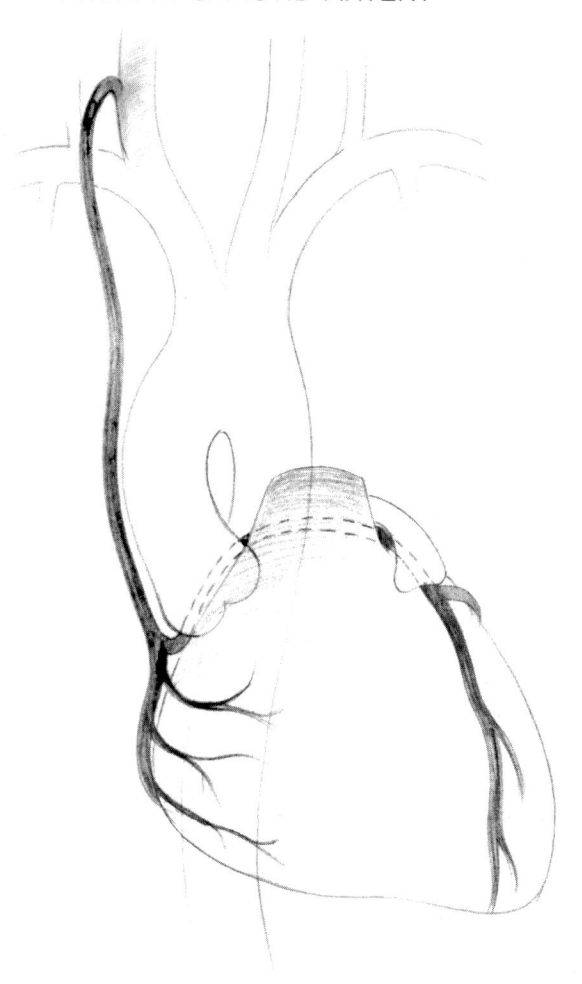

FIG 64–33.
Ectopic origin of single coronary artery from right *(R)* common carotid artery.

Other Congenital Causes of Impaired Coronary Flow

In patients with findings of impaired myocardial perfusion, several other congenital cardiac malformations must be considered:

1. Obstruction of the left coronary artery may occur in supravalvar aortic stenosis by a valvelike flap or adhe-

LAD FROM L. INTERNAL MAMMARY ARTERY

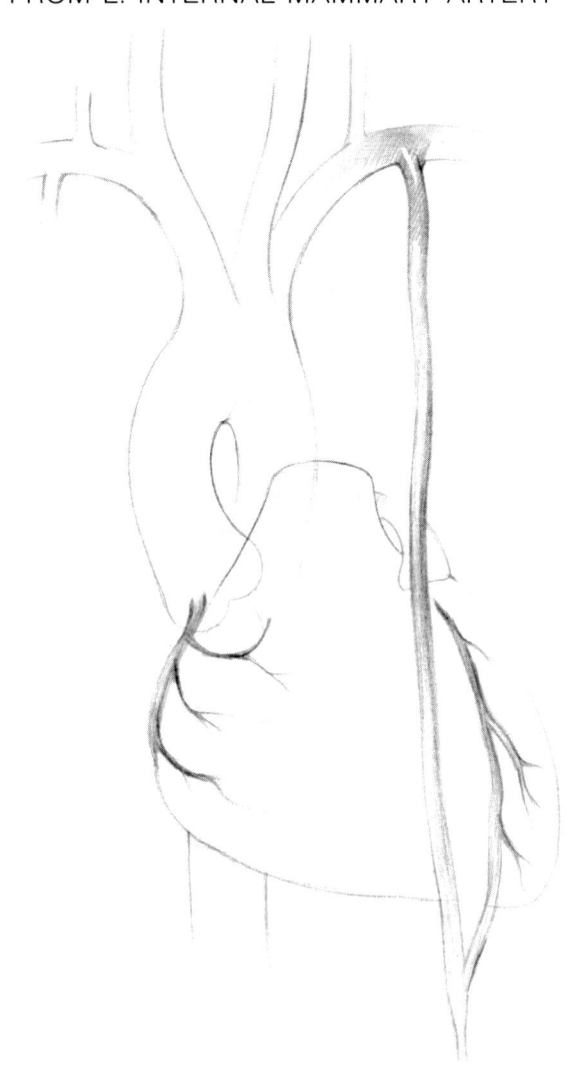

FIG 64–34.
Ectopic origin of left anterior descending artery *(LAD)* from left mammary artery.

sion of an aortic cusp to the wall occluding the orifice or by a discrete membrane arising from the aortic wall above the left sinus that attaches to the left coronary cusp (see Chapter 26).

2. Primary dissecting aneurysm of the coronary artery may occur (see Fig 64–39,A). This extremely rare complication occurs in individuals with cystic medial necrosis. The condition occurs most commonly in postpartum young adult females. It may result in sudden death. Ischemia is produced by compression of the coronary arterial lumen.

3. Secondary dissecting aneurysm may occur. In patients with cystic medial necrosis, aortic dissection may extend into the coronary arteries and compress the lumen (Fig 64–36,B).

4. Rupture of a congenital aneurysm of the coronary artery is an extremely rare cause of sudden death. Such aneurysms may also be a source of thrombosis and myocardial infarction because of embolism.

5. A rare anomaly is origin of the left anterior descending from the right coronary artery and tunneling through the ventricular septum, having therefore a long intramyocardial course (Fig 64–37). Symptoms caused by this rare abnormality are unclear.[14] They may be related to the length of the tunnel, the thickness of the myocardial bridge, the degree of systolic compression, and the cardiac rate.

The deeper and the longer the tunnel, the more pronounced is the systolic compression. Because coronary blood flow occurs primarily during diastole, compression during systole does not significantly decrease myocardial perfusion at rest. During exercise, however, with a markedly shortened diastolic filling period, the compressed arterial segment may not relax completely, and myocardial perfusion is impaired. If there is a history of angina and a positive stress test, the myocardial bridge should be operatively released, although bridges are commonly seen as incidental findings in asymptomatic patients.

If coronary angiography is entirely normal, variant angina should be considered; it may occur in children, leading to transient chest pain and electrocardiographic changes. Prinzmetal syndrome or variant angina is believed to be caused by coronary spasm. Ergonovine infusion has been used to provoke attacks, and coronary arteriography is repeated. Sometimes a history of migraine and concomitant chest pain can be elicited.

MYOCARDIAL BRIDGES

Myocardial bridges are a common finding at postmortem examination. On coronary angiography, they are detected in less than 10% of the patients on very careful review of excellent-quality arteriograms. Any left coronary branch may be involved. The midsegment of the left anterior descending branch is by far the most common site. The incidence of myocardial bridges detected at postmortem examination is approximately 30%. A similar incidence is found in heart transplant patients by selective coronary angiography. REASON: Probably increased stiffness of the myocardium and left ventricular hypertrophy secondary to hypertension caused by cyclosporin A therapy. There is a prevalence in men (70%). Myocardial bridges are also more commonly angiographically demonstrated in patients with idiopathic left ventricular hypertrophy (see Chapter 26).

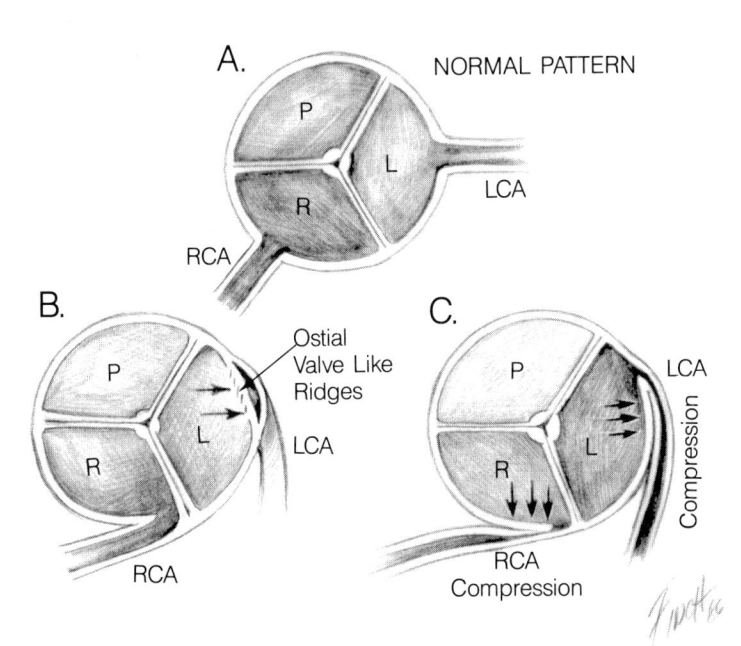

FIG 64-35.
Proposed mechanisms of coronary artery compression. **A,** normally coronary arteries arise at right angle from aorta. **B,** With acute origin of right *(RCA)* or left *(LCA)* coronary artery, a valvelike ridge forms, limiting coronary flow, thereby inducing myocardial ischemia. This mechanism may occur not only with coronary anomalies but also with ectopic high origin (see Fig 64-16). **C,** acute origin of coronary arteries may result in extrinsic compression of arterial lumen, particularly during exercise with increase of intraaortic pressure. Coronary arteries are vulnerable to extrinsic compression at the site of passage between right ventricular outflow tract and aorta.

Pathophysiology

Normally the coronary arteries and their major branches course in the epicardial fat, but occasionally they course beneath the myocardium for a various length (Fig 64-38). This occurrence is termed a myocardial bridge.

Myocardial bridges commonly cross the left anterior descending coronary artery and less frequently over left ventricular muscular branches. Bridges over right coronary arterial system should not cause systolic compression, because right ventricular systolic pressure is less than aortic pressure.

The clinical significance of myocardial bridges is unknown. The coronary artery is compressed by the bridge during systole, and this event can be demonstrated angiographically. Although coronary blood flow occurs primarily during diastole, blood flow may be significantly hampered by the bridges during tachycardia.

Most cases do not have typical symptoms of angina and have negative exercise stress tests results, suggesting that the myocardial bridge is not physiologically significant.

Occasionally typical findings of myocardial ischemia are found in a patient with a myocardial bridge. Such a pa-

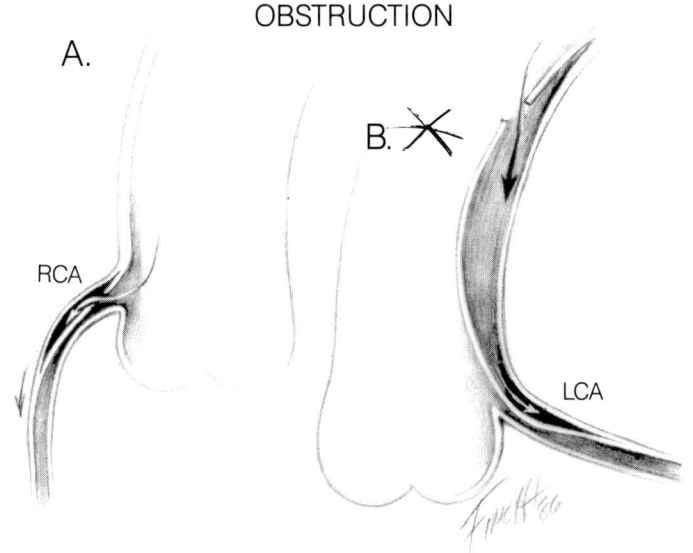

FIG 64-36.
Dissecting aneurysms. **A,** primary dissecting aneurysm arising in right coronary artery *(RCA)* compressing its lumen. Rare occurrence. **B,** dissecting aneurysm arising in ascending aorta in patient with cystic medial necrosis. Intramural hematoma has dissected into left coronary artery *(LCA),* compressing its lumen, resulting in ischemia, myocardial infarction, or both.

SOLITARY RIGHT CORONARY ARTERY WITH ITS THREE DIVISIONS

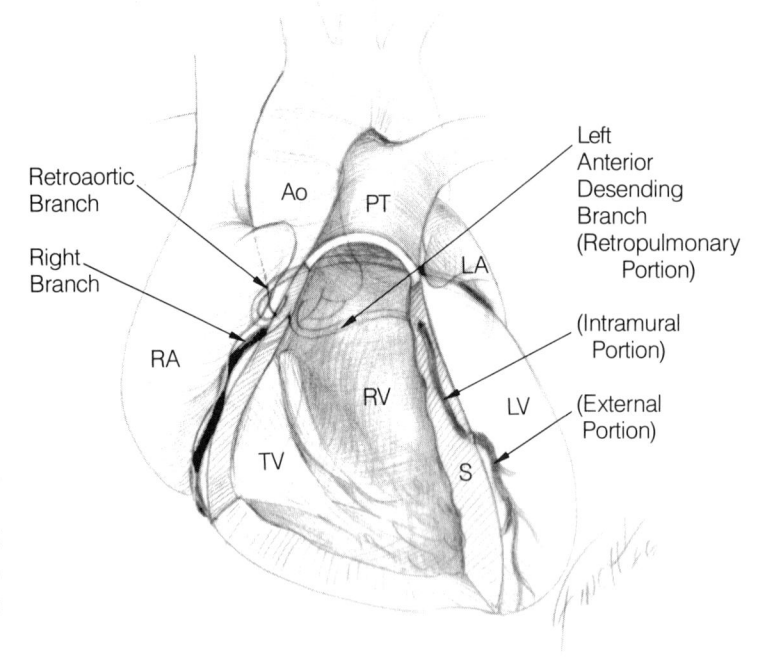

FIG 64–37.
Single coronary artery arising above right aortic cusp. Left anterior descending branch has long intramyocardial course in ventricular septum and finally reaches the epicardial surface near the apex. This is an example of an unusually long myocardial bridge, causing symptoms of myocardial ischemia. *Ao* = aorta; *PT* = pulmonary trunk; *LA* = left atrium; *RA* = right atrium; *RV* = right ventricle; *LV* = left ventricle; *TV* = tricuspid valve; *S* = septum.

tient may benefit from operative division of the bridging muscle band.

Myocardial bridges are most commonly an incidental angiographic finding because of the following:

1. The anomaly is present from birth, but symptoms usually occur later in life. We have had, however, a well-documented case in a child who was operated, with relief of symptoms.

2. Maximal stenosis occurs for a very short period during each systole when normally little blood flow occurs through the coronary arterial system (Fig 64–39,A and B). However, during exercise and tachycardia, the compressed coronary artery has to fill first before peripheral coronary perfusion occurs during diastole. Because the diastolic interval is very short, myocardial ischemia may result (Fig 64–39,C).

3. Myocardial bridges are a common incidental finding during a postmortem examination and are unassociated with evidence of myocardial ischemia.

MYOCARDIAL SINUSOIDS

Myocardial sinusoids provide an important regress of blood from both ventricles in aortic and pulmonary atresia. The anatomy of sinusoids is discussed in Chapter 34.

In normal patients the sinusoids are nonfunctioning. Rarely, for unknown reasons, they may remain patent, and a small amount of blood may enter through numerous small openings the left ventricle.

During selective coronary arteriography, faint puffs of contrast medium can be seen in the left ventricular cavity (Fig 64–40). By careful inspection of good-quality selec-

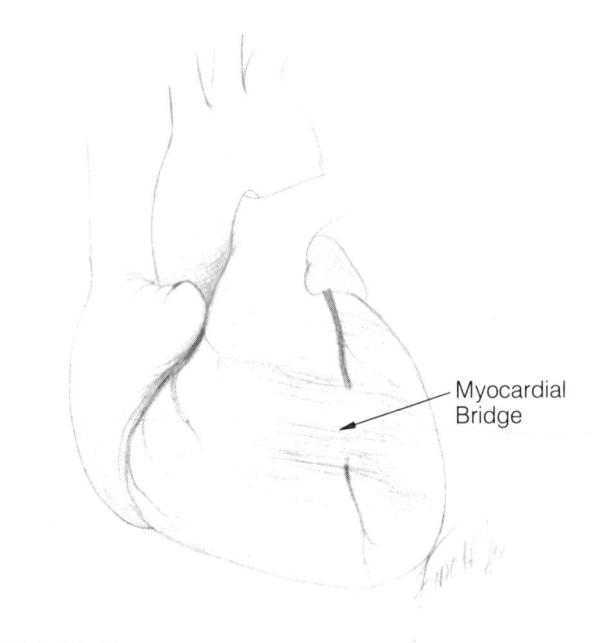

FIG 64–38.
Myocardial bridge. Muscle band crosses midportion of left anterior descending coronary artery. Variable degree of arterial compression occurs during systole.

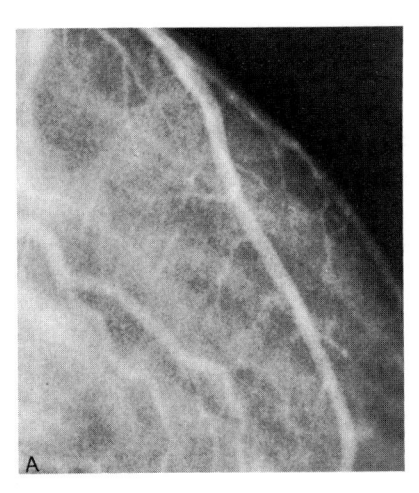

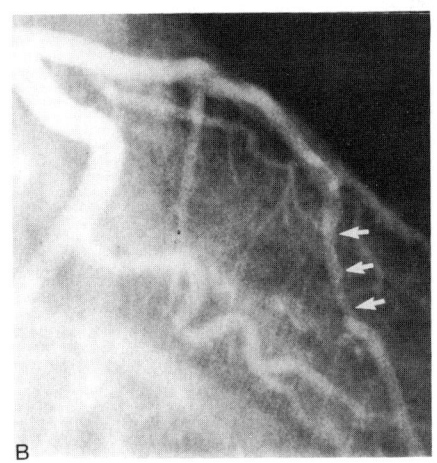

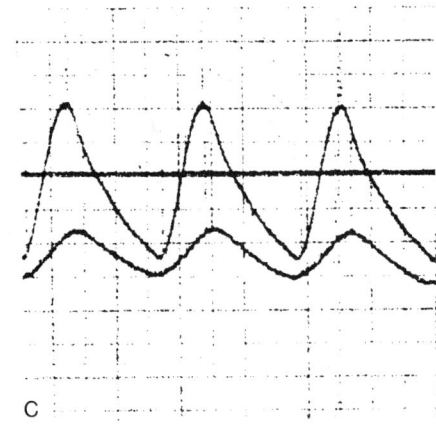

FIG 64–39.
Left coronary arteriogram. Asymptomatic patient. **A,** diastole. Normal caliber of left anterior descending artery. **B,** systole. Compression and bowing of left anterior descending artery by myocardial bridge *(arrows)*. Intermittent compression and change in caliber prove nonatherosclerotic narrowing. **C,** simultaneous pressure recording from aorta and coronary artery distal to myocardial bridge during tachycardia demonstrates a significant pressure gradient.

tive coronary arteriograms, myocardial sinusoids can be seen in less than 1% of the patients. There is some evidence that myocardial sinusoids are more common in transplanted hearts.

INFANTILE CORONARY ARTERY DISEASE

Symptomatic coronary artery disease in infancy is extremely rare and is usually part of a systemic arterial disease in which coronary arteries are involved.

Among the condition affecting the coronary arteries of infants are vasculitis, atherosclerosis, storage diseases, mucocutaneous lymph node syndrome (see Chapter 65), infantile polyarteritis nodosa, progressive arterial occlusive disease, neurofibromatosis, tuberous sclerosis, rubella, moyamoya disease, chronic arsenic poisoning, fibromuscular dysplasia, and idiopathic arterial calcification of infancy. Most of these generalized arterial diseases are diagnosed by their systemic manifestations, such as lymph node involvement (Kawasaki disease), skin lesions (progressive arterial occlusive disease), neurologic manifestations (moyamoya disease), gangrenous extremities (arsenic poisoning, black foot disease), and systemic stigmata (neurofibromatosis and tuberous sclerosis). Only fibromuscular dysplasia[15] and idiopathic arterial calcification of infancy[16] may not show obvious clinical manifestations, except for the findings of coronary artery disease.

FIBROMUSCULAR DYSPLASIA

Fibromuscular dysplasia is a nonatherosclerotic vascular disease of unknown etiology that involves virtually all small- and medium-sized arteries, particularly the renal arteries. The affected arteries are replaced by irregularly alternating segments of constriction and dilatation, giving the characteristic beaded angiographic appearance. The constrictions are caused by localized protuberance of hypoplastic arterial media, and the dilatations result from focally absent muscular media forming aneurysms of the ar-

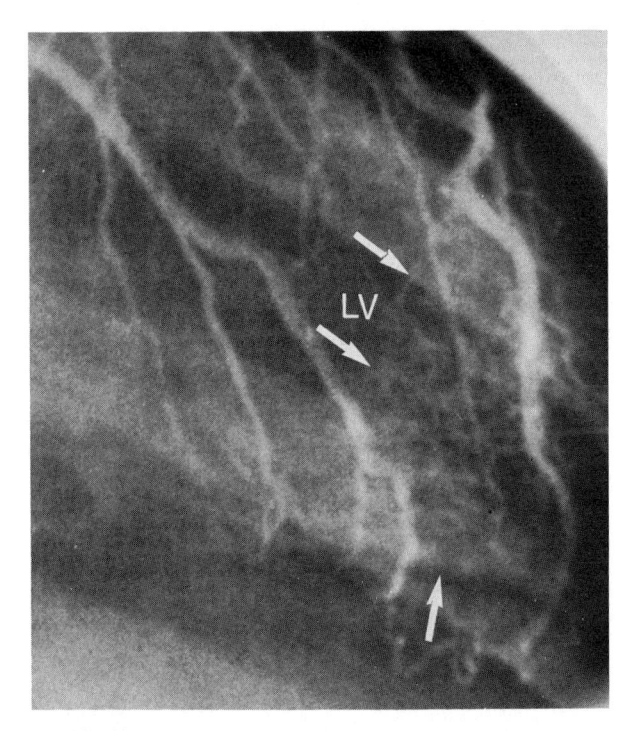

FIG 64–40.
Left coronary arteriogram. Right anterior oblique projection. Puffs of contrast medium *(arrows)* are seen in left ventricular cavity.

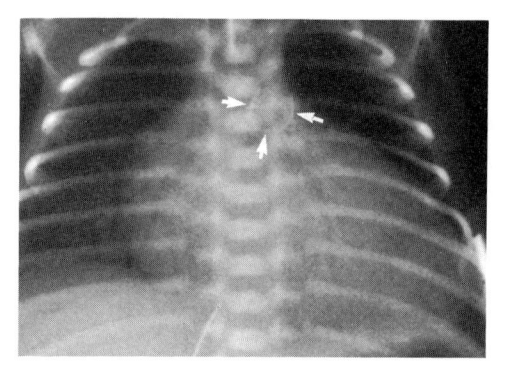

FIG 64-41.
Idiopathic infantile arterial calcification. Thoracic roentgenogram. Posteroanterior projection. Severe cardiomegaly from left ventricular enlargement. Dense calcification *(arrows)* in pulmonary artery. Coronary artery calcification is not seen.

tery. The hemodynamic consequence of the disease is arterial stenosis and spontaneous dissection.

Rarely, fibromuscular dysplasia involves the coronary arteries, leading to signs of coronary artery insufficiency, myocardial infarction, mitral regurgitation from papillary muscle infarction, left ventricular myopathy, or sudden death because of spontaneous dissection.

IDIOPATHIC INFANTILE ARTERIAL CALCIFICATION

This rare congenital arterial disease has also been termed idiopathic infantile calcinosis, generalized arterial calcification of infancy, infantile atherosclerosis, calcific arteriopathy, or Stryker disease.

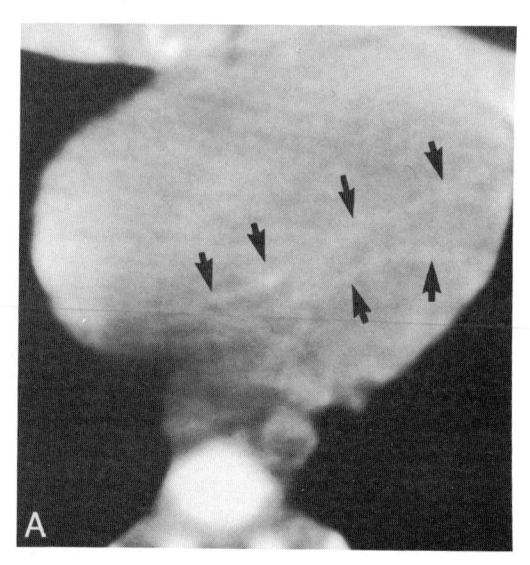

Pathologic Manifestations

The disease is characterized by deposition of calcific material in the walls of medium-sized systemic arteries, particularly in the coronary arteries. Absence of coronary calcifications does not exclude the disease. Intimal hyperplasia, in addition to coronary calcifications, leads to coronary artery occlusion with myocardial ischemia, myocardial infarction, myocardial fibrosis with left ventricular enlargement, and mitral insufficiency. The pathologic features resemble anomalous origin of the left coronary artery from the pulmonary artery. The disease may involve all medium-sized arteries, but involvement of the cerebrovascular arterial tree is very rare. Most patients die before the age of 6 months, although survival to adulthood has been reported.

Clinical Features

Most frequently, the presenting clinical features are respiratory distress, tachycardia, hepatomegaly, vomiting, regurgitation, and refusal of feeding. Continued crying after feeding is interpreted as angina pectoris.

On physical examination there may be evidence for cardiac enlargement and a systolic murmur of mitral insufficiency may be heard along the left sternal border. Serum calcium levels are typically normal.

Radiographic Features

Depending on the degree of myocardial damage, cardiac size varies from normal to severe cardiomegaly (Fig 64-41). Cardiac enlargement results from dilatation of the

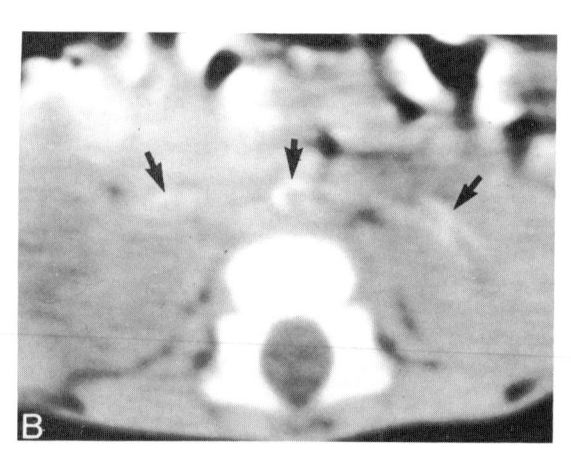

FIG 64-42.
Idiopathic infantile arterial calcification. **A,** computed tomography scan of heart. Coronary artery calcifications *(arrows)*. These calcifications were not seen on plain films or by cinefluorography. **B,** calcifications in abdominal aorta and both renal arteries *(arrows)*.

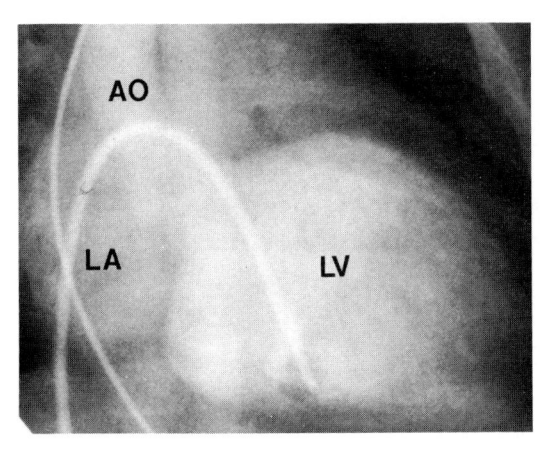

FIG 64–43.
Idiopathic infantile arterial calcification. Left ventriculogram. Anteroposterior projection. Mild mitral regurgitation. Severe left ventricular enlargement.

left ventricle. The left atrium is enlarged from increased left ventricular end-diastolic pressure or mitral regurgitation, as in anomalous origin of the left coronary artery from the pulmonary artery. The diagnosis can be established radiographically by identifying coronary artery calcifications, which occur in most cases.

Calcifications in coronary arteries and peripheral arteries such as the abdominal aorta and renal arteries may not be visible on roentgenograms but may become obvious by computed tomography examination (Fig 64–42).

Angiographic Features

1. Left ventriculography demonstrates a dilated, poorly contracting left ventricle with regional contraction abnormalities such as hypokinesia or akinesia caused by myocardial infarction.

2. The end-diastolic volume is increased, and the ejection fraction is typically decreased.

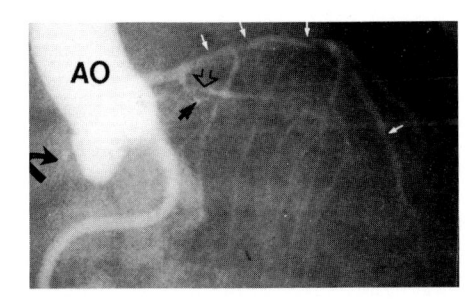

FIG 64–44.
Idiopathic infantile arterial calcification. Aortogram. Balloon occlusion technique. Anteroposterior projection. Diffuse stenoses throughout left anterior descending artery *(small arrows)*. Occlusion of circumflex artery *(black arrow)* and almost complete occlusion of first obtuse marginal branch *(open arrows)*. Occlusion of right coronary artery *(curved arrow)*. Ao = aorta.

3. There is a various degree of mitral regurgitation.
REASON: Relative mitral insufficiency secondary to dilatation of the left ventricle and papillary muscle infarction (Fig 64–43).

4. Selective coronary angiography demonstrates diffuse coronary lesions and typically calcifications in coronary arterial walls. Diffuse attenuation of the left coronary arterial tree, identical to adult atherosclerosis, occurs (Fig 64–44).

5. Coronary occlusions and collaterals may be present (see Fig 64–44).

Treatment

Treatment with corticosteriods, estrogens, and thyroid hormone has questionable efficacy. Treatment with etidronate disodium, a synthetic diphosphonate analogue of pyrophosphate, may enable complete reversal of the calcifications and prevent death.[17] The drug has been previously used for treatment of myositis ossificans and Paget's disease.

REFERENCES

1. Roberts WC: Major anomalies of coronary arterial origin seen in adulthood, *Am Heart J* 111:941, 1986.
2. Blake HA, Manion WC, Mattingly TW, et al: Coronary artery anomalies, *Circulation* 30:927, 1964.
3. Alexander RW, Griffith GC: Anomalies of the coronary arteries and their clinical significance, *Circulation* 14:800, 1956.
4. Mullins CE, El-Said G, McNamara DG, et al: Atresia of the left coronary artery ostium: repair by saphenous vein graft, *Circulation* 46:989, 1972.
5. Liberthson RR, Dinsmore RE, Bharati S, et al: Aberrant coronary artery origin from the aorta: diagnosis and clinical significance, *Circulation* 50:774, 1974.
6. Liberthson RR, Dinsmore RE, Fallon JT: Aberrant coronary artery origin from the aorta: report of 18 patients, review of literature and delineation of natural history and management, *Circulation* 59:748, 1979.
7. Chaitman BR, Lesperance J, Saltiel J, et al: Clinical, angiographic, and hemodynamic findings in patients with anomalous origin of the coronary arteries, *Circulation* 53:122, 1976.
8. Barth CW III, Roberts WC: Left main coronary artery originating from the right sinus of Valsalva and coursing between the aorta and pulmonary trunk, *J Am Coll Cardiol* 7:366, 1986.
9. Murphy DA, Roy DL, Sohal M, et al: Anomalous origin of left main coronary artery from anterior sinus of Valsalva with myocardial infarction, *J Thorac Cardiovasc Surg* 75:282, 1978.
10. Page HL Jr, Engel HJ, Campbell WB, et al: Anomalous origin of the left circumflex coronary artery: recognition,

angiographic demonstration and clinical significance, *Circulation* 50:768, 1974.
11. Bett JHN, O'Brien MF, Murray PJS: Surgery for anomalous origin of the right coronary artery, *Br Heart J* 53:459, 1985.
12. Chaitman BR, Bourassa MG, Lesperance J, et al: Aberrant course of the left anterior descending coronary artery associated with anomalous left circumflex origin from the pulmonary artery, *Circulation* 52:955, 1975.
13. Virmani R, Chun PKC, Goldstein RE, et al: Acute takeoffs of the coronary arteries along the aortic wall and congenital coronary ostial valve-like ridges: association with sudden death, *J Am Coll Cardiol* 3:766, 1984.
14. Kramer JR, Kitazume H, Proudfit WL, et al: Clinical significance of isolated coronary bridges: benign and frequent condition involving the left anterior descending artery, *Am Heart J* 103:283, 1982.
15. Siegel RJ, Dunton SF: Systemic occlusive arteriopathy with sudden death in a 10-year-old boy, *Hum Pathol* 22:197, 1991.
16. Moran JJ, Becker SM: Idiopathic arterial calcification of infancy: report of 2 cases occurring in siblings, and review of the literature, *Am J Clin Pathol* 31:517, 1959.
17. Meradji M, de Villeneuve VH, Huber J, et al: Idiopathic infantile arterial calcification in siblings: radiologic diagnosis and successful treatment, *J Pediatr* 92:401, 1978.

CHAPTER 65

Kawasaki Disease

Kawasaki disease, also called "mucocutaneous lymph node syndrome," was initially described in Japan in 1960 by Dr. Kawasaki (a contemporary Japanese pediatrician) and has been recognized in the United States since 1971. This acute and severe febrile illness, principally of young children, has widespread cardiovascular involvement.[1-3] Coronary arterial aneurysms develop frequently as a result of the inflammatory process and may lead to myocardial infarction. Myocarditis, pericarditis, and valvulitis occur less frequently. In many ways it resembles infantile periarteritis nodosa.[1] The disease is probably an acute immunologic reaction to an unidentified agent or agents. It tends to occur in clusters, more commonly in children of Asian background, and most commonly in late winter or spring. Antibody-antigen complexes and other immunoregulatory abnormalities have been identified. Because of these major and serious cardiovascular complications and the increasing frequency of Kawasaki disease, it is described here.

PATHOLOGIC ANATOMY

The primary pathologic process is a nonspecific vasculitis.[1-5] The involvement of the vasa vasorum of major arterial branches leads to secondary changes in the intima and adventitia, causing aneurysm formation, thrombosis, and their complications. Aneurysms do not form in all patients. Involvement may occur in coronary, renal, mesenteric, vertebral, splenic, hepatic, and iliac arteries. Aneurysms may cause local arterial obstruction and embolization, resulting in ischemia or rupture. However, asymptomatic healing is common.

The vascular pathologic changes of the heart have been divided into four stages. Stage I occurs during the first 10 days of the illness. Widespread perivasculitis of microvessels, arterioles, capillaries, venules, and small arteries are present. Acute pericarditis, interstitial myocarditis, valvulitis, and endocarditis occur. Stage II occurs from day 10 to day 25 of the illness. Arteritis and pericarditis are present, and these can lead to aneurysm formation or obstruction from thrombosis. Pancarditis persists.

Stage III occurs from 25 to 40 days of the illness and has been observed in fatal cases. Coronary arterial occlusion from thrombosis or intimal proliferation is observed. Vasculitis of the microvasculature disappears, and inflammatory changes in myocardium and endocardium become less evident.

In stage IV after 40 days of illness, severe stenosis of coronary arteries may be found. Myocardial fibrosis is evident. Other late complications are aortic or mitral valvar insufficiency and cardiomyopathy. Acute myocardial infarction may occur as a late complication.

The coronary arterial aneurysms that so typify this lesion are generally fusiform or saccular.[6] The left coronary artery is more commonly involved than the right, particularly the left anterior descending branch. Usually more than one coronary artery is involved. Inflammatory or ischemic changes are common in the conduction system during acute stages.

The causes of death are rupture of aneurysm, inflammation of conduction system or myocardial ischemia in stage I and myocardial ischemia in stages II through IV. Healing of aneurysms occurs by two different pathologic processes and results in a normal-sized smooth arterial lumen (Fig 65–1).

1. Marked intimal proliferation (see Fig 65–1,A). The intima is rich in smooth muscle cells, shows marked hypertrophy, and is finally covered by a normal endothelium.

THE TWO MECHANISMS OF HEALING OF ANEURYSM IN KAWASKI'S DISEASE

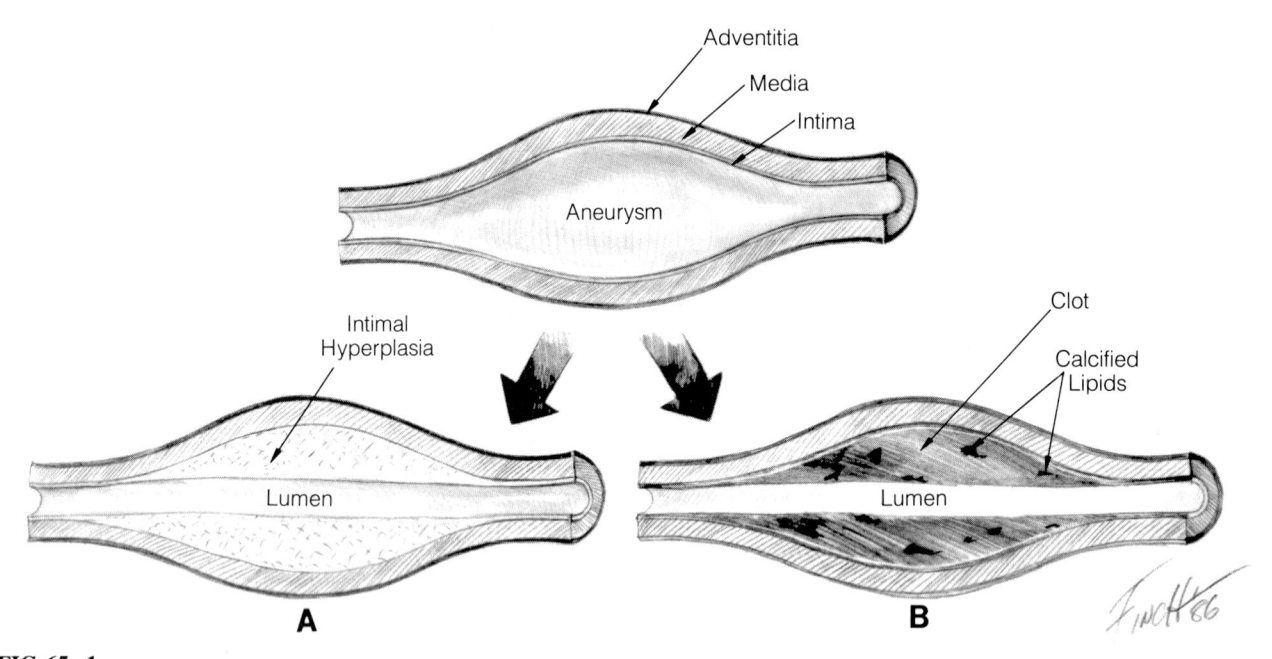

FIG 65–1.
Mechanism of "healing" of aneurysms with restoration of normal lumen. Aneurysm remains, but lumen becomes obliterated by (**A**) intimal hyperplasia or (**B**) thrombus formation. Lipids may become deposited, and calcifications may develop identical to atherosclerosis. "Healed" aneurysms appear angiographically normal, but artery remains less pulsatile.

2. Massive thrombus formation obliterating the space between the lumen and outside layer of the aneurysm (see Fig 65–1,B). Lipids may be deposited, which later may become calcified. Aspirin treatment may perhaps prevent or delay massive thrombus formation.

In either case, the outside of the aneurysm remains, but its lumen may become normal. Angiographically this is interpreted as "healing." Rarely the arterial lumen is restored by scarring and contraction of the arterial wall.

HEMODYNAMICS

Although myocardial anomalies from inflammation or infarction are found, and echocardiography shows increased left ventricular dimensions and reduced contractility, clinically evident hemodynamic abnormalities are rare.

CLINICAL FEATURES

The clinical findings are dominated by those of the acute febrile illness; although the cardiovascular aspects of the disease are serious in some patients, their clinical features are evident in only a few patients. One half of patients with cardiovascular involvement are less than 2 years of age, and 80% are less than 4 years old. Rarely are adults affected.

A diagnosis of Kawasaki disease can be made when five of the following six features are present[1–3]:

1. Fever of at least 5 days' duration. The fever is high (temperature > 40° C) and spiking. The fever starts on the first day of illness and may continue for 3 weeks. With the fever, the child appears lethargic and irritable.
2. Eyes. Bilateral congestion of the conjunctivae, without purulent discharge, is present. Discrete engorgement of bulbar conjunctival vessels begins on the first day of illness and persists for 2 weeks.
3. Oral cavity. Several changes occur, including erythema, dryness, fissuring of lips, erythema of tongue with prominence of papillae, and reddening of the oropharyngeal mucosa. These begin on the first day and last as long as 3 weeks.
4. Extremities. There is reddening of palms and soles and indurative edema of hands and feet beginning on the third day and lasting as long as 2 weeks. Desquamation of finger tips and toes follows.
5. Trunk. Beginning on the first day, a polymorphous macular erythematous rash spreads from the extremities to the trunk, lasting about 1 week.
6. Neck. Cervical lymph nodes. The nodes are present throughout the febrile course.

A number of other acute findings may be present:

1. Arthralgia or arthritis.
2. Vomiting, diarrhea, and abdominal pain.
3. Hydrops of gallbladder.
4. Mild jaundice.
5. Cough and rhinorrhea.
6. Signs of aseptic meningitis with lethargy, stiff neck, and cerebrospinal fluid pleocytosis.

Clinical cardiac findings occur in 20% of patients during the acute phase. The most common findings are tachycardia and gallop rhythm. More serious cardiovascular complications occur during the subacute phase from 9 to 21 days after the onset of fever. These include the findings of congestive cardiac failure, pericarditis or pericardial effusion, cardiac arrhythmia, or mitral insufficiency. Chest pain or findings of myocardial infarction may be present. Aneurysms may be palpated over major arteries, such as subclavian, axillary, or femoral arteries. About 1% to 2% of children die of cardiac complications during the acute phase.

After the acute and subacute phases, late sudden death or onset of myocardial infarction may occur,[7, 8] and there may be evidence of mitral or aortic insufficiency.[9]

LABORATORY STUDIES

A variety of laboratory abnormalities are also identified. Two are particularly striking. The leukocyte count is elevated and may reach 30,000/mm^3. There is a shift to the left. Thrombocytosis with levels exceeding 1,000,000/mm^3 is found during the acute phase.[10] The sedimentation rate is markedly elevated, as is the level of C-reactive protein.

Urinalysis shows mild to moderate pyuria and proteinuria. Results of other tests of renal function are normal. Mild elevation of transaminase is found, indicating hepatocellular damage.

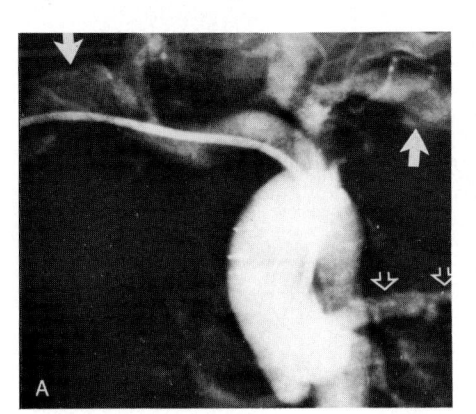

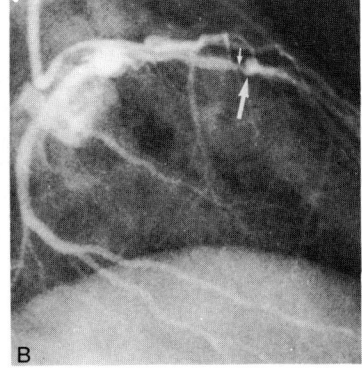

ELECTROCARDIOGRAPHIC FEATURES

Prolongation of PR interval, flattening of T waves, and ST-segment depression occur in 60% to 90% of cases.[5] Ventricular premature beats may be present, and QRS voltage increases, suggesting left ventricular hypertrophy may be present. Occasionally abnormal Q waves are present, indicating myocardial infarction.

ECHOCARDIOGRAPHIC FEATURES

Two-dimensional echocardiography has been extremely helpful in identifying coronary arterial aneurysms and following their course.[11-15] Because coronary arterial aneurysms may occur in as many as 20% of patients after the second week of illness, this technique is helpful in identifying the aneurysm in asymptomatic patients. Because some aneurysms tend to resolve during the first year of illness, serial studies should be performed. Since the major aneurysms occur predominantly in the proximal coronary arteries, they can usually be identified on a cross-sectional view of the aortic root. Aneurysms occurring beyond 1.5 cm from the aortic root are less accurately detected.[11]

Echocardiography is also used to identify abnormalities of left ventricular wall motion. The presence of abnormalities seems to be a sensitive indicator of myocardial involvement[12] These abnormalities occur in patients without identifiable coronary arterial aneurysms and may be present more than 1 year after the acute illness.[13] It is unknown whether these wall motion abnormalities are from ischemia or an inflammatory process involving the myocardium.

Finally, echo Doppler techniques may be used to identify regurgitation across insufficient valves.

RADIOGRAPHIC FEATURES

The diagnosis of Kawasaki disease cannot be suspected from thoracic roentgenograms in most cases, be-

FIG 65-2.
Kawasaki disease stage 2. **A.** Aortogram. Anteroposterior projection. Fusiform aneurysms of left main and left anterior descending arteries *(open arrows)*. Large aneurysms *(solid arrows)* of both subclavian arteries. **B,** selective left coronary arteriogram. Stenosis *(small arrow)* and saccular aneurysm *(large arrow)* of left anterior descending artery.

cause usually the radiographic findings are normal. REASON: Involvement of the myocardium, pericardium, and valves may be absent or of a minor degree not leading to cardiomegaly.

1. Cardiac silhouette may be entirely normal.
2. Cardiomegaly varying from a minor to massive may be observed, depending on the severity of the associated pancarditis with involvement of the myocardium and pericardium.
3. The radiographic findings may be indistinguishable from aortic and mitral regurgitation from other causes. REASON: Rarely Kawasaki disease also causes a valvulitis that leads to aortic and mitral regurgitation.
4. Aneurysms of the coronary arteries are usually not large enough to deform the cardiac silhouette and therefore cannot be suspected from a thoracic roentgenogram unless they are calcified.

CARDIAC CATHETERIZATION

The principal purpose of cardiac catheterization is to perform coronary angiography.

ANGIOGRAPHIC FEATURES

Whereas almost all autopsy cases of Kawasaki disease have aneurysms that may show thrombosis or rupture, only 25% are demonstrated angiographically. REASON: Depending on the stage of the disease process, the lumen of the aneurysms may have regressed to normal by either marked intimal proliferation or extensive thrombus formation.

Two-dimensional echocardiography is able to demonstrate aneurysms noninvasively, but if fusiform or located in the circumflex or right coronary artery, they may escape detection. Angiography remains the most reliable technique for detection of aneurysms in the acute stage, but in the later stages of the disease the coronary arteries may appear normal during the "healing" stage of the aneurysm.

Left ventriculography is indicated to demonstrate left ventricular size, contractility, and valvar insufficiency. REASON: The disease process may involve the myocardium, pericardium, or cardiac valves. Furthermore, myocardial infarction that affects ventricular contractility can occur.

Angiography may be indicated to demonstrate associated aneurysms and stenoses in the renal arteries that can produce hypertension or in the brachiocephalic, mesenteric, pancreatic, or iliofemoral arteries.

Aneurysms may occur in the right and left coronary arteries, particularly the left anterior descending branch.

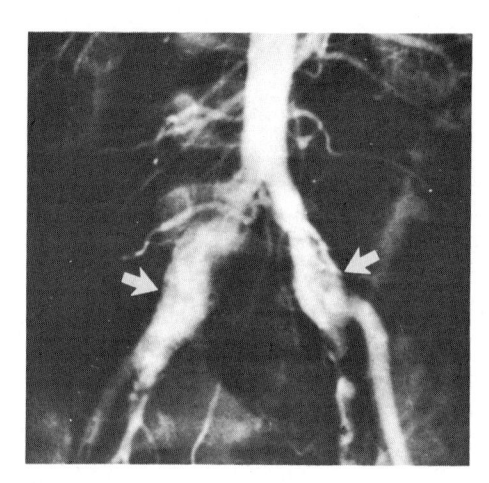

FIG 65–3.
Kawasaki disease. Abdominal aortogram. Anteroposterior projection. Large fusiform aneurysms of both iliac arteries.

The fusiform type (Fig 65–2,A) is more common than the saccular variety (Fig 65–2,B). Abdominal angiography should be added because of the common involvement of other arteries (Fig 65–3). Aneurysm formation may be the cause of hypertension (Fig 65–4).

Angiography as early as 1 year after the onset of the illness may demonstrate "healing." The previously noted aneurysm may have a smooth lumen and normal caliber, particularly if healing occurs with intimal proliferation. Slight irregularities may persist if the aneurysm has become filled with a thrombus that has a central channel.

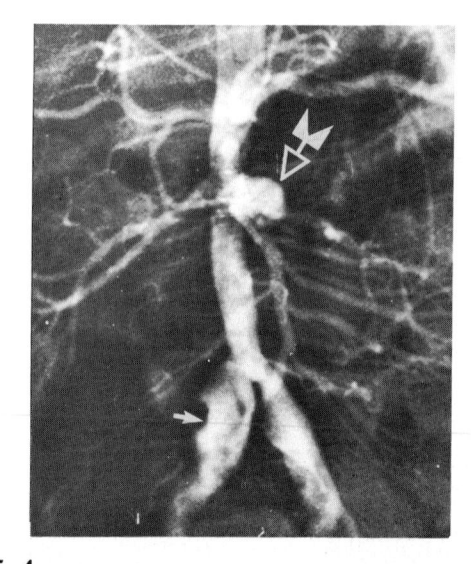

FIG 65–4.
Kawasaki disease and hypertension. Abdominal aortogram. Anteroposterior projection. Large saccular aneurysm (open arrow) involves left renal artery. Fusiform aneurysms in both common iliac arteries. Aneurysm of right iliac artery demonstrates mural thrombus (solid arrow), probably early stage of "healing" (see Fig 65–1) by mural thrombus formation.

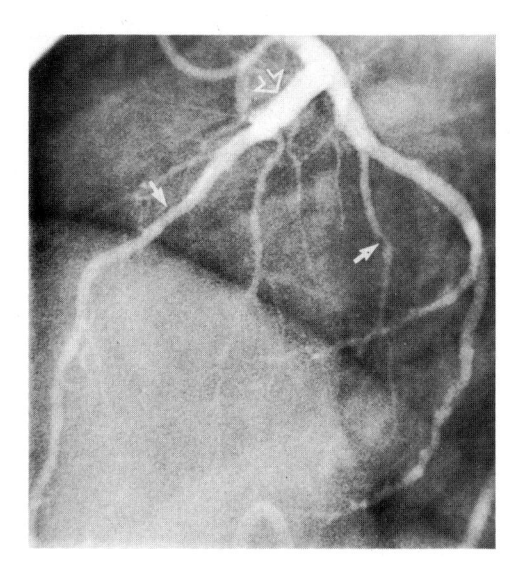

FIG 65-5.
Lupus erythematous and unstable angina. Selective coronary arteriogram. Left anterior oblique projection. Mild aneurysmal dilatation *(open arrow)* of proximal left anterior descending with distinct caliber changes in left anterior descending and smaller branches *(solid arrows)* consistent with arteritis.

The thrombus may progress and occlude the artery completely and lead to myocardial infarction and sometimes death.

If an aneurysm is demonstrated angiographically in the coronary arterial system, Kawasaki disease cannot be differentiated from other rare etiologies.

1. Congenital.
2. Atherosclerotic (most common in the older age group).
3. Mycotic.
4. Syphilitic.
5. Rheumatic.
6. Traumatic.
7. Polyarteritis nodosa.
8. Ehlers-Danlos syndrome.
9. Lupus erythematosus (Fig 65-5).

MANAGEMENT

During the acute phase, the patient is given large doses of aspirin to reduce the inflammatory process.[1-3, 16] After the acute illness, the aspirin dosage is reduced to a low level to achieve an antiplatelet effect. The duration of administration is uncertain, but aspirin should be continued as long as coronary aneurysms are present. Corticosteroids should not be given because their use may increase the incidence of aneurysms. High doses of γ-globulin administered in the early stages of the disease shorten the course, lessen the severity of symptoms, and probably also decrease the incidence of aneurysms.

Occasionally coronary arterial bypass operations have been performed in individuals with scarred and stenotic coronary arteries. The long-term course of the disease is unknown with the current methods of treatment, and further studies are needed to determine the prognosis and factors that influence it. Serial echocardiographic studies can better define the natural history of this rare disease.

REFERENCES

1. Morens DM: Kawasaki disease: a 'new' pediatric enigma, *Hosp Pract* 13:109, 1978.
2. Melish ME, Hicks RV, Reddy V: Kawasaki syndrome: an update, *Hosp Pract* 17:99, 1982.
3. Yanagihara R, Todd JK: Acute febrile mucocutaneous lymph node syndrome, *Am J Dis Child* 134:603, 1980.
4. Landing BH, Larson EJ: Are infantile periarteritis nodosa with coronary artery involvement and fatal mucocutaneous lymph node syndrome the same? Comparison of 20 patients from North America with patients from Hawaii and Japan, *Pediatrics* 59:651, 1977.
5. Fukushige J, Nihill MR, McNamara DG: Spectrum of cardiovascular lesions in mucocutaneous lymph node syndrome: analysis of eight cases, *Am J Cardiol* 45:98, 1980.
6. Onouchi Z, Shimazu S, Kiyosawa N, et al: Aneurysms of the coronary arteries in Kawasaki disease: an angiographic study of 30 cases, *Circulation* 66:6, 1982.
7. Ohyagi A, Hirose K, Tsujimoto S, et al: Kawasaki disease complicated by acute myocardial infarction 9 years after onset, *Am Heart J* 110:670, 1985.
8. Flugelman MY, Hasin Y, Bassan MM, et al: Acute myocardial infarction 14 years after an acute episode of Kawasaki's disease, *Am J Cardiol* 52:427, 1983.
9. Gidding SS, Shulman ST, Ilbawi M, et al: Mucocutaneous lymph node syndrome (Kawasaki disease): delayed aortic and mitral insufficiency secondary to active valvulitis, *J Am Coll Cardiol* 7:894, 1986.
10. Burns JC, Glode MP, Clarke SH, et al: Coagulopathy and platelet activation in Kawasaki syndrome: identification of patients at high risk for development of coronary artery aneurysms, *J Pediatr* 105:206, 1984.
11. Chung KJ, Brandt L, Fulton DR, et al: Cardiac and coronary arterial involvement in infants and children from New England with mucocutaneous lymph node syndrome (Kawasaki disease), *Am J Cardiol* 50:136, 1982.
12. Grenadier E, Allen HD, Goldberg SJ, et al: Left ventricular wall motion abnormalities in Kawasaki's disease, *Am Heart J* 107:966, 1984.
13. Anderson TM, Meyer RA, Kaplan S: Long-term echocardiographic evaluation of cardiac size and function in patients with Kawasaki disease, *Am Heart J* 110:107, 1985.

14. Capannari TE, Daniels SR, Meyer RA, et al: Sensitivity, specificity and predictive value of two-dimensional echocardiography in detecting coronary artery aneurysms in patients with Kawasaki disease, *J Am Coll Cardiol* 7:355, 1986.
15. Maeda T, Yoshida H, Funabashi T, et al: Subcostal 2-dimensional echocardiographic imaging of peripheral left coronary artery aneurysms in Kawasaki disease, *Am J Cardiol* 52:48, 1983.
16. Koren G, Rose V, Lavi S, et al: Probable efficacy of high-dose salicylates in reducing coronary involvement in Kawasaki disease, *JAMA* 254:767, 1985.

CHAPTER 66

Systemic Arteriovenous Fistulas

An arteriovenous fistula is a direct communication of an artery with a vein without an intervening capillary network. Fistulas may be either congenital or acquired. In either instance they tend to increase with time, because they offer less resistance to blood flow than the normal pathway. A systemic arteriovenous fistula may be located at various sites, and the clinical manifestations result from their location, size, and number.[1]

PATHOLOGIC ANATOMY

An arteriovenous fistula can result from either a direct connection or connections between an artery and vein or an angioma, in which the connections are between multiple small vessels. Fistulas may be single or multiple, and the size of the communication varies greatly between cases. The afferent artery and efferent vein are dilated and tortuous. The wall of the artery may be thinned, whereas that of the vein is thickened (arterialization).

With large communications, cardiac chambers and great vessels are dilated because of the associated increased cardiac output.

The most frequent locations are the brain,[2-6] neck,[7] thoracic wall,[8] liver,[9-12] and extremities. They may also occur in the heart between coronary artery and vein or in the lungs (see Chapters 25 and Chapter 48).

In the brain, fistulas usually involve the middle and posterior cerebral arteries, the vertebral artery, and the great vein of Galen.[2-6] Connections have been described between the left subclavian artery and innominate vein, between the internal mammary artery and ductus venosus,[8] hepatic artery and portal vein,[13] splenic artery and vein, pelvic arteries and veins,[14] skin, and peripheral arteries and veins in the extremities. In the latter, hypertrophy of the involved extremity and associated long bones and cutaneous or subcutaneous hemangiomas may be found.

Hepatic arteriovenous fistulas may be associated with hereditary hemorrhagic telangiectasis (Rendu-Osler-Weber syndrome) or hepatic hemangioendothelioma. The latter is a condition of multiple hepatic hemangiomas, associated with cutaneous hemangiomas.[9-12] The hemangiomas progressively enlarge during the first 6 months of life and then regress spontaneously.

HEMODYNAMICS

The major hemodynamic abnormality results from the shunt of blood directly from the artery to the vein, with the amount of shunt being proportional to the caliber of the communication or communications. Arteriovenous fistulas lower systemic vascular resistance, which has three effects: (1) increased stroke volume, (2) increased cardiac rate, and (3) increased pulse pressure. Cardiac output increases because of the combined effects of increased stroke volume and cardiac rate. Therefore, systemic venous return is increased, and the volume of blood carried by each cardiac chamber is increased.

If the volume load is excessive, congestive cardiac failure occurs. Although cardiac failure usually develops early in the neonatal period, it is not present at birth.[6] During fetal life, because of the placenta, systemic vascular resistance is normally low. Therefore, little blood flows through the fistula, although the cardiac chambers are dilated. With the elimination of the placenta from the circulation postnatally, systemic vascular resistance increases twofold, and blood flow through the fistula increases.

Therefore, the right ventricle receives augmented blood flow and ejects it into the pulmonary circulation, which has an elevated vascular resistance. Cardiac failure results. If the ductus arteriosus remains patent, a right-to-left shunt may occur, and there may also be a shunt in the same direction through the patent foramen ovale.

CLINICAL FEATURES

There are three clinical pictures of congenital systemic arteriovenous fistulas: (1) congestive cardiac failure, (2) hyperkinetic syndrome, and (3) local manifestations.

Neonates with a large fistula are often seen during the first day of life with features of profound congestive cardiac failure, manifested by tachypnea, tachycardia, and hepatomegaly. The peripheral pulses are bounding, unless cardiac failure is severe. Over the arteries supplying the fistula, if palpable, a thrill may be felt. The thrill disappears if the afferent artery is compressed. Cyanosis may be present.

There may be a murmur over the fistula, but we have seen several neonates with cerebral arteriovenous fistulas in whom a bruit could not be heard over the skull. When present, the murmur is continuous. On palpation of the thorax, cardiomegaly and increased cardiac activity are found. Nonspecific systolic ejection murmurs[15] and a third heart sound may be found. The pulmonary component of the second heart sound is accentuated because of the associated pulmonary hypertension. In children with a smaller fistula, cardiac failure does not occur, but there is tachycardia, wide pulse pressure, and soft systolic ejection murmur.

There may be local findings of the fistula. Arteriovenous fistulas have unique effects, depending on their location. When the renal artery and vein are involved, hypertension and hematuria result. Intracranial fistulas may cause neurologic findings, such as increased head circumference, diplopia, and hemiparesis. Increased extremity size has been previously mentioned to occur from fistulas involving extremities.

In any fistula, platelets may be consumed (Merritt-Kaselback syndrome), and bleeding problems may result.[16]

ELECTROCARDIOGRAPHIC FEATURES

In neonates with congestive cardiac failure, right-axis deviation, right atrial enlargement, and right ventricular hypertrophy are found, reflecting the combined effects of pulmonary hypertension and increased volume load. T waves may be inverted throughout the precordial leads.

Beyond infancy, the electrocardiogram shows a pattern of left ventricular hypertrophy, reflecting left ventricular dilatation in those with larger fistulae.

With a small fistula, the tracing is normal.

ECHOCARDIOGRAPHIC FEATURES

Both ventricles, the left atrium, and the great vessels are dilated. The vena cava draining the portion of the body with the fistula is enlarged. It may be possible to visualize a fistula involving major intrathoracic vessels. Continuous flow is present on Doppler analysis. The descending aorta is dilated.[17]

RADIOGRAPHIC FEATURES

A large arteriovenous fistula, whether congenital or acquired, causes a severe hemodynamic burden on the heart. Because of the excessive flow from the arterial to the venous side of the circulation (large pressure gradient), cardiac output is markedly increased. Cardiomegaly and sometimes cardiac failure develop. Because of the radiographic appearance of cardiomegaly and increased pulmonary vasculature, snapping pulses from a wide pulse pressure, the condition is commonly confused with an aortic runoff lesion, such as patent ductus arteriosus or aorticopulmonary window. No distinct radiographic clues allow differentiation between these lesions without angiography.

1. Depending on the size of the arteriovenous fistula, the heart shows a variable degree of enlargement.
2. In the most common forms seen in neonates, namely, arteriovenous fistulas of the brain (aneurysm of the great vein of Galen) or arteriovenous malformation in the liver, the heart is markedly enlarged (Fig 66–1).
3. The pulmonary vasculature is increased. REASON: The fistula results in a markedly increased blood flow through the lungs. Thus, pulmonary blood flow is increased and the left atrium is enlarged, as in conditions with a left-to-right shunt.

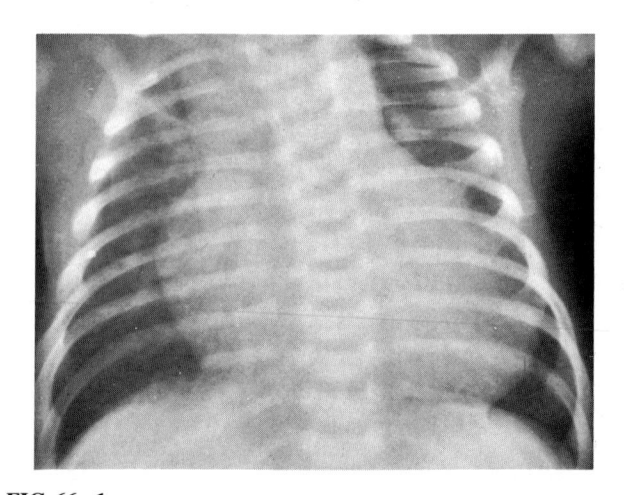

FIG 66–1.
Cerebral arteriovenous fistula (aneurysm of great vein of Galen). Thoracic roentgenogram. Posteroanterior projection. Markedly enlarged heart. Increased pulmonary vasculature. Findings are identical to large left-to-right shunt.

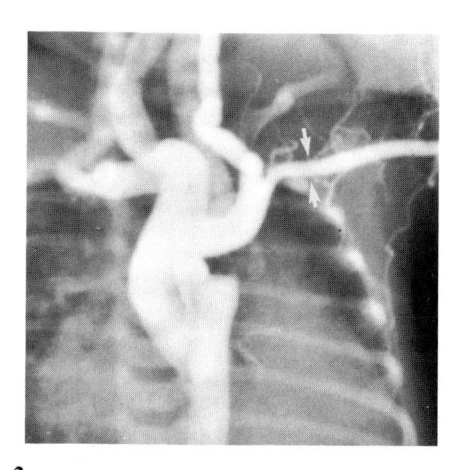

FIG 66–2.
Cerebral arteriovenous fistula (aneurysm of great vein of Galen). Aortogram. Anteroposterior projection. Marked enlargement and tortuosity of proximal left subclavian artery, left vertebral artery, both carotid arteries, and right vertebral artery. Left subclavian distal to origin of left vertebral artery *(arrows)* is normal. Angiographic findings are very characteristic of cerebral arteriovenous fistula in the brain.

CARDIAC CATHETERIZATION

Oxygen data show an elevated oxygen saturation of the venous blood from the area of the fistula and a marked discrepancy between the oxygen saturations of the superior and inferior vena cava, depending on the site of drainage.

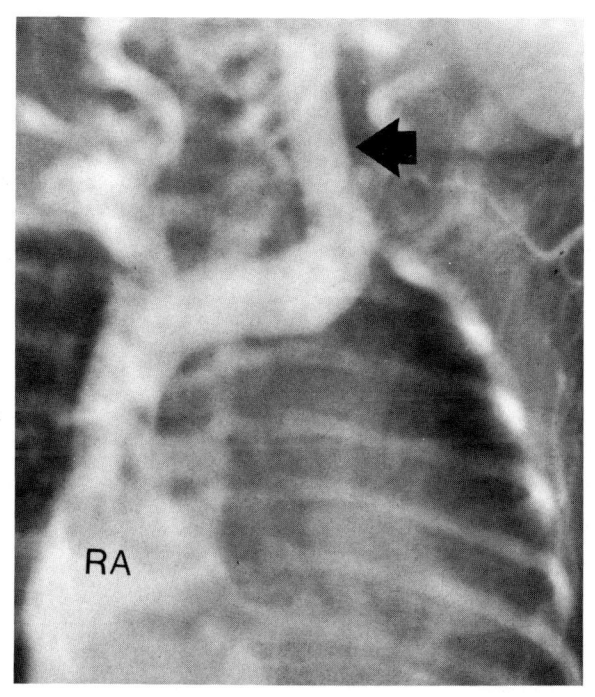

FIG 66–3.
Cerebral arteriovenous fistula. Aortogram. Anteroposterior projection. Venous phase. Early, dense return of contrast medium from brain through various veins, particularly enlarged left jugular vein *(arrow)*. RA = right atrium.

The arteriovenous oxygen difference is narrowed, in contrast to that expected in congestive cardiac failure. There may be mild systemic arterial desaturation.

In neonates, pulmonary arterial pressure is elevated to systemic levels. Right atrial and left atrial pressures are increased. Systemic arterial pulse pressure is widened.

ANGIOGRAPHIC FEATURES

Most arteriovenous fistulas have the following features in common:

1. The afferent arteries are enlarged.
2. The speed of blood flow through the afferent arteries is markedly increased, and, consequently, contrast medium is diluted.
3. The capillary phase of an angiogram is lacking because large draining veins opacify, immediately bypassing the capillary bed.

In neonates, angiography is usually performed to exclude an aortic runoff lesion. If a large artery arises from the aortic arch and there is a dense early venous phase, the suspicion of an arteriovenous fistula is high. Large arteriovenous fistulas are identified by injecting into the aorta a very rapid injection of a large amount of contrast medium, whereas smaller arteriovenous fistulas are usually diagnosed by selective injection of the afferent artery.

1. In patients with an aneurysm of the great vein of Galen, there is enlargement of both the carotid and the vertebral arteries associated with the arteriovenous fistula,

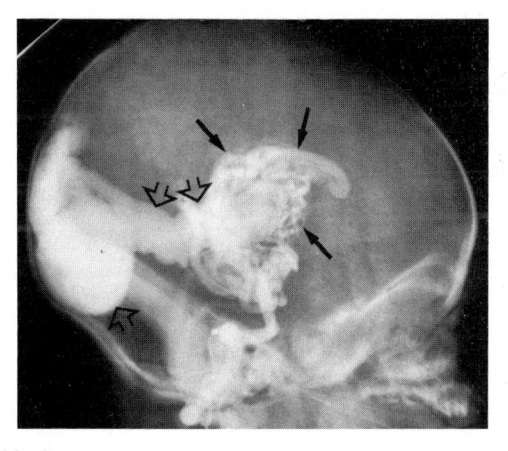

FIG 66–4.
Cerebral arteriovenous fistula. Vertebral arteriogram. Lateral projection. Tortuous arteries and veins *(arrows)* with immediate opacification of enlarged efferent vein *(open arrows)*. Aneurysmal enlargement of great vein of Galen is common; therefore the condition has been termed "aneurysm of the great vein of Galen."

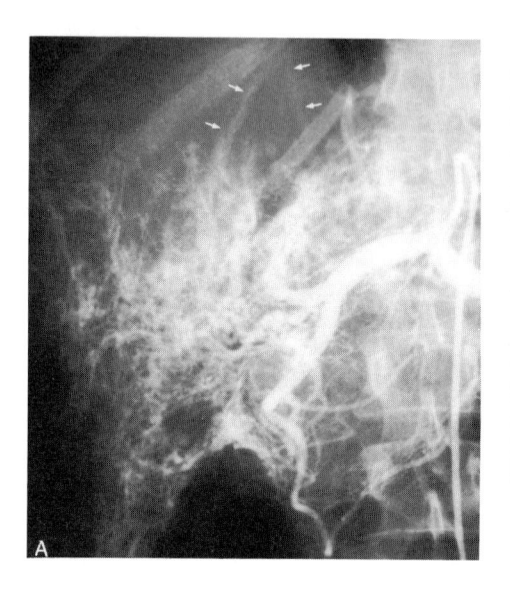

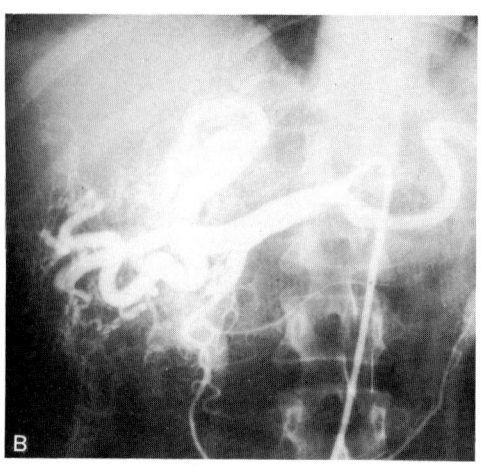

FIG 66-5.
Hemangiomatosis with massive shunting. Severe cardiac failure. **A,** selective balloon occlusion angiogram. Huge arteriovenous malformation of liver with early opacification of hepatic veins *(arrows).* **B,** successful obliteration of all major feeding branches after Ivalon embolization. One complication of this procedure is gangrene of gallbladder, which this patient developed. Cardiac size returned to normal, and cardiac failure disappeared.

but the size of the distal subclavian arteries is normal (Fig 66–2) because they are not involved in the fistula.

2. With an intracranial arteriovenous fistula, there is dense and early return of contrast medium from the brain through a dilated jugular venous system (Fig 66–3). Occasionally in a normal individual, contrast medium can be seen returning from the brain through the superior vena cava after aortography, but the return is delayed and faint.

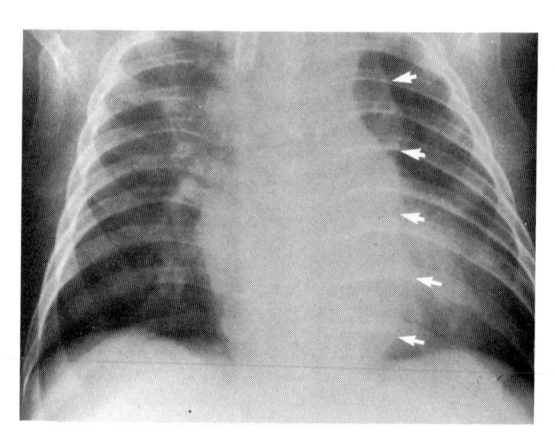

FIG 66-6.
Intra-abdominal and mediastinal hemangioma. Thoracic roentgenogram. Severe cardiomegaly, increased vasculature, and cardiac failure. Mass extends from cervical region to abdomen demonstrated by computed tomography scanning. Roentgenogram demonstrates intrathoracic extension (hemangioma) by double density *(arrows).* Aortography showed very rapid flow but no large afferent arteries, indicating a very diffuse arteriovenous shunt. (Courtesy of Dr. John Ring.)

In contrast with an arteriovenous fistula, contrast material returns quickly and densely.

3. An additional aortogram should be obtained with filming over the cranium to confirm the diagnosis (Fig 66–4).

4. A systemic arteriovenous fistula may occur at various sites in the systemic circulation, resulting in cardiac failure. Cerebral arteriovenous fistulas and hemangiomatous malformations in the liver are particularly prone to cause cardiac failure in infancy (Fig 66–5).

5. Typically pediatric hemangiomatosis may be self-involuting tumors, but a small fraction may not involute and may require aggressive intervention to prevent death secondary to cardiac failure.

6. Such tumors are most commonly located in the liver, but they may occur also extrahepatic (Fig 66–6).

7. Each chamber of the heart and both great vessels are enlarged. REASON: Increased blood flow through the systemic and pulmonary circulations.

OPERATIVE CONSIDERATIONS

Generally an arteriovenous fistula is difficult to treat by operation. REASON: Because of the multiple arteries supplying the fistula, the fistula recurs in a short time after arterial ligation. The recurrence occurs through very small arteries that were not ligated. Operation, however, is successful if the entire lesion can be excised, but this is rarely possible.

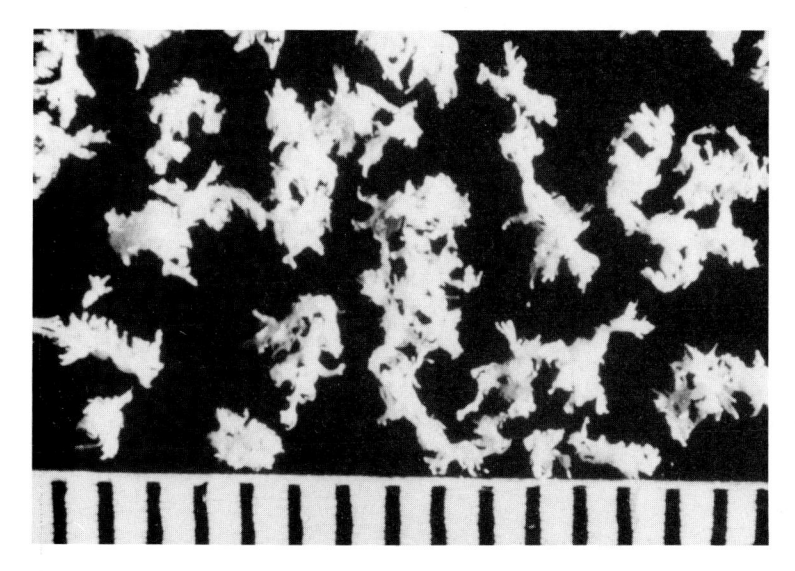

FIG 66–7.
Ivalon shavings used for embolization of peripheral arteriovenous fistula. Microscopic view. Ivalon shavings are suspended in saline solution and contrast medium.

An alternative and more successful treatment is embolic occlusion of various affluent arteries by the injection of particles of a specific size through a catheter. The size of the injected particles must be selected so they do not pass through the arteriovenous fistula into the venous side of the circulation but occlude the affluent branches as distal as possible. Numerous particulate materials have been used for embolization. These include coils, beads, powders, and shavings. A detailed description of various agents is beyond the scope of this book. Ivalon shavings of specific sizes are one of the most useful embolic agents (Fig 66–7). Ivalon is an open-pore, polyvinyl alcohol sponge, familiar to us as the kitchen sponge. Ivalon has been extensively tested[18] and is biocompatible. After embolization, fibrocytes grow into the open pores of the sponge, which becomes permanently incorporated in the vessel.

When embolization techniques are used, even very large arteriovenous malformations can be palliated (see Fig 66–5), and cardiac output returns to normal. These techniques have largely replaced operative ligation of afferent arteries. After successful treatment of large systemic arteriovenous fistulas by embolization or operation, cardiac size dramatically decreases, and supportive cardiac therapy is no longer necessary.

For an arteriovenous fistula with a large communication, particularly when acquired, embolization with metallic spiders and coils or detachable balloons are necessary for nonoperative occlusion.

In hepatic hemangiomatosis, a rare cause of peripheral arteriovenous fistulas that cause cardiac failure, the use of corticosteroids and ligation of the hepatic artery[19] have been described. Corticosteroids usually fail, but a few patients improve after hepatic artery ligation; recurrence has to be expected because of collateralization. The basic goal in the treatment is to palliate the infant during the critical stage of cardiac decompensation until spontaneous involution of the hemangioma occurs.

REFERENCES

1. Knudson RP, Alden ER: Symptomatic arteriovenous malformation in infants less than 6 months of age, *Pediatrics* 64:238, 1979.
2. Holden AM, Fyler DC, Shillito J Jr, et al: Congestive heart failure from intracranial arteriovenous fistula in infancy: clinical and pathologic considerations in eight patients, *Pediatrics* 49:30, 1972.
3. Levine OR, Jameson AG, Nellhaus G, et al: Cardiac complications of cerebral arteriovenous fistula in infancy, *Pediatrics* 30:563, 1962.
4. Gomez MR, Whitten CF, Nolke A, et al: Aneurysmal malformation of the great vein of Galen causing heart failure in early infancy: report of five cases, *Pediatrics* 31:400, 1963.
5. Glatt BS, Rowe RD: Cerebral arteriovenous fistula associated with congestive heart failure in the newborn: report of two cases, *Pediatrics* 27:596, 1960.
6. Cumming GR: Circulation in neonates with intracranial arteriovenous fistula and cardiac failure, *Am J Cardiol* 45:1019, 1980.
7. Suen JY, Boellner SW, Araoz CA, et al: Congenital arteriovenous fistula of the vertebral artery and internal jugular vein, *J Pediatr* 80:837, 1972.
8. Glass IH, Rowe RD, Duckworth JWA: Congenital arteriovenous fistula between the left internal mammary artery and the ductus venosus: unusual cause of congestive heart failure in the newborn infant, *Pediatrics* 27:604, 1960.
9. Touloukian RJ: Hepatic hemangioendothelioma during infancy: pathology, diagnosis and treatment with prednisone, *Pediatrics* 45:71, 1970.

10. Holden KR, Alexander F: Diffuse neonatal hemangiomatosis, *Pediatrics* 46:411, 1970.
11. McLean RH, Moller JH, Warwick WJ, et al: Multinodular hemangiomatosis of the liver in infancy, *Pediatrics* 49:563, 1972.
12. Cooper AG, Bolande RP: Multiple hemangiomas in an infant with cardiac hypertrophy: postmortem angiographic demonstration of the arteriovenous fistulae, *Pediatrics* 35:27, 1965.
13. Helikson MA, Shapiro DL, Seashore JH: Hepatoportal arteriovenous fistula and portal hypertension in an infant, *Pediatrics* 60:921, 1977.
14. Price AC, Coran AG, Mattern AL, et al: Hemangioendothelioma of the pelvis: a cause of cardiac failure in the newborn, *N Engl J Med* 286:647, 1972.
15. Falcone DM, Friedman S, Peker H: Precordial murmurs in high cardiac output states: differentiation from murmurs of congenital heart disease in infancy, *J Pediatr* 66:729, 1965.
16. Schum TR, Meyer GA, Grausz JP, et al: Neonatal intraventricular hemorrhage due to an intracranial arteriovenous malformation: a case report, *Pediatrics* 64:242, 1979.
17. Sapire DW, Casta A, Donner RM, et al: Dilatation of the descending aorta: a radiologic and echocardiographic diagnostic sign in arteriovenous malformations in neonates and young infants, *Am J Cardiol* 44:493, 1979.
18. Herrera M, Rysavy J, Kotula F, et al: Ivalon shavings, a new embolic agent: technical considerations, *Radiology* 144:638, 1982.
19. DeLorimier AA, Simpson EB, Baum RS, et al: Hepatic-artery ligation for hepatic hemangiomatosis, *N Engl J Med* 277:333, 1967.

PART ELEVEN

Other Conditions

In this section, ten conditions that cannot be easily grouped in any of the previous categories are discussed. Some represent distinct clinical entities and others may coexist with other congenital cardiac anomalies. In this section, Chapter 67 describes the common genetic problem of Marfan syndrome, which causes principally aneurysmal dilatation of the aortic root and mitral valve prolapse. The problem of mitral valve prolapse, which is commonly recognized echocardiographically as an isolated lesion, is explored further in Chapter 68. Other anomalies of the mitral valve that may be an incidental finding in other cardiac anomalies are discussed in Chapter 69. Congenital diverticula, which may arise from either ventricle, are considered in Chapter 70. In Chapters 71 and 72, two conditions, aneurysm of atrial appendage and pericardial defect, which may result in an abnormal cardiac silhouette on a thoracic roentgenogram, are discussed. Cardiac tumors are discussed in Chapter 73, because their clinical features may mimic a congenital lesion, and they have a unique angiographic appearance. Complete heart block (see Chapter 74) and pulmonary hypertension (see Chapter 75) may exist as either an isolated lesion or as a complicating factor of a congenital cardiac anomaly. Finally, two conditions, persistent fetal circulation and premature closure of the foramen ovale, are reviewed in Chapter 76.

CHAPTER 67

Marfan Syndrome (Cystic Medial Necrosis)

Marfan syndrome is a generalized connective tissue disease involving primarily elastic tissue, which results in characteristic ocular, skeletal, pulmonary, and cardiovascular anomalies.[1,2] The disease is presumed to result from a biochemical defect in protein synthesis of collagen or elastic tissue,[3] but the specific defect has not been identified. The condition is inherited as an autosomal dominant condition, but in 15% of instances no other member of the family has features of the syndrome.

PATHOLOGIC ANATOMY

By age 21 years, perhaps one half of patients have clinical evidence of cardiovascular anomalies, and all have histologic evidence of involvement.[1,2,4] The elastic media of the ascending aorta is disrupted and disorganized. Its fibers are separated by mucoid material (Fig 67–1). These features lead to the appearance of cysts and necrosis, but neither is actually present. In the mitral valve, to lesser degree aortic valve, and still less in the pulmonary and the tricuspid valves, myxomatous changes occur

The major cardiovascular anomalies are found in the aortic sinuses of Valsalva, the ascending aorta, and the mitral valve.[1,2] The aortic changes begin in the sinuses of Valsalva and progress with time to involve more of the ascending aorta. The sinuses of Valsalva show symmetric enlargement that may be extreme. Dilatation of the ascending aorta may reach aneurysmal proportions but rarely extends beyond the innominate artery. Small linear tears are often found in the intima immediately above the aortic valve (incomplete dissection). The incomplete dissections heal, accounting for the gradual enlargement of the aorta resulting in aneurysm. Small areas of calcifications may form at the site of incomplete dissections. Sometimes a dissecting hematoma may develop, which may lead to the typical complications of dissecting aneurysms.

The aortic valve leaflets may be thinned, show fenestrations, or prolapse. Marked aortic root dilatation leads to aortic regurgitation.

The mitral valve also shows several characteristic features. The chordae tendineae are elongated, allowing both the anterior and posterior leaflets to prolapse. In contrast, mitral valve prolapse usually involves most commonly the posterior leaflet. The degree of prolapse may be extreme. The free margin of the mitral valve billows between chordal attachments. When it is viewed from the left atrial aspect, it has been described as hemorrhoidal mitral valve (Fig 67–2). The valve leaflets are thickened. The mitral valve annulus is dilated, one of the few conditions in which this occurs. The valve can become calcified, perhaps from the degenerative myxomatous changes in the annulus.

The dilatation of mitral ring, abnormal valve cusps, and elongated chordae tendineae lead to mitral regurgitation, which may be severe, and the presenting clinical features (Fig 67–3,A). Ruptured chordae tendineae may further increase the regurgitation. Thus, the left atrium and left ventricle may be greatly dilated in this condition.

Myocardial infarction can occur in Marfan syndrome, even during childhood. Coronary blood flow may be compromised by aortic dissection, which compresses the origin of the coronary arteries, or an incomplete dissection of the coronary artery may occur. Also primary dissecting aneu-

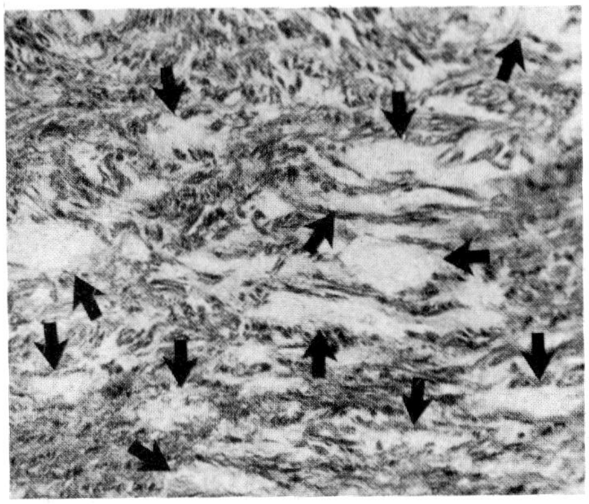

FIG 67-1.
Cystic medial necrosis. Aortic wall. Photomicrograph. Normal elements of aortic wall are disorganized, disrupted, and separated by mucoid material *(arrows)*.

rysm of the coronary arteries have been described (see Fig 61–33). If myocardial infarction is associated with dilatation of the left ventricle, the mitral prolapse may disappear. REASON: The elongated chordae tendineae are now of adequate length to allow apposition of the mitral valve leaflets. Previously they were too long and allowed the mitral valve to prolapse (Fig 67–3,B).

Similar pathologic changes may occur in the pulmonary trunk, pulmonary valve, and tricuspid valves as in the aortic and mitral valves, but the aortic and mitral valves are most consistently involved.

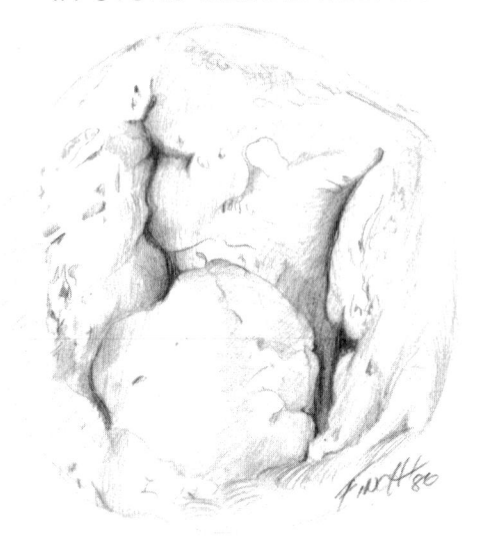

FIG 67-2.
Cystic medial necrosis. Mitral valve viewed from left atrial side. Mitral valve leaflets are redundant (hooded), giving appearance of hemorrhoids; therefore, "hemorrhoidal mitral valve."

HEMODYNAMICS

The principal hemodynamic alterations of Marfan syndrome relate to the development of aortic and mitral regurgitation. If these valvar anomalies allow little regurgitation, they are well tolerated, but if they are severe, left ventricular failure occurs. Similarly, if an aortic cusp or chordae tendineae rupture, the sudden regurgitation leads to the abrupt onset of cardiac failure with pulmonary congestion and cardiogenic shock because of the inability of the left ventricle to handle the increased volume load.

The changes in the pulmonary and tricuspid valves, although permitting regurgitation, are usually better tolerated, because the right-sided cardiac pressures are low.

CLINICAL FEATURES

In a typical case, the diagnosis is relatively easy, but in many cases, the diagnosis is less readily apparent, and the child is dismissed as merely being tall. Diagnosis still rests on clinical grounds, because a specific biochemical or other diagnostic test is unavailable.

Classically the involved individual is tall and thin and has arachnodactyly. Thoracic skeletal anomalies, particularly scoliosis,[1, 2] pectus carnivatum, or excavatum, may occur. Joints are hypermobile. Pes planus is frequently present. The palate is high and arched. In many patients these clinical stigmata are absent. These "forme fruste," idiopathic dilatations of the ascending aorta or Erdheim's cystic medial necrosis, escape clinical detection until aortic regurgitation ensues.

Ocular findings include ectopia lentis and myopia. Subluxation of the lenses occurs in 50% to 80% of involved individuals. The lens is most commonly displaced upward, permitting normal accommodation. The length of the globe is increased, contributing to a tendency to myopia. The risk of retinal detachment is increased.

At least 50% of patients have auscultatory evidence of cardiac involvement.[5-9] In children with Marfan syndrome, the major cardiac findings are those of mitral regurgitation, whereas in adults aortic regurgitation is the predominate lesion. In infants, mitral regurgitation occurs in both males and females, whereas aortic regurgitation usually occurs only in males.

Involvement of the mitral valve can lead to the findings of mitral valve prolapse with an apical click and late systolic murmur, which becomes longer and louder when the patient stands. In individuals with major mitral regurgitation, an apical pansystolic murmur is heard. The presence of aortic regurgitation is indicated by an early diastolic murmur along the midleft sternal border and an apical

IMPROVEMENT OF MITRAL REGIRGITATION

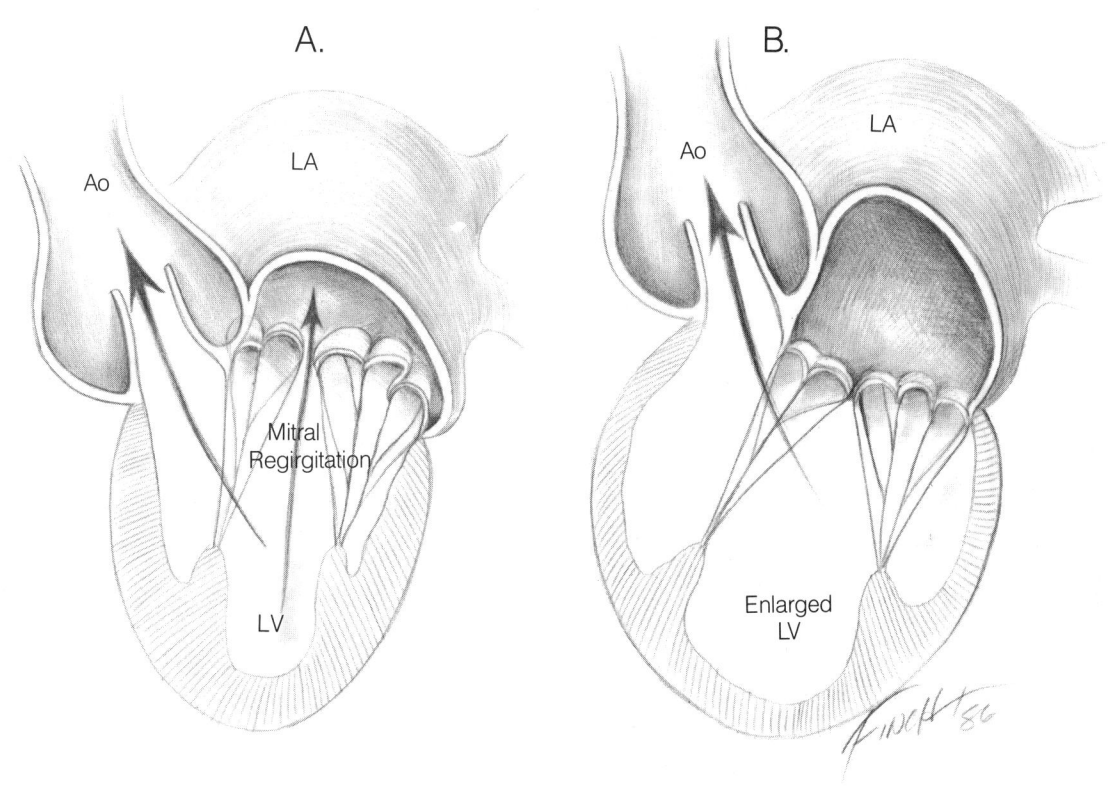

FIG 67–3.
Marfan syndrome. **A,** mechanism of mitral regurgitation is associated with elongated thinned chordae tendineae. Mitral valve prolapses deep into left atrium. Anterior and posterior leaflets no longer coapt, resulting in mitral regurgitation. **B,** mechanism of disappearance of mitral regurgitation after myocardial infarction and dilatation of left ventricle. Papillary muscles migrate because of left ventricular dilatation, and mitral prolapse diminishes, allowing coaptation of anterior and posterior leaflets. *Ao* = aorta; *LA* = left atrium; *LV* = left ventricle.

systolic ejection click, the latter reflecting the dilated ascending aorta.

Because of connective tissue abnormalities, there is a tendency to development of pneumothorax and inguinal hernias. Structural abnormalities of the lung such as bullous emphysema lead to spontaneous pneumothorax.[10, 11] Some patients have marked reduction in pulmonary capacity because of kyphoscoliosis and pectus excavatum.

ELECTROCARDIOGRAPHIC FEATURES

The electrocardiogram may be normal. If regurgitation of left-sided cardiac valves occurs, left ventricular hypertrophy and left atrial enlargement may develop.

The T waves may be inverted in the inferior limb leads (II, III, and aVF), particularly in those patients with mitral valve prolapse.

ECHOCARDIOGRAPHIC FEATURES

The echocardiogram has helped considerably in diagnosis, management, and understanding of the disease.[12–14] The abnormalities of the aorta, sinuses of Valsalva, and mitral valve are easily identified echocardiographically. About 60% of Marfan syndrome patients have dilatation of the proximal ascending aorta and aortic sinuses. These can be recognized much earlier by echocardiography than by thoracic roentgenograms. Accurate serial measurements of the diameter of the ascending aorta can be made and may show progressive enlargement. Based on the echocardiographic diameter, decisions are made regarding operation on the ascending aorta.

Echocardiography is also useful in detecting mitral valve anomalies. Prolapse of the posterior leaflet of the mitral valve is found and typically is pansystolic. Doppler interrogation may show mitral and aortic regurgitation.

Dissection of the ascending aorta may also be recognized by finding two parallel linear echoes within the as-

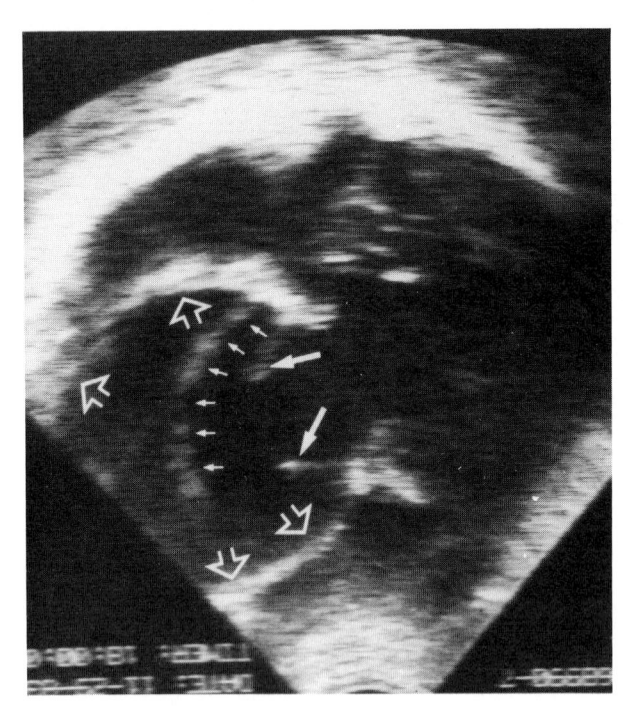

FIG 67–4.
Marfan syndrome. Echocardiogram. Long axis parasternal view. Dilated aortic sinuses *(open arrows)*. Aortic valve normal *(solid large arrows)*. Intimal flap *(small arrows)* indicating dissecting aneurysm.

cending aorta (Fig 67–4).[14] Whereas the ultrasound examination of the aorta is largely limited to the ascending aorta, nuclear magnetic resonance (NMR) studies may demonstrate dissections in the entire aorta (Fig 67–5). Furthermore, (NMR) can give important information about the blood flow in the false channel and indicate sites of reentry and decompression. Ultrasound examinations with color Doppler flow can also determine blood flow in the false channel.

RADIOGRAPHIC FEATURES

The diagnosis of Marfan syndrome is rarely made from radiographic findings of the thorax. REASON: The hallmark of the disease, dilatation of the aortic root, is usually not visible on a thoracic radiograph because the aorta lies within the center of the cardiac silhouette, and only structures that border on the lung are seen on a roentgenogram. Nevertheless, certain features may clinch the correct diagnosis, particularly in the advanced stages of the disease:

1. A narrow transverse diameter of the thorax, scoliosis, or carinatum pectus excavatum are commonly encountered in classic Marfan syndrome (Fig 67–6). In contrast, most patients with cystic medial necrosis (Erdheim's) do not have the skeletal stigmata of Marfan syndrome. Other characteristic skeletal anomalies of Marfan syndrome are not discussed here.

2. The incidence of calcification of the mitral valve annulus is higher, particularly in young patients (Fig 67–7). REASON: Unknown. Whereas mitral annular calcification occurs primarily in middle-aged women, it may be observed in Marfan syndrome in early adulthood.

3. Pulmonary abnormalities such as generalized emphysema and bullous emphysema (Fig 67–8) may be encountered. Spontaneous pneumothorax may result.

4. The cardiac hallmark of Marfan syndrome is dilatation of the sinuses of Valsalva. Without contrast medium, they are not visible on a thoracic radiograph (Fig 67–9). REASON: The sinuses of Valsalva occupy an intramediastinal position and are not surrounded by air.

5. With involvement of the ascending aorta and aorta reflux, prominence of the ascending aorta may be evident, suggesting aortic valvar disease (Fig 67–10).

6. If the aneurysmal dilatation and the sinuses of Valsalva are marked, it may still not be visible on a posteroanterior roentgenogram, but it may cause an unusual density in the retrosternal area of a lateral projection (Fig 67–11).

7. Incomplete dissection of the ascending aorta may heal by calcification, which may be seen on a lateral thoracic roentgenogram. Flecks of calcium in the ascending aorta of patients with Marfan syndrome are therefore common. Rarely, the entire aneurysm may be outlined by calcium (Fig 67–12). These calcifications should not be confused with the calcifications of the ascending aorta present in syphilis. In syphilis, the intima shows calcified athero-

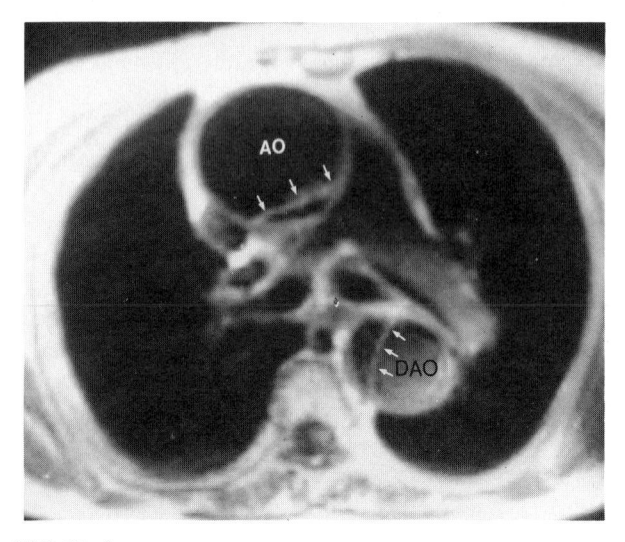

FIG 67–5.
Marfan syndrome. Magnetic resonance imaging study of thorax in transverse plane. Aneurysm of ascending aorta *(AO)* and dissecting hematoma *(arrows)* are demonstrated in ascending aorta and descending aorta *(DAO)*.

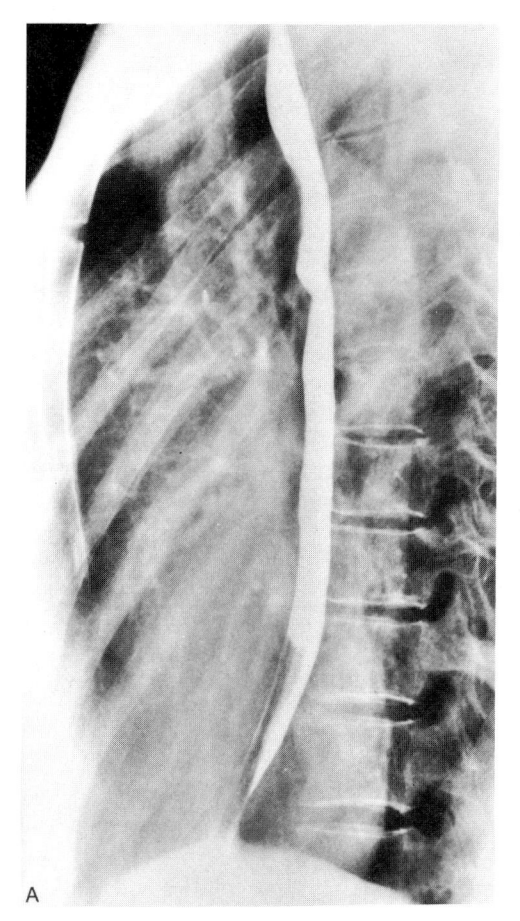

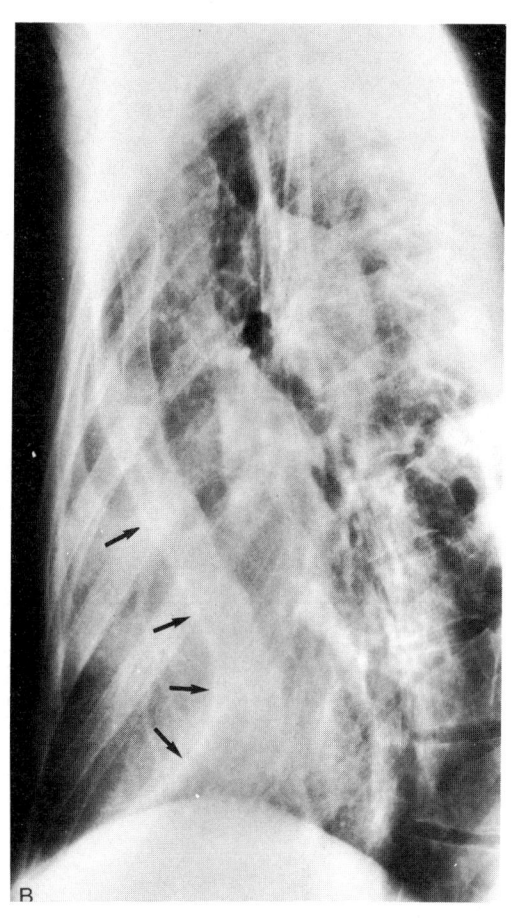

FIG 67–6.
Marfan syndrome. Thoracic roentgenogram. Lateral projection. Associated thoracic deformities. **A,** long narrow thorax. **B,** severe pectus excavatum deformity *(arrows).*

sclerotic plaques in the ascending aorta and dense calcifications of the thoracic and abdominal aorta. (Syphilis induces a rapidly progressing atherosclerosis through the entire aorta.) Calcifications in the descending aorta are absent in Marfan syndrome and consequently isolated calcifications in an ascending aortic aneurysm are more characteristic of calcified incomplete dissection in cystic medial necrosis.

8. Even though the posteroanterior roentgenogram may not suggest dilatation of the ascending aorta, it may be demonstrated on a lateral projection, where the retrosternal space is obliterated by the dilated aorta (Fig 67–13).

9. Marfan syndrome is a progressive condition. Initially there is dilatation of the sinuses of Valsalva, which is not visible on a thoracic roentgenogram. Subsequently, aneurysms form in the ascending aorta, which can be readily seen. Repeat thoracic roentgenograms are therefore valuable in patients suspected of the diagnosis of Marfan syndrome (Fig 67–14), but ultrasound examinations provide better information.

10. The formation of an ascending aortic aneurysm occurs by either dissection (dissecting aneurysm) or incomplete dissection where the aortic wall tears. The tear heals, and no extension of the dissection occurs. Areas of incomplete dissections may calcify (see Fig 67–12).

11. Typically the aneurysm of the ascending aorta becomes a visible density along the right cardiac contour, as in Figure 67–14. With scoliosis and pectus excavatum deformity causing displacement and rotation of the heart, the aneurysm may form the border of the left cardiac contour, simulating a prominent pulmonary arterial segment (Fig 67–15).

12. If mitral regurgitation is a major hemodynamic alteration, cardiomegaly and left atrial enlargement are found identical to other more common causes of mitral regurgitation. The degree of mitral regurgitation may be massive and may be the dominant presenting clinical feature.

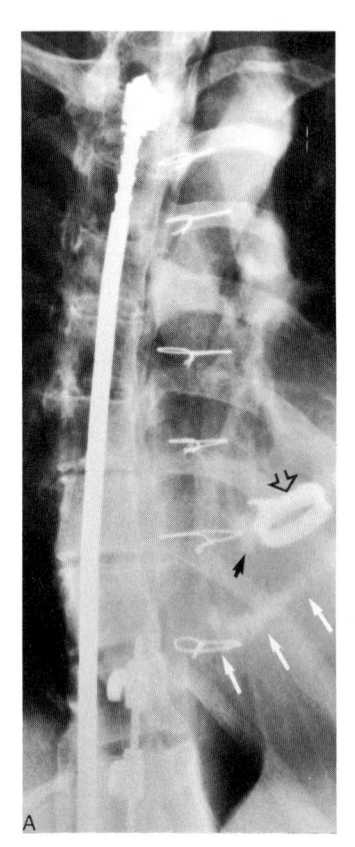

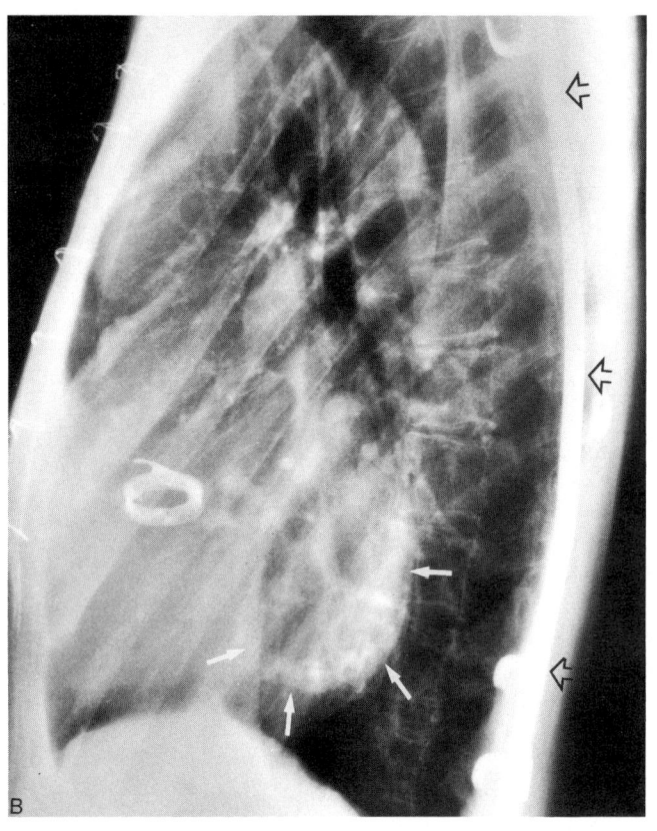

FIG 67–7.
Marfan syndrome. Thoracic roentgenogram. Anteroposterior and lateral projections. **A,** scoliosis was treated by Harrington rods. Aortic valve was replaced by a prosthesis and composite graft *(open arrow)*. Dense calcifications in mitral annulus *(white arrows)*, a very unusual finding in a young patient. Also calcifications in aortic annulus *(solid black arrow)*. **B,** Harrington rod *(open arrows)*. Characteristic C-shaped calcifications *(white arrows)* in mitral annulus.

ANGIOGRAPHY

Left ventriculography is indicated to assess left ventricular size and contractility and to determine the degree of mitral regurgitation. Aortography is performed to assess the size of the ascending aorta, the status of the coronary arteries, which may be compromised by aortic or coronary arterial dissection, and the degree of aortic regurgitation, which is commonly seen in advanced cases of Marfan syndrome. If a true dissection is present in the aortic arch, the brachiocephalic arteries and abdominal aorta should be studied angiographically as well. Because of the higher incidence of dissecting aneurysm with Marfan syndrome and other types of cystic medial necrosis, the catheter should be introduced into the right rather than left femoral artery, provided both femoral pulses are equal. REASON: Through the right femoral artery the catheter is more likely to enter the true channel, because most dissections extend into the left iliofemoral arterial system. If the true channel is injected, angiographic interpretation is easier, and the coronary arteries and aortic reflux can be evaluated.

Right ventriculography and pulmonary angiography may be indicated. REASON: The myxomatous degeneration may involve also the tricuspid valve and, less commonly, the main pulmonary artery and pulmonary valve. Tricuspid regurgitation may develop.

1. During cardiac catheterization the catheter course in the aorta may be unusual. REASON: In cases with a large aneurysm of the ascending aorta, the ascending aorta lies immediately behind the sternum, and the catheter may hug the sternum in the lateral projection (Fig 67–16).
2. It may be impossible to pass the catheter into the left ventricle in a retrograde fashion. REASONS:
   a. The catheter may have entered a false channel.
   b. The sinuses are so large that the catheters tend to coil in the right sinus of Valsalva (see Fig 67–15). Furthermore, there is incomplete systolic opening of the aortic valve.
3. The process of dilatation of the aorta starts at the level of the sinuses of Valsalva and progresses

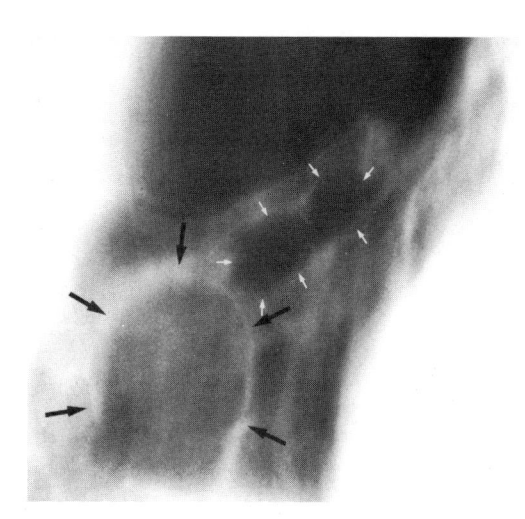

FIG 67–8.
Marfan syndrome. Tomograph of right lung base. Several small bulbae *(white arrows)* and a large bullus *(black arrows)*.

slowly into the ascending aorta. In the early stages of the disease the aortic valve is competent, and consequently the disease process is discovered accidentally by angiography or ultrasonography. It may be discovered in the neonatal period of life.

4. Enlargement of the aortic sinuses or ascending aorta may be demonstrated as an incidental finding during angiography (Fig 67–17), performed for coarctation of aorta, aortic stenosis, or patent ductus arteriosus. REASON: The incidence of cystic medial necrosis is slightly higher with these cardiac anomalies. Progressive dilatation of the sinuses of Valsalva and myxomatous changes in the aortic valve lead to aortic regurgitation of variable degree. The disease starts in infancy and progresses during life (Fig 67–18).
5. If aortic dissection has not occurred, the aortic arch is usually of near-normal caliber at the level of the innominate artery, even in the advanced stages of the disease (see Fig 67–9,B).
6. Dilatation of the sinuses of Valsalva has been unfortunately also termed "aneurysm of the sinuses of Valsalva," which is confusing because the pathologic features are entirely different from true sinus of Valsalva aneurysm (see Chapter 24).
7. During systole the aortic valve leaflets open incompletely. REASON: In a normal heart the size of the aortic annulus is about the size of the outflow tract, causing complete opening of the valve leaflets (see Chapter 2). With marked enlargement of the aortic annulus as in cystic medial necrosis, incomplete opening of the aortic valve is adequate to allow egress of a normal left ventricular stroke volume from the left ventricle (Fig 67–19).

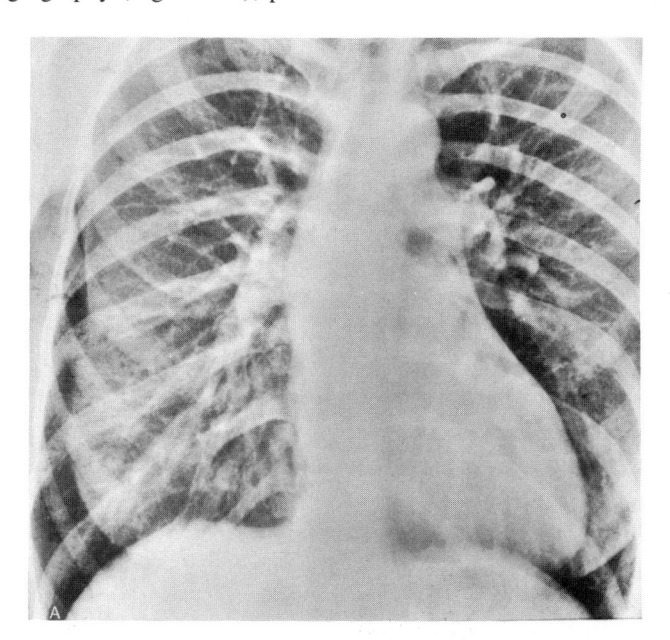

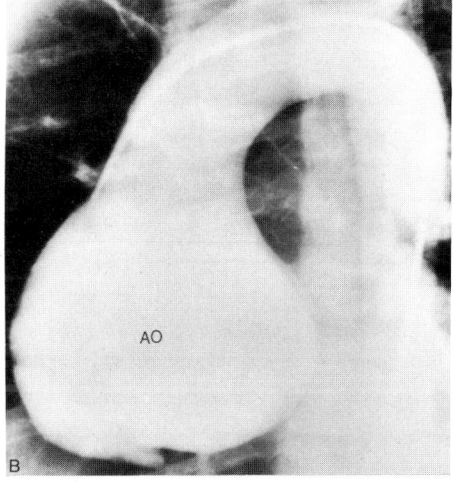

FIG 67–9.
Marfan syndrome. Huge sinuses of Valsalva without significant aortic regurgitation. **A,** thoracic roentgenogram. Posteroanterior projection. Mild scoliosis. Radiographic findings are within normal limits. Sinuses of Valsalva are not seen because they occupy an intracardiac position and do not form a cardiac border. Correct diagnosis cannot be suspected from this roentgenogram. **B,** aortogram *(AO)*. Lateral projection. Typical findings of cystic medial necrosis. Massive dilatation of sinuses of Valsalva. Minimal involvement of ascending aorta accounting for basically normal thoracic roentgenogram.

FIG 67-10.
Marfan syndrome. Massive enlargement of sinuses of Valsalva, involvement of ascending aorta, and aortic insufficiency. Thoracic roentgenogram. Posteroanterior projection. Prominence of ascending aorta *(arrows)*. Dilated sinuses of Valsalva cannot be suspected. Cardiomegaly due to aortic reflux.

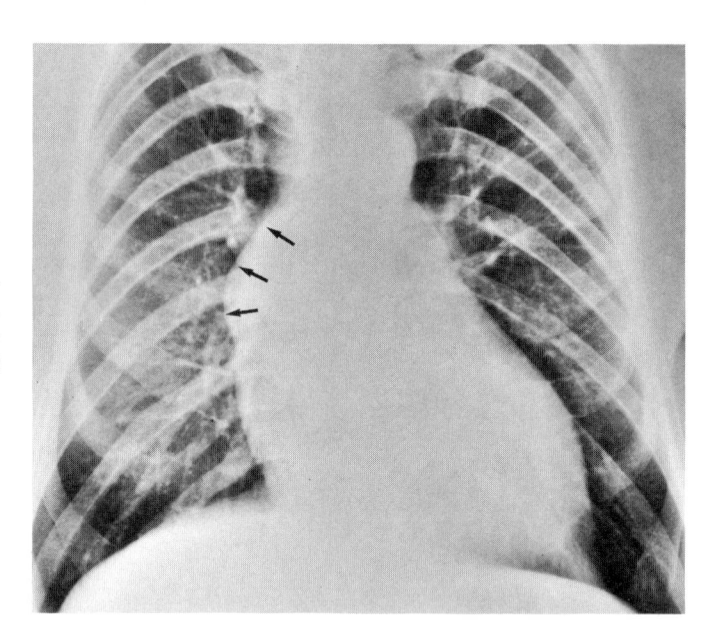

8. Because the incidence of cystic medial necrosis in aortic stenosis is increased, poststenotic dilatation must be differentiated from cystic medial necrosis. Poststenotic dilatation of the ascending aorta (see Chapter 26) is sometimes difficult to differentiate from Marfan syndrome either radiographically or during operation. When in doubt, the ascending aorta should be replaced by a graft. REASON: Cystic medial necrosis progresses and may ultimately be fatal. The process does not always involve the sinuses of Valsalva.
9. In the presence of valvar aortic stenosis with poststenotic dilatation, cystic medial necrosis can be diagnosed with certainty if a dissection is demonstrable (Fig 67-20).
10. If a dissection has occurred, the entire aorta must be studied angiographically (Fig 67-21). In contrast to dissecting aneurysms to hypertensive individuals, in

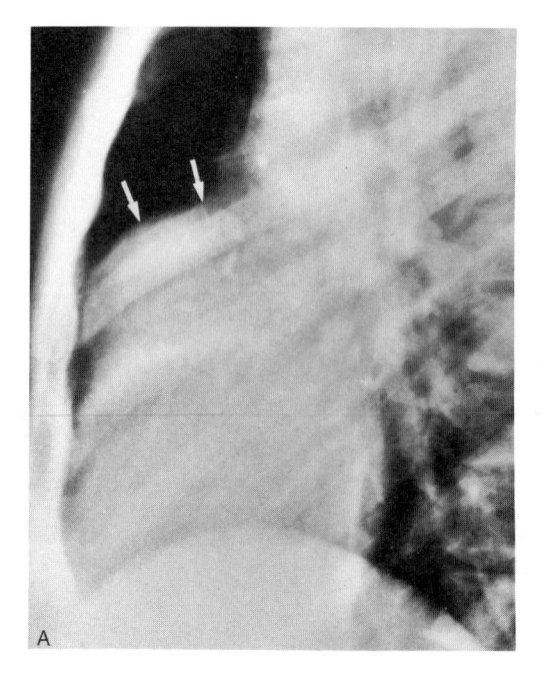

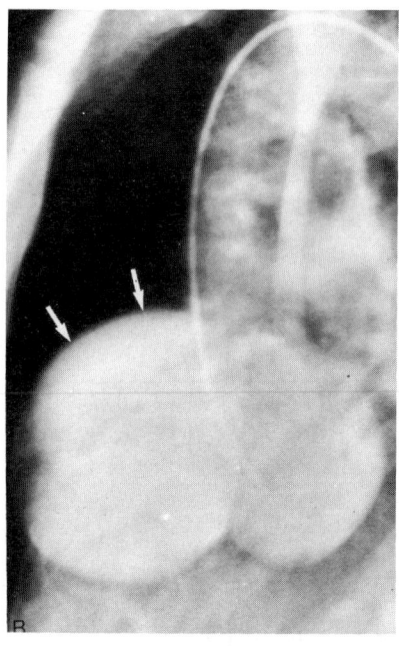

FIG 67-11.
Marfan syndrome. Massive dilatation of sinuses of Valsalva. **A,** thoracic roentgenogram. Lateral projection. Unusual density *(arrows)* in retrosternal space, simulating a dilated right ventricular outflow tract. **B,** Aortogram. Lateral projection. Huge sinuses of Valsalva. Density on roentgenogram is caused be massively dilated right sinus of Valsalva *(arrows)*.

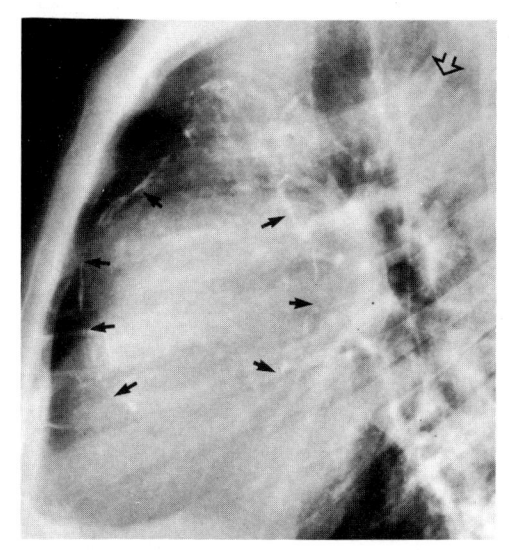

FIG 67–12.
Marfan syndrome. Massive dilatation of sinuses of Valsalva and ascending aorta. Thoracic roentgenogram. Lateral projection. Areas of incomplete dissection have become calcified, outlining entire aneurysm *(arrows)*. Aortic arch and descending aorta *(open arrow)* show no calcifications. Therefore, this does not represent a syphilitic aneurysm.

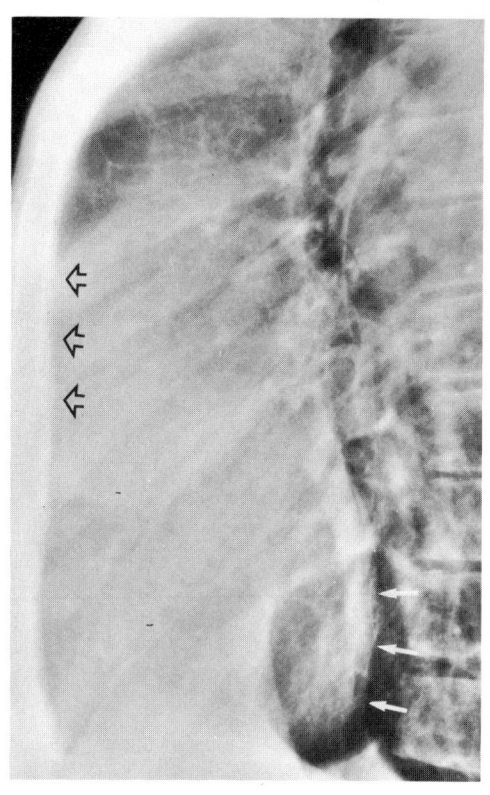

FIG 67–13.
Marfan syndrome. Aneurysm of the sinuses of Valsalva and ascending aorta. Thoracic roentgenogram. Lateral projection. Entire retrosternal space *(open arrows)* is filled by aneurysm of ascending aorta. Posteroanterior roentgenograms were normal. Left ventricular enlargement *(solid arrow)* is caused by aortic insufficiency.

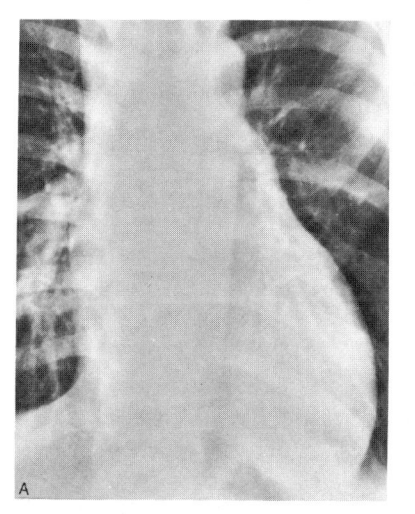

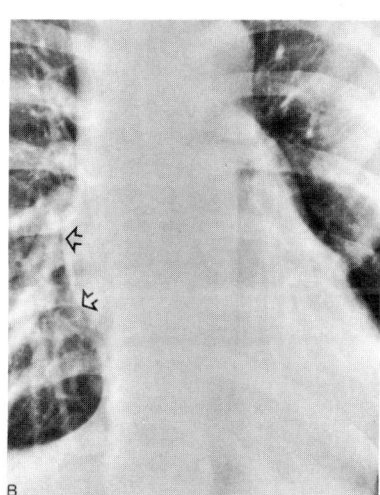

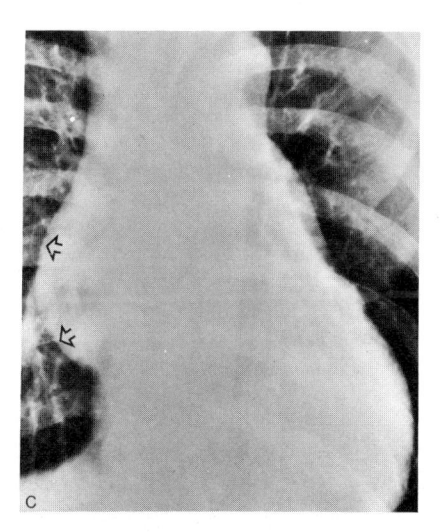

FIG 67–14.
Marfan syndrome. Progressive involvement of ascending aorta. Thoracic roentgenogram. Posteroanterior projection. **A,** minimal cardiomegaly and left ventricular prominence are caused by aortic insufficiency. Aneurysm of sinuses of Valsalva or ascending aorta cannot be suspected. **B,** bulge has appeared along right cardiac contour because of aneurysmal involvement of ascending aorta *(open arrows)*. **C,** bulge has become much larger, indicating progression with increasing involvement of ascending aorta. Typically aneurysm does not extend beyond origin of innominate artery.

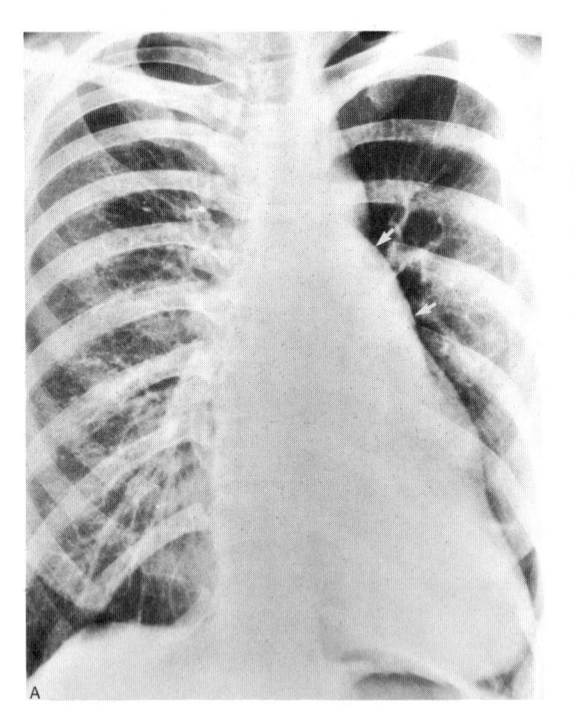

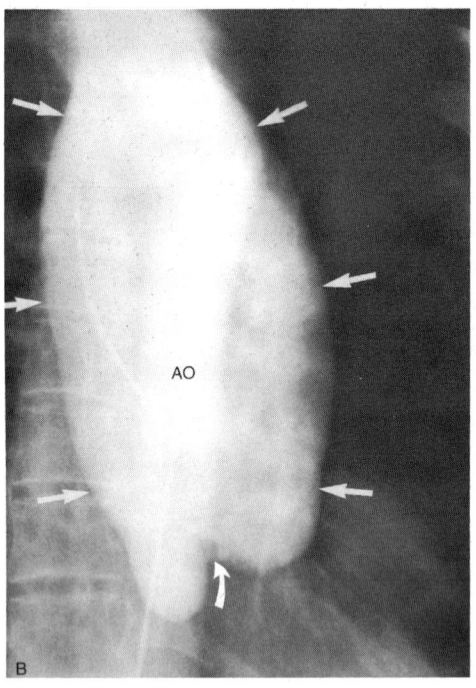

FIG 67–15.
Marfan syndrome. **A,** thoracic roentgenogram. Posteroanterior projection. Heart is displaced into left thoracic cavity because of pectus excavatum deformity. Prominent pulmonary arterial segment *(arrows)*. **B,** aortogram. Anteroposterior projection. Aneurysm of ascending aorta *(AO)* simulating prominent pulmonary arterial segment. Note aortic valve shows incomplete opening, which is normal in this condition and not to be mistaken for a subvalvar jet in subaortic stenosis.

Marfan syndrome the most common initial site of rupture is in the ascending aorta.

11. Cine angiography is preferable to cut-film recording of an aortogram. REASON: The thin intimal-medial flap of the dissection can be seen only if it lies parallel to the x-ray beam. Because considerable flutter of the flap occurs during systole, the flutter is better seen with cine recording than with cut-film techniques. (Sixty exposures per second compared with two to six exposures per second.)

12. The aortic arch should be studied in either a very steep left anterior oblique or a lateral projection. REASON: In the region of aortic arch, particularly the distal portion, the dissecting aneurysm is almost always located posteriorly (see Fig 67–21,B), the intramural pulsatile hematoma tends to progress in a straight course. Normally during the injection of contrast medium the catheter is in contact with the greater curvature of the aortic wall. With the dissecting hematoma located posteriorly along the greater curvature of the arch, the catheter is separated from the wall because the true channel is located along the lesser curvature of the aorta (Fig 67–21, B). This catheter sign is helpful in identifying the true and false channels. It is not infallible because (1) rarely the dissecting hematoma is located along the lesser curvature of the arch, and (2) some pigtail catheters with a large loop pull away from the greater curvature during a rapid injection.

13. In the abdominal aorta the false channel of the

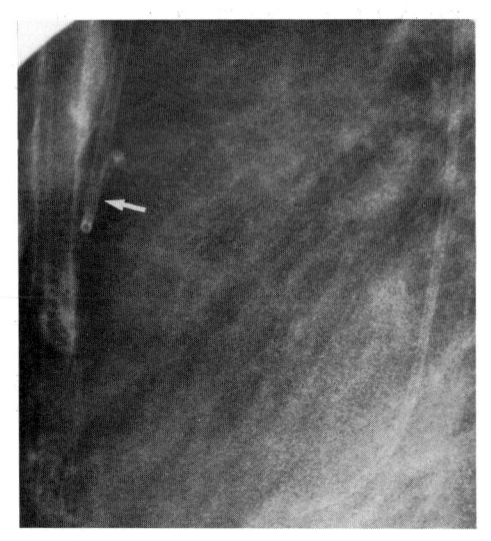

FIG 67–16.
Marfan syndrome. Aneurysm of ascending aorta. Thoracic roentgenogram before aortography. Lateral projection. Catheter *(arrow)* in immediate contact with sternum consistent with aneurysm of ascending aorta.

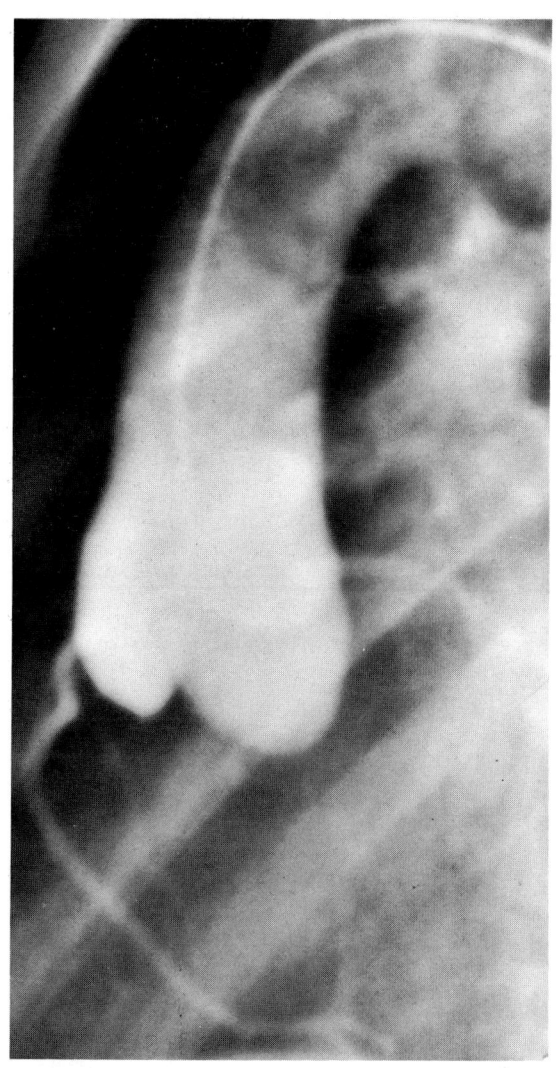

FIG 67–17.
Early stage of cystic medial necrosis. Aortogram. Lateral projection. Distinct dilatation of sinuses of Valsalva without involvement of ascending aorta. Competent aortic valve.

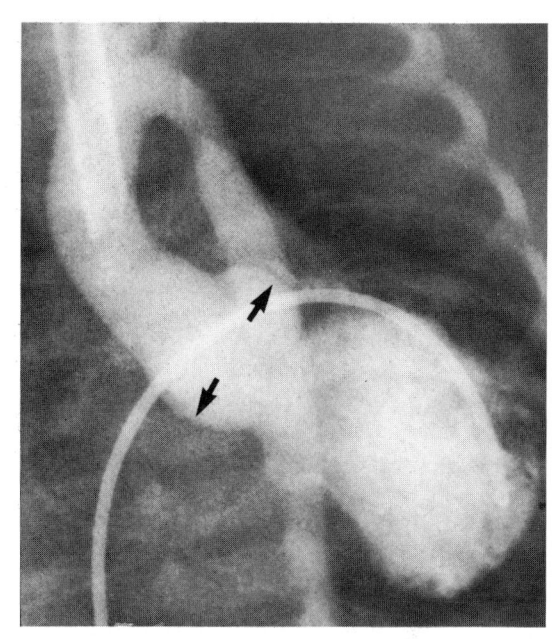

FIG 67–18.
Cystic medial necrosis in an infant. Early stage. Infant. Left ventriculogram. Anteroposterior projection. Distinct dilatation of sinuses of Valsalva (arrows). Beginning dilatation of ascending aorta.

dissection is most commonly located on the left side and consequently tends to dissect into the left renal artery and left iliofemoral arterial system (see Fig 67–21,C). REASON: The dissection tends to progress in the straightest direction. The abdominal aorta is usually slightly bowed towards the right. In the thoracic aorta compromise of the left intercostala arteries is more common.

Other Angiographic Features

1. Four angiographic features allow the diagnosis of mitral valvar involvement with Marfan syndrome (Fig 67–22):
   a. The mitral valve may be thickened, but this is not invariably the case.
   b. The valve is redundant and bubbly ("hooding," "hemorrhoidal mitral valve," "floppy mitral valve").
   c. The mitral valve prolapses into the left atrium because of elongation of chordae tendineae or chordal rupture. Prolapse usually involves both mitral leaflets contrary to the floppy mitral valve in patients without cystic medial necrosis who have involvement of primarily the posterior leaflet (see Chapter 68).
   d. Associated dilatation of the sinuses of Valsalva of the aorta strongly suggests Marfan syndrome as the underlying cause of the mitral valve prolapse (see Fig 67–22,B).
2. In most cases, hooding of the mitral valve is well seen angiographically as redundancy. The entire mitral valve prolapses into the left atrium (see Fig 67–22).
3. Involvement of the tricuspid valve is much less common than of the mitral valve. If it is suspected, right ventriculography should be performed to identify tricuspid regurgitation (Fig 67–23).
4. The main pulmonary artery and pulmonary valve are rarely involved in this condition. When they are involved, the pulmonary annulus and sinuses of Valsalva are dilated identical to the aortic involvement (Fig 67–24).

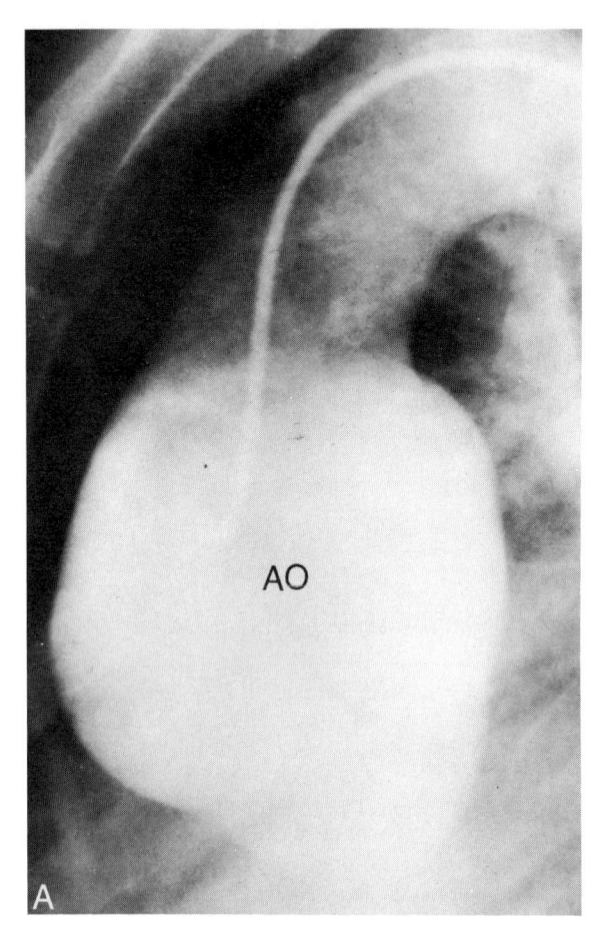

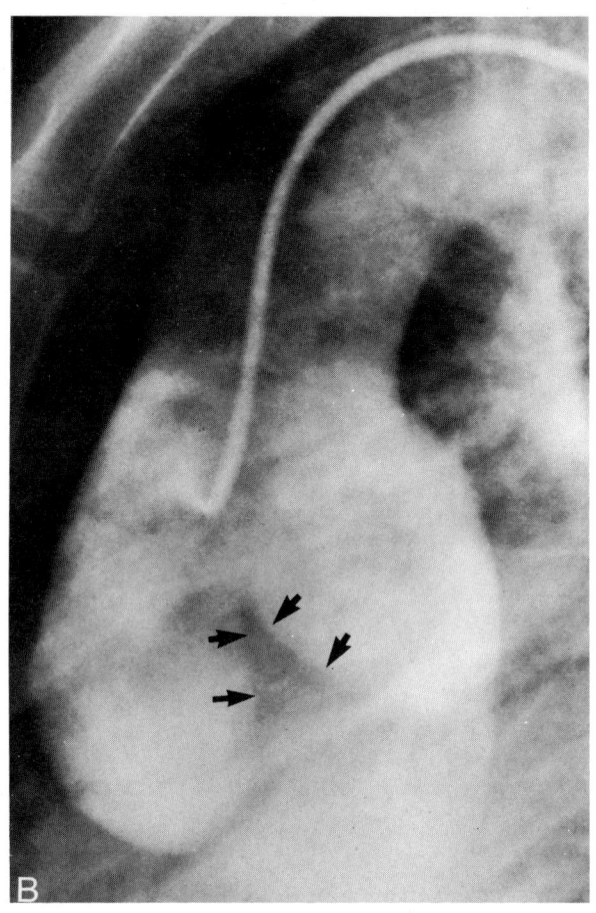

FIG 67–19.
Marfan syndrome. Aortogram *(AO)*. Lateral projection. **A,** diastole. Marked enlargement of sinus of Valsalva and beginning involvement of ascending aorta. **B,** systole. Aortic valve *(arrows)* opens incompletely because of huge annulus. Aortic valve does not dome, excluding aortic stenosis in spite of incomplete opening.

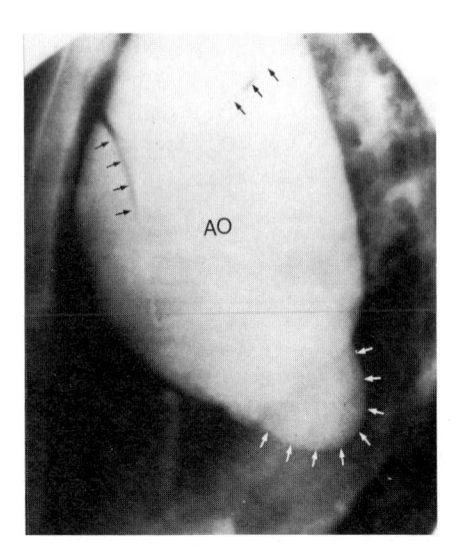

FIG 67–20.
Valvar aortic stenosis. Aortogram. Lateral projection. Sinuses of Valsalva are not dilated, but one cusp is oversized *(arrows)*, typical for congenital aortic stenosis (see Chapter 26). Intimal flaps *(black arrows)* are clearly visualized.

TREATMENT

There is no specific treatment for this disease. Propranolol has been given to individuals with a dilated ascending aorta in an effort to reduce the rate of further dilatation by reducing the ejection force into the aorta.[15]

Cardiac failure and aortic dissection are two complications of aortic involvement. These hazards are reduced by undertaking elective replacement of the ascending aorta[16–18] when the ascending aortic diameter exceeds 5.5 cm. The ascending aorta is incised, a Dacron graft is inserted, and then it is sutured proximally to the aortic annulus and distally to the aorta at the level of the origin of the innominate artery. Small openings are made in the graft, which are sutured to the coronary arterial orifices (Fig 67–25). The native aorta is then wrapped about the graft. Another approach is suturing the graft to the aorta above the level of the coronary arteries. If aortic insufficiency coexists, the aortic valve is replaced at the same time by a composite graft. In individuals with symptomatic mitral regurgitation, valve replacement is performed.

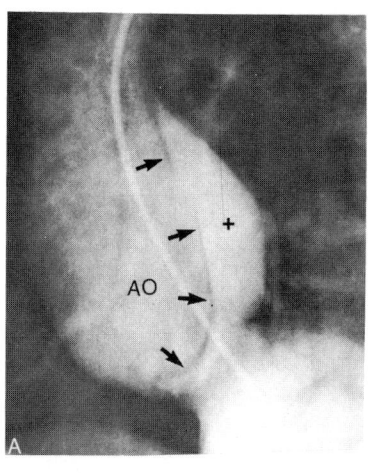

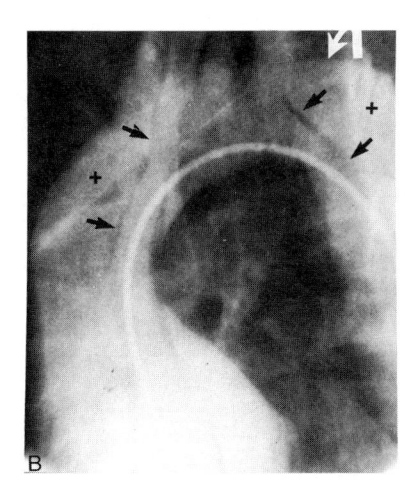

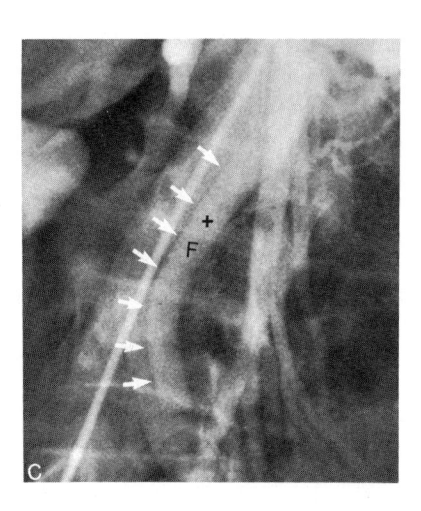

FIG 67–21.
Marfan syndrome. Dissecting aortic aneurysm. **A,** left ventriculography. Lateral projection. Dilatation of sinuses of Valsalva with excellent demonstration of dissecting flap *(arrows)*. False channel indicated by *plus sign*. **B,** aortography. Left anterior oblique projection. Dissection extends around aortic arch. Catherer is in true channel, which is located along lesser curvature of aortic arch. Dissecting hematoma *(curved arrows)* is densely opacified, indicating flow in both channels. Catheter is positioned along lesser curvature of arch in true channel. **C,** abdominal aortogram. Anteroposterior projection. Catheter is introduced into right femoral artery and in true channel. False channel *(F)* characteristically lies on left side of abdominal aorta and extends into left iliac artery. Dissection into left renal artery is more common than into right renal artery (exceptions exist). Both channels are opacified, indicating reentry with flow in both channels. False channel is marked by a plus sign.

POSTOPERATIVE FEATURES

1. After replacement of the aneurysmal ascending aorta by a graft, and, if necessary, replacement of the aortic valve by an artificial or tissue valve, the radiographic appearance changes drastically by showing a marked reduction in cardiac size.

2. The insertion of a composite graft is technically difficult and associated with complications, particularly leakage at one of the four anastomotic sites, proximal aorta, distal aorta, and two coronary arteries. Angiography is therefore indicated to exclude complications.

3. In an uncomplicated case with a composite graft, both coronary arteries fill normally, and extravasation of contrast medium does not occur (Fig 67–26).

4. In most cases the aortic arch is of normal diameter beyond the level of the innominate artery. When the aneurysm extends further around the arch, the graft may be sewn to the aneurysm. This is difficult technically; because of the cystic degeneration of the aortic wall, the sutures may tear.

5. The most common site of leakage from the graft is at site of anastomosis of the coronary arteries to the graft (Fig 67–27).

6. Leakage is visualized by cine angiography, because the size of the opening is usually small and the leakage minimal. REASON: The leak occurs into the false aneurysm (i.e., hematoma around the graft). The pressure in the graft and hematoma is the same. The native aorta that has been sewn around the graft, however, is distensible.

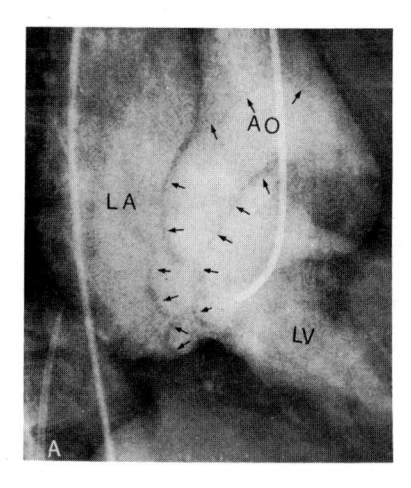

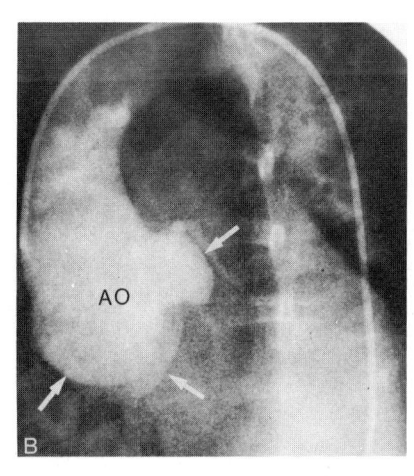

FIG 67–22.
Marfan syndrome. Marked involvement of mitral valve. **A,** left ventriculogram *(LV)*. Right anterior oblique projection. Slightly thickened redundant hooded hemorrhoidal valve. Anterior and posterior leaflets are involved. Significant mitral regurgitation with opacification of left atrium *(LA)*. **B,** Aortogram *(AO)*. Left anterior oblique projection. Distinct enlargement of sinuses of Valsalva *(arrows)*, indicating that mitral deformity and mitral regurgitation are caused by myxomatous degeneration in cystic medical necrosis in spite of absent aortic regurgitation.

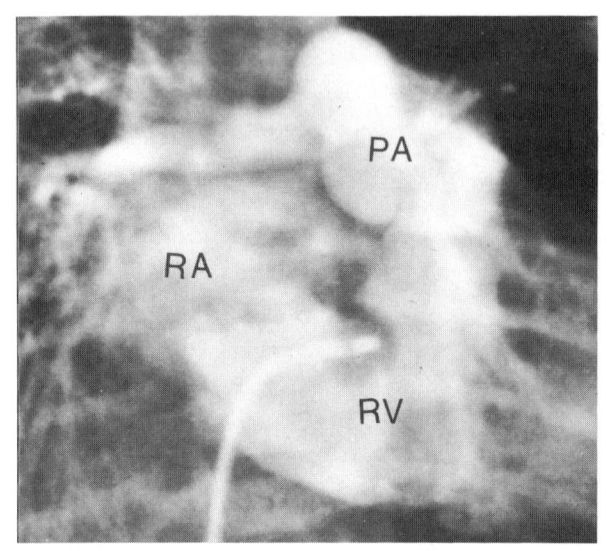

FIG 67-23.
Marfan syndrome. Right ventriculogram *(RV)*. Anteroposterior projection. Tricuspid regurgitation is likely caused by myxomatous involvement of tricuspid valve, but catheter is positioned too close to tricuspid valve to diagnose with certainty. *PA* = pulmonary artery; *RA* = right atrium.

Consequently, during systole, blood enters the false aneurysm. During diastole, blood flows backward into the aorta. Therefore, some pressure differential exists, and flow occurs through the leak, allowing angiographic detection.

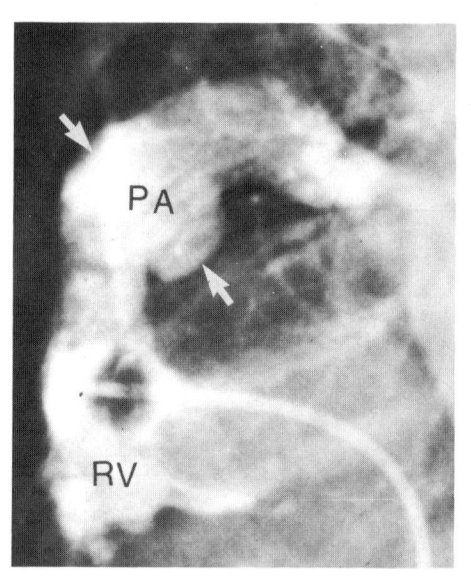

FIG 67-24.
Marfan syndrome. Right ventriculogram *(RV)*. Lateral projection. Distinct enlargement of sinuses of Valsalva *(arrows)* of pulmonary artery *(PA)*. This patient also had dilatation of sinuses of Valsalva of aortic valve.

7. Because of the small volume of flow through the leak, the entire false aneurysm does not opacify (see Fig 67-27).

8. Leakage may also occur at the proximal anastomotic site between graft and aorta. This is less common

SURGICAL REPAIR OF AORTIC ANEURYSM BY COMPOSITE GRAFT

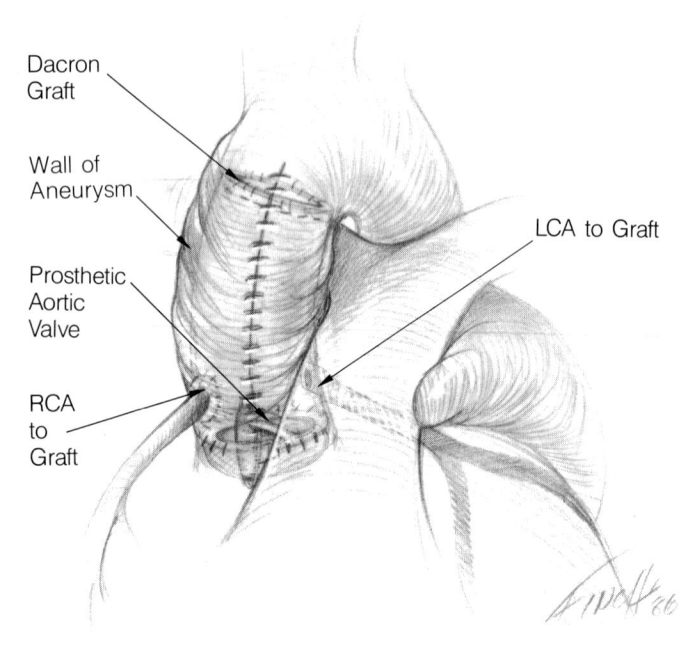

FIG 67-25.
Repair of aortic insufficiency and aneurysm of ascending aorta by composite graft. Aortic valve and ascending aorta are replaced. Coronary arteries (left *[LCA]* and right *[RCA]*) have been sewn to graft.

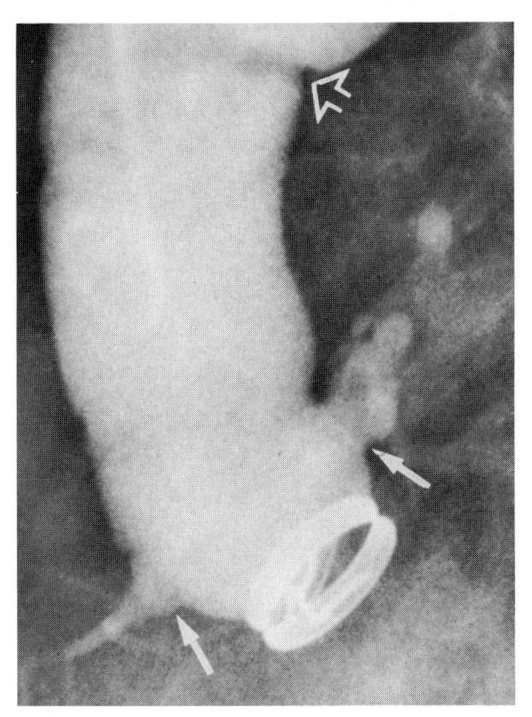

FIG 67–26.
Cystic medial necrosis after replacement of ascending aorta by composite graft. Aortogram. Lateral projection. Both coronary arteries *(arrows)* are sewn to graft containing an artificial valve. Distal anastomosis with native aorta *(open arrow)*. No extravasation of contrast material.

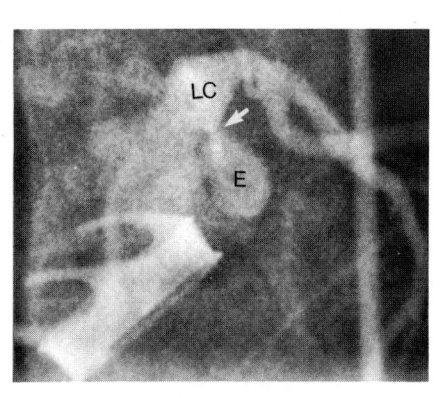

FIG 67–27.
Cystic medial necrosis after replacement of ascending aorta by composite graft. Selective coronary arteriogram. Left anterior oblique projection. Left coronary artery *(LC)* is well opacified. Artificial valve is present. Small leak *(arrow)* at site where coronary artery sewn to graft. Small amount of contrast medium *(E)* extravasates into space between graft and native aorta, which has been sewn around graft.

MECHANISM OF SYSTOLIC COLLAPSE OF COMPOSITE AORTIC GRAFT

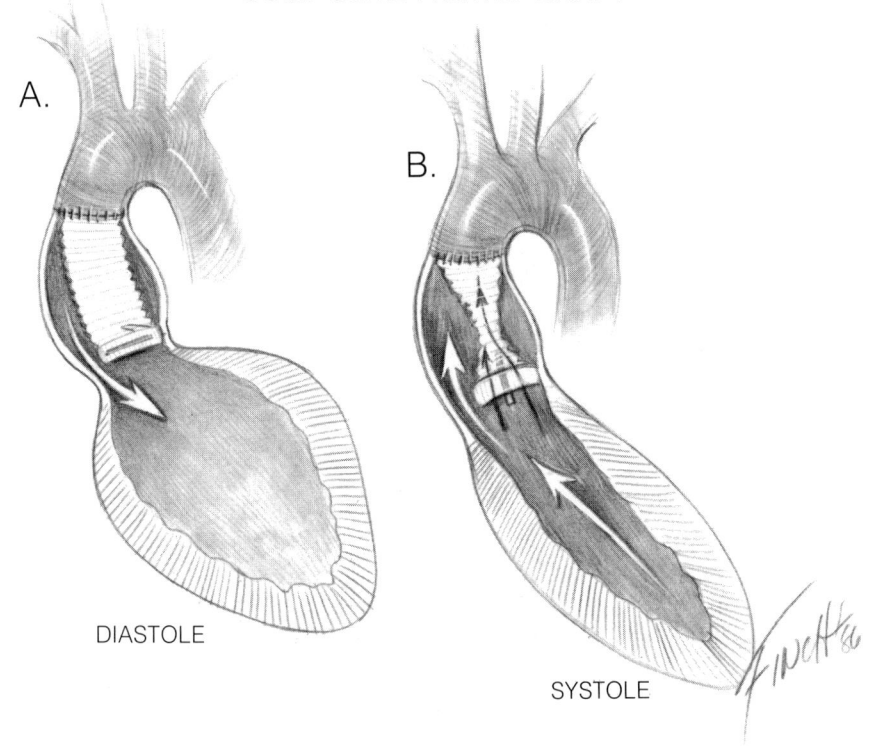

A. DIASTOLE

B. SYSTOLE

FIG 67–28.
Mechanism of systolic collapse of composite graft. Dehiscence of valve with communication of space around graft with left ventricle. Slightly higher left ventricular systolic pressure is transmitted to hematoma around graft, which causes its collapse **(B)**. In diastole **(A)**, diastolic pressure in graft is higher than in hematoma, causing distention.

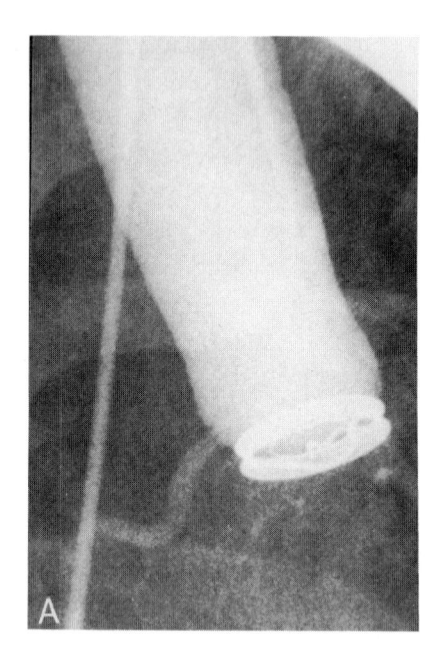

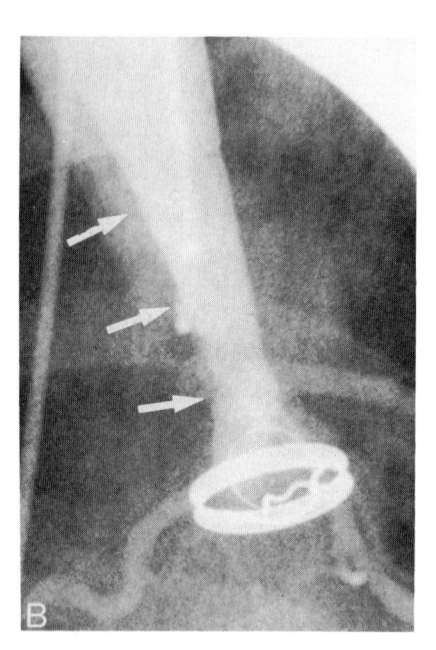

FIG 67-29.
Cystic medial necrosis after replacement of ascending aorta by composite graft. Aortogram. Right anterior oblique projection. **A,** diastole. Normal appearance of graft. Competent artificial valve. No extravasation of contrast medium. **B,** systole. Marked compression of graft because of free communication between left ventricle and hematoma around graft. Slightly higher left ventricular systolic pressure is transmitted to hematoma, causing collapse of graft *(arrows).*

because attachment of the coronary arteries to the graft is much more difficult.

9. A false communication may occur not only between the graft and the surrounding native aorta but also between the left ventricle and native aorta (the native aorta is usually sewn around the inserted graft). If a free communication exists between the left ventricle and the surrounding aorta, the graft collapses during systole (Fig 67–28). REASON: Left ventricular systolic pressure is transmitted to the collection of blood around the graft. Almost all artificial valves have a systolic pressure gradient. Therefore, during systole, a higher left ventricular pressure is transmitted to the hematoma around the graft, causing systolic compression of the graft (Fig 67–29). During diastole the aortic pressure is much greater than left ventricular pressure, resulting in distention of the graft.[19]

10. Similar angiographic findings can be found in

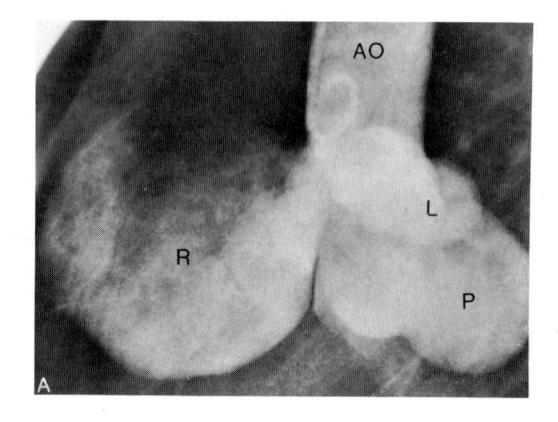

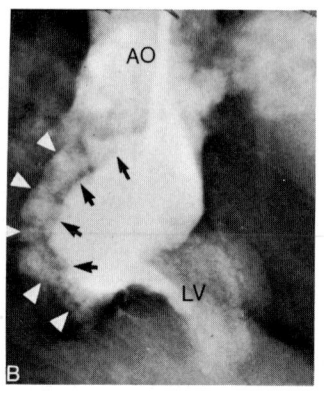

FIG 67-30.
Ehlers-Danlos syndrome. **A,** aortogram. Lateral projection. Left coronary sinus is fairly normal in size. Posterior sinus *(P)* is considerably dilated. Right sinus *(R)* is huge. Ascending aorta *(AO)* is normal. No aortic regurgitation. L = left sinus. **B,** left ventriculogram. Steep right anterior oblique projection. LV = left ventricle. Marked prolapse of redundant mitral valve. Prolapse of both leaflets *(white and black arrows).* No mitral regurgitation. Angiographic finding as in Marfan syndrome. (Courtesy of Dr. M. Tadavarthy.)

other collagen or elastic tissue disorders such as homocysteinuria, Ehlers Danlos disease, etc. (Fig 67–30).

REFERENCES

1. McKusick VA: The Marfan syndrome. In *Heritable disorders of connective tissue,* ed 4. St Louis, 1972, Mosby-Year Book, p 521.
2. Pyeritz RE, McKusick VA: The Marfan syndrome: diagnosis and management, *N Engl J Med* 300:772, 1979.
3. Boucek RJ, Noble NL, Gunja-Smith Z, et al: The Marfan syndrome: a deficiency in chemically stable collagen crosslinks, *N Engl J Med* 305:988, 1981.
4. Papaioannou AC, Matsaniotis N, Cantez T, et al: Marfan syndrome: onset and development of cardiovascular lesions in Marfan syndrome, *Angiology* 21:580, 1970.
5. Sisk HE, Zahka KG, Pyeritz RE: The Marfan syndrome in early childhood: analysis of 15 patients diagnosed at less than 4 years of age, *Am J Cardiol* 52:353, 1983.
6. Schaefer S, Peshock RM, Malloy CR, et al: Nuclear magnetic resonance imaging in Marfan's syndrome, *J Am Coll Cardiol* 9:70, 1987.
7. Bruno L, Tredici S, Mangiavacchi M, et al: Cardiac, skeletal, and ocular abnormalities in patients with Marfan's syndrome and in their relatives: comparison with the cardiac abnormalities in patients with kyphoscoliosis, *Br Heart J* 51:220, 1984.
8. Phornphutkul C, Rosenthal A, Nadas AS: Cardiac manifestations of Marfan syndrome in infancy and childhood, *Circulation* 47:587, 1973.
9. Gruber MA, Graham TP Jr, Engel E, et al: Marfan syndrome with contractural arachnodactyly and severe mitral regurgitation in a premature infant, *J Pediatr* 93:80, 1978.
10. Moothart RW, Spangler RD, Blount SG Jr: Echocardiography in aortic root dissection and dilatation, *Am J Cardiol* 36:11, 1975.
11. Bolande RP, Tucker A: Pulmonary emphysema and other cardiorespiratory lesions as part of the Marfan abiotrophy, *Pediatrics* 33:356, 1964.
12. Dwyer EM Jr, Troncale F: Spontaneous pneumothorax and pulmonary disease in the Marfan syndrome, *Ann Intern Med* 62:1285, 1965.
13. Come PC, Bulkley BH, McKusick VA, et al: Echocardiographic recognition of silent aortic root dilatation in Marfan's syndrome, *Chest* 72:789, 1972.
14. Brown OR, DeMots H, Kloster FE, et al: Aortic root dilatation and mitral valve prolpase in Marfan's syndrome: an echocardiographic study, *Circulation* 52:651, 1975.
15. Brown OR, Popp RL, Kloster FE: Echocardiographic criteria for aortic root dissection, *Am J Cardiol* 36:17, 1975.
16. Ose L, McKusick VA: Prophylactic use of propranolol in the Marfan syndrome to prevent aortic dissection, *Birth Defects* 13:163, 1977.
17. Helseth HK, Haglin JJ, Stenlund RR, et al: Evaluation of composite graft replacement of the aortic root and ascending aorta, *Ann Thorac Surg* 18:138, 1974.
18. Helseth, HK, Haglin JJ, Stenlund RR, et al: Ascending aorta aneurysms with associated aortic regurgitation, *Ann Thorac Surg* 16:368, 1973.
19. Gott VL, Pyeritz RE, Magovern GJ Jr, et al: Surgical treatment of aneurysms of the ascending aorta in the Marfan syndrome: results of composite-graft repair in 50 patients, *N Engl J Med* 314:1070, 1986.
20. Tadavarthy M, Castaneda-Zuniga W, Amplatz K, et al: Systolic collapse of an ascending aortic graft: an angiographic sign of perigraft hematoma communicating with the left ventricle. *AJR* 138:353, 1982.

CHAPTER 68

Mitral Valve Prolapse

Mitral valve prolapse (MVP) has been called by a variety of terms, including systolic click murmur syndrome, redundant cusp syndrome, ballooning mitral valve, myxomatous degeneration of the mitral valve, and floppy mitral valve. This is a relatively common condition, occurring in perhaps 7% of young adults.[1,2] Echocardiographic studies have aided our understanding of MVP and its frequency.[3] This is generally considered a benign condition, and one study showed a normal life expectancy of affected individuals.[4]

This disease is important because it probably accounts for most instances of severe mitral insufficiency,[5] 90% of ruptured chordae tendineae,[6] 40% of transient ischemic attacks or strokes in the young,[7] and perhaps 10% of instances of infective endocarditis.

PATHOLOGIC ANATOMY

The principal anatomic features involve the mitral valve leaflets and chordae tendineae.[4] The leaflets, particularly the posterior one, are voluminous and redundant (Fig 68–1). The chordae tendineae are thickened and elongated. Mitral annular dilatation and myxomatous transformation of the mitral valve are present. Two theories predominate regarding the etiology.[8,9] One implicates a primary myocardial problem, but the benign nature of this condition makes this an unlikely explanation. The second suggests an alteration in mitral valve collagen with subsequent myxomatous changes in the valve.

The specific anatomic features of a prolapsing mitral valve[4] include the following:

1. Thickening of the spongiosa, which encroaches and invades the fibrosa, causing focal interruption of the fibrosa.
2. Thickening of the spongiosa layer and secondary fibrosis.
3. Interchordal hooding. Prolapse of interchordal segments of the leaflet, causes hooding of the mitral valve. The degree of interchordal hooding of the floppy mitral valve has been classified:
   Grade 1: Interchordal hooding involving more than one half of the anterior leaflet or more than two thirds of the posterior leaflet.
   Grade 2: Interchordal hooding involving more than one half of the anterior leaflet and more than two thirds of the posterior leaflet (both leaflets involved).
   Grade 3: A significant magnitude of interchordal hooding greater than present in grade 2.

The posterior leaflet is always affected more than the anterior leaflet. If only a single leaflet is involved, it is always the posterior leaflet, and if one leaflet is more involved than the other, it is consistently the posterior leaflet. There is fibrosis of the valve leaflets involving the atrial or ventricular aspect or both. If the prolapse is so pronounced that the posterior leaflet contacts the left atrial wall, there is also fibrosis of the atrial wall.

The chordal length is normal in 75% of the cases and elongated in the remaining instances.[4,10] Chordae tendineae tend to be thin. Friction lesions caused by rubbing of chordae against the left ventricular endocardium cause localized fibrosis in 75% of the cases (Fig 68–2). Friction lesions are not necessarily always present and may also occur without prolapsed mitral valve. Chordae tendineae may become entrapped in fibrous tissue.

The chordae tendineae may rupture, causing acute and massive mitral regurgitation[6] and sudden death or pulmonary edema.

Mitral regurgitation varies in its severity among cases. It results from several abnormalities: (1) entrapment of chordae tendineae by fibrin, (2) failure of leaflet coaption from hooding or chordal elongation, or (3) chordal rupture

1119

FLOPPY MITRAL VALVE

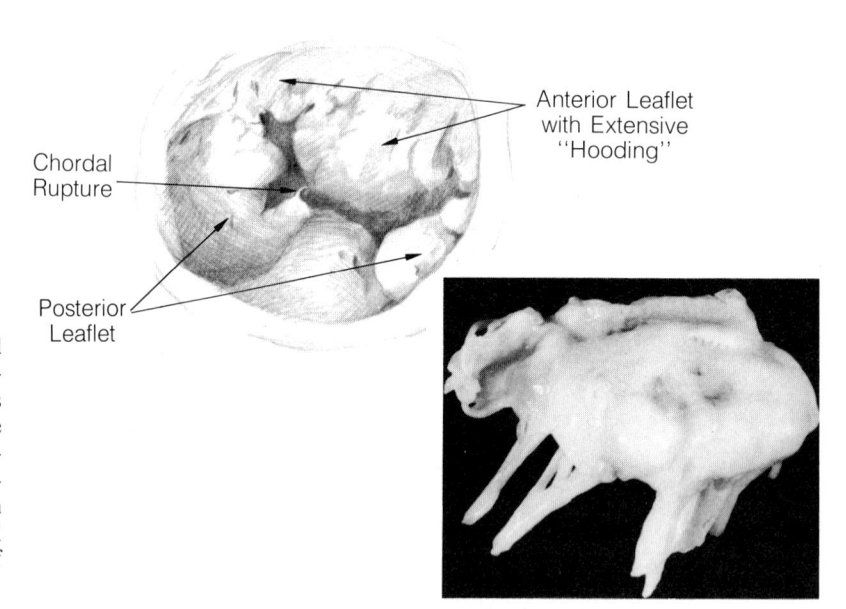

FIG 68–1.
Mitral valve prolapse. Viewed from left atrial side. Redundant valve leaflets. Dilated mitral annulus. Extensive billowing and hooding is caused by elongation of chordae tendineae. One chordal attachment has ruptured, allowing further prolapse of valve into left atrium. Gross appearance resembles hemorrhoids; thus, condition has also been termed "hemorrhoidal mitral valve." *Insert,* excised specimen. Hooding of mitral leaflets. (Courtesy of Dr. J Titus.)

or complications of infectious endocarditis. Ruptured chordae tendineae, bacterial endocarditis, anatomic evidence for mitral regurgitation, and thinning and elongation of the chordae tendineae are other complications.[4]

Several conditions are associated with an increased incidence of prolapsed mitral valve,[11] including:

1. Secundum atrial septal defect.[12]
2. Cystic medial necrosis.
3. Marfan syndrome (see Chapter 67). Prolapsed mitral valve is nearly always present.
4. Various collagen diseases.
5. Thoracic wall abnormality.

Prolapsed mitral valve may coexist with prolapsed tricuspid valve (40%) or redundant pulmonary (11%) and aortic valves.

Prolapse of mitral valve is a rare cause of death.[13, 14] In one study,[4] only 4 of 102 patients with anatomic evidence of MVP died of associated complications. Two of these four died of mitral regurgitation after rupture of chordae tendineae, and the two others died of bacterial endocarditis. None of the patients had a sudden unexpected death. Transient ischemic attacks and strokes have been found in young individuals with MVP. The etiology is unknown, but perhaps they represent embolic events from platelet thrombi on roughened areas of the mitral valve.[6]

CLINICAL FEATURES

Most patients with MVP are asymptomatic. The most frequent symptoms are chest pain, dyspnea, and fatigue.[15, 16] The chest pain is often ill defined but may be sharp, brief, and in the left precordial area or nonradiating substernally and last as long as several hours. It is rarely related to exercise and may be unrelated to auscultatory findings. It has been considered to be caused by papillary muscle ischemia from tension by the prolapsing mitral

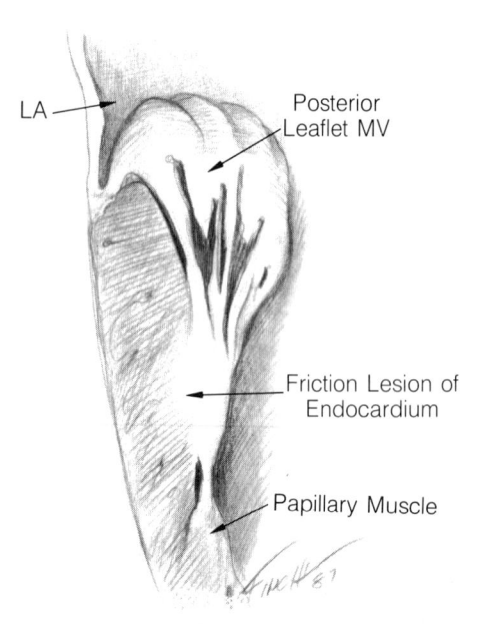

FIG 68–2.
Friction lesions of endocardium. Because of prolapse of mitral leaflet beyond annulus, chordae tendineae rub on endocardium, causing fibrotic friction lesions. Finally, chordae tendineae become entrapped and fixed in fibrous tissue, aggravating mitral regurgitation. *LA* = left atrium.

leaflets. Palpitations and syncope may occur which are related to arrhythmia.

On physical examination the individual may have thoracic abnormalities, such as scoliosis, pectus excavatum, or straight back syndrome. The typical auscultatory findings are found at the cardiac apex—a midsystolic click, followed by a late systolic murmur, being variable.[17-21] The click is a high-pitched sound usually occurring during the middle third of systole; this timing distinguishes it from the earlier appearing ejection clicks. Occasionally several clicks are present. The systolic murmur is typically midsystolic to late systolic and follows the click but may be pansystolic. Its quality varies and has been described as blowing, whooping, or honking.[22] The honking sound may be quite loud and can occur without evidence of mitral regurgitation. The origin of the click and murmurs are uncertain.

The onset and intensity of these two auscultatory findings vary according to left ventricular end-diastolic volume and velocity of contractions. Maneuvers decreasing left ventricular volume cause the findings to become more prominent and to begin earlier in systole. Such maneuvers include sitting, standing, or the Valsalva maneuver.[19, 20] When the patient squats or reclines, the murmur becomes softer and later may even disappear. Even between examinations the findings vary.

The peripheral pulses and other heart sounds are normal.

ELECTROCARDIOGRAPHIC FEATURES

The electrocardiogram (ECG) is often normal. The most frequently observed abnormality is flattened, biphasic, or inverted T waves in the inferior leads (II, III, and aVF) or lateral leads (V_5 and V_6).[15, 16] Associated ST-segment changes are uncommon. T-wave changes are variable. Their origin is unknown but have been ascribed to papillary muscle ischemia from tension by chordae tendineae.

Arrhythmias of a variety of types have been described in individuals with MVP. The cause of rhythm disturbances is unknown, but at least some can be ascribed to mere chance occurrence of two common conditions. The most common are ventricular premature beats and less common supraventricular beats. These may be induced during an exercise stress test. Patients' symptoms have been ascribed to arrhythmia, but this cannot always be established by 24-hour continuous ECG monitoring.

ECHOCARDIOGRAPHIC FEATURES

Echocardiography is a reliable, noninvasive technique that only confirms MVP and has been used as the noninvasive method of choice. Both M-mode and two-dimensional recordings have characteristic findings.[23-27]

On cross-sectional echocardiography, several features are present, including prolapse of both leaflets, more of the posterior leaflet, failure of coaption of mitral valve leaflets, or posterior displacement of site of coaption, and distortion of mitral valve annulus. Doppler analysis will show mitral regurgitation and its timing.

On M-mode recordings, mitral valve closure during systole is reflected by the C-D segment. Normally the C-D segment moves anteriorly and toward the ventricular septum during systole. In mitral prolapse, the C-D segment moves posteriorly. A variety of other M-mode echocardiographic features have been described, including late systolic posterior buckling of one or both leaflets, holosystolic hammocking of both leaflets, exaggerated anterior motion of the anterior leaflet during diastole, and paradoxical motion in early diastole of the posterior mitral valve.

RADIOGRAPHIC FEATURES

No specific radiographic findings allow distinction of a prolapsed mitral valve from other causes of mitral insufficiency. Absence of calcification in the mitral valve may support the diagnosis of prolapsed mitral valve. REASON: In rheumatic fever, the mitral valve may calcify, whereas a prolapsed mitral valve does not. The specific anatomic cause of mitral insufficiency is usually determined by other clinical means. There may be abnormalities of the thoracic cage, including pectus excavatum, scoliosis, and straight back with narrow anteroposterior diameter of the chest.[28]

The radiographic findings of prolapsed mitral valve are not uniform, because the degree of mitral regurgitation varies considerably, depending on the anatomical deformity of the mitral valve.

1. The appearance of the cardiac silhouette and pulmonary vasculature are identical to mitral insufficiency of other causes because the hemodynamics are similar.

2. In most patients, cardiac size is either normal or borderline enlarged. REASON: Most patients with a prolapsed mitral valve have either no or only a minor degree of mitral regurgitation.

3. In patients with sudden onset of severe mitral regurgitation from rupture of chordae tendineae, a complication of prolapsed mitral valve, the radiographic findings may show a prominent venous pattern only (Fig 68-3) or frank pulmonary edema without left atrial enlargement. REASON: Although mitral insufficiency causes left atrial and left ventricular enlargement, this takes considerable time to develop. Therefore, with acute mitral insufficiency, dilatation of the left atrium may be absent even in the presence of significant mitral regurgitation.

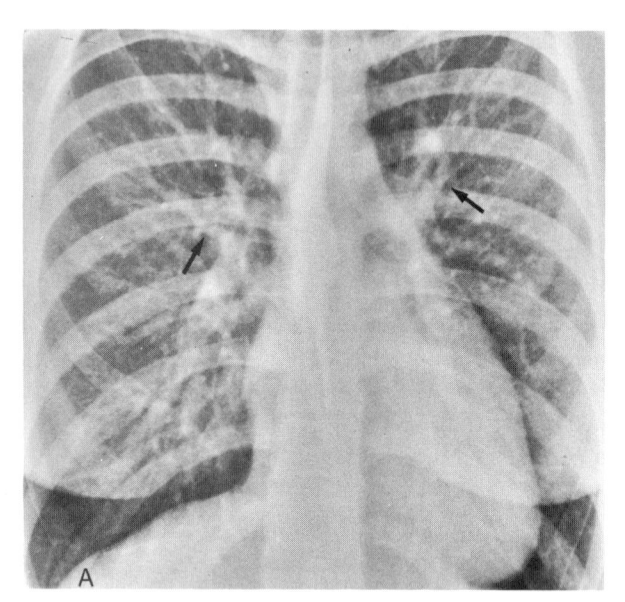

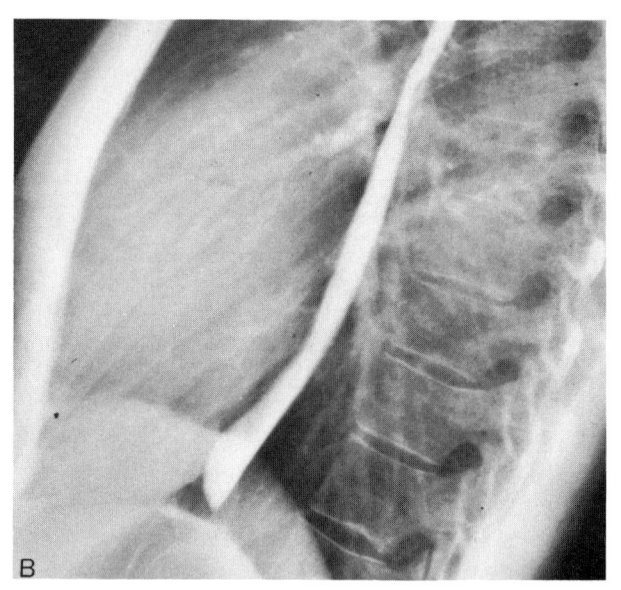

FIG 68–3.
Mitral valve prolapse with sudden onset of marked regurgitation because of chordal rupture. Thoracic roentgenogram. **A,** posteroanterior projection. Diffuse accentuation of venous pulmonary vasculature *(arrows)*. Straightening of left cardiac border may be caused by prominence of left atrial appendage. **B,** lateral projection. No significant left atrial enlargement because dilatation of left atrium and ventricle takes time to develop.

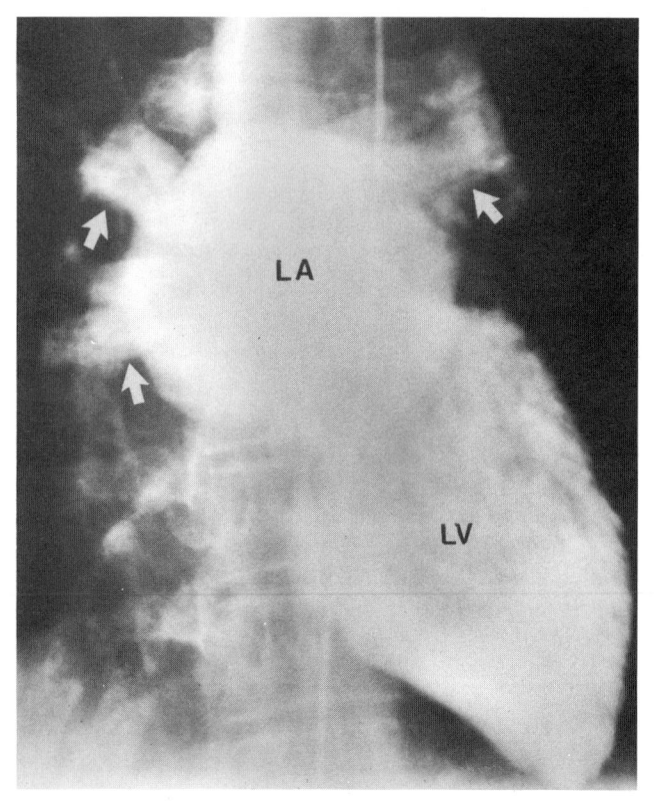

FIG 68–4.
Mitral valve prolapse. Same patient as in Figure 68–3. Left ventriculogram *(LV)*. Anteroposterior projection. Slightly enlarged left ventricle. Marked mitral regurgitation. Normal-sized left atrium *(LA)*. Dense opacification of pulmonary veins *(arrows)*, characteristic of recently acquired mitral regurgitation.

4. In acute and massive mitral regurgitation from chordal rupture, the left atrium is normal sized. It cannot accept the entire regurgitation blood volume. Consequently pulmonary veins opacify during systole on an angiogram (Fig 68–4).

5. The distended pulmonary veins may be seen on a thoracic roentgenogram (see Fig 68–3).

ANGIOGRAPHIC FEATURES

Left ventriculography performed in a right anterior oblique projection provides the best information about the degree of mitral regurgitation and mitral valve deformity. However, in this projection, because the anterior and posterior mitral leaflets are superimposed, the degree of involvement of the individual mitral valve leaflets cannot be determined. Either a very steep left anterior oblique or a lateral projection allows visualization of the individual leaflets to identify the nature of mitral valve anomaly. The posterior leaflet is invariably involved, but the anterior leaflet may be involved in advanced cases as well.

In most patients the angiographic findings are characteristic, allowing a firm diagnosis of prolapsed mitral valve.[29] Sometimes rupture of the chordae tendineae or papillary muscle with an otherwise normal mitral valve may result in prolapse and a similar angiographic appearance.

1. On an anteroposterior projection, a characteristic ring-like double density may be seen around the posterior

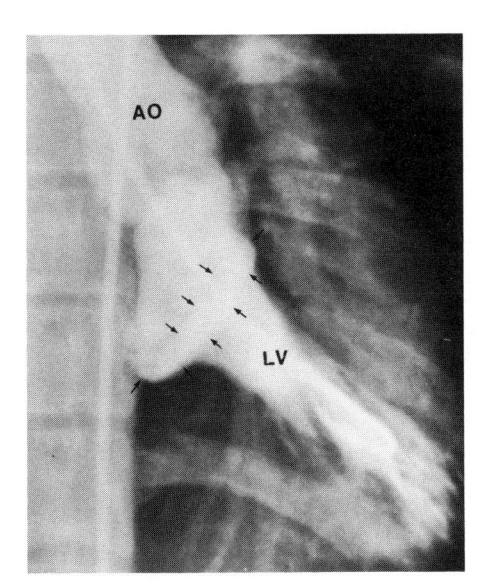

FIG 68–5.
Mitral valve prolapse. Left ventriculogram *(LV)*. Anteroposterior projection. Small left ventricular cavity is caused by ventricular extrasystoles. Ringlike double density along attachment of posterior mitral leaflet *(arrows)* because contrast medium is trapped behind prolapsing leaflet. No mitral regurgitation. *Ao* = aorta.

mitral annulus (Fig 68–5). REASON: Contrast medium is trapped beneath the ballooning prolapsed posterior leaflet of the mitral valve.

2. The steep left anterior oblique or lateral projection allows differentiation between posterior and anterior MVP (Fig 68–6).

3. On right anterior oblique left ventriculograms, both the grade of mitral insufficiency and the degree of mitral valve deformity can be determined. The degree of prolapse is graded by the distance between mitral annulus and prolapsing mitral valve leaflet during systole. The latter follows the anatomic classification.

4. With grade 1 deformity, only part of the posterior leaflet or anterior leaflet is involved. Interchordal hooding of the leaflets is of a minor degree (Fig 68–7). The valve extends only slightly beyond the annulus. There is a continuous spectrum from normal to grade 1 prolapse, because the mitral valve normally projects slightly beyond the annulus in systole.

5. With grade 2 deformity, interchordal hooding and prolapse are more pronounced (Fig 68–8).

6. With grade 3 deformity, there is marked hooding, which typically involves both leaflets, and there is significant mitral regurgitation (Fig 68–9).

7. Prolapse and hooding of the tricuspid valve (Fig 68–10) may occur, but it is much less common than MVP. Marked tricuspid insufficiency may be present. Tricuspid prolapse may be part of Marfan syndrome. The angiographic appearance is very similar to mitral valve prolapse.

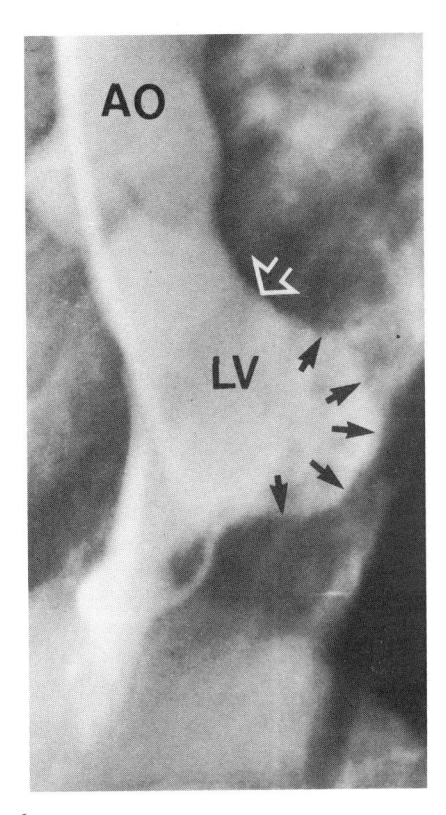

FIG 68–6.
Mitral valve prolapse. Left ventriculogram *(LV)*. Lateral projection. Marked prolapse of posterior leaflet *(white arrows)*. Anterior leaflet *(open arrow)* is not involved. *AO* = Aorta.

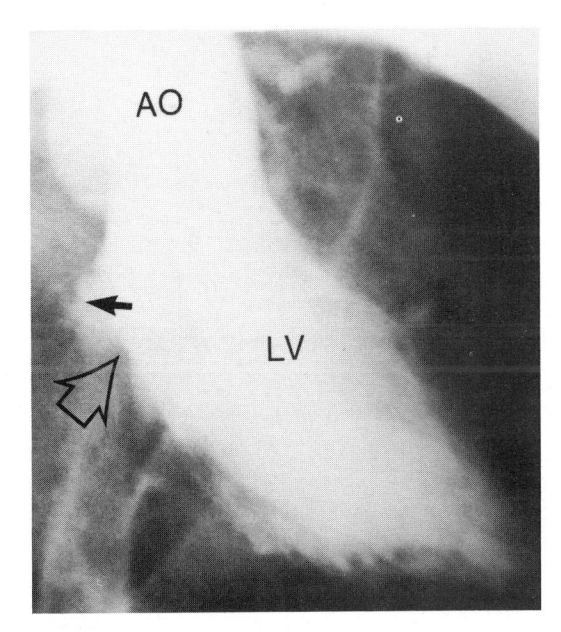

FIG 68–7.
Mitral valve prolapse grade 1. Left ventriculogram *(LV)*. Right anterior oblique projection. A small segment of mitral valve prolapses *(black arrow)* beyond mitral valve annulus *(open arrow)*. Degree of prolapse and interchordal hooding are minor. *AO* = aorta.

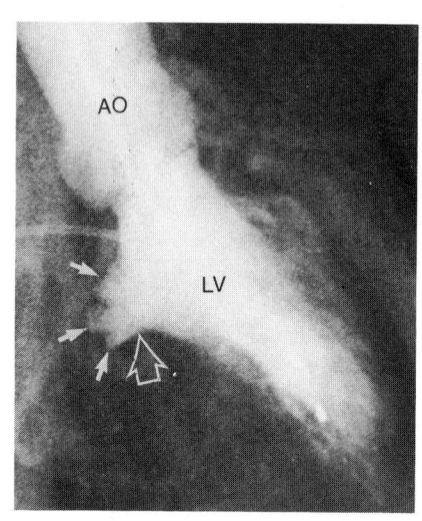

FIG 68-8.
Mitral valve prolapse grade 2. Left ventriculogram (LV). Right anterior oblique projection. Only part of mitral valve is involved. Distinct hooding (solid arrows) and systolic prolapse beyond mitral annulus (open arrow). No mitral regurgitation as yet. AO = aorta.

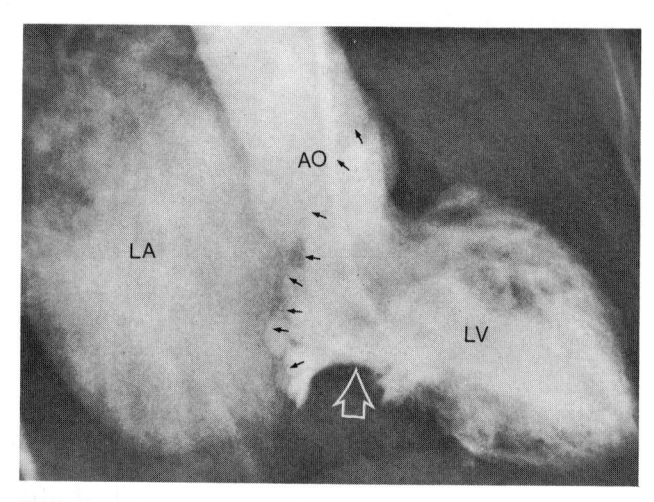

FIG 68-9.
Mitral valve prolapse grade 3. Left ventriculogram (LV). Right anterior oblique projection. Mitral valve prolapse far beyond mitral annulus (open arrow) deep into left atrium. Prolapse also involves anterior leaflets (arrows). Extensive intrachordal hooding of mitral valve. Marked mitral regurgitation outlines enlarged left atrium (LA). AO = aorta.

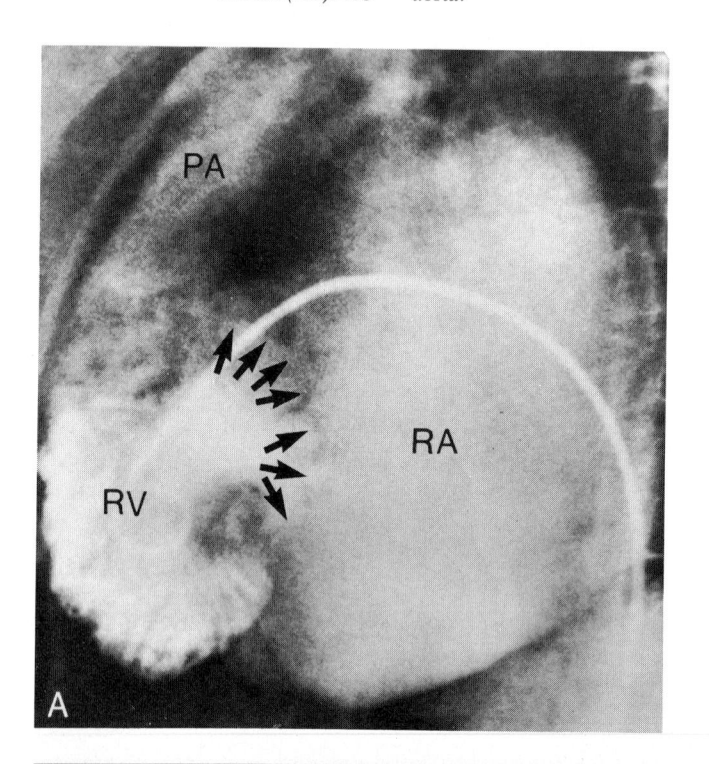

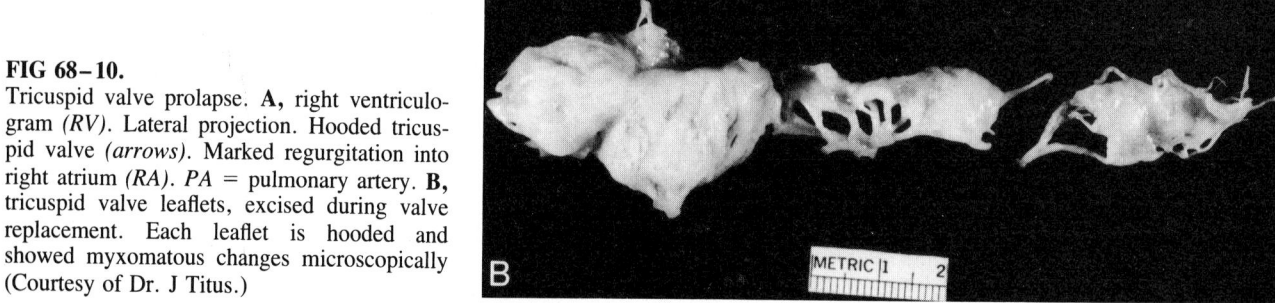

FIG 68-10.
Tricuspid valve prolapse. **A,** right ventriculogram (RV). Lateral projection. Hooded tricuspid valve (arrows). Marked regurgitation into right atrium (RA). PA = pulmonary artery. **B,** tricuspid valve leaflets, excised during valve replacement. Each leaflet is hooded and showed myxomatous changes microscopically (Courtesy of Dr. J Titus.)

MANAGEMENT

Mitral valve prolapse is generally a benign condition, and patients should be counselled accordingly. No restrictions need to be placed on activity of most patients. Bacterial endocarditis prophylaxis is administered to those with clinical findings of mitral insufficiency.[30] The risk of endocarditis is low among individuals with MVP and without mitral insufficiency.

Electrocardiograms should be performed periodically to detect ST-T wave abnormalities or arrhythmias. If present, an exercise stress test and 24-hour continuous ECG monitoring should be performed, especially to advise individuals regarding physical activities.

Therapy is recommended for patients with symptoms of palpitations, dizziness, or syncope associated with arrhythmias, those with frequent premature ventricular contractions, or those with ventricular tachycardia or fibrillation. β-Blocking agents have been used at times in combination with other antiarrhythmic agents. It is the group of patients with a history of syncope, abnormal exercise response, and ECG with ST-T wave changes suggesting ischemia or ventricular arrhythmia who are at risk of sudden death. Sudden death is a rare occurrence in this common condition,[31] and patients should be reassured regarding its rarity.

REFERENCES

1. Savage DD, Garrison RJ, Devereux RB, et al: Mitral valve prolapse in the general population: I, epidemiologic features: the Framingham study, *Am Heart J* 106:571, 1983.
2. Procacci PM, Savran SV, Schreiter SL, et al: Prevalence of clinical mitral-valve prolapse in 1169 young women, *N Engl J Med* 294:1086, 1976.
3. Alpert MA, Carney RJ, Flaker GC, et al: Sensitivity and specificity of two-dimensional echocardiographic signs of mitral valve prolapse, *Am J Cardiol* 54:792, 1984.
4. Lucas RV Jr, Edwards JE: The floppy mitral valve, *Curr Probl Cardiol* 7:1, 1982.
5. Waller BF, Morrow AG, Maron BJ, et al: Etiology of clinically isolated, severe, chronic, pure mitral regurgitation: analysis of 97 patients over 30 years of age having mitral valve replacement, *Am Heart J* 104:276, 1982.
6. Jeresaty RM, Edwards JE, Chawla SK: Mitral valve prolapse and ruptured chordae tendineae, *Am J Cardiol* 55:138, 1985.
7. Barnett HJM, Boughner DR, Taylor DW, et al: Further evidence relating mitral valve prolapse to cerebral ischemic events, *N Engl J Med* 302:139, 1980.
8. Perloff JK: Evolving concepts of mitral-valve prolapse, *N Engl J Med* 307:369, 1982.
9. King BD, Clark MA, Baba N, et al: "Myxomatous" mitral valves: collagen dissolution as the primary defect, *Circulation* 66:288, 1982.
10. Van Der Bel-Kahn J, Duren DR, Becker AE: Isolated mitral valve prolapse: chordal architecture as an anatomic basis in older patients, *J Am Coll Cardiol* 5:1335, 1985.
11. Malcolm AD: Mitral valve prolapse associated with other disorders: casual coincidence, common link, or fundamental genetic disturbance? *Br Heart J* 53:353, 1985.
12. Leachman RD, Cokkinos DV, Cooley DA: Association of ostium secundum atrial septal defects with mitral valve prolapse, *Am J Cardiol* 38:167, 1976.
13. Allen H, Harris A, Leatham A: Significance and prognosis of an isolated late systolic murmur: a 9- to 22-year follow-up, *Br Heart J* 36:525, 1974.
14. Nishimura RA, McGoon MD, Shub C, et al: Echocardiographically documented mitral-valve prolapse: long-term follow-up of 237 patients, *N Engl J Med* 313:1305, 1985.
15. Savage DD, Garrison RJ, Devereux RB, et al: Mitral valve prolapse in the general population: II, clinical features: the Framingham study, *Am Heart J* 106:577, 1983.
16. Bisset GS III, Schwartz DC, Meyer RA, et al: Clinical spectrum and long-term follow-up of isolated mitral valve prolapse in 119 children, *Circulation* 62:423, 1980.
17. Tei C, Shah PM, Cherian G, et al: The correlates of an abnormal first heart sound in mitral-valve-prolapse syndromes, *N Engl J Med* 307:334, 1982.
18. Barlow JB, Pocock WA: Mitral valve prolapse, the specific billowing mitral leaflet syndrome, or an insignificant non-ejection systolic click, *Am Heart J* 97:277, 1979.
19. Fontana ME, Wooley CF, Leighton RF, et al: Postural changes in left ventricular and mitral valvular dynamics in the systolic click—late systolic murmur syndrome, *Circulation* 51:165, 1975.
20. Fontana ME, Pence HL, Leighton RF, et al: The varying clinical spectrum of the systolic click-late systolic murmur syndrome: a postural auscultatory phenomenon, *Circulation* 41:807, 1970.
21. Barlow JB, Pocock WA, Marchand P, et al: The significance of late systolic murmurs, *Am Heart J* 66:443, 1963.
22. Felner JM, Harwood S, Mond H, et al: Systolic honks in young children, *Am J Cardiol* 40:206, 1977.
23. Chandraratna PAN, Tolentino AO, Mutucumarana W, et al: Echocardiographic observations on the association between mitral valve prolapse and asymmetric septal hypertrophy, *Circulation* 55:622, 1977.
24. DeMaria AN, King JF, Bogren HG, et al: The variable spectrum of echocardiographic manifestations on the mitral valve prolapse syndrome, *Circulation* 50:33, 1974.
25. Sahn DJ, Allen HD, Goldberg SJ, et al: Mitral valve prolapse in children: a problem defined by real-time cross-sectional echocardiography, *Circulation* 53:651, 1976.
26. Winkle RA, Goodman DJ, Popp RL: Simultaneous echocardiographic-phonocardiographic recordings at rest and during amyl nitrite administration in patients with mitral valve prolapse, *Circulation* 51:522, 1975.
27. Weiss AN, Mimbs JW, Ludbrook PA, et al: Echocardiographic detection of mitral valve prolapse: exclusion of false positive diagnosis and determination of inheritance, *Circulation* 52:1091, 1975.

28. Bon Tempo CP, Ronan JA Jr, deLeon AC Jr, et al: Radiographic appearance of the thorax in systolic click-late systolic murmur syndrome, *Am J Cardiol* 36:27, 1975.
29. Ranganathan N, Silver MD, Robinson TI, et al: Angiographic-morphologic correlation in patients with severe mitral regurgitation due to prolapse of the posterior mitral valve leaflet, *Circulation* 48:514, 1973.
30. Hickey AJ, MacMahon SW, Wilcken DEL: Mitral valve prolapse and bacterial endocarditis: When is antibiotic prophylaxis necessary? *Am Heart J* 109:431, 1985.
31. Chesler E, King RA, Edwards JE: The myxomatous mitral valve and sudden death, *Circulation* 67:632, 1983.

CHAPTER 69

Abnormalities of the Mitral Valve

Abnormalities of the mitral valve include a variety of conditions that may cause mitral obstruction, mitral regurgitation, or aortic outflow obstruction:

1. Mitral obstruction.
   a. Typical congenital mitral stenosis occurs with short chordae tendineae, reduction of intrachordal spaces, and reduction of intrapapillary distance.
   b. Congenital mitral stenosis caused by a hypoplastic valve almost always is associated with hypoplastic left heart syndrome.
   c. Supravalvar mitral ring.
   d. Parachute mitral valve.
   e. Duplication of the mitral valve.
   f. Abnormal mitral valve attachment. One or more chordae tendineae may insert directly into the free wall of the left ventricle, and the mitral valve may attach virtually directly into the papillary muscle with either very short or no chordae tendineae. This condition is probably the same as mitral arcade.
2. Left ventricular outflow obstruction by mitral valve anomalies.
   a. Redundant mitral valve tissue may cause left ventricular outflow tract obstruction. As pedunculated tissue attached to the mitral valve annulus, it moved through the aortic valve during systole and causes obstruction.
   b. Left ventricular outflow obstruction occurs from a parachute accessory mitral leaflet.
   c. Obstruction may occur when the anterior mitral valve leaflet attaches directly to the ventricular septum.
   d. Subaortic stenosis may be due to accessory valvar tissue, either mitral valve or tricuspid valve herniating through a ventricular septal defect.
3. Mitral regurgitation.
   a. Anatomically normal mitral valve.
   b. Abnormalities of the chordae tendineae.
   c. Inadequate mitral valve tissue.

CONGENITAL MITRAL INSUFFICIENCY

Mitral regurgitation with an anatomically normal mitral valve is usually caused by left ventricular enlargement (aortic valve regurgitation, myocarditis, and cardiomyopathies), which results in dilatation of the mitral annulus. The dilated annulus holds the anatomically normal valve leaflets apart during ventricular systole, resulting in mitral regurgitation. This type of mitral regurgitation is a secondary phenomenon and is also referred to as "relative mitral insufficiency." It frequently disappears if the left ventricle decreases in size.

Another cause of mitral regurgitation is dilatation of the left atrium. The endocardial surface of the mitral valve is continuous with the endocardial surface of the left atrium. If the left atrium enlarges, the leaflets of the mitral valve, particularly the posterior leaflet, are stretched and pulled downward against the free edge of the left ventricle (Fig 69–1). This stretching and tension of the posterior leaflet prevents normal mobility and results in mitral regurgitation. This type of mitral regurgitation is also relative and may disappear after the left atrium decreases in size.

The most common cause of congenital mitral regurgitation is chordal abnormalities. The chordae tendineae may

AGGRAVATION OF MITRAL REFLUX BY LEFT ATRIAL ENLARGEMENT

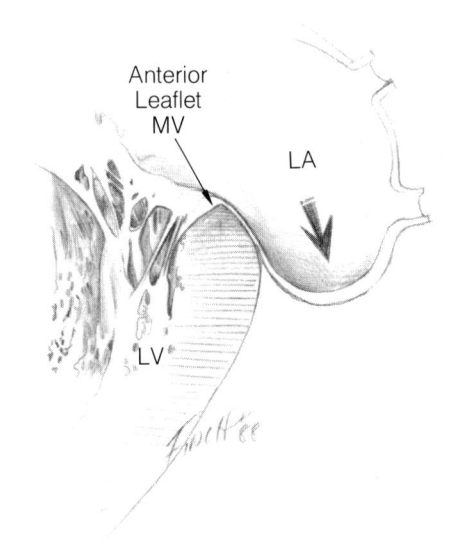

FIG 69–1.
Mechanism of aggravation of mitral regurgitation by marked left atrial enlargement. Posterior leaflet of mitral valve *(MV)* is pulled down draping over mitral annulus. This aggravates mitral regurgitation. *LA* = left atrium; *LV* = left ventricle.

insert anomalously into the septal or free wall of the left ventricle, and the chordae tendineae may be markedly thickened and shortened, interfering with adequate motion and closure of the mitral valve. This type of mitral regurgitation is commonly seen with endocardial sclerosis (see Chapter 56). Mitral regurgitation may also result when chordae tendineae are partially absent, thin, or elongated. Marked elongation of the chordae tendineae allows prolapse and overshoot of mitral leaflets, resulting in regurgitation.

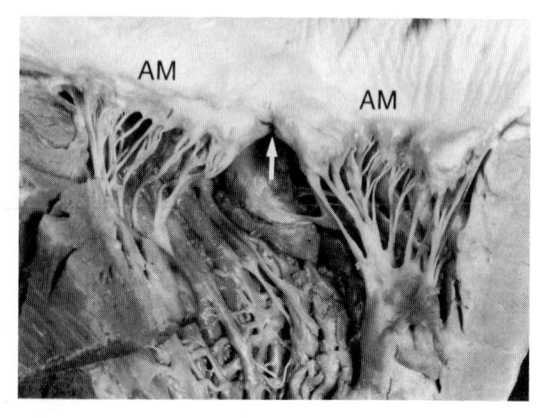

FIG 69–2.
Cleft anterior leaflet of mitral valve *(AM)*. Close-up view. Leaflet is split by a cleft *(arrow)* into superior and inferior halves. Typically atrial and ventricular septae are intact.

The valve tissues may be hypoplastic, retracted, or absent, particularly the anterior leaflet. Fibrotic thickening of valve tissue may increase valve rigidity and mitral regurgitation.

The mitral valve may be redundant and attached to thin elongated chordae tendineae, and these factors allow reflux and "hooding" (see Chapters 67, 68). A rare congenital mitral valve anomaly is an isolated cleft in the anterior leaflet of the mitral valve. Because this cleft is commonly associated with abnormal insertion of chordae tendineae (Fig 69–2), it is considered to be part of the endocardial cushion defect, in spite of an intact atrial and ventricular septum (see Chapter 23). An isolated cleft in the anterior leaflet of the mitral valve may result in a variable degree of mitral regurgitation, or the mitral valve may remain competent (rare).

A rare cause of mitral regurgitation is congenital duplication of the mitral valve or double-orifice mitral valve. In double-orifice mitral valve, an extra orifice is present in the midportion of the anterior leaflet of the mitral valve. From the circumference of this orifice, chordae tendineae pass to a set of papillary muscles in the left ventricle. Because of its anatomic location in the mitral valve, this anomaly has been considered a form of endocardial cushion defect. The papillary muscle–chordal mechanism may not close the orifice, so that mitral regurgitation results. Double-orifice mitral valve occurs as an isolated lesion or may coexist with another congenital cardiac anomaly (Fig 69–3).

DOUBLE ORIFICE OF THE MITRAL VALVE

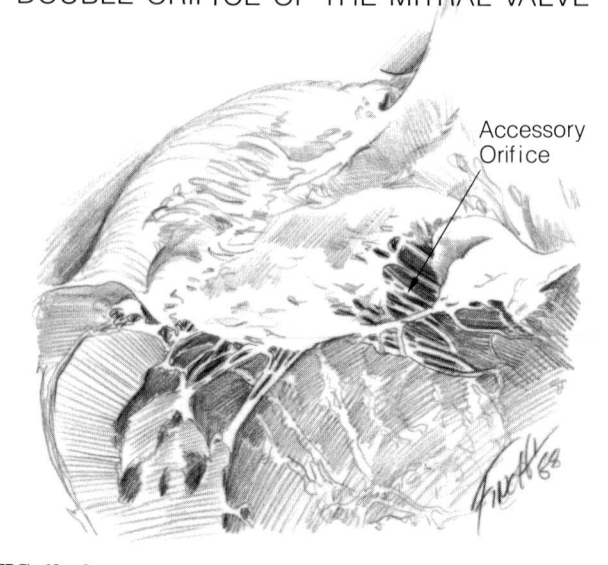

FIG 69–3.
Double-orifice mitral valve. One leaflet has accessory orifice, which may cause mitral insufficiency. Similar defect may occur in tricuspid valve, also leading to regurgitation.

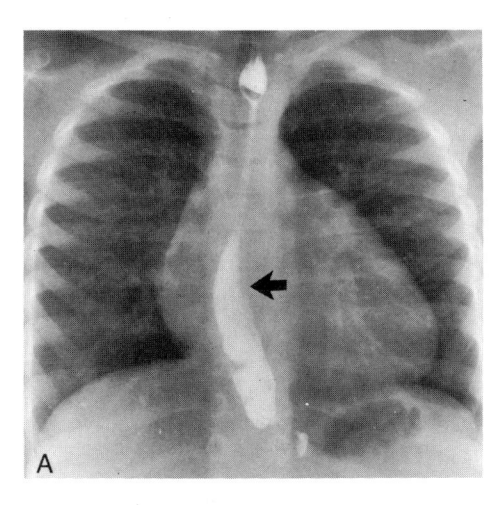

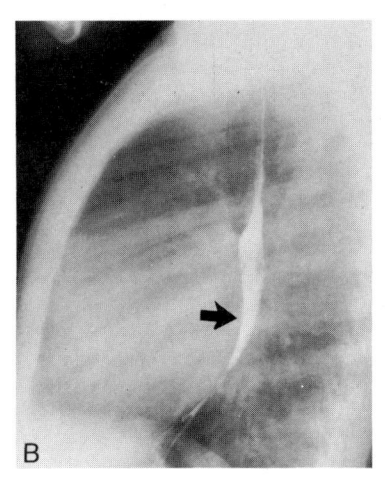

FIG 69–4.
Congenital mitral insufficiency from cleft mitral valve. Thoracic roentgenogram. **A,** posteroanterior projection. Cardiomegaly. Normal pulmonary vasculature. Kerley B lines and cephalization are absent. Barium-filled esophagus is displaced to left *(arrow)* by enlarged left atrium. **B,** lateral projection. Cardiac enlargement. Posterior displacement *(arrow)* of barium-filled esophagus by enlarged left atrium.

Radiographic Features

The degree of mitral regurgitation in this condition can be suspected from thoracic roentgenograms. The type of the mitral anomaly is, however, not apparent.

1. The cardiac silhouette shows a variable degree of enlargement (Fig 69–4,A). REASON: Mitral regurgitation results in left ventricular enlargement, which is well seen on a posteroanterior thoracic roentgenogram.

2. There is a variable degree of left atrial enlargement, as evidenced by displacement of the barium-filled esophagus (Fig 69–4,B). Generally the left atrium is larger in mitral regurgitation than in mitral stenosis. The largest left atria are produced by mitral regurgitation.

3. In contrast to mitral stenosis, radiographic signs of severe venous pulmonary hypertension, such as cephalization and Kerley B lines, are usually absent.

4. Slight increase of the venous pulmonary vasculature may be observed. REASON: Mitral insufficiency causes not only left atrial enlargement but also enlargement of the pulmonary veins.

Angiographic Features

Left ventriculography is indicated to assess the degree of mitral regurgitation. Careful placement of the catheter in a "quiet" zone in the left ventricle away from the mitral

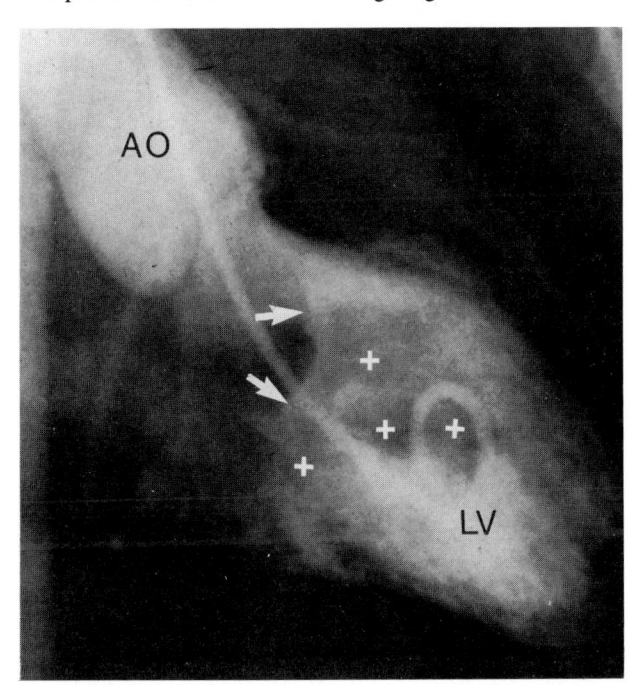

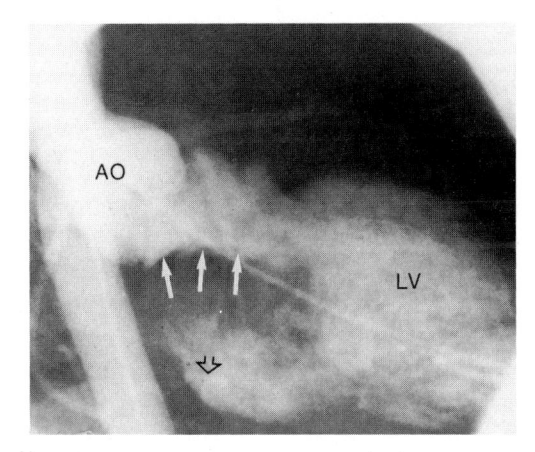

FIG 69–5.
Normal mitral valve. Left ventriculogram *(LV)*. Right anterior oblique projection. Diastole. Mitral valve leaflets are not seen because they are superimposed and viewed en face. Blood enters left ventricle and mixes freely with contrast medium, creating ill-defined radiolucency *(crosses)*. Posterior annulus is visible *(arrows)*. *AO* = aorta.

FIG 69–6.
Isolated cleft mitral valve. Left ventriculogram *(LV)*. Right anterior oblique projection. Diastole. Superior half of cleft anterior leaflet opens and is seen in profile *(arrows)*. It is outined by unopacified blood beneath and by contrast medium above. Inferior half of anterior leaflet is not well seen *(open arrow)*. *AO* = aorta.

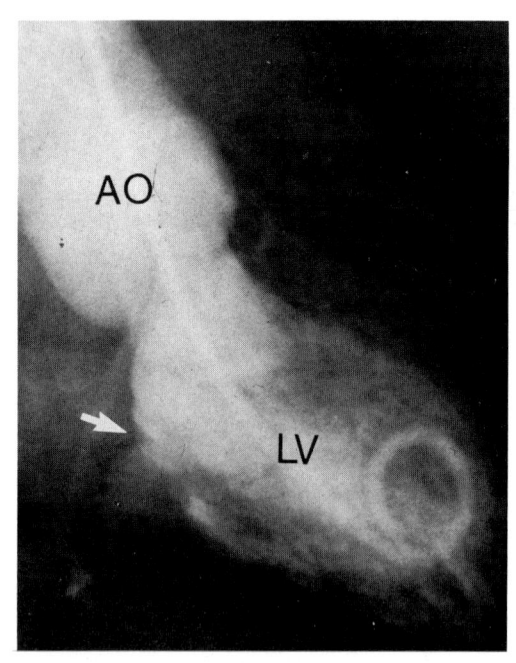

FIG 69–7.
Normal mitral valve. Left ventriculogram *(LV)*. Right anterior oblique projection. Systole. Small irregularity of mitral valve simulates cleft *(arrow)*. AO = aorta.

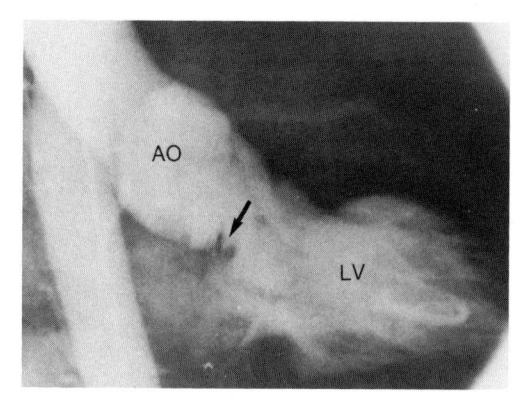

FIG 69–8.
Isolated mitral cleft. Left ventriculogram *(LV)*. Right anterior oblique projection. Mitral valve is closed. Edges of cleft anterior leaflet forms a distinct small filling defect *(arrow)*. AO = aorta.

valve is very important. The proximity of the catheter to the mitral valve or a prolonged burst of ventricular extrasystoles may induce mitral regurgitation. Because the incidence of ventricular extrasystoles is related to the contrast jets coming through the sideholes of the catheter striking the myocardium, a large-caliber catheter should be used. Thereby the jet energy is less, because a lower pressure is necessary to deliver the contrast medium. It is advantageous to use a balloon catheter, because it can hold the sideholes away from the endocardium, dissipating the energy of the jet by mixing with blood (see Chapter 8). A slower injection rate will also minimize extra systoles.

Relative mitral insufficiency and mitral regurgitation caused by deficient valve tissue can sometimes be diagnosed by angiography. All chordal anomalies, however, cannot be seen angiographically. The differentiation between regurgitation caused by chordal anomalies and deficient valve tissue, particularly cleft in the anterior leaflet of the mitral valve, is of practical importance, because a cleft can be repaired relatively simply surgically, whereas correction of chordal anomalies requires valve replacement or sophisticated valvuloplastic procedures, with generally poor results. Even with echocardiography, it is sometimes impossible to predict the exact valve anomaly, but angiography allows exclusion of a cleft or floppy mitral valve. This is accomplished by left ventriculography performed in the right anterior oblique position using an adequate amount of fairly rapidly injected contrast medium. REASON: Because of mitral regurgitation, the stroke volume of the left ventricle is increased; consequently, contrast medium tends to be markedly diluted. Careful observation of the mitral valve during both systole and diastole is important.

With an intact anterior leaflet, the diastolic inflow of blood during diastole can be observed as the blood mixes with contrast medium. The anterior mitral leaflet is seen en face (Fig 69–5) (see Chapter 2).

On the other hand, if the anterior leaflet of the mitral valve is cleft, its superior half opens similar to a door and is seen in profile, outlined on one side by unopacified blood entering the left ventricle, and on the other side by residual contrast medium (Fig 69–6). Unfortunately, only the anterior leaflet is usually seen in profile, but this angiographic finding (diastolic gooseneck deformity) is the best radiographic clue to diagnose an isolated cleft. The typical gooseneck deformity caused by foreshortening of the posterior septum is absent in this condition (see Chapter 23).

The systolic view with the closed mitral valve is less diagnostic, because a slight irregularity of the normal mitral valve may simulate a cleft (Fig 69–7). If the anterior leaflet of the mitral valve is cleft, the cleft can consistently be seen during systole as a characteristic filling defect (Fig 69–8). This defect is caused by the rolled, slightly thickened edges of both split anterior leaflets, which are coapted during systole.

CHAPTER 70

Congenital Diverticulum of the Ventricles

A congenital cardiac diverticulum is an outpouching from a ventricle, including in its wall, myocardium, endocardium, and occasionally the pericardium. Congenital diverticula are rare and usually coexist with an underlying congenital cardiac malformation. Generally no symptoms or abnormal clinical or laboratory findings result from the diverticulum, with the diverticulum being discovered during angiography or postmortem examination. Diverticula may occur from either the right, left, or both ventricles.

A cardiac diverticulum is probably an abnormal development during the embryonic life when the cardiac wall may become attached through the septum transversum to structures forming the yolk sac and then becomes drawn out as the embryo grows.

RIGHT VENTRICULAR DIVERTICULUM

Congenital diverticulum of the right ventricle may arise at either the apex or the lateral aspect of the base of the heart and project anteriorly. The composition of the wall is variable; both fibrous[1,2] and normal myocardial structures[1,3] have been reported. Rupture of a right ventricular diverticulum has been described in a 1 month old child.[4] Although the diverticulum may occur in individuals without other cardiac anomalies, most cases have coexistent congenital cardiac malformations, including tetralogy of Fallot,[1,3] double-outlet right ventricle,[5] truncus arteriosus,[4] atrial septal defect,[2] and left ventricular–right atrial shunt.[6] Both normal and paradoxical contractility of right ventricular diverticula have been described, depending on the histologic composition of its wall (fibrous or muscular). A fibrous diverticulum is perhaps more likely to rupture. It shows paradoxical systolic expansion.

Radiographic Features

Right ventricular diverticula are exceedingly rare. Like congenital left ventricular diverticula, they are usually not evident on a thoracic radiograph.

Angiographic Features

Angiographic visualization of a right ventricular diverticulum is important, because some consist principally of fibrous tissue and show paradoxical systolic expansion. Such a diverticulum represents a potential hemodynamic burden to the right ventricle and has the potential to rupture if right ventricular hypertension exists. Opacification is best accomplished by selective right ventriculography.

A diverticulum is usually seen as a broad-based outpouching from the right ventricle (Fig 70–1).

The composition of the diverticulum can be determined by the pattern of contraction during systole. Like a left ventricular diverticulum, contraction occurs during systole if the diverticulum contains muscle. A diverticulum composed of fibrous tissue demonstrates paradoxical systolic expansion (see Fig 70–1).

Operative Considerations

Operative extirpation (Fig 70–2,B) of the diverticulum, correction of intracardiac anomalies, if present, and closure of any interior body wall defect are performed as a single procedure.

LEFT VENTRICULAR DIVERTICULUM

Congenital left ventricular diverticula should not be confused with left ventricular aneurysms, which usually

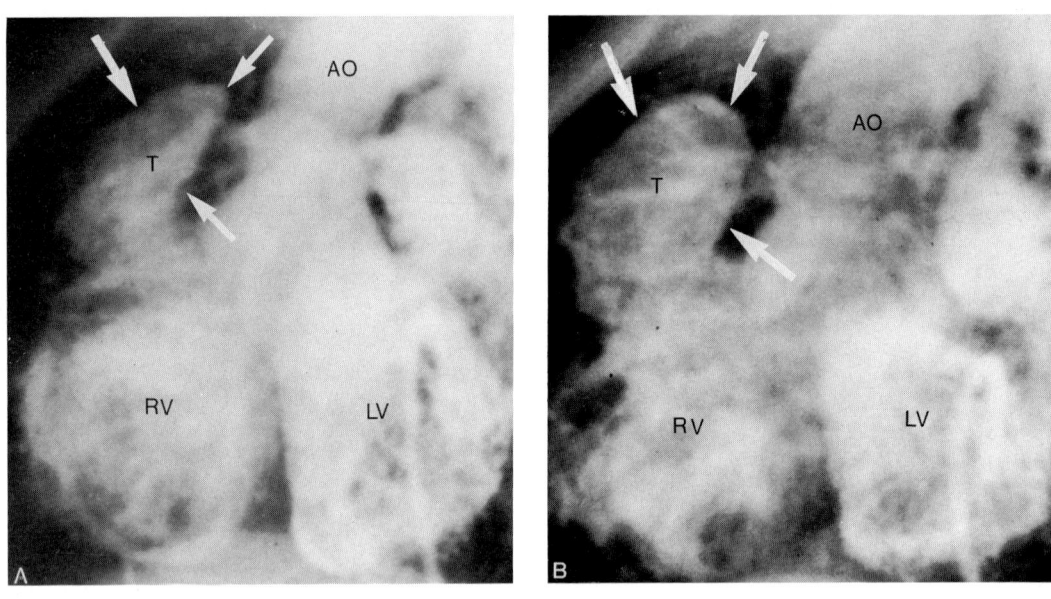

FIG 70–1.
Tetralogy of Fallot and right ventricular diverticulum. Right ventriculogram. Lateral projection. **A,** diastole. Both ventricles are opacified via ventricular communication. Large right ventricular diverticulum *(T)* along anterosuperior surface of right ventricle *(arrows)*. **B,** systole. Both ventricles are contracted, whereas diverticulum has expanded *(arrows)*, indicating fibrous rather than muscular tissue. At postmortem examination, diverticulum was fibrous and revealed endocardial fibroelastosis. It was considered to be congenital despite absence of muscle. *AO* = aorta; *LV* = left ventricle; *RV* = right ventricle.

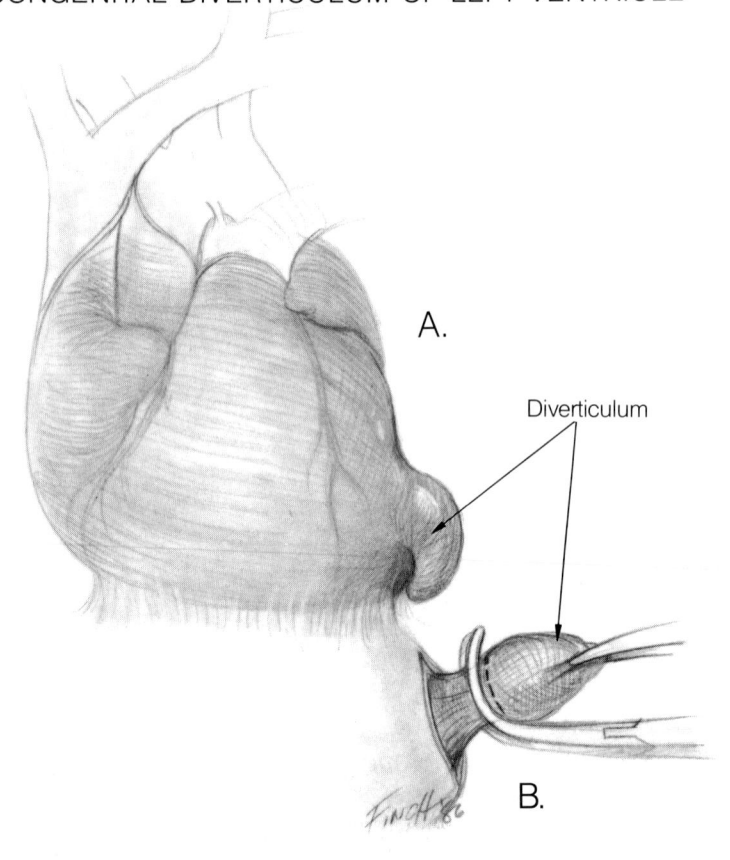

FIG 70–2.
Congenital diverticulum of left ventricle. **A,** apical location. **B,** insert. Surgical extirpation. Base of diverticulum is closed by sutures.

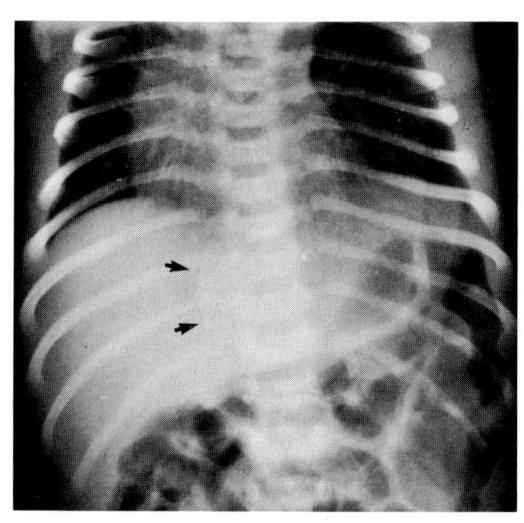

FIG 70-3.
Left ventricular diverticulum. Thoracic roentgenogram. Anterioposterior projection. Mass *(arrows)* in upper half of abdomen. Sharp margins of mass suggest it is surrounded by air and consequently outside thoracic cavity. Cardiac contour and pulmonary vasculature are normal. Minimal dextroposition of heart.

occur from myocardial infarction. Whereas congenital ventricular diverticula show either contraction or systolic expansion (dyskynesis), aneurysms caused by myocardial infarction tend to be broad based and akynetic (no wall motion). Muscular left ventricular diverticula generally arise from either of two sites—at the apex or at the base. When the diverticulum is located at the cardiac apex, it tends to be long and narrow and usually associated with a thoracic-abdominal defect. This has been described as part of a syndrome consisting of:[7-15]

1. A midline supraumbilical abdominal wall defect.
2. Short sternum.
3. Deficiency of the anterior diaphragm.
4. Defect of the diaphragmatic pericardium.
5. Congenital intracardiac anomalies.
6. Dextroposition of the heart.

Each of the components is not necessarily present in every case. The reported associated cardiac anomalies have been ventricular septal defect, tetralogy of Fallot, atrial septal defect, truncus arteriosus, and tricuspid atresia.[7-15]

The diagnosis is usually established by finding a pulsatile mass in the upper abdomen, because 60% of the cases have an associated omphalocele or hiatal hernia. Such cases have also been classified as partial ectopia cordis, but this is incorrect, because the heart remains within the thorax.

In contrast, fibrous diverticula of the left ventricle are generally located at the base rather than at the cardiac apex.[16-18] Fibrous diverticula may be located close to either the mitral or aortic valve annulus and may produce either mitral or aortic incompetence (submitral and subaortic aneurysm). These diverticula may be single or multiple, are subannular in position, and have a narrow connection with the left ventricle. Calcium deposits have been reported in the fibrous type but not in the muscular type. Most of the patients with a fibrous diverticulum have been either African Americans or Africans. The fibrous type is never associated with a midline defect or a congenital cardiac malformation. Mitral insufficiency probably results from involvement of papillary muscles, which may lead to symptoms. In this type the electrocardiogram may show findings of anterolateral myocardial infarction.

Left ventricular diverticula rarely rupture.[19] Left ventricular diverticula have also been described in coexistent hypoplastic right ventricle and ventricular septal defect[20] and in hypertrophic cardiomyopathy.[21] Routine left ventriculography in patients undergoing coronary angiography demonstrates left ventricular diverticula as an incidental finding. However, its occurrence is very rare.

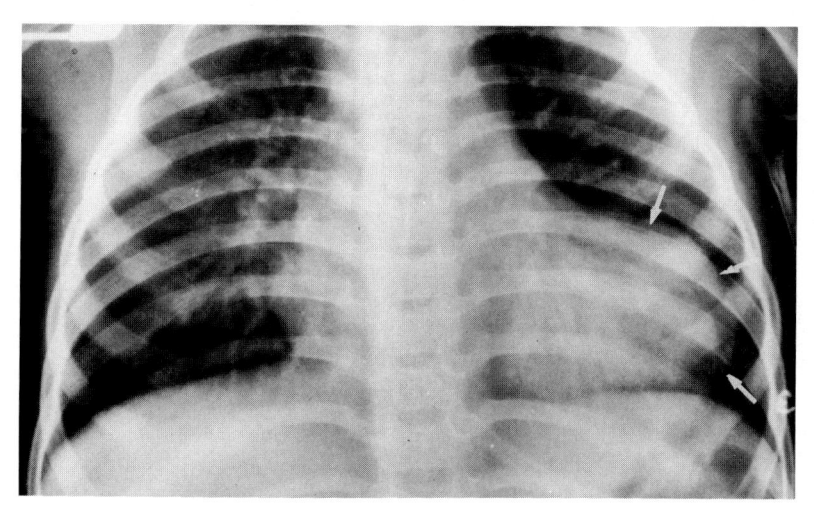

FIG 70-4.
Left ventricular diverticulum. Thoracic roentgenogram. Posteroanterior projection. Huge broad-based large left ventricular diverticulum *(arrows)* produces an abnormal left ventricular contour.

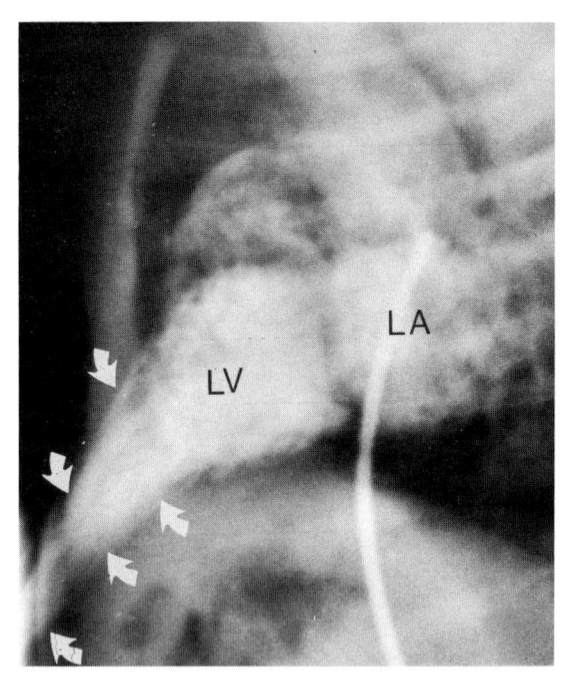

FIG 70–5.
Left ventricular diverticulum with thoracoabdominal defect. Same patient as in Figure 70–3. Left atriogram *(LA)*. Lateral projection. Long diverticulum of apex of left ventricle *(LV)* extends beyond thorax into hernial sac *(arrows)*.

Radiographic Features

When a left ventricular diverticulum occurs without a defect in the abdominal wall, the diagnosis cannot be suspected from a thoracic roentgenogram.

When it is associated with the thoracic-abdominal syndrome, the following radiographic features are common:

1. The left ventricular diverticulum extends through a defect of the abdominal wall and causes a mass density on an anteroposterior roentgenogram and an abdominal wall hernia (Fig 70–3).

2. During inspiration the heart shifts markedly into the right thoracic cavity. REASON: Lack of support of the heart because of the short sternum, defect of pericardium, and defect of anterior abdominal wall (see Fig 70–3).

3. The commonly associated short sternum is not apparent radiologically, because in most patients radiographs are obtained at an age when the sternum is not yet ossified.

4. When a left ventricular diverticulum is unassociated with thoracic or abdominal defects, the radiographic findings are either very subtle or normal, in spite of the obvious extension beyond the angiographically demonstrated ventricle.

5. With the very rare huge diverticulum, an abnormal cardiac contour can be seen (Fig 70–4).

Angiography

Angiography is important in the delineation of a left ventricular diverticulum, and its size, and its histologic composition. Most congenital left ventricular diverticula contain endocardium, myocardium, and epicardium and consequently show a normal contraction pattern. Commonly the contraction is slightly delayed from the left ventricle proper. Congenital ventricular aneurysms with a fibrous wall occur more frequently in the region of the mitral annulus and show either no or paradoxical contraction. Because this type of aneurysm may cause mitral regurgitation, significant hemodynamic burden is placed on the left ventricle. They can rupture spontaneously or with trauma; consequently, surgery must be performed in most cases. Left ventricular diverticulum can be well opacified by either left ventriculography or a left atrial injection.

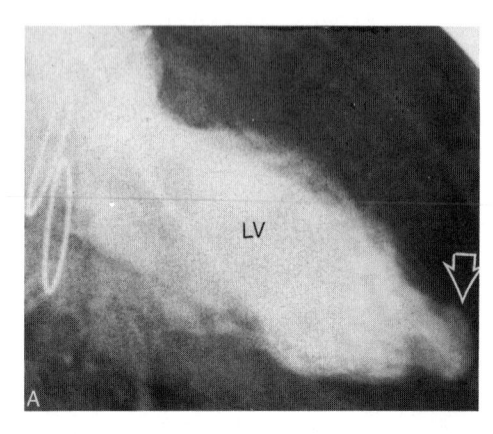

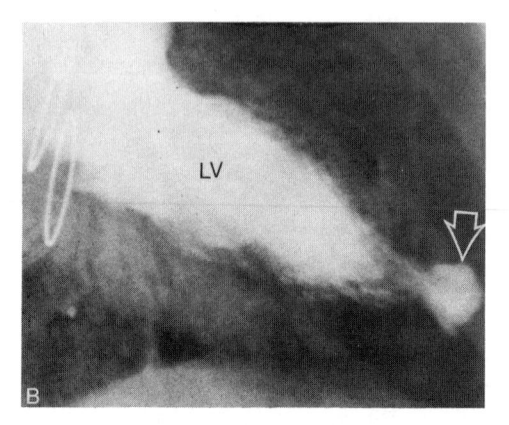

FIG 70–6.
Apical left ventricular diverticulum and no abdominal wall defect. Left ventriculogram *(LV)*. **A,** diastole and, **B,** systole. Aneurysm *(arrow)* is incidental finding and shows normal but slightly delayed contraction indicating fibrous composition.

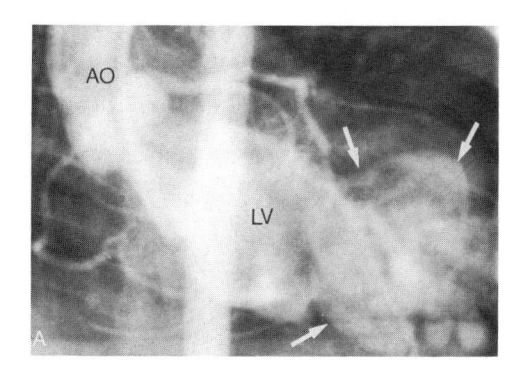

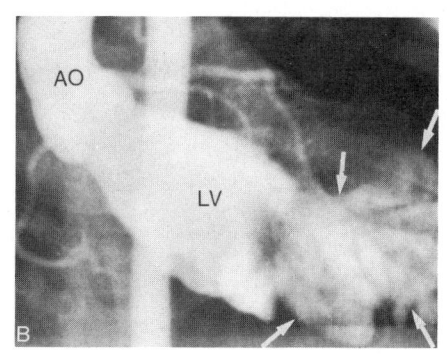

FIG 70–7.
Large broad-based congenital diverticulum of the left ventricle. Same patient as in Figure 70–4. Left ventriculograms *(LV)*. Anteroposterior projection. **A,** diastole. Aneurysm is well opacified *(arrows)*. **B,** systole. Left ventricle proper *(LV)* and congenital aneurysm are contracted, indicating normal musculature. Diverticulum has distinct internal architecture in contrast to an acquired aneurysm, which is smooth walled. *AO* = aorta.

Angiographic Appearance

1. When a congenital left ventricular diverticulum is associated with an abdominal wall defect, the diverticulum extends into a midline hernial sac.

2. Delineation of the diverticulum and the left ventricle is best seen on a lateral projection (Fig 70–5).

3. Most congenital left ventricular diverticula occur in the region of the cardiac apex and have an elongated characteristic shape and neck like connection with the main ventricle (Fig 70–6). The larger diverticula are also called "congenital aneurysms."

4. Rarely left ventricular diverticula are broad based and very large (Fig 70–7), deserving the connotation of "congenital left ventricular aneurysm."

5. Congenital aneurysms may have a trabeculated internal architecture and tend to show contraction. It is the contraction that is most helpful to exclude an aneurysm on an ischemic basis. If the diverticulum contains only fibrous tissue, it shows systolic expansion. REASON: The fibrous diverticula are very thin. In contrast, aneurysms caused by ischemia tend to be thick and thus are commonly akinetic.

6. Such huge diverticula may be visible on a thoracic roentgenogram (see Fig 70–4).

7. A congenital left ventricular diverticulum may also occur along the base of the heart, usually arising at the base posterolaterally (Fig 70–8).

8. Most congenital left ventricular diverticula occur in the region of the cardiac apex, but they also may be found anywhere along the free surface of the left ventricle.

9. The congenital nature of a diverticulum can be proved by the normal contraction pattern or a slightly delayed contraction (Fig 70–9). The reason for this delay is unknown.

CONGENITAL ANEURYSMS OF THE LEFT VENTRICLE

A very rare form of congenital aneurysm of the left ventricle is subvalvar aneurysms. They are considered to be congenital in nature, occurring primarily in blacks, particularly in the South African Bantu, in black races in Central and South Africa and the United States, and extremely rarely in a white patient. Approximately 50 cases have been reported. The condition should not be confused with the usually asymptomatic condition, congenital left ventricular diverticulum. The aneurysm forms immediately beneath either the mitral annulus or the aortic annulus. Submitral aneurysms are located beneath the posterior mitral leaflet, and subaortic aneurysms are located immediately beneath the left aortic cusp. The aneurysm probably forms because of a congenital weakness in the fibromuscu-

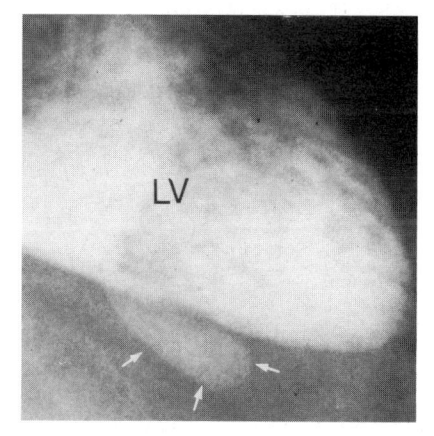

FIG 70–8.
Left ventricular diverticulum. Left ventriculogram *(LV)*. Right anterior oblique projection. Diverticulum posterolateral aspect of base of heart. Characteristic contour. Diverticulum showed a normal simultaneous contraction pattern. (Courtesy of Dr. T. Ovitt.)

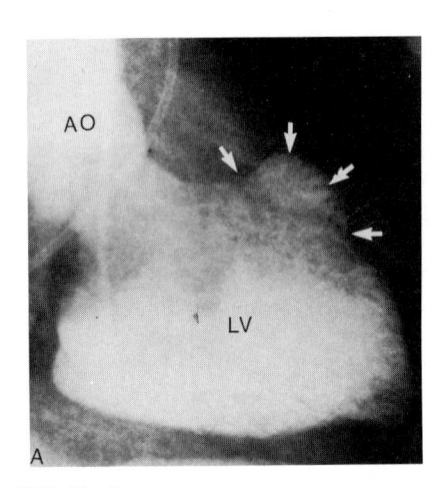

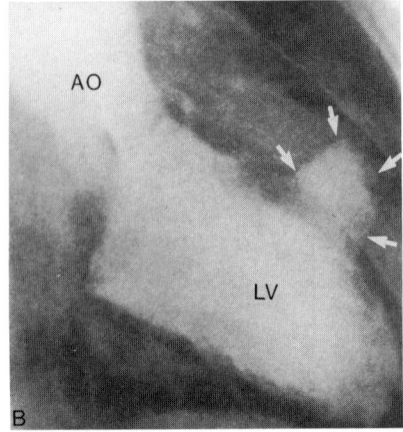

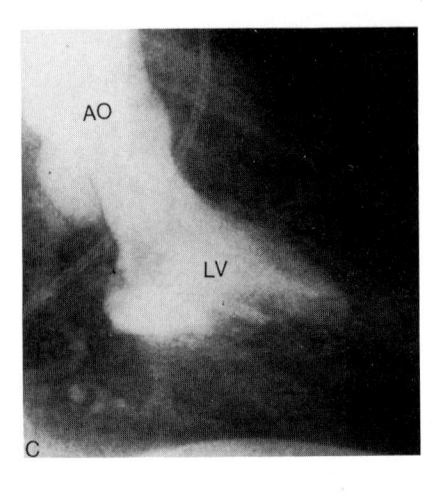

FIG 70–9.
Congenital diverticulum left ventricle. Anterolateral surface. Left ventriculogram (LV). Right anterior oblique projection. **A,** diastole. Left ventricle and diverticulum are fully distended (arrows). **B,** early systole. Ventricle is beginning to contract. Left ventricular diverticulum is still distended. Because of contraction of left ventricle, diverticulum becomes more obvious. **C,** end-systole. Left ventricle has completely contracted. Diverticulum has also contracted, indicating normal musculature in its wall. AO = aorta.

SUBMITRAL ANEURYSM

SUBAORTIC ANEURYSM

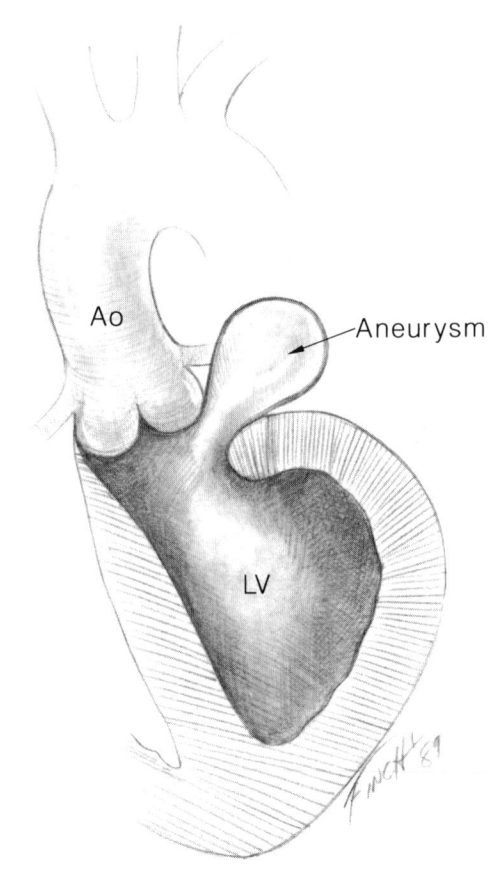

FIG 70–10.
Submitral left ventricular aneurysm. False aneurysm is located immediately beneath posterior mitral leaflet (MV) and connected by small communication with left ventricle (LV). Aneurysm tends to be large and commonly contains mural thrombus and calcifications. Distortion of mitral valve may cause mitral regurgitation. AO = aorta; LA = left atrium.

FIG 70–11.
Subaortic left ventricular aneurysm. Located immediately beneath left aortic cusp. Aneurysm tends to be smaller, but distortion of aortic valve may cause aortic regurgitation. AO = aorta; LV = left ventricle, MV = mitral valve. (Courtesy of Dr. E. Chesler.)

lar junction between valve annulus and myocardium. The pathologic condition is probably identical to that in sinus of Valsalva aneurysm, which occurs above the aortic valve (see Chapter 24). Congenital dehiscence allows the formation of a false aneurysm. Submitral aneurysms tend to be large and are connected to a left ventricle by a small communication (Fig 70–10). Subaortic aneurysms tend to be small (Fig 70–11).

The exact nature or cause of the defect in subaortic aneurysms is unknown. Factors such as myocardial infarction, syphilis, polyarteritis, and other conditions have not been identified.

The physiologic consequences of these aneurysms are as follows:

1. Distortion of the aortic or mitral valves, depending on location, resulting in aortic or mitral insufficiency, respectively.

2. Cardiac failure, particularly with large submitral aneurysms. REASON: The aneurysm is connected with the left ventricle and accepts a large amount of blood during systole. Thus, cardiac output is decreased because of paradoxical expansion of the aneurysm.

3. Coronary insufficiency caused by compression and distortion of the coronary arteries.

4. Peripheral embolization. Although the aneurysm commonly contains thrombotic material and may be calcified, peripheral embolization is very rare because of the small neck connecting the aneurysm with left ventricle.

5. Arrhythmias caused by compression of the conduction system.

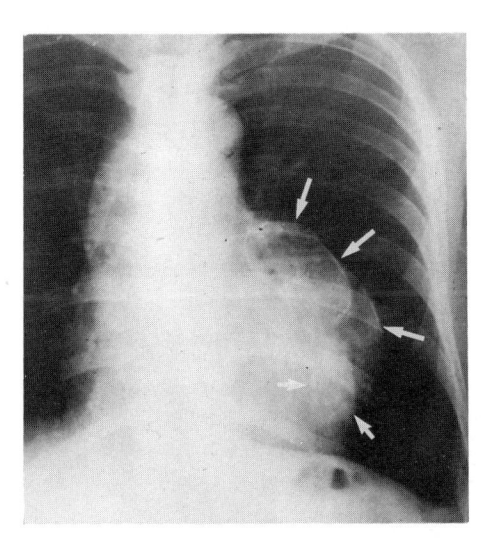

FIG 70–12.
Submitral left ventricular aneurysm. Thoracic roentgenogram. Posteroanterior projection. Large bulge along left cardiac border with dense shell-like calcifications *(arrows)* representing aneurysm. (Courtesy of Dr. E. Chesler.)

Clinical Manifestations

Clinical manifestation varies considerably. There may be cardiac failure and pulmonary edema because of left ventricular failure or a murmur of aortic or mitral insufficiency. Consequently, the condition is commonly confused with rheumatic heart disease or bacterial endocarditis. Rare clinical manifestations are arrhythmias caused by compression of the conducting system, signs of coronary insufficiency, or evidence for peripheral embolization.

Electrocardiography may show evidence of myocardial ischemia, and echocardiography may suggest the correct diagnosis. In a patient, particularly one from Africa with aortic or mitral insufficiency, signs of coronary insufficiency, or peripheral systemic emboli, the diagnosis of subvalvar aneurysms should be strongly considered. Diagnosis can be confirmed by angiocardiography and echocardiography.

Radiographic Findings

The radiographic findings are an important part of the clinical evaluation and may clinch the correct diagnosis. Whereas the radiograph in a subaortic aneurysm may be normal, the cardiac silhouette in a submitral aneurysm is usually abnormal because of the large size of the aneurysm. Fluoroscopy and cine fluoroscopy are helpful in demonstrating the paradoxical systolic expansion of the aneurysm along the posterior cardiac border. Fluoroscopic observation in various projections is advisable.

1. In submitral aneurysms the heart is usually greatly enlarged (Fig 70–12).

2. An abnormal bulge is commonly seen along the left cardiac border and forms a double density because of its posterior location. A ringlike calcification or calcifications within thrombi may be seen.

3. Findings of cardiac failure such as pulmonary congestion and pleural effusion may be present.

Subaortic aneurysms may have either normal radiographic findings or cardiomegaly and pulmonary congestion secondary to aortic insufficiency.

Angiographic Findings

The diagnosis can be established with certainty by angiocardiography. On left ventriculography the aneurysm may not readily opacify. Preferably an injection into the aneurysm itself should be performed.

1. In the left anterior oblique view, the left ventricle and large posterior aneurysm form a bilocular density.

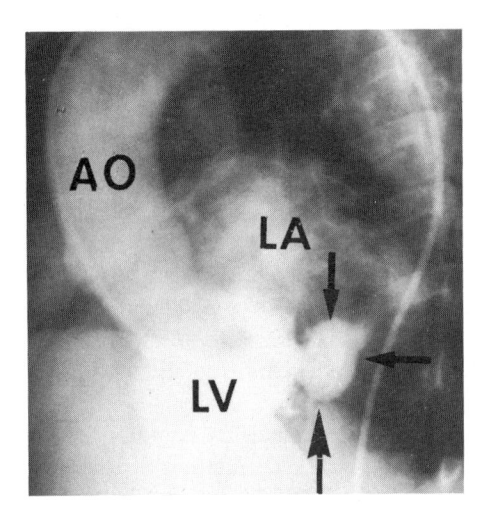

FIG 70-13.
Submitral left ventricular aneurysm. Left ventriculogram. Left anterior oblique projection. Aneurysm *(arrows)* is filled with mural thrombus and therefore the opacified cavity is small. Aneurysm is connected with left ventricle *(LV)* by a neck. Left atrium *(LA)* is opacified because function of leaflet of mitral valve is impaired by aneurysm. AO = aorta.

2. Characteristically the posterior collection of contrast medium represents the aneurysm, which is connected by a narrow neck with the ventricle.

3. If a large mural thrombus is present, the opacified aneurysmal cavity may be small (Fig 70-13).

4. One or more communications with the ventricle may be present.

5. During systole, the aneurysm shows characteristic expansion because its wall does not contain muscle tissue.

6. With an extensive mural thrombus no systolic expansion occurs.

Surgical Treatment

The aneurysm is opened and resected, and the orifice of the aneurysm is closed with a Dacron patch. If the function of the aortic and mitral valves is significantly compromised, valve replacement is carried out.

REFERENCES

1. Carter JB, VanTassel RA, Moller JH, et al: Congenital diverticulum of the right ventricle: association with pulmonary stenosis and ventricular septal defect, *Am J Cardiol* 28:478, 1971.
2. Cumming GR: Congenital diverticulum of the right ventricle, *Am J Cardiol* 23:294, 1969.
3. Magrassi P, Chartrand C, Guerin R, et al: True diverticulum of the right ventricle: two cases associated with tetralogy of Fallot, *Ann Thorac Surg* 29:357, 1980.
4. Rajs J, Thoren C, Kjellman NI: Spontaneous rupture of a congenital diverticulum of the right ventricle in a 1-month-old child, *Eur J Cardiol* 6:131, 1977.
5. Folger GM Jr, Hajar HA: The right ventricular outflow pouch with double-chambered right ventricle, *Am Heart J* 112:423, 1986.
6. Copeland J, Higgins C, Hayden W, et al: Congenital diverticulum of the right ventricle, *J Thorac Cardiovasc Surg* 70:536, 1975.
7. Cantrell JR, Haller JA, Ravitch MM: A syndrome of congenital defects involving the abdominal wall, sternum, diaphragm, pericardium, and heart, *Surg Gynecol Obstet* 107:602, 1958.
8. Ossandon F: Congenital diverticulum of the left ventricle extending into exomphalos, *Z Kinderchir* 30:265, 1980.
9. Toyama WM: Combined congenital defects of the anterior abdominal wall, sternum, diaphragm, pericardium, and heart: a case report and review of the syndrome, *Pediatrics* 50:778, 1972.
10. Edgett JW Jr, Nelson WP, Hall RJ, et al: Diverticulum of the heart: part of the syndrome of congenital cardiac and midline thoracic and abdominal defects, *Am J Cardiol* 24:580, 1969.
11. Crittenden IH, Adams FH, Mulder DG: A syndrome featuring defects of the heart, sternum, diaphragm, and anterior abdominal wall, *Circulation* 20:396, 1959.
12. Knight L, Neal WA, Williams HJ, et al: Congenital left ventricular diverticulum: part of a syndrome of cardiac anomalies and midline defects, *Minn Med* 59:372, 1976.
13. Murphy DA, Aberdeen E, Dobbs RH, et al: The surgical treatment of a syndrome consisting of thoracoabdominal wall; diaphragmatic, pericardial, and ventricular septal defects; and a left ventricular diverticulum, *Ann Thorac Surg* 6:528, 1968.
14. Gula G, Yacoub M: Syndrome of congenital ventricular diverticulum and midline thoraco-abdominal defects, *Thorax* 32:365, 1977.
15. Toyama WM: Combined congenital defects of the anterior abdominal wall, sternum, diaphragm, pericardium and heart: a case report and review of the syndrome, *Pediatrics* 50:778, 1972.
16. Gueron M, Hirsch M, Opschitzer I, et al: Left ventricular diverticulum and mitral incompetence in asymptomatic children, *Circulation* 53:181, 1976.
17. Chesler E, Joffe N, Schamroth L, et al: Annular subvalvular left ventricular aneurysms in the south African Bantu, *Circulation* 32:43, 1965.
18. Dimich I, Steinfeld L, Baron M, et al: Calcified left ventricular aneurysm in children, *Am J Cardiol* 23:739, 1969.
19. Pettersson G, Bergstrom T: A case of ruptured diverticulum of the left ventricle with hemopericardium in a neonate, treated successfully by surgery, *Scand J Thorac Cardiovasc Surg* 3:203, 1969.
20. Orsmond GS, Joffe HS, Chesler E: Congenital diverticulum of the left ventricle associated with hypoplastic right ventricle and ventricular septal defect, *Circulation* 48:1135, 1973.
21. Tecklenberg PL, Alderman EL, Billingham ME, et al: Di-

verticulum of the left ventricle in hypertrophic cardiomyopathy, *Am J Med* 64:707, 1978.

ADDITIONAL READINGS

Chesler E: Aneurysms of the left ventricle, *Cardiovasc Clin* 20:188, 1972.

Chesler E, Joffe N, Schamroth L, et al: Annular subvalvular left ventricular aneurysms in the South African Bantu, *Circulation* 32:43, 1965.

Chesler E, Mitha AS, Edwards JE: Congenital aneurysms adjacent to the anuli of the aortic and/or mitral valves, *Chest* 82:334, 1982.

Chesler E, Outim L, Dubb A: Ventricular tachycardia due to subvalvular left ventricular aneurysms, *S Afr Med J* 41:518, 1967.

Chesler E, Tucker RBK, Barlow JB: Subvalvular and apical left ventricular aneurysms in the Bantu as a source of systemic emboli, *Circulation* 35:1156, 1967.

Lewis BS, Van Der Horst RL, Rogers NMA, et al: Cine radiology in subvalvular left ventricular aneurysm, *S Afr Med J* 47:1677, 1973.

CHAPTER 71

Aneurysm of Atrial Appendage

Aneurysm of an atrial appendage is a very rare anomaly, which usually also involves the left atrium.[1,2] In most instances the aneurysmal dilatation is confined to the atrial appendage, but the adjacent left atrial wall may be involved, in which case the aneurysm is broad based (Fig 71–1). It is considered related to a congenital weakness of the left atrial wall.

Only one third of cases are recognized by the time the patient is 10 years of age. Typically the condition is discovered during the second, third, or fourth decades of life. Stasis in the aneurysm leads to thrombus formation and subsequent embolism. Symptoms result from either systemic embolization or supraventricular tachycardia. Nonspecific systolic murmurs may be heard. The electrocardiogram may show supraventricular tachycardia, interventricular conduction defect, or signs of left atrial hypertrophy.

Resection of the aneurysm stops the systemic embolization. If it is recognized, operation is performed prophylactically to prevent death from embolization.

RADIOGRAPHIC FEATURES

Thoracic radiographs are very abnormal and suggest a cardiac tumor, pericardial cyst, or partial absence of the pericardium. The radiographic appearance of partial absence of the left pericardium and of congenital aneurysm of the left atrial appendix are very similar. The conditions are commonly confused and cannot be differentiated with certainty on analysis of thoracic radiographs. Noninvasive techniques and creation of a left-sided pneumothorax are required to diagnose aneurysm of left atrial appendage and exclude partial absence of the left pericardium. Differentiation between these two conditions is of no practical importance.

1. The heart and mediastinum are in a midline position (Fig 71–2) in contrast to most patients with partial absence of the left pericardium, where cardiac rotation and shift occur toward the left (see Chapter 72).

2. Even if the aneurysm is huge (Fig 71–3), cardiac shift and rotation are not present. Therefore, partial absence of the left pericardium is unlikely, and congenital aneurysm of the left atrial appendage is more likely.

3. A variable-sized bulge is found in the region of the left atrial appendage simulating a large pulmonary arterial segment or mediastinal mass. The bulge is identical to that in partial absence of the left pericardium.

4. For diagnostic purposes, creation of a left-sided pneumothorax with the injection of carbon dioxide allows differentiation between these two conditions. The pericardial sac is not filled with gas, because the pericardium is intact with a left atrial aneurysm.

5. Because aneurysm of left atrial appendage causes a very atypical radiograph, many diagnostic possibilities might be considered. A left anterior oblique projection is helpful to identify that the abnormal bulge is associated with the left atrium (Fig 71–4) and exclude a large pulmonary artery as a cause of the bulge.

6. Congenital aneurysm of the left atrial appendage may involve not only the appendage but also the adjacent part of the left atrium and result in a very atypical broad-based bulge along the left cardiac contour. The bulge may be huge (see Figs 71–3 and 71–4).

7. Because the left atrial appendage is located laterally and the aneurysmal dilatation involves only the lateral

1142   Other Conditions

CONGENITAL ANEURYSM OF LEFT ATRIAL APPENDAGE

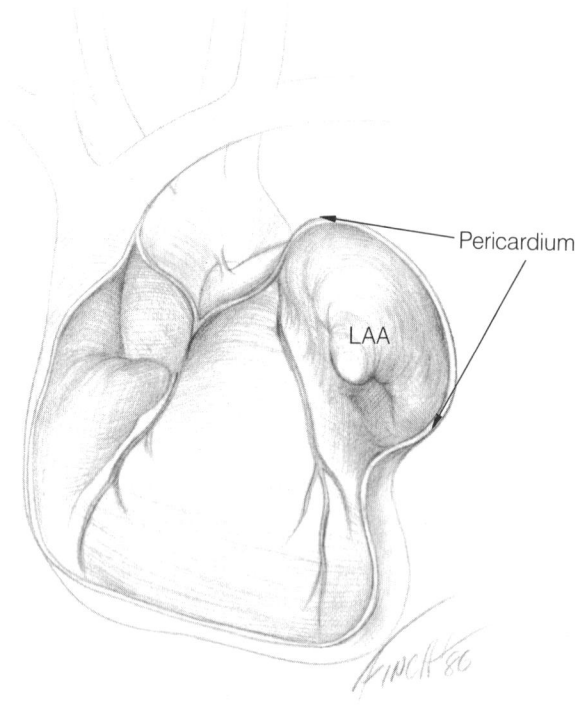

FIG 71–1.
Aneurysm of left atrial appendage *(LAA)*. Broad-based aneurysm partially involves left atrium. Intact pericardial sac in distinction to partial absence of left pericardium.

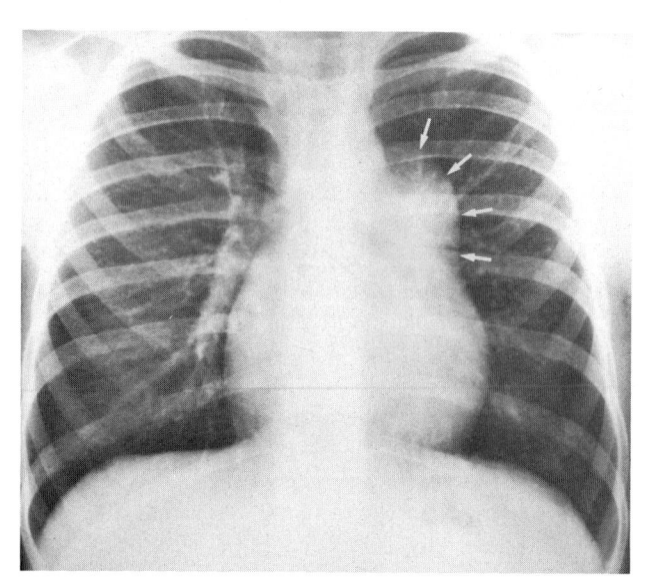

FIG 71–2.
Aneurysm of left atrial appendage. Thoracic roentgenogram. Posteroanterior projection. No mediastinal shift. Large bulge *(arrows)* in area of pulmonary arterial segment is caused by aneurysm of left atrial appendage.

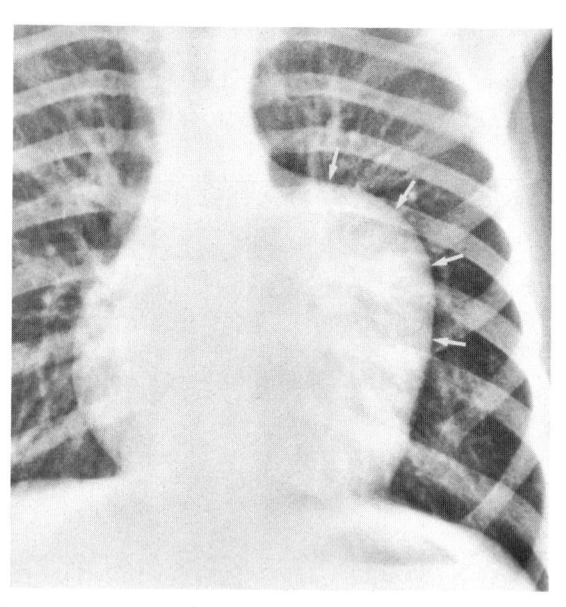

FIG 71–3.
Aneurysm of left atrial appendage. Thoracic roentgenogram. Posteroanterior projection. Huge bulge *(arrows)* in area of left atrial appendage overshadows pulmonary arterial segment. Because of large size of left atrial appendage and absence of cardiac shift and rotation of heart, diagnosis of congenital aneurysm of left atrial appendage is more likely than partial absence of pericardium.

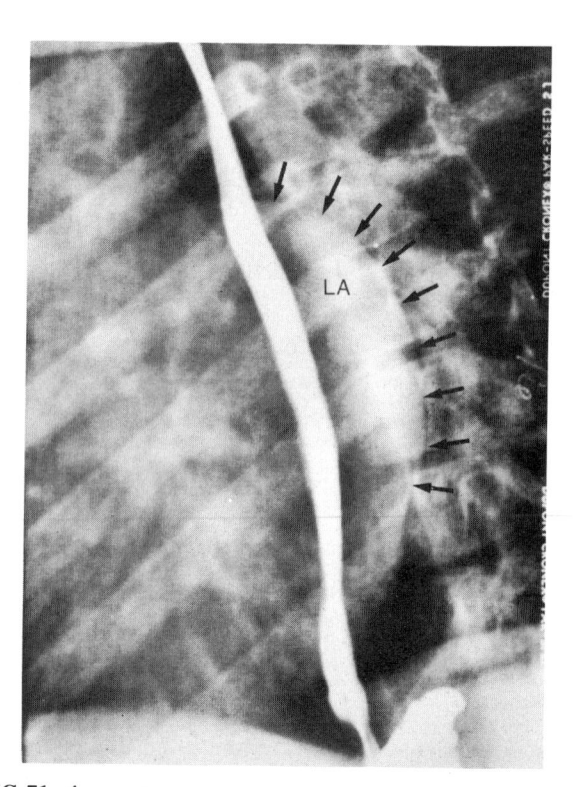

FIG 71–4.
Aneurysm of left atrial appendage. Same patient as in Figure 71–3. Left anterior oblique projection. Huge bulge in Figure 71–3 lies posteriorly and is part of left atrium *(LA)*. Therefore, aneurysm of left atrial appendage is the most likely diagnosis.

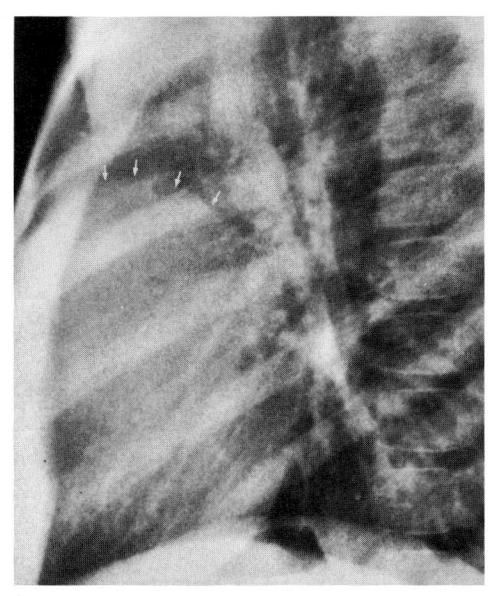

FIG 71–5.
Aneurysm of left atrial appendage. Same patient as in Figure 71–4. Lateral projection. Left atrium is not enlarged because aneurysmal dilatation involves only lateral aspect of left atrium and left atrial appendage. Lateral projection is normal except for density in anterior superior mediastinum *(arrows)* related to huge aneurysm of left atrial appendage. (Left atrium lies posteriorly, but appendage projects anteriorly at same level as pulmonary artery.)

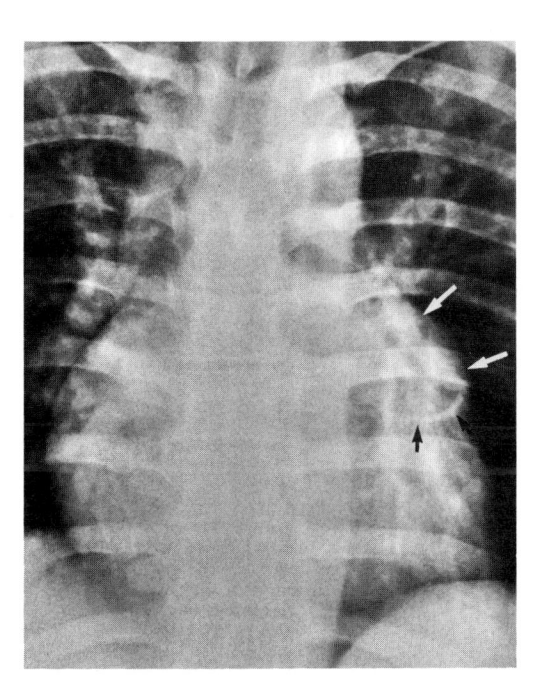

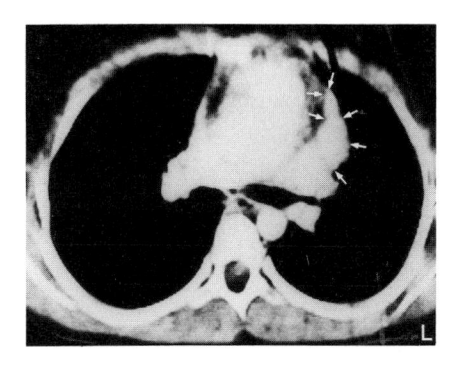

FIG 71–7.
Aneurysm of left atrial appendage. Computer tomography section. Huge appendage *(arrows)*. No displacement or rotation of heart. Diagnosis of aneurysm of left atrial appendage is more likely than partial absence of pericardium. L = left.

aspect of the left atrium, a lateral view does not show left atrial enlargement (Fig 71–5).

8. Long-standing thrombosis of a congenital aneurysm of the left atrial appendage may result in mural thrombus with calcifications. (Fig 71–6).

9. Computer tomography (CT) scanning allows the recognition of an enlarged left atrial appendage (Fig 71–7) but does not distinguish this condition from partial absence of the pericardium.

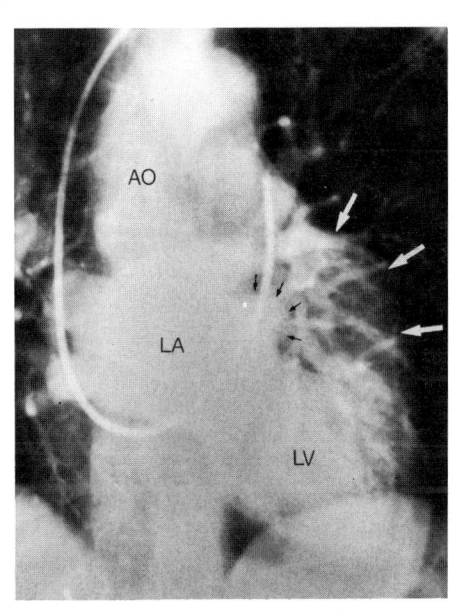

FIG 71–6.
Aneurysm of left atrial appendage and long-standing thrombosis. Thoracic roentgenogram. Posteroanterior projection. Calcifications *(arrows)* are demonstrated.

FIG 71–8.
Aneurysm of left atrial appendage. Same patient as in Figure 71–2. Pulmonary arteriogram. Late phase. Anteroposterior projection. Neck of left atrial appendage *(black arrows)* but not left atrial appendage opacifies. This appearance is consistent with either partial absence of left pericardium or aneurysm of left atrial appendage with thrombosis. Lack of cardiac shift is more consistent with aneurysm. Left-sided pneumothorax failed to fill the pericardial sac. At operation pericardium was intact, and a congenital aneurysm of the left atrial appendage with thrombosis was found. AO = aorta; LA = left atrium; LV = left ventricle.

10. Congenital aneurysm of the left atrial appendage may be confirmed by other techniques such as angiography (Fig 71–8) or contrast-enhanced CT scanning. These techniques are not infallible because a thrombus may completely obliterate the aneurysm. The calcification of a long-standing thrombus is well seen by CT scanning.

The most reliable noninvasive technique to recognize this abnormality is magnetic resonance scanning, but experience with this newer imaging modality is very limited with this condition.

REFERENCES

1. Krueger SK, Ferlic RM, Mooring PK: Left atrial appendage aneurysm: correlation of noninvasive with clinical and surgical findings: report of a case, *Circulation* 52:732, 1975.
2. Hougen TJ, Mulder DG, Gyepes MT, et al: Aneurysm of the left atrium, *Am J Cardiol* 33:557, 1974.

CHAPTER 72

Pericardial Defect

Pericardial defects are uncommon and usually first recognized by abnormalities discovered on a thoracic roentgenogram. Pericardial defects occur in a spectrum ranging from a small defect to total absence of the pericardium. Pericardial defects occur three times more commonly in males than females. Thirty percent of cases occur with another congenital anomaly, but the association is perhaps coincidental.

PATHOLOGIC ANATOMY

More than 75% of cases involve absence of the entire left side of the pericardium.[1,2] The remainder represent partial defects (also called "foramen defect") (Fig 72-1). Isolated right-sided defect,[3] total absence of the pericardium, and diaphragmatic pericardial defects are very rare.

Associated congenital anomalies have been left diaphragmatic hernia, bronchogenic cysts, and pulmonary sequestration. Cardiac anomalies reported are tetralogy of Fallot, mitral stenosis, tricuspid insufficiency, atrial septal defect, and patent ductus arteriosus.

Herniation of cardiac structures or portions of the lung may occur through the defect.[3-5] Herniation of the heart through a large pericardial defect may result in sudden death. Herniation of the left atrial appendage through a smaller defect (see Fig 72-1) may cause infarction of the left atrial appendage and chest pain simulating coronary artery disease. With large pericardial defects, the rim of the window may compress the left coronary artery, causing myocardial ischemia, particularly during exercise (Fig 72-2). In one patient with partial absence of the pericardium and tetralogy of Fallot,[4] herniation of the right upper lobe of the lung occurred through the defect into the pericardial space.[5] A case of partial absence of the right pericardium with herniation of the normal lung into the pericardial sac has also been described.[3] Besides symptoms related to herniation, emboli may occur from mural thrombi in the left atrial appendage.

Premature atrophy of the left duct of Cuvier, which supplies nourishment to the pleural-pericardial membrane, is thought to be the cause of incomplete formation of the left pericardium.

Although most instances are congenital, pericardial defects are created often at cardiac operation. Herniation of a ventricle through an operatively created defect after pneumonectomy has been described. Isolated pericardial rupture may occur from nonpenetrating injury to the thorax.[6]

Pericardial defects also occur with ectopia cordis and ventricular diverticulum, but these conditions are discussed separately (see Chapters 60 and 70).

PHYSIOLOGY

Patients may have chest pain indistinguishable from that of coronary arterial insufficiency. Particularly during exercise, the left atrial appendage may become partially incarcerated through the pericardial defect and ischemia results. Partial thrombosis and adhesion formation may develop as a result. In a patient with a larger defect, the left anterior descending coronary artery may be intermittently compressed by the pericardial foramen, again, particularly during exercise (see Fig 72-2). Patients with this mechanism of chest pain may respond to nitroglycerin as other patients with coronary arterial insufficiency.

Other possible causes of chest pain are torsion or strain on great vessels that serve to anchor the heart, tension on the pleural-pericardial adhesions, or pressure of

PARTIAL ABSENCE OF THE LEFT PERICARDIUM

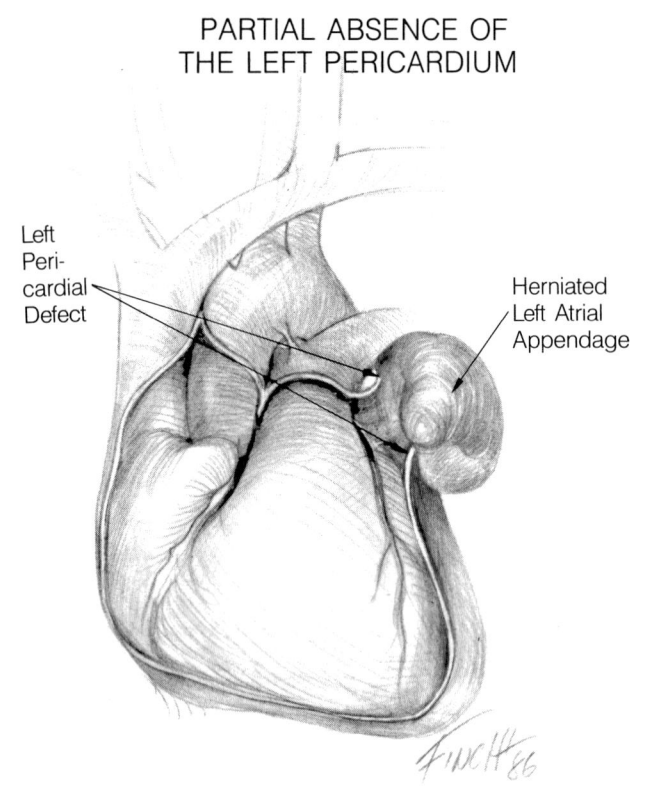

FIG 72–1.
Partial absence of pericardium. Typical small defect of pericardium allows herniation of left atrial appendage. Infarction of appendage and thrombosis may ensue.

the rim of the remaining pericardium on other cardiac structures.

CLINICAL FEATURES[2]

Total absence of left pericardium is often asymptomatic and may not decrease life expectancy. A portion of the heart can herniate and transiently incarcerate, particularly during exercise. This could lead to symptoms of chest pain, dyspnea, dizziness, and syncope. Herniation of the left ventricle may lead to sudden death.

Clinical manifestations of herniation of the left atrial appendage may resemble pericarditis with sharp precordial pain because of strangulation of the left atrial appendage with infarction.

Auscultatory findings are not specific. A systolic murmur is often heard, presumably from deformation of the heart or great vessels because of displacement of the heart.

ELECTROCARDIOGRAPHIC FEATURES

The electrocardiogram may show marked changes of the QRS axis because of distortion with a tendency toward right-axis deviation.

TOTAL ABSENCE OF LEFT PERICARDIUM

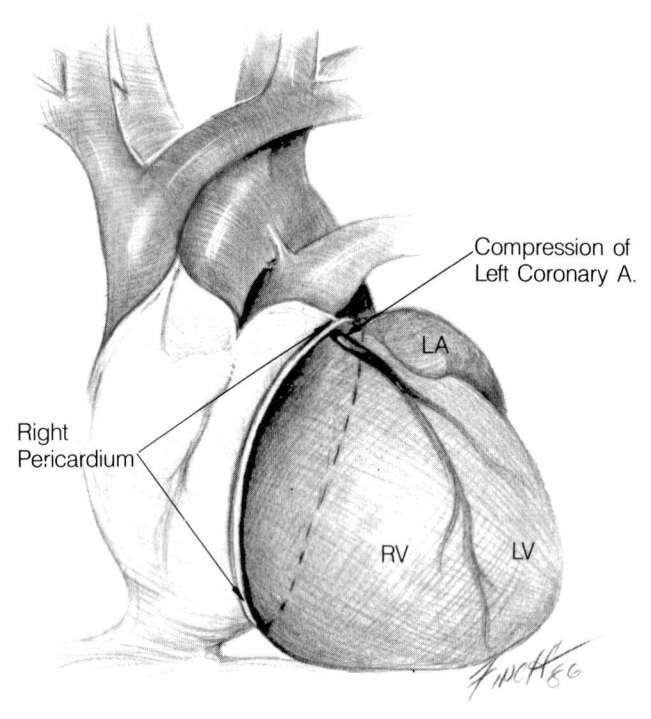

FIG 72–2.
Absence of entire left pericardium. Rim of defect causes compression of left anterior descending artery, producing angina-like symptom or sudden death. A = artery; LA = left atrium; LV = left ventricle; RV = right ventricle.

ECHOCARDIOGRAPHIC FEATURES

Few echocardiograms have been reported in this condition.[2, 7] These show findings of right ventricular volume overload.

RADIOGRAPHIC FEATURES

In most cases the radiographic findings of partial absence of the pericardium are characteristic. From careful analysis of thoracic radiographs, a correct diagnosis can usually be made. The diagnosis can be confirmed by noninvasive means such as ultrasound, computer tomography (CT), or nuclear magnetic resonance (NMR) or by more invasive tests such as angiography and by inducement of a left-sided pneumothorax. The differentiation between absence of the entire left pericardium and partial absence (foramen defects, which most commonly occur in the region of the left atrial appendage) cannot be made on thoracic radiographs. Fluoroscopy is unrewarding but may show paradoxical pulsation of the left atrial appendage, which may help to exclude an enlarged pulmonary arterial segment that shows expansion during systole.

The differential radiographic diagnosis includes many

conditions such as an atypical thymus, enlarged lymph nodes, cardiac or other tumors, pulmonary infarction, pericardial fat necrosis, idiopathic and poststenotic pulmonary artery dilatation, aneurysm of the pulmonary artery, or bronchogenic or pericardial cysts.

A difficult differential diagnosis is with aneurysm of the left atrial appendage. In this condition the left atrial appendage is enlarged, but the pericardial sac is intact. Partial absence of the left pericardium shows characteristic radiographic findings: levoposition of the heart, midline trachea, prominent pulmonary artery segment, indistinct right cardiac border hidden behind the spine, and interposition of the lung between left hemidiaphragm and inferior border of heart.

In partial absence the characteristic findings are prominence of pulmonary artery segment, left atrial appendage or both, and variable shift and rotation of the heart toward the left.

1. In most cases the radiographic findings are typical enough to suggest the correct radiograph diagnosis. These findings include shift of the heart into the left thoracic cage, bulge in the region of the pulmonary artery area, and right atrium superimposed on the spine.

2. Although in most patients the radiographic abnormalities are obvious, rarely they may be subtle (Fig 72–3).

3. Before the development of noninvasive techniques, a diagnostic pneumothorax was performed to confirm the diagnosis. A left-sided pneumothorax was created by the injection of carbon dioxide into the pleural space with the patient placed in a left lateral decubitus position (Figs 72–4 and 72–5). REASON: The gas (preferably CO_2) rises and enters the pericardial space through a invariably coexisting defect in the pleura. A radiograph is obtained in the left lateral decubitus position and studied carefully for gas in the pericardium. This may not be obvious because the pericardial sac is thin (see Figs 72–4). If after injection of a gas, both pleural spaces show gas, total absence of the pericardium or a defect in the left and right pericardium can be diagnosed.

The test is not infallible. REASON: Adhesions from repeated incarceration of the left atrial appendage in a foramen defect and inflammation may seal the atrial appendage to the foramen defect and obliterate the communication; thus, CO_2 is prevented from entering into the pericardium.

4. The lateral projection is helpful to exclude a mediastinal mass, because an abnormal mass density is not demonstrated (Fig 72–6).

5. In most patients with congenital absence of the pericardium, the heart is displaced into the left thoracic cavity. Typically the trachea shows no shift (Fig 72–7).

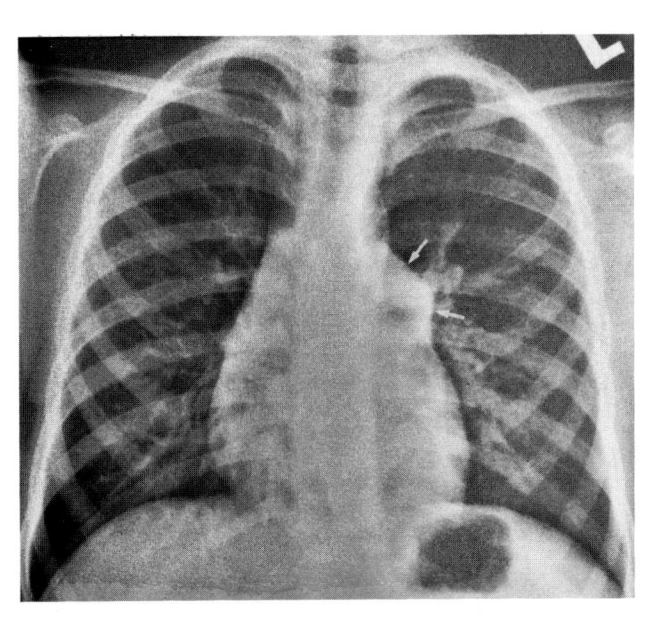

FIG 72–3.
Partial absence of pericardium. Thoracic roentgenogram. Posteroanterior projection. Angina-like symptoms during weight lifting. Two normal cardiac catheterizations were performed at another center. Normal cardiac size and pulmonary vasculature. No cardiac shift to left. An unusually shaped "pulmonary artery segment," which is actually a herniated left atrial appendage *(arrow)*, is seen. In spite of atypical appearance, because mediastinal shift was not present, a pneumothorax was performed because of clinical history. Diagnosis was proved (see Fig 72–4). At operation a foramen defect and incarcerated left atrial appendage were found. Patient was asymptomatic after operation.

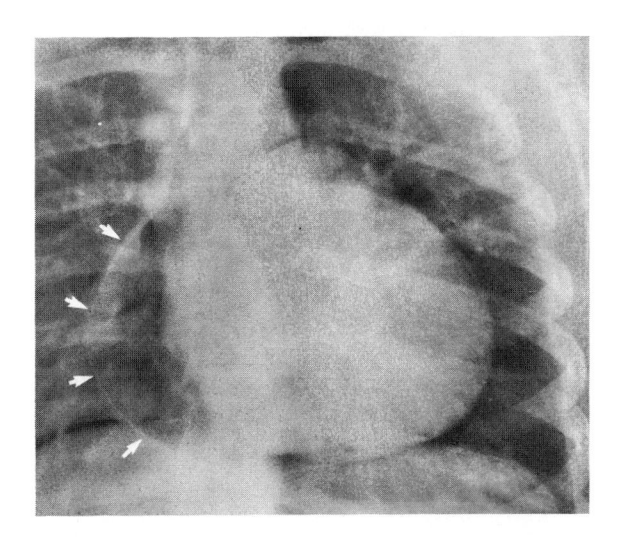

FIG 72–4.
Partial absence of pericardium. Same patient as Figure 72–3. Thoracic roentgenogram. Left lateral decubitus projection after left pneumothorax. Carbon dioxide has entered pericardial sac, proving defect in pericardium. Thin pericardium is well outlined *(arrows)*.

**LEFT LATERAL DECUBITUS
FILM FOLLOWING LEFT SIDED PNEUMOTHORAX**

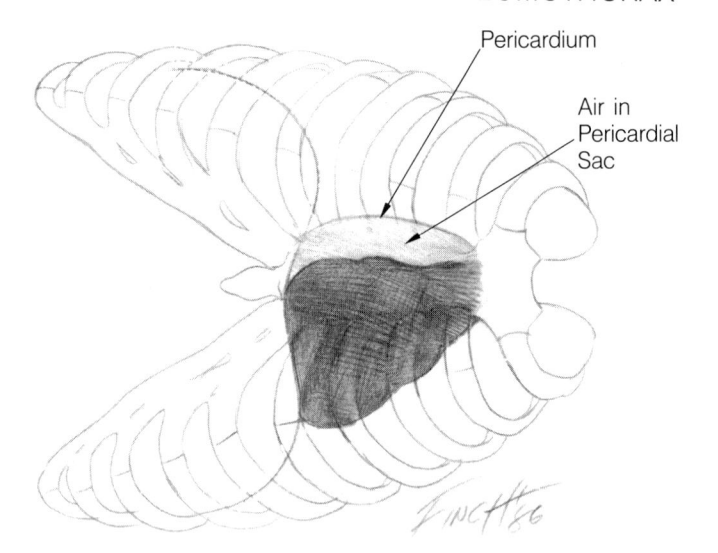

FIG 72–5.
Principle of diagnosis of pericardial defect with induction of left pneumothorax. Carbon dioxide was introduced into left pleural space, which passes through defects in parietal pleura and pericardium into pericardial space if patient is placed in left lateral decubitus position.

6. Clockwise rotation of the heart occurs. Therefore, the right atrium is not prominent and is indistinct because it may be partially superimposed on the spine (see Fig 72–7).

7. The pulmonary arterial segment becomes prominent because of clockwise cardiac rotation. However, the main bulge in the area of the pulmonary artery is usually formed by an enlarged herniated left atrial appendage (see Fig 72–7).

8. The pulmonary arterial segment cannot be distinguished from the prominent density caused by the left atrial appendage (see Fig 72–7).

9. With marked clockwise rotation the heart may be rotated off the dome of the diaphragm, and the flat undersurface of the heart may become visible (Fig 72–8).

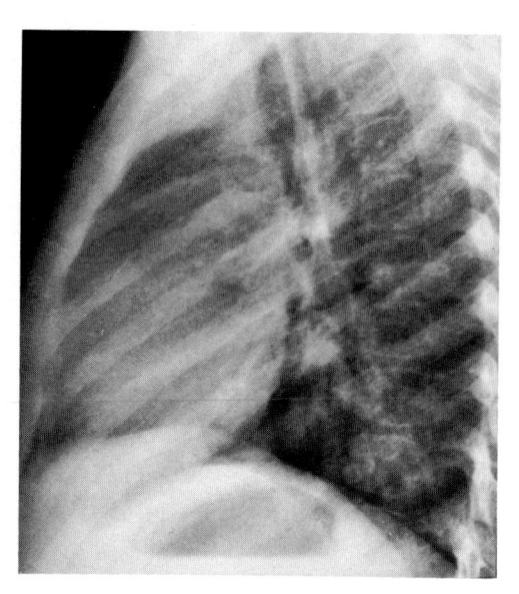

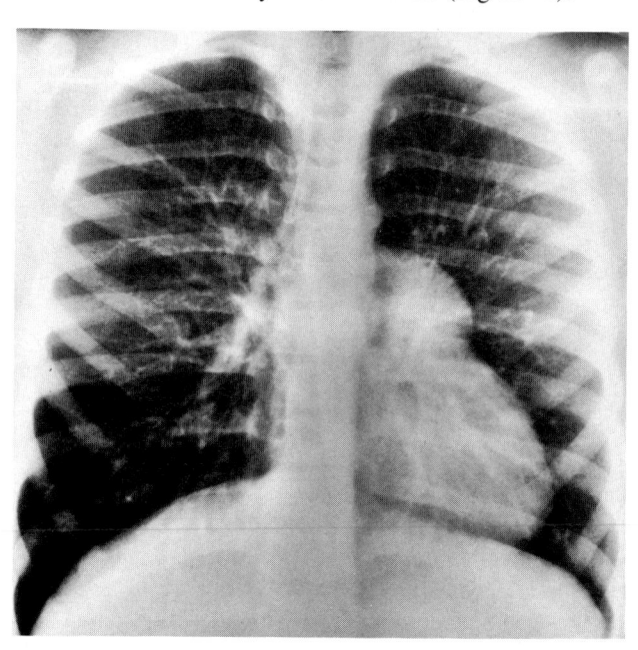

FIG 72–6.
Partial absence of pericardium and herniation of left atrial appendage. Thoracic roentgenogram. Lateral projection. No abnormal density is demonstrated. Therefore, mediastinal mass unlikely.

FIG 72–7.
Partial absence of pericardium. Thoracic roentgenogram. Posteroanterior projection. Heart is rotated and displaced toward left. Right atrium is superimposed on spine. Bulge along upper left cardiac border is formed by pulmonary arterial segment (clockwise rotation) and predominantly by enlarged herniated left atrial appendage. These two structures cannot be separated. Trachea is not shifted.

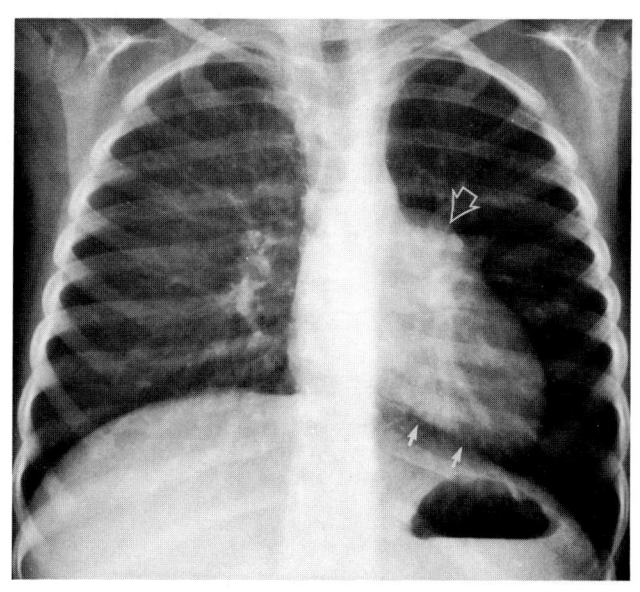

FIG 72–8.
Partial absence of left pericardium. Thoracic roentgenogram. Posteroanterior projection. Marked clockwise rotation. Enlarged herniated left atrial appendage *(open arrow)*. Ascending aorta and right superior vena cava are not seen (clockwise rotation). Heart is rotated off dome of diaphragm. Flat undersurface of heart is visible *(solid arrows)*.

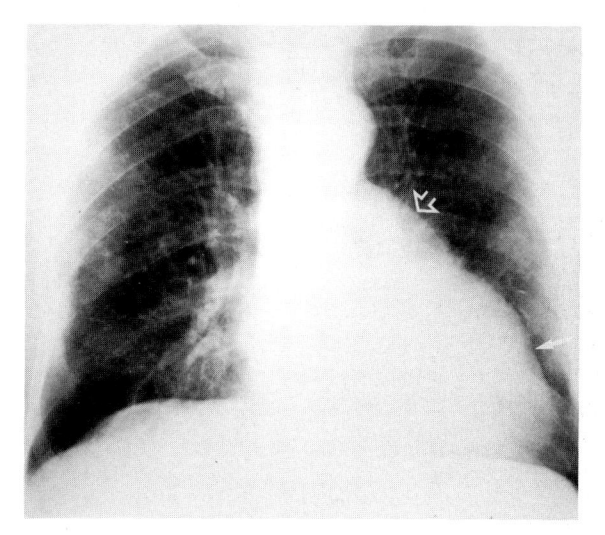

FIG 72–9.
Large foramen-type left pericardial defect. Thoracic roentgenogram. Mild shift of heart toward left. Large bulge along upper left cardiac border is caused by herniated left atrial appendage *(open arrow)*. Subtle notch along lower left cardiac border *(solid arrow)* suggests larger foramen-type defect. Notch is caused by pressure of rim of defect on myocardium.

10. An additional notch along the left cardiac contour may suggest a larger pericardial defect, although this finding is not reliable (Fig 72–9).

11. The diagnosis can be confirmed noninvasively by CT or NMR imaging. These show the cardiac rotation and the large left atrial appendage (Fig 72–10).

12. Whereas a diagnostic pneumothorax demonstrates the defect in the pericardium, CT and NMR do not. Thus, if cardiac rotation is lacking, differentiation from aneurysm of left atrial appendage cannot be made.

13. Displacement of the heart toward the left is not always present (Fig 72–11), and in such an instance the diagnosis is more difficult.

14. The herniated left atrial appendage may closely mimic an enlarged pulmonary arterial segment. Sometimes an atypical contour may suggest the correct diagnosis of partial absence of the pericardium (see Fig 72–11).

15. In patients with partial absence of the left-sided pericardium, cardiac structures tend to herniate through the defect. Herniation of lung into the pericardium may occur with partial right-sided absence of the pericardium (extremely rare).

16. The radiographic findings of complete absence of the pericardium are normal.

ANGIOGRAPHIC FEATURES

Angiography for pericardial defect is no longer indicated, but it is valuable in explaining the radiographic findings (Fig 72–12). Partial absence of the pericardium

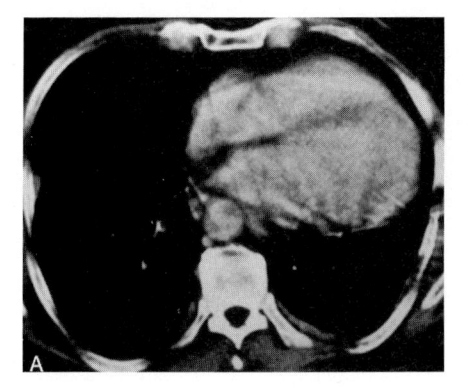

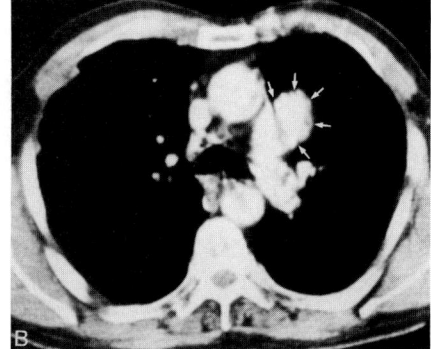

FIG 72–10.
Left pericardial defect and patent ductus arteriosus. Same patient as in Figure 72–9. Computer tomography study of heart. **A,** shift and rotation of heart into left thoracic cavity. **B,** enlarged left atrial appendage *(arrows)*.

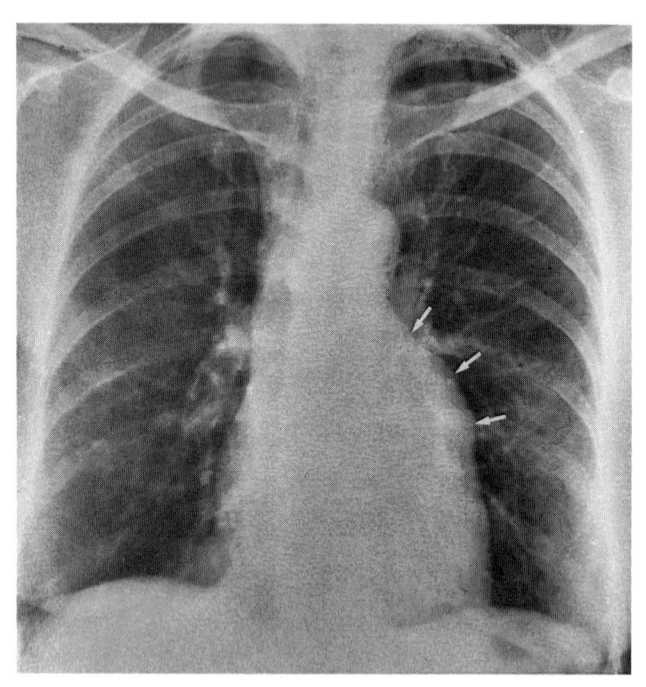

FIG 72–11.
Partial absence of pericardium. Thoracic roentgenogram. Posteroanterior projection. Radiographic findings are not typical because shift of heart is absent. Herniated atrial appendage mimics prominent pulmonary arterial segment, which extends unusually low *(arrows)*, suggesting a herniated left atrial appendage.

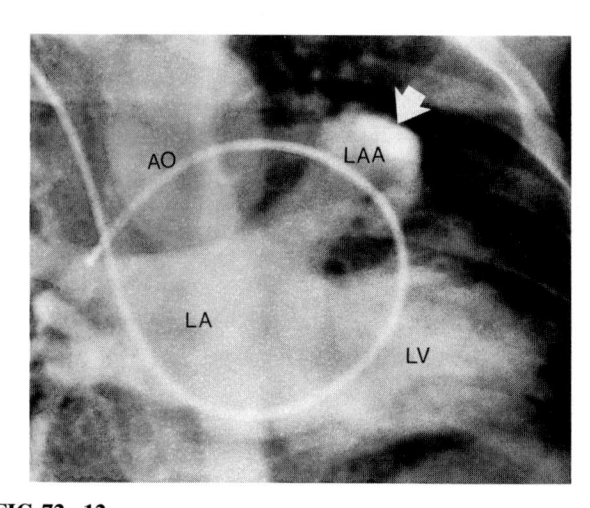

FIG 72–12.
Partial absence of pericardium. Pulmonary arteriogram. Late phase. Anteroposterior projection. Left atrium opacified. Elongated left atrial appendage *(LAA)* is herniated through foramen defect. Bulge on radiograph is formed exclusively by left atrial appendage *(arrow)*. AO = aorta; LA = left atrium; LV = left ventricle.

may be associated with other congenital cardiac anomalies that may require angiography, and the diagnosis may be made incidentally in asymptomatic patients. Angiography is also not infallible. REASON: The left atrial appendage may have become infarcted and thrombosed. Under these

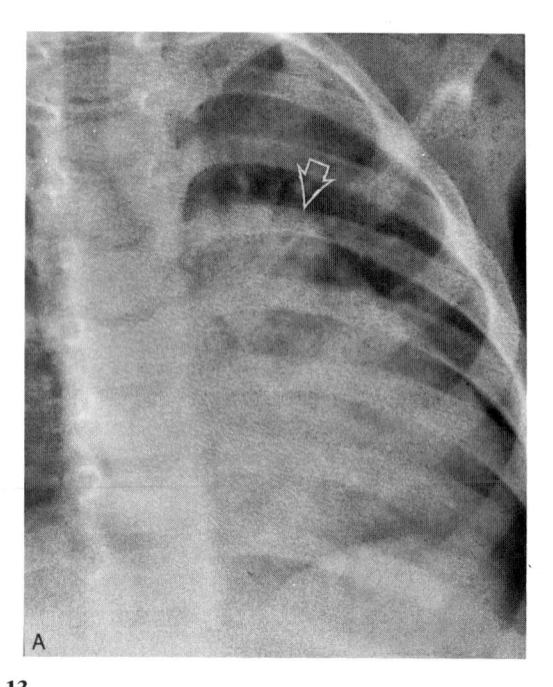

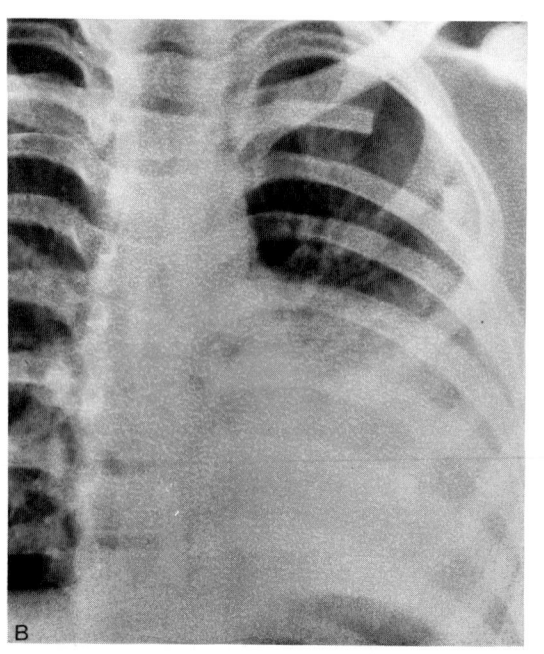

FIG 72–13.
Partial absence of left pericardium. **A,** thoracic roentgenogram. Posteroanterior projection. Typical findings. Midline trachea. Marked shift of heart into left hemithorax. Right atrial border is superimposed on spine. Herniated left atrial appendage mimics enlarged pulmonary arterial segment *(open arrow)*. **B,** thoracic roentgenogram. Posteroanterior projection. Postoperative view after left thoracotomy and partial resection of fourth rib. Previous bulge along left cardiac border is absent because of operative amputation of left atrial appendage.

circumstances it will not opacify with contrast medium. However, angiographic nonvisualization of the left atrial appendage with a large bulge in this region is consistent with partial absence of the pericardium and thrombosis of a herniated left atrial appendage.

OPERATIVE CONSIDERATIONS

An operation is indicated because of the various complications of the disease such as systemic embolization, angina pectoris, myocardial infarction, arrhythmias, and sudden death.

The pericardium is widely opened, and the herniated enlarged left atrial appendage is amputated. Operative closure of a congenital pericardial defect is contraindicated because of the possibility of compressing the heart in the pericardial sac.

POSTOPERATIVE FEATURES

After amputation of the herniated left atrial appendage and operative closure of the pericardial defect, the previously present bulge is not present, and the cardiac silhouette becomes normal (Fig 72–13).

PERICARDIAL FAT NECROSIS

Pericardial fat necrosis is a rare clinical entity that may be confused with myocardial infarction, tumor, or pulmonary embolism.[8] Radiographically, a well-delineated mass is found at the right cardiophrenic angle. Pain is abrupt in onset and pleuritic in nature and may radiate to the shoulder because of phrenic nerve irritation.

The pathogenesis is obscure, but obesity may be a predisposing factor. Patients are otherwise in excellent health. Clinically and pathologically there is a great resemblance of this condition to infarction of the epiploic appendages of the colon.

REFERENCES

1. Nasser W, Feigenbaum H, Helmen C: Congenital absence of the left pericardium, *Circulation* 34:100, 1966.
2. Nasser WK, Helmen C, Tavel ME, et al: Congenital absence of the left pericardium: clinical, electrocardiographic, radiographic, hemodynamic, and angiographic findings in six cases, *Circulation* 41:469, 1970.
3. Moene RJ, Dekker A, van der Harten HJ: Congenital right-sided pericardial defect with herniation of part of the lung into the pericardial cavity, *Am J Cardiol* 31:519, 1973.
4. Hipona FA, Crummy AB Jr: Congenital pericardial defect associated with tetralogy of Fallot: herniation of normal lung into the pericardial cavity, *Circulation* 29:132, 1964.
5. Duffie ER Jr, Moss AJ, Maloney JV Jr: Congenital pericardial defects with herniation of the heart into the pleural space, *Pediatrics* 30:746, 1962.
6. Andersen M, Fredens M, Olesen KH: Traumatic rupture of the pericardium, *Am J Cardiol* 27:566, 1971.
7. Payvandi MN, Kerber RE: Echocardiography in congenital and acquired absence of the pericardium: an echocardiographic mimic of right ventricular volume overload, *Circulation* 53:86, 1976.
8. Behrendt DM, Scannell JG: Pericardial fat necrosis: an unusual case of severe chest pain and thoracic "tumor," *N Engl J Med* 279:473, 1968.

CHAPTER 73

Cardiac Tumors

Cardiac tumors are rare, and an autopsy incidence of 0.0017% has been reported. Eighty-five percent of the primary cardiac tumors are benign, and myxoma is the most common of these tumors, consisting of 30% to 50% of all benign cardiac tumors. Metastatic tumors to the heart occur approximately 20 to 40 times as frequently as primary ones.

CLINICAL PRESENTATION

Cardiac tumors can present in a variety of ways, depending on their type and location. Because of their rarity and the diverse clinical features, cardiac tumors may be undiagnosed or diagnosed late. The methods of clinical presentation can be divided into three categories,[1,2] which are discussed later on. In patients with these presenting symptoms, cardiac tumor should be considered in the differential diagnosis:

1. Hemodynamic disturbances
   a. Cardiac arrhythmias. Cardiac arrhythmias, particularly ventricular tachycardia, can occur most notably in infants and children. Atrial fibrillation may occur with atrial myxoma.
   b. Pericardial involvement, perhaps with effusion. Pericardial effusion or diffuse involvement of the pericardium by tumor can produce cardiac tamponade.
   c. Cardiac obstruction. Myxoma in either atrium may produce inflow obstruction and fibromas, or rhabdomyomas may occasionally produce outflow obstruction. Clinical features of obstructive tumors may be those of valvar obstruction, pulmonary edema, syncope, or congestive cardiac failure.
   d. Embolism, either systemic, as from myxoma, or pulmonary as from right-sided cardiac tumors.
   e. Myocardial damage reflected by angina or electrocardiographic changes may develop from myocardial invasion or emboli to coronary arteries.
2. Mechanical hemolysis from atrial myxoma.
3. Constitutional features. With atrial myxoma, associated fever, anorexia, weight loss, and elevated erythrocyte sedimentation rate may suggest chronic illness. The clinical picture may mimic acute rheumatic fever or bacterial endocarditis if anemia or signs of embolization coexist.

CLASSIFICATION

Cardiac tumors may be classified in various ways,[1-5] but any classification has its limitations because of the variety of histologic types and clinical manifestations. We discuss cardiac tumors according to their location within the heart, because the clinical, hemodynamic, and laboratory features are often similar among different types of tumors located at the same site. Thus, primary cardiac tumors may be intracavitary, mural, or pericardial.

Intracavitary Tumors

Myxoma is the most frequently occurring intracavitary tumor.[6] Ninety percent of myxomas are located in the atria and 10% in other cardiac structures. Seventy-five percent of myxomas are located in the left atria and originate from the atrial septum in the region of the fossa ovalis. This location has been attributed to the presence of myxoid tissue at this site, but others deny this relationship. The next most common location is in the right atrium (20%). Occasionally an atrial myxoma exists in both atria and has a dumbbell appearance. Uncommon sites are in the ventricle, usually right ventricular free wall, or ventricular septum. Rarely, they arise on the mitral, tricuspid, or pulmonary valves and obstruct blood flow. The tumors may be multicentric, with more than one tumor coexisting in a patient.

Most myxomas are pedunculated. The pedicle may be short, allowing little movement of the tumor, or long, resulting in prolapse of the tumor across a valve. Those without a pedicle are sessile. The tumor may be solid and spherical or lobulated with villous projections. Myxomas may be either gelatinous or mucoid, and often they contain areas of hemorrhage. Rarely, myxomas calcify. Two percent of right atrial myxomas and 1% of left atrial myxomas show calcification. Myxomas have malignant potential by local extension and invasion.[7] Metastases may occur with invasion of vessel walls and result in aneurysmal changes. Histologic studies have shown that the tumor usually does not extend beyond the endothelial layers of the endocardium. Atrial myxomas are considered tumors rather than organized thrombi. Although they have similar histochemical staining properties, such as cutaneous myxomas and umbilical cord tissue, they stain differently from thrombi.

Fragments of myxomas may embolize and cause muscle necrosis and secondary inflammatory changes in muscle and arterial walls.[8] They may be the source of peripheral myxomas.[9] Because of their prolapse through atrioventricular valves, they may cause trauma and secondary changes of the valve leaflets.[10]

Right atrial myxoma may lead to pulmonary hypertension because of repeated pulmonary embolism. Death may occur suddenly from obstruction of the main pulmonary artery by a tumor embolus. A left atrial myxoma may embolize and disappear from the left atrium entirely. Systemic embolization from a left atrial myxoma may be to any organ and produce various clinical signs. Left atrial myxomas may recur as long as 6 years after resection, perhaps from incomplete resection of the tumor. During operation the underlying atrial tissue should be resected, because under rare circumstances the tumor may have infiltrated the septum or even have extended into the right atrium ("dumbbell tumor").

Clinical Features

Several important clinical features of atrial myxoma lead to the diagnosis:[1, 2, 4]

1. Absence of history of rheumatic fever; signs and symptoms of rheumatic fever in the absence of criteria to diagnose that disease.

2. Sudden onset or exaggeration of symptoms such as dizziness, syncope, or respiratory distress, particularly with change in body position. Symptoms may change with position in 25% of the cases.

3. Physical examination and radiologic findings that do not correlate with degree of failure or mitral obstruction.

4. The character of a murmur changing with body position.

5. Rapid progression of symptoms of cardiac failure and no response to medical therapy.

6. Peripheral emboli in the absence of cardiac arrhythmia.

7. Clinical features of subacute endocarditis or intermittent fever but with repeatedly negative blood cultures and normal-sized spleen.

8. Systemic reactions such as leukocytosis, fever, anemia, increased sedimentation rate, and hypergammaglobulinemia.

Left atrial myxoma has variable clinical presentations and a tendency to mimic other cardiac conditions. The clinical picture may be dominated by the obstructive features of the tumor, by embolic phenomena, or by constitutional symptoms.

If pedunculated, the tumor may prolapse through an atrioventricular valve.[11, 12] Obstruction by the tumor, usually of the mitral valve, causes syncope, vertigo, and dyspnea, but syncope is present in less than 20% of the cases. Obstruction usually leads to diastolic murmurs characteristic of either mitral or tricuspid obstruction. The diastolic murmur may be accompanied by an early diastolic sound. This sound, thought to be an opening snap, appears to be related to the checking of the tumor in the left ventricle ("tumor plop"). The auscultatory findings are commonly mistaken for rheumatic mitral stenosis. The murmur, however, changes with position, a finding highly suggestive of an atrial myxoma rather than either mitral or tricuspid valvar stenosis.

At least one half of the instances of atrial myxomas show evidence of systemic embolization. In a patient with evidence of embolization, the emboli should be examined histologically to identify if atrial myxoma is the source.[8, 9] Severe symptoms may result from embolization, including stroke and hematuria. False aneurysms may form in the cerebral circulation at sites of embolization.

Finally, atrial myxomas often present clinical findings consistent with bacterial endocarditis. This picture is usually caused by embolization and occlusion of small vessels by sterile tumor emboli. Myxomas may become infected, and such emboli may contain organisms. Infected emboli are extremely rare and usually diagnosed only at autopsy. The situation is confusing because blood cultures may be negative. A case was reported where the diagnosis of infected myxoma was made; the patient was treated with antibiotics but died of a ruptured cerebral mycotic aneurysm.

Constitutional features are common and include: fever, 50%; elevated erythrocyte sedimentation rate, 70%; weight loss, 50%; anemia, 40%; and abnormal serum protein levels, 50%.

In right atrial myxoma, the history is usually one of syncope and progressive dyspnea without orthopnea, and the symptoms are refractory to digitalis and diuretics. Prominent A waves are found in the jugular venous pulse, and a presystolic murmur is heard. The clinical findings are easily confused with tricuspid stenosis. The myxoma may be biatrial in location and may mimic combined tricuspid and mitral valvar disease.

An obstructing right atrial myxoma may increase right atrial pressure and cause a right-to-left atrial shunt.[12] The resulting cyanosis simulates a congenial cardiac anomaly.

Left atrial myxoma is usually a sporadic disease, but one family has been described where the mother and three of seven children had myxomas.[13] The mother's father and brother died suddenly without the tumor being diagnosed. Family data were consistent with dominant transmission. Because myxomas may be familial, all members of a family with an individual with myxoma should be screened by echocardiography.

Echocardiographic Features

Left atrial myxoma appears as a mass of echoes, within the left atrium or prolapsing through the mitral valve during diastole. The echocardiogram is a very reliable method of diagnosis.

Radiographic Features

The radiographic findings are nonspecific. Occasionally the discrepancy between radiographic and clinical features is suggestive of the diagnosis.

Intracavitary neoplasms are not visible on a thoracic roentgenogram unless they are calcified, which is rare. The films are usually normal until the tumor alters the hemodynamics by obstructing a cardiac valve. If valvar obstruction develops, the cardiac silhouette and the secondary changes in the lung are identical to those of other obstructive lesions of the mitral valve.

Cardiac tumors that obstruct the left ventricular outflow tract may mimic closely aortic valvar stenosis or those obstructing the tricuspid valve, tricuspid stenosis, or atresia. Hemodynamic mitral stenosis may be caused by obstruction of the mitral valve and result in secondary radiographic signs of pulmonary venous hypertension identical to other mitral obstructive lesions. Rarely, pulmonary arterial hypertension may be evident on a thoracic roentgenogram. REASON: A tumor in a right-sided cardiac chamber may induce repeated pulmonary emboli, which obstruct pulmonary arterial branches and cause secondary pulmonary arterial hypertension. Furthermore, malignant intracavitary cardiac tumors may metastasize to the lung, causing tumor implants by embolization.

Calcifications of a cardiac tumor, although rare, occur sometimes in rhabdomyomas, teratomas, or myxomas (2%); calcification is a helpful radiographic clue. If calcification occurs in a pedunculated tumor, the excessive motion of the calcification can be observed by either fluoroscopy or cine fluorography. Even if the tumor is calcified and relatively immobile, its presence can be suspected by the unusual location of calcium at a site other than in the coronary arterial circulation or a valvar structure. In older patients, calcified mural thrombi must be considered in the differential diagnosis of cardiac calcification, but this occurs extremely rarely in childhood. Calcified thrombi in adults occur usually in the region of the left atrial appendage rather than the atrial septum. Commonly there are concomitant calcifications of the atrial wall.

1. The radiographic manifestations of an intracavitary cardiac tumor results from secondary hemodynamic changes primarily because of valvar obstruction.

2. If the obstructing mechanism of the tumor is minimal, the cardiac silhouette is normal.

3. With severe hemodynamic impairment, particularly with mitral obstruction or insufficiency caused by left atrial myxoma, the radiographic findings are identical to other mitral obstructive lesions, particularly rheumatic mitral stenosis (Fig 73–1).

Cardiac Catheterization

Because the diagnosis can be made easily by echocardiography, nuclear magnetic resonance imaging, or other means,[14] cardiac catheterization is rarely needed. If it is performed, transseptal catheterization is contraindicated because the left atrial myxoma usually attaches close to the foramen ovale.[15] One case of peripheral embolization after transseptal catheterization was described. Diagnosis can be made by left ventriculography if mitral insufficiency is present or by pulmonary angiography.

Hemodynamic findings at time of catheterization show variation of the end-diastolic gradient between left ventricle and pulmonary wedge position caused by the tumor prolapsing across the mitral valve.

A notch in the upstroke of the left ventricular pressure curve may be observed in addition to a prominent C wave. The loud late element of the first heart sound occurring when the tumor prolapses through the mitral valve is associated with an abrupt diminution in left atrial volume, thus creating a rapid Y descent.

The tumor may remain in the left atrium during the entire cardiac cycle but still impede flow across the mitral

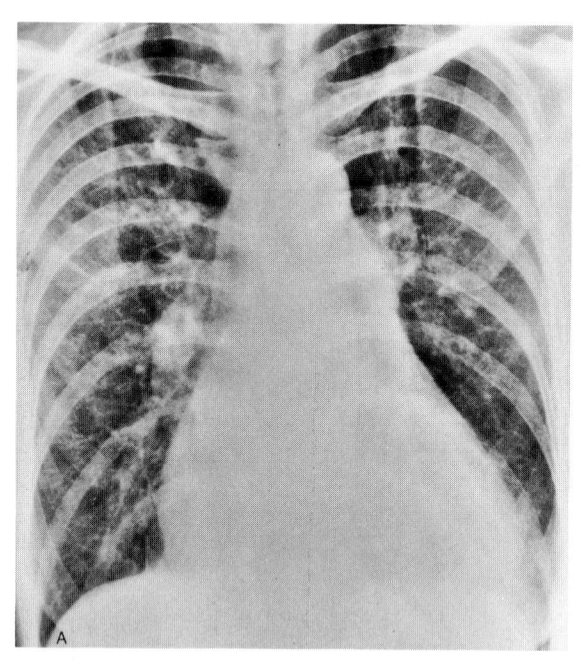

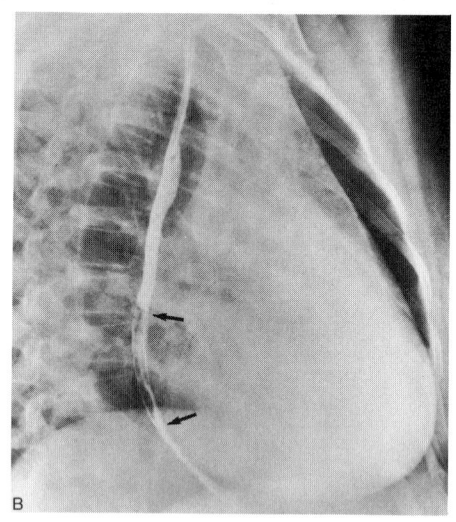

FIG 73–1.
Left atrial myxoma. Thoracic roentgenogram. **A,** posteroanterior projection. Pattern of pulmonary venous and arterial hypertension. Moderately enlarged heart. Diffuse exaggeration of interstitial venous markings. Prominence of upper lobe pulmonary veins. Mild prominence of main pulmonary artery segment. **B,** right anterior oblique projection. Barium swallow. Distinct left atrial enlargement *(arrows)*.

valve. The Y descent is slow, and the findings are indistinguishable from mitral stenosis.

Angiographic Features

Before the development of echocardiography, angiography was the only means to diagnose intracardiac tumors. With the perfection of echocardiography and nuclear magnetic resonance (NMR), angiocardiography has lost some of its importance, particularly in the diagnosis of left atrial myxomas. Nuclear magnetic resonance imaging, echocardiography and computer tomography are excellent means of diagnosing a cardiac tumor, particularly if it is intracavitary (Fig 73–2).

During catheterization, tumors in the right side of the heart can be demonstrated by the injection of contrast medium at a site proximal to the tumor.[16] Placement of a catheter close to a tumor, followed by selective delivery of contrast medium at this site, is unadvisable because of the risk of tumor embolization.

Tumors in the left side of the heart can be safely demonstrated on delayed films after pulmonary angiography (Fig 73–3). The opacification of the left-sided chambers may be suboptimal because the obstruction by an intracavitary tumor may decrease cardiac output and cause pulmonary venous distention. Transseptal catheterization and selective angiography of the left atrium should be avoided in atrial myxomas. REASON: Almost all left atrial myxomas are attached to the atrial septum near the fossa ovalis where the atrial septum is punctured. Left ventricular tumors can be demonstrated by careful injection of the left ventricular cavity or, better yet, via transseptal placement of a catheter into the left atrium with injection at that site. Some left atrial myxomas are visualized after left ventric-

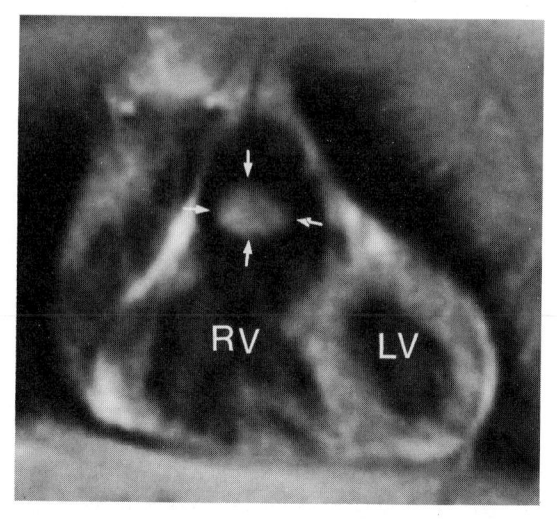

FIG 73–2.
Right ventricular myxoma. Nuclear magnetic resonance image. Anteroposterior projection. Coronal plane. Well-defined mass *(arrows)* in outflow tract of right ventricle. At operation, tumor was pedunculated and attached to crista supraventricularis. *RV* = right ventricle; *LV* = left ventricle. (Courtesy of Dr. F. Stone.)

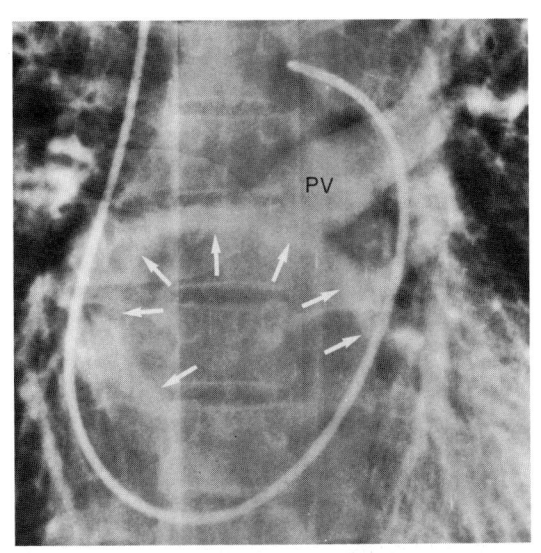

FIG 73-3.
Left atrial myxoma. Chevophase of pulmonary arteriogram. Anteroposterior projection. Left atrium is well delineated. Large smooth mass *(arrows)* in left atrial cavity.

ulography if mitral insufficiency is induced by the injection.

1. Angiography is a sensitive means to demonstrate intracavitary tumors. REASON: The lesion is outlined by contrast medium. Because NMR and ultrasonography can demonstrate the tumor and its anatomic relationship, angiography is performed only in doubtful cases.
2. Left atrial myxomas can be demonstrated angiographically by pulmonary angiography and viewing the late films as the left atrium is opacified. A filling defect is present in the left atrium (see Fig 73-3). If the tumor is on a stalk, it may be seen to prolapse through the mitral valve during diastole.
3. Pulmonary angiography may be disappointing. REASON: Some left atrial myxomas cause severe mitral obstruction. The resultant slow blood flow, increased pulmonary venous, and left atrial blood volume markedly dilute the contrast medium.
4. If the tumor produces mitral insufficiency, left ventriculography may demonstrate the tumor (Fig 73-4). REASON: Mitral regurgitation allows reflux of contrast material into the left atrium with opacification of the left atrium and delineation of the tumor (see Fig 73-4).
5. Characteristically left atrial myxomas are mobile and prolapse through the mitral valve during diastole and cause mitral obstruction. During systole the mass returns to the left atrium, and the filling defect in the left ventricle disappears (see Fig 73-4,B).
6. Pedunculated intraventricular tumors tend to prolapse through the semilunar valves (Fig 73-5). The impact of the tumor on the valve leaflets may cause valvar thickening and finally valvar insufficiency.
7. There are no angiographic clues as to the nature of an intracavitary mass. Histology is variable (Fig 73-6).
8. With the development of ultrasonography and NMR imaging, intracavitary tumors can be readily demonstrated noninvasively. A common intracavitary tumor is myxoma, which is usually found in the atria but may also occur in the ventricles (see Fig 73-4).
9. In older patients, intracavitary tumors are commonly extensions of malignancies. Hypernephroma, hepatoma, and lymphomas tend to grow along the venae cavae into the right-sided cardiac chambers (Fig 73-7).
10. In older patients with superior vena caval syndrome caused by extrinsic compression, a thrombus may form in the right atrium and ventricle. These are indistinguishable angiographically from tumor invasion (Fig 73-8).

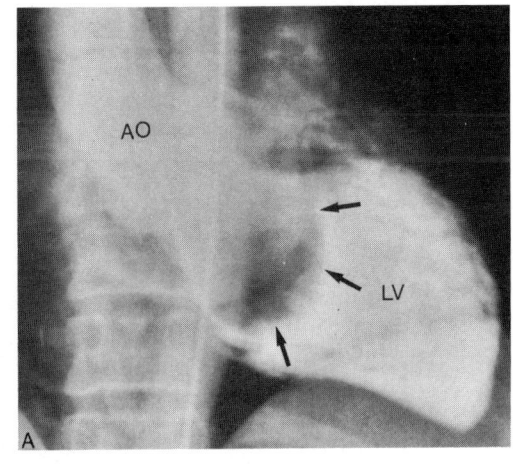

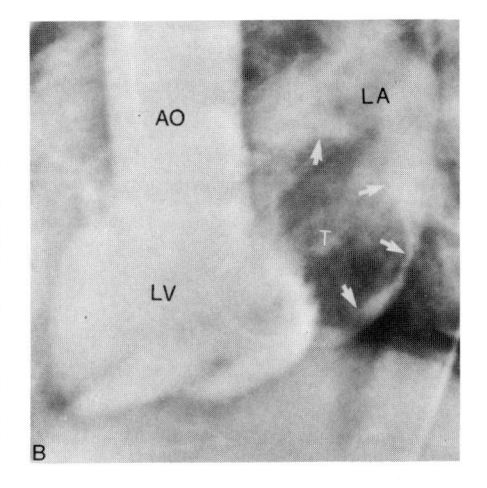

FIG 73-4.
Left atrial myxoma. Left ventriculogram *(LV)*. Anteroposterior projection. **A,** diastole. Large filling defect *(arrows)* visualized in left ventricle by atrial myxoma. **B,** systole. Lateral projection. Tumor *(T)* is outlined in left atrium *(LA)* because of mitral regurgitation. *AO* = aorta. *LV* = left ventricle; *LA* = left atrium.

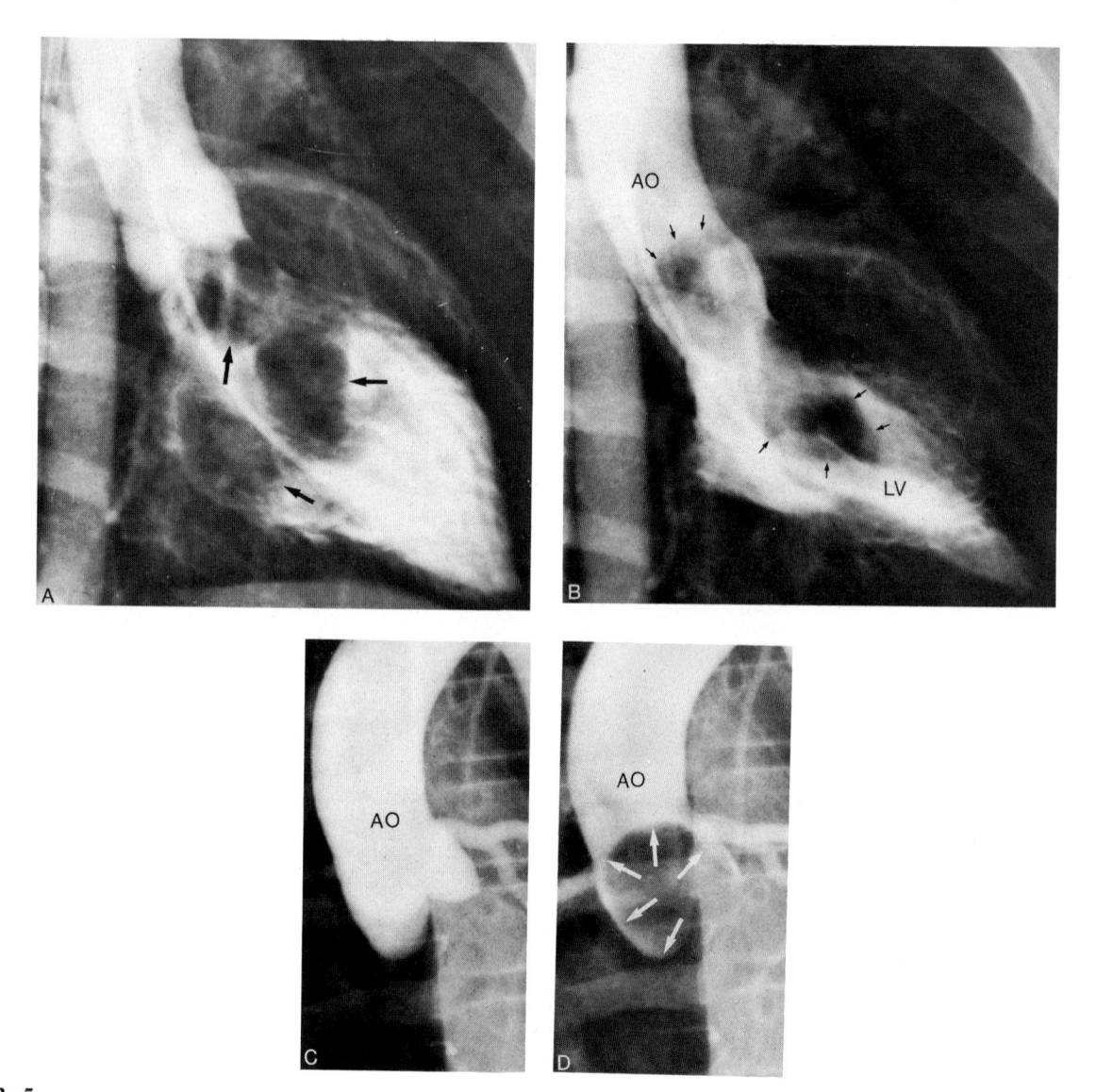

FIG 73–5.
Large rhabdomyosarcoma in left ventricle *(LV)*. **A,** left ventriculogram. **A,** diastole and, **B,** systole. Large lobulated filling defect *(arrows)* in left ventricle is caused by huge tumor mass. **B,** pedunculated tumor prolapses through aortic valve *(arrows)*. **C** and **D,** aortogram. **C,** diastole. Normal competent aortic valve. **D,** systole. Tumor mass protrudes through aortic valve *(arrows)*, causing aortic outflow obstruction. *AO* = aorta.

Treatment

Atrial myxoma should be treated by resection of the tumor. For a left atrial myxoma, the left atrium is incised and the point of attachment of the tumor is determined by finger exploration. If the tumor is attached to the septum, as it usually is, a right atriotomy is made. The atrial septum is incised, and a sufficient amount of atrial septum is excised, including the tumor attachment. The tumor is removed, and the atria are irrigated with saline solution to remove smaller fragments; the septum is closed by direct suture or with a pericardial or synthetic patch.

For right atrial myxomas, the left atrium is not opened. The right atrium is incised, and after the tumor attachment has been identified, the adjacent portion of the atrial septum beyond the attachment is resected. The defect in the septum is repaired identical to left atrial myxomas.

Recurrence may occur because of incomplete resection or growth of tumor implants.

Intramural Tumors

Intramural mesenchymal neoplasms of the heart are similar to other connective tissue tumors. Sarcomas are the most common and usually involve the right atrial wall. In 30% of the cases, distant metastases are present. Among

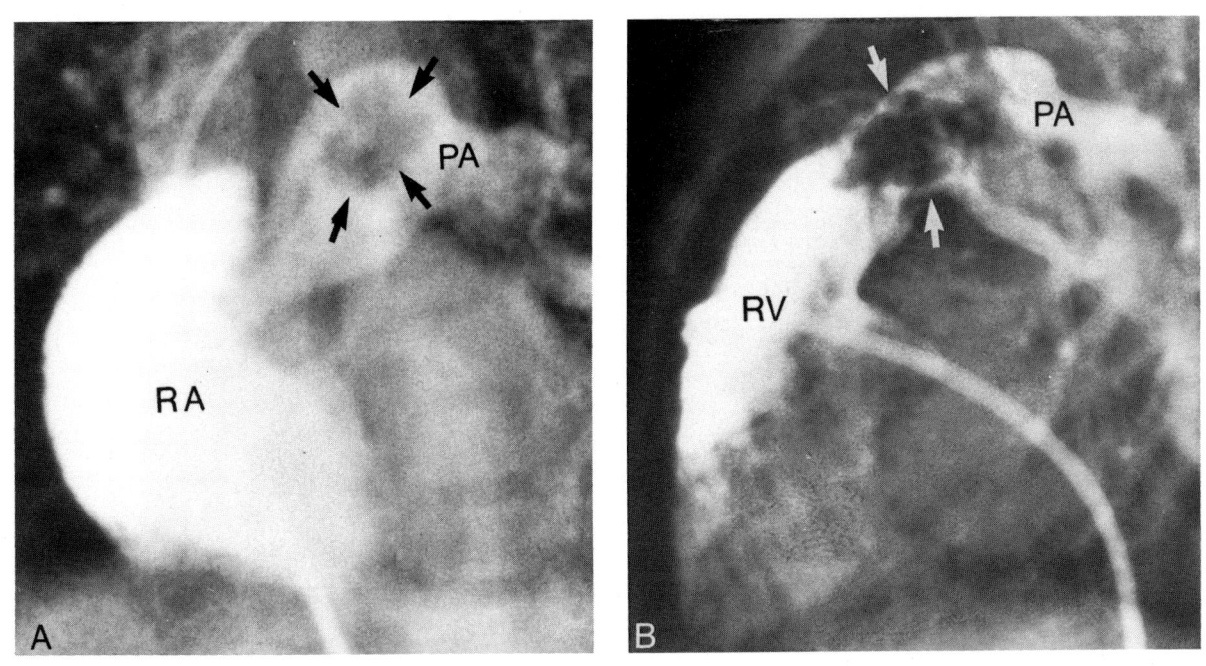

FIG 73–6.
Pulmonary arterial mass is caused by fungal infection. **A,** right atriogram *(RA).* Anteroposterior projection. Densely opacified right atrium. Well-defined filling defect in pulmonary artery **(PA)** proved to be fungal mass. **B,** right ventriculogram *(RV).* Lateral projection. Lobulated mass *(arrows)* in pulmonary artery.

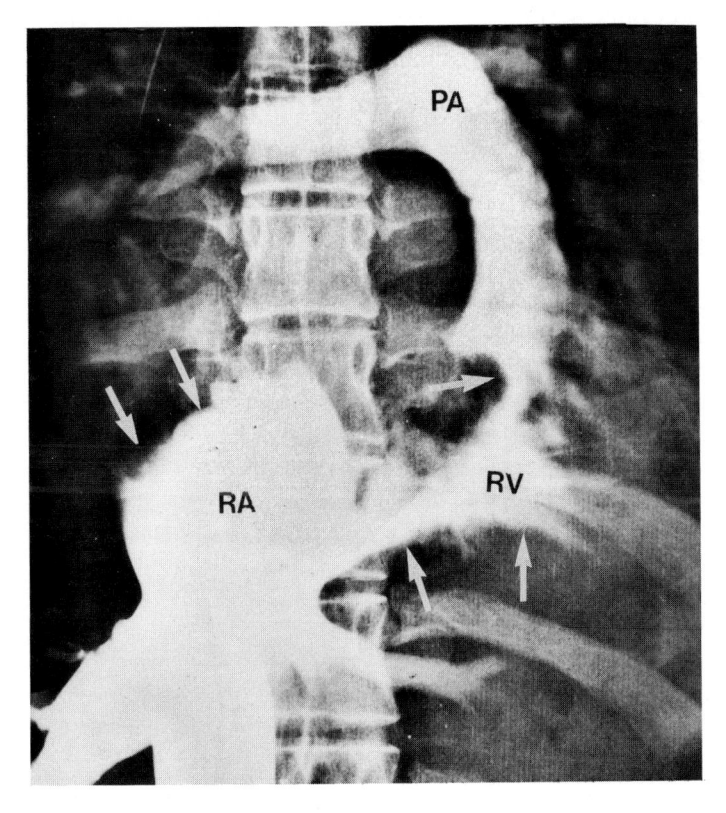

FIG 73–7.
Lymphoma. Inferior vena cavogram. Anteroposterior projection. Tumor mass *(arrow)* in right atrium *(RA)* and right ventricle *(RV)* is caused by tumor extension. PA = pulmonary artery.

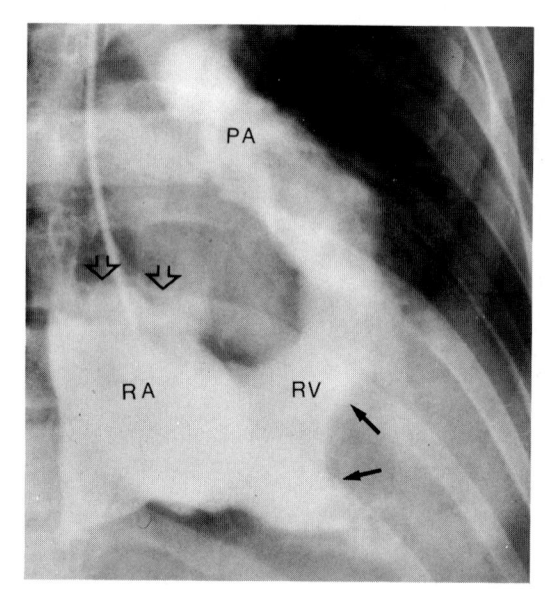

FIG 73-8.
Superior vena cava syndrome is caused by carcinoma of lung. Right atriogram (RA). Right anterior oblique projection. Occlusion of superior vena cava (open arrows). Large filling defect (solid arrow) in right ventricle (RV). Filling defects in atrium and ventricle are indistinguishable from primary tumor. Mass proved to be thrombus. PA = pulmonary artery.

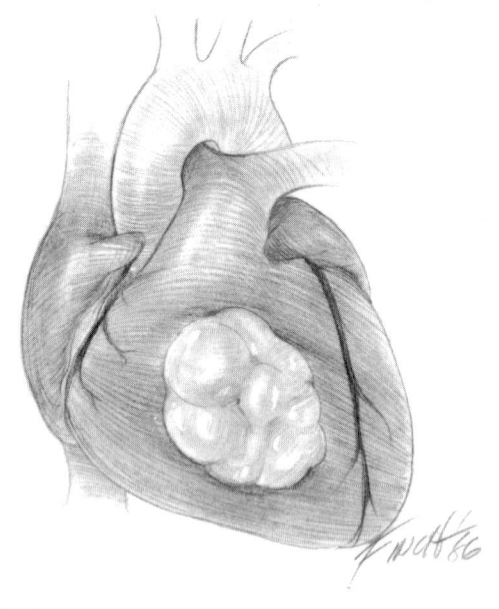

FIG 73-9.
Intramural rhabdomyosarcoma of right ventricle protruding through epicardium. Tumor may also protrude into ventricle and cause outflow obstruction.

the less frequent benign mural tumors are angiomas, lipomas, rhabdomyomas, and fibromas. Fibromas, which constitute about 5% of the primary cardiac tumors, are similar to desmoid tumors but are not commonly considered to be rhabdomyomas. Intramural tumors may cause an abnormal thoracic radiographic appearance, but calcifications are rare. Consequently, calcium in the cardiac silhouette of a young patient is suggestive of a calcified intramural tumor.

Rhabdomyomas

Whereas rhabdomyoma is the second most common benign cardiac tumor, rhabdomyosarcoma of the heart is rare. Less than 100 cases of cardiac rhabdomyosarcoma have been reported, and the most common sites are right ventricle, left atrium, and right atrium. The tumor may protrude into a ventricular cavity and obstruct blood flow or may protrude through the epicardial surface (Fig 73-9).

Rhabdomyomas usually occur as multiple discrete intramural tumors involving any or each of the cardiac chambers.[3, 14] The neoplastic origin of these tumors is uncertain, and some consider these tumors as hamartomas. The cells of these tumors contain large amounts of glycogen and have been called "spider cells" because of their spongy vacublated appearance.[17]

Usually rhabdomyomas occur in individuals with tuberous sclerosis, a complex of mental retardation, epilepsy, and adenoma sebaceum.[4, 18, 19] In such patients hamartomas may occur in other organs, particularly the kidney. Because of its predominate intramural location, this tumor can interfere with myocardial function and present as a cardiomyopathy or can cause an arrhythmia because of interference with the conduction system. Large tumors represent space-occupying masses within the heart, and those in the intraventricular septum may cause either subaortic (see Fig 73-4) or subpulmonary obstruction. Rarely, the tumor may obstruct an atrioventricular valve, and in one case this resulted in a clinical picture of tricuspid atresia.[20]

The presentation is usually from the cardiac symptoms, and the features of tuberous sclerosis, if recognized, are found secondarily. Often the cardiac involvement becomes evident in the neonatal period as cardiac failure or murmurs. Supraventricular or ventricular arrhythmias may be the presenting feature in infancy. The electrocardiogram may show prolonged P-R interval or evidence of intraventricular conduction delay or ST-T wave changes.

Echocardiographic Features.—Intramural rhabdomyomas, like other mural tumors, appear as localized, excessive thickening of the cardiac wall and may encroach on or obliterate a cardiac cavity.[21]

Radiographic Features.—The radiographic appearance of cardiac tumors is not uniform, and, consequently, the correct radiographic diagnosis is virtually never made.

Certain radiographic features, however, are consistent with the various types of cardiac tumors. Depending on the location of the tumor, the anatomic and hemodynamic consequences vary greatly so that the radiographic appearance depends largely on the location of the tumors. The cardiac contour is often normal.

Intramural tumors may enlarge and distort the cardiac chambers, giving the heart a bizarre radiographic appearance. In most cases cardiomegaly is nonspecific and is mistaken radiographically for cardiomyopathy. Rarely, an intramural tumor such as a fibroma calcifies. This radiographic finding of calcification clinches the diagnosis (Fig 73–10).

Cardiac Catheterization and Angiography.—Cardiac catheterization is performed principally to outline the tumor angiographically. Intramyocardial tumors are angiographically manifested by the impingement of the opacified ventricular cavities that distorts the ventricular chambers (Fig 73–11). Angiography is not the most sensitive means to diagnose these tumors. Magnetic resonance imaging is the preferred imaging modality because the signal from the tumor is different from the surrounding muscle. Intramyocardial tumors do not show significant motion because they are not pedunculated.[22]

1. Whereas angiography allows only visualization of one ventricular cavity at a time, both ventricular cavities can be depicted simultaneously by NMR imaging. Consequently, intramural tumors involving the ventricular septum become much more obvious by this imaging modality than by angiography (Fig 73–12).

2. Occasionally the histologic tumor type can be suggested by NMR imaging, particularly in a fatty tumor, because of its characteristic intense signal (Fig 73–13).

Treatment.—Rhabdomyomas may protrude into either the right or the left ventricular cavity. These can be removed under cardiopulmonary bypass by excision. Removal is accomplished by both blunt and sharp dissection.

Intrapericardial Tumors

Usually intrapericardial tumors occur secondary to metastatic disease. Benign pericardial tumors are about

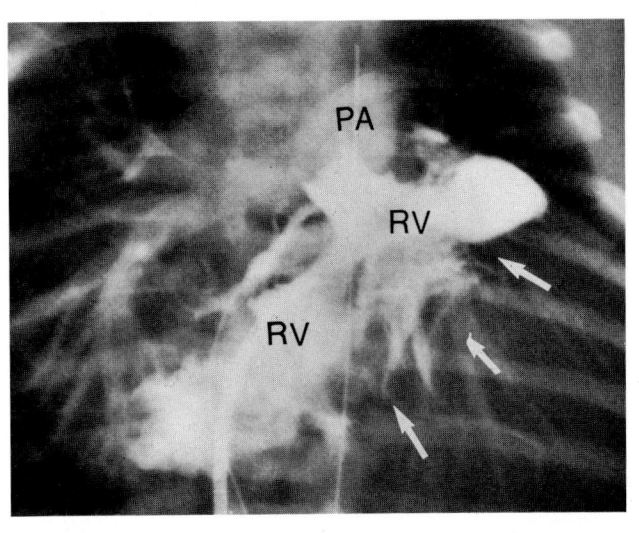

FIG 73–11.
Rhabdomyosarcoma of right ventricle. Right ventriculogram (RV). Anteroposterior projection. Right ventricular cavity is markedly narrowed and distorted by huge intramural tumor mass (arrows). PA = pulmonary artery.

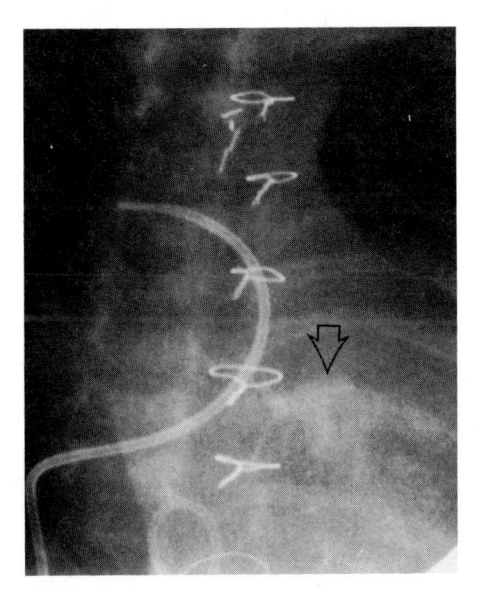

FIG 73–10.
Recurrent fibroma of heart. Thoracic roentgenogram. Anteroposterior projection. Calcified tumor (open arrow). Fluoroscopy is useful to exclude more common valvar calcifications. Catheter is in right pulmonary artery.

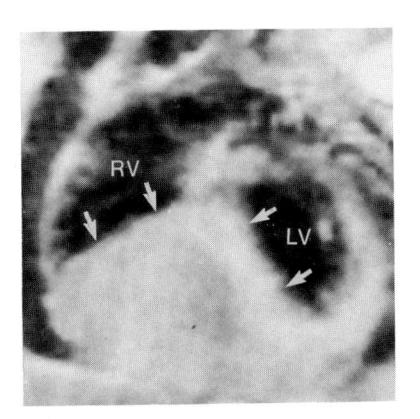

FIG 73–12.
Fibroma. Nuclear magnetic resonance image. Left anterior oblique projection. Huge tumor (arrows) involves ventricular septum impinging on right (RV) and left ventricular (LV) cavities.

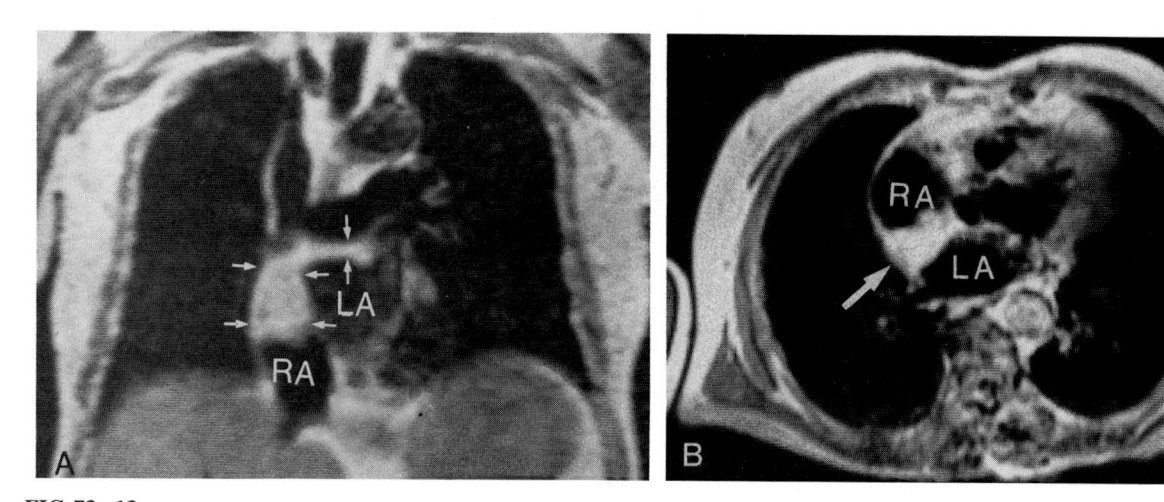

FIG 73–13.
Cardiac tumor. Nuclear magnetic resonance image of thorax. **A,** coronal plane. Tumor mass *(arrows)* in right atrium *(RA)* extends along roof of left atrium *(LA)*. Signal intensity of mass is identical to fat (compare with signal from subcutaneous fat of thorax). **B,** transverse plane. Fatty tumor is located in atrial septum, being characteristic of benign lipoma.

one half as common as benign tumors of other cardiac structures. Benign tumors are usually teratomas that are pedunculated and attached to the origin of the great vessels.[4, 23, 24] Composed of cells from each germinal layer, they may be larger than the size of the heart itself. Pericardial effusion, which may be bloody, is usually present.

Intrapericardial teratoma manifests in infancy with an enlarged cardiac silhouette on a thoracic roentgenogram or evidence of cardiac tamponade because of pericardial effusion.

Echocardiographic Features

There is evidence of pericardial effusion, with an echo-free space not found posteriorly but often anteriorly to the heart. The tumor is recognized anteriorly as an echo-dense mass that displaces the heart posteriorly and distorts the pulmonary artery and right ventricle.

Radiographic Features

1. In most patients primary intrapericardial tumors cause pericardial effusion, which may be bloody (in most reported cases of intrapericardial teratomas, the fluid is straw colored), and the thoracic roentgenogram is identical to pericardial effusion (very rare in infancy).

2. Radiographically the condition is commonly mistaken for more common causes of gross enlargement of the cardiac silhouette, such as Ebstein's malformation and trilogy of Fallot (Fig 73–14).

3. If a diagnostic pericardial tap is performed, a large amount of carbon dioxide should be introduced into the pericardial sac (see Fig 73–14). Upright, right, and left lateral decubitus projections, as well as cross-table lateral films obtained in prone and supine positions, should be obtained to outline the tumor mass.

4. The tumors are usually attached by a pedicle to the

FIG 73–14.
Intrapericardial teratoma. Thoracic roentgenogram. **A,** posteroanterior projection. Massively enlarged cardiac silhouette is caused by pericardial effusion. Radiographically, Ebstein's malformation or trilogy of Fallot have to be considered. **B,** lateral projection. Density is located mostly anteriorly. Heart *(arrows)* does not appear to be enlarged. Differentiation cannot be made radiographically.

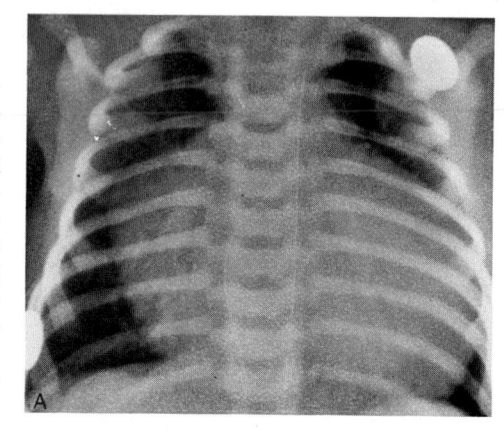

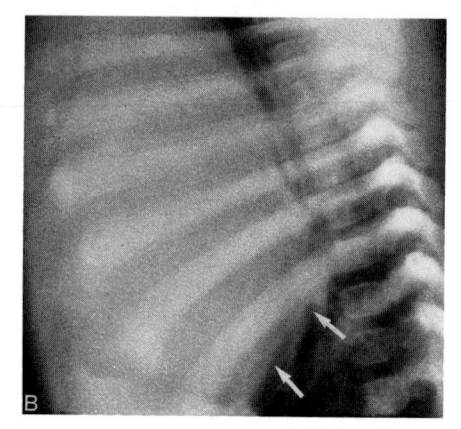

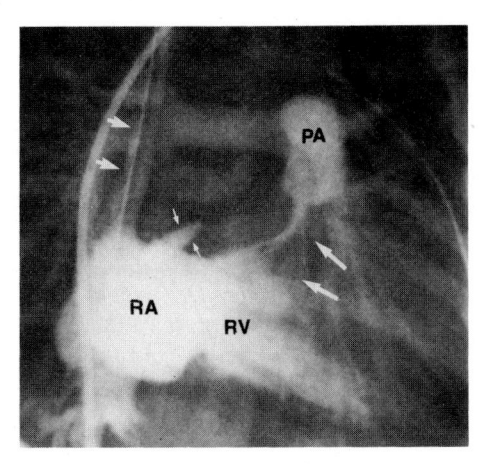

FIG 73-15.
Intrapericardial teratoma. Superior vena cavogram. Anteroposterior projection. Severe compression and distortion of cardiac chambers. Marked compression of superior vena cava *(short white arrows),* right atrial *(RA)* appendage *(small arrows)* and right ventricular *(RV)* outflow tract *(long arrows).* Entire right atrium is markedly compressed. At operation tumor was attached by a pedicle to proximal aorta. *PA* = pulmonary artery. *RA* = right atrium.

proximal aorta. They manifest as cardiac tamponade or by compression of various cardiovascular structures such as the superior vena cava, right atrium, right ventricle, pulmonary artery, or, less frequently, the left side of the heart (Fig 73-15).

Angiographic Features

1. Angiocardiography is less rewarding for intrapericardial and intramural tumors than for intracavitary tumors. REASON: Because the tumor lies outside the cardiac chambers, it is evident only by compression of opacified structures. In contrast, intracavitary tumors are surrounded by contrast medium and are obvious angiographically.

2. Intrapericardial tumors, particularly large teratomas, can be diagnosed angiographically by observing compression of the aorta or the right atrium (see Fig 73-15). Compression of the right-sided cardiac chambers and the aorta are most common, because these tumors are usually attached to one of the great vessels.

Treatment

The tumor should be removed by resecting its stalk from the great vessels. The results are excellent, and recurrence is rare.

Postoperative Features

After removal of an intracavitary cardiac tumor, the radiographic appearance does not change. With a large intramural tumor, operation may result in a decrease in cardiac size. The most striking radiographic postoperative change occurs with intrapericardial tumors. REASON: There is usually massive cardiomegaly because of a large pericardial effusion (Fig 73-16).

Other Tumors

Angiosarcoma is a rare tumor of the heart.[25] Primary leiomyosarcoma of the pulmonary artery has been described.[26] Tumors may originate from valve leaflets. Lipomas may occur anywhere in the heart but primarily in the atrial septum (see Fig 73-13). Papillary tumors of the tricuspid valve cause obstruction and simulate tricuspid atre-

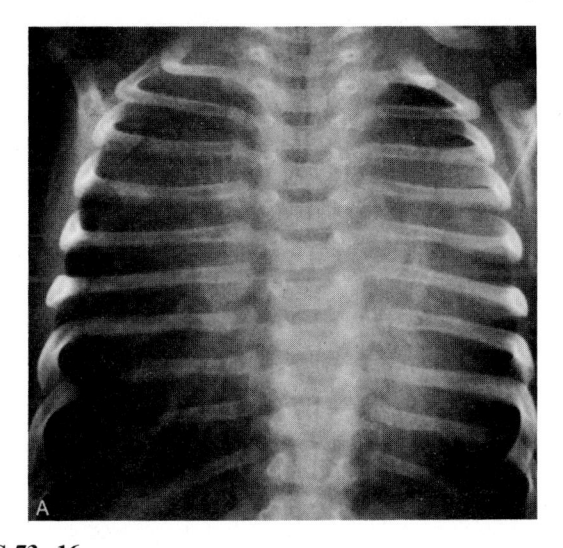

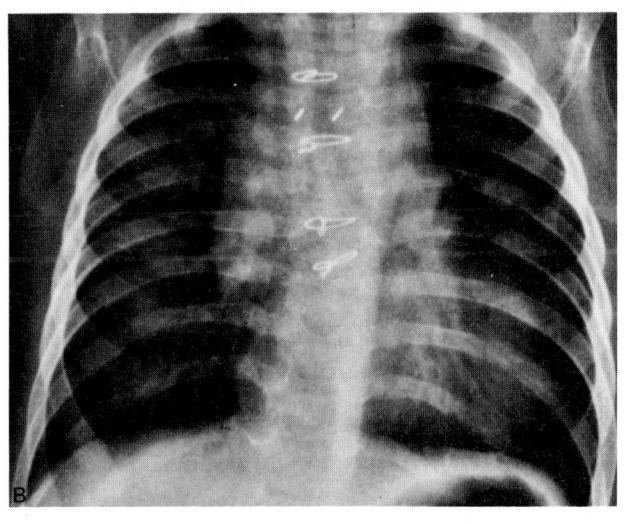

FIG 73-16.
Intrapericardial teratoma. Thoracic roentgenogram. Posteroanterior projection. **A,** massive enlargement of cardiac silhouette is caused by pericardial effusion. **B,** after operative removal of tumor mass and pericardial effusion. Normal cardiac size.

sia. Other intraventricular tumors are intramural cardiac fibromas and myxomas. Atrioventricular block may also be seen if tumors such as fibroma[27] or mesothelioma[28] are situated in the region of the bundle of His. Fibromas may also occur in the ventricular septum (see Fig 73–12).[29]

REFERENCES

1. Goodwin JF: Symposium on cardiac tumors: introduction: the spectrum of cardiac tumors, *Am J Cardiol* 21:307, 1968.
2. Harvey WP: Clinical aspects of cardiac tumors, *Am J Cardiol* 21:328, 1968.
3. Heath D: Pathology of cardiac tumors, *Am J Cardiol* 21:315, 1968.
4. Nadas AS, Ellison RC: Cardiac tumors in infancy, *Am J Cardiol* 21:363, 1968.
5. Arciniegas E, Hakimi M, Farooki ZQ, et al: Primary cardiac tumors in children, *J Thorac Cardiovasc Surg* 79:582, 1980.
6. St John Sutton MG, Mercier LA, Giuliani ER, et al: Atrial myxomas: a review of clinical experience in 40 patients, *Mayo Clin Proc* 55:371, 1980.
7. Walton JA Jr, Kahn DR, Willis PW III: Recurrence of a left atrial myxoma, *Am J Cardiol* 29:872, 1972.
8. Huston KA, Combs JJ Jr, Lie JT, et al: Left atrial myxoma simulating peripheral vasculitis, *Mayo Clin Proc* 53:752, 1978.
9. Balk AHM, Wagenaar SS, Bruschke AVG: Bilateral cardiac myxomas and peripheral myxomas in a patient with recent myocardial infarction, *Am J Cardiol* 44:767, 1979.
10. Carter JB, Cramer R Jr, Edwards JE: Mitral and tricuspid lesions associated with polypoid atrial tumors, including myxoma, *Am J Cardiol* 33:914, 1974.
11. Sung RJ, Ghahramani AR, Mallon SM, et al: Hemodynamic features of prolapsing and nonprolapsing left atrial myxoma, *Circulation* 51:342, 1975.
12. Goldschlager A, Popper R, Goldschlager N, et al: Right atrial myxoma with right to left shunt and polycythemia presenting as congenital heart disease, *Am J Cardiol* 30:82, 1972.
13. Powers JC, Falkoff M, Heinle RA, et al: Familial cardiac myxoma: emphasis on unusual clinical manifestations, *J Thorac Cardiovasc Surg* 77:782, 1979.
14. Pohost GM, Pastore JO, McKusick KA, et al: Detection of left atrial myxoma by gated radionuclide cardiac imaging, *Circulation* 55:88, 1977.
15. Pindyck F, Pierce EC II, Baron MG, et al: Embolization of left atrial myxoma after transseptal cardiac catheterization, *Am J Cardiol* 30:569, 1972.
16. Chandraratna PAN, Pedro SS, Elkins RC, et al: Echocardiographic, angiocardiographic, and surgical correlations in right ventricular myxoma simulating valvar pulmonic stenosis, *Circulation* 55:619, 1977.
17. Fenoglio JJ Jr, McAllister HA Jr, Ferrans VJ: Cardiac rhabdomyoma: a clinicopathologic and electron microscopic study, *Am J Cardiol* 38:241, 1976.
18. Shaher RM, Mintzer J, Farina M, et al: Clinical presentation of rhabdomyoma of the heart in infancy and childhood, *Am J Cardiol* 30:95, 1972.
19. Tsakraklides V, Burke B, Mastri A, et al: Rhabdomyomas of heart a report of four cases, *Am J Dis Child* 128:639, 1974.
20. Neal WA, Knight L, Blieden LC, et al: Clinical pathologic conference, *Am Heart J* 89:514, 1975.
21. Spooner EW, Farina MA, Shaher RM, et al: Left ventricular rhabdomyoma causing subaortic stenosis—the two-dimensional echocardiographic appearance, *Pediatr Cardiol* 2:67, 1982.
22. Orsmond GS, Knight L, Dehner LP, et al: Alveolar rhabdomyosarcoma involving the heart: an echocardiographic, angiographic and pathologic study, *Circulation* 54:837, 1976.
23. Arciniegas E, Hakimi M, Farooki ZQ, et al: Intrapericardial teratoma in infancy, *J Thorac Cardiovasc Surg* 79:306, 1980.
24. Reynolds JL, Donahue JK, Pearce CW: Intrapericardial teratoma: a cause of acute pericardial effusion in infancy, *Pediatrics* 43:71, 1969.
25. Glancy DL, Morales JB Jr, Roberts WC: Angiosarcoma of the heart, *Am J Cardiol* 21:413, 1968.
26. Hayes WL, Farha SJ, Brown RL: Primary leiomyosarcoma of the pulmonary artery, *Am J Cardiol* 34:615, 1974.
27. James TN, Carson DJL, Marshall TK: De subitaneis mortibus: I, fibroma compressing His bundle, *Circulation* 48:428, 1973.
28. Lewman LV, Demany MA, Zimmerman HA: Congenital tumor of atrioventricular node with complete heart block and sudden death: mesothelioma or lymphangioendothelioma of atrioventricular node, *Am J Cardiol* 29:554, 1972.
29. Geha AS, Weidman WH, Soule EH, et al: Intramural ventricular cardiac fibroma: successful removal in two cases and review of the literature, *Circulation* 36:427, 1967.

CHAPTER 74

Complete Heart Block

Complete heart block indicates total interruption of the normal transmission of atrial impulses into the ventricles. This can result from a variety of causes. Because of the slow ventricular rate and increased stroke volume, cardiomegaly is present. Radiologists must be aware of this rare cause of cardiomegaly.

PATHOLOGIC ANATOMY

Complete heart block results from a variety of identifiable causes, but frequently no etiology can be determined. Among the causes are the following:

1. Postoperative.[1-4] Although common during the early era of cardiac operations, with better understanding of the location of the conduction system, complete heart block is currently a rare complication. During the repair of a ventricular septal defect, either isolated or with more complex conditions such as tetralogy of Fallot, the bundle of His may be damaged, because its course frequently is along the rim of the defect. In operative replacement of a calcific aortic valve, removal of calcified material may damage the conduction system. Postoperative complete heart block has been associated with sudden death; thus, a pacemaker is generally placed even in asymptomatic patients.

2. Myocardial infarction.

3. Congenital cardiac malformations. Although individual cases of a variety of conditions have been reported to be associated with complete heart block, congenital corrected transposition of the great vessels[5] has an incidence of 10% of complete heart block.

4. Infectious disease. Myocarditis[6] and (rarely) bacterial endocarditis[7,8] have been associated with complete heart block, the latter by extension of the infection below the aortic valve into the conducting system.

5. Collagen-vascular disease. Rarely, polymyositis[9] and rheumatic carditis[10] are associated with complete heart block. Maternal lupus erythematosis is associated with the development of complete heart block in utero,[11] presumably from transplacental passage of antibodies. Involved neonates show evidence of other lupus antibodies, but these disappear during infancy. Complete heart block persists, however.

6. Congenital. In these cases several types of anomalies have been found, including lack of communication between atrial tissue and the atrioventricular node, discontinuity of the atrioventricular bundle, and absence of the atrioventricular node.[12]

PHYSIOLOGY

The cells in the atrioventricular node depolarize spontaneously but at a lower rate than the sinoatrial node and often between 45 and 65 beats/min.

Despite a slow ventricular rate, resting cardiac output is maintained by an increased stroke volume. End-diastolic volumes of the ventricles are increased, but end-systolic volumes are normal. Ventricular filling is partially impaired because atrial contraction is asynchronous with the ventricle. Atrial contraction normally contributes approximately 15% to ventricular filling. In congenital complete heart block, cardiac output increases to some extent with pharmacologic agents or exercise. Congestive cardiac failure may develop if cardiac anomalies that augment ventricular volume, such as left-to-right shunts, valvar insufficiency, or increased ventricular pressure, coexist. Without associated conditions, cardiac failure is rare.

Symptoms are also determined by the site of the ventricular pacemaker. If the ventricular pacemaker is stable and originates at the atrioventricular node, the cardiac rate ranges usually between 45 and 65 beats/min. If it originates in the His bundles, the rate is slower, and the QRS complex is often wide. The major symptoms are Adam-Stokes attacks or sudden death. The etiology of these events is unknown but may be related to failure of the idioventricular pacemaker or development of a ventricular tachyarrhythmia.

CLINICAL FEATURES

Congenital complete heart block may be recognized in utero, when a slow fetal cardiac rate is detected. Fetal distress is suspected, but the complete heart block can be recognized by fetal echocardiography, which shows discordance between atrial and ventricular contractions.[13] Most children with congenital complete heart block without other abnormalities grow and develop normally.

Most children and adults are asymptomatic and lead active lives and may even participate in competitive athletics.[14] Episodes of sudden loss of consciousness (Adams-Stokes) may occur[14, 15] and should prompt expeditious evaluation and treatment.

The history may reveal the underlying cause of the complete heart block, such as maternal lupus erythematous or myocardial infarction.

PHYSICAL EXAMINATION

The principal finding is a slow cardiac rate. The jugular venous pulse shows intermittent large pulsations (cannon waves), which occur as the atrium contracts against a closed tricuspid valve. On auscultation the intensity of the first heart sound varies, because the atrioventricular valves are closing at different intervals after atrial contraction, and the extent of their excursion to closure also varies. Soft systolic ejection murmurs are heard in both the aortic and pulmonary areas from the increased stroke volume across the outflow tracts. Low-pitched middiastolic murmurs may be heard because of the increased volume of blood flowing into the ventricles.

The pulse pressure is wide, the systolic pressure is elevated from the increased stroke volume, and diastolic pressure is lowered because of the prolonged period of diastole.

ELECTROCARDIOGRAPHIC FEATURES

There is no relationship between the P waves and the QRS complexes, and the QRS complexes occur at a slower rate. The atrial rate is variable and responds to the various factors such as exercise or vagal tone that influence the rate of sinoatrial node discharge.

The QRS complex may be of normal duration and occur at a regular R-R interval, indicating a stable pacemaker, or the QRS may be prolonged and resemble left or, less commonly, right bundle branch block. When the QRS complex is prolonged, the cardiac rate is usually slower (35–45 beats/min). A ventricular rate less than 30 beats/min with multiform QRS complexes suggests coexistent myocardial inflammatory disease.

There may be associated findings of the underlying cardiac conditions, such as congenitally corrected transposition of the great vessels.

ECHOCARDIOGRAPHIC FEATURES

The atria contract independently at a faster rate than the ventricles. Both ventricles are dilated, and the ejection fraction is increased. Both great vessels are likewise dilated. With a slower cardiac rate, the stroke volume is greater, and the cardiac chambers and great vessels show a proportional increase.

RADIOGRAPHIC FEATURES

The radiographic findings are nonspecific, and therefore the diagnosis can rarely be suggested from thoracic roentgenograms.

1. Each cardiac chamber is enlarged to a variable degree, depending on cardiac rate and status of the myocardium (Fig 74–1).
2. There is biventricular enlargement, but this diagno-

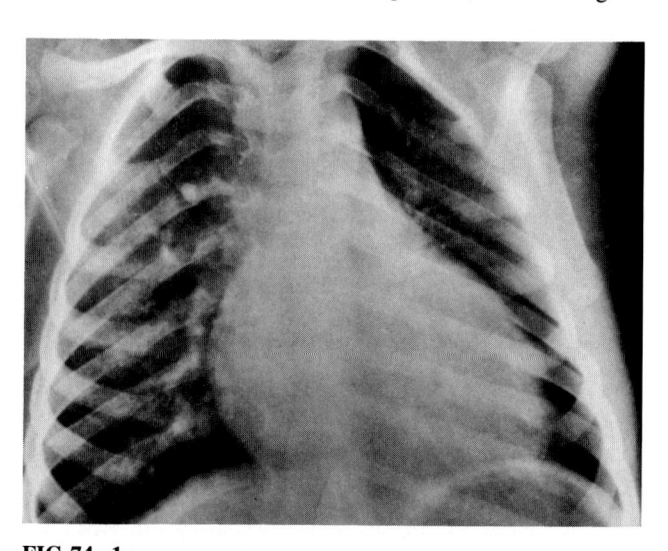

FIG 74–1.
Complete heart block. Thoracic roentgenogram. Posteroanterior projection. Nonspecific diffuse enlargement of cardiac silhouette. Normal pulmonary vasculature. Radiographic appearance is indistinguishable from cardiomyopathy or left-sided obstructive lesion.

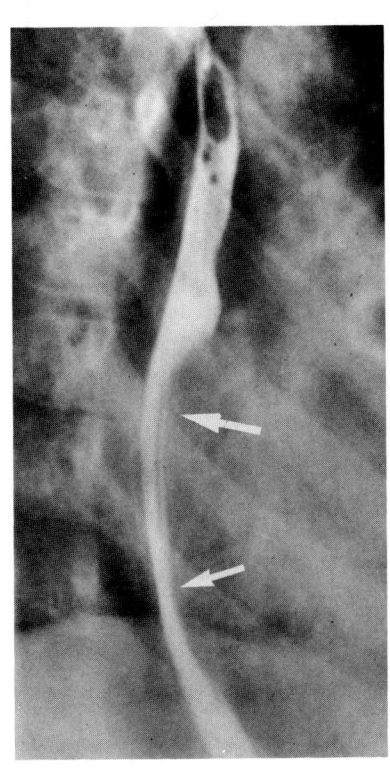

FIG 74–2.
Thoracic roentgenogram. Right anterior oblique projection. Barium swallow. Displacement of barium-filled esophagus by enlarged left atrium. Appearance changes depending on whether film is exposed during systole or diastole.

sis is difficult to make on standard thoracic radiographs. Left anterior oblique views are helpful in the demonstration of biventricular enlargement.

3. The left atrium tends to be enlarged, which can be detected by displacement of the barium-filled esophagus (Fig 74–2). REASON: The slow heart rate allows prolonged inflow of blood, resulting in overdistention of all cardiac chambers.

4. There may be mild prominence of the main pulmonary arterial segment and proximal branch pulmonary arteries. REASON: The increased stroke volume of the right ventricle dilates the pulmonary arteries.

5. The peripheral pulmonary vasculature is within normal limits.

6. Because of the large stroke volume, the appearance of the pulmonary arterial segment and cardiac size varies, depending on whether the radiograph was exposed during systole or diastole. Left atrium enlargement may also be absent if exposure is made during diastole.

7. The slow cardiac rate and very active pulsations of all cardiac chambers and both great vessels can be observed fluoroscopically and recorded by cine radiography, but the underlying cause cannot be determined.

CARDIAC CATHETERIZATION

During cardiac catheterization, intracardiac pressures are normal. Resting cardiac index is normal.[16] Stroke volume is increased. Ventricular pacing increases cardiac index by 26%. Isoproterenol infusion results in a greater rise

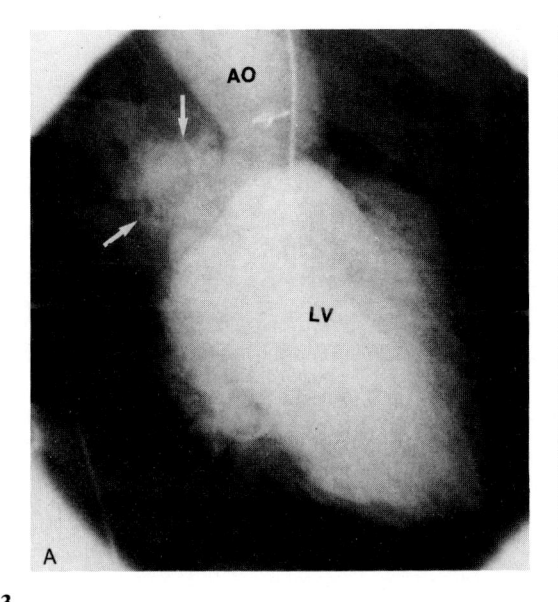

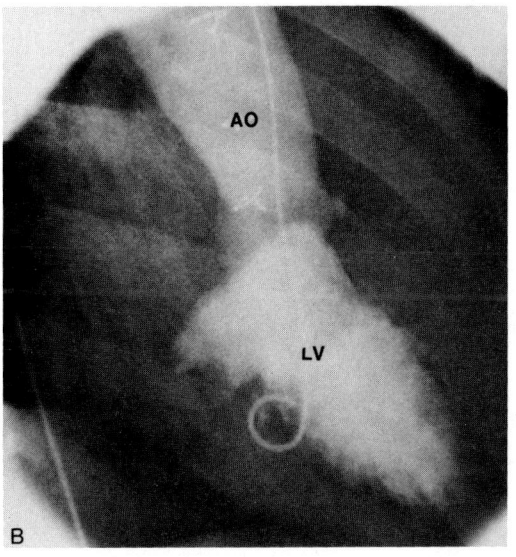

FIG 74–3.
Congenital heart block. Left ventriculogram. Right anterior oblique projection. **A,** diastole. Fully distended ventricle increased endystolic(LV). Contrast medium being injected escapes through open mitral valve into left atrium (arrow) (diastolic backflow). **B,** systole. Forceful contraction of left ventricle. Increased stroke volume. Normal endystolic volume. No mitral regurgitation. Competent mitral valve. AO = aorta.

in cardiac index and left ventricular ejection fraction. It also reduces systemic vascular resistance. The hemodynamic improvement is caused by combined inotropic, chronotropic, and peripheral vasodilatory effects.

ANGIOGRAPHIC FEATURES

The abnormally slow cardiac rate can be observed during cine angiocardiography, although the underlying electrocardiographic abnormality is not apparent.

Both ventricles are considerably distended during diastole. REASON: (1) prolonged diastolic filling time causes dilatation and complete distention of the ventricular chambers, and (2) both ventricles show a large stroke volume. Contrary to the findings in cardiac failure, there is a very forceful contraction and relatively normal to small end-systolic volume. On left ventriculography during diastole, contrast material may pass in a retrograde direction through the atrioventricular valves. REASON: During the prolonged ventricular filling period, contrast medium is being injected, and some escapes through the open atrioventricular valves into the atria (Fig 74–3). Such diastolic back flow may also be observed in a normal heart during a long compensatory pause after a ventricular extrasystole. However, patients with congenital heart block may have true end-diastolic backflow through an abnormal atrioventricular valve, which can be proven by other means such as echocardiography.

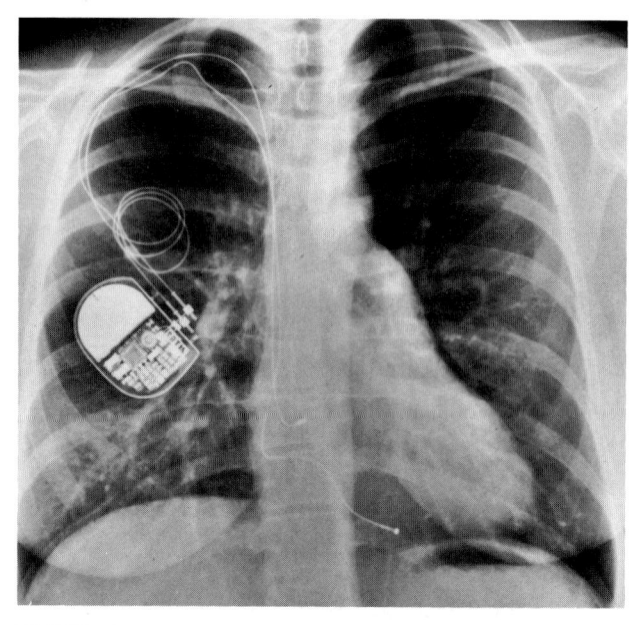

FIG 74–4.
Complete heart block was treated by permanent pacemaker. Thoracic roentgenogram. Posteroanterior projection. Cardiac size has returned to normal. Main pulmonary artery segment is still somewhat prominent.

TREATMENT

Whereas congenital complete heart block is usually stable and is well tolerated, postoperative heart block is not.[1, 2, 4] Operative heart block may occur with closure of a ventricular septal defect, particularly in tetralogy of Fallot or with repair of endocardial cushion defects. This form of heart block may be associated with sudden death. Permanent cardiac pacemakers are almost always implanted for persistent postoperative heart block, whereas they are rarely needed for congenital heart block. After a period of time, pacing may result in a significant decrease in cardiac size (Fig 74–4). Temporary pacemakers are not satisfactory for treatment of chronic pacing in infants. Once the pacemaker is implanted, a commitment is made for lifetime pacing.

REFERENCES

1. Driscoll DJ, Gillette PC, Hallman GL, et al: Management of surgical complete atrioventricular block in children, *Am J Cardiol* 43:1175, 1979.
2. Squarcia U, Merideth J, McGoon DC, et al: Prognosis of transient atrioventricular conduction disturbances complicating open heart surgery for congenital heart defects, *Am J Cardiol* 28:648, 1971.
3. Gannon PG, Sellers RD, Kanjuh VI, et al: Complete heart block following replacement of the aortic valve, *Circulation* 33–34(suppl 1):152, 1966.
4. Hofschire PJ, Nicoloff DM, Moller JH: Postoperative complete heart block in 64 children treated with and without cardiac pacing, *Am J Cardiol* 39:559, 1977.
5. Anderson RC, Lillehei CW, Lester RG: Corrected transposition of the great vessels of the heart: a review of 17 cases, *Pediatrics* 20:626, 1957.
6. Johnson JL, Lee LP: Complete atrioventricular heart block secondary to acute myocarditis requiring intracardiac pacing, *J Pediatr* 78:312, 1971.
7. Wang K, Gobel F, Gleason DF, et al: Complete heart block complicating bacterial endocarditis, *Circulation* 46:939, 1972.
8. Kleid JJ, Kim ES, Brand B, et al: Heart block complicating acute bacterial endocarditis, *Chest* 61:301, 1972.
9. Schaumburg HH, Nielsen SL, Yurchak PM: Heart block in polymyositis, *N Engl J Med* 284:480, 1971.
10. Stocker FP, Czoniczer G, Massell BF, et al: Transient complete A-V block in two siblings during acute rheumatic carditis in childhood, *Pediatrics* 45:850, 1970.
11. McCue CM, Mantakas ME, Tingelstad JB, et al: Congenital heart block in newborns of mothers with connective tissue disease, *Circulation* 56:82, 1977.
12. Anderson RH, Wenick ACG, Losekoot TG, et al: Congenitally complete heart block. Developmental aspects, *Circulation* 56:90, 1977.
13. Madison JP, Sukhum P, Williamson DP, et al: Echocardi-

ography and fetal heart sounds in the diagnosis of fetal heart block, *Am Heart J* 98:505, 1979.
14. Wright FS, Adams P Jr, Anderson RC: Congenital atrioventricular dissociation due to complete or advanced atrioventricular heart block, *Am J Dis Child* 98:72, 1959.
15. Molthan ME, Miller RA, Hastreiter AR, et al: Congenital heart block with fatal Adams-Stokes attacks in childhood, *Pediatrics* 30:32, 1962.
16. Thilenius OG, Chiemmongkoltip P, Cassels DE, et al: Hemodynamic studies in children with congenital atrioventricular block, *Am J Cardiol* 30:13, 1972.

CHAPTER 75

Pulmonary Hypertension

Pulmonary hypertension without an identifiable underlying cause (primary pulmonary hypertension) was first described by Romberg in 1891. It occurs rarely (17/10,000 individuals) in all age groups and in both sexes, but predominately in young females. Other names for the condition are idiopathic, essential, or solitary pulmonary hypertension.

PATHOLOGIC ANATOMY

A variety of conditions are associated with the development of pulmonary hypertension. These conditions must be excluded before a diagnosis of primary pulmonary hypertension can be made. Furthermore, the study of these conditions may provide a clue about the development of pulmonary vascular disease.

I. Pulmonary Parenchymal Disease
   A. Emphysema
   B. Asthma, bronchitis, bronchiectasis
   C. Cystic fibrosis
   D. Infiltrative disease
II. Ventilatory problems
   A. Kyphoscoliosis
   B. Central hypoventilation
III. Disease of pulmonary arterioles
   A. Collagen disease
IV. Cardiac anomalies
   A. Associated with increased pulmonary venous pressure
   B. Associated with increased pulmonary blood flow
V. Increased blood viscosity

The etiology of primary pulmonary hypertension is unknown.[1] Two general theories have been proposed. One theory holds that vasoconstriction of the pulmonary vascular bed occurs and that occlusive pulmonary vasculature changes occur secondary to the vasoconstriction. Another theory attributes primary pulmonary hypertension to recurrent pulmonary embolism, although early in the disease there may be a component of vasoconstriction secondary to the thrombosis.

Pathologically three types of primary pulmonary hypertension have been identified:[2,3]

1. Plexogenic pulmonary arteriopathy.
2. Recurrent pulmonary thromboembolism.
3. Pulmonary veno-occlusive disease.

Plexogenic Pulmonary Arteriopathy

Plexogenic pulmonary hypertension is characterized initially by pulmonary arterial vasoconstriction with medial hypertrophy. Subsequently, secondary proliferative intimal lesions, including plexiform lesions, develop (Fig 75–1). In the disease of muscular arteries and arterioles, an underlying factor, probably prolonged vasoconstriction of unknown etiology, is present. Pulmonary vasoconstriction may also be found in individuals residing at high altitudes, with obesity, musculoskeletal disorders, or chronic airway obstruction.[4-6] The common factor may be hypoxia producing vasoconstriction. Muscularization of the arterioles occurs, but the vascular bed may respond to vasodilators, indicating neurogenic reactive vasospasm. In children, plexogenic hypertension may have a rapid clinical course. In older children and in almost all adults, the pathologic lesions are located in the arterial intima and consist of cellular proliferation and concentric laminar fibrosis (Fig 75–2). Lesions are obstructive, causing pulmonary hypertension. The plexogenic type usually involves the smaller muscular arteries. Sometimes thrombosis is superimposed on plexiform lesions.

Recurrent Pulmonary Thromboembolism

In this form, thromboembolism in various stages of organization are found in muscular pulmonary arteries and in pulmonary arterioles.[2,3] Older organized thromboembo-

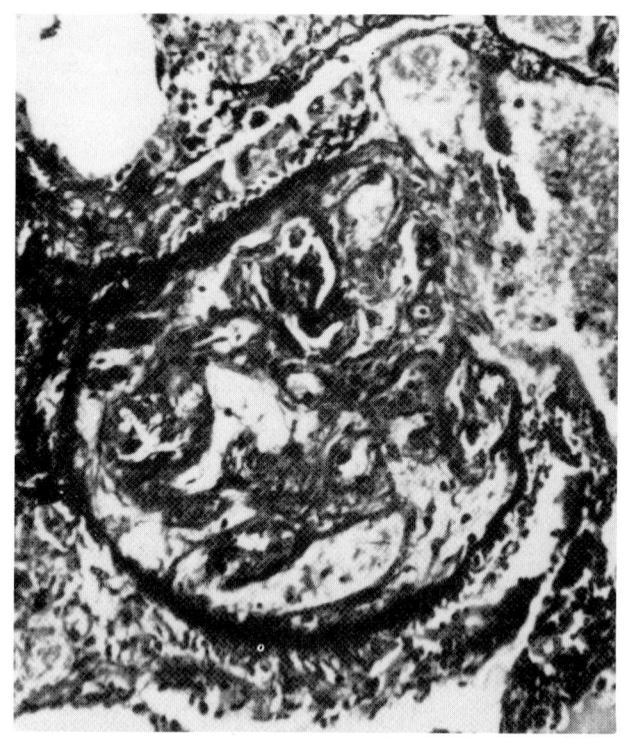

FIG 75-1.
Pulmonary hypertension. Photomicrograph. Small muscular pulmonary artery with characteristic plexogenic lesions. Within the lumen is a plexus of tortuous channels separated by cellular and fibrous strands.

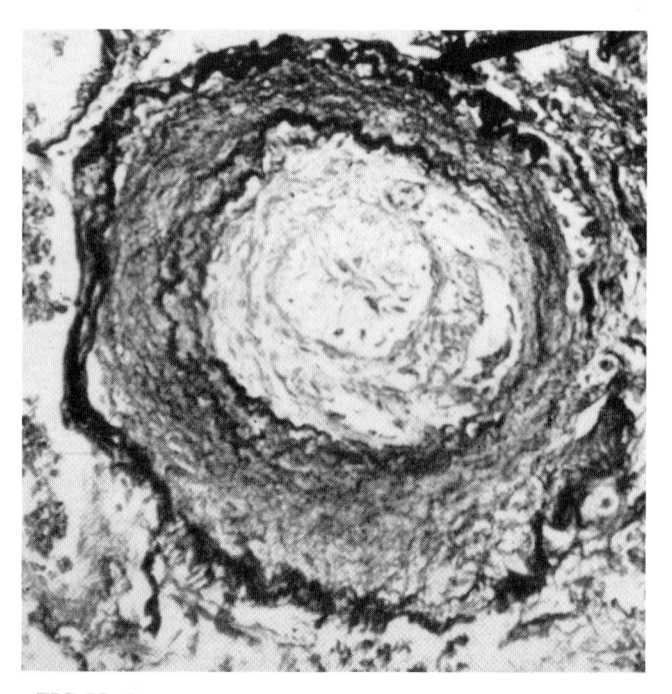

FIG 75-2.
Pulmonary hypertension. Photomicrograph. Intimal fibrosis of pulmonary artery.

lism may manifest as recanalized thrombi, as eccentric intimal fibrosis, or as intimal pads. Plexiform lesions are absent. The capillaries and veins are normal.

This disease of small muscular arteries and arterioles has to be differentiated from gross pulmonary embolism.

Pulmonary Veno-occlusive Disease

Pulmonary veno-occlusive disease is most likely thrombotic in origin and involves small pulmonary veins and venules.[2, 3] Organized thrombi become canalized but may result in intimal pads and fibrosis of veins. The pulmonary veins become dilated and hypertrophied proximal to the thrombi. The pathologic changes in the lungs resemble those in mitral stenosis. Pulmonary capillaries are engorged and tortuous. Signs of hemorrhage may be present. Pulmonary hemosiderosis may be excessive. Pulmonary and pleural lymphatics and those in intralobular septa are dilated. Thus, Kerley B lines may be present.

HEMODYNAMICS

Pulmonary arteriolar narrowing is the principal hemodynamic problem. This may initially occur because of vasoconstriction.[7, 8] Hypoxia is a potent pulmonary vasoconstrictor, at least in the neonatal period. Indeed, the condition persistent fetal circulation[9] occurs in diseases or situations with impaired oxygenation. Observations of individuals living at high altitude show them to have higher pulmonary arterial pressure than individuals living at sea level. Furthermore, exercise in high-altitude residents prompts a further rise in pressure. Hypoxia may occur with pulmonary parenchymal disease or diseases that affect ventilation, such as extreme obesity (Pickwickian syndrome), musculoskeletal disorders, or chronic upper airway obstruction. Factors other than hypoxia causing pulmonary arteriolar vasoconstriction remain to be defined. Even instances of pulmonary hypertension occurring from thromboembolism may also result from vasoconstriction secondary to the release of vasoconstrictor substances from platelets.

Because of the arteriolar changes, pulmonary vascular resistance is elevated. Pulmonary arterial and right ventricular systolic pressures also become elevated, and the right ventricle hypertrophies. Because of the elevated pulmonary vascular resistance, the cardiac output is limited at rest, and during exercise little increase occurs, so the patient experiences fatigue.

As the pulmonary vascular disease progresses, or if pulmonary vasoconstriction increases suddenly, cardiac failure may develop slowly or occur quickly. The symptoms of fatigue, syncope, and chest pain are probably related to inadequate cardiac output.

Arterial desaturation may be present from right-to-left atrial level shunt through a probe patent foramen ovale or from ventilation-perfusion maldistribution as in thromboembolism. In individuals with pulmonary disease, it can also result from hypoventilation or diffusion abnormalities.

Dyspnea is also a major symptom when pulmonary vascular resistance exceeds 10 mm Hg/L/min/m.[2] It probably results from a reflex induced by distention of the pulmonary artery.

CLINICAL FEATURES

The disease has an insidious onset and is progressive. The interval between onset of symptoms and death is variable and may extend from a few months to 5 years. Survival for more than 5 years is uncommon. Occasionally the disease resolves.[10] Dyspnea, weakness, and fatigue are prominent and are probably related to the limited cardiac output. Substernal chest pain ("right-sided angina"),[11] similar to angina pectoris, occurs, perhaps as a result of inadequate coronary arterial perfusion. The afferent nerves of the pulmonary artery enter the nervous system by the same pathways as those from the heart (the vagus and upper four dorsal sympathetic routes). Furthermore, there are many interconnecting fibers between the pulmonary plexus and the cardiac plexus. Thus, the chest pain may originate from the pulmonary artery as it becomes distended because of increased pressure. Syncope is a grave prognostic sign;[12] this perhaps occurs as a consequence of an abrupt increase in pulmonary vascular resistance and resultant decrease in cardiac output. Agitation, anxiety, and other psychologic symptoms have been described. When congestive cardiac failure develops, it indicates a poor prognosis. Cyanosis may occur from either an atrial right-to-left shunt or a ventilation-perfusion mismatch.

On physical examination, the critical finding is a loud pulmonary component of a narrowly split S_2.[13] Often there are no murmurs, but a murmur of pulmonary regurgitation may be present. A right ventricular heave is found, and there may be prominence of the sternum, both features indicative of right ventricular hypertrophy. A pulmonary systolic ejection click may be present because of the dilated pulmonary artery. Elevated right atrial pressure is evident as prominent neck veins and cyanosis.

ELECTROCARDIOGRAPHIC FEATURES

The electrocardiogram shows right-axis deviation and right ventricular hypertrophy.[12, 13] The P waves are often tall, peaked, and pointed, reflecting right atrial enlargement. Right ventricular strain, indicated by deeply inverted T waves and depressed ST segments in the right precordial leads, reflects a poor prognosis.

ECHOCARDIOGRAPHIC FEATURES

Echocardiography has aided considerably in the diagnosis of primary pulmonary hypertension and in the determination of pulmonary arterial pressure. When a patient with pulmonary hypertension is evaluated, associated cardiac conditions, such as intracardiac shunts and obstructive lesions at the level of the mitral valve, left atrium, and pulmonary veins, have to be considered. These can generally be excluded with certainty by this diagnostic technique.

In primary pulmonary hypertension, the pulmonary trunk is dilated, and the right ventricle hypertrophied. The right ventricle and right atrium may be dilated as well.

If either pulmonary or tricuspid insufficiency is present, Doppler measurement of the regurgitant jet can be used to estimate the level of systolic pressure. The time interval from onset to peak velocity of pulmonary arterial flow when corrected for variations in cardiac rate also correlates well with the pulmonary arterial pressure.[14, 15]

RADIOGRAPHIC FEATURES

Thoracic roentgenograms of patients with primary pulmonary hypertension are indistinguishable from those of patients with a left-to-right shunt and pulmonary vascular obstructive disease. In most cases a radiographic diagnosis of pulmonary hypertension can be suggested. However, the radiographic signs of increased pulmonary arterial pressure can be misleading. The most reliable radiographic finding is calcified plaques (pulmonary atherosclerosis), which appear later on in life.

The radiographic appearance of primary pulmonary hypertension is not uniform. It varies considerably according to age. If typical radiographic findings of increased pulmonary arterial pressure are present, idiopathic pulmonary hypertension is the last in the differential diagnosis, because it is extremely rare and can be diagnosed only if the other causes of secondary pulmonary hypertension have been excluded.

Radiographs of the plexogenic type and thromboembolic type are identical, but with the veno-occlusive disease, peripheral pulmonary venous markings are increased and Kerley B lines are present.

1. The heart may be of normal size, or cardiomegaly of varying degrees may be present. Cardiac enlargement occurs from decompensation of the right ventricle. This is progressive and occurs later in the course of the disease.

2. In a newborn the cardiac silhouette is normal. REASON: The fetal circulation is normal. Also in infancy, cardiac size remains commonly normal (Fig 75–3). REASON: Decompensation of the right ventricle and cardiomegaly appear gradually.

3. In early childhood typically mild cardiomegaly appears from beginning right ventricular decompensation (Fig 75–4).

4. The peripheral pulmonary vasculature remains normal or low normal (see Fig 75–4).

5. The right atrium is enlarged because of increased end-diastolic right ventricular pressure (Fig 75–5).

6. The cardiac silhouette may have a left ventricular contour from hypertrophy of the right ventricle (see Fig 75–5), causing counterclockwise rotation as in pulmonary stenosis (see Chapter 29).

7. With time, dilatation of the main pulmonary artery occurs. REASON: Long-standing increased pulmonary arterial pressure stretches the arterial wall, leading to dilatation.

8. Typically the dilatation of the pulmonary artery involves the main pulmonary artery and proximal right and left pulmonary arteries (Fig 75–6).

9. If the dilatation of the pulmonary artery involves primarily the main pulmonary artery, the radiographic appearance is identical to pulmonary valvar stenosis (see Fig 75–6).

10. A distinguishing feature between primary pulmonary hypertension and pulmonary valvar stenosis may be the demonstration of an increased number of vessels seen on end in pulmonary hypertension (see Fig 75–6). REASON: The increase in pulmonary arterial pressure causes not only dilatation but also elongation of arteries as peripherally in systemic hypertension. The pulmonary arteries therefore become tortuous and wavy, resulting in an increased number of nodular densities throughout both lung fields (see Fig 75–6).

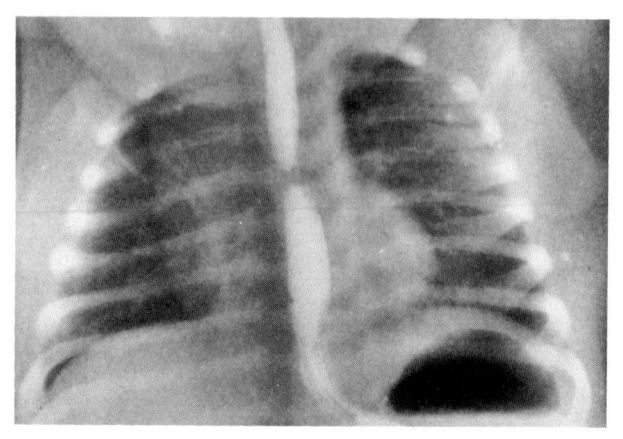

11. Whereas pulmonary valvar stenosis classically causes dilatation of the main pulmonary artery and usually the left pulmonary artery, (see Chapter 29), in pulmonary hypertension the main pulmonary artery and right and left

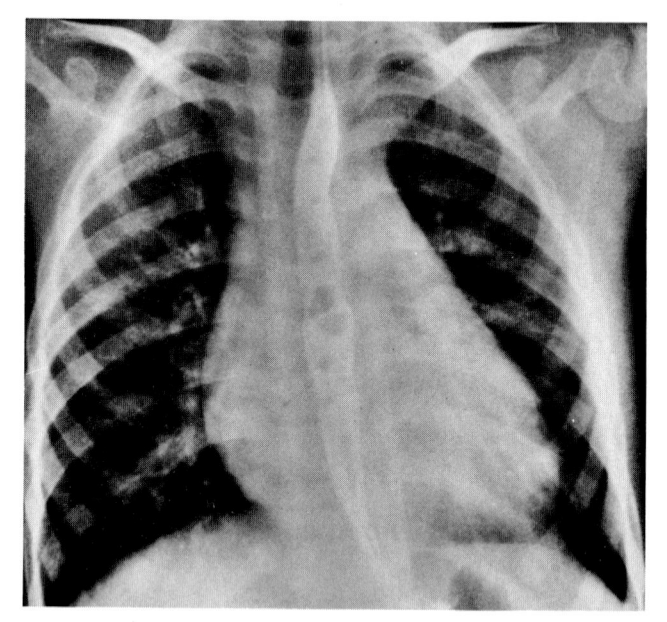

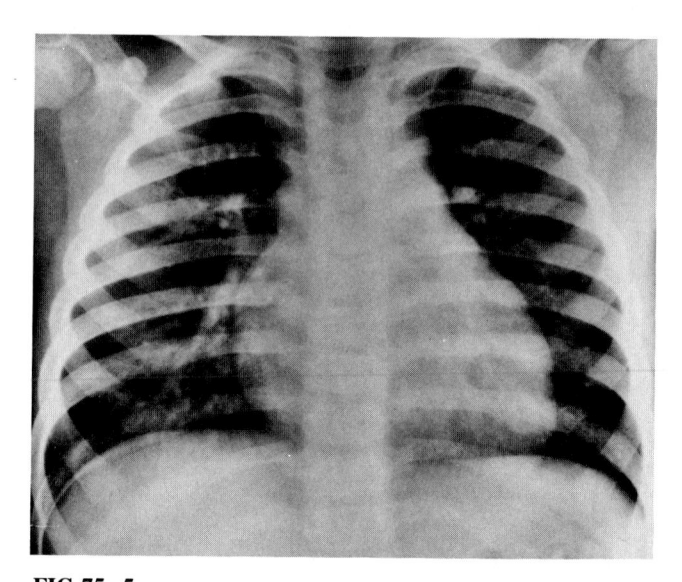

FIG 75–4.
Primary pulmonary hypertension in a 2-year-old. Thoracic roentgenogram. Posteroanterior projection. Mild cardiomegaly. Peripheral pulmonary vasculature is at lower limits of normal.

FIG 75–3.
Severe primary pulmonary hypertension. Infant. Thoracic roentgenogram. Posteroanterior projection. Normal pulmonary vasculature and cardiac size.

FIG 75–5.
Primary pulmonary hypertension in a 2-year-old child. Thoracic roentgenogram. Posteroanterior projection. Mild cardiomegaly. Left ventricular contour. Slight prominence of right atrium. Normal pulmonary vasculature. Correct diagnosis of primary pulmonary hypertension cannot be suggested radiographically.

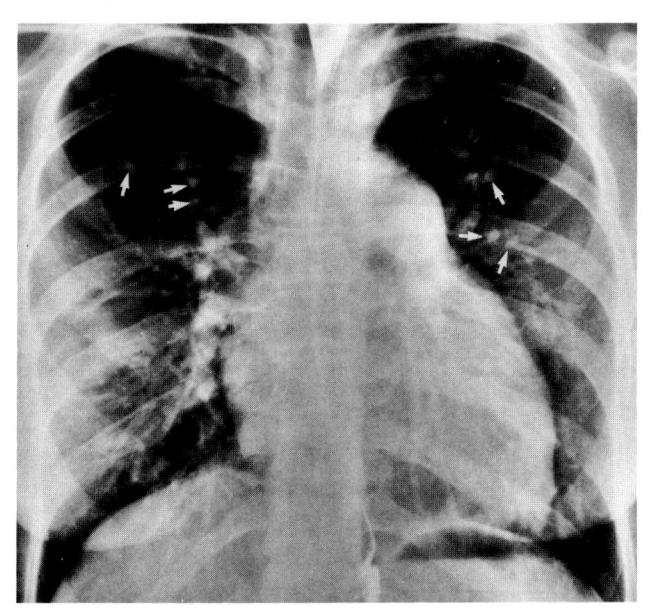

FIG 75-6.
Severe primary pulmonary hypertension. Thoracic roentgenogram. Posteroanterior projection. Slightly enlarged heart. Enlarged main pulmonary arterial segment. Enlarged pulmonary arteries in right hilum. Sparse peripheral pulmonary artery branches (pruning) increase number of pulmonary arteries seen on end (arrows) because of tortuosity.

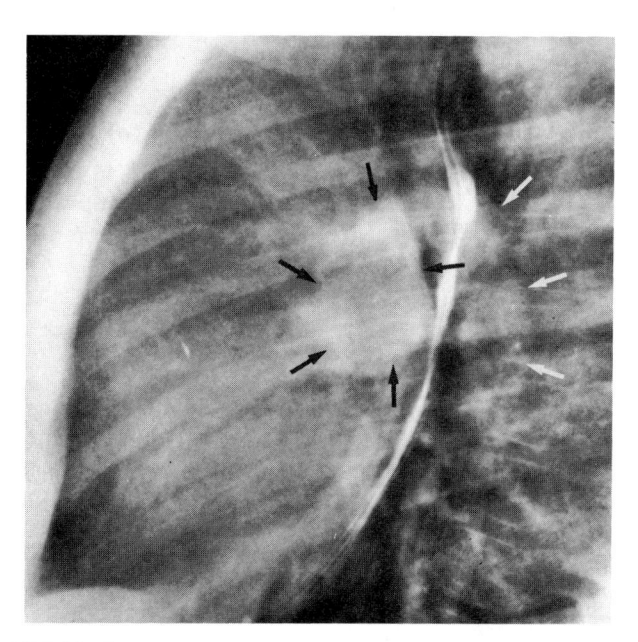

FIG 75-7.
Primary pulmonary hypertension. Thoracic roentgenogram. Lateral projection. Dilatation of main pulmonary artery. Concomitant dilatation of right pulmonary artery *(black arrows)*. This finding is more consistent with pulmonary hypertension than pulmonary valvar stenosis, which classically causes poststenotic dilatation of left pulmonary artery. Mild dilatation of left pulmonary artery *(white arrows)*.

pulmonary arteries become dilated. Dilatation of the left pulmonary artery may not be readily visible on a posteroanterior roentgenogram, but dilatation of the right pulmonary artery is usually well seen on the lateral projection as a large round density in front of the trachea (Fig 75-7).

12. The classical discrepancy between the size of the hilar vessels and the peripheral pulmonary arterial branches causes the radiographic picture of "pruning" (see Chapter 5).

13. In most patients with primary pulmonary hypertension, however, the dilatation of the pulmonary artery is confined mainly to the pulmonary trunk (see Fig 75-7). Consequently, radiographs are indistinguishable from pulmonary valvar stenosis. If the peripheral pulmonary arteries are dilated as well, pulmonary hypertension is most likely on the basis of a left-to-right shunt.

14. Rarely dilatation of the pulmonary arteries occurs beyond the hila (Fig 75-8). REASON: Unknown. Under those circumstances, differentiation from a left-to-right shunt with pulmonary hypertension cannot be made.

15. Enlargement of the pulmonary arteries progresses.

16. Left atrial enlargement is absent. REASON: Blood flow to the left side of the heart is normal or decreased.

17. The ascending aorta is inconspicuous. REASON: With enlargement of the right ventricle against the ster-

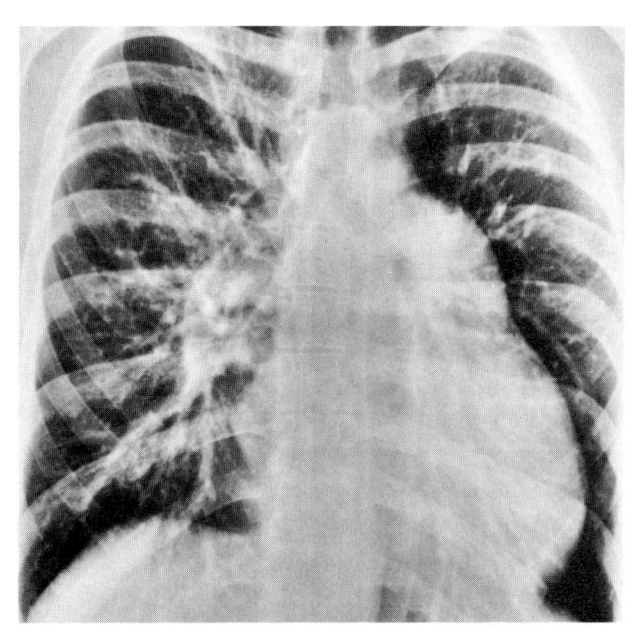

FIG 75-8.
Primary pulmonary hypertension. Thoracic roentgenogram. Posteroanterior projection. Dilatation involves main pulmonary artery, hilar arteries, and peripheral pulmonary arteries. Differentiation from left-to-right shunt with or without pulmonary hypertension is not feasible.

num, clockwise rotation of the heart occurs identical to atrial septal defect (see Chapter 19).

18. In the end stage of the disease, the cardiac silhouette is huge because of massive right ventricular decompensation and sometimes associated tricuspid and pulmonary insufficiency (relative). Tortuosity of the pulmonary arteries occurs by elongation of arteries secondary to long-standing increased pressure.

CARDIAC CATHETERIZATION

In the past, cardiac catheterization has been the method of choice for the diagnosis of primary pulmonary hypertension and for the exclusion of other conditions that might result in elevated pulmonary arterial pressure. Echocardiography can provide much of the necessary information, thereby eliminating the hazards of catheterization in individuals with primary pulmonary hypertension. Death may occur during or after cardiac catheterization in these patients, because they are hemodynamically unstable.[16] The development of bradycardia or a tachyarrhythmia has profound effects by lowering cardiac output because of the elevated pulmonary vascular resistance. The occurrence of ventricular fibrillation during catheterization has also been reported.

If a patient's heart is catheterized, the pulmonary arterial wedge pressure must be measured to exclude pulmonary venous obstruction. The pulmonary arterial and right ventricular systolic pressures are elevated, at times exceeding systemic levels.[13, 16] Right atrial pressures are elevated.

The cardiac output is low and consequently the oxygen saturations in right-sided cardiac chambers reduced. During cardiac catheterization, drug infusion studies may be performed to observe effects on cardiac output and pulmonary arterial pressure. Several agents, including hydralazine, captopril, and diazoxide, have lowered pulmonary vascular resistance in some patients with primary pulmonary hypertension.[17–25]

ANGIOGRAPHIC FEATURES

Angiography should be performed during cardiac catheterization, although it carries a higher risk than in patients with other congenital cardiac malformations and secondary pulmonary hypertension. REASON: Whereas contrast media cause vasodilatation in the systemic vascular bed, they induce vasoconstriction in the pulmonary arterial bed. During angiography, therefore, pulmonary arterial pressure increases because of increased vascular resistance. In patients with suprasystemic pressure in the pulmonary artery and fixed pulmonary resistance, a further increase in resistance may result in a precipitous decrease of cardiac output, with consequent underperfusion of the coronary arteries resulting in arrhythmias or death. The risk is minimized by injecting each pulmonary artery separately.

The purpose of angiography is to determine the degree of associated pulmonary insufficiency. This can be accomplished with a comparatively small amount of contrast medium using cine angiography in the lateral projection. Furthermore, angiography can be carried out during the inhalation of 100% oxygen. Right ventriculography should be performed to determine the degree of associated tricuspid insufficiency.

1. In younger patients with compensated right ventricle and in the early stage of the disease, right pulmonary arteriography and right ventriculography are normal (Fig 75–9).

2. As the process progresses, pulmonary angiography

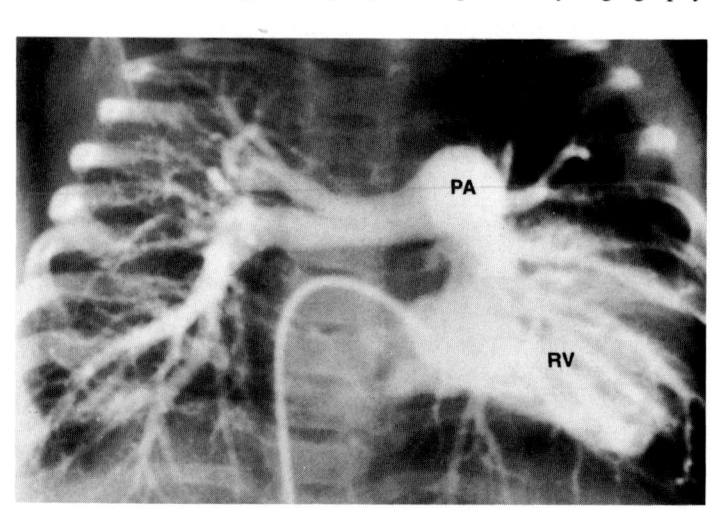

FIG 75–9.
Primary pulmonary hypertension in a 1-year-old. Right ventriculogram. Anteroposterior projection. Normal right ventricle *(RV)* and right pulmonary artery. Minimal tortuosity of peripheral pulmonary arterial branches. No significant dilatation of main pulmonary artery *(PA)*. Hypoplasia of left pulmonary artery.

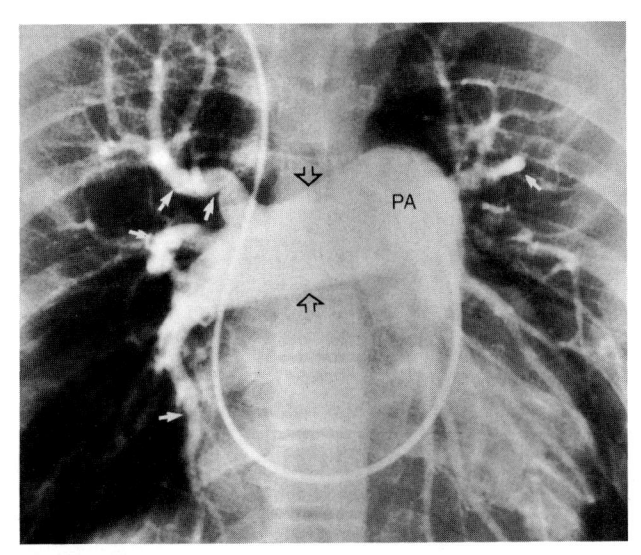

FIG 75-10.
Primary pulmonary hypertension. Pulmonary arteriogram *(PA)*. Anteroposterior projection. Main pulmonary artery and intramediastinal portion of right pulmonary artery *(open arrows)* are dilated. Hilar arteries are slightly dilated. Tortuosity of peripheral pulmonary arterial branches *(arrows)*. Sparse peripheral pulmonary vasculature, particularly in right lower lobe (pruning).

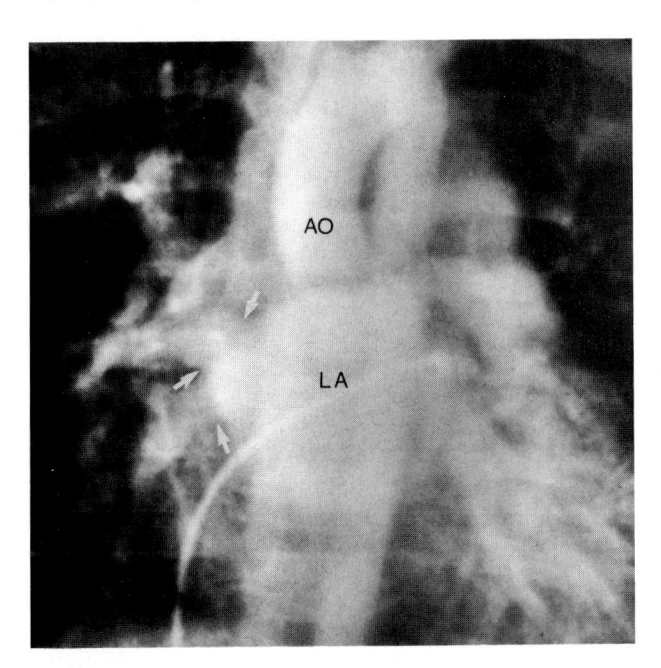

FIG 75-11.
Primary pulmonary hypertension. Pulmonary arteriogram. Anteroposterior projection. Late phase. Normal pulmonary veins in right side *(arrows)* exclude stenosis of individual pulmonary veins. Normal left atrium *(LA)* excludes obstruction at mitral valve level. *AO* = aorta.

demonstrates the dilated main pulmonary artery, tortuosity of the peripheral branches, and peripheral pruning (Fig 75-10).

3. It is advisable to demonstrate the pulmonary veins and left atrium to exclude left-sided obstruction (Fig 75-11).

MANAGEMENT

In virtually all patients, primary pulmonary hypertension progresses, although exceptions occur.[26, 27] Treatment is generally supportive, with anticongestive measures if cardiac failure ensues. A trial with vasodilators should be attempted, because in an occasional patient the pulmonary vasculature may respond.[17, 28] No single vasodilator is preferred, but the choice of a specific agent is guided by observations made during drug trials at the time of cardiac catheterization. Most of the agents that have been used in an attempt to treat pulmonary hypertension are systemic antihypertensive agents.[17-25] Thus, one of the major side effects in patients with pulmonary hypertension is the production of systemic hypotension.

REFERENCES

1. Haworth SG: Primary pulmonary hypertension, *Br Heart J* 49:517, 1983.
2. Edwards WD, Edwards JE: Recent advances in the pathology of the pulmonary vasculature. In *The lung: IAP monograph no. 19.* Baltimore, 1978, Williams & Wilkins, pp 235-261.
3. Edwards WD, Edwards JE: Clinical primary pulmonary hypertension: three pathologic types, *Circulation* 56:884, 1977.
4. Levy AM, Tabakin BS, Hanson JS, et al: Hypertrophied adenoids causing pulmonary hypertension and severe congestive heart failure, *N Engl J Med* 277:506, 1967.
5. Cox MA, Schiebler GL, Taylor WJ, et al: Reversible pulmonary hypertension in a child with respiratory obstruction and cor pulmonale, *J Pediatr* 67:192, 1965.
6. Menashe VD, Farrehi C, Miller M: Hypoventilation and cor pulmonale due to chronic upper airway obstruction, *J Pediatr* 67:198, 1965.
7. Wood P: Pulmonary hypertension with special reference to the vasoconstrictive factor, *Br Heart J* 20:557, 1958.
8. Wood P: Pulmonary hypertension, *Mod Concepts Cardiovasc Dis* 28:513, 1959.
9. Fox WW, Gewitz MH, Dinwiddie R, et al: Pulmonary hypertension in the perinatal aspiration syndromes, *Pediatrics* 59:205, 1977.
10. Fujii A, Rabinovitch M, Matthews EC: A case of spontaneous resolution of idiopathic pulmonary hypertension, *Br Heart J* 46:574, 1981.

11. Viar WN, Harrison TR: Chest pain in association with pulmonary hypertension: its similarity to the pain of coronary disease, *Circulation* 5:1, 1952.
12. Thilenius OG, Nadas AS, Jockin H: Primary pulmonary vascular obstruction in children, *Pediatrics* 36:75, 1965.
13. Sleeper JC, Orgain ES, McIntosh HD: Primary pulmonary hypertension: review of clinical features and pathologic physiology with a report of pulmonary hemodynamics derived from repeated catheterization, *Circulation* 26:1358, 1962.
14. Friedman DM, Bierman FZ, Barst R: Gated pulsed Doppler evaluation of idiopathic pulmonary artery hypertension in children, *Am J Cardiol* 58:369, 1986.
15. Serwer GA, Cougle AG, Eckerd JM, et al: Factors affecting use of the Doppler-determined time from flow onset to maximal pulmonary artery velocity for measurement of pulmonary artery pressure in children, *Am J Cardiol* 58:352, 1986.
16. Keane JF, Fyler DC, Nadas AS: Hazards of cardiac catheterization in children with primary pulmonary vascular obstruction, *Am Heart J* 96:556, 1978.
17. McGoon MD, Vlietstra RE: Vasodilator therapy for primary pulmonary hypertension, *Mayo Clin Proc* 59:672, 1984.
18. Leier CV, Bambach D, Nelson S, et al: Captopril in primary pulmonary hypertension, *Circulation* 67:155, 1983.
19. Ikram H, Maslowski AH, Nicholls MG, et al: Haemodynamic and hormonal effects of captopril in primary pulmonary hypertension, *Br Heart J* 48:541, 1982.
20. Rich S, Martinez J, Lam W, et al: Reassessment of the effects of vasodilator drugs in primary pulmonary hypertension: guidelines for determining a pulmonary vasodilator response, *Am Heart J* 105:119, 1983.
21. Young TE, Lundquist LJ, Chesler E, et al: Comparative effects of nifedipine, verapamil, and diltiazem on experimental pulmonary hypertension, *Am J Cardiol* 51:195, 1983.
22. Daoud FS, Reeves JT, Kelly DB: Isoproterenol as a potential pulmonary vasodilator in primary pulmonary hypertension, *Am J Cardiol* 42:817, 1978.
23. Rubin LJ, Peter RH: Oral hydralazine therapy for primary pulmonary hypertension, *N Engl J Med* 302:69, 1980.
24. Klinke WP, Gilbert JAL: Diazoxide in primary pulmonary hypertension, *N Engl J Med* 302:91, 1980.
25. Shettigar UR, Hultgren HN, Specter M, et al: Primary pulmonary hypertension: favorable effect of isoproterenol, *N Engl J Med* 295:1414, 1976.
26. Reeves JT: Hope in primary pulmonary hypertension? *N Engl J Med* 302:112, 1980.
27. Rozkovec A, Montanes P, Oakley CM: Factors that influence the outcome of primary pulmonary hypertension, *Br Heart J* 55:449, 1986.
28. Suarez LD, Sciandro EE, Llera JJ, et al: Long-term follow-up in primary pulmonary hypertension, *Br Heart J* 41:702, 1979.

CHAPTER 76

Fetal Circulatory Problems

The two conditions discussed in this chapter, persistent fetal circulation and premature closure of the foramen ovale, represent abnormalities occurring in the fetal circulation or in the transition from the fetal to neonatal circulation. Each is associated with pulmonary hypertension and major cardiopulmonary problems in the neonatal period.

PERSISTENT FETAL CIRCULATION SYNDROME

This established syndrome occurring in neonates is characterized by persistent cyanosis caused by a right-to-left shunt at the atrial or the ductal level or both. The syndrome is also known as "persistent pulmonary vascular obstruction" or "persistent pulmonary hypertension."

Pathophysiology

In affected neonates the exact cause for persistent pulmonary hypertension is unknown. There is fairly convincing evidence, particularly from animal studies, that the syndrome may be caused by asphyxia in utero or at the time of birth. The hypoxia produces vasoconstriction, which induces excessive medial thickening in the pulmonary arterioles.

Clinical Features

The syndrome usually involves full-term neonates and manifests itself a few hours after birth as cyanosis and moderate respiratory distress. In distinction to the much more common respiratory distress syndrome, pulmonary infiltrations are characteristically absent. Before the syndrome was recognized, such infants frequently underwent cardiac catheterization to exclude a cyanotic congenital cardiac anomaly. The syndrome is clinically evidenced by severe cyanosis, tachypnea, and moderate respiratory distress. There may be an abnormally prominent right ventricular impulse on palpation of the thorax and a loud pulmonary component of the second heart sound suggesting pulmonary hypertension. Significant cardiomegaly and hepatomegaly are characteristically absent.

Electrocardiographic Features

The electrocardiogram shows right ventricular hypertrophy.

Radiographic Features

The radiographic findings are not characteristic but are helpful in excluding the much more common respiratory distress syndrome. Cardiac size and pulmonary vasculature are normal, and the characteristic granular pattern of respiratory distress syndrome is absent.

The diagnosis can be made without cardiac catheterization by the administration of 100% oxygen for 5 to 10 minutes (hyperoxia test). The oxygen diffuses in poorly ventilated pulmonary areas and abolishes the ventilation-perfusion mismatch. Consequently, arterial Po_2 increases. If the Po_2 does not increase, a right-to-left shunt caused by a congenital cardiac malformation must be assumed.

Echocardiographic Features

Echocardiography and nuclear radiography have largely replaced cardiac catheterization in the diagnosis of this syndrome. The right ventricular cavity may be enlarged. The right-to-left shunt at the atrial or ductus level can be confirmed by Doppler and contrast echocardiography. Furthermore, intrinsic anatomic cardiac anomalies can be excluded.

Cardiac Catheterization

Cardiac catheterization was previously used to establish the diagnosis. Currently it is rarely performed. The pulmonary arterial pressure equals systemic pressure if the patent ductus is large and patent, or it may exceed systolic pressure if the ductus is small or closed. In patients with an atrial level shunt, desaturation occurs in the left atrium. With the administration of 100% oxygen, peripheral P_{O_2} increases.

PREMATURE CLOSURE OF FORAMEN OVALE

The term premature closure of foramen ovale refers to closure before birth of the channel that allows passage of blood from right to left atrium during fetal life. This condition may be associated with coexistent anomalies on the left side of the heart with hypoplasia of the left ventricle and stenosis or atresia of the mitral valve, aortic valve, or both. Often the right ventricle is enlarged, and the tricuspid valve may become insufficient. The pulmonary venous pressure is elevated and probably contributes to the increased medial musculature of the pulmonary arterioles. Premature closure of the foramen ovale is associated with fetal or neonatal cardiac failure and death.

Index

A

Abdomen
  echocardiography, subcostal plane, 204
  heterotaxia in single atrium, 829
Acoustic wavefront: compression and rarefaction, 197
Acrocyanosis: in congenital heart disease classification, 55
Allergic reactions: to contrast media, 181
Anastomosis
  Blalock-Taussig, 581
    pulmonary atresia and, 640
    in tetralogy of Fallot, 567
  Potts, in tetralogy of Fallot, 567–568, 570, 577–578
  Waterston-Cooley, in tetralogy of Fallot, 579
Anatomy: of heart, 13–47
Aneurysm
  aorta, ascending, in Marfan syndrome, 1110
  aortic
    dissecting, in Marfan syndrome, 1113
    surgical repair by composite graft, 1114
  atrial appendage, 1141–1144
    CT in, 1143
    radiographic features, 1141–1144
    with thrombosis, 1143
  "healing," mechanism of, 1088
  pulmonary artery, with patent ductus arteriosus, 298
  sinus of Valsalva, 395–405
    angiography in, 403–405
    aortography of, 402
    catheterization in, cardiac, 400–403
    causing right ventricular outflow obstruction, 528
    clinical features, 396–397
    echocardiographic features, 399
    electrocardiographic findings, 397–398
    in Marfan syndrome, 1109
    operative repair, diagram of, 404
    pathologic anatomy, 395–396
    radiographic appearance, postoperative, 405
    radiographic features, 399–400
    rupture, 400
    rupture, central circulation in, 400
    rupture repair, 405
    surgical approach, 405
  subaortic, 1136
  submitral, 1136, 1137, 1138
  vein of Galen, 1094
  vena cava, superior, 1054
  ventricular, left, 1135–1138
    angiographic findings, 1137–1138
    clinical manifestations, 1137
    radiographic findings, 1137
    surgical treatment, 1138
  ventricular septum, membranous, 279–283
    angiographic appearance, 281–282
    clinical findings, 281
    clues to presence of, 283
    complications, 279–280
    laboratory findings, 281
    operative considerations, 283
    prominence change during cardiac cycle, 281
    radiographic features, 281
Angina: unstable, and lupus erythematosus, 1091
Angiocardiography: pulmonary vein, 32
Angiography, 157–194
  aneurysm, ventricular septum, membranous, 281–282
  aorta, thoracic, 192
  in aortic arch
    cervical, 1030–1031
    double, with both arches patent, 1012
    double, with left arch atresia, 1015
    interruption distal to innominate artery, 1026–1028
    left, right descending aorta and, 1003
    with retroesophageal arterial vessel, 1002
    right, with left descending aorta, 1010
    right, with retroesophageal segment or vessel, 1009
    sixth, interruption, 1037–1039
  in aortic stenosis
    supravalvar, 440–446
    valvar, 421–426, 427
  in aortico left ventricular tunnel, 465–467
  aorticopulmonary septal defect, 313–314
  in asplenia syndrome, 963–965
  atrial appendages, right, 22
  in atrial identification, right, 22
  of atrial ring, supravalvar stenosing, 890
  in atrial septal defect, 330–335
  in atrium, single, 829
  balloon occlusion, 174–175
  in cardiomyopathy, 918–920
  cine
    biplane, 142

1181

Angiography (cont.)
  single-plane, 142
  in coarctation of aorta, 486–490
    abdominal, 495–496
  contraindications, 177–178
  contrast media, ionic, 177–178
  in cor triatriatum, 900–902
  in coronary artery anomalous origin from pulmonary trunk, 935–938
  in coronary artery calcification, idiopathic, in infant, 1085
  in coronary artery fistula, 409–411
  in coronary sinus-left atrial window, 343–344
  in criss-cross heart, 977–979
    normal, 979
  in transposition of great vessels, complete, 983
  in transposition of great vessels in, corrected, 984
  in cyanosis with increased pulmonary arterial vasculature, 672–673
  in dextroposition of heart, 951
  in dextroversion of heart, 952–953
  in double outlet ventricle, systemic, 748
  in Ebstein's malformation, 659–662
  in ectopia cordis, 987–988
  in endocardial cushion defect, 373–375
  in endocardial fibroelastosis, 922–924
  equipment, 131–156
  in glycogen storage disease, 925–926
  in heart block, complete, 1168
  in heart tumors
    intracavitary, 1156–1157
    intrapericardial, 1163
  in Kawasaki disease, 1090–1091
  in Marfan syndrome, 1106–1112
  in mitral atresia, 870–871
  in mitral insufficiency, 1129–1130
  in mitral stenosis, 882–886
  mitral valve, 35–37, 41–42
  in mitral valve cleft, 392–393
  in mitral valve prolapse, 1122–1124
  patent ductus arteriosus, 300–304
  in pericardial defect, 1149–1151
  in polysplenia syndrome, 973–976
  positioning, 144–152
    principles, 144–148
    with standard fixed biplane equipment, 149–152
  practical hints, 190–192
  in pseudocoarctation, 494–495
  in pulmonary arteriovenous fistula, 838–839
  in pulmonary artery dilatation, idiopathic, 531
  in pulmonary artery origin from ascending aorta, 317–319
  pulmonary artery sling, 1041
  in pulmonary artery stenosis, 514–515
  in pulmonary atresia, ventricular septum intact, 632–640
  in pulmonary hypertension, 1176–1177
  in pulmonary stenosis
    dome shaped, 504–508
    infundibular, 519
  in pulmonary valve, absence, 533–534
  in pulmonary valve, dysplastic, 512
  in pulmonary vein, anomalous connection, partial, 352–354
  in pulmonary vein, anomalous connection, total, 816–821
  in pulmonary vein atresia, 849–851
  in pulmonary vein stenosis, 908–910
  in Raghib syndrome, 341–342
  in rhabdomyoma, 1161
  in scimitar syndrome, 362–363
  in sinus of Valsalva aneurysm, 403–405
  in situs solitus levoposition, 955
  in subaortic stenosis
    discrete membranous, 430–434
    muscular, 451–455
  in subclavian artery isolation, 1017
  in systemic arteriovenous fistula, 1095–1096
  in tetralogy of Fallot
    pulmonary atresia in, 589–594
    pulmonary valve absence in, 602–604
  in tetralogy of Fallot (see Tetralogy of Fallot, angiography)
  in thoracopagus, 991–992
  in transposition of great vessels, complete, 684–693
    postoperative, 698–707
  in transposition of great vessels, corrected, 715–724
  in tricuspid atresia
    with normally related great vessels, 614–615
    with normally related great vessels, postoperative, 620–623
    with transposition of great vessels, 772–774
  in tricuspid insufficiency, 23, 667–668
  in truncus arteriosus, 796–800
  in ventricle
    diverticulum, left, 1134–1135
    diverticulum, right, 1131
    double inlet, 779–780
    double inlet, right, 783
    double outlet, 737–743
    inversion, 729–730
    left, 40
    left, communication with right atrium, 288–290
    left, double outlet, 749–750
    left, hypoplastic syndrome, 858–860
    right, 26–27
    right, hypoplasia, isolated, 649–651
    right, with muscle bundle anomalies, 521–522
    single, 759–763
  in ventricular aneurysm, left, 1137–1138
  in ventricular septal defect, 259–265
    aortic insufficiency in, 275–276
Angioplasty: balloon, of mitral valve, 887
Angle-dependent reflector, 197
Anomalies
  aortic arch, 995–1048
  coronary artery, 1061–1086
  coronary sinus, allowing intracardiac shunts, 339–344
  Ebstein's (see Ebstein's malformation)
  pulmonary vein connection (see Pulmonary vein, anomalous connection, partial)
  pulmonary vein (see Pulmonary vein, anomalous connection)
  vessels, major, 993–1098
  (See also Malformation)
Antecubital vein: contrast medium injected into, 342
Aorta
  abdominal
    in aortic stenosis, supravalvar, 445
    coarctation (see Coarctation of aorta, abdominal)
  anatomy, 47
  ascending
    aneurysm in Marfan syndrome, 1110
    in Marfan syndrome, 1109
    origin of pulmonary artery from (see Pulmonary artery origin from ascending aorta)

buckling (see Pseudocoarctation)
circumflex, 1002–1003, 1005
coarctation (see Coarctation of aorta)
descending, in aortic stenosis, supravalvar, 445
elongation, 1030
filling through ventricular septal defect, 319
kinking (see Pseudocoarctation)
persistent dorsal aortae, 1003–1004
persistent of dorsal aortae right and left, 1002–1004
suprasternal notch view, 211
tetralogy of Fallot overriding, 541, 543
thoracic, angiography, 192
transposition (see Transposition of aorta)
Aortic
anatomy, 40–42
aneurysm (see Aneurysm, aortic)
arch
anomalies, 995–1048
cervical, 1028–1031, 1032, 1033, 1034
in coarctation of aorta, 480
development, 7–8, 995–996
double (see below)
elongation, 495
embryology, 1035
fifth, abnormality, 1031–1033
fifth, persistent, 997, 1034
fourth, abnormalities, 996–1008
identification in tetralogy of Fallot, 554–556
interruption, 1017–1021
interruption, aorticopulmonary septal defect in, 314
interruption, between left carotid and left subclavian arteries, 1021, 1023
interruption, beyond left carotid artery, 1024, 1027
interruption, beyond left subclavian artery, 1022, 1023, 1026
interruption, beyond right carotid artery, 1025
interruption, distal to innominate artery, 1021–1028
interruption, distal to left subclavian artery, 1018–1021
interruption, in truncus arteriosus, 790, 798
interruption, surgical correction, 1029
interruption, transposition of great vessels and, repair, 703
interruption, truncus arteriosus and, 1029
interruption, ventricular septal defect and subaortic stenosis, 1028
left (see below)
normal, 998
right (see below)
sixth, abnormality, 1033–1039
sixth, interruption, proximal, 1033–1039
system, development, 11
third, abnormality, 1028–1031
arch, double, 997, 1010–1016
with both arches patent, 1011–1015
with left aortic arch atresia, 1015–1016, 1018
operative considerations, 1015–1016
operative correction, 1016, 1017
arch, left, 998–1004
atresia, in double aortic arch, 1015, 1018
cervical, 1032, 1034
double, 1014
double, and left descending aorta, 1013
mirror-image, 1004
normal, 1001
origin of major vessels from, common variations, 999
with retroesophageal arterial vessel, 1000–1002
right descending aorta and, 1002–1003, 1005
with subclavian artery aberrancy, right, 1000, 1003
without retroesophageal arterial vessel, 998
arch, right, 91, 1004–1010
cervical, 1031, 1032, 1033
circumflex, 1009, 1011
in coarctation of aorta, 489
innominate artery isolation in, 1020
interrupted, 306
with left descending aorta, 1009, 1011, 1012
with retroesophageal segment or vessel, 1004–1009
with subclavian artery aberrancy, left, 1007–1008, 1010
in tetralogy of Fallot, 543–546, 579
tricuspid atresia in, 612
truncus arteriosus and, 1001
without retroesophageal segment or vessel, 1004
arch., right
in tetralogy of Fallot, 574
atresia, 854, 856, 857, 858–859, 861
circulation in, central, 855
coarctation of aorta and, 859
Norwood procedure in, 862
Norwood procedure in, modified, 863
operative palliation, 862
ventricular septal defect and, 861
cusp
both coronary arteries from left cusp, 1073
demonstrating nodules of Arantius, 42
herniated and prolapsing into ventricular septal defect, 276
prolapse causing right ventricular outflow obstruction, 528
prolapse through ventricular septal defect, 527
right, both coronary arteries from, 1077
right, single coronary artery arising from, 1082
in single coronary artery, 1064–1065, 1065–1070, 1067, 1070
cusps, spatial relations of, 41
dissection in coarctation of aorta, 492
graft, composite, systolic collapse, 1115
insufficiency in ventricular septal defect (see Septal defect, ventricular, aortic insufficiency in)
sinus, 397
stenosis (see Stenosis, aortic)
valve
in anteroposterior projection, 42
bicuspid, MRI of, 230
cusp prolapse, 274
doming, jet through, 424
normal, 43–44
stenosis (see Stenosis, aortic, valvar)
thickening, aortography of, 434
valvotomy, 426
Aortico left ventricular tunnel, 461–467
angiographic features, 465–467
aorta in, diagram of, 462
catheterization in, cardiac, 465
clinical features, 461–462
echocardiographic features, 462
electrocardiographic features, 462
operation, 467
origin theories, 461
pathologic anatomy, 461
pathophysiology, 461
postoperative findings, 467
radiographic features, 462–465

Aortico left ventricular *(cont.)*
  ventricles in, diagram of, 462
  ventriculography in, left, 466
Aorticopulmonary
  septal defect *(see* Septal defect, aorticopulmonary)
  window *(see* Septal defect, aorticopulmonary)
Aortography
  in aortic stenosis, valvar, 428
  in aortic valve thickening, 434
  in atrioventricular canal, complete, 385
  in coarctation of aorta, atypical, 486
  in coronary artery fistula, 412
  in double outlet right ventricle, 740–743
  in lateral projection, 45
  in Marfan syndrome, 1112
  pulmonary atresia in, ventricular septum intact, 639–640
  in pulmonary vein atresia, 850
  retrograde, in coarctation of aorta, 487–488
  in sinus of Valsalva aneurysm, 402, 405
  subaortic membrane, 433
  in tetralogy of Fallot, 563–565
  in transposition of great vessels, complete, 695–696
  in truncus arteriosus, 797–799
Aprons: lead, for radiation protection, 51
Arteries
  brachiocephalic *(see* Brachiocephalic artery)
  carotid, in aortic arch interruption, 1021
  conal, separate origin, 1062
  coronary *(see* Coronary artery)
  epigastric, in coarctation of aorta, 473
  great *(see* Great arteries)
  innominate *(see* Innominate artery)
  pulmonary *(see* Pulmonary artery)

  spinal, in coarctation of aorta, 473
  subclavian *(see* Subclavian artery)
  switch operation in transposition of great vessels, complete, 699
    modified, 706
    modified Rastelli, 700
  thoracic, lateral, in coarctation of aorta, 473
  trunks, development, 996
Arteriography
  coronary
    in aortic stenosis, supravalvar, 448
    in transposition of great arteries, 410
  pulmonary, 179
    in anteroposterior projection, 29
    balloon, 175
    in lateral projection, 28
    levophase, 82
    in pulmonary artery banding, 270, 531
    in tetralogy of Fallot, 561
Arteriopathy: pulmonary plexogenic, 1171
Arteriovenous fistula
  cerebral, 1094
  peripheral, embolization of, 1097
  pulmonary, 833–843
    angiographic features, 838–839
    catheterization in, cardiac, 837–838
    clinical features, 834
    devices to occlude, 839
    electrocardiographic features, 834
    embolization of, 840
    hemodynamics, 833
    pathologic anatomy, 833
    radiographic features, 834–837
    telangiectasia and, hemorrhagic hereditary, 841
    treatment, 839–842
    unique forms, 842–843
  systemic, 1093–1098
    angiographic features, 1095–1096
    catheterization in, cardiac, 1095
    clinical features, 1094

    echocardiographic features, 1094
    electrocardiographic features, 1094
    hemodynamics, 1093
    operative considerations, 1096–1097
    pathologic anatomy, 1093
    radiographic features, 1094
Arteriovenous malformation: pulmonary, saccular, 834
Arteritis: mesenteric, complicating coarctation of aorta, 490–492
Asplenia
  with pulmonary atresia, 304
  vena cava in, double superior, 1053
Asplenia syndrome, 957–965, 967, 968
  angiographic features, 963–965
  bronchi in, 958
  dextrocardia in, 957
  diagnosis, 960
  differentiation from polysplenia, 960–963
  pulmonary atresia in, 641
  radiographic features, 960–963
  single atrium in, 829
Atelectasis: bronchography of, 112
Atresia
  aortic *(see* Aortic atresia)
  atrioventricular valve, corrected transposition and, 769
  coronary artery, left, 1065
  coronary sinus, 1053
  infundibular *(see* Infundibular atresia)
  mitral *(see* Mitral atresia)
  pulmonary artery, pulmonary atresia and, 643
  pulmonary *(see* Pulmonary atresia)
  pulmonary valve, 643
  pulmonary vein *(see* Pulmonary vein atresia)
  tricuspid *(see* Tricuspid atresia)

Atrial
  appendage
    aneurysm *(see* Aneurysm, atrial appendage)
    atrioventricular valve atresia and, 772
    juxtaposition with tricuspid atresia, 614
    left, selective injection of, 33
    right, angiography of, 22
    in tricuspid atresia and transposition of great vessels, 769–770
  enlargement
    aggravating mitral regurgitation, 1128
    left, radiography of, plain-film, 109–112
    right, diagrams of, 104
    right, radiography of, plain-film, 102–103
    right, severe, 106
  myxoma, 1156, 1157
  septal defect *(see* Septal defect, atrial)
  septum
    development, 367
    differentiation, 8
    viewed through opened right atrium, 20
  (See also Atrium)
Atriography, right, 20
  in pulmonary atresia, ventricular septum intact, 633
Atrioventricular canal
  complete, 368, 372–373
    aortography in, 385
    mitral regurgitation in, 384
    pulmonary stenosis and, 564
    repair, 390, 391, 393
    type C repair, 389
    ventriculography in, 378
    ventriculography in, left, 377, 386
  partial, 371–372
    cardiomegaly in, 371
    with mitral regurgitation, 372
    polysplenia syndrome and pulmonary stenosis, 971
    tetralogy of Fallot and, 554
  (See also Ostium primum defect)

Atrioventricular connection:
  in univentricular heart, type of, 754
Atrioventricular valve
  atresia
    with corrected transposition, 768–769
    juxtaposition of atrial appendages in, 772
  insufficiency, and transposition of great vessels, corrected, 718, 722
Atrium
  common (see single below)
  coronary sinus-left atrial window (see Coronary sinus-left atrial window)
  development, 4–6
  left
    anatomic features, 946
    anatomy, 31–34
    bronchus compressing, 247
    coronary artery fistula with, 412
    fistulous communication to pulmonary artery, 841
    pulmonary incorporation into, 10
    pulmonary vein anomalous course to, 350
    pulmonary vein incorporation into, 10
    relations to carina and esophagus, 33
    ring, supravalvar stenosing, 889–890
    vena cava connecting to, 344
    vena cava connecting to, inferior, 1059
    vena cava connecting to, right superior, 1054
  primitive, 5
  right
    anatomic features, 16–22, 946
    anatomy, 18
    angiographic identification, 22
    cast of, 25
    communication with left ventricle (see Ventricle, left, communication with right atrium)
  in posteroanterior projection, 77
  pulmonary vein anomalous connection to, total, 821
  pulmonary vein anomalous connection to, total, surgical correction, 823
  sinus venosus incorporation into, 6
  vena cava high insertion into, inferior, 1059
  single, 827–830
    angiographic features, 829
    in asplenia syndrome, 829
    catheter course in, 828
    catheterization in, cardiac, 828–829
    clinical features, 827
    echocardiographic features, 828
    electrocardiographic features, 827–828
    hemodynamics, 827
    operative considerations, 829–830
    pathologic anatomy, 827
    radiographic features, 828
    uncomplicated, 830
  (See also Atrial)
Azygos vein, pulmonary vein anomalous connection to, total, 813
  surgical correction, 823

B

Bacterial endocarditis: in coarctation of aorta, 492
Balloon
  angiography, occlusion, 174–175
  angioplasty of mitral valve, 887
  catheters, 172–174
    for ventriculography, 173
  dilatation technique for pulmonary artery stenosis, 517
  pulmonary arteriography, 175
  septostomy in transposition of great vessels, complete, 683
Barium-filled esophagus: in coarctation of aorta, 481–482
Berman catheter, 174
Bernheim phenomenon, 456
Blalock-Hanlon procedure, 697
Blalock-Taussig
  anastomosis, 581
  pulmonary atresia and, 640
  in tetralogy of Fallot, 567
Blalock-Taussig shunt, 569
Block
  heart, complete, 1165–1169
    angiographic features, 1168
    catheterization in, cardiac, 1167–1168
    clinical features, 1166
    collagen vascular disease and, 1165
    echocardiographic features, 1166
    electrocardiographic features, 1166
    myocardial infarction and, 1165
    pacemaker in, 1168
    pathologic anatomy, 1165
    physical examination, 1166
    physiology, 1165–1166
    postoperative, 1165
    radiographic features, 1166–1167
    treatment, 1168
    ventriculography, 1167
Blood
  flow
    in atrial septal defect, 322
    coronary, impairment, congenital causes of, 1079–1080
    pulmonary, in ventricular septal defect, 250, 258
    pulmonary, increase in transposition of great vessels, complete, 680–681
    pulmonary, obstruction and tricuspid atresia, 616
    pulmonary, obstruction in transposition of great vessels, complete, 682
  pool imaging, gated, 215–219
  pressure
    aortic, 126
    atrial, left, 126
    atrial, right, 124–125
    atrial, tracing with ECG, simultaneous, 125
    measurements, 124–127
    pulmonary vessels, 125–126
    ventricular, left, 126
    ventricular, right, 125
    ventricular, right, with ECG, simultaneous, 125
    withdrawal, 126
Bony abnormalities: in congenital heart disease, 85–86
Brachiocephalic
  artery, development, 996
  vessels, 425
    ectopic origin, 1044–1048
Bronchi
  artery enlargement in tetralogy of Fallot, 547
  in asplenia syndrome, 958
  compressing atrium and pulmonary artery, 247
  in polysplenia, 969
  situs, reflecting atrial situs, 23
  vessels, radiography of, plain-film, 69–71
Bronchography
  of atelectasis, 112
  oblique projection, left anterior, 30
  in scimitar syndrome, 362
Bulbar inversion: isolated, 768–769
Bypass: saphenous, coronary ostium atresia after, 448

C

Calcification: coronary artery (see Coronary artery calcification)
Camera: cine, 140–141
Carbon dioxide: injection, 176

Carcinogenic effects: of repeated ionizing radiation exposure, 50
Carcinoma: lung causing superior vena cava syndrome, 1160
Cardiac (*see* Heart)
Cardiomegaly
 aorticopulmonary septal defect and, 311
 in atrioventricular canal, partial, 371
 radiography of, plain-film, 88, 99
 in tetralogy of Fallot, 554
Cardiomyopathy, 911–927
 conditions showing, 913
 dilated, 918, 919
  angiographic features, 918
  catheterization in, cardiac, 917
  clinical features, 913
  echocardiographic features, 914
  electrocardiographic features, 913
  hemodynamics, 912
  radiographic features, 914–916
 early, 915
 hypertrophic
  catheterization in, cardiac, 917
  clinical features, 912–913
  echocardiographic features, 914
  electrocardiographic features, 913
  hemodynamics, 912
 idiopathic, gated blood pool study, 219
 myocarditis causing, 915
 operative considerations, 920
 pathologic anatomy, 911–912
 restrictive, 917, 920
  angiographic features, 918–920
  catheterization in, cardiac, 917–918
  clinical features, 913
  echocardiographic features, 914
  electrocardiographic features, 913
  hemodynamics, 912
  radiographic features, 917

specific forms, 920–926
 ventricular decompensation in, left, 916
Cardiovascular
 complications of contrast media, 180–181
 structures in chest, 18
Carotid artery: in aortic arch interruption, 1021
Catheterization, cardiac, 115–130
 in aortic stenosis
  supravalvar, 440
  valvar, 421
 in aortico left ventricular tunnel, 465
 aorticopulmonary septal defect, 311–313
 in atrial septal defect, 327–330
 in atrium, single, 828–829
 in cardiomyopathy, 917–918
 catheter course, 115–124
 catheters most often used for, 171
 in coarctation of aorta, 484–486
 in cor triatriatum, 899–900
 in coronary artery anomalous origin from pulmonary trunk, 935
 in coronary artery fistula, 409
 in coronary sinus-left atrial window, 343–344
 in Ebstein's malformation, 658–659
 in endocardial cushion defect, 373
 in fetal circulation syndrome, persistent, 1179–1180
 in heart block, complete, 1167–1168
 in heart tumors, intracavitary, 1155–1156
 in Kawasaki disease, 1090
 laboratory electric clock hazards in, 185–190
 in mitral atresia, 869–870
 in mitral stenosis, 882
 in mitral valve cleft, 392
 in patent ductus arteriosus, 298–300

positions in various types of congenital heart disease, characteristic, 116–123
 in pulmonary arteriovenous fistula, 837–838
 in pulmonary artery dilatation, idiopathic, 529
 in pulmonary artery origin from ascending aorta, 317
 in pulmonary artery stenosis, 514
 in pulmonary atresia, ventricular septum intact, 632
 in pulmonary hypertension, 1176
 in pulmonary stenosis
  dome shaped, 504
  infundibular, 519
 in pulmonary valve, dysplastic, 511–512
 in pulmonary vein
  anomalous connection, partial, 352
  anomalous connection, total, 815–816
  atresia, 849
  stenosis, 908
 in Raghib syndrome, 341
 retrograde, with sidewinder catheter, 172
 in rhabdomyoma, 1161
 in scimitar syndrome, 362
 in sinus of Valsalva aneurysm, 400–403
 in subaortic stenosis
  discrete membranous, 430
  muscular, 450
 in systemic arteriovenous fistula, 1095
 in tetralogy of Fallot, 556
  pulmonary atresia and, 588
  pulmonary valve absence in, 601–602
 in transposition of great vessels
  complete, 682–684
  corrected, 714–715
 in tricuspid atresia and transposition of great vessels, 772
 in tricuspid atresia with normally related great vessels, 612–614

in tricuspid insufficiency, 667
 in truncus arteriosus, 796
 in ventricle
  double inlet, 779
  double outlet, 736–737
  left, communication with right atrium, 288
  left, double outlet, 749
  left, hypoplastic syndrome, 857–858
  right, hypoplasia, isolated, 649
  right, with muscle bundle anomalies, 521
  single, 758–759
 in ventricular septal defect, 257–265
  with aortic insufficiency, 275–276
Catheterization, laboratories
 medical technologist recording data in, 52
 radiation protection in, 51–52
  protection by distance, 52
  protection by proper coning, 52
  protective barriers, 51–52
Catheters, 157–170
 balloon, 172–174
  for ventriculography, 173
 Berman, 174
 cobra, 170
 course, 115–124
  in atrial septal defect, 330
  in atrium, single, 828
  in transposition of great vessels, corrected, 718
 extruded, 160–161
 extruder, screw-type, 161
 flow dynamics, 164–166
 Goodale-Lubin, 170
 historical background, 157–158
 mechanical properties of, 161–166
 methods for making, 160
 NIH, 170
 nonthrombogenic, 169–170
 perforation by, 189
 pigtail, 170

plastic, 158
    steam kettle to meet specific need, 159
    during power injection, pressure relations of, 186
    recoiling during injection, 192
    sidewinder configuration, 170
        for retrograde catheterization, 172
    soft tip, 161
    surface of, 161
        scanning electron microscopy of, 162
    thrombogenicity, 166–170
        guidewire, 169
        testing for, 168–169
    torque, 163–164
    wire-reinforced, 161
    types of, 170
        most often used, 171
        for ventriculography, 173
    woven, 160
        braiding process of inner core, 160
Caudal beam angulation: diagram demonstrating, 30
Cavography: after Mustard procedure, 705
Central nervous system: complications of contrast media, 181–182
Cerebral arteriovenous fistula, 1094
Cerebrovascular complications:in coarctation of aorta, 492
Chest
    bony, in tetralogy of Fallot, 554
    cardiovascular structures in, 18
    in congenital heart disease, 84–91
    heart orientation in, 16
    heart position in, 13–16
        postoperative, in congenital heart disease, 86–89
    rotation in heart size and shape, 81
Chordal rupture: regurgitation causing, in mitral valve prolapse, 1122

Chylothorax: bilateral, after Mustard procedure in transposition of great vessels, complete, 707
Cine
    angiography (see Angiography, cine)
    camera, 140–141
    equipment, basic, 142–152
    film (see Film, cine)
    fluorography (see Fluorography, cine)
    fluoroscopy (see Fluoroscopy, cine)
    frames, 134
        radiation dose per, 140
    magnetic resonance imaging, 236–239
    projectors, 153–155
    pulsing system, 135
    trouble-shooting the system, 155–156
Circulation
    central
        in aortic atresia, 855
        in mitral atresia, 868
        in pulmonary atresia, ventricular septum intact, 627
        in sinus of Valsalva aneurysm rupture, 400
        in tricuspid atresia, 608
        in tricuspid atresia with complete transposition of great vessels, 768
        in truncus arteriosus, persistent, 792
    coronary artery, in pulmonary atresia, 628
    fetal, 8–10, 626
        persistent (see below)
        problems, 1179–1180
    in pulmonary atresia, ventricular septum intact, 625
    fetal, persistent syndrome, 1179
        catheterization in, cardiac, 1179–1180
        clinical features, 1179
        echocardiographic features, 1179
        electrocardiographic features, 1179
        pathophysiology, 1179
        radiographic features, 1179
    postnatal, 12

pulmonary, demonstration in tetralogy of Fallot, 589–594
    transitional, 10–12
    in ventricular septal defect, 251
Circumflex: left, aberrancy, arising from right coronary artery, 1073
Clavicle: and angulation of x-ray beam, 74
Cleft
    mitral, isolated, 1130
    mitral valve (see Mitral valve, cleft)
    tricuspid valve, 393
Coarctation of aorta, 469–497
    abdominal, 495–496
        anatomy, 495
        angiographic appearance, 495–496
        clinical features, 495
        electrocardiographic features, 495
        hemodynamics, 495
        radiographic features, 495
    treatment, 496
    anatomy, 469–471
    angiographic appearance, 486–490
    aortic arch in, 480
        right, 489
    aortic atresia and, 859
    aortic dissection in, 492
    aortography of, retrograde, 487–488
    arteries in, major collateral, diagram of, 474
    associated conditions, 474–475
    atypical, aortography of, balloon occlusion, 486
    beyond left subclavian artery with marked poststenotic dilatation, 484
    catheterization in, cardiac, 484–486
    cerebrovascular complications, 492
    clinical features, 475–476
    complications, 490–492
    correction, radiography after, plain-film, 89
    diffuse, 469–470, 471
    double aortic arch in, 489
    echocardiographic features, 476

electrocardiographic features, 476
embryology, 471–473
epigastric arteries in, 473
esophagus in, barium-filled, 481–482
    with heart failure, congestive, 477
hypertension after surgery, systemic, 490
hypoplasia, tubular, 469–470
    of aortic isthmus, 471
    and normal origin of subclavian artery, 482
incidence, 469
intercostal collaterals in, 473
juxtaductal, 472
localized, 469, 470
"low arch sign," 479
management, 488–490
    asymptomatic child, 490
    symptomatic newborn or young infant, 488–490
mediastinum in, 481–482
mesenteric arteritis complicating, 490–492
MRI of, 235
    with normal origin of left subclavian artery and tubular hypoplasia, 482
    and well-developed aortic knob, 482
operations for, three types, 490
    with origin of subclavian artery and level of coarctation, 482
patent ductus arteriosus in, 493
pathophysiology, 473–474
periscapular network in, 473–474
radiography, 476–484
    nonspecific features, 476–480
    nonspecific features, infants, 476–477
    nonspecific features, older children and adults, 477–480
    specific features, 480–482
recoarctation, 492

Coarctation of aorta—cont'd
  relation
    to ductus arteriosus, 470
    to subclavian arteries, 472
  repair
    radiography after, plain-film, 90
    by subclavian flap technique, 491
  rib notching in, 479, 480–481
  spinal artery in, 473
  spinal cord complications in, 492
  subclavian artery
    left, dilated, 483
    left, low origin, 484
    low origin, 484
    normal origin, 482
    origin at level of coarctation, 482
  subclavian flap technique repair, 494
  thoracic artery in, lateral, 473
  vascular complications, 492
  without tubular hypoplasia and with no poststenotic dilatation, 484
Cobra catheter, 170
Collagen vascular disease: and heart block, complete, 1165
Color flow imaging, 202–203
"Comma" shadow: of pulmonary artery, 82
Computed tomography
  of atrial appendage aneurysm, 1143
  of heart, 105
Conal artery: separate origin, 1062
Conduit: in tricuspid atresia with normally related great vessels, 620
Congenital heart disease
  bony abnormalities in, 85–86
  chest in, 84–91
    postoperative, 86–89
  classification, 55–58
    by cyanosis, 55
    by hemodynamics, 58–59
    methods, 55–58
  cyanotic, 1006
  hemodynamics, 58–60
    classification by, 58–59
    clinical implications, 59
    physical principles, 59
    pulmonary considerations, 59–60
  incidence, 57–58
  radiography of, plain-film (see Radiography, plain-film, of congenital heart disease)
  subclassification, 56–57
Contrast media, 175–182
  allergic reactions to, 181
  angiographic, ionic, 177–178
  cardiovascular complications, 180–181
  choice of, 177–178
  CNS complications of, 181–182
  death after, 179
  dose, 191–192
  effects on coronary artery bed and myocardium, 180–181
  embolism after, 180
  extravasation, paravascular, 190
  gastrointestinal complications, 180
  injection
    into antecubital vein, 342
    into femoral vein, 191
    into myocardium, 188
  kidney complications of, 182
  pericardial space injection, 189
  power injectors for, complications associated with, 184–185
  pulmonary complications, 179–180
  reactions
    adverse, 178–182
    prevention of, 175–177
  side effects, minor, 179
  subendocardial deposition of, 187
  subepicardial deposition, 188
Conus
  double, in transposition of great vessels, corrected, 721
  double coni and complete transposition, 741
  subpulmonary, in double inlet right ventricle, 783
Cor triatriatum, 891–903
  angiographic features, 900–902
  atrial septal defect and, 895
  catheterization in, cardiac, 899–900
  clinical features, 896–897
  diaphragmatic type, 893, 901, 902
  echocardiographic features, 897
  electrocardiographic features, 897
  hemodynamics, 892–896
  hourglass type, 893, 900
  imperforate membrane in, 897
  obstruction in, severe, 898, 899
  operative considerations, 903
  partial, 895, 896
  pathologic anatomy, 891–892
  radiographic features, 897–899
    postoperative, 903
  tubular type, 894
Coronary
  arteriography (see Arteriography, coronary)
  artery
    anatomy, 42–47
    anomalies, 1061–1086
    anomalies in tetralogy of Fallot, 546–547
    anomalous origin from pulmonary trunk (see below)
    atresia, left, 1065
    bed, effects of contrast media on, 180–181
    both coronaries from left aortic cusp, 1073
    both coronaries from right aortic cusp, 1077
    calcification, idiopathic, in infant (see below)
    circulation in pulmonary atresia, 628
    communicating with right ventricle, 413
    compression, proposed mechanisms of, 1081
    disease in infant, 1083
    distribution variation, 1071–1080
    fistula (see Fistula, coronary artery)
    left, anomalous, reimplantation, 938
    left, anomalous, surgical correction, 937
    left, anomalous, tunnel repair, 939
    left, separate origin above right aortic cusp, 1076
    left, system, 46
    number variations, 1061–1070
    obstruction, medial disease leading to, 1081
    origin, aberrancy, myocardial ischemia and, 1077–1079
    origin, ectopic, 1077
    origin, variation, 1071–1080
    pattern, in transposition of great vessels, complete, 679, 691–693
    pattern, in transposition of great vessels, corrected, 725
    right, origin, high and ectopic, 1070, 1071
    right, system, 46
    single, 548, 1061–1064
    single, arising above left aortic cusp, 1064–1065, 1070
    single, arising above left aortic cusp, variation, 1067
    single, arising above right aortic cusp, 1064, 1065, 1082
    single, arising above right aortic cusp, variation, 1067
    single, ectopic origin from right innominate artery, 1079
    single, interfering with ventriculotomy, 1070
    single, with hemodynamic consequences, 1065
    single, with operative implications, 1065
    single, without hemodynamic consequences, 1064–1070
    single, without operative implications, 1064–1070

system, in transposition
of great vessels,
corrected, 710
artery anomalous origin
from pulmonary
trunk, 929–942
angiographic features,
935–938
catheterization in,
cardiac, 935
clinical features, 932
echocardiographic
features, 932
electrocardiographic
features, 932
hemodynamics, 930–932
operative
considerations,
938–941
pathologic anatomy,
929–930
radiographic features,
932–935
radiographic features,
postoperative, 941
artery calcification,
idiopathic, in infant,
1084–1085
angiographic features,
1085
clinical features, 1084
pathologic
manifestations, 1084
radiographic features,
1084–1085
treatment, 1085
blood flow, impairment,
congenital causes,
1079–1080
fistula with pulmonary
artery, 410
ostia
atresia with saphenous
bypass injection, 448
four separate, 1063
position variation,
1070–1071
sinus
absence, 1054
anomalies allowing
intracardiac shunts,
339–344
atresia, 1053
catheter passed from
right atrium into vena
cava, 341
catheter passed through
vena cava into, 344
development, 340
fenestration of, 1053
fenestration of,
pathologic anatomy,
342

pulmonary vein
anomalous
connection to, total,
812
pulmonary vein
anomalous
connection to, total,
surgical correction,
822
stenosis, 1053
vena cava to, superior,
left, persistent,
1052
sinus, left atrial window,
342–344
angiography of,
343–344
catheterization in,
cardiac, 343–344
clinical features,
342–343
hemodynamics, 342
mitral atresia and vena
cava connecting to
left atrium in,
344
radiographic features,
342–343
Criss-cross heart, 977–986
angiographic features,
977–979
clinical features, 977
comparison with normal
heart, 978
normal
angiographic features,
979–980
concordance
atrioventricular and
ventriculoarterial
connections,
979–980
with transposition of great
vessels
complete, 980–983
complete, angiographic
features, 983
corrected, 983–984
without great vessel
malposition, 979,
980
Cyanosis
in congenital heart disease
classification, 55
in liver disease, chronic,
838
peripheral, in congenital
heart disease
classification, 55
with pulmonary artery
vasculature
decreased, 537–669
increased, 671–803

pulmonary blood flow
normal in, 831–843
pulmonary vein
vasculature increase
and, 845–872
radiography of, plain-film,
69
Cystic medial necrosis (*see*
Marfan syndrome)

D

D transposition of great
vessels: with single
ventricle, 758
Damus-Kaye-Stansel repair:
for transposition of
great vessels,
complete, 702
Death: after contrast media,
179
Development: of heart,
3–12
Dextrocardia, 950–954
in asplenia syndrome, 957
Dextroinversion: of situs
solitus in
transposition of great
vessels,
corrected, 717
Dextroposition: of heart,
950–951
Dextroversion
of heart, 951–953
MRI of, 233
in transposition of great
vessels, corrected,
721
Diaphragm
motordriven
semitransparent, 137
position influencing heart
size, 73
subaortic, 431
Diatrizoate, 177–178
clinical experience with,
178
Diverticulum
ductus, 296
of pulmonary artery,
306
ventricle, 1131–1139
left (*see* Ventricle, left,
diverticulum)
right, 1131
Doppler
aliasing, time axis, 201
high pulse
repetition-frequency,
202
Down syndrome: sternum in,
88

Ductus
arteriosus
anatomic closure, 12
patent (*see* Patent
ductus arteriosus)
relation to coarctation
of aorta, 470
diverticulum, 296
of pulmonary artery,
306
venosus, development, 10
Dysplasia
fibromuscular, 1083–1084
of pulmonary valve (*see*
Pulmonary valve,
dysplastic)

E

Ebstein's malformation,
653–664
angiographic features,
659–662
atrial enlargement due to,
right, 103
catheterization in, cardiac,
658–659
clinical features, 656
echocardiographic
features, 657
electrocardiographic
features, 656–657
hemodynamics, 654–656
late stage, 659
mild, 658
pathologic anatomy,
653–654
in pulmonary atresia,
ventricular septum
intact, 632
radiographic features,
657–658
postoperative, 663
severe, 654, 655
treatment, 662
tricuspid regurgitation in,
659
Echo sector: 30-degree, 199
Echocardiography, 102
abdomen, subcostal plane,
204
in aortic arch
interruption distal to
innominate artery,
1025
sixth, interruption, 1036
in aortic stenosis
supravalvar, 439
valvar, 418
in aortico left ventricular
tunnel, 462
aorticopulmonary septal
defect, 310

Echocardiography (cont.)
  in atrial septal defect, 324
  in atrium, single, 828
  in cardiomyopathy, 913–914
  in coarctation of aorta, 476
  in cor triatriatum, 897
  in coronary artery anomalous origin from pulmonary trunk, 932
  in coronary artery fistula, 408
  in Ebstein's malformation, 657
  in endocardial cushion defect, 371
  in fetal circulation syndrome, persistent, 1179
  in heart block, complete, 1166
  in heart tumors
    intracavitary, 1155
    intrapericardial, 1162
  in Kawasaki disease, 1089
  locations, 204–213
    precordial, 207–210
    precordial, apical, 210–213
    precordial, apical, aortic outflow plane, 211
    precordial, apical, four chamber plane, 210–211
    precordial, apical, two-chamber plane, 211–213
    precordial, parasternal long-axis plane, 207–208
    precordial, parasternal short-axis plane, 208–210
    precordial right upper sternal border, 213
    subcostal, 204–207
    subcostal, frontal plane, 205
    subcostal, long axial oblique plane, 205–207
    subcostal, right anterior oblique plane, 207
    subcostal, sagittal plane, 206, 207
    suprasternal notch, 213
    suprasternal notch, coronal plane, 213
    suprasternal notch, sagittal plane, 213
  M-mode, 208
  in Marfan syndrome, 1103–1104
  in mitral atresia, 869
  in mitral stenosis, 879–880
  in mitral valve cleft, 392
  in mitral valve prolapse, 1121
  patent ductus arteriosus, 293
  in pericardial defect, 1146
  pulmonary artery origin from ascending aorta, 316
  in pulmonary artery stenosis, 514
  in pulmonary atresia, ventricular septum intact, 630
  in pulmonary hypertension, 1173
  in pulmonary stenosis
    dome shaped, 501
    infundibular, 519
  in pulmonary valve, dysplastic, 510
  in pulmonary vein anomalous connection, partial, 349
  in pulmonary vein anomalous connection, total, 811
  in pulmonary vein atresia, 848
  in pulmonary vein stenosis, 905
  in rhabdomyoma, 1160
  in scimitar syndrome, 359
  in sinus of Valsalva aneurysm, 399
  in subaortic stenosis
    discrete membranous, 428
    muscular, 450
  in systemic arteriovenous fistula, 1094
  in tetralogy of Fallot, 550
    pulmonary atresia in, 586
    pulmonary valve absence in, 600
  in transposition of great vessels, complete, 680
  in tricuspid atresia and transposition of great vessels, 770
  in tricuspid atresia with normally related great vessels, 610
  in tricuspid insufficiency, 666
  in truncus arteriosus, 793
  in ventricle
    double inlet, 779, 782–783
    left, communication with right atrium, 287
    left, double outlet, 749
    left, hypoplastic syndrome, 856
    right, hypoplasia, isolated, 648
    right, with muscle bundle anomalies, 520
    single, 757
  in ventricular septal defect, 253
    aortic insufficiency in, 274–275
    worksheet for laboratory, 212
Ectopia cordis, 987–989
  angiographic features, 987–988
  postoperative features, 989
  radiographic features, 987
Edema, pulmonary, 65
  radiography of, plain-film, 68
Ehlers-Danlos syndrome, 1116
Eisenmenger's syndrome, 255
Electric shock hazards
  and catheterization laboratory, 185–190
  prevention, 185–186
Electrocardiography, 102
  in aortic arch
    interruption distal to innominate artery, 1022
    sixth, interruption, 1036
  in aortic stenosis
    supravalvar, 439
    valvar, 418
  in aortico left ventricular tunnel, 462
  aorticopulmonary septal defect, 310
  atrial pressure tracing and, simultaneous, 125
  in atrial septal defect, 323–324
  in atrium, single, 827–828
  in cardiomyopathy, 913
  in coarctation of aorta, 476
    abdominal, 495
  in cor triatriatum, 897
  in coronary artery anomalous origin from pulmonary trunk, 932
  in coronary artery fistula, 408
  in Ebstein's malformation, 656–657
  in endocardial cushion defect, 370–371
  in fetal circulation syndrome, persistent, 1179
  in heart block, complete, 1166
  in Kawasaki disease, 1089
  in Marfan syndrome, 1103
  in mitral atresia, 869
  in mitral stenosis, 879
  in mitral valve prolapse, 1121
  patent ductus arteriosus, 293
  in pericardial defect, 1146
  pulmonary arteriovenous fistula, 834
  of pulmonary artery dilatation, idiopathic, 529
  pulmonary artery origin from ascending aorta, 316
  in pulmonary artery stenosis, 514
  in pulmonary atresia, ventricular septum intact, 630
  in pulmonary hypertension, 1173
  in pulmonary stenosis
    dome shaped, 500–501
    infundibular, 519
  in pulmonary valve, dysplastic, 510
  in pulmonary vein anomalous connection, partial, 349
  in pulmonary vein anomalous connection, total, 811
  in pulmonary vein atresia, 848
  in pulmonary vein stenosis, 905
  in Raghib syndrome, 341
  in scimitar syndrome, 359
  in sinus of Valsalva aneurysm, 397–398
  in subaortic stenosis
    discrete membranous, 428
    muscular, 449–450

in systemic arteriovenous
fistula, 1094
in tetralogy of Fallot, 550
pulmonary atresia in,
586
pulmonary valve
absence in, 600
in transposition of great
vessels
complete, 680
corrected, 713
in tricuspid atresia and
transposition of great
vessels, 770
in tricuspid atresia with
normally related great
vessels, 610
in tricuspid insufficiency,
666
in truncus arteriosus, 793
in ventricle
double inlet, 779
double outlet, 735
left, communication
with right atrium,
287
left, double outlet, 749
left, hypoplastic
syndrome, 856
right, hypoplasia,
isolated, 647
right, with muscle
bundle anomalies,
520
single, 757
ventricular pressure
tracing with, right,
simultaneous, 125
of ventricular septal
defect, 252–253
aortic insufficiency in,
274
Electrocution: basic
principles, 185
Electron microscopy:
scanning, of catheter
surfaces, 162
Embolism
after contrast media, 180
in atrial septal defect, 335
Embolization
of peripheral arteriovenous
fistula, 1097
of pulmonary
arteriovenous fistula,
840
Embryogenesis: of ventricle,
right, double outlet,
733
Embryology
of aortic arch, 1035
in coarctation of aorta,
471–473

in endocardial cushion
defect, 365–366
of heart, 3–10
pulmonary artery origin
from ascending aorta,
315
in pulmonary vein
anomalous
connection, total, 805
in Raghib syndrome, 339
ventricular loops, 948
Endocardial cushion defect,
365–393
angiographic appearance,
373–375
angiographic findings,
380–386
angiographic technique,
380–386
associated conditions, 369
catheterization in, cardiac,
373
clinical features, 370
echocardiographic
features, 371
electrocardiographic
features, 370–371
embryology, 365–366
gooseneck deformity in,
374
hemodynamics, 369–370
mitral anatomy in,
380–381
mitral regurgitation in,
quantification of
degree of, 386–388
operative considerations,
388
pathologic anatomy,
366–369
postoperative appearance,
388–390
radiographic anatomy,
375–380
radiographic features,
371–373
ventriculography, left
anterior oblique
projection, systole,
378–380
anteroposterior
projection, 375–377
lateral projection,
diastole, 380
left anterior oblique
projection, diastole,
377–378
Endocardial fibroelastosis,
920–924
angiographic features,
922–924
catheterization, 923
contracted type, 921, 924

dilated type, 921
late stage, 923
mitral regurgitation in,
924
radiographic features,
921–922
Endocardial friction lesions,
1120
Endocarditis: bacterial, in
coarctation of aorta,
492
Epigastric arteries: in
coarctation of aorta,
473
Equipment: angiography,
131–156
Esophagus: barium-filled, in
coarctation of aorta,
481–482

F

Facies: in aortic stenosis,
supravalvar, 440
Fat
necrosis, pericardial, 1151
pad, pericardial,
radiography of,
plain-film, 92
Femoral vein: contrast
medium injected into,
191
Fetus, circulation (see
Circulation, fetal)
Fibroelastosis, endocardial
(see Endocardial
fibroelastosis)
Fibroma
of heart, recurrent, 1161
MRI of, 1161
Fibromuscular dysplasia,
1083–1084
Film, cine, 152–153
characteristics, 153
processing, 153
quality control, 153
strip exposed, 152
First-pass imaging, 219–221
Fistula
arteriovenous (see
Arteriovenous fistula)
coronary
with left atrium, 412
with pulmonary artery,
410
coronary artery, 407–414
angiographic
appearance, 409–411
aortography in, 412
catheterization in,
cardiac, 409
clinical features,
407–408

echocardiographic
features, 408
electrocardiographic
features, 408
hemodynamics, 407
operative
considerations,
411–413
pathologic anatomy, 407
postoperative
appearance, 413
radiographic features,
408–409
termination sites, 408
Floppy mitral valve, 1120
Flow-controlled injectors,
182–183
pressure limitation, 183
rise time, 183
Fluorocarbons, 159
Fluorography, cine,
132–142
brightness control,
automatic, 135
exposure time, variable,
136–137
framing, 139
optical system, 138–139
pulse width, variable,
136–137
quantum noise, 140
secondary radiation
emission during, 50
Fluoroscopy
cine, 131
of heart, 112–113
Fontan conduit, 620
Fontan modification: of large
main pulmonary
arteries, 619
Fontan procedure, 618
modified, 620
MRI of, 239
Foramen
bulboventricular, stenosis
of, and single
ventricle, 764
ovale
development, 10
premature closure, 1180
stenosis, and pulmonary
vein anomalous
connection, total, 820
ovalis
premature closure, 864
Fossa ovalis
diagram, 19
herniation, 854
tricuspid atresia in, 615
Framing: in cine
fluorography, 139
Frequency shift velocity:
calculation of, 200

Fungal infection: causing pulmonary artery mass, 1159

G

Gastrointestinal complications: of contrast media, 180
Gated blood pool imaging, 215–219
Gating: range, 201
Generator: x-ray, 132
Genetic effects: of repeated ionizing radiation exposure, 50
Glenn anastomosis, 621
Glenn procedure, 617
Glycogen storage disease, 924–926
  angiographic features, 925–926
Goodale-Lubin catheter, 170
Gooseneck deformity: in endocardial cushion defect, 374
Graft
  aortic, composite, systolic collapse, 1115
  composite, in aortic aneurysm surgical repair, 1114
  in tetralogy of Fallot, 570
Gray scale two-dimensional image: traditional, 199
Great arteries: development, 6
Great vessels
  abnormalities of, congenital, MRI of, 234–235
  normally related in tricuspid atresia (see Tricuspid atresia with normally related great vessels)
  orientation of, diagram demonstrating, 689
  transposition (see Transposition of great vessels)
Guidewire thrombogenicity: of catheters, 169

H

Heart
  anatomy, 13–47
  anomalies
    in asplenia syndrome, 957
    in polysplenia syndrome, 966
  block (see Block, heart)
  catheterization (see Catheterization, cardiac)
  chambers
    anatomic features, 946
    enlargement, radiography of, plain-film, 100–112
  conditions associated shunt, left-to-right, 241–414
  contour
    effect of heart rotation on, 107
    radiography of, plain-film, 72–79
    transposition of great vessels and, corrected, 715
  criss-cross (see Criss-cross heart)
  CT of, 105
  development, 3–12
  dextroposition, 950–951
  dextroversion, 951–953
  disease, congenital (see Congenital heart disease)
  embryology, 3–10
  enlargement
    radiography of, plain-film, 86
    right-sided, radiography of, plain-film, 104
  failure, congestive, in coarctation of aorta, 477
  fibroma, recurrent, 1161
  fluoroscopy of, 112–113
  Holmes', 756
  long axis
    foreshortening, elimination of, 150, 151
    inclination to each three major body planes, 146
  lymphatics, 47
  lymphoma, 1159
  malposition, 943–992
    radiography of, 955–957
  orientation in chest, 16
  position in thorax, 13–16
  radiography, plain-film
    anterior oblique view, left, 95–96, 97
    anterior oblique view, right, 95
    en face view, 92
    end-on view, 92
    four views, 91–98
    lateral projection, 96–98
    posteroanterior view, 93–95
  rotation
    clockwise, 79
    effect on heart contour, 107
  septum, development, 7
  shape, chest rotation in, 81
  size
    change and contour with rotation, 75
    change with breathing, 71–72
    chest rotation in, 81
    diaphragm position influencing, 73
    estimation, 91
    radiography of, plain-film, 71–72
  Taussig-Bing, double outlet right ventricle and, 739, 742
  tube, development, 4
  tumors, 1153–1164
    classification, 1153–1164
    clinical presentation, 1153
    intracavitary (see below)
    intramural, 1158–1161
    intrapericardial (see below)
    right ventricular outflow obstruction due to, 528–529
  tumors, intracavitary, 1153–1158
    angiographic features, 1156–1157
    catheterization in, cardiac, 1155–1156
    clinical features, 1154–1155
    echocardiographic features, 1155
    radiographic features, 1155
    treatment, 1158
  tumors, intrapericardial, 1161–1163
    angiographic features, 1163
    echocardiographic features, 1162
    postoperative features, 1163
    radiographic features, 1162–1163
    treatment, 1163
  version, 951
Hemangioma
  intra-abdominal, 1096
  mediastinal, 1096
Hemangiomatosis: with shunting, 1096
Hemitruncus (see Pulmonary artery origin from ascending aorta)
"Hemodynamic vise," 809
Hemodynamics: of congenital heart disease (see Congenital heart disease, hemodynamics)
Hemorrhagic telangiectasia, hereditary, 836
  pulmonary arteriovenous fistula and, 841
Herniation
  fossa ovalis, 854
  tricuspid atresia and, 615
Heterotaxia: abdominal, in single atrium, 829
Holmes' heart, 756
Hurler's syndrome, 914
Hydraulic forces: hazards from, 186–190
Hypertension
  Kawasaki disease and, 1090
  pulmonary (see Pulmonary hypertension)
  pulmonary vein, radiography of, plain-film, 63, 65, 66, 67
  systemic, after coarctation of aorta surgery, 490
Hypertrophy: interventricular septum with subpulmonary stenosis, 526, 527–528
Hypoplasia
  in coarctation of aorta (see Coarctation of aorta, hypoplasia)
  pulmonary artery, 1040
    in tetralogy of Fallot, 573
  ventricle
    right (see Ventricle, right, hypoplasia)
  ventricle (see Ventricle, hypoplasia)

Hypoplastic left ventricle syndrome (*see* Ventricle, left, hypoplastic syndrome)

I

Image intensifiers
 basic principles, 132–135
 dual-image field, diagram of, 138
 multiple-mode, 138
 quality control, 139–140
 single-mode, 137–138
 size, 137–138
 tube, basic principle, 133
Imaging
 first-pass, 219–221
 gated blood pool, 215–219
 isotope, 215–227
 magnetic resonance (*see* Magnetic resonance imaging)
 myocardial perfusion, 221–224
Indicator dilution techniques, 129–130
Infant
 coronary artery calcification (*see* Coronary artery calcification, idiopathic, in infant)
 coronary artery disease, 1083
Infarction: myocardial, and heart block, complete, 1165
Infundibular atresia
 pulmonary, 640
 in pulmonary atresia, ventricular septum intact, 636
 pulmonary valve atresia and, 643
Innominate artery
 aberrant origin, 1046
 single coronary artery ectopic origin from, 1079
Intercostal collaterals: in coarctation of aorta, 473
Interventricular septum, 244
 deficiency, 374
 hypertrophy with subpulmonary stenosis, 526, 527–528
 rhabdomyoma, 527

Intraabdominal hemangioma, 1096
Ionizing radiation (*see* Radiation, ionizing)
Iothalamates, 178
Ischemia: myocardial, in coronary artery origin aberrancy, 1077–1079
Isotope scanning, 215–227
Ivalon shavings: in peripheral arteriovenous fistula, 1097

J

Jet
 collapse, vascular, diagram of mechanism, 191
 through doming aortic valve, 424

K

Kartagener's syndrome, 954
Kawasaki disease, 1087–1092
 angiographic features, 1090–1091
 catheterization in, cardiac, 1090
 clinical features, 1088–1089
 echocardiographic features, 1089
 electrocardiographic features, 1089
 hemodynamics, 1088
 hypertension and, 1090
 laboratory studies, 1089
 management, 1091
 pathologic anatomy, 1087–1088
 radiographic features, 1089–1090
 stage 2, 1089
Kidney complications: of contrast media, 182
Kilovoltage: variable, 135–136

L

L loop: transposition, corrected, 949
L-transposition of great vessels (*see* Transposition of great vessels, corrected)

Lead aprons: for radiation protection, 51
Levocardia, 954–957
 in polysplenia, 958
Levoversion: with situs inversus, 955, 956
Liver disease: chronic, cyanosis in, 838
Lung
 overexpansion, 362
 perfusion studies, quantitative, 224–226
 in scimitar syndrome, 359
 transplantation, 225
 (*see also* Pulmonary)
Lupus erythematosus: and unstable angina, 1091
Lymphangiography: in Noonan syndrome, 534
Lymphatics: of heart, 47
Lymphoma: of heart, 1159

M

Magnetic resonance imaging, 229–240
 advantages of, 231
 applications to heart, 231–232
 cine, 236–239
 fibroma, 1161
 of great vessels, congenital abnormalities, 234–235
 in Marfan syndrome, 1104
 physical principles, 229–231
 pulmonary vascular abnormalities, 235–236
 visceroatrial situs and, 232–234
Malformation
 Ebstein's (*see* Ebstein's malformation)
 pulmonary arteriovenous, saccular, 834
 (*See also* Anomalies)
Malrotation: and L loop, 949
Marfan syndrome, 1101–1117
 aneurysm of ascending aorta in, 1110
 angiography in, 1106–1112
 aorta in, ascending, 1109
 aortic aneurysm in, dissecting, 1113
 aortic stenosis in, valvar, 1112

 aortography, 1112
 clinical features, 1102–1103
 early stage, 1111
 echocardiographic features, 1103–1104
 electrocardiographic features, 1103
 hemodynamics, 1102
 mitral regurgitation in, 1103
 mitral valve in, 1102, 1113
 MRI of, 1104
 pathologic anatomy, 1101–1102
 postoperative features, 1113–1117
 radiographic features, 1104–1105
 sinus of Valsalva aneurysm in, 1109
 sinus of Valsalva in, 1107
 treatment, 1112
 ventriculography in, 1114
Mediastinum
 in coarctation of aorta, 481–482
 enlargement, radiography of, plain-film, 102
 hemangioma, 1096
 shift to right, 363
Mesenteric arteritis: in coarctation of aorta, 490–492
Metrizoates, 178
Microscopy: electron, scanning, of catheter surfaces, 162
Mitral
 anatomic features, 34–35
 anatomy in endocardial cushion defect, 380–381
 angiographic features, 35–37, 41–42
 atresia, 344, 854, 867–872
 angiographic features, 870–871
 catheterization in, cardiac, 869–870
 circulation in, central, 868
 clinical features, 868–869
 echocardiographic features, 869
 electrocardiographic features, 869
 hemodynamics, 867–868
 MRI of, 232

Mitral (cont.)
   operative considerations, 871–872
   pathologic anatomy, 867
   polysplenia syndrome and, 973
   pulmonary stenosis and, infundibular, 870
   radiographic features, 869
   surgical correction, 871
   transposition of great vessels and, 869
  cleft, isolated, 1130
  disease, radiography of, plain-film, 112
  insufficiency, 1127–1130
   angiographic features, 1129–1130
   radiographic features, 1129
   radiography of, plain-film, 111
  oblique projection, right anterior, 36
  regurgitation
   aggravation by atrial enlargement, 1128
   in atrioventricular canal, complete, 384
   with atrioventricular canal, partial, 372
   in endocardial cushion defect, quantification of degree of, 386–388
   in endocardial fibroelastosis, 924
   in Marfan syndrome, 1103
  stenosis (see Stenosis, mitral)
  valve
   abnormalities, 1127–1130
   anatomy, 34–37
   angioplasty of, balloon, 887
   arcade, 887
   cleft (see below)
   double orifice, 1128
   floppy, 1120
   leaflet, 455
   leaflet, attached to ventricular septum, 374
   leaflet, cleft, 1128
   leaflet, open, 384
   leaflet, ventriculography of, left, 385
   in Marfan syndrome, 1102, 1113
   normal, 876, 877, 1129
   parachute, 878, 882, 884, 886
   prolapse (see below)
   prosthetic, in atrioventricular canal repair, complete, 391
   redundant, atypical, 887
   Starr-Edwards prosthetic, 390
  valve, cleft, 390–393
   anatomy, 390–391
   angiographic appearance, 392–393
   catheterization in, cardiac, 392
   clinical features, 392
   echocardiographic features, 392
   hemodynamics, 392
   isolated, 1129
   management, 393
   ostium primum defect and, 368
   radiographic features, 392
   repair, 388
  valve prolapse, 1119–1126
   angiographic features, 1122–1124
   clinical features, 1120–1121
   echocardiographic features, 1121
   electrocardiographic features, 1121
   grade 1, 1123
   grade 2, 1124
   grade 3, 1124
   management, 1125
   pathologic anatomy, 1119–1120
   radiographic features, 1121–1122
   regurgitation due to chordal rupture, 1122
   ventriculography in, 1123
Monitoring: of radiation, requirements, 50–51
Mucopolysaccharidosis: Hurler's syndrome, 914
Muscle bundle anomalies in right ventricle (see Ventricle, right, muscle bundle anomalies in)
  in ventricular outflow tract, right, 265
  ventricular septal defect in, 523
Mustard procedure, in transposition of great vessels, 698
  complete, 704–707
Myocarditis, 916
  cardiomyopathy due to, 915
Myocardium
  bridges, 1080–1082
   pathophysiology, 1081–1082
  effects of contrast media on, 180–181
  infarction in heart block, complete, 1165
  injection of contrast medium into, 188
  ischemia in coronary artery origin aberrancy, 1077–1079
  perfusion imaging, 221–224
  sinusoids, 1082–1083
Myxoma
  atrial, 1156, 1157
  ventricular, right, 1156

N

Necrosis
  cystic medial (see Marfan syndrome)
  pericardial fat, 1151
Newborn
  tricuspid insufficiency in, 668
   transient, 665, 666, 667
NIH catheter, 170
Noonan syndrome, 533, 534–535
  characteristic features, 533
  lymphangiography in, 534
Norwood procedure in aortic atresia, 862
  modified, 863

O

Osmolar agents: low, 178
Ostium primum: development, 5
Ostium primum defect, 371, 374
  cleft mitral valve and, 368
  repair, diagram of, 388
  in systole, 376
  ventriculography in, left, 381, 383, 384
  (See also Atrioventricular canal)
Outflow obstructive lesions, 415–536
Oximetry, 127–129
  derived data, 128–129

P

Pacemaker: in heart block, complete, 1168
Paint: spray gun with insufficient number of paint droplets, 140
Parallelogram mounting, 144, 145
Patent ductus arteriosus, 291–308
  in adult, 297
  anatomy, 291–292
  angiographic appearance, 300–304
  catheterization in, cardiac, 298–300
  clinical features, 292–293
  coarctation of aorta in, 493
  correction, 307
  echocardiographic features, 293
  electrocardiographic features, 293
  etiology, 291
  hemodynamics, 292
  incidence, 291
  management, 304–308
  pathology, 291–292
  pericardial defect and, 1149
  pulmonary vascular disease and right-to-left shunt, 297
  radiographic features, 293–298
   postoperative, 308
  respiratory distress syndrome and prematurity in, 299
  reversing
   aortic stenosis and, 860
   aortography of, 302
   with pulmonary artery aneurysm, 298
  rubella syndrome and, 303, 516
  transposition of great vessels and, complete, 688
  ventricular septal defect and, 300
Pectus excavatum: radiography of, plain-film, 80

Pericardial
  absence
    partial, 1146, 1147, 1148–1149, 1150
    total, 1146
  anatomy, 17
  defect, 1145–1151
    angiographic features, 1149–1151
    clinical features, 1146
    diagnosis, 1148
    echocardiographic features, 1146
    electrocardiographic features, 1146
    foramen-type, 1149
    operative considerations, 1151
    patent ductus arteriosus and, 1149
    pathologic anatomy, 1145
    physiology, 1145–1146
    postoperative features, 1151
    radiographic features, 1146–1149
  fat necrosis, 1151
  fat pad, radiography of, plain-film, 92
  space, contrast medium injected into, 189
  teratoma, 1162, 1163
Periodic wave: various components of, 196
Phasic dye injection, 183
Piezoelectric effect, 196
Pigtail catheter, 170
Pink tetrad, 551
Placenta: development, 9–10
Plastics
  for catheters, 158
    steam kettle to meet specific need, 159
  memory, 163
    test results, 164
  physical characteristics, 158–160
Plexogenic pulmonary arteriopathy, 1171
Pneumothorax: in pericardial defect, 1148
Polyolefins, 158
Polysplenia
  bronchi in, 969
  differentiation from asplenia syndrome, 960–963
  levocardia in, 958
  spleen in, 969
  syndrome, 966–976
    angiographic features, 973–976
    atrioventricular canal and pulmonary stenosis, 971
    diagnosis, 968–970
    mitral atresia in, 973
    radiographic features, 970–973
    vena cava duplication in, 975
    vena cava interruption in, 974
Polyurethane, 163
  for catheters, 159
Potts anastomosis: in tetralogy of Fallot, 567–568, 570, 577–578
Power injectors, 182–185
  complications associated with contrast media, 184–185
  flow-controlled, 182–183
    pressure limitation, 183
    rise time, 183
  pressure-controlled, 182
Prematurity
  patent ductus arteriosus and respiratory distress syndrome in, 299
  radiography in, plain-film, 62
Prenatal development: effect of repeated ionizing radiation exposure, 50
Pressure-controlled injectors, 182
Projectors: cine, 153–155
Prosthesis
  mitral valve in atrioventricular canal repair, complete, 391
  Starr-Edwards prosthetic mitral valve, 390
  valve, obstructing left ventricle outflow area, 437
Pseudocoarctation, 493–495, 1030
  angiographic appearance, 494–495
  radiographic features, 494
Pulmonary
  annulus, patch in tetralogy of Fallot, 576
  anomalies
    in asplenia syndrome, 957
    in polysplenia syndrome, 967–968
  arteriography, 179
    in anteroposterior projection, 29
    balloon, 175
    in lateral projection, 28
  arteriopathy, plexogenic, 1171
  arteriovenous fistula (see Arteriovenous fistula, pulmonary)
  arteriovenous malformation, saccular, 834
  artery
    absence in tetralogy of Fallot, 547–548, 580
    anatomy, 27–31
    aneurysm, with patent ductus arteriosus, 298
    atresia, pulmonary atresia and, 643
    band, arteriography of, pulmonary, 531
    band, in truncus arteriosus, 801
    band, removal, stenosis after, 529
    band, ventriculography of, 530
    banding, 259
    banding, arteriography in, 270–271
    banding, in ventricular septal defect, 269
    banding, ventriculography of, 270
    biventricular origin, 742
    "comma" shadow of, 82
    coronary fistula with, 410
    development, 1035
    dilatation (see below)
    ductus diverticulum, 306
    fistulous communication to left atrium, 841
    Fontan modification for, 619
    fungal infection, 1159
    hypoplasia, 1040
    hypoplasia in tetralogy of Fallot, 573
    interruption, 1037, 1038, 1039, 1040, 1041
    left, bronchus compressing, 247
    left, hypoplastic, in tetralogy of Fallot, 569
    muscular, maturation of, 246
    origin, bilateral ductal, 1040
    origin, from ascending aorta (see below)
    pressure in ventricular septal defect, 250
    projections, 31
    pulsations increased in atrial septal defect, 329
    reopacification, 301
    right, absence, 1036
    right, interruption, 1036
    sling, 1039–1044, 1045
    sling, operative correction, 1045
    stenosis (see Stenosis, pulmonary artery)
    tree, 32
    vasculature, decreased, cyanosis and, 537–669
    vasculature, increased, cyanosis and, 671–803
  artery, dilatation, idiopathic, 529–531
    angiographic appearance, 531
    catheterization in, cardiac, 529
    electrocardiographic features, 529
    radiographic features, 529–531
  artery, origin from ascending aorta, 315–320
    anatomy, 315
    angiographic appearance, 317–319
    associated conditions, 315
    catheterization in, cardiac, 317
    clinical features, 316
    diagram of, 316
    echocardiographic features, 316
    electrocardiographic features, 316
    embryology, 315
    hemodynamics, 316
    management, 319–320
    pathology, 315
    pulmonary atresia in, 319
    radiographic features, 317
  atresia
    asplenia and, 304
    in asplenia syndrome, 641

Pulmonary *(cont.)*
    Blalock-Taussig
        anastomosis and, 640
    infundibular, 640
    pulmonary artery atresia
        and, 643
    in pulmonary artery
        origin from ascending
        aorta, 319
    radiography of,
        plain-film, 69, 70
    in tetralogy of Fallot
        (*see* Tetralogy of
        Fallot, pulmonary
        atresia in)
    transposition of great
        vessels and,
        complete, 686
    ventricle in, right,
        hypoplasia, 636
    ventricular septal defect
        and, 583, 587, 590,
        799
    ventricular septal defect
        and, types of atresia,
        584
    ventricular septum
        intact in (*see below*)
atresia, ventricular septum
    intact in, 625–645
    angiographic features,
        632–640
    aortography in,
        639–640
    atriography of, right,
        633
    catheterization in,
        cardiac, 632
    central circulation in,
        627
    clinical features,
        629–630
    coronary artery
        circulation in, 628
    Ebstein's malformation
        in, 632
    echocardiographic
        features, 630
    electrocardiographic
        features, 630
    fetal circulation in, 625
    hemodynamics, 629
    infundibular atresia in,
        636
    operative
        considerations,
        640–642
    pathologic anatomy,
        625–629
    radiographic features,
        630–632
    radiographic features,
        postoperative,
        642–644
    tricuspid insufficiency
        in, 642
    tricuspid regurgitation
        in, 631, 638
    ventricle in, right,
        enlargement,
        626–629
    ventricle in, right,
        hypoplastic, 626
    ventriculography in,
        right, 633–638
blood flow in ventricular
    septal defect, 250
capillary bed, systemic
    collateral arteries that
    reach, 586
carcinoma causing
    superior vena cava
    syndrome, 1160
circulation demonstration
    in tetralogy of Fallot,
    589–594
disease, aorticopulmonary
    septal defect in, 314
edema, radiography of,
    plain-film, 68
flow, normal, radiography
    of, plain-film, 83
hemodynamic
    considerations in
    congenital heart
    disease, 59–60
hypertension, 1171–1178
    angiographic features,
        1176–1177
    catheterization in,
        cardiac, 1176
    clinical features, 1173
    echocardiographic
        features, 1173
    electrocardiographic
        features, 1173
    hemodynamics,
        1172–1173
    management, 1177
    pathologic anatomy,
        1171
    radiographic features,
        1173–1176
    radiography of,
        plain-film, 85, 86
    ventricular hypertrophy
        and, 313
stenosis (*see* Stenosis,
    pulmonary)
thromboembolism,
    recurrent,
    1171–1172
trunk
    absence, 1040
    biventricular origin,
        transposition of aorta
        and, 745–747
    coronary artery
        anomalous origin
        from (*see* Coronary
        artery anomalous
        origin from
        pulmonary trunk)
valve
    absence (*see below*)
    anatomy, 27–31
    atresia, 643
    bicuspid, 531–532
    bicuspid, in tetralogy of
        Fallot, 531
    dysplastic (*see below*)
    normal, 500
    projections, 31
    quadricuspid, 533
valve, absence, 532,
    533–534
    angiographic features,
        533–534
    clinical features, 533
    complete, 604
    partial, without
        tetralogy of Fallot,
        604
    radiographic features,
        533
    systolic view, 532
    in tetralogy of Fallot
        (*see* Tetralogy of
        Fallot, pulmonary
        valve absence in)
valve, dysplastic,
    509–513
    angiographic
        appearance, 512
    catheterization in,
        cardiac, 511
    clinical features, 509
    echocardiographic
        features, 510
    electrocardiographic
        features, 510
    hemodynamics, 509
    operative
        considerations, 513
    pathology, 509
    physical examination,
        510
    radiographic features,
        510–511
vein
    anatomy, 31–34
    angiocardiography, 32
    anomalous connection
        (*see below*)
    anomalous course to
        left atrium, 350
    atresia (*see below*)
    connection to right
        upper lobe vein, 336
    development, 7
    development, normal,
        892
    hypertension,
        radiography of,
        plain-film, 63, 65,
        66, 67
    incorporation into left
        atrium, 10
    increase, radiography
        of, plain-film, 62–68
    obstruction,
        radiography,
        plain-film, 64
    stenosis (*see* Stenosis,
        pulmonary vein)
    tree, 32
    vasculature, increased,
        cyanosis and,
        845–872
    vasculature, increased,
        heart conditions
        associated with,
        without cyanosis,
        873–942
vein, anomalous
    connection, MRI of,
    236
vein, anomalous
    connection, partial,
    333, 345–355, 895
    after atrial septal defect
        closure, 354
    anatomic forms of,
        various, 346
    anatomic pathology,
        345–346
    angiographic
        appearance, 352–354
    catheterization in,
        cardiac, 352
    clinical features,
        348–349
    echocardiographic
        features, 349
    electrocardiographic
        features, 349
    hemodynamics,
        346–347
    incidence, 345
    operations for, 353
    operative
        considerations,
        354–355
    postoperative features,
        355
    radiographic features,
        349–352
    to vena cava, 352
vein, anomalous
    connection, total,
    805–825
    anatomic types with
        sites of connection,
        807–808
    angiographic features,
        816–821

to atrium, 821
to atrium, right,
  surgical correction,
  823
to azygos vein, 813
to azygos vein, surgical
  correction, 823
catheterization in,
  cardiac, 815–816
clinical features,
  810–811
to coronary sinus,
  surgical correction,
  822
echocardiographic
  features, 811
electrocardiographic
  features, 811
embryology, 805
to foramen ovale,
  stenotic, 820
hemodynamics,
  809–810
infradiaphragmatic type,
  824
mixed type, 818
operative
  considerations,
  821–823
pathologic anatomy,
  805–809
pulmonary artery
  pressure elevation
  with vein connection
  obstructed, 814–815
pulmonary artery
  pressure normal and
  vein connection
  nonobstructed,
  811–814
pulmonary vein
  obstruction in, 811
radiographic features,
  postoperative,
  823–825
to vena cava, superior,
  810, 813
to vena cava, superior,
  surgical correction,
  822
without pulmonary vein
  obstruction, 810–811
vein, atresia, 847–851
angiographic features,
  849–851
aortography in, 850
catheterization in,
  cardiac, 849
clinical features,
  847–848
collateral flow to
  mediastinal veins in,
  848

echocardiographic
  features, 848
electrocardiographic
  features, 848
hemodynamics, 847
operative
  considerations, 851
pathologic anatomy,
  847
radiographic features,
  848–849
unilateral, 851
veno-occlusive disease,
  1172
venography with catheter
  wedged, 187
vessels
  abnormalities, MRI of,
    235–236
  admixture, radiography
    of, plain-film, 68
  decrease, radiography
    of, plain-film, 69
  disease, atrial septal
    defect in, 328
  disease, patent ductus
    arteriosus in, 297
  disease in ventricular
    septal defect, 255,
    257
  patterns, 55–56
  radiography of,
    plain-film, 61,
    79–84
  resistance in ventricular
    septal defect, 250
  resistance increase in
    truncus arteriosus,
    794
(See also Lung)

Q

Quality
  assurance for automatic
    film processors, 153
  control
    cine film, 153
    for image intensifiers,
      139–140

R

Radiation
  doses
    in diagnostic
      procedures, typical,
      50
    per cine frame, 140
  exposure of women of
    reproductive
    potential, 52

ionizing
  exposure, repeated,
    effects of, 50
  nature of, 49–50
  monitoring requirements,
    50–51
protection
  basic principles, 49–51
  in catheterization
    laboratories (see
    Catheterization
    laboratories, radiation
    protection in)
safety, 49–53
secondary
  emission during cine
    fluorography, 50
  shielding against, 52
Radiography
  aneurysm, ventricular
    septum,
    membranous, 281
  angulation of x-ray beam,
    effect on clavicle and
    ribs, 74
  in aortic arch
    cervical, 1030
    double, both arches
      patent, 1011–1012
    double, with left arch
      atresia, 1015
    interruption distal to
      innominate artery,
      1025–1026
    left, right descending
      aorta and, 1002–1003
    left, with
      retroesophageal
      arterial vessel,
      1001–1002
    left, without
      retroesophageal
      arterial vessel, 998
    with retroesophageal
      segment or vessel,
      1007–1009
    right, without
      retroesophageal
      segment or vessel,
      1004
    sixth, interruption,
      1036–1037
  in aortic stenosis
    supravalvar, 440
    valvar, 419–421
    valvar, postoperative,
      427
  in aortico left ventricular
    tunnel, 462–465
  aorticopulmonary septal
    defect, 310–311
  in asplenia syndrome,
    960–963

in atrial appendage
  aneurysm,
  1141–1144
of atrial ring, supravalvar
  stenosing,
  889–890
atrial septal defect,
  324–327
in atrium, single, 828
beam angulation along
  long axis of body,
  148
in brachiocephalic vessel
  ectopic origin,
  1047–1048
in cardiomyopathy,
  914–917
chest
  in ventricular septal
    defect, 253–257
  in ventricular septal
    defect, postoperative,
    269–271
in coarctation of aorta (see
  Coarctation of aorta,
  radiography)
in cor triatriatum,
  897–899
  postoperative, 903
in coronary artery
  anomalous origin
    from pulmonary
    trunk, 932–935
  postoperative, 941
in coronary artery
  calcification,
  idiopathic, in infant,
  1084–1085
in coronary artery fistula,
  408–409
in coronary sinus–left
  atrial window,
  342–343
in dextroposition of heart,
  951
in dextroversion of heart,
  952
in Ebstein's malformation,
  657–658
  postoperative, 663
in ectopia cordis, 987
in endocardial cushion
  defect (see
  Endocardial cushion
  defect, radiography)
of endocardial
  fibroelastosis,
  921–922
in fetal circulation
  syndrome, persistent,
  1179
in heart block, complete,
  1166–1167

Radiography (cont.)
  in heart malposition, 955–957
  in heart tumors
    intracavitary, 1155
    intrapericardial, 1162–1163
  in Kawasaki disease, 1089–1090
  in Marfan syndrome, 1104–1105
  in mitral atresia, 869
  in mitral insufficiency, 1129
  in mitral stenosis, 880–882
  in mitral valve cleft, 392
  in mitral valve prolapse, 1121–1122
  patent ductus arteriosus, 293–298
    postoperative, 308
  in pericardial defect, 1146–1149
  plain-film
    atrial enlargement, left, 109–112
    of atrial enlargement, right, 102–103
    of bronchial vessels, 69–71
    in cardiomegaly, 88, 99
    in coarctation of aorta correction, 89
    in coarctation of aorta repair, 90
    of congenital heart disease, 61–113
    of congenital heart disease, physiologic considerations, 61–79
    of congenital heart disease, technical considerations, 61–79
    of cyanosis, 69
    of heart (see Heart, radiography of, plain-film)
    mediastinal enlargement, 102
    of mitral disease, 112
    of mitral insufficiency, 111
    of mitral stenosis, 67
    of pectus excavatum, 80
    of pericardial fat pad, 92
    in prematurity, 62
    of pulmonary atresia, 69, 70
    of pulmonary edema, 68
    of pulmonary flow, normal, 83
    in pulmonary hypertension, 67, 85, 86
    of pulmonary vein, increase, 62–68
    of pulmonary vein hypertension, 63, 65, 66
    of pulmonary vein obstruction, 64
    of pulmonary vessels, 61–62, 79–84
    of pulmonary vessels, admixture, 68
    of pulmonary vessels, decrease, 69
    of shunt, left-to-right, 84
    in sternotomy, 89
    of subpleural edema, 65
    of tetralogy of Fallot, sternum in, 87
    in thoracotomy, left-sided, 89–90
    in thoracotomy, right-sided, 90–91
    of thymus, 98–100
    of thymus asymmetry, 100
    of thymus enlargement, 100, 101
    in trisomy 21, sternum in, 88
    of ventricular enlargement, left, 107–109
    of ventricular enlargement, right, 103–106
  in polysplenia syndrome, 970–973
  in pseudocoarctation, 494
  in pulmonary arteriovenous fistula, 834–837
  in pulmonary artery dilatation, idiopathic, 529–531
    origin from ascending aorta, 317
    sling, 1041
    stenosis, 514
  in pulmonary atresia, ventricular septum intact, 630–632
    postoperative, 642–644
  in pulmonary hypertension, 1173–1176
  in pulmonary stenosis
    dome shaped, 501–504
    infundibular, 519
  in pulmonary valve
    absence, 533
    dysplastic, 510–511
  in pulmonary vein
    anomalous connection
      partial, 349–352
      total, 811–815
      total, postoperative, 823–825
  in pulmonary vein atresia, 848–849
  in pulmonary vein stenosis, 905–908
  in Raghib syndrome, 341
  in rhabdomyoma, 1160–1161
  in scimitar syndrome, 359–361
  in sinus of Valsalva aneurysm, 399–400
    postoperative, 405
  in situs inversus, 953
  in situs solitus
    levoposition, 955
  in subaortic stenosis
    discrete membranous, 428–430
    muscular, 450
  in subclavian artery isolation, 1017
  in systemic arteriovenous fistula, 1094
  in tetralogy of Fallot, 550–556
    pulmonary atresia in, 586–588
    pulmonary valve absence in, 600–601
  in transposition of great vessels, complete, 680–682
    postoperative, 697–698
  in transposition of great vessels, corrected, 713–714
  in tricuspid atresia and transposition of great vessels, 770–771
    postoperative, 775
  in tricuspid atresia with normally related great vessels, 610–612
    postoperative, 619
  in tricuspid insufficiency, 666–667
  in truncus arteriosus, 793–796
    postoperative, 802
  tube for, 131–142
  in ventricle
    aneurysm, left, 1137
    diverticulum, left, 1133–1134
    diverticulum, right, 1131
    double inlet, 779
    double inlet, right, 783
    double outlet, 735–736
    double outlet, postoperative features, 744
    inversion, 727–729
    left, communication with right atrium, 287–288
    left, double outlet, 749
    left, hypoplastic syndrome, 856–857
    right, hypoplasia, isolated, 648
    right, with muscle bundle anomalies, 520–521
    septal defect, aortic insufficiency in, 275
    single, 757–758
Radiology (see Radiography)
Radionuclide scanning, 215–227
Raghib syndrome, 339–344, 1054
  angiographic appearance, 341–342
  catheterization in, cardiac, 341
  clinical features, 339–341
  electrocardiographic features, 341
  embryologic development, 339
  hemodynamics, 339
  operative considerations, 342
  pathologic anatomy, 339
  radiographic features, 341
  variants, 342–344
Range gating, 201
Rastelli procedure
  modified arterial switch, in transposition of great vessels, complete, 700
  in transposition of great vessels complete, 706
  ventricular septal defect and pulmonary stenosis, 701
Recoarctation of aorta, 492
Reflectors: angle-dependent and specular, 197

Respiratory distress
    syndrome, 305
  with patent ductus
    arteriosus in
    prematurity, 299
Rhabdomyoma,
    1160–1161
  angiography in, 1161
  catheterization in, cardiac,
    1161
  echocardiographic
    features, 1160
  interventricular septum,
    527
  radiographic features,
    1160–1161
  treatment, 1161
  ventricle
    left, 438
    right, 1160
Rhabdomyosarcoma,
    ventricle, 1161
  left, 1158
Rib
  and angulation of x-ray
    beam, 74
  notching in coarctation of
    aorta, 479, 480–481
Rubella syndrome: and
    patent ductus
    arteriosus, 303, 516
Rupture
  chordal, regurgitation
    causing, in mitral
    valve prolapse, 1122
  sinus of Valsalva
    aneurysm (see
    Aneurysm, sinus of
    Valsalva, rupture)

S

Saphenous bypass: and
    coronary ostium
    atresia, 448
Scanning (see Imaging)
Scimitar syndrome,
    357–364, 950
  angiographic features,
    362–363
  associated anomalies,
    357–358
  bronchographic features,
    362
  catheterization in, cardiac,
    362
  clinical features, 358–359
  echocardiographic
    features, 359
  electrocardiographic
    features, 359
  hemodynamics, 358
  lung in, 359

operative considerations,
    364
  pathologic anatomy, 357
  radiographic features,
    359–361
Sensitometric control record:
    for automatic cine
    processor, 154
Septal defect
  aorticopulmonary,
    309–314
  angiographic
    appearance,
    313–314
  anomalies associated
    with, 309
  cardiomegaly and, 311
  catheterization in,
    cardiac, 311–313
  clinical features, 310
  echocardiographic
    features, 310
  electrocardiographic
    features, 310
  embryology, 309
  hemodynamics,
    309–310
  locations, common, 310
  operative
    considerations, 314
  pathologic anatomy,
    309
  pulmonary disease and
    aortic arch
    interruption in, 314
  radiographic features,
    310–311
  atrial, 321–338
  angiographic
    appearance, 330–335
  associated conditions,
    321
  blood flow in, 322
  catheter course through,
    330
  catheterization, cardiac,
    327–330
  clinical features, 323
  closure, pulmonary vein
    anomalous
    connection after,
    partial, 354
  cor triatriatum and, 895
  during diastole, 332
  echocardiographic
    features, 324
  electrocardiographic
    features, 323–324
  embolism in, 335
  gated blood study, 220
  hemodynamics,
    322–323
  incidence, 321

location of various
    types, 322
  operative
    considerations,
    335–337
  ostium secundum
    defect, 334
  pathology, 321
  pathophysiology,
    322–323
  physical examination,
    323
  postoperative status,
    337
  pulmonary artery
    increased pulsations
    in, 329
  pulmonary vascular
    disease in, 328
  radiographic features,
    324–327
  shunt and, left-to-right,
    329
  during systole, 332
  tetralogy of Fallot and,
    546
  vena caval type,
    cyanosis after repair,
    337
  vena caval type,
    inferior, suture
    closure of, 335
  ventricular compliance
    in, 322
  ventricular enlargement,
    right, 326
ventricular, 243–272
  abnormalities associated
    with, 245–246,
    247–248
  anatomic changes in,
    secondary, 247
  anatomy, 243–248
  angiography in,
    259–265
  aortic arch interruption
    and subaortic
    stenosis, 1028
  aortic atresia and, 861
  aortic cusp prolapse
    through, 527
  aortic filling through,
    319
  aortic insufficiency in
    (see below)
  aortic stenosis in, 277
  beneath right aortic
    cusp, 265
  catheterization in,
    cardiac, 257–265
  circulation in, 251
  classification,
    244–245

clinical features,
    252–253
  closure, 267, 268
  double outlet right
    ventricle and,
    737–738, 740, 741
  double outlet right
    ventricle and,
    operative correction,
    745, 746
  ECG features, 252–253
  echocardiography of,
    253
  hemodynamics, 248–250
  management, 265–271
  MRI of, 238
  muscle bundle
    anomalies in, 523
  natural history,
    250–251
  operation, 268–269
  patent ductus arteriosus
    and, 300
  physical examination
    in, 252
  postoperative, 269
  pulmonary artery
    banding in, 269
  pulmonary atresia and,
    583, 587, 590–597,
    799
  pulmonary blood flow
    in, 258
  pulmonary stenosis and
    left-to-right shunt,
    551
  in pulmonary vascular
    disease, 255, 257
  radiography of, chest,
    253–257
  radiography of, chest,
    postoperative,
    269–271
  Rastelli procedure for,
    701
  in shunt, left-to-right,
    253
  in shunt, right-to-left,
    256
  subaortic stenosis and,
    249, 266
  supracristal, 264
  in tetralogy of Fallot,
    541
  in tetralogy of Fallot,
    location of defect and
    closure method with
    patch, 572
  transposition of great
    vessels and, 717
  transposition of great
    vessels and,
    complete, 688, 690

Septal defect *(cont.)*
   transposition of great vessels and, corrected, 714, 716, 723
   tricuspid atresia and, 613, 616–617
   true membranous ventriculography of, 262
   ventricular, aortic insufficiency in, 273–277
     angiographic appearance, 275
     angiographic findings, 275–276
     angiographic indications, 275–276
     aortic cusp herniated and prolapsing into, 276
     catheterization in, cardiac, 275–276
     clinical features, 274
     echocardiographic features, 274–275
     electrocardiographic features, 274
     operation, 276–277
     pathology, 273–274
     physical examination, 274
     radiographic features, 275
Septostomy: balloon, in transposition of great vessels, complete, 683
Septum
   of heart, development, 7
   primum, development, 5
   secundum, development, 5
Shone's syndrome, 879
Shunt
   Blalock-Taussig, 569
   central, in tetralogy of Fallot, 568–570
   hemangiomatosis with, 1096
   intracardiac, coronary sinus anomalies allowing, 339–344
   left-to-right
     atrial septal defect and, 329
     heart conditions associated with, 241–414
     radiography of, plain-film, 84
     in ventricular septal defect, 253
     ventricular septal defect and pulmonary stenosis, 551
   left ventricular-right atrial, 287
   right-to-left
     atrial, after pulmonary artery stenosis repair, 332
     patent ductus arteriosus in, 297
     pulmonary stenosis and, valvar, 637–638
     in tetralogy of Fallot (*see* Tetralogy of Fallot, shunt in, right-to-left)
     in ventricular septal defect, 256
   Waterston-Cooley, 571
   in tetralogy of Fallot, 568, 578
     occluded, 580
Siamese twins (*see* Thoracopagus)
Sidewinder configuration of catheters, 170
   for catheterization, retrograde, 172
Sinus
   aortic, 397
   coronary (*see* Coronary sinus)
   of Valsalva
     aneurysm (*see* Aneurysm, sinus of Valsalva)
     in Marfan syndrome, 1107
   venosus
     defect, 336
     development, 4, 5
     incorporation into right atrium, 6
"Sinusoids," 644
   myocardial, 1082–1083
Situs
   ambiguous, 946, 953–954, 955, 956
   inversus, 945, 953, 954
     levoversion in, 955, 956
     radiographic features, 953
   solitus, 149, 945, 950–953
     dextroversion, transposition of great vessels and, corrected, 717
     levocardia, 955
     levoposition in, 955
   visceroatrial, 945–946
Specular reflector, 197
Spine
   artery in coarctation of aorta, 473
   cord complications in coarctation of aorta, 492
Spinnaker origination, 524
Spleen: in polysplenia, 969
Spray gun: with insufficient number of paint droplets, 140
Starr-Edwards prosthetic mitral valve, 390
Stenosis
   aortic, 417–459
     bicuspid, diastole in, 426
     decompensated, 420–421
     general considerations, 417
     patent ductus arteriosus and, reversing, 860
     supravalvar (*see below*)
     valvar (*see below*)
     with ventricular decompensation and enlargement, left, 420
     ventricular septal defect in, 277
   aortic, supravalvar, 437–446
     anatomic considerations, 438
     angiographic appearance, 440–446
     aorta, abdominal, 445
     arteriography of, coronary, 448
     catheterization in, cardiac, 440
     clinical features, 438
     echocardiographic features, 439–440
     electrocardiographic features, 439
     facies in, 440
     hemodynamic considerations, 438
     hourglass type, 441, 443, 444
     hypoplastic type, 447
     hypoplastic type, diffuse, 441, 442, 444
     operative considerations, 446
     operative correction, 447
     physical examination, 439
     pressure tracing in, 441
     radiographic features, 440
   aortic, valvar, 417–427
     angiographic anatomy, 421–423
     angiographic appearance, 423–426, 427
     aortography in, 428
     catheterization in, cardiac, 421
     clinical features, 418
     complications, 427
     echocardiographic features, 418
     electrocardiographic features, 418
     in Marfan syndrome, 1112
     operative considerations, 426–427
     pathology, 421–423
     physical examination, 418
     pressure tracing in, 423
     radiographic appearance, postoperative, 427
     radiographic features, 419–421
   of atrial ring, 889–890
   bulboventricular foramen, and single ventricle, 764
   coronary sinus, 1053
   dilatation in coarctation of aorta after, 484
   foramen ovale and pulmonary vein anomalous connection, total, 820
   mitral, 875–888
     angiographic features, 882–886
     catheterization in, cardiac, 882
     clinical features, 878–879
     echocardiographic features, 879–880
     electrocardiographic features, 879
     fused dome-shaped valve causing, 883
     hemodynamics, 877–878

from mitral arcade, 881
operative
considerations,
886–887
pathologic anatomy,
875–876
radiographic features,
880–882
radiography of,
plain-film, 67
ventricular
decompensation in,
right, 881
pulmonary, 499–536
pulmonary,
atrioventricular canal
and, complete, 564
pulmonary, dome shaped,
499–509
angiographic
appearance, 504–508
clinical features,
499–500
echocardiographic
features, 501
electrocardiographic
features, 500–501
operative
considerations,
508–509
postoperative
appearance, 509
radiographic features,
501–504
pulmonary, double outlet
right ventricle and,
737, 740, 744–745
pulmonary, infundibular,
518–519
angiographic
appearance, 519
catheterization in,
cardiac, 519
clinical features, 518
echocardiographic
features, 519
electrocardiographic
features, 519
hemodynamics, 518
mitral atresia and, 870
operative
considerations, 519
pathology, 518
physical examination,
518–519
radiographic features,
519
various types, 544
pulmonary, polysplenia
syndrome and
atrioventricular canal,
971

pulmonary, Rastelli
procedure for, 701
pulmonary, single
ventricle and, 758
pulmonary,
subinfundibular,
519–523
pulmonary, supravalvar,
localized, 515
pulmonary, tetralogy of
Fallot and, 541–543
pulmonary, transposition
of great vessels and,
complete, 683
pulmonary, transposition
of great vessels and,
corrected, 714
pulmonary, tricuspid
atresia in, 612
pulmonary, valvar,
499–513
MRI of, 238
shunt and, right-to-left,
637–638
ventricle and, right,
hypoplasia, 650
pulmonary, ventricular
septal defect and
left-to-right shunt,
551
pulmonary artery, 225,
513–518
angiographic
appearance, 514–515
catheterization in,
cardiac, 514
clinical features, 514
diffuse type, 514
echocardiographic
features, 514
electrocardiographic
features, 514
hemodynamics, 514
operative
considerations,
515–518
pathology, 513–514
peripheral, 516
peripheral, balloon
dilatation technique
for, 517
physical examination,
514
radiographic features,
514
repair, shunt after,
right-to-left, 332
in tetralogy of Fallot,
573
pulmonary vein, 905–910
angiographic features,
908–910

catheterization in,
cardiac, 908
clinical features, 905
echocardiographic
features, 905
electrocardiographic
features, 905
hemodynamics, 905
hypoplastic type, 906
operations, 909
operative
considerations, 910
pathologic anatomy,
905
perfusion scan, 908
radiographic features,
905–908
unilateral, 907
residual, after pulmonary
arterial band
removal, 529
subaortic, 880
discrete membranous
(*see below*)
membranous,
ventriculography of,
409
muscular (*see below*)
rare causes of,
436–437
ventricular septal defect
and, 249, 266
subaortic, discrete
membranous,
427–436
anatomic
considerations,
427–428
angiographic
appearance, 430–434
catheterization in,
cardiac, 430
clinical features, 428
echocardiographic
features, 428
electrocardiographic
features, 428
hemodynamic
considerations,
427–428
operative considerations
and procedure,
434–437
physical examination,
428
pressure tracing in, 430
radiographic features,
428–430
subaortic, muscular,
446–457
angiographic
appearance, 451–455

aortic arch interruption
and ventricular septal
defect, 1028
catheterization in,
cardiac, 450–451
clinical features, 449
double outlet right
ventricle and, 738
echocardiographic
features, 450
electrocardiographic
features, 449–450
hemodynamic
considerations,
448–449
operation, 455–457
pathologic features, 448
physical examination,
449
radiographic features,
450
treatment, 455–457
ventricular septum
thickening in, 456
subpulmonary,
hypertrophied
interventricular
septum in, 526,
527–528
valve, diagrams of, 423
Sternotomy: radiography
after, plain-film, 89
Sternum
in tetralogy of Fallot, 87
in trisomy 21, 88
Subaortic aneurysm, 1136
Subaortic diaphragm, 431
Subaortic membrane, 430,
432, 433
aortography of, 433
resection, left
ventriculography of,
437
Subclavian
artery
aberrant in tetralogy of
Fallot, 545
aortic arch and (*see
under* Aortic arch)
in coarctation of aorta
(*see* Coarctation of
aorta, subclavian
arteries)
interruption in tetralogy
of Fallot, 1022
isolation, 1016–1017,
1019, 1020–1021
flap technique in
coarctation of aorta
repair, 491, 494
vein, right, diaphragm in,
1055

Subendocardial deposition:
of contrast medium, 187
Subepicardial deposition: of contrast medium, 188
Submitral aneurysm, 1136, 1137, 1138
Subpleural edema, 65
Systemic arteriovenous fistula (*see* Arteriovenous fistula, systemic)

T

Taussig-Bing heart: and double outlet right ventricle, 739, 742
Telangiectasia: hemorrhagic hereditary, 836
Teratoma: intrapericardial, 1162, 1163
Tetralogy of Fallot, 541–582, 651
  angiographic appearance, 557–563
  angiographic features, 556–557
  angiographic positioning, 557
  aortic arch and, right, 574
  aortic arch identification in, 554–556
  aortic arch in, right, 543–546, 579
  aortography in, 563–565
  arteriography in, pulmonary, 561
  atrial septal defect and, 546
  atrioventricular canal and, 554
  balanced and slightly cyanotic, 551
  Blalock-Taussig anastomosis in, 567
  bony thorax in, 554
  bronchial artery enlargement in, 547
  cardiomegaly in, 554
  catheterization in, cardiac, 556
  clinical features, 549–550
  conditions simulating, 605
  coronary artery anomalies in, 546–547
  echocardiographic features, 550
  electrocardiographic features, 550
  during extrasystole series, 558
  four components of, diagram, 542
  graft in, 570
  hemodynamics, 548–549
  management, 565–572
  MRI of, 237
  operations
    corrective, 570–572
    corrective, postoperative radiographic features, 572–574
    palliative, 565–570
    palliative, postoperative radiographic features, 574–582
  overriding aorta, 541, 543
  pathologic anatomy, 541–548
  physical examination, 550
  postoperative views, 565
  Potts anastomosis in, 567–568, 570, 577–578
  pulmonary annulus patch in, 576
  pulmonary artery absence in, 547–548, 580
  pulmonary artery hypoplasia, 573
    left, 569
  pulmonary artery stenosis in, 573
  pulmonary atresia in, 583–598
    angiographic features, 589–594
    catheterization in, cardiac, 588
    clinical features, 585–586
    echocardiographic features, 586
    electrocardiographic features, 586
    hemodynamics, 584–585
    MRI of, 234, 236
    operative considerations, 594–597
    pathologic anatomy, 583–584
    postoperative findings, 597–598
    radiographic features, 586–588
    systemic collateral arteries in, 585
    pulmonary circulation demonstration in, 589–594
  pulmonary size estimation for operative correction, 562
  pulmonary stenosis and, 541–543
  pulmonary valve, bicuspid, 531
  pulmonary valve absence in, 599–606
    angiographic features, 602–604
    catheterization in, cardiac, 601–602
    clinical features, 599–600
    echocardiographic features, 600
    electrocardiographic features, 600
    hemodynamics, 599
    management, 604–605
    partial, 602, 604
    pathologic anatomy, 599
    radiographic features, 600–601
  radiographic features, 550–556
    postoperative, 572–582
  severe, 553
  shunt in
    central, 568–570
    right-to-left, 551
    right-to-left, anteroposterior projection, 551–553
    right-to-left, lateral projection, 553–554
    right-to-left, left anterior oblique projection, 553
    Waterston-Cooley, 568
  sternum in, 87
  subclavian artery aberrancy in, left, 545
  subclavian artery interruption in, 1022
  tricuspid insufficiency and, 548
  variations of, 549
  vena cava and, superior, left, 546
  ventricular diverticulum and, right, 1132
  ventricular septal defect and, 541
    location of defect and closure method with patch, 572
  ventriculography in, right, 557–563
  Waterston-Cooley anastomosis in, 579
  Waterston-Cooley shunt in, 578
    occluded, 580
Thallium 201 imaging, 222–223
Thoracic artery: lateral, in coarctation of aorta, 473
Thoracopagus, 991–992
  angiographic features, 991–992
  ventriculography in, 992
Thoracotomy
  left-sided, radiography of, plain-film, 89–90
  right-sided, radiography of, plain-film, 90–91
Thorax (*see* Chest)
Thromboembolism
  prevention and catheters, 167–168
  pulmonary, recurrent, 1171–1172
Thrombogenicity of catheters (*see* Catheters, thrombogenicity)
Thrombosis: in atrial appendage aneurysm, 1143
Thrombus
  encasement, guidewire retrieval, 170
  formation, factors determining, 167
  retrieval system to collect, 169
  retrieving, in thrombogenicity testing, 168
Thymus
  asymmetric, radiography of, plain-film, 100
  enlargement, radiography of, plain-film, 100, 101
  radiography of, plain-film, 98–100
Torque transmission studies: results, 165
Trachea: vascular compression, 1047
Transplantation: lung, 225
Transposition: clinical (*see* Ventricle, inversion)
Transposition of aorta
  with pulmonary artery biventricular origin, 742
  pulmonary trunk biventricular origin and, 745–747

Index 1203

Transposition of great arteries: arteriography in, coronary, 410
Transposition of great vessels, 947
 anatomic relationships, diagram showing, 676
 complete, 675–708
  angiographic appearance, postoperative, 698–707
  angiographic features, 684–693
  aortic arch interruption and, repair, 703
  aortography in, 695–696
  arterial switch operation, 699
  arterial switch operation, modified, 706
  arterial switch operation, modified Rastelli, 700
  Blalock-Hanlon procedure, 697
  catheterization in, cardiac, 682–684
  clinical features, 679–680
  coni and, double, 741
  coronary artery pattern in, 679, 691–693
  criss-cross heart and, 980–983
  Damus-Kaye-Stansel repair for, 702
  echocardiographic features, 680
  electrocardiographic features, 680
  hemodynamics, 677–679
  management, 693–697
  Mustard procedure in, 698, 704–707
  natural history, 677–679
  patent ductus arteriosus and, 688
  pathologic anatomy, 675–677
  pulmonary atresia and, 686
  pulmonary blood flow increase in, 680–681
  pulmonary stenosis in, 683
  radiographic features, 680–682
  radiographic features, postoperative, 697–698
  Rastelli procedure for, 701, 706
  during septostomy, balloon, 683
  ventricle, right, hypoplasia, 685
  ventricular outflow obstruction in, left, anatomic causes, 678
  ventricular outflow obstruction in, left, demonstration of, 689–691
  ventricular septal defect and, 688–689, 690
  ventriculography in, left, 686–693
  ventriculography in, right, 684–686
  without pulmonary stenosis, 680
 corrected, 709–726
  angiographic features, 715–724
  atrioventricular valve insufficiency and, 718, 722
  catheter course in, 718
  catheterization in, cardiac, 714–715
  clinical features, 712–713
  coexistent cardiac malformations, 711–712
  coronary artery pattern in, 725
  coronary artery system in, 710
  criss-cross heart and, 983–984
  development of, 712, 713
  dextroversion and, 721
  double conus and, 721
  double outlet ventricle and, 737
  heart contours in, 715
  hemodynamics, 712
  intracardiac relationships in, 715
  inverted malformations and, 711–712
  operative considerations, 724–725
  pathologic anatomy, 709–711
  radiographic features, 713–714
  single ventricle and, 758
  situs solitus dextroversion and, 717
  variants of, 712
  ventricular hypoplasia and, 722, 723
  ventricular inversion and, 728
  ventricular septal defect and, 716, 717, 723
  ventricular septal defect and pulmonary stenosis in, 714
  ventriculography in, 719–721
 D loop, 980–983
 D transposition of great vessels with single ventricle, 758
 forms of, comparison of, 982
 L loop, 983–984
 L transposition (see corrected above)
 mitral atresia and, 869
 pulmonary blood flow obstruction in, 682
 single ventricle and, 756
 tricuspid atresia and (see Tricuspid atresia and transposition of great vessels)
 ventricular hypoplasia in, 711
 ventriculography in, right, 21
Tricuspid
 atresia
  aortic arch and, right, 612
  atrial appendage juxtaposition and, 614
  bulbar inversion and, isolated, 768
  circulation in, central, 608
  fossa ovalis herniation and, 615
  with normally related great vessels (see below)
  pulmonary blood flow obstruction and, 616
  pulmonary stenosis, 612
  transposition of great vessels in (see below)
  ventricular septal defect and, 613, 616
 atresia, and transposition of great vessels, 767–775
  angiographic features, 772–774
  catheterization in, cardiac, 772
  clinical features, 770
  complete transposition, 767
  corrected transposition, 767–770
  D transposition, 771
  echocardiographic features, 770
  electrocardiographic features, 770
  hemodynamics, 770
  management, 774–775
  pathologic anatomy, 767–770
  radiographic features, 770–771
  radiographic features, postoperative, 775
 atresia with normally related great vessels, 607–623
  angiographic appearance, postoperative, 620–623
  angiographic features, 614–615
  catheterization in, cardiac, 612–614
  clinical features, 609–610
  conduits in, 620
  echocardiography, 610
  electrocardiographic features, 610
  Fontan procedure, 618
  Fontan procedure, modified, 620
  Glenn anastomosis, 621
  Glenn procedure in, 617
  hemodynamics, 609
  management, 615–619
  pathologic anatomy, 607–609
  radiographic features, 610–612
  radiographic features, postoperative, 619
 insufficiency, 665–669
  angiographic features, 667–668
  angiography of, right atrial, 23
  catheterization in, cardiac, 667
  clinical features, 666
  echocardiographic features, 666

Tricuspid (cont.)
  electrocardiographic features, 666
  hemodynamics, 665–666
  management, 668
  pathologic anatomy, 665
  pulmonary atresia and, ventricular septum intact, 642
  radiographic features, 666–667
  tetralogy of Fallot and, 548
  transient, in newborn, 665, 666, 667, 668
  regurgitation
    in Ebstein's malformation, 659
    pulmonary atresia and, ventricular septum intact, 631, 638
  valve
    anatomy of membranous septum in relation to, 40
    cleft of, 393
    pouches, 525
Truncus arteriosus, 787–803
  angiographic features, 796–800
  aortic arch in, right, 1001
  aortic arch interruption in, 790, 798
  aortography in, 797–799
  catheterization in, cardiac, 796
  clinical features, 792–793
  development process as dividing, 788
  echocardiographic features, 793
  electrocardiographic features, 793
  hemodynamics, 791–792
  operative considerations, 800–801
  pathologic anatomy, 787–791
  persistent
    aortic arch interruption and, 1029
    bronchial arteries from descending aorta supply pulmonary arterial tree, 789
    circulation in, central, 792
    coronary arteries arise from separate orifice from truncus posterior wall, 789
    operative correction, 800
    pulmonary arteries arise adjacent to one another from truncus, 789
    pulmonary arteries arise from truncus through short common vessel, 789
    pulmonary artery proximal interruption, left, 790
    pulmonary artery proximal interruption, right, 790
    truncal valve variations in, 791
  pulmonary artery banding in, 801
  pulmonary resistance low in, 794
  pulmonary vascular increased resistance in, 794
  radiographic features, 793–796
  postoperative, 802
  variants, development processes, 788
  ventriculography in
    left, 797
    right, 797
Tube
  current, variable, 136
  image-intensifying, basic principle, 133
  radiographic, 131–142
  x-ray (see X-ray tube)
Tumors, heart (see Heart tumors)
Twins, conjoined (see Thoracopagus)

U

Ultrasound, 195–213
  methods, current, 203
  physical principles, 195–203
  techniques, 203–204

V

Valve
  anatomic relations of valves, 34
  aortic (see Aortic)
  atrioventricular (see Atrioventricular valve)
  mitral (see Mitral)
  prosthetic, obstructing ventricular outflow area, 437
  pulmonary (see Pulmonary valve)
  stenosis, diagrams of, 423
  tricuspid (see Tricuspid)
Valvotomy: aortic, 426
Vein
  antecubital, contrast medium injected into, 342
  azygos (see Azygos vein)
  cardinal
    anterior, 3
    posterior, system, 3–4
    system, 3
  femoral, contrast medium injected into, 191
  of Galen aneurysm, 1094
  posterocardinal, 3
  precardinal, 3
  pulmonary (see Pulmonary vein)
  systemic, system, 3–4
Vena cava
  abnormalities, 1051–1060
  anatomic features, 16–22
  inferior
    abnormalities, 1059–1060
    connection into left atrium, 1059
    diaphragm in, 1060
    duplication in polysplenia syndrome, 975
    hemiazygous continuation, MRI of, 233
    interruption, 970, 1056, 1057
    interruption, polysplenia syndrome and, 974
    left, connecting to right inferior vena cava, 1058
    valves of, 19
  superior
    abnormalities, 1051–1059
    aneurysm, 1054
    catheter passed through, into coronary sinus, 344
    connecting to left atrium, 344
    dilation, idiopathic, 1054
    double, 1053
    double, in asplenia, 1053
    left, persistent, 1051–1058
    left, persistent, after obliteration by coils, 1054
    left, persistent, with right superior vena cava absence, 1058
    left, tetralogy of Fallot and, 546
  pulmonary vein anomalous connection to, partial, 352
  pulmonary vein anomalous connection to, total, 810, 813
  pulmonary vein anomalous connection to, total, surgical correction, 822
  right, connecting to left atrium, 1054
  syndrome, lung carcinoma causing, 1160
Venography: pulmonary, with catheter wedged, 187
Ventricle
  anatomy
    normal, 243–244
  cast of, 25
  compliance in atrial septal defect, 322
  development, 6
  diverticulum, 1131–1139
  double inlet, 777–785
  double outlet, 731–751
    operative considerations, 743–744
    radiography of, postoperative, 744
    systemic ventricle, 748
  hypoplasia, transposition of great vessels and, 711
  corrected, 722, 723
  inversion, 727–730, 947
    angiographic features, 729–730
    radiographic features, 727–729
    transposition of great vessels and, corrected, 728
  left
    anatomic features, 946
    anatomy, 35, 37–40
    aneurysm (see Aneurysm, ventricular, left)

angiographic
  identification, 40
aortico left ventricular
  tunnel (see Aortico
  left ventricular
  tunnel)
communication with
  right atrium (see
  below)
decompensation in
  aortic stenosis, 420
decompensation in
  cardiomyopathy, 916
diverticulum (see
  below)
double inlet (see below)
double outlet (see
  below)
ejection fraction,
  calculation, effect of
  background position
  on, 218
enlargement,
  radiographic signs of,
  diagrams of, 108
enlargement,
  radiography of,
  plain-film, 107–109
enlargement in aortic
  stenosis, 420
hypoplastic syndrome
  (see below)
isolated, right atrial
  shunt, 287
in oblique and angled
  projection, 37
outflow area, prosthetic
  valve obstructing,
  437
outflow obstruction,
  mechanism, 525
outflow obstruction in
  transposition of great
  vessels (see
  Transposition of great
  vessels, complete,
  ventricular outflow)
outflow tract filling
  defect, 455
rhabdomyoma, 438
rhabdomyosarcoma,
  1158
left, communication with
  right atrium,
  285–290
angiographic
  appearance, 288–290
catheterization of,
  cardiac, 288
echocardiographic
  features, 287
electrocardiographic
  features, 287

management, 290
natural history,
  285–286
pathologic anatomy,
  285
physical examination,
  286–287
radiographic features,
  287–288
signs, 285–286
symptoms, 285–286
varieties of, diagram of,
  286
left, diverticulum,
  1131–1135, 1136
angiography in,
  1134–1135
radiographic features,
  1133–1134
with thoracoabdominal
  defect, 1134
left, double inlet,
  777–781
angiographic features,
  779–780
catheterization in,
  cardiac, 779
clinical features,
  777–779
echocardiographic
  features, 779
electrocardiographic
  features, 779
hemodynamics, 777
operative
  considerations,
  780–781
operative correction,
  780
pathologic anatomy,
  777
radiographic features,
  779
ventriculography, right,
  779
ventriculography in,
  left, 779–780
left, double outlet,
  748–750
angiographic features,
  749–750
catheterization in,
  cardiac, 749
clinical features, 749
echocardiographic
  features, 749
electrocardiographic
  features, 749
hemodynamics, 749
intact ventricular
  septum in, 749
operative conditions,
  750

radiographic features,
  749
left, hypoplastic
  syndrome, 853–865
angiographic features,
  858–860
catheterization in,
  cardiac, 857–858
clinical features,
  855–856
echocardiographic
  features, 856
electrocardiographic
  features, 856
hemodynamics, 854–855
operative
  considerations,
  860–861
pathologic anatomy,
  853–854
postoperative features,
  861–864
radiographic features,
  856–857
loops, embryology, 948
outflow tracts, diagram
  showing crossing of,
  39
right
  anatomic features,
    22–25, 946
  angiographic features,
    26–27
  angiographic
    identification, 27
  atrialized, progressive
    thinning and
    enlargement of, 655
  coronary artery
    communicating with,
    413
  cross-section pattern,
    552
  decompensation, in
    mitral stenosis, 881
  diverticulum, 1131
  diverticulum, tetralogy
    of Fallot and, 1132
  double inlet (see below)
  double outlet (see
    below)
  drawing with anterior
    wall removed, 24
  enlargement, diagrams
    of, 105
  enlargement, in atrial
    septal defect, 326
  enlargement, in
    pulmonary atresia,
    626–629
  enlargement,
    radiography of,
    plain-film, 103–106

enlargement, severe,
  106
filling defect, 530
hypertrophy due to
  pulmonary
  hypertension, 313
hypoplasia, in
  pulmonary atresia,
  626
hypoplasia, isolated
  (see below)
hypoplasia, pulmonary
  atresia and, 636
hypoplasia,
  transposition of great
  vessels and,
  complete, 685
muscle bundle
  anomalies in (see
  below)
myxoma, 1156
outflow obstruction,
  mechanism, 525
outflow obstruction,
  rare causes, 523–529
outflow tract,
  anomalous muscle
  bundle in, 265
outflow tract,
  foreshortening,
  elimination of, 150
pouchlike structures in,
  523–527
rhabdomyosarcoma,
  1160, 1161
trabeculated apical
  portion, 24
right, double inlet,
  781–783
angiographic features,
  783
clinical features, 782
echocardiographic
  features, 782–783
hemodynamics, 782
operative
  considerations, 783
pathologic anatomy,
  781–782
radiographic features,
  783
surgical correction, 784
right, double outlet,
  731–743
angiographic features,
  737–743
aortography in,
  740–743
associated conditions,
  732–733
catheterization in,
  cardiac, 736–737
clinical features, 735

Ventricle (cont.)
　　double inlet right ventricle and, 745, 747
　　echocardiographic features, 735
　　electrocardiographic features, 735
　　embryogenesis, 733
　　hemodynamics, 733–735
　　with intact ventricular septum, 733
　　operative correction, 745
　　operative correction by intraventricular patch, 746
　　pathologic anatomy, 731–732
　　pulmonary stenosis and, 737, 740, 744–745
　　radiographic features, 735–736
　　subaortic stenosis and, muscular, 738
　　Taussig-Bing heart and, 739, 742
　　transposition of great vessels and, corrected, 737
　　types of, 734
　　ventricular septal defect and, 740, 741
　　ventricular septal defect and, location, 737–738
　　ventricular septal defect and, operative correction, 746
　　ventriculography in, left, 739–743
　　ventriculography in, right, 738–739
　right, hypoplasia, isolated, 647–651
　　anatomic features, 648
　　angiographic features, 649–651
　　catheterization in, cardiac, 649
　　clinical features, 647
　　echocardiographic features, 648
　　electrocardiographic features, 647–648
　　hemodynamics, 647
　　operative considerations, 651
　　pathologic anatomy, 647
　　postoperative features, 651
　　pulmonary stenosis and, valvar, 650
　　radiographic features, 648–649
　right, muscle bundle anomalies in, 520–523
　　angiographic appearance, 521–522
　　catheterization, cardiac, 521
　　clinical features, 520
　　echocardiographic features, 520
　　electrocardiographic features, 520
　　operative considerations, 522
　　pathology, 520
　　radiographic features, 520–521
　septal defect (see Septal defect, ventricular)
　septum, 39
　　aneurysm (see Aneurysm, ventricular septum)
　　concavity, 260
　　curvature of, 39
　　mitral valve leaflet attached to, 374
　　thickening in subaortic stenosis, muscular, 456
　　views of, 245
　single, 753–766
　　angiographic features, 759–763
　　bulboventricular foramen and, stenotic, 764
　　catheterization in, cardiac, 758–759
　　clinical features, 756–757
　　D transposition of great vessels and, 758
　　echocardiographic features, 757
　　electrocardiographic features, 757
　　hemodynamics, 755–756
　　normally related great vessels in, 756, 763
　　operative considerations, 763–766
　　operative repair, 765
　　operative repair, by septation technique, 765
　　pathologic anatomy, 753–755
　　pulmonary stenosis and, 758
　　radiographic features, 757–758
　　transposition of great vessels and, 756
　　transposition of great vessels and, corrected, 760
　　types of, 755
Ventriculography
　catheters for, 173
　in endocardial cushion defect (see Endocardial cushion defect ventriculography)
　left, 38
　　anterior oblique projection with beam angulation, 378
　　in aortico left ventricular tunnel, 466
　　in atrioventricular canal, complete, 377, 378, 386
　　caudal beam angulation, 39
　　in double outlet right ventricle, 739–743
　　injection of large amount of air in, 180
　　inverted, in transposition of great vessels, corrected, 719–721
　　of mitral valve leaflet, 385
　　in ostium primum defect, 381, 383, 384
　　in subaortic membrane resection, 437
　　transposition of great vessels, complete, 686–693
　　in truncus arteriosus, 797
　　in ventricle, double inlet, 779–780
　　of ventricular septal defect, 262
　in Marfan syndrome, 1114
　mechanics of, 170–175
　in mitral valve prolapse, 1123
　right, 25
　　in anteroposterior projection, 31
　　with balloon catheter, 173
　　catheter recoiled during injection, 192
　　in double outlet right ventricle, 738–739
　　in lateral projection, 26, 27, 29
　　in pulmonary artery banding, 270, 530
　　in pulmonary atresia, ventricular septum intact, 633–638
　　in tetralogy of Fallot, 557–563
　　in transposition of great vessels, 21
　　in transposition of great vessels, complete, 684–686
　　in transposition of great vessels, corrected, 721–724
　　in truncus arteriosus, 797
　　in ventricle, double inlet, 779
　　in subaortic stenosis, membranous, 409
　　in thoracopagus, 992
Ventriculotomy: single coronary artery interfering with, 1070
Venturi effect, 429
Vessels
　brachiocephalic, 425
　ectopic origin, 1044–1048
　bronchial, radiography of, plain-film, 69–71
　complicating coarctation of aorta, 492
　great (see Great vessels)
　jet collapse, diagram of mechanism, 191
　major, anomalies, 993–1098
　pulmonary (see Pulmonary vessels)
　trachea compressed by, 1047
Visceral anomalies
　in asplenia syndrome, 959–960
　in polysplenia syndrome, 967–968
Visceroatrial situs, 945–946
　and MRI, 232–234

W

Waterston-Cooley anastomosis: in tetralogy of Fallot, 579

Waterston-Cooley shunt, 571
  in tetralogy of Fallot, 568, 578
  occluded, 580

X

X-ray
  tube, fixed biplane arrangement, 143
  tube mounting, 142–148
    C-arm mounting, 142–143
    L/U system, 143
    parallelogram mounting, 144, 145
    standard biplane technique, 142